EDITED BY

ROBERT W. KIRK, D.V.M.

Professor of Medicine, Emeritus
New York State College of Veterinary Medicine
Cornell University
Ithaca, New York

ASSOCIATE EDITOR

JOHN D. BONAGURA, D.V.M.

Associate Professor
College of Veterinary Medicine
The Ohio State University
Columbus, Ohio

Consulting Editors

CARL A. OSBORNE
Special Therapy

GARY D. OSWEILER
Chemical and Physical Disorders

JOHN D. BONAGURA
Cardiopulmonary Diseases

BRUCE R. MADEWELL
Hematology, Oncology, and Immunology

DANNY W. SCOTT
Dermatologic Diseases

THOMAS J. KERN and RONALD E. RIIS
Ophthalmologic Diseases

MURRAY E. FOWLER
Diseases of Caged Birds and Exotic Pets

JOE N. KORNEGAY
Neurologic and Neuromuscular Disorders

DAVID C. TWEDT
Gastrointestinal Disorders

MARK E. PETERSON
Endocrine and Metabolic Disorders

CRAIG E. GREENE
Infectious Diseases

JEANNE A. BARSANTI
Urinary Disorders

PATRICIA N. OLSON
Reproductive Disorders

CURRENT VETERINARY THERAPY

X

SMALL ANIMAL PRACTICE

1989

W.B. SAUNDERS COMPANY

Harcourt Brace Jovanovich, Inc.

Philadelphia   London   Toronto   Montreal   Sydney   Tokyo

W. B. SAUNDERS COMPANY
Harcourt Brace Jovanovich, Inc.

The Curtis Center
Independence Square West
Philadelphia, PA 19106

Library of Congress Cataloging-in-Publication Data

Current veterinary therapy. 1964/65-

Philadelphia, W. B. Saunders.

v. 26 cm.

"Small animal practice."

Editor: 1964/65-   R. W. Kirk.

Key title: Current veterinary therapy, ISSN 0070–2218.

1. Veterinary medicine—Periodicals.   2. Pets—Diseases—
   Periodicals.   I. Kirk, Robert Warren, 1922–   ed.
   [DNLM: W1 CU823]

SF745.C8   636.0896   64–10489
                                MARC-S

Library of Congress   [8308]

Editor: W. B. Saunders Staff
Developmental Editor: Linda Mills
Designer: Ellen Bodner
Production Manager: Peter Faber
Manuscript Editor: Gina Scala
Illustration Coordinator: Peg Shaw
Indexer: Julie Schwager

Current Veterinary Therapy   ISBN 0–7216–2858–3

Last digit is the print number: 9   8   7   6   5   4   3

CONTRIBUTORS

LARRY G. ADAMS, D.V.M. Veterinary Medical Associate, Department of Small Animal Clinical Sciences, College of Veterinary Medicine, University of Minnesota, St. Paul, Minnesota
Section 1

ZEINEB ALHAIDARI, D.V.M. Clinique Vétérinaire, Roquefort les Pins, France
Section 5

TIMOTHY A. ALLEN, D.V.M. Associate in Clinical Nutrition, Mark Morris Associates, Topeka, Kansas
Section 12

DONNA WALTON ANGARANO, D.V.M., Dipl. A.C.V.D. Associate Professor of Dermatology, Department of Small Animal Surgery and Medicine, College of Veterinary Medicine, Auburn University, Auburn, Alabama
Sections 5 and 6

P. JANE ARMSTRONG, D.V.M., M.S., Dipl. A.C.V.I.M. (Internal Medicine). Assistant Professor of Internal Medicine, Department of Companion Animal and Special Species Medicine, School of Veterinary Medicine, North Carolina State University; Internist, Veterinary Teaching Hospital, North Carolina State University, Raleigh, North Carolina
Sections 1 and 10

DENNIS N. ARON, D.V.M., Dipl. A.C.V.S. Associate Professor, Department of Small Animal Medicine, College of Veterinary Medicine, University of Georgia, Athens, Georgia
Section 3

E. MURL BAILEY, JR., D.V.M. Professor of Toxicology, Department of Veterinary Physiology and Pharmacology, College of Veterinary Medicine, Texas A&M University, College Station, Texas
Section 2

STEVEN C. BARR, B.V.Sc., M.V.S., M.S. Graduate Associate, Department of Veterinary Microbiology and Parasitology, Louisiana State University, School of Veterinary Medicine, Baton Rouge, Louisiana
Section 4

JEANNE A. BARSANTI, D.V.M., M.S., Dipl. A.C.V.I.M. Professor, Department of Small Animal Medicine, University of Georgia; Internist, University of Georgia Teaching Hospital, Athens, Georgia
Sections 12 and 13

R. RANDY BASINGER, D.V.M., Dipl. A.C.V.S. Director, South Carolina Surgical Referral Service, Columbia, South Carolina
Section 12

M. BATTISTA, D.V.M. Research Assistant, Department of Physiology, New York State College of Veterinary Medicine, Cornell University of Ithaca, New York
Section 13

TIMOTHY G. BAUER, D.V.M. Clinical Affiliate, Department of Surgery, Division of Cardiothoracic Surgery; Department of Medicine, Division of Cardiology; Department of Medicine, Division of Animal Medicine, University of Washington School of Medicine, Seattle, Washington. Private practice.
Section 3

VAL RICHARD BEASLEY, D.V.M., PH.D. Co-Director, Illinois Animal Poison Information Cen-

ter, and Assistant Professor of Toxicology, College of Veterinary Medicine, University of Illinois, Urbana, Illinois
Section 2

FORD WATSON BELL, D.V.M. Clinical Instructor, Internal Medicine, Department of Small Animal Clinical Sciences, College of Veterinary Medicine, University of Minnesota, St. Paul, Minnesota
Section 1

JOHN BENTINCK-SMITH, D.V.M. Visiting Professor of Clinical Pathology, College of Veterinary Medicine, Mississippi State University, Mississippi State, Mississippi
Appendices

DIANE BEVIER-TOURNAY, D.V.M., Dipl. A.C.V.D. Clinical Assistant Professor, Tufts University, North Grafton, Massachusetts; Staff Dermatologist, Angell Memorial Animal Hospital, Boston, Massachusetts
Section 5

STEPHEN J. BIRCHARD, D.V.M., M.S. Assistant Professor, College of Veterinary Medicine, The Ohio State University, Columbus, Ohio
Section 3

PATRICIA BLANCHARD, D.V.M., PH.D. Assistant Adjunct Professor, Department of Veterinary Pathology, University of California, Davis, California; California Veterinary Diagnostic Laboratory, Tulare Branch, University of California-Davis, Tulare, California
Section 11

JOHN D. BONAGURA, D.V.M., M.S. Dipl. A.C.V.I.M. (Internal Medicine, Cardiology). Associate Professor, Department of Veterinary Clinical Sciences, College of Veterinary Medicine, The Ohio State University; Cardiologist, Veterinary Teaching Hospital, The Ohio State University, Columbus, Ohio
Section 3

GERALD R. BRATTON, D.V.M., PH.D. Professor and Head, Department of Veterinary Anatomy, College of Veterinary Medicine, Texas A&M University, College Station, Texas; Professor of Neurology, Veterinary Teaching Hospital, Texas Veterinary Medical Center, College Station, Texas
Section 2

KYLE G. BRAUND, D.V.M., M.V.Sc., PH.D., F.R.C.V.S., Dipl. A.C.V.I.M. Director, Neuromuscular Research Laboratory, Scott-Ritchey Research Program; Professor, Department of

Small Animal Surgery and Medicine, College of Veterinary Medicine, Auburn University; Consultant Clinical Neurologist, Department of Small Animal Medicine and Surgery, College of Veterinary Medicine, Auburn University, Auburn, Alabama
Section 8

PATRICK T. BREEN, D.V.M., Dipl. A.C.V.D. Adjunct Assistant Professor, Department of Laboratory Animal Medicine, College of Medicine, University of Cincinnati, Cincinnati, Ohio; Owner and Director, Veterinary Dermatology Services, Cincinnati, Ohio
Section 5

SCOTT A. BROWN, V.M.D. Allen Products Fellow, College of Veterinary Medicine, University of Georgia, Athens, Georgia; Nephrology Fellow, School of Medicine, University of Alabama at Birmingham, Birmingham, Alabama
Section 12

DAVID S. BRUYETTE, D.V.M. West Los Angeles Veterinary Medical Group, Los Angeles, California
Section 10

ROBERT G. BUERGER, D.V.M., Dipl. A.C.V.D. Staff Dermatologist, Veterinary Dermatology Center, Baltimore, Maryland
Section 5

SUSAN E. BUNCH, D.V.M., PHD., Dipl. A.C.V.I.M. Associate Professor of Medicine, College of Veterinary Medicine, North Carolina State University; Internist, Veterinary Teaching Hospital, North Carolina State University, Raleigh, North Carolina
Section 9

JANICE L. CAIN, D.V.M. Postgraduate Research Associate, Department of Reproduction, School of Veterinary Medicine, University of California, Davis, California; Private practitioner, Alamo Animal Hospital, Vacaville, California
Section 13

GEORGE H. CARDINET III, D.V.M., PHD. Professor, Department of Anatomy, School of Veterinary Medicine, University of California; Neurology Service, Veterinary Medical Teaching Hospital, University of California, Davis, California
Section 8

LELAND E. CARMICHAEL, D.V.M., PH.D. Professor of Virology, New York State College of New York
Section 11

MARCIA CAROTHERS, D.V.M. Resident in Internal Medicine, The Ohio State University; Resident, Veterinary Teaching Hospital, Department of Clinical Sciences, College of Veterinary Medicine, The Ohio State University, Columbus, Ohio
Section 3

THOMAS L. CARSON, D.V.M., M.S., PH.D. Professor of Veterinary Pathology, College of Veterinary Medicine, Iowa State University; Veterinary Toxicologist, Veterinary Diagnostic Laboratory, College of Veterinary Medicine, Iowa State University, Ames, Iowa
Section 2

DENNIS D. CAYWOOD, D.V.M., M.S., Dipl. A.C.V.S. Associate Professor of Surgery, Department of Small Animal Clinical Sciences, College of Veterinary Medicine, University of Minnesota, St. Paul, Minnesota
Section 12

SHARON A. CENTER, D.V.M. Associate Professor, Department of Clinical Sciences, New York State College of Veterinary Medicine, Cornell University, Ithaca, New York
Section 9

DENNIS J. CHEW, D.V.M. Associate Professor, Department of Veterinary Clinical Sciences, College of Veterinary Medicine, The Ohio State University; Small Animal Clinician, Veterinary Teaching Hospital, The Ohio State University, Columbus, Ohio
Section 12

SCOTT B. CITINO, D.V.M. Staff Veterinarian and Head, Department of Veterinary Sciences, Miami Metro Zoo, Miami, Florida
Section 7

ROGER M. CLEMMONS, D.V.M., PH.D. Associate Professor, Department of Small Animal Clinical Sciences, College of Veterinary Medicine, University of Florida; Veterinary Medical Teaching Hospital, College of Veterinary Medicine, University of Florida, Gainesville, Florida
Section 8

CHRIS W. CLINTON, M.T. Supervisor, Crystallography, Urolithiasis Laboratory, Houston, Texas
Section 12

P. W. CONCANNON, M.S., PH.D. Senior Research Associate, Department of Physiology, New York State College of Veterinary Medicine, Cornell University, Ithaca, New York
Section 13

PENNIE L. COOLEY, D.V.M., Dipl. A.C.V.O. Staff Ophthalmologist, Animal Eye Clinic, Seattle, Washington
Section 6

ROBERT W. COPPOCK, D.V.M., M.S., PH.D. Dipl. A.B.V.T., Dipl. A.B.T. Head, Clinical Investigation Branch, Alberta Environmental Centre, Vegreville, Alberta, Canada
Section 2

LARRY M. CORNELIUS, D.V.M., PH.D., Dipl. A.C.V.I.M. (Internal Medicine). Professor of Small Animal Medicine, College of Veterinary Medicine, University of Georgia; Small Animal Internist, University of Georgia Veterinary Teaching Hospital, Athens, Georgia
Section 9

SUSAN M. COTTER, D.V.M., Dipl. A.C.V.I.M. (Internal Medicine/Oncology). Associate Professor of Medicine, School of Veterinary Medicine, Tufts University, North Grafton, Massachusetts
Section 4

C. GUILLERMO COUTO, D.V.M., Dipl. A.C.V.I.M. (Internal Medicine/Veterinary Medical Oncology). Associate Professor, Department of Veterinary Clinical Sciences, College of Veterinary Medicine, The Ohio State University; Associate Professor, Internal Medicine/Oncology, Veterinary Teaching Hospital, The Ohio State University; Full Member, The Ohio State University Comprehensive Cancer Center, The Ohio State University, Columbus, Ohio
Sections 3 and 4

LAINE A. COWAN, D.V.M., Dipl. A.C.V.I.M. Clinical Resident, Department of Small Animal Medicine, University of Georgia, Athens, Georgia
Section 13

PAUL A. CUDDON, B.V.SC. Assistant Professor, Neurology/Small Animal Internal Medicine, University of Wisconsin School of Veterinary Medicine, Madison, Wisconsin
Section 8

DEBORAH J. DAVENPORT, D.V.M., M.S., Dipl. A.C.V.I.M. Assistant Professor, Virginia-Maryland Regional College of Veterinary Medicine, Virginia Polytechnic Institute and State University; Internist, Veterinary Teaching Hospital, Virginia Polytechnic Institute and State University, Blacksburg, Virginia
Sections 9 and 12

MARIAN P. DAVENPORT, M.L.T. Crystallographer, Urolithiasis Laboratory, Houston, Texas
Section 12

LLOYD E. DAVIS, D.V.M., Ph.D. Professor of Clinical Pharmacology, Departments of Veterinary Biosciences and Veterinary Clinical Sciences, College of Veterinary Medicine, University of Illinois; Clinical Pharmacologist, Veterinary Teaching Hospital, College of Veterinary Medicine, University of Illinois, Urbana, Illinois
Section 1

MELISA A. DEGEN, D.V.M., Dipl. A.C.V.I.M. Staff Internist, Coast Pet Clinic, Animal Cancer Center, Hermosa Beach, California
Section 4

ROBERT C. DeNOVO, Jr., D.V.M., M.S., Dipl. A.C.V.I.M. Associate Professor of Medicine, Department of Urban Practice, College of Veterinary Medicine, University of Tennessee, Knoxville, Tennessee
Section 9

STEPHEN P. DiBARTOLA, D.V.M. Associate Professor of Medicine, Department of Veterinary Clinical Sciences, College of Veterinary Medicine, The Ohio State University; Small Animal Clinician, Veterinary Teaching Hospital, The Ohio State University, Columbus, Ohio
Section 12

PAUL F. DICE II, V.M.D., M.S., Dipl. A.C.V.O. Staff Ophthalmologist, Animal Eye Clinic, Seattle, Washington
Section 6

RAY DILLON, D.V.M., M.S., Dipl. A.C.V.I.M. (Internal Medicine). Professor and Head, Section of Medicine, Department of Small Animal Surgery and Medicine, Scott-Ritchey Research Program, College of Veterinary Medicine, Auburn University, Auburn, Alabama
Section 9

DAVID C. DORMAN, D.V.M. Visiting Instructor in Toxicology, College of Veterinary Medicine, University of Illinois, Urbana, Illinois
Section 2

STEVEN W. DOW, D.V.M., M.S., Dipl. A.C.V.I.M. Graduate Fellow, Feline Leukemia Virus Research Laboratory, Department of Pathology, College of Veterinary Medicine and Biomedical Sciences, Colorado State University, Fort Collins, Colorado
Sections 8, 10, and 11

IAN D. DUNCAN, B.V.M.S., Ph.D., M.R.C.V.S., M.R.C.Path. Professor, Department of Medical Sciences, University of Wisconsin School of Veterinary Medicine, Madison, Wisconsin
Section 8

JOAN DZIEZYC, D.V.M., Dipl. A.C.V.O. Assistant Professor, Department of Small Animal Medicine and Surgery, College of Veterinary Medicine, Texas A&M University, College Station, Texas
Section 6

MARK ALJIAN EDWARDS, M.A., D.V.M. Formerly Director, Atlanta Humane Society Veterinary Hospital, Atlanta, Georgia
Section 1

WILLIAM C. EDWARDS, D.V.M., M.S. Professor of Medicine and Surgery, College of Veterinary Medicine, Oklahoma State University; Toxicologist, Oklahoma Animal Disease Diagnostic Laboratory, College of Veterinary Medicine, Oklahoma State University, Stillwater, Oklahoma
Section 2

PETER P. EMILY, D.D.S., Dipl. A.V.D.C. Director of Animal Dentistry, School of Veterinary Medicine, Colorado State University, Fort Collins, Colorado
Section 9

JAMES F. EVERMANN, Ph.D. Clinical Virologist, Department of Veterinary Clinical Medicine and Surgery, College of Veterinary Medicine, Washington State University, Pullman, Washington
Section 13

BERNARD F. FELDMAN, D.V.M., Ph.D. Associate Professor of Veterinary Clinical Hematology and Biochemistry, Department of Clinical Pathology, School of Veterinary Medicine, University of California; Service Chief, Cytologic Services, and Director, Comparative Hemostasis Laboratory, Veterinary Medical Teaching Hospital, University of California, Davis, California
Section 4

EDWARD C. FELDMAN, D.V.M., Dipl. A.C.V.I.M. Professor, Department of Reproduction, School of Veterinary Medicine, University of California; Clinician, Small Animal Clinic, Veterinary Medical Teaching Hospital, University of California, Davis, California
Sections 10 and 13

DELMAR R. FINCO, D.V.M., Ph.D., Dipl. A.C.V.I.M. Professor, Department of Physiology and Pharmacology, College of Veterinary

Medicine, University of Georgia, Athens, Georgia
Section 12

ROGER B. FINGLAND, D.V.M., M.S. Assistant Professor, Department of Surgery and Medicine, College of Veterinary Medicine, Kansas State University; Head, Section of Small Animal Surgery, College of Veterinary Medicine, Kansas State University, Manhattan, Kansas
Section 3

SUSAN T. FINN, D.V.M. Radiology Resident, Department of Radiology and Radiation Biology, Colorado State University, Fort Collins, Colorado
Section 13

KEVEN FLAMMER, D.V.M. Assistant Professor, College of Veterinary Medicine, North Carolina State University; Veterinary Teaching Hospital, College of Veterinary Medicine, North Carolina State University, Raleigh, North Carolina
Section 7

JENS M. FOGH, D.V.M. Head, Department of In Vitro Biology, Nordisk Gentofte A/S, Gentofte, Denmark
Section 4

RICHARD B. FORD, D.V.M., M.S., Dipl. A.C.V.I.M. Associate Professor of Medicine, College of Veterinary Medicine, North Carolina State University, Raleigh, North Carolina
Sections 3 and 10

THERESA W. FOSSUM, D.V.M., M.S., Dipl. A.C.V.S. Assistant Professor, Department of Small Animal Medicine and Surgery, College of Veterinary Medicine; Surgeon, Department of Small Animal Medicine and Surgery, Texas A&M University, College Station, Texas
Section 3

MURRAY E. FOWLER, D.V.M., Dipl. A.C.Z.M., A.C.V.I.M., A.B.V.T. Professor of Veterinary Medicine, Department of Medicine, School of Veterinary Medicine, University of California; Chief, Zoological Medicine Service, Veterinary Medical Teaching Hospital, School of Veterinary Medicine, University of California, Davis, California
Section 7

PHILIP R. FOX, D.V.M., M.Sc., Dipl. A.C.V.I.M. (Cardiology). Staff Cardiologist, Department of Medicine, and Director of Clinics, The Animal Medical Center, New York, New York
Section 3

TRACY W. FRENCH, D.V.M., Dipl. A.C.V.P. Assistant Professor, Department of Pathology, New York State College of Veterinary Medicine, Cornell University, Ithaca, New York
Appendices

JONI L. FRESHMAN, D.V.M., M.S. Previous Resident in Small Animal Medicine, College of Veterinary Medicine and Biomedical Sciences, Colorado State University, Fort Collins, Colorado; Staff Veterinarian, Santa Anita Small Animal Hospital, Monrovia, California
Section 13

FREDRIC L. FRYE, D.V.M., M.S. Clinical Professor of Medicine, Department of Medicine, School of Veterinary Medicine, University of California, Davis, California; Attending Staff Clinician, Davis Animal Hospital, Davis, California; Attending Staff Clinician, Sacramento Animal Medical Group, Sacramento, California
Section 7

CATHY E. GABER, D.V.M., M.S., Dipl. A.C.V.I.M. (Cardiology). Assistant Professor, Department of Small Animal Clinical Sciences, Michigan State University, East Lansing, Michigan
Section 3

LAURA GALLAGHER, D.V.M., M.S. Assistant Professor, University of Sydney, Sydney, Australia
Section 3

PETER W. GASPER, D.V.M., PH.D. Assistant Professor of Hematopathology, Department of Pathology, College of Veterinary Medicine and Biomedical Sciences, Colorado State University; Clinical Pathologist, Veterinary Teaching Hospital, Colorado State University, Fort Collins, Colorado
Section 4

HOWARD B. GELBERG, D.V.M., PH.D. Associate Professor, Department of Veterinary Pathobiology, College of Veterinary Medicine, University of Illinois, Urbana, Illinois
Section 12

DIANE F. GERKEN, D.V.M., PH.D., Dipl. A.B.V.T., A.B.T. Associate Professor, Veterinary Physiology and Pharmacology, College of Veterinary Medicine, The Ohio State University, Columbus, Ohio
Section 2

URS GIGER, Dr.Med.Vet., F.V.H., Dipl. A.C.V.I.M. (Internal Medicine). Assistant Professor of Medicine and Medical Genetics, School

of Veterinary Medicine, University of Pennsylvania; Staff Clinician in Small Animal Medical Genetics, Section of Medical Genetics, Department of Clinical Studies, Veterinary Hospital of the University of Pennsylvania, Philadelphia, Pennsylvania
Section 4

MARY B. GLAZE, D.V.M., M.S., Dipl. A.C.V.O. Associate Professor of Veterinary Ophthalmology, Veterinary Clinical Sciences, Louisiana State University; Veterinary Ophthalmologist, Veterinary Teaching Hospital and Clinics, Louisiana State University, Baton Rouge, Louisiana
Section 6

J. L. GRANDY, D.V.M., Dipl. A.C.V.A. Assistant Professor, Department of Clinical Sciences, College of Veterinary Medicine and Biomedical Sciences, Colorado State University; Clinical Anesthesiologist, Veterinary Teaching Hospital, Colorado State University, Fort Collins, Colorado
Section 13

CHRIS K. GRANT, Ph.D., D.Sc. Adjunct Associate Professor, Division of Animal Medicine, School of Medicine, University of Washington, Seattle, Washington; Affiliate Associate Professor, Department of Microbiology, School of Veterinary Medicine, Cornell University, Ithaca, New York; Scientific Director, Immunology and Retrovirus Research, Pacific Northwest Research Foundation, Seattle, Washington
Section 4

GREGORY F. GRAUER, D.V.M., M.S. Associate Professor, Department of Medical Sciences, School of Veterinary Medicine, University of Wisconsin; Staff Internist, Veterinary Medical Teaching Hospital, School of Veterinary Medicine, University of Wisconsin, Madison, Wisconsin
Section 2

DEBORAH S. GRECO, D.V.M., M.S., Dipl. A.C.V.I.M. Research Associate, Department of Veterinary Physiology and Pharmacology, Texas A&M University, College Station, Texas
Section 10

CRAIG E. GREENE, D.V.M., Dipl. A.C.V.I.M. Professor, Department of Small Animal Medicine, College of Veterinary Medicine, University of Georgia, Athens, Georgia
Section 11

RUSSELL T. GREENE, D.V.M., Ph.D., Dipl. A.C.V.I.M. (Internal Medicine). Microbiology, Pathology, and Parasitology Department, College of Veterinary Medicine, North Carolina State University, Raleigh, North Carolina
Section 11

CLARE R. GREGORY, D.V.M., Dipl. A.C.V.S. Assistant Professor, Department of Surgery, School of Veterinary Medicine, University of California; Chief, Small Animal Surgical Services, Veterinary Medical Teaching Hospital, University of California, Davis, California
Section 4

CRAIG E. GRIFFIN, D.V.M., Dipl. A.C.V.D. Clinical Instructor, College of Medicine, University of California, Irvine, California; Director, Animal Dermatology Clinics, Garden Grove and San Diego, California
Section 5

IAN R. GRIFFITHS, B.V.M.S. Titular Professor, Department of Veterinary Surgery, University of Glasgow Veterinary School, Glasgow, Scotland
Section 8

ERIC GUAGUERE, D.V.M. Clinique Vétérinaire Saint-Bernard, Lomme, France
Section 5

DENNIS V. HACKER, D.V.M., Dipl. A.C.V.O. Assistant Clinical Professor, School of Veterinary Medicine, University of California, Davis, California; Berkeley Animal Eye Clinic, Berkeley, California
Section 6

ROBERT L. HAMLIN, D.V.M., Ph.D., Dipl. A.C.V.I.M. (Cardiology; Internal Medicine). Stanton Youngberg Professor of Veterinary Physiology and Pharmacology, College of Veterinary Medicine, The Ohio State University; Consulting Cardiologist, Veterinary Teaching Hospital, The Ohio State University, Columbus, Ohio
Section 3

ROBERT M. HARDY, D.V.M., Dipl. A.C.V.I.M. Associate Professor, Department of Small Animal Clinical Sciences, College of Veterinary Medicine, University of Minnesota, St. Paul, Minnesota
Section 1

ANN M. HARGIS, D.V.M., M.S., Dipl. A.C.V.P. Associate Professor, Department of Veterinary Microbiology and Pathology, and Washington Animal Disease Diagnostic Laboratory, College of Veterinary Medicine, Washington State University, Pullman, Washington
Section 5

NEIL HARPSTER, V.M.D., Dipl. A.C.V.I.M. (Cardiology). Clinical Associate Professor, Department of Medicine, Tufts University School of Veterinary Medicine, North Grafton, Massachusetts; Director of Cardiology, Angell Memorial Animal Hospital, Jamaica Plain, Massachusetts
Section 3

GARY HARWELL, D.V.M. Southeast Animal Clinic, Houston, Texas
Section 7

STEVE C. HASKINS, D.V.M., M.S., Dipl. A.C.V.A. Professor, Department of Veterinary Surgery, School of Veterinary Medicine, University of California; Director, Small Animal Intensive Care Unit, Veterinary Medical Teaching Hospital, University of California, Davis, California
Section 3

KIRK H. HAUPT, D.V.M., Dipl. A.C.V.I.M. Staff Veterinarian, Cats Exclusive Veterinary Hospital, Edmonds, Washington
Section 5

ELEANOR C. HAWKINS, D.V.M., Dipl. A.C.V.I.M. Assistant Professor, Internal Medicine, Department of Veterinary Clinical Sciences, School of Veterinary Medicine, Purdue University, West Lafayette, Indiana
Section 11

WILLIAM H. HAY, D.V.M., M.S. Chief Resident, Small Animal Medicine, Veterinary Teaching Hospital, Virginia-Maryland Regional College of Veterinary Medicine, Virginia Polytechnic Institute and State University, Blacksburg, Virginia
Section 9

STUART C. HELFAND, D.V.M., Dipl. A.C.V.I.M. Assistant Professor, Medicine/Oncology, Department of Clinical Studies, School of Veterinary Medicine, University of Pennsylvania, Philadelphia, Pennsylvania
Section 4

KOHLE HERRMANN, D.V.M., Dipl. A.C.V.O. Gulf Coast Animal Eye Clinic, Houston, Texas
Section 6

DWIGHT C. HIRSH, D.V.M., Ph.D. Professor of Microbiology, School of Veterinary Medicine, University of California; Chief, Microbiology Service, Veterinary Medical Teaching Hospital, School of Veterinary Medicine, University of California, Davis, California
Sections 1 and 11

PETER E. HOLT, B.V.M.S., Ph.D., M.I.Biol.,

M.R.C.V.S. Lecturer in Veterinary Surgery, University of Bristol, Langford, Bristol, United Kingdom
Section 12

ASTRID HOPPE, D.V.M. Clinical Professor, Department of Medicine and Surgery, University of Agricultural Sciences, Uppsala, Sweden
Section 12

PATRICK E. HOPPER, D.V.M. Small Animal Medical Resident, University of California, Davis, California; Staff Internist, Encina Veterinary Hospital, Walnut Creek, California
Section 4

WILLIAM E. HORNBUCKLE, D.V.M., Dipl. A.C.V.I.M. Associate Professor of Medicine, New York State College of Veterinary Medicine, Cornell University, Ithaca, New York
Section 13

JOHNNY D. HOSKINS, D.V.M., Ph.D., Dipl. A.C.V.I.M. Professor, Veterinary Internal Medicine, Department of Veterinary Clinical Sciences, School of Veterinary Medicine, Louisiana State University; Internist, Veterinary Teaching Hospital and Clinics, School of Veterinary Medicine, Louisiana State University, Baton Rouge, Louisiana
Sections 2 and 11

THOMAS N. HRIBERNIK, D.V.M. Associate Professor, Veterinary Internal Medicine, Department of Veterinary Clinical Sciences, School of Veterinary Medicine, Louisiana State University; Veterinary Teaching Hospital and Clinics, School of Veterinary Medicine, Louisiana State University, Baton Rouge, Louisiana
Sections 3 and 4

KATHARINE F. JACKSON, B.V.M.S., M.S., M.R.C.V.S. School of Veterinary Medicine, University of Wisconsin, Madison, Wisconsin
Section 8

GILBERT JACOBS, D.V.M., Dipl. A.C.V.I.M. (Cardiology). Assistant Professor of Medicine, College of Veterinary Medicine, University of Georgia; Staff Internist, Veterinary Teaching Hospital, University of Georgia, Athens, Georgia
Section 9

N. C. JAIN, M.V.Sc., Ph.D. Professor of Clinical Pathology, School of Veterinary Medicine, University of California; Chief, Hematology Section, Veterinary Medical Teaching Hospital, School of Veterinary Medicine, University of California, Davis, California
Section 4

CHERI A. JOHNSON, D.V.M., M.S., Dipl. A.C.V.I.M. Associate Professor, Michigan State University, E. Lansing, Michigan; Chief of Medicine, Department of Small Animal Clinical Sciences, College of Veterinary Medicine, Michigan State University, E. Lansing, Michigan
Section 13

GARY S. JOHNSON, D.V.M., PH.D. Associate Professor, Department of Veterinary Pathology, College of Veterinary Medicine, University of Missouri, Columbia, Missouri
Section 4

SUSAN E. JOHNSON, D.V.M., M.S., Dipl. A.C.V.I.M. Assistant Professor of Veterinary Medicine, College of Veterinary Medicine, The Ohio State University; Internist, Veterinary Teaching Hospital, The Ohio State University, Columbus, Ohio
Section 9

GARY R. JOHNSTON, D.V.M., M.S., Dipl. A.C.V.R. Associate Professor of Radiology, Department of Small Animal Clinical Sciences, College of Veterinary Medicine, University of Minnesota, St. Paul, Minnesota
Section 12

SHIRLEY D. JOHNSTON, D.V.M., PH.D. Associate Professor, Department of Small Animal Clinical Sciences, College of Veterinary Medicine, University of Minnesota, St. Paul, Minnesota
Sections 1 and 13

I. B. JOHNSTONE, D.V.M., M.SC., PH.D. Associate Professor, Department of Biomedical Sciences, Ontario Veterinary College, University of Guelph, Guelph, Ontario, Canada
Section 4

KIM LORRAINE JOYNER, D.V.M. Staff Veterinarian, Florida Agricultural Breeding and Research Center, Loxahatchee, Florida
Section 7

BRUCE W. KEENE, D.V.M., M.S., Dipl. A.C.V.I.M. (Cardiology). Assistant Professor, North Carolina State University, School of Veterinary Medicine, Raleigh, North Carolina
Section 3

MICHAEL J. KELLY, D.V.M., Dipl. A.C.V.I.M. Head of Medicine, Main Street Small Animal Hospital, San Diego, California
Section 10

ROBERT J. KEMPPAINEN, D.V.M., PH.D. Director, Endocrine Diagnostic Laboratory, Department of Physiology and Pharmacology, College of Veterinary Medicine, Auburn University, Auburn, Alabama
Section 10

THOMAS J. KERN, D.V.M., Dipl. A.C.V.O. Assistant Professor of Ophthalmology, New York State College of Veterinary Medicine, Cornell University, Ithaca, New York
Section 6

W. RANDAL KILGORE, D.V.M. Manager of Technical Services, Beecham Laboratories, Bristol, Tennessee
Section 1

PETER P. KINTZER, D.V.M. Resident, Department of Medicine, School of Veterinary Medicine, Tufts University, North Grafton, Massachusetts
Section 10

ROBERT W. KIRK, D.V.M., Dipl. A.C.V.I.M., A.C.V.D. Professor of Medicine, Emeritus, Department of Clinical Sciences, New York State College of Veterinary Medicine, Cornell University, Ithaca, New York
Appendices

MARK D. KITTLESON, D.V.M., PH.D., Dipl. A.C.V.I.M. (Cardiology). Assistant Professor, Department of Medicine, School of Veterinary Medicine, University of California; Staff Cardiologist, Veterinary Medical Teaching Hospital, University of California, Davis, California
Section 3

GARY J. KOCIBA, D.V.M., Dipl. A.C.V.P. Professor, Department of Veterinary Pathobiology, The Ohio State University; Clinical Pathologist, Veterinary Teaching Hospital, The Ohio State University, Columbus, Ohio
Section 4

JOE N. KORNEGAY, D.V.M., PH.D. Professor of Neurology, College of Veterinary Medicine, North Carolina State University; Clinical Neurologist, Veterinary Teaching Hospital, North Carolina State University, Raleigh, North Carolina
Section 8

DAVID F. KOWALCZYK, V.M.D., PH.D. Manager of Regulatory Affairs, Monsanto Company, St. Louis, Missouri
Section 2

KARL H. KRAUS, D.V.M. Resident in Surgery, Department of Veterinary Medicine and Surgery, College of Veterinary Medicine, University of Missouri, Columbia, Missouri
Section 4

DONALD R. KRAWIEC, D.V.M., M.S., PH.D. Associate Professor, Department of Veterinary Clinical Medicine, College of Veterinary Medicine, University of Illinois; Associate Professor, Veterinary Medical Teaching Hospital, College of Veterinary Medicine, University of Illinois, Urbana, Illinois
Section 12

SHERYL GREVE KROHNE, D.V.M., M.S. Postdoctoral Associate, Comparative Ophthalmology, Veterinary Clinical Sciences, Purdue University; Staff, Veterinary Teaching Hospital, School of Veterinary Medicine, Purdue University, West Lafayette, Indiana
Section 6

JOHN M. KRUGER, D.V.M., PH.D. Clinical Research Associate, Department of Small Animal Clinical Sciences, College of Veterinary Medicine, University of Minnesota, St. Paul, Minnesota
Section 12

GAIL A. KUNKLE, D.V.M., Dipl. A.C.V.M. Associate Professor, College of Veterinary Medicine, University of Florida, Gainesville, Florida
Section 5

KENNETH W. KWOCHKA, D.V.M., Dipl. A.C.V.D. Assistant Professor of Dermatology, Department of Veterinary Clinical Sciences, College of Veterinary Medicine, The Ohio State University; Staff Dermatologist, Veterinary Teaching Hospital, College of Veterinary Medicine, The Ohio State University, Columbus, Ohio
Section 5

MARY ANNA LABATO, D.V.M. Clinical Instructor, Department of Medicine, School of Veterinary Medicine, Tufts University; Staff Clinician, Foster Hospital for Small Animals, Tufts University, North Grafton, Massachusetts
Section 12

ARTHUR L. LAGE, D.V.M., Dipl. A.C.V.I.M. Assistant Professor of Veterinary Medicine, Harvard Medical School, Boston, Massachusetts; Adjunct Clinical Associate Professor of Medicine, School of Veterinary Medicine, Tufts University, North Grafton, Massachusetts; Urologist, Pembroke Animal Hospital, Pembroke, Massachusetts
Section 12

MICHAEL R. LAPPIN, D.V.M., PH.D., Dipl. A.C.V.I.M. Assistant Professor, Department of Clinical Sciences, College of Veterinary Medicine and Biomedical Sciences, Colorado State University, Fort Collins, Colorado
Sections 11 and 12

SUSAN M. LaRUE, D.V.M., M.S. NIH Fellow in Radiation Biology, Department of Radiology and Radiation Biology, Colorado State University, Fort Collins, Colorado
Section 4

DENNIS F. LAWLER, D.V.M. Research Veterinarian, Ralston Purina Company, St. Louis, Missouri
Sections 1 and 13

RICHARD A. LeCOUTEUR, B.V.SC., PH.D. Dipl. A.C.V.I.M. (Neurology). Associate Professor, Neurology, Department of Clinical Sciences, College of Veterinary Medicine and Biomedical Sciences, Colorado State University; Clinical Neurologist, Veterinary Teaching Hospital, Colorado State University, Fort Collins, Colorado
Sections 8 and 10

GEORGE E. LEES, D.V.M., M.S., Dipl. A.C.V.I.M. (Internal Medicine). Professor of Medicine, Department of Small Animal Medicine and Surgery, College of Veterinary Medicine, Texas A&M University; Chief of Small Animal Medicine Service, Texas Veterinary Medical Center, Texas A&M University, College Station, Texas
Section 12

ALFRED M. LEGENDRE, D.V.M., M.S., Dipl. A.C.V.I.M. Professor of Medicine, College of Veterinary Medicine, University of Tennessee; Director of Medical Services, Veterinary Teaching Hospital, University of Tennessee, Knoxville, Tennessee
Section 11

MICHAEL S. LEIB, D.V.M., M.S., Dipl. A.C.V.I.M. Associate Professor, Department of Small Animal Clinical Sciences, Virginia-Maryland Regional College of Veterinary Medicine, Virginia Polytechnic Institute and State University; Chief, Small Animal Medicine, Veterinary Teaching Hospital, Virginia-Maryland Regional College of Veterinary Medicine, Virginia Polytechnic Institute and State University, Blacksburg, Virginia
Section 9

DONALD H. LEIN, D.V.M., PH.D., Dipl. A.C.V.P. Associate Professor of Pathology and Theriogenology, New York State College of Veterinary Medicine, Cornell University; Consultant in Theriogenology, Small Animal Clinic, New York State College of Veterinary Medicine, Cornell University; Director, Diagnostic Laboratory, New York State College of Veterinary Medicine, Cornell University, Ithaca, New York
Section 13

L. E. LILLIE, D.V.M., M.Sc., Ph.D., Dipl. A.C.V.P. Director, Animal Sciences Division, Alberta Environmental Centre, Vegreville, Alberta, Canada
Section 2

AUNNA C. LIPPERT, D.V.M., M.S. Instructor/ Resident, Internal Medicine, Michigan State University; Instructor/Resident, Veterinary Clinical Center, Michigan State University, East Lansing, Michigan
Section 1

CLINTON D. LOTHROP, Jr., D.V.M., Ph.D. Assistant Professor, Department of Environmental Practice, College of Veterinary Medicine, University of Tennessee, Knoxville, Tennessee
Section 10

JODY P. LULICH, D.V.M. Veterinary Medical Associate, Department of Small Animal Clinical Sciences, College of Veterinary Medicine, University of Minnesota; Resident, Small Animal Medicine, Lewis Hospital for Companion Animals, University of Minnesota, St. Paul, Minnesota
Sections 1 and 12

DENNIS W. MACY, D.V.M., M.S., Dipl. A.C.V.I.M. (Internal Medicine). Associate Professor of Medicine, College of Veterinary Medicine and Biomedical Sciences, Colorado State University, Fort Collins, Colorado
Sections 1, 9, and 11

BRUCE R. MADEWELL, V.M.D., Dipl. A.C.V.I.M. Professor, Department of Veterinary Surgery, University of California; Chief of Oncology Service, Veterinary Medical Teaching Hospital, University of California, Davis, California
Section 4

MICHAEL L. MAGNE, D.V.M., M.S., Dipl. A.C.V.I.M. Santa Rosa Veterinary Specialty Group, Santa Rosa, California
Section 9

RONALD E. MANDSAGER, D.V.M. Resident, Division of Comparative Anesthesiology, Department of Small Animal Clinical Sciences, College of Veterinary Medicine, University of Minnesota, St. Paul, Minnesota
Section 1

CHARLES L. MARTIN, D.V.M., M.S. Professor, Small Animal Medicine, College of Veterinary Medicine, University of Georgia; Director,

Veterinary Teaching Hospital, University of Georgia, Athens, Georgia
Section 6

DAVID T. MATTHIESEN, D.V.M., Dipl. A.C.V.S. Staff Surgeon, Orthopedics, The Animal Medical Center, New York, New York
Section 12

ROBERT E. MATUS, D.V.M., M.S., Dipl. A.C.V.I.M. (Internal Medicine, Oncology). Head, Donaldson Atwood Cancer Clinic, The Animal Medical Center; Staff Oncologist, The Animal Medical Center, New York, New York
Sections 4 and 10

BARBARA H. McGUIRE, D.V.M. Resident in Small Animal Internal Medicine, Department of Clinical Sciences, College of Veterinary Medicine and Biomedical Sciences, Colorado State University; Resident in Small Animal Internal Medicine, Veterinary Teaching Hospital, Colorado State University, Fort Collins, Colorado
Section 1

ROSEMARY E. McKERRELL, M.R.C.V.S., Vet. M.B. Research Associate, Wellcome Laboratory for Comparative Neurology, Department of Clinical Veterinary Medicine, University of Cambridge, Cambridge, England
Section 8

BRENDAN C. McKIERNAN, D.V.M. Associate Professor, Department of Veterinary Clinical Medicine, College of Veterinary Medicine, University of Illinois, Urbana, Illinois
Section 3

SUSAN A. McLAUGHLIN, D.V.M., M.S., Dipl. A.C.V.O. Assistant Professor, College of Veterinary Medicine, University of Illinois, Urbana, Illinois
Section 6

LINDA MEDLEAU, D.V.M., M.S., Dipl. A.C.V.D. Associate Professor, Department of Small Animal Medicine, College of Veterinary Medicine, University of Georgia; Dermatologist, Veterinary Medical Teaching Hospital, College of Veterinary Medicine, University of Georgia, Athens, Georgia
Sections 5 and 11

GAVIN L. MEERDINK, D.V.M., Dipl. A.B.V.T. Chief Diagnostician, Veterinary Diagnostic Laboratory, University of Arizona, Tucson, Arizona
Section 2

V.N. MEYERS-WALLEN, V.M.D., Ph.D., Dipl. A.C.T. Assistant Professor of Reproduction in

Medical Genetics, School of Veterinary Medicine, University of Pennsylvania, Philadelphia, Pennsylvania
Section 13

MATTHEW W. MILLER, D.V.M., Dipl. A.C.V.I.M. (Cardiology). Assistant Professor, Texas A&M University, College of Veterinary Medicine; Staff Cardiologist, Veterinary Teaching Hospital, College of Veterinary Medicine, Texas A&M University, College Station, Texas
Section 3

WILLIAM H. MILLER, Jr., V.M.D., Dipl. A.C.V.D. Assistant Professor of Medicine, New York State College of Veterinary Medicine, Cornell University, Ithaca, New York
Section 5

N. SYDNEY MOISE, D.V.M., M.S. Assistant Professor of Medicine, New York State College of Veterinary Medicine, Cornell University, Ithaca, New York
Section 3

CECIL P. MOORE, D.V.M., M.S., Dipl. A.C.V.O. Associate Professor, Department of Veterinary Medicine and Surgery, College of Veterinary Medicine, University of Missouri; Section Head, Ophthalmology Service, Veterinary Teaching Hospital, University of Missouri, Columbia, Missouri
Section 6

PHILIPPE M. MOREAU, D.V.M., M.S. Clinique Vétérinaire de Vanteaux, Limoges, France
Section 12

SCOTT D. MOROFF, V.M.D. Associate Staff Pathologist, The Animal Medical Center, New York, New York
Section 12

M. S. MOSTROM, D.V.M., M.S. Candidate in Veterinary Toxicology, Western College of Veterinary Medicine, University of Saskatchewan, Saskatoon, Saskatchewan, Canada
Section 2

WILLIAM W. MUIR, D.V.M., Ph.D. Chairman/ Professor, Department of Veterinary Clinical Sciences; Professor, Department of Veterinary Physiology and Pharmacology; College of Veterinary Medicine; Professor, Division of Cardiology, College of Medicine, The Ohio State University, Columbus, Ohio
Section 3

THOMAS W. MULLIGAN, D.V.M., Dipl. A.V.D.C., A.B.V.P. President, Main Street Small Animal Hospital, San Diego, California
Section 9

MICHAEL J. MURPHY, D.V.M., Ph.D., Dipl. A.B.V.T. Assistant Professor, Veterinary Diagnostic Investigation, College of Veterinary Medicine, University of Minnesota, St. Paul, Minnesota
Section 2

R. J. MURTAUGH, D.V.M., M.S., Dipl. A.C.V.I.M. Assistant Professor, Department of Medicine, School of Veterinary Medicine, Tufts University, North Grafton, Massachusetts
Section 3

MARJORIE H. NEADERLAND, D.V.M. Animal Eye Clinic, Norwalk, Connecticut
Section 6

REGG D. NEIGER, D.V.M. Assistant Professor, Department of Veterinary Science, South Dakota State University, Brookings, South Dakota
Section 2

RICHARD W. NELSON, D.V.M., Dipl. A.C.V.I.M. Associate Professor, Department of Small Animal Clinics, School of Veterinary Medicine, Purdue University; Internist, Small Animal Clinic, Purdue University, West Lafayette, Indiana
Sections 10 and 13

RHETT NICHOLS, D.V.M., Dipl. A.C.V.I.M. Staff Clinician, Department of Medicine, Animal Medical Center, New York, New York
Section 10

PAUL NICOLETTI, D.V.M., M.S. Professor, Department of Infectious Diseases, College of Veterinary Medicine, University of Florida, Gainesville, Florida
Section 13

JAMES O. NOXON, D.V.M. Associate Professor, Department of Veterinary Clinical Science, College of Veterinary Medicine, Iowa State University, Ames, Iowa
Section 11

TIMOTHY D. O'BRIEN, D.V.M., Ph.D., Dipl. A.C.V.P. Assistant Professor, Department of Veterinary Pathobiology, College of Veterinary Medicine, University of Minnesota, St. Paul, Minnesota
Section 12

RICHARD G. OLSEN, PH.D. Professor, Department of Veterinary Pathobiology, The Ohio State University, Columbus, Ohio
Section 11

PATRICIA N. OLSON, D.V.M., PH.D., Dipl. A.C.T. Associate Professor, College of Veterinary Medicine and Biomedical Sciences, Colorado State University, Fort Collins, Colorado
Section 13

CARL A. OSBORNE, D.V.M., PH.D., Professor, Department of Small Animal Clinical Sciences, College of Veterinary Medicine, University of Minnesota, St. Paul, Minnesota
Sections 1 and 12

GARY D. OSWEILER, D.V.M., M.S., PH.D., Dipl. A.B.V.T. Professor, Veterinary Pathology, Veterinary Diagnostic Laboratory, College of Veterinary Medicine, Iowa State University, Ames, Iowa
Section 2

RICHARD L. OTT, D.V.M., Dipl. A.C.V.I.M. Professor Emeritus, Department of Clinical Medicine and Surgery, College of Veterinary Medicine, Washington State University, Pullman, Washington; Consultant in Hematology and Oncology, Division of Hematology, Department of Medicine, School of Medicine, University of Washington, Seattle, Washington
Section 11

ANGELA M. PACITTI, B.V.M.S.M., PH.D., M.R.C.V.S. Postdoctoral Research Fellow, Department of Veterinary Pathology, University of Glasgow, Bearsden, Glasgow, Scotland
Section 4

MARK G. PAPICH, D.V.M., M.S. Associate Professor, Clinical Pharmacology, Departments of Veterinary Physiological Sciences and Veterinary Internal Medicine, Western College of Veterinary Medicine; Clinical Pharmacologist, Veterinary Teaching Hospital, Western College of Veterinary Medicine, Saskatoon, Saskatchewan, Canada
Sections 1, 3, 9, and 13

MANON PARADIS, D.V.M., M.V.Sc. Assistant Professor, Faculté de Médecine Vétérinaire, Université de Montréal, St. Hyacinthe, Québec, Canada
Section 4

MARY LOU PARKER, B.S., M.B.A., M.T. (A.S.C.P.). Associate Director, Urolithiasis/

Urochemistry Laboratory, Baylor College of Medicine, Houston, Texas
Section 12

COLIN R. PARRISH, PH.D. Assistant Professor of Virology, New York State College of Veterinary Medicine, Cornell University, Ithaca, New York
Section 11

DONALD F. PATTERSON, D.V.M., D.SC. Professor of Veterinary Medicine and Human Genetics, Schools of Veterinary Medicine and Medicine, University of Pennsylvania; Chief, Section of Veterinary Medical Genetics, Veterinary Hospital of the University of Pennsylvania, Philadelphia, Pennsylvania
Section 13

ALLAN PAUL, D.V.M., M.S. Associate Professor, Small Animal Extension Veterinarian, College of Veterinary Medicine, University of Illinois, Urbana, Illinois
Section 2

MARK E. PETERSON, D.V.M., Dipl. A.C.V.I.M. Staff Endocrinologist, Department of Medicine, The Animal Medical Center; Director, Endocrinology Diagnostic Laboratory, The Animal Medical Center, New York, New York; Director of Clinical Medicine, Research Animal Resource Center, Cornell University Medical College, New York, New York
Section 10

MICHAEL E. PETERSON, D.V.M. Chief of Staff, Wiseman Animal Hospital; Staff Clinician, Animal Emergency Service, Tucson, Arizona
Section 2

LYNDSAY G. PHILLIPS, Jr., D.V.M., Dipl. A.C.Z.M. Department of Animal Health, National Zoological Park, Washington, D.C.
Section 7

PAUL D. PION, D.V.M., Dipl. A.C.V.I.M. (Cardiology). Postgraduate Researcher, School of Veterinary Medicine, University of California, Davis, California
Section 3

ROY V. H. POLLOCK, D.V.M., PH.D. Director, Center for the Study of Medical Informatics; Assistant Professor, Medical Informatics, Section of Epidemiology, Department of Clinical Sciences, New York State College of Veterinary Medicine, Cornell University, Ithaca, New York
Section 1

DAVID J. POLZIN, D.V.M., PH.D. Associate Professor, Department of Small Animal Clinical Sciences, College of Veterinary Medicine, University of Minnesota, St. Paul, Minnesota
Section 12

MARC R. RAFFE, D.V.M., M.S. Associate Professor, Division of Comparative Anesthesiology, Department of Small Animal Clinical Sciences, College of Veterinary Medicine, University of Minnesota, St. Paul, Minnesota
Section 1

SARAH L. RALSTON, M.S., V.M.D., PH.D. Assistant Professor, Mark Morris Chair of Clinical Nutrition, Colorado State University, Ft. Collins, Colorado
Sections 1 and 3

R. WAYNE RANDOLPH, V.M.D., Dipl. A.B.V.P. Owner and Director, Countryside Veterinary Hospital, Flemington, New Jersey
Section 7

JOHN R. REED, M.S., D.V.M., Dipl. A.C.V.I.M. (Cardiology). Staff Cardiologist, Sacramento Animal Medical Group, North Highlands, California
Section 3

THOMAS J. REIMERS, PH.D. Associate Professor of Endocrinology and Director of the Endocrinology Laboratory, Diagnostic Laboratory, New York State College of Veterinary Medicine, Cornell University, Ithaca, New York
Section 10

KEITH P. RICHTER, D.V.M., Dipl. A.C.V.I.M. Staff Clinician in Internal Medicine, Helen Woodward Specialty Referral Hospital, Santa Fe, California
Section 12

RONALD C. RIIS, D.V.M., M.S., Dipl. A.C.V.O. Associate Professor, Veterinary Medicine, New York State College of Veterinary Medicine, Cornell University; Comparative Ophthalmologist, New York State College of Veterinary Medicine, Cornell University, Ithaca, New York
Section 6

J. EDMOND RIVIERE, D.V.M., PH.D. Professor of Pharmacology and Toxicology, Laboratory of Toxicokinetics, Department of Anatomy, Physiological Sciences, and Radiology, North Carolina State University, Raleigh, North Carolina
Section 1

KENITA S. ROGERS, D.V.M., M.S., Dipl. A.C.V.I.M. (Internal Medicine). Assistant Professor of Medicine, Department of Small Animal Medicine and Surgery, College of Veterinary Medicine, Texas A&M University; Internist, Small Animal Medicine and Surgery, Texas Veterinary Medical Center, Texas A&M University, College Station, Texas
Section 12

QUINTON R. ROGERS, PH.D. Professor of Physiological Chemistry, School of Veterinary Medicine, University of California, Davis, California
Section 3

WAYNE ROSENKRANTZ, D.V.M., Dipl. A.C.V.D. Assistant Clinical Instructor, Perceptorship Program, University of California, Davis, California; Associate Dermatologist, Animal Dermatology Clinic, Garden Grove and Santa Monica, California
Section 5

ROBERT C. ROSENTHAL, D.V.M., M.S., PH.D., Dipl. A.C.V.I.M. Assistant Professor, Medicine/Oncology, Department of Medical Sciences, School of Veterinary Medicine, University of Wisconsin, Madison, Wisconsin
Section 4

LINDA A. ROSS, D.V.M. Assistant Professor, Department of Medicine, Tufts University School of Veterinary Medicine; Clinician, Foster Hospital for Small Animals, Tufts University, North Grafton, Massachusetts
Section 12

EDMUND J. ROSSER, JR., D.V.M., Dipl. A.C.V.D. Assistant Professor, Dermatology, Department of Small Animal Clinical Sciences, Veterinary Clinical Center, Michigan State University, East Lansing, Michigan
Section 5

LOIS ROTH, D.V.M., PH.D., Dipl. A.C.V.P. Assistant Professor, Department of Pathobiology, Virginia-Maryland Regional College of Veterinary Medicine, Virginia Polytechnic Institute and State University; Diagnostic Pathologist, Veterinary Teaching Hospital, Virginia-Maryland Regional College of Veterinary Medicine, Virginia Polytechnic Institute and State University, Blacksburg, Virginia
Section 9

STANLEY I. RUBIN, D.V.M. M.S. Associate Professor, Internal Medicine, Department of

Veterinary Internal Medicine, Western College of Veterinary Medicine, University of Saskatchewan; Attending Clinician, Small Animal Clinic, Veterinary Teaching Hospital, Western College of Veterinary Medicine, University of Saskatchewan, Saskatoon, Saskatchewan, Canada
Section 1

VICKI J. SCHEIDT, D.V.M., Dipl. A.C.V.D. Assistant Professor, Dermatology, College of Veterinary Medicine, North Carolina State University, Raleigh, North Carolina
Section 5

ERIC R. SCHERTEL, D.V.M., PH.D. Clinical Instructor, Department of Veterinary Clinical Sciences, College of Veterinary Medicine, The Ohio State University; Clinical Instructor, Veterinary Teaching Hospital, The Ohio State University, Columbus, Ohio
Section 3

STEPHEN M. SCHUCHMAN, D.V.M. Boulevard Pet Hospital, Castro Valley, California
Section 7

DANNY W. SCOTT, D.V.M., Dipl. A.C.V.D. Professor of Medicine, New York State College of Veterinary Medicine, Cornell University, Ithaca, New York
Section 5

FREDERIC W. SCOTT, D.V.M., PH.D. Professor of Virology, Department of Microbiology, New York State College of Veterinary Medicine, Cornell University; Director, Cornell Feline Health Center, Cornell University, Ithaca, New York
Appendices

HOWARD B. SEIM, III, D.V.M., Dipl. A.C.V.S. Associate Professor of Veterinary Surgery, Department of Clinical Sciences, Colorado State University; Staff Member, Department of Surgery, Veterinary Medical Teaching Hospital, Colorado State University, Fort Collins, Colorado
Section 8

DAVID F. SENIOR, B.V.SC., Dipl. A.C.V.I.M. (Internal Medicine). Associate Professor, Department of Medical Sciences, Veterinary Medical Teaching Hospital, University of Florida; Chief, Small Animal Medicine, Veterinary Medical Teaching Hospital, College of Veterinary Medicine, University of Florida, Gainesville, Florida
Section 12

WAYNE SHAPIRO, M.S., D.V.M. Clinical Assistant Professor of Medicine, Tufts University

School of Veterinary Medicine, North Grafton, Massachusetts; Staff Oncologist, Angell Memorial Animal Hospital, Jamaica Plain, Massachusetts
Section 4

NICHOLAS SHARP, B.Vet.Med., Dipl. A.C.V.S. Research Associate, College of Veterinary Medicine, North Carolina State University, Raleigh, North Carolina
Section 11

G. DIANE SHELTON, D.V.M., PH.D., Dipl. A.C.V.I.M. Postdoctoral Fellow, Receptor Biology Laboratory, The Salk Institute, La Jolla, California
Section 8

GRADY H. SHELTON, D.V.M. Affiliate Assistant Professor, Division of Animal Medicine, School of Medicine, University of Washington, Seattle, Washington; Clinical Director, Feline Retrovirus Clinic, Pacific Northwest Research Foundation, Seattle, Washington
Section 4

VICTOR M. SHILLE, D.V.M., PH.D., Dipl. A.C.T. Associate Professor, College of Veterinary Medicine, University of Florida, Gainesville, Florida
Section 13

ANDY SHORES, D.V.M., PH.D. Associate Professor, Neurology/Neurosurgery, College of Veterinary Medicine, Michigan State University; Department of Small Animal Clinical Sciences, Veterinary Clinical Center, Michigan State University, East Lansing, Michigan
Section 8

SAM SILVERMAN, D.V.M., PH.D., Dipl. A.C.V.R. Clinical Professor of Veterinary Radiology, School of Veterinary Medicine, University of California, Davis, California
Section 7

ERIC R. SIMONSON, A.H.T., R.L.A.T. Clinical Oncology, Department of Nursing, Veterinary Medical Teaching Hospital, University of California; Chemotherapy Instructor, Department of Nursing, Veterinary Medical Teaching Hospital, University of California, Davis, California
Section 4

STEPHEN T. SIMPSON, D.V.M., M.S., Dipl. A.C.V.I.M. (Neurology). Associate Professor, College of Veterinary Medicine, Auburn University; Staff Neurologist, Small Animal Clinic, College of Veterinary Medicine, Auburn University, Auburn, Alabama
Section 8

MICHAEL H. SIMS, PH.D. Associate Professor, College of Veterinary Medicine, University of Tennessee; Department of Urban Practice, College of Veterinary Medicine, University of Tennessee, Knoxville, Tennessee
Section 8

D. DAVID SISSON, D.V.M. Assistant Professor, College of Veterinary Medicine, University of Illinois; Staff Cardiologist, Veterinary Medical Teaching Hospital, University of Illinois, Urbana, Illinois
Section 3

ROBERT J. SLAPPENDEL, D.V.M., PH.D. Associate Professor of Internal Medicine, Department of Small Animal Medicine, Faculty of Veterinary Medicine, State University of Utrecht; Clinical Hematologist and Head of Intensive Care, Small Animal Clinic, State University of Utrecht, Utrecht, The Netherlands
Section 4

E. ELIZABETH SPARGER, D.V.M., M.S., Dipl. A.C.V.I.M. NIH Postdoctoral Research Fellow, Department of Medicine, School of Veterinary Medicine, University of California, Davis, California
Section 4

GLEN L. SPAULDING, D.V.M., Dipl. A.C.V.I.M. Assistant Professor, Department of Medicine, Tufts University School of Veterinary Medicine, North Grafton, Massachusetts
Section 3

JAMES F. SWANSON, D.V.M., M.S. Dipl. A.C.V.O. General Ophthalmology Practice, Gulf Coast Animal Eye Clinic, Houston, Texas
Section 6

JAY C. SWEENEY, V.M.D. Chief Veterinarian, Veterinary Consultant Services, San Diego, California
Section 7

TODD R. TAMS, D.V.M., Dipl. A.C.V.I.M. Medical Director, West Los Angeles Veterinary Medical Group, West Los Angeles, California
Sections 3 and 9

JAMES P. THOMPSON, D.V.M., PH.D., Dipl. A.C.V.I.M. Assistant Professor, College of Veterinary Medicine, University of Florida; Head, Oncology Service; Head, Clinical Immunology Laboratory; Veterinary Teaching Hospital, University of Florida, Gainesville, Florida
Section 4

LARRY P. THORNBURG, D.V.M., PH.D. Associate Professor, Department of Veterinary Pathology, University of Missouri, Columbia, Missouri
Section 9

HAROLD L. TRAMMEL, B.S.Pharm., Pharm.D. Co-Director, Illinois Animal Poison Information Center, College of Veterinary Medicine, University of Illinois, Urbana, Illinois
Section 2

WILLIAM TRANQUILLI, D.V.M., M.S., Dipl. A.C.V.A. Associate Professor, Veterinary Clinical Medicine (Anesthesiology), College of Veterinary Medicine, University of Illinois, Urbana, Illinois
Section 2

JANE M. TURREL, D.V.M., M.S. Radiation Oncologist, Veterinary Tumor Institute, Santa Cruz, California
Section 12

DAVID C. TWEDT, D.V.M., Dipl. A.C.V.I.M. Associate Professor, Department of Clinical Sciences, College of Veterinary Medicine and Biomedical Sciences, Colorado State University; Staff Internist, Veterinary Teaching Hospital, Colorado State University, Fort Collins, Colorado
Section 9

SHELLY VADEN, D.V.M. Medical Resident, Department of Companion Animal and Special Species Medicine, North Carolina State University; Medical Resident, Teaching Hospital, North Carolina State University, Raleigh, North Carolina
Sections 3 and 12

WILLIAM M. VALENTINE, PH.D., D.V.M. Postdoctoral Research Associate, Department of Veterinary Biosciences, College of Veterinary Medicine, University of Illinois, Urbana, Illinois
Section 2

W. A. VESTRE, D.V.M., M.S., Dipl. A.C.V.O. Veterinary Ophthalmic Consulting, Indianapolis, Indiana
Section 6

DANIEL A. WARD, D.V.M. Ophthalmology Resident, Department of Small Animal Medicine, College of Veterinary Medicine, University of Georgia, Athens, Georgia
Section 6

WENDY A. WARE, D.V.M., M.S. Assistant Professor, Department of Veterinary Clinical Sciences, Iowa State University; Staff Cardiologist, Veterinary Teaching Hospital, Iowa State University, Ames, Iowa
Section 3

ELEANOR C. WEIR, B.V.M.S., M.R.C.V.S., Dipl. A.C.V.I.M. (Internal Medicine) Assistant Professor, Comparative Medicine, Yale University School of Medicine; Head, Veterinary Clinical Sciences, Section of Comparative Medicine, Yale University School of Medicine, New Haven, Connecticut
Section 10

LYNN G. WHEATON, D.V.M., Dipl. A.C.V.S. Assistant Professor, Department of Veterinary Clinical Medicine, College of Veterinary Medicine, University of Illinois; Staff Surgeon, Small Animal Clinic, College of Veterinary Medicine, University of Illinois, Urbana, Illinois
Section 13

STEVEN L. WHEELER, D.V.M., M.S., Dipl., A.C.V.I.M.(Internal Medicine) Assistant Professor, Department of Clinical Sciences, College of Veterinary Medicine and Biomedical Sciences, Colorado State University; Intensive Care Unit, Veterinary Teaching Hospital, Colorado State University, Fort Collins, Colorado
Section 1

JERRY V. WHITE, D.V.M. Research Associate, Department of Physiology and Pharmacology, College of Veterinary Medicine, University of Georgia, Athens, Georgia
Section 12

MAURICE E. WHITE, D.V.M., Dipl. A.C.V.I.M., A.S.V.P. Associate Professor of Medicine, New York State College of Veterinary Medicine, Cornell University, Ithaca, New York
Section 13

STEPHEN D. WHITE, D.V.M., Dipl. A.C.V.D. Assistant Professor, Department of Clinical Sciences, College of Veterinary Medicine and Biomedical Sciences, Colorado State University, Fort Collins, Colorado
Section 5

ELIZABETH L. WHITNEY, D.V.M. Staff Member, Welsh Animal Clinic, Fort Collins, Colorado
Section 9

MICHAEL D. WILLARD, D.V.M., M.S., Dipl. A.C.V.I.M. Professor of Small Animal Medicine and Surgery, College of Veterinary Medicine,

Texas A&M University; Internist, Texas Veterinary Medical Center, College of Veterinary Medicine, Texas A&M University, College Station, Texas
Sections 1 and 9

DAVID A. WILLIAMS, M.A., VET.M.B., PH.D., M.R.C.V.S., Dipl. A.C.V.I.M. Assistant Professor, Department of Small Animal Clinical Studies, University of Florida; Small Animal Medicine, Veterinary Medical Teaching Hospital, University of Florida, Gainesville, Florida
Section 9

MELANIE M. WILLIAMS, D.V.M., Dipl. A.C.V.O. Assistant Professor, Ontario Veterinary College, University of Guelph, Guelph, Ontario, Canada; Veterinary Ophthalmologist, Vernale Veterinary Services, Campbellville, Ontario, Canada
Section 6

DENNIS WILSON, D.V.M., PH.D. Assistant Professor, Department of Veterinary Pathology, University of California, Davis, California
Section 11

KAREN J. WOLFSHEIMER, D.V.M., PH.D. Assistant Professor, School of Veterinary Medicine, Louisiana State University; Clinician, Veterinary Medical Teaching Hospital, Louisiana State University, Baton Rouge, Louisiana
Section 10

ROBERT H. WRIGLEY, B.V.SC., M.S., D.V.R., M.R.C.V.S., Dipl. A.C.V.R. Associate Professor, Department of Radiology and Radiation Biology, College of Veterinary Medicine and Biomedical Sciences, Colorado State University; Chief, Radiology Section, Veterinary Teaching Hospital, Colorado State University, Fort Collins, Colorado
Section 13

JANET K. YAMAMOTO, PH.D. Assistant Research Immunologist, Department of Medicine, School of Veterinary Medicine, University of California, Davis, California
Section 4

DENNIS A. ZAWIE, D.V.M., Dipl. A.C.V.I.M. Staff Internist, Co-Director, Farmingville Animal Hospital, Farmingville, New York
Section 9

CAROLE A. ZERBE, D.V.M., M.S. Resident, Department of Physiology and Pharmacology, College of Veterinary Medicine, Auburn University, Auburn, Alabama
Section 10

PREFACE

Current Veterinary Therapy X marks a special milestone—the twenty-fifth anniversary of publication of the first edition. In the preface to that fledgling edition, we stated: "This book has been written to provide the small animal clinician with easily accessible information on the latest accepted methods of treating medical conditions encountered in a pet practice." The subsequent series has been successful, since veterinarians have continued to use it in the front line of daily practice as a quick, authoritative source of help. We are pleased too, because it also helps our profession provide the public with better veterinary service. Over the years, we have tried to keep the "Current" in the title true by shortening deadlines and rotating topics, authors, and editors.

The time is fast approaching for this editor to rotate, too. With that in mind, John Bonagura has joined us as associate editor. John's expertise in internal medicine is well known from his outstanding reputation as a speaker, writer, and faculty member at The Ohio State University, and from his management of the cardiopulmonary section in recent editions of *Current Veterinary Therapy*. He brings a wealth of fresh, new ideas to the series.

In this edition, we continue our efforts to make the *CVT* series a continuum of reference texts. The dosage list in the appendices contains cross references to pages in the ninth as well as the tenth edition where more information can be found about individual drugs. The index in this edition also contains a complete listing of all articles in the ninth edition and notation of a few special topics from *CVT VIII*, which are still current. These references are appropriately highlighted in the index by the placing of Roman numeral VIII or IX before the appropriate page numbers. We hope that these changes will help busy practitioners find complete information more easily.

In this volume, the immunology and oncology, cardiopulmonary, gastrointestinal, endocrinology, dermatology, and reproduction sections reflect particularly active development. However, all sections are completely new, and we are proud to present this tenth edition for your use. We appreciate your acceptance of previous editions and hope that you will continue to use *Current Veterinary Therapy* as the "Bible" for your practice. As always, suggestions for additions and improvements are genuinely welcomed.

To each person involved in the preparation of this edition, we owe our deep appreciation. The authors of topics in the text are outstanding, dynamic clinical investigators who make the book authoritative. The section editors have skillfully planned their chapters to include pertinent new material, refereed the contents, and worked to coordinate the subject matter with other chapters. Darlene Pedersen, Linda Mills, and their colleagues at the W. B. Saunders Company have excelled in producing this book. Our most sincere thanks to all.

ROBERT W. KIRK, D.V.M.

Ithaca, New York

NOTICE

Extraordinary efforts have been made by the authors, the editors, and the publisher of this book to ensure that dosage recommendations are precise and in agreement with standards officially accepted at the time of publication.

It does happen, however, that dosage schedules are changed from time to time in the light of accumulating clinical experience and continuing laboratory studies. This is most likely to occur in the case of recently introduced products.

It is urged, therefore, that you check the manufacturer's recommendations for dosage, especially if the drug to be administered or prescribed is one that you use only infrequently or have not used for some time.

In addition, some drugs mentioned have been used by the authors as experimental drugs. Others have been used after official clearance for use in one species but not in others described here. This is particularly true for rare and exotic species. In these cases, the authors have reported their own considerable experience, but readers are urged to view the recommendations with discretion and precaution.

THE EDITORS

CONTENTS

SECTION

1

SPECIAL THERAPY

Carl A. Osborne
Consulting Editor

COMPUTER-AIDED DIAGNOSIS 2
  Roy V. H. Pollock

UNDERSTANDING CLINICAL STUDIES 8
  Jody P. Lulich,
  Carl A. Osborne, and
  Shirley D. Johnston

CAUSE AND CONTROL OF DECREASED
APPETITE 18
  Dennis W. Macy and
  Sarah L. Ralston

PARENTERAL NUTRITIONAL SUPPORT 25
  Aunna C. Lippert and
  P. Jane Armstrong

ENTERAL NUTRITIONAL SUPPORT 30
  Steven L. Wheeler and
  Barbara H. McGuire

MAINTENANCE FLUID THERAPY 37
  Ford Watson Bell and
  Carl A. Osborne

HYPOPHOSPHATEMIA 43
  Robert M. Hardy and
  Larry G. Adams

NONSTEROIDAL ANTI-INFLAMMATORY
DRUGS 47
  Stanley I. Rubin and
  Mark G. Papich

GLUCOCORTICOID THERAPY 54
  Mark G. Papich and
  Lloyd E. Davis

CHEMICAL RESTRAINT TECHNIQUES IN
DOGS AND CATS 63
  Ronald E. Mandsager and
  Marc R. Raffe

ANTIMICROBIAL SUSCEPTIBILITY TESTS 70
  Dwight C. Hirsh

CEPHALOSPORINS 74
  J. Edmond Riviere

CLAVULANATE-POTENTIATED ANTIBIOTICS ... 78
  W. Randal Kilgore

TREATMENT OF FUNGAL AND ENDOCRINE
DISORDERS WITH IMIDAZOLE
DERIVATIVES 82
  Michael D. Willard

THE PRACTICE OF VETERINARY MEDICINE
IN HUMANE SOCIETY FACILITIES 85
  Mark Aljian Edwards

DISINFECTION OF ANIMAL
ENVIRONMENTS 90
  Dennis F. Lawler

SECTION

2

CHEMICAL AND PHYSICAL DISORDERS

Gary D. Osweiler
Consulting Editor

INCIDENCE OF POISONINGS IN SMALL
ANIMALS 97
  Val Richard Beasley and
  Harold L. Trammel

COMPANION ANIMAL FORENSIC
TOXICOLOGY 114
   William C. Edwards

EMERGENCY AND GENERAL TREATMENT
OF POISONINGS 116
   E. Murl Bailey, Jr.

TOXICANT-INDUCED ACUTE RENAL
FAILURE 126
   Gregory F. Grauer

THIACETARSAMIDE AND ITS ADVERSE
EFFECTS 131
   Johnny D. Hoskins

ORGANOPHOSPHORUS AND CARBAMATE
INSECTICIDE POISONING 135
   Gavin L. Meerdink

PYRETHRINS AND PYRETHROIDS 137
   William M. Valentine and
   Val Richard Beasley

IVERMECTIN 140
   Allan Paul and
   William Tranquilli

THE ANTICOAGULANT RODENTICIDES 143
   Michael J. Murphy and
   Diane F. Gerken

BROMETHALIN POISONING 147
   Thomas L. Carson

DIAGNOSIS OF AND THERAPY FOR
CHOLECALCIFEROL TOXICOSIS 148
   David C. Dorman and
   Val Richard Beasley

LEAD POISONING 152
   Gerald R. Bratton and
   David F. Kowalczyk

ARSENIC POISONING 159
   Regg D. Neiger

TOXICOLOGY OF DETERGENTS, BLEACHES,
ANTISEPTICS, AND DISINFECTANTS 162
   Robert W. Coppock,
   M. S. Mostrom, and
   L. E. Lillie

ETHANOL AND ILLICIT DRUGS OF ABUSE 171
   Robert W. Coppock,
   M. S. Mostrom, and
   L. E. Lillie

BITES AND STINGS OF VENOMOUS
ANIMALS 177
   Michael E. Peterson and
   Gavin L. Meerdink

SECTION

3

CARDIOPULMONARY DISEASES
John D. Bonagura
Consulting Editor

DIAGNOSTIC APPROACH TO
CARDIOPULMONARY DISORDERS 188
   Timothy G. Bauer

INITIAL MANAGEMENT OF RESPIRATORY
EMERGENCIES 195
   R. J. Murtaugh and
   Glen L. Spaulding

ECHOCARDIOGRAPHY: THERAPEUTIC
IMPLICATIONS 201
   N. Sydney Moise

BRONCHOSCOPY IN THE SMALL ANIMAL
PATIENT 219
   Brendan C. McKiernan

CONGENITAL HEART DISEASE 224
   Matthew W. Miller and
   John D. Bonagura

ACQUIRED VALVULAR HEART DISEASE IN
THE DOG 231
   John R. Reed

CANINE CARDIOMYOPATHY 240
   Bruce W. Keene

CARDIOMYOPATHY IN THE CAT AND ITS
RELATION TO TAURINE DEFICIENCY 251
   Paul D. Pion,
   Mark D. Kittleson, and
   Quinton R. Rogers

CANINE AND FELINE HEARTWORM
DISEASE 263
   Thomas N. Hribernik

ATRIAL ARRHYTHMIAS 271
   John D. Bonagura

THERAPY FOR VENTRICULAR
ARRHYTHMIAS 278
    Wendy A. Ware and
    Robert L. Hamlin

BRADYARRHYTHMIAS AND CARDIAC
PACING 286
    D. David Sisson

THERAPY FOR FELINE AORTIC
THROMBOEMBOLISM 295
    Paul D. Pion and
    Mark D. Kittleson

DIETARY CONSIDERATIONS IN THE
TREATMENT OF HEART FAILURE 302
    Sarah L. Ralston

COMPLICATIONS OF CARDIOPULMONARY
DRUG THERAPY 308
    Philip R. Fox and
    Mark G. Papich

SHOCK: PATHOPHYSIOLOGY, MONITORING,
AND THERAPY 316
    Eric R. Schertel and
    William W. Muir

CARDIOPULMONARY RESUSCITATION 330
    Steve C. Haskins

MEDICAL MANAGEMENT OF UPPER
RESPIRATORY TRACT DISEASE 337
    Shelly Vaden and
    Richard B. Ford

LARYNGEAL PARALYSIS 343
    Dennis N. Aron

TRACHEAL COLLAPSE 353
    Roger B. Fingland

CHRONIC RESPIRATORY DISEASE IN THE
DOG 361
    John D. Bonagura,
    Robert L. Hamlin, and
    Cathy E. Gaber

PULMONARY HYPERSENSITIVITY
DISORDERS 369
    Timothy G. Bauer

PNEUMONIA 376
    Todd R. Tams

PULMONARY EDEMA 385
    Neil Harpster

CHYLOTHORAX 393
    Theresa W. Fossum and
    Stephen J. Birchard

RESPIRATORY NEOPLASIA 399
    Marcia Carothers and
    C. Guillermo Couto

PLEURODESIS 405
    Stephen J. Birchard,
    Theresa W. Fossum, and
    Laura Gallagher

SECTION

4

HEMATOLOGY, ONCOLOGY, AND IMMUNOLOGY

Bruce R. Madewell

Consulting Editor

SAMPLE PREPARATION FOR THE
LABORATORY 410
    Bruce R. Madewell

PARASITIC BLOOD DISEASES OF DOGS
AND CATS 419
    Thomas N. Hribernik and
    Steven C. Barr

FELINE ANEMIA 425
    Gary J. Kociba

HEREDITARY DISORDERS OF CANINE
ERYTHROCYTES 429
    Urs Giger

DIAGNOSTIC APPROACH TO THE BLEEDING
PATIENT 436
    I. B. Johnstone

FACTOR VIII (HEMOPHILIA A) AND
FACTOR IX (HEMOPHILIA B)
DEFICIENCIES IN SMALL ANIMALS 442
    Jens M. Fogh

VON WILLEBRAND'S DISEASE IN DOGS 446
    Karl H. Kraus and Gary S. Johnson

DISSEMINATED INTRAVASCULAR
COAGULATION 451
    Robert J. Slappendel

DISORDERS OF PLATELETS 457
    Bernard F. Feldman

CYTOCHEMISTRY OF CANINE AND FELINE
LEUKOCYTES AND LEUKEMIAS 465
    N. C. Jain

ACUTE PHASE PROTEINS 468
    N. C. Jain

ANTINEOPLASTIC AGENTS IN CANCER
THERAPY 472
    James P. Thompson

SPECIAL CONSIDERATIONS IN DRUG
PREPARATION AND ADMINISTRATION 475
    Bruce R. Madewell and
    Eric R. Simonson

CHEMOTHERAPY OF LYMPHOMA AND
LEUKEMIA 482
    Robert E. Matus

CHEMOTHERAPY OF SOLID TUMORS 489
    Stuart C. Helfand

CHEMOTHERAPY-INDUCED
MYELOSUPPRESSION 494
    Robert C. Rosenthal

CISPLATIN CHEMOTHERAPY 497
    Wayne Shapiro

RADIATION THERAPY 502
    Susan M. LaRue

BIOLOGICAL RESPONSE MODIFIERS 507
    Chris K. Grant and
    Grady H. Shelton

CYCLOSPORINE 513
    Clare R. Gregory

BONE MARROW TRANSPLANTATION 515
    Peter W. Gasper

CONGENITAL AND ACQUIRED
NEUTROPHIL FUNCTION ABNORMALITIES
IN THE DOG 521
    C. Guillermo Couto and
    Urs Giger

THE RISK OF TRANSMISSION OF FeLV
FROM LATENTLY INFECTED CATS 526
    Angela M. Pacitti

FELINE IMMUNODEFICIENCY VIRUS
INFECTION 530
    E. Elizabeth Sparger and
    Janet K. Yamamoto

FELINE LYMPHOID HYPERPLASIA 535
    Susan M. Cotter

ACUTE HYPERSENSITIVITY REACTIONS 537
    Melisa A. Degen

IMMUNE-MEDIATED NONEROSIVE
ARTHRITIS IN THE DOG 543
    Patrick E. Hopper

SECTION

5

DERMATOLOGIC DISEASES
Danny W. Scott
Consulting Editor

RETINOIDS IN DERMATOLOGY 553
    Kenneth W. Kwochka

IVERMECTIN IN SMALL ANIMAL
DERMATOLOGY 560
    Manon Paradis

FATTY ACID SUPPLEMENTS AS ANTI-
INFLAMMATORY AGENTS 563
    William H. Miller, Jr.

NONSTEROIDAL ANTI-INFLAMMATORY
AGENTS IN THE MANAGEMENT OF CANINE
AND FELINE PRURITUS 566
    William H. Miller, Jr.

IMMUNOMODULATING DRUGS IN
DERMATOLOGY 570
    Wayne Rosenkrantz

IMIDAZOLES AND TRIAZOLES 577
    Linda Medleau

LASERS IN DERMATOLOGY 580
    Patrick T. Breen

MILIARY DERMATITIS, EOSINOPHILIC
GRANULOMA COMPLEX, AND SYMMETRIC
HYPOTRICHOSIS AS MANIFESTATIONS OF
FELINE ALLERGY 583
    Gail A. Kunkle

FLEAS AND FLEA CONTROL 586
    Diane E. Bevier-Tournay

RAST AND ELISA TESTING IN CANINE
ATOPY 592
    Craig E. Griffin

SEX HORMONE–RELATED DERMATOSES IN DOGS 595
William H. Miller, Jr.

HORMONAL REPLACEMENT THERAPY IN VETERINARY DERMATOLOGY 602
Stephen D. White

FAMILIAL CANINE DERMATOMYOSITIS 606
Kirk H. Haupt and
Ann M. Hargis

STAPHYLOCOCCI AND GERMAN SHEPHERD PYODERMA 609
Robert G. Buerger

LICHENOID DERMATOSES IN DOGS AND CATS 614
Danny W. Scott

DERMATOSES OF THE NOSE AND THE FOOTPADS IN DOGS AND CATS 616
Donna Walton Angarano

DERMATOSES OF THE PINNAE 621
Vicki J. Scheidt

CANINE CUTANEOUS HISTIOCYTOSES 625
Danny W. Scott

FELINE CUTANEOUS MAST CELL TUMORS ... 627
Robert G. Buerger

DISORDERS OF MELANIN PIGMENTATION IN THE SKIN OF DOGS AND CATS 628
Eric Guaguere and
Zeineb Alhaidari

SPOROTRICHOSIS AND PUBLIC HEALTH 633
Edmund J. Rosser, Jr.

OPHTHALMIC USAGE OF NONSTEROIDAL ANTI-INFLAMMATORY AGENTS 642
Sheryl Greve Krohne and
W. A. Vestre

SUDDEN BLINDNESS 644
Marjorie H. Neaderland

MEDICAL THERAPY FOR GLAUCOMA 647
Charles L. Martin and
Daniel A. Ward

UVEITIS 652
James F. Swanson

ULCERATIVE KERATITIS 656
Joan Dziezyc

NEONATAL OPHTHALMIC DISORDERS 658
Melanie M. Williams

CONJUNCTIVAL DISORDERS 673
Cecil P. Moore

DERMATOLOGIC DISORDERS OF THE EYELID AND PERIOCULAR REGION 678
Donna Walton Angarano

OCULAR DISORDERS OF RABBITS, RODENTS, AND FERRETS 681
Thomas J. Kern

THE OPHTHALMOLOGY REFERRAL PATIENT 686
Pennie L. Cooley and
Paul F. Dice, II

NEURO-OPHTHALMOLOGY 687
Mary B. Glaze

ADNEXAL TUMORS OF DOGS AND CATS 692
Dennis V. Hacker

SECTION

6

OPHTHALMOLOGIC DISEASES

Thomas J. Kern and Ronald C. Riis
Consulting Editors

OCULAR EMERGENCIES 636
Susan A. McLaughlin

THERAPEUTIC USE OF HYDROPHILIC CONTACT LENSES 640
Kohle Herrmann

SECTION

7

DISEASES OF CAGED BIRDS AND EXOTIC PETS

Murray E. Fowler
Consulting Editor

ZOONOSES OF CONCERN TO VOLUNTEERS AND STAFF OF WILD ANIMAL REHABILITATION CENTERS 697
Murray E. Fowler

BASIC ORNAMENTAL FISH MEDICINE 703
  Scott B. Citino

WHAT PRACTITIONERS SHOULD KNOW
ABOUT WHALE STRANDINGS 721
  Jay C. Sweeney

PREVENTIVE MEDICINE IN NONDOMESTIC
CARNIVORES 727
  Lyndsay G. Phillips, Jr.

LLAMA BASICS 734
  Murray E. Fowler

INDIVIDUAL CARE AND TREATMENT OF
RABBITS, MICE, RATS, GUINEA PIGS,
HAMSTERS, AND GERBILS 738
  Stephen M. Schuchman

MEDICAL AND SURGICAL CARE OF THE
PET FERRET 765
  R. Wayne Randolph

UPDATE ON AVIAN ANESTHESIA 776
  Keven Flammer

MICROBIOLOGIC TECHNIQUES FOR THE
AVIAN PRACTITIONER 780
  Kim Lorraine Joyner

ADVANCES IN AVIAN AND REPTILIAN
IMAGING 786
  Sam Silverman

REPAIR OF INJURIES TO THE CHELONIAN
PLASTRON AND CARAPACE 789
  Gary Harwell

VITAMIN A SOURCES, HYPOVITAMINOSIS A,
AND IATROGENIC HYPERVITAMINOSIS A
IN CAPTIVE CHELONIANS 791
  Fredric L. Frye

SEXUAL DIMORPHISM AND
IDENTIFICATION IN REPTILES 796
  Fredric L. Frye

SECTION

8

NEUROLOGIC AND NEUROMUSCULAR DISORDERS

Joe N. Kornegay
Consulting Editor

HEARING LOSS IN SMALL ANIMALS:
OCCURRENCE AND DIAGNOSIS 805
  Michael H. Sims

HYPOKALEMIC POLYMYOPATHY OF CATS 812
  Steven W. Dow and
  Richard A. LeCouteur

CANINE MASTICATORY MUSCLE
DISORDERS 816
  G. Diane Shelton and
  George H. Cardinet, III

HEREDITARY MYOPATHY OF LABRADOR
RETRIEVERS 820
  Rosemary E. McKerrell and
  Kyle G. Braund

SENSORY NEUROPATHY 822
  Ian D. Duncan and
  Paul A. Cuddon

PROGRESSIVE AXONOPATHY OF BOXER
DOGS 828
  Ian R. Griffiths

DEGENERATIVE MYELOPATHY 830
  Roger M. Clemmons

HYPOMYELINATION IN DOGS 834
  Katharine F. Jackson and
  Ian D. Duncan

CONGENITAL CEREBELLAR DISEASES OF
DOGS AND CATS 838
  Joe N. Kornegay

HYDROCEPHALUS 842
  Stephen T. Simpson

CRANIOCEREBRAL TRAUMA 847
  Andy Shores

GRANULOMATOUS
MENINGOENCEPHALOMYELITIS 854
  Kyle G. Braund

WOBBLER SYNDROME IN THE
DOBERMAN PINSCHER 858
  Howard B. Seim, III

SECTION

9

GASTROINTESTINAL DISORDERS

David C. Twedt
Consulting Editor

ENDOSCOPY 864
  Todd R. Tams

FELINE HEPATIC LIPIDOSIS 869
Larry M. Cornelius and
Gilbert Jacobs

SERUM BILE ACID CONCENTRATIONS FOR
HEPATOBILIARY FUNCTION TESTING IN
CATS 873
Sharon A. Center

DRUG-INDUCED HEPATIC DISEASE OF
DOGS AND CATS 878
Susan E. Bunch

CHOLELITHIASIS AND CHOLANGITIS 884
Susan E. Johnson

COPPER METABOLISM DEFECT IN WEST
HIGHLAND TERRIERS 889
Larry P. Thornburg

MANAGEMENT OF HEPATIC COPPER
TOXICOSIS IN DOGS 891
David C. Twedt and
Elizabeth L. Whitney

FELINE PANCREATITIS 893
Dennis W. Macy

EFFECTS OF GLUCOCORTICOIDS ON THE
GASTROINTESTINAL SYSTEM 897
Ray Dillon

ESOPHAGEAL STRICTURES 904
Dennis A. Zawie

REFLUX ESOPHAGITIS 906
Todd R. Tams

MEDICAL THERAPY FOR
GASTROINTESTINAL ULCERS 911
Mark G. Papich

ANTRAL PYLORIC HYPERTROPHY
SYNDROME 918
Robert C. DeNovo

CANINE LYMPHOCYTIC-PLASMACYTIC
ENTERITIS 922
Michael L. Magne

EXOCRINE PANCREATIC INSUFFICIENCY 927
David A. Williams

CHRONIC INTESTINAL BACTERIAL
OVERGROWTH 933
Michael D. Willard

PLASMACYTIC-LYMPHOCYTIC COLITIS IN
DOGS 939
Michael S. Leib,
William H. Hay, and
Lois Roth

CAMPYLOBACTER ENTERITIS 944
Deborah J. Davenport

EXTRACTION AND ORAL-NASAL FISTULA 948
Peter P. Emily

ORAL DIAGNOSIS 951
Peter P. Emily

ENDODONTICS 954
Thomas W. Mulligan

SECTION

10

ENDOCRINE AND METABOLIC DISORDERS

Mark E. Peterson
Consulting Editor

COMMON ENDOCRINE DIAGNOSTIC TESTS:
NORMAL VALUES AND INTERPRETATION 961
Robert J. Kemppainen and
Carole A. Zerbe

GUIDELINES FOR COLLECTION, STORAGE,
AND TRANSPORT OF SAMPLES FOR
HORMONE ASSAY 968
Thomas J. Reimers

DIABETES INSIPIDUS 973
Rhett Nichols

CANINE GROWTH HORMONE–RESPONSIVE
DERMATOSIS 978
Clinton D. Lothrop, Jr.

FELINE ACROMEGALY (GROWTH
HORMONE EXCESS) 981
Mark E. Peterson

CANINE PRIMARY HYPERPARATHYROIDISM ... 985
Edward C. Feldman

HYPERCALCEMIA OF MALIGNANCY 988
Robert E. Matus and
Eleanor C. Weir

TREATMENT OF CANINE HYPOTHYROIDISM .. 993
Richard W. Nelson

CANINE MYXEDEMA STUPOR AND COMA 998
Michael J. Kelly

FELINE HYPOTHYROIDISM 1000
  Mark E. Peterson

TREATMENT OF FELINE
HYPERTHYROIDISM 1002
  Mark E. Peterson

DIETARY THERAPY FOR CANINE DIABETES
MELLITUS 1008
  Richard W. Nelson

INSULIN-RESISTANT DIABETES MELLITUS .. 1012
  Karen J. Wolfsheimer

MEDICAL TREATMENT OF NEUROENDOCRINE
TUMORS OF THE GASTROENTEROPANCREATIC
SYSTEM WITH SOMATOSTATIN 1020
  Clinton D. Lothrop, Jr.

THERAPY FOR SPONTANEOUS CANINE
HYPERADRENOCORTICISM 1024
  Edward C. Feldman,
  David S. Bruyette, and
  Richard W. Nelson

RADIATION THERAPY FOR CANINE ACTH-
SECRETING PITUITARY TUMORS 1031
  Steven W. Dow and
  Richard A. LeCouteur

MITOTANE (O,P'-DDD) TREATMENT OF
CORTISOL-SECRETING ADRENOCORTICAL
NEOPLASIA 1034
  Peter P. Kintzer and
  Mark E. Peterson

FELINE HYPERADRENOCORTICISM 1038
  Carole A. Zerbe

FELINE HYPOADRENOCORTICISM 1042
  Deborah S. Greco and
  Mark E. Peterson

HYPERLIPIDEMIA 1046
  P. Jane Armstrong and
  Richard B. Ford

SECTION
11
INFECTIOUS DISEASES
Craig E. Greene
Consulting Editor

PANEL ON FELINE LEUKEMIA VIRUS
VACCINATION

    INTRODUCTION 1052
      Craig E. Greene

DISCUSSION 1 1052
  Alfred M. Legendre

DISCUSSION 2 1056
  Richard L. Ott

DISCUSSION 3 1060
  Richard G. Olsen

ALTERNATIVE TESTING PROCEDURES FOR
FeLV 1065
  Eleanor C. Hawkins

MANAGEMENT OF THE FeLV-POSITIVE
PATIENT 1069
  Dennis W. Macy

CLINICAL SIGNIFICANCE OF ANTIGENIC
VARIATION IN CANINE PARVOVIRUS 1076
  Leland E. Carmichael and
  Colin R. Parrish

BACTEREMIA IN DOGS AND CATS 1077
  Steven W. Dow

ANAEROBIC INFECTIONS IN DOGS AND
CATS 1082
  Steven W. Dow

CANINE LYME BORRELIOSIS 1086
  Russell T. Greene

PLAGUE 1088
  Dennis W. Macy

GROUP G STREPTOCOCCAL INFECTIONS IN
KITTENS 1091
  Patricia Blanchard and
  Dennis Wilson

GROUP A STREPTOCOCCAL INFECTIONS IN
DOGS AND CATS 1094
  Craig E. Greene

CLINICAL AND PUBLIC HEALTH
SIGNIFICANCE OF ANTIMICROBIAL-
RESISTANT ENTERIC BACTERIAL
INFECTIONS 1096
  Dwight C. Hirsh

CAT-SCRATCH FEVER 1099
  Johnny D. Hoskins

SYSTEMIC ANTIFUNGAL CHEMOTHERAPY 1101
  James O. Noxon

NASAL ASPERGILLOSIS 1106
  Nicholas Sharp

FELINE CRYPTOCOCCOSIS 1109
Linda Medleau

FELINE TOXOPLASMOSIS 1112
Michael R. Lappin

SECTION

12

URINARY DISORDERS

Jeanne A. Barsanti
Consulting Editor

DIAGNOSTIC APPROACH TO CANINE AND
FELINE HEMATURIA 1117
Arthur L. Lage

CLINICAL EVALUATION OF RENAL
FUNCTION 1123
Delmar R. Finco and
Jeanne A. Barsanti

CRYSTALLURIA: CAUSES, DETECTION, AND
INTERPRETATION 1127
Carl A. Osborne,
Timothy D. O'Brien,
Marian P. Davenport, and
Chris W. Clinton

SPECTRUM OF CLINICAL AND LABORATORY
ABNORMALITIES IN UREMIA 1133
David J. Polzin

DIAGNOSTIC APPROACH TO PROTEINURIA 1139
Jerry V. White

POSITIVE-CONTRAST
VAGINOURETHROGRAPHY FOR DIAGNOSIS
OF LOWER URINARY TRACT DISEASE 1142
Peter E. Holt

USE OF URODYNAMICS IN MICTURITION
DISORDERS IN DOGS AND CATS 1145
Keith P. Richter

URODYNAMIC ABNORMALITIES
ASSOCIATED WITH CANINE PROSTATIC
DISEASES AND THERAPEUTIC
INTERVENTION 1151
R. Randy Basinger and
Jeanne A. Barsanti

FELINE VESICOURACHAL DIVERTICULA 1153
Carl A. Osborne,
John M. Kruger, and
Gary R. Johnston

RENAL EFFECTS OF NONSTEROIDAL ANTI-
INFLAMMATORY DRUGS 1158
Scott A. Brown

INFILTRATIVE URETHRAL DISEASES IN THE
DOG 1161
David T. Matthiesen and
Scott D. Moroff

FANCONI'S SYNDROME 1163
Scott A. Brown

RENAL FAILURE IN YOUNG DOGS 1166
Stephen P. DiBartola,
Deborah J. Davenport, and
Dennis J. Chew

CHRONIC RENAL DISEASE IN CATS 1170
Donald R. Krawiec and
Howard B. Gelberg

MEDICAL MANAGEMENT OF CANINE
GLOMERULONEPHROPATHIES 1174
Jeanne A. Barsanti,
Delmar R. Finco, and
Shelly Vaden

MEDICAL MANAGEMENT OF URATE
UROLITHS 1178
David F. Senior

CANINE CALCIUM OXALATE UROLITHIASIS .. 1182
Jody P. Lulich,
Carl A. Osborne,
Mary Lou Parker,
Chris W. Clinton, and
Marian P. Davenport

MEDICAL DISSOLUTION AND PREVENTION
OF CYSTINE UROLITHIASIS 1189
Carl A. Osborne,
Astrid Hoppe, and
Timothy D. O'Brien

MANAGEMENT OF PROSTATIC NEOPLASIA 1193
Jane M. Turrel

MANAGEMENT OF ADVANCED CHRONIC
RENAL FAILURE 1195
Timothy A. Allen

NEWER CONCEPTS AND CONTROVERSIES
ON DIETARY MANAGEMENT OF RENAL
FAILURE 1198
Delmar R. Finco and
Scott A. Brown

USE OF DRUGS TO CONTROL
HYPERTENSION IN RENAL FAILURE 1201
Linda A. Ross and
Mary Anna Labato

MANAGEMENT OF URINARY TRACT
INFECTIONS 1204
    Kenita S. Rogers and
    George E. Lees

FELINE PERINEAL URETHROSTOMY 1209
    Carl A. Osborne,
    Dennis D. Caywood,
    Gary R. Johnston, and
    John M. Kruger

PHARMACOLOGIC MANAGEMENT OF
URINARY INCONTINENCE 1214
    Philippe M. Moreau and
    Michael R. Lappin

SECTION

13

REPRODUCTIVE DISORDERS

Patricia N. Olson
Consulting Editor

DRUGS AFFECTING FERTILITY IN THE
MALE DOG 1224
    Joni L. Freshman

ULTRASONOGRAPHY AND ULTRASOUND-
GUIDED BIOPSY OF THE CANINE
PROSTATE 1227
    Susan T. Finn and
    Robert H. Wrigley

ULTRASONOGRAPHY OF THE CANINE
UTERUS AND OVARY 1239
    Robert H. Wrigley and
    Susan T. Finn

CHRONIC BACTERIAL PROSTATITIS IN THE
DOG 1243
    Laine A. Cowan and
    Jeanne A. Barsanti

CANINE SEMEN FREEZING AND
ARTIFICIAL INSEMINATION 1247
    P. W. Concannon and
    M. Battista

PREPUTIAL DISCHARGE IN THE DOG 1259
    William E. Hornbuckle and
    Maurice E. White

DISORDERS OF SEXUAL DEVELOPMENT IN
DOGS AND CATS 1261
    V. N. Meyers-Wallen and
    Donald F. Patterson

HORMONAL AND CLINICAL CORRELATES
OF OVARIAN CYCLES, OVULATION,
PSEUDOPREGNANCY, AND PREGNANCY IN
DOGS 1269
    P. W. Concannon and
    Donald H. Lein

DYNAMIC TESTING IN REPRODUCTIVE
ENDOCRINOLOGY 1282
    Victor M. Shille and
    Patricia N. Olson

INDUCTION OF ESTRUS AND OVULATION IN
THE BITCH 1288
    Janice L. Cain

EFFECTS OF DRUGS ON PREGNANCY 1291
    Mark G. Papich

DRUGS THAT AFFECT UTERINE MOTILITY ... 1299
    Lynn G. Wheaton

VAGINAL PROLAPSE 1302
    Shirley D. Johnston

DIAGNOSIS AND TREATMENT
ALTERNATIVES FOR PYOMETRA IN DOGS
AND CATS 1305
    Edward C. Feldman and
    Richard W. Nelson

VULVAR DISCHARGES 1310
    Cheri A. Johnson

DIAGNOSIS OF CANINE HERPETIC
INFECTIONS 1313
    James F. Evermann

DIAGNOSIS AND TREATMENT OF
CANINE BRUCELLOSIS 1317
    Paul Nicoletti

ANESTHETIC CONSIDERATIONS FOR
CESAREAN SECTION 1321
    J. L. Grandy

CARE AND DISEASES OF NEONATAL
PUPPIES AND KITTENS 1325
    Dennis F. Lawler

APPENDICES

Robert W. Kirk
John D. Bonagura
Consulting Editors

A ROSTER OF NORMAL VALUES FOR DOGS
AND CATS 1335
    John Bentinck-Smith and
    Tracy W. French

TABLES OF NORMAL PHYSIOLOGIC DATA 1346

63-DAY PERPETUAL GESTATION CHART 1347

RECOMMENDED NUTRIENT ALLOWANCES
FOR DOGS (PER LB OR KG OF BODY
WEIGHT PER DAY) 1348

CALORIC REQUIREMENTS FOR ADULT
DOGS BASED ON PHYSICAL ACTIVITY AND
BREED SIZE 1349

RECOMMENDED DAILY CALORIC INTAKE
DURING FIRST FOUR WEEKS OF LIFE 1350

COMPOSITION OF MATERNAL MILK AND
SUBSTITUTES 1351

NUTRITIONAL REQUIREMENTS (AMOUNTS
SUBSTITUTES 1351
OF ADULT CATS AND 10-WEEK-OLD
KITTENS 1352

RECOMMENDED DAILY METABOLIZABLE
ENERGY ALLOWANCES FOR CATS 1353

COMPENDIUM OF CANINE VACCINES, 1988 .. 1354
        Frederic W. Scott

COMPENDIUM OF FELINE VACCINES, 1988 .. 1356
        Frederic W. Scott

COMPENDIUM OF ANIMAL RABIES
CONTROL, 1989 1357

IMMUNIZATION PROCEDURES 1361

USE OF ANTIMICROBIAL AGENTS FOR
TREATMENT OF INFECTIONS 1363

CONVERSION TABLE OF WEIGHT TO BODY
SURFACE AREA (IN SQUARE METERS) FOR
DOGS 1365

EQUIVALENTS AND CONVERSION FACTORS ... 1366

ANTINEOPLASTIC AGENTS IN CANCER
THERAPY 1367
        James P. Thompson

TABLE OF COMMON DRUGS: APPROXIMATE
DOSES 1370

INDEX 1381

Section
1

SPECIAL THERAPY

CARL A. OSBORNE, D.V.M.
Consulting Editor

Computer-Aided Diagnosis 2
Understanding Clinical Studies 8
Cause and Control of Decreased Appetite 18
Parenteral Nutritional Support 25
Enteral Nutritional Support 30
Maintenance Fluid Therapy 37
Hypophosphatemia 43
Nonsteroidal Anti-Inflammatory Drugs 47
Glucocorticoid Therapy 54
Chemical Restraint Techniques in Dogs and Cats 63
Antimicrobial Susceptibility Tests 70
Cephalosporins 74
Clavulanate-Potentiated Antibiotics 78
Treatment of Fungal and Endocrine Disorders with Imidazole
    Derivatives 82
The Practice of Veterinary Medicine in Humane Society Facilities 85
Disinfection of Animal Environments 90

COMPUTER-AIDED DIAGNOSIS

ROY V. H. POLLOCK, D.V.M.

Ithaca, New York

The past two decades have witnessed unprecedented growth in the number and kinds of diagnostic techniques available to veterinarians. Ultrasonography, serologic tests performed in the office, increasingly sophisticated biochemistry, and a host of other techniques allow greater accuracy and sensitivity in the detection and classification of diseases. Concomitant advances in our knowledge of pathophysiology, infectious agents, immunology, and pharmacology have enormously broadened both the number of diagnostic possibilities to be considered and the number that can be managed successfully.

However, these increases themselves have become a problem. The number of diagnostic possibilities that must be considered and the number of potentially useful diagnostic and therapeutic strategies that could be employed now greatly exceed human recall. As a result, care suffers because a condition must be considered before it can be diagnosed, and must be detected before it can be successfully managed. Thus, there is the need for a new medical tool, one that can help veterinarians formulate differential diagnoses and select appropriate tests and treatment regimens. Computer-aided diagnosis (CAD) programs have been designed to meet this need. Several systems are already available commercially, and others are being developed. This article considers their potential and their pitfalls.

THE DIAGNOSTIC PROCESS

Diagnosis—the assignment of a label to a patient's condition—is not an end in itself; it is an essential intermediate step toward the ultimate goal of curing or mitigating the patient's medical problem. A diagnosis, even a tentative or very general one, determines which additional diagnostic tests will be ordered and which therapy will be tried. The effectiveness of that therapy, and even the predictive value of the diagnostic tests employed, depend on the correctness of the working hypothesis. For these reasons, substantial research effort has been expended to understand how clinicians make diagnoses (Schwartz and Griffin, 1986).

Although there is disagreement about the specific details, most studies suggest that the basic process of making a diagnosis is a hypothetico-deductive one. That is, a clinician formulates a series of hypotheses about the patient's condition and then collects additional information in order to decide among them. This process begins almost immediately, so that before the first few minutes of the encounter with the patient have elapsed, the clinician has already established a number of competing explanations for the patient's condition (Barrows and Tamblyn, 1980). Ideally, these are fairly broad and general concepts ("an infectious process") that are successively refined as additional information is collected and analyzed.

There are several inherent pitfalls to the hypothetico-deductive approach, however. One is that later hypotheses tend to be elaborations of earlier ones, rather than new constructs (Elstein et al., 1978). The practical result is that if a possibility is overlooked initially, it may never surface later. Data tend to be evaluated only for their effect on existing hypotheses. As the workup proceeds, it becomes more and more difficult to evaluate the patient from a fresh point of view.

Another pitfall is that the hypotheses under consideration strongly influence which data will be collected and how they will be interpreted In general, this is an efficient problem-solving strategy. However, a consequence of this strategy is that if a potential diagnosis is not considered initially, data to suggest its presence will not be sought, and the likelihood of the later discovery of the diagnosis is further reduced. This is more likely to occur with rare diseases. Since common diseases occur frequently, the clinician's overall "batting average" will be good, even if his or her diagnostic list contains only a few of the most common diagnoses. However, owners expect clinicians to find the rare and unusual as well as the common, and it is the infrequent diseases that often offer the greatest potential for intellectual challenge and professional growth. Moreover, it is not only new or rare diseases that are misdiagnosed. Well-known or common conditions can be missed if the diagnostic plan starts on the wrong track (as in the case of Jeep, the dog with chronic emesis who was treated unsuccessfully for food allergy by several different veterinarians over two years, until radiographs taken for another reason revealed gastric foreign bodies, two tennis balls).

This article was supported in part by grant R23 LM04484 from the National Library of Medicine.

A mechanism that would aid clinicians in considering the full range of diagnostic possibilities has the potential to improve medical care substantially. One possibility is a textbook of differential diagnoses, several of which are available for small animal medicine. These can be helpful in expanding the clinician's differential diagnosis for a given clinical sign or problem, but they are of limited utility in helping the clinician decide which of the diagnostic possibilities are the most profitable to pursue in a particular patient. The problem was neatly summarized by Nash (1960): "A book will give the causes of a single symptom or sign, but . . . it cannot deal with combinations. Yet it is just by considering the causes of combinations of symptoms, etc., that the most rapid narrowing down of range of possibilities is secured." Nash's solution was his "logoscope," a huge slide-rulelike device in which one lined up symptoms on two scales and read diagnostic possibilities from a third.

Nash's ideas were ahead of available technology. His device was able to consider only a relatively small number of symptoms simultaneously and, like textbooks, was difficult and costly to update or revise. Then, beginning in the 1960's, the capabilities of computers began an increasingly rapid upward spiral. It became apparent that computers could very rapidly evaluate an extensive list of clinical findings against an enormous number of potential diseases. Computer scientists confidently predicted diagnostic programs that would far surpass clinicians in both speed and accuracy. Such programs have yet to be written. The problems of medical diagnosis turned out to be far subtler than initially conceived, and the available data from which to build computer-based diagnostic systems proved to be scarce and unreliable.

Several successful diagnostic programs have been developed for circumscribed medical problems in human medicine (e.g., the acute abdomen), but there is no practical system capable of rendering a reliable final diagnosis in either human or veterinary general internal medicine. While diagnosis by computer has proved to be an elusive goal, computer-*aided* diagnosis, in which the computer acts as a resource and a consultant, is steadily gaining acceptance. It now appears that the combination of human and machine diagnostic skills is the most productive approach and has the greatest potential to improve medical care.

HOW COMPUTERS CAN ASSIST

Adlassnig and coworkers (1985) summarized the advantages of computer-based expert systems:

Medical expert systems take into account an enormous number of diseases that the individual diagnostician cannot simultaneously keep in mind; they can support the physician by displaying rare as well as frequent diseases with the only criterion given that the diagnoses explain the patient's symptom pattern; they can accelerate the diagnostic process by offering proposals for further examinations of the patient in order to confirm or deny diagnostic hypotheses as fast as possible; and they can act as instructional systems for medical students, young physicians, and non-specialists.

To that list could be added the potential to act as an up-to-date source of diagnostic tests and treatments and as access to a far broader sample of the biomedical literature than is usually available to practitioners.

The current emphasis is on the ability of such systems to *aid* the clinician and to present relevant information, rather than to make autonomous decisions. Barnett (1982), commenting on computer-based diagnostic systems in human medicine, concluded that their greatest potential was their "ability to remind the user of diagnoses that should be considered, given a specific set of signs and symptoms; and to suggest the collection of additional data that might be of diagnostic value."

KINDS OF SYSTEMS

A number of CAD systems are, or soon will be, available to practicing veterinarians. The author is the principal developer of PROVIDES; the illustrations and many of the examples in this article are taken from this work. Several other systems are used as examples, but they do not constitute an exhaustive list, nor does their mention constitute endorsement. How well a CAD system supports a clinician's professional activities is determined mainly by its architecture and data base, but the clinician's personal preferences and work habits may make some features more important than others.

An expert system has three main components: (1) a user interface, (2) a medical data base, and (3) a system or set of rules (called the inference engine) by which it compares a patient's symptoms to its knowledge base and derives a list of diagnostic suggestions (Fig. 1).

The User Interface

As its name suggests, the user interface is the way in which the computer interacts with the clinician. This is typically by means of a keyboard and computer console, although future systems may make increasing use of "mice" or touch-sensitive screens. There are two general methods of data collection: (1) menu-driven and (2) open-entry.

In menu-driven systems (e.g., PROVIDES, Animed Computer Systems, Oshkosh, WI; Veterinary

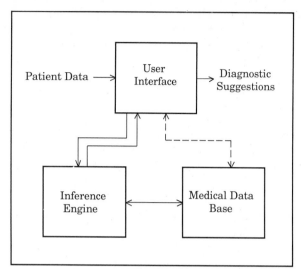

Figure 1. The three components of a computer-aided diagnostic system. (1) The user interface, through which clinical findings are entered and medical information is received; (2) the inference engine, the logic the computer uses to generate its differential; and (3) the medical knowledge base of information about diseases, tests, treatments, and so forth on which the inference engine bases its suggestions. In some systems, the user is also able to access the data base directly (dashed line).

Problem-Knowledge Couplers, PKC Corp., South Burlington, VT; AQUAMEDIC, N-Squared Computing, Silverston, OR), the user selects findings from a menu of available choices. The advantages of this approach are that the clinician is reminded to look for findings that have diagnostic significance but that might not otherwise be noted (especially if the clinician has forgotten about, or is unaware of the possibility of, a specific diagnosis). In addition, a minimum of typing is required. The disadvantage is that more time is required for data entry, since all possible findings must be reviewed.

Open-entry systems (e.g., CONSULTANT, New York State College of Veterinary Medicine, Ithaca, NY) allow the user simply to type in one or more findings. To manage the virtually limitless ways of expressing clinical observations, such systems use a controlled vocabulary, codes for specific signs and symptoms, or both. An advantage of open-entry systems is that data entry and the generation of diagnostic suggestions are fast. The principal disadvantage is that the computer's differential diagnosis is strongly influenced by the findings the clinician chooses to enter, which, as noted earlier, are determined by the diseases the clinician already has under consideration.

Systems also differ in the information they can accept and analyze. For example, HEMO (VetSoft, Inc., Davis, CA) is designed specifically to aid in interpreting clinical laboratory data and does not take into account the history or physical findings. CONSULTANT considers only clinical signs, whereas PROVIDES and Knowledge Couplers encompass historical, physical, laboratory, and other findings as well as environmental predispositions, age, breed, and sex.

For special applications (e.g., CARDIO, an electrocardiography analysis aid, VetSoft, Inc., Davis, CA), the user is asked to supply specific measurement values. A system in which the computer reads and analyzes the electrocardiogram (ECG) directly is available (ECG Analyzer, Vetronics, Inc., Lafayette, IN), and the potential to analyze clinical chemistry data directly from a computer-generated file is being explored. RORI, an experimental and freely distributed CAD system developed by Dr. Fred Smith at the College of Veterinary Medicine, University of Georgia, can be used in "query" mode, in which the computer asks questions according to which disease is currently ranked most probable. While this approach is mathematically most efficient and results in the fewest number of questions, experience in human medicine suggests that clinicians are frustrated by the seemingly haphazard order of data collection this technique produces.

Regardless of the specific means by which the CAD system collects data, clinicians should look for systems in which the user interface is straightforward (requires little or no knowledge of computers), efficient (responsive), easy to interpret, and forgiving (allows errors to be corrected without having to start over). They should try to look beyond "bells, whistles, and flashing lights" to day-in, day-out function and usefulness.

The Data Base

The principal advantage of using a computer-aided diagnostic system derives from the size and the nature of its data base; the computer can "know" about and rapidly "consider" far more diseases than can a clinician. It can recall a myriad of details about frequencies, predispositions, contraindications, test interpretations, sample collections, and so forth. Moreover, it can be frequently and readily updated so that its "knowledge" remains current.

Clinicians considering acquiring a CAD system should critically evaluate the system's data base, since no amount of elegant programming at the user interface or mathematical manipulation in the diagnostic process can compensate for a fundamentally flawed data base. Key questions include (1) How extensive is the data base? (2) What is the depth of the information? (3) Does it contain only clinical findings, or does it also include test, treatment, and prognostic information? (4) How much detail is provided? (5) Are the sources of information identified? (6) Are references cited that refer the practitioner to additional information?

Currently available systems vary widely in the answers to these questions. Illustrative of one end of the spectrum is AQUAMEDIC, a diagnostic program for fish diseases that currently (July 1988) contains no information beyond the name and clinical signs associated with each of the more than 100 fish diseases that it covers; no references or sources of additional information are given. CONSULTANT, a time-sharing system developed by Dr. Maurice White at Cornell University, has information on an enormous number of diseases (approximately 1500 listings for dogs and cats). For each disease, there is a three- to twenty-line description, one to five bibliographic citations, and a list of clinical signs the disease may produce. The veterinary versions of the Problem-Knowledge Coupler concept developed by Dr. Lawrence Weed contain on-line lists of findings, tests, and treatment options. A printed copy of relevant abstracts accompanies each Coupler (diagnostic program).

PROVIDES contains detailed information on clinical findings, tests, treatments, and expected outcomes, each of which is supported by one or more outline synopses of current articles or books (Fig. 2). These synopses can be stored on disk and displayed virtually instantaneously. A typical problem is documented by 300 to 600 synopses. Reprints of the journal articles cited in both PROVIDES and CONSULTANT are available for a fee to users of these systems.

Specific disease information can be retrieved directly by disease name as well as from the differential diagnosis, a feature also available in CONSULTANT. The diseases listed in the PROVIDES data base are limited to specific problem areas in small animal medicine, whereas the data base in CONSULTANT is much broader, covering virtually all known diseases of domestic animals.

The Inference Engine

The inference engine (i.e., the decision rules that the computer uses to generate its differential diagnosis) is the brain of a diagnostic system. The optimal method of deriving probable diagnoses from clinical data is the subject of intense research in medical informatics; there is no agreement on the best method. Every approach has advantages and disadvantages. The intelligent use of a CAD system requires that the clinician understand the method used, its strengths, and its shortcomings.

Complex diagnostic schemes are not necessarily superior. Simple systems have the advantage of being fast and easy to understand. More complicated systems have the potential to produce better predictions but are dependent on the exact method used and the accuracy of the disease profiles in the data base. The more complicated the diagnostic strategy, the more difficult it becomes for the clinician to identify and compensate for shortcomings in the computer's analysis.

A straightforward matching system is the simplest method of generating, from a set of clinical findings, a list of possible diseases that should be ruled out. For example, a list of all the diseases that could account for the clinical findings entered could be displayed. This is the system used by CONSULTANT. Its major advantages are speed, understandability, and generation of a relatively short list of diseases. Its major disadvantages are that (1) all findings receive equal weight and (2) since only diseases that can account for *every* entered finding are displayed, any single finding can eliminate a disease from consideration. In CONSULTANT, the author purposely left the list of diseases unranked,

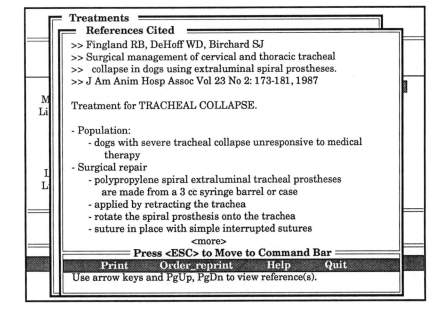

Figure 2. An example of a literature citation and treatment abstract in PROVIDES. The user has requested additional information on the surgical correction of collapsed trachea. Additional information on technique, efficacy, and complications, as well as other abstracts, would be viewed by pressing the page down (PgDn) key. Pressing P would generate a printed copy for later reference.

Treatments
References Cited
>> Fingland RB, DeHoff WD, Birchard SJ
>> Surgical management of cervical and thoracic tracheal
>>   collapse in dogs using extraluminal spiral prostheses.
>> J Am Anim Hosp Assoc Vol 23 No 2: 173-181, 1987

Treatment for TRACHEAL COLLAPSE.

- Population:
    - dogs with severe tracheal collapse unresponsive to medical
        therapy
- Surgical repair
    - polypropylene spiral extraluminal tracheal prostheses
        are made from a 3 cc syringe barrel or case
    - applied by retracting the trachea
    - rotate the spiral prosthesis onto the trachea
    - suture in place with simple interrupted sutures
                    <more>
            Press <ESC> to Move to Command Bar
        Print   Order_reprint   Help   Quit
Use arrow keys and PgUp, PgDn to view reference(s).

arguing that all ranking systems were suspect, and that the clinician could and should rapidly scan the entire list (White and Lewkowicz, 1987).

An alternative approach is to list all diseases that could account for *any* of the entered findings and rank them according to how many of the findings the disease would be likely to produce. This is probably advantageous, in that it avoids premature exclusion of a disease. However, its utility depends on the accuracy and completeness of the disease descriptions in the data base. Such a system is unwieldy if the number of diseases to be considered is very large.

A somewhat different matching algorithm, developed by Dr. Lawrence Weed, is used in Problem-Knowledge Couplers. The data base is organized by *problem* (e.g., cough, diarrhea, polyuria-polydipsia). An exhaustive list of diseases is prepared for each problem, and the patient findings are used to rank these. The disease that accounts for the greatest number of findings is listed first. This is similar to the approach used by clinicians in solving clinicopathologic conference cases (Eddy and Clanton, 1982). The advantage of this approach is that it limits the search sphere to a specific problem, which, in turn, allows more detailed characterization and, hence, finer distinctions to be made between diseases than is possible with a program that spans all of internal medicine. The disadvantages are that (1) the system can be used only for cases that fall within one of its problem sets, (2) all findings are weighted equally, and (3) because diseases are ordered according to the total number of findings they could explain, it is difficult for diseases that produce only a few findings to rank near the top of the list. As in all CAD systems, the clinician must scan the entire diagnostic list and combine his or her clinical judgment with the computer's predictions.

PROVIDES and RORI use a similar algorithm, except that diseases are ranked according to the *ratio* of findings displayed by the patient to those *expected* for the disease (Fig. 3). Findings for which there are no data are not taken into consideration (e.g., radiographic findings in a patient who has not yet been radiographed). This approach avoids bias against diseases that produce few or vague clinical signs, but the definition of "expected" findings for each disease, created by the system designer, greatly affects performance.

All the aforementioned methods evaluate findings as if they had equal importance, even though common sense and clinical experience indicate that this is not the case. Assigning different values to various combinations of clinical findings should, at least in theory, improve the system's diagnostic ability. Various schemes have been proposed to incorporate this feature. In the human diagnostic system called INTERNIST-I, expert opinion is used to assign scores to concepts such as the frequency with which certain findings occur, and the evoking strength (how often the manifestation is associated with the disease) (Miller et al., 1982). Next, these are combined by an empirical formula to determine the most probable diagnosis. A more precise formulation of the process is bayesian inference, in which the conditional probability of the disease is calculated from unconditional incidence estimates and the probabilities of different findings occurring in association with each of the competing hypotheses. Unfortunately, there are few data on which to base the estimates of required probabilities. For most diseases, the probabilities used are little more than rough estimates based on expert opinion; this should be considered when one reviews output from such systems. The reported estimates on the probability of various diseases are frequently misleading because they imply a degree of precision far greater than that of the estimates from which they were derived.

THE PLACE FOR CLINICAL JUDGMENT

CAD systems are neither omniscient nor infallible. They are, as their name suggests, only aids—albeit potentially very powerful ones. Their recommendations should never be followed slavishly. CAD systems are categorical in their approach; they cannot distinguish shades of meaning or degree or the goals and concerns of the owner. Thus, their recommendations must always be tempered by human experience and judgment. They can never replace the clinician; the final responsibility for diagnosis and patient care must, and should, depend on the professional judgment of the veterinarian.

Clinical judgment is best applied, however, after a thorough, systematic workup and rigorous analysis of the full range of diagnostic possibilities. It should be augmented by a sophisticated information delivery system to ensure that decisions are made in the context of complete and current information. Computers have the potential to augment the clinician's judgment in all these ways. As early as 1952, the physicist L. N. Ridenour suggested that "computer" was really a misnomer and that "information machine" was a better description (Kleinmuntz, 1984). That observation was never more aptly applied than to CAD systems in veterinary medicine as we move into the last decade of the twentieth century. Computers may well become our primary sources of medical information in the next ten years. They also have enormous potential as sources of continuing education, because (1) they could constantly present new, previously unknown, or formerly forgotten information to the clinician in the context of active patient care, (2) they could serve as full-time mentors, and (3) the information they provide is better

Figure 3. An example of a CAD differential. The patient was a seven-year-old Old English mastiff that lived on a pig farm and suffered from chronic, intermittent diarrhea, coprophagia, polyphagia, steatorrhea, weight loss, dependent edema, and palpably thickened intestine. Causes are listed in order of the ratio of observed to expected findings. No laboratory work had yet been done; hence, there are no data for some findings. Note that a number of the suggested diagnoses are not necessarily mutually exclusive.

PROVIDES - Differential Diagnosis - Canine Diarrhea/Vomiting

	Cause	Findings:	Present/ Known	no data
↑ More Likely	1: lymphocytic-plasmacytic enteritis		4/4	1
	2: exocrine pancreatic insufficiency		6/7	0
	3: lymphangiectasia		5/6	2
	4: chronic ancylostomiasis		4/5	1
	5: granulomatous enteritis		4/5	1
	6: protein-losing gastroenteropathy		4/6	1
	7: short bowel syndrome		4/6	0
Less Likely	8: intestinal bacterial overgrowth		3/5	0
	9: gastrinoma		3/5	1
↓	10: idiopathic intestinal pseudoobstruction		3/5	0

Untreated Fatality: High   **Treatment: Non-Specific**

Press <ESC> to Move to Command Bar

Findings   Treatments   DxTests   Outcome   Help   Quit

remembered than that obtained from reading or lectures.

SUMMARY

Computer-based diagnostic (CAD) systems have significant potential to increase the quality of small animal clinical practice. They can help ensure that diagnostic possibilities are not overlooked, suggest diagnostic tests and treatment strategies, and clarify the probable disease outcomes. As the amount of medical information increases at an exponential rate, the need for more efficient methods of storing, indexing, and retrieving that information likewise increases. Although computer-aided diagnosis is still in the early stages of its development in veterinary medicine, its potential appears almost unlimited.

References and Supplemental Reading

Adlassnig, K-P., Kolarz, G., Scheithauer, W., et al.: CADIAG: Approaches to computer-assisted diagnosis. Comput. Biol. Med. 15:315, 1985.

Barnett, G. O.: Computers and clinical judgment. N. Engl. J. Med. 307:493, 1982.

Barrows, H. S., and Tamblyn, R. M.: *Problem Based Learning: An Approach to Medical Education*. New York: Springer Publishing Co., 1980, pp. 42–47.

Blois, M. S.: Clinical judgment and computers. N. Engl. J. Med. 303:192, 1980.

Eddy, D. M., and Clanton, C. H.: Solving the clinicopathological exercise. N. Engl. J. Med. 306:1263, 1982.

Elstein, A. S., Shulman, L. S., and Sprafka, S. A.: *Medical Problem Solving*. Cambridge, MA: Harvard University Press, 1978.

Fessler, A. P.: Computer-assisted decision-making in veterinary medicine. Vet. Med. 79:409, 558, 1984.

Kleinmuntz, B.: Diagnostic problem solving by computer: A historical review and the current state of the science. Comput. Biol. Med. 14:255, 1984.

Miller, R. A., Pople, H. E., and Myers, J. D.: *INTERNIST-I*, An experimental computer-based diagnostic consultant for general internal medicine. N. Engl. J. Med. 307:468, 1982.

Nash, F. A.: The mechanical conservation of experience, especially in medicine. IRE Trans. Med. Electronics 7:240, 1960.

Pollock, R. V. H.: Anatomy of a diagnosis. Comp. Contin. Ed. 7:621, 1985.

Pollock, R. V. H.: Diagnosis by calculation. Comp. Contin. Ed. 7:1019, 1985.

Pollock, R. V. H.: Computers as medical management tools. Vet. Clin. North Am. [Small Anim. Pract.] 16:669, 1986.

Schwartz, S., and Griffin, T.: *Medical Thinking: The Psychology of Medical Judgment and Decision Making*. New York: Springer-Verlag, 1986.

Stevens, F.: Special medical applications of computers. Vet. Clin. North Am. [Small Anim. Pract.] 16:685, 1986.

White, M. E.: Computer-assisted diagnosis: Experience with the CONSULTANT program. J.A.V.M.A. 187:475, 1985.

White, M. E., and Lewkowicz, J. M.: The CONSULTANT database for computer-assisted diagnosis and information management in veterinary medicine. Automedica 8:135, 1987.

UNDERSTANDING CLINICAL STUDIES

JODY P. LULICH, D.V.M.,
CARL A. OSBORNE, D.V.M.,
and SHIRLEY D. JOHNSTON, D.V.M.
St. Paul, Minnesota

STATISTICS: THE LANGUAGE OF CLINICAL STUDIES

Why should practicing veterinarians become familiar with statistics? Because knowledge and conceptual understanding of statistical principles will improve the quality of care we provide to our patients. Such training will alert us to the pitfalls associated with premature generalizations based on a few uncontrolled observations. Too frequently we practice veterinary medicine by utilizing empirical knowledge and hypotheses based on personal experiences, conversations, and poorly designed clinical reports. We often unconsciously force conclusions on facts rather than strive to allow reproducible observations (i.e., facts) to force the conclusions.

Understanding the enormous conceptual difference between random clinical observations and results of controlled clinical trials should be a prerequisite for every reader of veterinary journals. Rational scientific treatment, rather than empirical therapy, emerged when clinical research changed from anecdotal documentation to prospective randomized controlled double-blind studies. We recognize that randomized trials are not methods of discovery but rather a means of validation. We realize that empirical observations are extremely important. However, the therapist who accepts the results of uncontrolled studies in lieu of properly controlled ones may be responsible for the perpetuation of medical myths. A treatment may lack acceptable evidence of therapeutic efficacy, but the occasional dramatic result is vividly remembered, the failures are forgotten, and folklore therapy often becomes established.

Traditionally, the burden of data collection and analysis has been the province of "researchers." However, researchers who collect clinical data and clinicians who use it have a great deal in common. Both are dependent on the accuracy and meaningful interpretation of information. Consequently, *clinicians are researchers*, and therefore they must understand basic principles of data collection and analysis to interpret clinical reports.

The practice of modern medicine has become inseparable from the use of statistics. For example, statistics are used to deal with common clinical problems such as (1) In a dog with radiodense urocystoliths, alkaline urine pH, and a staphylococcal urinary tract infection, what is the likelihood that the uroliths are composed of magnesium ammonium phosphate? (2) What is the appropriate dose of potassium chloride to correct severe hypokalemia? and (3) What is the yearly cost of evaluation and treatment of a 20-lb poodle dog with diabetes mellitus?

As the volume of quantitative information increased in the medical literature, a new vocabulary was developed to ensure proper description of that information. Thus, learning statistical principles is analogous to learning a new language. One must learn the vocabulary and then the rules to understand the concepts of design, reporting, and interpretation of modern clinical studies.

The goal of this discussion is to familiarize the reader with statistical terms and concepts utilized daily in the evaluation of clinical data. Additionally, guidance is provided to help assess the advantages, reliability, and pitfalls of statistical inferences by answering three consecutive questions common to all clinical studies: (1) How were the data collected? (2) How were the data analyzed? and (3) What do the answers mean? (Fig. 1).

The section entitled Clinical Studies answers the question, How were the data collected? This section describes various study designs relevant to clinical medicine and their ability to provide meaningful answers. The question, How were the data analyzed? is answered in the section entitled Methods of Statistical Analysis. This section provides guidelines for selection of appropriate methods of analysis. The section entitled Statistical Inference deals with the interpretation of outcomes of statistical tests. Since proper inference from data is the goal of clinical studies, this section is of greatest interest to veterinarians and their patients.

OVERVIEW OF STATISTICS

Statistics is derived from the Latin word *statisticus*, meaning status or standing. Its modern-day meaning encompasses the status of facts that are systematically collected, numerically and categorically grouped, and then analyzed to describe a particular phenomenon. Statistics are numeric expressions of events; in a medical context, they are numeric expressions of biologic phenomena.

Based on their application, statistics are divided into two fundamental categories: *descriptive statistics* and *inferential statistics*. Descriptive statistics are concerned with the description and summarization of a sample of data (e.g., numbers describing the average life span of dogs with lymphocytic leukemia evaluated at the University of Minnesota Veterinary Hospital, or the breeds of cats developing renal amyloidosis between the years 1980 and 1990). In contrast, inferential statistics are related to making decisions (estimations, predictions, or generalizations) about larger populations of animals, based on information contained in a sample. Typical examples include the probability that cats with aseptic peritoneal exudates have feline infectious peritonitis and the probability that neutering at an early age decreases the occurrence of mammary gland neoplasia later in life. The type of statistical application (descriptive or inferential) is dependent on questions the investigator is attempting to answer (i.e., description of data, or extrapolation of results of sample data to a larger population at risk).

CLINICAL STUDIES

Definitions

Clinical studies encompass reproducible examinations and analyses of a variety of biologic phenomena. Such studies are essential to confirm our present understanding of diseases and to verify "clinical dogma" addressed in such questions as Does megestrol acetate always cause diabetes mellitus in cats? Is renal failure always progressive? and Are diverticulectomies always appropriate therapy in cats with hematuria and dysuria? To help answer questions such as these, two general categories of clinical studies are frequently used: *descriptive* studies and *explanatory* studies (Table 1). Descriptive studies, as the name implies, describe findings associated with a disease and its treatment, its prevention, or both. For example, the occurrence and severity of vomiting, anemia, hypertension, and hyperkalemia in cats with chronic renal failure represents a typical format for reporting data from descriptive studies. On the other hand, explanatory studies compare two or more different groups of animals, in an attempt to demonstrate that true differences occur and to identify processes that explain why the groups are different.

Types of Descriptive Studies

Descriptive studies are used to describe observed phenomena. They represent accounts of events, observations, and laboratory findings associated with a disease. Types of descriptive studies include case reports and case series (Table 1).

Descriptive studies are relatively inexpensive and easy to conduct. These studies often utilize pre-existing data from case records. Prospective data may also be reported.

Summary statistics (Table 2) are often used to describe results of descriptive studies. These include measures of the clustering, or centering, of data (mean, median, mode), measures of the spread of data (range, variance, standard deviation), and a measure of the relative standing of data (percentile).

One disadvantage of descriptive studies is their poor ability to prove a relationship between cause and effect. Consider the following example: Contrast urethrocystography was performed on 20 cats with hematuria, dysuria, and intraluminal urethral obstruction of unknown cause. It was discovered that 18 of the cats had urachal diverticula. Obstructions were alleviated and diverticula were surgically excised. Six months after surgery, all 18 cats were reported free from disease during this period. Based on these results, investigators concluded that diverticula were a contributing cause of lower urinary tract disease in cats and recommended diverticulectomy as the therapy of choice. Are these conclusions correct? No, they are overstatements. The only statement that can be made with certainty is that diverticula are commonly seen in cats with hematuria, dysuria, and urethral obstruction. The occurrence of diverticula in normal cats remains unknown. Likewise, it is unknown whether diverticula are a cause or a result of urethral obstruction. Would clinical signs resolve without diverticulectomy? A follow-up clinical study using medical therapy revealed that diverticula were self-limiting. This example emphasizes the fact that descriptive studies cannot address such questions because they lack *internal control groups* (comparison groups followed simultaneously with treatment groups). Consequently, statements of inference should be avoided in descriptive studies. If reported, they should be stated as theory rather than fact and interpreted with appropriate caution.

In some instances, descriptive studies are compared with external control groups. A variety of *external control groups* are used for comparison, including those from another time period or another clinical trial. They may even be as ill-defined as "common knowledge."

Even without control groups, descriptive studies provide valuable scientific information. For example, they are usually the first account of clinical phenomena from which hypotheses can be developed and investigated.

Table 1. Some Characteristics of Various Types of Clinical Studies

Type of Study	Ease of Investigation	Relationship to Time of Disease Occurrence	Use of a Control Group	Random Allocation to Groups Evaluated	Ability to Provide Proof of Relationship	Relevance to Natural Disease Process
Descriptive						
Case report	Easy	Retrospective	None or external	NA	Low	Low to high
Case series	Easy	Retrospective	None or external	NA	Low	Low to high
Explanatory						
Observational						
Case control	Moderate	Retrospective	Internal	No	Low to moderate	Moderate to high
Cohort	Difficult	Prospective	Internal	No	High	High
Experimental						
Laboratory	Difficult	Prospective	Internal	Yes	Very high	Low to moderate
Clinical trial	Difficult	Prospective	Internal	Yes	High	High

NA, not applicable; descriptive studies involve only one study group. All animals within the group have the character being investigated.

Internal controls are comparison groups followed simultaneously with the treated group and by the same investigators.

External controls are comparison groups from another time period or a study different from the treated group being studied.

Types of Explanatory Studies

Unlike descriptive studies, results of explanatory studies are based on comparisons between two or more different groups. Comparison is important because it minimizes *bias*. Bias is defined as any effect, at any stage of an investigation, tending to produce results that depart from their actual values. Thus, explanatory studies help explain clinical phenomena by comparing disease groups with control groups. Based on the degree of control designed by the investigator, explanatory studies can be divided into two subcategories: (1) *observational studies* and (2) *experimental studies*. In experimental studies, the investigator randomly allocates animals to either a study or a control group. The ability to randomly assign individuals to either group helps eliminate bias. Observational studies lack this feature.

OBSERVATIONAL STUDIES

Case control studies and cohort studies are common types of observational studies used in clinical medicine (Table 1). Neither study affords the investigator the opportunity to allocate patients to the study group or the control group.

CASE CONTROL STUDIES. Case control studies are unique in that they begin after animals have devel-

Table 2. Definitions and Concepts of Terms Used in the Numeric Description of Data

Measures of Central Tendency

MEAN is the statistical term for average. It is calculated by adding all measurements in a data set and then dividing this value by the number of measurements.

MEDIAN is the measurement in the middle of the data set, when all data points are arranged in descending or ascending order. Unlike the mean, the median is affected minimally by very large or very small measurements. Consequently, the median may represent a more appropriate measure of centering tendency in data sets with extremely large or extremely small values.

MODE is the measurement that occurs most frequently. The mode indicates where data tend to cluster.

Measures of Variability

RANGE is equal to the largest measurement minus the smallest measurement. It is not a sensitive measure of variability; it is affected by extreme values in the data set.

VARIANCE is a more sensitive measure of the variability of measurements in a data set. The variance is obtained by averaging the squared differences between the mean and the measurements.

STANDARD DEVIATION is the square root of the variance. In contrast to variance, standard deviations are commonly used to describe variability of a data set because standard deviations are expressed in the units of the original data and provide a relative basis for comparison with other groups of data. In addition, standard deviations have the unique advantage of rapid assessment of the percentage of data points spread around the mean. From samples that are normally distributed (see below, The Normal Distribution), (1) approximately 68% of the data points will lie within one standard deviation of the mean (one standard deviation on either side of the mean), (2) approximately 95% of the data points will lie within two standard deviations of the mean, and (3) approximately 99% of all the data points will lie within three standard deviations of the mean.

Measure of Relative Standing

PERCENTILE reflects the percentage of data points lower in value than the datum point of interest. A 90th percentile implies that 90% of the data points are lower in value and 10% of the data points are higher in value than the one of interest.

The Normal Distribution

Distributions reflect the relative number of measurements in various categories of the population. The shape of the *NORMAL DISTRIBUTION* approximates a bell-shaped curve. It is symmetric and continuous, and the mean value lies at the highest point of the curve. The normal distribution is statistically important because it is assumed to represent the infinite population of measurements from which samples are drawn.

oped the disease in question. As the name implies, they are studies of cases (case records). The study group consists of case records of patients that have a disease; the control group consists of case records of similar (e.g., breed, sex, age, weight) patients that do not have the disease. Data in case records are then compared to determine if certain factors (causes) can be associated with disease occurrence.

Case control studies offer the advantage of being relatively inexpensive and rapid, and there is no risk to patients. In addition, they provide an opportunity to study uncommon diseases. However, these studies are susceptible to many biases, including difficulty in assessing that the "accepted" cause actually preceded a disease process.

COHORT STUDIES. A *cohort* is defined as a group of individuals (e.g., animals, patients) who share a common exposure, experience, or characteristic. Thus, a cohort study consists of patients who share a common characteristic compared with a similar group without that characteristic.

In contrast to case-controlled studies, which are retrospective, cohort studies begin before patients develop disease. Individual patients are then followed prospectively (forward in time) to determine if disease develops. Cohort studies offer the advantages of consistent and complete evaluation, in addition to establishment of the proper time sequence between cause and outcome. It is unfortunate that such studies are often time consuming and expensive.

EXPERIMENTAL STUDIES

Experimental studies can be classified as *laboratory studies* or *clinical trials* (Table 1). Experimental studies offer the greatest ability to provide proof of a relationship between causes and the occurrence of disease.

LABORATORY STUDIES. These have the advantage of providing an investigator with the ideal opportunity to control the environment necessary to investigate a hypothesis. Both study and control groups share all the same environmental factors except the one being studied. Although this setting provides the best opportunity to test a hypothesis with the least bias, its relevance to naturally occurring disease is often low.

CLINICAL TRIALS. These allow the evaluation of various diseases in their natural setting. One disadvantage of clinical trials is the difficulty in controlling variables in the natural environment that affect the outcome of the study (e.g., diet, activity, consistency of treatment administration). Perhaps the most significant disadvantage is the unpredictable loss of patients. Thus, one must use appropriate caution when interpreting results of clinical trials.

METHODS OF STATISTICAL ANALYSIS

Conceptual understanding of statistical methods commonly used in medical literature does not require mathematical sophistication. It does require an understanding of (1) the completeness of the population being analyzed and (2) whether the study is designed to evaluate associations or differences.

The Population of Interest

The common denominator of every statistical problem is a population. Statisticians use the term *population* to define a set of data that characterizes some phenomenon. Thus, the term population is used to represent a set of measurements rather than a group of animals. For example, if one were discussing the average life span of cats in the United States, the statistical population would refer to the life span value rather than the cats in the United States. The statistical population often is an infinitely large collection of measurements. When populations are infinitely large, only a *sample* (subset of data selected from the population) is subjected to statistical analyses. Thus, the majority of statistical analyses are performed on smaller sets of measurements (samples) in an attempt to make decisions (estimations, predictions, or generalizations) about the whole set of measurements (the population). Based on the completeness of the population analyzed (remember, population refers to a set of all the measurements), statistics may be divided into population statistics or sample statistics.

POPULATION STATISTICS

Population statistics describe populations (i.e., when all measurements of the population are included in the investigation). The important advantage of studying the entire population is that observed differences are actual differences. They are not inferences based on samples of the population. As a result, population statistics need only report the differences or associations detected. When the entire population is used, there is no sampling variation and, therefore, no need for tests of statistical significance. Significance tests are designed to measure the probability of obtaining the observed sample results in the population, under the assumption that no actual differences or associations exist in the population.

SAMPLE STATISTICS

It is unfortunate that analyzing the entire population of measurements is usually impractical, if not

Table 3. *Types of Data Commonly Analyzed by Statistical Methods*

NOMINAL DATA fit into one of a limited number of categories. As the term implies, these categories are not numeric but represent names. For example, the sex of a patient would be categorized as female, female-neutered, male, or male-neutered. Because nominal data are not numeric, they cannot be ordered (i.e., from lowest to highest).

ORDINAL DATA also fit into a limited number of categories but can be ordered one above the other. Examples include the stages of heart failure (stage 1 to stage 4) and the severity of proteinuria as measured with test strips (0 to 4 +). Although ordinal data can be ordered, the distance between each datum may not be equal.

CONTINUOUS DATA implies that there is an unlimited number of equally spaced categories. Serum concentrations of creatinine or glucose are examples of continuous data. Like ordinal data, continuous data can be ordered.

impossible. Therefore, most studies are based on samples of a particular population.

The validity of sample statistics rests on the fundamental assumption that the samples are randomly drawn from the larger population. That is, both the study group and the control group are representative of all those in the true population. If this assumption of random samples is not true, results from the study cannot be reliably extrapolated to the larger population. This does not imply that statistical methods cannot be used to evaluate samples selected in a nonrandom fashion. However, if samples are not randomly selected, clinical judgment must be used in addition to statistical analyses when extrapolating results to individuals not included in the original study group.

Association Between Variables

Statistical associations imply that two characteristics occur together more often than would be expected by chance alone. To study associations, two or more characteristics of the patient are measured. If an association exists, changes in the magnitude of one variable should reflect changes in the magnitude of the other variable.

What questions should be considered when evaluating problems of statistical association? To help formulate questions, consider the following example. A study was conducted in normal cats to evaluate the relationship between daily protein consumption and serum urea nitrogen concentration. The investigator sampled 100 cats that consumed various amounts of protein and determined that serum concentrations of urea nitrogen rose with the quantity of protein ingested. Thus, the investigator concluded that serum urea nitrogen concentrations were influenced by the quantity of protein consumed. In order to state inferences about the population of all normal cats, the investigators would have to answer three fundamental questions: (1) What is the "strength" of the association between the variables (serum urea nitrogen concentration and protein consumption)? (2) Is the association observed in the sample data statistically significant? and (3) How much of the variation in serum urea nitrogen concentration is due to protein consumption?

The type of statistical methods used to answer these questions depends on the type of data (Table 3) analyzed, and the presence or absence of a linear association between the variables evaluated (Table 4). If a linear association is present, a straight line can be used to describe the relationship between the variables (serum urea nitrogen concentration and quantity of protein ingested).

In the previous example of 100 cats fed various quantities of protein, assume the data are continuous and linearly associated. In this situation, Pearson's correlation methods can be used to answer the three questions of interest (Table 4). The degree of association is measured by the correlation coefficient, denoted as "r." The absolute value of r varies between 0 and 1. A value of 0 indicates no linear correlation; a value of 1 indicates a perfect linear correlation between the quantity of protein fed and the serum concentration of urea nitrogen. Let's assume that r = 0.9. This value indicates that the strength of a linear correlation between daily protein consumption and serum urea nitrogen concentration is high. Tests of significance of r can be performed to determine if the linear correlation of the sample is likely to represent an actual linear association in the larger population. Also, by multiplying r by itself (in this case, $0.9 \times 0.9 = 0.81$), investigators obtain the coefficient of determination, denoted "r squared" (r^2). The value of r^2 specifies the proportion of variation in serum urea nitrogen concentration that is attributable to the quantity of protein consumed. As a result, 81 per cent of the changes in serum urea nitrogen in normal cats can be explained by the amount of protein consumed.

Differences Between Groups

Clinicians are frequently interested in measuring the differences between groups of data. For example, the effectiveness of ivermectin compared with that of diethylcarbamazine in the prevention of *Dirofilaria immitis* infection represents a difference between groups. Likewise, the daily urine calcium excretion in dogs with calcium oxalate urolithiasis compared with that in normal dogs is a difference between groups. To determine if differences observed in these sample data are likely to occur in the larger population, one must answer two impor-

Table 4. Common Statistical Procedures Used to Assess Associations Between Variables

Type of Data*	Linear Association	Tests of Degree of Association	Tests of Statistical Significance	Tests of Extent of Variation Attributed to Independent Variable
Nominal	NA	Odds ratio	Significance test of odds ratio	Attributable risk
		Relative risk	Significance test of relative risk	Attributable risk
Ordinal	NA	Spearman's rho	Significance test of rho or tau	$(rho)^2$ or $(tau)^2$
		Kendall's tau		
Continuous	Linear	Pearson's correlation coefficient (r)	Significance test of r	r^2
	Nonlinear	Spearman's rho	Significance test of rho or tau	$(rho)^2$ or $(tau)^2$
		Kendall's tau		

NA, not applicable.
*See Table 3.

tant questions: (1) What is the magnitude of the difference observed in the sample data? and (2) Is this difference statistically significant? *Statistical significance* indicates that differences observed in the study reflect actual differences in the larger population.

The type of statistical method used to answer these questions depends on (1) the type of data analyzed (Table 3), (2) the number of comparisons made, and (3) whether data points are matched or unmatched (Tables 5 and 6). For illustration, consider the previous example comparing daily urine calcium excretion in dogs with calcium oxalate urolithiasis with that in normal control dogs. Twenty-four–hour urine excretion studies were performed on 40 dogs with calcium oxalate urolithiasis. Likewise, 24-hour urine excretion studies were performed on 40 dogs without urolithiasis that were matched for age, sex, breed, and weight. The average difference in calcium excretion for each pair of dogs was 33 mg/day. Thus, 33 mg/day is the answer to the first question, What is the magnitude of the difference observed?

Are the findings statistically significant? The data are continuous, only one comparison is considered,

and animals in the study group are paired with animals in the control group. What statistical method can be used to assess whether or not the difference of 33 mg/day is likely to reflect an actual difference in the larger population (Table 5)? The concept of statistical significance is discussed in the next section, entitled Statistical Inference.

STATISTICAL INFERENCE

Results of clinical studies, which are only samples of a population, must be properly interpreted. Interpretation requires inference; an inference is a conclusion based on logical reasoning. Statistical inferences are conclusions based on calculated probabilities and likelihoods that events will occur. In terms of application, *statistical inferences* are decisions (estimations, predictions, or generalizations) about a population (the set of all measurements) based on analysis of information obtained from a sample (a subset of the measurements of the population). Because the entire population is not analyzed, inferences are associated with a degree of uncertainty. As a consequence, statements of infer-

Table 5. Common Statistical Procedures Used to Assess Differences Between Groups

Type of Data*	No. of Comparisons	Matching† of Data	Test of Statistical Significance
Nominal	One or more	Unmatched	Chi-squared test‡
	One or more	Matched	McNemar's test§
Ordinal	One	Unmatched	Mann-Whitney U or median test
	One	Matched	Wilcoxon's signed-rank test
	More than one	Unmatched	Kruskal-Wallis one-way analysis of variance
	More than one	Matched	Friedman's two-way analysis of variance
Continuous	One	Unmatched	T-Test
	One	Matched	Paired t-test
	More than one	Unmatched	F-test for analysis of variance
		Matched	F-test for analysis of variance with blocking or analysis of covariance

*See Table 3.
†Investigators may match or pair individuals in the study group with individuals in the control group. This procedure may decrease variability and increase the power of a significance test.
‡Use Fisher's exact test for studies with small sample size.
§Use Sign test for studies with small sample size.

Table 6. *Definitions and Concepts of Some Terms Associated with Methods of Statistical Analysis*

MATCHING is the process of pairing patients in the study group with patients in the control group. Patients are matched according to factors (e.g., age, sex, breed) likely to affect the outcome of a study. Appropriate matching of patients increases the statistical power of a test (Table 7).

RELATIVE RISK is a measure of the "strength" of the association between variables (i.e., cause and effect). It is calculated by dividing the probability of developing the disease if the factor is present, by the probability of developing the disease if the factor is not present. For example, a relative risk of 3 implies that patients with the factor are 3 times more likely to develop disease than patients without the factor. Relative risks are applicable to cohort (prospective) studies. In contrast, the *ODDS RATIO* is used as a measure of the "strength" of association for case control (retrospective) studies.

ATTRIBUTABLE RISK is a measure of the risk explained by (attributed to) the factor studied.

ANALYSIS OF VARIANCE (ANOVA) is a statistical method used to analyze differences between two or more groups of data. This method is appropriately named, because it compares the variability within groups to the variability between groups.

LINEAR REGRESSION is a statistical method used to analyze linear associations between variables. Linear regression techniques are used for fitting lines to data and evaluating how well a line describes the data.

INDEPENDENT VARIABLE is a factor the investigator can control and manipulate. Independent variables are synonymous with treatments factors. In contrast, *DEPENDENT VARIABLES* represent outcome variables. Dependent variables are synonymous with treatment effects.

COEFFICIENT OF CORRELATION ("r") is a measure of the strength of a linear relationship between variables. The absolute value of r varies between 0 and 1. A value of 0 indicates no linear correlation; a value of 1 indicates a perfect linear correlation.

COEFFICIENT OF DETERMINATION ("r^2") specifies the proportion of variation of the dependent variable that is attributable to variation in magnitude of the independent variable.

ence should also include measures of their reliability (or reproducibility). These measures of reliability are commonly referred to as *p*-values and confidence levels.

The process of statistical inference may be thought of as asking and answering questions about data obtained from a sample. For example, when an investigator is interested in comparing the differences between two groups, three questions should be answered: (1) What is the magnitude of the difference? (2) How accurately does the magnitude of the sample difference reflect the actual difference in the larger population? and (3) Is the difference statistically significant?

The first two questions are concerned with estimating a population parameter (Fig. 1). In the first question, the magnitude of the difference is called a *point estimate*. The second question asks how likely it is that the point estimate reflects the magnitude of the actual difference in the larger population. This probability is referred to as the *confidence interval*. Confidence intervals are calculated to determine a range of point estimates for the population. The last question (Is the difference statistically significant?) is called a *hypothesis test*. A yes or no answer based on probability is expected.

Point Estimate

Point estimates answer the question, What is the magnitude of the difference between two or more groups of data? They are obtained by calculating the difference between the groups studied. For example, to determine the point estimate for the numeric means of two groups, the smaller value is subtracted from the larger value. In the previous example, dogs with calcium oxalate uroliths excreted more calcium (33 mg) per day than normal

dogs. The point estimate is 33 mg; it represents the magnitude of difference between the two groups. Because it is not feasible to evaluate all dogs, this point estimate is used as an estimate of the actual difference between comparisons of all dogs with calcium oxalate urolithiasis and control dogs.

Confidence Interval

A *confidence interval* is the range of probable values that encompass a point estimate. The range is calculated in such a manner that there is a high probability that the actual value of the population difference lies within the range. It follows that confidence intervals answer the previous question, How likely is the point estimate to reflect the magnitude of the actual difference in the larger population?

Statisticians have coined the term *confidence coefficient* to indicate the reliability of confidence intervals. A confidence coefficient represents the probability that intervals obtained from samples taken repeatedly from a population will contain the actual population difference. For example, a confidence coefficient of 0.95 implies that 95 per cent of confidence intervals measured from repeatedly chosen samples will contain the true estimate for the population. The point estimate, 33 mg, expressed the difference in urine calcium excretion between two groups of dogs (dogs with calcium oxalate urolithiasis and normal dogs). A 95 per cent confidence interval was calculated: The numeric limits of the interval ranged between 21 mg and 55 mg. From a practical viewpoint, this interval means that the difference between the two groups may be as little as 21 mg/day or as great as 55 mg/day in the larger population.

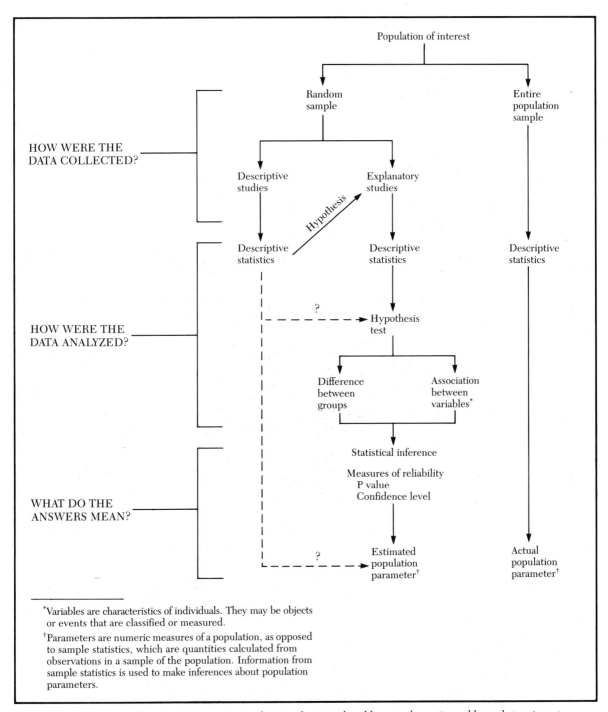

Figure 1. Flow diagram illustrating the stepwise evaluation of statistical problems, and questions addressed at various steps.

Hypothesis Tests

Hypothesis tests answer the commonly asked question, Is the difference statistically significant? *Statistical significance* implies that the difference observed in the sample data represents an actual difference in the population. This question is answered through statistical evaluation of sample data to determine whether data are consistent or incon-sistent with the null hypothesis. *Hypotheses* are not statements of fact but assumptions brought forward as a basis for reasoning and argument. Two hypotheses are essential to statistical problems: the research hypothesis and the null hypothesis.

The concept of "consistent with the null hypothesis" is essential to understanding hypothesis tests. Suppose that an investigator assumes that all Labrador retriever dogs in the world are black and that his or her assumption represents a null hypothesis. According to the null hypothesis (all Labrador retriever dogs are black), what is the likelihood that the next Labrador retriever dog seen is black? According to the hypothesis, the likelihood is very high. Assume that the next Labrador retriever dog seen is black. Seeing a black dog is *consistent* with the null hypothesis (all Labrador retriever dogs are black). According to the null hypothesis, what is the likelihood that the next Labrador retriever dog seen is not black? To be consistent with the null hypothesis, it would have to be zero. Assume that the next Labrador retriever dog was yellow, and so were the third and the fourth ones. Are these findings consistent with the null hypothesis? No, yellow Labrador retriever dogs are *inconsistent* with the null hypothesis. Therefore, one would infer that the null hypothesis is incorrect, and it would be rejected.

Identical to this illustration, hypothesis tests are used to assess the probability that sample data are consistent with the null hypothesis. If the sample data are consistent with the null hypothesis, the null hypothesis is not rejected. If sample data are inconsistent with the null hypothesis, the null hypothesis is rejected, and the study is considered statistically significant.

Hypothesis tests consist of several elements: hypotheses, a level of significance, the test statistic, the outcome, and a measure of outcome reliability. Each of these characteristics (Table 7) is described in the following discussion.

HYPOTHESES

The *research hypothesis* represents the theory that the study is trying to prove (e.g., dogs with calcium oxalate urolithiasis excrete more urine calcium per day than normal dogs, or daily protein consumption influences the magnitude of serum urea nitrogen in cats). The *null hypothesis* is stated such that it opposes the research hypothesis (e.g., dogs with calcium oxalate urolithiasis excrete the same level of urine calcium per day as normal control dogs, or daily protein consumption does not alter the magnitude of serum urea nitrogen). Support for the research hypothesis is gained by producing evidence that the null hypothesis is false (i.e., sample data are inconsistent with the null hypothesis).

LEVEL OF SIGNIFICANCE

The level of significance represents the probability of an event. In this context, that sample data are consistent with the null hypothesis. The most commonly used levels of statistical significance are 0.05 or 0.01.

Consider the following example. The results of a study of dogs with calcium oxalate uroliths reveal that they excrete more calcium in their urine than do control dogs (p-value = 0.05). This means that there is a 5 percent probability that dogs with calcium oxalate uroliths will excrete the same amount of calcium in their urine as control dogs. Actually a p-value of 0.05 means that 5 per cent of samples repeatedly chosen from the population will not be different from those of normal dogs (i.e., they are consistent with calcium excretion of normal dogs). In this example assume that the level of statistical significance was equal to the p-value (to be discussed). The significance level (0.05) was established during planning phases of the study

---

Table 7. *Common Definitions and Terms Associated with Hypothesis Tests*

PROBABILITY is a measure of the chance or likelihood that an event will occur. The "classic" interpretation of probability is the number of outcomes in favor of an event, divided by the total number of possible outcomes. For example, the probability of choosing an ace from a deck of 52 cards is 4/52, or 0.077. Likewise, the probability of choosing the ace of hearts is 1/52, or 0.019. Since extrapolation of sample results to the population of interest involves uncertainty, probability serves as a useful tool by which statistical inferences are made and assessed.

HYPOTHESIS TESTS are calculations and decisions used to address the question, Are study results statistically significant?

RESEARCH HYPOTHESIS is the theory the study is attempting to prove.

NULL HYPOTHESIS is also a theory but is stated in such a manner that it directly opposes the research hypothesis.

SIGNIFICANCE LEVEL is a probability that reflects the investigator's tolerance of the sample data being consistent with the null hypothesis, when the null hypothesis is false. By convention significance levels are commonly set at 0.05 or 0.01. Above these limits (probabilities), the investigator concludes that one does not have enough evidence to reject the null hypothesis.

POWER OF A STUDY is the probability of rejecting the null hypothesis if the research hypothesis is true. Power is directly related to the sample size and magnitude of the difference or association between groups compared. Powerful studies are analogous to very sensitive tests; few false-negative results occur.

P-VALUE is the probability that sample data will occur, under the assumption that the null hypothesis is true.

TYPE I ERROR is the probability that study results are statistically significant (rejection of the null hypothesis when it is false), if the null hypothesis is true.

TYPE II ERROR is the probability that study results are not statistically significant (failing to reject the null hypothesis), if the research hypothesis is true.

TEST STATISTIC is the statistical procedure used to calculate the p-value of a study.

STATISTICAL SIGNIFICANCE implies that a difference or an association detected in sample data reflects an actual difference in the larger population.

and, therefore, prior to the use of statistical methods to calculate the p-value. The level of significance (0.05 in this example) is related to the null hypothesis, which is the exact opposite of the hypothesis being tested (the research hypothesis). Thus, level of significance defines a limit (in the example, it was 5 per cent) above which the investigator concludes that the sample data are consistent with the null hypothesis. If the p-value is equal to or less than the previously established level of significance, the null hypothesis is rejected, and the value is accepted as statistically significant.

TEST STATISTIC

A test statistic is a numeric quantity calculated from the observations or measurements in a sample. Information from a test statistic (e.g., p-values) is used to make inferences about the population. Methods of obtaining a test statistic were presented in the section entitled Methods of Statistical Analysis.

OUTCOME

Hypothesis tests result in one of two possible outcomes: (1) rejection of the null hypothesis (in favor of the research hypothesis), or (2) failure to reject the null hypothesis. The decision is based on the magnitude of the p-value in relation to a level of significance.

A p-value represents the probability that the sample data will occur under the assumption that the null hypothesis is true. Since the goal of hypothesis tests is to reject the null hypothesis, sample data should be as inconsistent with the null hypothesis as possible. Consequently, very low p-values are desired. Recall the study comparing urine calcium excretion in dogs having calcium oxalate urolithiasis with that in control dogs. Instead of a p-value of 0.05, assume that the p-value for the difference in urine calcium excretion is 0.50. This means that there is a 50 per cent probability that dogs with calcium oxalate urolithiasis excrete the same amount of calcium in their urine as do normal dogs. The null hypothesis is not rejected, and the study is not statistically significant.

To summarize, the null hypothesis is rejected if the p-value is smaller than the significance level of the hypothesis test. In this situation, the study is considered statistically significant; the difference observed in the sample data probably reflects an actual difference in the larger population. If the p-value is larger than the significance level, one cannot reject the null hypothesis. In this situation, there is not enough evidence to demonstrate that

differences occur in the population at the specified significance level.

One disadvantage of some hypothesis tests is an inability to detect real differences (i.e., that the null hypothesis is false). This is commonly referred to as a type II error (Table 7). This occurs in studies with inadequate power (see following discussion).

The *power of a study* is the probability that the null hypothesis is rejected, if the research hypothesis is true. Power is directly related to sample size and the magnitude of the difference between groups compared. Studies with large sample sizes are more powerful. Likewise, studies with greater differences between groups are also more powerful.

Powerful studies are analogous to very sensitive tests; few false-negative results occur. Consequently, negative results (i.e., results that are not statistically significant) from powerful studies support the null hypothesis. In contrast, negative results from studies with inadequate power may not provide enough evidence to disprove a null hypothesis. As a result, failing to reject the null hypothesis is not the same as accepting the null hypothesis. It may be related to a study with insufficient power.

MEASURE OF RELIABILITY

P-values measure the reliability of outcome of hypothesis tests (see previous section entitled Outcome). P-values represent the probability of rejecting the null hypothesis, if the null hypothesis is true (type I error; see table 7). Using the p-values from the previous illustration of the difference in daily calcium excretion in calcium oxalate dogs and controls, a p-value of 0.50 means that there is a 50 per cent probability that dogs with calcium oxalate uroliths will excrete the same amount of calcium as control dogs. It thus follows, that there is a 50 per cent chance of erroneously rejecting the null hypothesis, if it is true. In contrast, a p-value of 0.05 means that there is only a 5 per cent probability that dogs with calcium oxalate urolithiasis will excrete the same amount as normal dogs. In this situation, there is a 5 per cent chance of erroneously rejecting the null hypothesis, if it is true. If the null hypothesis is rejected in both situations, it follows that the lower p-values provide greater evidence of statistical significance.

At the end of the section entitled Differences between Groups, you were encouraged to answer the question, What statistical method can be used to assess the probability that the finding of a 33 mg/day difference in calcium excretion reflects an actual difference in the larger population (Table 5)? A significance level was set at 0.05. The data are continuous, only one comparison is considered, and the animals in the study group are paired with animals in the control group. The data should be analyzed using a *paired t-test*. Statistical analysis resulted in a *p*-value of 0.02.

You were also asked if the findings were statistically significant. You have the knowledge to answer this question. You can also determine the probability that the null hypothesis is erroneously rejected, if it is true (yes, it is 2 per cent).

Are all statistically significantly data *clinically important?* Three questions must be considered in determining the clinical importance of a statistically significant study: (1) Can the needed procedures be used to evaluate animals in a clinical setting? (2) Are differences or associations between groups large enough to be clinically useful? and (3) Is the degree of overlap between different groups small enough to accurately separate normal animals from animals with disease? Further evaluation of the research techniques and data is necessary to answer these questions. Consultation with statisticians is recommended.

In this discussion, we used differences between groups to illustrate the principles of statistical inference. Confidence intervals and hypothesis tests can also be performed on correlation coefficients (r), coefficients of determination (r^2), slopes of lines, and other statistically useful variables. Calculations may be different, but concepts and interpretations remain the same.

References and Supplemental Reading

Bailar, J. C., Louis, T. A., Lavori, P. W., et al.: Studies without internal controls. N. Engl. J. Med. 311:156, 1984.

Bellamy, J. E. C.: Coming to grips with statistics. Can. J. Comp. Med. 47:385, 1983.

Berry, G.: Statistical significance and confidence intervals. Med. J. Aust. 144:618, 1986.

Browner, W. S., Newman, T. B.: Are all significant p values created equal? J.A.M.A. 257:2459, 1987.

Dohoo, I. R., Walter-Toews, D.: Interpreting clinical research, Part I. General considerations. Comp. Cont. Ed. 7:473, 1985.

Dohoo, I. R., Walter-Toews, D.: Interpreting clinical research, Part II. Descriptive and experimental studies. Comp. Cont. Ed. 7:513, 1985.

Dohoo, I. R., Walter-Toews, D.: Interpreting clinical research, Part III. Observational studies and interpreting results. Comp. Cont. Ed. 7:605, 1985.

Godfrey, K.: Comparing the means of several groups. N. Engl. J. Med. 313:1450, 1985.

Godfrey, K.: Simple linear regression in medical research. N. Engl. J.Med. 313:1629, 1985.

Ingelfinger, J. A., Mosteller, F., Thibodeau, L. A., et al.: *Biostatistics in Clinical Medicine.* New York: Macmillan Publishing Co., Inc., 1987.

Jorgensen, R. R.: Data, dilemma, decision: The biometric approach. J.A.V.M.A. 166:915, 1975.

McClave, J. T., Dietrich, F. H.: *Statistics.* Riverside, NJ: Dellen Publishing Company, 1985.

Riegelman, R. K.: *Studying a Study and Testing a Test.* Boston: Little, Brown, and Company, 1981.

Simon R.: Confidence intervals for reporting results of clinical trials. Ann. Intern. Med. 105:429, 1986.

CAUSE AND CONTROL OF DECREASED APPETITE

DENNIS W. MACY, D.V.M.,
and SARAH L. RALSTON, V.M.D.

Fort Collins, Colorado

Many diseases of dogs and cats are frequently accompanied by anorexia. Although the medical management of these patients is usually directed toward the primary disorder, there is increasing recognition of the importance of nutritional supplementation. Some disease states (e.g., hyperthyroidism, cancer, and fever) result in above-normal caloric requirements, which enhance the effect of even partial anorexia.

Prolonged inadequate nutritional intake may be more detrimental to the patient than the underlying disorder. For example, extended periods of anorexia can result in significant alterations in the immune system. Decreases in cell-mediated immunity, immunoglobulin production, complement levels, and phagocytic activity have been noted following rapid loss of body weight due to anorexia. It is fortunate that these abnormalities in the immune system are reversible with nutritional supplementation. Inadequate protein intake in itself may result in slower wound healing, alteration in the intestinal-epithelial barrier, and a greater likelihood of septicemia due to increased risk of entrance of enteric organisms. In addition to these aberrations, there is a lowering of the ability of the liver to metabolize or detoxify drugs and toxins, which may make some drugs less effective or more toxic when administered to cachectic patients. Cats appear to be especially susceptible to the detrimental effects of short-term anorexia because of their special requirements for amino acids (especially arginine to prevent hyper-ammoniemia) and B vitamins. Vitamin B requirements for cats are eight times those for dogs. B vitamin deficiency alone can precipitate or perpetuate an anorexic episode.

CONTROL OF FOOD INTAKE

Whether or not an animal will eat voluntarily is influenced by a complex interplay of metabolic, gastrointestinal (GI), and sensory cues. The resultant neural, metabolic, and hormonal stimuli are integrated and modified in the central nervous system (CNS), based on the animal's current energy status, motivational state, and previous experience with the food. A single factor, such as palatability, may override all other inputs. However, the relative strength of a cue is usually modulated by other exogenous and endogenous stimuli. There are many factors that can be manipulated to stimulate food intake in hospitalized animals.

The taste, odor, and texture of a food determine to some degree its acceptability to a patient motivated to eat. Flavor preferences differ between species and may also be modified by previous experience. For example, cats usually do not prefer sweet foods, whereas dogs do. Foods or flavors associated with rewards such as petting or a sense of well-being are preferred. Both cats and dogs frequently develop preferences for food items that normally would be rejected, such as tomatoes, celery, and chili, owing to conditioning in the home environment. A food (especially one with a novel flavor, odor, or texture) that has previously been associated with nausea, vomiting, or cramping will be avoided by dogs in the future (learned aversion). Cats do not appear to avoid foods previously associated with GI disturbances as quickly as dogs.

The act of eating (chewing and swallowing) and associated sensory stimuli generate neural and hormonal cues that facilitate absorption and utilization of the food. For example, the insulin response to voluntarily ingested glucose is greater than the insulin response to the same amount of glucose infused directly into the stomach or given intravenously (IV). Therefore, voluntary consumption of food facilitates digestion and metabolism. It is the safest and most effective mode of alimentation in hospitalized animals.

Nutrients in the GI tract also stimulate vagal nerves and the release of hormones (e.g., insulin, bombesin, cholecystokinin, and gastrin), which have been strongly implicated in the control of food intake. Infusion of glucose, fat, or protein into the stomachs of dogs, rats, and monkeys reduces subsequent feeding activity in proportion to the caloric content of the infusion. In dogs, nonpainful GI distention does not influence normal eating activity

Table 1. Neural Pathways and Substances That Influence CNS Control of Feeding Activity

System	Effect on Food Intake
Serotonin Agonists	
5-Hydroxytryptamine	Inhibits
Fenfluramine	Inhibits
8-OH-DPAT (low-dose)	Stimulates
(high-dose)	Inhibits
Serotonin Antagonists	
Cyproheptadine (central action)	Stimulates
Xylamide (peripheral action only)	Stimulates
Methysergide	Stimulates
Pizotifen	Stimulates
Metergoline	Stimulates
Chlorimipramine	Stimulates
Opioids	
Naloxone	Inhibits
Endorphins (beta- and gamma-endorphins, D-Ala-enkephalin, alpha-neoendorphin)	Stimulate
Morphine (low-dose)	Stimulates
Catecholamines	
Alpha-adrenergic agonists	
Norepinephrine (low-dose)	Stimulates
Clonidine	Stimulates
Trazodone	Stimulates
Amphetamines (low-dose)	Stimulate
(high-dose)	Inhibit
Dopaminergic/GABA	Stimulates
Benzodiazepines (low dose)	Stimulate
Lithium chloride (low-dose)	Stimulates
(high-dose)	Inhibits; produces malaise
Corticotropin-releasing factor	Inhibits

as much as the nutrient content of the foods. Most amino acids (especially tryptophan) stimulate release of cholecystokinin, which inhibits appetite. However, arginine is a strong stimulus for insulin release, which may, in turn, enhance subsequent food intake if adequate carbohydrate calories are not given at the same time. Fats slow gastric emptying to a much greater degree than do other classes of nutrients and appear to reduce subsequent intake to a greater degree than an equal amount of other (although calorically less dense) food. Cats are unique in that they are relatively insensitive to the caloric content of their food and ingest relatively constant dry-matter volumes (2 to 3 per cent of their body weight) regardless of nutrient content. Therefore, foods with high caloric density should be used in cats with exceptional caloric needs due to disease.

Postabsorptive stimuli generated by nutrients also influence subsequent feeding activity. Peripheral blood glucose concentrations per se do not regulate feeding activity but only reflect the degree of hunger a normal animal is experiencing. The availability of glucose for metabolism in the cells does influence the degree of hunger or satiety an animal experiences. For example, phloridzin blocks peripheral utilization of glucose. Animals treated with this drug tend to be hyperglycemic and yet have increased appetites. Similar situations are seen in hyperglycemic diabetic animals that still have increased appetites and often become obese. The point is that infusion of glucose resulting in hyperglycemia reduces appetite only if the animal is capable of utilizing the sugar. This may explain why some critically ill animals may be relatively glucose-intolerant and hyperglycemic and yet still eat if other factors do not inhibit their appetite.

Vagal stimuli generated by nutrients in the liver also influence subsequent feeding activity. Metabolic stimuli that regulate the motivation to eat have not been well-defined. However, anabolic agents (e.g., steroids) tend to stimulate appetite, whereas strong catabolic stimuli (e.g., interleukin-1; also called cachexin) reduce the motivation to eat. Interleukin-1 is released from mononuclear cells during autoimmune or infectious processes and is a factor in the anorexia frequently seen in severe sepsis or hemolytic crisis. Since the interleukins are synthesized from prostaglandin precursors, antiprostaglandin drugs such as aspirin may stimulate appetite by inhibition of interleukin-1 as well as by reducing fever.

All stimuli that influence feeding are integrated in the brain via hormonal and neuronal pathways and, in this way, ultimately determine the motivational state of the animal and whether or not it will eat. A number of neurotransmitters and substances have a physiologic role in the control of food intake (Table 1; Fig. 1). The systems are not mutually exclusive. For example, adrenalectomized rats do not eat in response to centrally administered opioids or alpha-adrenergic agonists unless an exogenous source of corticosterone is provided. Therefore, cortisol appears to have a permissive action for appetite stimulants such as morphine and epinephrine. The effect of a given system also is not constant. Corticotropin-releasing factor is a potent satiety agent, but corticosteroids administered peripherally frequently stimulate appetite. Similarly, mixed adrenergic agents (amphetamines) reduce feeding activity, whereas alpha-adrenergic agonists (norepinephrine, clonidine) stimulate eating in rats. It is thought that the increased feeding activity observed after a mild stressor (such as a tail pinch in rats and strong petting over the back of cats) is due to alpha-adrenergic stimulation. Presynaptic serotonin agonists usually reduce appetite, but 8-hydroxy-

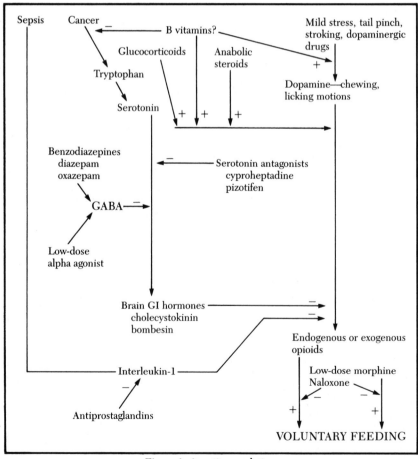

Figure 1. Appetite regulation.

2-(di-N-propylamino-tetrahydronaphthalene) (Tetralin, Du Pont) (8-OH-DPAT), a postsynaptic serotonin agonist, stimulates feeding.

Tryptophan concentrations are elevated in the serum of cancer patients and are thought to play a role in causing inappetance. Reduction of the dietary intake of tryptophan in patients with cancer, hepatic dysfunction, or renal dysfunction often reduces the sense of malaise and increases food intake.

The hypothalamus is considered to be the major integrative center for appetite control. The lateral portion generates sensations of hunger; the ventromedial section regulates satiety. However, other loci influence feeding activity as much as, or more than, the hypothalamus (Table 2).

Nausea, vomiting, cramping, fever, severe stress, and pain all cause anorexia via activation of a variety of known and hypothesized pathways. Pain, nausea, vomiting, intestinal cramping, and stress cause release of catecholamines and serotonin, whereas fever-induced anorexia is thought to be mediated via interleukin-1 and other prostaglandins. Certain hormones or transmitters increase intake of specific nutrients. Opioids stimulate increases in fat intake, whereas dopamine stimulates enhanced protein intake. Mild alpha-adrenergic stimulation increases intake of foods high in carbohydrates. Since the benzodiazepine derivatives appear to act primarily as antiserotoninergic agents or as dopamine pathways, animals treated with diazepam (Valium, Lemmon) should be fed foods relatively high in protein to maximize their food intake.

STIMULATION OF APPETITE IN DOGS AND CATS

Knowledge of the factors that influence normal feeding activity in dogs and cats enables the selection of feeding regimens and foods that maximize intake in clinically ill patients. Normal feeding patterns and sensory, GI, and metabolic stimuli that regulate the motivation to eat all should be considered when feeding a sick dog or cat that has reduced appetite.

Cats

Cats are true carnivores. Carnivores eat infrequent meals that vary little in nutritional value; have a high water, protein, and fat content; and frequently are still warm when consumed. Cats prefer food served at 78 to 103°F (25.6 to 39.4°C). Some cats are social eaters, consuming more if other animals are present, whereas others prefer to eat alone. Cats especially prefer meat and fat flavors; they have little interest in sweets, as a rule. Low pH foods are also usually preferred over alkaline or neutral substances. Cats usually prefer moist foods, although some are addicted to dry or semimoist texture, having been fed only one type of food throughout their lives. It is important to recognize that cats, more than most other domestic animals, are strongly influenced by habit in their selection of foods and are less likely to switch easily from one type of food to another.

Cats tend to be extremely sensitive to the odor and the texture of food. Any change in the texture, flavor, or odor of a diet usually reduces a cat's total intake for three to four days. Cats rely heavily upon their sense of smell in the selection of foods and prefer strong meat, fish, or cheese odors. Cats that were made anosmic experimentally would eat but became more finicky about the texture and the taste of their foods. Butter-flavored lard (with a strong butter odor) is more readily accepted than plain lard as a food additive.

Cats do not appear to be able to regulate their energy intake when given foods that vary in energy density, relying instead upon a fairly constant dry-matter intake. Therefore, in order to get a cat to ingest more calories, energy-dense foods must be used. However, cats will "sample" small amounts of a new food that has an attractive odor or texture,

Table 2. CNS Loci Implicated in the Control of Food Intake

Locus	Effect of Stimulation	Effect of Ablation	Pathways or Neurotransmitters Affecting Response
Hypothalamus			
lateral	Hunger	Anorexia	Norepinephrine, dopamine
ventromedial	Satiety	Obesity	Norepinephrine, opioids
Caudate nucleus	Anorexia	?	Gamma-aminobutyric acid (GABA)
Paraventricular nucleus (requires presence of corticosterone)	Hunger	Anorexia	Opioids, norepinephrine, neuropeptide Y
Nucleus of the solitary tract	Feeding activity	Lack of glucoprivic feeding response	Taste afferents, metabolic cues
Area postrema	Learned aversion; nausea, vomiting	Failure to regulate body weight; no learned aversions	Vagal afferents, metabolic cues

especially when offered in conjunction with positive stimuli such as petting.

Based on the preceding knowledge of the normal factors that influence feeding in cats, several avenues of stimulating food intake are apparent. Acidic foods with a high moisture, protein, and fat content are most likely to be accepted. These include meats, fish, dairy products (especially yogurt), eggs, and poultry. Warming the food to body temperature to volatilize odors and simulate recently killed prey also enhances the likelihood of its being accepted. Keep the cat's nasal passage as clear as possible, using humidifiers and topical anti-inflammatory agents if nasal discharge is a problem.

Always determine the types of foods the cat preferred at home, as many often develop eating habits that are not usually expected in Felidae. For example, some cats readily consume fruits such as avocados and bananas or vegetables such as cooked green beans and carrots.

The mode in which the food is presented is also important. An advantage of foods with the texture of baby food is that they can easily be force-fed or placed on the cat's paws. Putting a small amount of food on the cat's lips or paws usually stimulates a licking response. If palatable food is then placed directly in front of the mouth, licking may be continued (possibly owing to dopaminergic stimulation), resulting in ingestion.

Many cats initially reject food held directly in front of their faces but consume it if it is then placed on the floor or in a dish in front of them. Bowls used for feeding should be wide and shallow, so the sides do not touch the cat's whiskers as it is eating. Many cats do not tolerate having their whiskers touched and, therefore, lift food out of a bowl with their paws. This is not a problem if the floor of the cage is solid and the cat is able to lift the food out, but it results in food wastage on mesh floors. Offering small amounts of fresh food frequently encourages greater intake (not exceeding the normal total of 2 to 3 per cent of body weight in dry matter per day) than if a single bowl of food were offered once a day and left in the cage.

Mild stimulation of a cat by petting and stroking its back frequently stimulates eating if a palatable food is present. However, severe stress should be minimized. If the environment outside the cage is noisy and the cat appears to be disturbed by other cats or dogs, placing the food in a cardboard box or hanging a towel over the front of the cage may reduce these anorexigenic stimuli.

Alleviating other causes of anorexia also enhances food intake. Antipyretic, anti-inflammatory, analgesic, and antiemetic agents should be used when appropriate to reduce fever, pain, and GI disturbances. Food should never be offered immediately before or after administration of a drug or treatment known to cause malaise and vomiting, especially if the food is a new type that you are attempting to get the cat to eat. The association of the food with the feeling of sickness may induce a learned aversion to that food that will be difficult to overcome. Wait until the nausea has passed before offering food.

Strained chicken, lamb, veal, and beef baby foods are frequently accepted when more solid foods are rejected. However, these should not be fed as the sole source of nutrition for more than a few days, since they are deficient in calcium and are not balanced in their vitamin or trace mineral content. Puddings, yogurt, or milk-based baby foods are more balanced and are often accepted as readily as the baby foods. Even these should not be fed for more than a few days without vitamin and mineral supplementation.

Dogs

Dogs eat more types of foods than do cats and are attracted to sweet foods in addition to protein and fat. They, too, prefer infrequent meals. LeBlanc and Diamond report that dogs fed small meals derived less net energy from their food than if the same amount were ingested as a single large meal. The difference was attributed to a higher heat increment apparently induced by hormonal changes associated with the anticipation of eating. However, in the case of a sick dog, feeding small amounts frequently (as in cats) may stimulate greater intakes than if a large amount of food were presented only once. The novelty and the stimulation of presentation may overcome other anorexigenic stimuli. Some dogs tend to be solitary in their feeding habits and do not eat if a human is watching them; others eat only if fed by hand. Dogs are more able to adapt their total intake to the varying energy density of foods and are not as restricted to a given dry-matter intake per day as cats. However, dogs are apparently more sensitive to GI stimuli than are cats. Fats delay gastric emptying to a greater degree than proteins or carbohydrates; they tend to reduce subsequent intake more than the latter two nutrients. Dogs rapidly learn to avoid foods, especially novel flavors or odors, that have been associated with nausea, vomiting, or GI cramping. Therefore, they should not be fed just before or after giving a drug or treatment known to induce vomiting.

Dogs also rely upon olfaction in the selection of foods. Therefore, use of foods that have strong odors (e.g., canned cat or dog foods), warming the food to volatilize the odors, and keeping the nasal passages clear of discharge are important when enticing a sick dog to eat. As in cats, odiferous canned cat foods, strained meat baby food, and high protein meat, dairy, and poultry products are often preferred by dogs. Carbohydrate-rich foods such as pasta, rice, and breads may also be readily accepted.

Dogs appear to be attracted to non-nutritive flavors such as garlic. They are not usually as bound by habit to a single food or type of food as are cats. However, older pampered dogs may be extremely finicky. Therefore, it is important to get an accurate history of the animal's normal diet and preferred foods.

Dogs are not as sensitive as cats about their whiskers being touched and usually eat readily out of a bowl. Small amounts of food offered frequently may stimulate greater intakes but will also cause a greater heat increment. Petting and speaking to the dog may encourage eating, but some dogs may prefer to eat alone.

In both dogs and cats, liquid supplements such as Ensure Plus, Vivonex, and Criticare HN (all available through human hospitals and some grocery stores) may be imbibed by an animal that refuses all solid and semisolid foods. If enteral alimentation is being considered, always offer the fluid to the animal to see if it will voluntarily consume it. Voluntary consumption of food results in better assimilation of the nutrients than if it is delivered by an enteral or an intravenous route.

If a dog or cat refuses to eat voluntarily, any or all of the prior suggestions may be tried in conjunction with chemical stimulation of appetite.

CHEMICAL STIMULATION OF APPETITE

A variety of drugs have been used clinically and experimentally to stimulate appetite in a number of species. Appetite stimulation plays an important role in the management of debilitated animals by inducing voluntary eating, thus improving their nutritional status, their chances of recovering from illness or surgery, or their ability to respond to specific forms of therapy. However, appetite stimulation should not be used as a substitute for accurate diagnosis and specific treatment of a disease.

Chemical stimulants of appetite may be divided into (1) proven short- and long-term active agents and (2) agents that have yet to be evaluated in dogs and cats but are effective in other species.

Proven short-term appetite-stimulating agents include the benzodiazepine derivatives and the antiserotonin agents, cyproheptadine (Periactin, Merck, Sharp & Dohme), and pizotifen. The benzodiazepine derivatives stimulate appetite in a variety of species, including humans, rats, dogs, pigs, sheep, cattle, horses, and chickens. There is wide variation in the efficacy of benzodiazepine appetite stimulation, depending on the structure of the derivative used and upon the species in which it is administered. The most frequently used benzodiazepine appetite stimulant is diazepam. Diazepam is most effective when given intravenously; its appetite-stimulating ability following intramuscular (IM) and oral (PO) administration appears to be decreased. Following intravenous administration of diazepam, feeding usually starts within a minute and may continue for 20 minutes to half an hour. In one study of anorexic cats, voluntary consumption of up to 25 per cent of the total daily caloric requirements was observed following each IV administration of diazepam. In dogs and cats, an IV dose of 1 mg/10 lb (0.2 mg/kg) of diazepam, with a maximum dose of 5 mg/patient, appears to be most effective. Reduced dosages should be considered in severely depressed or debilitated animals, since they are extremely sensitive to the sedative properties of the benzodiazepine derivatives. Oxazepam (Serax, Wyeth Labs) is another benzodiazepine derivative used for appetite stimulation; it is available for oral administration only. Oxazepam is most frequently administered to cats at a dose of 2.5 mg/cat and usually results in eating within 20 minutes after administration. Although oxazepam is regarded as a more powerful appetite stimulant than diazepam, its oral administration tends to make it less effective clinically. Most benzodiazepine derivatives have the potential to cause sedation and ataxia. It is not uncommon to find animals asleep, with their heads in their food bowls, following a short feeding episode. Diazepam may be administered twice daily; however, the appetite-stimulating properties appear to wane with time when used in sick animals. This is in contrast to its effect in normal animals, in whom continued use of diazepam does not result in reduction of its appetite-stimulating qualities.

Cyproheptadine, a serotonin and histamine antagonist, has been shown to stimulate the appetites of cats and humans but not dogs. Although the drug is inexpensive and readily available, it has not had extensive clinical use in veterinary medicine. The experimental dose used in cats is 4 mg/kg/day. However, extreme excitability and aggression were reported in one fifth of the cats treated with this drug. In human medicine, cyproheptadine is used principally for its antihistaminic effects in asthmatic patients, but it has also been success in increasing the appetite of underweight patients with pulmonary tuberculosis. Pizotyline (pizotifen) is another antiserotonin agent that has been shown to stimulate the appetite of cats. It is available in Europe, Canada, and Australia but not in the United States.

Glucocorticoids have long been used clinically in veterinary medicine and recently in human medicine for nonspecific stimulation of appetite. The specific mechanism of glucocorticoid stimulation of appetite has not been clearly defined. When there are no contraindications for glucocorticoid use, patients who have poor appetite or who are losing weight may benefit from relatively low doses of prednisolone (0.25 to 0.5 mg/kg/day or every other day, or intermittently as needed).

The anabolic steroids stanozolol (Winstrol, Winthrop-Breon) (1 to 2 mg b.i.d. orally or 25 to 50 mg IM weekly) or nandrolone decanoate (Deca-Durabolin, Organon Pharmaceuticals) (5 mg/kg maximum dosage or 200 mg/patient IM weekly) have been used to stimulate appetite. These drugs tend to produce more prolonged stimulation of appetite than the benzodiazepine derivatives or glucocorticoids. The positive nitrogen balance associated with use of anabolic steroids in debilitated animals has been shown to be associated with the increase in the patient's appetite rather than alterations in metabolism. Although the appetite-stimulating properties of the anabolic steroids are usually not as pronounced as seen with glucocorticoids or benzodiazepines, they are usually devoid of the polydipsia, polyuria, and adrenal suppression associated with glucocorticoid therapy. Prolonged use of oral anabolic steroids may result in hepatotoxicity.

Megestrol acetate (Ovaban Schering), 1 mg/kg/day/PO is used primarily for birth control or dermatologic conditions in domestic animals. An inconsistent side effect noticed with this drug is an increase in appetite and weight gain in both domestic animals and humans. The appetite-stimulating properties of megestrol acetate are less consistently observed than are those of the other agents; however, it has been used by some veterinarians to stimulate appetite in debilitated animals. The mechanisms of stimulation of appetite with anabolic steroids and progesterone compounds such as megestrol acetate have not been defined but appear to be different from those with glucocorticoids; thus, cross-resistance between the two agents may not exist.

B vitamins have been used in clinical practice for some time to stimulate appetite. Experimental evidence of their efficacy is hard to find; however, B vitamin deficiencies result in anorexia. Cats have a particularly high requirement for B vitamins, which makes supplementation especially important in anorexic cats. The addition of B vitamin complex to intravenous fluids (1 cc/L) is an easy way of ensuring an adequate source of B vitamins for these anorexic patients.

Lithium, morphine, and phenobarbital have been used experimentally to stimulate appetite in other species but have not been thoroughly evaluated in dogs and cats. Because of the wide range of species susceptibility to appetite stimulation and other properties of these drugs, they cannot be recommended at this time for nonspecific appetite stimulation.

References and Supplemental Reading

Beauchamps, G. K., Maller, O., and Rogers, J. G.: Flavor preferences in the cat (Felis catus and panthera spp). J. Comp. Physiol. Psych. 91:1118, 1977.

Burt, G. S., and Smotherman, W. P.: Amygdalectomy-induced deficits in conditioned taste aversion: Possible pituitary-adrenal involvement. Physiol. Behav. 24:651, 1980.

Copeland, E. M., Daly, J. M., and Dudrick, S. J.: Nutrition as an adjunct to cancer treatment in the adult. Cancer Res. 37:2451, 1977.

Della Fera, M. A., Baily, C. A., and McLaughlin, C. L.: Feeding elicited by benzodiazepine-like chemicals in puppies and cats: Structure-activity relationships. Pharmacol. Biochem. Behav. 12:195, 1980.

Dowrish, C. T., Hutson, D. H., and Curzon, G.: Characteristics of feeding induced by the serotonin agonist 8-hydroxy-2-(di-N-propylamine) Tetralin (8-OH-DPAT). Brain Res. Bull. 15:377, 1985.

Garattini, S., Mennini, J., Bendotti, C., et al.: Neurochemical mechanism of action of drugs which modify feeding via the serotonergic system. Appetite 7:15, 1982.

Heber, D., Byerly, L. O., and Chlebowski, R. T.: Metabolic abnormalities in the cancer patient. Cancer 55:225, 1985.

Hirsch, E., Dubose, C., and Jacobs, H. L.: Dietary control of food intake in cats. Physiol. Behav. 20:287, 1978.

Kanarek, R. B.: Determinants of dietary self-selection in experimental animals. Am. J. Clin. Nutr. 42:940, 1985.

LeBlanc, J., and Diamond, P.: Effect of meal size and frequency on postprandial thermogenesis in dogs. Am. J. Physiol. 250:E144, 1986.

Lundholm, K., Edström, S., Ekman, L., et al.: Metabolism in peripheral tissues in cancer patients. Cancer Treat. Rep. 65:79, 1981.

Macy, D. W., and Gasper, P. W.: Diazepam-induced eating in anorexic cats. J. Am. Anim. Hosp. Assoc. 21:17, 1985.

Morley, J. E.: The neuroendocrine control of appetite: The role of endogenous opiates, cholecystokinin, hydrotropic-releasing hormone, gamma-aminobutyric acid and the diazepam receptor. Life Sci. 27:355, 1980.

Ralston, S. L.: Patterns and control of food intake in domestic animals. Compend. Cont. Ed. 6:S628, 1984.

Roland, C. R., Bhakthavatsalam, P., and Leibowitz, S. F.: Interaction between corticosterone and alpha-2-noradrenergic system of the paraventricular nucleus in relation to feeding behavior. Neuroendocrinology 42:296, 1986.

Toates, F. M.: The control of ingestive behavior by internal and external stimuli—a theoretical review. Appetite 2:35, 1981.

Weischer, M. L., and Opitz, K.: Orexigenic effects of pizotifen and cyproheptadine in cats. I. R. C. S. Med. Sci. 7:55, 1979.

Willox, J. C., Corr, J., Shaw, J., et al.: Prednisolone as an appetite stimulant in patients with cancer. Br. Med. J. 288:27, 1984.

Woods, J. S., and Leibowitz, S. F.: Hypothalamic sites sensitive to morphine and naloxone: Effects on feeding behavior. Pharmacol. Biochem. Behav. 23:431, 1985.

PARENTERAL NUTRITIONAL SUPPORT

AUNNA C. LIPPERT, D.V.M.,
East Lansing, Michigan

and P. JANE ARMSTRONG, D.V.M.
Raleigh, North Carolina

INTRODUCTION AND DEFINITION OF TERMS

Although most critically ill patients can be maintained using enteral nutrition, a small number are temporarily unable to assimilate nutrients administered into the gastrointestinal tract. Parenteral nutrition may be beneficial for selected patients for whom withholding or limiting nutrients given enterally allows time for the resolution of disease.

There is some confusion surrounding the terms that refer to parenteral nutrition. Total parenteral nutrition (TPN) is the provision of all essential nutrients by an intravenous route. TPN is almost always administered into a central vein, most commonly the cranial vena cava, because of the hyperosmolarity of the solutions. Partial parenteral nutrition (PPN) supplies part of the nutritional requirements, but a negative energy or nitrogen balance may result if the remainder is not provided enterally. Parenteral nutrition administered into a peripheral vein is almost always PPN, because of volume and osmolarity constraints. Intravenous hyperalimentation (IVH) is an outdated term that describes the parenteral administration of nutrients in excess of individual requirements in order to promote anabolism. This practice is no longer customary in human medicine because it carries a great risk of metabolic complications.

INDICATIONS FOR PARENTERAL NUTRITIONAL SUPPORT

The principal advantage of parenteral nutrition is that it can be used when the gastrointestinal tract is nonfunctional. There is a greater probability that the administered nutrients will reach the tissues, without being subject to inconsistencies in digestion and absorption. In most cases, a shorter period is required for the transition to a full nutrient load than with enteral nutritional support.

Disadvantages of the parenteral route of nutrition include the requirements for comparatively expensive specialized products, asepsis in preparation and administration, and skilled personnel. There is some risk of septic and metabolic complications. In addition, gastrointestinal atrophy may occur in animals receiving TPN with nothing per os (PO). Following return of enteral intake, gastrointestinal atrophy subsides.

The nutritional assessment and selection of patients in need of nutritional support is discussed in the following article, Enteral Nutritional Support. For the reasons outlined previously, parenteral nutrition should *not* be selected as a method of nutritional support unless it is clearly indicated. TPN should be considered in any animal in whom one anticipates an inability to absorb enterally administered nutrients for longer than 3 to 5 days. The exact time is dependent on the patient's initial nutritional status. Examples include patients undergoing massive small bowel resection and patients with impaired small intestinal motility or function, severe diarrhea, or intractable vomiting. TPN may also be indicated in patients with severe prolonged pancreatitis and in those with severe malnutrition or catabolism associated with a temporarily nonfunctional gastrointestinal tract. Parenteral nutrition is less correctly used, often out of necessity, in animals judged to be unable to tolerate anesthesia for a surgically placed "ostomy," and those who are poor candidates for nasogastric, repeated orogastric, or force-feeding.

The general goal of parenteral nutrition in veterinary patients is the prevention of further deterioration in nutritional status until the patient can return to full enteral intake, at which time weight gain can be more safely achieved if necessary.

CALCULATION OF NUTRITIONAL REQUIREMENTS FOR TPN

Worksheets are used in the authors' hospitals for the calculation of nutritional requirements for TPN (Figs. 1 and 2). The basal energy requirement (BER) is calculated using the actual body weight, as de-

Worksheet for Calculation of Nutritional Requirements for TPN

1. Basal energy requirement (BER):
   = 70 × weight in kg$^{0.75}$ (for all patients).
   or
   = 30 × weight in kg + 70 (for patients weighing >2 kg).
   = _____ Kcal/day.
2. Illness energy requirement (IER):
   —healthy animal, cage rest = 1.25 × BER.
   —trauma or major surgery = 1.3–1.6 × BERT.
   —sepsis or major burns = 1.5–2.0 × BER.
   IER = _____ × BER = _____ Kcal/day (provide
   as nonprotein calories).
3. Protein requirement:
   = 4 gm/kg in adult dogs.
   = 6 gm/kg in dogs with extraordinary protein loss.
   = 1.5 gm/kg in dogs with renal or hepatic failure.
   Protein requirement = _____ gm/day.
4. Volumes of nutrient solutions required:
   a) 8.5% amino acid solution = 85 mg protein/ml.
      To supply _____ gm of protein, need _____ ml.
   b) 20% lipid solution = 2 Kcal/ml.
      To supply 40–60% of IER (_____ Kcal), need _____
      ml (do not use in lipemic patients).
   c) 50% dextrose solution = 1.7 Kcal/ml.
      To supply 40–60% of IER (_____ Kcal), need _____
      ml (use ½ this volume on 1st day and increase to full
      volume on 2nd day if no glucosuria).
5. Total volume of TPN solution = _____ ml.
   Administer at _____ ml/hr.
6. Electrolyte requirement:
   dependent on patient status and products selected.
7. Vitamin requirement:
   administer 0.5 mg/kg vitamin K SC on 1st day, and weekly
   add 3 ml/10 kg/day multivitamin (up to 10 ml) to TPN
   solution.

Figure 1. TPN worksheet for dogs.

scribed in the article, Enteral Nutritional Support, using the exponential formula (valid for all patients) or the linear approximation (valid only for patients weighing more than 2 kg). For dogs, the illness/injury/infection energy requirement (IER) is derived from the BER by multiplying it by "stress factors" extrapolated from human studies. For sick cats, the factor 1.4 has been used successfully for determining the IER. Certain modifications are made for the administration of nutrients by the parenteral route. It is customary in the authors' hospitals to provide dogs with nonprotein calories in meeting the calculated IER. Generally, 40 to 60 per cent of the nonprotein calories are provided as lipid, and the remainder as dextrose. Recent work in cats by one of the authors (ACL) indicates that this method results in complications associated with overfeeding. For cats, the protein calories are calculated (4 Kcal/gm of protein), and the result is subtracted from the IER. The remaining calories are provided as a 50:50 mixture of lipid and dextrose.

The amount of protein administered is decreased if renal or hepatic insufficiency or failure is present and is increased if extraordinary protein loss is occurring, as in septic peritonitis with an open abdomen. Laboratory monitoring is very important in patients given TPN; nutrient intake may be

modified, depending on the response to therapy. Specialized amino acid formulations are available for specific disease states, but they are generally more expensive than basic mixtures.

COMPONENTS OF PARENTERAL NUTRITION

The three basic components of parenteral nutrition are dextrose, amino acids, and lipids. Dextrose has traditionally been the major source of calories in TPN, but hyperglycemia and hyperosmolarity may occur if large volumes of concentrated dextrose solution are given without an adequate transition period. Some patients may require exogenous insulin. Dextrose, widely available in concentrations of 2.5 to 75 per cent, is inexpensive and compatible with most other solutions.

The protein source in TPN was originally the product of acid or enzymatic hydrolysis of casein, fibrin, or meat products and contained a heterogeneous mixture of amino acids, dipeptides and tripeptides, and larger proteins. Three to 15 per cent crystalline amino acid solutions, with or without added electrolytes, have replaced protein hydrolysates as nitrogen sources. The basic solutions available contain all essential amino acids for dogs and cats, except taurine. If TPN is administered to cats

Worksheet for Calculation of Nutritional Requirements for TPN

1. Basal energy requirement (BER):
   = 70 × weight in kg$^{0.75}$ (for all patients).
   or
   = 30 × weight in kg + 70 (for patients weighing >2 kg).
   = _____ Kcal/day.
2. Illness energy requirement (IER):
   = 1.4 × BER = _____ Kcal/day
   (provide as protein and nonprotein calories).
3. Protein requirement:
   = 6 gm/kg in adult cats.
   = 3.5 gm/kg in cats with renal or hepatic failure.
   Protein requirement = _____ gm/day.
   Protein calories = 4 Kcal/gm = _____ Kcal.
   Nonprotein calories = IER − protein calories
   = _____ Kcal.
4. Volumes of nutrient solutions required:
   a) 8.5% amino acid solution = 85 mg protein/ml.
      To supply _____ gm of protein, need _____ ml.
   b) 20% lipid solution = 2 Kcal/ml.
      To supply 50% of nonprotein calories (_____ Kcal),
      need _____ ml (do not use in lipemic patients).
   c) 50% dextrose solution = 1.7 Kcal/ml.
      To supply 50% of nonprotein calories (_____ Kcal),
      need _____ ml (use ½ this volume on 1st day and
      increase to full volume on 2nd day if no glucosuria).
5. Total volume of TPN solution = _____ ml.
   Administer at _____ ml/hr.
6. Electrolyte requirement:
   dependent on patient status and products selected.
7. Vitamin requirement:
   administer 0.5 mg/kg vitamin K SC on 1st day, and weekly
   add 3 ml/day multivitamin to TPN solution.

Figure 2. TPN worksheet for cats.

for longer than 1 week, taurine supplementation may be advisable as plasma and myocardial taurine concentrations are rapidly depleted if cats are deprived of this amino acid.

The addition of lipid emulsions to TPN remains optional. Unless pathologic hyperlipidemia exists, the authors use them routinely to provide some portion of the nonprotein calories. Lipids are an excellent concentrated energy source and supply essential fatty acids. Commercially available products contain soybean or safflower oil, egg yolk phospholipids, and glycerol in concentrations of 10 or 20 per cent. Because the emulsion is isotonic, it can be given peripherally or centrally, separately, or mixed with the other components in an "all-in-one" approach. Unlike the case with dextrose, no transition period is required for the administration of lipids; the emulsion need not be started and discontinued gradually. When lipids provide some of the nonprotein calories, hyperglycemia is less likely to occur.

Electrolytes are conveniently included in the TPN solutions by using amino acid products with added electrolytes (Travasol with Electrolytes, Clintec Nutrition Co., Deerfield, IL). The composition will be appropriate for the majority of patients, with the addition of calcium gluconate alone. Other approaches include addition of a concentrated electrolyte mixture (TPN Electrolytes [multiple electrolyte additive], Abbott Laboratories, North Chicago, IL) or use of multiple individual electrolyte solutions. The routine electrolyte concentrations for TPN solution are listed in Table 1. These will maintain normal electrolyte status in most patients not experiencing extraordinary losses.

Multivitamin additives, which provide all fat- and water-soluble vitamins with the exception of vitamin K, are usually combined with the TPN solution. Vitamin K is given subcutaneously once weekly at a dose of 0.5 mg/kg. Trace elements such as zinc, iron, copper, chromium, manganese, selenium, cobalt, and iodine are not added routinely unless the duration of TPN administration exceeds one week.

TPN generally provides water in excess of maintenance requirements, but extra crystalloids may be necessary if there are continuing losses due to vomiting, diarrhea, exudation, or diuresis. These may be added to the TPN solution or may be given separately through a peripheral catheter.

The cost of TPN components varies greatly with

Table 1. *Common Electrolyte Concentrations** *of TPN Solutions*

Sodium = 35–45 mEq/L	Chloride = 35–45 mEq/L
Potassium = 35–45 mEq/L	Phosphate = 10–15
Calcium = 4–5 mEq/L	mmole/L
	Magnesium = 4–5 mEq/L

*Concentrations are those found in the final solution given to patients.

the source from which they are obtained. The least expensive approach is to obtain them from institutions that purchase them under a state contract or buy large quantities at one time.

COMPOUNDING PARENTERAL NUTRITION

For economic reasons, the "all-in-one," or total nutrient admixture, approach to compounding has recently become popular in human medicine. It is also the simplest and most convenient method in veterinary medicine. The three basic components are pooled in a sterile container (preferably made of ethylene vinyl acetate [EVA] plastic), and additives are mixed just prior to administration. The lipid emulsion and dextrose should not be added directly to each other (i.e., mix them in the sequence: (1) dextrose, (2) amino acids, (3) lipids, or vice versa) during compounding. Always check the manufacturer's recommendations regarding solution compatibility. To prevent septic complications, asepsis must be maintained during compounding. Compounding is best performed under a laminar flow hood, but a surgical suite is a practical alternative. Compounding is facilitated by pooling bags equipped with three lead transfer sets and vented filters (All-in-One Bag, Clintec Nutrition Co., affiliated with Baxter Healthcare Corp., Deerfield, IL). Containers and injection ports should be swabbed with 70 per cent isopropyl alcohol prior to penetration with needles or transfer sets. Nothing should be vented to the outside without a bacterial filter unless a flow hood is being used. Air should not be injected into vials to facilitate withdrawal of their contents.

The initiation of a TPN program can be simplified considerably if the pharmacist at a local hospital is willing to assist and advise the novice. Sales representatives of the companies manufacturing the components may be another valuable resource (Table 2).

ADMINISTRATION OF PARENTERAL NUTRITION

The administration of TPN need not be complicated. An established protocol supervised by experienced and interested members of a Nutritional Support Service (NSS) appears to be the best approach. Only a superficial discussion of the vital topic of central venous catheter placement and care is possible here. The TPN catheter is placed using aseptic and atraumatic technique by the most experienced operator available. The authors prefer to use a percutaneously placed single-lumen polyurethane catheter (L-Cath, Luther Medical Products Inc., Santa Ana, CA). It should be changed only

Table 2. *Manufacturers of Parenteral Nutrition Products*

Clintec Nutrition Co.
Affiliated with Baxter Healthcare Corp.
Deerfield, IL 60015
Clintec Parenteral Nutrition Technical Hotline
1-800-422-ASK2
Alternate Care Services (for ordering information)
1-800-222-0488 ext. 550

Hospital Products Division
Abbott Laboratories
North Chicago, IL 60064
1-312-937-3829

Kendall McGaw Laboratories Inc.
Irvine, CA 92714
1-800-854-6851

Table 3. *Composition of a Parenteral Nutrition Solution for Short-term Peripheral Use*

100 ml 20% lipid emulsion*
200 ml 8.5% amino acids with electrolytes†
400 ml 10% dextrose
300 ml lactated Ringer's solution
20 mEq potassium chloride

Provides 337 nonprotein calories (59% as lipid) and 17 gm of protein in 1 liter of solution.
Calculated osmolality = 546 mOsm/L

Electrolyte concentrations:

Sodium = 53 mEq/L	Chloride = 67 mEq/L
Potassium = 33 mEq/L	Phosphate = 6 mmol/L
Calcium = 0.9 mEq/L	Magnesium = 2 mEq/L

*20% Intralipid, Clintec Nutrition Co., affiliated with Baxter Healthcare Corp., Deerfield, IL 60015.
†8.5% Travasol with Electrolytes, Clintec Nutrition Co., Deerfield, IL 60015.

when indicated, not at set time intervals. The catheter is "dedicated" to TPN administration, is handled only by members of the NSS, and is not used for blood sampling, medication administration, or central venous pressure (CVP) monitoring. Multilumen catheters allow multipurpose access to the central vein but increase the cost of TPN and generally must be placed by surgical cut-down. The catheter bandage and intravenous sets used for TPN administration are changed every other day.

Initiation of TPN is simplified when lipids provide a percentage of the nonprotein calories. One half of the calculated volume of dextrose is included in the TPN solution on the first day. If glucosuria is not a problem, the dextrose is increased to the full amount on the second day. If dextrose provides all the nonprotein calories, 25 per cent of the anticipated load is given initially, and the administration rate is increased stepwise based on urine and blood glucose monitoring.

Use of an intravenous infusion pump is mandatory for TPN unless supervision is continuous. The authors find that constant infusion over 24 hr is simple and convenient. If round-the-clock observation is unavailable, TPN can be administered over a 15-hr period. However, extra care must be taken to prevent hyperglycemia and hypoglycemia; there may be a heightened risk of septic complications and catheter occlusion.

PPN may be an alternative to TPN if limited enteral intake is possible, if the anticipated period of fasting is short, or if use of a central venous catheter is impossible or is considered to be too great a risk. It is difficult to provide the IER using peripheral administration, but the BER may be given if the patient is able to tolerate a large volume of solution. A parenteral nutrition solution appropriate for short-term peripheral use is described in Table 3.

Discontinuation of TPN is ideally considered when enteral intake has increased to provide greater than 50 per cent of the IER. Dilute (5 to 10 per cent) dextrose solutions may be administered for a

few hours after stopping TPN. Alternatively, the rate of the infusion may be reduced stepwise over several hours to prevent the development of hypoglycemia.

Monitoring

The intensity of monitoring required for patients receiving TPN is at a level similar to that required for any critically ill animal. Routine protocol in the authors' hospitals is described in Table 4. To this may be added other laboratory and critical care monitoring as indicated by the patient's disease and condition. Alterations in the TPN solution are often made on the basis of laboratory results or clinical response.

Complications

The most common type of complication occurring in a retrospective study of 35 animals receiving TPN was mechanical and included (1) catheter occlusion or other malfunction, (2) line disconnection or breakage, and (3) an inability to recatheterize the animal after accidental or intentional catheter removal. The best way to prevent mechanical com-

Table 4. *Monitoring during Parenteral Nutrition*

Variable	Frequency
Vital signs (attitude, hydration, body temperature, pulse, respiration, mucous membrane color, capillary refill time)	b.i.d. to q.i.d.
Urine glucose	b.i.d. to q.i.d.
Body weight	Daily
PCV/TS	Daily
Serum electrolytes	24 to 48 hr after initiating TPN
CBC, biochemical profile	1–2 times weekly

plications is by using meticulous catheter placement and maintenance technique and by closely supervising the animals receiving TPN. If the patient is likely to chew the intravenous set, adhesive tape can be applied to the line and sprayed with a bitter-tasting deterrent (Bitter Apple, Valhar Chemical Corp., Greenwich, CT).

Catheter- or solution-related sepsis is a very serious complication of TPN. If an obvious source of infection other than the catheter is present, TPN may be continued as long as the infection appears to be responding to therapy. Pyrexia or leukocytosis that cannot be ascribed to another septic process indicates the need to consider the TPN catheter. The bandage is removed, and the vein is examined for evidence of phlebitis (swelling, heat, tenderness, or exudation). If this condition is present, the catheter is removed, and the tip is collected aseptically for bacterial culture. If absent, blood may be collected through the catheter for culture and then compared with a sample collected percutaneously from a peripheral vein. An absolute indication to remove the TPN catheter exists only when the culture obtained through the catheter is positive; but in most cases, the catheter is removed once the cultures are collected. The animal usually becomes afebrile within hours after catheter removal. TPN may be resumed after the animal has been normothermic for 24 hr. Septic complications are rarely encountered when catheter placement and maintenance, and solution compounding and administration, are strictly supervised by members of an NSS. Compromise may have serious consequences; parenteral nutrition should not be administered casually!

Metabolic abnormalities are another type of complication that may be associated with TPN administration. Hyperglycemia and glucosuria are rarely a problem in dogs, except those with pancreatic disease. These conditions occur commonly in cats with any disease process. This is probably due to this species's susceptibility to stress-induced hyperglycemia. If glucosuria of greater than 500 mg/dl occurs on the first day of TPN administration, the inclusion of only half of the calculated dextrose calories is continued on the second day. If significant glucosuria persists, insulin therapy is initiated. Ten units (U) of regular insulin are added to each liter of TPN solution. This amount is adjusted according to the result of blood and urine glucose monitoring. If more than 60 U of insulin/L are required to control hyperglycemia, provision of fewer calories as dextrose and more as lipid should be considered. Alternatively, regular insulin may be given subcutaneously as needed. Although not recommended, abrupt discontinuation of the TPN infusion rarely results in clinical signs of hypoglycemia unless exogenous insulin is being given.

Electrolyte abnormalities may be encountered during TPN administration but are generally mild and easily corrected by adjusting the electrolyte composition of the solution. Hypokalemia develops most commonly, since glucose and insulin accelerate intracellular movement of potassium. When administering high concentrations of potassium intravenously, the rate should not exceed 0.5 mEq/kg/hr.

Mild elevations in serum urea nitrogen (SUN) concentration may be seen occasionally after the initiation of TPN. The azotemia is probably prerenal in origin and is often related to the amount of protein being administered. If hypovolemia is not present and if the creatinine is within normal limits, the calculated protein requirement is reduced by 1 gm/kg/day; the SUN concentration should be reassessed in 24 hr. In patients with renal compromise prior to the initiation of TPN, an increase in SUN associated with stable or decreasing serum creatinine concentrations is an indication to decrease the calculated protein requirement by 0.5 gm/kg/day. This patient will already have been receiving restricted protein TPN (Figs. 1 and 2). Further research may result in a revision of the recommendations regarding protein requirements for dogs and cats receiving TPN.

Moderate lipemia is common for one to two days after initiating TPN. However, if the serum triglyceride concentration exceeds 300 mg/dl after three days, the calories provided by lipid should be decreased and replaced by dextrose calories. If lipemia is severe or is accompanied by clinical signs, supply all nonprotein calories as dextrose.

SUMMARY

Parenteral nutrition is not heroic, fraught with complications, or outrageously expensive. TPN can be of considerable benefit to selected patients in need of nutritional support because they are temporarily unable to assimilate enterally administered nutrients. The use of TPN in veterinary medicine will grow as critical and intensive care units proliferate and as owners demand increasingly sophisticated therapy for their pets.

References and Supplemental Reading

Adamkin, D. H., Gelke, K. N., and Andrews, B. F.: Fat emulsions and hypertriglyceridemia. J.P.E.N. 8:563, 1984.
ASPEN Board of Directors: Guidelines for the use of total parenteral nutrition in the hospitalized adult patient. J.P.E.N. 10:441, 1986.
Brown, R., Quercia, R., and Sigman, R.: Total nutrient admixture: A review. J.P.E.N. 10:650, 1986.
Caprile, K. A., and Spears, K. E.: Long-term, cyclic total parenteral nutrition in the growing canine. Proceedings of the American College of Veterinary Internal Medicine, San Diego, CA, 1987, p. 906.
Cerra, F. B.: Pocket Manual of Surgical Nutrition. St. Louis: C.V. Mosby Co., 1984.

Krey, S. H., and Murray, R. L. (eds.): *Dynamics of Nutritional Support.* Norwalk, CT: Appleton-Century-Crofts, 1986.

Lewis, L. D., Morris, M. L., and Hand, M. S.: *Small Animal Clinical Nutrition,* 3rd ed. Topeka, KS: Mark Morris Associates, 1987.

Lippert, A. C.: Total parenteral nutrition in dogs and cats. Proceedings of the American College Veterinary Internal Medicine, San Diego, CA, 1987, p. 905.

Murphy, L. M., and Lipman, T. O.: Central venous catheter care in parenteral nutrition. J.P.E.N. 11:190, 1987.

Raffe, M. R.: Total parenteral nutrition. *In* Slatter, D. H. (ed.): *Textbook of Small Animal Surgery,* Vol I. Philadelphia: W.B. Saunders Co., 1985, pp. 225–241.

Rombeau, J. L., and Caldwell, M. D. (eds.): *Parenteral Nutrition.* Philadelphia: W.B. Saunders Co., 1986.

ENTERAL NUTRITIONAL SUPPORT

STEVEN L. WHEELER, D.V.M.,
and BARBARA H. McGUIRE, D.V.M.

Fort Collins, Colorado

Despite significant advances in veterinary medical and surgical care during the last decade, nutritional support of ill and injured animals remains virtually unchanged. Protein and caloric malnutrition (PCM), defined as inadequate intake of protein and energy resulting in negative energy and protein balance, is a significant problem in hospitalized human patients, with a reported incidence as high as 50 per cent. The adverse effects of PCM in humans include anemia, hypoproteinemia, delayed wound healing, compromised immunity, increased susceptibility to infections, and compromised cardiovascular, pulmonary, and gastrointestinal function. The end result is an increase in morbidity and mortality in patients with PCM. Since inadequate nutritional intake is also a problem in hospitalized dogs and cats, PCM is often a significant problem in veterinary hospitals. With appropriate nutritional support via enteral or parenteral routes, the detrimental effects of PCM in hospitalized dogs and cats can be minimized. Enteral nutrition is defined as the provision of liquid formula diets by tube (tube feeding) or mouth into the gastrointestinal tract. In parenteral nutrition, nutrients are provided by means other than the gastrointestinal tract, usually via catheters, directly into a central or a peripheral vein. This review focuses on enteral nutritional support, a practical, cost-effective, physiologic method of safely providing nutritional support to ill or traumatized dogs and cats.

PATHOPHYSIOLOGY OF FASTING

In order to utilize enteral nutritional support, it is necessary first to understand the consequences of inadequate nutrient intake in both normal animals and those suffering from the stresses of illness, trauma, or burns. Fasting in a healthy animal results in decreased glucose, amino acid, and fatty acid concentrations in the portal blood. In response, there are increases in insulin and counter-regulatory hormones (glucagon, cortisol, growth hormone, and catecholamines). A decrease in the ratio of insulin to counter-regulatory hormone results in accelerated hepatic glycogenolysis and gluconeogenesis in order to maintain normal blood glucose concentrations. Maintenance of a normal blood glucose concentration is essential, because red blood cells, white blood cells, the renal medulla, and the central nervous system during the initial 7 to 10 days of fasting absolutely require glucose as an energy substrate. Other body tissues can rapidly adapt to utilization of fatty acids and fatty acid metabolites (ketone bodies) for energy. After only a few days of fasting, hepatic glycogen stores are depleted; only gluconeogenesis maintains blood glucose concentration in the normal range. Since fatty acids cannot serve as substrates for gluconeogenesis, amino acids become the primary gluconeogenic precursor. The carbon chains of amino acids are used for gluconeogenesis, forming ammonia, which is then converted to urea and is excreted by the kidneys. Thus, in starvation, body protein is catabolized to provide glucose, resulting in a negative nitrogen balance. Since there is no storage form of protein in the body and all protein is associated with function, loss of protein results in loss of function. In the absence of illness or injury (nonstressed starvation), there is decreased energy expenditure as a result of loss of cells, decreased metabolic rate of the remaining cells, and decreased physical activity. This adaptive decrease in energy expenditure results in conservation of proteins. Also, after about 1 week of starvation, the central nervous system is able to utilize ketone bodies for energy instead of glucose.

This beneficial adaptation results in decreased glucose requirements and further conserves functional protein. Without these adaptive responses, only brief periods of starvation could be tolerated. By day 10 of fasting, 30 to 50 per cent of total body nitrogen would be depleted, and death would occur.

When starvation is accompanied by illness or injury (stressed starvation), the metabolic consequences are more devastating than those of nonstressed starvation. The stressed patient displays an increase in metabolic rate and a marked negative nitrogen balance rather than the decrease in metabolic rate and the protein sparing associated with nonstressed starvation. Additionally, injured body tissue preferentially utilizes glucose rather than fatty acids or ketone bodies as an energy substrate. The increases in energy expenditure and the negative nitrogen balance are proportional to the degree of injury. Thus, protein catabolism is accelerated in the stressed anorectic animal, compared with that in the nonstressed animal. Loss of functional protein, in turn, results in a significant compromise of organ function. Decreases in cardiac muscle mass and cardiac function have been demonstrated in starving humans and rodents. Decreases in pulmonary function (as evidencd by a decreased hypoxic ventilatory response) have been reported in malnourished humans. In the gastrointestinal tract, there is loss of mucosal integrity, resulting in increased translocation of bacteria and endotoxin from the gastrointestinal tract into the portal circulation. This mechanism accounts for the septic complications observed in many critically ill hospitalized patients. Additionally, villous blunting and decreased disaccharidase activity occur in the gastrointestinal tracts of experimental rodents and humans undergoing stressed starvation. Finally, stressed starvation results in compromise of nonspecific, cellular, and humoral immunity, contributing to an increased incidence of septic complications in both rodents and humans. Nutritional support can prevent PCM and the resulting compromise in organ function. Once an animal develops PCM, nutritional support can be used to re-establish positive protein and energy balances and to reverse the compromises that occur in organ function.

INDICATIONS FOR NUTRITIONAL SUPPORT

Not all hospitalized dogs and cats require nutritional support. However, in order to prevent the morbidity and mortality associated with PCM, it is essential that patients requiring nutritional support be recognized early during their hospital stay, so that appropriate nutritional support may be administered. It is unfortunate that no single clinical sign or laboratory test exists to identify animals that require nutritional support. The clinician must carefully examine the data obtained from the history,

physical examination, and appropriate laboratory tests to recognize when nutritional support is indicated. Mature dogs or cats that have a history of insignificant nutrient intake for 5 days or that have lost more than 10 per cent of lean body weight in a relatively short period (1 to 2 weeks) are candidates for nutritional support. Since neonates have increased nutritional requirements and decreased hepatic stores of glycogen, nutritional support should be instituted in these patients after 1 to 2 days of anorexia or when lean body weight loss exceeds 5 per cent. Nutritional support should also be given to animals with conditions that result in direct protein and energy losses, such as malabsorption states, protein-losing nephropathies, peritonitis or pleuritis with effective drainage, and large wounds or burns. Animals with diseases and those receiving treatments (surgery, chemotherapy, and radiation therapy) that prevent oral feedings for longer than 3 to 5 days should receive nutritional support. Lack of body fat, muscle wasting, poor haircoat, pressure sores, and general debilitation are signs that indicate the need for nutritional support. Unfortunately, pre-existing obesity may make it very difficult to recognize PCM in overweight dogs and cats. Nutritional support should not be withheld from these animals, since PCM and the accompanying increase in morbidity and mortality will occur just as quickly in obese as nonobese patients. Hypoalbuminemia, lymphopenia, and anemia may be detected in animals with PCM. However, the changes associated with these conditions are insensitive measures of nitrogen and energy balance, since they cannot be detected until severe PCM has occurred.

Anorectic dogs and cats that are capable of eating but simply refuse to do so should be tempted to eat prior to initiating nutritional support (see the preceding article, Cause and Control of Decreased Appetite). In human patients, the preferred route of nutritional support is the gastrointestinal tract if nutrients can be administered safely and effectively by this means. Compared with parenteral nutrition, enteral nutrition is associated with fewer complications and is more physiologic, less expensive, and technically easier to accomplish. In both humans and rodents, enteral nutritional support is more effective than parenteral nutritional support in preventing compromised gastrointestinal function and septic complications resulting from this compromise. For these reasons, "If the gut works, use it." It is unfortunate that there are situations in which enteral nutritional support should not be used or is of limited value. For example, it is recommended that the enteral route not be used in human patients with complete mechanical intestinal obstruction unless nutrients may be administered distal to the site of obstruction and there is a significant length of nonobstructed intestine for adequate absorption. Since human patients with ileus or intestinal hypomotility tolerate enteral nutrition poorly and are at increased risk for aspiration and infectious enteritis, the enteral route should not be used in veterinary patients with this disorder. Patients with severe diarrhea are also difficult to treat by the enteral route. Animals with acute pancreatitis requiring nutritional support should receive parenteral rather than enteral nutrition, if possible. In these cases, nutrients administered by the enteral route will stimulate pancreatic exocrine secretion and will exacerbate the pancreatitis. Finally, patients with hypovolemic or septic shock should not receive either enteral or parenteral nutrition until hemodynamic stability is restored. When the enteral route cannot be used in dogs and cats that require nutritional support, they should receive parenteral nutritional support (see the preceding article, Parenteral Nutritional Support). However, even when the parenteral route will be used primarily, supplemental enteral feeding can also be considered, since enteral nutrition is superior to parenteral nutrition in maintaining the integrity of the gastrointestinal epithelial barrier to bacteria and endotoxin.

In addition to nutritional therapy, it is essential that appropriate medical and surgical therapies be instituted. Even though nutritional therapy reduces morbidity and mortality rates, a poor outcome is probable if other aspects of case management are ignored.

ROUTES OF ENTERAL FEEDING

Enteral nutritional support can be achieved by the oral, orogastric, nasogastric, or pharyngostomy route or via gastrostomy or jejunostomy. Forced oral feeding may be used for very short-term (1 to 2 days) support but is usually not well-tolerated. Repeated orogastric intubation may also be performed, but it is time consuming and stressful to the patient, may induce vomiting if large quantities are given at a single feeding, and entails the risk of endotracheal intubation leading to aspiration pneumonia. Since forced oral feeding and orogastric tube feeding are stressful to the patient, these methods should not be used for critically ill patients. Pharyngostomy tubes may be used but require anesthesia and are associated with hemorrhage, infection, and airway aspiration. Because of these disadvantages, the authors do not recommend the use of pharyngostomy tubes.

The authors most commonly use nasogastric, gastrostomy, and jejunostomy tubes for enteral nutritional support. Tube selection, contraindications for use, placement, management, and potential complications will be briefly discussed, but the reader is referred to other works (Crowe, 1986; Lewis et al., 1987; Orton, 1986) for more extensive discussions of these techniques.

Nasogastric Tubes

Nasogastric tubes are ideal for the short-term (less than 7 days) nutritional support of small animal patients. However, this route should not be used if the animal is vomiting, has gastric paresis (commonly occurs following gastric surgery), has gastric outlet obstruction, or is stuporous or comatose and therefore at risk for aspiration. When a patient has esophageal dilation, this method of enteral support is a poor choice because it is extremely difficult to pass nasogastric tubes into the stomach.

A wide variety of nasogastric tubes are available. Polyurethane (Silk Bullet Tip —Nonweighted, with stylet, Corpak, Inc., Wheeling, IL) is preferred over polyvinyl chloride (Infant Feeding Tube, Argyle, St. Louis, MO) for nasogastric tubes because it is less irritating to the nasal mucous membranes and is therefore better tolerated by the animal. In cats and smaller dogs (less than 5 to 7 kg), a tube no larger than a no. 6 French should be used; in larger dogs, a no. 8 French tube is usually well-tolerated. Especially in larger dogs, it is much easier to pass nasogastric tubes equipped with stylets to increase their stiffness.

Prior to passing the tube, local anesthesia is induced by holding the dog's or the cat's head upward and instilling 0.5 to 1.0 ml of 2 per cent lidocaine into the nostril of the dog, or 0.5 ml of 2 per cent mepivacaine into the nostril of the cat. In most dogs, sedation is not required; if needed, 1 mg/kg of diazepam, up to a maximum of 20 mg, may be given intravenously. Unless the cat is severely debilitated, ketamine, at a dose of 2 mg/kg, should be given to cats to facilitate tube passage.

In dogs, the distance from the external nares to the thirteenth rib is measured, so that intragastric intubation may be accomplished. In cats, vomiting is a more frequent complication with intragastric tube placement than with tube placement into the distal esophagus. For this reason, the distance from the nares to the ninth rib is measured in cats to ensure esophageal placement.

The end of the tube should be lubricated with water-soluble jelly to facilitate passage. In dogs, the tube is initially passed in a dorsal direction, to allow passage over a small ventral ridge and into the nasal vestibule. At this point, the tube should be passed in a ventromedial direction and into the ventral meatus. Because there is no ventral ridge in cats, the tube should be directed in a ventromedial direction at the start of tube placement. If resistance to passage of the tube is encountered after passage to the level of the eyes, the tube is likely to be located in the dorsal meatus and to be coming into contact with the ethmoid turbinate. If this problem occurs, the tube should be withdrawn and reinserted. Once the tube reaches the nasopharynx, the animal's head should be held in a neutral position (avoid extreme flexion or extension) to facilitate passage of the tube into the esophagus rather than the trachea. After passing the tube for the previously measured distance, the stylet is withdrawn. To check placement of the tube, inject 5 to 10 ml of air while auscultating over the cranial abdominal region for gurgling sounds. If there is any question about the location of the tube, a radiograph should be taken to ensure that it has not been placed into an airway. In humans, nasopulmonary intubation occurs most commonly in debilitated or neurologically impaired patients who cannot swallow. Nasopulmonary intubation has also been described in human patients despite the presence of a cuffed endotracheal tube or tracheostomy tube.

After proper placement has been determined, the tube should be secured. In cats, the tube should be passed dorsally over the bridge of the nose and secured onto the frontal region of the head by attaching the tube to the head with a permanent adhesive (Superglue, Loctite Corp., Cleveland, OH). It is also necessary to secure the tube with a single suture on the bridge of the nose, as close to the nares as possible. Because contact between the tube and the whiskers is poorly tolerated in cats, it should be avoided. In dogs, use a permanent adhesive to secure the tube to the side of the face that is ipsilateral to the intubated nostril. Again, a single suture should be placed to secure the tube as close to the nares as possible along with gluing the tube to the hair on the side of the animal's face. To prevent the animal from dislodging the tube, an Elizabethan collar should be used. Minor complications associated with nasogastric tubes include vomiting, rhinitis, and gastroesophageal reflux. Major complications include aspiration pneumonia, either due to nasopulmonary intubation or secondary to vomiting, and pneumothorax secondary to nasopleural intubation.

Gastrostomy Tubes

For nutritional support of a greater duration (longer than 7 days), gastrostomy and jejunostomy tubes are preferred. Gastrostomy tubes are usually well-tolerated, but they should not be used in animals with uncontrolled vomiting, gastric paresis, or gastric outflow obstruction. Since animals with esophageal dilation may have an incompetent lower esophageal sphincter, allowing regurgitation of gastric contents, gastrostomy tubes should not be used. If a gastrostomy tube is used in an animal with esophageal disease, the animal should be kept in a sitting position for at least 30 minutes following each feeding period to help prevent regurgitation.

SURGICAL PLACEMENT

Gastrostomy tubes may be placed surgically or with endoscopic guidance. For surgical placement

of gastrostomy tubes, balloon-tipped urethral catheters (Foley Catheter, Bardex, Murray Hill, NJ) are used. In dogs weighing less than 5 to 7 kg and in cats, nos. 18 to 24 French catheters should be used; in larger animals, nos. 26 to 30 French tubes are appropriate. For all tube diameters, a 5-ml rather than a 30-ml balloon should be used. Following general anesthesia, the left paracostal area is shaved and is prepared for surgery. A 2- to 3-cm incision is made through the skin and subcutaneous tissue, just behind and parallel to the last rib. The dorsal limit of the incision should be just below the ventral edge of the paravertebral epaxial musculature. A bluntly dissected grid incision is placed through the external and internal oblique and transverse muscles of the abdominal wall. In order to facilitate location of the stomach, a stomach tube is passed by an assistant. Inflation of the stomach with 10 to 15 ml of air/kg will allow it to be easily located through the small grid incision. Once the stomach is located, temporary traction stay sutures are placed in its seromuscular layers, at the 12 o'clock and 6 o'clock positions. Two concentric full-thickness purse-string sutures of 2-0 nylon are then sewn through all layers of the gastric wall. The feeding tube is prepared by cutting off the tip and checking the patency of the balloon. Once the tube has been prepared, a small stab incision is made into the center of the purse-string sutures, and the tube is placed into the stomach through this incision. After inflating the balloon with 5 ml of water, the innermost purse-string suture is tightened and tied. Next, tie the outermost purse-string suture while inverting the stomach in the region adjacent to the tube. To close the incision around the tube, the free ends of one of the purse-string sutures are used to close the muscle layers, while the subcutaneous tissues are closed with the free ends of the other purse-string suture. The skin is closed in the routine manner, and the tube is secured to the skin with sutures. An abdominal wrap is placed on the animal to further secure the feeding tube. Dogs with gastrostomy tubes should wear an Elizabethan collar to prevent chewing of the gastrostomy tube. Elizabethan collars are not required for cats.

Complications seen with surgically placed tubes include pyloric obstruction, peritonitis, and cellulitis. Pyloric obstruction is more common if 30-ml balloon catheters are used. Peritonitis can result from rupture of the balloon and extravasation of gastric contents into the peritoneal space. However, if the stomach is secured to the abdominal wall, only localized peritonitis is likely to result. After 7 to 10 days, the feeding-tube balloon may spontaneously rupture. By this time, the stomach should be adhered to the body wall, so that a new balloon-tipped tube may be passed percutaneously into the stomach.

To remove the tube, simply deflate the bulb, and

apply traction on the tube. The gastrocutaneous fistula that is formed after gastrostomy tube removal will spontaneously heal in 3 to 7 days.

PERCUTANEOUS PLACEMENT

For percutaneous placement of gastrostomy tubes, with the aid of endoscopy, specialized tubes (Dubhoff PEG, Biosearch, Somerville, NJ) designed for use in humans are preferred. One end of the tube is tapered; there is a disk-shaped bumper on the opposite end. A no. 20 French is the largest diameter available, but this size can be used for all animals. Included with the tube are all other materials necessary for placing and securing the tube, including a polyvinylchloride catheter, traction wire, and retaining ring.

First, the endoscope is passed into the stomach, and the stomach is distended with air, so that the gastric wall comes into contact with the body wall. Then, an assistant firmly presses in on the abdomen with one finger, in the area caudal to the last rib. The endoscopist visualizes the depression in the fundus of the stomach. After making a 1-cm skin incision, the assistant passes an over-the-needle polyvinylchloride catheter percutaneously into the gastric lumen. After removing the stylet, the traction wire is passed through the catheter and into the stomach. Using a biopsy snare, the endoscopist grasps the free end of the wire, and the endoscope and biopsy snare are withdrawn, bringing the wire out through the animal's mouth. The tapered end of the tube is attached to the wire, as described in the instructions provided by the manufacturer. Then, the assistant pulls the other end of the line back through the incision, so that the tapered end of the tube enters the stomach and begins to exit through the skin incision. The assistant pulls the tube through the abdominal wall so that the disk-shaped phalange is adjacent to the gastric wall. The assistant slides the retainer ring over the tube, so that it is adjacent to the body wall. To prevent inadvertent slippage, use a permanent adhesive to glue the retainer ring to the feeding tube. Then, cut the tube so that there is about 20 cm of free tube extending from the body wall; place a cap on the free end of the tube. Next, the tube is secured to the animal with an abdominal wrap. After 7 days, the gastric wall will be adhered to the body wall, and the tube can be safely removed by transecting the tube flush with the skin and endoscopically retrieving the disk-shaped end of the tube from the gastric lumen.

Complications associated with percutaneous endoscopic gastrostomy tubes include peritonitis, cellulitis, and pressure necrosis adjacent to the tube. The advantages of percutaneous as compared with surgically placed gastrostomy tubes are ease and speed of placement and less tissue trauma. The disadvantages of percutaneous tubes are that an endoscope is required for tube placement and removal of the disk-shaped end of the tube. Unless there is another reason to perform a laparotomy, percutaneous tubes are preferred over surgically placed tubes.

Needle Catheter Jejunostomy

Needle catheter jejunostomy can be used in the vomiting patient who will not tolerate nasogastric intubation or gastrostomy. It is indicated in the nutritional support of patients undergoing surgery of the proximal gastrointestinal tract. The only requirement for the use of jejunostomies is a functional intestinal tract. A no. 5 French polyvinyl infant nasogastric feeding tube (Infant Feeding Tube, Argyle) is preferred for this procedure. A loop of the distal portion of the duodenum or proximal portion of the jejunum may be utilized. If bowel surgery is performed, the tube should be placed distal to the surgical site. Next, a purse-string suture of 3-0 polyglactin 910 is placed in the antimesenteric border of the isolated loop of bowel. With the bevel up, a 12-gauge needle is advanced 1 to 2 cm subserosally before being directed through the mucosa into the bowel lumen. The catheter is introduced into the bowel lumen through the hypodermic needle and is advanced 20 to 30 cm aborally from the enterostomy site. The needle is removed, and the purse-string suture is tightened and tied. Using a second hypodermic needle, the catheter is exteriorized through the abdominal wall. The enterostomy site is fixed to the abdominal wall, using four interrupted 3-0 polyglactin sutures. The catheter is secured to the skin with sutures and is incorporated into an abdominal bandage. When enteral feeding is completed, the external sutures are cut, and the catheter is slowly withdrawn. Complications of jejunostomy feeding include abdominal cramping, diarrhea, and peritonitis. See Figure 1 for a summary of selection of routes of nutritional support.

NUTRITIONAL REQUIREMENTS

The goal of enteral nutrition is to provide caloric, protein, electrolyte, vitamin, and mineral requirements for the animal. Basal energy requirement (BER) is the energy utilized by an animal in the postabsorptive state, at rest, with a neutral ambient temperature. Maintenance energy expenditure (MEE) equals BER plus energy expenditure to support physical activity, nutrient digestion and absorption, and temperature homeostasis. In the normal animal, MEE is about two times BER.

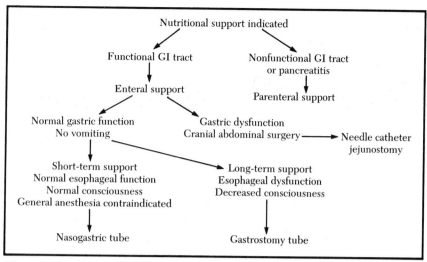

Figure 1. Flow diagram for choosing the route of nutritional support in small animal patients.

Smaller animals have a larger surface-area-to-body-weight ratio and, therefore, have larger heat losses by radiation and convection. Consequently, they have a higher energy requirement on a per kilogram basis. Kleiber's formula estimates BER to be:

$$BER\ (Kcal) = 70 \times body\ wt.\ (kg)^{0.75}$$

For animals weighing more than 2 kg, BER may be estimated by using the following formula:

$$BER\ (Kcal) = 30 \times body\ wt.\ (kg) + 70$$

Until indirect calorimetry studies are performed to accurately measure the energy requirements of ill and injured animals, energy requirements can only be estimated. Currently, guidelines established for humans are used to estimate energy requirements for animals. The MEE for mature hospitalized dogs and cats is equal to about 1.25 times their BER. Major surgery or trauma is thought to increase energy requirements by 30 to 60 per cent over BER, depending on the severity of the insult. Severe infections, sepsis, and burns can increase nutritional requirements by 50 to 100 per cent over BER. To determine the amount of nutrients to feed the patient, first calculate BER, then calculate MEE, using the aforementioned stress factors, and then divide MEE by caloric density to arrive at the diet dosage.

Until nitrogen balance studies are performed on ill and injured animals, exact protein requirements remain unknown. Currently, it is recommended that dogs receive 5.0 to 7.5 gm of protein per 100 Kcal of calculated energy needs. For cats, 6.0 to 9.0 gm of protein per 100 Kcal of calculated energy need is recommended. In dogs with severe renal or hepatic insufficiency or failure, protein should not exceed 3.0 gm per 100 Kcal; in similarly affected cats, protein should not exceed 4.0 gm per 100 Kcal. See Table 1 for a summary of calculation of nutritional requirements.

It is not necessary to supplement enteral diets with vitamin, mineral, or electrolyte supplements when using the enteral feeding products described in the following section.

ENTERAL FEEDING PRODUCTS AND FEEDING METHODS

The choice of what product to feed enterally depends largely on the type of enteral access util-

Table 1. *Calculation of Nutritional Requirements*

1. Calculation of basal energy requirement (BER):
   Body weight < 2 kg: $BER(Kcal) = 70 \times BW_{kg}^{0.75}$
   Body weight > 2 kg: $BER(Kcal) = 30 \times BW_{kg} + 70$
2. Multiply BER by stress factor to determine maintenance energy expenditure (MEE):
   Hospitalized animals: BER × 1.25
   Major surgery or trauma: BER × 1.3 to 1.6
   Severe infection, sepsis, or   BER × 1.5 to 2.0
   burns:
3. Divide MEE by caloric density of diet (Tables 2 and 3) to calculate amount of food to feed:
   MEE/caloric density = amount of food to be fed
4. Calculate protein requirements:
   Dogs: 5.0 to 7.5 gm protein/100 Kcal MEE
   Cats: 6.0 to 9.0 gm protein/100 Kcal MEE
   With severe renal or hepatic failure
   Dogs: <3.0 gm protein/100 Kcal MEE
   Cats: <4.0 gm protein/100 Kcal MEE
5. Calculate gm of protein fed (Tables 2 and 3):
   ml or oz of food × protein content = gm of protein fed
6. Calculate gm of protein to be supplied as a protein supplement (Table 3):
   gm of protein supplemented = gm of protein required − gm of protein fed
7. Calculate amount of ProMod protein supplement to be fed:
   gm of ProMod = gm of protein supplemented × 1.3
   (one 6.6 gm scoop of ProMod provides 5 gm of protein)

Table 2. Nutritional Content of Canned Pet Foods for Enteral Feeding

Product	Manufacturer	Kcal/oz	Protein (gm/oz)
p/d (canine)	Hill's	42.1	2.7
i/d (canine)	Hill's	36.8	2.2
k/d (canine)	Hill's	38.9	1.2
h/d (canine)	Hill's	41.1	1.4
c/d (feline)	Hill's	40.3	3.6
p/d (feline)	Hill's	45.0	4.5
k/d (feline)	Hill's	45.3	2.4

ized. Gruels of dog or cat foods put through a blender are used with large-bore gastrostomy tubes. Feeding should be delayed for 24 hr after placing a gastrostomy tube, to allow gastric motility to return and to allow formation of a fibrin seal. Usually, bolus feedings are given four to six times daily. After each feeding, the tube should be flushed with 20 ml of lukewarm water to prevent occlusion of the tube. On the first day of feeding, only one fourth of the animal's caloric requirements should be administered. This amount should be increased gradually so that the animal's entire caloric requirements are met by the third day following initiation of feeding. See Table 2 for the caloric and protein content of various canned dog and cat foods. For nasogastric and jejunostomy feeding, human enteral nutrition products should be used.

Either continuous or bolus feeding may be used with nasogastric feeding. However, continuous feeding is preferred over bolus feeding because vomiting occurs less frequently with continuous feeding. If continuous feeding is employed, it should be interrupted every 6 to 8 hr, and suction should be applied to the nasogastric tube to determine residual volume. In dogs, if the residual volume is greater than twice the volume infused in 1 hr, feeding should be discontinued for 2 hr, and the rate of infusion decreased by 25 per cent to prevent vomiting. If vomiting or excessive residual volumes remain a problem, a constant infusion of metoclopramide, given at a dose of 1 to 2 mg/kg/24 hr, may be used to stimulate gastric emptying and to prevent vomiting. Following an episode of vomiting, proper placement of the nasogastric tube should be ensured before feeding is resumed. In cats, if the residual volume is greater than 50 per cent of the hourly infused volume, the same guidelines should be followed. To prevent occlusion,

nasogastric tubes should be flushed with 5 ml of lukewarm tapwater after each feeding, or every 6 to 8 hr if continuous feeding is used. If peristalsis is present following jejunostomy tube placement, feeding can usually be started within 6 hr. Bolus feeding should never be used with jejunostomy feeding, since it results in abdominal cramping and diarrhea. Jejunostomy tubes should be flushed with 5 ml of lukewarm water every 6 hr to prevent occlusion.

The nutritional content of human nutrition products for enteral feeding is summarized in Table 3. Osmolite HN (Ross) is the product the authors prefer to administer through small-bore (nasogastric and jejunostomy) feeding tubes. The authors have also used Ensure (Ross) and Ensure Plus (Ross). Both are available at supermarkets and drugstores. To increase the protein content of these products, ProMod Protein Supplement (Ross) should be added to the feeding formula selected. ProMod (Ross) provides 5 gm of protein for every 6.6-gm scoop supplemented. Osmolite and Osmolite HN have the advantage of being isosmotic; they are well-tolerated when fed in an undiluted form. Enteral feeding products of high osmolality are poorly tolerated if initially fed undiluted to animals (Table 3). If hyperosmolar solutions are used, they should be diluted so that the osmolality of the final product is between 200 and 350 mOsm/kg. On the first day of supplementation, only one fourth of the animal's caloric requirements should be administered. Over the next 2 to 3 days, the volume and strength should be gradually increased so that the animal's entire nutritional requirements are satisfied using a full-strength solution. If vomiting, diarrhea, or cramping develops, the concentration of the infused product and the volume infused should be decreased to previously tolerated levels. Diarrhea may be controlled in some patients by using an enteral product containing fiber (Enrich, Ross). To prevent bacterial contamination, enteral formulations should be reformulated every 24 hr.

PATIENT MONITORING

Body weight, packed cell volume (PCV), total protein, and blood glucose should be monitored daily. Urine should be tested daily for glucosuria.

Table 3. Nutritional Content of Human Enteral Feeding Products

Product	Manufacturer	Kcal/ml	Protein (gm/ml)	Osmolality (mOsm/kg)
Ensure	Ross	1.06	0.037	470
Osmolite	Ross	1.06	0.037	300
Ensure HN	Ross	1.4	0.059	470
Osmolite HN	Ross	1.06	0.059	300
Ensure Plus	Ross	1.5	0.055	690
Enrich	Ross	1.53	0.055	480

Critically ill animals may initially develop carbohydrate intolerance as a result of concentrations of counter-regulatory hormones. If hyperglycemia or glucosuria are seen, the amount of calories fed should be decreased. Also, serum electrolytes should initially be monitored every 3 to 4 days, and then every 7 days if the patient is stable.

References and Supplemental Reading

ASPEN Board of Directors: Guidelines for the use of enteral nutrition in the adult patient. J.P.E.N. 11:435, 1987.

Crowe, D. T., Jr.: Enteral nutrition for critically ill or injured patients—Part I. Comp. Cont. Ed. 8:603, 1986.
Crowe, D. T., Jr.: Enteral nutrition for critically ill or injured patients—Part II. Comp. Cont. Ed. 8:719, 1986.
Crowe, D. T., Jr.: Enteral nutrition for critically ill or injured patients—Part III. Comp. Cont. Ed. 8:826, 1986.
Lewis, L. D., Morris, M. L., and Hand, M. S.: Small Animal Clinical Nutrition III. Topeka, KS: Mark Morris Associates, 1987.
Orton, E. C.: Enteral hyperalimentation administered via needle catheter jejunostomy as an adjuvant to cranial abdominal surgery in dogs and cats. J. Am. Vet. Med. Assoc. 188:1406, 1986.
Rombeau, J. L., and Caldwell, M. D. (eds.): Enteral and Tube Feeding. Philadelphia: W.B. Saunders Co., 1984.

MAINTENANCE FLUID THERAPY

FORD WATSON BELL, D.V.M.,
and CARL A. OSBORNE, D.V.M.
St. Paul, Minnesota

Parenteral fluid therapy is an established therapeutic modality in small animal practice. Often, attention is focused on the acute patient, whose fluid needs may be immediate and dramatic. Concerns about fluid type, rate, replacement volume, and maintenance requirements for such patients are usually given careful consideration. Patients in a more chronic state of fluid imbalance—those receiving maintenance fluid therapy—may be subjected to less careful scrutiny and monitoring. However, the same concerns are equally critical in formulation of maintenance fluid therapy. "Maintenance" implies a static state. However, maintenance fluid therapy is a dynamic state that, like all other therapies, must be planned, implemented, and monitored with care, if the patient is to consistently benefit.

BASIC CONCEPTS

The physiology of normal body fluid balance has been reviewed extensively (Muir and DiBartola, 1983; Haskins, 1984; Raffe 1985). Water represents 60 to 70 per cent of total body weight in the adult animal. Total body water (TBW) is divided into intracellular fluid (ICF) and extracellular fluid (ECF) compartments. ICF and ECF each constitute about 50 per cent of TBW. ECF is subdivided into plasma and interstitial fluid volumes. Plasma volume represents about 5 per cent of body weight, while interstitial fluid volume makes up 25 to 30 per cent of body weight.

Water distributed between the intravascular and extravascular spaces is maintained in equilibrium by a combination of factors generating osmotic and hydrostatic pressure gradients. Plasma proteins create oncotic pressure, which attracts fluid into the vascular space; hydrostatic pressure generated by the heart opposes intravascular fluid movement.

Intracellular fluid volume is maintained primarily by osmotic forces generated by the intracellular cations, potassium and magnesium. The principal extracellular ions are sodium, chloride, and bicarbonate. Sodium is maintained extracellularly by the sodium-potassium ATPase pump. Variations in extracellular sodium concentration have marked effects on transcellular fluid movement. Hyponatremia and resultant hypo-osmolality cause intracellular movement of water and cellular swelling. By the opposite mechanism, hypernatremia results in a net extracellular movement of water, with consequent cellular dehydration (Haskins, 1984; Raffe, 1985).

The kidneys are responsible for regulation of extracellular water balance and osmotic pressure. Minimal increases in plasma osmolality stimulate pituitary antidiuretic hormone (ADH) release, which, in turn, causes increased water permeability of collecting tubule segments. The result is greatly enhanced water reabsorption in excess of solute. ADH release is also mediated by hypovolemia and by a number of other nonosmotic factors including stress, cranial trauma, hyperthermia, and a variety of drugs.

Whereas osmoregulation is maintained by changes in water balance, primarily mediated by ADH release, volume regulation is the province of volume receptors located in the cardiopulmonary circulation, carotid sinuses, aortic arch, and kidneys. Decreases in volume sensed by the receptors activate effector mechanisms, principally the renin-angiotensin system (RAS). Activation of the RAS causes aldosterone release, leading to renal conservation of sodium and increased renal excretion of potassium. Increased sympathetic tone in response to volume depletion also has a direct effect on compensatory renal sodium reabsorption (Rose, 1984; Raffe, 1985).

Routes of water loss in the healthy animal include sensible and insensible components. Sensible losses consist of urinary and gastrointestinal losses and constitute over two thirds of maintenance fluid requirements. Insensible losses (cutaneous and pulmonary losses) are quantitatively less important.

THERAPEUTIC PLAN

A therapeutic plan for maintenance fluids should be constructed prior to initiation of therapy. Plans are usually based on a 12- or 24-hr interval. The patient's fluid needs for that period are calculated and fluid administered in conjunction with orders providing for ongoing monitoring of the patient's fluid, electrolyte, and acid-base status. Collection of baseline data prior to initiation of therapy is critical for accurate patient monitoring. The minimum data base should include packed cell volume, total plasma proteins, body weight, and urine specific gravity. It may be wise to save and freeze small aliquots of serum and urine for potential future use, especially in patients with undiagnosed illnesses or patients with rapid changes in fluid, electrolyte, and acid-base status.

Optimal patient care is facilitated when original orders, subsequent changes in orders, and monitoring parameters are clearly written in an organized, systematic form. An example of a Fluid Order–Flow Sheet is given in Figure 1. Such a form provides a record of all pertinent baseline data, indicates fluid type and additives used, and gives calculated fluid rate. The type of drip set is indicated (regular or minidrip) as well as whether oral fluids are allowed and how often. Hourly fluids can be recorded if desired, and provision is made for recording urine output. The clinician can indicate which parameters should be monitored, and how often, by placing checks in the appropriate time boxes.

The advantage of such a system is that it minimizes the likelihood of haphazard fluid plans and patient monitoring. Thus, maintenance fluid therapy can be consistently implemented in a systematic and repeatable fashion. The Fluid Order–Flow Sheet provides cues for appropriate baseline data, orders, and monitoring parameters.

Types of Maintenance Fluids

A number of multiple-electrolyte maintenance fluids are available commercially. Maintenance fluids differ from replacement fluids in that they have a much lower sodium concentration (generally 40 mEq/L vs. 130 mEq/L in lactated Ringer's) and a higher potassium concentration (13 mEq/L vs. 4 mEq/L). The reason for this is that maintenance requirements are not directly related to the serum concentrations of sodium and potassium. Some maintenance fluids are available with 5 per cent dextrose, which is the same as supplying free water. The calorie contribution from such fluids is negligible. One liter of 5 per cent dextrose supplies only 170 calories. Table 1 shows a comparison of several different fluid types.

Fluids designed for replacement purposes should not be used as maintenance fluids. For example, use of lactated Ringer's as a maintenance fluid cause patients to become hypernatremic and hypokalemic. If commercial maintenance fluids are not available, a homemade maintenance fluid can be concocted by combining one part lactated Ringer's with two parts 5 per cent dextrose in water. Potassium is supplemented as needed. The resulting solution will have a sodium concentration of 43 mEq/L (Haskins, 1984).

Maintenance-type fluids should not be used as replacement fluids to treat hypovolemic conditions, since their compositions differ greatly with regard to plasma electrolyte values (Haskins, 1984). Large volumes of hyperosmolar maintenance fluids (e.g., Plasma-Lyte 56 and 5% Dextrose, Travenol) should not be administered subcutaneously because the relatively slow rate of glucose absorption may cause diffusion of intracellular water into the injection site before administered fluid is absorbed. In addition, these fluids may be irritating as a result of low pH (Cohen, 1982).

Maintenance Fluid Volumes

Maintenance fluid volumes range from 20 to 30 ml/lb/day (44 to 66 ml/kg/day), depending on the size of the patient. Larger dogs tend toward the lower extreme, whereas smaller dogs and cats need the higher volume. These rough guidelines take into account sensible (urinary and fecal) and insensible (cutaneous and respiratory) losses. Fluid needs will be greater if contemporary losses are ongoing (vomiting, diarrhea). Volumes of contemporary losses due to gastrointestinal disease should be estimated. The estimated volume is doubled, and this value is added to the calculated maintenance fluid volume, thereby reducing the risk of under-replacing lost fluids (Twedt and Grauer, 1982). Other factors may also contribute to increased main-

FLUID ORDER/FLOW SHEET

This sheet is for ONE fluid type only. If orders (other than rate) are changed, a new sheet must be used. This sheet is not valid and orders it contains will NOT be recognized unless COMPLETELY filled out.

Patient SMITH, SHATZIE Case # 20-00-00 Date 2/19/88

Clinician/Student BELL/BACHMAN Clinical Problem VOMITING, DIARRHEA

20 00 00
SMITH, JANE
K9 TERR X 1/80

Admission Data Weight 36 LBS. PCV 51 TPP 8.3 Usg 1.048

FLUID TYPE LACTATED RINGER'S **ADDITIVES** 15 MEQ KCL/L

RATE (1st) ~~116~~ ml/hr = ~~19~~ drops/min Date & Time ~~2/19/88, 08:30~~ FWB 2/19, 16:00

To cancel, draw line through orders and initial; indicate date & time.

RATE (2nd) 75 ml/hr = 12 drops/min Date & Time 2/19/88; 16:15

To cancel, draw line through orders and initial; indicate date & time.

RATE (3rd) ______ ml/hr = ______ drops/min Date & Time ______

To cancel, draw line through orders and initial; indicate date & time.

Drip set type REG. Oral fluids? X No ___ YES How often? ______

Record hourly fluids? ___ No X Yes Measuring outs X Metab. cage ___ Estimate ___ Free catch

CLINICIAN COMMENTS PLEASE USE FLUID PUMP.

Hour	Ml/Hr	Wt	PCV	TPP	Outs	Hour	Ml/Hr	Wt	PCV	TPP	Outs
08:00		X 36	X 51	X 8.3		21:00					
09:00	116					22:00					
10:00	116/232					23:00					
11:00	116/348					24:00					
12:00	50/398	(OFF FLUIDS FOR RADS)				01:00					
13:00	100/498					02:00		X			X
14:00	116/614	X 37	48	8.0	X	03:00					
15:00	116/730					04:00					
16:00	116/846	(CHANGE IN FLUID RATE)				05:00					
17:00	70/916					06:00					
18:00	75/991					07:00					
19:00	75/1066					08:00		X	X	X	
20:00	75/1141	X 38	X 46	X 7.5	X 150	09:00					

Figure 1. Example of a combined order and flow sheet for fluid therapy.

Table 1. *Commercially Available Parenteral Fluid Solutions*

Solution	Ionic Concentration (mEq/L)				Calories (Kcal/L)	Tonicity	Osmolality (mOsm/L)
	Na^+	K^+	Cl^-	HCO_3^-			
Lactated Ringer's	130	4	109	28 (as lactate)	9	Isotonic	273
Ringer's solution	147	4	156	0	0	Isotonic	310
0.9% Saline	155	0	155	0	0	Isotonic	308
5% Dextrose	0	0	0	0	170	Hypotonic	250
0.45% Saline	77	0	77	0	0	Hypotonic	154
5% Dextrose/0.45% saline	77	0	77	0	170	Hypertonic	404
Plasma-Lyte 56 and 5% Dextrose (Travenol)	40	13	40	16 (as acetate)	170	Hypertonic	363

tenance fluid volumes, such as heavy panting and pyrexia. It has been suggested that for every 1°C rise in body temperature, there is a 13 per cent increase in metabolic rate. This would require an increase in maintenance fluid volumes of 10 per cent for each degree Celsius (Wingfield, 1987). However, such guidelines do not obviate the need for careful monitoring to avoid excessive, or inadequate, fluid therapy.

Required maintenance fluid volumes are related to daily caloric requirements. Therefore, fluid needs may be calculated from graphs that relate body weight to basal metabolic rate. Figure 2 provides a means for determining caloric needs and fluid requirements based on body weight. Administered fluid volumes may need to be increased, depending on patient activity level and intercurrent disease processes such as fever and inflammation (Haskins, 1984).

Calculated maintenance fluid volumes are only estimates; actual needs vary greatly from patient to patient. Therefore, ongoing maintenance fluid volumes must be reasessed daily in light of routine patient evaluation.

Monitoring

Periodic, systematic monitoring of patients receiving maintenance fluid therapy is essential. To do otherwise is the medical equivalent of "flying blind." Packed cell volume, total plasma proteins, and body weight should be monitored on at least a daily basis. More frequent monitoring may be indicated, depending on patient status. These three important parameters require no sophisticated equipment or expertise and are readily available to all. Recording of values on a flow sheet is also of utmost importance, so that the clinician can readily perceive and evaluate trends during therapy.

Changes in body weight of animals receiving adequate caloric intake are reflective principally of variations in fluid balance. In animals not receiving adequate caloric intake, a weight loss of 0.1 to 0.3 kg/day/1000 calories can be attributed to tissue catabolism (Raffe, 1985). It is helpful if animals are weighed on the same scale every day. Small dogs and cats should be weighed on a pediatric-type scale. Precision in weighing is important, since variations in body weight of only 1 lb (0.5 kg) reflect gain or loss of 454 ml of fluid.

Urine output is also an important variable in monitoring animals receiving parenteral fluid therapy. If renal function is adequate, quantitation of output is not necessary. However, urination should be noted with estimates of urine volume. Where renal function is compromised or of unknown status, measurement of urine output becomes an important monitoring parameter. Urine output can be measured in a metabolic cage or in a grate and pan designed for conventional cages. Alternatively, urine output can be estimated from free-catch specimens, on the basis of pre- and post-urination body weight, or from subjective evaluation of urine volume.

In patients with uncertain renal function, fluids should be administered on an interval basis (e.g., six 4-hr intervals). The administered volume should be equal to urine output during the previous interval, plus allowance for estimated insensible losses. Such correlation of fluid administration with urine output prevents overhydration even in oliguric patients. With persistent oliguria, fluid volume can be increased on a daily basis by an amount equal to 5 per cent of body weight, in the event that original assessment of patient dehydration was underestimated (Muir and DiBartola, 1983). Measurement of serum urea nitrogen (SUN) and serum creatinine concentrations and urine specific gravity indicates whether oliguria is physiologic or pathologic.

In selected cases, measurement of central venous pressure (CVP) may be of benefit, especially if concerns about fluid overload develop. Normal CVP values range from 0 to 5 cm H_2O. Values greater than 16 cm H_2O are likely to be associated with formation of edema. It has been recommended that CVP not exceed 10 to 12 cm H_2O during fluid replacement therapy (Bonagura, 1982; Raffe, 1985). Others recommend a decrease in the rate of fluid administration or cessation of treatment if an increase in CVP of 2 cm H_2O above baseline values occurs during fluid therapy (Muir and DiBartola,

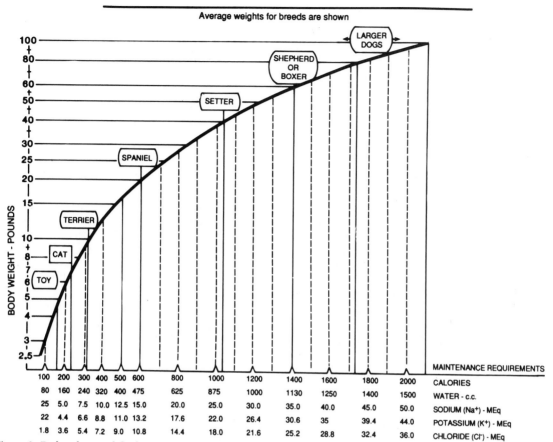

Figure 2. Daily caloric and fluid requirements for hospitalized small animal patients. (Reprinted with permission from Harrison, J. B.: Fluid and electrolyte therapy in small animals. J.A.V.M.A. 137:637–645, 1960.)

1983). CVP is measured via a jugular catheter positioned at the level of the right atrium. The technique for measurement of CVP has been described (Haskins, 1983).

Biochemical monitoring should be performed at regular intervals, with frequency of monitoring depending on patient status. Increases in SUN and serum creatinine concentrations may herald development of prerenal azotemia, suggesting inadequacy of maintenance fluid volumes. Alterations in levels of electrolytes, particularly potassium, are of special concern during chronic fluid therapy. Potassium abnormalities are examined further in the discussion on fluid additives that follows.

With the increasing availability and the decreasing cost of new and used automated infusion pumps, their use in veterinary medicine can be expected to grow. Such pumps are convenient to use; they enhance high-quality patient care by ensuring that a set volume of fluid is administered over a predetermined period. Fluid pumps are not a substitute for careful patient monitoring, however.

Equipment and the Patient

Catheter care is of major concern in fluid therapy patients. Catheters should be installed as aseptically as possible. A povidone-iodine ointment applied to a small gauze patch should cover the catheter entry site, and the catheter should be bandaged in place. The catheter bandage should be checked regularly and should be changed if it is found to be wet or damaged. Evidence of swelling or erythema is an indication for removal of the catheter. If phlebitis develops, the catheter tip should be submitted for bacterial culture and antimicrobial susceptibility tests. The catheter should also be removed if it becomes occluded. In general, catheters should not be allowed to remain in place for more than 3 days.

Fluid bags should always be labeled to indicate fluid additives. The fluid bag and administration set should be replaced after 48 hr in order to minimize iatrogenic sepsis.

Jugular catheters offer numerous advantages over cephalic or saphenous catheters. For example, patients are not as able to dislodge them or disrupt protective bandages. They are not as prone to getting wet as are distal limb catheters, which have an undesirable proximity to water bowls. Jugular catheters provide convenient access for sampling in small dogs and cats, in whom repeated venipunctures (e.g., blood glucose) may be difficult or inadvisable. When jugular catheters are used to obtain diagnostic blood samples, the first milliliter of blood should be discarded, before collecting blood for sample submission.

The new breakaway cannula catheters (L-CATH, Luther Medical Products, Inc.) are particularly useful for jugular installation. The needle breaks away after insertion, leaving only the plastic hub protruding above the entry point. Because there is less weight above the skin, these catheters are much less prone to kinking at the insertion site. Aseptic installation and meticulous maintenance are especially important with jugular catheters.

Fluid Additives

POTASSIUM. Hypokalemia is a common iatrogenic complication of fluid therapy. Underlying disease processes (vomiting, diarrhea), anorexia, and therapeutic measures (alkalinizing therapy, diuretics, and dextrose or insulin administration) all predispose to potassium loss and lowered serum potassium. Therefore, prolonged use of fluids with low concentrations of potassium is likely to result in hypokalemia.

Maintenance fluids contain higher levels of potassium (usually 13 mEq/L) than do replacement fluids (usually 4 mEq/L), but potassium supplementation is usually required beyond this level. Table 2 provides guidelines for potassium supplementation, based on serum potassium levels.

Oral potassium supplementation is used much less commonly in veterinary medicine than in human medicine. Numerous preparations are available. Oral potassium chloride solutions (Potassium Chloride Oral Solution, 10%, Barre) should be diluted in water before administration. Palatability

Table 2. Guidelines for Intravenous Potassium Supplementation*

Serum Potassium (mEq/L)	mEq KCl to Add per 250 ml of Fluid†	Maximal Infusion Rate (ml/kg/hr)‡
<2.0	20	6
2.1 to 2.5	15	8
2.6 to 3.0	10	12
3.1 to 3.5	7	16

*From R. C. Scott, Animal Medical Center, New York, NY.
†Assume a potassium-free fluid (e.g., 0.9% NaCl). Adjust amount of potassium added according to potassium content of fluid used.
‡Do not exceed 0.5 mEq/kg/hr.

may still be a problem. Because of the potential for gastric irritation, these solutions should be administered in conjunction with meals. Supplements are also available in tablet form, such as 10 mEq (750 mg) extended-release potassium chloride tablets (K-Tab, Abbott). Management of hypokalemia has been reviewed elsewhere (Bell and Osborne, 1986).

Hyperkalemia may also develop during fluid therapy if potassium supplementation, rate of administration, or both is excessive. Use of potassium-sparing diuretics such as spironolactone in conjunction with potassium supplementation predisposes to hyperkalemia. Diagnosis and treatment of hyperkalemia has recently been reviewed (Willard, 1986).

BICARBONATE. Bicarbonate supplementation is normally initiated during the early, replacement phase of fluid therapy. Addition of bicarbonate to maintenance fluids is rarely indicated. Persistent acidemia suggests failure to identify and control underlying disease processes. Determination of the anion gap may be of benefit in identifying the cause of ongoing acidemia. Persistent diarrhea, early stages of renal failure, and renal tubular acidosis are examples of hyperchloremic (normal anion gap) acidoses. Lactic acidosis (e.g., due to failure to correct dehydration) and uncontrolled diabetic ketoacidosis are examples of high anion gap acidoses (Polzin and Osborne, 1986).

PHOSPHORUS. Hypophosphatemia may develop in diabetic dogs and cats treated with insulin. Deficits can be severe, leading to development of secondary hemolytic anemia. Phosphorus can be added to parenteral fluids using potassium phosphate (see the following article, Hypophosphatemia).

MAINTENANCE FLUID THERAPY AND DISEASE STATES

As with any other therapy, maintenance fluid therapy should be adjusted to the immediate needs of the patient. The principal components of fluid therapy—fluid type, volume, and rate—may need to be altered, singly or in combination, in response to changes in the patient's status. For example, the vomiting, alkalotic patient may need higher levels of chloride than are supplied by typical maintenance fluids. In this situation, either Ringer's solution or 0.9 per cent sodium chloride (with potassium supplementation as needed) may be the best fluid choice available.

The diabetic patient receiving maintenance fluids may not need the dextrose supplied by many commercial maintenance fluid preparations. Half-strength (0.45 per cent) sodium chloride without dextrose (with appropriate potassium supplementation) is often an excellent choice for maintenance fluid support.

Patients with cardiac failure have special fluid needs, because of their extreme intolerance of administered sodium loads. Five per cent dextrose in water is often used in such patients, with careful monitoring of the parameters previously discussed to ensure that overhydration is not occurring. Half-strength (0.45 per cent) sodium chloride in 2.5 per cent dextrose may also be used, but sodium intake should not exceed 12 mg/kg of body weight, approximately 0.5 mEq/kg (Bonagura, 1982).

CESSATION OF FLUID THERAPY

Because of the increased nursing care required and potential for complications associated with indwelling intravenous catheters, patients should be weaned off parenteral fluids as soon as practicable. Subcutaneous fluids are an easy, practical method of bridging the period between termination of intravenous fluids and return to 100 per cent oral intake. Hyperosmolar, low pH fluids are not recommended for subcutaneous use. Ringer's solution, lactated Ringer's, or 0.9 per cent sodium chloride all are good choices for subcutaneous fluid administration. They may be supplemented with potassium chloride, if necessary, up to a total of 30 mEq/L of fluid.

References and Supplemental Reading

Bell, F. W., and Osborne, C. A.: Treatment of hypokalemia. In Kirk, R. W. (ed.): Current Veterinary Therapy IX. Philadelphia: W.B. Saunders Co., 1986, pp. 101–107.

Bonagura, J. D.: Fluid management of the cardiac patient. In Schaer, M. (ed.): The Veterinary Clinics of North America—Fluid and Electrolyte Balance. Philadelphia: W.B. Saunders Co., 1982, pp. 501–513.

Cohen, J. S.: A summary of complications of fluid therapy. In Schaer, M. (ed.): The Veterinary Clinics of North America—Fluid and Electrolyte Balance. Philadelphia: W.B. Saunders Co., 1982, pp. 545–558.

Haskins, S. C.: Shock. In Kirk, R. W. (ed.): Current Veterinary Therapy VIII. Philadelphia: W.B. Saunders Co., 1983, pp. 2–27.

Haskins, S. C.: Fluid and electrolyte therapy. Comp. Cont. Ed. Prac. Vet. 6:244, 1984.

Muir, W. W., and DiBartola, S. P.: Fluid therapy. In Kirk, R. W. (ed.): Current Veterinary Therapy VIII. Philadelphia: W.B. Saunders Co., 1983, pp. 28–40.

Polzin, D. P., and Osborne, C. A.: Anion gap—diagnostic and therapeutic applications. In Kirk, R. W. (ed.): Current Veterinary Therapy IX. Philadelphia: W.B. Saunders Co., 1986, pp. 52–59.

Raffe, M. R.: Fluid therapy in the surgical patient. In Slatter, D. H. (ed.): Textbook of Small Animal Surgery. Philadelphia: W.B. Saunders Co., 1985, pp. 90–102.

Rose, B. D.: Clinical Physiology of Acid-Base and Electrolyte Disorders. New York: McGraw-Hill, 1984.

Twedt, D. C., and Grauer, G. F.: Fluid therapy for gastrointestinal, pancreatic, and hepatic disorders. In Schaer, M. (ed.): The Veterinary Clinics of North America—Fluid and Electrolyte Balance. Philadelphia: W.B. Saunders Co., 1982, pp. 463–485.

Willard, M.D.: Treatment of hyperkalemia. In Kirk, R. W. (ed.): Current Veterinary Therapy IX. Philadelphia: W.B. Saunders Co., 1986, pp. 94–101.

Wingfield, W.: Fluid therapy in emergency patients. In Scientific Presentations of the 54th Annual Meeting, American Animal Hospital Association, 1987, pp. 477–480.

HYPOPHOSPHATEMIA

ROBERT M. HARDY, D.V.M.,
and LARRY G. ADAMS, D.V.M.
Saint Paul, Minnesota

Hypophosphatemia (i.e., serum phosphorus of <2.5 mg/dl in dogs and <2.9 mg/dl in cats) is not commonly recognized in companion animal practice. However, in humans, 10 to 15 per cent of all hospitalized patients may have this biochemical abnormality (Agus and Goldfarb, 1981). Similar information for dogs and cats is currently unavailable. An increased recognition of this problem occurred in human medicine following the advent of routine biochemical screening of hospitalized patients as well as the development of new and more aggressive therapeutic techniques (Williams, 1975). This phenomenon is now occurring in the authors' practice as well. Hypophosphatemia is considered moderately severe when serum phosphorus levels are in the range of 1.0 to 2.5 mg/dl, and severe if levels are less than 1.0 mg/dl (Kurokawa et al., 1985). Because hypophosphatemia can result in a wide variety of clinical signs, some of which are life threatening (hemolytic anemia, seizures), it is important to become familiar with diseases likely to produce hypophosphatemia, and to develop a therapeutic approach for treatment of this potentially serious electrolyte abnormality.

APPLIED PHYSIOLOGY AND BIOCHEMISTRY

Phosphorus is widely available in nature; it is present in high concentrations in red meat, poultry, fish, eggs, dairy products, and legumes. A true phosphorus deficiency (total body depletion) is unknown in animals eating a normal diet (Williams, 1975). The jejunum is the primary site of addition of phosphorus to the body, while the kidney serves as both an organ for excretion of excess phosphorus and the main organ for conservation of phosphorus in depletion states. Most of the phosphorus in the body (85 per cent) is present in bone as calcium and magnesium phosphate salts; 15 per cent is in soft tissues. Less than 1 per cent is present in the extracellular fluid, as neutral inorganic phosphate ($HPO_4^{--}/H_2PO_4^-$) (Knochel, 1977; Korokawa et al., 1985; Nesbakken and Reinlie, 1985; Stoff, 1982). Phosphorus is a major intracellular anion; potassium is the major intracellular cation. The ratio of intracellular to extracellular phosphorus is 100:1 (Lenta et al., 1978). Thus, the extracellular serum concentration is a poor estimate of the total body phosphorus status. Hypophosphatemia may exist with a normal total body phosphorus level, while phosphorus depletion can be present when serum phosphorus concentrations are normal.

Phosphorus is a critical element in intermediary metabolism. It is an essential component of cell membrane phospholipids and nucleic acids, serves as a buffer system allowing for the excretion of fixed acids from the body, and is important in cellular defense mechanisms against infectious organisms (Knochel, 1977; Kurokawa et al., 1985; Nesbakken and Reinlie, 1985). Most intracellular phosphorus is present in high-energy phosphate compounds, such as adenosine triphosphate (ATP), which serve as cellular energy sources for processes such as muscle contraction, neurologic transmission, electrolyte transport, glycolysis, ammoniagenesis, and synthesis of red blood cell (RBC) 2,3-diphosphoglycerate (2,3-DPG) (Stoff, 1982). Extracellular inorganic phosphate constitutes a very small fraction of this total pool but is the sole source of phosphorus for ATP and other intracellular phosphorus-containing compounds. Thus, it is critical for maintenance of normal cellular functions.

ETIOPATHOGENESIS

In humans, clinically important hypophosphatemia has the potential to develop in multiple situations (Table 1). However, it has been reported to be of significance only in dogs and cats with diabetic ketoacidosis, and in a cat with hepatic lipidosis (Adams et al., 1988; Willard et al., 1987). Hypophosphatemia develops in these clinical states because one or more of the following is occurring: (1) phosphorus shifts *from* the extracellular space *into* the intracellular space, (2) decreased gastrointestinal absorption occurs, and (3) there is increased renal loss of phosphorus (Kurokawa et al., 1985). In diabetic ketoacidosis, the serum phosphorus con-

centration is usually normal prior to treatment, even though many of these patients have severe phosphorus depletion (Kurokawa et al., 1985). When insulin is given, (1) acidosis is corrected, (2) ketonuria is controlled, and (3) glucose and phosphorus move intracellularly and are utilized in formation of phosphorylated carbohydrates, which causes significant decreases in extracellular phosphorus concentrations. Hypophosphatemia becomes evident in the first 24 hr following insulin therapy and peaks in severity within 24 to 36 hr; if patients are starved or if cirrhosis is present, this effect is magnified (Knochel, 1977). A similar fall in the serum phosphorus level occurs if intravenous glucose is given to normal patients, since it causes endogenous insulin release, which, in turn, promotes glucose and phosphorus entry into cells. In this situation, the magnitude of the drop is usually less than 0.5 mg/dl (Knochel, 1977). If cachectic animals are refed diets relatively low in phosphorus, such as those used for total parenteral nutrition or renal failure, aggressive cellular uptake of nutrients occurs, with a shift toward anabolic pathways. The result is rapid depletion of extracellular phosphorus if adequate supplementation is not provided (Knochel, 1977). This is particularly likely to occur when glucose is used as the primary caloric source.

CLINICAL SIGNS

Clinical signs associated with hypophosphatemia fall into one of four main categories: (1) hematologic, (2) neuromuscular, (3) skeletal, and (4) hepatic (Table 2) (Adams et al., 1988; Knochel, 1977; Willard, 1987; Williams, 1975; Yawata et al., 1974). Only hematologic and neuromuscular manifestations have been documented in association with naturally occurring hypophosphatemia in dogs and cats (Adams et al., 1988; Willard, 1987).

Hypophosphatemia causes structural or functional abnormalities in RBCs, neutrophils, and platelets (Jacobs and Amsden, 1971; Knochel, 1977; Kurokawa et al., 1985; Williams, 1975; Yawata et al., 1974). The most striking abnormality documented in dogs and cats is development of severe hemolytic anemia in association with serum phosphorus concentrations of 1.5 mg/dl or less (Adams et al., 1988; Willard, 1987; Yawata et al., 1974). Adequate intracellular concentrations of ATP must be present in RBCs to maintain normal cell structure and function. As extracellular phosphorus concentrations fall, RBCs are unable to generate sufficient intracellular ATP to maintain normal cell membrane function. When intracellular ATP concentrations approach 15 to 20 per cent of normal, hemolysis occurs. In experimental dogs, hemolysis is consistently present when the serum phosphorus concentration falls to less than 0.5 mg/dl. It has been

Table 1. *Conditions Associated with Hypophosphatemia, Mechanisms That Induce It, and General Severity*

	Mechanisms			Severity*	
Cause	Transcellular Shifts	Increased Renal Loss and Decreased Renal Reabsorp.	Increased GI Loss Decreased GI Absorp.	M	S
IV glucose	+	+		+	
Diabetic ketoacidosis therapy	+	+		+	+
Starvation/refeeding	+			+	+
Diuretics		+		+	
Respiratory alkalosis	+			+	+
Oral antacid therapy			+	+	+
Hyperalimentation	+			+	+
Low phosphorus diets			+	+	
Renal tubular defects		+		+	
Glucocorticoid use		+		+	
Hyperparathyroidism		+		+	
Saline administration		+		+	
GI malabsorption		+	+	+	
Bicarbonate administration	+			+	
Androgen for cachexia	+			+	
Metabolic acidosis	+	+		+	
Sepsis	+			+	

*Severity: M, moderate hypophosphatemia (phosphorus level = 1.0–2.5 mg/dl); S, severe hypophosphatemia (phosphorus level < 1.0 mg/dl).

documented to occur in cats with phosphorus concentrations of less than 1.6 mg/dl (Adams et al., 1988; Willard, 1987; Yawata et al., 1974). Intracellular ATP is necessary for RBCs to maintain their normal plasticity and biconcavity. In hypophosphatemia, RBCs become microspherocytic and rigid, have decreased survival times, and are rapidly removed from the circulation by the spleen and other reticuloendothelial tissues. The precise mechanism responsible for hemolysis is unknown. However, ATP is necessary to maintain the normal intracellular sodium-potassium pump. Failure of this system would lead to intracellular accumulation of water and to lysis. Phosphorus is also an important component of RBC membrane phospholipids that may undergo structural alteration during hypophosphatemia. The RBC membrane contains actinomyosin-like microfilaments that are thought to be important in the maintenance of normal RBC deformability. If RBC ATP affects these membrane microfilaments as it does muscle actinomyosin elements, decreased ATP would lead to more rigid cell membranes and earlier removal of these cells from the circulation.

A functional change also occurs within hypophosphatemic RBCs. The affinity of RBC hemoglobin for oxygen is determined by the intracellular concentration of 2,3-DPG. Since phosphorus is required for synthesis of this compound, hypophosphatemia leads to decreased intracellular 2,3-DPG concentrations (Jacobs and Amsden, 1971; Kurokawa et al., 1985; Williams, 1975). This results in increased affinity of RBCs for oxygen and decreased availability of oxygen to tissues (a so-called "shift to the left" of the oxyhemoglobin dissociation curve). This may be particularly important for the central nervous system.

Important functional changes also occur in neutrophils. Experimental work in hypophosphatemic dogs indicates that a 50 per cent decrease in chemotaxis, phagocytosis, and bacteriocidal activity of canine neutrophils occurs at serum phosphorus concentrations of less than 1.0 mg/dl (Knochel, 1977). This may contribute to the rate of infection in diabetic patients and patients receiving parenteral hyperalimentation with low phosphorus solutions. These functional defects are reversed by phosphorus supplementation.

Table 2. *Clinical Signs Associated with Hypophosphatemia*

Hematologic	Neuromuscular	Skeletal	Hepatic
Hemolysis; decreased RBC 2,3-DPG*; thrombocytopenia; impaired neutrophil function	Neuroencephalopathy; paresthesias; seizures; coma; respiratory paralysis; cardiomyopathy; rhabdomyolysis; weakness	Bone pain; joint pain	Cirrhotics decompensate if hypophosphatemic

*2,3-diphosphoglycerate.

Platelet defects have also been identified in experimental studies of hypophosphatemic dogs (Yawata et al., 1974). Decreased platelet numbers and large-diameter platelets have been observed in their blood smears. Also, poor clot retraction and decreased platelet survival have been observed in these dogs. This may have clinical relevance if stored blood is given to animals with hypophosphatemic hemolytic anemia. Platelet numbers are often low in stored blood. In addition, anticoagulants low in phosphorus could impair platelet function and decrease 2,3-DPG concentrations in the transfused RBCs.

A multitude of neuromuscular signs are associated with hypophosphatemia (Knochel, 1977; Williams, 1975). Reported neurologic signs in humans included weakness, anorexia, paresthesias, dysarthria, confusion, obtundation, intention tremors, seizures, coma, and death. Seizures have been observed in one dog with severe hypophosphatemia (Willard, 1987). Clinical signs became evident at serum phosphorus concentrations below 2.0 mg/dl; the lower the serum phosphorus level, the more dramatic were the signs. In dogs with experimentally induced hypophosphatemia that resulted in ataxia, convulsions, and death (Williams, 1975), a 50 to 90 per cent decrease in neuronal ATP concentrations occurred.

Abnormalities of both skeletal and smooth muscle occur in association with hypophosphatemia. Respiratory failure due to diaphragmatic weakness, reversible cardiomyopathy, and rhabdomyolysis have been observed in humans (Darsu and Nutter, 1978; Fuller et al., 1978; Knochel, 1977, 1985; Stoff, 1982). Dramatic increases in serum creatine kinase concentrations can occur if serum phosphorus concentrations drop below 1.0 mg/dl. The authors have observed one cat with massive increases in creatine kinase concentrations associated with severe hypophosphatemia. A reversible form of congestive cardiomyopathy was observed in three humans with serum phosphorus concentrations of less than 1.0 mg/dl due to chronic antacid ingestion (Darsu and Nutter, 1978). In dogs with experimentally induced hypophosphatemia, decreased stroke volume and myocardial performance have been documented (Fuller et al., 1978).

THERAPY

Not all patients with hypophosphatemia need to be, or should be, specifically treated. This is particularly the case when the level of serum phosphorus is greater than 1.5 mg/dl (moderate hypophosphatemia). Correcting the cause of the hypophosphatemia generally results in normalization of phosphorus concentrations within several days. Clinicians must anticipate clinical situations in which serious

Table 3. Available Oral and Parenteral Sources of Phosphorus

Preparations	Phosphate (mmol/ml)	Dose
Oral		
Whole cow's milk	0.029	0.5–2 mmol/kg/day
Phospho-soda*	4.15	0.5–2 mmol/kg/day
Parenteral		
Sodium phosphate†	3.0	0.06–0.18 mmol/kg, given over 6 hr
Potassium phosphate†	3.0	0.06–0.18 mmol/kg, given over 6 hr

*Fleet Co. Inc., Lynchburg, VA 24505.
†Abbott Laboratories, North Chicago, IL 60064.

hypophosphatemia may already exist or is likely to develop (Table 1). This is particularly true for the untreated ketoacidotic diabetic and cachectic animals being refed diets low in phosphorus. Such patients should be monitored carefully to detect the presence of serious hypophosphatemia early in the clinical course of their illness, prior to the development of hemolysis or central nervous system derangement. Opinions are mixed regarding the value of phosphorus replacement in the management of hypophosphatemic human patients, particularly those with diabetes mellitus. Based on our limited clinical experience with this disorder, the authors believe that judicious phosphorus supplementation will benefit animals with serum phosphorus concentrations of less than 1.5 mg/dl and should be given if the serum phosphorus level is less than 1.0 mg/dl.

Both oral and parenteral phosphate preparations can be administered to animals with hypophosphatemia (Table 3). The safest and preferred method of phosphorus supplementation is the oral route, provided oral medications can be administered safely. If a balanced commercial diet is voluntarily consumed or can be force-fed, it should prevent moderate hypophosphatemia from worsening and should reverse severe hypophosphatemia. As an alternative to a balanced commercial diet, whole milk is a readily available source of phosphorus (it contains 0.29 mmol/ml) (Lenta et al., 1978). Oral sodium phosphate solutions (Phospho-Soda, Fleet) contain 4.5 mmol/ml but may induce diarrhea if it is not given in small, frequent amounts. In humans, oral doses of 0.5 to 2 mmol/kg/day are used to supplement TPN solutions low in phosphorus, and these doses are probably good starting doses in dogs and cats (Lenta et al., 1978; Takala et al., 1985).

Parenteral phosphate supplementation is the most controversial route of phosphorus administration because of the potential for serious complications to develop, and the fact that neither the size of the phosphorus deficit nor the dose to be given can be predicted with any certainty. Intravenous preparations of phosphorus may be given as either the sodium or the potassium salt (Table 3). Dosages should always be converted to mmol/L, since significant dosing errors can be made if mg/dl or mEq availability are used in dosing calculations (one mmol/l = 3.1 mg/dl = 1.7 mEq/L). Most commercially available parenteral phosphate solutions contain 3.0 mmol/ml. Intravenous dosages that the authors have used successfully in dogs and cats range from 0.06 to 0.18 mmol/kg, given over 6 hr (0.01 to 0.03 mmol/kg/hr). The level of serum phosphorus must be rechecked prior to administering more phosphorus, to avoid complications related to overdosage. Parenteral phosphate should be added to fluids that do not contain calcium (i.e., normal saline or dextrose and water) to avoid precipitation of calcium-phosphate salts. It is not necessary to continue phosphorus supplementation until the serum concentration is normal. Generally, once the serum phosphorus level reaches 2.0 mg/dl, supplementation can be stopped.

COMPLICATIONS

Potential complications of parenteral phosphorus therapy include hyperphosphatemia, hypocalcemia, soft tissue mineralization, hypotension, and renal failure (Knochel, 1977; Kurokawa et al., 1985; Lenta et al., 1978; Shackney and Hasson, 1967). Four of six hypophosphatemic cats treated at the authors' hospital developed significant hypocalcemia (Ca^{++} = 5.5 to 8.1 mg/dl). One had signs of mild tetany, weakness, and depression, which required treatment with calcium gluconate. Contraindications to the administration of phosphorus-containing fluids include hypercalcemia of any origin, hyperphosphatemia, oliguric renal failure, and evidence of tissue necrosis.

References and Supplemental Reading

Adams, L. G., Hardy, R. M., and Bartges, J.: Hypophosphatemic hemolytic anemia associated with diabetes mellitus and hepatic lipidosis in cats. University of Minnesota, College of Veterinary Medicine, 1988 (in preparation).

Agus, Z. S., and Goldfarb, S. N.: Clinical disorders of calcium and phosphate. Med. Clin. North Am. 65:385, 1981.

Darsu, J. R., and Nutter, D. O.: Reversible severe congestive cardiomyopathy in three cases of hypophosphatemia. Ann. Intern. Med. 89:867, 1978.

Fuller, T. J., Nichols, W. W., Brenner, B. J., et al.: Reversible depression in myocardial performance in dogs with experimental phosphorous deficiency. J. Clin. Invest. 62:1194, 1978.

Jacobs, H. S., and Amsden, T.: Acute hemolytic anemia with rigid red cells in hypophosphatemia. N. Engl. J. Med. 285:1446, 1971.

Knochel, J. P.: The pathophysiology and clinical characteristics of severe hypophosphatemia. Arch. Intern. Med. 137:203, 1977.

Knochel, J. P.: The clinical status of hypophosphatemia. N. Engl. J. Med. 313:447, 1985.

Kurokawa, D., Levine, B., Lee, D. B., et al.: Physiology of phosphorous metabolism and pathophysiology of hypophosphatemia and hyperphosphatemia. In Arieff, A. I., and DeFronzo, R. A. (eds.): Fluid, Electrolyte, and Acid-Base Disorders. New York: Churchill-Livingstone, 1985, p. 625.

Lenta, R. D., Brown, D. M., and Kjellstrand, C. M.: Treatment of severe hypophosphatemia. Ann. Intern. Med. 89:941, 1978.

Nesbakken, R., and Reinlie, S.: Magnesium and phosphorus: The electrolytes of energy metabolism. Acta Anesthesiol. Scand. 29:60, 1985.

Shackney, S., and Hasson J.: Precipitous fall in serum calcium, hypotension, and acute renal failure after intravenous phosphate therapy for hypercalcemia. Report of two cases. Ann. Intern. Med. 66:906, 1967.

Stoff, J. S.: Phosphate homeostasis and hypophosphatemia. Am. J. Med. 72:489, 1982.

Takala, J., Neuvonen, P., and Klossner, J.: Hypophosphatemia in hypercatabolic patients. Acta Anaesthesiol. Scand. 29:65, 1985.

Willard, M. D.: Severe hypophosphatemia: Significance and treatment. Proceedings of the 5th Annual Veterinary Medical Forum. Omnipress, Madison, WI, 1987, pp. 141–143.

Willard, M. D., Zerbe, C. A., Schall, S. D., et al.: Severe hypophosphatemia associated with diabetes mellitus in 6 dogs and 1 cat. J.A.V.M.A. 190:1007, 1987.

Williams, H. E.: Hypophosphatemia. West. J. Med. 122:487, 1975.

Yawata, Y., Hebber, R. P., Silvis, S., et al.: Blood cell abnormalities complicating the hypophosphatemia of hyperalimentation: Erythrocyte and platelet ATP deficiency associated with hemolytic anemia and bleeding in hyperalimented dogs. J. Clin. Lab. Med. 84:643, 1974.

NONSTEROIDAL ANTI-INFLAMMATORY DRUGS

STANLEY I. RUBIN, D.V.M.,
and MARK G. PAPICH, D.V.M.
Saskatoon, Saskatchewan

Nonsteroidal anti-inflammatory drugs (NSAIDs) have been described as substances other than steroids that suppress one or more elements of the inflammatory response. These agents act by inhibiting the enzyme system responsible for converting arachidonic acid to eicosanoids, some of the potent chemical mediators of inflammation. All NSAIDs have these similar modes of action, accounting for their therapeutic and toxic effects. By virtue of these actions, NSAIDs have anti-inflammatory, anti-

Table 1. Classification of NSAIDs

Enolic Acids	Carboxylic Acids
Pyrazolones	Salicylates
Phenylbutazone	Aspirin
Oxyphenbutazone	Sodium salicylate
Dipyrone	Diflunisal
Isopyrin	Propionic acids
Asapropazone	Naproxen
Benzothiazines	Ibuprofen
Piroxicam	Benoxaprofen
	Anthranilic acids
	Meclofenamic acid
	Mefenamic acid
	Aminonicotinic acids
	Flunixin
	Clonixin
	Quinolines
	Cinchophen
	Indolines
	Indomethacin

pyretic, and analgesic properties, for which they have been used in medicine for over 100 years.

The NSAIDs are enolic acid or carboxylic acid derivatives of several different classes. The chemical classification of NSAIDs is listed in Table 1. The most popular ones include the salicylates, pyrazolones, and the propionic acids.

The NSAIDs are a weakly acidic group of drugs (pKa 4.5 or less) and are characteristically bound to plasma proteins (primarily albumin). Some NSAIDs are 95 to 99 per cent protein-bound. Although many classes of NSAIDs are used in humans and horses, there are relatively few drugs that are appropriate for use in dogs and cats. This is attested to by the number of case reports that have documented NSAID toxicity in dogs and cats. Currently, the most commonly used NSAIDs in small animal medicine are aspirin and phenylbutazone.

THE INFLAMMATORY RESPONSE

Inflammation is one of the body's primary responses to an insult or injury. The inflammatory response may be initiated by infectious organisms, and chemical or physical agents that result in cell injury. Inflammation is characterized by four "cardinal signs," which were described by Celsus (35 A.D.). These are redness (rubor), swelling (tumor), heat (calor), and pain (dolor), with loss of function. These signs represent the interaction of vascular, immunologic, and cellular reactions involving many chemical mediators of inflammation. Factors that have been long implicated in the inflammatory process include histamine, 5-hydroxytryptamine, and the kinin, complement, and clotting systems. In the past 15 years, eicosanoids, another group of mediators, were discovered to be major components of the inflammatory process. Not only do these compounds play a direct role in inflammation, but also they act indirectly through synergism with other mediators such as the vasoactive amines and bradykinin. In addition, they may be a chemotactic, enhancing leukocyte accumulation at the site of injury.

Eicosanoids are derived from 20 carbon fatty acids, of which arachidonic acid is most common. Arachidonic acid is widely distributed in the body; it is usually stored (covalently bound in its esterified

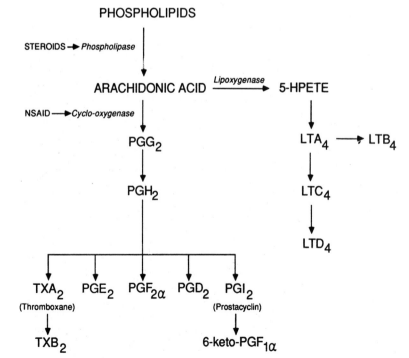

Figure 1. Schematic illustration of the cyclo-oxygenase and lipoxygenase pathways of arachidonic acid metabolism. Following an inflammatory stimulus, phospholipase acts to release arachidonic acid from the phospholipid pool. The enzyme cyclo-oxygenase converts arachidonate to intermediate cyclic endoperoxides (prostaglandin G_2 [PGG_2] and prostaglandin H_2 [PGH_2], which subsequently are converted to the prostaglandins (prostaglandin D_2 [PGD_2], prostaglandin E [PGE_2] and prostaglandin $F_{2\alpha}$ [$PGF_{2\alpha}$]); prostacyclin (PGI_2); and the thromboxanes (thromboxane A_2 [TXA_2] and thromboxane B_2 [TXB_2]). Prostacyclin (PGI_2) and thromboxane (TXA_2) are rapidly broken down to the stable, but biologically inert metabolites TXB_2 and 6-keto-$PGF_{2\alpha}$. The enzyme lipoxygenase converts arachidonic acid to a number of intermediates including 5-hydroperoxyeicosatetraenoic acid (5-HPETE), which gives rise to the leukotrienes (LTA_4, LTB_4, LTC_4, and LTD_4).

Table 2. *Products of Arachidonic Acid Cascade*

Eicosanoid	Primary Source	Response
PGD_2	Mast cells; multiple tissues	Vasodilation; bronchoconstriction
$PGF_{2\alpha}$		Vasoconstriction; uterine and bronchial smooth muscle contraction
TXA_2 (thromboxane)	Platelets; leukocytes	Vasoconstriction; platelet aggregation
PGI_2 (prostacyclin)	Vascular endothelium; macrophages	Vasodilation; inhibits platelet aggregation; acute inflammatory reactions
PGE_2	Leukocytes; multiple tissues	Vasodilation; acute inflammatory response; inhibits gastric acid secretion; pyrexia; analgesia; inhibits renal tubular sodium reabsorption; stimulates osteoclast activity
LTB_4	Leukocytes; mast cells; macrophages	Leukocyte chemotaxis; vascular permeability
LTG_4, LTD_4 (SRS-A)	Leukocytes; mast cells; macrophages	Bronchoconstriction; vasoconstriction

form) in the phospholipid fraction of the cell membranes of most body cells. Phospholipase-A_2, an acyl hydrolase, is activated by an inflammatory stimulus and acts to release arachidonic acid from its phospholipid pool. Arachidonate is then available for enzymes of the cyclo-oxygenase and lipoxygenase pathways (Fig. 1).

The enzyme cyclo-oxygenase converts arachidonate to intermediate cyclic endoperoxides (prostaglandin G_2 [PGG_2] and prostaglandin H_2 [PGH_2]). These metabolites are subsequently converted to the prostaglandins (prostaglandin D_2 [PGD_2]; prostaglandin E_2 [PGE_2]; prostaglandin $F_{2\alpha}$ [$PGF_{2\alpha}$]; and prostacyclin [PGI_2]) and the thromboxanes (thromboxane A_2 [TXA_2] and thromboxane B_2 [TXB_2]). These products, the prostanoids, have very short half-lives and are not stored in the tissues. Eicosanoids have been implicated in every phase of inflammation (Table 2).

The enzyme lipoxygenase converts arachidonate to hydroperoxy acids, which are metabolized to noncyclized eicosanoids called leukotrienes. Leukotriene B_4 (LTB_4) is one of the most potent endogenous chemotactic factors and is responsible for migration of leukocytes to sites of inflammation and release of lysosomal enzymes. Elevated concentrations of LTB_4 have been found in synovial fluid of humans afflicted with rheumatoid arthritis and also in inflamed joints and soft tissues of horses (Higgins, 1985). Leukotriene B_4 also potentiates bradykinin-induced vascular exudation and, together with vasodilatory prostaglandins, may mediate vascular permeability. Leukotrienes C_4 and D_4 account for most of what has been called Slow-Reacting Substance of Anaphylaxis (SRS-A), an important mediator of asthmatic bronchoconstriction in humans.

MECHANISM OF ACTION

OVERVIEW. All the NSAIDs have anti-inflammatory, analgesic, antipyretic activity and inhibit platelet aggregation. The NSAIDs also may be beneficial in the treatment of septic shock. Their activity is attributed to inhibition of conversion of arachidonic acid to the cyclic endoperoxide PGG_2, via inhibition of the cyclo-oxygenase enzyme. These drugs have no inhibitory effect on arachidonic acid metabolites already formed, but rather suppress further formation of PG and thromboxanes. Drugs such as acetylsalicylic acid (aspirin), phenylbutazone, and meclofenamic acid bind cyclo-oxygenase irreversibly, whereas many other NSAIDs are reversible inhibitors of cyclo-oxygenase. Aspirin acetylates serine at the active site of cyclo-oxygenase, which results in its irreversible inhibition. The majority of the NSAIDs do not block the lipoxygenase pathways.

ANTI-INFLAMMATORY ACTIVITY. Arachidonic acid metabolites play a role in vasodilation, increased vascular permeability, leukocyte chemotaxis, pain, bronchoconstriction, and platelet aggregation (Higgins and Lees, 1984). The clinical response to many NSAIDs seems to be prolonged despite the short half-lives of many of these drugs (Higgins, 1985). This may be related to a high percentage of tissue binding or irreversible binding of the drug to cyclo-oxygenase.

The anti-inflammatory activity exerted by NSAIDs appears to occur by virtue of inhibition of the cyclo-oxygenase pathway. Currently, there is active research to produce an effective "dual blocker," that is, a drug that effectively inhibits both the cyclo-oxygenase and lipoxygenase enzyme pathways. The only available drugs capable of dual blockade are the glucocorticoids (see the following article entitled Glucocorticoid Therapy). Benoxaprofen, a drug with dual action, was used for a short period in humans; however, it was subsequently withdrawn because of toxic side effects.

ANALGESIC ACTIVITY. The analgesic activity of NSAIDs is related to their ability to prevent PG release associated with inflammation. Prostaglandins of the E series enhance the pain-producing effects of bradykinin. NSAIDs prevent PG-induced sensitization of pain receptors, caused by mechanical stimulation or other chemicals.

ANTIPYRETIC ACTIVITY. Pyrogens such as bacterial endotoxin stimulate release of interleukin-1 (also known as endogenous pyrogen) by monocytes, macrophages, and Kupffer's cells. The endogenous pyrogen causes synthesis of prostaglandins (PGE_1 and PGE_2) in the preoptic areas of the hypothalamus, which, in turn, are responsible for raising the hypothalamic set point and causing fever. The antipyretic actions of NSAIDs occur by virtue of their inhibition of prostaglandin synthesis. Aspirin-like drugs reduce the body temperature in febrile states; however, these drugs do not reduce hyperthermia associated with heat stress or intense exercise. Suppressing fever caused by infectious agents is · of questionable benefit on the course of the disease. It is hypothesized that the febrile response actually enhances an animal's ability to suppress growth of infectious agents and enhances natural immunity. There is substantial evidence that supports the benefit of fever in infectious diseases.

OTHER PROPOSED EFFECTS OF NSAIDs. Although the greatest proportion of NSAID activity can be attributed to inhibition of arachidonic acid metabolism to prostaglandins, thromboxanes, and prostacyclin, other mechanisms of action for NSAIDs have been suggested. NSAIDs also may uncouple oxidative phosphorylation, scavenge oxygen-derived toxic radicals, inhibit leukocyte migration into tissues, inhibit local release of kinins, and facilitate cAMP-mediated membrane stabilization.

CLASSES OF DRUGS

SALICYLATES. Salicylates have been employed in medicine for centuries. This group of drugs includes aspirin (acetylsalicylic acid), sodium salicylate, and diflunisal (Dolobid, Merck, Sharpe and Dohme). Aspirin is the most widely prescribed analgesic-antipyretic and anti-inflammatory agent; it remains as the standard for comparison and evaluation of other NSAIDs. Diflunisal has not yet been evaluated clinically in dogs or cats.

Aspirin and sodium salicylate are readily absorbed from the stomach and intestine of dogs and cats. At an acidic pH, the drug is present predominantly in un-ionized form, which favors rapid absorption from the stomach. Following absorption, aspirin is deacetylated to salicylic acid. Salicylate is conjugated with glucuronate and glycine in the liver and is excreted in the urine.

There are both species and age differences in the rates of elimination of salicylates. The half-life of salicylate is 37.5 hr in cats, and 8.6 hr in dogs (Davis and Westfall, 1972). The reason for the prolonged half-life of salicylate in the cat is that cats are relatively deficient in the glucuronyl transferase responsible for conjugating the salicylate with glucuronic acid. Thus, the hepatic clearance of salicylate is slow in this species. Newborn animals are deficient in the microsomal enzymes necessary for the biotransformation of salicylate and also have limited ability to excrete these drugs in urine.

Therefore, salicylates have longer half-lives in neonates (Davis, Westfall, and Short, 1973). The plasma elimination rate of salicylate reaches adult values in the dog by 30 days of age. In addition, the half-life of salicylates is dose-dependent in dogs and cats; the higher the dose, the longer the half-life (Yeary and Brant, 1975).

Plain, buffered, and enteric-coated types of aspirin are capable of producing sustained therapeutic concentrations of salicylate in dogs. Plain aspirin was found to be most irritating to the gastric mucosa, while enteric-coated aspirin produced the greatest fluctuations in serum salicylate concentrations (Lipowitz et al., 1986). Doses of 25 mg/kg every 8 hr in dogs and 25 mg/kg every 24 hr in cats were found to produce salicylate concentrations within the therapeutic range (anti-inflammatory, analgesic). A recent investigation found that dosages of 1 to 10 mg/kg/day were effective in inhibiting platelet aggregation in dogs; however, animals with disease may not react in the same way as the normal animals used in the aforementioned study (Rackear et al., 1988).

PYRAZOLONE DERIVATIVES. This class of drugs includes phenylbutazone, oxyphenbutazone, antipyrine, aminopyrine, dipyrone, and apazone. Phenylbutazone is the most commonly used drug; apazone is the newest. The others are seldom used today. The anti-inflammatory effects of phenylbutazone are similar to those of the salicylates. These are highly protein bound (99 per cent) and, as such, have the potential to displace other highly protein-bound drugs such as warfarin. An increased fraction of free unbound drug elicits a more pronounced pharmacologic response (e.g., anticoagulation, in the case of warfarin). Metabolism of phenylbutazone may be accelerated by hepatic microsomal inducers, such as phenobarbital, griseofulvin, and phenytoin.

INDOMETHACIN. Indomethacin (Indocin, Merck, Sharp and Dohme) is one of the most potent inhibitors of cyclo-oxygenase. This drug has high potential for gastrointestinal toxicity in carnivores; cases of gastrointestinal hemorrhage following its use have been reported. Gastrointestinal toxicity is probably related to the extensive enterohepatic recirculation of the drug; it is recycled in the bile, resulting in repeated exposure of the gastrointestinal mucosa to the drug. A dose as low as 0.5 mg/kg may be toxic in dogs (Duggan et al., 1975). In contrast, the toxic dose in humans is approximately 20 mg/kg.

PROPIONIC ACID DERIVATIVES. The propionic acid derivatives include ibuprofen (Motrin, Upjohn; Advil, Whitehall) and naproxen (Naprosyn, Syntex; Equiproxen, Syntex). These drugs share the analgesic, antipyretic, and anti-inflammatory activities of aspirin. Ibuprofen is now widely available as an over-the-counter medication. Although its analgesic activity is less than that of aspirin in humans, it is preferred because of fewer gastrointestinal side effects. The drug appears to cause gastric irritation and ulcers more frequently in dogs than in humans. Gastrointestinal toxicity may be related to entero-hepatic circulation of this drug in dogs. There are reports of ibuprofen toxicity in dogs; after 2 to 6 days of treatment the drug consistently produced vomiting in dogs (Scherkl and Frey, 1987). It is rapidly absorbed following oral administration and is 96 per cent bound to plasm proteins. The elimination half-life of ibuprofen in dogs varies from 3.7 to 5.8 hr (Scherkl and Frey, 1987). This drug is not recommended for routine anti-inflammatory therapy because of the gastrointestinal toxicity and because it probably offers no advantages over other NSAIDs such as aspirin and phenylbutazone.

Naproxen is a relatively new NSAID. It is currently used in horses and humans, without a high incidence of adverse effects. However, dogs appear to be particularly sensitive to the gastrointestinal side-effects of this drug, a fact that may be accounted for by the tremendous interspecies variability in drug elimination. In humans, naproxen has an elimination half-life of approximately 12 hr; in horses, the half-life is 6 hr. In dogs, the half-life varies from 35 to 74 hr (Frey and Rieh, 1981). In dogs, the drug is rapidly absorbed following oral administration; peak plasma concentrations occur between 0.5 and 3 hr. The drug is greater than 99 per cent protein bound. Gastrointestinal changes were observed in dogs given 5 mg/kg daily; 15 mg/kg per day was clearly toxic. There are numerous reports of naproxen-induced hemorrhagic gastroenteropathy in dogs. However, this drug may be safely used in dogs at an initial dose of 5 mg/kg, followed by a daily maintenance dose of 2 mg/kg.

FLUNIXIN MEGLUMINE. Flunixin meglumine (Banamine, Schering) is a potent NSAID approved by the Food and Drug Administration (F.D.A.) for use in horses in the United States. Clinical trials of an oral preparation for dogs are currently under way for the treatment of acute exacerbations of chronic musculoskeletal disorders (hip dysplasia, osteoarthritis, and intervertebral disk disease). France has recently approved its use in dogs. The analgesic properties of flunixin are superior to those of aspirin and phenylbutazone. Flunixin has prolonged anti-inflammatory and analgesic efficacy despite its relatively short elimination half-life of 3.7 hr. It may have potential for the treatment of endotoxic shock in dogs.

PIROXICAM. Piroxicam (Feldene, Pfizer) is one of the newest NSAIDs for use in humans. In humans, this drug appears to be equivalent in efficacy to aspirin, indomethacin, and naproxen for treatment of osteoarthritis or rheumatoid arthritis. Its long half-life in humans (45 hr) permits administration of a single daily dose. It has a similar half-life in dogs. Like other NSAIDs, this drug may cause hemorrhagic gastroenteropathy. Until further safety and efficacy studies are available, use of piroxicam in dogs and cats is not recommended.

ACETAMINOPHEN. The para-aminophenol class of drugs, which includes acetaminophen and phenacetin, is widely used in humans and contains effective alternatives to aspirin as an analgesic-antipyretic. However, they possess weak anti-inflammatory activity by virtue of their weak cyclo-oxygenase inhibitory activity. Because cats are unable efficiently to metabolize and excrete acetaminophen (as is the situation with other phenolic drugs), acetaminophen causes a syndrome of acute toxicity in the cat, characterized by methemoglobinemia, hemolytic anemia, facial and forelimb edema, dyspnea, and death. One "extra-strength" acetaminophen capsule (Tylenol, McNeil, [500 mg]) produces toxic signs in cats, while two "extra-strength" capsules given within 24 hr can cause death.

THERAPEUTIC USES

The primary therapeutic indications for the NSAIDs include suppression of pain, inflammation, and platelet aggregation (Table 3). It is recommended that only familiar drugs, such as aspirin and phenylbutazone, that have been evaluated thoroughly in small animals be used. This recommendation is based on the potential toxicities of many of the newer NSAIDs in small animals and the lack of clinical data that demonstrate the superiority of the newer NSAIDs over traditional ones. In addition, the newer drugs are considerably more expensive in comparison with aspirin or phenylbutazone.

The NSAIDs are widely used in the management of arthritis (degenerative joint disease, immune-mediated disease), myositis, tendinitis, postsurgical inflammation, and other soft tissue and osseous inflammatory conditions. Both aspirin and phenylbutazone have been found to be successful in the treatment of symptoms of these conditions.

NSAIDs are effective in the relief of minor pain, particularly of musculoskeletal origin. These drugs are not effective in the treatment of severe somatic or visceral pain such as that associated with visceral distention or torsion.

Antiplatelet Therapy

Following a stimulus, arachidonic acid in platelets is preferentially metabolized to the prostanoid thromboxane, which is one of the most potent vasoconstrictor substances known. It is also a potent stimulus for platelet aggregation. NSAIDs inhibit thromboxane production and, thus, inhibit platelet aggregation and vasoconstriction. The effects of aspirin persist for the life of the platelet because platelets are unable to synthesize new enzymes, and acetylation of cyclo-oxygenase is permanent.

Table 3. NSAID Preparations and Dosages

Drug*	Dosage	Comments
Aspirin (many)	Dog: 25 mg/kg every 8 hr PO;	Anti-inflammatory; analgesic
	10 mg/kg once daily PO	Antiplatelet
	Cat: 25 mg/kg twice weekly PO;	Antiplatelet
	25 mg/kg once daily PO	Anti-inflammatory, analgesic
Phenylbutazone (many)	Dog: 22 mg/kg every 8 hr PO	Anti-inflammatory, analgesic
	Cat: Not recommended	
Naproxen (Naprosyn, Syntex; Equiproxen, Syntex)	Dog: 5 mg/kg initially PO; then 2.0 mg/kg every 24 hr	Anti-inflammatory; analgesic
	Cat: Not recommended	
Flunixin meglumine (Banamine, Schering)	Dog: 1.1 mg/kg daily IV for 3 days	Anti-inflammatory; analgesic (do not repeat course more often than every 2– weeks)
	Cat: Not recommended	

*Proprietary name in parentheses.
Key: PO, oral; IV, intravenous.

The ability of NSAIDs to inhibit platelet aggregation has been used in clinical medicine for a number of conditions including thromboembolism associated with feline cardiomyopathy, pulmonary vessel damage associated with canine dirofilariasis, thromboembolic disease, and disseminated intravascular coagulation.

Thrombus formation and embolization can occur in any of the forms of feline cardiomyopathy. Emboli may lodge and occlude any systemic artery but are usually found in the terminal aorta at the bifurcation of the iliac arteries. Platelets contribute to this disease by mechanical obstruction of the artery and by release of vasoactive substances. These substances, including thromboxane, cause vasoconstriction and promote further platelet aggregation. Aspirin inhibits platelet adhesion and aggregation, and has been recommended as therapy and prophylaxis for thromboemboli caused by feline cardiomyopathy. A dose of 25 mg/kg (one pediatric aspirin [90 mg]) twice weekly has been recommended for cats (Greene, 1985).

Adult heartworms (*Dirofilaria immitis*) cause damage to the endothelium of the pulmonary arteries. Following endothelial injury, platelets are activated, adhere, aggregate, and release platelet-derived growth factor. Platelet-mediated injury to pulmonary vessels has been extensively described in dogs. It is seen as extensive thromboembolism, villous proliferation, myointimal proliferation, and radiographic evidence of reduced blood flow to the caudal and accessory lung lobes. Treatment with aspirin lessened these deleterious changes via platelet inhibition and decreased synthesis of thromboxane A_2. Aspirin is given for 7 to 14 days prior to, and 21 to 28 days after, adulticide therapy (see p. 406, *Current Veterinary Therapy IX* for more information regarding the management of canine dirofilariasis).

Endotoxic Shock

Septic shock is a syndrome of cardiovascular collapse associated with severe overwhelming bacterial infection. Numerous early hemodynamic changes include portal hypertension, hepatosplanchnic pooling of blood, decreased cardiac output, and reduction in both central venous and systemic blood pressure. The early changes are transitory and are soon followed by a period in which values return to pre-shock levels. In the late phase of shock, blood pools in the gastrointestinal tract, followed by a life-threatening fall in cardiac output and systemic blood pressure.

Arachidonic acid metabolites such as thromboxane B_2 (the stable metabolite of thromboxane A_2) and 6-keto-prostaglandin $F_{1\alpha}$ (the stable metabolite of prostacyclin) are elevated in dogs with septic shock. Thromboxane B_2 concentrations increase in the early phases. Later, the 6-keto-prostaglandin $F_{1\alpha}$ concentrations rise in association with terminal hypotension. NSAIDs block the increases in prostanoids.

The role of NSAIDs in the treatment of overwhelming septic or endotoxic shock remains controversial. Experimental studies have demonstrated that these drugs increased systemic blood pressure and lessened metabolic acidosis in dogs (Hardie, Rawlings, and Collins, 1985). Increased cardiac output, increased stroke volume, increased plasma glucose concentration, decreased hemoconcentration, and improved respiratory function have been demonstrated. Short-term survival times are improved, but the effect on long-term survival has not been studied (Hardie, Rawlings, and Collins, 1985). There are no clinical studies that support the usefulness of NSAIDs in shock.

The clinical response to NSAIDs given to patients with naturally occurring endotoxic shock is difficult to predict because in experimental animals, NSAIDs were given before or shortly after administration of endotoxin or induction of peritonitis. Because early administration of NSAIDs appears to be an important factor for the efficacy of NSAIDs in endotoxic shock, the authors recommend that NSAIDs be administered early in the course of the disease.

Aspirin, phenylbutazone, and flunixin meglumine aid in the treatment of experimentally induced sepsis or endotoxemia in dogs. Flunixin has been recommended because of its greater potency in comparison with aspirin and phenylbutazone. In addition, there are no readily available injectable formulations of aspirin. Patients that receive NSAIDs for shock should be monitored for gastrointestinal hemorrhage and renal dysfunction.

Practitioners routinely give flunixin meglumine to dogs with parvovirus enteritis. NSAIDs may be beneficial in the management of secretory diarrheas in which prostaglandins play a role in stimulating intestinal fluid and electrolyte secretion via the activation of adenylate cyclase. However, the cause of diarrhea in canine parvovirus enteritis is increased permeability secondary to loss of villous epithelial cells. It is not caused by increased secretion. There have been no clinical studies supporting the benefit of flunixin in the treatment of canine parvovirus enteritis. The authors question whether flunixin meglumine provides an increased therapeutic response beyond what is achieved by aggressive fluid therapy and antibiotics.

ADVERSE EFFECTS

The NSAIDs share common toxicities, which usually can be attributed to their blockage of prostaglandin biosynthesis. These include gastric and intestinal ulceration, nephrotoxicity, decreased platelet aggregation, and prolongation of gestation. Less common effects include hypersensitivity reactions, methemoglobinemia, and Heinz body anemia. The overdosage of aspirin and acetaminophen produces acute intoxication, the clinical signs and treatment of which are described elsewhere (see pp. 188 and 524, *Current Veterinary Therapy IX*).

GASTROINTESTINAL TOXICITY. The most common adverse effect of NSAIDs is gastric or intestinal ulceration and, frequently, perforation. Anemia resulting from gastrointestinal blood loss may subsequently occur. Aspirin causes alterations in gastric mucosal ion transport and permeability, permitting backdiffusion of acid into the gastric interstitium. The latter results in microvascular damage, inflammation, and subsequent gastric ulceration and hemorrhage. All NSAIDs can cause this toxicity, but aspirin has been the most studied. The local effects of aspirin are via uptake into gastric epithelial cells; cellular damage probably results from shutdown of oxidative phosphorylation, decreased availability of adenosine triphosphate (ATP), decreased sodium-potassium transport, cell swelling, and necrosis. Local inflammation and necrosis are aggravated by decreased mucosal blood flow, decreased protective mucous secretion, decreased bicarbonate secretion, and decreased mucosal cell turnover and repair, all

of which can be attributed to impaired prostaglandin synthesis. These changes probably result from NSAID action on gastric PG synthesis. The gastric mucosa synthesizes PGE_2 and PGI_2, which inhibit acid secretion by the stomach and promote secretion of cytoprotective mucus and bicarbonate. Locally released PG may also maintain blood flow to the gastrointestinal mucosa and mediate gastric epithelial cell turnover and repair. There are numerous reports describing gastrointestinal ulceration and hemorrhage associated with the use of aspirin, naproxen, indomethacin, and piroxicam in dogs (see p. 911).

RENAL TOXICITY. Prostaglandins participate in a number of renal physiologic processes including autoregulation of renal blood flow, glomerular filtration, tubular ion transport, modulation of renin release, and water metabolism. Renal prostaglandin blockade from administration of NSAIDs is probably of little consequence in healthy animals. However, NSAIDs can markedly decrease renal blood flow, glomerular filtration rate, and sodium and water excretion in animals with (1) decreased circulating blood volume (such as occurs after water deprivation, diuretic administration, hemorrhage, and septic shock, or in association with the nephrotic syndrome), (2) other sodium-avid states (congestive heart failure, cirrhosis) or (3) pre-existing renal insufficiency. Acute renal failure in a dog, caused by administration of toxic doses of ibuprofen, has recently been described. Papillary necrosis has been described in horses given phenylbutazone. If treated with NSAIDs, patients may develop acute renal failure, papillary necrosis, or exacerbations of pre-existing renal insufficiency owing to ischemia resulting from blockade of prostaglandin synthesis.

HEMATOPOIETIC TOXICITY. Prolongation of bleeding time as a result of inhibition of platelet aggregation by NSAIDs may be a problem in patients with bleeding tendencies. This may be significant in patients with von Willebrand's disease, other coagulation disorders, or gastrointestinal ulceration.

Myelotoxicity associated with use of phenylbutazone has been reported in dogs. This reaction is common in humans, but is apparently rare in domestic animals. Toxicity is usually manifested by a severe agranulocytosis with milder suppression of erythrocytes and megakaryocytes.

References and Supplemental Reading

Calvert, C. A., and Rawlings, C. A.: Therapy of canine heartworm disease. *In* Kirk, R. W. (ed.): *Current Veterinary Therapy IX.* Philadelphia: W.B. Saunders Co., 1986, pp. 406–419.

Davis, L. E.: Clinical pharmacology of salicylates. J.A.V.M.A. 176:65, 1980.

Davis, L. E., and Westfall, B. A.: Species differences in biotransformation and excretion of salicylate. Am. J. Vet. Res. 33:1253, 1972.

Davis, L. E., Westfall, B. A., and Short, C. R.: Biotransformation and pharmacokinetics of salicylate in newborn animals. Am. J. Vet. Res. 34:1105, 1973.

Duggan, D. E., Hooke, K. F., and Noll, R. M.: Enterohepatic recirculation of indomethacin and its role in intestinal irritation. Biochem. Pharmacol. 25:1749, 1975.

Flower, R. J., Moncada, S., and Vane, J. R.: Analgesic-antipyretics and anti-inflammatory agents: Drugs employed in the treatment of gout. In Gilman, A. G., Goodman, L. S., Rall, T. W., et al. (eds.): The Pharmacologic Basis of Therapeutics, 7th èd. New York: Macmillan Publishing Co., 1986, pp. 674–715.

Frey, H. H., and Rieh, B.: Pharmacokinetics of naproxen in the dog. Am. J. Vet. Res. 42:1615, 1981.

Greene, C. E.: Effects of aspirin and propranolol on feline platelet aggregation. Am. J. Vet. Res. 46:1820, 1985.

Hangadama, P.: Salicylate toxicity. In Kirk, R. W. (ed.): Current Veterinary Therapy IX. Philadelphia: W.B. Saunders Co., 1986, pp. 524–527.

Hardie, E. M., Rawlings, C. A., and Collins, L. G.: Canine E. coli peritonitis: Long-term survival with fluid, gentamicin sulfate and flunixin meglumine treatment. J. Am. Anim. Hosp. Assoc. 21:681, 1985.

Higgins, A. J.: The biology, pathophysiology and control of eicosanoids in inflammation. J. Vet. Pharmacol. Ther. 8:1, 1985.

Higgins, A. J., and Lees, P.: The acute inflammatory process, arachidonic acid metabolism and the mode of action of anti-inflammatory drugs. Equine Vet. J. 16:163, 1984.

Lipowitz, A. J., Boulay, J. P., and Klausner, J. S.: Serum salicylate concentrations and endoscopic evaluation of the gastric mucosa in dogs after oral administration of aspirin-containing products. Am. J. Vet. Res. 47:1586, 1986.

Oehme, F. W.: Aspirin and acetaminophen. In Kirk, R. W. (ed.): Current Veterinary Therapy IX. Philadelphia: W.B. Saunders Co., 1986, pp. 188–190.

Rackear, D., Feldman, B., and Farver, T.: The effect of three different dosages of acetylsalicylic acid on canine platelet aggregation. J. Am. Anim. Hosp. Assoc. 24:23, 1988.

Ruckebusch, Y., and Toutain, P. L.: Nonsteroidal anti-inflammatory agents: Species differences in pharmacodynamics. Vet. Res. Com. 7:359, 1983.

Scherkl, R., and Frey, H. H.: Pharmacokinetics of ibuprofen in the dog. J. Vet. Pharmacol. Ther. 10:261, 1987.

Yeary, R. A., and Brant, R. J.: Aspirin dosages for the dog. J.A.V.M.A. 167:63, 1975.

Yeary, R. A., and Swanson, W.: Aspirin dosages for the cat. J.A.V.M.A. 163:1177, 1973.

GLUCOCORTICOID THERAPY

MARK G. PAPICH, D.V.M.,

Saskatoon, Saskatchewan

and LLOYD E. DAVIS, D.V.M.

Urbana, Illinois

METABOLIC EFFECTS

Carbohydrate, Protein, and Lipid Metabolism

Glucocorticoids, so named for their influence on carbohydrate metabolism, raise blood glucose concentrations via increased gluconeogenesis and insulin antagonism. There is a compensatory increase in insulin secretion to account for the corresponding hyperglycemia. Glucocorticoids may cause insulin resistance in tissues. Glucocorticoids inhibit insulin suppression of gluconeogenesis and induce the synthesis of hepatic enzymes that catalyze reactions of glucose synthesis (e.g., phosphoenolpyruvate carboxykinase and glucose-6-phosphatase).

Glucocorticoids also act to promote hepatic glycogen storage. Proteolytic and lipolytic effects of glucocorticoids produce free fatty acids and amino acids, substrates for hepatic glycogen. Increased protein breakdown, a well-known effect of glucocorticoids, is reflected during prolonged administration by muscle wasting, decreased fibroblast activity, osteoporosis, thin skin, and thin mucosal membranes. Lipolysis is also evident in peripheral tissues during prolonged glucocorticoid therapy.

Water and Electrolyte Balance

Cortisol and some synthetic glucocorticoids produce a mineralocorticoid response that promotes excretion of potassium, retention of sodium, and expansion of extracellular fluid volume. Synthetic glucocorticoids have been synthesized with minimal mineralocorticoid effects (Table 1). They are admin-

Table 1. Comparison of Various Glucocorticoid Bases

Drug	Duration of Action (hr)*	Comparative Potency†	Mineralo-corticoid Effects
Hydrocortisone (cortisol)	8–12	1	+2
Prednisolone	12–36	4	+1
Prednisone	12–36	4	+1
Methylprednisolone	12–36	5	0
Triamcinolone	12–36	5	0
Flumethasone	32–48	15	0
Dexamethasone	32–48‡	30	0
Betamethasone	32–48	30	0

*Based on duration of HPA-axis suppression.

†Potency is listed by arbitrarily assigning cortisol with a potency of 1.0. As value increases, so does potency.

‡Duration may be greater than 48 hr.

istered for systemic treatment of inflammatory conditions.

Commonly recognized side effects of glucocorticoid therapy are polydipsia and polyuria. Polyuria-polydipsia occurs in over 90 per cent of dogs administered glucocorticoids but is not observed in cats, even at high doses (Scott, 1980). Although the exact mechanism of polyuria-polydipsia in dogs given glucocorticoids is not known, increased glomerular filtration rate, inhibition of antidiuretic hormone action, or a direct action of glucocorticoids to decrease permeability of the renal distal tubules to water may account for this effect.

Adrenal Suppression

Glucocorticoids control their endogenous secretion via negative feedback on the anterior pituitary and hypothalamus. In dogs and cats, cortisol is the major adrenal glucocorticoid; its secretion is estimated to be approximately 1 mg/kg/day. In dogs, 24-hr cortisol secretion variations may be under circadian control, with highest secretion rates occurring in the morning. Results of studies establishing this rhythm have conflicted, as in some a circadian rhythm has been observed, whereas in other studies it was subtle (Kemppainen, 1986). It has been suggested that cats also have a circadian rhythm (Scott, 1980), but in cats the highest secretion occurs in the evening.

One intravenous injection of 0.1 mg/kg of dexamethasone can suppress the hypothalamic-pituitary-adrenal (HPA) axis for 32 hr in healthy dogs. The effect is dose-related, as suppression persisted for only 16 hr after a dose of 0.01 mg/kg (Kemppainen and Sartin, 1984). Prednisolone suppresses the HPA axis for 24 to 36 hr, while cortisol suppresses it for 12 to 24 hr (Table 1). Administration of glucocorticoids to dogs and cats for 1 to 2 weeks is unlikely to have a prolonged effect on the adrenal cortex. However, following prolonged administration, adrenal cortical atrophy is possible.

Recovery of adrenal function occurs relatively quickly in dogs and cats after chronic steroid administration. Adrenocorticotropin (ACTH) response tests have returned to normal three months after long-term steroid therapy was terminated (Scott, 1980). Cats are the most resistant domestic species with respect to adrenal glucocorticoid suppression. They recover more quickly than dogs and are very resistant to iatrogenic hyperadrenocorticism.

Recommendations to slowly reduce steroid doses in dogs and cats over several months were apparently based on studies in humans, who recover from adrenal suppression more slowly. In humans, one dose of dexamethasone can suppress the HPA axis for as long as 10 days; adrenal atrophy can occur following doses of prednisolone as low as 0.5 mg/

kg/day for 1 week (Kehrl and Fauci, 1983). Recovery of adrenal function after chronic therapy may take as long as 9 to 12 months in humans. Although adrenocortical insufficiency following long-term glucocorticoid therapy has been demonstrated in dogs and cats, via ACTH stimulation test results, clinical signs of iatrogenic hypoadrenocorticism have been uncommon. If signs of hypoadrenocorticism appear after terminating steroid therapy, hydrocortisone (1.0 mg/kg every 12 hr) or prednisolone (0.25 mg/kg/day) supplementation may be initiated. If a patient is stressed (e.g., requires surgery, goes on a trip) the doses should be doubled until the "stress" is relieved. Return of healthy adrenal function is best determined by an ACTH response test.

Adrenal suppression can also occur as a result of local or topical therapy with glucocorticoids. For example, ocular applications of prednisolone acetate (1.0 per cent) suppressed the HPA axis for 2 weeks (Roberts et al., 1984). Likewise, application of glucocorticoids to the skin of healthy dogs for 5 consecutive days suppressed ACTH response for 3 to 4 weeks following the last treatment (Zenoble and Kemppainen, 1987). Based on results of these studies, the possibility of iatrogenic hypoadrenocorticism should be considered when discontinuing long-term topical steroid therapy.

Because mineralocorticoid secretion is only minimally affected by ACTH, mineralocorticoid secretion is not normally suppressed by glucocorticoid therapy. Angiotensin II is the primary stimulus for mineralocorticoid secretion; hypoaldosteronemia is unlikely following prolonged glucocorticoid therapy.

ANTI-INFLAMMATORY AND IMMUNOSUPPRESSIVE EFFECTS

Overview

The exact nature of anti-inflammatory action of glucocorticoids in dogs and cats is not precisely understood. One reason is that much of the research on the anti-inflammatory and immunosuppressive effects of glucocorticoids has been carried out in glucocorticoid-sensitive species such as rats, rabbits, and mice; results of these studies may not apply to domestic animals. Because humans are more sensitive to steroids than are dogs and cats, similar cautions apply to results from studies in humans. In addition, experimental studies usually are performed in normal animals, and it has not been determined whether steroids affect animals with hyperimmune syndromes and inflammatory disease differently from normal animals. Also, in vitro studies utilizing tissue preparations or blood cells involved use of glucocorticoid concentrations that were higher than those achieved in vivo. The steroid effects observed during *in vitro* studies may not occur at usual therapeutic concentrations.

The anti-inflammatory and immunomodulating effects of the glucocorticoids have been reviewed (Cupps and Fauci, 1982; Kerhl and Fauci, 1983; Dannenberg, 1979; Fauci, 1978–1979; Meuleman and Katz, 1985). In general, the following effects have been observed:

1. Polymorphonuclear neutrophils (PMNs): decreased migration and egress into inflammatory tissue.

2. Lymphocytes: decreased circulation of T-cell lymphocytes and suppressed lymphocyte activation.

3. Blood Vessels: decreased vascular permeability.

4. Arachidonic acid metabolites: decreased prostaglandin, prostacyclin, thromboxane, and leukotriene synthesis.

Polymorphonuclear Neutrophils

MEMBRANE EFFECTS. Decreased migration of PMNs from blood vessels into inflammatory tissue is a profound anti-inflammatory effect of glucocorticoids. Shortly after administration of a pharmacologic dose, neutrophilia occurs as a result of increased release of cells from the maturation pool of the bone marrow, and decreased egress of cells from vessels via diapedesis. Because neutrophils mature within hours, inhibition of their egress results in a rapidly developing mature neutrophilia. The mechanism for decreased egress may be related to a cell surface configurational change that results in decreased vessel margination and adherence.

Cell membranes may be stabilized by glucocorticoids. However, stabilization of lysosomal membranes occurs only at suprapharmacologic concentrations, which are not achieved *in vivo* following conventional dosages. Therefore, lysosomal membrane stabilization may not be a true anti-inflammatory effect of glucocorticoids (Meuleman and Katz, 1985; Fauci, 1978–1979; Cupps and Fauci, 1982).

PHAGOCYTOSIS. The influence of steroids on phagocytosis and destruction of bacteria is incompletely understood. There appears to be species differences in the effect of glucocorticoids on phagocytosis, and the assay techniques used have been variable. In humans and cattle, corticosteroids depress or have no effect on bacterial phagocytosis. In horses and goats, bacterial phagocytosis does not appear to be affected by corticosteroids. Corticosteroids may impair the ability of neutrophils to kill ingested bacteria. However, use of different assay techniques and species differences preclude such specific statements. Corticosteroids may hinder microbicidal activity by decreasing oxidative metabolism in cattle and humans. However, in other animals, the mechanism for decreased microbicidal activity has not been identified. It may be related to impaired respiratory burst, decreased fusion of neutrophil granules to lysosomes, or an effect on the pH in the lysosomes of phagocytes. Regardless of the mechanism involved, corticosteroids render a patient more susceptible to infection because of impaired bacterial killing.

Lymphocytes

Following administration of pharmacologic doses of glucocorticoids, lymphopenia occurs. In steroid-sensitive animals (mice, rats, and rabbits), lymphocytolysis contributes to the lymphopenia. In steroid-resistant animals (humans, horses, cattle, dogs, and cats) lysis of normal lymphocytes does not occur. A notable exception is neoplastic lymphocytes.

Lymphopenia is the result of changes in lymphocyte migration. The lymphocyte population is composed of a circulating pool and a noncirculating pool (Fauci, 1978–1979). The circulating pool freely moves between the intravascular compartment and the extravascular compartment (lymph nodes, spleen, bone marrow, and thoracic duct). Following glucocorticoid administration, lymphocytes of the circulating pool redistribute to the extravascular compartment. T-cell lymphocytes are affected more than B-cells (T-cells constitute approximately 70 per cent of the circulating pool). The discrepancy in lymphocyte responses is not easily explained, but the ability of B-cells to metabolize glucocorticoids faster than T-cells may be involved (Kehrl and Fauci, 1983; Cupps and Fauci, 1982).

A decrease in circulating lymphocytes reduces their participation in immunologic and inflammatory reactions. The proliferative response of lymphocytes is also suppressed by glucocorticoids. Decreased response to mitogens, suppressed lymphokine synthesis, suppressed proliferation, and decreased transformation, antigen recognition, and cytotoxic ability all have been observed (Meuleman and Katz, 1985; Cupps and Fauci, 1982).

The response of B-cell lymphocytes to glucocorticoids is more complicated. Glucocorticoids have few direct effects on B-cells but affect B-cell function indirectly by modulating the accessory cells. Full expression of lymphocyte function requires a complex series of interactions between T-cells (helper), macrophages, antigens, and cell mediators (Nossal, 1987). Therapeutic doses of glucocorticoids do not decrease an animal's ability to mount a normal immunologic response (e.g., from vaccinations) (Nara et al., 1979; Meuleman and Katz, 1985). However, as doses increase, concentrations of immunoglobulin G (IgG), IgA, and, to a lesser extent, IgM are decreased. Synthesis of IgE is not affected. Studies in humans suggest that repeated daily doses of long-acting corticosteroids (e.g., dexamethasone) suppress antibody synthesis, but alternate-day administration of anti-inflammatory doses of an intermediate-acting glucocorticosteroid (e.g., prednisolone) does not.

Macrophages

Lymphocyte accessory cells (monocytes and macrophages) appear to be more sensitive to glucocorticoid effects than PMNs. Therapeutic doses of glucocorticoids decrease phagocytosis and bactericidal activity and diminish the cells' ability to process antigens for presentation to B-cells. Synthesis of cell mediators (specifically, interleukin-1) also may be suppressed. Glucocorticoids are potent inhibitors of both lymphokine synthesis and the cellular response to lymphokines (Dinarello and Mier, 1987; Cupps and Fauci, 1982).

Arachidonic Acid Metabolism

The arachidonic acid cascade and its role in inflammation has been reviewed (see pp. 47–54). The prostaglandin-leukotriene cascade begins with injury to cell membranes, which triggers the activity of a specific phospholipase (phospholipase-A_2) in cell membranes to form arachidonic acid. The enzymes cyclo-oxygenase and lipoxygenase form prostacyclin, thromboxane, and leukotrienes from arachidonic acid. Cells exposed to pharmacologic concentrations of glucocorticoids synthesize phospholipase A_2–inhibitory proteins (lipomodulin and macrocortin), which suppress arachidonic acid metabolism (Hirata, 1980, 1983). An immediate antiprostaglandin effect may not be observed for several hours after glucocorticoid administration, the time necessary for cell induction and synthesis of phospholipase inhibitors.

Effects on Vessels

Stabilization of microvascular integrity occurs following administration of glucocorticoids. The benefits of glucocorticoids in shock, central nervous system edema, and other diseases are associated with their ability to improve microvascular stability, which, in turn, reduces edema formation and extravasation of cells from the vasculature to tissues.

The beneficial effects on the vasculature are attributed to suppressed PMN action and decreased prostaglandin synthesis. It has been suggested that glucocorticoids also antagonize vasoactive substances (e.g., histamine, kinins) and thereby protect against the toxic effects of free oxygen radicals released during inflammation. Additionally, glucocorticoids appear to decrease the synthesis of plasminogen activator by macrophages (Kehrl and Fauci, 1983). Macrophages release a plasminogen activator as part of the cascade of reactions during inflammation. Activated plasmin digests supporting tissue of vessels and enhances vascular permeability.

Summary of Anti-inflammatory Effects

The anti-inflammatory and immunosuppressive effects of glucocorticoids are attributed to complete or partial suppression of a complex interaction of cells and cell mediators. It is clear that the potent effects of glucocorticoids on leukocytes are responsible for most of the anti-inflammatory activity. These effects are also immunosuppressive, which accounts for their efficacy in immune-mediated disease. However, use of glucocorticoids can lead to increased susceptibility to infection.

GLUCOCORTICOID PREPARATIONS

Structure—Activity Relationships

An understanding of the basic ring structure of glucocorticoids and the essential features that are responsible for glucocorticoid action has led to the synthesis of several preparations. The modifications of cortisol (hydrocortisone) are shown in Figure 1. The essential features of the structure for glucocorticoid activity are (1) the C-11 hydroxyl, (2) a ketone at C-20 and at C-3, and (3) a double bond between the fourth and fifth carbons. Additions of a double bond between the first and second carbons, methyl groups at C-6 or C-16, and fluorine to C-9 are examples of additions that increase the biologic half-life of glucocorticoids, decrease their mineralocorticoid potency, and substantially increase their anti-inflammatory action (Table 1; Fig. 1). Corticosteroids are not active unless they possess the proper functional groups. For example, activation of prednisone and cortisone requires hydroxylation at C-11 by hepatic reductive enzymes to form either prednisolone or cortisol.

When choosing systemic glucocorticoid therapy, it is not critical whether prednisolone or prednisone is used. They are equal therapeutically. However, prednisone and cortisone are not effective when applied topically, because they have not been converted to the active molecule. If an animal has hepatic dysfunction, conversion from prednisone to prednisolone may be delayed. However, because drug protein binding may be decreased, and because elimination of the active drug may be slowed, it has not been possible to demonstrate a disadvan-

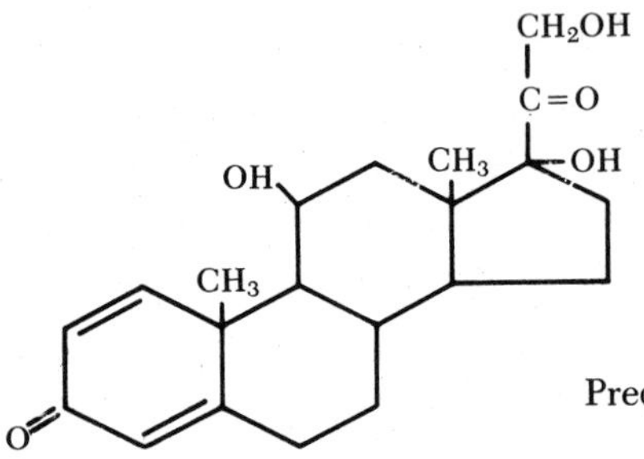

Prednisolone

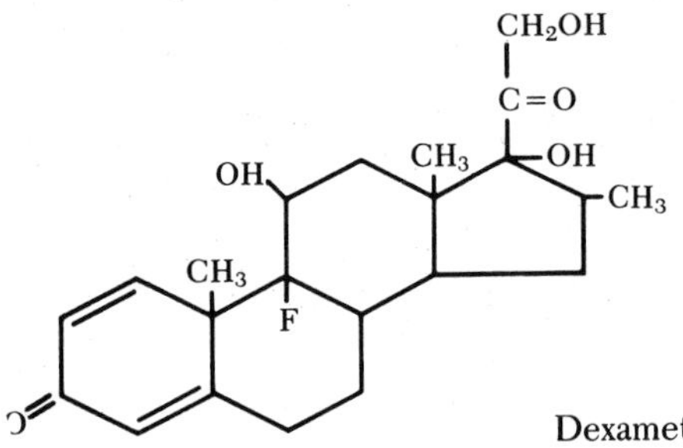

Figure 1. Synthetic corticosteroids. Structural differences between synthetic prednisolone and dexamethasone.

Dexamethasone

tage in administering prednisone instead of prednisolone to patients with liver disease.

Comparison of Glucocorticoids

The comparative potencies and duration of HPA suppression for commonly used glucocorticoids are listed in Table 1. As the biologic half-life increases, the anti-inflammatory potency increases, and mineralocorticoid potency diminishes. Failure to recognize the potency of glucocorticoids can result in serious problems in dosing. For example, if an animal was stabilized on 1 mg/kg of dexamethasone and then was switched to prednisolone, 7 to 8 mg/kg of prednisolone would have to be administered to give an equivalent anti-inflammatory dose.

The pharmacokinetics of various glucocorticoid preparations have been examined in several species. In dogs, the plasma half-life of hydrocortisone has been reported to be 52 minutes; for prednisolone, it has been reported to be 80 minutes (Frey et al., 1980) and 166 to 197 minutes (Hankes et al., 1985); and for dexamethasone, it was 119 to 136 minutes (Toutain et al., 1983). The rate of plasma elimination does not appear to account for the observed differences in the biologic duration of action of these drugs in dogs (Table 1).

Steroid Esters

As there are various glucocorticoid bases available, so too are there different injectable formula-

tions of each base. Some of the forms available for administration to animals are listed on Table 2, and some of the substitutions made on the steroid base are shown in Figure 2.

Formulations used for acute conditions should be administered via an intravenous injection or infusion and must be water soluble. The sodium phosphate and sodium succinate esters are polar and highly water soluble and can be administered in concentrated solutions. Glucocorticoid esters must be converted to the parent drug to become active. This occurs rapidly; the half-life of conversion is 9 to 11 min (Coppoc, 1984). Dexamethasone base is poorly soluble in water but is available as an injectable preparation in solution with propylene glycol (Azium, Schering Animal Health).

Table 2. Injectable Preparations of Glucocorticoids

Hydrocortisone sodium succinate (Solu-Cortef, Upjohn)
Prednisolone sodium succinate (Solu-Delta-Cortef, Upjohn)
Prednisolone sodium phosphate (Cortisate-20, Schering Animal Health)
Prednisolone acetate (Neo-Delta-Cortef, Upjohn)
Prednisolone suspension (Meticorten, Schering Animal Health)
Methylprednisolone sodium succinate (Solu-Medrol, Upjohn)
Methylprednisolone acetate (Depo-Medrol, Upjohn)
Triamcinolone acetonide (Vetalog, Squibb)
Betamethasone dipropionate and betamethasone sodium phosphate (Betasone, Schering Animal Health)
Dexamethasone solution (Azium, Schering Animal Health)
Dexamethasone sodium phosphate (Azium SP, Schering Animal Health)

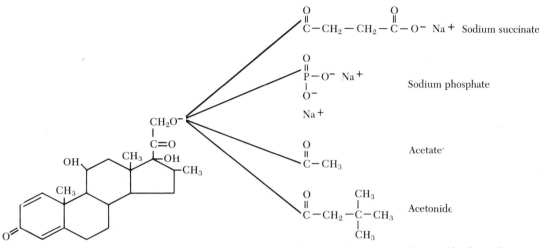

Figure 2. Esters of glucocorticosteroids. Glucocorticoid structure illustrating various esters that may bind to carbon 21.

There has been considerable debate as to which corticosteroid and steroid salt is the most rapidly acting and is therefore best suited for acute needs. Most experimental studies utilizing methylprednisolone sodium succinate for shock and central nervous system trauma have shown that this ester is effective. Other studies have demonstrated the effectiveness of dexamethasone solution (in propylene glycol) (Ferguson et al., 1978; Grinstein-Nadler and Bottoms, 1976). In comparative studies, it has been difficult to demonstrate differences between sodium phosphate and sodium succinate esters. However, Hoerlein and coworkers (1985) reported that methylprednisolone sodium succinate performed better than dexamethasone sodium phosphate for treatment of spinal cord trauma in cats. Shatney and colleagues (1982) reported no difference between the two esters in canine models of septic shock; however, methylprednisolone sodium succinate was more effective than dexamethasone sodium phosphate in models of cardiogenic shock.

Other injectable steroid preparations include the acetate and acetonide esters (Table 2; Fig. 2). These preparations are very insoluble, release steroids slowly, and exert an anti-inflammatory effect and HPA-axis suppression for days to weeks. After one injection, triamcinolone acetonide's effect persists for 7 to 15 days, while methylprednisolone acetate's effect persists for 14 to 21 days.

CLINICAL USES OF CORTICOSTEROIDS

Adverse Effects

Corticosteroids may have adverse effects on metabolism, protein synthesis, host defense mechanisms, and the HPA-axis. There are a number of other adverse effects that have been recognized in animals (Table 3).

Central Nervous System Diseases

Glucocorticoids are used for treatment of both brain and spinal cord disease. Most often, they are administered following trauma, but they have also been used to temporarily decrease edema associated with brain neoplasms.

The benefits of glucocorticoids in central nervous system disease are associated with protection of cellular membranes from the toxic effects of oxygen-derived free radicals, improvement in microvascular integrity, stabilization of central nervous system intercellular tight junctions, decreased edema formation, and decreased intracranial pressure as a result of decreased cerebrospinal fluid formation.

Table 3. *Potential Adverse Effects of Glucocorticoids*

Central Nervous System	Metabolic
Polyphagia	Hyperlipidemia
Euphoria	Lipolysis
Musculoskeletal System	Protein catabolism
Osteoporosis	Fatty infiltration of liver
Myopathy	Steroid hepatopathy
Fibroblast inhibition	**Endocrine**
Decreased intestinal calcium	HPA-axis suppression
absorption	Diabetogenic
Gastrointestinal System	Decreased thyroid synthesis
GI ulceration	Increased parathyroid hormone
Pancreatitis	mone
Colonic perforation	**Host Defenses**
Fluid Balance	Decreased bacterial killing
Sodium and fluid retention	Increased risk of septicemia
Polyuria and polydipsia	Recurrent septic cystitis

BRAIN TRAUMA. Metz and coworkers (1982) reviewed the distinction between various forms of edema that can occur in the brain. Steroids appear to be ineffective for treatment of cytotoxic and interstitial edema but may be beneficial for vasogenic edema associated with neoplasia, trauma, hemorrhage, contusion, or abscesses. Veterinary textbooks recommend dexamethasone for the management of acute head injury, although studies in humans have not demonstrated a beneficial effect (Cooper et al., 1979).

SPINAL CORD TRAUMA. Glucocorticoids may be effective in diminishing the pathologic effects of spinal trauma. Effects of trauma on the spinal cord include (1) hypoxia and (2) generation of oxygen radicals in cell membranes. Lipid peroxidation of cell membranes leads to a loss of membrane enzyme function (sodium and potassium ATPase) and cellular swelling (Hall and Braughler, 1982). Release of catecholamines may play a role in producing spinal cord vasoconstriction as well. Glucocorticoids may improve function by interfering with norepinephrine-induced ischemia and by preventing oxygen free radical peroxidation in myelin, neuronal, glial, and vessel membranes.

SIDE EFFECTS. Toombs and colleagues (1986) summarized the gastrointestinal complications associated with glucocorticoid administration in dogs. Neurosurgical patients with spinal cord disease received dexamethasone at relatively high doses (2.7 to 15.5 mg/kg). The mortality rate was high. Neurologic injury and dysfunction, surgical stress, and glucocorticoids may be interrelated in the development of gastrointestinal ulceration and perforation. The exact sequence of pathologic events is uncertain, but it is believed that a compromise in bowel motility and blood supply compounded by decreased mucous production, and decreased mucosal cell turnover by glucocorticoids contribute to the lesions (Sorjonen et al., 1983). There are no reports available that assess the efficacy of gastric acid–suppressing drugs (e.g., cimetidine, ranitidine) or mucosal protectants (e.g., sucralfate, kaolin-pectin) in the prevention of gastrointestinal complications associated with glucocorticoid administration.

DOSAGES. If corticosteroids are administered for spinal cord trauma, there should be convincing evidence that the benefits of therapy outweigh potential adverse effects. The benefits of steroids have been demonstrated only in experimental studies in which the drugs were administered within 1 hr of spinal cord trauma. There are no clinical studies that demonstrate a benefit. Nevertheless, available reports suggest that relatively high doses are necessary. Hall and Braughler (1982) compared various doses used for spinal cord trauma in cats; they concluded that doses of methylprednisolone of at least 15 to 30 mg/kg were needed to prevent spinal cord lipid peroxidation. These doses correspond to 2.5 to 5.0 mg/kg of dexamethasone. Further work (Braughler and Hall, 1982) suggested that animals should be retreated 3 to 4 hr after a dose of glucocorticoids because methylprednisolone had a half-life of approximately 3 hr. Hoerlein and coworkers (1985) treated cats with experimentally induced spinal cord lesions with tapering doses of methylprednisolone. Cats that received methylprednisolone showed a significant improvement in comparison with cats that underwent other medical and surgical treatment. They noted that daily doses of at least 30 mg/kg were necessary for a beneficial effect.

In veterinary textbooks, there has been a lack of consistency respecting corticosteroid dosage recommendations; dosages for dexamethasone have varied from 2.5 mg/kg every 8 hr to 0.2 mg/kg/day. Currently, the authors recommend the use of prednisolone or methylprednisolone because these drugs are less potent and have a shorter duration of action than dexamethasone. A glucocorticoid with a short duration of action (e.g., prednisolone) may decrease the adverse effects seen with long-acting corticosteroids. Initial dosages may range from 15 to 30 mg/kg of prednisolone or methylprednisolone, followed by gradual reduction to an anti-inflammatory dosage of 1 to 2 mg/kg every 12 hr. There is no information to support their administration for longer than 5 to 7 days.

CANINE ASEPTIC MENINGITIS. A group of canine meningitides deserves special mention because these diseases are responsive to steroids (Meric, 1988). The steroid-responsive diseases are granulomatous meningoencephalitis (GME), steroid-responsive suppurative meningitis, and necrotizing vasculitis of the central nervous system. All are of unknown etiology. Affected dogs respond to prednisolone at dosages of 2 to 4 mg/kg/day, followed by gradual reduction of dose until it is administered on an every-other-day basis. Following the induction period, tapering to a lower dose should occur over 1 to 2 months. Their response to corticosteroids can be dramatic. Dogs with GME often respond to a slightly lower dose of 1 to 2 mg/kg/day, which often can be tapered slowly and administered every other day.

Immune-Mediated Disease

Common indications for glucocorticoid administration include immune-mediated skin disease, hemolytic anemia, and thrombocytopenia. In a hemolytic or thrombocytopenic crisis, glucocorticoids can be life saving. Doses suggested for immune-mediated diseases are 2.2 to 6.6 mg/kg of prednisolone or prednisone (total daily dose). For the initial induction period, the daily dose is divided and administered every 8 or 12 hr. An initial dose of a rapid-acting formulation may be given parenterally and doses thereafter can be administered PO. High induction doses should be administered for 7 to 10 days, or as needed, depending on the patient's response. It appears that cats require higher doses than dogs, sometimes almost double the canine dose. In a recent review of the management of immune-mediated dermatoses (Scott et al., 1987), the best results (i.e., best remission with least adverse effects) were achieved with doses within the range of 2.2 to 6.6 mg/kg. Induction doses were 4.4 mg/kg/day for dogs and 6.6 mg/kg/day for cats. Once induction therapy has been completed, the dose of glucocorticoids should be gradually reduced. Following an initial dose administered every 12 hr, first lengthen the dose interval to every 24 hr for another 7 to 10 days. Next, decrease the dose by one half for another 7 to 10 days, followed by increasing the dose interval to every 48 hr. Thereafter, the dose should be progressively decreased until the animal is stable on as low a dose as possible. For many diseases (e.g., systemic lupus erythematosus, pemphigus, and hemolytic disorders) do not expect a dose reduction below 1 mg/kg of prednisolone every 48 hr, unless the animal's disease spontaneously regresses. Some patients cannot be maintained on therapy given every other day; others may require adjunctive immunosuppressive therapy (e.g., cyclophosphamide, azathioprine, aurothioglucose).

Glucocorticoids in the Treatment of Shock

Shock is characterized by poor perfusion of organs and tissues; the goal of treatment is the maintenance or re-establishment of normal intravascular volume and tissue perfusion. Therefore, therapy should be focused on volume replacement and correcting the underlying cause of shock. In spite of this logical approach, there have been hundreds of studies examining the pros and cons of corticosteroids, their doses, timing, and the most effective steroid ester.

Shock can be cardiogenic, hypovolemic, or septic (endotoxic) in origin. Effective therapy for cardiogenic shock requires restoration of cardiac function and cardiac output. Despite slight positive inotropic effects associated with corticosteroid therapy, they are not indicated for cardiogenic shock.

HEMORRHAGIC SHOCK. Glucocorticoids used in the treatment of hemorrhagic shock in dogs were associated with a dramatic positive benefit, as they demonstrated an improvement in blood pressure as early as 3 min after steroid administration (Grinstein-Nadler and Bottoms, 1976; Ferguson et al., 1978). Large doses of steroids were required (5 mg/kg of dexamethasone). Other studies also support the use of large doses to reverse the signs of shock.

The reported benefits of glucocorticoids in hemorrhagic shock are (1) improved integrity of microcirculation and blood flow in viscera, (2) stabilization of cell membranes against the toxic effects of oxygen radicals that are produced during ischemia, and (3) increased gluconeogenesis. Ferguson and associates (1978) reported that beneficial effects occurred independent of an increase in blood pressure.

The use of glucocorticoids for hemorrhagic shock (prednisolone or methylprednisolone, 15 to 30 mg/kg; and dexamethasone, 4 to 8 mg/kg) may be beneficial, but they should not be used as a substitute for aggressive fluid therapy and other support. Timing is critical. Many studies have demonstrated that glucocorticoid treatment initiated later than 30 min after the onset of shock was too late for optimum effectiveness.

SEPTIC SHOCK. Results of several studies have demonstrated the benefits of glucocorticoids in experimental shock; however, controversy surrounds their clinical use. The reported beneficial effects of glucocorticoids include (1) improved vascular integrity, (2) increased regional blood flow, and (3) decreased synthesis of arachidonic acid metabolites. Glucocorticoids at high doses can prevent mortality from gram-negative sepsis that is not preventable by antibiotics alone (Greisman, 1982; Hinshaw et al., 1982). If administered with antibiotics, steroids may facilitate antibiotic delivery to tissues by improving microvascular circulation.

The following points about steroid use in septic shock are emphasized:

1. Optimum doses must be used. Beneficial results have been associated with doses of 15 to 30 mg/kg of methylprednisolone or prednisolone, and of 4 to 6 mg/kg of dexamethasone. Lower doses are inconsistently associated with a positive effect.

2. Timing is critical. The earlier the steroid is given after bacterial or endotoxin challenge, the greater its protective effect. Delays in steroid use longer than 1 hr following administration of toxin greatly annulled their protective effect. When treatment was delayed longer than 4 hr, there was a marked reduction in benefit.

3. Additional doses may be necessary. Additional steroid treatments for shock at 4- to 6-hr intervals improved survival. However, improvement associated with each additional dose became progressively less.

While glucocorticoids can prevent death in laboratory animals when administered before, or concurrently with, lethal doses of endotoxin, studies that demonstrate a benefit in preventing death from overwhelming gram-negative bacterial sepsis are less conclusive. Moreover, one must be aware of the potential adverse effects. Experimental studies rarely are long enough to evaluate adverse effects from secondary infections. Results from clinical studies in humans suggest that this is an important complication (Bone et al., 1987; Hinshaw et al.,

1987). In a veterinary survey (Calvert and Greene, 1986), administration of glucocorticoids was the most common single factor that contributed, or predisposed dogs, to bacteremia.

References and Supplemental Reading

Bone, R. C., Fisher, C. J., Clemmer, T. P., et al.: A controlled clinical trial of high-dose methylprednisolone in the treatment of severe sepsis and septic shock. N. Engl. J. Med. 317:653, 1987.

Braughler, J. M., and Hall, E. D.: Correlation of methylprednisolone levels in cat spinal cord with its effects on sodium potassium ATPase, lipid peroxidation and alpha motor neuron function. J. Neurosurg. 56:838, 1982.

Calvert, C. A., and Greene, C. E.: Bacteremia in dogs: Diagnosis, treatment, and prognosis. Compend. Cont. Ed. 8:179, 1986.

Cooper, P. R., Moody, S., Clark, W. K., et al.: Dexamethasone and severe head injury. J. Neurosurg. 51:307, 1979.

Coppoc, G. L.: Relationships of the dosage form of a corticosteroid to its therapeutic efficacy. J.A.V.M.A. 185:1098, 1984.

Cupps, T. R., and Fauci, A. S.: Corticosteroid-mediated immunoregulation in man. Immunol. Rev. 65:133, 1982.

Dannenberg, A. M.: The anti-inflammatory effects of glucocorticoids: A review of the literature. Inflammation 3:329, 1979.

Dinarello, C. A., and Mier, J. W.: Lymphokines. N. Engl. J. Med. 317:940, 1987.

Fauci, A. S.: Mechanism of the immunosuppressive and anti-inflammatory effects of glucocorticoids. J. Immunopharmacol. 1:1, 1978–1979.

Ferguson J. L., Bottoms, G. D., Corwin, D., et al.: Dexamethasone treatment during hemorrhagic shock: Effects independent of increased blood pressure. Am. J. Vet. Res. 39:825, 1978.

Frey, F. J., Frey, B. M., Gireither, A., et al.: Prednisolone clearance at steady state in dogs. J. Pharmacol. Exp. Ther. 215:287, 1980.

Greisman, S. E.: Experimental gram-negative bacterial sepsis: Optimal methylprednisolone requirements for prevention of mortality not preventable by antibiotics alone. Proc. Soc. Exp. Biol. Med. 170:436, 1982.

Grinstein-Nadler, E., and Bottoms, G. D.: Dexamethasone treatment during hemorrhagic shock: Changes in extracellular fluid volume and cell membrane transport. Am. J. Vet. Res. 37:1337, 1976.

Hall, E. D., and Braughler, J. M.: Effects of intravenous methylprednisolone in spinal cord peroxidation and sodium and potassium ATPase reactivity. J. Neurosurg. 57:247, 1982.

Hankes, G. H., Lazenby, L. R., Raves, W. R., et al.: Pharmacokinetics of prednisolone sodium succinate and its metabolites in normovolemic and hypovolemic dogs. Am. J. Vet. Res. 46:476, 1985.

Hinshaw, L. B., Beller-Todd, B. K., and Archer, L. T.: Review update: Current management of the septic shock patient: Experimental basis for treatment. Circ. Shock 9:543, 1982.

Hinshaw, L., Peduzzi, P., Young, E., et al.: Effect of high-dose gluco-

corticoid therapy on mortality in patients with clinical signs of systemic sepsis. N. Engl. J. Med. 317:659, 1987.

Hirata, F.: Lipomodulin: A possible mediator of the action of glucocorticoids. In Samuelsson, B., Paoletti, R., and Ramwell, P. (eds.): Advances in Prostaglandin, Thromboxane, and Leukotriene Research. New York: Raven Press, 1983, pp. 73–78.

Hirata, F., Schiffmann, E., Venkatasubramanian, K., et al.: A phospholipase A-2 inhibitory protein in rabbit neutrophils induced by glucocorticoids. Proc. Natl. Acad. Sci. (USA) 77:2533, 1980.

Hoerlein, B. F., Redding, R. W., Hoff, E. J., et al.: Evaluation of naloxone, crocetin, thyrotropin-releasing hormone, methylprednisolone, partial myelotomy, and hemilaminectomy in the treatment of acute spinal cord trauma. J. Am. Anim. Hosp. Assoc. 21:67, 1985.

Kehrl, J. H., and Fauci, A. S.: The clinical use of glucocorticoids. Ann. Allergy 50:2, 1983.

Kemppainen, R. J.: Glucocorticoids. In Kirk, R. W. (ed.): Current Veterinary Therapy IX. Philadelphia: W.B. Saunders Co., 1986.

Kemppainen, R. J., and Sartin, J. L.: Effects of single intravenous doses of dexamethasone on baseline cortisol concentrations and responses to synthetic ACTH in healthy dogs. Am. J. Vet. Res. 45:742, 1984.

Meric, S.: Canine meningitis: A changing emphasis. J. Vet. Int. Med. (in press).

Metz, S. R., Taylor, S. R., and Kay, W. J.: The use of corticosteroids for treatment of neurologic disease. Vet Clin North Am. [Small Animal Pract] 12:41, 1982.

Meuleman, J., and Katz, P.: The immunologic effects, kinetics and use of glucocorticoids. Med. Clin. North Am. 69:805, 1985.

Nara, P. L., Krahwoka, S., and Powers, T. E.: Effect of prednisolone on the development of immune response to canine distemper virus in beagle pups. Am. J. Vet. Res. 40:1742, 1979.

Nossal, G. J. V.: The basic components of the immune system. N. Engl. J. Med. 316:1320, 1987.

Roberts, S. M., Lavach, J. D., Macy, D. W., et al.: Effect of ophthalmic prednisolone acetate on the canine adrenal gland and hepatic function. Am. J. Vet. Res. 45:1711, 1984.

Scott, D. W.: Systemic glucocorticoid therapy. In Kirk, R. W. (ed.): Current Veterinary Therapy VII. Philadelphia: W.B. Saunders Co., 1980, pp. 988–994.

Scott, D. W., Walton, D. K., Slator, M. R., et al.: Immune-mediated dermatoses in domestic animals: Ten years after—Parts I and II. Compend. Cont. Educ. 9:424, 539, 1987.

Shatney, C. H., Lillehei, R. C., Dietzman, R. H., et al.: Influence of the salt moiety on the effectiveness of corticosteroid therapy in cardiogenic shock. Circ. Shock 9:247, 1982.

Sorjonen, D. C., Dillon, A. R., Powers, R. D., et al.: Effects of dexamethasone and surgical hypotension on the stomach of dogs: Clinical, endoscopic, and pathologic evaluations. Am. J. Vet. Res. 44:1233, 1983.

Toombs, J. P., Collins, L. G., Graves, G. M., et al.: Colonic perforation in corticosteroid-treated dogs. J.A.V.M.A. 188:145, 1986.

Toutain, P. L., Alvinerie, M., and Ruckebusch, Y.: Pharmacokinetics of dexamethasone and its effect on adrenal gland function in the dog. Am. J. Vet. Res. 44:212, 1983.

Zenoble, R. D., and Kemppainen, R. J.: Adrenocortical suppression by topically applied corticosteroids in healthy dogs. J.A.V.M.A. 191:685, 1987.

CHEMICAL RESTRAINT TECHNIQUES IN DOGS AND CATS

RONALD E. MANDSAGER, D.V.M.,
and MARC R. RAFFE, D.V.M.

St. Paul, Minnesota

Chemical restraint is often necessary in small animal practice to facilitate diagnostic or therapeutic procedures. Chemical restraint should be considered in (1) painful procedures (e.g., dental work, wound débridements), (2) procedures that require patient cooperation (e.g., pelvic radiographs), and (3) intractable patients. Although all pharmacologic agents for chemical restraint have the potential for adverse effects, their use in the uncooperative patient is justified to reduce pain, fear, or physical injury that may occur with manual restraint. Human safety is an additional consideration. The goal of this article is to review the agents available for chemical restraint in small animals and to compare their advantages and disadvantages. Manufacturers and formulations are shown in Table 1.

AGENTS AVAILABLE FOR CHEMICAL RESTRAINT

The agents utilized in chemical restraint (Table 2) include tranquilizers, sedative-hypnotics, opioids, opioid antagonists, dissociatives, and inhalation agents.

Tranquilizers

By definition, tranquilizers are agents that produce a calm, tranquil state. There are a large number of tranquilizers available; however, only a few are widely used in veterinary medicine. Three classes of tranquilizers are available: phenothiazines, butyrophenones, and benzodiazepines.

PHENOTHIAZINES (ACEPROMAZINE, PROMAZINE). Acepromazine and promazine are the phenothiazine tranquilizers most commonly used in veterinary medicine. Phenothiazine tranquilizers share several characteristics, including mild to moderate tranquilization, slow onset of action (30 to 60 min to peak effect), long duration of action, antiemetic qualities, hypotension, protection against epinephrine-induced arrhythmias, and the potential for unmasking seizure activity. Phenothiazine tranquiliz-

ers have no inherent analgesic properties, a characteristic of all tranquilizers. Since they are eliminated by hepatic metabolism, prolonged duration of effect may be expected in patients with compromised liver function. Acepromazine and promazine can be administered intravenously, intramuscularly, or orally.

BUTYROPHENONES (DROPERIDOL, LENPERONE). Butyrophenones have properties similar to those of phenothiazines, but they generally are not used alone for chemical restraint. Butyrophenones have a larger therapeutic index (the ratio of effective dose to lethal dose) compared with phenothiazines. Their administration may cause tremors, catalepsy, and behavioral changes. The degree of hypotension following administration may be less than that associated with phenothiazines. Of the many drugs that are available in this class, two are used in small animal practice. Droperidol is combined with the narcotic fentanyl in Innovar-Vet and is generally used in this combination. Lenperone is marketed as a single agent but has not achieved widespread popularity.

BENZODIAZEPINES (DIAZEPAM, MIDAZOLAM, ZOLAZEPAM). Benzodiazepines are widely used in humans but have limited use in veterinary medicine. Following benzodiazepine administration, a variety of effects can be seen, ranging from mild tranquilization to excitement and agitation. It is unfortunate that the type of response is unpredictable when these agents are administered to healthy animals. Debilitated animals generally respond favorably to benzodiazepine treatment.

Benzodiazepines are useful for chemical restraint when given in combination with other agents. They are also employed to manage seizures and may be beneficial for appetite stimulation. Benzodiazepines are generally safe drugs; they have minimal cardiovascular and pulmonary effects. They are relatively short-acting, but duration of effect depends on the speed of hepatic metabolism.

Diazepam is the most widely used member of this group but has the disadvantage of being insoluble in water. Diazepam is marketed in a propylene glycol base, which makes it poorly absorbable from

Table 1. Manufacturers and Formulations

Generic Name	Trademark	Manufacturer	Concentration (mg/ml)
Acepromazine	PromAce	Ft. Dodge	10
Lenperone	Elanone-V	A. H. Robins	5
Diazepam	Valium	Hoffmann-LaRoche	5
	—	Elkins-Sinn	5
Midazolam	Versed	Hoffmann-LaRoche	5
Thiopental	Pentothal	Abbott	Variable
Thiamylal	Bio-tal	Bio-Ceutic	Variable
	Surital	Parke-Davis	Variable
Methohexital	Brevital	Lilly	Variable
Xylazine	Rompun	Haver	20 or 100
	Gemini	Vet-A-Mix	100
	—		
Yohimbine	Yohimix*	Vet-A-Mix	—*
Morphine	—	Lilly	15
	—	Elkins-Sinn	15
	—	Wyeth	15
Oxymorphone	Numorphan	DuPont	1.5
	—	Pitman-Moore	1.5
Meperidine	Demerol	Wyeth	50
	—	Winthrop-Breon	50
	—	Elkins-Sinn	50
Butorphanol	Torbutrol	Ft. Dodge	0.5
	Torbugesic	Ft. Dodge	10
Nalbuphine	Nubain	DuPont	10 or 20
Naloxone	Narcan	Pitman-Moore	0.4
	—	Elkins-Sinn	0.4
Ketamine	Ketaset	Ft. Dodge	100
	Vetalar	Parke-Davis	100
Halothane	Fluothane	Ft. Dodge, Ayerst	—
	—	Halocarbon Lab.	—
Isoflurane	Aerrane	Anaquest	—
Fentanyl + droperidol	Innovar-Vet	Pitman-Moore	0.4 Fentanyl + 20 droperidol
Tiletamine + zolazepam	Telazol	A. H. Robins	50 tiletamine and 50 zolazepam, or 50 of each
Atropine	—	Ft. Dodge	0.5
	—	Astra	0.5
	—	Elkins-Sinn	0.5
Glycopyrrolate	Robinul-V	A. H. Robins	0.2
	—	LyphoMed	0.2

*Not yet available.

intramuscular or subcutaneous sites of injection. An additional concern is that propylene glycol may induce adverse cardiac effects following rapid intravenous administration.

Midazolam is a recently introduced benzodiazepine that is water soluble. It may be safely and effectively administered via intramuscular or intravenous routes. Midazolam is two to three times as potent as diazepam and has a shorter half-life.

Zolazepam is another benzodiazepine that is marketed in combination with tiletamine, a dissociative agent. Zolazepam appears to have effects similar to those of other benzodiazepines.

Sedative-Hypnotics

ULTRASHORT-ACTING BARBITURATES (THIOPENTAL, THIAMYLAL, METHOHEXITAL). Ultra short-act-

ing barbiturates are frequently used for brief periods of chemical restraint. These drugs have a rapid onset of action, provide a dependable response, and generally are associated with rapid recovery following single-dose administration. However, there are several disadvantages in their use for chemical restraint. The alkaline pH of barbiturates irritates tissues when these drugs are given extravascularly. A small margin of safety between an effective dose and a lethal dose is characteristic. Apnea and marked respiratory depression following bolus administration often occur. A high percentage of animals exhibit cardiac arrhythmias following administration. The distribution of barbiturates depends on the degree of ionization and the amount of protein binding of the drug. Acidosis decreases barbiturate ionization, resulting in greater cell membrane permeability and increased drug effect. Barbiturates are normally highly protein bound, but

Table 2. *Agents Used for Chemical Restraint*

Agent	Dose	Route	Species
Tranquilizers			
Acepromazine	0.11 mg/kg	IM, SC	Dog, cat
Diazepam*	0.11–0.22 mg/kg	IV	Dog, cat
Droperidol†	0.5–1.0 mg/kg	IM, IV	Dog, cat
Lenperone	0.22–1.5 mg/kg	IM, IV	Dog, cat
Midazolam	0.06–0.22 mg/kg	IM, IV	Dog, cat
Promazine	2.2–6.6 mg/kg	IM, SC	Dog, cat
Zolazepam‡		IM, IV	Dog, cat
Sedative-hypnotics§			
Methohexital§	10–12 mg/kg	IV	Dog, cat
Pentobarbital§	15–30 mg/kg	IV	Dog, cat
Thiopental§	15–22 mg/kg	IV	Dog, cat
Thiamylal§	15–22 mg/kg	IV	Dog, cat
Xylazine	1–2 mg/kg	IV, IM	Dog, cat
Opioid Agonists			
Butorphanol	0.44–0.88 mg/kg	IM, SC	Dog, cat
Innovar-Vet (fentanyl + droperidol)	1 ml/7–9 kg	IM	Dog, cat
	1 ml/20–30 kg	IV	
Meperidine	2.2–6.6 mg/kg	IM, SC	Dog, cat
Morphine	1.1–2.2 mg/kg	IM, IV	Dog
Oxymorphone	0.11–0.22 mg/kg	IM, IV	Dog, cat
Opioid Antagonists			
Naloxone	0.06 mg/kg	IM, IV	Dog, cat
Nalbuphine	0.3 mg/kg	IM, IV	Dog, cat
Dissociative Agents			
Ketamine‖	2.2–11 mg/kg	IV	Dog, cat
	6.6–30 mg/kg	IM	Cat
Inhalation Agents			
Halothane	5% induction, 1–2% maintenance		Dog, cat
Isoflurane	5% induction, 1.5–2.5% maintenance		

*To be used with opioids or ketamine.
†Mainly used with fentanyl as Innovar-Vet.
‡Used with tiletamine as Telazol.
§Dose may be reduced with tranquilizers and narcotics.
‖Also used in combination with tranquilizers.
IM, intramuscular; IV, intravenous; SC, subcutaneous

decreased protein binding with increased drug effect can be seen in patients with hypoproteinemia, with renal or hepatic disease, or receiving concomitant drug therapy (e.g., certain sulfonamides or nonsteroidal anti-inflammatory drugs). Barbiturates provide little analgesia; thus, high doses are required in performing painful procedures.

Recovery from ultra short-acting barbiturates is associated mainly with drug redistribution from the brain to other tissues, followed by hepatic metabolism. Methohexital, an oxybarbiturate, is more rapidly metabolized than the thiobarbiturates; metabolism plays a greater role in clinical recovery from methohexital administration. Methohexital differs from thiobarbiturates in that recovery is stormy following single-dose administration unless a tranquilizer or sedative, such as acepromazine or oxymorphone, is given prior to use.

XYLAZINE. Xylazine, an alpha-2 adrenergic receptor agonist, is used widely in veterinary medicine as a sedative-hypnotic agent. It causes marked sedation and also has analgesic qualities. However, there are significant adverse effects associated with this drug. Marked effects on the cardiovascular system are noted, including bradycardia and bradyarrhythmias, sensitization to epinephrine-induced ventricular arrhythmias, decreased cardiac output, and blood pressure fluctuations. Bradycardia may be prevented by administration of anticholinergics such as atropine or glycopyrrolate. Anticholinergics do not entirely inhibit the cardiovascular effects of xylazine. A recent study in cats indicated that anticholinergics may not prevent the reduction in cardiac output noted with xylazine. Other effects of xylazine administration include emesis (particularly in cats), decreased gastrointestinal motility, mild respiratory depression, increased uterine pressure, hyperglycemia, glycosuria, and polyuria. Xylazine has a rapid onset and a long duration of action. Doses of other anesthetic agents must be markedly reduced when used in conjunction with xylazine. One potential advantage of xylazine is the ability to reverse its effects with alpha-2 receptor antagonists, such as yohimbine or tolazoline. Yohimbine may soon be readily available as an injectable solution; however, its effects have not been well documented in clinical situations.

Opioids

The opioids (narcotics) are a large class of drugs that can be used for chemical restraint. The property that sets opioids apart from other tranquilizers and sedatives is that they relieve pain; thus, they are useful in performing painful procedures. Among the opioids (particularly opioid agonists/antagonists) there is variation in the degree of sedation and restraint obtained following administration. One major advantage of opioids is that their effects can be reversed with opioid antagonists.

In general, opioids are safe and have minimal adverse effects on the cardiovascular system. However, they generally produce bradycardia and may produce bradyarrhythmias. Anticholinergics readily reverse this effect. Opioids are generally considered to be respiratory depressants; hypoventilation results in increased carbon dioxide levels (hypercapnia). Hypercapnia, in turn, can increase cerebrospinal fluid pressure by causing dilation of the cerebral vasculature. Because of this effect, opioids should be used with caution in patients with cranial trauma, unless ventilation is controlled. Opioids also have emetic activity. Another drawback is the addictive potential of these drugs in humans, and the associated regulations involved in their use. Opioids can be used successfully in cats; appropriate doses or concurrently administered tranquilizers should be used to prevent excitement. The agonists/antagonists are generally well-tolerated by cats, without excitement. Although the opioids are a large class of drugs, only a few are commonly used in small animal practice (Table 3).

OPIOID AGONISTS (MORPHINE, OXYMORPHONE,

FENTANYL, MEPERIDINE, BUTORPHANOL). *Morphine* is a well-known opioid agonist with a moderate duration of action. It provides good analgesia and a moderate degree of sedation. Morphine has a minimal effect on the cardiovascular system but may cause hypotension due to histamine release following intravenous administration. Morphine commonly produces bradycardia; an anticholinergic may be needed to maintain heart rate. Respiratory depression may be noted following administration. In dogs being treated with the drug, emesis commonly occurs.

Oxymorphone is similar to morphine in many respects but has several advantages. It is more potent than morphine and has a shorter duration of action. Oxymorphone does not cause histamine release, may be safely administered intravenously, and is associated with a lower incidence of emesis than is morphine. Oxymorphone has positive cardiac effects in dogs with hemorrhagic shock; it is a relatively safe drug to use in very ill or debilitated patients.

Fentanyl is a short-acting narcotic that is combined with droperidol in Innovar-Vet. Alone, fentanyl causes excitement rather than sedation in dogs. It provides stable cardiovascular performance, although it can cause marked bradycardia. Fentanyl does not induce histamine release; however, it does cause respiratory depression.

Meperidine is a short-acting narcotic that has several disadvantages. It has minimal sedative effects and, therefore, is seldom useful in providing chemical restraint. Meperidine is the only narcotic with depressant effects on the heart and may also cause histamine release. Therefore, it should be used with extreme caution in debilitated patients.

Butorphanol is a narcotic agonist/antagonist that provides analgesia with few adverse effects. It has minimal effects on the cardiovascular system and causes only slight respiratory depression. Alone, it

Table 3. *Opioid and Dissociative Agent Combinations Used in Chemical Restraint*

Drug Combination	Dosage (mg/kg)	Route	Species
Opioid Combinations			
Butorphanol/acepromazine	0.88/0.11	IM, IV	Dog, cat
Morphine/acepromazine	1.0/0.11	IM	Dog
Oxymorphone/acepromazine	0.22/0.11	IM	Dog, cat
	0.11/0.05	IV	
Oxymorphone/midazolam	0.11/0.11	IV	Dog
Butorphanol/xylazine	0.4/0.5	IV, IM	Dog
Dissociative Agent Combinations			
Ketamine/xylazine	11/1.0	IM	Dog, cat
Ketamine/acepromazine	6.6–11/0.11	IV	Dog
	6.6–30/0.11	IM	Cat
Ketamine/diazepam	6.6–11/0.22	IV	Dog
Ketamine/midazolam	11/0.11	IV	Dog
	6.6–11/0.06–0.22	IM	Cat
Ketamine/acepromazine + diazepam	6.6–11/0.11/0.22	IV	Dog
Tiletamine + zolazepam	5–10 mg/kg	IM	Dog, cat

has little sedative effect. Therefore, butorphanol must generally be combined with a tranquilizer to provide restraint. It can be used as an antagonist to narcotic agonists such as morphine and oxymorphone.

OPIOID ANTAGONISTS (NALBUPHINE, NALOXONE). Naloxone is a pure opioid antagonist and rapidly reverses all clinical effects of opioids. Nalbuphine is an agonist/antagonist that the authors use clinically as an opioid reversal agent. It has a longer duration of action than naloxone, reverses sedation and respiratory depression, and provides some degree of analgesia. Both naloxone and nalbuphine may be administered via intravenous, intramuscular, or subcutaneous routes. However, if rapid reversal is necessary, the intravenous route is preferred.

Dissociative Agents

KETAMINE, TILETAMINE. Dissociative agents (Table 3) have been widely employed in veterinary medicine for restraint or anesthesia. Ketamine has been utilized for many years, but tiletamine, in combination with zolazepam, has just recently become available. Dissociative agents are useful because they have positive cardiovascular effects, produce minimal respiratory depression, and are rapidly absorbed after intramuscular injection. However, several drawbacks exist. They generally produce little or no muscle relaxation, often increase respiratory secretions, increase intraocular and cerebrospinal fluid pressures, and generally result in stormy recoveries. In dogs, dissociative agents often are associated with seizure activity. The positive cardiac effects of ketamine are due to release of endogenous catecholamines. However, negative cardiac effects may become evident in severely debilitated patients. Because of the drawbacks noted with dissociative agents, they are often administered in combination with anticholinergics, sedatives, or tranquilizers. Combined routes of administration using low doses intramuscularly for restraint followed by additional doses administered intravenously, as needed, result in small drug doses and quick recoveries.

Inhalants

HALOTHANE, ISOFLURANE. Many chemical restraint agents are available in injectable form, but inhalant agents offer several advantages and should not be overlooked. Both halothane and isoflurane can be successfully employed for short procedures. These agents are particularly useful in two groups of patients. In debilitated patients with impaired hepatic or renal function, inhalant drugs can be administered by mask for induction and maintenance of anesthesia. In fractious cats or small dogs, use of an induction chamber permits induction of a light anesthetic plane without touching the patient. Inhalation anesthesia can then be maintained by use of either a mask or an endotracheal tube. When sufficient restraint is not initially achieved, inhalants may also be used in combination with other techniques covered in this article.

Although both isoflurane and halothane possess properties that make them suitable for chemical restraint, isoflurane has several advantages. Isoflurane reaches anesthetic levels more rapidly than does halothane, shortening induction time. It is also more rapidly eliminated, resulting in quick recovery. Cardiovascular status is better maintained with isoflurane; therefore, it is preferable in the compromised patient. Isoflurane does not sensitize the heart to epinephrine-induced arrhythmias as does halothane. This may prove safer in the patient with arrhythmias or with the potential for developing them during anesthesia. For this reason, isoflurane may also be safer for chamber inductions of highly stressed patients. Isoflurane also is more resistant to degradation than is halothane, resulting in fewer potential toxic reactions.

Drug Combinations

INNOVAR-VET. Innovar-Vet is a combination of fentanyl (0.4 mg/ml) and droperidol (20.0 mg/ml) that produces neuroleptanalgesia, a state of marked sedation and analgesia. It results in profound, reliable chemical restraint in aggressive dogs. Innovar-Vet may be administered by either the intravenous or the intramuscular route. However, pain is often associated with intramuscular administration. Neuroleptanalgesia from Innovar-Vet lasts for only 30 to 60 min because of the short duration of action of fentanyl. Maximum drug effect occurs 20 to 30 min following intramuscular injection.

Innovar-Vet is a safe drug that has minimal effects on cardiovascular function. Mild hypotension may result from droperidol. Fentanyl may cause bradycardia and bradyarrhythmias. To inhibit the bradycardic effect of Innovar-Vet, anticholinergics (e.g., atropine) are generally also administered. Respiratory depression is commonly associated with fentanyl administration. Long recovery times and behavioral changes may be noted in patients receiving Innovar-Vet. Both of these effects are due to the relatively high dose of droperidol in the combination product.

TELAZOL. Telazol is a one-to-one combination of tiletamine and zolazepam. Telazol produces dissociative anesthesia and analgesia, similar to a combination of ketamine and a benzodiazepine. Telazol may be effectively administered by intramuscular injection. Zolazepam is included in this combination to prevent seizures and provide muscle relaxation. Following intramuscular administration, effects may be seen within 3 to 5 min. Cardiovascular effects are similar to those of ketamine and benzodiazepine combinations. This combination does appear to cause significant respiratory depression for a short time after administration. Excessive salivary and respiratory secretions may be a problem; anticholinergics (e.g., atropine) may be useful as antisialogogues.

RECOMMENDATIONS FOR CHEMICAL RESTRAINT TECHNIQUES

Dogs

BARBITURATES. Thiobarbiturates, such as thiopental or thiamylal, are successfully used for short-term anesthesia (Table 4). They should be administered only to effect. Barbiturates should be used very cautiously in patients with pre-existing arrhythmias, acidosis, electrolyte disturbances, hepatic insufficiency, and hypoalbuminemia. Apnea and respiratory depression are common following administration of barbiturates; therefore, one should be prepared to assist ventilation.

NEUROLEPTANALGESIC TECHNIQUES. Neuroleptanalgesia can be successful in dogs. The ability to reverse the opioid effect of the combination assists in quick recoveries. Residual tranquilizer effects may be noted for several hours following reversal. Innovar-Vet has been used for many years. Acepromazine and oxymorphone are a combination that provides a similar degree of sedation and restraint. The duration of oxymorphone is longer than that of fentanyl, so neuroleptanalgesia is present for a longer time. Morphine also can be used with ace-

promazine, but the potential for histamine release following intravenous morphine administration, along with the hypotension from acepromazine, could lead to cardiovascular compromise. Butorphanol and acepromazine is effective and produces a surprising degree of sedation. Alone, butorphanol has minimal sedative effects; however, marked sedation occurs when it is combined with acepromazine. This combination seems to work best in medium-sized to large breed dogs; toy breeds do not seem to become as sedate. Respiratory depression should not be as significant a problem with this combination. The occurrence of behavioral changes following administration of these drug combinations is unique to Innovar-Vet. Recovery from these combinations is slow because of the prolonged effect of acepromazine or droperidol.

To achieve more rapid and complete recovery, benzodiazepines can be substituted in place of acepromazine. The combination of oxymorphone with either diazepam or midazolam works well. However, the degree of sedation in young healthy dogs is not as profound as that achieved with other narcotic-tranquilizer combinations. In old or debilitated dogs, this combination works well; recovery is rapid following oxymorphone reversal. Either diazepam or midazolam can be intravenously administered, but midazolam is preferred for intramuscular injection. Full recovery is faster from midazolam than from diazepam. Anticholinergics, such as atropine or glycopyrrolate, are generally indicated with any of these combinations to maintain heart rates.

The combination of butorphanol and xylazine provides profound chemical restraint. Significant bradycardia and respiratory depression are often noted. With xylazine, negative cardiovascular effects will be present. Anticholinergics, such as atropine or glycopyrrolate, may be used to maintain

Table 4. *Chemical Restraint Techniques Grouped by Time*

Duration	Restraint Technique	Species
5–15 min	10–15 mg/kg thiobarbiturate IV	Dog, cat
	6–11 mg/kg ketamine, IM, with or without 0.11 mg/kg midazolam IM	Cat
	Halothane	Dog, cat
	Isoflurane	Dog, cat
15–30 min	15–22 mg/kg thiobarbiturate IV	Dog, cat
	1 ml/15 kg Innovar-Vet (fentanyl + droperidol), IM	Dog, cat
	1 ml/30 kg Innovar-Vet, IV	Dog
	Oxymorphone + tranquilizer IV, IM	Dog, cat
	Butorphanol + acepromazine IV, IM	Dog, cat
	10 mg/kg ketamine with or without 0.11 mg/kg acepromazine or 0.11 mg/kg diazepam	Dog, cat
	Halothane	Dog, cat
	Isoflurane	Dog, cat
30–45 min	15–22 mg/kg thiobarbiturate IV	Dog, cat
	1 ml/10 kg Innovar-Vet IM	Dog
	1 mg/kg xylazine + 10 mg/kg ketamine	Dog, cat
	1 mg/kg morphine + 0.11 mg/kg acepromazine	Dog, cat
	Halothane, isoflurane	Dog, cat

heart rate. A potential advantage with this combination is that both components can be reversed with a combination of naloxone and yohimbine. Recovery is slow when reversal agents are not used.

KETAMINE COMBINATIONS AND TELAZOL. Ketamine is not approved for use in dogs; when used alone, it frequently results in seizures. Acepromazine or xylazine, used in combination with ketamine, decreases the incidence of seizure activity. These two drugs also provide some muscle relaxation and facilitate a smooth recovery. However, positive cardiovascular effects of ketamine are negated by the use of xylazine and acepromazine. Substituting diazepam or midazolam for xylazine or acepromazine abolishes seizure activity and maintains cardiovascular performance. The use of either midazolam or diazepam with ketamine intravenously provides a short period of chemical restraint, with minimal effect on cardiovascular function. The depth of anesthesia obtained with diazepam or midazolam is not as profound as that with ketamine and xylazine in combination. The authors also have used ketamine and midazolam, administered intramuscularly. Although dogs receiving this combination appear fairly rigid, it provides good chemical restraint. Use of an anticholinergic to reduce salivary and pulmonary secretions may be indicated with any of these combinations; in the authors' experience, secretions have rarely been a severe problem.

Telazol has profound effects in dogs. Therefore, patients should be observed closely following drug administration. Onset of action is very rapid. Because respiratory depression may occur quickly, ventilatory support may be necessary. In the authors' limited experience with this new drug combination, use of the low end of the recommended doses provides marked restraint, but recoveries may be prolonged and rough.

INHALANTS. The inhalants work well in dogs for chemical restraint; however, in larger dogs, periods of excitement during induction can be difficult to manage unless the patient is debilitated or is sedated prior to induction.

Cats

BARBITURATES. In cats, thiobarbiturates work very well; however, the necessity for intravenous administration makes these agents difficult to use in fractious patients. Use of a low dose (5–10 mg/kg) of ketamine intramuscularly, followed by thiobarbiturates, intravenously, to effect, for additional restraint, works well (Table 4).

NEUROLEPTANALGESIC TECHNIQUES. Neuroleptanalgesic techniques have not been widely used in cats but may be of potential benefit. Narcotic-tranquilizer combinations do not appear to give the same degree of restraint and sedation in cats as they do in dogs. However, Innovar-Vet as well as acepromazine and oxymorphone has been used successfully to produce some sedation and restraint in cats. Butorphanol and acepromazine may also be used to provide mild restraint.

KETAMINE, KETAMINE COMBINATIONS, AND TELAZOL. Alternative drug combinations have not been widely used in cats because of the success of ketamine and ketamine combinations. Unlike the effect in dogs, seizure activity is rarely noted following ketamine administration in cats. For this reason, ketamine alone is often used for chemical restraint. Other agents are combined with ketamine to reduce undesirable side effects, such as muscle rigidity and stormy recoveries. Anticholinergics (e.g., atropine, glycopyrrolate) are often used to decrease salivary and pulmonary secretions, which may be more of a problem in the small airways of cats. Xylazine and ketamine have been widely employed in cats. However, recent reports document adverse cardiovascular effects of xylazine associated with this drug combination. Acepromazine and ketamine also may be used, with less detrimental cardiovascular effects. Midazolam and ketamine, administered either intramuscularly or intravenously, provide dependable chemical restraint with minimal cardiovascular effects.

The effects of telazol are similar to those of ketamine combinations in cats. Onset of action is very rapid following intramuscular administration, respiratory depression may be significant, and recovery may be prolonged if large doses are used. Cats should be observed closely following drug administration, and ventilatory assistance should be given if necessary.

INHALANTS. The use of inhalants in cats for chemical restraint may be of value. Using an induction chamber, it is possible to chemically restrain a fractious cat without direct contact, providing safety for the clinician and attendants. However, one should closely observe the cat during induction, and it should be removed from the chamber as soon as restraint is achieved. Anesthesia may be maintained with a tightly fitting mask or an endotracheal tube. This technique, or the use of mask induction alone, also is satisfactory for use with debilitated patients.

DRAWBACKS TO CHEMICAL RESTRAINT TECHNIQUES

The safe use of chemical restraint agents requires appropriate evaluation of the animal prior to drug administration. In young healthy patients, this may require only a thorough physical examination. In geriatric or debilitated patients, additional diagnostic information, such as hematologic and biochemical profiles, radiographs, and electrocardiograms should be obtained as indicated. Correction of fluid deficits, acid-base imbalances, electrolyte disturbances, or other derangements should be attempted before restraint agents are administered. If a fractious patient requires chemical restraint before diagnostics or therapy are possible, restraint agents should be chosen that have minimal detrimental effects.

References and Supplemental Reading

Allen, D. G., Dyson, P. J., Pascoe, P. J., et al.: Evaluation of a xylazine-ketamine hydrochloride combination in the cat. Can. J. Vet. Res. 50:23, 1986.

Copland, V. S., Haskins, S. C., and Patz, J. D.: Oxymorphone: Cardiovascular, pulmonary, and behavioral effects in dogs. Am. J. Vet. Res. 48:1626, 1987.

Dunkle, N., Moise, N. S., Scarlett-Kranz, J., et al.: Cardiac performance in cats after administration of xylazine or xylazine and glycopyrrolate: Echocardiographic evaluations. Am. J. Vet. Res. 47:2212, 1986.

Gleed, R. D.: Tranquilizers and sedatives. In Short, C. E. (ed.): *Principles and Practice of Veterinary Anesthesia.* Baltimore: Williams and Wilkins, 1987, pp. 16–27.

Granby, J. L., and Heath, R. B.: Cardiopulmonary and behavioral effects of fentanyl-droperidol in cats. J.A.V.M.A. 191:59, 1987.

Haskins, S. C., Patz, J. D., Copland, S. V., et al.: A Comparison of the Cardiopulmonary Effects of Oxymorphone and Ketamine in Hypovo-lemic Dogs. Proceedings of the American College of Veterinary Anesthesiologists, 1987, Atlanta, GA, p. 1.

Knight, A. P.: Xylazine. J.A.V.M.A. 176:454, 1980.

Lumb, W. V., and Jones, E. W.: *Veterinary Anesthesia.* Philadelphia: Lea and Febiger, 1984.

Raffe, M. R., and Lipowitz, A. J.: Evaluation of Butorphanol Tartrate Analgesia in the Dog. Proceedings of the 2nd International Congress of Veterinary Anesthesiologists. Sacramento, CA, October, 1985, p. 155.

Reves, J. G., Fragen, R. J., Vinik, H. R., et al.: Midazolam: Pharmacology and uses. Anesthesiology 62:310, 1985.

Short, C. E.: Pain, analgesics, and related medications. In Short, C. E. (ed.): *Principles and Practice of Veterinary Anesthesia.* Baltimore: Williams and Wilkins, 1987, pp. 28–46.

Short, C. E.: Neuroleptanalgesia and alpha-adrenergic receptor analgesia. In Short, C. E. (ed.): *Principles and Practice of Veterinary Anesthesia.* Baltimore: Williams and Wilkins, 1987, pp. 47–57.

Short, C. E.: Barbiturate anesthesia. In Short, C. E. (ed.): *Principles and Practice of Veterinary Anesthesia.* Baltimore: Williams and Wilkins, 1987, pp. 58–69.

Short, C. E.: Inhalant anesthesia. In Short, C. E. (ed.): *Principles and Practice of Veterinary Anesthesia.* Baltimore: Williams and Wilkins, 1987, pp. 70–90.

Short, C. E.: Dissociative anesthesia. In Short, C. E. (ed.): *Principles and Practice of Veterinary Anesthesia.* Baltimore: Williams and Wilkins, 1987, pp. 158–169.

Taylor, P.: Analgesia in the Dog and Cat. In Practice 7:5, 1985.

Weiskopf, R. B., Bogetz, M. S., Roizen, M. F., et al.: Cardiovascular and metabolic sequelae of inducing anesthesia with ketamine or thiopental in hypovolemic swine. Anesthesiology 60:214, 1984.

Wright, M.: Pharmacological effects of ketamine and its use in veterinary medicine. J.A.V.M.A. 180:1462, 1982.

Wright, M., Heath, R. B., and Wingfield, W. E.: Effects of xylazine and ketamine on epinephrine-induced arrhythmias in the dog. Vet. Surg. 16:398, 1987.

ANTIMICROBIAL SUSCEPTIBILITY TESTS

DWIGHT C. HIRSH, D.V.M.

Davis, California

Antimicrobial drugs are used to treat or prevent disease produced by an infectious agent. These drugs are chosen according to the results of susceptibility tests, which determine the susceptibility of pathogenic bacteria to antibiotics. Susceptibility tests provide measurements of the effectiveness of a drug in killing or suppressing an infectious agent at the site(s) of disease or expected compromise. Susceptibility test results determine the actual amount of antimicrobial drug needed to inhibit or kill the infectious agent (minimal inhibitory or bactericidal concentration [MIC or MBC]) or offer a qualitative prediction of the effectiveness of a particular drug.

This is not to suggest that each isolate from an infectious process be tested for susceptibility to antimicrobial drugs. On the contrary, the antimicrobial susceptibility test should be performed only when the susceptibility of an infectious agent cannot be predicted with any degree of certainty. For example, it would be inappropriate to measure the susceptibility of a beta-hemolytic streptococcus to penicillin.

TYPES OF SUSCEPTIBILITY TESTS

Dilution Tests

The *minimal inhibitory concentration (MIC)* is the smallest concentration of antibiotic that will inhibit the growth of an infectious agent *in vitro.* The *minimal bactericidal concentration (MBC)* is the smallest concentration of antibiotic that will kill the infectious agent *in vitro.*

Agar or broth dilution tests are used to determine

the MIC. Various amounts of an antimicrobial agent are dissolved in broth or are incorporated into an agar medium. In most instances, serial twofold dilutions are made because they are easy to do. However, this technique has difficulty with antimicrobial agents that have a narrow therapeutic index (e.g., gentamicin), because the differences in concentration per dilution are too large. For example, assume that the true MIC of gentamicin is 2.5 μg/ml for a particular isolate. The MIC of gentamicin as measured in a twofold dilution scheme, however, would be 4 μg/ml, since most dilution schemes use 1 μg/ml as a benchmark concentration.

The standard medium is Mueller-Hinton broth or agar, depending upon the method of assay. If broth medium is used, supplementation with calcium and magnesium is necessary because the amounts of these cations are too small to give an accurate assessment of the susceptibility of *Pseudomonas* to aminoglycosides (recommended amount of calcium is 50 mg/L, and of magnesium, 25 mg/L). The amounts of calcium and magnesium in Mueller-Hinton agar are adequate.

The amount of thymidine in the medium is important for testing some organisms for susceptibility to trimethoprim-sulfonamides. With most microorganisms, the amount present is too low for concern. However, if it is of concern, thymidine phosphorylase or lysed ("laked") horse blood (which contains high concentrations of this enzyme) may be added to the medium. Alternatively, a medium that is normally low in thymidine (e.g., Diagnostic Sensitivity Test Agar, Oxoid Ltd, Basingstoke, England) may be used. The suitability of the medium in this regard should be tested with *Streptococcus faecalis* (ATCC 29212). The MIC of trimethoprim should be less than 0.25 μg/ml, and that for sulfonamides, less than 4.75 μg/ml.

Most microorganisms grow adequately in or on Mueller-Hinton medium. It is sometimes necessary to add supplements in order for sufficient growth to occur, as may be the case with some streptococci and pasteurellae. Blood is sometimes used; no special problems have been noticed, except with those antimicrobial agents that are tightly bound to protein (novobiocin and nafcillin) and with trimethoprim and sulfonamides, which are antagonized by blood (except for horse blood cells, as previously noted). Some of these problems can be circumvented by adding supplements (e.g., IsoVitaleX, BBL Microbiology Systems, Cockeysville, MD; Supplement VK, Difco Laboratories, Detroit, MI).

In order to detect staphylococci resistant to methicillin and oxacillin, the medium should contain 2 per cent sodium chloride.

After the antimicrobial agent is diluted in agar or broth, a standardized suspension (final concentration of 10^5–10^6 microorganisms/ml) of the isolate is added to each tube (or well of a microtiter plate) of broth or is spotted on the surface of an agar plate (0.001–0.002 ml of a solution containing 10^6–10^7 microorganisms/ml). Plates or tubes are incubated at 35°C (methicillin-resistant staphylococci do not express resistance at temperatures above 35°C) for 16 to 20 hr. An atmosphere of air is preferable, since an increased concentration of carbon dioxide changes the pH of the medium, especially on an agar surface. The activity of some antimicrobial agents is affected by pH.

The MIC is the lowest concentration of an antimicrobial drug that will inhibit the growth of an isolate. In agar dilution tests, the MIC is the lowest concentration of antimicrobial drug on agar plates that show no growth or only a barely discernible haze.

The MBC is measured from tubes used in the broth dilution assay. The purpose of the test is to determine the ability of the antimicrobial drug to kill a particular microorganism. The MBC is defined as the lowest concentration of antimicrobial drug to reduce the inoculum by 99.9 per cent. Using the broth dilution assay for the MIC, the MBC can be estimated by sampling the fluid from tubes with no growth. Briefly, after incubation of inoculated tubes containing the drug, aliquots (moistened swab) of the fluid of the tubes with no growth are inoculated onto the surface of agar plates, and the plates are incubated at 35°C overnight, with or without carbon dioxide. The concentration of drug in the tube (well) from which three or fewer colonies grow is the MBC.

Disk Diffusion Assay

A standardized suspension of microorganisms is inoculated onto agar plates. Disks containing an antimicrobial agent are applied to the surface of the agar. The media are incubated overnight. There is a linear relationship between the MIC of the antimicrobial agent and the diameter of the zones of inhibition around the disks. For each antimicrobial agent, a regression curve has been constructed, relating the MIC and the diameter of the zone of inhibition. An inverse relationship exists between the MIC and zone diameter.

The categories of "susceptible," "intermediate," and "resistant" were established first by determining the concentrations of a particular antimicrobial agent that are routinely achieved in serum. Then, these concentrations were adjusted (upward or downward), depending on the drug (distribution) and clinical experience. The upper limit, the highest concentration acceptable or attainable, corresponds to the last zone diameter not included in the "resistant" category.

The slope of the regression curve is directly related to the conditions under which the assay is performed. Variations from standard conditions result in errors in interpreting whether a particular zone diameter translates to a concentration of drug that is "attainable" or not (i.e., calling an isolate resistant when it is susceptible, and vice versa). The important parameters affecting the disk diffusion assay are (1) inoculum size, (2) medium, (3) disk potency, and (4) conditions of incubation.

The inoculum size is difficult to manage in small, in-house clinical laboratories. Yet, in the authors' estimation, this parameter produces the biggest errors in this assay. There are two acceptable ways in which the inoculum size is adjusted to conform to the standard method (refer to any modern manual of clinical microbiology for specific details). Briefly, the first involves adjustment of a suspension of the isolate to a particular density; the second comprises dilution of a stationary suspension of the isolate. Both are cumbersome for small laboratories. It is fortunate that there is a commercially available system whereby these maneuvers can be done quickly and easily (Prompt Inoculation System, Medical Products Division/3M, St. Paul, MN, 55144). This system employs a wand that is designed to pick up a calibrated amount of growth when a colony of the isolate is touched. The growth is then inoculated into a premeasured volume of buffered saline (supplied), which serves as the inoculum for the plate.

Mueller-Hinton agar must be used for the disk diffusion method. Blood (defibrinated sheep blood, 5 per cent) may be added, but variations in zone size may occur with the sulfonamides and trimethoprim as well as with oxacillin, nafcillin, and methicillin (a reduction in zone size of about 2 mm). Chocolate blood agar should not be used; supplements containing the needed growth factor(s) (IsoVitaleX, or Supplement VK, see preceding) may be used if necessary.

Plates are incubated at 35°C, in air. Incubation in carbon dioxide results in change in pH on the surface, which, in turn, causes a change in the zone diameters of some antimicrobial agents. At temperatures higher than 35°C, heteroresistant staphylococci do not express resistance to methicillin or nafcillin.

Each batch of Muller-Hinton agar should be tested to ascertain that there are acceptable amounts of thymidine (use *S. faecalis* ATCC 29212, see preceding). Plates should contain 2 per cent sodium chloride to ensure detection of heteroresistant staphylococci. There is no need to add calcium or magnesium, since most agar-containing media contain adequate amounts of these ions.

Disk potency is regulated by the Food and Drug Administration. The potency used is strictly determined by the standard method. Storage of disks is important. Long-term storage should be at −14°C, especially for drugs belonging to the penicillin and cephalothin families. Disks may safely be kept at refrigerator temperatures for no longer than 1 week. Be especially careful of methicillin disks (it is better to use oxacillin as the class disk because the drug is more stable).

SUSCEPTIBILITY TESTING OF ANAEROBES

Tests to measure the antimicrobial susceptibility of anaerobes *in vitro* are very similar to those used for aerobic microorganisms. Such tests include agar dilution, broth dilution, and broth–disk elution. There is no disk diffusion assay that predicts susceptibility of anaerobes *in vivo*. As with all anaerobic procedures, these tests may add a financial burden to the clinical laboratory. For this reason, testing anaerobic bacteria for susceptibility to antimicrobial agents may be an unnecessary luxury. In the authors' experience, resistance to penicillin (cephalosporins) presents the only therapeutic problem with this group of microorganisms. Whether an anaerobic isolate secretes a cephalosporinase (enzyme that inactivates first- and second-generation cephalosporins, penicillin, and ampicillin) can be determined by using a disk assay (Cefinase, B.B.L., Cockeysville, MD 21030; PADAC, Carr-Scarborough Microbiologicals, Inc., Stone Mountain, GA 30086). The test is performed by rubbing a portion of a colony on a disk containing a chromogenic cephalosporin (changes color when degraded).

When performing susceptibility tests on anaerobes, good anaerobic technique must be followed. All media should be freshly made or prereduced and anaerobically sterilized. All inoculations not done in an anaerobic environment should be performed as quickly as possible. Every effort should be made to prevent the entrance of molecular oxygen into the media (e.g., by using tubes with soft rubber stoppers that can be inoculated with syringe and needle).

Agar Dilution

Serial twofold dilutions of antimicrobial agents are made in freshly prepared Wilkens-Chalgren agar (with or without lysed blood cells to improve growth of some microorganisms). The inoculum is prepared in fluid thioglycolate broth supplemented with hemin and vitamin K_1, to a density matching a McFarland 0.5 (approximately 10^5 microorganisms per spot), and 0.001 to 0.005 ml are spotted on the plate. (Use of a Steers's replicating device [Craft Machine, Inc., Chester, PA] is an easy way to transfer the microbes.) The plates are then incubated for 24 to 48 hr in an anaerobic atmosphere.

The MIC is read as described for aerobic microorganisms.

Broth Dilution

Serial twofold dilutions of antimicrobial agents are made in Schaedler's broth, West-Wilkins broth, Wilkens-Chalgren broth (without agar), or brain-heart infusion broth. All should be freshly made or prereduced and anaerobically sterilized. Each tube (well) is inoculated to achieve a final concentration of 10^5 to 10^6 microorganisms/ml. The tubes are incubated for 24 to 48 hr and are read as previously described for aerobic microorganisms.

Disk Elution

Disks containing antimicrobial agents are added to freshly prepared or prereduced and anaerobically sterilized broth. The number of disks per tube depends on the final concentration of antimicrobial agent desired. The concentration of the drug depends on the antimicrobial agent and its achievable concentration in the animal. Brain-heart infusion, Wilkins-West, Schaedler's, Wilkens-Chalgren (without agar) or thioglycollate broth should be used. The inoculum consists of 1 drop of a fresh culture of the isolate (isolate taken from chopped meat broth is sufficient). Whether an isolate is susceptible or resistant is determined by whether or not growth occurs. If growth occurs, the isolate is resistant.

Special mention is made concerning testing of members of the genus *Fusobacterium*. It has been the authors' experience that members of this genus are very efficient in scavenging thymidine; if there are sufficient amounts in the medium, these isolates will test resistant to trimethoprim-sulfonamides even though they may be susceptible. For this reason, addition of thymidine phosphorylase (by way of lysed horse red blood cells) or use of a medium low in thymidine (e.g., Diagnostic Sensitivity Test agar, see preceding) is recommended. Brain-heart broth or thioglycollate broths have unacceptable amounts of thymidine.

QUALITY CONTROL

It is crucial that some attempt at quality control be made. For each of the tests previously described, a set of performance standards has been established to test the reliability of the assay being used. A susceptibility test that gives unreliable results is useless. A quality control series should be run at least once a week. Guidelines have been set by the National Committee for Clinical Laboratory Standards. Strains used in the testing of the quality of

the assay are available through the American Type Culture Collection (12301 Parklawn Drive, Rockville, MD 20852).

INTERPRETATION

A microorganism is susceptible to a particular antimicrobial agent if the drug achieves sufficient concentration at the site of infection to kill or inhibit microbial growth. In this equation, the only parameter that has been measured is the amount of drug needed to kill or inhibit the growth of the isolate *in vitro*. Virtually nothing is known about the concentration achievable at the site of infection. However, there are data that allow for an approximation. The first approximation comes from knowledge of the blood (cerebrospinal fluid, urine, synovial fluid) concentration of a drug achieved following administration of a certain dose by a certain route. The second approximation comes from knowledge of clinical response in the past (i.e., relating certain MIC values, the isolate, dose and route, and blood [cerebrospinal fluid, urine, joint fluid] concentration with clinical response). An "achievable level" is agreed upon; isolates with MIC values above this level are termed resistant, those with MIC values below it are labeled susceptible. Uncertainties still are present, including dilution errors, distribution and absorption differences from patient to patient, and other unknowns. To account for these influences, an isolate must have an MIC of at least one fourth the achievable level (and perhaps lower than for isolates obtained from immunocompromised patients) to be interpreted as susceptible.

Disk diffusion assays account for these variables, but only in infectious processes that freely communicate with blood (no central nervous system or prostate barrier; no excretion effects, as in urine). For this reason, results of diffusion assays must be interpreted with care. Isolates from the urine that test "resistant" by this assay may be susceptible. Likewise, isolates from the cerebrospinal fluid may test "susceptible" but may be resistant.

There are numerous antimicrobial agents; therefore, a laboratory cannot test an isolate against each one. However, certain antimicrobial agents can be used as "class drugs." The results of "class" tests may be used for all antimicrobial agents that belong to that class. Penicillin G is the best drug for testing staphylococci for resistance to ampicillin, amoxicillin, and hetacillin. Ampicillin is the class representative for testing susceptibility of members of the family Enterobacteriaceae. Cephalothin is the class representative for the first-generation cephalosporins (cephalothin, cefaclor, cefadroxil, cephalexin, cephapirin, cefazolin, cephaloridine, and cephradine). Cefazolin should not be used to predict isolate susceptibility to other first-generation cephalosporins because a significant number of isolates give false "susceptible" errors (especially *Escherichia coli*). There are no class representatives for the second- and third-generation cephalosporins; each has to be tested separately. Tetracycline is the representative for all the tetracyclines (chlortetracycline, doxycycline, minocycline, and oxytetracycline). Methicillin or oxacillin (preferred because of stability) are class representatives for the penicillinase-resistant penicillins.

Caution should be exercised in interpreting test results with the so-called heteroresistant staphylococci. These strains are resistant to methicillin and oxacillin and, therefore, are resistant to all the penicillinase-resistant penicillins. However, cloxacillin does not predict isolate resistance to methicillin or oxacillin. Likewise, cephalothin does not detect cephalothin resistance in these strains. If they are resistant to methicillin or oxacillin, they should be assumed to be resistant to cephalosporin, as well as to amoxicillin–clavulanic acid and to ticarcillin–clavulanic acid, regardless of *in vitro* test results.

Interpretation of staphylococcal resistance to penicillin G also presents a problem. Isolates with an MIC of less than 0.03 μg/ml usually lack beta-lactamase; those with an MIC of greater than 0.25 μg/ml produce it. Isolates with an MIC between these values may or may not produce beta-lactamase. The authors test all isolates with an MIC between 0.03 and 0.25 μg penicillin G/ml for the production of beta-lactamase by using a disk test (Beta Lactam Reagent Disk, Marion Scientific Corporation, Kansas City, MO 64114). A colony is rubbed on a disk containing a penicillin and a pH indicator. Beta-lactamase breaks down penicillin to penicilloic acid, which changes the color of the pH indicator. This problem does not occur if the disk diffusion assay is used.

References and Supplemental Reading

Alternative Methods for Antimicrobial Susceptibility Testing for Anaerobic Bacteria, Vol. 5, no. 18. Villanova, PA: National Committee for Clinical Laboratory Standards, 1985.

Lennette, E. H., Balows, A., Hausler, W. J., et al.: *Manual of Clinical Microbiology*, 4th ed. Washington, D.C.: American Society for Microbiology, 1985.

Methods for Dilution Antimicrobial susceptibility Tests for Bacteria that Grow Aerobically, Vol. 5, no. 22. Villanova, PA: National Committee for Clinical Laboratory Standards, 1985.

Performance Standards for Antimicrobial Disk Susceptibility Tests, 3rd ed. Villanova, PA: National Committee for Clinical Laboratory Standards, 1984.

CEPHALOSPORINS

J. EDMOND RIVIERE, D.V.M.
Raleigh, North Carolina

Cephalosporins are a class of beta-lactam antibiotics that are clinically effective against infections caused by gram-positive and gram-negative bacteria. They are pharmacologically similar in mechanism of action and clinical use to the more widely utilized beta-lactams, the penicillins. In order to optimally utilize them, an understanding of their mechanism of action, pharmacology, toxicology, and antimicrobial properties is essential. Although cephalosporins are often referred to in the clinical literature as a single group of drugs sharing similar properties, the overview presented in this article will demonstrate that three specific classes exist. This fact must be taken into consideration when one selects a cephalosporin for treatment of an infectious disease process. The data put forward are tabulated for the dog, since little information exists on cephalosporin pharmacology in the cat.

MECHANISM OF ACTION

Both cephalosporins and penicillins have a beta-lactam ring. In penicillin it is coupled to a thiazolidine ring; in cephalosporins, the beta-lactam ring is coupled to 7-amino-cephalosporanic acid. The beta-lactam moiety confers antimicrobial activity on the molecule, because it is a structural analogue of D-alanine/D-alanine, normally present in the peptide crosslinks of bacterial peptidoglycan cell walls. Like penicillins, cephalosporins prevent bacterial peptidoglycan cell wall synthesis by competitively inhibiting the bacterial transpeptidase responsible for crosslinking of the linear peptidoglycan polymers. The bacterial transpeptidase preferentially binds to the drug. In order for antimicrobial activity to occur, beta-lactams must have access to the extracellular site of cell wall synthesis. The cell wall structure of gram-positive bacteria has an "accessible" peptidoglycan network. However, the cell walls of gram-negative bacteria are more complex and have an outer coat of lipoprotein and lipopolysaccharide through which the beta-lactam must penetrate. Once inhibition of bacterial cell wall synthesis is complete, the effects on bacteria include rapid lysis or production of oval, bulbous, spherical, or filamentous forms prior to lysis. The effect on bacteria observed and the ultimate outcome are dependent on pH, availability of nutrients, and osmolarity of the local environment. If the environment is iso-osmotic with the intracellular cytoplasm (i.e., renal medulla with 1200 mOsm/L), L-forms of the organism may persist despite the presence of effective drug concentrations. This phenomenon helps explain why chronic renal infections are difficult to eradicate, since a beta-lactam antibiotic may suppress but not eradicate the infectious locus. If the environment is hypo-osmotic with the interior of the bacterial cell (i.e., normal extracellular fluid), the cells will swell and burst when cell wall synthesis is impaired.

Development of resistance is a common problem associated with penicillin use. Penicillin-resistant bacteria produce and liberate enzymes (beta-lactamases) that are capable of inactivating beta-lactam drugs. Gram-positive bacteria liberate the enzymes into the environment, whereas gram-negative bacteria produce them in the periplasmic space between the cell membrane and the peptidoglycan network. It is fortunate that most gram-positive bacteria are still sensitive to penicillin G. The major exception is penicillinase-producing *Staphylococcus*. Beta-lactamases are a heterogeneous group of enzymes: some have activity limited to penicillins, some have activity limited to cephalosporins, and some may inactivate both classes. The major direction of cephalosporin drug development has been to produce compounds that are resistant to beta-lactamase activity, bestowing on these drugs activity against gram-negative organisms that liberate these enzymes. This drug development effort has produced three "generations" of cephalosporin drugs (Table 1) Later (newer) generations tend to have (1) increased activity against gram-negative organisms, (2) decreased activity against gram-positive organisms, (3) decreased susceptibility to beta-lactamase inactivation, (4) a more selective spectrum of activity against specific micro-organisms, and (5) increased cost. In addition to these differences in the spectrums of antimicrobial activity, individual drugs in this class differ in routes of administration and pharmacokinetic properties.

PHARMACOLOGY

Cephalosporins are generally well-absorbed after intramuscular, subcutaneous, or oral administra-

Table 1. *Selected Cephalosporin Antibiotics*

Generic Name	Route	Dosage Range (mg/kg q 8 hr)	Half-life (min)
First-generation			
Cephalothin	IV,IM,SC	10–30	40–50
Cefazolin	IV,IM,SC	10–30	50–90
Cephapirin	IV,IM,SC	10–30	25–30
Cephalexin	PO	10–30	80–150
Cefadroxil	PO	10–30	80–120
Cephradine	PO,IM,SC	10–30	80–90
Cephaloridine	IM,SC	10–15	50–150
Second-generation			
Cefoxitin*	IV	10–20	45–60
Cefotetan*	IV	10–20	50–60
Cefamandole	IM,IV	15–30	30–55
Cefaclor	PO	10–25	100–120
Third-generation			
Cefotaxime	IV,IM,SC	25–50	45–60
Moxalactam†	IV	25–50	60–70

The dosages and half-lives tabulated are estimated based on the author's assessment of the literature.

*Classified as a cephamycin.

†Classified as an oxalocephalosporin.

tion, with bioavailability being greater than 75 per cent. Since many of these compounds are not stable in an acid environment, only a selected number are useful for oral administration. However, the rate of absorption is rapid, making available oral preparations a convenient dosage form.

The distribution of the cephalosporins is limited to the extracellular fluid space, with volumes of distribution for most drugs ranging from 0.25 to 0.5 L/kg. Protein binding is primarily to albumin, with the extent of binding being a function of the specific drug. These compounds are weak organic acids with pKa's ranging from 2.1 to 3.5. Significant concentrations can be found in the liver, kidneys, intestine, bile, lymph, and semen. There is generally poor distribution to the cerebrospinal fluid and ocular fluids, although some of the third-generation compounds have good distribution to the cerebrospinal fluid.

The elimination rate of the cephalosporins is very rapid, as can be appreciated from their short half-lives. This suggests that dosages must be administered on a divided daily basis to maintain effective serum and tissues concentrations of the drug. The dosages tabulated are estimates for a regimen in which drug administration is every 8 hr. In cases of severe infections in debilitated patients, a shorter dosage interval may be appropriate. Most compounds are eliminated primarily in urine, by glomerular filtration and active transport in proximal tubules. Because cephalosporins are eliminated almost exclusively by the kidney, urine concentrations are of an order of magnitude greater than serum concentrations. Therefore, they are pharmacologically well-suited for treatment of urinary tract infections. Renal tubular secretion is by the organic acid transport pathway; inhibition by probenecid may prolong the elimination half-life.

The exception to the aforementioned generalities are the cephalosporins that undergo hepatic biotransformation; they include cephalothin, cephapirin, cefaclor, and cefotaxime. A significant percentage of the systemic dose of these drugs may be metabolized before elimination. Because most cephalosporins are eliminated by the kidneys, dosages must be adjusted for patients with significant renal impairment. The preferred method is to extend the dosage interval in proportion to the degree of renal impairment. However, for compounds that are also eliminated by hepatic mechanisms, dosage adjustment is not required until severe renal insufficiency is present. Cefaclor is especially useful in these situations, since it is eliminated primarily by the liver in dogs. Since these compounds are relatively nontoxic, dosage adjustment is not critical. The exception is cephaloridine (a compound no longer available), which is contraindicated in renal failure because of its nephrotoxic potential.

Many extrapolations of the clinical utility of cephalosporins in dogs and cats are based on results obtained in human trials, since few data exist in the veterinary literature. This is especially true with the newer third-generation drugs; almost all the available information is based on studies conducted in humans. Cephalosporin elimination in humans may differ from that in canines. For example, the half-lives of elimination of moxalactam, cefotetan, cefoperazone, cephapirin, and cefpiramide may be significantly longer (two to four times) in humans than in canines. Deacetylation is a primary metabolic pathway for cephalosporin biotransformation, a pathway that consistently shows greater activity in dogs compared with humans. Interspecies differences in extent of protein binding also appear to contribute to differences in disposition. For many cephalosporins, the percentage of serum protein binding is much less in dogs than in humans. These interspecies differences are difficult to quantitate and are not a simple function of body surface area. Prolonged elimination half-life is a major therapeutic advantage of the newer cephalosporins in humans. For example, ceftriaxone has a half-life in humans of approximately 8 hr, and thus, less frequent dosing is required. Data on the half-life of this drug are not available for dogs. In spite of the canine tendency for enhanced elimination of many cephalosporins, the pharmacokinetics of cefotaxime is similar in dogs, cats, and humans. Nonetheless, species differences and the inability to accurately make consistent predictions preclude extrapolation of advantages cited in the human medical literature to small animal therapeutics.

TOXICOLOGY

Cephalosporins are a relatively nontoxic group of antibiotics, a fact that facilitates their clinical use in a wide variety of patients. The primary reported adverse effect is hypersensitivity, a very rare event. Crossallergenicity with penicillins may also occur. Mild nausea and vomiting may also be encountered. Because some drugs produce pain following intramuscular injection, specific formulations have been developed to minimize this problem (i.e., lidocaine is incorporated into the formulation). Thrombophlebitis can also occur after intravenous administration.

Cephalosporins may interact with various clinical laboratory tests. Elevations in the activity of serum alkaline phosphatase, alanine aminotransferase, aspartate aminotransferase, and lactate dehydrogenase as well as increased serum urea nitrogen concentrations have been reported. False-positive results of Coombs's tests and false-positive urinary glucose reactions have also been reported. Cephalothin sodium should not be mixed with other drugs prior to administration.

The major toxic manifestation discussed in the literature is nephrotoxicity. However, nephrotoxicity is primarily an attribute of cephaloridine, a drug no longer marketed for clinical use. Like other cephalosporins, cephaloridine is actively transported from the renal peritubular fluid into the tubules by the probenecid-sensitive acid transport system. However, unlike the situation with the other cephalosporins, there is no lumenal transport mechanism to allow cephaloridine to have a net secretion into the tubular fluid. The resulting active accumulation of cephaloridine in tubule cells produces cytotoxic intracellular concentrations. For the other cephalosporins, lumenal transport is present, net tubular secretion occurs, and toxicity is not seen. Some reports have suggested that cephalothin may be nephrotoxic in a small number of cases; however, supportive evidence is lacking to make a firm statement. Controversy still exists as to the effects of concurrent cephalosporin dosing on the nephrotoxic potential of aminoglycoside antibiotics. Data for dogs are not available. Thus, an assessment of risk is not possible, since potentiation occurs in some species, while protection occurs in others.

THERAPEUTIC USE

The primary criterion for selecting a cephalosporin antibiotic is the spectrum of its antimicrobial activity. It is in this context that the classification by generations is useful. It is beyond the scope of this section to discuss the comparative pharmacology of cephalosporins relative to other classes of antimicrobial agents. However, if a penicillin-sensitive gram-positive bacterium is responsible for the disease process, then a penicillin should be utilized as the first-line drug. Cephalosporins should not be administered unless resistance develops. For many serious gram-negative infections, the only alternatives are newer cephalosporins or an aminoglycoside. The choice between these two classes must be based on the assessment of relative sensitivities, local resistance patterns, cost, and the potential for inducing aminoglycoside toxicity. Each case must be considered on the basis of the individual data at hand.

First-generation cephalosporins have a very similar spectrum of activity. In fact, *in vitro* sensitivity to cephalothin is the reference standard for all first-generation cephalosporins. Because of this fact, there is no microbiologic basis for selecting one drug over another if sensitivity to the group is indicated. Only differences in availability, route of administration, pharmacokinetics, or "clinical experience" are valid criteria. First-generation cephalosporins have activity primarily against gram-positive bacteria and have excellent resistance to inactivation by beta-lactamases produced by penicillin-resistant *Staphylococcus intermedius* and *S. aureus*. However, these cephalosporins are NOT resistant to inactivation by gram-negative beta-lactamases. Therefore, their spectrum of activity against gram-negative bacteria is very similar to that of ampicillin, with first-generations cephalosporins having a slightly higher activity against *Proteus vulgaris*, *P. mirabilis*, and *Klebsiella* species. Such generalizations concerning gram-negative bacterial susceptibilities may be suspect, since individual patient history and geographic patterns of antimicrobial resistance may be predominant factors in the selection of a cephalosporin over an aminopenicillin such as ampicillin or amoxicillin. However, first-generation cephalosporins are NOT the drugs of choice for gram-negative bacterial infections, although they are for penicillin-resistant (including aminopenicillin-resistant) *Staphylococcus* infections.

First-generation cephalosporins designed for oral administration tend to have a slower rate of bactericidal action than parenteral products. This phenomenon may be related to the phenylglycine side group, which confers oral bioavailability. The final decision in selecting a first-generation cephalosporin depends on clinical diagnosis and antimicrobial susceptibility testing. This decision can only be used to select a cephalosporin over a different antibiotic group and not to select one first-generation drug over another.

Second-generation cephalosporins have greater resistance to degradation by gram-negative beta-lactamases. The cephamycins also have activity against many anaerobic infections. Some workers classify cefaclor as a first-generation drug, although its activity against *Haemophilus influenzae* is justification for not including it in this group. Since antimicrobial activity is not similar for all second-generation cephalosporins, individual susceptibility testing is required. The activity of cephamycins (cetoxitin and cefotetan) against indole-positive *Proteus* and some *Enterobacter* species is especially good. These drugs may be indicated for ampicillin-resistant *Escherichia coli* infections. Cefamandole does not share this activity against ampicillin-resistant enteric organisms. It is classified in this group because of activity against *Haemophilus influenzae* and *Neisseria* species (primarily human pathogens). These drugs retain activity against gram-positive organisms, although penicillins would be the preferred choice as a first-line antimicrobial agent.

Third-generation cephalosporins have moderate activity against gram-positive organisms; however, they have excellent activity against gram-negative microbes, especially *Pseudomonas*, *Proteus*, *Enterobacter*, and *Citrobacter* species. They are highly resistant to inactivation by beta-lactamases produced by gram-negative pathogens and *Staphylococcus*. Although documented clinical experience in veterinary medicine is lacking, they are probably the drugs of choice for severe, multiple resistant Enterobacteriaceae genera. Newer members of this group (for which very limited data exist) include cefoperazone, ceftizoxime, ceftazidime, and ceftriaxone.

References and Supplemental Reading

Aronson, A. L., and Aucoin, D. P.: Antimicrobial Drugs. *In* Ettinger, S., (ed.): *Textbook of Veterinary Internal Medicine*, 3rd ed. Philadelphia: W. B. Saunders Co. (in press).

Davis, L. E.: *Handbook of Small Animal Therapeutics*. New York: Churchill Livingstone, 1985.

Goldberg, D. M.: The cephalosporins. Med. Clin. North Am. 71:1113, 1987.

Johnston, D. E.: *The Bristol Veterinary Handbook of Antimicrobial Therapy, 2nd Edition*, Veterinary Learning Systems, Lawrenceville, NJ, 1987.

Mandell, G. L., and Sande, M. A.: Antimicrobial agents: Penicillins, cephalosporins and other beta-lactam antibiotics. *In* Gilman, A. G., Goodman, L. S., Rall, T. W., and Murad, F. (eds.): *Goodman and Gilman's The Pharmacological Basis of Therapeutics, 7th ed.* New York: Macmillan Publishing Co., 1985, pp. 1115–1149.

Neu, H. C.: New antibiotics: Areas of appropriate use. J. Infect. Dis. 155:403, 1987.

Powers, T. E., and Garg, R. C.: Pharmacotherapeutics of newer penicillins and cephalosporins. J.A.V.M.A. 176:1054, 1980.

Quintiliani, R., Nightingale, C. H., Rossi, J. G., and Ristuccia, A. M.: Cephalosporins: An overview. *In* Ristuccia, A., and Cunha, B. A. (eds.): *Antimicrobial Therapy*. New York: Raven Press, 1984, pp. 289–303.

Riviere, J. E., Craigmill, A. L., and Sundlof, S. F.: *Handbook of Comparative Pharmacokinetics and Tissue Residues of Antimicrobial Drugs*. Boca Raton, FL: CRC Press (in press).

Salton, M. R. J., and Shockman, G. D.: *Beta Lactam Antibiotics*. New York: Academic Press, 1981.

Sawada, Y., Hanano, M., Sugiyama, Y., et al.: Prediction of the disposition of beta-lactam antibiotics in humans from pharmacokinetic parameters in animals. J. Pharmacokinet. Biopharm. 12:241, 1984.

Thomson, T. D., Quay, J. F., and Webber, J. A.: Cephalosporin group of antimicrobial drugs. J.A.V.M.A. 185:1109, 1984.

CLAVULANATE-POTENTIATED ANTIBIOTICS

W. RANDAL KILGORE, D.V.M.

Bristol, Tennessee

Since its inception, antibiotic therapy has been hampered by bacterial resistance. A bacterial enzyme capable of destroying penicillin was described even before penicillin could be developed as a useful therapeutic agent. Remarkable advances have been made in the battle to overcome resistance, allowing medicine to maintain an advantage over most bacterial pathogens. Yet, the continued emergence of bacterial resistance has been, and will continue to be, a major motivation for the development of new and better antimicrobial agents.

BACTERIAL RESISTANCE TO BETA-LACTAM ANTIBIOTICS

No group of antibiotics has had greater impact on chemotherapy of infection than beta-lactam 'antibiotics. This family of antimicrobial agents, which comprises the penicillins and the cephalosporins, was named for the chemical structure common to all its members. As a class, beta-lactams continue to be extremely safe and effective antibiotics.

The most important means of bacterial resistance to beta-lactams is production of beta-lactamase. Beta-lactamases are enzymes that destroy antibiotic activity of both penicillins and cephalosporins by hydrolyzing the beta-lactam ring.

Beta-lactamases are a diverse, expanding family of enzymes. This is not surprising, considering most bacteria and fungi are thought to be capable of beta-lactamase production. The ability of pathogens to transmit genetic information for production of beta-lactamase from one organism to another continues to contribute to the increasing incidence of beta-lactamases. Classification systems can be based on many criteria. One classification schema is shown in Figure 1.

Beta-lactamases are generally found in the periplasmic space of intact gram-negative bacteria and are excreted as exoenzymes in gram-positive bacteria. The phenomenon of indirect pathogenicity is of significance in some mixed infections, particularly with reference to exoenzymes. Therapeutic failure can occur when the primary pathogen is protected from the antibiotic by a secondary organism that produces large quantities of beta-lactamase.

The most recent success in the battle against resistance was the introduction of beta-lactamase inhibitors, which protect the antibiotic from destruction by beta-lactamases. The first to be introduced to clinical practice was clavulanic acid (CA). Other inhibitors are in various stages of development for use in both humans and animals.

CLAVULANIC ACID

Clavulanic acid was isolated from *Streptomyces clavuligerus* in the late 1960's (Fig. 2). Despite its beta-lactam ring structure, it possesses little intrinsic antibacterial activity. However, it does inhibit a broad spectrum of beta-lactamases, including Richmond-Sykes types II, III, IV, and V. Beta-lactamases such as those produced by *Staphylococcus aureus* and *Bacteroides fragilis* are also inhibited. The only enzymes not well inhibited are most of the narrow-spectrum cephalosporinases of the type I category, which are not adept at destroying penicillins. CA readily penetrates both gram-negative and gram-positive bacteria.

Pharmacology and toxicology studies conducted during both preclinical and clinical phases of development, together with several years of field use, demonstrated that CA possesses a wide margin of safety not unlike those of other beta-lactams. The combination of amoxicillin and CA (AM/CA) (Augmentin, Beecham Laboratories) for oral use in humans first became available in the United States in 1984. Food and Drug Administration (FDA) approval for its use in dogs followed 3 months later (Clavamox, Beecham Laboratories). A parenteral combination of ticarcillin and CA (TI/CA) (Timentin, Beecham Laboratories) for human use, approved in 1985, is the latest CA potentiated antibiotic to become available.

Clavulanic acid, supplied as the potassium salt, possesses a pharmacokinetic profile similar to that of many beta-lactam antibiotics. It is well-absorbed orally and is not significantly affected by food in the stomach. There is poor penetration into the CSF in the absence of meningeal inflammation. Excretion is primarily by glomerular filtration, with high levels of the active drug in the urine. Probenecid does not significantly increase excretion time.

An oral CA dose of 2.75 mg/kg of body weight

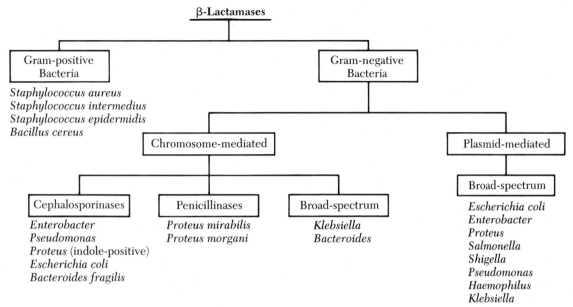

Figure 1. Classification of beta-lactamases. (Reprinted with permission from Kilgore, W. R., Simmons, R. D., Jackson, J. W.: Compend. Cont. Ed. Prac. Vet. 8:325, 1986.)

every 12 hr has been established through preclinical and clinical studies in dogs and cats as providing adequate inhibition of beta-lactamases. The drug is supplied in a fixed combination with an antibiotic partner. Should alteration of the antibiotic dosage be desired in certain clinical situations, the demand for CA will not be increased or decreased. CA has been classified as a "suicide" inhibitor; that is, a stable complex is formed between enzyme and inhibitor. Therefore, extended tissue levels of CA are not required. Relatively low levels of less than 1 μg are required to inhibit beta-lactamases.

Safe use of CA in pregnant or breeding animals has not been determined, although laboratory animal studies have not demonstrated any reproductive problems. Oral suspension formulations should be stored under refrigeration following reconstitution and should be used within 10 days.

Potentiation of Amoxicillin

Considerable improvement in the *in vitro* spectrum of activity of amoxicillin (AM) is attained

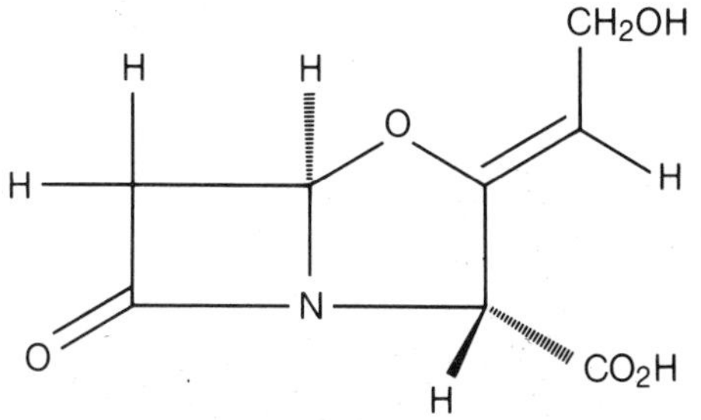

Figure 2. Clavulanic acid (CA).

through addition of CA. Oral use of AM/CA is approved for canine skin and soft tissue infections caused by susceptible *Staphylococcus* species including *S. aureus*, *Streptococcus* species, and *Escherichia coli*. AM/CA is also approved for skin and soft tissue infections in cats, including those caused by susceptible *Pasteurella*. Feline urinary tract infections caused by susceptible *E. coli* have also received FDA approval for treatment. The compound is supplied in a fixed dosage of 5 mg of amoxicillin for every 1.25 mg of CA. The recommended canine dosage for the combination is 13.75 mg/kg of body weight twice a day. A cat of average size receives a unit dose of 62.5 mg twice daily.

In human medicine, AM/CA is indicated in the treatment of otitis media or sinusitis and of infections of the lower respiratory tract, urinary tract, and skin and skin structures. A number of anaerobes from human infections have displayed *in vitro* susceptibility to AM/CA. As with the veterinary product, the various formulations of the human product contain 5 mg of amoxicillin for every 1.25 mg of CA acid, with one exception. There are two tablet forms for adults, one containing a higher amoxicillin content (500 mg), and the other a lower level (250 mg). Since each tablet contains 125 mg of CA, the "250" tablet contains 2.5 mg of amoxicillin for every 1.25 mg of CA. The larger tablet size is intended for more severe infections or less susceptible pathogens.

The prevalence of beta-lactamase is not well known in veterinary medicine. Therefore, bacterial susceptibility to AM/CA is best predicted by *in vitro* methods. A study encompassing 1524 unselected clinical isolates from dogs and cats compared

Table 1. *Sensitivity of 1524 Canine Clinical Isolates by Standard Disk Method*

Organism	Am/Cl[a] % (n)	AMPI[b] % (n)	CEPH[c] % (n)	CHLOR[d] % (n)	ERYTH[e] % (n)	GENT[f] % (n)	LINC[g] % (n)	PEN[h] % (n)	TETRA[i] % (n)	SXT[j] % (n)
Bordetella bronchiseptica	93 (14)	7 (14)	86 (14)	92 (13)	67 (3)	100 (14)	0 (2)	0 (3)	93 (14)	21 (14)
Escherichia coli	81 (277)	45 (288)	60 (285)	73 (269)	6 (127)	92 (287)	1 (172)	1 (134)	54 (287)	82 (288)
Klebsiella pneumoniae	66 (80)	1 (84)	64 (84)	45 (75)	0 (11)	59 (82)	0 (32)	0 (24)	43 (81)	49 (84)
Pasteurella spp.	98 (58)	97 (58)	95 (58)	95 (56)	90 (52)	98 (58)	12 (42)	98 (46)	89 (56)	95 (58)
Proteus mirabilis	91 (84)	76 (86)	88 (86)	71 (78)	0 (9)	95 (85)	0 (28)	5 (21)	7 (85)	88 (86)
Proteus spp.	90 (41)	83 (41)	76 (41)	81 (41)	3 (39)	98 (41)	0 (40)	18 (40)	7 (41)	85 (41)
Pseudomonas aeruginosa	2 (90)	1 (92)	2 (92)	2 (88)	12 (26)	79 (92)	0 (29)	4 (25)	4 (92)	6 (91)
Staphylococcus aureus	99 (309)	34 (308)	99 (307)	94 (287)	84 (291)	100 (307)	81 (298)	33 (290)	61 (307)	96 (309)
Staphylococcus intermedius	100 (106)	38 (118)	99 (118)	89 (118)	75 (118)	98 (118)	67 (79)	33 (72)	45 (118)	86 (118)
Staphylococcus (coagulase positive)	100 (81)	37 (82)	99 (81)	85 (82)	77 (82)	96 (82)	87 (77)	32 (81)	50 (82)	88 (80)
Streptococcus (beta-hemolytic)	98 (94)	91 (98)	93 (98)	96 (97)	88 (92)	76 (97)	83 (80)	94 (83)	40 (97)	81 (98)

[a]Am/Cl = amoxicillin/clavulanate potassium.   [e]ERYTH = erythromycin.   [h]PEN = penicillin.
[b]AMPI = ampicillin.   [f]GENT = gentamicin.   [i]TETRA = tetracycline.
[c]CEPH = cephalothin.   [g]LINC = lincomycin.   [j]SXT = sulfa/trimethoprim.
[d] CHLOR = chloramphenicol.
(Reprinted with permission from Kilgore, W. R., Simmons, R. D., Jackson, J. W.: Beta-lactamase inhibition: A new approach in overcoming bacterial resistance. Compend. Cont. Ed. Pract. Vet. 8:325, 1986.)

AM/CA to other commonly used veterinary antibiotics, using the disk method (Table 1) (Kilgore et al., 1986). Comparison of ampicillin and AM/CA susceptibilities correlates well with production of beta-lactamase. When seen, resistance to AM/CA is usually the result of a permeability barrier to amoxicillin, as in the case of *Pseudomonas aeruginosa*.

Potentiation of Ticarcillin

Ticarcillin (TI) is an extended-spectrum parenteral penicillin similar to, but more potent in activity than, carbenicillin. Approved veterinary use is limited to intrauterine treatment of endometritis.

Therefore, the broad spectrum of *in vitro* and *in vivo* activity demonstrated in human medicine is little known to many small animal practitioners.

Ticarcillin is more adept than amoxicillin in overcoming the permeability barrier gram-negative bacteria employ to resist some beta-lactam antibiotics. However, it is unstable in the presence of many beta-lactamases, including those produced by *Staphylococcus* and *Klebsiella*. Therefore, CA potentiation of ticarcillin represents a significant improvement in antibiotic activity. *In vitro* minimal inhibitory concentration (MIC) data from human bacterial isolates are summarized in Table 2. Susceptibilities of veterinary isolates to TI/CA have been examined in at least one study. Results were similar to those obtained with human isolates

Table 2. *Effect of Clavulanic Acid on Ticarcillin Minimal Inhibitory Concentrations (MICs) of Bacterial Isolates from Humans*

Organism	Number	Ticarcillin MIC_{50}[†]	Ticarcillin MIC_{90}[†]	TI/CA MIC_{50}	TI/CA MIC_{90}	Percent Susceptible* Ticarcillin	Percent Susceptible* TI/CA
GRAM-NEGATIVE							
Klebsiella pneumoniae	908	>64	>64	4	32	25	93
Proteus vulgaris	49	8	32	≤1	≤1	94	100
Escherichia coli	1875	2	>64	2	64	79	93
Enterobacter aerogenes	259	2	64	2	64	90	93
Serratia marcescens	311	4	>64	4	64	85	90
Proteus mirabilis	617	≤1	≤1	≤1	≤1	98	100
Pseudomonas aeruginosa	1385	16	>64	16	>64	89	88
Bacteroides fragilis	56	32	>64	≤1	4	79	100
GRAM-POSITIVE							
Staphylococcus aureus	1137	4	8	2	4	—	—
Coagulase-negative staphylococci	689	4	64	2	32	—	—
Enterococci	1138	>64	>64	64	64	—	—
Other streptococci	60	2	8	2	8	—	—

Percentage of strains tested susceptible to ≤64 µg/ml of ticarcillin alone and ticarcillin with 2 µg/ml of clavulanic acid (TL/CA).
[†]MIC at which growth of 50 and 90 per cent of strains tested are inhibited.
Adapted from Fuchs, P. C., Barry, A. L., and Jones, R. N.: In vitro activity and disk susceptibility of Timentin: Current status. Am. J. Med. 79:25, 1985.

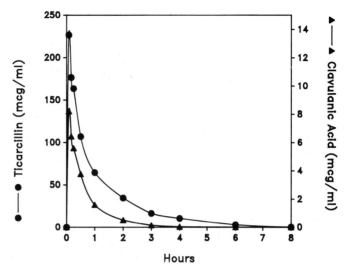

Figure 3. Canine serum levels following intravenous administration of TI/CA (ticarcillin, 50 mg/kg; CA, 1.7 mg/kg). (Adapted from Garg, R. C., Keefe, T. J., and Vig, M. M.: J. Vet. Pharmacol. Therap. 10:324, 1987.)

(Sparks et al., 1987). The pharmacokinetics of TI/CA in dogs have been investigated (Garg et al., 1987).

A canine dose of TI/CA (50 mg/kg of ticarcillin, 1.7 mg/kg of CA) has been proposed (Garg et al., 1987). As with humans, higher doses of ticarcillin than typically used for penicillins are needed, because MICs of many gram-negative isolates are high. Serum levels of TI/CA following intravenous administration in dogs are depicted in Figure 3. Ticarcillin is not absorbed following oral administration. Therefore, TI/CA is supplied for injection as a sterile, soluble powder for reconstitution. Depending on the MIC of the pathogen, frequency of administration may be three to four times daily. Intramuscular administration may cause discomfort at the injection site.

TI/CA has not been FDA approved for use in veterinary medicine. Veterinary clinical efficacy and safety studies have not been conducted with the combination. As with AM/CA, the combination should not be used in individuals known to be hypersensitive to penicillin. In human medicine, TI/CA is indicated in the treatment of bacterial septicemia, lower respiratory tract infections, bone and joint infections, skin and skin structure infections, and urinary tract infections caused by susceptible strains.

In summary, the availability of CA has done more than rejuvenate antibiotic activity against microbes with newly acquired resistance. The spectra of amoxicillin and ticarcillin have been enhanced to include pathogens historically resistant to these antibiotics. With a wide margin of safety and a reasonable cost, CA is a significant addition to the clinician's antimicrobial armamentarium.

References and Supplemental Reading

Bywater, R. J., Palmer, G. H., Buswell, J. F., et al.: Clavulanate-potentiated amoxycillin: Activity in vitro and bioavailability in the dog. Vet. Rec. 115:33, 1985.

Fuchs, P. C., Barry, A. L., and Jones, R. N.: In vitro activity and disk susceptibility of Timentin: Current status. Am. J. Med. 79:25, 1985.

Garg, R. C., Keefe, T. J., and Vig, M. M.: Serum levels and pharmacokinetics of ticarcillin and clavulanic acid in dogs following parenteral administration of Timentin. J. Vet. Pharmacol. Ther. 10:324, 1987.

Kilgore, W. R., Simmons, R. D., and Jackson, J. W.: Beta-lactamase inhibition: A new approach in overcoming bacterial resistance. Compend. Cont. Ed. Pract. Vet. 8:325, 1986.

Richmond, M. H., and Sykes, R. B.: The beta-lactamases of gram-negative bacteria and their possible physiological role. In Rose, A. H., Tempest, D. W. (eds.): Advances in Microbial Physiology, Vol. 9. London: Academic Press, 1973, pp. 31–88.

Sparks, S. E., Jones, R. L., and Kilgore, W. R.: In vitro susceptibility of bacteria to ticarcillin–clavulanic acid combination. Am. J. Vet. Res. (in press).

TREATMENT OF FUNGAL AND ENDOCRINE DISORDERS WITH IMIDAZOLE DERIVATIVES

M. D. WILLARD, D.V.M.
College Station, Texas

KETOCONAZOLE

Applied Pharmacology

Ketoconazole, itraconazole, and enilconazole are imidazole derivatives with significant antifungal activity. They are similar to miconazole, an older but less commonly used drug. Although not currently approved for use in dogs and cats, ketoconazole is a popular treatment for various mycoses in these species. The canine dosage usually ranges from 10 to 30 mg/kg/day, although 40 mg/kg/day is recommended for nasal and central nervous system problems. Feline doses usually range from 10 to 30 mg/kg/day, although as much as 70 mg/kg/day has been administered without significant side effects. There is debate as to whether simultaneous feeding alters the bioavailability of orally administered ketoconazole. Theoretically, food stimulates the release of gastric acid, which should increase bioavailability. Simultaneous oral administration of sodium bicarbonate or antacids seem to decrease ketoconazole absorption. After oral administration, significant concentrations of ketoconazole occur in the liver, adrenal, lungs, kidneys, bone marrow, bladder, milk, fur, sebum, and connective tissue, whereas skin, brain, testes, bone, and bile have minimal concentrations. There are conflicting data as to ketoconazole concentrations in cerebrospinal fluid (CSF) and urine, although CSF concentrations clearly tend to be less than those found in other organs. Ketoconazole has the potential to produce birth defects.

Maximal canine blood ketoconazole concentrations occur 1 to 5 hr after oral administration. Following ingestion of 10 mg of ketoconazole/kg, peak plasma concentrations of 8.9 μg/ml with a half-life of 2.8 hr are expected in most dogs; however, bioavailability varies considerably among patients. Absorption can sometimes be enhanced by administering the drug as an oral solution. In most dogs, approximately 50 per cent of the drug can be recovered unchanged from the feces. Most of the absorbed drug is metabolized by the liver into inactive fragments. Eventually, 80 per cent of these inactive fragments will be excreted via the biliary tract, whereas less than 10 per cent will be excreted in the urine. Total metabolism and excretion of a dose of ketoconazole requires 24 to 72 hr in dogs. At commonly used dosages, ketoconazole slows the hepatic metabolism of methylprednisolone and chlordiazepoxide. Ketoconazole interacts with few drugs (e.g., warfarin and rifampin), but it may increase serum cyclosporin concentrations into the toxic range.

Treatment of Fungal Disorders

Ketoconazole inhibits fungal ergosterol biosynthesis 30 to 70 times more readily than mammalian cholesterol metabolism. This inhibition is probably responsible for ketoconazole's fungistatic effect, as it weakens the fungal cell wall and causes C-14 methylsterols to accumulate. These affect membrane permeability and inhibit growth. Finally, hydrogen peroxide accumulates in the fungal cell, causing subcellular degeneration.

Ketoconazole has been used for the treatment of *Candida* species, *Blastomyces dermatitidis*, *Histoplasma capsulatum*, *Coccidioides immitis*, *Cryptococcus neoformans*, dermatophytes, and other fungi. It is preferred over amphotericin B in patients with renal dysfunction. Ketoconazole is effective against *Candida* species, in which it prevents the leukocyte-engulfed yeasts from producing mycelium and pseudomycelium, structures that survive in white blood cells (WBCs). Ketoconazole also has reasonable activity against *C. immitis*. Histoplasmosis and blastomycosis can be treated with ketoconazole, but 1 to 2 weeks of therapy may be required before a clinical response is seen. Blastomycosis may progress significantly during that time; therefore, patients with ocular or severe pulmonary involvement are best treated initially with amphotericin B. Increased relapse rates can occur when ketoconazole is the only drug used to treat blastomycosis. Therefore, long treatment periods (e.g., at least 3 to 4 and up to 6 to 8 months) are recommended.

Cutaneous cryptococcosis can be cured with ketoconazole; however, extensive nasal lesions may be more difficult to cure. Patients with central nervous system (CNS) cryptococcosis have a poor prognosis. Nasal aspergillosis has been treated with ketoconazole, with mixed results. Ketoconazole inhibits the fungi but is often unable to cure the infection. Nasal aspergillosis may be controlled as long as ketoconazole is administered, only to relapse when therapy ceases. Finally, various other organisms have been successfully treated with ketoconazole, such as *Blastocystis hominis*, *Trypanosoma cruzi*, *Trichinella spiralis*, and *Prototheca* and *Leishmania* species, although the last two have not always responded.

Ketoconazole is typically the sole therapeutic agent used in mycoses, but ketoconazole and amphotericin B have been combined in some cases. Amphotericin B can be used initially to quickly obtain control, after which ketoconazole is substituted to resolve the infection. This approach is convenient because ketoconazole is administered orally and is not nephrotoxic. Amphotericin B therapy can also follow ketoconazole. While such therapy has often been successful, caution is warranted. Exposing certain fungi (e.g., *Candida* and *Aspergillus* species) to ketoconazole may render them resistant to amphotericin B, even though they were previously sensitive to it, ostensibly owing to lessened amounts of ergosterol. Simultaneous use of ketoconazole with other antifungal drugs has also been tried. In experimental *Histoplasma* and *Cryptococcus* infections, most combinations offer only a modest advantage over ketoconazole alone. Clinical canine blastomycosis and histoplasmosis seem to respond as well or perhaps better to ketoconazole plus amphotericin B compared with either agent alone.

Treatment of Endocrine Disorders

Even though ketoconazole inhibits principally plant ergosterol biosynthesis, it affects mammalian cholesterol synthesis if present in sufficient concentrations. High doses (e.g., 30 mg of ketoconazole/kg) decrease cholesterol synthesis and lower serum cholesterol concentrations. Ketoconazole also inhibits certain enzymes responsible for synthesis of hormones from cholesterol (e.g., cortisol). However, this inhibition only exists as long as blood ketoconazole concentrations persist. The inhibitory effect disappears when the concentration wanes. Therefore, once daily administration of ketoconazole rarely causes clinical adrenal suppression. Even though the plasma cortisol concentrations are decreased each day, the serum ketoconazole concentration decreases 8 to 10 hr after administration, allowing the pituitary-adrenal axis to be re-established. However, if constant blood ketoconazole concentrations are attained by multiple daily administrations or high dosages, there may be persistent

plasma cortisol suppression. This does not seem to be coupled with increased adrenocorticotropic hormone (ACTH) secretion. Ketoconazole can also directly antagonize cortisol by occupying glucocorticoid receptors in some cells. Suppression of cortisol production can be used in the treatment of spontaneous hyperadrenocorticism resistant to mitotane (*o,p'*-DDD), or when rapid control of adrenal disease is desirable. Although the drug is not expected to destroy adrenal tumors, there is one report of adrenal tumor regression after ketoconazole therapy. (For further information on treatment of hyperadrenocorticism with ketoconazole, see p. 1027.) The typical dosage of ketoconazole used in treating canine hyperadrenocorticism is 30 mg/kg, divided 2 to 3 times per day.

Ketoconazole has been used to lower serum testosterone concentrations in humans with prostatic carcinoma. Dogs with prostatic carcinoma are usually castrated; however, many dogs develop this neoplasm years after having been neutered. Ketoconazole therapy might be useful in these dogs as well as those with prostatitis, because it transiently reduces serum testosterone concentrations. However, there seems to be a tendency for serum testosterone concentrations to rebound after ketoconazole therapy.

The same enzymatic inhibition that lowers testosterone and cortisol concentrations may elevate concentrations of other steroidal hormones. In male dogs, serum progesterone and 17-hydroxyprogesterone concentrations greatly increase during ketoconazole therapy. Interestingly, both of these hormones are potent antipruritics. This may explain why some dermatophytosis patients treated with ketoconazole become nonpruritic before the fungal infection is controlled.

Ketoconazole's effects on other hormones are unclear. Plasma aldosterone response to ACTH may be slightly inhibited, while effects on estrogen appear to be inconsistent. In normal male humans, ketoconazole decreases 1,25-dihydroxyvitamin D concentrations, but not concentrations of serum 25-hydroxyvitamin D, calcium, and phosphorus. The clinical significance of these findings is currently speculative. Finally, ketoconazole has been shown to inhibit leukotriene formation in some species, offering protection against certain aspects of anaphylaxis.

Cats treated with similar dosages of ketoconazole have minimal changes in plasma cortisol and serum progesterone concentrations, while changes in serum testosterone concentrations are difficult to predict. These findings may be due to differences in drug absorption and metabolism or adrenal gland physiology.

Ketoconazole has few significant side effects in dogs and cats. Anorexia or vomiting may occur, but these signs usually resolve when the dosage is reduced or when the drug is given twice a day with food. Cats in particular may benefit from the latter. The acute canine oral median lethal dose (LD_{50}) is greater than 500 mg/kg. The typically used dosage of 10 to 40 mg/kg/day usually does not cause significant problems even when used for 12 months. However, 60 mg/kg/day may cause severe illness in dogs after several months, and 80 mg/kg/day typically causes death within a month. A dosage of 30 mg/kg/day has been used in cats for one month without problems, and some reports describe longer treatment periods with higher dosages (e.g., 70 mg/kg/day). Hepatic enzymes can transiently increase. Rarely, there may be a dose-independent hepatopathy with icterus and increased hepatic enzyme activities. This hepatopathy seems similar to that reported in humans, being reversible if the drug is withdrawn. There are several reports of humans with symptomatic hypoadrenocorticism due to ketoconazole therapy. This has not yet been reported in pets, but some dogs treated with ketoconazole for hyperadrenocorticism have shown transient signs of hypoadrenocorticism, ostensibly from the rapid decrease in plasma cortisol concentrations. Finally, azoospermia, lack of libido, and gynecomastia have been reported in humans and might occur in dogs.

ITRACONAZOLE AND ENILCONAZOLE

Itraconazole and enilconazole are related to ketoconazole. Administered orally, itraconazole is more potent against *Aspergillus* species, *Blastomyces dermatitidis*, and *Cryptococcus neoformans* in *in vitro* studies than equal amounts of ketoconazole. It also has significant activity against dermatophytes, *Candida* species, and *Trypanosoma cruzi*. Itraconazole causes necrosis of invasive *Aspergillus* hyphae at less than one tenth the concentration required for ketoconazole. Subjectively, itraconazole seems to be at least as effective as ketoconazole in the treatment of blastomycosis. Although it kills *Coccidioides immitis* more slowly than does

ketoconazole, itraconazole reduces the number of colony-forming units in pulmonary parenchyma. Minimal toxicity has been seen in dogs given itraconazole, although rare gastrointestinal upset and vasculitis have been anecdotally reported. Finally, itraconazole has minimal effects upon mammalian steroidal hormone concentrations.

Enilconazole is a topically administered wettable powder. It is fungicidal and sporicidal, having activity against *Aspergillus* and *Penicillium* species and dermatophytes. For the latter, the patients are dipped in a solution of 2000 ppm enilconazole. For nasal aspergillosis, 20 mg/kg of enilconazole is divided into two treatments/day and flushed through the sinuses and nostrils every day for 7 to 10 days. Enilconazole currently appears to be the most effective therapy for canine nasal aspergillosis. The acute oral LD_{50} is greater than 500 mg/kg in dogs. Dogs chronically given a dosage of enilconazole of 5 mg/kg/day suffered only a slight decrease in weight.

References and Supplemental Reading

Baxter, J. G., Brass, C., Schentag, J. J., et al.: Pharmacokinetics of ketoconazole administered intravenously to dogs and orally as tablets and solution to humans and dogs. J. Pharm. Sci. 75:443, 1986.

Cutsen, J. V., Gerven, F. V., VanDeVen, M., et al.: Itraconazole, a new triazole that is orally active in aspergillosis. Antimicrob. Agents Chemother. 26:527, 1984.

Dieperink, H., and Moller, J.: Ketoconazole and cyclosporin. Lancet 2:1217, 1982.

Dunbar, M., Jr.: Ketoconazole: Oral absorption, serum clearance, and tissue distribution in the dog. Master's thesis, Texas A&M University, May 1983.

Intraconazole, Basic Medical Information Brochure. Washington Crossing, NJ: Pitman-Moore, Inc., August 1984.

Levine, H. B. (ed.): *Ketoconazole in the Management of Fungal Disease.* New York: ADIS Press, 1982.

Odds, F. C.: Interactions among amphotericin-B, 5-fluorocytosine, ketoconazole, and miconazole against pathogenic fungi *in vitro.* Antimicrob. Agents Chemother. 22:763, 1982.

Schaffner, A., and Frick, P. G.: The effect of ketoconazole on amphotericin-B in a model of disseminated aspergillosis. J. Infect. Dis. 151:902, 1985.

Sonino, N.: The use of ketoconazole as an inhibitor of steroid production. N. Engl. J. Med. 317:812, 1987.

Technical Information on Enilconazole. Washington Crossing, NJ: Pitman-Moore, Inc., 1985.

Wilson, G., and Peacock, J. E., Jr.: Imidazoles, ketoconazole, amphotericin-B, and *Candida guilliermondii.* Ann. Intern. Med. 102:866, 1985.

THE PRACTICE OF VETERINARY MEDICINE IN HUMANE SOCIETY FACILITIES

MARK ALJIAN EDWARDS, D.V.M.

Brighton, South Australia

Today, modern humane societies in large cities are complex organizations consisting of the humane society adoption facilities, veterinary hospitals, and animal control facilities. Community animal control may be provided on a contract basis by the humane society to the municipality or by a separate government agency that relies on the humane society medical expertise through consultation. The humane society as the central point of the organization typically consists of a board of directors, an executive committee, an executive director, an operations director, and head and staff veterinarians, along with the supervisors of the various departments (public education/public relations, bookkeeping, maintenance, and animal control). Working staff, volunteers, and auxiliary personnel may bring the total number of people directly involved with some operations to over 200.

The role of veterinarians in this organization varies with its size and diversity and with the medical, management, and administrative skills of the veterinarians. In this unique practice environment the veterinarian, being an educated and respected professional member of the humane society management team, will be called upon to provide direction in three distinct areas: medicine, management, and administration.

MEDICAL ASPECTS

The Clients

To manage the patient, the veterinarian must first understand the client. The veterinarian is frequently dealing with members of lower socioeconomic levels who mistrust or are apprehensive of medical and societal institutions in general. The veterinarian must overcome these apprehensions and improve or protect the health of the animal patients. Accordingly, there is a need for interpersonal skills in addition to veterinary skills. Most clients of a humane society veterinary hospital located near a lower socioeconomic level often do not seek veterinary services. They have limited disposable income and, therefore, do not want expensive diagnostics or therapies. They are apprehensive about what they perceive as unnecessary costs, and if oversold, will refuse therapy and not return. The approach to this type of client should be to conduct a proper physical examination of the patient, but it should begin by addressing the primary concerns of the owner. Many clients become apprehensive and defensive when the veterinarian appears to be "searching" for problems that will make the bill higher. After the primary problems have been discussed, other areas of medical concern can be addressed. The veterinarian should suggest probable causes, outline recommended treatment and options, and give estimates of prices. Success of therapy should be discussed in terms of probability so that clients can decide what is affordable. In some cases, deferred payment or discount service may be discussed. However, in the author's experience, one should not supply gratis medical service or products, since this diminishes the impetus for preventive medicine.

The Animals

On the basis of a defined history and physical examination, a list of problems should be developed and refined. Presumptive diagnoses (rule-outs) for the problems should then be formulated. In the usual humane society clinic, a huge volume of cases provide statistical data of the probability rates of many disorders. Utilizing this information, the clinician can thus "play the odds" in making a presumptive diagnosis.

Once the list of rule-outs is constructed, treatment may be initiated for the disease of highest probability. The rule-outs are then accepted or rejected based on the patient's response to treatment.

Most general humane society hospitals see a broad range of cases. Some diseases that are encountered at these facilities include distemper, canine respiratory disease complex, upper respiratory infections, kennel cough, parvovirus enteritis, die-

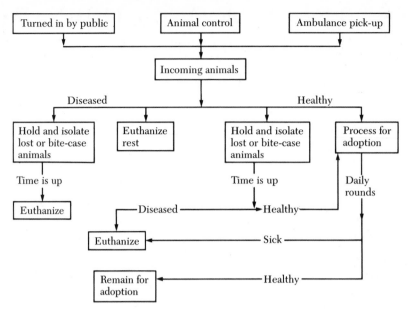

Figure 1. Humane Society flow chart.

tary and foreign body enteritis, malnutrition, ingrown collars, untreated trauma and open wounds, heartworm disease, ectoparasites, intestinal parasites, feline respiratory disease complex, and feline leukemia. Treatment of these diseases has been described elsewhere. Distemper requires special mention because it is seen and treated with disproportionate frequency in humane shelters as compared with many private practices.

Distemper commonly affects puppies and unvaccinated adults. It is important to differentiate this disease from upper respiratory infection as early as possible because of the prognosis, especially if the animal has been adopted from the humane society. The author has found that the earliest clinical sign of both diseases usually is a slight serous nasal discharge that precedes a cough. The discharge in distemper becomes mucopurulent in 2 to 3 days, and presumptive diagnosis may be made upon this sequence of signs. It has been the author's experience that distemper can be treated successfully in many instances if early treatment is initiated in an animal that has received some protection from colostral antibodies or vaccination and, most importantly, if signs are confined to the respiratory system. When gastrointestinal and nervous system signs appear, the prognosis is less favorable. Amoxicillin/clavulanic acid, 14 mg/kg b.i.d. can be effective for secondary bacterial infection if given for 3 to 4 weeks.

Always address preventive medicine when the client visits the hospital with any health problem. Many clients will not return for preventive medicine after the animal gets well unless the veterinarian has impressed them with its importance. The preventive medicine discussion should include the rationale for vaccination schedules, routine fecal examinations and deworming, heartworm prevention, and ectoparasite control. Spaying and neutering should receive special emphasis, since 10 to 13 million unwanted animals are euthanized at humane societies in the United States each year.

Preventive medical procedures are an essential function of the humane society veterinary staff and are initiated and carried out under its guidance. Management of a facility housing 300 to 400 puppies, dogs, kittens, and cats requires proficiency in preventive medicine and epidemiology. Approximately 100 animals from unknown backgrounds may be admitted each day; none are turned away. Animals arriving at the humane society come from three major sources: (1) the public, (2) the police or animal control officers, and (3) animals involved in automobile accidents or strays picked up by the humane society ambulance. Preventive medicine begins with an examination to separate diseased from healthy animals (see flow chart, Fig. 1).

Special circumstances arise regularly. The police bring in animals from owners who are in jail. These animals are held for an indefinite period until a humane society representative can obtain written permission from the owner that it is in the best interests of the animal to turn it over to the humane society, or a family member claims the animal.

The veterinary staff performs daily rounds to observe all individuals in the adoption facility in order to detect early signs of disease. A slight ocular or nasal discharge today may become an upper respiratory infection or distemper 7 to 10 days after the puppy is adopted. This results in embarrassment, poor public relations, and a consequent drop in adoption rates. It also involves emotional trauma for the adopting family, especially when children are involved and the puppy must be replaced. Signs of illness detected by humane society staff should immediately be reported to the veterinarian. Many diseases for which animals are "pulled" from the adoption ward are treatable. Whether an individual animal is treated or not depends on several factors including sociability of the animal, time, space, and the probability of future adoption.

The healthy individuals that make up the standing population of animals for adoption remain in the "pool" until they are adopted or become sick. Humane societies may have a few animals that have been there longer than some of the employees.

Stress has been well-established as a factor contributing to disease. It is very difficult to minimize stress at an animal shelter. There is a constant inflow of new animals, with attendant disruption and testing of the established social hierarchies, change of environment and food, constant flow of people, handling, and noise. Although stress is inevitable, efforts should be made to reduce it. For example, animals are spayed or neutered only after they are adopted and will be going to a loving home following surgery. The author has found that most animals that were pre-spayed or neutered at the shelter before being sent to the adoption wards became ill within 5 days. One can also limit stress by limiting the number of animals per cage or run and by keeping the membership within a particular run stable. Limited access to food and water contributes significantly to intra-run stresses and fights. Food and water should be constantly available from multiple sources to avoid a single source being guarded by a dominant animal. If this is not possible, food should be given at the same time each day and left long enough to ensure that each member has had enough to eat.

Accurate record keeping is an essential part of preventive medicine. It is necessary in order to evaluate the efficacy of the preventive medical procedures. A standardized form is completed for each animal as it is admitted; the form should include the usual descriptive statistics, a medical-vaccination history, and a behavioral history. (Does the animal bite? Is it particularly aggressive? Is it particularly friendly?) This information is notably important in today's litigious society. An animal adopted from the humane society with a predilection to biting or even chewing on the furniture can put the humane society in a vulnerable position. This information is used to prevent antisocial animals from being adopted. Where does one draw the line? Animals that possess negative traits by someone's standards will inevitably be put up for adoption. Pertinent information should be clearly marked on the form and should be available to the potential adopter. Under no circumstances should such information be withheld.

CRITERIA FOR UNADOPTABLE ANIMALS

Humane societies euthanize 10 to 13 million animals each year. Those humane facilities that accept all animals are forced to euthanize many because the national adoption rate is only 25 to 30 per cent. Generally, in adopting animals, the public makes its choice on the basis of health, physical appeal, personality, and age.

The veterinarian examines incoming animals for disease, pregnancy, poor socialization, age (animals 7 years and older are not readily adopted), and legal requirements. Lost animals must be held for a minimum of 4 days, depending on local statutes. Abandoned animals may be placed for adoption or euthanized immediately. However, determining that they are abandoned is not easy. The veterinarian must make a decision based on whether a collar or I.D. is present, the condition of the animal, and other information gained from the person admitting the animal. If the animal has been held for less than 2 weeks by the admitting person, the veterinarian should consider it lost, in order to protect himself. Animals that are otherwise not suitable for adoption should be euthanized as soon as possible to minimize their suffering and fear, to prevent the spread of disease, and to make space.

Animals that are to be made available for adoption are "processed" prior to their introduction to the adoption wards. This includes the standard vaccination for age and species. The author does not recommend intranasal vaccinations for the respiratory diseases. Although rapid local and systemic immunity is developed, a large percentage of the animals develop mild upper respiratory signs characterized by ocular and nasal discharge and sneezing 2 to 7 days after vaccination. This interferes greatly with the accurate assessment of illness during daily rounds and further contaminates the adoption facility. All animals are routinely treated for roundworms and hookworms with pyrantel pamoate. Other intestinal parasites are treated when indicated. Puppies, kittens, and cats are sprayed with a mild flea spray. Dogs are sprayed or dipped in standard flea and tick preparations. Dogs older than 4 months are tested for heartworms. Cats are tested for feline leukemia. An identification collar with the date of entry is put on the animal, and it is designated for adoption. An isolation period for these animals would allow the vaccination time to take effect and would enhance detection of individuals incubating disease. However, this is usually not practical, since this group is the largest category of animals entering the system each day.

MANAGEMENT

Management consists of judicial assignment and utilization of people and materials in an effort to meet the organization's goals. Selection, training, supervision, and employee turnover are major areas of concern facing humane society veterinary supervisors. Success in handling these problems determines the level of animal care provided. The importance of this should be underscored. Lay staff (including kennel workers, desk personnel, adoption facilitators, ambulance drivers, animal control officers, and the myriad volunteers) are in direct and constant contact with the animals, the public, or both. They care for animals and impart information to the public regardless of their level of knowledge.

Because humane societies customarily have less funds than private enterprise, they often use varied sources of personnel. Along with the more traditional sources for staff and volunteers, more humane societies are utilizing court-ordered community service programs and prison half-way house programs to obtain both paid and volunteer workers.

A well-organized effective training program is essential. The program should present

1. The general history, present function, and future goals of the humane society.

2. Information on the inter-relationship of the various parts of the humane society (hospital, public education, adoption facility, animal control) and the community functions they perform.

3. The general flow of animals through the facility.

4. The importance of disease control within the shelter and strict adherence to established and demonstrated procedures of preventive medicine.

5. Information on the common early signs of infectious disease, with emphasis on the need to report them to the medical staff immediately.

6. An understanding of the role of euthanasia. Many people come to work at a humane society because of their emotional concern for animals.

7. Emphasis that the individual volunteer or employee is representing the humane society to the public. He or she should always give correct information to the public in response to a question or should direct the questioner to someone who can.

The initial orientation program takes 1 to 2 working days and is composed of a film, personal presentations, visits to various departments, and discussion of hand-out literature. The author has found that such a comprehensive orientation is a good investment. New employees become better representatives of the humane society and work with pride.

All employees and volunteers are presented with detailed job descriptions and operational procedures. These are reviewed and demonstrated by the veterinarian. The veterinarian should provide this initial orientation because he or she has the greatest ability to impress new personnel with the necessity of following established operational procedures. Follow-up training may then be assigned to experienced members of the staff.

After the employee becomes proficient at a specific job, further training at conferences and seminars is a good motivator. Participants are often rewarded with a certificate at completion, which gives them a sense of accomplishment. Information on the place and the date of national and local training seminars can be obtained from Community Animal Control Magazine, P.O. Box 22599, Kansas City, MO, 64113; The Human Society News, 2100 L Street N.W., Washington, D.C., 20037; and National Animal Control Association News, 3353 S. Main Street, Suite 303, Salt Lake City, UT, 84115.

Because training is an ongoing process, the veterinarian will obtain the best results by fostering an esprit de corp among the staff with appropriate reinforcement for a difficult job well done. Within the humane society structure, pay is not the major reward. Rather, a sense of helping, caring, learning, and personal satisfaction is the motivating factor. The veterinarian who creates a positive working environment will motivate and keep his or her best employees longer and will solve the most difficult and prevalent problem in the humane society, employee turnover.

Procurement of materials and supplies at a favorable price is important to the success of a nonprofit animal facility. Food is a special case. It is a major expense to feed 300 to 500 animals each day. Good quality should be maintained. The author has found that consistency of diet is important. Changing from one brand of food to another or from dried to canned food on a daily basis, even if quality is maintained, may result in transitory gastroenteritis, simulating infectious diseases. A contributing factor may be overeating by all dogs or by the dominant dogs when more palatable foods are given. Thus, other dogs may be underfed. The following day these may overeat in compensation. The author has found dog and cat food manufacturers to be a fine source of reasonably priced food. In many instances, the humane society can make an arrangement to give free samples of food with each adoption, and the pet food company will supply the sample as well as free food for the rest of the shelter. Distributors and wholesalers who maintain large stores of food that may be purchased at a discount are also a source of reasonably priced food. Supermarkets and other retailers are generally less desirable sources of food because it may be of mixed quality, mixed brands, and mixed consistency and, thus, may produce digestive upsets.

ADMINISTRATION

Administration is the stewardship of the humane society in its relationship to the community, its agencies, and organizations. The humane society is a community resource of information. The veterinarian is the source of the information. In large humane societies, there will be a director of public education who works closely with the veterinarian to disseminate knowledge.

The media and the humane society have a symbiotic relationship. The media uses humane society expertise to complement current news events and to provide informative and appealing filler material for broadcasts. The humane society uses the media to give the public information about its services, animal care, and preventive medicine. The veterinarian prepares public service announcements. These are concise 30 to 45 sec of reading material addressing common health topics such as heartworm prevention, vaccination, and animal behavior. The public education department sends the public service announcement to all radio, television, and print media in its metropolitan area. Radio stations are usually the most obliging group, with a 35 per cent on-air rate.

Today, more and more clients have come to view the humane society as a resource to help with animal care. This enlightenment has been achieved by word of mouth from clients who have been impressed with the importance of animal care and preventive medicine. Other important factors are public service announcements and educational programs prepared and presented by the veterinary staff and humane society public education department to schools, civic organizations, and the media. Also, establishing an efficient, consistent, and up-to-date client reminder card system based on rabies vaccination certificates has been helpful. Since rabies vaccination is the only legally required and enforced system of pet registration in many areas, it has the broadest base. The humane society should foster local legislation requiring mandatory rabies vaccination for cats as well, because reported cases of rabies in cats in the United States now outnumber those in dogs. In addition, mandatory vaccination resulting in registration of cats will allow better access to owners.

The veterinarian is an integral part of the society's fund-raising team. As a professional, he or she is essential in establishing credibility in relationships with large donors such as foundations and corporations.

The humane society provides animal control to the community on a contract basis or works closely with governmental animal control. The humane society veterinarian often is required to provide medical assistance to animal control officers and police in the field. This generally takes one of three forms: (1) emergency care for injured animals, (2) overseeing animal capture and restraint, and (3) field euthanasia. In the field, most domestic and companion animals can be captured and restrained by well-planned and coordinated efforts of trained personnel. However, there are times when chemical capture is indicated. For large animals at long range (35–100 yd), the Pneu-Dart Model 171 Cartridge Fired Rifle (Pneu-Dart, Williamsport, PA) is effective. Capture and restraint of small animals at short range (<30 yd) is effectively accomplished by use of the Telinject Vario System Blowpipe Rifle (Telinject, U.S.A., Newhall, CA).

When the veterinarian is called upon to perform field euthanasia of large and small animals, pentobarbital sodium (Euthanasia-6-Solution II), 1 ml/5 kg IV, is recommended. Use of firearms for field euthanasia and chemical rifles for capture, although acceptable, may produce public relations problems in an urban setting. What is perceived as a nuisance stray dog by one citizen may be perceived by neighbors and portrayed by the media as someone's maligned pet.

Animal control officers perform cruelty investigations. In this instance, the role of the humane society veterinarian is twofold. He or she examines the animal and discusses the case with the investigating officers to determine if cruelty in fact has occurred. In addition, he or she may be required to present his or her conclusions to the court during a trial. The area of cruelty and cruelty legislation is a complex one. The veterinarian should be aware that cruelty investigation and prosecution require much time and effort.

In deciding which cases to prosecute, we divide cruelty into three categories: (1) intentional cruelty, (2) cruelty by neglect, and (3) cruelty by ignorance.

INTENTIONAL CRUELTY. The following is an example of a statute dealing with this category.

> *Any person who shall maliciously, either out of a spirit of revenge or wanton cruelty or who shall mischievously kill, maim or wound, or injure any horse, mare, gelding, mule, sheep, cattle, hog, dog, poultry or other livestock or cause any person to do the same, shall be fined not more than $1,000 or imprisoned not exceeding six months, or both.*

These cases have a high probability of being prosecuted successfully.

CRUELTY BY NEGLECT. Under this category we place long-standing cases of medical neglect. Severe cases of mange, internal parasites, and untreated open wounds are common examples. The probability of successful prosecution of these cases is moderate. The determining factor is whether the owner eventually sought medical attention on his own initiative. If the animal has been impounded by the animal control officer, the likelihood of successful prosecution is high. On the other hand, if the owner has come for help of his or her own free will, even belatedly, the likelihood of successful prosecution is poor. The case is best handled by educating and warning the owner.

CRUELTY BY IGNORANCE. Although there is some overlap with the other categories, cases that involve an element of home remedies and treatment are placed in this group. Common examples are attempts at home neutering, leaving the animal maimed, and poisons given as treatment for worms. These cases have a poor likelihood of being prosecuted successfully. They are best dealt with by educating the client.

Veterinarians working in humane society facilities have special problems and opportunities. Hope-fully, this discussion has helped to clarify these issues.

References and Supplementary Reading

Curtis, P.: *The Animal Shelter.* New York: Lodestar Books, E. P. Dutton, 1984.

Favre, D. S., and Loring, M.: *Animal Law.* West Port, CT: Quorum Books, 1983.

McPartland, B.: Distemper treatment. *In* Control and Therapy Series. Postgrad. Comm. Vet. Sci. Univ. of Sydney, Sydney, August 1988.

Wilson, M.: *Effective Management of Volunteer Programmes.* Boulder, CO: Volunteer Management Associates, 1981.

Wilson, M.: *Survival Skills for Managers.* Boulder, CO: Volunteer Management Associates, 1976.

DISINFECTION OF ANIMAL ENVIRONMENTS

DENNIS F. LAWLER, D.V.M.

St. Louis, Missouri

During the nineteenth century, it was proposed and eventually accepted that microorganisms cause disease in animals and humans. The development of the concepts of antisepsis and disinfection followed, as mankind began the search for new ways of controlling infectious diseases. Refinement of disinfectant chemistry in the twentieth century has resulted in the availability of an array of products for the control of pathogenic microorganisms.

Many disease-causing organisms are resistant to at least some drugs; some are resistant to many or most drugs. Therefore, a working knowledge of preventive management procedures designed to exclude infectious agents or to reduce their concentration is necessary. Likewise, this information is needed for effective use of disinfectants. Four interrelated types of information should be considered when choosing the proper disinfectant: the physical and chemical properties of the agent(s) under consideration, the identity of offending microorganisms, the type of environment, and some general principles of disinfection. These primary aspects of environmental sanitation are the subject of this discussion.

TYPES AND CHARACTERISTICS OF DISINFECTANTS

Overview

Choosing an appropriate product among available disinfectants is usually not difficult if pertinent issues are considered in an orderly fashion. Confusion may arise over terminology, which can lead to incorrect choices and, therefore, misuse of chemical products. Some of the most commonly used terms are defined in Table 1.

Broad classification of the many kinds of chemical agents having antimicrobial activity includes organic acids, amines, alcohols, halogens, quaternary ammonium compounds, organometallics, aldehydes, phenolics, and biguanides. Currently, most disinfecting agents used in the environment are substituted phenolics, quaternary ammoniums, or halogens. The biguanide chlorhexidine is frequently used in veterinary hospitals.

An ideal disinfecting agent acts rapidly, has a broad spectrum of activity, and penetrates adequately (as contrasted with simply superficial activ-

Table 1. *Definitions*

Disinfectants—Chemical agents applied to inanimate objects or surfaces to kill pathogenic microorganisms. This includes vegetative bacteria but usually not bacterial spores. Fungi and at least some viruses are often susceptible to effective disinfectants.

Antiseptics—Chemical agents applied to living tissue (such as wounds) to prevent growth and reproduction of microorganisms.

Sanitizing Agents—Chemicals that reduce the bacterial population of inanimate objects or surfaces. Ordinarily, this involves killing over 99 per cent of viable bacteria.

Sterilization—The process of complete destruction of all forms of microbial life.

Germicide—A broad term applied to chemical agents that kill microorganisms.

Bactericide, Fungicide, and Virucide—Chemical agents that kill bacteria, fungi, or viruses.

Bacteriostat, Fungistat—Chemical agents that inhibit the growth and reproduction of bacteria or fungi.

Detergents—Combinations of compounds that act by emulsifying grease and suspending dirt particles.

Soaps—Combinations of fat with alkali.

---

ity). In addition, such an agent is (1) nonirritating, (2) nontoxic to animals and humans, (3) nonstaining, (4) noncorrosive, (5) chemically stable, and (6) inexpensive and (7) is not readily inactivated after application. It is unfortunate that no agent totally fulfills these criteria and is completely suitable in every situation. Thus, understanding the general characteristics of the primary classes of products is essential.

Phenolics

The primary effect of phenolic disinfectants is denaturation of intracellular enzymes. Secondarily, destructive effects on the cell membrane and nuclear material also occur. These multiple, nonspecific cellular effects make it unlikely that most organisms would develop resistance (as they do to antibiotics with more specific actions). There are three principal groups of phenolic disinfectants: higher alkylphenols, arylphenols, and chlorinated phenols. The importance of these chemical differences is that increasing length of side chains increases the lipophilic nature of the disinfectant, facilitating more effective isolation and penetration of the target microorganisms' lipid cell membrane in aqueous media. Halogenation of the phenol ring increases the activity of the molecule, resulting in faster destruction of intracellular enzyme systems.

Phenolics are relatively fast-acting and tend to retain their activity in hard water. They are generally least effective at alkaline pH. Some require longer surface contact time but may be corrosive. Loss of activity in the presence of organic material (e.g., feces, urine, soil) occurs but is often less than that noted with other types of disinfectants.

Newer substituted phenolics possess greater activity and less tissue toxicity than older forms and have a less offensive odor. Usually, substituted phenolics are formulated with soaps, alcohols, alkalies, or nonionic wetting agents, which help to maintain solubility. Other types of phenolic compounds are acidic solutions with detergent-sanitizers, which give higher activity at lower concentrations, thus decreasing the potential for tissue toxicity.

Halogens

The use of halogens in disinfectants is based on chemical carrier agents for the inorganic halogen. These agents provide slower release, greater stability, and longer duration of activity.

Chlorine and iodine are commonly used halogen disinfectants in this class. Elemental iodine is the active agent of iodine-containing halogen preparations, while hypochlorous acid ($HOCl$) is generally considered to be the source of the activity in those that contain chlorine. The primary effect of iodine is destruction of cellular enzyme systems by iodination and salt formation. The effect of chlorine-containing products is oxidation of sulphydryl enzymes. Secondarily, toxic intracellular compounds are produced as a result of reaction with proteins in the cell membrane and cytoplasm.

Iodophors are among the most frequently used iodine compounds. These compounds consist of iodine combined with surface-active agents (e.g., nonionic detergents) for solvent purposes, as wetting agents, and to effect the slow release of the iodine. Iodophors act rapidly, with low tissue toxicity. They are somewhat compromised by organic material, are least effective at alkaline pH and less active than phenolics in hard water. Over time, corrosion of some metal surfaces can occur.

Chlorine-containing disinfectants are readily inactivated by organic material and thus may not deliver the desired effectiveness without proper environmental management. Surfaces to be disinfected must be very clean. Chlorine disinfectants are more active in weakly acidic solutions. They are inexpensive and act rapidly. Tissue toxicity is low, but they do have an offensive odor, which is a disadvantage in confined or poorly ventilated areas. They are less active then phenolics in hard water. They are corrosive to many metal surfaces, but less so to stainless steel.

Quaternary Ammonium Compounds

These agents affect intracellular enzymes, especially those involving oxidative pathways that produce energy. In addition, they attack the cell membrane and cell wall, causing loss of permeability barriers by inducing charge reversal. Alkyl side chain lengths of about 14 carbon atoms optimize lipophilic activities of the molecule, enhancing penetration of bacterial cells while maintaining the necessary ionic binding properties for germicidal activity.

Quaternary ammonium compounds are most effective in alkaline environments. They act rapidly, with low tissue toxicity and minimal corrosiveness. Soaps and ionic detergents readily inactivate quaternary ammonium compounds, as does organic matter. Considerable effect is lost in hard water.

Biguanides

Chlorhexidine is the biguanide disinfectant most commonly used in veterinary hospitals. The properties of biguanides are generally similar to those of quaternary ammonium compounds. Precipitation of intracellular compounds is believed to be their mode of action. Alkaline pH and formulation with a nonionic detergent favor activity. Anionic compounds, hard water, and organic matter compromise biguanides to some extent. Tissue toxicity is low.

For most disinfectants, exposure time, temperature, and concentration are interrelated. If any one is held constant, the other two vary inversely. The importance of pH is that it changes the charge density on the surface of the bacteria and changes the degree of ionization (and thus the effectiveness) of the disinfectant.

Additives

The characteristics of environments and surfaces to be disinfected rarely are ideal. Often, surfaces are rough, porous, or soiled, with microorganisms in less accessible locations. To overcome these problems, germicidal compounds can be combined with other chemicals, particularly surfactants, solubilizers, and chelating and peptizing agents.

Surfactants may be anionic agents such as soaps and some alcohols. They may also be nonionic agents such as ethoxylate compounds. Surfactants lower surface tension and emulsify organic material, resulting in more rapid and thorough penetration. The physical and chemical properties of the agent determine the type of accompanying surfactant. For example, anionic surfactants are commonly used with phenolics, since nonionic agents complex with phenolic compounds by hydrogen bonding, resulting in loss of effectiveness. Iodophors and quaternary ammonium compounds contain nonionic detergents to act as the iodine carrier (iodophors) and to avoid formation of inactive salts (quaternary ammonium compounds). Chlorine compounds are used with both types of surfactants.

Solubilizers are mainly used with phenolics and quaternary ammonium compounds to produce a product that is sold as a concentrate and diluted for use. Halogen disinfectants are less limited in this respect and usually do not require solubilizers.

Chelating and peptizing agents are used to remove divalent cations, which otherwise might compromise the antimicrobial effect of the disinfectant. This is especially true for quaternary ammonium compounds. The peptizing action is desirable to break down soil particles, thus improving the surfactant activity. Commonly used agents include EDTA, carbonates, phosphates, silicates, and sodium hydroxide.

MICROORGANISMS

Among chemical disinfectant agents of a particular class, a degree of variability may be found in their effects against microorganisms. However, some generalizations about microorganism susceptibility can be considered as guidelines.

Gram-positive and gram-negative bacteria are readily killed by most disinfectants, with gram-positive bacteria being slightly more susceptible. Exceptions are (1) mycobacteria that are more resistant and are best managed by substituted phenolics; (2) bacterial spores of *Bacillus* and *Clostridium*, which are quite insensitive to disinfectants generally; and (3) *Pseudomonas aeruginosa*, which is more resistant than other gram-negative bacteria when hard water is used. In one study, more than one half of the products tested were not effective against *P. aeruginosa* in water as soft as 100 ppm of calcium carbonate. Clearly, manufacturers would need to be aware of this problem in formulating products. Although fungi are spore producers, their sensitivity to disinfectants more closely parallels that of vegetative bacteria.

Viruses also present differential susceptibility to common disinfectants. In general, viruses can be categorized into two groups for purposes of discussion of disinfectant effectiveness. The lipophilic viruses have lipoprotein outer envelopes. These viruses are usually more labile in the environment. Important enveloped viruses of dogs and cats include canine parainfluenza virus, rabies virus, canine and feline coronaviruses, canine distemper virus, feline leukemia virus, and canine and feline herpesviruses. Nonenveloped viruses are termed hydrophilic. Nonenveloped viruses include canine and feline parvoviruses, feline caliciviruses, and canine adenoviruses. Nonenveloped viruses are generally more resistant and have a greater tendency to persist in the environment.

In general, the targets of disinfection of the various microorganisms present the following order of increasing resistance to disinfection: vegetative bacteria, fungi, enveloped viruses, tuberculosis organisms, nonenveloped viruses, protozoan cysts, bacterial spores *(Bacillus, Clostridium)*. Greater concentrations of microorganisms may require longer contact time for killing with any particular temperature and disinfectant dilution.

Phenolics are effective against many lipophilic viruses, vegetative bacteria, and fungi. Orthophenyl phenol is highly effective against acid-fast organisms. Ordinarily, bacterial spores are unaffected.

In the absence of organic material, halogens containing chlorine are effective against vegetative bacteria, hydrophilic and lipophilic viruses, and fungi. Killing of bacterial spores is possible with prolonged contact. Halogens containing iodine have a generally similar range of activity, but may be slightly more efficient sporicidal and bactericidal agents, and are slightly less effective against hydrophilic viruses.

Quaternary ammonium compounds are effective against vegetative bacteria, most lipophilic viruses, and fungi. Spores are generally unaffected, and only minimal effects on acid-fast bacteria may be noted.

The spectrum of microbes against which biguanides are effective includes gram-negative bacteria, lipophilic viruses, and fungi. Bacterial spores, gram-positive bacteria, and hydrophilic viruses tend to be more resistant.

Zoonotic Considerations

Veterinarians must be conscious of the zoonotic potential of many members of the various groups of microorganisms. For all zoonotic diseases, strict environmental sanitation and personal hygiene are paramount. Also, monitoring of recovery or carrier states for these agents is a necessity. Practical steps, such as prompt removal of all fecal material, washing of hands between animal pens, wearing gloves when removing feces, and food storage in cool, dry areas are important. In addition, insect and rodent control plays an important role in the prevention of disease dissemination.

Recently, specific disinfectant recommendations have been reviewed for several zoonotic agents. For bacteria (including *Salmonella, Campylobacter,* and *Yersinia*), standard disinfectants such as sodium hypochlorite, iodophors, 70 per cent alcohol, phenolics, and quaternary ammonium compounds are effective. For *Cryptosporidium*, formalized saline and 5 to 10 per cent ammonia are reported to be effective disinfectants. *Giardia* cysts are not resistant to freezing, boiling, or drying. Quaternary ammoniums are reported to be effective, as well as 1 per cent sodium hypochlorite, and 2 to 5 per cent pine tar. However, with unsealed concrete surfaces, *Giardia* cysts probably do survive most disinfecting agents, underscoring the importance of routine sanitation.

THE ENVIRONMENT

In addition to the types of microorganisms present and the particular disinfectant(s) being considered, the environment and sanitation program also influence the effectiveness of the disinfection process.

Drainage of water and waste material is critical to the maintenance of a clean, dry, and sanitary environment, which in turn depends upon the nature of the facility. Dirt floors are generally unsatisfactory because disinfection and parasite control are virtually impossible. The water puddles and mud that result from wet weather, along with fecal and urine contamination, are aesthetically undesirable. In addition, in cold weather especially, the ability to maintain freedom from respiratory and enteric disorders appears to be compromised by this type of environment. In climates that are usually warm and humid, the added parasite burden can be devastating. Facilities with grass ultimately present the same problems unless they can be rotated or replenished regularly.

Some types of gravel runs are popular because they offer a pleasing appearance when clean, construction is relatively inexpensive, and sanitation can be reasonably well-managed for a small number of dogs with minimal population turnover. However, for larger or high-turnover facilities, proper maintenance and disease control are more difficult. Movement of gravel by digging and running necessitates frequent raking to cover underlying dirt. Even with frequent removal of fecal matter and an aggressive worming program, control of infectious agents requires careful monitoring. Retention of urine and resulting odor may also occur. Regular application of agents to control these problems is often only partially effective, and exposure of residents to potentially harmful quantities of disinfectant chemicals is possible if accumulation with time is allowed. Complete replacement of the gravel material at intervals may solve these problems but requires an investment of time, money, and labor.

In many situations, the most effective kennel flooring is concrete. Even here, however, design and maintenance are important. A concrete surface with a light broom brush is most desirable. Cracks, rough areas, and depressions all harbor moisture and provide shelter for parasite ova and other infectious organisms. A very rough surface can abrade dogs' foot pads, causing bleeding and discomfort. On the other hand, a surface that is too smooth becomes slippery when wet with water or urine and may lead to injury. Combinations of the aforementioned systems can also be effective, but appropriate preventive medicine practices are necessary.

Cage maintenance is practiced in some facilities. Provided the temptation to overcrowd to save construction costs is resisted, this system can be very effective in achieving environmental control when used with an appropriately designed preventive medicine program. While many types of caging materials may be encountered, stainless steel or good quality galvanized metal are probably the most durable and easiest to keep clean.

The extent to which actual field results with disinfectants agree with laboratory evaluations of products is largely dependent upon correct identification of offending microorganisms, the type of disinfectant used, and complicating environmental or management factors. Therefore, target organisms, the environment (and the potential for environmental contamination), and the type of disinfectant should be considered together. For example, chlorine-containing agents are effective against some fairly resistant viruses, such as parvoviruses. However, they can be corrosive to surfaces over time. Odor can be a problem in confined areas, organic material greatly reduces their effectiveness, and hard water and soaps also reduce activity to a degree. Nevertheless, the persistence of certain organisms may indicate that a chlorine-containing disinfectant is the most appropriate choice if used with the correct management system (i.e., vaccination, worming, ventilation, proper cleaning, and temperature).

Monitoring the Environment

Five factors are involved in the assessment of the effectiveness of the sanitation portion of the management program:

AIR. For indoor facilities, properly filtered, circulated air should not present a problem if airborne infectious agents are controlled by proper health programs and animal management. Wide variations in temperature and humidity aggravate health problems, especially in crowded or rapid turnover situations. Total microorganism counts need to be interpreted in light of activity levels and should be conducted over several weeks to yield the maximum usefulness. Regular and frequent changing of filters on air-handling systems is recommended. For catteries, about 15 air changes per hour are desirable.

WATER. Municipal water is not usually a problem. Wells, ponds, and nonstandard water systems should be monitored for microorganism and mineral content.

FEED. The primary infectious problems with feed arise from rodent or insect access as a result of improper storage after purchase (commercial feeds)

or from improperly acquired and prepared ingredients of home-formulated feeds.

BEDDING. Bedding must be dry, odorless, insect free, and clean. Access to bedding by rodents, birds, and insects must be prevented.

SURFACES. The importance of cleaning and disinfection of floors, walls, tables, and so forth is emphasized in preceding and following discussions.

PRINCIPLES OF DISINFECTION

In general, surfaces to be disinfected must first be cleaned to maximize effectiveness of disinfectants. Organic material, such as feces, urine, and soil, decreases the effectiveness of many products. Undesirable combinations that may occur between different products or product and environment must also be considered. For example, some soaps may combine chemically with some disinfectants, inactivating both. Unless prepared by the manufacturer or indicated for simultaneous use, agents should not be combined.

Management programs must be devised to maximize the effectiveness of the disinfectant chosen. In general, the following concepts apply in kennel and cattery situations:

1. There is no substitute for vigorous physical cleaning.

2. A regular, written schedule should be established, so that important steps are not overlooked.

3. Manufacturers' directions for chemical agents should be followed exactly.

4. Pens should be dry and sheltered from drafts. Animals should be removed from pens when the pens are flushed or hosed and when disinfectants are applied.

5. Bedding should be clean, dry, odorless, and insect-free. It should be changed frequently (at least daily). For litters of puppies, multiple changes per day may be necessary.

6. Accessory equipment, such as vacuums, should be cleaned regularly. Disregard for cleaning and servicing of such equipment creates a habitat for microorganisms.

7. Heaters or air conditioners should be cleaned regularly and serviced by qualified professionals. This equipment, along with duct work, can also provide a habitat for microorganisms.

8. Many products are more effective in hot water (180°F; 82.2°C), less effective in hard water, or neutralized by inappropriate chemical combinations. Organic material reduces the effectiveness of many products.

9. Drawers, cabinets, counters, and so forth should be kept free of clutter, which provides shelter for rodents and insects. The same is true for the kennel exterior. Removal of stored equipment,

debris, and weeds from the kennel exterior reduces available habitat for pests.

10. Animal contact with potentially harmful chemical agents must be avoided.

11. Waste containers should be cleaned and disinfected frequently, and fecal matter should be promptly disposed.

12. In large or high-turnover facilities, animal handling should follow some type of priority basis, such as youngest first and progressing through successively older groups. Some attempt at spatial isolation by age and isolation of ill animals are also desirable.

13. A workable disinfecting system should include pickup of solid debris, followed in succession by detergent application and scrub, thorough rinse, disinfection (observing the indicated surface contact time), thorough rinse (as appropriate), drying, and replacing the animals.

SUMMARY

The necessity for adequate vaccination and parasite control programs is a commonly recognized aspect of animal management systems. The same is true for proper nutrition, genetic selection in breeding programs, and general sanitation and environmental management. Less well understood is the concept that disinfectant agents are not a substitute for proper attention to other details of animal care. The time and ability of the veterinarian will be well spent and substantially rewarded when invested in this educational process.

References and Supplemental Reading

Bebiak, D. M., Lawler, D. F., and Reutzel, L. F.: Nutrition and Management of the Dog. Vet. Clin. North Am. 17:3, 505–533, 1987

Disinfectants: Their Chemistry, Use, and Evaluation. (Publication 74-5). Proceedings, 23rd Annual Session, American Association for Laboratory Animal Science, 1974.

Huber, W. G.: Antiseptics and disinfectants. *In* Jones, L. M., Boothe, N. H., and McDonald, L. E. (eds.): *Veterinary Pharmacology and Therapeutics,* 4th ed. Ames, IA: Iowa State University Press, 1977.

Kowalski, J. J., and Mallman, W. L.: Is Your Disinfection Practice Effective? J. Am. Anim. Hosp. Assoc. 9:3, 1973.

Lawler, D. F.: Practical Disinfection. Nutrition and Management of Dogs and Cats. 3rd ed. Ralston Purina Company, 1987.

Lawler, D. F., and Bebiak, D. M.: Nutrition and management of reproduction in the cat. Vet. Clin. North Am. 16:3, 495–519, 1986.

Scott, E. W.: Virucidal disinfectants and feline viruses. Am. J. Vet. Res. 41:3, 410–414, 1980.

Zimmer, J. F., and Pollock, R. V. H: Esophageal, gastric, and intestinal disorders of young dogs and cats. Vet. Clin. North Am. 17:3, 641–661, 1987.

Section

2

CHEMICAL AND PHYSICAL DISORDERS

GARY D. OSWEILER, D.V.M.
Consulting Editor

Incidence of Poisonings in Small Animals 97
Companion Animal Forensic Toxicology 114
Emergency and General Treatment of Poisonings 116
Toxicant-induced Acute Renal Failure..................................... 126
Thiacetarsamide and Its Adverse Effects 131
Organophosphorus and Carbamate Insecticide Poisoning 135
Pyrethrins and Pyrethroids 137
Ivermectin... 140
The Anticoagulant Rodenticides 143
Bromethalin Poisoning... 147
Diagnosis of and Therapy for Cholecalciferol Toxicosis 148
Lead Poisoning... 152
Arsenic Poisoning 159
Toxicology of Detergents, Bleaches, Antiseptics, and Disinfectants........ 162
Ethanol and Illicit Drugs of Abuse 171
Bites and Stings of Venomous Animals..................................... 177

INCIDENCE OF POISONINGS IN SMALL ANIMALS

VAL RICHARD BEASLEY, D.V.M.,
and HAROLD L. TRAMMEL, Pharm.D.

Urbana, Illinois

It is essential to have an idea of the incidence of a given toxicosis in order to rank it by probability in a list of differential diagnoses. This article reflects the recent experiences of an animal poison information center at the College of Veterinary Medicine of the University of Illinois. The center changed its name from the National Animal Poison Control Center to the Illinois Animal Poison Information Center (IAPIC) as it began to serve as part of the National Animal Poison Information Network (NAPINet). The second NAPINet center is now fully operational at the College of Veterinary Medicine, University of Georgia; several veterinary toxicology groups in the United States and Canada are working toward similar involvement. Ideally, all centers will acquire case and call data in a uniform, coordinated manner for subsequent computer-assisted analysis. This will result in more broad-based information on the likelihood of various toxicoses and the nature of the associated adverse effects. The telephone numbers for the Georgia and Illinois centers are 404-542-6751 and 217-333-3611, respectively.

Calls to the Illinois center pertaining to small animals increased from less than 8000 in 1984 to roughly 20,000 in 1986 and 25,000 in 1987. This chapter reflects the 1986 and 1987 calls. The information derived from these calls has some epidemiologic bias in that

1. The telephone number has been publicized primarily among veterinarians.

2. People may hesitate to call long distance, depending upon their location.

3. Calls are more probable when exposure is followed by clinical signs than when no effects are apparent.

4. Calls from owners are more probable after exposure to substances believed to be particularly toxic. Factors such as media attention given a toxicant tend to increase the likelihood of calls to the center.

5. Calls from owners and veterinarians are more common when exposure is followed by unexpected effects (e.g., as in the case of pyrethrins).

6. Once veterinarians have become familiar with a given toxicosis, they no longer find it necessary to call regarding that toxicosis.

7. Calls pertaining to animals that are still under

veterinary care may be emphasized, whereas if the animal has died, veterinarians may be more likely to contact local diagnostic laboratories for assistance.

8. Calls regarding suspected cases of toxicosis are assessed strictly on the basis of information available at the time of the call. Most of these cases are not confirmed by chemical analysis. Only a very limited number of follow-up calls can be made at this time. The net result is an underestimation of poisoning rates, since many exposures would be likely to cause clinical signs, given sufficient time.

9. Some packages of rodenticides formulated with brodifacoum or bromethalin have listed the telephone number of the Illinois center, causing calls regarding these rodenticides to be over-represented.

Despite these limitations, the patterns of species involvement and clinical signs reported tend to be quite reproducible over a period of years for products and natural toxicants that are widely available. As a result, the acquired data begin to take on the nature of population statistics and serve as a useful baseline to gauge the toxicologic hazard of other products to domestic animals.

Most calls to the center are from the North Atlantic area, the Midwest, and the West Coast (Fig. 1), which influences the cross-section of toxicant exposures involved. Thus, problems in the North Atlantic area may be over-represented and significant toxicoses in the Midsouth may be unrecognized. Examples of regional differences in toxicant availability include (1) poisonous plants that grow in different climates, (2) animals bearing zootoxins that live in different habitats, and (3) pesticides used in varying ways and amounts in response to regional pest control problems.

Based on the probability, degree, and route of exposure, the toxicologic potential of the agent, and the consistency of both time factors and clinical findings, each call is assessed as one of the following:

1. Toxicosis: All criteria are met (high degree of assurance of adequate toxicant exposure).

2. Suspected toxicosis: Criteria are met, but a limited amount of confirming information is unobtainable.

3. Exposure: No clinical signs at the time of the call.

97

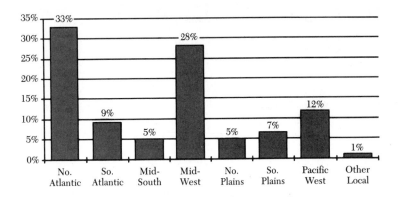

Figure 1. Percentage of calls in 1986 by USDA Research Area.

4. Doubtful toxicosis: Findings not appropriate for the toxicant, timeframe, or degree of exposure in question. Opportunity for exposure is low, or another explanation is more probable.

5. Information only (no exposure).

6. Other problem (includes various diseases and nutritional deficiencies).

7. Residue concern (regarding food-producing animals only).

Tables 1, 3, and 5 represent the 1986 assessments of calls by class of agent for dogs, cats, and birds (all species), respectively. Similarly, Tables 2, 4,

and 6 display the most prevalent generics represented in calls to the center in these animals. Tables 1 to 6 indicate that the majority of anticoagulant rodenticide calls were exposures. The numbers were influenced by the bias regarding *brodifacoum*. The telephone number on brodifacoum-containing products resulted in many calls shortly after exposure. In many cases, subtoxic levels were involved. However, exposures to potentially toxic amounts were also common, and recommendations often included measures to limit absorption, and a month-long course of prophylactic administration of vitamin

Table 1. *1986 Canine Inquiry Distribution by Class and Reason*

Class	Total No.	Total %	Toxicosis No.	Toxicosis %	Suspected No.	Suspected %	Doubtful No.	Doubtful %	Exposure No.	Exposure %	Information No.	Information %	Other No.	Other %	Residue No.	Residue %
Avicide	7	0.0	0	0.0	3	42.9	1	14.3	2	28.6	0	0.0	1	14.3	0	0.0
Biotoxin	187	1.3	34	18.2	72	38.5	43	23.0	29	15.5	5	2.7	4	2.1	0	0.0
Combination	95	0.6	11	11.6	14	14.7	13	13.7	54	56.8	1	1.1	2	2.1	0	0.0
Construction	560	3.8	51	9.1	109	19.5	96	17.1	285	50.9	11	2.0	8	1.4	0	0.0
Cosmetic	112	0.8	9	8.0	19	17.0	15	13.4	65	58.0	1	0.9	3	2.7	0	0.0
Fertilizer	347	2.4	34	9.8	87	25.1	69	19.9	144	41.5	12	3.5	1	0.3	0	0.0
Fungicide	58	0.4	3	5.2	10	17.2	18	31.0	22	37.9	2	3.4	3	5.2	0	0.0
Herbicide	356	2.4	13	3.7	115	32.3	162	45.5	41	11.5	21	5.9	4	1.1	0	0.0
Hotline information	6	0.0	0	0.0	0	0.0	0	0.0	0	0.0	6	100.0	0	0.0	0	0.0
Household product	927	6.3	119	12.8	170	18.3	136	14.7	474	51.1	8	0.9	20	2.2	0	0.0
Human medicine	2498	17.0	516	20.7	411	16.5	121	4.8	1368	54.8	35	1.4	47	1.9	0	0.0
Insecticide	1771	12.0	227	12.8	414	23.4	386	21.8	613	34.6	90	5.1	41	2.3	0	0.0
Metal	191	1.3	23	12.0	38	19.9	35	18.3	80	41.9	11	5.8	4	2.1	0	0.0
Misc. chemical	661	4.5	94	14.2	141	21.3	90	13.6	295	44.6	18	2.7	23	3.5	0	0.0
Molluscacide	55	0.4	16	29.1	14	25.5	6	10.9	16	29.1	3	5.5	0	0.0	0	0.0
NA	379	2.6	11	2.9	140	36.9	127	33.5	21	5.5	9	2.4	71	18.7	0	0.0
Nutritional agent	543	3.7	128	23.6	101	18.6	80	14.7	203	37.4	24	4.4	7	1.3	0	0.0
Other	29	0.2	0	0.0	0	0.0	1	3.4	1	3.4	14	48.3	13	44.8	0	0.0
Petroleum	259	1.8	41	15.8	77	29.7	36	13.9	100	38.6	2	0.8	3	1.2	0	0.0
Physical agent	202	1.4	10	5.0	18	8.9	25	12.4	138	68.3	3	1.5	8	4.0	0	0.0
Plant	1449	9.8	182	12.6	328	22.6	301	20.8	558	38.5	51	3.5	29	2.0	0	0.0
Rodenticide	3345	22.7	88	2.6	303	9.1	231	6.9	2597	77.6	47	1.4	79	2.4	0	0.0
Veterinary medicine	684	4.6	124	18.1	129	18.9	124	18.1	252	36.8	28	4.1	27	3.9	0	0.0
TOTALS	14721	100.0	1734	11.8	2713	18.4	2116	14.4	7358	50.0	402	2.7	398	2.7	0	0.0

NA, specific agent not available.

Table 2. *1986 Canine Inquiry Distribution by Top Generics and Reason*

Class	Total No.	Total %	Toxicosis No.	Toxicosis %	Suspected No.	Suspected %	Doubtful No.	Doubtful %	Exposure No.	Exposure %	Information No.	Information %	Other No.	Other %	Residue No.	Residue %
Brodifacoum	2058	30.9	26	1.3	110	5.3	132	6.4	1727	83.9	20	1.0	43	2.1	0	0.0
NA	903	13.5	31	3.4	245	27.1	225	24.9	254	28.1	30	3.3	118	13.1	0	0.0
Caffeine	454	6.8	165	36.3	80	17.6	38	8.4	144	31.7	18	4.0	9	2.0	0	0.0
Warfarin	388	5.8	6	1.5	10	2.6	24	6.2	337	86.9	6	1.5	5	1.3	0	0.0
Theobromine	316	4.7	93	29.4	62	19.6	33	10.4	107	33.9	17	5.4	4	1.3	0	0.0
Ibuprofen	239	3.6	71	29.7	42	17.6	13	5.4	107	44.8	3	1.3	3	1.3	0	0.0
N-P-K (fertilizer)	214	3.2	21	9.8	56	26.2	37	17.3	89	41.6	10	4.7	1	0.5	0	0.0
Cholecalciferol	161	2.4	10	6.2	38	23.6	10	6.2	94	58.4	9	5.6	0	0.0	0	0.0
Acetaminophen	157	2.4	17	10.8	18	11.5	15	9.6	102	65.0	4	2.5	1	0.6	0	0.0
Propoxur	155	2.3	8	5.2	18	11.6	14	9.0	113	72.9	1	0.6	1	0.6	0	0.0
Hydramethylnon	140	2.1	5	3.6	14	10.0	20	14.3	99	70.7	1	0.7	1	0.7	0	0.0
2,4-D	136	2.0	5	3.7	47	34.6	57	41.9	18	13.2	9	6.6	0	0.0	0	0.0
Boric acid	134	2.0	9	6.7	23	17.2	18	13.4	81	60.4	1	0.7	2	1.5	0	0.0
Diazinon	134	2.0	10	7.5	30	22.4	43	32.1	36	26.9	8	6.0	7	5.2	0	0.0
Diethylcarbamazine	129	1.9	11	8.5	7	5.4	14	10.9	85	65.9	4	3.1	8	6.2	0	0.0
Ethylene glycol	128	1.9	23	18.0	41	32.0	8	6.3	46	35.9	3	2.3	7	5.5	0	0.0
Diphacinone	121	1.8	11	9.1	24	19.8	7	5.8	74	61.2	2	1.7	3	2.5	0	0.0
Chlorpyrifos	115	1.7	6	5.2	36	31.3	43	37.4	17	14.8	9	7.8	4	3.5	0	0.0
Pyrethrins	109	1.6	6	5.5	34	31.2	37	33.9	20	18.3	10	9.2	2	1.8	0	0.0
Zinc oxide	104	1.6	49	47.1	19	18.3	5	4.8	27	26.0	1	1.0	3	2.9	0	0.0
Bromadiolone	102	1.5	1	1.0	10	9.8	8	7.8	80	78.4	0	0.0	3	2.9	0	0.0
Aspirin	99	1.5	19	19.2	21	21.2	8	8.1	47	47.5	2	2.0	2	2.0	0	0.0
Silica gel	93	1.4	0	0.0	2	2.2	6	6.5	83	89.2	1	1.1	1	1.1	0	0.0
Cannabis sativa	81	1.2	41	50.6	30	37.0	2	2.5	6	7.4	1	1.2	1	1.2	0	0.0

NA, specific agent not available.

Table 3. *1986 Feline Inquiry Distribution by Class and Reason*

Class	Total No.	Total %	Toxicosis No.	Toxicosis %	Suspected No.	Suspected %	Doubtful No.	Doubtful %	Exposure No.	Exposure %	Information No.	Information %	Other No.	Other %	Residue No.	Residue %
Avicide	7	0.1	0	0.0	0	0.0	2	28.6	3	42.9	2	28.6	0	0.0	0	0.0
Biotoxin	41	0.8	8	19.5	13	31.7	12	29.3	5	12.2	1	2.4	2	4.9	0	0.0
Combination	20	0.4	1	5.0	5	25.0	4	20.0	7	35.0	2	10.0	1	5.0	0	0.0
Construction	212	4.2	32	15.1	50	23.6	34	16.0	88	41.5	1	0.5	7	3.3	0	0.0
Cosmetic	27	0.5	2	7.4	9	33.3	8	29.6	8	29.6	0	0.0	0	0.0	0	0.0
Fertilizer	76	1.5	2	2.6	15	19.7	31	40.8	25	32.9	3	3.9	0	0.0	0	0.0
Fungicide	24	0.5	0	0.0	4	16.7	15	62.5	4	16.7	1	4.2	0	0.0	0	0.0
Herbicide	84	1.7	5	6.0	16	19.0	49	58.3	7	8.3	4	4.8	3	3.6	0	0.0
Hotline information	1	0.0	0	0.0	0	0.0	0	0.0	0	0.0	1	100.0	0	0.0	0	0.0
Household product	381	7.5	52	13.6	111	29.1	110	28.9	91	23.9	9	2.4	8	2.1	0	0.0
Human medicine	503	9.9	111	22.1	115	22.9	63	12.5	186	37.0	20	4.0	8	1.6	0	0.0
Insecticide	1303	25.7	341	26.2	410	31.5	309	23.7	133	10.2	81	6.2	29	2.2	0	0.0
Metal	29	0.6	3	10.3	10	34.5	7	24.1	6	20.7	2	6.9	1	3.4	0	0.0
Misc. chemical	147	2.9	16	10.9	45	30.6	36	24.5	35	23.8	12	8.2	3	2.0	0	0.0
Molluscacide	9	0.2	0	0.0	1	11.1	4	44.4	4	44.4	0	0.0	0	0.0	0	0.0
NA	159	3.1	3	1.9	42	26.4	69	43.4	6	3.8	5	3.1	34	21.4	0	0.0
Nutritional agent	51	1.0	3	5.9	5	9.8	13	25.5	24	47.1	3	5.9	3	5.9	0	0.0
Other	11	0.2	0	0.0	0	0.0	0	0.0	0	0.0	9	81.8	2	18.2	0	0.0
Petroleum	151	3.0	30	19.9	38	25.2	15	9.9	65	43.0	0	0.0	3	2.0	0	0.0
Physical agent	35	0.7	0	0.0	5	14.3	11	31.4	18	51.4	0	0.0	1	2.9	0	0.0
Plant	1086	21.4	54	5.0	200	18.4	307	28.3	248	22.8	253	23.3	24	2.2	0	0.0
Rodenticide	426	8.4	10	2.3	49	11.5	83	19.5	245	57.5	26	6.1	13	3.1	0	0.0
Veterinary medicine	292	5.8	63	21.6	80	27.4	60	20.5	67	22.9	16	5.5	6	2.1	0	0.0
TOTALS	5075	100.0	736	14.5	1223	24.1	1242	24.5	1275	25.1	451	8.9	148	2.9	0	0.0

NA, specific agent not available.

Table 4. 1986 Feline Inquiry Distribution by Top Generics and Reason

Class	Total No.	%	Toxicosis No.	%	Suspected No.	%	Doubtful No.	%	Exposure No.	%	Information No.	%	Other No.	%	Residue No.	%
NA	349	17.9	16	4.6	100	28.7	114	32.7	47	13.5	23	6.6	49	14.0	0	0.0
Pyrethrins	271	13.9	68	25.1	97	35.8	71	26.2	21	7.7	8	3.0	6	2.2	0	0.0
Brodifacoum	223	11.4	0	0.0	12	5.4	42	18.8	150	67.3	15	6.7	4	1.8	0	0.0
Chlorpyrifos	184	9.4	80	43.5	57	31.0	25	13.6	6	3.3	15	8.2	1	0.5	0	0.0
Acetaminophen	125	6.4	47	37.6	25	20.0	10	8.0	38	30.4	5	4.0	0	0.0	0	0.0
Boric acid	76	3.9	5	6.6	26	34.2	22	28.9	17	22.4	6	7.9	0	0.0	0	0.0
Limonene	58	3.0	17	29.3	19	32.8	17	29.3	3	5.2	2	3.4	0	0.0	0	0.0
Philodendron	56	2.9	5	8.9	15	26.8	11	19.6	13	23.2	12	21.4	0	0.0	0	0.0
Diazinon	54	2.8	6	11.1	15	27.8	20	37.0	6	11.1	7	13.0	0	0.0	0	0.0
Warfarin	50	2.6	2	4.0	6	12.0	5	10.0	33	66.0	2	4.0	2	4.0	0	0.0
N-P-K (fertilizer)	49	2.5	1	2.0	10	20.4	24	49.0	14	28.6	0	0.0	0	0.0	0	0.0
Carbaryl	48	2.5	7	14.6	19	39.6	15	31.3	3	6.3	4	8.3	0	0.0	0	0.0
Ibuprofen	45	2.3	8	17.8	14	31.1	9	20.0	14	31.1	0	0.0	0	0.0	0	0.0
Propoxur	45	2.3	2	4.4	15	33.3	16	35.6	10	22.2	2	4.4	0	0.0	0	0.0
Phosmet	44	2.3	17	38.6	13	29.5	11	25.0	0	0.0	1	2.3	2	4.5	0	0.0
Sodium arsenate	41	2.1	16	39.0	9	22.0	2	4.9	13	31.7	0	0.0	1	2.4	0	0.0
Rotenone	39	2.0	13	33.3	16	41.0	6	15.4	2	5.1	1	2.6	1	2.6	0	0.0
Aspirin	38	1.9	10	26.3	5	13.2	9	23.7	11	28.9	3	7.9	0	0.0	0	0.0
Ethylene glycol	36	1.8	3	8.3	15	41.7	8	22.2	8	22.2	2	5.6	0	0.0	0	0.0
2,4-D	33	1.7	0	0.0	8	24.2	20	60.6	3	9.1	1	3.0	1	3.0	0	0.0
Motor oil	31	1.6	7	22.6	6	19.4	4	12.9	13	41.9	0	0.0	1	3.2	0	0.0
Dieffenbachia	30	1.5	2	6.7	4	13.3	9	30.0	10	33.3	5	16.7	0	0.0	0	0.0
Piperazine	30	1.5	8	26.7	15	50.0	6	20.0	1	3.3	0	0.0	0	0.0	0	0.0

NA, specific agent not available.

Table 5. 1986 Avian Inquiry Distribution by Class and Reason

Class	Total No.	%	Toxicosis No.	%	Suspected No.	%	Doubtful No.	%	Exposure No.	%	Information No.	%	Other No.	%	Residue No.	%
Avicide	4	0.7	0	0.0	3	75.0	0	0.0	0	0.0	1	25.0	0	0.0	0	0.0
Biotoxin	8	1.3	0	0.0	4	50.0	0	0.0	0	0.0	3	37.5	1	12.5	0	0.0
Combination	3	0.5	0	0.0	2	66.7	0	0.0	0	0.0	0	0.0	0	0.0	1	33.3
Construction	28	4.6	0	0.0	4	14.3	6	21.4	8	28.6	10	35.7	0	0.0	0	0.0
Cosmetic	5	0.8	0	0.0	1	20.0	1	20.0	3	60.0	0	0.0	0	0.0	0	0.0
Fertilizer	7	1.1	0	0.0	1	14.3	2	28.6	2	28.6	2	28.6	0	0.0	0	0.0
Fungicide	2	0.3	0	0.0	2	100.0	0	0.0	0	0.0	0	0.0	0	0.0	0	0.0
Herbicide	8	1.3	0	0.0	1	12.5	3	37.5	1	12.5	2	25.0	1	12.5	0	0.0
Hotline information	1	0.2	0	0.0	0	0.0	0	0.0	0 (24)	0.0	1	100.0	0	0.0	0	0.0
Household product	50	8.2	5	10.0	8	16.0	7	14.0	10 (16)	48.0	4	8.0	2	4.0	0	0.0
Human medicine	17	2.8	1	5.9	3	17.6	0	0.0	6 (7)	58.8	2	11.8	1	5.9	0	0.0
Insecticide	87	14.2	9	10.3	16	18.4	12	13.8	0	18.4	32	36.8	2	2.3	0	0.0
Metal	21	3.4	2	9.5	7	33.3	2	9.5	2	28.6	4	19.0	0	0.0	0	0.0
Misc. chemical	36	5.9	6	16.7	8	22.2	5	13.9	0	19.4	10	27.8	0	0.0	0	0.0
NA	15	2.5	0	0.0	7	46.7	6	40.0	1	0.0	1	6.7	1	6.7	0	0.0
Nutritional agent	11	1.8	0	0.0	4	36.4	2	18.2	4	18.2	1	9.1	2	18.2	0	0.0
Other	2	0.3	0	0.0	0	0.0	0	0.0	113	0.0	2	100.0	0	0.0	0	0.0
Petroleum	6	1.0	1	16.7	2	33.3	0	0.0	24	16.7	2	33.3	0	0.0	2	0.0
Physical agent	7	1.1	0	0.0	0	0.0	3	42.9	5	57.1	0	0.0	0	0.0	0	0.0
Plant	242	39.5	3	1.2	26	10.7	23	9.5		46.7	74	30.6	3	1.2		0.0
Rodenticide	39	6.4	0	0.0	7	17.9	4	10.3		61.5	2	5.1	0	0.0		5.1
Veterinary medicine	13	2.1	3	23.1	3	23.1	1	7.7		38.5	1	7.7	0	0.0		0.0
TOTALS	612	100.0	30	4.9	109	17.8	77	12.6	226	36.9	154	25.2	13	2.1	3	0.5

NA, specific agent not available.

Table 6. 1986 Avian Inquiry Distribution by Top Generics and Reason

Class	Total		Toxicosis		Suspected		Doubtful		Exposure		Information		Other		Residue	
	No.	%	No.	%	No.	%	No.	%	No.	%.	No.	%	No.	%	No.	%
Philodendron	30	4.9	1	3.3	2	6.7	5	16.7	20	66.7	2	6.7	0	0.0	0	0.0
NA	23	3.8	0	0.0	7	30.4	7	30.4	0	0.0	8	34.8	1	4.3	0	0.0
Brodifacoum	20	3.3	0	0.0	4	20.0	3	15.0	12	60.0	0	0.0	0	0.0	1	5.0
Diazinon	13	2.1	4	30.8	3	23.1	0	0.0	0	0.0	6	46.2	0	0.0	0	0.0
p-dichlorobenzene	10	1.6	0	0.0	3	30.0	1	10.0	5	50.0	1	10.0	0	0.0	0	0.0
Teflon fumes	8	1.3	2	25.0	2	25.0	1	12.5	0	0.0	3	37.5	0	0.0	0	0.0
Dieffenbachia	7	1.1	1	14.3	0	0.0	2	28.6	4	57.1	0	0.0	0	0.0	0	0.0
Hypochlorite	7	1.1	1	14.3	1	14.3	1	14.3	3	42.9	1	14.3	0	0.0	0	0.0
Warfarin	7	1.1	0	0.0	0	0.0	0	0.0	7	100.0	0	0.0	0	0.0	0	0.0
Ficus	6	1.0	0	0.0	1	16.7	0	0.0	1	16.7	4	66.7	0	0.0	0	0.0
Lead	6	1.0	1	16.7	3	50.0	0	0.0	1	16.7	1	16.7	0	0.0	0	0.0
2,4-D	5	0.8	0	0.0	0	0.0	3	60.0	0	0.0	1	20.0	1	20.0	0	0.0
Bendiocarb	5	0.8	0	0.0	2	40.0	2	40.0	0	0.0	1	20.0	0	0.0	0	0.0
Boric acid	5	0.8	0	0.0	0	0.0	0	0.0	4	80.0	1	20.0	0	0.0	0	0.0
Christmas cactus	5	0.8	0	0.0	0	0.0	0	0.0	5	100.0	0	0.0	0	0.0	0	0.0
Ilex	5	0.8	0	0.0	0	0.0	0	0.0	5	100.0	0	0.0	0	0.0	0	0.0
Persea americana	5	0.8	0	0.0	1	20.0	1	20.0	2	40.0	1	20.0	0	0.0	0	0.0
Pyrethrins	5	0.8	0	0.0	0	0.0	2	40.0	0	0.0	3	60.0	0	0.0	0	0.0
Amaryllis	4	0.7	0	0.0	1	25.0	0	0.0	3	75.0	0	0.0	0	0.0	0	0.0
Graphite	4	0.7	0	0.0	0	0.0	2	50.0	2	50.0	0	0.0	0	0.0	0	0.0
Paint	4	0.7	0	0.0	1	25.0	1	25.0	0	0.0	2	50.0	0	0.0	0	0.0
Saintpaulia	4	0.7	0	0.0	0	0.0	1	25.0	3	75.0	0	0.0	0	0.0	0	0.0
Sansevieria	4	0.7	0	0.0	0	0.0	1	25.0	3	75.0	0	0.0	0	0.0	0	0.0

NA, specific agent not available (unknown).

K. Without such intervention, toxicosis would have been probable in a significant fraction of the patients exposed to this extremely persistent anticoagulant.

Much of the following discussion centers on compounds represented in a large number of calls in 1987. Other toxicants are listed because they are repeatedly encountered, but information on their toxicity is not widely available in the veterinary literature. Treatment recommendations address only some of the most common concerns for the toxicants involved.

AVICIDES

Poisoning due to bird-killing agents is a relatively infrequent problem. However, multiple animals may be involved, since large amounts of bait are often used to kill a flock of birds. In 1987, the center received 8 calls with regard to *4-aminopyridine*, the active ingredient in Avitrol (Avitrol Corp.). The compound has been previously investigated as an antagonist of certain anesthetics in small animals. Toxicosis due to 4-aminopyridine can result in involuntary muscle contractions and seizures. Affected pigeons (the target species) are commonly presented to diagnostic laboratories after flying about awkwardly and suffering traumatic injury. Formulations of Rid-A-Bird (Rid-A-Bird, Inc.) may contain *endrin*, a highly toxic cyclodiene organochlorine compound that is toxicologically similar to, but more potent than, chlordane. More recent Rid-A-Bird formulas may contain the organophosphorus cholinesterase inhibitor, *fenthion*. Another avicide, *3-chloro*-p-*toluidine hydrochloride* (Ralston Purina Starlicide), is reportedly a cause of methemoglobinemia and cardiovascular collapse, but poisoning is apparently infrequent.

INSECTICIDES

It is unfortunate that many companies list only chemical names on containers of insecticidal products rather than generic terms. This delays establishing the agent involved and is a cause of erroneous information, as owners unfamiliar with chemical names attempt to give the information on the label to poison control center staffers. Most toxicologic data needed to assess the seriousness of an insecticide exposure are listed by generic, not by chemical names.

For most groups of toxicants, poisoning is relatively uncommon in patients undergoing topical exposures. This is not true with insecticides. Of 440 cases in which pets were exposed via the topical route and had clinical signs compatible with the toxicant in question, 82 per cent were due to insecticides.

Organophosphorus (OP) Insecticides

Products bearing chemical names containing "phosphoro" and recommendations to use atropine plus pralidoxime (2-PAM) as an antidote for poisoning can be assumed to contain OP insecticides. Commonly reported effects of OP toxicosis include tremors, vomiting, salivation, ataxia, anorexia, diarrhea, seizures, dyspnea, weakness, and death. Diagnosis of OP toxicosis rests upon a toxic level of exposure, appropriate clinical signs, and cholinesterase inhibition. In the cat, diagnosis is made more difficult because of the extreme sensitivity of feline whole blood cholinesterase to inhibition by OP insecticides. This is, in part, a result of the extremely low cholinesterase activity of feline red blood cells. For example, oral doses of chlorpyrifos of only 0.1 mg/kg abolished detectable whole blood cholinesterase activity, whereas deaths were not observed until an oral dose of 40 mg/kg was given.

When OP insecticides are considered as a group, the more toxic dip solutions dispensed by veterinarians cause a disproportionately large share of serious poisonings. Major problems commonly result when canine preparations are used on cats.

Among dogs, *chlorpyrifos* and *diazinon* (*dimpylate*) were the OP insecticides most often involved in the telephone calls. Although chlorpyrifos is in many products approved for use in dogs while diazinon is not, the number of toxicoses plus suspected toxicoses in dogs for these two generics was essentially the same. However, in 1987, there were 25 deaths from chlorpyrifos in cats (more than those from any other generic) and two chlorpyrifos-related deaths in dogs. Yet, only one cat and one dog died of diazinon toxicosis. Historically, a large proportion of chlorpyrifos-associated deaths have been attributable to dip solutions. Toxicosis in cats undergoing topical exposive to chlorpyrifos can be unusual in that onset may be delayed and toxicosis may persist for weeks. Behavioral aberrations and anorexia may be marked.

Dichlorvos (DDVP) was the third most commonly reported organophosphorus insecticide, with over 100 calls per year pertaining to all types of animals. Some calls were associated with anthelmintic medications, but most pertained to insecticides. Roughly one third of canine and two thirds of feline calls were assessed as a toxicosis or a suspected toxicosis. Foggers containing DDVP as well as products containing both DDVP and another cholinesterase inhibitor were associated with some of the more severe problems. DDVP-based flea collars were occasionally involved with toxicoses and suspected toxicoses, especially in cats. In one instance, three 7-week-old kittens died within 12 hr of initial exposure to a DDVP-containing flea collar.

Perhaps, because some formulations are more concentrated than many other organophosphorus-based insecticides, a number of toxicoses and suspected toxicoses were associated with *malathion.* Among 62 calls involving dogs in 1986 and 1987, 31 per cent were assessed as either a toxicosis or suspected toxicosis. Of 46 calls involving cats, over half were assessed as a toxicosis or suspected toxicosis.

Phosmet (Vet-Kem Paramite Flea and Tick Dip, Zoecon), sometimes called *prolate,* is used in dips for dogs or at half-strength for cats. It was associated with a total of 129 calls in 1986 and 1987. Approximately half of the canine and 60 per cent of the feline calls were assessed as toxicosis or suspected toxicosis. Death was reported in 5 per cent of these calls in dogs and cats in 1987.

Dichlorvos and chlorpyrifos should not be confused with *chlorfenvinphos* (supona). Chlorfenvinphos, which is the active ingredient in Dermaton II (Burroughs Wellcome Co.) dip, was associated with a total of 22 calls during the period 1986 to 1987. It appears that poisoning from chlorfenvinphos occurs most often in cats. Another commonly encountered OP with a similar name is *tetrachlorvinphos* (Gardona or Rabon). It is found in many products by Hartz labeled with the chemical name 2-chloro-1-(2,4,5-trichlorophenyl)-vinyl dimethyl phosphate. From 1986 through 1987, there were a total of 35 tetrachlorvinphos calls pertaining to dogs and cats. Although this compound is much less toxic than most other OP insecticides, assessments of calls as related to toxicosis or suspected toxicosis did occur. These tetrachlorvinphos toxicoses were primarily the result of exposure of cats to flea spray and powder formulations.

The emerging OP insecticide, *propetamphos* (Safrotin, Sandoz), is restricted to use by pest control operators, who commonly apply it to homes. Of the 30 to 40 calls per year that pertained to dogs and cats, roughly 40 per cent were assessed as toxicosis or suspected toxicosis in both species.

Cythioate (Proban, Haver-Lockhart), an orally administered systemic insecticide, was involved in a total of 40 calls in 1986 and 44 in 1987. Less than 25 per cent of the canine and approximately 50 per cent of the feline calls were assessed as toxicosis or suspected toxicosis. Another 25 per cent of the calls pertained to inadvertently exposed, asymptomatic humans who accidentally consumed their animal's recommended dose of cythioate. This reinforces the concern for human exposure to veterinary drugs and the importance of using warning labels and child-resistant containers.

Fenthion was involved in a total of 101 calls in dogs and cats in 1986 and 1987. Dogs were involved more than twice as often as cats. However, roughly 50 per cent of the canine and 70 per cent of the feline calls were assessed as either toxicosis or suspected toxicosis. Poisoning was more commonly reported with Spotton (Mobay) than with Pro-Spot (Haver-Lockhart), possibly reflecting differences in dosage. Some forms of Rid-A-Bird (mentioned under the section on avicides), as well as the large animal products Lysoff Pour-On and Tiguvon (Haver-Lockhart) containing fenthion, have been associated with occasional toxicoses in dogs. In 1987 calls, three cases involving death in dogs and two in cats were attributed to fenthion toxicosis.

Another OP, *disulfoton* (Disyston, Mobay; various types of Jobe's Spikes for outdoor plants; International Spike), was associated with a total of 45 calls in all species in 1986 and 1987. Disulfoton is an extremely toxic, systemic insecticide for use on plants. Most of the 1987 small animal calls assessed as toxicosis or suspected toxicosis pertained to dogs. Deaths were reported in one canine and one feline case.

DIFFERENT FORMULATIONS WITH THE SAME NAME. The oxime 2-PAM chloride (Protopam, Ayerst, Fort Dodge) is often of value in OP toxicosis, although it is believed to be of little value in carbamate insecticide toxicosis. Therefore, it is necessary to differentiate formulations of Golden Malrin or Golden Malrin products that contain *DDVP, other organophosphorus insecticides*, or both from Golden Maldrin containing only the carbamate *methomyl* (all these products by Zoecon). It is unfortunate that there are many other instances in which a single product name is used for multiple formulations.

Carbamate Insecticides

The clinical effects of carbamate insecticides are similar to those of the OP insecticides. In 1986 and again in 1987, *propoxur* (Baygon, Mobay) was involved in over 125 calls pertaining to dogs. Ant traps were the products most commonly involved, but these typically contain such a small amount of propoxur that exposure ordinarily represents a negligible risk for cats and dogs. Thus, in both years, almost 75 per cent of the canine calls were classified as exposures only. Toxicoses plus suspected toxicoses, attributed almost exclusively to formulations other than those in ant traps, amounted to fewer than 15 per cent of the propoxur calls. In cats, this compound was involved in a total of 55 calls for the 2-year period. Effects compatible with a toxicosis were present in 38 per cent of the feline cases.

Carbaryl (Sevin, Union Carbide) was the toxicant in question in 94 calls pertaining to dogs and 88 pertaining to cats in the 2-year period. In dogs 32 per cent and in cats 40 per cent of the cases were assessed as toxicosis or suspected toxicosis. *Bendiocarb* is the active ingredient in Ficam (Mallinckrodt, Inc., or Schering AG), a formulation applied to homes by pest control operators. In 1986, the IAPIC handled a total of 54 bendiocarb calls involving dogs, but this number increased to 132 in 1987. The large increase in canine calls coincided with a tendency toward exposure only calls and was an apparent result of the introduction of bendiocarb-containing ant traps, such as Raid Ant Trap II (S.C.

Johnson & Sons). In both years, the number of bendiocarb calls pertaining to cats was just over 20. Toxicoses and suspected toxicoses accounted for 9 per cent of the canine and 27 per cent of the feline calls.

Aldicarb is a highly toxic agriculturally applied carbamate insecticide. There were 20 calls pertaining to aldicarb for all species in the 2-year period. In 1987, there were nine calls pertaining to dogs and none involving cats. Most were classified as toxicoses or suspected toxicoses.

From 1986 through 1987, there were 21 *carbofuran* (Furadan, FMC Corp.) inquiries pertaining to dogs but only three involving cats. Almost all carbofuran calls were assessed as toxicosis or suspected toxicosis. Moreover, death was reported in 8 of the 30 calls pertaining to carbofuran in all species in 1987, again reflecting the extreme hazard of this granular insecticidal product.

Methomyl is another carbamate that is extremely hazardous to dogs and cats. This is due to its inherent toxicity (LD_{50} of 17 mg/kg) and the apparent palatability of the sugar baits in which it is often formulated, such as Golden Maldrin (Zoecon). It appears that dogs are poisoned far more often than all other species of domestic animals. Of 146 methomyl calls in dogs and cats from 1986 through 1987, 105 were assessed as either a toxicosis or a suspected toxicosis. Predominant clinical signs included salivation, tremors, vomiting, seizures, diarrhea, and ataxia. Deaths had already occurred in 11 per cent of the total methomyl calls.

Organochlorine Insecticides

Lindane, also called gamma isomer of benzene hexachloride (a misnomer), is commonly encountered in Kwell products (Reed & Carnrick) for human scabies, Ralston Purina Mange Control, Happy Jack Kennel Dip (Happy Jack, Inc.), and Zema Dip. It should be noted that not all Zema Dip products contain lindane. Some are a combination of malathion and lindane, and others are chlorpyrifos based. Of 56 canine calls pertaining to lindane from 1986 through 1987, 33 were assessed as toxicosis or suspected toxicosis. Although not recommended for the feline, 49 calls regarding cats were received, with 37 of these classified as toxicosis or suspected toxicosis. The principal clinical signs included seizures, salivation, vomiting, and tremors.

Chlordane is a cyclodiene organochlorine insecticide. Members of this group (which also includes endrin, aldrin, dieldrin, heptachlor, and an active constituent of toxaphene) are believed to exert their toxic effects primarily as a result of interference with gamma-aminobutyric acid (GABA)–associated inhibition in the central nervous system. Chlordane was involved in a total of 40 calls pertaining to dogs and cats in 1986 and 30 in 1987, possibly reflecting a gradual reduction in use. In 77 per cent of the calls, dogs were involved. In both dogs and cats, the cases were assessed as a toxicosis or a suspected toxicosis 25 to 33 per cent of the time. The most commonly reported clinical signs for this termiticide were tremors, vomiting, seizures, and salivation, with a lesser number showing hyperthermia and ataxia.

In 1987, nine *endosulfan* calls pertained to dogs or cats, and 78 per cent were assessed as a toxicosis or a suspected toxicosis. Toxicosis from endosulfan was most often characterized by seizures, and two of the cases involved deaths.

The organochlorine insecticide p-*dichlorobenzene* is occasionally used in mothballs, although less often than is naphthalene. It is formulated especially in moth crystals, and as a deodorant "cake" for diaper pails, closets, and urinals. Apparently, dogs find p-dichlorobenzene less aversive than do cats. Of the 47 calls involving dogs from 1986 through 1987, 36 per cent were assessed as a toxicosis or a suspected toxicosis. However, in cats, there were only ten calls altogether, and of these, only one was assessed as a suspected toxicosis. Signs in dogs most often included tremors, fasciculations, ataxia and incoordination, depression, paresis, mydriasis, hypersalivation, vomiting, and diarrhea.

Pyrethrin and Pyrethroid Insecticides

In 1986, *pyrethrin* calls to the center with regard to cats were more numerous than for any other generic; over 60 per cent of these calls were regarded as toxicosis or suspected toxicosis. Six of the feline calls assessed as suspected toxicoses were accompanied by deaths. Dogs appear to be affected less often. For all species, there were a total of 401 pyrethrin-related calls to the center in 1987. *Allethrin* calls totaled 45 in 1987. Cats were involved in the greatest number of toxicosis and suspected toxicosis assessments; the common clinical signs, from most to least commonly reported, were tremors or fasciculations, hypersalivation, altered behavior, depression, anorexia, hyperthermia, mydriasis, and miosis.

The active ingredients in Hartz Blockade, a heavily marketed product, are the pyrethroid *fenvalerate* and the insect repellant *N,N-diethyl-m-toluamide (DEET)*. As a result of the poisoning problems and the associated publicity involving this product, 1135 calls were received in 1987. Forty per cent of the calls were assessed as toxicosis or suspected toxicosis. Cats were most often affected. Part of the problem may have been insufficient clarity in the directions for application. Also, adequate toxicity testing on the domestic cat had not been carried out prior to mass marketing. Deaths in both dogs and cats were reported. In canine cases assessed as toxicosis or suspected toxicosis, the most common clinical signs were vomiting, tremors, ataxia and incoordination, hyperactivity, hypersalivation, depression, anorexia, seizures, and dyspnea. In feline cases, the most common clinical signs were hypersalivation, tremors, ataxia and incoordination, vomiting, depression, hyperactivity, seizures, and anorexia. Other effects in cats included hypothermia, mydriasis, vocalization and altered behavior, disorientation, dyspnea, and death.

Miscellaneous Insecticides

Naphthalene is the most commonly used agent in moth balls. As is the case with p-dichlorobenzene, dogs are more often affected than cats. Naphthalene was involved in a total of 90 calls in dogs and 22 in cats from 1986 through 1987. In each of the species, roughly 25 per cent of the calls involved toxicosis or suspected toxicosis. The clinical signs of naphthalene toxicosis, from most to least often reported, were vomiting, depression, tremors, anorexia, diarrhea, and mydriasis. In past years, the center has also encountered calls involving signs suggestive of hemolysis and methemoglobinemia (effects also documented in humans). Therapy for naphthalene-exposed animals often includes measures to limit absorption from the gastrointestinal tract. If methemoglobinemia is present to a clinically significant degree, cats or dogs may be given vitamin C (ascorbic acid) orally or parenterally at a dose of 20 mg/kg (efficacy not experimentally established); or dogs only may be given methylene blue at a dose of 5 mg/kg (1 per cent solution as a maximum concentration; use one time only; efficacy and safety not established). When hemolysis occurs (as a result of any toxicosis), fluid therapy with judicious use of bicarbonate is usually recommended to diminish the chance of hemoglobin-associated nephrosis. When serious anemia or unresponsive, life-threatening methemoglobinemia occurs, blood transfusions may be of value. Exchange transfusions should be considered in some life-threatening cases because of the need to avoid volume overload polycythemia. Oxygen therapy may be of value until measures to correct methemoglobinemia or anemia are successful.

Highly hazardous and widely available, the *sodium arsenate*-based, liquid sugar-bait insecticides (e.g., Terro Ant Killer, Senoret) still cause considerable suffering and death among small animals. This type of bait was the most common formulation involved in the over 100 calls regarding sodium arsenate in both 1986 and 1987. All but six of the calls from that period involved dogs and cats; approximately half were assessed as toxicosis or suspected toxicosis. Cats appear somewhat less likely to be exposed but are nevertheless more prone to be poisoned. Vomiting, the most common sign, occurred in 50 per cent of the cases. Most arsenic calls in general, and all those that involve clinical signs, should be handled as urgent emergencies with measures (1) to prevent absorption (activated charcoal and enterogastric lavage; the latter is used only in the absence of marked clinical signs); (2) to combat shock (fluid and other supportive therapy); and (3) to chelate absorbed arsenic with BAL (British antilewisite or dimercaprol) until better chelation agents are available. Generally, chelation therapy should be continued until 24 hr after the cessation of clinical signs. Continued fluid and nutritional support is often called for in sodium arsenate toxicosis.

A minority of the *rotenone* calls involved a single generic insecticide. Many times pyrethrins were concurrently involved. Overall, rotenone was involved in a total of 55 canine and 66 feline calls from 1986 through 1987. Approximately 47 per cent of the canine and 76 per cent of the feline calls were assessed as toxicosis or suspected toxicosis. Predominant signs in affected dogs were vomiting and depression. In cats, clinical signs from most to least commonly reported were depression, tremors, seizures, mydriasis, salivation, vomiting, ataxia and incoordination, miosis, hypothermia, and recumbency. There is no specific antidote for rotenone poisoning. The primary aim is removal of any insecticide from the skin by bathing in detergent. Activated charcoal and a saline or osmotic cathartic may be of value for both orally and topically exposed animals. Anticonvulsants such as diazepam or barbiturates may be given according to need.

There were over 200 *borate* or *boric acid* calls for all species in both 1986 and 1987. For insecticide calls involving dogs, boric acid was the third most commonly mentioned generic compound in 1986. In insecticide calls regarding cats, boric acid was the fourth most common generic involved. Exposure to this agent (often by ingestion) was associated with clinical signs of toxicosis or suspected toxicosis in approximately 25 per cent of the canine and 35 per cent of the feline calls. The most frequently reported effects were vomiting, depression and lethargy, anorexia, and diarrhea. Evidence of oral damage (stomatitis or oral ulcers) and especially anorexia were also mentioned repeatedly. Seizures occurred infrequently in suspected toxicosis cases in both dogs and cats in 1987. Treatment involves (1) measures to limit absorption, (2) demulcents, (3) treatment of symptoms, including anticonvulsants when required, and (4) fluid therapy to minimize renal tubular injury.

Testing on cats of the d-*limonene* product Hill's Holiday Flea and Tick Dip (Pet Chemicals, Inc.) revealed a relatively wide margin of safety, since no deaths or persistent effects were observed at 15 times the recommended dilution rate. Signs of toxicosis included salivation, hypothermia (sometimes marked), ataxia, and, in some highly exposed males, scrotal and perineal dermatitis. Apart from the skin effects, all clinical signs subsided within 6 hr of exposure. In d-limonene calls to the center, salivation, tremors, and ataxia have been the most common effects, followed by vomiting, mydriasis, and hypothermia. In 9 of 85 d-limonene calls in 1986, death was listed. However, nearly all such deaths were believed not to be attributable to d-limonene because of a long delay before death occurred, which would be inconsistent with the physical and toxicologic properties of this compound, or because of simultaneous exposure to other more toxic agents.

When tested on cats at 10 or 20 times the normal concentration, a pump spray product consisting of *linalool*, d-*limonene*, and *piperonyl butoxide* caused the animals to be unable to stand for up to 5 days. Hypothermia and tremors were observed, with severe mydriasis and delayed to absent pupillary light reflexes. At five times the normal concentration, ataxia was present for up to 13 hr postdosing; while at the recommended dilution and at two times the normal concentration, the only signs were hypersalivation and shivering. When used according to the label directions, neither d-limonene nor the combination of linalool plus d-limonene plus piperonyl butoxide appears to be as toxic as a previously available *crude citrus oil extract*–based product, Pet's Pride (Vin-Dotco Inc.). One of three cats died after being experimentally dipped, using the recommended dilution rate for this product.

Hydramethylnon (American Cyanamid) is very low in toxicity, with an LD_{50} of over 1 gm/kg. However, because it has been used so widely in recent years, for dogs it is one of the most commonly reported generic insecticides, with 312 calls in the 2-year period of 1986 through 1987. Although consumption of relatively large quantities of Amdro Fire Ant Insecticide or Combat Fire Ant Killer can result in hydramethylnon toxicoses, lethal poisoning is extremely rare. In 1987, seizures were associated with hydramethylnon exposure in one dog and two cats. By far, the most common clinical sign of this toxicosis was vomiting. When dogs or, very rarely, cats ingest parts of Max-Force or Combat Roach Control Systems, or Combat Ant Control Systems, the amount of hydramethylnon consumed is so small that the primary concern pertains to the possibility that the bait-containing plastic disk may act as a gastrointestinal foreign body.

Methoprene (Precor, Altosid, Pharorid, Zoecon) is a very safe insecticide that acts as an insect hormone mimic to prevent development of flea pupae. It was the compound of primary concern in 64 small animal calls from 1986 through 1987.

However, in each case of associated toxicosis or suspected toxicosis, concurrent exposure to more toxic compounds was deemed more likely to be responsible for the clinical signs.

MOLLUSCACIDES

Metaldehyde, primarily in snail bait and mainly through exposures in yards or gardens, was responsible for a total of 100 canine and 17 feline calls from 1986 through 1987, most of which came from California. The most common clinical signs, listed in decreasing frequency, were tremors, vomiting, seizures, hypersalivation, diarrhea, and hyperthermia. Ataxia, nystagmus, mydriasis, anisocoria, and blindness were also reported. For recent exposures, therapy is comprised of (1) activated charcoal and a saline or osmotic cathartic, or enterogastric lavage with instillation of activated charcoal; (2) diazepam or, as a second choice, a barbiturate to control seizures as needed; (3) fluid therapy and bicarbonate, as needed to control acidosis and shock; and (4) monitoring and supporting the animal to minimize hepatic or renal toxicity.

RODENTICIDES

Anticoagulants

Although known exposure to a specific agent could not be confirmed in over 100 calls during both 1986 and 1987, anticoagulant rodenticide involvement was suspected, based on the history, clinical signs, and laboratory findings. In 7 per cent of such calls, deaths had occurred.

Experimental data and experience (Tables 2 and 4) clearly indicate that dogs are much more likely to consume a toxic amount of *brodifacoum*-containing rodenticide (e.g., D-Con Mouse Prufe II, Havoc, and Talon) than are cats. The need for prolonged vitamin K therapy in cases of toxicosis with this compound has become apparent in many instances in which premature cessation of antidotal treatment has been followed by signs of hemorrhage or even death. The recent mass marketing of this generic in D-Con Mouse Prufe II has greatly increased the frequency of small animal exposure.

With 779 calls pertaining to dogs and 88 calls pertaining to cats from 1986 through 1987, *warfarin* was the generic rodenticide associated with the second highest number of calls to the center. However, only 4 per cent of the canine and 11 per cent of the feline calls were assessed as either toxicosis or suspected toxicosis. The warfarin and brodifacoum data, when considered in view of the bias with regard to brodifacoum, indicate that the present trend away from the marketing of warfarin in favor of the use of brodifacoum will result in a substantial increase in anticoagulant toxicoses among dogs. Moreover, the problems will probably be amplified when the emergency telephone number for animal exposures is no longer listed on the label, unless consumers appreciate the importance of acquiring the recommended antidotal therapy.

Another anticoagulant that constitutes a considerable hazard to dogs is *diphacinone*. The compound was involved in 127 small animal calls in 1986 and 161 in 1987; only 5 per cent of these involved cats. Almost 28 per cent of the canine calls were assessed as toxicosis or suspected toxicosis. As in the case of brodifacoum, prolonged vitamin K therapy is essential for animals exposed to potentially toxic amounts of diphacinone.

With 185 total calls in 1987, *bromadiolone* was sixteenth among generics of all classes in terms of calls to the center. The increase from 102 canine and 21 feline calls in 1986 to 173 canine and 26 feline calls in 1987 probably indicates both increasing usage and the growth in workload of the center. Over the 2-year period, only two of the canine calls were assessed as toxicosis, while almost 13 per cent were assessed as suspected toxicosis. In 1987, death was believed to be related to bromadiolone ingestion in only one small animal case, which involved a dog. In cats, 5 per cent of the calls were assessed as suspected toxicosis.

Miscellaneous Rodenticides

From 1986 to 1987, 46 per cent of the 83 canine calls regarding *strychnine* were assessed as toxicosis or suspected toxicosis. Nearly all were manifested by seizures. Cats were involved in only seven calls in the 2-year period, and only one of these cases was assessed as a suspected toxicosis. For all species, deaths were reported in 19 per cent of the calls. It is difficult to rationalize the continued use of strychnine in view of the safer pesticides available.

Bromethalin is a new generic ingredient present in Assault (Purina) and Vengeance (Velsicol) rodenticides. Because of the presence of the IAPIC telephone number on packages of Vengeance, the total of only 34 calls pertaining to small animals in 1986 and the 129 calls in 1987 indicate that the product is being gradually introduced into the marketplace. Approximately 12 per cent of the 112 canine calls were assessed as toxicosis or suspected toxicosis, whereas in the more susceptible feline animal, almost 30 per cent of the 17 cats involved displayed clinical signs compatible with poisoning. Clinical signs in dogs and cats believed to be affected by bromethalin most often included ataxia and incoordination, seizures, tremors, weakness, coma, vomiting, depression, extensor rigidity, blindness, and mydriasis.

Apparently, the sales of rodenticides containing *cholecalciferol* (vitamin D_3) are increasing at a rapid pace. In 1986, 12 of 24 feline cases were assessed as toxicosis or suspected toxicosis; in 1987, 17 of 41 feline cases were given these designations. For dogs, in 1986, 46 of 153 cases were assessed as toxicosis or suspected toxicosis, while in 1987, the ratio was 107 of 310 cases. Thus, as discussed in another article, these rodenticide formulations constitute a new *major hazard* to dogs (see pp. 148–152). Extrapolation from studies with technical material rather than data obtained with the bait itself was responsible for the inaccurate prediction of a lack of problems in small domestic animals.

When animals become attached to *sticky traps* used for rodents or insects, removal can usually be achieved by dissolving the material in a hand degreaser or with butter (margarine may not be as effective), followed by bathing in a mild liquid dish detergent. There were over 55 calls pertaining to adhesives in 1986 alone.

HERBICIDES

The center received 281 calls pertaining to small animals and *2,4-D* from 1986 through 1987. Of these, approximately one third in both dogs and cats were assessed as toxicosis or suspected toxicosis. The predominant clinical signs include vomiting, diarrhea, anorexia, ataxia and incoordination, hypersalivation, and tremors. In acute 2,4-D toxicosis, the electromyogram (EMG) almost invariably displays marked aberrations (especially prolonged insertional activity and harmonic potentials). The EMG effects induced by 2,4-D and residues in serum and urine are often readily detectable, even when concentrations in the body are too low to cause clinical toxicosis. Thus, when available, either EMG or analytic studies can serve as a reliable indicator of exposure to the herbicide. Only when given massive doses of phenoxy herbicides will healthy dogs experience seizures. Other phenoxyacetic acid derivatives (*MCPP, MCPA*) and the benzoic acid herbicide *dicamba* (Banvel, Velsicol and Sandoz) seem to affect dogs similarly. In acutely exposed animals, measures should be taken to prevent gastrointestinal absorption. Because of the water solubility and acidic character of phenoxy and benzoic acid herbicides, their elimination after they have already been absorbed may be hastened somewhat by administration of fluids and of bicarbonate.

Glyphosate (Roundup; Kleenup [Monsanto]) was involved in 126 canine and 41 feline calls from 1986 through 1987. Roughly 12 to 15 per cent of the calls in either species were assessed as toxicosis or suspected toxicosis. However, the compound is not highly toxic, so relatively few of such calls involved marked effects (these calls generally involved exposure to concentrates). The predominant clinical signs consist of vomiting and diarrhea.

Almost half the 25 canine and each of the three feline *paraquat* calls from 1986 through 1987 were assessed as toxicosis or suspected toxicosis. The most common clinical signs were as follows: dyspnea, vomiting, depression, hypersalivation, oral ulcers, hyperthermia, hypothermia, and seizures. Because of the potentially irreversible or lethal pulmonary effects of paraquat and its high affinity for clays, recent oral ingestions should be treated with immediate oral or intragastric administration of liberal amounts of kaolin and activated charcoal (Toxiban, Vet-A-Mix) or another source of finely divided clay. If clays are not immediately available, activated or superactivated charcoal should be administered. Oxygen therapy is generally contraindicated, since the increased oxygen concentration is likely to aggravate free radical–induced injury to the lungs. Supportive care includes forced diuresis to minimize renal injury and to promote excretion with care to avoid overhydration and exacerbation of pulmonary edema. Paraquat is also an eye irritant. The compound is poorly absorbed through intact skin, but human poisoning has resulted from absorption through broken skin; thus, precautions are advised for persons removing paraquat from topically exposed animals.

FERTILIZERS

N-P-K, meaning nitrogen, phosphorus, and potash, is the primary entry for fertilizers in the center's data base. Dogs are significantly more likely than are cats to be exposed; when they are exposed, they are more prone to consume enough to be affected. A total of 84 of 274 canine calls and 9 of 55 feline calls from 1986 through 1987 were assessed as toxicosis or suspected toxicosis. The major effect was vomiting, with diarrhea about half as often. Most exposed animals are treated by immediate dilution of the ingested fertilizer with milk or water and supportive care to minimize the effects of gastrointestinal irritation or associated dehydration. Fertilizers containing added herbicides or insecticides are more likely to cause serious toxicoses.

HUMAN MEDICINES

Dogs commonly ingest quantities of human medications that have spilled or have been left lying about, frequently resulting in exposure to toxic doses. Cats are not as often involved but sometimes consume significant quantities of human drugs without provocation. However, most feline cases of *acetaminophen* toxicosis continue to result from deliberate administration by well-meaning but uninformed owners. In 1986, 67 of 117 feline calls involved effects compatible with poisoning and, in 1987, the ratio was 76 of 131 feline calls. Affected cats commonly displayed cyanosis or other evidence of methemoglobinemia, compensatory dyspnea or tachypnea, vomiting, and edema most often affecting the face and paws. In dogs, there were even more calls: 142 in 1986 and 170 in 1987. However, at the time of the calls, only 18 per cent of the dogs displayed clinical signs compatible with poisoning. Most toxicoses in dogs involved ingestion of approximately 100 mg/kg or more. Vomiting and depression were the two most common clinical signs in acetaminophen-poisoned dogs. These may be accompanied by hepatic injury.

In both species, treatment consists of attempts to limit gastrointestinal absorption (which occurs quite rapidly) with activated charcoal when the patient is presented quite early as well as administration of acetylcysteine (Mucomyst, Bristol), which helps detoxify reactive metabolites and facilitates their excretion. Acetylcysteine is administered in solution at 140 to 280 mg/kg for the first dose, followed by 70 mg/kg q.i.d. for 4 or more days as needed. The drug is preferably given orally, but if activated charcoal has been administered or if severe respiratory distress is present, it may be given intravenously, slowly over a period of approximately 15 min. For cats that develop methemoglobinemia, treatment is suggested as previously described for naphthalene. Many severely affected cats recover.

IAPIC data suggest that *aspirin* is currently causing more concern with regard to toxicoses in dogs than in cats, which is a possible reflection of differences in eating habits between the two species. Poisoning of either species generally involves significant clinical effects. There were 162 calls involving dogs from 1986 through 1987, and 44 per cent were assessed as toxicosis or suspected toxicosis. There were 64 calls pertaining to cats during the same period, with 34 per cent believed to involve poisoning. In aspirin-poisoned cats, liver damage has been demonstrated experimentally; however, in calls to the center, clinical signs were more nonspecific and included vomiting, retching and gagging, dyspnea, and tachypnea and panting. In dogs, vomiting was the most common clinical sign, followed by depression, ataxia and incoordination, diarrhea, and tachypnea and panting. Tachypnea is likely to be due to metabolic acidosis induced by the acetylsalicylic acid itself, in conjunction with the metabolic effects of the toxic syndrome. Measures to limit the rapid absorption of aspirin are employed when possible. Correction of acidosis with fluids and judiciously administered bicarbonate may be needed.

Recently developed *nonsteroidal anti-inflamma-tory drugs* (NSAIDs) have become important toxicants in small animal practice. Although the half-lives and relative toxicities of different NSAIDs vary widely, most of the clinical poisoning syndromes involve two organs: the stomach and the kidneys. *Ibuprofen*, the NSAID in Motrin and Rufen, which has recently become available without prescription as Advil and Nuprin, is currently the most common agent involved. Serious toxic effects appear to occur at ibuprofen doses as low as 50 mg/kg of body weight. In both dogs and cats, the number of calls in 1987 was approximately 50 per cent greater than in 1986. The totals for the 2-year period were 585 calls involving dogs and 119 for cats. The relative proportions of toxicoses and suspected toxicoses have been consistent at approximately 45 per cent of the canine and 50 per cent of the feline calls. In 1987, the clinical signs reported in ibuprofen poisoning of dogs, listed in order of decreasing frequency, were vomiting, depression or stupor, diarrhea, anorexia, ataxia and incoordination, bloody stool and melena, polyuria, and polydipsia. Hemorrhagic gastritis can be severe, and perforation is a possibility. Cats seem to develop hemorrhagic gastroenteritis less often than dogs but may display tachypnea and panting somewhat more frequently. Therapy may involve emetics; activated charcoal and a saline or osmotic cathartic to minimize absorption (for animals presented early); fluids to facilitate perfusion of target organs; bicarbonate (in the fluids—slowly administered) to promote elimination of the acidic drug; and cimetidine (Tagamet, SmithKline) as well as the "ulcer-coating agent" sucralfate (Carafate, Marion) for gastritis. Other NSAIDs commonly involved in calls included *naproxen* (Naprosyn, Syntex), *piroxicam* (Feldene, Pfizer), and *indomethacin* (Indocin, Merck, Sharp & Dohme).

In 1987 alone, the *benzodiazepine alprazolam* (Xanax, Upjohn) was the source of 42 calls in small animals; *diazepam* (Valium, Roche) was involved in 25; *triazolam* (Halcion, Upjohn) in 19; *flurazepam* (Dalmane, Roche) in 8; and *lorazepam* (Ativan, Wyeth) in 8. The clinical signs pertaining to the effects of these benzodiazepines in canine cases assessed as toxicosis or suspected toxicosis (from most common to least) were ataxia and incoordination, depression, and hyperactivity. Although other clinical signs were occasionally mentioned, no deaths had occurred at the time of the calls. This finding is consistent with the experience in most human exposures, and none of the drugs was unique in the spectrum of clinical signs described.

There were roughly 100 small animal calls pertaining to *zinc oxide* in both 1986 and 1987; the overwhelming majority involved dogs. Most of the poisonings were due to ingestion of diaper rash products such as Desitin ointment (Leeming). Over half were assessed as either toxicosis or suspected toxicosis, with vomiting reported in 66 per cent of the calls. Depression and lethargy or, less often, diarrhea occurred, but other signs were only rarely observed. Acute zinc oxide ingestion must not be confused with subacute or chronic toxicosis, which can result from ingestion of zinc hardware or pennies or from repeated exposure to zinc oxide. In subacute or chronic zinc toxicosis, hemolysis, regenerative anemia, and hemoglobin-associated renal failure may be seen. Diagnosis of zinc foreign body ingestion may be augmented by radiographs, and recognition of any zinc toxicosis is facilitated through the use of special blood tubes for mineral analysis (free of zinc stearate, which is commonly present on rubber stoppers of other commonly available types of tubes). Appropriate supportive and chelation therapy (systemic edetate calcium disodium) may be needed for animals with subacute or chronic toxicoses.

Topical creams such as Efudex (Roche) that contain 5-*fluorouracil* (5-FU) are used for human solar and actinic keratoses and superficial skin tumors. Ingestion of such products was associated with a total of 21 calls in 1986 and 1987. This antimetabolite acts by inhibition of enzymes involved in DNA synthesis and by inhibiting or altering the processing of RNA. It has been postulated that neurotoxicity in cats is a result of production of fluorocitrate, the metabolite responsible for the effects of fluoroacetate (Compound 1080, Tull Chemical Co.). Clinical signs in dogs may develop within 1 hr of exposure, and *death* may occur within 6 to 16 hr. Gastrointestinal and neurotoxic syndromes have been reported to the Illinois center more frequently than other effects. Clinical signs often include vomiting, seizures, depression, hypersalivation, ataxia, tremors, and death. Other effects may include respiratory distress, cyanosis, bradycardia, depression, and lacrimation.

Therapy includes measures to limit absorption (emetic when not contraindicated, and, in all cases, activated charcoal with either a saline or osmotic cathartic, with care to avoid aspiration), gastrointestinal protectants, and supportive care. Phenobarbital or pentobarbital appear to be more effective in controlling seizures than is diazepam. Phenothiazine tranquilizers have been associated with seizures when administered to humans being given 5-FU chemotherapy. Secondary bacterial infections are an indication for antibiotic therapy. In humans, subcutaneous infusions of uridine or intravenous infusions of allopurinol have been used to limit the toxic effects of 5-FU chemotherapy. Their effectiveness in acute toxicosis in the dog is unknown.

Pseudoephedrine was the most commonly involved alpha-adrenergic agent in the period 1986 to 1987, with 135 canine calls, of which 77 were assessed as either toxicosis or suspected toxicosis. However, of 15 calls pertaining to cats in the same period, only two were believed to represent poisoning. The primary clinical manifestations at the time of the calls, from most to least commonly reported, were hyperactivity, mydriasis, depression, vomiting, hyperthermia, disorientation, bradycardia, and tachycardia. Toxicosis or suspected toxicosis due to *phenylpropanolamine* was assessed in 23 of 52 canine and 1 of 8 feline calls from 1986 to 1987; the signs were similar to those reported with pseudoephedrine toxicosis. *Oxymetazoline* was the agent in question in 23 calls to the center in 1987. The most frequent clinical signs were vomiting and depression. Therapy to alleviate toxicosis from alpha-adrenergic agents is directed toward prevention of absorption with activated charcoal and a saline or osmotic cathartic when feasible; control of tachyarrhythmias with lidocaine (dogs only) or, if it fails, with procainamide (also dogs only); and control of seizures with diazepam or, if it fails, phenobarbital or pentobarbital. Sympathomimetic agents are contraindicated.

The beta-2-agonist *albuterol* (Ventolin, Glaxo) is a bronchodilator that was involved in 28 calls in 1987, all of which involved dogs. Clinical signs may appear shortly after exposure. The signs, listed from most to least often reported, were tachycardia, tremors, vomiting, tachypnea and panting, and depression. The most common management measures involve steps to (1) limit gastrointestinal absorption; (2) control seizures (with diazepam, phenobarbital, or pentobarbital); and (3) counteract serious tachyarrhythmias with metoprolol or, if it is not immediately available, with propranolol. Monitoring for hypokalemia may be needed.

Illegal *marijuana* was associated with assessments of toxicosis or suspected toxicosis in 101 of 175 canine calls from 1986 to 1987 and 6 of 12 feline calls for the same period. The predominant clinical signs are related to sedation, which may persist for more than a day in the affected canine. Supportive care and activated charcoal are usually successful.

VETERINARY MEDICINES

Veterinarians often receive requests for information when medications intended for animals are consumed by humans. Rather than assessing the risk of the medication to the exposed person, when possible the veterinarian should provide information directly to the physician or poison control professional. In many instances, equivalent human products exist. When this is not the case, it is often helpful to provide information on animal toxicity if it is known. When this information is provided, the caller should be told of its source.

Despite its relatively high degree of safety, the generic veterinary medicine responsible for the greatest number of calls in 1987 was *diethylcarbam-*

azine, with a total of 249 calls in all species. Of a total of 188 calls in 1986, 41 involved humans; most were regarded as exposure only. Use of this drug in humans is described in readily available pharmacology texts. Ingestion of large quantities of chewable products was a common factor in the 1987 canine calls pertaining to diethylcarbamazine that were assessed as toxicosis or suspected toxicosis. The predominant clinical sign was vomiting. Depression was the only other clinical sign mentioned repeatedly, and no deaths were reported. Therapy includes measures to terminate absorption (activated charcoal and a saline cathartic), and symptomatic and supportive care when needed.

After initially considering many *piperazine* calls as doubtful, it gradually became apparent that toxicoses occur in a small fraction of the exposed animals. From 1986 to 1987, 32 of 44 canine calls and 52 of 69 feline calls were assessed as toxicosis or suspected toxicosis. The most common clinical signs, in order of decreasing frequency, were tremors, ataxia, seizures, vomiting, and weakness. A range of other clinical effects suggestive of disorientation were commonly reported. For recent ingestions, activated charcoal and a saline or osmotic cathartic are recommended. Since piperazine is eliminated partly in the urine, fluid therapy may be of some value. Also, renal dysfunction may predispose an animal to piperazine-induced neurotoxicity. Other therapeutic measures are aimed at treatment of symptoms and supportive care.

In spite of toluene's many uses, the majority of calls about this compound involved *toluene*-containing anthelmintics. Most of these products also contain dichlorophen. In 1987, the clinical signs reported in 39 canine and feline calls assessed as toxicosis or suspected toxicosis, from most to least often reported, were ataxia and incoordination, disorientation, hypersalivation, vomiting, tremors, and mydriasis. Death had occurred in one suspected toxicosis case.

Ivermectin calls increased from 75 canine and 13 feline calls in 1986 to 161 canine and 19 feline in 1987. Over half the dogs and nearly all the cats displayed signs compatible with the toxic effects of ivermectin. Although collies and related breeds are predisposed to toxicosis, ivermectin can cause problems when sufficient doses are given to other breeds of dogs as well as cats and birds.

Although there were only 15 calls regarding *metronidazole* (Flagyl, Barr, Danbury, Lederle, or Zenith) in 1987, the effects of this drug (used against enteric diseases) were relatively consistent and included a large number of nervous system or neuromuscular effects. The following clinical signs were reported for toxicosis and suspected toxicosis calls in dogs and cats: ataxia and incoordination, headtilt, proprioceptive deficits, seizures, anorexia, tremors, joint knuckling, disorientation, rigidity and stiffness, paresis, depression, mydriasis, nystagmus, bradycardia, colic, and vomiting. Although the recommended dose for adult dogs is 60 mg/kg and the canine will reportedly tolerate doses of 100 mg/kg per day for 1 month, the levels of exposure at which these effects were observed ranged from 6 mg/kg, t.i.d. for 6 months, to a single ingestion of 3800 mg/kg. Management of acute metronidazole toxicosis involves measures to limit absorption (activated charcoal and a saline or osmotic cathartic), with fluids to promote elimination in the urine; control of seizures; treatment of other symptoms; and supportive care. Recovery of neurologic function may take several days.

In both 1986 and 1987, there were approximately 35 calls to the center with regard to *amitraz* (Mitaban, Upjohn). Most involved amitraz-treated dogs. The predominant clinical sign was ataxia or depression, which was sometimes severe (eyes rolled back in one dog; headpressing in another), followed by hypothermia or hyperthermia, vomiting, diarrhea, and, occasionally, bradycardia. Although young puppies are especially sensitive, dogs of all ages were affected, including numerous 3- to 4-month-old puppies, young adult dogs, and some aged individuals. Cats, including those treated only in the external ears, have also been reportedly poisoned.

Pentobarbital toxicosis as a result of feeding on carcasses of animals previously subjected to euthanasia is a recurrent cause of poisonings in dogs. Prolonged general anesthesia is the predominant clinical effect. Measures to minimize absorption of the anesthetic from the digestive tract, including activated charcoal and an osmotic cathartic, are often indicated in many such patients when they are presented sufficiently early. Magnesium sulfate is not recommended as the cathartic because of the possibility of further central nervous system depression. Good nursing care is needed, including keeping the animal warm, dry, well-hydrated, and in a positive energy balance. Alkalinization of the urine modestly enhances the elimination of pentobarbital.

In calls from 1987 pertaining to *benzocaine*, 9 of 17 involving dogs and 7 of 7 involving cats, were assessed as a toxicosis or a suspected toxicosis. Problems typically result from excessive oral exposures in dogs and cats. The following clinical signs are listed from most to least often reported: evidence suggestive of methemoglobinemia, depression, vomiting, dyspnea, diarrhea, pallor, anemia, ataxia and incoordination, seizures, and cyanosis. For methemoglobinemia or hemolysis, therapy is similar to that for naphthalene toxicosis. Other local anesthetics sometimes exert similar effects.

Of 25 *methionine*-related calls in 1987, 18 involved cats, and of these, 12 were assessed as toxicosis or suspected toxicosis. Of the seven canine calls, four were believed to represent a poisoning problem. Most toxicoses resulted from ingestion of quantities of chewable formulations, such as Methioform, Vet-A-Mix. In small animal cases assessed as toxicosis or suspected toxicosis, ataxia and incoordination, and vomiting, were mentioned most often, followed by depression, and tachypnea and panting. Animals with liver failure are predisposed to neurotoxic effects of metabolites of methionine, but most calls to the center do not seem to involve hepatic insufficiency. However, in the 1987 calls, each of the following nervous system or neuromuscular effects were reported: seizures, tetany, extensor rigidity, dysmetria, and disorientation.

The ionophore feed additive and coccidiostat *lasalocid* (Bovatec, Hoffman-LaRoche) is commonly used for cattle and sheep. It is also occasionally responsible for toxicoses in dogs that ingest it in concentrated form. Initial signs include weakness and paralysis in an otherwise alert animal. An affected dog may be unable to lift its head or body yet may wag its tail and follow humans about the room with its eyes. In dogs, death results from respiratory paralysis. Although suggested treatment includes enterogastric lavage, activated charcoal, vitamin E and selenium, and artificial respiration as needed, the value of therapeutic intervention remains to be demonstrated.

MISCELLANEOUS CHEMICALS

In 1986, there were 37 calls pertaining to *lead* and dogs, and of these, 21 were assessed as toxicosis or suspected toxicosis. Of the three cases involving cats, one was assessed as a suspected toxicosis.

Ethylene glycol, primarily in automotive antifreeze, commonly poisons dogs and cats. Of 269 calls to the center pertaining to dogs from 1986 through 1987, 132 were assessed as either toxicosis or suspected toxicosis. Similarly, of 78 calls regarding cats, 41 were believed to represent poisonings. Toxicologically significant exposures to ethylene glycol must be handled as emergencies. Rational therapy may involve measures intended to (1) prevent absorption; (2) inhibit alcohol dehydrogenase–mediated metabolism of the parent compound to more toxic metabolites (when presented within the first 18 hr after exposure); and (3) correct dehydration and acidosis as well as promote excretion of the parent compound and metabolites via fluid therapy with added bicarbonate.

There were almost 100 calls from 1986 through 1987 pertaining to ingestion of *cyanoacrylate*, the primary constituent in various brands of Superglue or Krazy Glue. The product generally causes no harmful effects apart from occasional panic or other difficulty associated with sticking of the lips to the gingival tissue or similar attachment. Careful separation of the tissues is all that is ordinarily necessary.

When swallowed, there are generally no problems observed, apparently because of rapid polymerization of the glue and the protective mucous coating of the membranes. Solvents are *not* recommended to facilitate the removal of cyanoacrylate from the oral or pharyngeal cavities of exposed animals.

There were more than 570 *petroleum distillate* calls in all species in 1986. Petroleum distillates were the only ingredients involved in 171 of these calls. Because of their use in products containing more toxic compounds, such as pesticides, the petroleum distillates were believed to be the principal toxicant in only 70 of the remaining 401 calls. Similar trends were apparent in the 1987 calls. Of 246 petroleum distillate calls in 1987 pertaining to dogs, 39 per cent were assessed as toxicosis or suspected toxicosis. The most common effects were gastrointestinal upset (especially vomiting), central nervous system depression, signs referable to skin irritation (a probable result of defatting of the skin in topically exposed animals), and hypersalivation. Respiratory signs were occasionally present and included dyspnea, tachypnea and panting, abnormal lung sounds, and cough. Fifty-seven of 124 exposed cats were believed to be poisoned by petroleum distillates, and similar signs were observed. However, ataxia and incoordination and depression were more common in cats than in dogs. Hyperactivity, tremors, and, infrequently, seizures were also reported.

Gasoline was the primary generic entry in another 38 calls in 1987. Both dogs and cats were involved, with clinical signs, from most to least commonly reported, including vomiting, hypersalivation, ataxia and incoordination, hyperactivity, altered behavior, depression, hyperthermia, vocalizing (cats), dyspnea, coma, and seizures. Management of animals that have ingested any form of petroleum distillate depends upon the type of hydrocarbon involved, its volatility, and any other substances present therein. Emesis is usually contraindicated in cases of ingestion of lighter-weight hydrocarbons because of the risk of aspiration. If toxic pesticides or other toxic compounds are present, an adsorbent such as activated charcoal, an emetic, or a lavage procedure may be warranted. Mineral seal oil is especially prone to be aspirated. Used motor oil from engines burning leaded gasoline is a potential cause of lead poisoning.

Accidental exposure of dogs and cats to *turpentine* is a common cause of significant toxicosis. There were a total of 55 calls regarding turpentine in 1987. Common clinical signs included vomiting, salivation, dyspnea, diarrhea, dermatitis (with significant associated pain and sometimes lameness because of involvement of the feet), and hyperactivity, perhaps in response to dermatitis in some cases. Activated charcoal is recommended for recent ingestions, followed by supportive care for an irritated upper gastrointestinal tract. For topical exposure, applying a hand degreaser, followed by bathing with detergent, may be of value. Thereafter, if dermatitis is present, an emollient may be needed to prevent drying of the skin.

There were 46 canine and 45 feline calls regarding *pine oil*–containing products from 1986 through 1987. Approximately one half of the dogs and two thirds of the cats displayed adverse effects attributed to the pine oil. The primary effect was vomiting, followed by salivation, ataxia, and, occasionally, seizures, coma, stomatitis, polyuria, miosis, hypothermia or hyperthermia, and diarrhea.

For *hypochlorite*, 36 per cent of 130 canine calls and 30 per cent of 46 feline calls from 1986 through 1987 were assessed as toxicosis or suspected toxicosis. Most calls involved liquid bleach products. Hypochlorite was sometimes encountered in toilet bowl–sanitizing products, which can be much more hazardous when concentrated forms are ingested. Few ingestions of liquid bleach are life-threatening. Vomiting is the most commonly reported effect, and significant stomatitis and gastroenteritis can readily occur. The primary therapeutic measures for ingestion of hypochlorite (as well as for strong acids or alkali) include immediate dilution with milk or water, followed by supportive care including a bland semisolid or liquid diet, and fluid therapy if needed. Animals should be monitored for severe mucosal damage or perforation, which is improbable but may follow ingestion of highly concentrated forms of hypochlorite. Perforations often require surgical intervention, whereas deep circumferential burns of the esophageal mucosa without perforation are treated with glucocorticoids to lessen the severity of stricture formation.

PHYSICAL AGENTS

In 1986, the center received 54 calls about *fiber glass insulation*, 39 of which pertained to dogs, and 11 to cats. The predominant clinical signs were vomiting and diarrhea. Lubricant cathartics may be of value if large ingestions result in partial obstruction of the intestine.

SILICA GEL. Silica gel packets used as desiccants are commonly consumed by pet animals. Despite the warning labels on these packets, silica gel is nontoxic. The only concern pertains to the abrasive effects of the crystals themselves, or the unlikely possibility of a foreign body problem if the intact packet is swallowed. Usually, no clinical signs are observed, and the only remedial measures generally involve feeding the animal a bulky diet such as bran cereal mixed with a palatable pet food.

POISONOUS PLANTS

A few of the plants responsible for a large number of calls are mentioned. Poinsettia (*Euphorbia pul-*

cherrima) was the agent involved in over 200 calls in 1987. Most calls are exposures only, but toxicoses sometimes resulted when animals consumed large amounts of the plant. Cats seem to be affected about as frequently as dogs. In 1987, in cases assessed as toxicosis and suspected toxicosis, the most common clinical sign by far was vomiting, followed by depression, anorexia, and diarrhea.

Of 135 *Philodendron* species calls involving dogs from 1986 through 1987, 36 per cent were assessed as toxicosis or suspected toxicosis. In cats, 23 per cent of 105 calls were assessed as toxicosis or suspected toxicosis. The most common clinical signs, listed in order of decreasing frequency, were vomiting, diarrhea, anorexia, dyspnea, hypersalivation, ataxia, tremors, hypothermia, and dehydration. There were over 85 calls pertaining to dogs or cats with regard to *Dieffenbachia* in both 1986 and 1987, and approximately 50 per cent of canine and 20 per cent of feline calls were assessed as toxicosis or suspected toxicosis. In these calls, vomiting, hypersalivation, and anorexia were reported most often. Treatment for these and other calcium oxalate crystal–containing plants includes activated charcoal, milk given orally, and supportive care according to need.

METHYLXANTHINES

Chocolate and, to a lesser degree, *caffeine* toxicoses are quite common in dogs. In 1987, theobromine, the primary active constituent of chocolate, was the twelfth most common generic overall, with 230 calls. There were 144 calls pertaining to caffeine. Toxicoses caused by these agents are discussed on page 191 of *Current Veterinary Therapy IX*. A misprint may be included there with regard to maintenance therapy with lidocaine. The correct maintenance (IV drip) dose of lidocaine is given in the Appendix (see Table of Common Drugs, p. 1370). When using antiarrhythmic drugs such as lidocaine, monitoring the electrocardiogram can be used to reduce the likelihood of serious overdose.

ETHANOL

Beverages containing *ethanol* are commonly consumed by pet animals. Of 71 calls involving dogs from 1986 through 1987, 69 per cent were assessed as toxicosis or suspected toxicosis. Of 30 calls pertaining to cats, 43 per cent were assessed as toxicosis or suspected toxicosis. Clinical signs were largely compatible with human alcohol intoxication, including most often depression and stupor, and less often ataxia and incoordination, pulmonary problems including dyspnea, vomiting or retching, and abnormal lung sounds.

CLINICAL TOXICOLOGY AND CAGE BIRDS

In 1987, there were 441 calls regarding pet birds. Psittacines, especially parrots, were most often involved, with lesser numbers pertaining to canaries, finches, and, rarely, racing pigeons. Because of the range of species involved and the much lower total number of calls, the data on the relative importance of various toxicants are much less reliable than those for dogs and cats. Accordingly, only some of the more notable syndromes are mentioned.

Philodendron, Spathiphyllum, Dieffenbachia, and similar calcium oxalate crystal–containing plants are very commonly consumed and may cause signs suggestive of digestive tract (oral or abdominal) pain and upset. Occasionally, depression or disorientation were reported. Often, no signs were present at the time of the calls. Deaths were reported after birds ingested green onions (*Allium cepa*). Onion ingestion has previously been associated with hemolysis in dogs.

Bleach (*hypochlorite*) fumes were associated with coughing 90 min after exposure. The following are believed to have affected the respiratory systems of birds, sometimes resulting in deaths: the refrigerant gas *Freon*, the propellant gas *trifluoroethylene*, and especially fumes and particulate matter from over-heated nonstick cookware coated with *Teflon* or *Silverstone.*

Lead weights and lead solder were associated with fecal abnormalities including bloody diarrhea, as well as polydipsia, dyspnea, depression, disorientation, weakness, and, possibly, anemia. *Zinc oxide* ointment ingestion resulted in vomiting as in dogs.

Ivermectin was associated with two cases of depression and stupor; one involved signs of blindness. *Dimetridazole* (Emtryl, Salsbury) soluble powder, when administered in water at eight times the intended concentration, was associated with anorexia, weakness, depression, seizures, and oliguria in two cockatiels beginning less than 2 days after initial exposure. One of the birds died.

Carbamate and *organophosphorus insecticides* were associated with diarrhea, weakness, recumbency, curled toes, and death. The organochlorine *lindane* (in Kwell) was associated with seizures less than 8 hr after exposure in one case. The anticoagulant rodenticides *diphacinone* and *brodifacoum* have been associated with hemorrhage and death.

Many *felt-tip* and *ball-point pens* as well as other writing instruments were mouthed and broken by various birds with essentially no adverse effects noted at the time of the calls.

COMMENT

Because of the limited number of animal poison information centers currently in existence, the best use of these services is likely to result when the veterinarian obtains a thorough history and then calls the center directly. However, asking clients to call animal poison information centers directly is sometimes appropriate, as in cases in which the practitioner has tried but has been unable to associate a probable toxicant with the signs involved. Commonly, measures to reduce exposure are of utmost urgency, and the client and the practitioner both can be involved in the call when made from the veterinary facility during or after the initial examination.

References and Supplemental Reading

Barton, J., and Oehme, F. W.: The incidence and characteristics of animal poisonings seen in Kansas State University from 1975 to 1980. Vet. Hum. Toxicol. 23:101, 1981.
Beasley, V. R.: Prevalence of Poisonings in Small Animals. *In* Kirk, R. W. (ed.): *Current Veterinary Therapy IX.* Philadelphia: W. B. Saunders Co., 1986, pp. 120–129.
Humphreys, D. J.: A review of recent trends in animal poisoning. Br. Vet. J. 134:128, 1978.
Maddy, K. T., and Winter, J.: Poisoning of animals in the Los Angeles area with pesticides during 1977. Vet. Hum. Toxicol. 22:409, 1980.
Maddy, K. T., Peoples, S. A., and Riddle, L. C.: Poisoning in dogs in California with pesticides. Calif. Vet. 31:9, 1977.
Osweiler, G. D.: Incidence and diagnostic considerations of major small animal toxicoses. J.A.V.M.A. 155:2011, 1969.
Osweiler, G. D.: Common poisonings in small animal practice. *In* Kirk, R. W. (ed.): *Current Veterinary Therapy VIII.* Philadelphia: W. B. Saunders Co., 1983, pp. 76–82.
Osweiler, G. D.: Potential sources of small animal poisonings. *In* Kirk, R. W. (ed.): *Current Veterinary Therapy VIII.* Philadelphia: W. B. Saunders Co., 1983, pp. 93–98.
Yeary, R. A.: Oral intubation of dogs with combinations of fertilizer, herbicide, and insecticide chemicals commonly used on lawns. Am. J. Vet. Res. 45:288, 1984.

COMPANION ANIMAL FORENSIC TOXICOLOGY

WILLIAM C. EDWARDS, D.V.M.

Stillwater, Oklahoma

Forensic veterinary toxicology encompasses the legal aspects of veterinary pathology and toxicology. It is the study of the conditions and circumstances by which animals of any species may be poisoned and the subsequent legal ramifications under civil or criminal law. Forensic veterinary toxicology involves such broad areas of the disciplines of law, pathology, and toxicology that it often requires the coming together of specialists and experts from these different disciplines to satisfactorily conclude a case.

Animal poisonings, unlike human poisonings, are not generally regulated by state laws or investigated under the medical examiner or coroner systems. When poisoning is suspected as a cause of animal illness or death, the attending veterinarian may seek assistance from state animal disease diagnostic laboratories or commercial laboratories. In most instances, the cost of pathologic and toxicologic testing must be borne by the animal owner; in some special cases, an insurance company will cover the expense. Thus, it is unfortunate that for strictly economic reasons many cases are not investigated. However, there is a current generation of animal owners who seek to learn the cause of death when foul play is suspected or when there is the possibility of collecting damages from a second party.

Cases of poisoning from pesticide applications, contaminated feed, improperly labeled commercial products, pharmaceuticals, and industrial waste have resulted in actual and punitive damages being awarded to animal owners in civil suits when a second party has been proved to be negligent or liable. The veterinary practitioner may be called as a witness of fact or as an expert witness in such civil suits. The burden of proof in civil cases is generally less stringent than in criminal cases and requires only a reasonable degree of medical certainty.

In cases in which criminal charges may be brought against an individual for animal cruelty or malicious poisoning, the burden of proof must be much greater. Prosecuting attorneys quite often do not pursue such cases unless they believe they have sufficient evidence for conviction. The classic case is a neighbor threatening to poison a dog, followed by confirmation of the pet's death by strychnine poisoning. Such a case is often regarded as circumstantial evidence at best. Unless caught in the act, the culprit may never be prosecuted and may continue such malevolent acts.

Veterinary practitioners may occasionally find themselves as defendants in civil actions involving alleged malpractice or negligence. These cases often involve anesthetic accidents, drug idiosyncrasies, drug interactions, and drug or pesticide toxicoses.

Another area of companion animal forensic toxicology involves animal doping. There have been cases of doping of competitors' animals at dog shows to make them show poorly. Less common is the doping of dogs to improve performance, with the exception of greyhound racing. Companion animals have also been poisoned from controlled substances such as cocaine, marijuana, and heroin. Some of these cases have involved attempts to use companion animals to smuggle controlled substances, while others have been accidental exposures or experimentation by drug abusers.

When companion animal poisoning is suspected, particularly in those cases with potential for litigation, it is recommended that the intact animal be transported to a qualified animal disease diagnostic laboratory. Under conditions in which excessive postmortem degeneration may occur, the veterinary practitioner may wish to conduct the gross necropsy and submit tissues, both frozen and in formalin, to a diagnostic laboratory.

Diagnostic laboratory submissions should include a comprehensive case history along with properly collected and preserved tissues.

Abnormal organs should be sectioned for histopathologic examination as well as all organs that may be related to the clinical signs. Abnormal organs should be described in detail on the necropsy report. In addition, organs with no visible gross changes should be reported.

Essential specimens for a toxicology investigation include

1. Urine, all available.
2. Serum, with clot removed.
3. Heart blood, 10 to 20 ml.
4. Brain, one half in formalin and one half frozen.
5. Liver, 200 gm if possible.
6. Kidney, 200 gm if possible.
7. Stomach contents, generally all available.
8. Intestinal contents, generally all available.
9. Intact eyeball (or aspirated aqueous humor).

Because storage problems exist at most diagnostic laboratories and the legal system is extremely slow, it is highly recommended that duplicate samples be collected and retained by the attending veterinarian.

Accurate records documenting the collection, identification, transportation, and storage of specimens are essential in maintaining a chain of evidence.

Nonanimal samples that relate to suspected poisoning cases may include feed, water, suspected bait, pesticides, and chemicals. When dealing with commercial products, label information and lot numbers should be submitted with the samples.

Diagnostic veterinary medicine is a science of interpretation that is dependent upon the quality (and sometimes quantity) of submitted specimens and the economic feasibility of pursuing an exact diagnosis. In correlating the pathologic and toxicologic findings, it is soon apparent that varying degrees of subjective interpretation are required to arrive at a conclusion. Generally speaking, lawyers and the courts are not interested in technical descriptions of lesions observed, they want to know the cause of death. However, the technical descriptions are important because they help substantiate the practitioner's interpretations and conclusions.

Conclusions will be based upon interpretative probability or what constitutes a "reasonable degree of medical certainty." Thus when serving as an expert witness, the veterinary practitioner or diagnostician has the obligation of formulating an opinion or conclusion based upon this reasonable degree of medical certainty. It is the obligation of the expert to educate the court as to the facts of the case and to express his or her conclusion or expert opinion based on these facts. The comprehensive toxicologic testing that may be required to meet the legal aspects of a case is costly and may require several weeks, particularly if screening tests indicate evidence of suspected toxins or chemical agents that require special testing for confirmation. The conditions under which the veterinary practitioner may be involved in litigation concerning companion animal poisoning are as varied as the conditions under which animals have been maliciously or accidentally poisoned.

In most instances, when veterinary practioners serve as expert witnesses, the emphasis is on their specialized knowledge rather than their general knowledge. Guidelines for the expert witness are

1. Know your limitations, and do not accept a case against your better judgment.

2. Do your homework, and know what is expected of you.

3. Establish your fees in advance. You are entitled to a reasonable fee for your time.

4. During a deposition or trial, dress with dignity, and speak with candor.

5. When possible, give concise answers in simple terms. Do not ramble or respond in complicated medical terminology.

6. Do not let the opposing attorney get your goat. Likewise, do not play word games with attorneys. When you do not understand a question, ask that it be restated.

In some instances, a subpoena may be served, requiring the presence of the veterinary practitioner for deposition or trial. The *subpoena ad testificandum* compels the person served to appear and testify. The *subpoena duces tecum* may specify certain medical records, books, or radiographs to be produced in court. Subpoenas should not be taken lightly. Failure to appear and testify in obedience to a legal subpoena may result in criminal prosecution.

Preparing and following a thorough course of action is the best way for the veterinarian to provide the court with as complete a medical record as possible, in order that any future legal action will be easier to resolve.

References and Supplemental Reading

Bell, R. H., and Meerdink, G. L.: *Medical-Legal Aspects of Veterinary Medicine. Part I*. American Association of Veterinary Laboratory Diagnosticians, 25th Annual Proceedings, 1982, pp. 491–498.

Edwards, W. C.: Animal doping. Vet. Med. Small Anim. Clin. 78:3, 317–318, 1983.

Taylor, R. J., and Sexton, J. W.: *Medical-Legal Aspects of Veterinary Medicine. Part II*. American Association of Veterinary Laboratory Diagnosticians, 25th Annual Proceedings, 1982, pp. 499–519.

EMERGENCY AND GENERAL
TREATMENT OF POISONINGS

E. MURL BAILEY, Jr., D.V.M.

College Station, Texas

Cases of intoxication in animals continually confront veterinary practitioners with therapeutic and prophylactic problems. Many acutely ill animals are diagnosed as poisoned when no other diagnosis can be readily ascertained. The veterinary clinician should direct efforts toward treating the signs exhibited by the affected animal unless the correct diagnosis is obvious. Pre-existing conditions and the diagnosis should be determined following stabilization of the patient.

Special goals of therapy in cases of intoxication are as follows:

1. Emergency intervention and prevention of further exposure.
2. Preventing further absorption.
3. Application of specific antidotes.
4. Hastening elimination of the absorbed toxicant.
5. Supportive measures.
6. Client education.

PRELIMINARY INSTRUCTIONS TO CLIENTS

Veterinarians are frequently contacted by telephone concerning an intoxicated animal. The preliminary instructions given at this time are very important to the success of subsequent therapeutic measures.

The client should be instructed to protect the affected animal as well as the people in contact with it. This may include keeping the animal warm and not allowing it to be exposed to any other stressful stimuli. Onlookers should be warned about the condition of the animal, and it may be desirable to muzzle the animal.

If the animal's exposure was topical, the animal owner should be instructed to cleanse the animal's skin or eyes with copious amounts of water. The client should also be instructed to be careful to avoid self-exposure to the toxicant and to use some type of protective clothing (e.g., rubber gloves, apron) if available.

In many instances, the client will be concerned about inducing emesis in the animal. The clinician should cite the contraindications to emesis (e.g., central nervous system [CNS] depression; ingestion of petroleum distillates, acids, or alkalis). Emetic preparations and techniques easily available to lay individuals (e.g., hydrogen peroxide, table salt, copper sulfate, and sticking the finger in the back of the animal's mouth) are generally ineffective and sometimes dangerous. One-half to two teaspoons of syrup of ipecac may be administered if the animal is fully awake.

If the client is very insistent about administering medication, he or she should be advised to allow the animal to drink as much water as it wants. This will act as a diluent. In most cases, one may also advise the administration of milk or egg whites. Activated charcoal tablets may also be administered. The client should be cautioned not to administer anything by mouth if the animal is convulsing, depressed, or unconscious.

It is imperative that the client not waste time. The animal should be taken to the veterinarian as soon as possible (or the veterinarian should be summoned). The owner should be instructed to bring vomitus or suspected toxic materials or their containers with the animal. The client should be advised to bring the specimens in clean plastic containers or glass jars and should be cautioned not to contaminate the material. In many instances, valuable time can be saved by applying the proper therapeutic measure if the suspected intoxicant is known. However, the clinician should not be biased in the diagnosis and treatment of an animal based on labels or material brought with the animal. In some cases, the signs exhibited by the affected animal do not correspond with suspected ingredients. This suspected material may also be valuable from a medicolegal aspect.

EMERGENCY INTERVENTION

The most important aspect of emergency treatment in cases of intoxication is to ensure adequate physiologic function. All the antidotal procedures available to the clinician will be of no avail if the animal has lost one or all of its vital functions. Emergency intervention may include establishment

Supported in part by the Texas Agricultural Experiment Station, Project no. H-6255. Published as TAES Pub. no. TA-23256.

of a patent airway, artificial respiration, cardiac massage (external or internal), and perhaps the application of defibrillation techniques. Following stabilization of the vital signs, the clinician may proceed with subsequent therapeutic measures.

PREVENTING FURTHER ABSORPTION

Preventing the animal from absorbing additional intoxicant is a major factor in treating intoxicated patients. In many instances, intoxication may be prevented in this manner if the animal was actually observed ingesting or coming in contact with suspected material. Removal of the animal from the affected environment is a necessary first step in preventing further absorption. It is hoped that bringing the animal to the veterinary clinic or hospital will suit this purpose. Prevention of absorption may also entail washing the animal's skin to remove the noxious agent. If an external toxicant is involved, caution must be exercised to avoid contamination of persons handling the animal. In addition, the judicious use of emetics, gastric lavage techniques, adsorbents, and cathartics aids in the prevention of further absorption of toxic materials that are ingested.

Induction of Emesis

Emesis may be considered as a method of emptying the stomach of toxic materials. Some commonly available agents are not very reliable, and emesis may be of little value after 4 hr following exposure to a toxicant.

Syrup of ipecac is considered a general emetic. Its mechanism is gastric irritation as well as central stimulation. The dose of ipecac for small animals is 1 to 2 ml/kg. However, it is only about 50 per cent effective, and not more than 15 ml (1 tablespoon) should be used with even the largest dog. The dose may be repeated in 20 min if emesis does not occur. However, if the patient does not vomit, lavage procedure should be instituted to recover the ipecac. Syrup of ipecac can exert a cardiotoxic effect. This agent should never be used when activated charcoal is part of the therapeutic regimen, since it markedly reduces the effectiveness of the charcoal. *The drug should not be confused with ipecac fluid extract, which is 14 times stronger than the syrup.* Outdated syrup of ipecac can still be used as it is now considered effective.

Other agents such as *copper sulfate, table salt,* or *hydrogen peroxide* have been advocated as locally acting emetics. However, the effectiveness of these agents is highly questionable.

Apomorphine (Eli Lilly & Co.) is the most effective and most reliable emetic available for dogs and cats. Although Apomorphine is no longer a controlled drug, it is not widely available. The effective dose in most small animals is 0.04 mg/kg IV or 0.08 mg/kg IM or SC. Apomorphine may cause respiratory depression, and protracted emesis may develop following its use. These signs may be effectively controlled with appropriate narcotic antagonists injected intravenously, such as naloxone (Narcan, Endo), 0.04 mg/kg; levallorphan (Lorfan, Roche), 0.02 mg/kg; and nalorphine (Nalline, Merck), 0.1 mg/kg. In addition to the general contraindications of emetics, apomorphine may be further contraindicated in cases in which additional CNS depression must be avoided. The contraindications for induction of emesis are unconscious or severely depressed animals; ingestion of strong acids or bases; and intoxication by petroleum distillates, tranquilizers, or other antiemetics. If the time interval following exposure to the toxicant is greater than 4 hr, most of the toxicant will have passed the duodenum.

Intoxication with acids or alkalis may be diagnosed when corrosive changes are present in and around the mouth, forepaws, and other areas on the cranial portions of the body. If emesis is induced, caustic agents could cause additional damage to the esophagus and oral cavity. In addition, these agents generally weaken the gastric wall, which could easily be ruptured during forceful emesis.

Activated charcoal may increase the efficacy of emesis. If charcoal is to be used, first induce emesis with apomorphine. Then, administer the charcoal, and reinduce emesis with a subsequent IV dose of apomorphine (0.04 mg/kg). Syrup of ipecac should never be used if activated charcoal is used, since the agent negates the adsorbent activity of the charcoal.

Any vomitus should be saved for analysis, especially if there are medicolegal considerations. The clinician should conduct treatment accordingly.

Gastric Lavage

Gastric lavage is an emergency procedure that has at times been maligned as being relatively inefficient. Changes in technique (e.g., using a larger tube, more volume, and more frequent lavages) have made this a very reliable procedure when undertaken within 2 hr of exposure to an ingested toxicant.

The animal should be unconscious or under light anesthesia. A cuffed endotracheal tube should be placed within the trachea. The distal end of the tube should extend 2 in (5 cm) beyond the teeth. This increases the animal's dead space but is required to prevent any inhalation of lavage fluid. The head and thorax should be lowered slightly but not enough to compromise respiration owing to the weight of the abdominal viscera. The stomach tube should be premeasured from the tip of the animal's nose to the xiphoid cartilage. In all cases, as large a stomach tube as possible should be used. A good rule is to use the same size stomach tube as cuffed endotracheal tube (1 mm = no. 3 French). The volume of water or lavage solution to be used for each washing is 5 to 10 ml/kg body weight. Following infusion of the solution, the fluid should be aspirated from the stomach via the stomach tube, with either a large aspirator bulb or a 50-ml syringe. The infusion and aspiration cycle of the lavage solution should be repeated 10 to 15 times. Activated charcoal in the solution enhances the effectiveness of this procedure.

Some precautions to be taken with this technique are (1) using low pressure to prevent forcing the toxicant into the duodenum, (2) reducing the infused volume in obviously weakened stomachs, and (3) making sure not to force the stomach tube through either the esophagus or the stomach wall.

Adsorbents

Activated charcoal is probably the best adsorbing agent available to the practitioner. Although it does not detoxify toxicants, it effectively prevents absorption of a toxicant when properly used. Activated charcoal can be effectively combined with emetic and gastric lavage techniques.

The proper type of activated charcoal for treatment of intoxication is of petroleum or vegetable, not mineral or animal, origin. The new, highly activated charcoal made from petroleum is available and is two to three times more adsorptive than activated charcoal (SuperChar-Vet, Gulf Biosystems). There are several commercial types of activated charcoal available, and these are listed in Table 1. Also available are the compressed activated charcoal tablets (5 gm, B.C. Crowley Co. and Requa Mfg. Co.). These tablets may be easier to handle than the powdered charcoal and are apparently as effective as activated charcoal.

A bathtub or some other easily cleansed area is the best place to administer activated charcoal to small animals. Activated charcoal is used as follows: (1) Make a slurry of the charcoal with water. A proper dose is 1 to 5 gm/kg body weight in a concentration of 1 gm charcoal/5 to 10 ml water. (2) Administer the charcoal by a stomach tube, using either a funnel or a large syringe. (3) A cathartic of sodium sulfate should be administered 30 min after administration of the charcoal. This technique may be modified if the charcoal is used in conjunction with emetic or lavage techniques. However, with either technique some charcoal should remain in the stomach and should be followed by a cathartic to prevent desorption of the toxicant. Newer methods suggest the administration of activated charcoal

three to four times a day for 2 to 3 days after occurrence of an intoxication.

Activated charcoal is highly adsorptive for many toxicants, including mercuric chloride, strychnine, other alkaloids (morphine and atropine), barbiturates, and ethylene glycol. It is ineffective against cyanide.

Syrup of ipecac negates some of the adsorptive characteristics of the activated charcoal. The "universal antidote," consisting of two parts activated charcoal, one part magnesium oxide, and one part tannic acid, is very inefficient, since the mangesium oxide and tannic acid decrease the adsorptive capability of the charcoal. Burned or charred toast as described in some emergency texts is ineffective as an adsorbing agent.

Cathartics

Sodium sulfate is a more efficient agent for evacuation of the bowel than is magnesium sulfate and is the preferable agent to use, especially with activated charcoal. There is some danger of CNS depression due to the magnesium ion, although the sodium ion may also precipitate a sodium ion intoxication or water-deprivation syndrome. However, either agent may be used in an emergency. The oral dose of sodium sulfate is 1 gm/kg.

Mineral oil or vegetable oils are of value if lipid-soluble toxicants are involved. Mineral oil (liquid petrolatum) is inert and is unlikely to be absorbed. Vegetable oil, however, is more likely to be absorbed and therefore may be contraindicated. Regardless of the type of oil used, it should be followed by a saline cathartic in 30 to 40 min.

A colonic lavage or high enema may be of value to hasten the elimination of toxicants from the gastrointestinal tract. Warm water with castile soap makes an excellent enema solution. Hexachlorophene soaps should be avoided. There are several commercially available enema preparations that act as osmotic agents. Care should be taken to avoid the induction of dehydration and electrolyte imbalances with overzealous treatment (see *Current Veterinary Therapy IX*, pp. 212–216).

APPLICATION OF ANTIDOTES

LOCALLY ACTING ANTIDOTES. There are numerous locally acting antidotes and therapeutic regimens reported for preventing the absorption of toxicants. The nonspecific antidotal procedures for some of the more common toxicants are described in Table 2.

SPECIFIC ANTIDOTES. There are a few specific antidotal agents available for some of the more

Table 1. *Some Available Activated Charcoal Products*

Trade Name	Ingredients	Manufacturer or Distributor	Address
Acta-Char	Activated charcoal powder, 30 gm in wide-mouth plastic bottle (400 ml capacity)	Med-Corp, Inc.	5310 Harvest Hill Road Dallas, TX 75230
Activated Charcoal, USP, Humco	Activated charcoal powder, 30 gm in 8-oz wide-mouth plastic jar (unit dose); 120 gm in 16-oz wide-mouth jar; 240 gm in 32-oz wide-mouth jar	Humco Laboratories	1008 Whitaker Texarkana, TX 75504
Activated Charcoal, USP, Mallinckrodt	Activated charcoal powder, 454 gm (1 lb) in wide-mouth jar	Mallinckrodt, Inc.	Box M Paris, KY 40361
Activated charcoal, USP, in liquid base	Activated charcoal, in liquid base containing water and propylene glycol (amount of propylene glycol unspecified); 12.5 gm in 60-ml wide-mouth bottle; 25 gm in 120-ml squeeze bottle with spout; 50 gm in 240-ml squeeze bottle with spout	Bowman Pharmaceuticals, Inc.	119 Schroyer Ave., S.W. Canton, OH 44702
Bowman Poison-Antidote Kit	1. Activated charcoal, in liquid base containing water and propylene glycol (amount of propylene glycol unspecified); 4 bottles, 12.5 gm each, of activated charcoal in liquid base, 60 ml 2. 1 bottle, ipecac syrup, 30 ml	Bowman Pharmaceuticals, Inc.	119 Schroyer Ave., S.W. Canton, OH 44702
Charoaid	Activated charcoal, 30 gm in sorbitol solution; 150 ml in squeeze bottle with spout	Requa Mfg. Co.	1 Seneca Place Greenwich, CT 06830
Charcolantidote	Activated charcoal powder; 15-gm bottle (150-ml capacity); 30-gm bottle (200-ml capacity)	U.S. Products, Inc.,	16636 N.W. 54th Ave. Miami Lakes, FL 33014
Insta-Char	Activated charcoal, in aqueous suspension (water is the sole liquid ingredient); 15 gm in 120-ml squeeze bottle with spout; 50 gm in 250-ml squeeze bottle with spout	Frank W. Kerr Chemical Co.	43155 S.W. Nine Mile Rd. Northville, MI 48167
Liquid-Antidose	Activated charcoal, in liquid base containing carboxymethylcellulose, sodium benzoate (preservative), and water; 40 gm in liquid base, 200 ml	U.S. Products	16636 N.W. 54th Ave. Miami Lakes, FL 33014
Norit USP XX	Activated charcoal powder, in bulk 15-kg containers (Norit XX is the activated charcoal used in all products listed above)	American Norit Co.	6301 Glidden Way Jacksonville, FL 32201
SuperChar-Vet	Highly activated charcoal. Liquid: 30 gm in 8-oz squeeze bottle. Powder: 227 gm in pouch for reconstitution	Gulf Bio-Systems, Inc.	5310 Harvest Hill Rd Dallas, TX 75230
Toxiban	Granules 47% activated charcoal, 10% kaolin, 42% wetting and dispensing agents, 5-kg pail	Vet-A-Mix	604 W. Thomas Ave. Shenandoah, IA 51601

Adapted from Activated charcoal products for medicinal (antidote) use. Vet. Hum. Toxicol. 25:294, 1983.

common animal toxicants. A list of these specific antidotal procedures is presented in Table 3.

Caution should be exercised with the use of some of the more specific antidotes, since many of these agents are themselves toxic. In certain chronic metallic intoxications such as lead poisoning, chelating agents have precipitated an acute metallic intoxication. Consequently, the dosage of chelating agents should be reduced in some chronic metal intoxications.

HASTENING ELIMINATION OF ABSORBED TOXICANTS

Absorbed toxicants are generally excreted via the kidneys. Some toxicants may be excreted by other routes (bile-feces, lung, other body secretions). Renal excretion can be manipulated in many instances. Urinary excretion of toxicants may be enhanced by the use of diuretics or by altering the pH of the urine.

Table 2. *Locally Activating Antidotes Against*
Unabsorbed Poisons and Principles of Treatment

Toxicant	Antidote and Dose or Concentration
Acids, corrosives	Weak alkali–magnesium oxide solution (1:25 warm water) internally. *Never give sodium bicarbonate!!* Milk of magnesia, 1 to 15 ml. Flush externally with water. Apply paste of sodium bicarbonate.
Alkalis, caustics	Weak acid: vinegar (diluted 1:4); 1% acetic acid or lemon juice given orally. Dilute albumin (4 to 6 egg whites to 1 qt warm water), or give whole milk followed by activated charcoal and then a cathartic, because some compounds are soluble in excess albumin. Local: Flush with copious amounts of water and apply vinegar.
Alkaloids	Potassium permanganate (1:5000 to 1:10,000) for lavage or oral administration Tannic acid or strong tea (200 to 500 mg in 30 to 60 ml of water) except in cases of poisoning by cocaine, nicotine, physostigmine, atropine, and morphine Emetic or purgative should be used for prompt removal of tannates.
Arsenic	Sodium thiosulfate, 10% solution given orally (0.5 to 3.0 gm for small animals). Followed by lavage or emesis Protein (e.g., evaporated milk, egg whites). Tannic acid or strong tea (see specific antidote in Table 3)
Barium salts	Sodium sulfate and magnesium sulfate (20% solution given orally). Dosage: 2 to 25 gm
Bismuth salts	Acacia or gum arabic as mucilage
Carbon tetrachloride	Empty stomach, give high-protein and carbohydrate diet; maintain fluid and electrolyte balance. Hemodialysis is indicated in anuria. Epinephrine is contraindicated (ventricular fibrillation!).
Copper	Albumin (see Alkalis, above) Sodium ferrocyanide in water (0.3 to 3.5 gm for small animals) (see specific antidote in Table 3) Magnesium oxide (see Acids, above)
Detergents, anionic (Na, K, NH_4^+ salts)	Milk or water followed by demulcent (oils, acacia, gelatin, starch, egg white)
Detergents, cationic (chlorides, iodides)	Soap (castile) dissolved in four times its bulk of hot water Albumin (see Alkalis, above)
Fluoride	Calcium (milk, limewater, or powdered chalk mixed with water) given orally
Formaldehyde	Ammonia water (0.2% orally) or ammonium acetate (1% for lavage) Starch, 1 part to 15 parts hot water added gradually Gelatin soaked in water for ½ hr Albumin (see Alkalis, above) Sodium thiosulfate (see Arsenic, above)
Iron	Sodium bicarbonate, 1%, for lavage (see specific antidote in Table 3)
Lead	Sodium or magnesium sulfate, given orally Sodium ferrocyanide (see Copper, above) See specific antidote (Table 3) Albumin (see Alkalis, above)
Mercury	Protein: milk, egg whites (see Alkalis, above) Magnesium oxide (see Acids, above) Sodium formaldehyde sulfoxylate, 5% solution for lavage Starch (see Formaldehyde, above) Activated charcoal, 5 to 50 gm (see specific antidote in Table 3)
Oxalic acid	Calcium: calcium hydroxide as 0.15% solution. Other alkalis are contraindicated because their salts are more soluble. Chalk or other calcium salts Magnesium sulfate as cathartic Maintain diuresis to prevent calcium oxalate deposition in kidney.
Petroleum distillates (aliphatic hydrocarbons)	Olive oil, other vegetable oils, or mineral oil given orally. After ½ hour, sodium sulfate as cathartic. Emesis and lavage are contraindicated for ingested volatile solvents, but petroleum distillates are used as carrier agents for more toxic agents.
Phenol and cresols	Soap-and-water or alcohol lavage of skin. Sodium bicarbonate (0.5%) dressings. Activated charcoal, mineral oil, or both, given orally
Phosphorus	Copper sulfate (0.2 to 0.4% solution) or potassium permanganate (1:5000 solution) for lavage. Turpentine (preferably old oxidized) in gelatin capsules or floated on hot water. Give 2 ml 4 times at 15-min intervals. Activated charcoal. Do not give vegetable oil cathartic. Remove all fat from diet.
Silver nitrate	Normal saline for lavage. Albumin (see Alkalis, above)
Unknown (e.g., toxic plants or other materials)	Activated charcoal (replaces universal antidote). For small animals—via stomach tube, as a slurry in water. Follow by emetic or cathartic, and then repeat procedure.

Table 3. *Specific Systemic Antidotes and Dosages*

Toxic Agent	Systemic Antidote	Dosage and Method of Treatment
Acetaminophen	Beta-acetylcysteine (Mucomyst, Mead Johnson)	150 mg/kg loading dose, orally or IV, then 50 mg/kg every 4 hr for 17 to 20 additional doses
Amphetamines	Chlorpromazine	1 mg/kg IM, IP, IV; administer only half dose if barbiturates have been given; blocks excitation
Arsenic, mercury, and other heavy metals except cadmium, lead, silver, selenium, and thallium	Dimercaprol (BAL, Hynson, Wescott & Dunning)	10% solution in oil; give small animals 2.5 to 5.0 mg/kg IM (0.025 to 0.05 ml/kg) every 4 hr for 2 days; b.i.d. for the next 10 days or until recovery. *Note:* In severe acute poisoning, 5 mg/kg dose should be given only on first day.
	D-Penicillamine (Cuprimine, Merck & Co.)	Developed for chronic mercury poisoning, now seems most promising drug; no reports on dosage in animals. Dosage for humans is 250 mg orally, every 6 hr for 10 days (3 to 4 mg/kg).
Atropine, belladonna alkaloids	Physostigmine salicylate	0.1 to 0.6 mg/kg (do not use neostigmine)
Barbiturates	Doxapram	2% solution: give small animals 3 to 5 mg/kg IV only (0.14 to 0.25 ml/kg); repeat as necessary.
		Note: The above is reliable only when depression is mild; in animals with deeper levels of depression, artificial respiration (and oxygen) is preferable.
Bromides	Chloride (sodium or ammonium salts)	0.5 to 1.0 gm orally daily for several days; hasten excretion.
Carbon monoxide	Oxygen	Pure oxygen at normal or high pressure; artificial respiration; blood transfusion
Cholinergic agents	Atropine sulfate	0.02 to 0.04 mg/kg, as needed
Cholinesterase inhibitors	Atropine sulfate	Dosage is 0.2 mg/kg, repeated as needed for atropinization. Treat cyanosis (if present) first. Blocks only muscarinic effects. Atropine in oil may be injected for prolonged effect during the night. *Avoid atropine intoxication!*
Cholinergic agents and cholinesterase inhibitors (organophosphates, some carbamates, but not carbaryl, dimethan, or carbam piloxime)	Pralidoxime chloride (2-PAM)	5% solution; give doses of 20 to 50 mg/kg IM, or by slow IV (0.2 to 1.0 mg/kg) injection (maximum dose is 500 mg/min). Repeat as needed. 2-PAM alleviates nicotinic effect and regenerates cholinesterase. Morphine, succinylcholine, and phenothiazine tranquilizers are contraindicated.
Copper	D-Penicillamine (Cuprimine)	See arsenic
Coumarin-derivative anticoagulants	Vitamin K_1 (MEPHYTON, Merck, 5-mg caps) (VITA K_1, Eschar, 25-mg caps)	Give 3 to 5 mg/kg/day with canned food. Treat 7 days for warfarin-type, treat 21 to 30 days for second-generation anticoagulant rodenticides. Oral therapy is more efficacious than IV.
	Whole blood or plasma	Blood transfusion, 25 ml/kg
Curare	Neostigmine methylsulfate	Solution: 1:5000 for 1:2000 (1 ml = 0.2 or 0.5 mg/ml). Dose is 0.005 mg/5 kg, SC. Follow with IV injection of atropine (0.04 mg/kg).
	Edrophonium chloride (Tensilon, Roche), Artificial respiration	1% solution; give 0.05 to 1.0 mg/kg IV.
Cyanide	Methemoglobin (sodium nitrite is used to form methemoglobin)	1% solution of sodium nitrate; dose is 16 mg/kg IV (1.6 ml/kg).
	Sodium thiosulfate	Follow with: 20% solution at dose of 30 to 40 mg/kg (0.15 to 0.2 ml/kg) IV. If treatment is repeated, use only sodium thiosulfate.
		Note: Both of the above may be given simultaneously as follows: 0.5 ml/kg of combination consisting of 10 gm sodium nitrate, 15 gm sodium thiosulfate in distilled water q.s. 250 ml. Dose may be repeated once. If further treatment is required, give only 20% solution of sodium thiosulfate at level of 0.2 ml/kg.
Digitalis glycosides, oleander, and *Bufo* toads	Potassium chloride	Dog: 0.5 to 2.0 gm, in divided doses orally; or in serious cases, as diluted solution given IV by slow drip (ECG control is essential)
	Phenytoin	25 mg/min IV until control is established.
	Propranolol (beta-blocker)	0.5 to 1.0 mg/kg IV or IM as needed to control cardiac arrhythmias (ECG control is essential)
	Atropine sulfate	0.02 to 0.04 mg/kg as needed for cholinergic control

Table continued on following page

Table 3. *Specific Systemic Antidotes and Dosages* Continued

Toxic Agent	Systemic Antidote	Dosage and Method of Treatment
Fluoride	Calcium borogluconate	3 to 10 ml of 5 to 10% solution
Fluoroacetate (Compound 1080)	Glyceryl monoacetin (Sigma)	0.1 to 0.5 mg/kg IM hourly for several hours (total 2 to 4 mg/kg); or diluted, 0.5 to 1.0% IV (danger of hemolysis). Monoacetin is available only from chemical supply houses.
	Acetamide	Animal may be protected if acetamide is given prior to or simultaneously with Compound 1080 (experimental).
	Pentobarbital	May protect against lethal dose (experimental).
	Note: All treatments are generally unrewarding.	
Hallucinogens (LSD, phencyclidine [PCP])	Diazepam (Valium, Roche)	As needed; avoid respiratory depression (2 to 5 mg/kg).
Heparin	Protamine sulfate	1% solution; give 1.0 to 1.5 mg to antagonize each 1 mg of heparin; slow IV injection. Reduce dose as time increases between heparin injection and start of treatment (after 30 min give only 0.5 mg).
Iron salts	Deferoxamine mesylate (Desferal, Ciba)	Dosage for animals not yet established. Dose for humans is 5 gm of 5% solution given orally, then 20 mg/kg IM every 4 to 6 hr. In case of shock, dose is 40 mg/kg by IV drip over 4-hr period; may be repeated in 6 hr, then 15 mg/kg by drip every 8 hr.
Lead (Pb)	Calcium disodium edetate (CaEDTA)	Dosage: Maximum safe dosage is 75 mg/kg/24 hr (only for severe case). EDTA is available in 20% solution; for IV drip, dilute in 5% glucose to 0.5%; for IM, add procaine to 20% solution to give 0.5% concentration of procaine.
	EDTA and dimercaprol (BAL)	BAL is given as 10% solution in oil. Treatment: 1. In severe case (CNS involvement with > 100 μg Pb/100 ml whole blood) give 4 mg/kg. BAL only as initial dose; follow after 4 hr, and every 4 hr for 3 to 4 days, with BAL and EDTA (12.5 mg/kg) at separate IM sites; skip 2 or 3 days and then treat again for 3 to 4 days. 2. In subacute case with < 100 μg Pb/100 ml whole blood, give only 50 mg EDTA/kg/24 hr for 3 to 5 days.
	Penicillamine (Cuprimine, Merck & Co.)	3. May use after treatments nos. 1 or 2 with 100 mg/kg/day orally for 1 to 4 weeks.
	Thiamine hydrochloride	Experimental for nervous signs; 5 mg/kg IV b.i.d., for 1 to 2 weeks; give slowly and watch for untoward reactions.
Metaldehyde	Diazepam (Valium, Roche)	2 to 5 mg/kg IV to control tremors
	Triflupromazine	0.2 to 2.0 mg/kg IV
	Pentobarbital	To effect
Methanol and ethylene glycol	Ethanol	Give IV, 1.1 gm/kg (4.4 ml/kg) of 25% solution. Give 0.5 gm/kg (2.0 ml/kg) every 4 hr for 4 days. To prevent or correct acidosis, use sodium bicarbonate IV, 0.4 gm/kg. Activated charcoal: 5 gm/kg orally if within 4 hr of ingestion
Methemoglobinemia-producing agents (nitrites, chlorates)	Methylene blue	1% solution (maximum concentration), given by *slow* IV injection, 8.8 mg/kg (0.9 ml/kg), repeat if necessary. To prevent fall in blood pressure in case of nitrite poisoning, use a sympathomimetic drug (ephedrine or epinephrine). Not recommended for cats
Morphine and related drugs	Naloxone chloride (Narcan, Endo)	0.1 mg/kg IV. Do not repeat if respiration is not satisfactory.
	Levallorphan tartrate (Lorfan, Roche)	Give IV, 0.1 to 0.5 ml of solution containing 1 mg/ml. *Note:* Use either of the above antidotes only in acute poisoning. Artificial respiration may be indicated. Activated charcoal is also indicated.
Oxalates	Calcium	Treatment: 23% solution of calcium gluconate IV. Give 3 to 20 ml (to control hypocalcemia).

Table 3. *Specific Systemic Antidotes and Dosages* Continued

Toxic Agent	Systemic Antidote	Dosage and Method of Treatment
Phenothiazine	Methylamphetamine hydrochloride (Desoxyn, Abbott)	0.1 to 0.2 mg/kg IV; also transfusion. Only available in tablet form
	Diphenhydramine hydrochloride	For CNS depression, 2 to 5 mg/kg IV for extrapyramidal signs
Phytotoxins and botulin	Antitoxins not available commercially	As indicated for specific antitoxins. Examples of phytotoxins: ricin, abrin, robin, crotin
Plants		Treat signs as necessary
Red squill	Atropine sulfate, propranolol, potassium chloride	As for digitalis and oleander
Snake bite: rattlesnake, copperhead, water moccasin	Antivenin (Wyeth) (Trivalent Crotalidae)	Caution: equine origin. Administer 1 to 2 vials IV, slowly, diluted in 250 to 500 ml of saline. Also administer antihistamine. Corticosteroids are contraindicated.
Coral snake	Antivenin (Wyeth)	Caution: equine origin
Spider bite (black widow)	Antivenin (Merck & Co.)	Caution: equine origin. Administer IV slowly, do not dilute.
	Dantrolene sodium (Dantrium, Norwich-Eaton)	1 mg/kg IV. Followed by 1 mg/kg PO every 4 hr
Strontium	Calcium salts	Usual dose of calcium borogluconate
	Ammonium chloride	0.2 to 0.5 gm orally, 3 to 4 times daily
Strychnine and brucine	Pentobarbital	Give IV to effect; higher dose is usually required than that required for anesthesia. Place animal in warm, quiet room.
	Amobarbital	Give by slow IV; inject to effect. Duration of sedation is usually 4 to 6 hr
	Methocarbamol (Robaxin, Robins)	10% solution; average first dose is 149 mg/kg IV (range: 40 to 300 mg). Repeat half dose as needed.
	Glyceryl guaiacolate (Geocolate, Summit Hill Labs)	110 mg/kg IV, 5% solution. Repeat as necessary.
	Diazepam (Valium, Roche)	2 to 5 mg/kg, control convulsions, induce emesis, then use other agents.
Thallium	Diphenylthiocarbazone	1. Dog: 70 mg/kg, orally, t.i.d. for 6 days. Hastens elimination but is partially toxic. or
	Prussian blue	2. 0.2 mg/kg orally in 3 divided doses daily
	Potassium chloride	Give simultaneously with thiocarbazone or Prussian blue, 2 to 6 gm orally daily in divided doses.

The use of diuretics to enhance urinary excretion of toxicants requires adequate renal function and hydration of the affected animal. Once these requisites are established, diuretics are indicated. Monitoring of urinary output is essential in these animals, and a minimum urinary flow of 0.1 ml/kg/min is necessary. The diuretics of choice are mannitol and furosemide (Lasix, Hoechst-Roussel). Both of these agents are very potent diuretics. The dosage for mannitol is 2 mg/kg/hr and for furosemide is 5 mg/kg every 6 to 8 hr. Again, hydration must be maintained for proper renal excretion.

Alteration of urinary pH to expedite the excretion of toxicants and foreign chemicals is a classic pharmacologic technique. The technique relies on the physiochemical phenomenon that ionized compounds do not readily traverse cell membranes and hence are not reabsorbed by the renal tubules. Consequently, acid compounds such as acetylsalicylic acid (aspirin) and some barbiturates remain ionized in alkaline urine, and alkaline compounds such as amphetamines remain ionized in acidic urine. As a result, urinary excretion of many toxic compounds may be enhanced by modifying the urine pH. Urinary acidifying agents include ammonium chloride, 200 mg/kg/day in divided doses, and ethylenediamine dihydrochloride (Chlor-Ethamine, Pitman-Moore), 1 to 2 tablets t.i.d. for the average-sized dog. Sodium bicarbonate, 5 mEq/kg/hr, may be used as an alkalinizing agent. (There are numerous human preparations available for acidifying or alkalinizing urine.)

Peritoneal dialysis is indicated when an intoxicated animal exhibits oliguria or anuria. It is a rather time-consuming but effective technique in many conditions. The process of peritoneal dialysis involves the infusion of 10 to 20 ml/kg of a dialyzing solution into the peritoneal cavity, waiting the prescribed length of time (usually 1 to 2 hr), withdrawing the dialyzing solution, and reinfusing a fresh solution. The infusion and withdrawal cycles should be maintained for 12 to 24 hr or until normal renal function is restored. The pH of the dialyzing solutions may be altered to maintain the ionized state of the offending compound. (For additional information on peritoneal dialysis, see *Current Veterinary Therapy VIII*, pp. 1028–1033.)

SUPPORTIVE MEASURES

Supportive measures are very important in cases of intoxication. These measures include control of body temperature, maintenance of respiratory and cardiovascular function, control of acid-base imbalances, alleviation of pain, and control of CNS disorders.

BODY TEMPERATURE CONTROL. Hypothermia may be controlled with the use of blankets and by keeping the animal in a warm, draft-free cage. Infrared lamps or heating pads should be used with caution and under constant observation. A pad with circulating warm water may be of greater value and is less dangerous than lamps or conventional heating pads. This type of pad is convenient for both emergency and surgical use (Aquamatic K Pad, American Hospital Supply).

Hyperthermia is controlled through the use of ice bags, cold water baths, cold water enemas, or cold peritoneal dialysis solution. Regardless of the type of temperature control required, it is vitally important that the animal's body temperature be constantly monitored to ensure that overcorrection does not occur.

RESPIRATORY SUPPORT MEASURES. Adequate respiratory support requires the presence of an adequate, patent airway, which may be obtained with either a cuffed endotracheal tube in an unconscious animal or a tracheostomy performed with the patient under local anesthesia. An emergency tracheostomy tube may be made from a cuffed endotracheal tube that has been shortened to reduce the dead space.

A respirator such as a Bird Respirator (Bird Corp.) or Ohio Ventilator (Ohio Medical Products) is of great value in cases of respiratory depression; however, an anesthetic machine may be used with manual compression of the bag. A mixture of 50 per cent oxygen and 50 per cent room air is generally adequate unless there is a thickened respiratory membrane, in which case 100 per cent oxygen is necessary.

The use of analeptic drugs in cases of severe respiratory depression or apnea is questionable, owing to the short duration of their effects and to other undesirable side effects. Positive pressure ventilatory support is of greater value.

CARDIOVASCULAR SUPPORT. Cardiovascular support requires the presence of an adequate circulating volume, adequate cardiac performance, adequate tissue perfusion, and adequate acid-base balance. Volume and cardiac activity are of immediate concern; perfusion and acid-base balance, although of no lesser importance, are not of immediate concern.

In the presence of hypovolemia due to loss of both cells and volume, whole blood is the necessary agent. A good rule is to give a sufficient quantity of whole blood to raise the packed cell volume to 75 per cent of the animal's estimated normal level (minimum of 20 ml/kg).

Hypovolemia due to fluid loss alone can be treated with the administration of lactated Ringer's solution or plasma expanders. In these patients, central venous pressure should be monitored to prevent overloading the heart with too much volume too rapidly.

Tissue perfusion should also be monitored periodically to determine the adequacy of the replacement therapy. In some patients, it may be necessary to administer massive doses of IV corticosteroids to restore adequate tissue perfusion, such as dexamethasone (Azium, Schering), 2 to 10 mg/kg. Caution should be exercised in the use of these steroids since hypovolemia may ensue. Therefore, large IV doses of corticosteroids should never be administered unless volume replacement therapy is ongoing.

Cardiac activity can be aided by the application of closed-chest cardiac massage for immediate requirements, but the administration of pharmaceutical agents that can stimulate inotropic and chronotropic activity must also be undertaken in most instances. One of these agents is 10 per cent calcium gluconate; 10 to 30 ml can be infused intravenously *very slowly*. This agent is also reported to be a good nonspecific treatment in many toxicities. Other agents include glucagon, 25 to 50 µg/kg IV, and digoxin, 0.02 to 0.04 mg/kg IV. Care must be taken to avoid overdosage with cardioactive agents, since they are highly toxic to the myocardium. The electric activity of the heart should be closely monitored during administration of cardioactive agents.

ACID-BASE IMBALANCE. Control of acid-base balance problems is primarily a matter of physiologically maintaining an animal in a homeostatic condition. The most common acid-base disturbance seen in animals is acidosis, mainly of metabolic origin. However, acidosis or alkalosis may occur in cases of intoxication.

In correcting acidosis not of respiratory origin, sodium bicarbonate, administered IV at a dosage rate of 2 to 4 mEq/kg every 15 min. is the drug of choice. Other alkalinizing solutions include 1/6 molar sodium lactate, 16 to 32 ml/kg; lactated Ringer's solution, 120 ml/kg; and tromethamine (THAM) buffer, 300 mg/kg. Bicarbonate is generally the easiest to administer with respect to volume and requires no metabolic conversion. Caution must be exercised when administering all alkalinizing agents to avoid the induction of alkalosis.

Alkalosis, unless drug-induced, does not generally occur in animals. However, if alkalosis is present, the IV administration of 0.9 per cent sodium chloride (physiologic saline), 10 ml/kg, is usually sufficient for initial therapy. This should be followed by the oral administration of ammonium chloride, 200 mg/kg/day in divided doses. As in the case of acidosis, the clinician should be cautioned about overtreatment of the alkalotic patient.

PAIN CONTROL. Another important supportive measure in cases of intoxication is the control of pain. A minimal dose of morphine (dogs, 1 to 2 mg/kg; cats, 0.1 to 0.2 mg/kg) or meperidine (Demerol, Winthrop) (dogs, 5 to 10 mg/kg; cats, 1 to 2 mg/kg) is indicated in animals showing pain as a result of intoxication. Meperidine has an extremely short action in dogs and cats and, thus, may be of minimal benefit.

CENTRAL NERVOUS SYSTEM (CNS) DISORDERS. Management of CNS disorders in cases of intoxication is simple in appearance but complex in actuality. The type of therapy depends on the presence of depression or hyperactivity. Either disorder can easily be turned into the opposite problem by overzealous therapeutic measures.

CNS DEPRESSION. CNS depression can also be considered respiratory depression, since the management of the two conditions is very similar. Although the IV administration of analeptic agents such as doxapram (Dopram, Robins), 3 to 5 mg/kg, or pentylenetetrazol (Metrazol, Knoll), 6 to 10 mg/kg, is reported to be efficacious in these conditions, their actions are short-lived, and CNS depression can return if the animals are not monitored continuously. Another disadvantage is that analeptics can also induce convulsions. Artificial respiration or respiratory support is of greater value in animals exhibiting CNS depression and is the treatment of choice for most CNS depression syndromes.

CNS HYPERACTIVITY. Cases of CNS hyperactivity including convulsions can be managed by the administration of CNS depressants or tranquilizers. Pentobarbital sodium is generally the agent of choice for convulsions and hyperactivity. Care must be taken, since in many patients a respiratory depressing dose may be required to alleviate the signs. In these patients, respiratory support is mandatory. Inhalant anesthetics have been reported as excellent for long-term management of CNS hyperactivity, but this removes the anesthetic machine from operating-room use for extended periods. Central-acting skeletal muscle relaxants and minor tranquilizers have been reported for use with convulsant intoxicants. These include methocarbamol (Robaxin, Robins), 110 mg/kg IV; glyceryl guaiacolate (Gecolate, Summit Hill Labs), 110 mg/kg IV; and diazepam* (Valium, Roche), 0.5 to 1.5 mg/kg IV or IM. In other cases of CNS stimulation due to amphetamines and some hallucinogens such as lysergic acid diethylamide (LSD) and phencyclidine, phenothiazine tranquilizers have produced adequate control. Regardless of the regimen of therapy for CNS hyperactivity, the animals should be placed in a quiet, dark room to prevent additional stimulation from auditory or visual stimuli.

POISON CONTROL CENTERS AND DIAGNOSTIC LABORATORIES

Poison control centers and animal diagnostic laboratories can be of great value to the clinician in cases of suspected intoxication, especially when labels or containers are presented with the acutely ill animal. *When the suspected compound and the signs exhibited by the animal do not concur, the signs should be treated and the label should be disregarded.*

The diagnosis should be confirmed by chemical analysis, even though this may occur after the fact. An accurate diagnosis, as well as detailed records, may help the veterinarian faced with subsequent cases from the same intoxicant. Detailed records also are invaluable considerations in any medicolegal proceedings.

References and Supplemental Reading

Klaassen, C. D., Amdur, M. O., and Doull, J. (eds.): *Casarett and Doull's Toxicology, The Basic Sciences of Poisons,* 3rd ed. New York: Macmillan, 1986.
Oehme, F. W. (ed.): Symposium in clinical toxicology for the small animal practitioner. Vet Clin. North Am. 5:737, 1975.
Osweiler, G. D., Carson, T. L., Buck, W. B., et al.: *Clinical and Diagnostic Veterinary Toxicology,* 3rd ed. Dubuque, IA: Kendall/Hunt, 1984.

*Editor's Note: Many clinicians find diazepam IV to be highly effective in convulsive emergencies such as *status epilepticus.*

TOXICANT-INDUCED ACUTE RENAL FAILURE

GREGORY F. GRAUER, D.V.M.

Madison, Wisconsin

Acute renal failure (ARF) results from an abrupt decline in renal function and is characterized by impaired regulation of water and solute balance. Toxic and ischemic insults are the most common causes of acute renal dysfunction, usually resulting in damage to the epithelium of the proximal tubules. Nephrotoxicants interfere with essential tubular cell functions and cause cellular injury and death, which result in renal vasoconstriction and decreased glomerular filtration. However, toxicant-induced tubular lesions are often reversible.

MECHANISMS OF NEPHROTOXICITY

The kidneys are susceptible to toxicants because of their unique anatomic and physiologic features (Table 1). The disproportionately large renal blood flow (approximately 20 per cent of the cardiac output) can result in increased delivery of blood-borne toxicants to the kidney as compared with other organs. The renal cortex is especially vulnerable to toxicant exposure because it receives 90 per cent of the renal blood flow and contains the large endothelial surface area of the glomerular capillaries. Within the renal cortex, the proximal tubular epithelial cells are frequently affected by toxicant-induced injury and hypoxia because of their transport functions and high metabolic rate. In the process of reabsorbing water and electrolytes from the glomerular filtrate, proximal tubular epithelial cells may be exposed to increasingly high concentrations of toxicants. Toxicants that are either secreted or reabsorbed by tubular epithelial cells (e.g., gentamicin) may accumulate in high concen-

trations within these cells. Similarly, in the medulla, the countercurrent system may concentrate toxicants. The kidneys also play a role in the biotransformation of many drugs and toxicants. Biotransformation usually results in the formation of metabolites that are less toxic than the parent compound; however, in some cases (e.g., ethylene glycol), metabolites are more toxic.

Table 2 contains a partial list of potential nephrotoxicants. It should be noted that toxic insults to the kidneys are often caused by therapeutic agents in addition to the more well-known nephrotoxicants. In the author's experience, gentamicin is the most common cause of toxicant-induced ARF, followed by ethylene glycol.

Nephrotoxicants damage tubular epithelium by interacting with cell membranes or intracellular organelles. Cell membrane function may be impaired by lipid peroxidation, decreased ATP-mediated transport, or disruption of normal sterol-lipid interactions. Changes in cell membrane permeability impair cellular osmoregulation and result in swelling and death. Toxicants may also act as haptens and initiate immune-mediated damage subsequent to cell membrane attachment. Toxicants that accumulate within epithelial cells may interact with

Table 1. *Factors That Predispose the Kidneys to Toxicant-induced Injury*

Kidneys receive 20% of cardiac output. The cortex receives 90% of the renal blood flow.

Large glomerular capillary endothelial surface area.

Proximal tubular cells have a high metabolic rate and are susceptible to hypoxia.

Tubular secretion and reabsorption may concentrate toxicants within cells.

Countercurrent multiplier system may concentrate toxicants within the medulla.

Xenobiotic metabolism within kidneys can create toxic metabolites.

Table 2. *Partial List of Potential Nephrotoxicants*

Therapeutic Agents	Heavy Metals
Antimicrobials	Lead
Aminoglycosides	Mercury
Cephalosporins	Cadmium
Polymyxins	Chromium
Sulfonamides	**Organic Compounds**
Tetracyclines	Ethylene glycol
Antifungals	Carbon tetrachloride
Amphotericin B	Chloroform
Anthelmintics	Pesticides
Thiacetarsamide	Herbicides
Anesthetics	**Mycotoxins**
Methoxyflurane	Citrinin
Analgesics	Ochratoxin A
Acetaminophen	**Pigments**
Ibuprofen	Myoglobin
Phenylbutazone	Hemoglobin
Intravenous Radiographic Contrast Agents	**Miscellaneous**
Chemotherapeutic agents	Hypercalcemia
Cis-platinum	Snake venom
Methotrexate	
Daunorubicin	

cellular proteins, nucleic acids, or lipids. Cellular injury or death can occur by uncoupling of the mitochondrial chain or by disruption of critical enzymatic activity. The result of tubular cell injury and death is nephron dysfunction and a decrease in glomerular filtration rate.

Nephron dysfunction and reduced glomerular filtration in toxicant-induced ARF are due to a combination of tubular obstruction, tubular backleak, renal vasoconstriction, and decreased glomerular permeability. Cellular debris within the tubule may inspissate and obstruct flow of filtrate through the nephron. Backleak of filtrate results from loss of tubular cell integrity, which allows filtrate to escape from the tubular lumen to the interstitial space, where it may be reabsorbed. Toxicant-induced tubular damage and tubuloglomerular feedback are thought to play a role in causing renal vasoconstriction. Decreased reabsorption by damaged proximal tubule segments increases solute delivery to the distal nephron and macula densa, which results in afferent glomerular artery constriction. The exact mediator of this vasoconstriction is not known, but renal prostaglandins, natriuretic factor, or the renin-angiotensin system may be involved. A decrease in the permeability of the glomerular capillary wall can also lead to a reduction of the glomerular filtration rate. Aminoglycosides have been shown to decrease both the number and the size of fenestrae in glomerular capillary endothelial cells, thereby reducing the available surface area for ultrafiltration.

Toxicant-induced ARF has three distinct phases, which are categorized as: (1) initiation, (2) maintenance, and (3) recovery. Toxicants that are responsible for initiating ARF may be present only for a matter of minutes or hours. During the initiation phase, therapeutic measures that reduce the renal insult can prevent development of established ARF. The maintenance phase is characterized by tubular lesions and established nephron dysfunction. Therapeutic intervention during the maintenance phase, although often life saving, usually does little to diminish renal lesions or improve function. The recovery phase is the period when renal lesions resolve and function improves. Even if renal function recovery is incomplete, adequate function may be re-established over a period of weeks or months.

CLINICAL PATHOLOGY AND DIAGNOSIS

The hallmark of ARF due to any cause is a decrease in glomerular filtration rate. However, azotemia is not evident until two thirds to three fourths of the nephrons are not functioning. Therefore, significant toxicant-induced tubular lesions and decreases in glomerular filtration are often present before the onset of azotemia. Urine volume may be normal or decreased, but the quality of the urine is always poor. For example, gentamicin-induced ARF is usually nonoliguric, whereas ARF induced by ethylene glycol is oliguric. However, both produce urine that is isosthenuric or minimally concentrated, containing high concentrations of sodium (> 40 mEq/L) and relatively low concentrations of creatinine. In addition, the urine may contain glucose, abnormal quantities of protein, and, depending on urine volume, casts and renal epithelial cells. Calcium oxalate crystals may be observed in the urine sediment in approximately 50 per cent of dogs and cats that have ingested ethylene glycol.

If there is no history of administration of potentially nephrotoxic drugs or exposure to nephrotoxicants, it is often difficult to establish a diagnosis of toxicant-induced ARF. Histologic examination of renal biopsy specimens reveals proximal tubular cell degeneration ranging from cloudy swelling to necrosis. The interstitium may be edematous and infiltrated by polymorphonuclear leukocytes. Although these changes are not specific for toxicant-induced ARF (tubular lesions due to renal ischemia exhibit similar changes), evaluation of renal histology is often helpful in establishing a prognosis. Evidence of tubular regeneration (flattened, basophilic epithelial cells with irregular nuclear size, mitotic figures, and high nucleus to cytoplasm ratios) and generally intact tubular basement membranes are good prognostic signs. Conversely, large numbers of granular casts and extensive tubular necrosis and interstitial mineralization and fibrosis are poor prognostic signs. The degree of functional impairment and the response to therapy should also be considered when formulating a prognosis.

MANAGEMENT CONSIDERATIONS

Since toxicant-induced ARF is frequently caused by therapeutic agents, prevention is the best therapy. Several risk factors have been identified that predispose dogs to gentamicin-induced ARF (Table 3). These factors may also predispose dogs and cats to other types of toxicant-induced ARF. Pre-existing

Table 3. *Toxicant-induced Acute Renal Failure: Risk Factors*

Pre-existing renal disease or renal insufficiency
Advanced age
Dehydration
Decreased cardiac output
Sepsis
Fever
Liver disease
Electrolyte abnormalities (e.g., hypokalemia, hypercalcemia)
Concurrent use of diuretics
Concurrent use of potentially nephrotoxic drugs (e.g., aminoglycosides, intravenous radiographic contrast agents, methoxyflurane)
Diabetes mellitus(?)

conditions associated with decreased glomerular filtration and renal blood flow increase the risk of ARF in animals exposed to nephrotoxicants. Renal disease or renal insufficiency, advanced age, dehydration, and reduced cardiac output decrease glomerular filtration and, thereby, renal excretion of nephrotoxicants. In addition, dehydration and decreased cardiac output may cause increased tubular reabsorption of nephrotoxicants. Fever, sepsis, liver disease, electrolyte abnormalities, and concurrent use of diuretics or other potential nephrotoxicants are additional predispositions. In particular, concurrent use of furosemide and gentamicin has been associated with heightened risk and severity of ARF. Furosemide probably potentiates gentamicin-induced nephrotoxicity by causing dehydration and a reduction in volume of distribution or by increasing the renal cortical concentration of gentamicin. In humans, diabetes mellitus has been identified as a risk factor for toxicant-induced ARF. When potentially nephrotoxic drugs are indicated, recognition of these risk factors should alert the clinician to assess the risk-benefit ratio for the patient.

If toxicant-induced renal damage is suspected, all potentially nephrotoxic drugs should be withdrawn. Induction of emesis or gastric lavage should be considered to decrease absorption of recently ingested toxicants. In addition, use of gastrointestinal adsorbents and cathartics (activated charcoal and sodium sulfate) may also be beneficial. Peritoneal dialysis can be used to lower blood concentrations of dialyzable toxicants (e.g., ethylene glycol and gentamicin), and diuresis initiated by intravenous administration of isotonic saline will help increase renal excretion of toxicants. Recognition and appropriate treatment of renal injury in the initiation phase of ARF is associated with improved prognosis. Therefore, patients receiving potentially nephrotoxic drugs should be monitored closely (see *Current Veterinary Therapy IX*, pp. 1142–1150, for discussions on amphotericin B and gentamicin nephrotoxicoses).

The goal of treatment of established toxicant-induced ARF is correction of renal hemodynamic disorders and alleviation of water and solute imbalances in order to "buy time" for renal repair and regeneration. A positive response to therapy is indicated by an increase in glomerular filtration rate and urine production. Induction of diuresis facilitates management of ARF by decreasing serum urea nitrogen and potassium concentrations and by lessening the tendency for overhydration to occur. Even though glomerular filtration rate and renal blood flow may improve with diuresis, these parameters are frequently unchanged and the increased urine production is actually a result of decreased tubular resorption of filtrate. Increased urine production alone does not indicate an improvement in renal excretory function.

INCREASING GLOMERULAR FILTRATION RATE AND URINE PRODUCTION

Volume replacement to reduce any prerenal component of the disease process is the first step of therapy for ARF. Mild volume expansion, in addition to volume replacement, has been recommended when replacement fluid therapy alone does not result in diuresis (mild dehydration that is, less than 3 to 5 per cent of body weight, is difficult to detect clinically). However, correction of fluid deficits and volume expansion seldom result in improved renal function in ARF, and therefore, additional therapeutic agents are often employed.

Mannitol has been widely studied in dogs with ischemic and toxic ARF. Improvement in renal blood flow and glomerular filtration rate is often demonstrated when mannitol is administered prior to, or concurrently with, the induction of toxic or ischemic ARF. The vasodilator response to mannitol is thought to be mediated in large part by increased renal prostaglandin activity. Mannitol is also frequently used in ARF patients to induce diuresis. Preservation of high tubular flow rates and increased intratubular hydrostatic pressure, along with the increase in renal hemodynamics, probably accounts for the protective effects of mannitol in experimental ARF. Caution should be used when administering mannitol, since expansion of the intravascular volume may precipitate pulmonary edema in oliguric patients.

Evidence for a protective effect of furosemide in experimental ARF is less consistent than that with mannitol. Like mannitol, furosemide probably increases renal blood flow though activation of the renal prostaglandin system; however, a diuresis often occurs without improvement in glomerular filtration rate. In dogs, furosemide has been shown to exert a protective effect against experimentally induced ischemic ARF but not toxicant-induced ARF. Although diuresis in general is thought to be beneficial, furosemide therapy seldom improves renal function and does not affect the duration of renal failure, the need for dialysis, or the mortality rate. However, furosemide therapy may contribute to deterioration of renal function by producing extensive water and solute loss. Furosemide should not be used in patients that have received aminoglycosides because of the potential for prolonged antibiotic retention and enhanced nephrotoxicity. Whether or not furosemide can potentiate the toxicity of other nephrotoxicants is not known.

Low-dose (subpressor) dopamine infusion induces renal and mesenteric vasodilatation with minimal systemic effects; therefore, recent interest has focused on the use of dopamine in the treatment of ARF. In some experimental models of ARF, dopamine or a dopamine precursor has been protective. In other studies, dopamine in combination with furosemide was protective, whereas dopamine alone was not. Vasodilatation induced by dopamine is thought to enhance intrarenal delivery of furosemide. Uncontrolled clinical studies in humans, using dopamine in combination with furosemide, have been effective in inducing diuresis. Many of these patients had established renal failure and had failed to respond to prior therapy with mannitol or furosemide alone. However, dopamine-induced diuresis is not always associated with an increase in glomerular filtration rate.

Hypertonic glucose is often recommended as a diuretic for dogs with ARF. However, there are no controlled comparisons between hypertonic glucose, mannitol, and furosemide with regard to preservation of urine production or influence on duration of ARF. Mannitol might be expected to be a superior osmotic diuretic because it is an impermeate solute and it is not reabsorbed by the tubular epithelium.

TREATMENT GUIDELINES

A list of treatment guidelines for toxicant-induced ARF is presented in Table 4. Identification and correction of any prerenal or postrenal abnormalities are essential. For fluid deficits, replacement fluid should be administered intravenously within 6 hr with 0.45 per cent saline and 2.5 per cent dextrose. Maintenance fluid needs and continuing-loss fluid needs should be met over a 24-hr period, again using 0.45 per cent saline and 2.5 per cent dextrose so as not to enhance hypernatremia and hyperkalemia. Oliguria is common with ARF and was once thought to be a hallmark of the syndrome; however, nonoliguric ARF is being recognized with increasing frequency. Urine production should be quantitated so that maintenance fluid needs can be properly

Table 4. *Treatment Guidelines for Toxicant-induced Acute Renal Failure*

Discontinue all potentially nephrotoxic drugs.
Start specific antidotal therapy (e.g., alcohol dehydrogenase inhibitors for ethylene glycol).
Identify and treat any prerenal or postrenal abnormalities.
Start intravenous fluid therapy: (1) rehydrate patient within 6 hr, (2) meet maintenance fluid needs and continuing-loss fluid needs.
Assess volume of urine production.
Correct acid-base and electrolyte abnormalities, rule out hypercalcemic nephropathy.
Provide mild volume expansion while monitoring urine volume, body weight, plasma total solids, hematocrit, and central venous pressure.
Administer vasodilators, diuretics, or both.
Consider peritoneal dialysis if there is no response to the above treatment.
Control hyperphosphatemia.
Treat gastroenteritis and gastric hyperacidity.
Provide caloric requirements (70–100 Kcal/kg/day).

Table 5. *Examples of Daily Maintenance Fluid Requirements*

	Normal Urine Production (ml/kg)	Oliguric ARF (ml/kg)	Nonoliguric ARF (ml/kg)
Insensible loss	20	20	20
Urine volume	40	8	110
TOTAL	60	28	130

assessed. Since two thirds of maintenance fluid needs are due to fluid loss in urine, oliguric and nonoliguric patients can have large variations in their fluid needs (Table 5). Measurement of urine volume also facilitates assessment of endogenous creatinine clearance, providing an estimation of glomerular filtration rate. If indwelling urinary catheters are used to measure urine volume, strict aseptic technique and closed collection systems must be employed. Uremic patients have depressed cellular immunity and phagocytic function, and infection is a leading cause of death in renal failure. Intermittent urinary bladder catheterization is usually recommended over indwelling catheterization.

During the period of rehydration, acid-base and electrolyte status should be evaluated and treated. Metabolic acidosis and hyperkalemia are common in oliguric ARF. The acidosis is usually partially compensated for by a respiratory alkalosis. Bicarbonate therapy should be reserved for patients whose blood pH is 7.1 or less. Overzealous sodium bicarbonate therapy can create ionized calcium deficits and sodium excesses, which may contribute to hypervolemia in the oliguric patient. Hyperkalemia can cause cardiac conduction abnormalities and is the most life-threatening electrolyte disturbance that occurs in ARF. Diagnosis of hyperkalemia is based on serum potassium concentrations; however, clinical signs frequently associated with hyperkalemia are bradycardia and the electrocardiographic changes of decreased P-wave amplitude, increased PR interval, widened QRS complexes, and tall, spiked T waves. If severe, hyperkalemia can cause atrial standstill, sinoventricular rhythms, ventricular tachycardia, fibrillation, and asystole. Hyperkalemia should be promptly treated with slow intravenous

Table 6. *Drugs and Dosages Used in Treatment of Acute Renal Failure*

Mannitol, 0.5 to 1.0 gm/kg as a 20 or 25% solution, given as a slow IV bolus
Furosemide, 2 to 4 mg/kg IV
Dopamine, 1 to 3 μg/kg/min IV (50 mg of dopamine in 500 ml of 5% dextrose results in a 100 μg/ml solution)
Cimetidine, 5 to 10 mg/kg every 6–12 hr IV or PO
Trimethobenzamide, 3 mg/kg every 8 hr IM
Metoclopramide, 0.2 to 0.4 mg/kg every 6–8 hr SC
Aluminum hydroxide, 500 mg at each feeding (pull capsule apart and mix contents into food)

bolus administration of 1 to 2 mEq/kg of sodium bicarbonate. Insulin, dextrose, and calcium gluconate may also be used to decrease or counteract hyperkalemia (see *Current Veterinary Therapy IX,* p. 94).

If signs of overhydration are not present and oliguria persists after apparent rehydration, mild volume expansion (3 to 5 per cent of the patient's body weight in fluid) may be tried. Monitoring body weight, plasma total solids, hematocrit, and central venous pressure helps protect against overhydration. When fluid therapy alone fails to induce diuresis, either mannitol or dopamine and furosemide in combination is the therapeutic strategy of choice (Table 6). If one regimen does not work, the other may be tried. Furosemide therapy is probably a better choice for overhydrated patients. However, it appears that furosemide is more efficacious in ischemic ARF compared with toxicant-induced ARF, and it can potentiate gentamicin-induced nephrotoxicosis. Whether or not diuresis occurs, maintenance fluid requirements should be derived from the volume of urine produced (Table 5). If diuresis occurs, polyionic solutions (e.g., lactated Ringer's) should be used for maintenance fluid requirements, and potassium supplementation is often necessary. The latter should be determined by measuring serum potassium concentrations.

Provision of daily caloric requirements is an important aspect of conservative management of renal failure. Energy requirements have a higher priority than do protein requirements. Therefore, if caloric needs are not met, endogenous proteins will be catabolized for energy. Protein catabolism not only causes weight loss and muscle wasting but also increases blood urea nitrogen concentrations. Protein breakdown in humans can be reduced by providing as little as 100 gm of carbohydrate per day. Supplementation of essential amino acids in anephric dogs has been shown to stabilize serum urea nitrogen concentrations and increase survival time. Inappetence due to gastric hyperacidity and

vomiting can usually be controlled by the use of an H_2 receptor–blocker (cimetidine), aluminum-containing antacids, or antiemetics that act at the chemoreceptor trigger zone (trimethobenzamide or metoclopramide). Administration of food blended with water via a stomach tube may be tolerated by animals that are anorexic if they are not vomiting. Reduced protein diets and enteric phosphate binders (aluminum hydroxide) should be used to reduce increased serum urea nitrogen and phosphorus concentrations.

Dialysis should be considered in patients with severe, persistent uremia, acidosis, or hyperkalemia. Dialysis may also be used to treat overhydration and, in some cases, hasten elimination of toxicants. Renal biopsy should be performed if the diagnosis is in doubt, the patient does not respond to therapy within 4 to 5 days, or long-term dialysis is considered. The long-term prognosis for toxicant-induced ARF is usually fair to good if the patient survives the period of renal dysfunction. Several weeks may be required for renal function to improve. The severity of the azotemia and the histologic lesions and the response to therapy are the most important prognostic indicators.

References and Supplemental Reading

Brown, S. A., and Barsanti, J. A.: Gentamicin nephrotoxicosis in the dog. *In* Kirk, R. W. (ed.): *Current Veterinary Therapy IX.* Philadelphia: W. B. Saunders Co., 1986, pp. 1146–1150.

Brown, S. A., Barsanti, J. A., and Crowell, W. A.: Gentamicin-associated acute renal failure in the dog. J.A.V.M.A. 186:686, 1985.

Fox, L. E., Grauer, G. F., Dubielzig, R. R., et al.: Reversal of ethylene glycol–induced nephrotoxicosis in a dog. J.A.V.M.A. 191:1433, 1987.

Grauer, G. F., and Thrall, M. A. H.: Ethylene glycol (antifreeze) poisoning. *In* Kirk, R. W. (ed.): *Current Veterinary Therapy IX.* Philadelphia: W. B. Saunders Co., 1986, pp. 206–212.

Rubin, S. I.: Nephrotoxicity of amphotericin B. *In* Kirk, R. W. (ed.): *Current Veterinary Therapy IX.* Philadelphia: W. B. Saunders Co., 1986, pp. 1142–1146.

Willard, M. D.: Treatment of hyperkalemia. *In* Kirk, R.W. (ed.): *Current Veterinary Therapy IX.* Philadelphia: W. B. Saunders Co., 1986, pp. 94–101.

THIACETARSAMIDE AND ITS ADVERSE EFFECTS

JOHNNY D. HOSKINS, D.V.M.

Baton Rouge, Louisiana

Thiacetarsamide solution has been the preferred drug for the treatment of adult *Dirofilaria immitis* infection in dogs since its introduction in 1947. After its discovery by Otto and Maren during a World War II screening program for human filariasis, it was released for use in dogs at a dosage of 2.2 mg/kg/day for 11 to 15 days (Drudge, 1952; Otto and Maren, 1958). This schedule remained in use for nearly 10 years, until workers found that twice the daily dosage (4.4 mg/kg/day) given for 2 or 3 days was equally effective (Kume and Ohishi, 1957; Bailey, 1958). The 2- or 3-day treatment of 4.4 mg/kg once daily became increasingly popular, but shock-like reactions occasionally occurred soon after injection. Jackson reported that these shock-like reactions could be virtually eliminated by dividing the daily dosage into two doses of 2.2 mg/kg each (Jackson, 1963). This dosage protocol, 2.2 mg/kg body weight given intravenously twice daily for 2 days (a total of four injections), has subsequently become the standard treatment for adult *Dirofilaria immitis* infection in dogs.

CHEMISTRY AND EXCRETION

Thiacetarsamide is available as a 1 per cent aqueous solution of the neutral dibasic sodium salt of S,S-diester of *P*-carbamoyldithiobenzenearsonous acid with mercaptoacetic acid. Recently, high-performance liquid chromatography studies have determined that thiacetarsamide solution is a combination of thiacetarsamide and *P*-arsenosobenzamide. These compounds are trivalent arsenicals that can be oxidized to more stable pentavalent arsenic compounds when stored at room temperature or exposed to air. The reactivity of the trivalent arsenic and *P*-amide group present in thiacetarsamide and *P*-arsenosobenzamide is essential for the therapeutic efficacy of thiacetarsamide solution against the adult heartworm.

Upon exposure to oxygen and light, the clear, colorless thiacetarsamide solution deteriorates to a distinctly yellow or orange solution containing visible precipitates. When thiacetarsamide solution develops a yellow or an orange color or precipitates, it is probably ineffective and should be discarded (Leadbetter, 1984). Once a commercial bottle of

thiacetarsamide solution is opened and a needle is inserted, room air within the bottle can produce degradation of a minute amount of thiacetarsamide and a small amount of *P*-arsenosobenzamide as well as unidentified degradation products.

The toxicity and therapeutic activity of thiacetarsamide solution depend on reaction with sulfhydryl groups present in essential enzyme systems. Thiacetarsamide either transfers the *P*-arsenosobenzamide moiety directly to a sulfhydryl, or hydrolyzes to *p*-arsenosobenzamide, which subsequently reacts with a sulfhydryl. Therefore, this chemical reactivity of the thiacetarsamide solution is responsible for its action against adult heartworms and also for its instability (Leadbetter, 1984).

When a single dose of thiacetarsamide solution is injected intravenously (IV), about 50 per cent is excreted in the urine and feces within 24 hr. Although the thiacetarsamide solution is widely distributed throughout the dog's body, with higher concentrations in the organs of excretion, the liver and kidneys, its concentration is even greater in the adult heartworm (Knight, 1977). Since 1969, Jackson has stressed that the infected dog should be weighed accurately and a full dose of thiacetarsamide solution should be administered, regardless of its size (Jackson, 1969a). Any amount less than the prescribed dose will reduce adverse reactions to thiacetarsamide solution but cannot be relied on to kill all the adult heartworms, with efficacy ranging from 20 to 80 per cent. It is not necessary to space the two daily injections at 12-hr intervals; 6- to 8-hr intervals are sufficient. However, the full course of treatment should be given within 36 hr (i.e., within two successive days) (Jackson, 1969a).

EVALUATION BEFORE TREATMENT WITH THIACETARSAMIDE

The decision to administer thiacetarsamide solution to a dog with *Dirofilaria immitis* infection is often based on the animal's current health. It is always desirable to treat dogs as early in the course of the infection as possible. The risk of adverse reactions from thiacetarsamide therapy is diminished if treatment is performed before overt symptoms of heartworm disease develop or any evidence

131

of heart, lung, kidney, or liver damage is discernible (Jackson, 1969a). Since pretreatment diagnostic procedures have not been able to predict adverse reactions to thiacetarsamide solution, selection of dogs for therapy is generally based upon current health status as determined from the animal's case history, physical findings, and laboratory and radiographic evaluations (Hribernik and Hoskins, 1986).

An algorithm for the management of *Dirofilaria immitis* infection in dogs is presented in Figure 1. The algorithm can be modified according to the severity of infection seen in a veterinary practice area, and adherence to the algorithm may be adjusted to reflect professional judgment and experience (Rawlings, 1986). Thiacetarsamide solution should not be given, at least temporarily, to infected dogs with right heart failure, vena caval syndrome, pulmonary thromboembolism, disseminated intravascular coagulation (DIC), allergic pneumonitis, advanced hepatic disease, or azotemic, protein-losing nephropathy (Fig. 1). The diagnosis and management of these entities are described elsewhere (Jackson et al., 1977; Knight, 1983; Calvert and Rawlings, 1985).

Under ordinary circumstances, dogs judged to be in good health can receive thiacetarsamide solution with minimum risk at the time diagnosis is made. Many dogs older than 5 years of age or that have significant disease associated with the *Dirofilaria immitis* infection are successfully treated with thiacetarsamide solution. However, these dogs often require additional medical care through other types of treatment before thiacetarsamide solution is given (Fig. 1). The veterinarian and dog owner must use their judgment to weigh the risk of thiacetarsamide therapy against the benefits of the dog's potentially prolonged and enjoyable life after heartworm treatment (Rawlings, 1986). Furthermore, thiacetarsamide solution should not be administered until the dog's medical problems other than the heartworm disease are resolved or stabilized.

ADVERSE EFFECTS

The only thiacetarsamide solution that is currently used and is approved by the United States Food and Drug Administration (FDA) is Caparsolate Sodium (CEVA Laboratories, Inc., Overland Park, KS). *Caparsolate Sodium must be given intravenously.* If even a few drops are present perivascularly, an immediate painful, edematous swelling develops. Perivascular injections are promptly treated by dilution with sterile saline and lidocaine infiltration. If progressive swelling develops, apply topical dimethyl sulfoxide (DMSO), with anti-inflammatory steroid every 4 to 6 hr until pain subsides. It should be noted that the effect of DMSO

on thiacetarsamide solution action has not been evaluated (Rawlings, 1986).

The adverse effects of thiacetarsamide solution in dogs affected with *Dirofilaria immitis* infections may include anorexia, vomiting, lethargy, fever, diarrhea, tubular casts in urine sediment, elevated liver enzyme concentrations, icterus, bilirubinuria, and death (Jackson, 1969b; Carlisle et al., 1974; Hoskins et al., 1983). In a recent study of 276 thiacetarsamide-treated dogs with naturally occurring *Dirofilaria immitis* infection, a total of 39 dogs (14.1 per cent) reacted adversely to therapy (Hoskins et al., 1983). The adverse reactions were severe enough in ten dogs that thiacetarsamide therapy was suspended. Eight of the ten dogs were subsequently treated with a second course of thiacetarsamide solution and experienced no adverse reactions. Vomiting (38 dogs) was the most frequently seen reaction, followed by anorexia (11 dogs) and icterus (5 dogs). Most of these reactions occurred after the first and second thiacetarsamide injections. Vomiting was transient, and further toxic reactions did not appear in 31 of the 38 dogs. Treatment was suspended in dogs that developed icterus, vomited persistently, or vomited and were anorectic. Although not seen in this study, other potential, albeit less common, adverse reactions related to thiacetarsamide therapy may include bleeding, pulmonary thromboembolism, and right heart failure or an immediate worsening of a failure state (Hribernik and Hoskins, 1986).

In light of the aforementioned adverse reactions, one should, prior to each thiacetarsamide injection, monitor the dog's attitude, body temperature, appetite, and state of hydration and observe for evidence of vomiting, increased respiratory rate or respiratory distress, cough or increased coughing, abdominal distention, bleeding, or icterus (Hribernik and Hoskins, 1986). Urinalysis may show the presence of bilirubinuria and tubular casts; however, such findings alone seldom necessitate immediate suspension of thiacetarsamide therapy (Rawlings, 1986). Liver enzyme concentrations also seem to be of limited value. They are frequently elevated in dogs with and without adult heartworms, and their elevations do not correlate well with symptoms and physical appearance of treated dogs (Rawlings, 1986).

Thiacetarsamide therapy should be suspended in dogs in whom there is evidence of profuse vomiting, icterus, disseminated intravascular coagulation (DIC), or pulmonary thromboembolism (Rawlings, 1986). In addition, anorexia in combination with vomiting may be an indication to stop therapy. An episode of vomiting, especially within 1 hr of thiacetarsamide injection as a single symptom of an adverse reaction, is not an indication to suspend therapy. Dogs with symptoms of severe heartworm disease or coexisting disorders, such as renal dis-

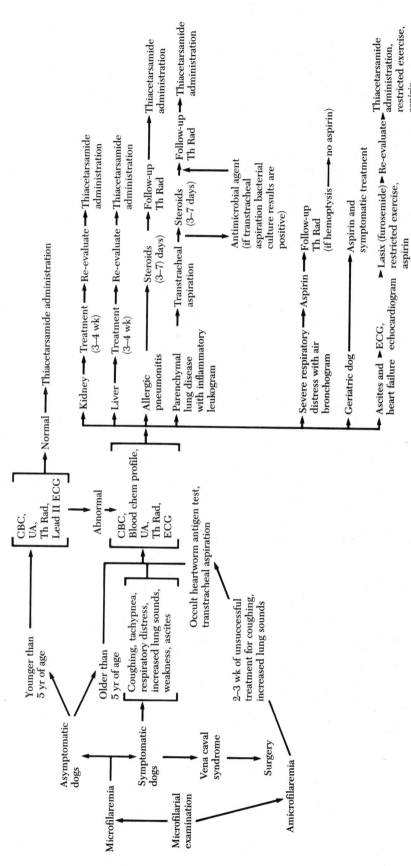

Figure 1. Algorithm for the management of heartworm disease in dogs. CBC, complete blood count; UA, urinalysis; Th Rad, thoracic radiographs; ECG, electrocardiogram; blood chem profile, serum chemistry determinations for blood urea nitrogen, hepatic enzymes, glucose, electrolytes, total protein, and albumin. (Modified from Rawlings, C. A.: Heartworm Disease in Dogs and Cats. Philadelphia, W.B. Saunders Company, 1986, and Proceedings of the Heartworm Symposium '86. Washington, D.C., American Heartworm Society, 1986.)

133

ease, diabetes mellitus, gastrointestinal disease, and hyperadrenocorticism, should be monitored more critically. In these dogs, an elevation of body temperature of only 1°F (0.6°C), depression, anorexia, or vomiting may be adequate justification for stopping thiacetarsamide therapy (Rawlings, 1986).

TREATMENT

The treatment for thiacetarsamide-induced adverse reactions is supportive; no specific antidote is available (Rawlings, 1986). A single episode of vomiting usually requires no treatment. Fluid therapy is indicated if the dog is dehydrated or is likely to develop prerenal azotemia. Persistently vomiting dogs should have food withheld and should be treated with balanced electrolyte-containing fluids. If a dog develops a body temperature of more than 103°F (39.4°C), anti-inflammatory doses of corticosteroids may be administered daily for 5 days. Antimicrobial agents, vitamins, corticosteroids, and "liver-sparing" drugs, such as those containing methionine, choline, and inositol, should not be routinely used during thiacetarsamide therapy (Calvert, 1986; Rawlings, 1986). However, multiple feedings of a nutritionally complete diet and restricted exercise should be prescribed. Symptoms related to adverse reactions to thiacetarsamide solution usually resolve within 2 or 3 days, although icterus may persist for up to 2 weeks (Calvert, 1986).

Dogs that experience adverse reactions or have thiacetarsamide therapy interrupted can usually be treated with thiacetarsamide solution 3 to 4 weeks later. During the intervening time, a dog should be maintained on a good diet and be treated for other coexisting disorders and parasites. Prior to re-treatment, a thorough physical examination, complete blood count, serum chemistry profile, and urinalysis should be performed (Rawlings, 1986). Most dogs will not experience adverse effects from the thiacetarsamide solution during the second treatment attempt (Hoskins et al., 1983).

References and Supplemental Reading

Bailey, R. W.: A comparison study of various arsenical preparations as filaricides of *Dirofilaria immitis*. J.A.V.M.A. 133:52, 1958.

Calvert, C. A.: Management of heartworm-infected dogs following thiacetarsamide treatment. Proceedings of Heartworm Symposium 1986, pp. 43–48, 1986.

Calvert, C. A., and Rawlings, C. A.: Diagnosis and management of canine heartworm disease. *In* Kirk, R. W. (ed.): *Current Veterinary Therapy VIII.* Philadelphia: W. B. Saunders Co., 1985, pp. 348–359.

Carlisle, C. H., Prescott, C. W., McCosker, P. J., et al.: The toxic effects of thiacetarsamide sodium in normal dogs and in dogs infested with *Dirofilaria immitis.* Aust. Vet. J. 50:204, 1974.

Drudge, J. H.: Arsenamide in the treatment of canine filariasis. Am. J. Vet. Res. 13:220, 1952.

Hoskins, J. D., Hagstad, H. V., and Hribernik, T. N.: Effects of thiacetarsamide sodium in Louisiana dogs with naturally occurring canine heartworm disease. Proceedings of Heartworm Symposium 1983, pp. 134–140, 1983.

Hribernik, T. N., and Hoskins, J. D.: Adulticide therapy in canine heartworm disease. Proceedings of Heartworm Symposium 1986, pp. 53–55, 1986.

Jackson, R. F.: Two-day treatment with thiacetarsamide for canine heartworm disease. J.A.V.M.A. 142:23, 1963.

Jackson, R. F.: Treatment of heartworm-infected dogs with chemical agents. J.A.V.M.A. 154:390, 1969a.

Jackson, R. F.: Complications during and following chemotherapy of heartworm disease. J.A.V.M.A. 154:393, 1969b.

Jackson, R. F., Seymour, W. G., Growney, P. J., et al.: Surgical treatment of caval syndrome of canine heartworm disease. J.A.V.M.A. 171:1065, 1977.

Knight, D. H.: Heartworm heart disease. *In* Brandly, C. A., and Jungherr, E. L. (eds.): *Advances in Veterinary Science and Comparative Medicine. Cardiovascular Pathophysiology.* New York: Academic Press, 1977, pp. 107–149.

Knight, D. H.: Heartworm disease. *In* Ettinger, S. J. (ed.): *Textbook of Veterinary Internal Medicine.* Philadelphia: W. B. Saunders Co., 1983, pp. 1097–1124.

Kume, S., and Ohishi, I.: Observations on the chemotherapy of canine heartworm infection with arsenicals. J.A.V.M.A. 131:476, 1957.

Leadbetter, M. G.: Storage considerations for thiacetarsamide sodium. J.A.V.M.A. 185:753, 1984.

Otto, G. F., and Maren, T. H.: Filaricidal activity of substituted phenylarsenoxides. Science 106:105, 1958.

Rawlings, C. A.: *Heartworm Disease in Dogs and Cats.* Philadelphia: W. B. Saunders Co., 1986.

ORGANOPHOSPHORUS AND CARBAMATE INSECTICIDE POISONING

GAVIN L. MEERDINK, D.V.M.

Tucson, Arizona

Chemical control of insects is essential and is likely to continue, given the estimate that 40 to 50 per cent of the world's food supply is lost to some form of pest. Over the last two decades, the organophosphorus (OP) and carbamate insecticides have largely replaced the organochlorine group of insecticides for agricultural, industrial, and home use. Although more acutely toxic, the OP and carbamate insecticides are less persistent in the environment than the organochlorines. Over a hundred OP and carbamate compounds are now manufactured under many trade names.

The OP and carbamate insecticides are discussed together because use, clinical syndrome, and treatment (with some exceptions) are identical. These compounds have a wide range of acute oral toxicity, 10 to 3000 mg/kg body weight; toxic doses are significantly higher for dermal exposure. The toxicity values given for each compound are not precise. Different values are derived from different tests, and, certainly, species, age, and sex affect the dose necessary for poisoning. With the exception of dichlorvos, most OP insecticides have comparatively low volatility. Generally, when used according to directions, environmental degradation of the OP and carbamate insecticides occurs rapidly by a variety of chemical or other mechanisms.

The small animal clinician will likely receive more questions regarding suspected or potential poisoning from these insecticides than actual toxicoses. Many, if not most, intoxications in domestic pets result from the ingestion of stored or spilled material or from access to improperly discarded containers. When these compounds are used as directed and pooling or other types of "accumulation" are avoided, the hazard is very low. For example, if a 1 per cent concentration of an insecticide (which could produce toxic effects at a dose of 50 mg active ingredient per kg of body weight) was sprayed over an area, a 2-kg pet would have to ingest (absorb) *ca.* 50 ml of the material to consume the toxic dose. When the insecticide is evenly dispersed, exposure to this amount of liquid is very remote. Other common causes of toxicosis are excessive dosage or prolonged use of OP or carbamate insecticides to control ectoparasites of small animals (consult a toxicologist or poison control center for further information).

These insecticides are generally readily absorbed but do not accumulate in body tissues. Numerous conjugation reactions follow the primary metabolic processes, and the phosphorus-containing residue is eliminated in 1 to 2 days via urine and, to a lesser degree, feces. Because of this reactivity, the amounts of unchanged OP and carbamate insecticides in food and animal tissues following poisoning are generally extremely low.

MECHANISM OF ACTION

Acetylcholine is the transmitter substance at cholinergic nerve synapses. Following the nerve axon release of acetylcholine for transfer of the impulse across the synapse, acetylcholinesterase (AChE) inactivates acetylcholine within 5 msec. OP and carbamate insecticides act by binding to AChE, which inactivates this enzyme and allows the uninhibited buildup of acetylcholine. This results in continual stimulation and fatigue of cholinergic end-organs and muscles. Death is due to respiratory failure.

Acetylcholinesterase is only one of several cholinesterases that are named according to their substrate affinity. Other cholinesterase enzymes (e.g., plasma cholinesterase, butyrylcholinesterase) can also (less efficiently) hydrolyze acetylcholine and are inhibited by OP and carbamate insecticides.

Reactivation of cholinesterase may occur when the bonded insecticide and the AChE enzyme separate. This reaction is more likely to happen with carbamates than with OPs. Conversely, with some OP insecticides, a process referred to as "aging" occurs in which a molecular change makes separation irreversible.

The delayed neuropathy syndrome can be caused by some OP insecticides, most of which are not in common use. The reaction with AChE is not involved. The syndrome requires at least 8 days to develop and involves a secondary metabolite that affects peripheral axons and myelin sheaths, resulting in sensory and motor neuropathy. This syndrome is extremely rare in small animals.

CLINICAL SIGNS

The clinical signs of OP and carbamate poisoning are characterized by overstimulation of the parasympathetic autonomic nervous system, skeletal muscles, and, to a limited degree, the central nervous system. Signs of intoxication can begin within minutes of exposure or can be delayed a few hours. For the most part, they will occur within 12 hr, unless some delay of absorption has occurred. The duration of clinical signs may be as short as a few minutes or as prolonged as several hours.

The earliest change observed is an appearance of anxiety or apprehension with an uneasiness due perhaps to abdominal discomfort. This subtle attitude change is quickly followed by mild, but progressively more copious salivation; frequent urination and defecation; and emesis. Fine muscle tremors in the facial region and head soon extend to the rest of the body. The muscle tremors (nicotinic effects) become more generalized and violent, progressing to a stiffened, jerky stance. By that time, the animal has difficulty in staying on its feet, and dyspnea is evident from increased bronchial secretions and bronchoconstriction. Convulsive seizures may or may not occur prior to coma, respiratory depression, and death.

The central nervous system effects are less obvious than the cholinergic signs described. Stimulation precedes depression, which is more pronounced in most cases. If convulsions do occur, clonic spasms are more prominent than tonic seizures.

DIAGNOSIS

Confirmation of OP or carbamate insecticide poisoning consists of (1) detection of the chemical compound in stomach contents and tissues (if possible) and (2) demonstration of the adverse biologic effect, cholinesterase (ChE) inhibition.

Detection of insecticide does determine intake. However, the degree of exposure cannot be determined by quantification of the chemical in tissues because of the rapid metabolism and excretion of these compounds. The demonstration of reduced cholinesterase activity is important in the confirmation of OP and carbamate insecticide poisoning. Interpretable cholinesterase activity can be determined on whole blood, blood clots, brain (particularly caudate nucleus), and retina. However, because of normal individual variation, interpretation can be difficult. Multiple samples, including serial blood samples at 24-hr intervals from clinical survivors, increase the validity of interpretation. A decrease in cholinesterase activity of at least 50 per cent is considered significant inhibition (less if the individual's pre-exposure level is known). For most cases of poisoning, cholinesterase activity is less than 25 per cent of normal activity. As post-mortem tissues decompose, the ChE activity of normal animal tissues gradually decreases. The ChE activity of tissues from poisoned animals tends to increase because of enzyme reactivation. Therefore, post-mortem decomposition escalates the difficulty of interpreting ChE activity.

Submit whole blood (EDTA or heparinized), vomitus, and suspect material from the clinical patient. Post-mortem samples should include whole blood or blood clots, brain, eyes, liver, and stomach contents. These samples should be chilled; if they cannot be received by the laboratory in a few days, the specimens can be frozen (after removal of the retinas from eyes). Contact the laboratory for further recommendations.

Necropsy lesions are usually unremarkable. Signs of cholinergic nervous system stimulation (e.g., salivation, tracheal fluid, diarrhea) may be observed. Gross evidence of pulmonary edema, which is usually reported in the literature, is variable and should not be a diagnostic determinant.

TREATMENT

Because of the rapid progression of OP and carbamate poisoning, the clinical case is an emergency and therapeutic measures should be instituted as soon as possible in animals with clinical signs. For those animals that are asymptomatic (although the owner is sure ingestion has occurred), induction of emesis followed by activated charcoal (see no. 2, following) may be indicated. Monitor the animal for at least 8 hr.

1. Administer atropine at a dose of 0.2 mg/kg of body weight intramuscularly (IM) or subcutaneously (SC). A fourth of the initial dose can be given intravenously (IV). Atropine has no effect on the bonded insecticide–ChE enzyme. Rather, the drug blocks the muscarinic (but not nicotinic) and some central nervous system effects at the nerve endings. Therefore, do not administer excess atropine; repeat only as needed to control clinical signs. If some reduction in the severity of clinical signs is not demonstrated by the patient within 10 to 15 min after atropine administration, the atropine dose or the diagnosis should be reviewed.

2. Activated charcoal can be given orally (PO) to prevent absorption of insecticide remaining in the alimentary tract. Understandably, this therapeutic adjunct is most beneficial when administered as early as possible.

3. Oximes (eg., Protopam Chloride, Ayerst) are ChE enzyme–reactivating agents that work directly on the insecticide-enzyme bond to deconjugate the union. They are probably of little benefit after 24 hr postexposure and appear to be most efficacious

within the first 12 to 18 hr. Excess administration is contraindicated, since the oximes have the molecular capability to inhibit ChE. The oximes are of no benefit in the treatment of carbamate poisoning.

4. Anticonvulsant drugs, particularly diazepam (Valium), have been used to supplement the effects of atropine or the atropine-oxime combination. By an unexplained mechanism, recovery has been hastened in some cases.

5. Diphenhydramine (Benadryl, Parke-Davis) (4 mg/kg of body weight PO every 8 hr) has been shown to block the effects of nicotine receptor overstimulation. Diphenhydramine does not alter inhibition of cholinesterases but appears to enhance nerve function and to prevent the receptor paralysis associated with OP-induced myasthenia-like syndrome.

6. Artificial respiration can be effective in maintaining life until the return of sufficient ChE activity. Respiratory failure is the principal cause of death with OP or carbamate insecticide poisoning.

7. Animals with dermal exposure should be washed with soap and water to prevent further absorption.

8. Other drugs that inhibit cholinesterase (eg., physostigmine, morphine, succinylcholine, phenothiazine, pyridostigmine, neostigmine) should be avoided.

References and Supplemental Reading

Buck, W. B., Osweiler, G. D., and Van Gelder, G. A.: *Clinical and Diagnostic Veterinary Toxicology.* Dubuque, IA: Kendall-Hunt Publishing Co, 1976.

Carson, T. L.: Organophosphate and carbamate insecticide poisoning. *In* Kirk, R. W. (ed.): *Current Veterinary Therapy VIII.* Philadelphia: W. B. Saunders Co., 1983.

Clark, E. G. C., and Clarke, M. L.: *Veterinary Toxicology.* London: Baillière Tindall, 1975.

Clemmons, R. M., Meyer, D. J. Sundlof, S. F., et al.: Correction of organophosphate-induced neuromuscular blockade by diphenhydramine. Am. J. Vet. Res. 45:2167, 1984.

Johnson, M. K. (ed.): Environmental Health Criteria 63, *Organophosphorus Insecticides: A General Introduction.* Geneva: World Health Organization, 1986.

Matsumura, F.: *Toxicology of Insecticides,* 2nd ed. New York: Plenum Press, 1985.

Radeleff, R. D.: *Veterinary Toxicology,* 2nd ed. Philadelphia: Lea & Febiger, 1979.

PYRETHRINS AND PYRETHROIDS

WILLIAM M. VALENTINE, D.V.M.,
and VAL RICHARD BEASLEY, D.V.M.
Urbana, Illinois

Pyrethrum has been produced as an insecticide for several centuries, its manufacture originating in the Middle East and moving to Europe, then Japan, and eventually Kenya, the major supplier today. In the United States, extracts of pyrethrum have been used for approximately 120 years. Pyrethrum is a combination of insecticidal compounds, termed pyrethrins, derived from flowers in the genus *Chrysanthemum.* Individual pyrethrin names are sometimes found on insecticide labels. The six naturally occurring pyrethrins all are esters and include pyrethrin I and II, cinerin I and II, and jasmolin I and II. Purified pyrethrins are viscous liquids that are soluble in organic solvents and oils and relatively insoluble in water. They are degraded by light and air and undergo hydrolysis, which can be catalyzed by acid or base. Because of their susceptibility to hydrolysis, as would occur in the alimentary canals of insects, they are primarily "contact poisons," having low "stomach poison" activity.

Currently available synthetic pyrethroids provide a broader spectrum of activity than that of pyrethrins with regard to insecticidal potency, environmental stability, and mammalian toxicity. Both pyrethrins and pyrethroids are used in numerous formulations including aerosols, sprays, dusts, dips, and shampoos for control of insects on animals as well as in the house and garden and in agriculture. Virtually all pyrethrin and many pyrethroid insecticides are formulated in combination with a synergist. Some formulations include additional insecticides, insect repellents, or both, and many contain hydrocarbon solvents. Flea control products constitute the primary source of exposure that leads to toxicosis in small animals. Historically, pyrethrins have been considered innocuous to domestic animals, thus most toxicologic investigations have involved invertebrates or laboratory rodents.

TOXICITY

Rat median lethal dose (LD_{50}) values for pyrethroids vary widely (Table 1). The low mammalian

Table 1. *Toxicity of Pyrethrins and Pyrethroids*

	*Rat LD$_{50}$ (mg/kg)	
	Oral	Intravenous
Type I Compounds		
Pyrethrin I	900	
Allethrin	680	
Tetramethrin (phthalthrin)	4,640	
Kadethrin	600	
Resmethrin	100	7
Phenothrin	10,000	>300
Permethrin	2,000	>135
cis-methrin		5
Bromophenothrin		> 30
Type II Compounds		
Fenpropathrin	25	1
Cypermethrin	500	6–9
Deltamethrin (decamethrin)	31	2
Fenvalerate	450	20
Fluorocyphenothrin		5–7
Fluvalinate	1,000	
Dowco 417	460	
Flucythrinate	67	
Bay-FCR	590	

*The values presented here pertain to the most toxic isomer and the lowest values found. (Values taken from *The Merck Index*, 10th ed., M. Windholz, ed., Rahway, NJ: Merck and Co., Inc., 1983, and *Agricultural Chemicals. Book 1, Insecticides*, W. T. Thomson, Fresno, CA: Thomson Publications, 1982.)

oral toxicity of these compounds has been attributed to their lability in the gastrointestinal tract and hepatic detoxification as a result of oxidation or ester cleavage. These processes contribute to the comparatively high selectivity (relative toxicity to insects versus that to mammals) of these compounds. In contrast, when administered intravenously (IV), intraperitoneally, or intracranially, the majority of the pyrethroids display significant inherent toxicity. Structural changes in either the alcohol or the acid component of pyrethroids that hinder ester cleavage increase mammalian toxicity. For example, compounds containing an alpha-S-cyano phenoxybenzyl alcohol group are generally five to ten times more toxic than pyrethroids not containing this modification. These compounds can generally be identified by an alpha-S-cyano or similar term within the chemical names used on pyrethroid-containing products.

Synergists are commonly combined with most pyrethrins and pyrethroids to enhance their insecticidal activity. The synergists in wide use all are inhibitors of microsomal oxidation and include piperonyl butoxide, N-octylbicycloheptene dicarboximide (MGK 264), sulfoxide, sesamin, and sesamolin. By inhibiting mixed function oxidases, synergists also potentiate mammalian toxicity, as has been observed in mice given piperonyl butoxide and various pyrethroids. Similarly, esterase inhibitors such as organophosphorus or carbamate insecticides can potentiate the toxicity of pyrethrin and pyrethroid compounds.

MECHANISM OF ACTION OF PYRETHRINS AND PYRETHROIDS

Syndromes

Pyrethroid syndromes have been designated as type I or type II based upon the *clinical signs* produced in rats. Although most of the clinical signs can be induced by intracranial injection, the fact that some compounds are less toxic when administered intracranially than by the intravenous route indicates a contribution of both central and peripheral components to the observed toxicosis.

Type I pyrethroids cause a syndrome in rats with increased aggressive sparring behavior and sensitivity to external stimuli. Next, fine muscle tremors progress in severity until the animals become prostrate and exhibit whole body tremors. Hyperthermia and a rapid onset of rigor commonly occur.

In rats, type II compounds cause a progressive increase in pawing and burrowing behavior, profuse salivation, coarse whole body tremors, increased startle responses, and abnormal locomotion involving the hind limbs. The coarse whole body tremors progress to "sinuous writhing of the entire body." Clonic seizures may occur as a terminal event. Although all pyrethroids that produce the type II effects contain the alpha-cyano phenoxybenzyl alcohol moiety, the converse does not hold; some alpha-cyano compounds can cause either type I or type II syndrome or a combination of the two, depending on the isomer involved.

Ion-channel Effects

The principal effects of allethrin, a type I pyrethroid, on nerve fibers are to (1) decrease peak sodium conductance, (2) prolong the inactivation of sodium conductance, and (3) suppress potassium conductance. This decreases the peak amplitude of the action potential and augments and prolongs the negative afterpotential, resulting in repetitive afterdischarges following a single stimulus. With increased concentration of allethrin or decreased temperature, there is an eventual block of nerve conduction. No major alterations of the resting membrane potential are ascribed to type I pyrethroids.

Type II pyrethroids differ only quantitatively from type I pyrethroids in respect to their action upon nerve axon sodium channels. There is a decrease in peak amplitude of the action potential, with extreme prolongation but only slight augmentation of the negative afterpotential. Also, a large depolarization of the resting membrane potential occurs, with ensuing conduction block. This depolarization of the resting membrane potential is believed to account for stimulation of sensory nerves, which causes the cutaneous paresthesia reported in humans and suggested by responses in guinea pigs.

GABA and Cyclic GMP Effects

Type II pyrethroids act as antagonists of the gamma-aminobutyric acid (GABA) receptor–ionophore complex. The interaction is mediated at the picrotoxin-binding sites and not the GABA or benzodiazepine sites of the receptor-ionophore complex. The result is a reduction in GABA-stimulated chloride influx. This difference from type I pyrethroids provides a possible explanation for the two distinct clinical syndromes observed. However, it appears that this interaction of type II pyrethroids at the GABA receptor–ionophore complex contributes to the overall symptoms but is not the principal molecular site of action.

Isoniazid, apomorphine, and several bicyclic phosphorous esters that cause hyperactivity, tremors, or convulsions increase brain cyclic guanosine monophosphate (cGMP) without affecting cyclic adenosine monophosphate (cAMP), suggesting that cGMP may play an intermediate role in producing seizures. Similarly, cypermethrin and decamethrin (type II pyrethroids) increase cerebellar cGMP without altering cAMP. The magnitude of the increases in cGMP are correlated with the severity of clinical signs. However, when incubated with slices of cerebellum, cypermethrin did not produce increases of cGMP, suggesting that the in vivo effect was indirect. Whether this effect is common to other pyrethroids is currently unknown.

CLINICAL SIGNS

There have been few studies on the toxicity of pyrethrins and pyrethroids to domestic animals. As a result, the clinical syndrome displayed in these animals has not been well characterized or clearly divided into two distinct categories. The clinical signs associated with toxicoses in dogs and cats are numerous. Mildly affected animals and those observed in early stages of the toxicosis often display hypersalivation, vomiting, diarrhea, mild tremors, and hyperexcitability or depression. More severely affected animals can present with hyperthermia, hypothermia, dyspnea, severe tremors, disorientation, and seizures. Generally, the onset of clinical signs is within a few hours of exposure but may be longer in cases of delayed ingestion that might result from grooming or in toxicosis from dermal absorption. Following termination of exposure, animals usually recover within 24 hr although individual animals may be affected for as long as 3 days.

DIAGNOSIS

There is no laboratory diagnostic test or characteristic lesion that can confirm a pyrethrin or synthetic pyrethroid as the definitive cause of an acute toxicosis. Clinical signs are numerous and varied, precluding a diagnosis on that basis alone. Since the clinical signs produced by organophosphorus, carbamate, and pyrethroid insecticides are similar, determination of cholinesterase activities can aid in making a diagnosis. In pyrethroid toxicosis, in the absence of concurrent exposure to a carbamate or an organophosphorus insecticide, cholinesterase values (whole-blood or brain) are expected to be in normal ranges. The history is instrumental in establishing (1) the time, nature, and degree of the exposure of the animal to an insecticide formulation; (2) the particular compounds involved; (3) the existence of any predisposing factors including exposure to synergists and other insecticides; and (4) the onset and the duration of clinical signs. In addition, the nature of the response of the patient to treatment may help support a diagnosis.

In cases involving fatalities, the analysis of skin, liver, fat, and brain for the presence and concentration of compounds in this class of insecticides may be possible, depending on the compound involved and the laboratory employed. Detection of pyrethrins or pyrethroids in tissue samples serves to establish exposure of an animal to the product, but concentrations supportive of a confirmed diagnosis have not yet been determined. In two cases in which cats died after treatment with a product containing the type II pyrethroid, fenvalerate, and the insect repellent, diethyltoluamide (deet), brain concentrations of the latter compound were approximately 130 ppm. In one case, fenvalerate was found at 0.01 ppm in brain. Whether the toxic effects of the pyrethroid or the repellant were responsible is currently unknown.

TREATMENT

Whenever possible, active ingredients of products should be confirmed by viewing labels to assess whether additional specific therapy is indicated (e.g., for organophosphorus or carbamate toxicosis). Treatment for pyrethrin or pyrethroid toxicosis involves preventing further absorption and instituting basic life-support measures, including control of seizures and symptomatic and supportive care. The initial examination of the patient should include assessment of respiratory and cardiovascular function.

Seizures represent the most probable severe complication and may result in irreversible brain damage or death from hyperthermia, lactic acidosis and shock, or, especially, hypoxia. A number of muscle relaxants that have a depressant action on spinal polysynaptic interneurons antagonize pyrethroid toxicosis in rats. Of these muscle relaxants, diazepam (Valium) and methocarbamol (Robaxin-V) are two readily available agents. Diazepam is preferred because of its safety and its ability to control seizures arising from a variety of causes. If the patient is having seizures or is displaying severe muscle tremors, diazepam should be administered to effect (0.2 to 2.0 mg/kg IV). If methocarbamol is administered, it is given at a dose of 55 to 220 mg/kg IV, at a rate not to exceed 200 mg/min. If the aforementioned treatment is unsuccessful or transient, phenobarbital (6 mg/kg) or pentobarbital (4 to 20 mg/kg) should be given intravenously, slowly to effect. Owing to the extrapyramidal stimulation induced by pyrethrins and pyrethroids, phenothiazine tranquilizers are contraindicated. When control of seizures is achieved, body temperature, blood glucose, hydration, and electrolytes should be assessed and any imbalances corrected.

For dermal exposure, thorough bathing with a mild detergent is needed, after which the patient should be kept warm to prevent hypothermia. In oral exposures, emesis is contraindicated (1) when products containing a high concentration of petroleum distillates are involved, such as some undiluted dip formulations, (2) when the animal is severely depressed, comatose, or likely to have a seizure or has lost the gag reflex, and (3) in certain species of animals (e.g., rodents and rabbits). In an animal that is severely depressed or comatose or has lost the gag reflex, an endotracheal tube should be placed and a gastric or enterogastric lavage with activated charcoal performed. Otherwise, in cases of oral exposure, emesis should be induced within 1 hr of ingestion when possible. Within 3 to 4 hr of ingestion, activated charcoal at 2 gm/kg and magnesium sulfate or sodium sulfate at 0.5 gm/kg (as a 10 per cent solution) should be administered orally. To avoid possible enterohepatic recirculation of some pyrethroids, in the presence of severe or protracted clinical signs (whether a result of oral or dermal exposure), administration of activated charcoal and a saline cathartic may prove efficacious even when it has been longer than 4 hr since exposure.

Basic symptomatic and supportive care may include correction of fluid and acid base balance if vomiting or diarrhea has been significant or if extreme exertion has occurred. Although atropine may prevent or relieve some clinical signs of pyrethroid toxicosis, it does not appear to enhance survival. Nutritional supplementation is sometimes desirable in the anorectic patient.

References and Supplemental Reading

Bloomquist, J. R., Adams, P. M., and Soderland, D. M.: Inhibition of gamma-aminobutyric acid–stimulated chloride flux in mouse brain vesicles by polychlorocycloalkane and pyrethroid insecticides. Neurotoxicology 7:11, 1986.

Casida, J. E., Gammon, D. W., Glickman, A. H., et al.: Mechanisms of selective action of pyrethroid insecticides. Ann. Rev. Pharmacol. Toxicol. 23:413, 1983.

Elliott, M. (ed.): *Synthetic Pyrethroids*. Washington, D.C.: American Chemical Society, 1977.

Gray, A. J.: Pyrethroid structure-toxicity relationships in mammals. Neurotoxicology 6:127, 1985.

Lock, E. A., and Berry, P. N.: Biochemical changes in the rat cerebellum following cypermethrin administration. Toxicol. Appl. Pharmacol. 59:508, 1981.

Metcalf, R. L., and McKelvey, J. J., Jr.: *The Future for Insecticides: Needs and Prospects*, Vol. 6. New York: John Wiley and Sons, 1976.

Narahashi, T.: Mode of action of pyrethroids. Bull. WHO 44:337, 1971.

Narahashi, T.: Cellular and molecular mechanisms of action of insecticides: Neurophysiological approach. Neurobehav. Toxicol. Teratol. 4:753, 1982.

Verschoyle, R. D., and Aldridge, W. N.: Structure-activity relationships of some pyrethroids in rats. Arch. Toxicol. 45:325, 1980.

IVERMECTIN

ALLAN PAUL, D.V.M.,
and WILLIAM TRANQUILLI, D.V.M.
Urbana Illinois

Ivermectin is a member of the family of compounds produced by the soil micro-organism *Streptomyces avermitilis*. It is structurally similar to the macrolide antibiotics but apparently lacks any antibacterial or antifungal activities. However, ivermectin has exhibited remarkably potent and broad-spectrum antiparasitic activity. Dosages at microgram levels have been effective against numerous external and internal parasites in a wide range of hosts including dogs, cats, horses, cattle, sheep, swine, and humans.

The compound was first introduced in the United States in 1983 and is currently approved for use in horses (Eqvalan, Merck), cattle (Ivomec, Merck), swine (Ivomec, Merck), and recently dogs (Heart-gard-30, Merck).

It is generally accepted that ivermectin produces its antiparasitic action by potentiating the release and binding of gamma-aminobutyric acid (GABA) at certain nerve synapses. The disruption of GABA-mediated transmission of nerve signals paralyzes susceptible nematodes and arthropods. The affected synapses are peripheral in both nematodes and arthropods, while in mammals, GABA-mediated neurotransmission occurs only in the central nervous system, where ivermectin does not readily or normally penetrate. This mode of action may explain the wide margin of safety that has been shown in mammalian species.

Acute signs of toxicity in dogs following oral administration of large doses of ivermectin were mydriasis, depression, tremors, ataxia, stupor, emesis, drooling, coma, and death (Seward et al., 1986). Acute toxicity was not observed after oral dosages of 2000 μ/kg or less. Single oral dosages of 2500 μ/kg produced mydriasis, those of 5000 μ/kg produced tremors, and those of 10,000 μ/kg produced more severe tremors and ataxia. Deaths occurred only after dosages exceeded 40,000 μ/kg. The approximate median lethal dose (LD_{50}) for beagles was 80,000 μ/kg. In another study, daily oral administration of ivermectin at 500 μ/kg for 14 weeks produced no signs of toxicity. Dogs receiving 1000 or 2000 μ/kg/day for 14 weeks developed mydriasis and lost a small amount of weight. However, tremors, ataxia, anorexia, dehydration, and depression were seen in four of eight dogs given 2000 μ/kg/day.

The recommended dose of Heartgard-30 of 6.0 μ/kg at monthly dosing intervals for the prevention of heartworm infections is well below the levels where toxic signs are manifested and should provide for a wide margin of safety. However, reports of adverse reactions in dogs following the unapproved (extra-label or off-label) use of ivermectin products formulated and marketed for horses and cattle continue to occur. Many of these reactions appear to be due to the accidental or erroneous administration of excessive amounts of ivermectin. One can visualize how easily an overdose can occur when owners attempt to accurately dose their dogs with the horse paste formulation.

It has become evident that certain dogs, particularly of the collie breed (both rough and smooth-coated), are unusually sensitive to the toxic effects of ivermectin. Reported adverse reactions and apparent toxicity at unexpectedly low doses of ivermectin have indicated that a breed idiosyncrasy exists. In some collies, the concentration of ivermectin in the central nervous tissues following treatment is apparently greater than observed in other dogs. This is possibly due to a more readily penetrated blood-brain barrier in these dogs or to sequestration.

There appears to be a wide range of susceptibility to ivermectin-induced toxicosis among collies. In two clinical trials (Paul et al., 1987; Pulliam et al., 1985), 50 per cent of the collies were found to display severe toxic signs following oral ivermectin doses of 200 μ/kg. No signs were observed in any of the dogs when they were given 50 or 100 μ/kg. Because the 200 μ/kg dose is many times greater than the recommended 6 μ/kg dose of ivermectin used for heartworm prevention, it appears that use of Heartgard-30 would be safe even in the most sensitive dogs. Signs of ivermectin-induced toxicosis in sensitive dogs or dogs massively overdosed include early signs of drooling, vomiting, ataxia, tremors, and disorientation, which may progress to weakness, recumbency, nonresponsiveness, stupor, and coma.

Treatment of ivermectin-induced toxicity can be successful. Although recovery may be slow and supportive care may be difficult, it has been the authors' experience that even severely affected dogs can recover completely.

At present, little is known about antagonism or reversal of ivermectin toxicity. One attempt to reverse ivermectin-induced toxicity with picrotoxin has been reported (Sivine, 1985). Picrotoxin was given by intravenous infusion at a rate of 1 mg/min for 8 min, and 30 min later the dog was observed to be in violent clonic seizures. These seizures were controlled with thiopental. This dog recovered over the ensuing 7 days. Because of its potentially serious side effects, questionable efficacy, and dangers of preparation, picrotoxin is not the drug of choice for treatment of ivermectin-induced toxicosis.

A commercially available product, physostigmine (Antilirium, O'Neal, Jones and Feldman Pharmaceuticals), has been shown to be of some therapeutic value in the treatment of ivermectin toxicity (Tranquilli et al., 1987). Collies that had progressed into severe depression or coma following ivermectin administration were given physostigmine by slow IV injection, at a dose of 1 mg every 12 hr for several days until toxic signs abated. Within a few minutes of each physostigmine injection, the dogs became more responsive, regained some muscle activity, showed increased respiration rate, and made attempts to drink and eat. This period of increased alertness ranged from 30 to 90 min, after which time the dogs would return to a severely depressed or comatose state. In this regard, the use of physostigmine to improve responsiveness not only may be of benefit to the patient but also may improve the client's willingness to continue long-term therapy. Physostigmine did not induce seizures in any treated comatose dog, but care was taken to deliver the drug slowly and at a relatively low dose. However, when physostigmine was administered to a dog exhibiting only minor ataxia and confusion, seizurelike activity was observed. Thus, it appears that physostigmine therapy would be beneficial in dogs with severe depression or in a coma, but not in dogs exhibiting minimal signs of toxicity. In this study, all dogs survived with no apparent long-term complications. However, these results should be interpreted cautiously. Other reported cases of ivermectin toxicity indicate that complete recovery can occur following symptomatic, supportive therapy without any attempts at specific reversal or antagonism.

In conclusion, although physostigmine may provide some temporary benefits, it cannot be recommended as an antidote, nor should it be used as the sole therapy for inadvertent ivermectin toxicity. Further research is needed to identify a more specific antagonist for ivermectin.

The mainstay of management of cases of ivermectin toxicity is supportive and symptomatic care. Proper fluid therapy and maintenance of electrolyte balance, nutritional support, and the prevention of secondary complications are important therapeutic goals. Since these animals may remain recumbent for long periods, appropriate bedding, frequent turning of the dog, and other standard treatment measures for a recumbent animal are of paramount importance. Because of the severe central depression produced in ivermectin toxicity, bradycardia and inefficient respiratory function can develop. Glycopyrrolate, 0.01 mg/kg (Robinul, Robins), can be given as needed to maintain a heart rate of more than 80 beats/min. Although there is no evidence that brain edema results from ivermectin toxicosis, dexamethasone (Azium, Schering), 0.25 mg/kg IV every 8 hr, may be beneficial. Antibiotics and vitamin supplementation may also be helpful in preventing complications associated with low caloric intake, debilitation, and secondary bacterial infection (e.g., aspiration pneumonia). However, it should be remembered that corticosteroid therapy can be associated with increased gastric acidity. Concomitant cimetidine (Tagamet, SmithKline) therapy should be instituted to help minimize gastric irritation when long-term dexamethasone administration is considered.

In conclusion, the prognosis and eventual outcome in cases of ivermectin toxicosis are dependent on a number of factors, including individual and breed sensitivity, the amount of drug ingested or injected, how rapidly severe clinical signs develop (the onset of severe depression within 1 to 2 hr following ingestion or injection should prompt a guarded prognosis), response to supportive therapy, and the overall health and condition of the animal. It must be emphasized that convalescence may be prolonged (several weeks). However, good supportive care in many seemingly hopeless cases has resulted in complete recovery.

References and Supplemental Reading

Campbell, W. C., and Benz, G. W.: Ivermectin: A review of efficacy and safety. J. Vet. Pharmacol. Ther. 7:1, 1984.

Paul, A. J., Tranquilli, W. J., Seward, R. L., et al.: Clinical observations in Collies given ivermectin orally. Am. J. Vet. Res. 48:684, 1987.

Pulliam, J. D., Seward, R. L., Henry, R. T., et al.: Investigating ivermectin toxicity in Collies. Vet. Med. 35–50, 1985.

Seward, R. L., Brokken, E. S., and Plue, R. E.: Ivermectin vs heartworms—a Status Update. Proceedings of the Heartworm Symposium '86. American Heartworm Society, Washington D.C., pp. 1–8, 1986.

Sivine, F.: Picrotoxin, the antidote to ivermectin in dogs? Vet. Rec. 116:195, 1985.

Tranquilli, W. J., Paul, A. J., Seward, R. L., et al.: Response to the physostigmine administration in collie dogs exhibiting ivermectin toxicosis. J. Vet. Pharmacal. Ther. 10:96, 1987.

THE ANTICOAGULANT RODENTICIDES

MICHAEL J. MURPHY, D.V.M.,
St. Paul, Minnesota

and DIANE F. GERKEN, D.V.M.
Columbus, Ohio

The anticoagulant rodenticides were developed following investigations of moldy sweetclover poisoning in cattle. In this well-known syndrome, the naturally occurring coumarin in the clover was converted by fungi to dicumarol—the toxic agent (Smith, 1938). Warfarin was synthesized during research efforts into the mechanism of action of dicumarol and subsequently became widely marketed as a rodenticide. After continued exposure from this widespread use, many rodent species developed a resistance to warfarin (Jackson et al., 1975). Other compounds of similar toxicity were utilized, but reports of inadequate rodent control (resistance) persisted. More recently, compounds effective against resistant rodents have been marketed. It is unfortunate that domestic animals are sometimes inadvertently, and occasionally maliciously, exposed to anticoagulant rodenticide baits. This article attempts to discuss briefly the therapeutic approaches available to the veterinary practitioner in dealing with these types of poisonings (for a more detailed discussion, *Current Veterinary Therapy IX*, p. 156).

MECHANISM OF ACTION

Considerable biochemical research is still under way to discern specific enzymes and chemical intermediates involved in the synthesis of vitamin K_1-dependent clotting factors. Nevertheless, the essential toxic event in anticoagulant rodenticide poisoning is depletion of active vitamin K_1.

The clotting factors II, VII, IX, and X must bind calcium to be active in clot formation. Dicarboxylic acid groups (similar to those on EDTA, oxalate, or citrate) present on these factors are responsible for this calcium binding. The actual biochemical step that requires vitamin K_1 is the synthesis of these dicarboxylic acid groups. In essence, one carboxylic acid group is added to each of 10 to 16 existing gamma-glutamyl amino acids on factor II, VII, IX, and X precursor proteins (Fig. 1). The oxidation of vitamin K_1 to vitamin K_1 epoxide (catalyzed by vitamin K_1 epoxidase) is associated with this step.

In the normal animal, vitamin K_1 is regenerated by the reduction of vitamin K_1 epoxide. The inhibition of this regenerative step by the anticoagulant rodenticides results in depletion of active vitamin K_1 (Suttie, 1987). Synthesis of new clotting factors (II, VII, IX, and X) is subsequently impaired. Since these factors have respective plasma half-lives of 41, 6.2, 13.9, and 16.5 hr in the dog, they are also rapidly depleted. Clinical coagulopathy soon follows the depletion of vitamin K_1 in the liver and the preformed clotting factors in the plasma.

This indirect mechanism of action explains the lag time commonly observed between ingestion of bait and onset of clinical signs. Normally this time is 3 to 5 days, although individual variations commonly occur.

TOXICITY

Eight different anticoagulant rodenticides are distributed in the United States over the counter and through pest control operators. These compounds are categorized as either first- or second-generation, based on their efficacy against warfarin-resistant rats. By definition, the compounds that are effective against warfarin-resistant rats are termed second-generation anticoagulant rodenticides.

The pest must generally ingest the first-generation compounds for a period of time before receiving a lethal dose. Since inconsistent bait ingestion may have contributed to the development of warfarin resistance, the second-generation compounds were designed to deliver a lethal dose in a single feeding. Single-dose efficacy was achieved by maximizing potency, biological duration of action, or both in these compounds. Thus, the second-generation anticoagulant rodenticides are more potent, longer acting, or both when compared with first-generation compounds. Therapeutically, this categorization suggests the dose and length of vitamin K_1 treatment necessary for successful recovery of poisoned animals (Table 1).

The likelihood of secondary toxicity occurring in

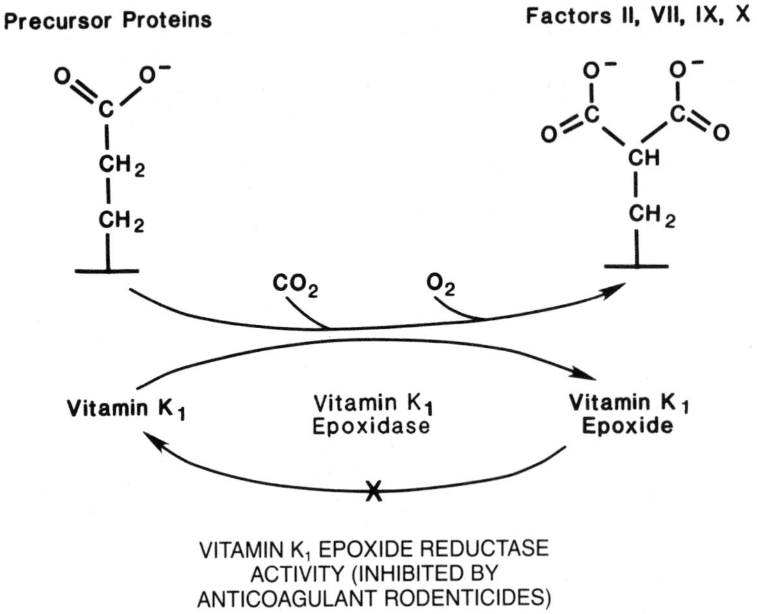
Precursor Proteins
Factors II, VII, IX, X
CH_2
CH_2
CH
CH_2
CO_2
O_2
Vitamin K_1
Vitamin K_1 Epoxidase
Vitamin K_1 Epoxide
VITAMIN K_1 EPOXIDE REDUCTASE ACTIVITY (INHIBITED BY ANTICOAGULANT RODENTICIDES)

Figure 1. Site of action of anticoagulant rodenticides.

a rodent-eating pet is of interest when anticoagulant rodenticides are used. This toxicity may be more probable with the second-generation compounds; however, the authors are not aware of any confirmed field cases.

CLINICAL CONSIDERATIONS

Signs

Animals may hemorrhage from virtually any traumatized site following depletion of active coagulation factors. Hemorrhage (melena, epistaxis, hematuria, or hematomas) is clinically consistent with coagulopathy, but it is not always the presenting sign. Dyspnea, lethargy, or anorexia may be the only clinical signs observed in many cases of anticoagulant rodenticide toxicity (DuVall et al., 1987).

Diagnosis

Some differential considerations of coagulopathies in small animals include disseminated intravascular

Table 1. Toxicity and Therapy of Anticoagulant Rodenticides

Chemical	Bait Concentration (ppm)	Acute Oral LD_{50} Compound (mg/kg) Dog	Acute Oral LD_{50} Compound (mg/kg) Cat	Acute Oral LD_{50} Bait* (oz/lb) Dog	Vitamin K_1 Therapy Dose (mg/kg)	Vitamin K_1 Therapy Length
Short-acting						
Warfarin	250	20–300	5–30	1.3	1	4–6 days
Unknown						
Fumarin	250	?	?	?	1	4–6 days†
Pindone	250	5–75	?	0.3	1	4–6 days
Valone	250	?	?	?	1	4–6 days
Long-acting						
Diphacinone	50	0.9–8	15	0.3	2.5–5.0	3–4 weeks§
Chlorophacinone	50	?	?	?	2.5–5.0	3–4 weeks
Brodifacoum	50	0.2–4	25‡	0.06	2.5–5.0	2–3 weeks
Bromadiolone	50	11–15	>25‡	3.5	2.5–5.0	?

*Ounces of finished bait per pound of body weight required to achieve the lowest LD_{50} value reported in the dog.
†Animals should be closely observed and re-examined at the end of therapy.
‡Limited data.
§Re-examination following therapy is strongly recommended.
?, No data available.

coagulopathy, congenital factor deficiencies, von Willebrand's disease, anticoagulant rodenticides, hyperviscosity syndromes, platelet deficiencies, functional defects, or both; and canine ehrlichiosis. Laboratory tests often employed to support a clinical diagnosis of the aforementioned disorders are circulating fibrin degradation products (FDPs); factor testing; prothrombin, partial thromboplastin, thrombin, and bleeding times; plasma fibrinogen; platelet counts; and serology. A prolonged prothrombin, partial thromboplastin, or thrombin time in the presence of normal fibrinogen, FDPs, and platelet counts is consistent with anticoagulant rodenticide toxicity. Additionally, a positive therapeutic response within 24 hr of adequate vitamin K_1 administration strongly suggests anticoagulant rodenticide toxicity.

Once a diagnosis of anticoagulant rodenticide coagulopathy is made, the specific compound involved may influence the therapeutic regimen chosen. It is unfortunate that no clinical sign or routine laboratory procedure can distinguish between first- and second-generation anticoagulant toxicity.

Although methods are available for the detection of a few anticoagulant rodenticides in the blood of a poisoned animal, the most expedient and, by far, the easiest means of determining the specific anticoagulant involved is via the history. Please note that numerous similarities exist in trade names, and one company may market rodent baits with different ingredients. For example, D-Con may contain warfarin, while D-Con Mouse Pruf II may contain brodifacoum. Proper identification of the anticoagulant involved may significantly affect therapeutic success. The most practical means of determining the involved compound is examining the ingredient listing on the box of bait or speaking with the pest control operator directly. The owner should be instructed to bring the suspect container to the clinic. In cases where it was consumed, a trip to the store to specifically identify the suspect bait is recommended. An alphabetical listing of some trade names is included for your convenience (Table 2). This list is by no means comprehensive.

TREATMENT

Vitamin K_1 is the treatment of choice for cases of anticoagulant rodenticide intoxication. This form of the vitamin is immediately available for synthesis of new clotting factors, whereas other chemical forms of vitamin K are not. Vitamin K_1 has no direct effect on coagulation, and clinically significant synthesis of new clotting factors commonly requires at least 6 to 12 hr. For this reason, emergency needs for circulating clotting factors can be met only via a transfusion. Animals with markedly reduced PCVs or signs of severe hypovolemic shock often require

Table 2. *Some Common Names of Anticoagulant Rodenticides*

Trade Name*	Chemical Name
Bromone	Bromadiolone
Caid	Chlorophacinone
Co-Dax	Warfarin
Cov-R-Tox	Warfarin
D-Con Pruf II	Warfarin
D-Con Mouse	Brodifacoum
Drat	Chlorophacinone
Enforcer Mouse Kill	Brodifacoum
Havoc	Brodifacoum
Just-One-Bite	Bromadiolone
Kill-Ko Rat	Fumarin
Kill-Ko Rat Killer	Diphacinone
Liphadione	Chlorophacinone
Liqua-Tox	Warfarin
Maki	Bromadiolone
P.C.Q. Rodent Cake	Diphacinone
Pival	Pindone
Pivalyl	Pindone
Ramucide	Chlorophacinone
Ratomet	Chlorophacinone
Raviac	Chlorophacinone
Rax	Warfarin
Rodex	Warfarin
Rodex-Blox	Warfarin
Rozol	Chlorophacinone
SuperCaid	Bromadiolone
Talon	Brodifacoum
Topitox	Chlorophacinone
Tox-Hid	Warfarin
Volid	Brodifacoum
Warfarin	Warfarin
Weather-Blok	Brodifacoum

*As listed in *Farm Chemicals Handbook*, 1987.
(*Note*: Specific trade names are included in the interest of assisting the practitioner in providing appropriate therapy to animals inadvertently exposed to anticoagulant rodenticides. The presence or absence of a product listing in no way implies endorsement or lack of support for that product.)

fresh plasma (9 ml/kg body weight) or whole blood (20 ml/kg body weight) (Mount et al., 1985; Osweiler et al., 1985). Animals with less severe clinical signs may be successfully treated with vitamin K_1, cage rest, and supportive therapy. Severely dyspneic animals in shock, with moderately reduced packed cell volumes (PCVs) (15 to 20 per cent), may be successfully treated with vitamin K_1, 5 mg/kg PO.

Vitamin K_1 may be administered by the intravenous (IV), intramuscular (IM), subcutaneous (SC), or oral (PO) route. Differences of minutes in the absorption of vitamin K_1 are probably not clinically significant, so individual patient factors determine the preferred route of vitamin K_1 administration. The IV route is not recommended for reasons of safety and efficacy. The potential for anaphylaxis is always present with IV administration of vitamin K_1 (Clark and Halliwell, 1963). An initial IM dose of vitamin K_1 may result in life-threatening IM hemorrhage, so this route is discouraged early in the therapeutic regimen. Animals in severe hypovolemic shock probably have poorly perfused peripheral tissues, which may affect vitamin K_1 absorption from a SC site. Oral administration of vitamin K_1 should be reconsidered in animals known to have a fat malabsorption problem.

The two most commonly recommended routes of vitamin K_1 administration are PO and SC. Oral absorption of vitamin K_1 may be significantly enhanced by coadministration of fat-containing foods. Administration of vitamin K_1 with canned dog food increased its relative bioavailability four to five times compared with vitamin K_1 given alone (Gerken, 1987). Feeding is likely to stimulate the availability of bile salts and the chylomicron formation necessary for vitamin K_1 absorption (Mandel and Cohn, 1985).

Recommended daily dosages of vitamin K_1 range from 0.25 to 2.5 mg/kg in warfarin exposure to 2.5 to 5.0 mg/kg for long-acting rodenticide intoxication (Mount et al., 1985). Loading doses are commonly given at the same dosage as that recommended for daily treatment. The higher dosages of vitamin K_1 may be necessary for successful treatment of second-generation anticoagulant toxicity. To illustrate, a small dog was observed to ingest approximately one half an LD_{50} of a second-generation anticoagulant. Vitamin K_1 therapy of 1 mg/kg administered SC was initiated on the day of ingestion. Dyspnea and ventral hematomas observed 3 days later were alleviated within 36 hr of increasing the dose to 2.5 mg/kg.

Since vitamin K_1 has no effect on the metabolism or elimination of the rodenticide, therapy must be maintained until toxic amounts of the compound are no longer present in the animal. For this reason, the length of the vitamin K_1 therapeutic regimen is dependent upon the dose and toxicokinetics of the specific rodenticide involved. Abnormal coagulation may last for 7 days with warfarin exposure, or 6 weeks with multiple-dose exposure to the long-acting rodenticides (Table 1). The length of therapy values in this table are based on dogs experimentally dosed with an LD_{50} of the respective rodenticide. In a given case, the length of therapy required will be directly related to the amount of anticoagulant ingested. Since, in clinical situations, this amount is rarely known, some practitioners may elect to evaluate patients periodically. In this approach, animals are treated for a period of time—often 7 to 10 days. Then, one-stage prothrombin time (OSPT) evaluations are performed 2 days after cessation of vitamin K_1 administration. If the OSPT is prolonged, therapy is commonly continued for another week. If the OSPT is normal, OSPT is repeated following an additional 2 to 3 days. If the OSPT remains normal for 5 to 6 days *following cessation of vitamin K_1 therapy*, the rodenticide may be adequately metabolized at that point to discontinue treatment. It must be noted that OSPT values may be normal even though individual clotting factors are still significantly reduced (Mount and Feldman, 1983). Also, keep in mind that numerous animals, to the disappointment of the veterinarian, have bled to death 4 to 6 days after the completion of a 7-day regimen of vitamin K_1.

Although vitamin K_3 given PO is used as a feed supplement, it was found to be ineffective in treating dogs experimentally intoxicated with warfarin (Clark and Halliwell, 1963) or dicumarol (Miller et al., 1950). (Production and marketing of injectable vitamin K_3 was suspended in 1985 by the Center for Veterinary Medicine of the Food and Drug Administration for safety and efficacy reasons.) Dogs dosed with 25 mg/kg or more of vitamin K_3 developed Heinz-body anemia, hemoglobinuria, urobilinuria, urobilinogenuria, methemoglobinemia, cyanosis, and hepatic damage (Nangeroni, 1986; Fernandez et al., 1984; Finkel, 1961).

The prognosis in patients with anticoagulant rodenticide poisoning is generally good to excellent. Predisposing liver disease or other complications may, of course, interfere with the animal's ability to respond to therapy or the veterinarian's success in controlling life-threatening hemorrhage.

References and Supplemental Reading

Clark, W. T., and Halliwell, R. E. W.: The treatment with vitamin K preparations of warfarin poisoning in dogs. Vet. Rec. 75:1210, 1963.

DuVall, M. D., Murphy, M. J., Ray, A. C., et al.: Case Studies of Second-Generation Anticoagulant Rodenticide Toxicities in Non-Target Species. Proceedings of the American Association of Veterinary Laboratory Diagnosticians, Salt Lake City, 1987.

Fernandez, F. R., Davies, A. P., Teachout, D. J., et al.: Vitamin K-induced Heinz-body formation in dogs. J. Am. Anim. Hosp. Assoc. 20:711, 1984.

Finkel, M. J.: Vitamin K_1 and the vitamin K analogues. Clin. Pharmacol. Ther. 2:794, 1961.

Gerken, D. F.: Unpublished data, 1987.

Jackson, W. B., Brooks, J. E., Bowerman, A. M., et al.: Anticoagulant resistance in Norway rats. Pest Control 5:14, 1975.

Mandel, H. G., and Cohn, V. H.: Fat-soluble vitamins. In Gilman, A. G., et al. (eds.): The Pharmacological Basis of Therapeutics. New York: MacMillan Publishing Co., 1985, pp. 1582–1589.

Miller, R., Harvey, W. P., and Finch, C. A.: Antagonism of dicumarol by vitamin K preparations. N. Engl. J. Med. 242:211, 1950.

Mount, M. E., and Feldman, B. F.: Mechanism of diphacinone rodenticide toxicosis in the dog and its therapeutic implication. Am. J. Vet. Res. 44:2009, 1983.

Mount, M. E., Woody, B. J., and Murphy, M. J.: The anticoagulant rodenticides. In Kirk, R. W. (ed.): Current Veterinary Therapy IX. Philadelphia: W. B. Saunders, 1985, pp. 156–165.

Nangeroni, L. L.: Injectable vitamin K_3. (letter) J.A.V.M.A. 189:850, 1986.

Osweiler, G. D., Carson, T. L., Buck, W. B., et al.: Anticoagulant rodenticides. In Osweiler, G . D., et al. (eds.): Clinical and Diagnostic Veterinary Toxicology, 3rd ed. Dubuque, IA: Kendall-Hunt, 1985, pp. 334–339.

Smith, W. K.: Relation of bitterness to the toxic principle in sweetclover. J. Agr. Res. 56:145, 1938.

Suttie, J. W.: Current Advances in Vitamin K Research. Proceedings of the Seventeenth Steenbock Symposium, June 21–25, 1987.

BROMETHALIN POISONING

THOMAS L. CARSON, D.V.M.

Ames, Iowa

SOURCE

Bromethalin is a new nonanticoagulant single-dose rodenticide that is commercially available in bait form as Assault (Purina Mills, Inc.) and Vengeance (Velsicol Chemical Corporation). These pelleted grain-base baits contain 0.01 per cent (100 ppm) bromethalin and are packaged in 1.5 oz (42 gm) paper place-pack envelopes. Vengeance is also available in bulk to commercial pest control operators. Assault bait pellets are colored green with a water-soluble dye.

TOXICITY

The acute oral median lethal doses (LD_{50}) for bromethalin for several animals are listed in Table 1. From this information, it can be calculated that a 30-lb dog would need to consume 642 gm of bait (15 place packs) to receive an LD_{50} dose. A minimum toxic dose of bromethalin for the dog is 1.67 mg/kg, whereas the minimum lethal dose is 2.5 mg/kg (25 gm of bait per kg).

Secondary poisoning of nontarget animals appears unlikely, as dogs that consumed 600 gm of ground rat carcass (killed by bromethalin) per day for 14 days did not show clinical signs of bromethalin toxicosis.

Bromethalin has not produced dermal or ocular irritation or inhalation hazards at the 0.1 and 0.005 per cent concentrations tested.

MECHANISM OF ACTION

Bromethalin is rapidly absorbed from the gastrointestinal tract, with peak plasma concentration in the rat occurring 4 hr after exposure. However, excretion is slow, with a half-life for plasma clearance of 5.6 days (Van Lier and Ottosen, 1981).

Bromethalin rodenticide is a neurotoxin, as it appears to uncouple oxidative phosphorylation in central nervous system mitochondria. This could lead to a decreased production of ATP, a diminished activity of $Na+/K+$ ATPase, and a subsequent fluid build-up manifested by fluid-filled vacuoles between the myelin sheaths. This vacuole formation in turn leads to an increased cerebrospinal fluid (CSF) pressure and increased pressure on nerve axons, yielding a decrease in nerve impulse conduction, paralysis, and death (Jackson et al., 1982).

CLINICAL SIGNS

Bromethalin toxicosis can be presented clinically as either an acute or a chronic syndrome, depending on the dose consumed. Acute effects follow a dose of at least 5.0 mg bromethalin/kg body weight and are usually associated with generous bait consumption. These acute signs appear about 10 hr after dosing and are characterized by hyperexcitability, severe muscle tremors, occasional running fits, grand mal seizures, hind limb hyper-reflexia, mild to severe depression, and death.

Chronic effects are seen with lower bromethalin dosages of 1.6 to 2.5 mg/kg body weight. Clinical signs may occur from 24 to 86 hr after dosing and may last for up to 12 days. This syndrome is characterized by tremors, mild to severe depression, ataxia, vomiting and lateral recumbency and has been the type of syndrome observed in dogs that have consumed bromethalin baits. These effects are generally reversible if exposure to the toxicant is discontinued.

PHYSIOPATHOLOGY

Cerebrospinal fluid pressure elevated to a level three to four times the normal pressure is clinical evidence of the cerebral edema. Light and electron microscopic examination of the brain and spinal cord show intramyelinic vacuolation of the white matter similar to that seen with trialkyltin or hexachlorophene toxicosis. Both water and sodium levels of these tissues are elevated (Cherry et al., 1982; Van Lier and Ottosen, 1981).

Table 1. *Acute Oral LD_{50} of Bromethalin and Amount of 0.01% Bait to Provide the LD_{50}*

Animal	LD_{50} (mg/kg)	Amount of Bait to Provide LD_{50} (gm of bait/lb body wt)
Norway rat	2	9.1
Mouse	5	22.7
Dog	4.7	21.4
Cat	1.8	8.2
Monkey	5	22.7
Rabbit	13	59.1

DIAGNOSIS

Bromethalin toxicosis should be considered in a differential diagnosis when clinical signs of cerebral edema or posterior paralysis are present. A history of exposure to bromethalin bait would be substantiating evidence. Although chemical analysis can be used to detect bromethalin in baits, little is known about tissue residues and their diagnostic significance.

TREATMENT

Treatment of bromethalin poisoning should emphasize blocking absorption from the gut and reducing cerebral edema. Use of an osmotic diuretic (e.g., mannitol) and corticosteroids (e.g., dexamethasone) has been beneficial in reducing CSF pressure in rats. However, recent work (Dorman et al., 1988) found this treatment regime to be ineffective in reversing the clinical signs in affected dogs. The survivability of bromethalin-poisoned dogs was increased, however, with early and continued (perhaps for several days) treatment with super-activated charcoal (Superchar-Vet, Gulf Biosystems, Dallas, Texas).

References and Supplemental Reading

Cherry, L. D., Gunnoe, M. D., and Van Lier, R. B. L.: The metabolism of bromethalin and its effects on oxidative phosphorylation and cerebrospinal fluid pressure. Toxicologist 2:108, 1982.

Dorman, D. C., Parker, A. J., and Buck, W. B.: Bromethalin toxicosis in the dog. Manuscript in preparation, 1988.

Jackson, W. B., Spaulding, S. R., Van Lier, R. B. L., et al.: Bromethalin—a promising new rodenticide. Proceedings of the Tenth Vertebrate Pest Conference, University of California, Davis, California, 1982.

Van Lier, R. B. L., and Ottosen, L. D.: Studies on the mechanism of toxicity of bromethalin, a new rodenticide. Toxicologist 1:114, 1981.

DIAGNOSIS OF AND THERAPY FOR CHOLECALCIFEROL TOXICOSIS

DAVID C. DORMAN, D.V.M.,
and VAL RICHARD BEASLEY, D.V.M.

Urbana, Illinois

For many years vitamin D toxicosis in dogs and cats has been infrequently associated with chronic dietary or therapeutic oversupplementation of vitamin D preparations. Recently, however, acute vitamin D intoxication has been frequently associated with the ingestion of rodenticides containing vitamin D_3 (cholecalciferol). Rodenticides containing cholecalciferol (0.075 per cent) have been marketed under the trade names Quintox (Bell Laboratories), Rampage (Ceva Laboratories), and Ortho Rat-B-Gone and Ortho Mouse-B-Gone (Chevron).

The acute oral median lethal dose (LD_{50}) of 100 per cent technical material in dogs has been reported to be 88 mg/kg body weight. However, the Illinois Animal Poison Information Center (IAPIC) has repeatedly received reports of toxicoses in dogs following ingestion of 1 gm bait/lb body weight (2 to 3 mg cholecalciferol/kg body weight). Of the 169 case calls in 1986 involving canine or feline exposures to cholecalciferol rodenticides, 58 were classed as toxicoses or suspected toxicoses. In these 58 calls, 48 dogs and 13 cats displayed compatible clinical signs. No breed predilection was noted, but the majority of dogs were of breeds that as adults have body weights generally under 12 kg. This finding probably represents a higher risk resulting from a greater relative dose. Animals younger than 9 months of age also appeared at high risk, since they represented 53 per cent of the cases. The increased sensitivity of these young animals may be the result of indiscriminate feeding habits, dose response effects due to smaller body size, or increased sensitivity to the action of cholecalciferol and especially its active metabolites.

Calcium homeostasis is under the control of (1) calcitonin, (2) parathyroid hormone (PTH), and (3) vitamin D metabolites. These agents regulate ionized calcium concentrations via control of intestinal uptake, renal excretion, and skeletal mobilization of calcium. Parathyroid hormone elevates serum calcium primarily by stimulating osteoclastic bone resorptive activity. Calcitonin inhibits osteoclastic activity, which lowers serum calcium by antagonism of the PTH effects. Cholecalciferol and especially its active metabolites increase intestinal absorption of calcium, stimulate bone resorption, and increase the renal tubular reabsorption of calcium.

Cholecalciferol, a fat-soluble vitamin, is absorbed with other neutral lipids via chylomicrons into the lymphatic system of mammals. The vitamin is then metabolized by the liver to 25-hydroxycholecalciferol (25-OH-D_3), which becomes the major circulating metabolite during vitamin D excess. Further metabolism of 25-OH-D_3 occurs in the kidney, where calcitriol (1,25-$(OH)_2$-D_3) is produced. Cholecalciferol and 25-hydroxycholecalciferol have limited biologic activity; calcitriol is the most potent cholecalciferol metabolite in terms of enhancing bone resorption and intestinal calcium transport. Cholecalciferol rodenticide poisoning results in an increase in circulating vitamin D metabolites, which causes the development of hypercalcemia (serum calcium > 12 mg/dl), and associated dystrophic calcification.

CLINICAL SIGNS

The clinical signs most commonly associated with cholecalciferol-induced hypercalcemia can be divided into neurologic, cardiovascular, gastrointestinal, and renal. Clinical signs generally develop within 18 to 36 hr following ingestion and include depression, anorexia, polyuria, and polydipsia. Clinical signs become more severe as serum calcium levels rise. Serum calcium concentrations in excess of 16.0 mg/dl are common and are associated with the most severe clinical signs. Metabolic acidosis increases the ionized (physiologically active) fraction of serum calcium via hydrogen ion–induced displacement of calcium from serum albumin. This increase in available calcium may intensify clinical signs.

Calcium is important in maintaining the stability and excitability of cellular membranes. In hypercalcemic states, cardiac conduction is slowed and automaticity is decreased. This is reflected by PR interval prolongation and shortening of the QT interval. With marked hypercalcemia, ventricular fibrillation may result from the associated impairment of conduction or from actual direct myocardial damage secondary to mineralization. In humans, cardiac depression and arrest have been reported with severe (> 20 mg/dl) hypercalcemia. Hypertension occurs in vitamin D toxicosis and may result from arteriolar vasoconstriction. Decreased gastrointestinal smooth muscle excitability is manifested by anorexia, vomiting, and constipation. Neurologic signs commonly include depression, although hypercalcemia-induced seizures occur rarely. Decreased neuromuscular excitability results in generalized weakness.

The renal effects of hypercalcemia depend on the severity, rate of development, and duration of the hypercalcemic state. Tubular injury may be the result of (1) hypercalcemia-induced vasoconstriction resulting in ischemia, (2) mineralization, or, possibly, (3) direct vitamin D nephrotoxicity. Loss of renal concentrating ability, possibly due to a loss of medullary hypertonicity, is the most frequent renal effect of hypercalcemia. The mechanism by which medullary washout occurs is not known but may involve a decrease in glomerular filtration rate (GFR), enhanced medullary blood flow, or inhibition of chloride reabsorption in the loop of Henle. The loss of renal concentrating ability results in the development of polyuria and polydipsia. As hypercalcemia persists, microscopic calcium deposits in the kidney may result in progressive renal insufficiency. However, acute renal failure can occur without the development of renal mineralization. As the toxic effects of hypercalcemia develop, the uremic syndrome usually becomes more severe.

Gastrointestinal and pulmonary hemorrhage sometimes occur as an apparent result of dystrophic calcification, and should not lead to a misdiagnosis of anticoagulant rodenticide toxicosis.

DIAGNOSIS

Diagnosis is based upon a history of a potentially toxic level of exposure to a cholecalciferol-containing rodenticide, appropriate clinical signs, and the development of hypercalcemia. Differential diagnosis of hypercalcemia includes normal juvenile hypercalcemia, cancer-associated (paraneoplastic) hypercalcemia, hypoadrenocorticism, primary renal failure, primary hyperparathyroidism, hemoconcentration (hyperproteinemia), and disuse osteoporosis.

Clinical laboratory evaluation of animals with vitamin D toxicosis generally reveals hypercalcemia, hyperphosphatemia, elevated blood urea nitrogen (BUN), and elevated serum creatinine. The presence of azotemia may be renal or prerenal (dehydration) in origin or due to a combined effect. Urinalysis may reveal hyposthenuria (urine specific gravity of 1.001 to 1.007), proteinuria, and glucosuria. Urine sediment examination occasionally reveals leukocytes, erythrocytes, and casts in variable numbers. Serum concentrations of cholecalciferol and its metabolites may support a diagnosis, but at this time the assays are not widely available.

Radiographic or ultrasonographic examination of affected individuals may reveal mineralization of the kidney and other tissues. In our laboratory, kidney calcium concentrations of animals that died of cholecalciferol toxicosis have ranged from 300 to 1000 ppm on a wet tissue weight basis. In contrast, kidney calcium values of normal animals have ranged from 100 to 150 ppm; in several cases of lethal ethylene glycol toxicosis, kidney calcium concentrations have ranged from 3000 to 12,000 ppm.

Gross lesions associated with cholecalciferol toxicoses commonly involve the kidneys, thyroid glands, gastrointestinal tract, cardiovascular system, and lungs. Kidneys may have irregularly pitted mottled-brown cortical surfaces. Thyroid glands may appear enlarged and pale. Diffuse hemorrhage in the gastric mucosa, duodenum, and jejunum of dogs poisoned with cholecalciferol-based rodenticides has been reported. Cardiovascular lesions include roughened, raised red plaques in the great vessels (e.g., aorta). Similar plaques may also be found on the parietal surface of the lungs and on the surfaces of abdominal viscera. Microscopically evident mineralization of soft tissues in dogs is most pronounced when the serum calcium value (mg/dl) multiplied by the serum phosphate value (mg/dl) exceeds 60. Renal changes are often the most prominent lesions found and include mineral deposition in the tubular epithelial cells.

TREATMENT

The goals of the clinician are (1) to decrease cholecalciferol absorption, (2) to correct fluid and electrolyte imbalances, and (3) to initiate specific therapy to prevent or reduce the hypercalcemic state. Seizure control, treatment of arrhythmias, and other symptomatic therapies may be required. Baseline serum calcium determinations are recommended for all cases of potentially toxic ingestions. These serve as a basis for comparison with subsequent time points. The calcium values obtained are likely to be within the normal range (even when potentially lethal doses are consumed) up to several hours after ingestion.

Detoxification procedures include emesis (apomorphine, 0.04 mg/kg IV) for cases involving recent (< 2 hr) ingestion if the patient is alert and ambulatory. This is generally followed by the administration of activated charcoal (1 to 2 gm/kg) and a saline cathartic (magnesium sulfate at 250 mg/kg in five to ten times as much water). To the authors' knowledge, the efficacy of activated charcoal and saline cathartics in vitamin D toxicosis has not been experimentally demonstrated.

The second phase of therapy is designed to prevent or control the development of a hypercalcemic state by promoting urinary calcium excretion and decreasing calcium influx into the extracellular fluid from the skeletal and gastrointestinal systems. Calciuresis may be enhanced by administering 0.9 per cent sodium chloride (normal saline) IV, because additional sodium presented to the renal tubules diminishes calcium reabsorption. Saline diuresis is recommended in significant (> 0.4 gm bait/kg body weight) ingestions of cholecalciferol-containing rodenticides. In the first 24 hr, diuresis can be accomplished by intravenous or subcutaneous administration of saline. Early diuresis is highly recommended

for individuals at highest risk, including juveniles, animals with pre-existing renal disease, and all animals that have ingested doses likely to cause renal damage or death.

Following significant exposures, serum calcium and BUN are checked 24 hr after exposure. If hypercalcemia (serum calcium > 12 mg/dl) is present or the animal is symptomatic, then further diuresis and additional therapies are indicated. As mentioned previously, a minor percentage of puppies have physiologic hypercalcemia that results in serum calcium values up to 14 mg/dl. When juvenile hypercalcemia is present, it may be difficult and unnecessary to lower the serum calcium value to the normal range for adults. This is an advantage of knowing preonset (< 8 hr after exposure) baseline values.

Calciuresis can be further increased by the use of furosemide. Furosemide, given intravenously at an initial bolus dose of 5 mg/kg followed by a maintenance infusion of 5 mg/kg/hr, has been shown experimentally to reduce serum calcium by a mean value of 2.7 mg/dl in hypercalcemic dogs. When this technique is used, fluid balances must be closely monitored. Unlike maintenance infusions, b.i.d. intravenous injections of furosemide failed to lower serum calcium levels. Experience with cholecalciferol rodenticide toxicoses indicates that furosemide, 2.5 to 4.5 mg/kg PO t.i.d. to q.i.d. in conjunction with saline infusions, can be beneficial in the lowering of hypercalcemia. Thiazide diuretics reduce the urinary excretion of calcium and, therefore, are contraindicated.

Glucocorticosteroids are another component of the regimen employed in treating patients with vitamin D toxicoses. Glucocorticoids work by inhibiting bone resorption, enhancing renal calcium excretion, and decreasing gastrointestinal absorption of calcium. Doses of prednisone, 2 to 3 mg/kg, divided twice daily, will lower serum calcium and can be effective within 24 to 48 hr of administration. Methylprednisolone, 1 mg/kg IV every 2 hr, has been reported to be beneficial in the acute (1 to 3 days postingestion) management of cholecalciferol-induced hypercalcemia. Prednisolone, 4 mg/kg PO, lowered serum calcium in vitamin D–treated rats. The use of prednisolone therapy was associated with an increase in renal calcium concentrations. Although this finding seems to suggest an increased risk of nephrocalcinosis, the use of glucocorticoids has been successful as part of the treatment protocol for vitamin D toxicosis in both humans and domestic animals. Therefore, glucocorticoids are recommended.

Other treatment modalities have been recommended in the acute management of the hypercalcemic crisis. The most commonly used additional treatment is salmon calcitonin, 4 to 6 IU/kg SC every 2 to 3 hr until serum calcium levels stabilize.

Calcitonin is an osteoclast inhibitor and can exert its effects on serum calcium within 12 hr of administration. It is recommended primarily for animals that fail to respond adequately to combined saline, furosemide, and glucocorticoid therapy. The maximal reduction of hypercalcemia in calcitonin-treated humans is approximately 3 mg/dl and occurs 4 to 12 hr after injection. Calcitonin has no effect on the vitamin D–enhanced absorption of calcium from the small intestine and has been of variable benefit in the management of cholecalciferol rodenticide toxicosis. Some hypercalcemic animals become refractory to treatment with calcitonin after several days and redevelop significant hypercalcemia. Concurrent administration of glucocorticoids may prolong the effective time period of calcitonin therapy.

Mithramycin is another potent inhibitor of osteoclastic activity and has been used in the control of cancer-associated hypercalcemia in humans. The use of mithramycin in the management of vitamin D toxicosis has been reported only rarely. In one clinical case involving a dog, mithramycin was used intravenously at a dose of 2 μg/kg/day. Mithramycin is cytotoxic and can cause severe hepatotoxicity, which may limit its usefulness in veterinary medicine at this time. Mithramycin is not recommended in the management of these poisonings.

Inorganic phosphate binds to calcium and, when given orally at 15 mg/kg divided every 6 hr, may be effective in decreasing intestinal calcium absorption. Dosage recommendations are based on the human literature, since approved dosages for dogs and cats are not available. When phosphate is given intravenously, the risk of soft tissue calcification is increased; therefore, administration by parenteral routes is not recommended.

Another treatment modality that has been used only for the management of life-threatening (> 20 mg/dl) hypercalcemia is sodium EDTA administered intravenously. EDTA is potentially nephrotoxic but has been recommended for human patients at a dose of 25 to 75 mg/kg/hr IV. In severely uremic or hypercalcemic animals, peritoneal dialysis with a calcium-free dialysate solution can be used to lower serum calcium concentrations even if other methods have failed. Sodium bicarbonate infusion at 1 to 3 mEq/kg can also be used in the management of the hypercalcemic crisis. The ionized portion of serum calcium is determined in part by acid-base status. By correcting acidosis or creating a slight alkalosis, a portion of the ionized calcium is shifted to the protein-bound fraction, which is less physiologically active. The most commonly employed methods of calcium analysis measure total serum calcium, which tends to remain constant during sodium bicarbonate therapy, despite the anticipated shift toward the bound state.

Cholecalciferol and its metabolites have long physiologic half-lives in affected animals. Vitamin D–induced hypercalcemia sometimes persists for several weeks, necessitating long-term management. After serum calcium is stabilized within the normal range, maintenance therapy consisting of furosemide, 2 to 4.5 mg/kg PO b.i.d., and prednisone, 4 mg/kg divided b.i.d., is advised to be continued for 2 to 4 weeks in animals that had been severely affected (serum calcium > 14 to 16 mg/dl). Adrenocortical suppression is not expected to occur with this dosage regimen. To prevent acute adrenocortical insufficiency, especially if therapy continues beyond 2 weeks, tapering dosages can be begun near the end of the 2-week treatment period.

It is also important to assess response to therapy based on resolution of clinical signs, azotemia, and a stable decrease to normal serum calcium ranges. In vitamin D–poisoned dogs, BUN may be a more sensitive indicator of renal function than creatinine. Since physiologic hypercalcemia of youth in dogs can be associated with normal serum calcium concentrations of 12 to 14 mg/dl, the animal's age and baseline values must be considered when assessing its response to therapy. Animals that develop renal mineralization may regain normal renal function with proper management of the acute renal failure and hypercalcemia. In general, the poorest prognoses for return to normal renal function are given for animals for which there has been a significant delay before the onset of treatment. Animals that ingest a potentially toxic dose (> 0.4 gm bait/kg body weight) of these rodenticides and are treated with fluid therapy alone often have a favorable prognosis, but the institution of emergency measures to prevent initial absorption from the digestive tract is emphasized. Once severe hypercalcemia develops, aggressive medical management is often required, and delays in the initiation of specific therapies are often met with little or no clinical response.

In all instances of significant exposure, a low calcium diet is provided. Low calcium diets include Hill's Prescription Diets s/d, u/d, and k/d. Milk and other dairy products and calcium supplements should be avoided.

TREATMENT SUMMARY

Current treatment recommendations include the use of emetics, activated charcoal, and a saline cathartic in recent exposures. If a potentially toxic amount of these rodenticides is consumed, fluid therapy with normal saline is begun and may need to be continued for 4 to 14 days. Serum calcium and BUN should be determined at the time of admission and 24 hr after exposure. If hypercalcemia (serum calcium > 12 to 14 mg/dl, depending upon age) is present at this time or if it redevelops, normal saline diuresis is continued. In addition, prednisone (2 to 6 mg/kg s.i.d.), furosemide (2.5 to 4.5 mg/kg PO t.i.d. to q.i.d.), and, if needed to maintain normal serum calcium values, salmon calcitonin (4 to 6 IU/kg SC every 2 to 3 hr until serum calcium levels stabilize) are used in the initial treatment. Corticosteroids and furosemide therapy should be continued for a minimum of 2 weeks in affected animals, along with ensuring adequate fluid intake (saline, parenterally, and food and water PO) and monitoring serum calcium and BUN. Animals should be placed on a low calcium diet.

References and Supplemental Reading

Allen, T. A., and Weingard, K.: The vitamin D (calciferol) endocrine system. Comp. Cont. Ed. 7:482, 1985.
Chew, D. J., and Capen C. C.: Hypercalcemic nephropathy and associated disorders. *In* Kirk, R. W. (ed.): *Current Veterinary Therapy VII.* Philadelphia: W. B. Saunders Co., 1980, pp. 1067–1072.
Chew, D. J., and Meuten, D. J.: Disorders of calcium and phosphorous metabolism. Vet. Clin. North Am. 12:411, 1982.
deCristofaro, J. D., and Tsang, R. C.: Calcium. Emerg. Med. Clin. North Am. 4:207, 1986.
Fraser, D. A.: Regulation of the metabolism of vitamin D. Physiol. Rev. 60:551, 1980.
Gunther, R., Felice, L. J., et al.: Toxicity of a vitamin D_3 rodenticide to dogs. J.A.V.M.A. 193:211, 1988.
Haschek, W. M., Krook, L., Kallfelz, F. A., et al.: Vitamin D toxicity: Initial site and mode of action. Cornell Vet. 68:324, 1978.
Kinberg, D. V., Baerg, R. D., Gershon, E., et al.: Effect of cortisone treatment on the active transport of calcium by the small intestine. J. Clin Invest. 50:1309, 1971.
Ong, S. C., Shalhoub, R. J., Gallagher, P., et al.: Effect of furosemide on experimental hypercalcemia in dogs. Proc. Soc. Exp. Biol. Med. 145:227, 1974.
Pages, J. P., and Troulit, J. L.: Nephropathie hypercalcemique: A propos de quatre intoxications aigues par la vitamine D chez le chien. Pratique Medical et Chirurgicale de l'animal de Compagnie 19:293, 1984.
Sjoden, G., and Lindgren, U.: The effect of prednisolone on kidney calcification in vitamin D–treated rats. Calcif. Tiss. Int. 37:613, 1985.
Streck, W. F., Waterhouse, C., and Haddad, J. G.: Glucocorticoid effects in vitamin D intoxication. Arch. Intern. Med. 139:974, 1979.

LEAD POISONING

GERALD R. BRATTON, D.V.M.,
College Station, Texas

and DAVID F. KOWALCZYK, V.M.D.
St. Louis, Missouri

Lead poisoning in animals has probably occurred since its recognition in humans almost 3000 years ago, but it was not until 1969 that the significance of lead poisoning in dogs was recognized. Zook and associates (1972) reported that 1 of every 25 dogs younger than 6 months of age hospitalized at the Angell Memorial Animal Hospital (Boston) had been poisoned by lead. Since 1973, lead poisoning has been the most common toxicity reported in dogs and cats at the School of Veterinary Medicine in Philadelphia, while at the Texas Veterinary Diagnostic Laboratory in College Station it ranked fourth most common in 1987 behind strychnine, antifreeze, and organic insecticides. Although the number of dogs poisoned by lead varies between the large urban and more rural settings, lead should still be a major consideration in animal poisonings in any area of the United States.

Currently there are no data to indicate whether lead poisoning in dogs and cats is increasing or decreasing, whether certain populations are more at risk, or whether the decreasing lead in gasoline and paint has had any effect on the incidence of lead poisoning in animals. The only safe assumption to be made is that any pet animal with signs of neurologic or gastrointestinal disturbance of several days duration could have had exposure to lead.

ABSORPTION, DISTRIBUTION, RETENTION, AND EXCRETION OF LEAD

There is no clearly established normal (safe) level for lead in blood or tissues; no established levels of lead absorption, retention, or excretion for age, breed, sex, or size of animals; no clearly established parameters for laboratory diagnosis; and no specific means of treatment. Moreover, the parameters often given in the literature for levels of absorption, distribution, retention, and excretion of lead in dogs have been extrapolated from studies in animals or humans. This dangerous and often unreliable practice is, however, necessary because specific data for dogs, cats, horses, and cattle are just not available.

The most common route of entry of lead is through the gastrointestinal tract. Inhaled lead particles of large size are cleared by ciliary action and are swallowed, adding to the ingested lead. Only in situations in which animals are exposed to air containing small aerial particles of lead ($< 10 \mu m$) should attention be given to respiratory lead intake. The absorption rate of lead reaching the respiratory alveoli is much higher (> 50 per cent) than that of lead entering the gastrointestinal tract (< 10 per cent). In all animals, the young (dogs and cats younger than 6 months of age) absorb much more of ingested lead than do adults. Absorption levels as high as 90 per cent have been reported for immature rats.

The diverse effects of many dietary factors on the bioavailability of lead have been well documented and probably account for the tremendous variability in measured lead-related parameters from both experimental and clinical case studies. An enhancement or inhibition of lead absorption has been demonstrated in various animals with dietary deficiencies or excesses of calcium, zinc, iron, phosphorus, selenium, copper, sulfur, magnesium, fat, protein, vitamin C, vitamin D, thiamine, B complex vitamins, vitamin E, milk, dietary fiber, and cellulose. Lead dissolves much faster in an acid environment, such as an empty stomach, which thus enhances absorption. In bottom-feeding water fowl, the ingestion of one to three shotgun pellets (which tend to remain in the gizzard) can be lethal.

Once lead has been absorbed, it enters the blood, where over 90 per cent of it becomes associated with the red blood cell (either absorbed into the cell and bound by hemoglobin or associated with the cell membrane). The free lead present in the plasma is rapidly distributed into the soft tissues of the body, with the blood cell–associated lead serving as a replenishing source of free lead over time. The presence of lead in the liver, kidneys, central nervous system, and bone marrow causes the major signs of lead toxicity. The penetration of lead across the blood-brain barrier occurs more readily in immature animals, accounting for the higher incidence of severe neurologic signs in young animals. Lead also directly crosses the placenta and can produce lead poisoning in the newborn. Eventually, lead redistributes from the blood and soft tissue to bone, where it is biologically inert until physiologic reabsorption of bone mineral occurs (acidosis, hyperparathyroidism, pregnancy, or calcium deficiency), which causes toxicity.

Lead is excreted very slowly from the whole body, predominantly into the bile, although the major route of excretion varies among species. The enterohepatic circulation of lead is not known. The elimination of lead through urine is minimal in dogs and cats unless chelating agents (e.g., calcium disodium edetate [$CaNa_2EDTA$]) are used. Liver and bone account for approximately 90 per cent of retained body lead levels. Liver levels have been reported to be from 2 to 25 per cent and bone levels from 60 to 98 per cent.

The concentration of lead in blood can fluctuate greatly, depending on the time of exposure. The blood lead concentration does not reflect tissue lead concentrations or the extent of lead toxicity; nor does it correlate with the severity of clinical signs or the success of chelation therapy. Even with treatment, it may require from 2 to 9 months for blood lead to return to levels below 15 μg/dl.

SOURCES OF LEAD

The sources of lead are numerous and varied, the most common being lead-containing paint. Interiors of dwellings painted before 1950 often contain layers of lead-based paint. Leaded paints are sometimes mistakenly used indoors even today and, thus, may be accessible to dogs in new as well as old houses. So-called lead-free paints can contain up to 1.0 per cent lead and still meet current government specifications. The lead salts in paint impart a sweet taste, making them quite palatable to animals. Lead paint continues to account for more than 50 per cent of lead toxicity in pet animals.

Other sources of lead include batteries, linoleum, solder, plumbing material and supplies, grease and lubricating compounds, putty, tar paper, lead foil, golf balls, roofing materials, caulking materials, plasterboard, rug pad, toys, lead pipes (especially when used with soft water), canned dog foods or cat foods, improperly glazed ceramic water or food bowls, lead window weights, fishing sinkers, drapery weights, insulation, lead emissions that settle out on soil or vegetation, house dust, burnt lubrication oil, shotgun pellets, ink (newsprint), and dyes. Lead bullets or shotgun pellets that are present subcutaneously or in muscle tissue usually become encapsulated and are biologically inert.

AGE

Lead poisoning may occur at any age, but most affected dogs are younger than 1 year old. Teething, curiosity, and the bizarre appetites of young dogs result in the gnawing on and ingestion of strange objects and play a role in the increased incidence of lead poisoning in young dogs.

SEASON

A seasonal occurrence (summer and fall) has been indicated in both children and pets, as the majority of clinical cases seem to occur between June and October in the United States. Vitamin D changes that increase lead absorption and the fact that animals are outdoors and roaming more during these months have been used to explain this finding.

However, lead poisoning in Australia also occurs during these same months, which represent winter and spring in that hemisphere.

CLINICAL SIGNS

Clinical signs of lead poisoning in dogs and cats are generally associated with the gastrointestinal and nervous systems. Usually, both systems are clinically involved, but one or the other may predominate. In some cases, only one system may be involved. As a rule, the nervous system signs predominate in acute, high levels of exposure to lead, whereas gastrointestinal signs result from lower, long-term exposures. Very often, gastrointestinal signs are present for several days before the dog is examined, and they frequently precede the neurologic signs. Such clinical signs in young dogs may be mistaken for canine distemper.

The most common gastrointestinal signs are vomiting, abdominal pain, tense abdomen, and anorexia. Diarrhea and constipation are less frequently observed. The presence of abdominal pain or "lead colic" is manifested by whining, restlessness, abdominal splinting, and crying when the abdomen is palpated. Many gastrointestinal disturbances display similar signs, but lead toxicity should be suspected if the signs persist for more than 3 days. Occasionally, megaesophagus has been associated with lead poisoning and is probably the result of esophageal paralysis.

The most common neurologic signs in order of frequency are convulsions, hysteria (characterized by barking and crying continuously, running in many directions without purpose, and indiscriminantly biting at animate and inanimate objects), and other behavioral changes. Ataxia, tremors, papillary changes, blindness, and clamping of the jaws are also observed. Many dogs with hysteria or convulsions have increased rectal temperatures that decrease after episodes subside.

LABORATORY FINDINGS

One of the most helpful screening tests for the diagnosis of lead poisoning in dogs, but not necessarily other animals, is examination of a stained blood smear. Of prime importance is the finding of large numbers of nucleated erythrocytes (5 to 40 nucleated erythrocytes/100 white blood cells) without evidence of severe anemia (packed cell volume less than 30 per cent). The nucleated erythrocytes are a relatively easy cell type to identify regardless of the staining procedure. However, other diseases can cause nucleated erythrocytes to appear in circulation, and lead toxicity does not always produce nucleated erythrocytes.

Other common abnormalities in red blood cell morphology are anisocytosis, polychromasia, poikilocytosis, target cells, and hypochromasia. Basophilic stippling is currently considered of little use by most authorities.

Red blood cell abnormalities usually precede clinical signs except in very acute poisoning. Once chelation therapy has been started, these changes disappear quickly.

The leukocyte counts are usually elevated because of a neutrophilic leukocytosis. It is important to correct the white blood cell count for the presence of nucleated erythrocytes; otherwise, falsely exaggerated white blood cell counts result.

Bone marrow examination discloses an increase of erythroid elements. Elevated reticulocyte counts and the finding of many immature red blood cells in peripheral blood smears indicate early release of erythroid cells from the hyperplastic bone marrow. The urine usually contains granular casts. Often, mild proteinuria and, sometimes, glycosuria are found. Lead levels in urine are so variable that single sample evaluation is of little value. The cerebrospinal fluid usually has normal pressure, protein, and cell count.

Other tests that have become very useful in cases of human lead poisoning are related to detection of abnormalities in heme synthesis. The interference of lead at several enzymatic steps has proved to be the most sensitive indicator of biologic change. Aminolevulinic acid dehydrase (ALAD) is extremely sensitive to lead, and its activity becomes depressed at a blood lead level of 15 μg/dl in humans. Currently, levels of ALAD in blood and delta-aminolevulinic acid (ALA) in urine are not practical indicators of clinical lead toxicosis in cats and dogs.

Zinc protoporphyrin (ZPP) accumulates in erythrocytes in lead poisoning owing to the inhibition of ferrochelatase, the enzyme responsible for the insertion of iron into the heme molecule. Zinc is substituted for iron and remains in the heme molecule for the life span of the erythrocyte. Blood lead levels above 50 μg/dl failed to alter blood ZPP levels until the eighth week of daily lead dosing, and clinical signs of lead poisoning occurred in one dog long before ZPP levels changed. The appearance of clinical signs was not well correlated with ZPP.

One of the major drawbacks of the laboratory tests previously described is the absence of normal data for dogs and cats. In addition, the effects of high-dose lead intake (acute exposure) and low-dose intake over long periods (chronic exposure) on these parameters have not been adequately evaluated. Until these data are available, the value of these tests in lead toxicity in dogs must remain questionable.

RADIOGRAPHIC FINDINGS

The most helpful radiographic finding is the presence of diffuse radiopaque material in the gastrointestinal tract or the finding of lead objects that should be surgically removed (fishing sinker, window weight). However, it should be emphasized that it is impossible to differentiate these radiodensities from bone chips or gravel. It is important to have radiographs taken of the animal, since chelation therapy may enhance intestinal absorption of lead.

The metaphyses of long bones in rapidly growing young dogs may develop lead lines (metaphyseal sclerosis). These radiopaque bands are best seen just proximal to the open epiphysis of the distal radius, ulna, and metacarpal bones. Lead lines are difficult to distinguish, even for radiologists and, as a diagnostic indicator, have not been useful.

DIAGNOSIS

Since the signs of lead poisoning are not pathognomonic, a history detailing the likelihood of exposure or the finding of many nucleated erythrocytes without anemia may be the first clue in dogs. Blood may be taken for lead analysis to confirm the diagnosis, but treatment for lead poisoning should be started.

The analysis of heparinized whole blood for lead content is the best single index for establishing a definitive diagnosis. Many laboratories can now perform a lead analysis with less than 2 ml of whole, oxalated, or heparinized blood collected in a clean, lead-free vial. However, it is wise to contact the laboratory toxicologist directly to determine the minimum volume required, as it is usually less than the amount stated in their brochure. Versenate (EDTA) anticoagulant interferes with some methods and should be avoided. Even though there is no established normal blood lead level, the non–lead-exposed dogs we have measured at Texas A&M University over the last year have had blood lead levels of 3 to 12 μg/dl (0.03 to 0.12 ppm). The finding of 60 μg/dl (0.6 ppm) or more of blood lead has been reported to be virtually diagnostic of lead poisoning in dogs. However, a diagnosis of lead poisoning should never be made based on blood lead values alone. In experimental situations, dogs with blood lead levels in excess of 100 μg/dl (1.0 ppm) frequently do not show signs, whereas dogs with blood lead levels lower than 60 μg/dl (< 0.6 ppm) on occasion display both gastrointestinal and neurologic signs. One must also keep in mind that a blood lead measurement reflects a static point in a system that constantly fluctuates. Blood lead values of 30 to 50 μg/dl (0.3 to 0.5 ppm) are abnormally high and indicate lead poisoning if associated with typical signs and hematologic findings. As a general rule, levels of blood lead below 25 μg/dl (0.25 ppm) are rarely associated with poisoning. The small difference between background and toxic blood lead levels make interpretation of this test difficult at the lower levels. It is important to remember that the severity of clinical signs, the levels of lead in the body tissues, the length of lead exposure, and the actual state of health of the animal have no correlation with the blood lead content.

Currently, the best means to assess the body lead burden is to use the calcium disodium ethylenediaminetetra-acetate (CaNa$_2$EDTA) mobilization test. It is unfortunate that this test requires a 24-hr urine collection and is time consuming and expensive; however, it can be a valuable aid to treatment. A 24-hr urine sample is taken, followed by treatment with 75 mg/kg of CaNa$_2$EDTA and collection of a second 24-hr urine sample. The level of lead excretion following chelation treatment compared with the pretreatment level correlates with the body burden of lead. Increases of 10- to 60-fold have been reported.

For post-mortem confirmation, analysis of liver for lead is the best diagnostic test. The upper limit of normal is 3.5 ppm (wet weight); 5 ppm or more is virtually diagnostic. Samples of hair or feces or single specimens of urine for lead analysis are not recommended. However, fecal levels correlated with blood lead levels may have merit. High levels of blood lead plus high levels of fecal lead may indicate very recent exposure, whereas high levels of blood lead plus low levels of fecal lead may indicate exposure 3 or 4 weeks prior to sampling. This two-way evaluation may become even more valuable if metabolic indicators of lead toxicity become better adapted for dogs.

TREATMENT

The purposes of therapy in lead poisoning are to (1) remove lead, if present, from the gastrointestinal tract so that further absorption is prevented, (2) remove lead from the blood and body tissues as rapidly as possible, (3) alleviate marked neurologic signs, and (4) identify the source of lead and prevent re-exposure. Prevention of re-exposure may be the most important point to emphasize to the client.

Lead should be removed from the gastrointestinal tract with enemas and emetics prior to chelation therapy because chelating agents (especially oral agents) can enhance the absorption of lead from the intestines. Magnesium sulfate (Epsom salt) or sodium sulfate are the drugs of choice, since they precipitate lead (as PbSO$_4$) and prevent further absorption during transit; they also possess mild and safe cathartic action. Large objects in the stomach or intestines may require surgery.

Chelating agents effectively remove heavy metals by forming nontoxic, water-soluble complexes with the metal that can, in turn, be rapidly excreted via the urine or bile. The chelating agent of choice is $CaNa_2EDTA$, which has been shown to be effective in treating lead poisoning in a wide variety of animals. This drug must be administered as the calcium chelate to prevent hypocalcemia. The need to purchase the calcium disodium salt (Calcium Disodium Versenate, Riker) cannot be overemphasized, because the disodium salt (Disodium Versenate, Riker) carries a similar name on a similar label and is available from the same company. This matter is further complicated by the various abbreviations and names given to $CaNa_2EDTA$. $CaNa_2EDTA$ is available for use in humans or small pets as a 20 per cent solution in 5-ml ampules (total of 1 gm) and for use in large dogs, horses, or cattle as a 6.6 per cent solution in 500-ml bottles (total of 33 gm) (Havidote, Haver-Lockhart). The larger volume is more economical for larger animals. However, since no preservatives are added, care should be exercised in multiple dosing from the same bottle, and fractional contents should not be saved for future use.

$CaNa_2EDTA$ is usually given at the rate of 100 mg/kg body weight daily for 2 to 5 days; although dosage levels of 75 to 110 mg/kg are published in the literature. The daily dose is divided into four equal portions and is administered subcutaneously (SC) after dilution to a concentration of about 10 mg $CaNa_2EDTA$/ml 5 per cent dextrose solution. High concentrations of $CaNa_2EDTA$ can cause pain at the injection site. Lidocaine can be mixed with the injection solution, if necessary, to further control pain. $CaNa_2EDTA$ can be given by slow intravenous (IV) drip, the common route of treatment in humans, and is probably more effective but much more time consuming and troublesome by that route. Dosing should never continue longer than 5 consecutive days, since $CaNa_2EDTA$ has been shown to produce renal damage; to depress DNA turnover, thus affecting normal growth of the intestinal epithelium; and to produce a 10- to 50-fold increase in the excretion of zinc. The total daily dose in dogs should not exceed 2 gm in order to minimize renal damage. Multiple treatments can be utilized in combinations of 5 days treatment followed by 5 days rest, if necessary, to alleviate lead poisoning. The 5-day rest period allows the body to recover its normal physiologic function. Experimentally, ZnCaEDTA has been shown to be as effective as $CaNa_2EDTA$ in removing lead and to alleviate the problem with zinc excretion; however, ZnCaEDTA is not commercially available. Consideration should be given to dietary zinc supplementation (2.0 mg/kg/day) in dogs being fed diets suspected to be low in zinc or in dogs given multiple chelation treatments. Dosing should be performed during the periods of $CaNa_2EDTA$ treatment. Copper and iron are also lost through chelation treatment, but usually not at significant levels.

There is a rapid drop in blood lead concentration over the first 1 to 3 days of treatment, depending on the initial blood lead concentration. However, it will then remain constant despite continued therapy and may remain in the toxic range (> 40 μg/dl). There is no correlation between the improvement in clinical signs and the decrease in blood lead; thus, the monitoring of blood lead levels during treatment is not valuable. The rapid change in blood lead levels is probably due to the fact that $CaNa_2EDTA$ removes lead primarily from the extracellular space and from bone rather than from intracellular stores. The lowering of tissue lead levels results as the lead in soft tissue redistributes to bone from which lead was removed. It is much more important to evaluate the animal's clinical condition than to rely on blood lead values as a guide to length of treatment. However, a blood lead determination taken 10 days after the initial day of treatment and again 2 to 3 weeks after cessation of chelation therapy can help determine when to stop chelation therapy or may indicate reexposure. The dangerous rebounds in blood lead levels that sometimes occur following chelation therapy would also be observed. These rebounds are dangerous only if they go undetected and are allowed to remain for long periods of time. The major reason for continuing to develop and evaluate metabolic assays of lead effects is the assessment of treatment effectiveness.

The use of $CaNa_2EDTA$ has been extremely effective. Clinical improvement occurs in 24 to 48 hr after $CaNa_2EDTA$ treatment has been started. Dogs that respond (clinically improve) slowly or that have a pretreatment blood lead level of more than 100 μg/dl (1.0 ppm) may need multiple treatments to recover completely. The additional treatments prevent recurrence of clinical signs, provided the animal is not allowed to consume more lead after discharge from the hospital. It is important that an all-out attempt be made to identify the source of lead and to send the animal home to an environment in which it will not be exposed to more lead.

$CaNa_2EDTA$ can produce acute necrotizing nephrosis of proximal convoluted tubules that is reversible; however, the renal changes appear to be more severe in rats and humans than in dogs. In dogs, $CaNa_2EDTA$ causes depression and gastrointestinal signs (e.g., vomiting, diarrhea) that precede the renal changes. Since these signs are similar to the gastrointestinal signs of lead poisoning, their occurrence after initiation of chelation therapy is difficult to interpret. However, zinc alleviates these signs if they are related to $CaNa_2EDTA$. When they occur during therapy, continued lead exposure and $CaNa_2EDTA$ toxicity should be considered.

Two precautions should be considered in the use of CaNa₂EDTA.

1. An adequate oral intake of fluids must be ensured, and CaNa₂EDTA should never be given in the absence of an adequate urine flow. If possible, urinalysis, BUN, serum creatinine, and liver function tests should be carefully monitored throughout the period of chelation therapy. These tests will signal impending renal failure, at which point alternative therapy can be considered.

2. Rapid mobilization of lead from bone can aggravate signs of lead poisoning or kill dogs with very high blood lead concentrations or dogs with extremely high body burdens of lead. Animals exposed to low or moderate levels of lead for extended periods of time may have moderately elevated blood lead levels (35 to 50 μg/dl), but their tissues may be loaded with lead. If possible, the urine lead levels should be measured prior to the initiation of chelation treatment and after the first 24 hr of therapy. If the increased lead excretion is extremely high (> 1000 μg/l), very careful monitoring of the animal should be initiated around the clock for the entire 5 day-treatment period.

Recent work in the authors' laboratory (Bratton et al., 1981) has shown that thiamine (vitamin B₁) may be effective in treating and preventing lead intoxication in ruminants. Both experimentally poisoned calves and clinically poisoned cattle have responded favorably to thiamine treatment. Flora and colleagues (1986) have further shown that thiamine used in conjunction with CaNa₂EDTA enhanced the chelation effectiveness of CaNa₂EDTA in lead-poisoned rats. The authors have observed similar enhancement in lead-poisoned cattle. The combination of thiamine and CaNa₂EDTA was particularly effective in reducing both the brain concentration of lead and the neurologic signs. However, thiamine must be used with caution, as its use is not entirely without risk. Intravenous use has caused anaphylactic shock and allergic reactions. Dosages of thiamine have not been evaluated in dogs, but 2 mg/kg of body weight given intramuscularly at the same time as CaNa₂EDTA (total thiamine dose 8 mg/kg/day) is effective in cattle. Until dosage has been established in dogs, it is recommended that the same dosages recommended for cattle be utilized in dogs. The authors have given dogs total doses of thiamine up to 5 gm/day for 7 days without adverse effects.

The only oral chelating agent is D-penicillamine, commercially available as 250-mg scored tablets (Depen Titratable Tablets, Wallace) or in 125-mg capsules (Cuprimine, Merck, Sharp & Dohme). The drug should be given to the patient only when the stomach is empty (30 min before a single daily feeding) to prevent chelation of dietary metals. The daily dose can be divided and given at 6- to 8-hr intervals to prevent some of the adverse effects,

such as vomiting, listlessness, and partial anorexia. Antiemetic drugs (e.g., phenothiazines and antihistamine) have been of benefit when given 30 min to 1 hr before the dose of D-penicillamine. Dimenhydrinate (Dramamine, Searle), 2 to 4 mg/kg PO, is the pre-medication of choice; D-penicillamine should be given at 110 mg/kg body weight daily for 2 weeks, followed by a week of no therapy. Multiple periods of therapy may be necessary for total recovery. Lower doses of D-penicillamine (33 to 55 mg/kg daily) seem to be better tolerated by dogs and may be just as efficacious in eliminating body stores of lead. The contents of the capsule or tablet can be dissolved in fluids (fruit juice) for ease of administration, since D-penicillamine is stable at acid pH. At present, this drug can be recommended for dogs that are not seriously ill or that do not have marked neurologic disorders or persistent vomiting. Also, D-penicillamine can be used as follow-up therapy to an initial 5-day treatment with CaNa₂EDTA if necessary, and the dog can be treated at home. If the owner refuses hospitalization for the dog, D-penicillamine can be prescribed for home treatment; however, the owner should be fully warned that side effects may occur and that additional lead ingested while on treatment will be highly absorbed and will result in severe consequences for the animal.

D-Penicillamine severely affects animals with penicillin allergies and can cause renal damage. Drastic decreases in neutrophil counts have been reported in humans, and vitamin B₆ deficiencies have resulted from multiple treatments in children and adults. Although these considerations have not been reported in dogs, the possibility of such problems should not be totally ignored.

D-Penicillamine might also be beneficial in combination with CaNa₂EDTA. It may be that CaNa₂EDTA needs to be given for only a few days followed by D-penicillamine. This regimen would be less likely to produce dehydration, would promote renal function, and would help reduce the time and cost of treatment. D-Penicillamine might also be useful in treating dogs that recover slowly after a 5-day course of CaNa₂EDTA or that had an initial blood lead of more than 100 μg/dl (1.0 ppm) and therefore should be treated again.

2,3-Dimercaptosuccinic acid (DMSA) (Succimer) is an antischistosomal drug that has been used for some time in the Soviet Union and China as an oral chelating agent for lead poisoning; however, it is still an experimental drug in the United States. This drug may quickly become the drug of choice for lead poisoning in animals and is expected to become commercially available in 1989.

Many pet birds, birds of prey, game birds, exotic birds, and water fowl that have ingested lead shot, paint chips, or lead objects retain the lead material in their ventriculus (gizzard) for extended periods, during which time lead is continuously being released and absorbed. A ventriculotomy is often necessary. However, the surgery may be delayed until the bird's condition improves with chelation therapy.

SUPPORTIVE TREATMENT

The gastrointestinal signs (e.g., vomiting, diarrhea, anorexia) do not usually require specific drug therapy because they subside quickly after chelation therapy. However, the severe neurologic signs (e.g., convulsions) are due to cerebral edema and thus require immediate attention. Mannitol, dimethyl sulfoxide (DMSO), and dexamethasone are the agents of choice. The use of barbiturates may also be indicated, since they decrease cerebral blood flow and cellular metabolism. Mannitol is given by slow intravenous injection (30-min infusion) at a dose of 1 to 2 gm/kg and should be repeated in 3 hr.

PROGNOSIS

The prognosis in the majority of lead poisoning patients (95 per cent) that undergo chelation therapy is favorable, with a dramatic improvement in 24 to 48 hr. Thus, chelation therapy may be used as a diagnostic tool in cases of high suspicion where a blood lead determination is impractical or delayed. Prognosis in patients treated promptly and adequately depends on the degree and duration of neurologic involvement and, to a lesser extent, on the amount of lead found in the blood. Continuous or uncontrolled convulsions warrant an unfavorable prognosis. Some dogs with blood lead levels of 100 μg/dl or greater tend to recover slowly, and signs may recur if a second course of therapy is not given. If there are no neurologic signs or if signs are mild or readily controlled by ancillary treatment, the prognosis is favorable regardless of the blood lead level.

The prognosis in untreated patients that are displaying only gastrointestinal signs should be favorable if further exposure to lead is prevented. If the economic situation does not permit treatment with CaNa$_2$EDTA, a course of oral D-penicillamine may be utilized.

PATHOLOGIC FINDINGS

Gross necropsy findings are generally not remarkable; however, careful examination may reveal chips of paint or other lead-containing substances in the gastrointestinal tract. White bands are sometimes found in transversely sectioned metaphyses

of immature dogs. Microscopic study may disclose acid-fast intranuclear inclusion bodies in renal proximal tubular cells and, less often, in hepatocytes. These inclusions are pathognomonic of lead poisoning but are seldom seen. They are rapidly removed by CaNa$_2$EDTA therapy and are often absent if the animal was treated for several days prior to death. Lesions in the brain include degenerative changes in small vessels, hemorrhages, laminar necrosis, and proliferation of capillaries and gliosis in chronic encephalopathies.

VETERINARIAN'S OBLIGATION

For detecting lead poisoning, young dogs are the most appropriate sentinel animals because they share the same environment and eating habits (e.g., pica) as children. A recent study from Illinois indicated that an abnormally high blood lead level in a family dog increased the probability sixfold of finding a child in the same family with an increased blood lead level.

When lead poisoning is diagnosed in pets belonging to owners who have small children, veterinarians should warn the family and family physician that a danger exists in all young children exposed to the same environment. Most urban centers have clinics for testing children for lead, free of charge.

LEAD POISONING IN OTHER PETS

Cats are rarely poisoned by lead because, unlike dogs, they are very selective eaters and seldom gnaw on or ingest nonfood substances. Therefore, they are not subject to most sources of lead. However, because of their fastidious fur-cleaning habits, they may ingest lead-containing dust, paint scrapings, or other substances that contaminate the coat. When lead poisoning does occur in the cat, the signs, diagnosis, treatment, and prognosis are similar to those previously described.

Parrots, and other caged birds, may pick at and ingest peeling paint, or if the bars of their cages are painted, they may ingest the paint while clambering about or trimming their beaks. Numerous pet and zoo parrots have died of lead poisoning. In Amazon parrots, hemoglobinuria associated with intravascular hemolysis has been associated with lead poisoning. Any curious pet with indiscriminate eating traits that is exposed to lead is a likely candidate for lead intoxication.

References and Supplemental Reading

Bratton, G. R., Childress, M., Zmudzki, J., et al.: Delta-aminolevulinic acid dehydrase activity in erythrocytes from cattle administered low concentrations of lead acetate. Am. J. Vet. Res. 47:2068, 1986.

Bratton, G. R., Zmudzki, J., Bell, M. C., et al.: Thiamin (vitamin B₁) effects on lead intoxication and deposition of lead in tissues: Therapeutic potential. Toxicol. Appl. Pharmacol. 59:164, 1981.

Center, S. A.: Suspected calcium EDTA intoxication in a dog. J.A.V.M.A. 183:884, 1983.

Flora, S. J. S., Singh, S., and Tandon, S. K.: Chelation in metal intoxication XVIII: Combined effects of thiamine and Calcium Disodium Versenate on lead toxicity. Life Sci. 38:67, 1986.

George, J. W., and Duncan, J. R.: The hematology of lead poisoning in man and animals. Vet. Clin. Pathol. 8:23, 1979.

Kowalczyk, D. F.: Lead poisoning in dogs at the University of Pennsylvania Veterinary Hospital. J.A.V.M.A. 168:428, 1976.

Kowalczyk, D. F.: Clinical management of lead poisoning. J.A.V.M.A. 184:858, 1984.

Schunk, K. L.: Lead poisoning in dogs. Small Anim. Vet. Med. Update 8:2, 1978.

Stowe, H. D., Goyer, R. A., Krigman, M. M., et al.: Experimental oral lead toxicity in young dogs. Arch. Pathol. 95:106, 1973.

Thomas, C. W., Rising, J. L., and Moore, J. K.: Blood lead concentrations of children and dogs from 83 Illinois families. J.A.V.M.A. 169:1237, 1976.

Zook, B. C., Carpenter, J. L., and Leeds, E. B.: Lead poisoning in dogs. J.A.V.M.A. 155:1329, 1969.

Zook, B. C., Kopito, L., Carpenter, J. L., et al.: Lead poisoning in dogs: Analysis of blood, urine, hair, and liver for lead. Am. J. Vet. Res. 33:903, 1972.

ARSENIC POISONING

REGG D. NEIGER, D.V.M.

Brookings, South Dakota

SOURCE

Arsenic is a ubiquitous element present naturally in many environmental sources that rarely cause a toxicologic problem. Smelters may release arsenic trioxide into the surrounding environment. There is a risk of poisoning with commercial arsenicals, especially pesticides. Arsenic poisoning is seen more frequently in cats than dogs. Roach and ant baits are common sources of arsenic poisoning in cats. The route of exposure is usually oral, but systemic toxicosis can result from percutaneous exposure (Evinger and Blakemore, 1984). In small animals, the organic arsenical thiacetarsamide is used for treatment of dirofilariasis. Systemic poisoning may occur when treating an apparently healthy dog (see pp. 131–134).

Toxicity of arsenicals is affected by many factors. Organic arsenicals in general are less hazardous than inorganic arsenicals. Trivalent arsenic is four to ten times more toxic than pentavalent compounds. Weak, debilitated, and dehydrated animals have greater susceptibility to arsenic toxicosis. Because many factors affect toxicity, the lethal oral dose of sodium arsenite in most species falls within a range of 1 to 25 mg/kg of body weight. Cats are one of the more susceptible species, with the lethal dosage being less than 5 mg/kg of sodium arsenite. Sodium arsenite is one of the most toxic arsenicals because it is inorganic, highly water soluble, and trivalent.

Trivalent arsenicals interact with sulfhydryl group compounds in biologic systems, especially by inactivation of enzymes, coenzymes, and substrates. Pentavalent arsenicals are reduced to more toxic trivalent forms *in vivo*. Pentavalent arsenic ion (arsenate) can substitute for phosphate in many important metabolic reactions. The arsenate esters formed undergo spontaneous hydrolysis, causing interruption of metabolic pathways (Squibb and Fowler, 1983).

TOXICOSIS

Inorganic and trivalent aliphatic arsenicals cause similar toxicoses (NAS, 1977). In general, signs and lesions are similar when arsenic is administered orally or parenterally.

ACUTE TO SUBACUTE TOXICOSIS. Peracute and acute oral poisonings have dramatic signs and high morbidity and mortality rates. Signs may occur within minutes, and death may occur in hours. Progression of signs includes intense abdominal pain; salivation; vomiting; staggering gait and weakness; diarrhea; rapid, weak pulse; prostration; subnormal temperature; collapse; and death.

Subacute oral poisoning results in death in several days. Anorexia and oliguria often develop. The urine contains protein, red blood cells, and casts (NAS, 1977; Osweiler et al., 1985).

Peracute poisoning causes death so rapidly that no gross or microscopic lesions may be present. Gross lesions of acute and subacute poisoning consist of diffuse reddening of the mucosa of the stomach and proximal small intestine; variable amounts of watery fluid in the gastrointestinal tract; a soft, yellow liver; and wet, red lungs. If the animal lives more than 18 hr, edema, hemorrhage, and necrosis of the gastrointestinal tract cause blood and shreds of mucosa to be present in the stool. Perforation of the stomach or intestine may occur. There is splanchnic congestion with petechial hemorrhage of serous membranes. Hemorrhages are especially prominent in the heart (NAS, 1977; Sullivan, 1985). Gastrointestinal lesions are the most consistent and prominent of those listed. The others may not be present.

If poisoning occurs by skin contact, many of the same systemic signs previously described occur. However, skin lesions are prominent, with blistering, edema, cracking, bleeding, and secondary infection (NAS, 1977; Evinger and Blakemore, 1984).

SUBCHRONIC TO CHRONIC TOXICOSIS. There is little documentation of spontaneous chronic arsenic poisoning in animals. Subchronic to chronic exposure to dietary inorganic arsenic causes a dose-dependent weight loss or reduced weight gain (Byron et al., 1967; Neiger, 1987). In the author's laboratory, weight loss in dogs was shown to be an effect of feed rejection, not a direct effect of arsenic.

Although the liver and the kidneys are major target organs in acute poisonings, only subtle changes occur consistently in chronic studies (Byron et al., 1967; Neiger, 1987). With regard to the liver and the kidneys, mild increases in leakage of the enzymes serum glutamic-oxaloacetic transaminase (SGOT) and serum glutamate pyruvate transaminase (SGPT) from the liver were the only clinical pathologic changes in dogs chronically exposed to dietary arsenic.

Anemia has been reported in cases of arsenic intoxication in dogs (Byron et al., 1967).

DIAGNOSIS

If an animal is presented with a clinical picture consistent with arsenic poisoning, as previously described, arsenic analyses should be used to confirm the diagnosis. Specimens of value include urine, liver, kidney, hair, gastrointestinal content, and the suspected source of contamination. To determine if poisoning has occurred, the arsenic concentrations in specimens must be evaluated in light of the circumstances of each case. One must take into account the signs exhibited by the animal, species of animal, type of specimen, time since exposure, exposure route, and type of arsenical.

Urine is the specimen of choice in the evaluation of current arsenic exposure. In poisoning cases, urine arsenic levels vary from 2 to 100 ppm, depending on the factors just listed (Osweiler et al., 1985). Urine arsenic levels drop dramatically within days of the end of exposure. Kidney and liver tissues are the next best choice after urine. Concentrations of elemental arsenic greater than 10 ppm on a wet weight basis in the liver and kidneys confirm arsenic poisoning (Osweiler et al., 1985; Clark et al., 1981). Normal liver and kidney arsenic values are less than 0.5 ppm. Liver and kidney arsenic concentrations

drop rapidly after arsenic exposure stops. Hair is an excellent indicator of chronic arsenic exposure. There is a dose-dependent relationship between hair, arsenic concentration, and chronic arsenic exposure. However, confirmation of poisoning from arsenic concentration in hair is not well documented. Beagles used as control subjects at the author's laboratory had hair concentrations of 0.4 ppm of elemental arsenic. With exposures of up to 4 mg of dietary sodium arsenite per kilogram of body weight per day for 6 months, hair concentrations were 25 ppm of elemental arsenic (dogs were asymptomatic). Blood arsenic concentration is not a useful indicator of exposure in domestic species.

PROGNOSIS AND TREATMENT

Prognosis is grave unless the diagnosis is made and treatment is started before clinical signs are advanced (Furr, 1977; Osweiler et al., 1985). Treatment should be designed to remove arsenic from the stomach, inactivate arsenic remaining in the gastrointestinal tract, protect the gastrointestinal tract, reverse the toxic syndrome, and reinstate the animal's homeostatic equilibrium (Furr, 1977).

If poisoning signs are not present, small animals should have their stomachs emptied. This can be accomplished using a warm water or 1 per cent sodium bicarbonate solution gastric lavage (Osweiler et al., 1985). Depending on the solubility and concentration of the arsenical ingested, the time before onset of vomiting can range from several minutes to several hours. Gastric lavage should not be used if vomiting has already occurred. In the author's experience, the rapid onset of vomiting protects dogs from severe toxicosis, depending on the amount of arsenic absorbed before the animal vomited. In other cases, especially in cats, if the arsenical ingested is highly concentrated and water soluble, a lethal dose will be absorbed even if vomiting starts within minutes of ingestion.

Dimercaprol (British anti-Lewisite, BAL) is a sulfhydryl-containing compound that chelates arsenic. BAL is not very effective in advanced cases, so it should be given early after exposure. BAL itself is toxic, and therapy should be administered with care and clinical judgment. Signs of BAL toxicosis are vomiting, tremors, convulsions, coma, and death. However, toxic effects of BAL at therapeutic levels are not severe and reverse as the drug is excreted. BAL is excreted rapidly over a period of 3 to 4 hr. Therefore, it is best to administer recommended doses of BAL at recommended (frequent) intervals to maximize therapeutic, and minimize toxic, effects (Hatch, 1982). Arsenic stored in tissues may be mobilized by chelator treatment, causing increased circulating arsenic and exacerbation of clinical signs of arsenic toxicosis. If this happens, a little extra chelator (BAL) might be given. If therapy makes the animal worse over 2 to 3 days, the BAL dose may be too large for that animal (Hatch, 1982). When BAL binds to arsenic, the resulting relatively nontoxic complex is water soluble, is readily excreted in the urine, and should be susceptible to dialysis. The literature on poisoning in humans suggests that hemodialysis is effective in removing arsenic and its BAL complex, but intraperitoneal dialysis is of questionable value (Gosselin et al., 1984). The main indication for dialysis should be arsenic-induced renal failure.

In small animals, the dose of BAL is 2.5 to 5 mg/kg of body weight, given intramuscularly as a 10 per cent solution in oil. The dosage of 5 mg/kg of body weight should be used only in acute cases and only on the first day of treatment. Injections should be repeated every 4 hr for the first 2 days, every 8 hr on the third day, and twice a day for the next 10 days until recovery (Szabuniewicz et al., 1971).

In addition to BAL therapy, sodium thiosulfate should be given. The initial intravenous dose of sodium thiosulfate for dogs is 40 to 50 mg/kg of body weight, in a 20 per cent solution (Bartik and Piskac, 1981). It should be repeated two to three times daily until recovery (usually 3 to 4 days). Sodium thiosulfate can be given orally, after gastric lavage, at a rate of 0.5 to 3 gm as an antidote against unabsorbed arsenic (Szabuniewicz et al., 1971).

Oral penicillamine has been advocated in humans as a follow-up to BAL treatment or as primary treatment in chronic poisonings. The dosage in humans is up to 1 gm per day divided into 4 doses, for no longer than 1 week. The dosage in animals is not established.

Other sulfhydryl-containing compounds that protect laboratory animals against arsenic include lipoic acid, cysteine, glutathione, and N-acetylcysteine (Hatch, 1982). Dimercaptosuccinic acid has been shown to be less toxic and just as effective as BAL in protecting rats from arsenic (Graziano et al., 1978). However, no definitive dosages are available for small animals.

Intensive supportive care is important. Appropriate fluid therapy is needed to reverse dehydration caused by vomiting and diarrhea. Whole blood should be given if loss of blood is significant. Renal failure, liver damage, and electrolyte abnormalities should be monitored and appropriate therapy administered as indicated. The animal should be kept warm and comfortable, and symptomatic care given. Veterinary literature repeatedly lists the administration of B-complex vitamins and amino acids as supportive care. Antibiotics are recommended to prevent secondary bacterial infections (Osweiler et al., 1985). When emesis has stopped, oral kaolin-pectin preparations can be given to aid in controlling diarrhea. Start feeding the animal a high-quality diet in small portions, and increase the amount given as the animal's gastrointestinal tract can tolerate it (Furr, 1977).

Treatment of chronic poisoning starts with the removal of the source of the arsenic. Chelation therapy is usually not needed because of the rapid excretion rate of arsenic (Gossel and Bricker, 1984).

References and Supplemental Reading

Bartik, M., and Piskac, A.: *Veterinary Toxicology.* New York: Elsevier, 1981.

Byron, W. R., Bierbower, G. W., Brouwer, J. B., et al.: Pathologic changes in rats and dogs from two-year feeding of sodium arsenite or sodium arsenate. Toxicol. Appl. Pharmacol. 10:132, 1967.

Clark, M. L., Harvey, D. G., and Humphreys, D. J.: *Veterinary Toxicology.* 2nd ed. London, Baillière Tindall, 1981.

Evinger, J. V., and Blakemore, J. C.: Dermatitis in a dog associated with exposure to an arsenic compound. J.A.V.M.A. 184:1281, 1984.

Furr, A.: Arsenic poisoning. *In* Kirk, R. W. (ed.): *Current Veterinary Therapy VI: Small Animal Practice.* Philadelphia: W. B. Saunders Co., 1977.

Gossel, T. A., and Bricker, J. D.: *Principles of Clinical Toxicology.* New York: Raven Press, 1984.

Gosselin, R. E., Smith, R. P., and Hodge, H. C.: *Clinical Toxicology of Commercial Products.* 5th ed. Baltimore, William & Wilkins, 1984.

Graziano, J. H., Cuccia, D., and Friedheim, E.: The pharmacology of 2,3-dimercaptosuccinic acid and its potential use in arsenic poisoning. J. Pharmacol. Exp. Ther. 207:1051, 1978.

Hatch, R. C.: Poisons causing abdominal distress or liver or kidney damage. *In* Booth, N. H., and McDonald, L. E. (eds.): *Veterinary Pharmacology and Therapeutics.* 5th ed. Ames, IA: Iowa State University Press, 1982.

National Academy of Sciences (NAS): *Arsenic.* Committee on Medical and Biological Effects of Environmental Pollutants, National Research Council, Washington, D.C., 1977.

Neiger, R. D.: Effects of Chronic Dietary Inorganic Arsenic in Dogs. Ph.D. dissertation, Iowa State University, Ames, Iowa, 1987.

Osweiler, G. D., Carson, T. L., Buck, W. B., et al.: *Clinical and Diagnostic Veterinary Toxicology.* Dubuque, IA: Kendall-Hunt Publishing Co., 1985.

Squibb, K. S., and Fowler, B. A.: The toxicity of arsenic and its compounds. *In* Fowler, B. A. (ed.): *Biological and Environmental Effects of Arsenic.* New York: Elsevier, 1983.

Sullivan, N. D.: The nervous system. *In* Jubb, K. V. F., Kennedy, P. C., and Palmer, N. (eds.): *Pathology of Domestic Animals.* New York: Academic Press, 1985.

Szabuniewicz, M., Bailey, E. M., and Wiersig, D. O.: Treatment of some common poisonings in animals. Vet. Med. Small Anim. Clin. 66:1197, 1971.

TOXICOLOGY OF DETERGENTS, BLEACHES, ANTISEPTICS, AND DISINFECTANTS

R. W. COPPOCK, D.V.M.,
Vegreville, Alberta

M. S. MOSTROM, D.V.M.,
Saskatoon, Saskatchewan

and L. E. LILLIE, D.V.M.
Vegreville, Alberta

INTRODUCTION

Cleaning agents, antiseptics, and disinfectants are commonly used in the home, in veterinary practices, and in kennels and catteries. Chemically, these products are often complex mixtures formulated to meet specific uses and marketing objectives. Toxicoses produced by these complex mixtures are not always predictable from the chemical and physical properties of the individual ingredients. Exposure is generally by ingestion or surface contact. Estimated exposure to surface-acting compounds, for example, may range from 0.3 to 3.0 mg/day.

It is beyond the scope of this chapter to provide a comprehensive list of ingredients of the various proprietary products and the toxicoses that may result from exposure to them. A few selected products are listed in Tables 1 through 3. The best single source of specific information is the Poisindex (Micromedex, Inc., Denver, CO 80204-4506). Information on proprietary products is also available in *Clinical Toxicology of Commercial Products* (Gosselin et al, 1986). Large veterinary hospitals and central emergency clinics should have reference information such as the Poisindex available in-house for use by emergency clinicians.

General Toxicology

Circumstances that result in small animal exposure incidents are essentially the same as for children. The most common route of accidental exposure is oral. Dogs and cats may ingest both dilute and concentrated forms of household cleaning products, antiseptics, and disinfectants that are left unattended. Oral exposure may also occur when animals groom soiled fur, skin, and, especially, their feet. Inappropriate use of these mixtures as enema agents may also induce intoxication.

Surface-active agents and alkalies may dissolve mucus and expose surface cells of mucous membranes to other xenobiotics or infectious agents. More concentrated solutions, especially alkalies, may cause liquefaction necrosis by dissolution of the lipoprotein matrix of cell membranes. Surfactants may also induce intravascular hemolysis by dissolution of erythrocyte membranes. Acids and other corrosive agents may produce coagulation necrosis; the coagulated cells then act as a barrier to further penetration. Formaldehyde and phenolic compounds produce a similar lesion. However, phenol itself may produce a penetrating lesion. Phenolics are also hepato-, neuro-, and nephrotoxic.

Other products such as oxalates may be toxic

Table 1. *Partial List of Phenolic Antiseptics and Disinfectants Used in Veterinary Medicine*

Phenolic	Trade Name	Use
Hexachlorophene	Septisol	Surgical hand scrub
o-Phenylphenol	Instracal, Dowicide 1, Lysol	Disinfectant
o-Benzyl-p-chlorophenol	Instracal	
Cresol	Cresylic Acid, Tricresol	Disinfectant
Saponated cresol		Antiseptic and disinfectant
Resorcinol	Resorcin	Antiseptic, disinfectant, otics

Table 2. Products That Contain Borates

Product Type	Trade Name
Over-The-Counter Products	
Mouth wash–gargle	Listerine
Eye drops	Murine Plus; Clear Eyes; Collyrium Eye Lotion
Vaginal douche	Massengill's Vaginal Douche Powder
Fungicides	Maseda Foot Powder; Dr. Scholl's Foot Powder; Star-Otic
Contact lens care	Boil N Soak; Flex-Care
Ointments	Beecham-Massengill Baby Ointment
Veterinary Products	
Ear drying solution	Panodry
Astringent	Tanisol
Eye powder	Tylan Plus Neomycin Eye Powder
Over-The-Counter Veterinary Products	
Antiseptics	Dr. Naylor's Antiseptic Dusting Powder
Eye drops	Dr. Daniel's Collyrium
Cleaners	
Hand soaps	Boraxo Hand Soap
Laundry aids	Boraxo; Borateem
Denture cleaners	
Photographic	Kodak F5A Hardener
Roach control	

because of the binding of cations such as calcium. For some ingredients, such as the borates, a toxic mechanism has not yet been established.

The majority of household products that present a significant hazard have warning labels, and some may be packaged in "child-proof" containers. Commercial products are generally more concentrated than those available for domestic use. In both cases, inadvertent or careless use markedly increases the risk of exposure.

General Patient Assessment

When an exposure incident is reported by telephone or the exposed patient is brought to the hospital, the clinician must immediately assess the probable severity of exposure and determine a course of action. Essential information includes (1) confirmation that an exposure has occurred; (2) the time, route, and other circumstances of the exposure; (3) the present condition of the patient, including clinical signs and changes in the overall health status as observed by the owner; (4) identification of the toxic agent(s); and (5) the estimated dose. Then, the clinician must decide whether the patient can be treated at home, or whether it should be brought to the clinic or hospital.

Because most cleaning agents and disinfectants are complex mixtures, the clinician must, for each proprietary product, determine the most probable toxic ingredient(s) and carefully evaluate the hazard resulting from exposure to those ingredients. If the patient is to be treated at home, explicit instructions must be given, and all recommendations should be charted in the patient's record or recorded in the hospital telephone log. If the owner is instructed to bring the patient to the hospital, he or she should be requested to bring the labeled container including some of the contents or, if the substance is a solid, large pieces of the suspected toxic agent. In the medical management of the patient at the hospital, each treatment regimen must be evaluated in the context of risk to the patient versus benefit.

The suspected poisoned patient must be given a thorough examination. Special attention should be paid to the eyes. Some surfactants have topical anesthetic properties and may also produce penetrating liquefaction of corneal tissue. However, clinical signs of corneal injury may not be present at the time of the initial examination. Conversely, other surfactants may produce intense blepharospasm, which is readily apparent but which makes examination of the cornea difficult. Initial patient evaluation should also include appropriate baseline radiographs, generally of the abdomen, thorax, or other specifically affected area. Such radiographs allow the clinician to monitor the development of subsequent lesions such as chemical pneumonia subsequent to ingestion of pine oil. Appropriate specimens for clinicopathologic evaluation should also be taken for use in monitoring the clinical course of the poisoned patient.

CLEANING AGENTS AND BLEACHES

Cleaning Agents

Cleaning agents are formulated to meet certain cleaning specifications and, thus, are usually complex mixtures. Soap, detergent (surface-active agent, or surfactant), or both are the principal organic ingredients. These ingredients lower the surface tension of water, enabling wetting to occur. Builders are added to detergents to condition the water by regulating pH and ionic concentrations. Some cleaning agents, such as automatic dishwash-

Table 3. Products That Contain Pine Oil

Trade Name	Pine Oil (%)
Pine Sol	35
Pine-O-Fect	—*
Parson's Pine-O-Lin	77
Pine Plus	—
Pine-O-Cide	—
Pinetene Disinfectant	10
Pinotol	80
C-Z Pinalene	73

*Information not available.

ing detergents, oven cleaners, and wax strippers (e.g., sodium metasilicate), have high alkalinity. Other cleaning agents contain pine oils, isopropyl alcohol, or other solvents. Products for removing rust from lavatories may be high in oxalates.

Soaps

A true soap is a specific salt of a fatty acid and is produced by reacting natural fatty acids with an alkali.

TOXICOLOGY. Essentially all true soaps, which do not contain an excess of alkali, have a low order of oral toxicity. Homemade soaps and laundry soaps can be an exception, as they may be very palatable to small animals and may contain an excess of alkali. Essential oils, used for fragrance, can be very irritating to the gastrointestinal tract. The use of soap enemas can result in severe irritation and possibly necrosis of the rectum and large bowel.

CLINICAL FEATURES. The most prominent feature of soap ingestion is emesis. Excess alkali usually produces diffuse irritation of the oral mucous membranes and ptyalism (excess salivation). The eyes should be carefully examined for loss of surface epithelium.

TREATMENT. If marked irritation of the oral and pharyngeal membranes, suggestive of alkali burn, is observed, induction of emesis is contraindicated. As a general rule for nonalkali soaps, if more than 20 gm of soap/kg body weight has been ingested and emesis has not occurred within 30 min, vomiting should be induced with Apomorphine (Lilly) (0.04 to 0.09 mg/kg SC) or ipecac (1.5 per cent syrup; 2.2 ml/kg, max. 15 ml, PO). If less than 20 gm of soap/kg has been ingested, activated charcoal antidote (2.0 gm/kg PO) should be given. Persistence of soap-induced emesis and retching may require medical management. Antiemetics should not be given until there is reasonable assurance that the stomach is empty. After vomiting has been controlled, Toxiban suspension (6 to 12 ml/kg PO q.i.d. for 24 hr) should be administered.

For treatment of alkali burns, see the discussion on alkalies.

Detergents

A detergent is broadly defined as any cleaning agent. However, in a historic sense, the term detergent is used to identify synthetic surface-active compounds. Detergents consist of an organic (hydrophobic) moiety attached to a hydrophilic group such as a sulfonate. Detergents are usually classified by the charge on the surface-active ions (hydrophilic groups) at neutral pH, namely, anionics, cationics, nonionics, and Zwitterionics. Anionic detergents have a negatively charged surface-active ion, cationics have a positive charge, nonionics carry no charge, and Zwitterionics (amphoteric) have both positive and negative charges.

ANIONIC DETERGENTS (SURFACTANTS)

Anionic detergents are used most commonly in household products such as laundry detergents, dish soaps, and shampoos.

TOXICOLOGY. All anionic detergents have a low order of oral toxicity. The emetic effects of anionic detergents generally prevent intoxication by the oral route. The skin is a good barrier against anionic surfactants. However, they are readily absorbed through the dermis and subcutaneous tissues, and intoxication may occur by this route. The liver appears to be the primary organ for biotransformation of anionic detergents. Hepatic biotransformation in dogs occurs rapidly by beta-oxidation to about the fourth carbon of the alkyl chain. The sulfonate residue is excreted primarily by the kidneys.

Anionic detergents may induce intravascular hemolysis. This phenomenon appears to be related to blood concentration. Anionic detergents should not be used in enemas because, in addition to damaging the large bowel, they may be absorbed and induce a hemolytic crisis, especially in patients with liver disease.

CLINICAL FEATURES. There are no specific clinical features of intoxication by anionic detergents. General clinical signs may include ptyalism and emesis. The clinician must be alert for routes of exposure that may result in intravascular hemolysis.

TREATMENT. The treatment of anionic detergent intoxication is the same as described for soaps.

CATIONIC DETERGENTS (INCLUDING QUATERNARY AMMONIUM DISINFECTANTS)

Cationic detergents, including the quaternary ammonium compounds, are used in specialty products such as fabric softeners and antiseptic agents and as disinfectants and sanitizers. Cationic detergents also have industrial use as rust inhibitors in petroleum products, in ore flotation, and as emulsifying agents for asphalt. Intoxication of small animals with cationic agents is not commonly reported.

TOXICOLOGY. Benzalkonium chloride (alkyl dimethyl-benzylammonium; Zephiran Chloride, Winthrop) is a mixture of linear saturated hydrocarbons that range from C8 to C16. Cationic detergents may produce both acute and delayed toxic syndromes. Delayed toxicity is reduced when the alkyl chain length is from C8 to C10. Delayed toxicity appears to occur more frequently with heterocyclic (e.g., cetyl pyridinium) quaternary ammonium compounds. As a general rule, cationics with low water solubility are less toxic.

Cationic surfactants may be readily absorbed from the gastrointestinal tract. Ethanol and isopropanol enhance gastrointestinal absorption. Chyme markedly reduces toxicity. Percutaneous absorption is minimal; however, cationics are absorbed through exposed dermal and subcutaneous tissues. Therefore, loss of epidermis, as occurs in trauma and burn patients, increases absorption.

Mammalian toxicity does not seem to be correlated with germicidal activity. The majority of quaternary ammonium compounds seem to have a curare-like activity that is more profound with parenteral routes of exposure. In acute exposures, central nervous system (CNS) depression and seizures have been attributed to these curare-like effects. Some cationics have topical anesthetic properties, and ocular exposure, which may result in significant corneal injury, may not be readily apparent.

CLINICAL FEATURES. There are no specific clinical features associated with intoxication by cationic detergents. Oral and pharyngeal membranes may be hyperemic, and, subsequently, ulceration of the oral membranes is frequently observed. Clinical signs may include ptyalism, emesis, muscular weakness, depression, and seizures. Ptyalism is generally profuse, vomiting and retching can be persistent, and hematemesis (vomiting blood) may occur.

Intoxication with quaternary ammonium compounds may mimic intoxication with organophosphorous insecticides. Muscular weakness may be accompanied by muscular fasciculation, especially of the antigravity muscles. Muscular weakness may also result in ptosis of the eyelids and depressed respiration. Depression of the CNS may be accompanied by transient intervals of seizurelike movements that may progress to frank convulsions.

Dermal exposure, especially of the feet, can result in clinical signs of systemic intoxication. Dermal exposure may also produce marked erythema of the skin, which can progress to purulent inflammation. Contact dermatitis may occur, and surface exposure may complicate healing of surgical wounds.

In cases of surface exposure of the face and head, the eyes should be carefully examined. Staining of the cornea with fluorescein is helpful in detecting loss or damage of corneal epithelium.

TREATMENT. There is no specific treatment or antidote for cationic surfactant intoxication. Within 2 hr of exposure, induction of emesis is indicated and should be followed with milk, egg white, or gelatin antidote. A slurry of powdered milk (100 ml PO) is a convenient antidote. Expectant (symptomatic) treatment of systemic intoxication appears to be the most successful.

Early superficial exposure may be treated by flushing the affected area with water. If ocular exposure has occurred, the eyes should be lavaged with isothermic, isotonic saline for 20 to 30 min. Corneal ulcers should be managed by generally accepted methods.

NONIONIC AND ZWITTERIONIC DETERGENTS

Nonionic detergents are used in dish soaps, shampoos, laundry detergents, and whiteners. The majority of nonionic detergents appear to have a low order of toxicity.

BUILDERS

Builders are added to detergents, especially granular detergents, to bind elements (calcium and magnesium) responsible for water hardness and, thereby, prevent inactivation of surface-active agents, particularly in the case of anionic detergents.

TOXICOLOGY. Builders are toxic because they inflict caustic burns (colliquative necrosis) and induce hypocalcemia by binding calcium. Builders, in descending order of causticity, include metasilicate, sodium carbonate or sesquicarbonate, polyphosphates, silicates, and bicarbonate. Hypocalcemia occurs most commonly following exposure to oxalates and may occur following polyphosphate ingestion.

Oxalate is highly corrosive (coagulation necrosis) and can produce severe injury to the oral, pharyngeal, esophageal, and gastrointestinal mucosae. Oxalate is readily absorbed from the digestive tract and has a high affinity for calcium, rapidly forming calcium oxalate. Hypocalcemia and renal damage from precipitation of calcium oxalate crystals may result from oxalate ingestion (see also discussion on acids).

Nitrilotriacetate (NTA) is very irritating to the eyes and can damage the cornea, but does not readily produce methemoglobinemia (see discussion on phenolics).

CLINICAL FEATURES. Clinical features of intoxication due to builders are covered in the discussions on alkalies and acids. In addition to determining the extent of chemical burns, blood calcium and magnesium levels must be monitored.

TREATMENT. Surface exposure may be treated by flushing the affected area with water. Ingestion of oxalates may require intravenous administration of calcium and induction of diuresis (see discussion on acids).

Bleaches

Pets occasionally ingest bleaches; however, intoxication due to bleaches is uncommon.

TOXICOLOGY. Liquid bleaches generally contain sodium hypochlorite at concentrations of 3 to 16 per cent. Concentrations of hypochlorite are frequently given in terms of "available chlorine," a term defined as grams of chlorine gas (Cl_2) produced per 100 ml of bleach solution, or grams of Cl_2 per 100 gm of solid bleach. Solutions of hypochlorite with acidic pH are unstable. Addition of acid to hypochlorite results in the formation of chlorine gas and hypochlorous acid.

The toxicity of hypochlorite appears to be limited to its corrosive action on skin and mucous membranes. The oxidative (corrosive) potential of hypochlorite bleaches can be determined by the available chlorine. Hypochlorous acid appears to penetrate the mucosa. Acid antidotes, which contribute to the formation of hypochlorous acid, can enhance the toxicity of hypochlorite. As with acids, the corrosive activity of hypochlorite appears to be related more to concentration than dose (concentration × volume).

Trichloroisocyanuric acid, used in bleaches, scouring powders, and sanitizing agents, has a low order of toxicity that is essentially limited to its corrosive action.

Sodium perborate decomposes to peroxide and boric acid. The alkalinity of perborate is irritating to mucous membranes but usually does not produce caustic burns. Borate poisoning can also occur subsequent to perborate ingestion (see discussion on borate intoxication).

CLINICAL FEATURES. Animals may have a bleach (chlorine) odor, and bleaching of the hair, especially of the head and feet, may be observed. Clinical signs are due to irritation and may include ptyalism, emesis, and abdominal pain, especially rebound tenderness of the anterior abdominal regions. Hematemesis can occur, and the vomitus may contain fresh blood or small clots of partially digested blood (coffee ground appearance). Edema of the pharynx, glottis, and larynx may be observed. Inhalation of hypochlorous acid vapors, chlorine gas, and powdered bleaches can produce signs of upper respiratory tract irritation and pulmonary edema. Assessment of corrosive injury is essential.

TREATMENT. Induction of emesis within 3 hr of exposure is generally indicated. Milk of magnesia (2 to 3 ml/kg PO) is considered the antidote of choice for hypochlorite and trichloroisocyanuric acid ingestion. Other demulcents, such as egg white, corn starch, and powdered milk slurry may also be used. Bicarbonate of soda (baking soda) produces distention of the stomach with carbon dioxide and enhances the formation of hypochlorous acid.

Automatic Dishwasher Detergents

Chemically, dishwasher detergents are complex mixtures of anionic, nonionic, and other detergents, and builders. Automatic dishwasher detergents range from moderately to very toxic. The primary toxic effect results from alkali burns inflicted by the builders. In dogs, the fatal oral toxic dose of high metasilicate dishwasher detergent ranges from 0.5 to 2.5 gm/kg body weight.

CLINICAL FEATURES AND TREATMENT. These are discussed under the sections on builders and cationic detergents.

ANTISEPTICS AND DISINFECTANTS

Antiseptics are chemicals that kill or prevent the growth of micro-organisms. The term is generally used to define preparations applied to living tissue but does not include antibiotics or chemotherapeutic agents. The same active ingredients may be used in the formulation of antiseptics, disinfectants, and sanitizers. However, antiseptics generally are formulated to minimize tissue irritation and damage. Sanitizers generally contain essential oils, such as pine oil, to give them a "clean" odor. Pine oil is also classed as a disinfectant.

Quaternary Ammonium Compounds

See discussion on cationic detergents.

Chlorhexidine

Chlorhexidine (Hibitane, Ayerst; Nolvasan, Fort Dodge Laboratories), a cationic bisbiguanide compound, is a commonly used antiseptic and disinfectant.

TOXICOLOGY. Chlorhexidine has a low order of acute oral toxicity. It is poorly absorbed from the gastrointestinal tract or through the intact skin. Chlorhexidine is absorbed across serous membranes and from the urinary bladder and uterus. Sufficient quantities can be absorbed to induce intravascular hemolysis due to a direct effect on the red blood cell membrane. Accidental direct injection of chlorhexidine into the cerebrospinal fluid can produce severe neurotoxicity. Deafness also can result from the use of chlorhexidine tincture to treat infections of the auditory canal.

CLINICAL FEATURES. Clinical signs of chlorhexidine intoxication are hemoglobinemia and hemoglobinuria. Deafness may also be observed.

TREATMENT. If hemoglobinuria is observed, diuresis should be induced to prevent precipitation of hemoglobin and renal damage.

Phenol and Phenolic Compounds

The phenolic compounds, also referred to as coal tar derivatives, are still commonly used in veterinary medicine (Table 1). Benzoic acid is used as a preservative in drugs and foods. Phenol is used in caustics and escharotics; phenol and resorcinol are used in keratolytics; and phenol and coal tar are used in antiseborrheics. The British Pharmacopoeia lists lysol as a synonym for cresol-soap solution, whereas in the United States, Lysol is a registered trademark.

TOXICOLOGY. Phenol is very corrosive and, unlike acids, produces a penetrating lesion. Phenol is rapidly absorbed percutaneously, and essentially all phenolic compounds are absorbed from the gastrointestinal tract. The phenolics may also be absorbed through the dermis and subcutaneous tissues in concentrations sufficient to produce intoxication. There are marked species differences in biotransformation of the phenolics. Cats, certain reptiles, and birds appear to be more susceptible to intoxication. Some over-the-counter preparations may contain phenol or other phenolics in concentrations sufficient to induce toxicity in these species.

The phenolic compounds are hepato-, nephro-, and neurotoxic. The primary target organ varies from compound to compound. As an example, exposure to hexachlorophene (a bisphenol) may induce liver damage and spongy degeneration of the brain. Intoxication with phenolics generally increases the metabolic demand for oxygen. Otic preparations containing phenolics should be used with caution.

Phenol is very caustic to oral and ocular membranes and generally produces visible corrosion. Domestic animals will not usually ingest phenolics in quantities sufficient to produce esophageal injury. Cutaneous exposure to phenol usually results in the formation of a dry eschar (area of exposed dermis). Ocular and cutaneous exposure is often accompanied by a short interval of intense pain, followed by local anesthesia. Phenol produces a penetrating corneal lesion.

CLINICAL FEATURES. There are no unique clinical features of intoxication with phenolic compounds. Careful evaluation of oral and pharyngeal membranes is essential. Although clinical signs may vary, profuse ptyalism, emesis, apprehension, panting, and ataxia are commonly the first signs observed. As clinical signs progress, the animal may develop marked fasciculations, followed by shock and unconsciousness. The mucous membranes may be dark as a result of respiratory depression and the formation of methemoglobin due to oxidation of Fe^{++} to Fe^{+++}.

Clinical signs of hepatic and renal damage generally become apparent within 12 to 24 hr following exposure. Changes in hepatic and renal clinicopathologic parameters are typical of hepatocellular and proximal tubular necrosis. Excretion of metabolites may discolor the urine green or black; the addition of ferric chloride turns the urine violet or blue.

Ocular exposure may not be apparent at the time the patient is examined because of the topical anesthetic effect of phenol.

TREATMENT. An intoxication known to be due to exposure to phenolics must be considered as a clinical emergency. If esophageal injury is suspected, emesis should not be induced nor gastric lavage attempted. Otherwise, gastric lavage with olive or mineral oil is considered the treatment of choice. Do not give ethanol or use an alcohol lavage. Olive oil (10 ml/kg PO) is preferred over activated charcoal antidotes.

N-acetylcysteine (Mucomyst, Mead-Johnson) (140 mg/kg loading dose; then 50 mg/kg IV every 4 hr for 15 doses) may help prevent hepatic and renal toxicity. Methemoglobinemia can be treated by reducing the methemoglobin (Fe^{+++}) to hemoglobin (Fe^{++}) with methylene blue (8.0 mg/kg, slow IV infusion) or ascorbic acid (10–50 mg/kg, slow IV infusion). Cats appear to be sensitive to methylene blue–induced Heinz body anemia; therefore, ascorbic acid is considered the drug of choice for this species. Acid-base imbalance, characterized by respiratory alkalosis followed by metabolic acidosis, may occur and is similar to aspirin overdose. Oxygen therapy may also be required.

In ocular exposure, the eyes should be flushed with isothermic-isotonic saline for 20 to 30 min. Corneal erosions should be managed by generally accepted procedures. Exposed skin should be washed with soap, and olive oil should be applied.

Isopropanol (Isopropyl Alcohol)

Isopropanol (isopropyl alcohol, 2-propanol, secondary propyl alcohol, dimethylcarbinol, petrohol) is an aliphatic alcohol widely used as a rubefacient, antiseptic, and disinfectant; in the formulation of skin lotions, hair tonics, and after-shave lotions; as a cleaning solvent; and as a solvent in window cleaners and in sanitizers, especially those containing pine oil. Although not common, intoxication may result from the use of isopropanol in home remedies. Isopropanol rubefacients may be formulated with camphor and methyl salicylate, and some products may contain naphthalenes.

TOXICOLOGY. Isopropanol is approximately twice as toxic as ethanol (ethyl alcohol). Oral exposure to less than 3.0 ml/kg can produce marked clinical signs of intoxication. Isopropanol is a potent CNS depressant, and clinical signs of intoxication are similar but more severe than those observed for ethanol. Isopropanol vapors are heavier than air, and inhalation exposure can produce coma. Pulmonary edema and chemical pneumonia can result from inhalation and hematogenous exposure.

Isopropanol is readily absorbed from the gastrointestinal tract. In most species, the rate of biotransformation and elimination of isopropanol is slower than that for ethanol.

CLINICAL FEATURES. The odor of isopropanol and clinical signs of intoxication generally alert the clinician to isopropanol intoxication. The first clinical sign is generally acute gastritis typified by emesis (including hematemesis), retching, and tenderness over the anterior abdominal regions. Gastritis is rapidly followed by CNS depression characterized by marked respiratory depression and deep coma. If the formulation contains camphor, methyl salicylate, or naphthalenes, CNS stimulation may be observed early in the toxicosis. Clinical signs of hypotensive shock may also be observed.

Ketonemia and ketosuria (usually without glucosuria) may be observed, along with high anion gap acidosis.

TREATMENT. In oral exposure, emptying the stomach within 2 hr following exposure by induction of emesis or by gastric lavage is the most important method of treatment. Maintenance of ventilation, fluid balance, and treatment of the acidosis are essential. Little is known about the use of ethanol to block the biotransformation of isopropanol to toxic metabolites. In human medicine, dialysis has been successful. Because isopropanol is widely distributed in body water, peritoneal dialysis or hemodialysis would have to be continued over 5 or more hr to be effective. In the medical management of the CNS stimulatory effects of methyl salicylate and naphthalene, the clinician must plan for subsequent long-term CNS depression induced by isopropanol.

Boric Acid and Borates

Boric acid and sodium borate are used as antiseptics and disinfectants and are listed as ingredients in a large number of consumer compounds (Table 2). Borates are also used as food preservatives and in laundry aids (borax), wood preservatives, roach killers, herbicides, and fertilizers. In small animals, the number of fatalities from borate intoxication appears to be low.

TOXICOLOGY. Boric acid and other borates are generally nonirritating to skin and mucous and serous membranes and are essentially isotonic in saturated solutions. The lethal oral dose of boric acid for small animals is approximately 0.20 to 0.50 gm/kg body weight. Borate-induced vomiting generally occurs only after a substantial quantity of borates has been absorbed.

Soluble borates are readily absorbed from the gastrointestinal tract, mucous and serous membranes, and abraded skin. Borates are excreted mainly in the urine, and approximately 40 to 60 per cent of the dose is excreted within 12 to 24 hr of exposure. Repeated exposure may result in borates

accumulating to toxic concentrations. Blood concentrations above 50 µg/ml are generally considered diagnostic for borate intoxication. Borates have a high order of toxicity to the kidneys and CNS and have a low order of hepatotoxicity. Borates also induce riboflavin depletion.

Poisoning can occur following a single dose, and chronic poisoning may result from repeated low doses. Iatrogenic poisonings have occurred following the use of boric acid to lavage serous cavities or in enema solutions and after application of boric acid to burned or abraded skin.

CLINICAL FEATURES. There are no outstanding features of borate intoxication. A detailed anamnesis (history) is absolutely essential for establishing a presumptive diagnosis.

Clinical signs of acute poisoning are progressive and may include ptyalism, emesis, diarrhea, abdominal pain (especially rebound tenderness over the anterior regions), ataxia, hyperesthesia, tremors, general muscular weakness, seizures, coma, and death. A moderate elevation in body temperature and Cheyne-Stokes respiration may also be observed. Shock and diffuse intravascular coagulation may also occur.

Clinicopathologic features of acute borate intoxication are those of acid-base and electrolyte imbalances and renal failure. Chronic borate poisoning may produce dry skin, patchy alopecia, and conjunctivitis.

TREATMENT. There is no specific antidote for borate intoxication. If ingestion has occurred within 2 hr, emesis should be induced with Apomorphine (Lilly) or gastric lavage followed by administration of activated charcoal. A saline or sorbitol (2.0 gm/kg PO p.r.n.) cathartic is recommended, but the effectiveness of this treatment has not been well-established. Persistent nonproductive vomiting, when there is reasonable assurance of complete gastric emptying, should be controlled medically. Seizures can be controlled with diazepam or barbiturates. Detoxification by hemodialysis and peritoneal dialysis is considered the treatment of choice in human medicine. Riboflavin (1 mg/kg IM 4 days, or 20 mg/day PO) should be given.

Pine Oil

Pine oil (alpha-terpineol, aromatic pine oil) is used as a sanitizer, disinfectant, rubefacient, expectorant, and urinary disinfectant.

TOXICOLOGY. Pine oil is a colorless to pale-yellow liquid, which boils at 200 to 220°C and has a turpentinelike odor.

The lethal oral dose of pine oil for small animals is estimated to range from 1.0 to 2.5 ml/kg of body weight, and a substantially lower dose can result in severe intoxication. Pine oil is readily absorbed from the intestinal tract and is rapidly distributed to lipoidal tissues. Intoxication causes severe gastrointestinal irritation, CNS depression, and damage to the renal cortex. Vomiting generally occurs subsequent to ingestion, but spontaneous vomiting does not prevent intoxication. Chemical pneumonia may also occur.

Pine oil is very irritating to the eyes and skin but does not appear to cause penetrating damage to the eye.

CLINICAL FEATURES. Pine oil can produce a fulminating toxicosis. The patient usually has the turpentinelike odor of pine oil. Generally, there is marked irritation of the mouth and oropharynx. Vomiting and retching are common signs. Progressive signs of CNS intoxication are hyperesthesia, ataxia, muscular weakness, and twilight to frank coma. Tachycardia, toxic nephritis, and hyperthermia are common.

Clinical signs of ocular exposure are marked blepharospasm, epiphora, photosensitivity, and erythema of the conjunctiva and sclera.

Following a thorough physical examination, radiographs should be taken of the chest, and clinicopathologic parameters determined. All patients with known oral exposure and patients with clinical signs of intoxication should be hospitalized and observed for at least 24 hr.

Clinicopathologic features of pine oil intoxication are those of acid-base and electrolyte imbalances and of damage to the renal cortex.

TREATMENT. No specific antidote for pine oil intoxication exists. Because many of the household and commercial products that contain pine oil are complex mixtures of several ingredients, defendable clinical judgment in choosing a treatment regimen is essential. Induction of vomiting is most effective if initiated within 30 min following oral exposure. Since the danger of aspiration pneumonia may exist, induction of emesis in patients that have ingested large quantities of pine oil may be contraindicated (see *Current Veterinary Therapy IX*, p. 201). Gastric lavage should also be considered. After ascertaining that the stomach is empty, activated charcoal antidote (2.0 gm/kg PO p.r.n.) and sorbitol cathartic (1.0 to 2.0 gm/kg PO n.r.) may be given to adsorb and remove pine oil from the gastrointestinal tract. Maintenance of fluid and electrolyte balance is essential.

Animals with dermal exposure (including the feet) should be bathed with soap. Eyes should be irrigated with copious amounts of isothermic-isotonic saline for 15 to 30 min.

ACIDS AND ALKALIES

Acids and Other Corrosives

A number of household and commercial products contain acids in sufficient concentration to produce corrosive burns (coagulation necrosis). Hydrochloric (muriatic), sulfuric, nitric, and phosphoric acids are used in a variety of products that are purchased for home use. Hobbyists may use a variety of acids including hydrofluoric acid and aqua regia (combination of nitric and hydrochloric acid). Toilet bowl cleaners frequently contain sodium bisulfide, which forms sulfuric acid upon contact with water. Antirust compounds contain hydrochloric acid and oxalates; soldering flux contains zinc chloride and hydrochloric acid. Substances that contain free halogens (iodine, bromine, chlorine) can also be corrosive. Inhalation of acid vapors can be very damaging to the respiratory tract.

TOXICOLOGY. The primary toxic effect of acids is coagulation necrosis. Acids produce a fulminating lesion at the point of contact, with severity directly related to concentration (acidity or pH).

Because of the intense pain produced when acids come in contact with mucous membranes, animals generally do not swallow concentrated acids. Ingestion of lower concentrations of acid on an empty stomach appears to induce pylorospasm, entrapping the acid in the pyloric region. Ingestion of acid on a full stomach produces a more diffuse gastric lesion. Although less common than with alkali, necrotizing lesions of the esophagus may also occur.

In addition to being corrosive, oxalates are readily absorbed from the gastrointestinal tract and rapidly deplete serum calcium. Precipitation of calcium oxalate in the kidneys can result in moderate to severe renal damage.

CLINICAL FEATURES. Ingestion of acids produces grossly visible lesions in mucous membranes. Necrotic areas are initially gray but rapidly become black. An exception is nitric acid, which gives tissues a yellow color. Irritation of the pharynx by acids can produce laryngeal spasm and a life-threatening blockage of the airway due to laryngeal edema. Inhalation of acid vapors can result in pulmonary edema and shock.

Ocular exposure generally results in intense pain and blepharospasm. Clinical signs can be deceiving, as the actual injury to the eye can be minimal. However, this should not preclude a thorough eye examination.

Oxalate is highly corrosive and produces a whitish opaque appearance of the mucous membranes. Emesis, including hematemesis, and profuse diarrhea can occur. However, emesis does not prevent fulminating oxalate intoxication. Delayed effects include nephrosis and renal failure.

TREATMENT. The treatment of acid ingestion is controversial. Alkali antacids, such as aluminum hydroxide, and water antidotes are generally contraindicated in cases in which considerable quantities of acid have been ingested, because the resulting exothermic reaction can produce thermic burns. Induction of emesis is also contraindicated.

If esophageal injury is minimal, gastric lavage followed by antacid (aluminum hydroxide) lavage is the treatment of choice. Prophylactic antimicrobial chemotherapy is generally indicated.

Exposed skin should be irrigated with water for 10 to 20 min. Medical management includes control of licking and of self mutilation, and appropriate topical ointments. In severe cases, surgical débridement may be necessary.

In ocular exposure, the eyes should be lavaged with isothermic-isotonic saline for 30 min. Appropriate management of corneal lesions is essential.

The corrosive actions of oxalates may be complicated by systemic oxalate intoxication. Pulverized chalk, slurry of powdered milk, lime water (150 to 200 ml), or other sources of calcium ions should be given (PO) to precipitate oxalates in the gastrointestinal tract. Serum calcium concentration must be monitored and, if necessary, controlled with calcium gluconate (23 per cent solution given IV to effect). Osmotic diuresis should be induced with mannitol (2 gm/kg/hr IV), and fluid and electrolyte balance should be maintained.

Alkalies and Other Caustics

TOXICOLOGY. Alkalies produce penetrating liquefaction necrosis of tissues by solubilizing cell membranes. Tissue penetration continues until the base excess of the alkali is neutralized. Ingested granules of lye and other caustic substances may produce focal to diffuse esophageal necrosis.

It appears that the routes of alkali exposure in small animals, in order of descending frequency, are cutaneous, oral, and ocular. The most caustic household products are solid drain cleaners, toilet bowl cleaners, "button" alkali batteries, dishwasher detergents, and ammonia. Because of the pain associated with exposure, small animals generally do not swallow enough material to produce esophageal lesions. Exposure to alkali batteries is the exception. These small batteries may become lodged in the esophagus and leakage of the alkali produces severe penetrating burns. Ingestion of small batteries generally goes unnoticed by the owner, and the clinician may not see the animal until clinical signs have developed.

CLINICAL FEATURES. The most prominent clinical sign of alkali ingestion is marked diffuse irritation of the oral mucous membranes and ptyalism. Since deep chest pain is often difficult to evaluate, chest radiographs should be taken during the initial examination of the patient, when there is evidence of oral exposure. Changes from baseline hematologic parameters are helpful in detecting esophageal infection. Because of the danger of esophageal perforation, the patient should be evaluated for 12 hr before initiating endoscopic evaluation of the esophagus.

The eyes should be carefully examined in all patients with known or suspected alkali exposure. Total reliance on the severity of clinical signs of eye irritation to evaluate deep corneal damage can result in serious diagnostic errors.

TREATMENT. Treatment is directed toward all known routes of exposure, including oral, cutaneous, and ocular. In oral exposure, the action of an alkali is immediate; therefore, milk or other antidotes are of limited benefit. Gastric secretions are generally sufficient to neutralize the excess base. Because of the danger of esophageal rupture or perforation, vomiting should not be induced, and gastric lavage is contraindicated. When esophageal burns are suspected, no food or water should be allowed until the extent of esophageal injury has been established. Administration of acids or water as an antidote is contraindicated, as the generation of exothermic heat can produce thermic burns of the esophagus and stomach. However, washing of externally exposed areas is indicated.

Ingested alkali batteries can be detected by radiography. The battery should be removed from the esophagus or stomach by endoscopy or surgery.

For ocular exposure, the eye should be irrigated with isothermic-isotonic saline for 30 min. Generally, petrolatum-based ointments are contraindicated.

SUMMARY

Exposures of small animals to household and other commercial products present the clinician with complex toxicologic incidents. The diagnosis of poisoning can be straightforward or very difficult. Owners may be embarrassed by their own negligence and withhold essential information.

In planning the medical management of poisoning incidents, the clinician must give priority to (1) emergency stabilization of the patient; (2) detailed clinical evaluation; (3) removal of the poison from the gastrointestinal tract (if not contraindicated), eyes, fur, or skin; (4) administration of an appropriate antidote; (5) if possible, removal of the absorbed substance; and (6) supportive therapy.

Reliable sources of toxicologic information are absolutely essential. The single most accessible source is your hospital library.

References and Suggested Readings

Atkins, C. E.: Hypertonic sodium phosphate enema intoxication. *In* Kirk, R. W. (ed.): *Current Veterinary Therapy IX: Small Animal Practice.* Philadelphia: W. B. Saunders Co., 1986, pp. 212–216.

Atkins, C. E., and Johnson, R. J.: Clinical toxicoses of cats. Vet. Clin. North Am. 5:632, 1975.

Block, S. S.: *Disinfection, Sterilization, and Preservation.* 3rd ed. Philadelphia: Lea & Febiger, 1983.

Coppock, R. W., Mostrom, M. S., and Smetzer, D. L.: Volatile hydrocarbons (solvents, fuels) and petrochemicals. *In* Kirk, R. W. (ed.): *Current Veterinary Therapy IX: Small Animal Practice.* Philadelphia: W. B. Saunders Co., 1986, pp. 197–202.

Davis, L. E., and Westfall, B. A.: Species differences in biotransformation and excretion of salicylates. Am. J. Vet. Res. 33:1253, 1972.

Fowler, M. E.: Disinfectant and insecticide usage around birds and reptiles. *In* Kirk, R. W. (ed.): *Current Veterinary Therapy VIII: Small Animal Practice.* Philadelphia: W. B. Saunders Co., 1983, pp. 606–611.

Gloxhuber, C.: *Anionic Surfactants: Biochemistry, Toxicology, Dermatology.* Vol. 10. New York: Marcel Dekker, 1980.

Gosselin, R. E., Hodge, H. C., Smith, R. P., et al.: *Clinical Toxicology of Commercial Products,* 4th ed. Baltimore: Williams & Wilkins, 1986.

Hardin, R. D., and Tedesco, F. J.: Colitis after Hibiclens enema. J. Clin. Gastroenterol. 8:572, 1986.

Huber, W. G.: Antiseptics and disinfectants. *In* Booth, N. H., and McDonald, L. E. (eds.): *Veterinary Pharmacology and Therapeutics.* 5th ed. Ames, IA: Iowa State University Press, 1982, pp. 693–716.

Koppel, C., Tenczer, J., Tonnesmann, U., et al.: Acute poisoning with pine oil: Metabolism of monoterpenes. Arch. Toxicol. 49:73, 1981.

Oehme, F. W.: Information resources for toxicology. *In* Kirk, R. W. (ed.): *Current Veterinary Therapy IX: Small Animal Practice.* Philadelphia: W. B. Saunders Co., 1986, pp. 129–132.

Osweiler, G. D.: Household and commercial products. *In* Kirk, R. W. (ed.): *Current Veterinary Therapy IX: Small Animal Practice.* Philadelphia: W. B. Saunders Co., 1986, pp. 193–196.

Rousseaux, C. G., Smith, R. A., and Nicholson, S.: Acute pinesol toxicity in a domestic cat. Vet. Hum. Toxicol. 28:316, 1986.

Winter, M. L., and Ellis, M. D.: Automatic dishwasher detergents: Their pH, ingredients and a retrospective look. Vet. Hum. Toxicol. 28:536, 1986.

ETHANOL AND ILLICIT DRUGS OF ABUSE

R. W. COPPOCK, D.V.M.,
Vegreville, Alberta

M. S. MOSTROM, D.V.M.,
Saskatoon, Saskatchewan

and L. E. LILLIE, D.V.M.
Vegreville, Alberta

INTRODUCTION

Use of Illicit Drugs

Illicit drugs are controlled substances that are illegally obtained, sold, or otherwise dispensed. The use of controlled substances, generally by self-administration, for which there is no medically based indication, is referred to as a nonmedical use. The nonmedical use of controlled substances is generally considered illegal.

Illegal drugs are sold under a variety of "street" names and formulations, frequently in complex mixtures. Street terminology used to identify illicit drugs is highly variable and continually changing. This presents the clinician with considerable difficulty in determining the actual active ingredient(s) in various street preparations. Because the street jargon for illicit drugs varies substantially among geographic locations, the clinicians may have considerable difficulty in otaining accurate information for their particular locations. Very reliable information can be obtained from police officers working in the narcotics squad.

Illicit drugs are usually diluted (cut) with a variety of substances before being sold on the street. Lactose, mannitol, corn starch, and talc are used as diluents for a variety of street drugs. Cocaine is frequently cut with procaine, lidocaine, other local anesthetic agents, and quinine.

Users of illicit drugs, especially cocaine and marihuana (marijuana) are primarily adults in all social, economic, and professional strata of society. Substances of abuse may be incorporated into foods (happy foods) such as brownies, cookies, candies, and other confectioneries, and various beverages (happy punch).

Exposure of Small Animals

Small animals are exposed to illicit drugs and ethanol (ethyl alcohol) in a variety of ways. Intoxicated owners may wish to share their experience with their pets. Dogs and sometimes cats will "help themselves" to "happy" foods or to the punch bowl. Drugs and drug paraphernalia left unattended are consumed or chewed by pets. Illicit drugs, hidden in "secret locations," are discovered and consumed by small animals. In other incidents, small animals may be given illicit drugs or ethanol maliciously or as a practical "joke."

In establishing a provisional diagnosis of intoxication by illicit drugs or ethanol, a complete history is absolutely essential. The owners may be very reluctant or may refuse outright to provide essential information. Owners may be in a state approaching hysteria when they find that their pet has consumed illicit drugs or edible substances containing illicit compounds. They are often reluctant to identify themselves or bring their animal to the clinic. In such situations, owners may demand that appropriate treatment be prescribed over the telephone. A friend, who has little or no knowledge of the incident, may bring the patient to the hospital. Veterinarians should be clearly aware that knowledge of illicit drug use by clients themselves or in incidents of poisoning of animal patients is not legally privileged information, and there may be a legal obligation to report such incidents to the police.

ETHANOL (ETHYL ALCOHOL)

Pets, especially dogs, may voluntarily consume ethanol, particularly wine, beer, and mixed drinks. Conditions of exposure vary considerably. Some individuals find it jocose to entice a pet to imbibe alcoholic beverages and thereby become intoxicated. Some dogs will quaff from a punch bowl left unattended, and the quantity of alcoholic beverage consumed can result in serious intoxication. Cats most frequently become intoxicated by grooming fur soiled with beverages or solvents with a high alcoholic content. Alcoholic beverages are also commonly used in a wide variety of home remedies.

Ingestion of commercial products containing denatured ethanol can result in ethanol intoxication or intoxication by complex chemical mixtures to which ethanol makes a significant contribution. These products include over-the-counter drugs, antiseptics, rubefacients, denatured ethanol-based solvents, and gasohol.

TOXICOLOGY

Chemically, ethanol (ethyl alcohol, grain alcohol) is an aliphatic alcohol. Ethanol is a yeast metabolite and is produced on a variety of substrates, which may include cereal grain mash, fruit juices, and potato water. The concentration of ethanol in beverages is also expressed as "proof" (twice the volume percentage), and the "fifth" (one fifth U.S. gal, or 760 ml) is a commonly used volumetric measure. Denatured ethanol is ethyl alcohol to which some substance (denaturant) has been added to make it unfit for human consumption. Therefore, it is tax exempt. Denaturants include methanol, benzene, isopropanol, amyl alcohol, acetone, gasoline, kerosene, terpineol, camphor, castor oil, brucine, aniline dyes, and diethyl phthalate (Table 1).

The pharmacokinetics of ethanol have been well-defined. Ethanol is rapidly absorbed following oral and inhalation exposure, and a small amount is absorbed through the intact skin. Following absorption, ethanol is widely distributed in body water. Detoxification is primarily by sequential biotransformation: Alcohol dehydrogenase metabolizes ethanol to acetaldehyde, and aldehyde dehydrogenase biotransforms acetaldehyde to acetate. Approximately 80 per cent of the dose is metabolized by the liver, 15 to 20 per cent is metabolized by the other tissues, and 3 to 5 per cent of the parent compound is excreted by the kidneys or blown off by the lungs. At blood concentrations sufficient to produce clinical signs of intoxication, ethanol is metabolized by zero-order kinetics; in other words, elimination is independent of dose. In dogs, the rate of ethanol detoxification ranges from 150 to 200 mg/kg/hr (the density of 95 per cent ethanol is approximately 816 mg/ml).

Alcohol causes many systemic effects. Ethanol is a general anesthetic. Selective inhibitory effects often give an appearance of central nervous system (CNS) stimulation. In small animals, enhanced inquisitiveness and loss of motor coordination are frequently observed. Peripheral vasodilation can result in hypothermia. Ethanol can induce emesis by gastric irritation and direct stimulation of the vomiting center. Emesis, if induced by ethanol, can protect the animal from fatal intoxication. As the dose of ethanol is increased, the anesthetic effects become progressively more apparent. Surgical anesthesia is accompanied by potentially lethal respiratory depression. The primary cause of death in ethanol intoxication is respiratory failure. Ethanol also interferes with intermediary metabolism. Hypoglycemia frequently occurs in acute intoxication, and metabolic acidosis may also be observed. In dogs, the oral median lethal dose (LD_{50}) of 95 per cent ethanol ranges from 5.5 to 6.6 ml/kg (2.5 to 3.0 ml/lb). At high concentrations, the dose response curve for ethanol is very steep. Life-threatening intoxication can occur at doses as low as one half the median lethal dose. Cats are less tolerant of ethanol than are dogs. Ethanol has local anes-

Table 1. *Examples of Compounds Used to Denature Ethanol*

Formula No.	Denaturing Agent
1A and 3A	5% Methanol
23A	10% Acetone
39C	1% Diethyl phthalate

thetic properties. Percutaneous exposure results in local vasodilation. Ethanol is irritating to the eyes; the severity of coagulation necrosis produced by ethanol is dependent on concentration.

In denatured ethanol, the interactions between ethanol and the denaturant must be evaluated. Denaturants, which are biotransformed into toxic substances by alcohol dehydrogenase, are generally rendered less toxic by the presence of ethanol. Conversely, ethanol generally has an additive, synergistic, or potentiating effect on denaturants, which are dependent on alcohol dehydrogenase or other hepatic biotransformation mechanisms for detoxification. Ethanol acts in a manner similar to that of denaturants that are CNS depressants.

CLINICAL FEATURES

The patient has an odor of ethanol in the expired air. Ethanol can induce emesis, and nonproductive emesis and retching may persist. Various stages of CNS depression, including an excitement phase, may be observed. Incoordination is frequently observed in ambulatory patients. Patients with ethanol-induced twilight consciousness may progress to frank coma with signs that include muscular fasciculations, extensor rigidity, trismus (tense to rigid jaw muscles), convulsions, and severe respiratory depression.

TREATMENT

If ingestion has occurred within 2 hr and the patient does not have marked CNS depression, emesis should be induced. Unabsorbed ethanol can also be removed by gastric lavage with isothermic tap water. Activated charcoal antidote also reduces ethanol absorption.

In patients with alcohol-induced coma, ventilation must be maintained. Naloxone (Narcan, Du Pont) (0.1 mg/kg) has been successfully used in human medicine to stimulate respiration and arouse individuals from acute alcoholic coma. However, the efficacy of naloxone has not been established in dogs. Unless the clinician is reasonably certain that CNS depression will not occur, or that it can be medically controlled, animals that are excited should not be given depressants. Body temperature must be maintained.

Blood acid-base, electrolyte, glucose, and fluid balances must be maintained. Intravenous fluids containing or amended with lactic acid are contraindicated, as lactic acid enhances ethanol-induced metabolic acidosis. Drugs that block ethanol biotransformation pathways, such as disulfiram, are contraindicated. Because ethanol is distributed in body water, induction of diuresis is of little benefit in increasing ethanol excretion.

In ocular exposure, the eyes should be irrigated with isotonic-isothermic saline for 20 to 30 min. The eyes should be thoroughly examined, and appropriate treatment should be prescribed.

PHENCYCLIDINE

Phencyclidine hydrochloride, 1-(1-phenylcyclohexyl)piperidine hydrochloride, is an arylcyclohexylamine. Old trade names for phencyclidine (CI-395) are Sernyl and Sernylan (Parke-Davis). It is a white crystalline powder that is readily soluble in water and ethanol. Concurrent with the introduction of phencyclidine as a veterinary anesthetic, it made its debut as "Peace Pill," an illicit street drug. However, essentially none of the legally marketed phencyclidine was used as a street drug. Because of illicit use, phencyclidine is a Schedule 1 Drug and is no longer available for the veterinary market.

Phencyclidine is sold on the street under a variety of names (Table 2). The concentration of phencyclidine in various illicit preparations varies greatly. Tablets and capsules generally contain approximately 1 to 15 mg. Leaf mixtures (parsley, mint, and marihuana) generally contain 1 mg of phencyclidine per 150 mg of leaves. Happy foods and beverages can contain varying amounts of phencyclidine.

TOXICOLOGY

The oral dose of phencyclidine required to produce marked clinical signs of intoxication ranges from 2.5 to 10.0 mg/kg and 1.1 to 12.0 mg/kg for dogs and cats, respectively. Being a weak base with a pKa of 8.5, phencyclidine is ionized at gastric pH

Table 2. *Street Nomenclature for Phencyclidine*

Name	Concentration* (%)
Angel dust; Crystal; Monkey Tranquilizer; Elephant Embalmer	30–90
PCP; Dust; Elephant Tranquilizer; Polar Bear Killer; THC	10–90
Peace Pill; Hog Dust	10–60
Magic Mist; Mist; Rocket Fuel	10–45
Goon; Scuffle; Surfer; Soma; Cadillac; CJs; Cyclones; Horse Tracks; Sheets	10–30
Crystal Joints; Crystal Weed; Goon Weeu; Killer Weed; Killer Joint (KJ); Super Grass; Super Weed; Super Cools; Wobble Weed	5–30

*Concentration of phencyclidine in preparations sold on the street is highly variable.

and, therefore, is poorly absorbed from the stomach. However, in the alkaline pH of the duodenum and jejunum, phencyclidine is readily absorbed. Chyme generally alters phencyclidine absorption. A carbohydrate meal decreases phencyclidine absorption, whereas a high-protein meal increases absorption of phencyclidine. In addition, ion trapping in the nephron occurs when urine pH is less than 5.5. Phencyclidine is also distributed in body lipids.

There are considerable species differences in the biotransformation of phencyclidine. In dogs, approximately 68 per cent of a single dose (given IV or IM) is metabolized by the liver, and 38 per cent (depending on urine pH) of the parent compound is excreted by the kidneys. In cats, approximately 88 per cent of a single dose (given IV or IM) of phencyclidine is excreted by the kidneys as the parent compound.

Phencyclidine is a CNS stimulant, depressant, hallucinogen, and analgesic. It disrupts CNS function by a variety of mechanisms, none of which have been well-defined. It interacts with the neurotransmitter system by blocking the re-uptake of dopamine, serotonin, and norepinephrine by synaptosomes, and it appears to interact with opioid receptors. New findings suggest that phencyclidine also partially blocks potassium conductance in certain neurons.

The CNS effects of phencyclidine include analgesia and anesthesia, central-acting antiemesis, and disruption of body temperature regulation. Phencyclidine can block the emetic effects of apomorphine and ipecac. Sequential changes in body temperature are generally observed. Initially, hyperthermia occurs. This is generally followed by hypothermia, depending on ambient temperature. Since phencyclidine increases muscle tone, intoxicated animals can be very susceptible to heat stroke. Protective spinal cord and cranial nerve reflexes are not inhibited, and muscular tone is increased.

CLINICAL FEATURES

In general, all the clinical signs observed with phencyclidine intoxication are an enhancement of those observed in animals anesthetized with ketamine. The most prominent features, even at lower doses, are profuse ptyalism, tachycardia, nystagmus, and mydriasis. Ambulatory patients are incoordinated, and hyperesthesia may be observed. At high doses, seizures may be observed.

In phencyclidine intoxication, the patient generally retains brisk reflexes and increased muscular tone. These observations can assist in differentiating phencyclidine intoxication from intoxication with sedatives or hypnotics, which generally result in flaccid muscular tone and a loss of reflexes.

Recovery, especially in cats, can be prolonged. Cats may have repeated episodes of phencyclidine intoxication for as long as 2 weeks following exposure. Prolonged hospitalization and supportive care may be required.

There are no distinct clinicopathologic features of phencyclidine intoxication. Profound muscular activity can induce hypoglycemia. Intense muscular activity can result in elevations of serum glutamic-oxaloacetic transaminase (SGOT) and creatine phosphokinase (CPK).

TREATMENT

Since absorption of phencyclidine occurs primarily in the intestinal tract, either or both induction of emesis and administration of activated charcoal antidote within 3 to 4 hr after ingestion is very beneficial. If clinical signs of phencyclidine intoxication are observed, induction of emesis or gastric lavage can be difficult. Therefore, repeated doses of apomorphine or ipecac should not be given. Gastric lavage is also difficult to accomplish because of trismus and persistence of the gag reflex. Administration of diazepam (Valium, Roche) generally reduces muscular rigidity, but the gag reflex frequently persists. Activated charcoal appears to prevent gastric-enteric recycling of phencyclidine.

Many drugs, in combination with phencyclidine, are potent respiratory depressants. Drugs that are contraindicated include the barbiturates, phenothiazine tranquilizers, and xylazine. Atropine and other parasympatholytics are contraindicated because they potentiate the sympathomimetic effects of phencyclidine and increase the viscosity of respiratory secretions.

Diazepam, given intravenously to maintain the desired effect, is the treatment of choice. Halothane can safely be used to anesthetize patients intoxicated with phencyclidine. Supportive care of the patient in a quiet darkened environment is recommended. The patient should be monitored for hypoglycemia.

Urinary acidifiers can be used to enhance excretion of phencyclidine. The object of urine acidification is to trap phencyclidine in the ionized form, which is achieved at urinary pH of less than 5.5, and then to increase urine flow. Ascorbic acid (2 gm/500 ml of intravenous fluids; IV over 6 hr) is given to achieve urinary pH of 5.5 or less. As soon as the urine reaches the desired pH, furosemide (Lasix, Hoechst-Roussel) (2.5 mg/kg, slow IV infusion) is given to increase urine flow. Care must be taken to ensure that blood pH, electrolyte and glucose concentrations, and fluid balance are maintained.

MARIHUANA (MARIJUANA)

Marihuana refers to a crude preparation made from the leaves and flowering tops of *Cannabis sativa*, varieties *indica* and *americana*. The term marihuana is also used to describe any part or extract of the plant that contains the active principle, primarily cannabinoids. Marihuana (cannabinoids) is listed as a Schedule 1 Substance and has no currently accepted medical use.

Marihuana is used in a variety of ways. In addition to being smoked, it is used as the active ingredient in "happy" foods. Marihuana is also used in a variety of ways with phencyclidine and other CNS-active drugs.

TOXICOLOGY

Marihuana (marijuana, grass, happy tobacco, pot, indian hemp, indian cannabis, hashish, charas, bhang, ganja, and kift) is an illicit substance that has common usage. The intoxicating principle is a complex mixture of cannabinoids, of which the best studied is delta 9-tetrahydrocannabinol (THC). Although all parts of *Cannabis sativa*, varieties *indica* and *americana*, contain cannabinoids, the highest concentrations are found in the flowering tops. The various illicit marihuana preparations contain differing concentrations of cannabinoids (Table 3). In descending order of cannabinoid concentration, they are hashish, or charas, dried resinous exudate from the flowering tops; bhang, dried leaves and flowering shoots; and ganja, dried resinous mass from small leaves, and brackets of inflorescence. The most common form of marihuana (grass, happy tobacco) sold on the street is used for making roll-your-own cigarettes (roaches, reefers). During smoking, cannabinoids are concentrated in the cigarette butt and smoking paraphernalia such as pipes.

Cannabinoids are readily absorbed following oral and inhalation exposure. The cannabinoids are readily detoxified by the liver, and only 6 to 20 per cent of the oral dose reaches the systemic circulation. Some cannabinoid metabolites are lipid soluble and retain their biological activity. However, the major-

Table 3. *Concentration of Cannabinoids in the Various Marihuana Products*

Product	Concentration of Cannabinoids* (%)
Average cigarette (0.5 to 1.0 gm)	1–2
Napo	2.81
Jamaica	2.80
Mexico	1.68
USA and Canada	0.35–2.0*
Average cigarette butt	10–15
Hashish	10–60
Hash oil	20–70

*Depending on the geographic region where the *Cannabis* species is grown.

ity are more polar and are excreted in bile and urine. Cannabinoid metabolites are also circulated in the hepatic-enteric loop.

The mechanisms by which the cannabinoids affect the CNS are unknown. Cannabinoids have a variety of pharmacologic effects. As a group, they are potent antiemetics, analgesics, anticonvulsants, and soporifics. Cardiovascular effects are tachycardia and hypotension.

In general, cannabinoids have a low order of acute toxicity and, in veterinary medicine, are not usually the cause of life-threatening intoxication incidents. Cats will seek out marihuana and will react to it in a manner very similar to catnip.

CLINICAL FEATURES

There are no distinct features of marihuana intoxication. The most common clinical features in ambulatory patients are ataxia, tachycardia, and increased auditory and olfactory sensitivity. Some animals have an obsession to investigate sounds, odors, and objects. Cats may be presented with a history of having been very destructive of household items. Generally, cats have not engaged in normal aggressive play but rather have knocked items from shelves. Owners may be very vexed because their cats have destroyed the household marihuana plants.

The patient may be presented in a state of sopor (deep sleep). The patient can be aroused by physical stimuli but does not appear to be aware of its surroundings. Profound analgesia can also be observed. If marihuana and phencyclidine were ingested, the patient may have varying degrees of catatonia. Ingestion of substances containing high concentrations of cannabinoids can result in hyperesthesia. However, hyperesthesia is almost always followed by sopor. Since marihuana smoke is generally more irritating than tobacco smoke, animals exposed to marihuana smoke for an extended time may develop chronic bronchitis.

There are no prominent clinicopathologic features of intoxication with cannabinoids. Blood glucose, acid-base, and electrolyte balances should be monitored.

TREATMENT

There is no specific treatment for intoxication with the cannabinoids. If ingestion has occurred within 2 hr and clinical signs of intoxication are not apparent, induction of emesis should be attempted. However, if apomorphine or ipecac do not induce emesis, repeat treatment is contraindicated. Activated charcoal (2 gm/kg PO) appears to be a suitable antidote. Supportive care and conservative treatment of clinical signs is recommended. Respiratory depression, if present, should be controlled with doxapram (Dopram, Robbins) 2.0 to 10.0 mg/kg given by slow IV infusion, to effect). If arrhythmogenic analeptic stimulants are given, the heart must be monitored for arrhythmias.

COCAINE ("COKE")

Cocaine has historically been used in veterinary and human medicine as a topical and local anesthetic, CNS stimulant, and mydriatic. As better drugs have become available, the medical use of cocaine has decreased.

Drug abusers self-administer cocaine by inhalation, all parenteral routes, and orally. Cocaine is absorbed buccally, and chewing of coca leaves or substances impregnated with cocaine takes advantage of this route of exposure. Cocaine powder or coca leaves are also added to alcoholic beverages or teas. Illicit cocaine is sold on the street under many different names and in various concentrations (Table 4).

TOXICOLOGY

Chemically, cocaine is benzoylmethylecgonine; it is the active principle in *Erythroxylon coca* and *E. monogynum*. The leaves of these plants contain approximately 1 per cent by weight of the active principle. Cocaine has a pKa of 8.7.

Cocaine is rapidly absorbed from the mucous membranes, gastrointestinal tract, all parenteral administration sites, and abraded skin. Absorption of cocaine from mucous membranes is enhanced by inflammation. Following oral administration, peak plasma concentrations of cocaine generally occur within 1 to 2 hr. The bioavailability of an oral dose is approximately 10 to 20 per cent, owing to first-pass hepatic biotransformation.

Cocaine is rapidly metabolized by hepatic and plasma esterases. Metabolites of cocaine are excreted primarily by the kidneys and, to a lesser extent, in the bile. The plasma half-life of cocaine in dogs administered 5 mg/kg body weight intravenously was 1.2 hr. The biotransformation products of cocaine in dogs are norcocaine, benzoylnorecgonine, benzoylecgonine, norecgonine, ecgonine methyl ester, and ecgonine. Norcocaine, formed by hepatic N-demethylation, appears to have more biologic activity than does cocaine. The majority of biotransformation products are excreted in the urine. Very little of the parent drug is excreted in urine or feces.

Surprisingly little is known about the pharmacodynamics of cocaine. However, it is generally accepted that cocaine stimulates the nervous system by complex mechanisms.

The acute LD_{50} of intravenously administered cocaine hydrochloride in dogs is 13 mg/kg (range of 11.9 to 14.2 mg/kg), and the acute LD_{99} is 20 mg/kg (16.5 to 24.4 mg/kg). The oral LD_{50} of cocaine for dogs appears to be two to four times that of the intravenous dose. Cats are more sensitive to cocaine than are dogs.

CLINICAL FEATURES

The most prominent clinical feature of cocaine intoxication is stimulation of the CNS. This includes profuse ptyalism, hyperesthesia, mydriasis, increased muscular tone, muscular fasciculations, tachycardia, hyperpnea, emesis, and hyperpyrexia. The degree of hyperesthesia varies with the amount of cocaine ingested and can range from mild excitation to clonic-tonic convulsions. Cocaine-induced mydriasis is generally light responsive. Contraction and rigidity of skeletal muscles can be severe enough to produce trismus and rhabdomyolysis (rupture of skeletal muscles and release of myoglobin).

The cardiopulmonary effects of cocaine can be life threatening. Cardiac effects are tachycardia, and increased cardiac output and left ventricular pressure. Generally, the mean blood pressure does not increase, and total peripheral resistance decreases. Constriction of the coronary vessels and cardiac arrest can occur. Stimulation of respiration results in increase in tidal and minute volume. However, the increase in respiration does not compensate for increased oxygen consumption, and, therefore, arterial P_{O_2} decreases. If the dose of cocaine is sufficient, severe respiratory depression, and pulmonary congestion and edema may occur. Persistent emesis

Table 4. Street Names and Measures for Cocaine

Street Name	Street Measures
Snow	Snort; line; hit; dose (2 to 200 mg)
Dama Blanca	
Green Gold	
Coke	
Blow	
Toot	
Snuff	Spoon (500 mg to 1 gm)
Her	
Girl	
Nose Crystals	
White Lady	
White Girl	
C-Lady	
C-Candy	
Leaf	
Highly pure (>90%) free-based cocaine	
Crack	
Rock	
Flake	

and retching can be observed. Body temperature can increase to 106.7° F (41.3°C).

There are no prominent clinical pathologic features of cocaine intoxication. Increased muscular activity can result in hypoglycemia, and a functional decrease in available oxygen can increase blood lactic acid. Rhabdomyolysis results in elevations of serum glutamic-oxaloacetic transaminase (SGOT) and creatine phosphokinase (CPK) and in myoglobinuria.

TREATMENT

There is no specific treatment for cocaine intoxication. If large amounts of cocaine are known to have been ingested and if advanced clinical signs of intoxication are not yet apparent, induction of emesis is indicated. The efficacy of activated charcoal in cocaine intoxication by oral exposure has not been established.

Diazepam (given IV to effect) is the drug of choice for controlling cocaine-induced seizures. Oxygen should be administered. If tachycardia and threatening cardiac arrhythmias are observed, propranolol (Inderal, Ayerst) (given by slow IV infusion to effect) appears to be the most effective therapy. Cocaine could potentiate the arrhythmogenic effects of halothane. Acidification of the urine does not increase the excretion of cocaine. If myoglobinuria occurs, diuresis should be induced to prevent precipitation of myoglobin in the renal tubules. Blood acid-base, electrolyte, glucose, and fluid balances must be maintained. Body temperature should be controlled by the use of ice packs, by immersing the patient in chilled water, or with cold enemas.

References and Suggested Readings

Catravas, J. D., Waters, I. W., Walz, M. A., et al.: Acute cocaine intoxication in the conscious dog: Pathophysiologic profile of acute lethality. Arch. Int. Pharmacodyn. 235:328, 1978.

Coppock, R. W.: Pharmacology of Phencyclidine. Unpublished report. Vegreville, Alberta, 1988.

Coppock, R. W., Mostrom, M. S., and Smetzer, D. L.: Volatile hydrocarbons (solvents, fuels) and petrochemicals. In Kirk, R. W. (ed.): Current Veterinary Therapy IX. Philadelphia: W. B. Saunders Co., 1986, pp. 197–202.

Jones, R. T.: The pharmacology of cocaine. In Grabowski, J. (ed.): Cocaine: Pharmacology, Effects and Treatment of Abuse. Washington, DC: National Institute on Drug Abuse, Res. Monograph 50, 1984, pp. 34–53.

Misra, A. L.: Disposition and biotransformation of cocaine. In Mule, S. J. (ed.): Cocaine: Chemical, Biological, Clinical, Social and Treatment Aspects. Cleveland, CRC Press, 1976, pp. 73–90.

Moreman, D. E.: Personal communication. Fort Royal, VA: Cedarville Clinic, 1987.

National Academy of Sciences. Marijuana and Health. Washington, DC: National Academy Press, 1985.

The drugs on the street where you live. (editorial) Emerg. Med. 18:129, 1986.

Wetli, C. V., and Mittleman, R. E.: The "body packer syndrome": Toxicity following ingestion of illicit drugs packaged for transportation. J. Forensic Sci. 26:492, 1981.

BITES AND STINGS OF VENOMOUS ANIMALS

M. E. PETERSON, D.V.M.,
and G. L. MEERDINK, D.V.M.

Tucson, Arizona

Many members of the animal kingdom produce toxins that are used offensively in the procurement of food or defensively for protection of themselves or the colony and, occasionally, as an aid in digestion. Venomous animals exist in all parts of North America, although species variations occur from one region to another. The veterinarian should become familiar with local venomous species, since the identity of the perpetrator is seldom known when the bitten victim is presented.

VENOMOUS SNAKES

An estimated 15,000 domestic animals are bitten by snakes annually in the United States. Rattlesnakes account for approximately 80 per cent of the deaths. The poisonous snakes of the United States belong to three groups: pit vipers, elapids, and the colubrids. Pit vipers are the largest group and include five subspecies of copperheads (*Agkistrodon contortrix*), three subspecies of cottonmouth water moccasins, or cottonmouths (A. piscivorus), three subspecies of pygmy rattlesnakes (Sistrurus miliaris), three subspecies of massassauga (S. catenatus), and at least 26 subspecies of rattlesnakes (Crotalus spp.). Pit vipers have special heat-sensing "pits" located between the eye and the nostril, retractable fangs, and triangle-shaped heads.

The elapids have fixed front fangs and include the Texas coral (Micrurus fulvius tenere), the eastern coral snake (M. fulvius fulvius), and the smaller species of Sonoran coral snake (Micruroides euryxanthus). Coral snakes are brightly colored, with full encircling bands (without belly scale interruption) that start with the black head and then alternate black, yellow (or white), and red. (Some nontoxic species mimic the color arrangement; however, in these, the red band is adjacent to black.)

The third group, the colubrids, with fixed hind fangs, include the vine snake (Oxybelis aeneus), the Sonoran lyre snake (Trimorphodon lambda), and the night snake (Hypsiglena torquata). The colubrids have been considered of minor significance; however, human illness from this species' envenomation has been documented. Colubrids are widely distributed throughout North America and may be more hazardous than previously assumed.

The dogmatic assignment of properties to venoms of particular snakes (i.e., hemolytic vs. neurotoxic) is an oversimplification that could be dangerous for your patient. Although pit viper venoms have been associated with hemolytic properties, several species contain neurotoxins (e.g., the Mojave rattlesnake, Crotalus scutulatus scutulatus). Species and venom toxicities are listed in Table 1.

Pit Vipers

PATHOPHYSIOLOGY

The primary function of venom is to immobilize the victim and predigest the victim's body tissues. Pit viper venoms consist of two major fractions: enzymes and nonenzymatic polypeptides. There are currently 26 known enzymes in snake venoms, ten of which are found in all pit viper venoms. Some major enzymes are hyaluronidase ("spreading factor"), which decreases the viscosity of connective tissue, allowing other fractions of the venom to penetrate the tissues, and phospholipase A, which disrupts membranes, uncouples phosphorylation, inhibits cellular respiration, and may release histamines, kinins, and serotonin. Major coagulation defects may occur with consumptive coagulopathies, and different areas of the coagulation cascade are attacked, depending upon the individual species of pit viper involved (Fig. 1). The nonenzymatic polypeptide fraction directly affects the cardiovascular and the respiratory systems. Crotalidae Crotalus venom causes blood pooling in the hepatosplanchnic bed in dogs; however, in cats, this pooling occurs in the lungs and the major vessels of the thorax. The net result in both species is severe hypotension. The marked edema that often accompanies envenomation can also be a major contributor to the shock state. Most pit viper venoms cause destruction of blood vessel walls, allowing for massive leakage of red blood cells and plasma. Up to one third of the total circulating fluid volume of the blood may be lost into an affected extremity within several hours of a severe envenomation.

Table 1. Venom Yields of Some North American Snakes

Snake	Dry Weight (mg/body weight)	Median Lethal Dose (LD$_{50}$)*
Rattlesnakes (Crotalus)		
Eastern diamondback (C. adamanteus)	200–850	1.68
Western diamondback (C. atrox)	176–600	2.18
Sidewinder (C. cerastes)	18–50	2.64
Timber (C. horridus horridus)	75–210	2.69
Red diamond (C. ruber ruber)	120–450	3.77
Mojave (C. scutulatus)	75–150	0.23
Prairie (C. viridis viridis)	35–110	1.62
Southern Pacific (C. viridis helleri)	75–250	1.60
Great Basin (C. viridis lutosus)	75–150	2.01
Pygmy rattlesnakes (Sistrurus)		
Pygmy (S. miliaris)	12–35	2.85
Massassauga (S. catenatus)	15–45	2.91
Moccasins (Agkistrodon)		
Copperhead (A. contortrix)	40–75	10.92
Cottonmouth (A. piscivorus)	90–170	4.19
Coral snakes (Micrurus and Micruroides)		
Western coral (M. euryxanthus)	1–6	0.90
Eastern coral (M. fulvius)	2–20	0.28

*All LD$_{50}$ determinations are intravenous for 18 to 26 gm mice.
(Reprinted with permission from Russell, F. E.: Snake Venom Poisoning. Great Neck, NY: Scholium International, Inc., 1983.)

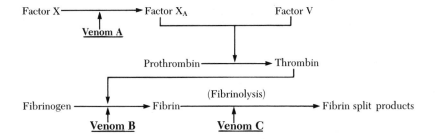

Venom A
  Crotalus viridis helleri (So. Pacific rattlesnake)
Venom B
  Agkistrodon contortrix (copperhead)
  A. piscivorus (cottonmouth)
  C. adamanteus (Eastern diamondback rattlesnake)
  C. horridus (timber rattlesnake)
  C. viridis helleri (So. Pacific rattlesnake)
Venom C
  C. atrox (Western diamondback rattlesnake)
  C. molossus molossus (black-tailed rattlesnake)

Figure 1. Venom effect on clotting mechanisms.

FACTORS INFLUENCING THE SEVERITY OF THE BITE. The severity of the bite depends primarily upon the quantity and the toxicity of the venom injected by the snake. However, the amount and composition of the venom available at any given time is dependent upon several factors:

1. Time of year—the peptide fraction is higher in relation to the enzymatic fraction in spring and lower in fall.

2. Regenerated volume since last bite.

3. Age of the snake—very young snakes have high peptide fractions.

4. Aggressiveness of the snake.

5. Motivation of the snake—offensive strikes are usually much more severe. Agonal strikes are most severe; a decapitated head is dangerous for up to 1½ hr.

FACTORS ASSOCIATED WITH THE VICTIM. These include (1) size of the victim, (2) site of the bite, (3) time elapsed since the bite, and (4) amount of physical activity after bite occurred (increasing the uptake of venom).

CLINICAL SIGNS AND DIAGNOSIS

Venomous snakebite is not always easy to diagnose, particularly if heavy hair and swelling obscure fang puncture wounds. It is prudent to clip the hair in the region while searching for wounds. Often bleeding puncture wounds can be found, indicating pit viper bite. One or more puncture wounds may be present, and the victim may have received multiple strikes. Local edema can obscure puncture wounds. The initial symptoms are often marked edematous swelling, resulting from increased vascular permeability, pain, and ecchymosis in the region. The initial swelling can be difficult to differentiate from angioedema due to allergic reactions to arthropod bites. Pain is often immediate and seems to subside after the first hour or two. Ecchymoses and discoloration of the skin often appear within several hours after bites by pit vipers, especially the Eastern or Western diamondbacks or the Pacific rattlesnakes. These reactions can also be seen with most other rattlesnakes and the cottonmouth but are less common following copperhead envenomations.

Severe hypotension is often present. Local edema can be dangerous with bites to the laryngeal region (e.g., a tracheotomy was required in one case of envenomation in the tongue that completely occluded the airway.) Edema is progressive for up to 36 hr following the bite. Other signs can include muscle fasciculations, increased salivation, and enlarged, painful regional lymph nodes.

The majority of dogs are bitten on the head (80 per cent of 300 cases); the remainder are bitten on the legs and, rarely, on the body. Cats are bitten more often on the front legs (44 per cent of 100 cases) and head (35 per cent). The other 21 per cent occur on the cat's body, usually on the shoulder or over the thorax. The bites to the body tend to involve much more severe envenomation. Dogs are presented for medical treatment earlier than cats, perhaps because of the reclusive nature of injured cats. Because of the venom:body weight ratio, smaller animals are at greater risk.

Clinical signs of severe envenomation may take several hours to appear; therefore, all patients should be hospitalized and monitored for at least 24 hr. Laboratory values can be a valuable aid in defining the severity of the envenomation. The severity of envenomation cannot be judged by the amount of local reaction. Biochemical profiles prove the fallacy of this clinical assumption. Experience indicates that severe envenomations can occur with little or no local edema (see preceding discussion on factors affecting the severity of the bite).

Obtain a laboratory data baseline upon presentation of the patient. Values to be acquired should include complete blood count (CBC), platelets, coagulation profile (prothrombin time [PT], partial thromboplastin time [PTT], fibrinogen), serum electrolytes, BUN, creatinine, creatine phosphokinase (CPK), and glucose. Measure the circumference of the affected body part above, below, and at the bite site. These measurements will quantify the progression of edema and should be recorded at 15-min intervals. Decreased platelet counts, prolonged clotting times, or both indicate envenomation severity with most pit viper bites. A persistent drop in platelet count suggests progressive venom activity. Hemoglobinuria or myoglobinuria (from severe rhabdomyolysis) is evidence of severity, as is marked, early (within first 12 hr) elevation of the CPK level. Electrocardiographic monitoring should be performed in cases of severe envenomation.

Common differential diagnoses include allergic reactions from bites of arthropods, cat fight wounds, or early abscesses. Failure to locate multiple puncture wound sites is a problem. Envenomation—the injection of venom—is necessary for toxic effect. Therefore, "snakebite" is not a valid medicolegal term to refer to the effects of snake venom.

TREATMENT

The bitten animal should be subdued and immobilized as much as possible to slow the uptake of venom. Most first-aid measures are ineffective and often increase the severity of the condition, especially in untrained hands. Therefore, rapid transport to a veterinary medical facility is the best advice that can be given to owners.

Controlled studies should prevail when therapeutic regimens are designed. The following treatment protocol is recommended:

1. Diphenhydramine (Benadryl, Parke-Davis). In small dogs and cats, administer 10 mg; in large dogs, give up to 25 mg IV or SC. Diphenhydramine has *no* effect upon the snake venom or body responses. It is used to calm the victim (half of this dose subcutaneously calms the fractious animal and eases catheterization) and to pretreat against allergic responses to antivenin.

2. IV fluids: Lactated Ringer's solution, 9 per cent sodium chloride or colloids. Remember that the primary cause of death is cardiovascular collapse due to hypovolemic shock, so aggressive fluid therapy is indicated.

3. Antivenin (Antivenin [Crotalidae] Polyvalent [equine origin], Fort Dodge or Wyeth)—at least one vial administered IV. (Reconstitution requires several minutes and is facilitated by warming the vial to body temperature and swirling but not shaking.) All animals should be skin tested before antivenin is given, even though many false-positive or false-negative test results are encountered. Follow the skin-test directions in the package insert. Injection of antivenin should be slow, as a complement reaction can occur if it is given too fast. Monitoring the inner pinna for hyperemia is a good indicator of systemic reactions. Epinephrine should be available. If the patient has a reaction to the antivenin, discontinue administration, give diphenhydramine intravenously, wait a few minutes, and then start antivenin more slowly under close observation. If a reaction recurs, stop injection and seek consultation. Antivenin should not be injected IM or around the bite site, as it is absorbed poorly. If the skin test is positive, it does not preclude antivenin use, but close monitorng is advised. This is the only proven treatment against pit viper envenomation. Several vials may be necessary. Repeated administration may be needed, depending on clinical and laboratory results. One vial should be administered as soon as the diagnosis is established. Antivenin is most effective when given early. The cost of this product often precludes the use of several vials.

4. Antibiotics. Broad-spectrum antibiotic therapy is recommended.

Corticosteroids are of questionable value. Steroids do not alter the course of envenomation, and marked increases in mortality may occur with their use. Corticosteroids alter laboratory results that can be extremely important in monitoring the patient's clinical progress. For these reasons, the use of corticosteroids is not advocated.

Elapids (Coral Snakes)

Bites by the coral snake are uncommon because of its reclusive behavior and nocturnal habits. However, if threatened, coral snakes can exhibit aggressive behavior, with pugnacious bites and vigorous chewing action.

The coral snake's venom is primarily neurotoxic; however, the mechanism of action is not well-understood. Cholinesterase is present but has been shown not to contribute significantly to the neuromuscular block produced by the venom.

Puncture wounds are difficult to find owing to their small size and the absence of local signs. Pain may be present initially after the bite but is transient. These factors, coupled with a heavy hair coat, create a significant diagnostic challenge. Usually, swelling is not detected at the bite site; however, small punctures can be found from which blood can be expressed.

Clinical signs may be delayed several hours. In one prospective study, the mean time from bite to onset of signs was 170 min, with a range of 30 to 780 min. Once signs develop, they progress with alarming rapidity. Therapeutic intervention may not be successful if antivenin is given after the onset of the syndrome. It is extremely difficult to assess the severity of the bite, since clinical signs may not develop for 12 hr or more. Bulbar paralysis with respiratory collapse is the primary cause of death. There is no evidence of cardiac failure or arrhythmias in severely envenomated patients. If complete paralysis does not occur, aspiration pneumonia is the primary complication and can account for marked increases in morbidity and mortality rates (Kitchens and Van Mierop, 1987).

TREATMENT

If coral snake bite is highly suspected, early and aggressive antivenin (Antivenin [*Micrurus fulvius*] [equine origin], Wyeth) administration is recommended before onset of clinical signs (see preceding discussion on antivenin administration for pit viper bite). The animal should be transported immediately to a facility that can provide respiratory support in a critical care setting. Experience has shown that once clinical signs appear, abatement of further progression of envenomation is not always possible. All victims should be hospitalized for 48 hr, and vital signs should be monitored closely.

If respiratory paralysis occurs, it can be managed with respiratory support and usually will subside within 48 hr. If the animal begins to demonstrate pharyngeal paralysis, intervention to prevent aspiration pneumonia should be instituted via intubation. Several weeks may be required for complete recovery. Successful intervention is achieved not by waiting for clinical signs to appear but by intervening early and aggressively (minimum of two vials antivenin) coupled with the administration of respiratory support if needed.

Note: Sonoran coral snake (*Micruroides euryxanthus*) venom is not inactivated by Antivenin (*Micrurus fulvius*, equine origin); therefore, treatment is largely supportive. Symptoms are less severe in humans bitten by this species of coral snake, but the practitioner should have respiratory support available. Also, this species of coral snake tends to be less aggressive, and bites are not common.

GILA MONSTER

The only species of poisonous lizards in the world are found in the southwestern United States and Mexico—the Gila monster (*Heloderma suspectum*) and the Mexican beaded lizard (*H. horridum*). These heavy-bodied lizards are easily recognized by the beadlike surface and the yellow or coral-colored pattern of their skin. These lizards are lethargic and nonaggressive, and thus animal envenomations are rare. They do not have fangs per se but are armed with grooved teeth that are bathed in venom from modified salivary glands located on each side of the lower jaw. Gila monsters and Mexican beaded lizards tenaciously hold onto the victim and, with chewing movements, increase the quantity of envenomation.

The *Heloderma* venom is less well characterized than many of the snake venoms. A neurotoxin, a hyaluronidase, peptides related to the vasoactive intestinal peptide-secretin family, and two arginine esterases have been described. The venom contains a heat-stable, noncholinergic, and nonhistaminic smooth muscle–stimulating factor. Also, recent work has isolated a kallikreinlike hypotensive enzyme from the venom of the Mexican beaded lizard.

The teeth of these lizards usually produce simple puncture wounds, which may vary from 1 to as many as 18. If envenomation has taken place, pain is usually present within several minutes. Intense pain may radiate from the periphery but seldom extends beyond the involved extremity. Some hemorrhage may occur at the site of the bite, but there is no clinical evidence to suggest that the venom alters blood coagulation. A rapid fall in blood pressure follows, with congestion of blood in the lungs, which can result in a life-threatening hypotensive crisis. Other symptoms seen are increased salivation, lacrimation, and frequent urination and defecation. Several laboratory studies have noted severe retrobulbar hemorrhage with resultant exophthalmus. Also of note was the production of aphonia in some cats.

The reptile may have to be disengaged by sticking a prying instrument between the jaws and pushing against the back of the mouth. A flame to the underside of the jaw seems to be very effective, as the lizard will usually release the victim. The teeth of the lizard are brittle and easily break off and remain embedded in the wound.

TREATMENT

Pain can be quite intense but generally can be controlled with aspirin; in more severe cases, morphine or meperidine may be required. Diazepam (Valium, Roche) reduces anxiety and the need for analgesia. The primary danger is hypotension: therefore, intravenous fluid therapy should be instituted whenever envenomation has occurred. A direct venom action upon cardiac muscle has been suggested, and electrocardiographic monitoring is prudent. Locally, the wound should be irrigated (not infused) with lidocaine, washed, and probed for broken teeth. Follow-up therapy of soaks with a solution similar to Burow's solution t.i.d., along with appropriate antibiotic therapy, is usually sufficient.

There is no commercial antivenin; therefore, treatment must be supportive. Neither antihistamines nor corticosteroids are of value. Anaphylactic reaction to *Heloderma* venom is rare.

SPIDERS

Practically all spiders are venomous; however, severe reactions are limited to two genera: *Latrodectus* (black widow and red widow spiders, females) and *Loxosceles* (brown recluse and common brown spiders). *Tegenaria agrestis* (Walckenaer [Hobo] spider) has also been associated with lesions of necrotic arachnidism (see discussion on brown recluse spider). The infamous tarantula (Eurytelma) is capable of a venomous bite, but serious reactions from natural bites in domestic animals have not been reported.

Spiders subsist on the body fluids of their prey and thus use their venom to immobilize the victim. Venom is injected through channeled bilateral head appendage fangs called chelicerae. Considering the inconspicuous size of the bite marks as well as the animal's hair cover, diagnosis of spider bites is difficult for the veterinarian and is usually dependent on clinical signs.

Latrodectus (Black and Red Widow Spiders)

The adult female may be recognized by an hourglass-shaped marking, red to orange, on the underside of her globose, shiny, black abdomen. It is equally important to identify the immature female, which has a colorful pattern of red, brown, and beige on the dorsal surface of her abdomen, as she has the same potential for envenomation. The male is usually much smaller, and his bite generally lacks the ability to penetrate the skin.

Found throughout the United States and Canada, the black widow lives in funnel-shaped webs in dry, dimly lit, secluded places, often around houses where outside lights attract prey insects. These spiders are small and nonaggressive, with the ex-

ception of the extreme aggression shown by some females when protecting egg masses.

Latrodectus venom is neurotoxic to presynaptic nerve processes by increasing calcium ion permeability through the nerve cell membrane, locking open cation exchange channels. This depolarization promotes calcium-independent release of the neurotransmitters acetylcholine and norepinephrine.

Seasonal variation occurs in toxicity (highest toxicity in the autumn and lowest toxicity in the spring). Approximately 86 per cent of all bites occur in the 4-month period of late summer and early autumn.

Using striated muscle, the black widow squeezes the venom glands, forcing a controlled and variable amount of venom into the wound. Therefore, the amount of envenomation is variable, and estimates indicate that up to 15 per cent of bites are dry.

DIAGNOSIS

Local tissue changes are absent, and swelling of the affected body part is uncommon. The bite site shows small puncture wounds and may exhibit a blanched central area surrounded by a slightly erythematous region. This is difficult to see in animal victims because of pigmented skin and dense hair coats.

Regional numbness with tenderness in the local lymph nodes may precede hyperesthesia, progressive muscle pain, and fasciculations in the affected region. Cramping of the musculature of the chest, abdomen, lumbar region, and other large muscle masses is common. Abdominal rigidity without tenderness is a hallmark sign of *Latrodectus* envenomation. The victim suffers a great deal of pain in a moderate to severe envenomation. Abdominal cramping may compromise respiration. There is often obvious restlessness, writhing, and contorted spasmlike activity; seizures are possible. Signs of motor restlessness may abate over 10 to 20 hr, with a possible onset of paralysis. Hypertension and tachycardia should be expected; in high-risk victims, these cardiovascular manifestations may lead to stroke, exacerbation of heart failure, and myocardial ischemia. Death is usually due to respiratory or cardiovascular collapse

The cat is extremely sensitive to black widow spider venom (in one study of 22 envenomated cats, 20 died). Severe pain, excessive salivation, and restlessness are common. Paralytic signs may appear early and are particularly marked, with the body becoming atonic and adynamic.

Patients at greatest risk are those at the extremes of age and those with hypertensive cardiovascular disease. Envenomations in domestic animals have rarely been reported, probably because of failure to recognize the condition. The true incidence and mortality in veterinary patients is unknown.

TREATMENT

First aid is essentially of no value in treating *Lactrodectus* envenomation, and constricting bands and tourniquets should not be used. Treatment is largely supportive and is directed at relieving the presenting symptoms. If no systemic signs are seen, treatment with mild analgesics, such as aspirin, can be instituted. The patient should be closely monitored, as systemic symptoms may be delayed for several hours after envenomation and have taken several days to become manifest in less severe envenomations.

In those patients with severe muscle cramping and fasciculation, high concentrations of calcium, as well as other agents that facilitate the entrance of calcium ion into the nerve endings, antagonize the releasing effect of the venom. Therefore, the mainstay of treatment has become intravenous calcium as 10 per cent calcium gluconate, 10 to 30 ml (dog) and 5 to 15 ml (cat), given very slowly, carefully monitoring cardiac rate and rhythm during infusion. Calcium infusion may have to be repeated (4–6 hr), and if it fails to maintain the patient for more than 1½ hr, subsequent infusions may not be effective.

Hypertensive crisis may need to be treated specifically. Convulsive seizures are rare but are best treated with intravenous diazepam. Morphine or meperidine may be needed to control pain.

Antivenin (Lyovac Antivenin [equine origin], Merck Sharp & Dohme) is available and, if used, should be administered as soon as possible. One vial is usually sufficient. Antivenin treatment is reserved for severe envenomations. Antivenin treatment has provided the quickest relief, within a half hour, and gives the most permanent relief in humans. Care should be used, as the product is of equine origin, but anaphylactic reactions are rare (11 of 2062 cases, but all patients were pretreated with antihistamine).

The prognosis with *Latrodectus* envenomation is uncertain for several days, and recovery may take a long time. Weakness, fatigue, insomnia, and impotence may persist for several months.

Loxosceles

Brown spiders (*Loxosceles arizona*), brown recluse spiders (*L. reclusa*), fiddleback spiders (*L. deserta*) and other small brown spiders, found primarily in the southern half of the United States, can be distinguished from other light-brown spiders by a violin-shaped marking on the dorsal surface of the cephalothorax. The neck of the violin points toward the spider's abdomen. These species are nocturnal, active, and rarely aggressive; they usually require provocation to bite. *Loxosceles* species are often found outdoors, under stationary objects, or indoors, in basements, storage areas, and other darkened, undisturbed areas.

Loxosceles species are known for their potent and enduring dermonecrotic effects, which result from a complex venom of necrotizing enzymes and other proteins. The venom injected during bites often produces a necrotic dermal ulceration that spreads from the original envenomation site into dependent adjacent areas. Without medical management, this ulceration can progress and possibly involve tissue as deep as the underlying muscle layer. These lesions can remain active for months and cause gross disfiguration.

The bite is usually not painful initially. However, if envenomation has occurred, localized pain and erythema develop within 2 to 6 hr. A bleb, or blister, forms as early as 12 hr after envenomation. This site evolves into what has classically been referred to as a "bull's-eye" lesion, with the characteristic dark necrotic center bordered by a white ischemic ring upon an erythematous background. Necrosis follows as a result of ischemia, and by 7 to 14 days, the focal ulceration is evident. The ulceration can enlarge and become indolent. Fever, joint pain, weakness, emesis, convulsive seizures, hemolysis, and thrombocytopenia can occur from some bites. Healing is slow. A minimum of 8 weeks and perhaps several months is necessary for complete resolution. Permanent scar tissue is not uncommon.

TREATMENT

There is no specific antidote. Dapsone has lately been highly recommended in the literature on human medicine. Excision of all affected tissues allows healing by primary intention. This may be delayed until after maximum lesion development. Conservative treatment in human patients consists of daily irrigation with hydrogen peroxide, and Burow's solution soaks t.i.d. with débridement as necessary. Hyperbaric oxygen, 1 to 2 atmospheres b.i.d. for 3 days, has shown promise. Prophylactic antibiotics may be advisable in some cases.

SCORPIONS

Common stinging scorpions in the United States are in the genera *Vejovis*, *Hadruruis*, *Androctonus*, and *Centruroides*. The only life-threatening North

American scorpion sting is that of *Centruroides sculpturatus (C. exilicauda)*. It is distinguished from other less toxic species by more slender pincers, the presence of a tubercle at the base of its stinger, and a yellowish cephalothorax. The last segment of the highly mobile tail of this eight-legged arthropod contains a hollow, curved stinging apparatus through which venom is injected. *C. sculpturatus* is nocturnal, approximately 1½ inches long, and endemic to the Southwest. Often found around buildings, these scorpions seek out daytime microenvironments that are moist and cool, under stones, bricks, and wood, thus deriving their common name "bark scorpions."

C. sculpturatus envenomations are not uncommon in humans and can produce fatalities; however, the incidence of envenomations in domestic animals is not known. Difficulty in recognizing the condition may account for its low recorded incidence in veterinary medicine.

North American scorpion stings by species other than *C. sculpturatus* are not a major medical threat and, in the early stages, are very difficult to differentiate from insect stings. In contrast, the sting site of *C. sculpturatus* is often initially unremarkable, with the onset of local signs delayed up to 1 hr.

The venom of *C. sculpturatus* contains five separate neurotoxins that activate sodium channels, resulting in prolonged action potentials and depolarization of the presynaptic terminal. This causes an excitatory neurotoxicity.

Systemic neurotoxic effects of *C. sculpturatus* include parasympathetic signs of excessive lacrimation, urination, defecation, and salivation. Sympathetic signs of hypertension, mydriasis, piloerection, and hyperglycemia can occur. Skeletal muscle fasciculations and perpetual restlessness with jerking, writhing, and contortions can be severe in humans. Roving eye movements have been reported in many human patients. Death results from respiratory collapse, cardiac conduction disturbances, or severe hypertension.

Routine laboratory data should include serum calcium levels.

Common misdiagnoses include organophosphorus or carbamate toxicity, respiratory distress, and idiopathic seizures.

TREATMENT

There are no first-aid measures of value. Medical management is generally supportive and should be directed by clinical signs. Aspirin can be used for minor discomfort. The majority of scorpion stings do not require treatment beyond pain relief; however, patients should be monitored for clinical progression of the syndrome. The attending clinician should be prepared to support respiration and combat severe hypertension. Electrocardiographic monitoring is recommended in moderate to severe envenomations. Pharyngeal spasms can lead to aspiration.

Ventricular tachycardia can be treated with propranolol, which may also lower blood pressure. Severe hypertension can be treated with nitroprusside, diazoxide, captopril, or hydrazine. Muscle spasms have been mitigated with slow intravenous infusion of methocarbamol, 150 mg/kg, or 10 per cent calcium gluconate, 10 to 30 ml IV for dogs or 5 to 15 ml IV for cats, followed by diazepam, 2.5 to 20 mg for dogs or 2.5 to 5 mg for cats, every 4 to 6 hr.

Atropine has been used in the treatment of scorpion envenomations, but its effectiveness is questionable. Corticosteroids and antihistamines are of no value. Meperidine, morphine derivatives, and epinephrine are contraindicated owing to a synergistic effect with scorpion venom.

If intravenous fluids are administered, extreme care should be used owing to the increased risk of pulmonary edema.

Severe envenomations by *C. sculpturatus* may require treatment with antivenin. Currently, available scorpion antivenin has not been approved by the FDA.

BEES, WASPS, HORNETS, AND ANTS

The order Hymenoptera contains the important stinging insects—bees, wasps, hornets, and ants. Many species of this order are more dangerous because of the colony's aggressive reaction to disturbance and its ability to inflict a multitude of stings within a few minutes, with resultant massive envenomation. The venom apparatus is located on the terminal portion of the abdomen. In a few species, including the honeybee, the stinger is barbed, and the entire venom apparatus is torn from the insect's body and left attached to the victim.

Insect stings cause more human deaths in the United States than all other venomous animals combined. The most common cause of death is hypersensitization to the venom and anaphylaxis from subsequent exposure. Multiple envenomations by social insects may cause systemic nonimmunologic intoxication, with possible neurotoxicity, deranged blood clotting, hemolysis, hepatotoxicity, rhabdomyolysis, acute renal tubular necrosis, and other systemic effects already reported in animal studies with various Hymenoptera species. Deaths from multiple stings (hundreds) have been reported in dogs.

The venoms within this order vary among species.

Phospholipase and hyaluronidase are common to most Hymenoptera venoms. Venoms of the honeybee, harvester ant, and paper wasp contain potent hemolysins. Fire ants have several alkaloids that are necrotizing and hemolytic, and field ants exude formic acid that causes short-lived, intense pain. Seasonal variations in venom fractions and antigens occur.

Stings of these insects cause local inflammation; local pain usually subsides within the first hour. Stings from these insects can cause intense regional edema (which may be important with buccal or pharyngeal stings). The intensity of the reaction can be increased by multiple stings, to the extent that shock becomes an important clinical problem.

TREATMENT

The first consideration in clinical management is the differentiation of shock from anaphylaxis or from multiple stings. Second, laboratory blood and urine values may alert the clinician to the possible systemic damage from multiple stings (e.g., hemolysis, rhabdomyolysis, hepatic or renal dysfunction).

If needed, 1 to 5 ml of 1:10,000 aqueous solution of epinephrine should be injected subcutaneously in dogs and cats, as well as corticosteroids and antihistamines. (Antihistamines are of little value in fire ant stings.) The clinician must be alert to the fact that in some cases anaphylaxis may be delayed. Oxygen may be necessary if dyspnea is evident.

TICKS

Tick paralysis is an ascending afebrile motor paralysis that appears most commonly in children, cattle, sheep, and dogs. The offending ticks from paralyzed victims in North America are usually females of the genera *Dermacentor* and *Amblyomma;* their saliva contains a neurotoxin that blocks conduction in terminal nerve fibers, which results in inhibition of neurotransmitter release at end plates. The neurotoxin exerts a more profound effect on the nodes of Ranvier; therefore, longer nerve fibers are more markedly influenced. Acetylcholine evidently is the neurotransmitter most affected.

The factors responsible for toxin production by ticks are unknown. Toxicity can vary with geographic location within the same species of tick. The engorged female tick has usually been attached for 5 to 9 days prior to onset of neurologic signs. First, ataxia is observed; a bilateral ascending motor paralysis soon follows. Within 36 hr after onset of symptoms, dyspnea may develop if paralysis ascends to the respiratory center. Death results from respiratory paralysis.

The condition is one of lower motor neuron paresis with intact sensory and cranial nerve function. The animal may demonstrate proprioception deficiency but maintain normal anal sphincter tone. Absence of fever, normal cerebrospinal fluid parameters, and evidence of normal sensory function help differentiate this condition from central nervous system infections, polyradiculoneuritis, botulism, and other similar conditions.

TREATMENT

Removal of the tick results in rapid recovery within hours, and the victim is usually asymptomatic within 48 hr. All ticks must be removed, since a single tick can cause the condition. Careful inspection around the head and neck, including the external ear canal, should be performed. The use of insecticide dips or sprays effective against ticks aids in the removal process.

Australian researchers have been able to stimulate dogs to high titers of neutralizing antibodies against the Australian tick neurotoxin with administration of a toxoid. A toxoid is not available against North American tick toxin.

CENTIPEDES

Centipedes are a group of arthropods all of which share the common features of an elongated, multisegmented body. Each segment (10 to 50) has a pair of legs. Size and coloration also vary among species. Species of large centipedes may reach 25 cm in length.

Envenomation occurs through punctures made by the gnathopods on the head segment. The toxic principle involved is a cytolysin. It usually produces localized pain, hyperemia, and inflammation and may cause a lymphangitis.

Symptoms usually abate within a few hours, although, in rare instances, a persistent tenderness can last for extended periods of time, up to several weeks.

TREATMENT

Usual treatment is symptomatic and conservative. This includes reassurance of the victim, promotion of bleeding at the envenomation site, washing of the bite site, and a cool compress. If marked edema develops, the victim should be monitored closely. Analgesics can be given, and the patient should be monitored for possible anaphylactic allergic reactions.

References and Supplemental Reading

Curry, S. C., Vance, M. V., Ryan, P. J., et al.: Envenomation by the scorpion *Centruroides sculpturatus*. J. Toxicol. Clin. Toxicol. 21:417, 1983–84.

Gladstone, A. M.: Wasps, bees and hornets: The nature of their threat and countermeasures available. Dangerous Properties of Industrial Materials Journal 6:2, 1986.

Kitchens, C. S., and Van Mierop, L. H. S.: Envenomation by the Eastern coral snake (*Micrurus fulvius fulvius*)—a study of 39 victims. J.A.M.A. 258:1615, 1987.

Pennell, T. C., Babu, S. S., and Meredith, J. W.: The management of snake and spider bites in the Southeastern United States. Am. Surg. 53:198, 1987.

Rachesky, I. J., Banner, W., Jr., Dansky, J., et al.: Treatments for *Centruroides exilicauda* envenomation. Am J. Dis. Child. 138:1136, 1984.

Russell, F. E.: *Snake Venom Poisoning*. Great Neck, NY: Scholium International, Inc., 1983.

Russell, F. E., and Bogert, C. M.: Gila monster: Its biology, venom, and bite—a review. Toxicon 19:341, 1981.

Smith, R. S.: Venomous Animals of Arizona. Coop Ext Serv, Coll. of Agriculture, Univ. of Arizona, Bull. 8245, 1982.

Stewart, M. E., Greenland, S., and Hoffman, J. R.: First-aid treatment of poisonous snakebite: Are currently recommended procedures justified? Ann. Emerg. Med. 10:331, 1981.

Wasserman, G. S., and Siegel, C.: Loxoscelism (brown recluse spider bites): A review of literature. Vet. Hum. Toxicol. 19:256, 1977.

Section

3

CARDIOPULMONARY DISEASES

JOHN D. BONAGURA, D.V.M.
Consulting Editor

Diagnostic Approach to Cardiopulmonary Disorders 188
Initial Management of Respiratory Emergencies........................... 195
Echocardiography: Therapeutic Implications............................... 201
Bronchoscopy in the Small Animal Patient............................... 219
Congenital Heart Disease........................ 224
Acquired Valvular Heart Disease in the Dog 231
Canine Cardiomyopathy 240
Cardiomyopathy in the Cat and Its Relation to Taurine Deficiency....... 251
Canine and Feline Heartworm Disease 263
Atrial Arrhythmias.. 271
Therapy for Ventricular Arrhythmias.................................... 278
Bradyarrhythmias and Cardiac Pacing................................... 286
Therapy for Feline Aortic Thromboembolism............................. 295
Dietary Considerations in the Treatment of Heart Failure................ 302
Complications of Cardiopulmonary Drug Therapy......................... 308
Shock: Pathophysiology, Monitoring, and Therapy 316
Cardiopulmonary Resuscitation.. 330
Medical Management of Upper Respiratory Tract Disease 337
Laryngeal Paralysis... 343
Tracheal Collapse.. 353
Chronic Respiratory Disease in the Dog 361
Pulmonary Hypersensitivity Disorders 369
Pneumonia.. 376
Pulmonary Edema.. 385
Chylothorax... 393
Respiratory Neoplasia 399
Pleurodesis 405

DIAGNOSTIC APPROACH TO CARDIOPULMONARY DISORDERS

TIMOTHY BAUER, D.V.M.

Seattle, Washington

In cardiopulmonary medicine, as in every medical discipline, the establishment of a precise diagnosis is of paramount importance. Although this is not always possible in every patient, recommendations regarding treatment and prognosis should be based on the most precise morphologic and etiologic diagnosis obtainable by reasonable diagnostic methods. Just as retrieval and identification of an infectious agent from the lung provides important diagnostic and therapeutic information, recognition of degenerative, neoplastic, or immunologic processes will have prognostic and therapeutic implications.

This article outlines the diagnosis of cardiothoracic disorders. It is not designed to cover every subject in depth, rather it outlines the methods available and their indications, diagnostic potential, and limitations. Two major areas, pulmonary function testing and blood gas analysis, are not included (see *Current Veterinary Therapy VIII*, p. 201). Although pulmonary function testing may eventually become an important part of diagnostic veterinary pulmonary medicine, its clinical application and availability are limited at this time.

DIAGNOSTIC APPROACH

Clinicians dealing with thoracic disorders have a variety of diagnostic techniques at their disposal. How and when each is employed depends on the clinician's knowledge of and skill with each technique, as well as his or her understanding of the patient and the disease process.

Diagnostic methods can be divided into categories based on their invasiveness and diagnostic yield; it would clearly be preferable to utilize procedures with minimal invasiveness and high diagnostic yield. Unfortunately, in the field of cardiopulmonary medicine, few procedures possess both of these characteristics.

Some procedures that require minimal invasiveness but usually do not produce a definitive diagnosis are (1) history, (2) physical examination, (3) thoracic radiography, (4) electrocardiography, (5) hematologic evaluation, (6) biochemical evaluation, and (7) blood gas analysis. These may suggest a disease process; however, reliance on them as the only diagnostic studies may lead to serious misdiagnoses. Other procedures that require minimal invasiveness and may yield a definitive diagnosis when combined with procedures from the aforementioned group include (1) serologic tests, (2) urine culture, (3) blood culture, (4) Gram stain, (5) peripheral lymph node aspiration, and (6) ultrasonography. Invasive procedures may place some patients at significant risk but have the highest diagnostic yields. These procedures may provide the most valuable information and, in most instances, carry less risk than thoracotomy. They are listed in increasing order of invasiveness.

1. Pulmonary scintigraphy (ventilation-perfusion scanning).
2. Transtrachial aspiration.
3. Thoracentesis.
4. Laryngoscopy.
5. Bronchoscopy.
6. Bronchography.
7. Percutaneous pleural needle biopsy.
8. Bronchoalveolar lavage.
9. Fine-needle aspiration of the lungs.
10. Transbronchial lung biopsy.
11. Cardiac catheterization and angiography.
12. Cutting-needle lung biopsy.
13. Mediastinoscopy.
14. Thoracoscopy.
15. Open lung biopsy.

The decision to proceed from noninvasive procedures to invasive techniques depends on the clinical situation. In a seriously ill patient, a definitive diagnosis should be obtained as rapidly as possible, and the early use of invasive procedures may be justified. The patient's clinical progress should dictate the techniques used; changes in the clinical condition should prompt appropriate changes in the diagnostic approach.

HISTORY AND PHYSICAL FINDINGS

Clinical Signs

There are relatively few specific clinical signs exhibited by animals with thoracic disorders. These signs, which may occur acutely or develop insidiously over several days or weeks, are often alarming to the client and cause variable degrees of discomfort to the patient. In addition to the complete review of systems, it is important to obtain from the client a detailed description of the clinical signs and their progression. Cough, dyspnea, and abnormal respiratory sounds are the most important clinical signs of thoracic disorders.

COUGH. Cough is one of the most frequent signs of pulmonary disease in the dog and is one of the most specific indicators of airway or pulmonary parenchymal disease, although it occasionally occurs as a primary sign of other thoracic disorders (e.g., pleural disease). Cough is a normal defense mechanism that is often the first sign of a wide variety of unrelated pulmonary disorders in the dog. Although it is caused by similar mechanisms, cough in cats is a much less common sign with thoracic disorders other than airway-oriented processes.

Cough may be characterized as productive or nonproductive and dry or moist. Although nocturnal cough may be reported with some disorders and early-morning cough with others, the timing and frequency of the cough are often unreliable in determining the nature and severity of the chest disorder.

DYSPNEA. Although dyspnea is a subjective feeling of difficulty in breathing and, therefore, is not detectable objectively, the term is usually used in veterinary medicine to encompass abnormalities of respiratory rate and character, such as tachypnea and hyperpnea. Dyspnea may result from a variety of disorders, many of which are extrapulmonary; its presence is significant and warrants immediate investigation. It may be the result of muscular or neurologic disorders, pain, anemia, fever, sepsis, hypotension, or abdominal disorders (masses or ascites), as well as primary pulmonary, pleural, and cardiac disorders. Patients with upper airway obstruction often exhibit acute dyspnea with hypoxia that may approach asphyxiation. Difficult breathing at rest should be distinguished from that following exertion or excitement, and the presence or absence of cyanosis should be identified.

The primary studies undertaken in the patient with cough or dyspnea as the primary sign include historical and physical examination, thoracic radiography, and basic laboratory evaluation, including complete blood count, serum chemistries, and urinalysis. Patients can be arbitrarily grouped into those with radiographic evidence of cause and those without radiographic evidence of cause. In patients with radiographic change that will require further diagnostic procedures to establish cause, interventions will be dictated by results of initial laboratory tests and the pertinent physical findings.

ABNORMAL RESPIRATORY SOUNDS. Hoarseness and changes in vocal character are signs of an upper airway or laryngeal abnormality. Such a finding, especially when accompanied by stridor or dyspnea, should prompt examination by direct visualization of the upper airway. Neurologic disorders, either central or peripheral, may result in laryngeal dysfunction. In addition, local, neoplastic, or inflammatory disorders may be responsible for such signs.

Wheeze, a sound produced by air being forced through a narrowed airway, may become audible as a result of either upper or lower airway obstruction and may occur either at rest or with exertion. Inspiratory wheezing with stridor suggests narrowing of an extrathoracic airway (larynx or trachea), whereas expiratory wheezing usually indicates intrathoracic obstruction. However, because airway obstruction at the laryngeal level is often fixed rather than variable, this differentiation can be confusing.

Physical Examination

The detailed physical examination remains the most important foundation for thoracic diagnosis, with other studies dictated by the results of the examination. Examination of the chest requires knowledge of regional anatomy, as well as the range of normal variation encountered with different species, breeds, and somatotypes within a species. Accurate interpretation of physical findings requires patience, a quiet environment, a cooperative patient, and, most important, experience. Because the animal's posture may affect one's ability to evaluate heart and lung sounds as well as extrathoracic features, patients should be evaluated in their normal standing posture whenever possible.

EXTERNAL EVALUATION OF THE THORAX. The first determination should be whether respiration is normal or abnormal. If respiratory effort is increased, one must ascertain whether it is mainly inspiratory, expiratory, or both. Audible respiratory sounds should be noted and described. The visible upper respiratory tract passages, including external nares and oral pharanx, should be examined.

General thoracic configuration should be observed for symmetry of structure and motion. Patients with either acute or chronic obstructive airway disorders, a large pleural effusion, or other space-occupying thoracic lesions may appear to have enlarged or barrel-shaped thoraces.

PALPATION. The larynx and neck should be inspected for swelling or tracheal displacement. The larynx should be lightly compressed, and the quality of respirations should be observed. Patients with partial laryngeal obstruction by vocal cords or masses may become completely obstructed or develop stridor with minimal compression. Similarly, palpation of the cervical trachea may reveal deformity, collapse, or sensitivity. Diminished or asymmetric thoracic motion observed initially may be confirmed by direct palpation. The cardiac impulse should be evaluated for location, intensity, and thrills. The jugular vein should be examined and palpated for distention and abnormal pulsations, which are usually a sign of right-sided heart disease or pericardial effusion, either primary or caused by pulmonary disorders.

MEASUREMENT OF CENTRAL VENOUS PRESSURE. Exact measurement of venous pressure requires direct vascular cannulation; this, however, is infrequently necessary, as clinically relevant estimates may be obtained by visual and digital inspection of the neck veins. Findings may be obtunded in the severely volume-depleted patient or a patient given diuretics; thus, re-examination should be undertaken following adequate rehydration.

Distended neck veins without pulsation are most frequently associated with venous obstruction at various levels. Superior vena cava syndrome is perhaps the most frequent cause, followed by right atrial inflow obstruction.

Distended veins with pulsation may be caused by a wide variety of disorders, both cardiac and pulmonary. Consideration must be given to the following diagnoses: any cause of right-sided heart failure, pericardial effusion, large pleural effusion, hyperthyroidism, any pulmonary disorder associated with profound small airway obstruction, and tricuspid valve disorders with or without overt congestive heart failure (CHF).

EXAMINATION OF ARTERIAL PULSES. Routine examination of the arterial pulses should include both the femoral and carotid arteries. The neck arteries are frequently unobservable; however, when abnormalities are present they may be profound.

Weak pulses with a narrow pulse pressure are a prominent finding in the disorders of decreased cardiac output, peripheral vasoconstriction, or mechanical obstruction such as aortic stenosis or distal aortic obstruction. Causes include hypovolemia, shock, cardiac tamponade, and myocardial failure.

Hyperkinetic or bounding pulses with a wide pulse pressure may be present in disorders of increased cardiac output, increased stroke volume, or increased vasomotor tone. Hypertension, hyperthyroidism, fever, anemia, heart block, aortic regurgitation, patent ductus arteriosus, and arteriovenous fistulas all are potential causes.

PERCUSSION. Percussion of the chest serves two major functions: to identify the normal anatomic borders of thoracic and extrathoracic structures and to ascertain if there is aerated lung in appropriate sites. Because interpretation of percussed sound is subjective, considerable practice is required to develop a reliable percussion technique.

Percussion over normal lung produces a low-frequency vibration with a resonant note. When underlying structures are dense, such as over the cardiac region, consolidated lung, pleural fluid, or other thoracic masses, characteristic dulling of the vibration is noted. The character of the note obtained will vary with the area of the chest examined, amount of subcuticular tissue, and depth of breathing or body posture. It is sufficient to characterize the sounds as normal or full. Hyper-resonance has been reported with emphysema or pneumothorax, but this is more difficult to recognize.

AUSCULTATION. The major force in the generation of normally heard breath sounds is the turbulent flow of gas in the major airways, including the trachea and large bronchi. As air passes peripherally in the normal lung, flow becomes more laminar and the diameter of the airways prevents the transmission of sound to the surface. When there is a lung consolidation with patent airways, the major airway sounds may be better transmitted to the chest wall, producing more peripheral bronchial sounds. Pleural fluid, air, other mass lesions, or lung consolidation with airway obstruction inhibits sound transmission and causes diminished lung sounds.

Although debate continues regarding the correct terminology for abnormal lung sounds, continuous sounds are usually referred to as wheezes or rhonchi, whereas intermittent sounds are referred to as rales or crackles. Other terms used to further describe the sounds include dry, moist, and harsh. Crackles (rales) are short, randomly distributed sounds often audible during both inspiration and expiration. Initially, they may be heard only with deep inspiration or following cough. Crackles are usually caused by disorders that result in filling or collapsing of air spaces, including edema, pneumonia, lung fibrosis, and diffuse bronchial disease. The crackling is generated by the initial increase in pressure on residual air, forcing it toward adjacent air spaces. Wheezes (rhonchi) are continuous sounds with a musical character. The sound is generated by narrowing the airway, forcing air to pass through a narrow region abruptly into a wider region. The timing may be inspiratory or expiratory, depending on the location of the obstructive lesion.

Although diastolic gallops and the splitting of heart sounds invariably indicate pathologic changes in small animals, the finding of cardiac murmurs may not be referable to the patient's thoracic signs. A loud cardiac murmur of mitral regurgitation may be an impressive finding; however, careful evaluation of radiographic, electrocardiographic (ECG), and echocardiographic studies must corroborate the clinical diagnosis of symptomatic heart disease. Frequently, elderly patients with valvular heart disease will have concurrent airway or pulmonary parenchymal disease as the cause of their clinical signs.

Thoracic Radiography

Thoracic radiography remains a major tool in the investigation of chest disease. Although there are limited numbers of ways in which the lung or heart can react to injury (and produce radiographic patterns), the chest radiograph is invaluable when interpreted in light of other clinical information. Whenever possible, previous studies should be evaluated, as they may document progression of disorder and in some cases provide a normal study for comparison. The attending clinician is usually best qualified to interpret these studies, but it is useful to obtain a second opinion from a colleague or radiologist. Objectivity and unfamiliarity with the patient and client may allow useful observations overlooked on initial evaluations.

Proper technique is critical in thoracic radiography. A technically poor study may be worse than no study at all. Owing to the nature of the air-tissue interface in the lungs, an overexposed film may mask pulmonary lesions, whereas an underexposed film may create a false impression of infiltrates or masses. For this reason, it is advisable to develop a technique for a wide variety of patient sizes. Radiographic examination should always consist of lateral and dorsoventral views, using high kilovolt peak (kVp) and short (1/60 second or less) exposure time. Standard thoracic radiographs interpreted in conjunction with the patient's physical findings will dictate the progression of diagnostic maneuvers. Recognition of radiographic change will allow diagnostic management to be dictated by specific anatomic involvement of patients' disease.

DIAGNOSTIC MANAGEMENT

Cough or Dyspnea Without Pulmonary Opacification

Although patients with diffuse small airway disease may not have "normal" radiographic findings, frequently pulmonary opacification (increased density) is absent. Air trapping with hyperlucency and large lung volumes may be evident with flattening of the diaphragm in patients with acute bronchial asthma. Central airway obstruction (e.g., laryngeal obstruction, foreign body, or tumor) may mimic these findings; however, the clinical feature of stridor should easily help distinguish the two.

Patients with cough frequently will have near-normal radiographic studies; however, in others there may be associated bronchial thickening or increase in interstitial density. Decisions regarding further diagnostic studies such as bronchial secretion retrieval are governed by the duration and severity of clinical signs and response to prior therapy.

Pulmonary hypertension, with or without thrombosis, is characterized by clear lung fields and profound dyspnea. Lobar pulmonary arteries may be distended, but this is variable. In all but young patients with congenital pulmonary hypertension, the differentiation between thrombosis and primary pulmonary hypertension may be impossible without nuclear scintigraphy or pulmonary arteriography.

Pulmonary Nodules, Single or Multiple

The goals of diagnosis are threefold: (1) to allow early resection of malignancy; (2) to avoid needless thoracotomy or resection of metastatic lesions; and (3) to avoid needless thoracotomy for identification of benign or infectious lesions.

Pulmonary nodules often are unexpected in the asymptomatic patient, and many lesions are recognized on survey radiographs undertaken for unrelated reasons. Re-evaluation of the patient's history and physical examination may yield new findings. If previous radiographic studies exist, they should be reviewed.

Calcification of a solitary lesion, although uncommon, almost always denotes a benign cause such as granuloma. Metastatic spread of tumors with calcification rarely occurs without the obvious presence of an adjacent primary lesion (e.g., local invasion by osteo- or chondrosarcoma).

Lesion size and growth rate may indicate its nature; if previous studies confirm the lesion's existence and no change is observed, exploration or biopsy is probably not warranted. If the lesion has enlarged, but not doubled in size over a relatively long period of time (e.g., months), it is likewise not likely to represent malignancy. It would be advisable to follow such patients radiographically for an additional year, repeating studies quarterly.

In the converse situation, if significant lesion growth is observed, early intervention is warranted, by either closed needle biopsy or aspiration. Open biopsy and resection may be preferable if fluoroscopically guided pulmonary biopsy or aspiration is not possible. If tomography or computed tomography (CT) scan is available, such studies may help identify small metastasis or mediastinal node invasion, obviating the need for surgical intervention. Long-term survival following resection of pulmonary malignancy is not frequently observed, suggesting that the majority of these malignancies have spread prior to surgical intervention.

The presence of previously diagnosed extrathoracic neoplasia greatly increases the prospect that pulmonary nodules represent metastasis. If the etiology of the pulmonary lesions is unclear, intervention, both diagnostic and therapeutic, should be governed by the natural history of the probable primary malignancy (e.g., mammary gland carcinoma).

Pulmonary Mass Lesions

The recognition of a pulmonary or pleural mass lesion in any patient is an obviously disturbing finding. As with any malady, the appropriate laboratory evaluation should be obtained, including indicated parasitic or fungal serologic studies. If associated pleural effusion is present, it should be examined via thoracentesis. If available, nuclear or CT scan should be obtained. The majority of pulmonary mass lesions will be malignant. This knowledge may adversely affect a clinician's motivation to initiate other diagnostic or therapeutic maneuvers; however, large, benign lesions, such as lung lobe torsion, pleuropulmonary cysts, or lung abscesses, may then be missed.

Bronchoscopy and biopsy or needle biopsy may be important in some instances and may yield the diagnosis, obviating the need for diagnostic thoracotomy. Biopsy or needle aspiration is relatively contraindicated under a number of circumstances: (1) pre-existing respiratory distress; (2) fever or other findings suggestive of primary lung abscessation or secondary abscessation of a malignancy; (3) pulmonary hypertension; and (4) bullous lung disease or pulmonary cavitation abutting the pleura.

Although the aggressive nonsurgical pursuit of a diagnosis may well be warranted, serious consideration should be given to early thoracotomy. It may be interesting to provide a definitive diagnosis by minimally invasive means; however, it may be solely of academic interest. The author's opinion remains that the finding of a pulmonary mass in a symptomatic patient requires surgery, regardless of the etiology. All diagnostic maneuvers must have some therapeutic relevance; thus, in a disorder necessitating surgical intervention, thoracotomy ultimately will be diagnostic and potentially therapeutic. The questions that need to be answered prior to surgery relate to (1) survival: whether the patient will have increased longevity following resection as compared with that with the natural course of the disease; (2) resectability: whether the patient is a reasonable candidate for the magnitude of the proposed procedure, or whether other aspects of the patient's medical status prohibit the procedure (e.g., concurrent renal failure, sepsis, or congestive heart failure); (3) operability: whether, following pulmonary resection, the patient will have enough pulmonary tissue to function reasonably. The last-named can usually be ascertained without sophisticated pulmonary function testing by simply determining how much, if any, function the affected pulmonary segment currently has. In most instances, it has none.

Lobar Consolidation and Associated Fever

As with all clinical problems, re-evaluation of the patient's history and physical examination is advisable, as are routine hematologic, serologic, biochemical, and bacteriologic studies. Microbiologic evaluation of respiratory secretions retrieved by transtracheal aspiration should be done in the patient with probable lobar pneumonia. In addition, blood and urine cultures should be performed in any patient with a septic clinical syndrome. If pleural effusion is demonstrated on routine radiographic evaluation, samples are obtained by thoracentesis for both culture and cytopathologic evaluation. Samples should be cultured aerobically and anaerobically. Although it will take 24 to 48 hours for organisms to grow, Gram stains should be immediately evaluated and utilized as a guide for the initiation of antimicrobial therapy. None of these procedures should be used as a sole diagnostic tool, rather their results should be considered in concert.

Failure of antibiotic therapy to obtain complete resolution of a presumed pneumonic process may indicate a number of phenomena: (1) multiple disorders (e.g., secondary infection of a pre-existing neoplasm or foreign body); (2) inappropriate antimicrobial therapy; (3) frank lung abscess; or (4) inappropriate diagnosis. In such cases, it should be assumed that misinterpretation of data has occurred or that there have been errors in laboratory assessment. Such patients should be re-evaluated, and further diagnostic studies should be initiated, such as bronchoscopy, needle aspiration, or lung biopsy.

If initial evaluation does not yield an infectious agent, lung biopsy may be required to definitively diagnose the problem. An inability to demonstrate organisms may be related to (1) concurrent or previous antimicrobial use; (2) failure to culture material anaerobically; or (3) bronchial obstruction that has prevented access to sites of infection. Although these may be plausible explanations, another consideration must be that the pulmonary consolidation is not referable to a bacterial cause. The primary diagnostic clue that will suggest that the process is not a primary lobar pneumonia is complete failure of therapy without radiographic proliferation.

Neoplasia, both discrete and infiltrative, must be a consideration in such patients. Bronchogenic carcinoma may affect the lung in both these ways, the former causing bronchial obstruction with a secondary obstructive pneumonitis and the latter resulting in infiltration of an entire lung lobe. Pulmonary lymphosarcoma may produce a similar picture; however, airway obstruction and resorption of bronchial air are not prominent features of this disorder. Noninfectious pneumonitis associated with lipid or water aspiration may mimic lobar pneumonia. These disorders are difficult to definitively diagnose with bronchoalveolar lavage; transbronchial lung biopsy or open lung biopsy may be required for definitive diagnosis. Pulmonary eosinophilia associated with angiitis and granulomatosis frequently demonstrates radiographic consolidation of a lung lobe. This disorder will require biopsy for definitive diagnosis. However, the probability of misdiagnosing this disorder as lobar pneumonia is unlikely, particularly if profound circulating eosinophilia is present.

Pulmonary Cavitation or Cystic Pulmonary Lesions

As a wide variety of benign and malignant disorders may produce pulmonary cavitation or cysts, the differential diagnosis is complex. Historical features of environmental exposure may aid in identifying patients with fungal disorders; this group may often be noninvasively evaluated with thoracic radiography and the appropriate serologic studies. Organisms may be retrieved in bronchial secretions or fine-needle lung aspirates, making the necessity for lung biopsy less probable. As with the fungal causes of cavitation, both lung abscesses and cavitary neoplasia typically drain debris into the airway; this usually makes bronchoscopy and bronchoalveolar lavage high-yield procedures. Any of the above causes may go undiagnosed with less invasive means of evaluation. An increased yield can be expected with bronchoscopic bronchial brushings or biopsy. Needle biopsy may be a useful technique; however, fluoroscopic guidance is necessary because the risk of pneumothorax appears to be increased when such procedures are done blindly.

Even when the diagnosis appears evident, there are some disorders in which thoracotomy is advisable. Examples include pneumothorax due to radiographically discernible rupture of cavitary or cystic lesions, with associated bronchopleural fistula; operable neoplasia; lung abscesses; pneumatoceles; or pulmonary cysts. Any thick-walled cavity in a symptomatic patient that is assumed to be infectious is an indication for resection if preceded by ineffective appropriate antimicrobial therapy.

Hilar Enlargement

The primary diagnostic problem associated with hilar mass lesions is the differentiation among (1) dilation of the great vessels, (2) left atrial enlargement, and (3) hilar adenopathy. In most cases, the determination can be made by assessment of the two standard views of survey radiographs. Distinction of vascularized structures may be easily made by angiography, although this is rarely necessary. Left atrial enlargement can be readily identified by echocardiographic evaluation. Tomography or CT scans can be helpful in identifying equivocal hilar node enlargement.

Hilar adenopathy is a prominent finding in a number of neoplastic, infectious, and immune disorders; among these are histoplasmosis, coccidioidomycosis, actinomycosis, lymphoma, metastatic carcinoma, and pulmonary eosinophilia associated with angiitis and granulomatosis. As nonsurgical access to the hilum is anatomically prohibitive, biopsy is not a rational option in most cases. All the aforementioned disorders typically also affect extrahilar or extrathoracic sites that can more easily be examined; hematologic, serologic, and amenable biopsy sites should be examined prior to consideration of thoracotomy.

Acute Air Space (Bronchoalveolar) Infiltrates

Following initial evaluation, patients may be arbitrarily divided into two diagnostic groups: (1) those that have distinctive physical, laboratory, and radiographic findings, with primary examinations strongly suggesting a diagnosis; and (2) those patients with acute signs, with physical findings and radiographs not suggesting a cause.

Although there are many potential causes for air space disease with frank hemoptysis, the overwhelming majority of patients will have either an endobronchial foreign body or coagulopathy. As such, all patients with these findings should have activated coagulation time (ACT), prothrombin time (PT), partial thromboplastin time (PTT), platelet counts, or specific factor analysis evaluated prior to any consideration of bronchoscopic evaluation.

In most patients with overt congestive heart failure (CHF) and pulmonary edema, the diagnosis is readily apparent when a complete evaluation has been obtained. The physical findings of murmur, gallop, and tachycardia, associated with cardiomegaly and bronchoalveolar infiltrate, should alert the clinician to the likelihood of this diagnosis. These findings should prompt both electrocardiographic and echocardiographic evaluation. With the strong clinical presumption of left-sided heart failure and pulmonary edema, any residual questions as to a cardiac etiology of the air space disease should be answered by a therapeutic trial with diuretic. If there is no demonstrable resolution of the infiltrate, the diagnosis of CHF should be re-evaluated. Although not diagnostic, the historical features associated with smoke inhalation, near-drowning, trauma, transfusion reactions, and iatrogenic overhydration should serve to differentiate these causes of pulmonary edema from those of primary cardiogenic etiology.

Fever, cough, and associated pulmonary infiltrates, in conjunction with purulent respiratory secretions, would suggest pneumonia. The appropriate diagnostic course has been previously discussed. Careful cytopathologic evaluation will allow infectious disorders to be differentiated from immunologic or eosinophilic pulmonary disorders.

When cardiac failure is ruled out by the appropriate studies and a primary pulmonary disorder is suspected, the aggressiveness of diagnostic investigation is governed by the patient's clinical condition. In the minimally symptomatic patient in whom a tentative diagnosis is likely, an appropriate therapeutic trial is warranted. In patients with rapidly progressive disease or those with significant respiratory distress on presentation, the early use of needle aspiration, bronchoscopy, or lung biopsy is warranted.

Pleural Effusion

Under most circumstances, the radiographic recognition of a pleural effusion merits thoracentesis and pleural fluid analysis. This should include both aerobic and anaerobic cultures if the cytopathologic evaluation is suggestive of infection. The only exception is a patient with previously diagnosed disease in which pleural effusion is a predictable sequela (i.e., CHF or hypoproteinemia). When previously diagnosed patients develop effusions that are atypical or coexist with unexplained exacerbation of their disease, diagnostic thoracentesis should be performed to rule out concurrent disorders such as CHF with coexisting pneumonia or parapneumonic effusion. The risks of attempting to sample small pleural effusions by needle thoracentesis are largely related to iatrogenic pneumothorax. Such risks must be weighed against inability to provide patient care owing to lack of a specific diagnosis.

Often thoracentesis is both diagnostic and therapeutic in the dyspneic patient. When a significant pleural effusion prevents radiographic evaluation of the thorax, a new study is always obtained following bilateral pleural drainage. Should fluid analysis and radiographic evaluation not suggest a cause for the effusion, choice of further diagnostic maneuvers is dictated by the character of the pleural fluid.

True hemothoraces rarely occur for reasons other than trauma, hemorrhagic diathesis, previous thoracic surgery, or rupture of a vascular tumor such as hemangiosarcoma. It should be noted that many disorders will produce a bloody fluid that does not truly represent intrathoracic bleeding; most notably, cats with a combination of cardiac and renal failure will frequently have bloody effusions. Previously clear effusions may become bloody following a traumatic thoracentesis. Patients with lung torsion will typically have bloody pleural effusions.

When laboratory evaluation of pleural fluid classifies it as a true transudate, the scope of the differential diagnosis is distinctly narrowed, and consideration should be given to the following diagnoses: heart failure, vena caval or right atrial inflow obstruction, constrictive pericarditis, lymphangiectasias, and disorders resulting in hypoproteinemia, such as nephrotic syndrome or cirrhosis.

The etiology of noninfected exudates may be more obscure and may well require the use of more invasive techniques to define the problem. When postdrainage chest radiographs and pleural fluid analysis fail to render a diagnosis, needle biopsy (Cope and Bernhardt, 1963) of the pleura is indicated. This procedure will have a variable yield, dependent on the disorder and its anatomic distribution. Disorders most frequently producing pleural effusion diagnosable by pleural biopsy include metastatic carcinoma, mesothelioma, feline infectious peritonitis, and actinomycosis. There are variable findings with lymphoma, bronchogenic carcinoma, fibrosarcoma, alveolar cell carcinoma, and fungal disorders. Under most circumstances, there is radiographic evidence of mediastinal or pulmonary involvement with these disorders, suggesting alternative methods of diagnosis.

References and Supplemental Reading

Andersen, H. A., and Fontana, R. S.: Transbronchoscopic lung biopsy for diffuse pulmonary diseases; techniques and results in 450 cases. Chest 62:125, 1972.

Bookstein, J. J., and Silver, T. M.: The angiographic differential diagnosis of acute pulmonary embolism. Radiology 110:254, 1974.

Braunwald, E.: *Heart Disease: A Textbook of Cardiovascular Medicine*, 3rd ed. Philadelphia: W. B. Saunders Co., 1988.

Cope, C., and Bernhardt, H.: Hook-needle biopsy of pleura, pericardium, peritoneum and synovium. Am. J. Med. 35:189, 1963.

Ferrari, M., Paez, A., Lopez Soto, C., et al.: Basic physiopathological patterns of perfusion and inhalation pulmonary scintigraphy. Thorax 24:695, 1969.

Kalinske, R. W., Parker, R. H., Brandt, D., et al.: Diagnostic usefulness and safety of transtracheal aspiration. N. Engl. J. Med. 276:604, 1967.

Light, R. W., MacGregor, W. I., Luchsinger, P. C., et al.: Pleural effusions; the diagnostic separation of transudates and exudates. Ann. Intern. Med. 77:507, 1972.

Ramirez, R. J.: Bronchopulmonary lavage. Dis. Chest 50:581, 1966.

Suter, P. F., and Lord, P. F.: *Thoracic Radiography: A Text Atlas of Thoracic Diseases of the Dog and Cat*. Wettswil, Switzerland: Peter F. Suter, 1984.

INITIAL MANAGEMENT OF RESPIRATORY EMERGENCIES

R. J. MURTAUGH, D.V.M.,
and GLEN L. SPAULDING, D.V.M.
North Grafton, Massachusetts

NON–LIFE-THREATENING RESPIRATORY EMERGENCIES

The problems of intractable cough and severe sneezing, along with epistaxis, are not usually medical emergencies from the perspective of veterinarians. However, these conditions are disturbing to the animals' owners and frequently result in their consulting the veterinarian for immediate assistance.

Uncontrolled paroxysms of coughing can be debilitating for an animal, can be associated with syncopal episodes, and can result in self-perpetuating airway inflammation. The most common scenario usually involves a dog with infective or nonspecific tracheobronchitis. In the emergency room setting, the most important determination to be made based on physical examination findings and chest radiographs is to rule out causes for the cough that should not be treated with cough suppressants (e.g., pulmonary edema and bronchopneumonia). Having excluded these possibilities, emergency treatment should be directed at suppression of the cough through sedation (acepromazine, 0.1 mg/kg SC) of the animal or administration of cough suppressants (butorphanol, 0.5 to 1.0 mg/kg b.i.d. or q.i.d. PO; hydrocodone, 0.25 to 0.5 mg/kg b.i.d. or q.i.d. PO; or both). Corticosteroid administration and antibiotic and bronchodilator therapy may be indicated following further evaluation of radiographs or transtracheal aspirate samples by culture and cytologic study. Collection of these samples can usually be delayed until regular, nonemergency hours.

Acute onset of severe sneezing in dogs and cats is usually associated with the passage of a foreign body (e.g., plant awn or sliver of wood) through the nostrils into the nasal cavity. Hypocalcemia and focal epilepsy may manifest similarly. Acute upper respiratory tract infections can have similar clinical signs, usually in association with bilateral seromucoid oculonasal discharge, fever, and oral ulcers (especially in cats). Animals with nasal foreign bodies will often appear agitated and paw at their faces. Epistaxis may result from direct mucosal damage by the foreign material or indirectly from rupture of small blood vessels caused by violent sneezing.

Treatment in these cases of nasal foreign material involves use of general anesthesia and removal of the offending material via rhinoscopy with an otoscope or small fiberoptic endoscope/arthroscope and an alligator forceps.

Epistaxis can occur as a result of facial trauma, neoplasia, inhalation of a foreign body, or a coagulopathy (e.g., thrombocytopenia, disseminated intravascular coagulation, intoxication with a vitamin K antagonist, multiple myeloma, and congenital coagulation factor deficiency). The most common cause in small animals is trauma. Foreign body–induced epistaxis is often accompanied by severe paroxysmal sneezing. Epistaxis associated with a coagulopathy rarely has concomitant signs of nasal cavity disease, but other clinical signs may suggest a systemic disease process.

Epistaxis associated with trauma is often self-limiting, requiring only cage rest and careful observation of the patient. Sedation of the animal to relieve anxiety and decrease activity that could exacerbate hemorrhaging may be indicated in some animals. The benefits of using tranquilizers to keep patients quiet during the time necessary for endogenous hemostatic mechanisms to become effective must be weighed against risks of inducing hypotension in animals potentially prone to development of shock.

Severe epistaxis associated with trauma or a coagulopathy requires more specific or aggressive treatment measures. The use of intravenous fluid therapy and possibly fresh whole blood transfusions may be required in animals with severe blood loss from epistaxis. When placed or sprayed into the nostrils (with muzzle pointed toward ceiling), dilute epinephrine (1:100,000) can be beneficial in decreasing epistaxis by vasoconstricting blood vessels (Norris and Laing, 1985). Severe hemorrhage (arterial bleeding) should be treated by packing the internal and external nares with gauze (which may be epinephrine soaked) with the animal intubated and under general anesthesia (Norris and Laing, 1985). This bandage material is generally left in place for 24 to 48 hours and is removed when hemorrhage has ceased. The evaluation of these patients is discussed elsewhere (see pp. 337–343).

LIFE-THREATENING RESPIRATORY EMERGENCIES

Cyanosis

Cyanosis can develop when blood is insufficiently oxygenated in the lungs, when hemoglobin is unable to carry oxygen, and when blood flow stagnates in peripheral capillary beds (Table 1). Unoxygenated hemoglobin concentration must be greater than 5 gm/dl of blood for cyanosis of mucous membranes to be appreciated clinically. Considerable hypoxemia can be present before cyanosis is detected (Pa_{O_2} often less than 50 mm Hg). In addition, anemic animals may not develop cyanosis despite marked hypoxemia (Amis and Haskins, 1986). Oxygen administration and rapid identification and treatment of the underlying cause of respiratory compromise is vitally important (Table 1). Important respiratory causes of cyanosis are discussed below.

Respiratory Distress

Identification of respiratory distress requires careful observation for characteristic clinical signs of anxious expression, extended head and neck, openmouth breathing with retraction of the corners of the mouth during inspiration, abducted elbows, tachycardia, and the animal's minimal concern for events going on in the immediate vicinity (Amis and Haskins, 1986). The nature of the ventilatory effort as well as ventilatory rate should be characterized to help categorize potential underlying causes of respiratory distress (e.g., slow, deep inspiration suggests upper airway obstruction and

Table 1. Causes of Cyanosis

Central	Peripheral*
Right-to-left shunting congenital heart defects and pulmonary AV shunting	Arterial thromboembolism
	Venous obstruction
	Arteriolar vasoconstriction
Hypoventilation CNS disease	Low cardiac output states
Respiratory muscle paralysis Pleural disease	Shock
Airway obstruction	
Ventilation-perfusion mismatch—pneumonia, pulmonary edema, pulmonary contusion, most generalized bronchial, interstitial, and alveolar lung diseases	
Methemoglobinemia†—chemical poisoning (many compounds; see Krotje, 1987)	

*Results from increased peripheral extraction of oxygen from normally saturated blood (low cardiac output—generalized cyanosis) or decreased delivery of blood to a peripheral area (thromboembolism—localized cyanosis).

†Blood sample will remain chocolate brown when shaken and exposed to air.

Reprinted with permission from Krotje, L. J.: Comp. Cont. Ed. Pract. Vet. 9:271, 1987.

rapid, shallow breathing suggests the possibility of pleural cavity disease). Nonrespiratory disorders can result in increased respiratory efforts that could be misinterpreted as suggesting respiratory distress. These conditions include hyperthermia, shock, metabolic acidosis, fear/anxiety, pericardial tamponade, anemia, abdominal organ enlargement or ascites, and drug-induced, metabolic, or central nervous system (CNS) disease effects on respiration (Amis and Haskins, 1986). Respiratory distress can result from airway obstruction, pleural cavity disease, chest wall abnormalities, pulmonary parenchymal disease (e.g., contusion, edema, and pneumonia), pulmonary arterial disease, and other causes.

GENERAL AIRWAY OBSTRUCTION

Evaluation of animals with airway compromise must be rapid, thorough, and minimally distressing to the patient. Assessment should include identification of the level and the severity of the obstruction. The major errors in the initial management of upper airway problems include underestimation of the degree of respiratory distress, overzealous examination, and performance of diagnostic procedures that disturb the patient and worsen the patient's clinical condition (Aron and Crowe, 1985). The patient should be allowed to maintain a position that is least stressful for it, and minimal restraint should be used when performing palpation and auscultation. An oxygen mask may be helpful to the patient or may induce further anxiety or distress. Observation from a distance for the pattern of breathing, evidence of stridorous breathing, and color of mucous membranes, followed by auscultation of the thorax, often provides reliable information from which to formulate an initial clinical treatment regimen without severely compromising the patient (Aron and Crowe, 1985). Animals with mild to moderate respiratory distress from airway obstruction usually respond well to sedation (with neuroleptanalgesic agents) (Aron and Crowe, 1985) and oxygen administration for stabilization prior to definitive treatment (e.g., partial laryngectomy or foreign body retrieval under general anesthesia). For animals with severe respiratory distress from upper airway obstruction, an adequate airway should be established by tracheostomy or endotracheal tube placement following induction of general anesthesia.

SPECIFIC CAUSES OF AIRWAY OBSTRUCTION

NASAL CAVITY. Trauma to the nasal cavity can result in obstruction of the airway as a result of edema, hemorrhage, and compromise of the nasal passages by fracture fragments. Postural drainage (head lower than body) and suction of the pharynx may be required to remove blood clots that may be contributing to airway occlusion, especially in obtunded patients with severe nasal bleeding. In patients that have significant nasal obstruction without adequate compensation by mouth breathing, sedation with narcotics or tracheostomy may be required to ensure adequate ventilation. Nasal obstruction usually resolves spontaneously over several days following nasal trauma as inflammation, edema, and hemorrhage subside. Surgical reconstruction is almost never required to re-establish a patent airway following severe nasal trauma.

Acute viral upper respiratory tract infections may result in a similar compromise to flow of air through the nasal passages. Useful supportive therapy may include administration of oxygen (O_2 cage), frequent cleaning of the nostrils, maintenance of adequate hydration by administration of intravenous or subcutaneous fluids, humidification of inspired gases to prevent inspissation of airway secretions and drying or inflammation of mucous membranes, intranasal administration of decongestants (phenylephrine, ephedrine), and use of antibiotics if secondary bacterial infection occurs.

LARYNX. For a more detailed discussion on treatment of laryngeal disease, the reader is referred to page 343.

In general, airway compromise in dogs with brachiocephalic airway disease, laryngeal trauma, laryngeal paralysis, or laryngeal masses is initially managed by cage rest, sedation, and oxygen supplementation. If significant laryngeal edema is present, the use of rapidly acting corticosteroids (prednisolone sodium succinate, 10 to 20 mg/kg IV) may be beneficial. Severe laryngeal edema, trauma, collapse, paralysis, or obstruction by tumor may require a temporary tracheostomy or general anesthesia and orotracheal intubation to stabilize the patient and ensure an adequate airway pending definitive surgical treatment.

Attempts to remove foreign objects lodged in the larynx can be made by suspending an animal by its hindlimbs, shaking the animal, and applying sharp compression to the abdomen (simulating a cough) (Amis and Haskins, 1986).

External palpation/massage of the larynx and pharynx in a caudal-to-rostral direction followed by a sharp blow to the back of the head and neck with the animal suspended may also dislodge foreign objects from the larynx. If these maneuvers are not *rapidly* successful in clearing the airway, the animal should be anesthetized (with neuroleptanalgesic agents) and a tracheostomy should be performed, followed by forceps retrieval of the foreign material with aid of laryngoscopy.

Laryngospasm commonly occurs in cats recovering from general anesthesia following endotracheal intubation and in dogs and cats undergoing laryngeal manipulation with an inadequate (too light) plane of anesthesia. Treatment involves sedation, topical application of lidocaine to the larynx, and temporary orotracheal intubation to maintain the airway and stabilize the animal.

TRACHEA. Dogs with tracheal collapse may require emergency treatment for reasons of intractable cough or airway obstruction. Airway obstruction is due to a combination of the anatomic defect, mucosal inflammation and edema, and anxiety in the animal (increased respiratory efforts result in further dynamic compromise of airway). Treatment involves use of short-acting corticosteroids, cage rest with sedation, and oxygen supplementation; rarely, tracheal intubation may be required. (For a more extensive discussion of management of tracheal collapse, see p. 353.)

Tracheal foreign bodies can occasionally be removed by manipulations similar to those recommended for laryngeal foreign bodies, but more commonly they require endoscopically guided retrieval or tracheotomy. Initial management of the airway in these patients requires general anesthesia and passage of small-bore catheters around the tracheal foreign body to ensure adequate ventilation and oxygenation of the patient pending definitive therapeutic intervention. If the foreign body is in the cervical trachea, percutaneous placement of a catheter into the trachea or a "slash" tracheostomy at the thoracic inlet will allow oxygenation of the patient for short-term management. These patients require a quick diagnosis and rapid definitive treatment!

SMALL AIRWAYS. Asthmatic cats often have coughing, wheezing, severe respiratory distress, and cyanosis. These animals may require empiric therapy based on a physical examination, as diagnostic procedures (radiography, bronchoscopy, or transtracheal aspiration) may be too stressful to undertake. However, radiographs should be obtained prior to therapy whenever possible. The primary differential diagnoses for acutely dyspneic cats would include acute viral/bacterial pneumonia (expect fever), pleural effusions or pneumothorax (dull lung sounds), cardiomyopathy (gallop rhythms/murmurs, pulmonary crackles), and thoracic trauma. Emergency treatment involves administration of oxygen; corticosteroids (prednisolone sodium succinate, 10 to 20 mg/kg IV); bronchodilators (aminophylline, 4 mg/kg IM or *slowly* IV); and possibly epinephrine (0.5 to 1 ml, 1:10,000 dilution IM or SC), beta-adrenergic agonists (terbutaline, 1.25 to 2.5 mg PO), and parasympatholytics (atropine, 0.04 mg/kg SC or IM). A dramatic response is commonly seen in 15 to 30 minutes. Failure of the animal to respond to treatment should prompt reassessment of the diagnosis. Airway foreign body and occult heartworm disease also should be considered in these cats. Additional discussion on management of asthmatic cats and chronic airway disease in dogs is available in this (see pp. 188–194 and 361–368) and other texts (Moses and Spaulding, 1985).

Trauma

PNEUMOTHORAX

The diagnosis of closed chest pneumothorax in an animal can be made by careful observation of a characteristic respiratory pattern and by auscultation (decreased dorsal lung sounds) and percussion (dorsal hyper-resonance) of the thorax. Respirations are usually rapid and shallow with an increase in respiratory rate. Tension pneumothorax is evidenced by hyper-resonance on percussion accompanying a severely exaggerated respiratory effort ("air hunger") in conjunction with minimal movement of the chest wall.

Treatment of closed chest pneumothorax depends on the severity of clinical signs of respiratory compromise. Mild pneumothorax, usually diagnosed on chest radiographs, can often be treated conservatively with observation and cage rest. Moderate to severe pneumothorax should be treated with bilateral therapeutic thoracentesis (using 22-gauge needle, extension set, stopcock, and syringe) and continued observation of the animal for evidence of recurrence of pneumothorax, indicating a persistent air leak from pulmonary parenchyma. Repeated needle aspirations can be performed with minimal risk, provided the amount of air appears to be decreasing over the course of several hours following trauma. Rapid recurrence or failure of the air accumulation to decrease in amount over time requires treatment with a tube thoracostomy and continuous suction through a three-bottle system (Double Sealed Chest Drainage Unit, Argyle, St. Louis, MO). In large dogs, a Heimlich valve can be used for continuous evacuation of a persistent pneumothorax requiring chest tube placement. Tension pneumothorax requires rapid diagnosis and immediate placement of a tube thoracostomy.

Pneumothorax associated with an open chest wound requires application of an occlusive (petrolatum) dressing and bandage over the wound, with needle aspirate thoracentesis or placement of a chest tube for draining air from the pleural space. These wounds should be explored and closed as soon as the patient is stable from any concomitant shock or other injuries associated with the trauma.

Subcutaneous emphysema and pneumomediastinum may occur as isolated events, or they may be associated with pneumothorax following trauma. If these conditions are isolated events they rarely require treatment, as they do not result in significant respiratory or hemodynamic compromise to the patient. Esophageal tear should be considered in these patients.

FLAIL CHEST

These injuries are often associated with significant pulmonary contusions (see next section). Hypoxemia and respiratory distress result from a combination of hypoventilation (related to paradoxical movement of the flail segment and pain from the rib fractures) along with intrapulmonary shunting and ventilation-perfusion mismatch associated with the contusion to the lung. The most important factor associated with the respiratory distress is the underlying pulmonary contusion (Bjorling et al., 1982). Initial treatment should consist of cage rest, oxygen administration, and careful observation. Tracheostomy and positive pressure ventilation may be required in cases unresponsive to a more conservative approach.

The animal's level of activity and manipulation of the patient should be kept to a minimum for several days (until the flail segment is surgically stabilized) to prevent further damage to the lungs by fractured rib segments. External bandaging results in minimal stabilization of the flail segment and may further restrict ventilatory capabilities of the patient. Assuming that the pulmonary contusions on the side of the thorax with the flail segment are more severe than those on the opposite side, it may be advisable to position the animal in lateral recumbency with the flail side up the majority of the time (for best matching of perfusion with ventilation); however, this potential benefit may vary from patient to patient.

Following stabilization of the patient, stabilization of the flail segment should be attempted. Stabilization of the flail segment will improve ventilation, decrease chest wall pain, minimize the risk of ongoing lung damage, and improve chances for proper healing by creating anatomic realignment. External fixation with sutures placed around involved ribs and tied through an external brace (plaster or fiber glass cast material or padded metal rod device) molded to fit the thorax is recommended. This technique minimizes anesthetic time, is generally well tolerated by animals, and can also be performed during the initial treatment phase in an obtunded patient with a flail segment.

PULMONARY CONTUSION

Pulmonary contusions are common sequelae to trauma in small animals. A 40 to 50 per cent prevalence following motor vehicle trauma was reported in one study of dogs and cats sustaining long-bone fractures (Tamas et al., 1985). The full extent of pulmonary injury may not be apparent clinically or radiographically for several hours following injury. Most animals sustaining pulmonary contusion will have minimal evidence of respiratory distress. Treatment is generally conservative with use of cage rest and careful observation for evidence of respiratory difficulty. Crystalloid fluid administration for treatment of concomitant shock in these patients has been reported to result in worsening of pulmonary lesions (Fulton and Peter, 1973). Conflicting evidence exists, and until definitive studies confirm the detrimental effects on respiratory function associated with aggressive fluid therapy, erring on the side of aggressive shock therapy is recommended. The use of the smaller volumes of hypertonic saline for shock treatment presents interesting possibilities (see pp. 316–330). Arterial blood gas analysis can be helpful in determining the functional extent of the injury (radiographic evaluation and clinical signs are not uniformly sensitive indicators). Supplemental oxygen therapy (O_2 cage or nasal O_2 catheter) may be helpful in providing respiratory support in patients with mild to moderate hypoxemia (P_{O_2}, 75 to 90 mm Hg). Occasionally pulmonary contusions can result in significant respiratory compromise. Animals with severe, fulminant pulmonary hemorrhage may require intubation and ventilatory support (intermittent positive pressure ventilation [IPPV], positive end-expiratory pressure [PEEP], or both). The prognosis in these cases is often poor.

BITE WOUNDS

Extensive soft tissue damage, tracheal rupture with extensive subcutaneous emphysema, pneumothorax, pulmonary contusion, and rib fractures are possible injuries that can occur following bite wounds to the neck and chest in dogs and cats. These animals, even those with tracheal rupture, may or may not have respiratory distress. Careful evaluation for neurologic injury to the cervical spine is an important consideration in these animals. Establishment of a patent airway and occlusion of any open chest wounds are initial considerations in therapy. Tracheostomy may be required in animals with tracheal tears. Extensive surgical exploration and debridement of cervical and thoracic wounds is recommended as soon as the animal has been stabilized. Extensive tissue devitalization and internal injuries (to thoracic viscera) are often associated with these injuries. Antibiotic therapy is indicated, as these are contaminated wounds.

DIAPHRAGMATIC HERNIA

Similar to animals with flail segments, animals with traumatic diaphragmatic hernias have significant concomitant pulmonary contusions. The respiratory distress manifested initially in these animals is associated with a combination of factors—pulmonary chest wall and cardiac contusions, shock, pain, ruptured diaphragm, and often rib fractures or pleural effusion or both. The ruptured diaphragm is probably of minor significance in contributing to respiratory distress in most cases. These are not surgical emergencies, as animals with chronic diaphragmatic hernias often show little evidence of respiratory distress. Data from a recent retrospective study suggest that early operations (within the first 24 hours) of diaphragmatic hernias may be associated with increased mortality (Boudrieau and Muir, 1987). Animals with diaphragmatic hernias have a significant risk for mortality under anesthesia when pulmonary contusions and shock injury are absent, and the risks are greater when they are present. Initial treatment of these animals should include cage rest, oxygen supplementation, intravenous fluid administration for shock treatment, thoracentesis to remove air or fluid (if substantial accumulations are present), and tracheostomy for administration of positive pressure ventilation (if severe respiratory distress is unresponsive to more conservative treatments).

Confirmation of a diaphragmatic hernia can occasionally be a diagnostic challenge. Positive contrast peritoneography (Stickle, 1984) and two-dimensional ultrasound evaluation of the diaphragm are more sensitive techniques than the upper gastrointestinal barium study for obtaining the diagnosis.

Pleural Effusion

Pleural effusions are a common cause of respiratory emergencies in dogs and cats. Treatment involves removal of the fluid from the chest cavity by needle aspiration thoracentesis or placement of a tube via thoracostomy. Regardless of character of fluid or etiology of the pleural effusion the clinical signs are directly related to the presence of fluid in the pleural space, resulting in compression atelectasis and restriction of ventilation. As with pneumothorax, diagnosis can be made during physical examination. Empiric use of thoracentesis to exclude or confirm presence of pleural effusion is the preferred diagnostic approach in the dyspneic patient when compared with the potential for death of the patient associated with the stress of radiography. Definitive treatment during the initial stabilization or subsequent management of animals with pleural effusion requires a specific diagnosis of the character of the effusion and its etiology (Suter and Zinkl, 1983; Haskins, 1986).

Heartworm Disease

Dogs and cats with heartworm disease may have signs of respiratory distress (coughing, tachypnea, and hemoptysis). Pulmonary thromboembolism and the inflammatory reaction in the pulmonary parenchyma associated with heartworm disease can cause significant respiratory compromise. Cats may have eosinophilic pleural effusion.

Treatment for acute respiratory manifestations of heartworm disease includes cage rest, oxygen administration, corticosteroid administration (prednisone, 0.5 mg/kg b.i.d. PO), aspirin (5 to 10 mg/kg daily in dogs and every 3 days PO in cats), and bronchodilators (aminophylline, 6 to 10 mg/kg b.i.d. PO). These animals are occasionally febrile as a result of pulmonary thromboembolism, but antibiotics are indicated only when an infectious bacterial component is confirmed by cultures of a transtracheal aspirate. A more detailed discussion of treatment of heartworm disease is presented on pages 263 to 270.

Pulmonary Parenchymal Diseases

Respiratory distress associated with pulmonary parenchymal disorders is described elsewhere in this text, including pneumonia (see pp. 376–384), pulmonary edema (see pp. 385–392), and interstitial disease and bronchitis (see pp. 361–368). For information on treatment of near-drowning, please refer to Farrow's complete discussion in *Current Veterinary Therapy VIII* (pp. 167–173).

ADDITIONAL CONSIDERATIONS

Arterial Blood Gas Evaluation

Arterial blood gas analysis can define characteristics of respiratory distress, provide objective data concerning the need for ventilatory support, and monitor the response to treatment. Detection of hypoxemia in conjunction with hypercapnia suggests hypoventilation (e.g., CNS or neuromuscular disease, restrictive pleural disease, pain response to rib fractures and chest wall trauma, drug effects on respiration, and airway obstruction), whereas hypoxemia accompanying normocapnia or hypocapnia usually suggests pulmonary parenchymal disease. Clinical signs of respiratory distress may not be readily evident on casual observation (e.g., in a pneumonia or heartworm patient at cage rest), but arterial blood gas data may demonstrate significant hypoxemia (P_{O_2}, 75 to 80 mm Hg) that may warrant oxygen administration. Likewise, an animal on oxygen treatment that continues to demonstrate "relative" hypoxemia compared with expected value for the known FI_{O_2} should be considered for IPPV or PEEP. Animals on ventilator therapy require serial evaluation of arterial blood gases to tailor treatment appropriately.

Animals with less severe signs of respiratory distress undergoing more conservative treatment also benefit from serial arterial blood gas analysis to assess progress. For a more detailed discussion of specifics related to blood gas analysis, *Current Veterinary Therapy VIII* (pp. 201–215).

Tracheostomy

In addition to using tracheostomy for treatment of some cases of airway obstruction, other indications include hypoventilation associated with CNS and neuromuscular diseases and hypoxemia associated with severe pulmonary disease (e.g., acute lung edema or pneumonia) requiring ventilatory support. Procedures for placement of tracheostomy tubes have been recently reviewed (Harvey, 1986; Aron and Crowe, 1985; Haskins, 1986).

If placement of a tracheostomy tube appears indicated, *do it*. In many instances, patients give ample warning, if the clinician is attentive to monitoring for worsening respiratory distress. It is better to anticipate and place a tracheostomy under controlled conditions than to delay interventions and have to place one in the less than ideal circumstances of respiratory arrest.

Proper maintenance of tracheostomies involves careful attention to hygiene around the tracheostomy site, frequent suctioning of the tube and the airway, and proper attention to humidification of inspired gases to prevent excess drying out of tracheal membranes (Haskins, 1986). Tracheostomy tubes with disposable internal cannulas (tracheostomy tube with inner cannula, Portex Inc., Wilmington, MA) that can be removed and cleaned or replaced help ease problems associated with maintenance of tracheostomy tubes.

Ventilatory Support and Inhalation Therapy

For information on ventilatory support and oxygen administration, see *Current Veterinary Therapy IX* (pp. 269–277).

References and Supplemental Reading

Amis, T. C., and Haskins, S. C.: Respiratory failure. Semin. Vet. Med. Surg. 1:261, 1986.
Aron, D. N., and Crowe, D. T.: Upper airway obstruction: General principles and selected conditions in the dog and cat. Vet. Clin. North Am. [Small Anim. Pract.] 15:891, 1985.
Bjorling, D. E., Kolata, R. J., and DeNovo, R. C.: Flail chest: Review, clinical experience and new method of stabilization. J. Am. Anim. Hosp. Assoc. 18:269, 1982.

Boudrieau, R. J., and Muir, W. W.: Pathophysiology of traumatic diaphragmatic hernia in dogs. Comp. Cont. Ed. Pract. Vet. 9:379, 1987.

Fulton, R. L., and Peter, E. T.: Physiologic effects of fluid therapy after pulmonary contusion. Am. J. Surg. 126:773, 1973.

Harvey, E.: Tracheotomy and tracheostomy. In Kirk, R. W. (ed.): Current Veterinary Therapy IX. Philadelphia, W. B. Saunders Co., 1986, pp. 262–264.

Haskins, S. C.: Physical therapeutics for respiratory disease. Semin. Vet. Med. Surg. 1:276, 1986.

Krotje, L. J.: Cyanosis: Physiology and pathogenesis. Comp. Cont. Ed. Pract. Vet. 9:271, 1987.

Moses, B. L., and Spaulding, G. L.: Chronic bronchial disease of the cat. Vet. Clin. North Am. [Small Anim. Pract.] 15:929, 1985.

Noone, K. E.: Pleural effusions and diseases of the pleura. Vet. Clin. North Am. [Small Animal Pract.] 15:1069, 1985.

Norris, A. M., and Laing, E. J.: Diseases of the nose and sinuses. Vet. Clin. North Am. [Small Anim. Pract.] 15:865, 1985.

Stickle, R. L.: Positive-contrast celiography (peritoneography) for the diagnosis of diaphragmatic hernia in dogs and cats. J.A.V.M.A. 185:295, 1984.

Suter, P. F., and Zinkl, J. G.: Mediastinal, pleural, and extrapleural diseases. In Ettinger, S. J. (ed.): Textbook of Veterinary Internal Medicine, 2nd ed. Philadelphia: W. B. Saunders, 1983, pp. 840–883.

Tamas, P. M., Paddleford, R. R., and Krahwinkel, D. J.: Thoracic trauma in dogs and cats presented with limb fractures. J. Am. Anim. Hosp. Assoc. 21:161, 1985.

ECHOCARDIOGRAPHY: THERAPEUTIC IMPLICATIONS

N. SYDNEY MOISE, D.V.M.

Ithaca, New York

Echocardiography is now well accepted as an integral part of the diagnostic investigation of many patients with cardiac disease. In conjunction with the physical examination, electrocardiogram, and radiograph, the echocardiogram has facilitated diagnosis by shortening the workup (i.e., angiography is not as frequently required), improving the diagnostic accuracy, and lessening the stress and risk to the patient. Simply because the echocardiogram can render a specific diagnosis in most cases, it has therapeutic implications. In some diseases the echocardiographic results can quickly direct or change therapy. The purpose of this chapter is to describe and illustrate selected M-mode, two-dimensional, and Doppler echocardiograms that most specifically influence therapy.

PREREQUISITES FOR INTERPRETING THE ABNORMAL ECHOCARDIOGRAM

This article assumes that the reader has an understanding of the structural abnormalities and hemodynamic consequences of most cardiac diseases. For introductory information and general principles of echocardiographic interpretation the reader is directed to the references and supplemental reading. Table 1 lists the information that should be mastered. Table 2 lists the major principles of echocardiographic interpretation. Figures 1 and 2 provide examples of M-mode and two-dimensional echocardiograms at the ventricular level for common abnormalities.

VALVULAR AND SUBVALVULAR LESIONS

Atrioventricular (AV) valve insufficiency due to endocardiosis (valve degeneration) is a common lesion studied echocardiographically. Thickened nodular valve leaflets are seen (Fig. 3). The severity of regurgitation can be indirectly appreciated by the degree of ventricular and atrial enlargement. The amount of chamber dilation in concert with physical and other diagnostic findings dictates the aggressiveness of therapy. The percentage of fractional shortening (FS) may indicate the need for positive inotropic therapy. However, the meaning of the FS in mitral insufficiency must be understood before generalizations about therapy are made. With mitral insufficiency the FS may be low, normal (usual range: dog, 30 to 40 per cent; cat, 35 to 60 per cent), or high (Fig. 1B and C). In early mitral insufficiency, with a low regurgitant fraction, the FS will be normal. As the regurgitant fraction increases and myocardial function is preserved, the FS increases; however, it must be remembered that a high FS is not a guarantee that myocardial failure is absent. With mitral insufficiency the left ventricle (LV) faces a decreased afterload (left atrial pressures are lower than systemic arterial pressures) and it is easier to unload the blood into the left atrium. Additionally, because of ventricular filling, an exaggerated septal motion toward the right ventricle (RV) occurs during diastole (Fig. 4) and an increased preload contributes to a stronger contraction. These factors contribute to a high FS. When myocardial failure develops, the fractional shortening declines

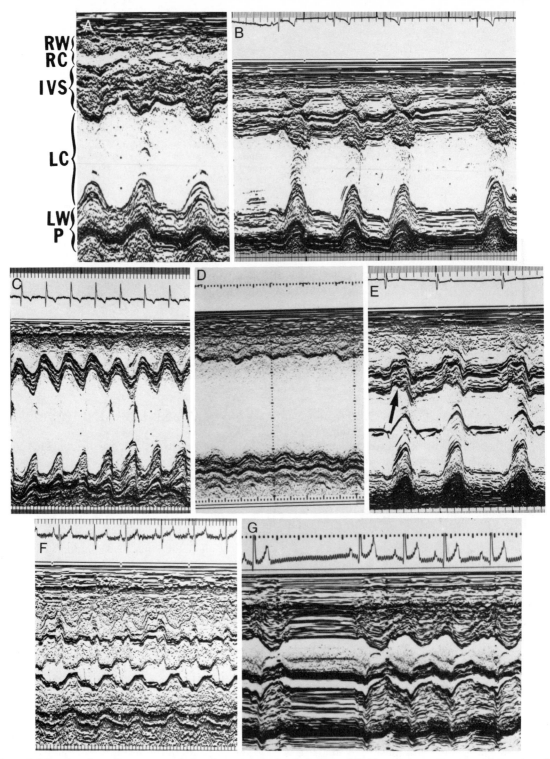

Figure 1. M-mode echocardiograms recorded at the ventricular level. *A,* Normal Golden retriever. Note the relative sizes of the right and left ventricles (normally left ventricular size is approximately four times the right ventricular size) and the thicknesses and motion of the interventricular septum (IVS) and the left ventricular free wall (LW). *B,* Asymptomatic cocker spaniel with grade II/VI systolic murmur due to mild mitral insufficiency. The fractional shortening (FS) is elevated (58 per cent). Minimal left atrial enlargement was present. *C,* Poodle with severe mitral insufficiency. The left ventricle is markedly dilated, and the FS is normal (44 per cent). The normal FS may indicate that the dog is also suffering from myocardial failure. *D,* Doberman pinscher with dilated cardiomyopathy and a FS of only 14 per cent. *E,* German shepherd with heartworm disease demonstrating paradoxical motion of the IVS (arrow). During systole the IVS moves toward the right side of the heart instead of toward the LVFW. *F,* Two-year-old Yorkshire terrier with severe valvular pulmonic stenosis. Marked hypertrophy of the right ventricular wall is seen, and the left ventricular chamber is reduced in size. *G,* Four-month-old cocker spaniel with hypertrophic cardiomyopathy demonstrating marked thickening of the IVS and the LVFW. Distance between markers, 1 cm; paper speed, 50 mm/sec.

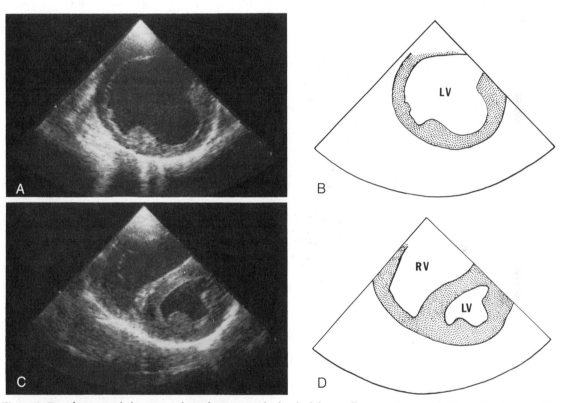

Figure 2. Two-dimensional short-axis echocardiograms at the level of the papillary muscles recorded from the right hemithorax. *A* and *B*, Dog with volume overload to the left heart due to dilation cardiomyopathy. The left ventricle (LV) is globoid in shape. *C* and *D*, Dog with volume and pressure overload to the right heart (RV) due to heartworm disease. The left ventricle (LV) is abnormal in shape owing to a flattened interventricular septum. Compare the relative sizes of the right and left ventricles.

Table 1. Knowledge Necessary for the Proper Interpretation of the M-Mode and Two-Dimensional Echocardiogram

Pattern recognition of echocardiographic images for the identification of structures
What constitutes a technically satisfactory image
Standard views that should be obtained
  M-mode echocardiogram
    Ventricles
    Mitral valve
    Aorta/left atrium (auricle)
  Two-dimensional echocardiogram
    Views recorded from the right hemithorax
      Long axis 4 and 5 chamber
      Long axis left ventricular outflow region
      Short axis at level of apex, papillary muscle, chordae tendineae, AV valves, aortic and pulmonic valves
    Views recorded from the left hemithorax
      4 and 5 chamber
      Left ventricular inflow and outflow regions
      Short axis at ventricular level
      Right atrium and auricle with caudal vena cava
      Great vessels
Echocardiographic measurement techniques and standards
  Chamber sizes
  Wall thicknesses
  Aortic and pulmonic root sizes
  Mitral valve (excursion, E-F slope, E-point septal separation)
  Calculated values (percentage of fractional shortening, percentage of wall thickening, velocity of circumferential shortening)
  Qualitative features of echocardiogram (cardiac situs, echogenicity of myocardium, character of valves, septal and free wall motion, presence of abnormal structures, continuity of cardiac structures)

Some common terms used in echocardiography:

Ultrasound	Acoustic shadow
Echogenicity	Acoustic enhancement
Hyperechoic	Acoustic impedance
Hypoechoic	Resolution
Anechoic	Pulse repetition
Hyperkinesis	Transducer frequency
Hypokinesis	Reverberation
Dyskinesis	Contrast echocardiogram
Attenuation	Slide lobe artifact

gram (Fig. 5) and may explain a sudden cardiac decompensation despite proper therapy. Doppler echocardiography can be used to identify jets of regurgitant blood flow.

Aggressive antibiotic therapy is indicated when the echocardiogram renders a diagnosis of vegetative endocarditis. Abscesses within the myocardium can be seen as hypoechoic irregular areas. Lesions must be approximately 2 mm in diameter to be identified. Generally, the vegetative lesions are more irregular in shape than those of endocardiosis. With time and successful therapy the masses tend to become smaller and lessen in irregularity. The shape and size of the mass may also change if embolization occurs. With long-standing disease, calcification occurs and hyperechoic valvular masses are seen to cast an acoustic shadow. Valvular stenosis and insufficiency of the affected valve can develop (Fig. 6).

The severity and location of pulmonic or aortic stenosis determine the prognosis and the therapeutic recommendations. With pulmonic valvular stenosis thickened immobile leaflets are seen with varying degrees of poststenotic dilation of the pulmonary trunk (Fig. 7). The degree of dilation of the pulmonary trunk is not indicative of the severity of the valvular stenosis. The amount of right ventricular and septal hypertrophy is proportional to the severity of stenosis (pressure gradient) (Fig. 1F). Paradoxical motion of the septum during systole and diastole means marked right ventricular pressure overload. In addition, with severe stenosis signs of right-sided heart failure are seen by echocardiography to include dilated right atrium, dilated cranial and caudal venae cavae, dilated hepatic veins, pleural fluid, ascites, or spontaneous contrast. With subvalvular aortic stenosis (SAS) the degree

such that the animal with mitral regurgitation and decreased pump power has a normal to decreased FS. The bottom line is this: with mitral insufficiency the FS gives an idea of myocardial function but should not be used exclusively as an assurance of preservation of inotropic strength because preload and afterload markedly affect this index of pump strength. The overall value of calculated left ventricular end-systolic volume index in guiding inotropic therapy remains undefined. These same principles apply to congenital AV insufficiencies. The E-point septal separation (EPSS) indicates the inotropic state (as well as chamber diameter), and it is usually normal with left AV insufficiency. Decreases in myocardial contractility may be shown by an increase in EPSS (> 0.5 to 0.6 cm for dogs, > 0.3 to 0.4 cm for cats). Rupture of one of the chordae tendineae may be diagnosed from the echocardio-

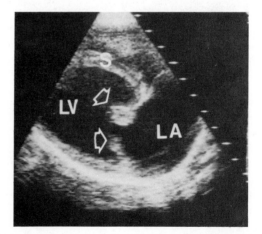

Figure 3. Long-axis view recorded from the right hemithorax of the ventricular inflow of a dog with mitral insufficiency due to endocardiosis. Dilation of the left ventricle (LV) and atrium (LA) are seen with marked thickening of the mitral leaflets (arrows). S, interventricular septum.

Table 2. Principles of Interpretation

Determination of Cardiac Rhythm
Arrhythmias will alter cardiac motion

Determination of Image Plane and Structure Identification
Presence or absence of anticipated structures, cardiac situs
Identification of cardiac mass lesions and thrombi
Identification of abnormal structures (for example, dilated coronary sinus, heartworms)

Cardiac Mensuration
Ventricular dilation or hypertrophy
Atrial enlargement
Aortic/pulmonary artery dilation or attenuation
Abnormally small chamber or great vessel

Mitral/Tricuspid Valves
Identification of valve cusps, motion during cardiac cycle
Reduced diastolic (E-F) slope—rule out stenosis, decreased AV flow
Increased echogenicity—rule out vegetation, degenerative thickening, dysplasia
Diastolic mitral fluttering—rule out aortic insufficiency
Systolic fluttering—rule out AV valve insufficiency
Chaotic motion—rule out arrhythmias, ruptured chordae tendineae
Prolapse into atrium—rule out degenerative disease, ruptured chordae tendineae
Lack of diastolic separation—rule out stenosis, inflammation, dysplasia
Premature (diastolic) closure—rule out severe semilunar valve insufficiency or long P-R interval
Delayed (systolic) closure—rule out LV failure
Increased mitral E-point septal separation—rule out LV dilation, myocardial failure
Cleft—rule out endocardial cushion defect

Aortic/Pulmonic Valves
Identification of valve leaflets, motion during cardiac cycle
Narrowing of the LV or RV outflow tracts—rule out stenosis, hypertrophy
Diastolic fluttering—rule out semilunar valve insufficiency
Systolic fluttering—rule out normal or high-flow state
Increased echogenicity—rule out vegetation, degeneration, dysplasia
Prolapse into ventricle—rule out endocarditis
Lack of systolic separation—rule out low cardiac output, arrhythmia, stenosis
Premature (midsystolic) closure— rule out outflow tract obstruction, ventricular septal defect
Systolic doming—rule out valvular stenosis

Left Ventricular Wall and Chamber
Hypertrophy—rule out hypertension, aortic or subaortic stenosis, hyperthyroidism, hypertrophic cardiomyopathy
Dilation—rule out causes of volume overload, cardiomyopathy, valvular disease, left-to-right shunts, AV fistula

Hyperkinesis—rule out mitral or aortic insufficiency, volume overloads (e.g., left-to-right shunts), hyperthyroidism, sympathetic stimulation, hypertrophic cardiomyopathy, aortic stenosis
Hypokinesis—rule out dilated cardiomyopathy
Dyskinesis—rule out cardiomyopathy, ischemia, infarct
Giant papillary muscle—rule out hypertrophy, AV valve dysplasia

Ventricular Septum
Hypertrophy—rule out aortic or pulmonic stenosis, pulmonary hypertension, tetralogy of Fallot, hypertrophic cardiomyopathy
Hyperkinesis, as per left ventricular chamber
Flat or reduced systolic motion—rule out RV pressure or volume overload
Paradoxical motion—rule out moderate to severe RV pressure or volume overload such as atrial septal defect, heartworm disease, tricuspid regurgitation
Echo "dropout"—rule out septal defect
Discontinuity of septum and aortic root—rule out septal defect, tetralogy of Fallot, pulmonary artery atresia, truncus arteriosus

Right Ventricular Wall and Chamber
Hypertrophy—rule out pulmonary hypertension, pulmonic stenosis, tetralogy of Fallot, heartworm disease
Dilation—rule out tricuspid insufficiency, chronic RV pressure overload, atrial septal defect, heartworm disease

Left Atrium
Decreased size—rule out right-to-left shunting, hypovolemia
Dilation—rule out mitral regurgitation, cardiomyopathy, left-sided heart failure, left-to-right shunts, mitral stenosis
Increased density—rule out thrombus or tumor

Right Atrium
Dilation—rule out tricuspid regurgitation, cardiomyopathy, right-sided heart failure, atrial septal defect, hyperthyroidism, tricuspid stenosis
Increased density—rule out tumor thrombus

Atrial Septum
Marked "bowing"—rule out volume overload of one atrium
Echo "dropout"—rule out septal defect

Pulmonary Artery
Absence—rule out atresia
Dilation—rule out pulmonic stenosis, intracardiac left-to-right shunt, pulmonary hypertension

Aorta
Decreased diameter—rule out low cardiac output
Dilation—rule out subaortic or aortic stenosis, tetralogy of Fallot, pulmonary artery atresia with or without patent ductus arteriosus, systemic hypertension

Pericardium
Rule out pericardial effusion, constriction, or mass lesion

With permission from Bonagura, J. D., O'Grady, M. R., and Herring, D. J.: Vet. Clin. North Am. 15:1177, 1985
Doppler echocardiography can be used to identify abnormal flow, estimate cardiac pressures, and assess severity of valvular diseases.

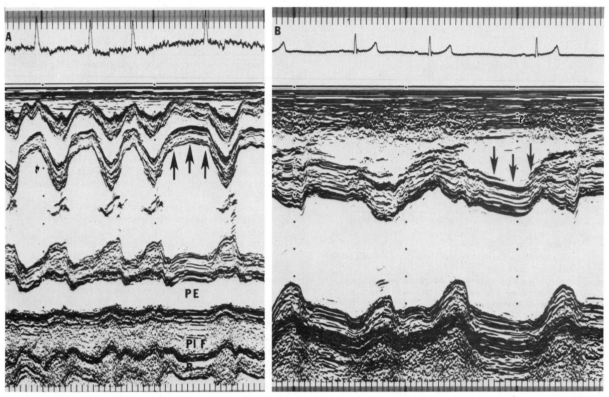

Figure 4. M-mode echocardiograms at the ventricular level. *A*, Volume overload to the left heart is seen in this dog with severe left and right atrioventricular insufficiency. Arrows point to the exaggerated septal motion toward the right side of the heart during diastole. Pericardial effusion (PE) and pleural fluid (Pl F) are present. A reverberation (R) artifact can be seen. *B*, Exaggerated motion of the septum toward the left ventricle is seen during diastole in this dog with heartworm disease. Distance between markers, 1 cm; paper speed, 50 mm/sec.

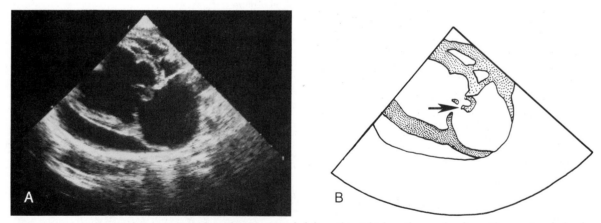

Figure 5. *A*, Four-chamber long-axis echocardiogram recorded from the right hemithorax of a dog with a ruptured chordae tendineae. *B*, The flail leaflet (arrow) is seen prolapsing into the left atrium (LA). Other specific features of a ruptured chordae tendineae include chaotic diastolic motion of the mitral leaflets, systolic fluttering of the mitral valve, the presence of left atrial echoes during ventricular systole, evidence of a mobile echo in diastole situated between the anterior and posterior mitral leaflets, or paradoxical posterior mitral valve movement.

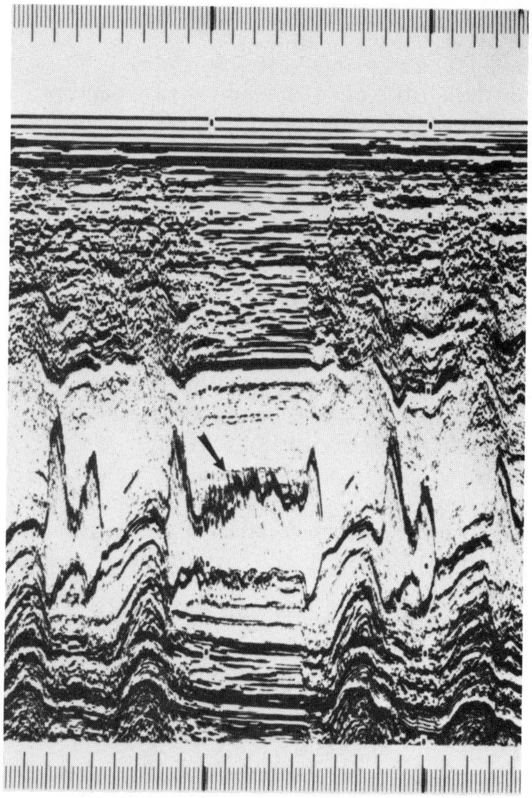

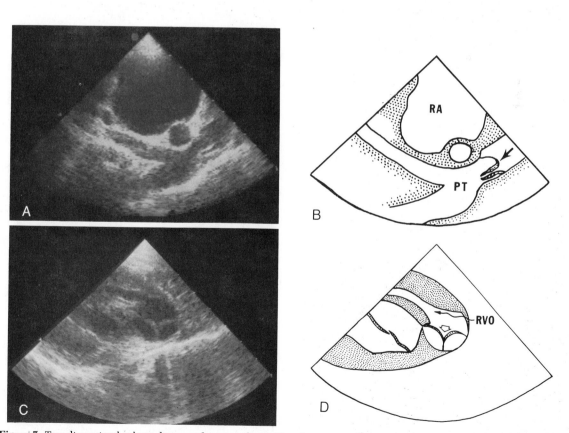

Figure 6. M-mode echocardiogram recorded at the level of the mitral valve. Fine and rapid fluttering is seen during diastole, indicating aortic insufficiency. As the jet of blood hits the open mitral leaflet, it causes it to vibrate dramatically.

Figure 7. Two-dimensional echocardiograms from two dogs with pulmonic stenosis. A and B, Short-axis view recorded from the right hemithorax of the heart base. A markedly dilated right atrium (RA) is seen. The pulmonic valve (arrow) is thickened, and the pulmonary trunk (PT) is dilated. C and D, The right ventricular outflow tract (RVO) is narrow and the pulmonic valve (open arrow) is normal in this dog with subvalvular pulmonic stenosis. Doppler echocardiography and angiography confirmed the locations of both lesions.

of left ventricular hypertrophy indicates the severity of the obstruction. The subvalvular band of fibrous tissue can be identified (Fig. 8), except in mild cases. Dilation of the aortic root, aortic arch, and descending aorta frequently will be seen. Some animals may actually have premature closure of the aortic valve because of systolic anterior motion of the mitral leaflet (Fig. 9) blocking the left ventricular outflow tract. When this or other signs of severe SAS are identified, beta-blocking drugs may lessen the obstruction. Some animals with SAS also have left atrial dilation due to the lack of ventricular compliance or a cleft mitral valve causing regurgitation. In severe cases of SAS in which myocardial perfusion is reduced, causing ischemia, necrosis, and fibrosis, the echogenicity of the myocardium will vary. Hypoechoic areas appear where necrosis or fluid is present and hyperechoic areas where fibrosis is present.

The degree of semilunar valve stenosis can more accurately be determined by Doppler echocardiography. Briefly, with Doppler echocardiography sound waves are directed parallel to blood flow. When the ultrasound strikes the flowing blood cells it is bounced back, giving information via a shift in sound wave frequency as to the velocity and direction of blood flow. Because blood flow velocity can be determined with the Doppler equation, the pressure gradient across a stenosis can be calculated using a modified Bernoulli equation:

$$\text{pressure gradient} = 4 \times (\text{maximum velocity})^2$$

Pulsed, color flow mapping, and continuous wave are all forms of Doppler echocardiography. Pulsed and color flow Doppler techniques send and receive sound waves with the same transducers and are used to locate turbulence and abnormal blood flow and, therefore, the level of structural abnormality. The maximum velocity that can be measured with pulsed Doppler technology is limited (velocity am-

biguity) (Fig. 10A). If blood flow is too fast, the velocity and direction of flow cannot be determined with pulsed Doppler echocardiography. This occurs because the frequency shift is higher than one half the frequency of the pulsed Doppler sound wave; this is termed the Nyquist limit and results in aliasing. Aliasing is recognized on the Doppler spectral display as a band with no identifiable beginning or end. When this is seen, continuous wave Doppler method is used to determine direction and blood flow velocity. Continuous wave Doppler technique simultaneously sends and receives sound waves. Therefore, the exact location for blood flow direction or velocity analysis cannot be determined (range ambiguity), but a limit on the maximum velocity that can be measured does not exist, and, therefore, with high flow states (e.g., pressure gradient in stenotic lesions), the continous wave Doppler is used (Fig. 10B). With this technique an accurate assessment of the instantaneous pressure gradient will dictate the need for surgical correction or medical management. Because Doppler echocardiography is noninvasive, animals may be repeatedly evaluated during treatment or after surgery.

SHUNTS

The most common shunt identified in small animal practice is a patent ductus arteriosus (PDA). Although auscultation of the continuous murmur is usually adequate for accurate diagnosis, identification of the severity of cardiac compromise, the presence of coexisting anomalies, and the PDA by echocardiography (Fig. 11) completes the cardiac workup. Dilation of the cardiac chambers (primarily the left side of the heart) and great vessels is seen. Postoperative follow-up imaging and Doppler echocardiographic examination may provide useful information as to cardiac improvement or complication (Fig. 12). Many dogs with a PDA have a reduced

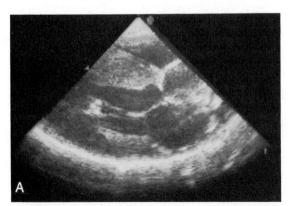
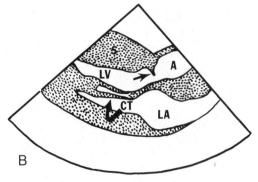

Figure 8. *A,* Long-axis view of the left ventricular outflow tract recorded from the right hemithorax. *B,* Straight arrow points to subaortic fibrous band. Left ventricular hypertrophy is present. LV, left ventricle; LA, left atrium; S, interventricular septum; A, aorta; CT, chordae tendineae.

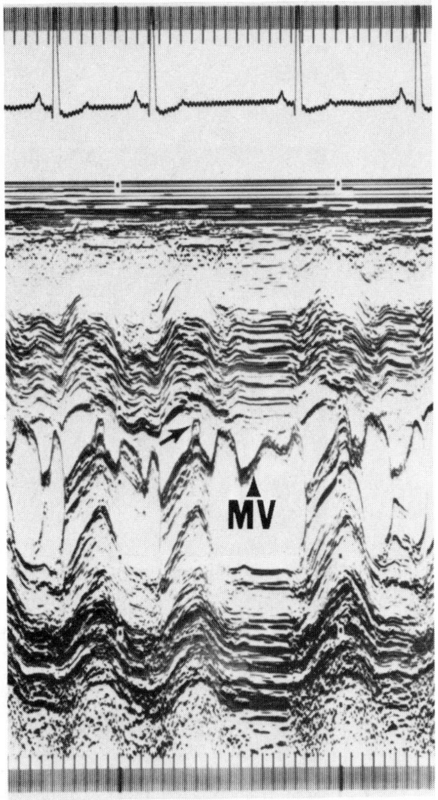

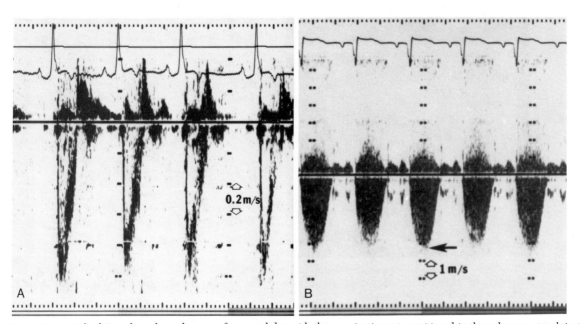

Figure 9. M-mode echocardiogram of a Newfoundland puppy with subaortic stenosis. Systolic anterior motion of the mitral leaflet (arrow) is seen. Because of this abnormal motion during systole, premature closure of the aortic valve was also present. MV (arrowhead), mitral valve. Distance between markers, 1 cm; paper speed, 50 mm/sec.

Figure 10. *A*, Pulsed Doppler echocardiogram of a normal dog with the examination gate positioned in the pulmonary trunk just distal to the pulmonic valve. When echocardiogram is recorded from the right cranial position, providing a long-axis view of the pulmonary trunk, blood flow is away from the transducer and therefore below the baseline. Maximum blood flow velocity is approximately 1 m/sec. *B*, Continuous wave Doppler echocardiogram of a dog with valvular pulmonic stenosis. Dedicated continuous wave Doppler transducer beam directed craniodorsal from the right hemithorax. Flow is away from the transducer with a maximum blood flow velocity of approximately 4.25 m/sec. Using the modified Bernoulli equation (see text), the pressure gradient across the stenosed valve is estimated at $4(4.25)^2$ or 72 mm Hg.

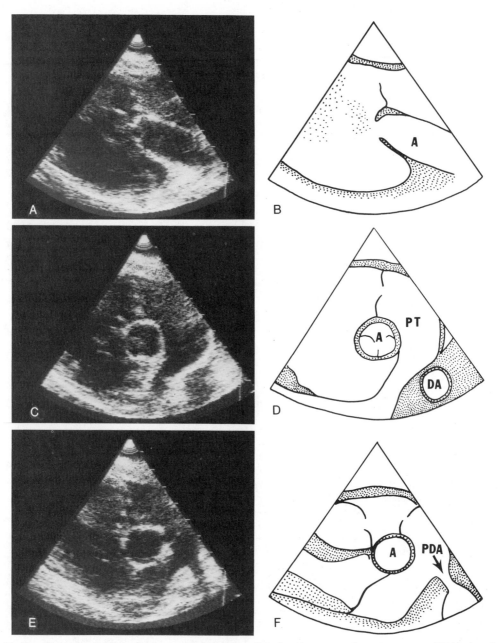

Figure 11. Two-dimensional echocardiograms recorded from a Briard with a patent ductus arteriosus (PDA). *A* and *B*, Partial long-axis view of the aorta (A) recorded from the left cranial position. *C* and *D*, The transducer is rotated in plane with the long axis of the pulmonary trunk (PT) and short axis of the descending aorta (DA). A, aorta. *E* and *F*, With slight angulation the PDA is seen. A, aorta.

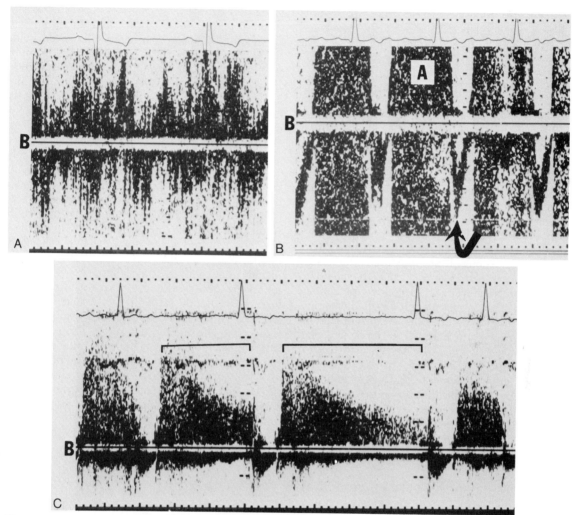

Figure 12. Doppler echocardiogram from the same dog described in Figure 11. *A,* With the gate of the pulsed wave positioned near the PDA, continuous turbulence is identified. B, baseline. Distance between markers, 20 cm/sec; paper speed, 100 mm/sec. *B,* After surgical ligation of the PDA the dog developed atrial fibrillation and aortic insufficiency. Fine fluttering of the mitral valve during diastole was present; with the gate of the pulsed wave positioned in the left ventricular outflow tract (imaging from the left apical five-chamber view), turbulence and a regurgitant jet that aliased during diastole (A) is identified. Left ventricular outflow tract systolic blood flow is also seen (arrow). B, baseline. Distance between markers, 20 cm/sec; paper speed, 100 mm/sec. *C,* Continuous wave Doppler echocardiography directed from the left apical position reveals the diastolic blood flow returning to the left ventricle (brackets). Because of angulation the systolic flow is not well seen. B, baseline. Distance between markers, 1 meter/sec; paper speed, 100 mm/sec.

FS. These dogs tend to be animals with long-standing or large shunts. Some dogs will actually have a reduction in the FS after surgical ligation of the vessel. Pulsed Doppler and color flow mapping may identify intracardiac shunts as well.

Identification of shunts with contrast echocardiography is easy if an intracardiac right-to-left shunt exists (Fig. 13). Identification of extracardiac shunts such as a right-to-left PDA can also be made and can direct therapeutic recommendations.

MYOCARDIAL DISEASE

Echocardiography has been exceedingly important in the rapid diagnosis of the cardiomyopathies in dogs and cats (Fig. 1D and G). The quick differentiation of dilated (DCM) and hypertrophic cardiomyopathies (HCM) in the cat has served well in allowing the proper therapy to be chosen. Dilation of all cardiac chambers, with the left side of the heart more severely affected; reduced pump power as evidenced by a decreased FS; and velocity of circumferential fiber shortening, increased EPSS, decreased excursions of the mitral valve, abnormal delayed closure of the mitral valve (B shoulder), decreased aortic amplitude, decreased percentage of septal and left ventricular free-wall thickening, and normal to thin wall thicknesses are all features of DCM. In cats with taurine deficiency and dogs with carnitine deficiency, the response to therapy can be monitored (Fig. 14). The appearance of improved cardiac function with administration of positive inotropic agents (digoxin, milrinone) can be detected in some cases; although the echocardiogram can display evidence of improved function, it is not a sensitive indicator. Dilated cardiomyopathy

can be identified with echocardiography in animals treated with adriamycin.

Hypertrophic cardiomyopathy is characterized on the echocardiogram by myocardial hypertrophy (cat: interventricular septum and left ventricular free wall, > 0.55 cm). Other features include normal to elevated FS, enlarged left atrium, and normal to small left ventricular chamber size. Intracardiac thrombi can be identified in cats with cardiomyopathy and indicate a poor prognosis; however, pooled blood that has not yet organized into a thrombus should not be mistaken for a clot (Fig. 15), as anticoagulant therapy and supportive care can more likely reverse the latter situation. Other cardiac diseases classified as cardiomyopathies (excessive moderator bands, restrictive cardiomyopathy) can also be identified.

It should be stated that with the advent of echocardiography veterinary cardiologists began identifying a variety of other cardiac abnormalities in cats that may previously have been confused with the formerly thought more common DCM and HCM. Adult cats with AV insufficiency (AV dysplasia or possibly acquired valve disease) have echocardiographic features similar to those in the dog with AV insufficiency, and disease in these cats is now being identified. Many of the cats with echocardiographic features common to both DCM and HCM are geriatric (older than 12 years) and exhibit signs of right- and left-sided heart failure. Some geriatric cats will have cardiomegaly with mild myocardial hypertrophy and mild atrial enlargement. The role of systemic hypertension caused by chronic renal disease may be important in these animals. These cats have normal serum thyroxin concentrations; however, abnormal echocardiograms are found in many cats with hyperthyroidism (Fig. 16). The

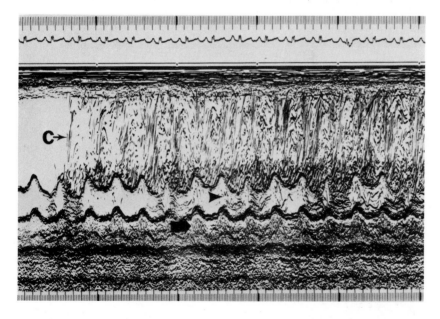

Figure 13. Contrast M-mode echocardiogram performed on a 3-month-old chocolate Labrador retriever with tricuspid dysplasia and a patent foramen ovale causing right-to-left shunting. Agitated 0.9 per cent saline was rapidly injected into the cephalic vein. The linear lines of saline contrast (C) are seen within the right inflow tract, as well as in the left auricle (arrow) and aorta (arrowhead).

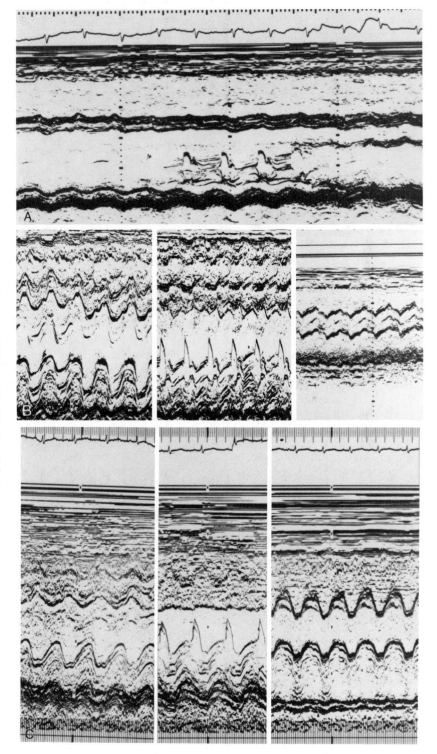

Figure 14. M-mode echocardiograms recorded from a cat with taurine-responsive dilated cardiomyopathy. *A,* Initial echocardiographic sweep from the left ventricle to the aorta and left atrium reveals the typical echocardiogram of dilated cardiomyopathy with a dilated left ventricle and atrium, reduced fractional shortening (FS) of 10 per cent, and an increased E point septal separation (EPSS) of 0.8 cm. *B,* Echocardiograms recorded on and after day 8 of treatment with 250 mg of taurine twice daily. The left ventricle and atrium gradually reduced in size. *C,* On day 32 after taurine administration the FS had increased to 42 per cent and the EPSS had decreased to 0.2 cm. Distance between markers, 1 cm; paper speed, 50 mm/sec.

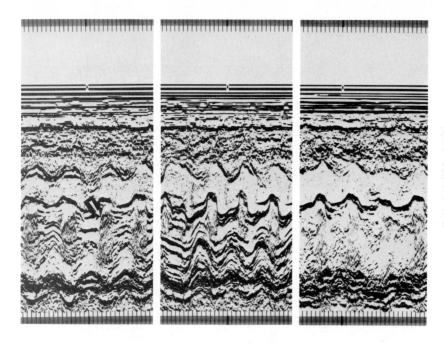

Figure 15. M-mode echocardiogram of a cat with abnormal echoes (arrow) present in the left ventricular inflow tract and left atrium. These echoes could indicate a thrombus, however, in this case they were evidence of spontaneous contrast due to static blood. Distance between markers, 1 cm; paper speed, 50 mm/sec.

frequency of abnormalities varies with the population examined. The echocardiogram of the hyperthyroid cat can be normal or abnormal. Some cats have severe cardiac changes with left and right atrial dilation, marked myocardial hypertrophy, hyperkinetic wall motion, and extracardiac signs of congestive heart failure. Many hyperthyroid cats only have mild myocardial hypertrophy, and whether this is secondary to the effects of thyroxin or other causes such as renal insufficiency or normal age-related changes is debatable. A few cats with hyperthyroid-

ism will have echocardiograms similar to those of cats with DCM; however, the presence of coexisting taurine deficiency is not known. After successful treatment of hyperthyroidism, most of the cardiac changes seen echocardiographically resolve or lessen.

Infiltrative myocardial diseases can be detected when attention is directed to the echogenicity of the myocardium. Thickening of the myocardium is usually detected as well. Inflammatory disease such as pyogranulomatous myocarditis (Figs. 17 and 18)

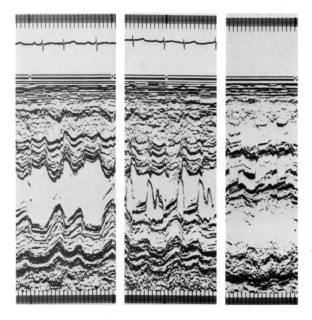

Figure 16. M-mode echocardiogram of a cat with hyperthyroidism. Left ventricular hypertrophy and left atrial enlargement are seen. Atrial premature beats disrupt the mitral valve motion. Distance between markers, 1 cm; paper speed, 50 cm/sec.

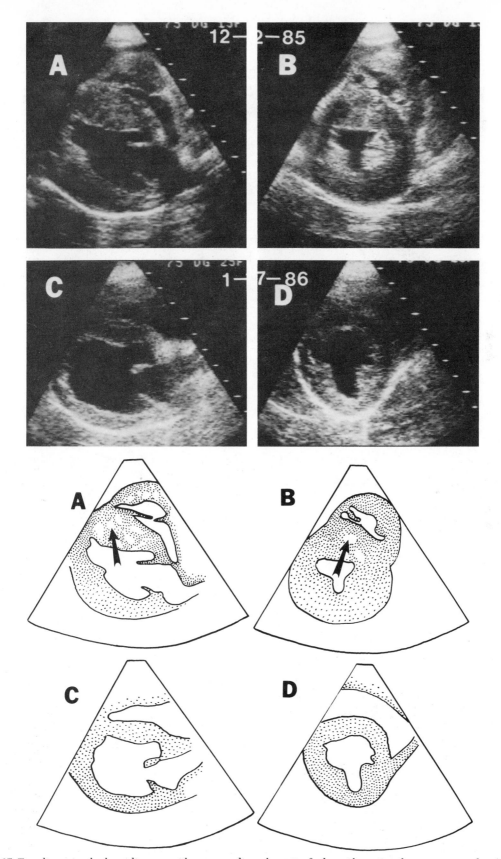

Figure 17. Two-dimensional echocardiograms with corresponding schematic of a dog with pyogranulomatous myocarditis (confirmed by cardiac biopsy) of unknown etiology. *A* and *B*, Initial long-axis four-chamber and short-axis views recorded from the right hemithorax show thickened walls and mottled myocardium (arrows). *C* and *D*, Same echocardiographic views as in *A* and *B* recorded after 6 weeks of antibiotic therapy. Wall thickness and mottling of the myocardium have notably lessened. See Figure 18 for M-mode echocardiograms of this dog.

215

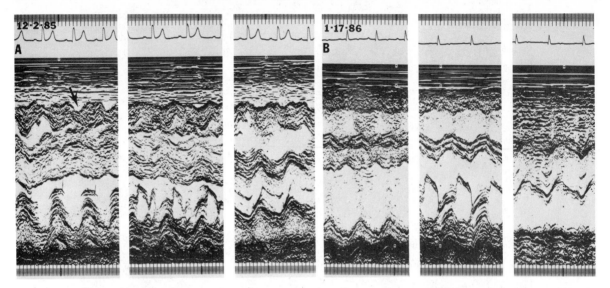

Figure 18. M-mode echocardiograms recorded from dog described in Figure 17. *A*, Initial echocardiogram showing thickened right ventricular wall and interventricular septum (IVS). The IVS is hypoechoic compared with the ventricular free walls, and its motion is reduced. Mild pericardial effusion is present (arrow). *B*, Echocardiogram recorded 6 weeks after *A* demonstrating a reduction in the thickness of the IVS and the ventricular free walls. The low fractional shortening (27 per cent) and increased E point septal separation suggest some myocardial pump failure. Distance between markers, 1 cm; paper speed, 50 mm/sec.

and neoplastic disease such as lymphoma are examples in which follow-up echocardiography has demonstrated resolution of the myocardial infiltrate.

HEARTWORM DISEASE

Echocardiography can be beneficial in selected cases of *Dirofilaria immitis* infection in which occult heartworm disease exists and adequate numbers of worms are present (approximately 25) to be visible in chambers and vessels that can be imaged. It is of even more value when occult tests are negative,

yet heartworms are seen. The worms appear as specs or flashes of short lines on the two-dimensional image and as lines on the M-mode echocardiogram. If large numbers of worms are present, a large echodense structure will be seen (Fig. 19). The worms may be noted in the caudal vena cava (obstruction of this vessel with a thrombus of worms in the right atrium will be identified in animals with postcaval syndrome), right atrium, right ventricle, pulmonary trunk, or the right or left pulmonary vessels. In addition to possibly providing the diagnosis and the indication for adulticide therapy, the severity of cardiac compromise and need for sup-

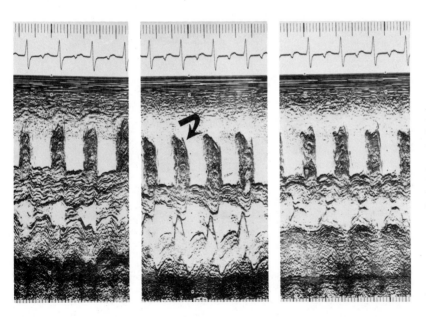

Figure 19. M-mode echocardiogram recorded from a German shepherd with heartworms. A large mass of worms (arrow) is seen in each echocardiographic view of the right ventricular inflow tract. As the tricuspid valve opens, the mass of worms falls into the ventricle from the right atrium. Note the reduced size of the left ventricular chamber. Distance between markers, 1 cm; paper speed, 50 mm/sec.

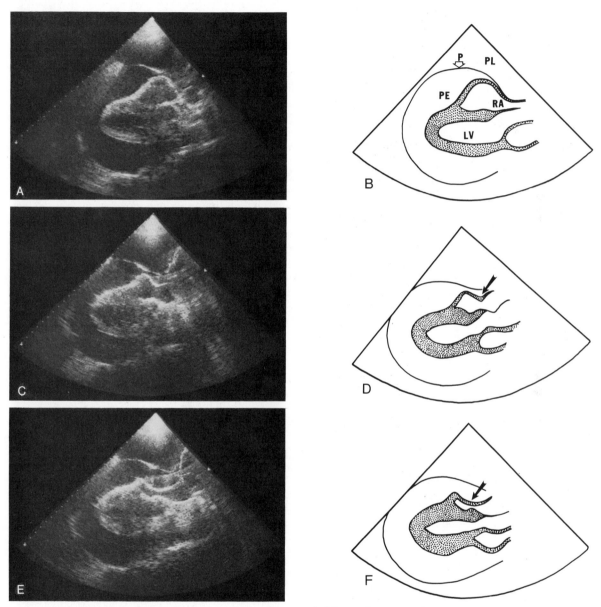

Figure 20. A through F, Two-dimensional echocardiograms recorded from a dog with cardiac tamponade during different phases of the cardiac cycle to illustrate the collapse of the right atrium (RA; arrow in D and F). P (open arrow), pericardium; PE, pericardial effusion; PF, pleural fluid; LV, left ventricle.

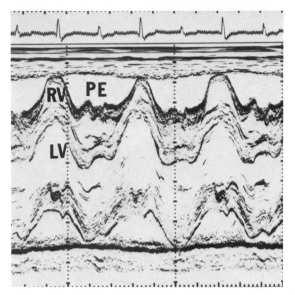

Figure 21. M-mode echocardiogram recorded from a dog with pericardial effusion (PE). The to-and-fro motion of the heart and corresponding electrical alternans is illustrated. RV, right ventricle; LV, left ventricle.

portive therapy can be ascertained by the degree of right ventricular hypertrophy and dilation, presence of paradoxical septal motion (Fig. 1E) and tricuspid regurgitation (using Doppler techniques), amount of pulmonary artery dilation and tortuosity, degree of reduction in left ventricular and atrial chamber size, estimation of pulmonary artery pressures by Doppler, and extracardiac signs of right-sided heart failure. After adulticide treatment when clinical signs persist or an inability to rid the dog of microfilaria is encountered, persistent identification of worms will confirm an inadequate kill of worms.

PERICARDIAL EFFUSION

Echocardiography can provide life-saving information in the identification of cardiac tamponade. Emergency pericardiocentesis can even be guided by ultrasound, although it is most commonly performed blindly. With cardiac tamponade the ultrasound image displays a "convulsing" heart. The

right side of the heart, especially the right atrium, will wiggle and collapse (Fig. 20). A to-and-fro motion that is responsible for electrical alternans may be seen (Fig. 21). The chaotically moving heart is surrounded by the pericardial fluid, which may be anechoic or hypoechoic, depending on the cellularity of the fluid. The echocardiographic differentiation between pericardial effusion and cardiac tamponade rests in the identification of the erratic right-sided heart motion. In addition, the greater the intrapericardial pressure, the more compromise occurs in cardiac filling and the smaller the heart size is. After pericardiocentesis dramatic increases in chamber sizes will be appreciated. The pericardium can be investigated for its thickness and contour. The pericardium is more easily identified when pleural effusion also is present. The cause of pericardial effusion can be determined by echocardiography in many cases of heart base tumors. The origin of the echogenic mass assists in suggesting the type of tumor (hemangiosarcoma, chemodectoma, or ectopic thyroid carcinoma). Hematomas or periaortic fat should not be misidentified as cardiac tumors because a dog with benign pericardial effusion will be mistreated. This mistake is most likely to happen if echocardiographic examination for tumor presence is conducted soon after pericardiocentesis.

References and Supplemental Reading

Bonagura, J. D.: M-mode echocardiography: Basic principles, cardiopulmonary diagnostic techniques. Vet. Clin. North Am. 13:299, 1983.

Bonagura, J. D., and Herring, D. S.: Echocardiography: Congenital heart disease. Vet. Clin. North Am. 15:1195, 1985.

Bonagura, J. D., and Herring, D. S.: Echocardiography: Acquired heart disease. Vet. Clin. North Am. 15:1209, 1985.

Bonagura, J. D., O'Grady, M. R., and Herring, D. S.: Echocardiography: Principles of interpretation. Vet. Clin. North Am. 15:1177, 1985.

DeMadron, E., Bonagura, J. D., and Herring, D. S.: Two-dimensional echocardiography in the normal cat. Vet. Radiol. 26:149, 1985.

Feigenbaum, H.: *Echocardiography*, 4th ed. Philadelphia: Lea & Febiger, 1986.

Moise, N. S., Dietze, A. E., Mezza, L. E., et al.: Echocardiography, electrocardiography, and radiography of cats with dilatation cardiomyopathy, hypertrophic cardiomyopathy, and hyperthyroidism. Am. J. Vet. Res. 47:1476, 1986.

Moise, N. S.: Echocardiography. *In* Fox, P. R. (ed.): *Canine and Feline Cardiology.* New York: Churchill Livingstone, 1988, pp. 113–154.

Thomas, W. P.: Two-dimensional, real-time echocardiography in the dog: Technique and anatomic validation. Vet. Radiol. 25:50, 1984.

BRONCHOSCOPY IN THE SMALL ANIMAL PATIENT

BRENDAN C. MCKIERNAN, D.V.M.

Urbana, Illinois

Rigid bronchoscopy has been used in human medicine since the late 1890's, but the introduction of the flexible fiberscope by Ikeda in 1967 marked a major development. Bronchoscopy is widely used in veterinary medicine, both in the clinical setting and as a research tool. A recent search of the literature revealed nearly 150 articles on bronchoscopy in dogs published since 1966, including 15 during the past 2 years alone.

Bronchoscopy has been used to diagnose various diseases in veterinary medicine, including bronchitis, bronchiectasis, pneumonia, primary parasitic diseases (e.g., infection with *Paragonimus* or *Oslerus osleri*), foreign body aspiration, lung lobe torsion, both dynamic (e.g., collapse) and fixed airway caliber changes (e.g., extramural compression from lymph nodes, granuloma, or tumor). Both rigid and flexible bronchoscopic techniques have been a part of respiratory specialty practices in veterinary medicine since at least the early 1970's, providing the clinician with valuable information about the patient's respiratory system.

EQUIPMENT

There are a wide variety of instruments available for bronchoscopy. For the purpose of discussion they can be easily divided into two groups: rigid and flexible systems. There are specific advantages and disadvantages of each type of system. For the most part endoscopes are *not* specifically made for veterinary use, and species differences (for example, in airway length and diameter) result in certain limitations in the use and application of "human bronchoscopes" and often necessitate the selection of other endoscopes (e.g., the flexible pediatric gastroscope) for use as a "veterinary bronchoscope." Although in human medicine it is recommended that both rigid and flexible systems be available to the bronchoscopist (to utilize the advantages of each), the cost of the individual systems will usually limit the veterinary practitioner to purchasing only one.

RIGID BRONCHOSCOPES. The currently available rigid fiberoptic bronchoscopes (Holinger Ventilating Fiberoptic Bronchoscope, Pilling Co., Fort Washington, PA) technically provide the bronchoscopist with a number of distinct advantages over flexible systems. Rigid systems, by design, have a larger channel for biopsy, suction, and instrumentation. This is important in situations of excessive bleeding or thick secretions and for the manipulation of large foreign bodies. Because of the clarity of view, they also allow for exceptional photographic documentation. Finally, these instruments cost less than the flexible bronchoscope systems but are more limited in their potential for other endoscopic applications when compared with flexible systems.

Rigid bronchoscopes have the disadvantage of limiting the viewing area to the more central regions of the tracheobronchial tree. Older rigid bronchoscope systems were unable to control patient ventilation, but newer bronchoscopes incorporate a Venturi ventilating system for administering oxygen, anesthetic gases, or both.

FLEXIBLE ENDOSCOPES. Because of the shorter length of the human tracheobronchial tree one endoscope may be satisfactory for bronchoscopy. However, two different flexible endoscopes may be required in veterinary practice to perform bronchoscopy in all sizes of small animals. (This is also true for the rigid instruments.) At the University of Illinois, both the small-caliber gastroscope (7.9-mm diameter by 1025-mm working length) (Olympus GIF-XP10 OES Small Caliber Gastrointestinal Fiberscope, Olympus Corp., New Hyde Park, NY) and the thin bronchoscope (5.0-mm diameter by 550-mm working length) (Olympus BF type P-10 Bronchofiberscope, Olympus Corp.) are used for bronchoscopy in small animals. These two endoscopes will allow for excellent bronchoscopic evaluation in patients weighing from 1.0 to over 75 kg and also have enough versatility to be used in other endoscopic procedures, such as rhinoscopy, esophagoscopy, gastroscopy, and cystoscopy.

Flexible endoscopes have distinct advantages over the rigid endoscopes, including greater maneuverability and an increased viewing area within the tracheobronchial tree. They also have disadvantages in comparison with the rigid endoscopes; these include increased purchase and repair costs, a decreased quality of image transmission (noted primarily with endoscopic photography), decreased durability (the greater flexibility also can result in more optical bundle breakage), and less suction and instrumentation capability (the channel is usually between 1.8 and 2.6 mm in diameter, depending on the endoscope model). In the author's opinion, the greater maneuverability and increased viewing area of flexible endoscopes, as well as the potential for use in other endoscopic procedures, are distinct benefits and with few exceptions outweigh the potential disadvantages mentioned.

The lack of a specific ventilating capability in flexible endoscopes, which potentially can lead to hypoxemia and, if severe, cardiac arrhythmias, can be minimized (see discussion of anesthesia below).

Recent microelectronic technology advancements have allowed the development of a microchip that can transmit an image electronically from the tip of the endoscope to a television viewing monitor. These new endoscopes are reported to present a high-quality image, while avoiding problems (breakage and clouding) that may be encountered with flexible glass fiber bundle instruments. Instruments are currently too large in diameter for small animal bronchoscopy; the smallest videoendoscope (Video Gastroscope, Welch Allyn, Inc., Skaneateles Falls, NY) is 9.5 mm in diameter. However, microelectronic applications are likely to expand and be useful in veterinary practice in the future.

SOURCES OF ENDOSCOPIC EQUIPMENT. New endoscopes (both rigid and flexible) are available from several manufacturers. Veterinarians have purchased good quality used endoscopes from a local hospital or endoscope salesperson. These sources should be investigated by those who are interested in performing endoscopy in animals but are unable to afford the cost of a new system.

CARE AND CLEANING

All endoscopes, *especially* flexible ones, are delicate, expensive instruments, which should be handled, used, and cleaned with the utmost care. Improper handling (e.g., forceful insertion or bending) or cleaning (e.g., some instruments can be totally immersed, others should be gas sterilized) can result in instrument damage and expensive repair costs. Maintenance of sterility is often hampered by humidity. *Pseudomonas* is a common contaminant of respiratory equipment of all types, including endoscopic equipment. Various gas (ethylene oxide), steam, and cold soaking techniques have been successfully used to sterilize endoscopes and biopsy equipment. All manufacturers include detailed use, care, and cleaning instructions with their instruments; this information is prerequisite reading material for anyone who will handle the endoscope.

INDICATIONS AND CONTRAINDICATIONS

Bronchoscopy is indicated for both diagnostic and therapeutic purposes. Clinical indications for bron-

choscopy are investigation of chronic cough or parenchymal disease of undetermined etiology; evaluation of hemoptysis; foreign body aspiration; evaluation of airway caliber changes, either fixed or dynamic (especially in the absence of fluoroscopy); presurgical staging (e.g., to determine presence of single versus multiple lobe disease); evaluation of persistent halitosis when oral, nasal, and pharyngeal examinations are nondiagnostic; and when therapy fails or relapses occur.

Diagnostic bronchoscopy is used to obtain visual information concerning the airways (e.g., compression, collapse, and dilation) and to obtain samples (biopsy, cytology, and, with certain restrictions, culture) to help establish a specific etiologic diagnosis. Bronchoscopy assumes a therapeutic role less often but can be used for the removal of a foreign body or copious bronchial secretions.

Other than the risks associated with anesthesia/sedation required for the procedure, there is no absolute contraindication to bronchoscopy in veterinary medicine. Zavala (1978) has proposed both relative and absolute contraindications to bronchoscopy in human medicine. A modification of this list for veterinary use is presented, along with a summary of the indications for bronchoscopy, in Table 1.

ANESTHESIA, MONITORING, AND PATIENT POSITIONING

The insertion of an endoscope into the airways results in strong reflex stimulation, including sneez-

Table 1. *Indications and Contraindications for Bronchoscopy in Small Animals*

Indications
Diagnostic: for sample acquisition, visual assessment, or both
Chronic cough or parenchymal disease of undetermined etiology
Hemoptysis
Evaluation of airway caliber disorders
Dynamic changes (tracheobronchial collapse)
Fixed changes (compression, bronchiectasis)
Presurgical staging
Persistent halitosis, not of upper airway origin
Therapeutic
Removal of a foreign body
Removal of copious/retained secretions
Contraindications*
Relative: evaluation on individual patient basis
Uremia—increased risk of hemorrhage
Poor cardiopulmonary reserve—increased risk of arrhythmias
Absolute
Uncorrected bleeding diathesis
Nonreversible hypoxemia ($Pa_{O_2} \leq 65$ mm Hg while receiving oxygen)—increased risk of arrhythmias
Serious pre-existing cardiac arrhythmias

*Modified in part from Zavala (1978).

Editor's Note: Evaluation of patients with chronic alveolar-interstitial diseases and patients with persistent pneumomediastinum may be additional indications.

ing, head shaking, paroxysmal coughing, and airway constriction. General anesthesia, or neuroleptanalgesia, is necessary to control these reflexes, to prevent trauma to the airways, and also to protect the endoscope.

The necessity for general anesthesia is a potential drawback of bronchoscopy, although the information that may be obtained from bronchoscopy (i.e., a definitive diagnosis) may override this concern. The availability of the newer injectable anesthetics (e.g., oxymorphone) has allowed bronchoscopy to be performed on narcotized animals and has provided the ability to reverse the patient's anesthesia following completion of the procedure. Because many of the chronic conditions for which bronchoscopy is indicated occur in older patients, this form of anesthesia has been beneficial. In most cases, it not only provides adequate anesthesia for bronchoscopy but also allows for rapid patient recovery, an important factor in geriatric patients.

There are a variety of anesthetic protocols that are satisfactory for bronchoscopy. Selection of a particular protocol should be based on the patient's condition, the bronchoscopic equipment to be used (e.g., can the animal be ventilated through the bronchoscope?), and the veterinarian's familiarity with the anesthetic agent. The ideal protocol should provide adequate patient restraint, have minimal adverse effects on the cardiorespiratory system, and be either reversible or of short duration.

Anesthesia is usually induced with a short-acting barbiturate such as thiamylal or thiopental. Depending on the size of the patient, the bronchoscope, and the endotracheal tube, anesthesia can be maintained with gas anesthetics (e.g., halothane, or halothane–nitrous oxide mixture, or isoflurane) while the bronchoscope is passed through a bronchoscopic T piece connected to the endotracheal tube. This technique has the distinct advantage of allowing adequate ventilation during the bronchoscopic procedure. In patients too small to allow the bronchoscope to be passed through an endotracheal tube, some form of injectable anesthesia is indicated. Short-acting barbiturates, ketamine-diazepam combination, or reversible narcotic agents (e.g., oxymorphone) are typically used in these animals. Although flexible endoscopes will not allow true ventilation in these cases, a high oxygen flow (e.g., 1 to 5 L/min) may be provided to the patient through the endoscope when suction is not being used. Gas anesthesia should not be passed through the endoscopic port, as positive pressure ventilation may result, with rapid development of apnea and bradycardia, and expose operating room personnel to anesthetic gases.

The cardiovascular systems of all patients should be monitored during the bronchoscopy procedure. Irritation of the respiratory mucosa during endoscopy can be stimulating and may give rise to an occasional premature ventricular contraction (PVC). In the author's experience, these arrhythmias are more common with *deep* rhinoscopic rather than with bronchoscopic procedures but in either instance usually subside as soon as the stimulation stops. In humans, Pa_{O_2} decreases of between 10 and 20 mm Hg have been reported during bronchoscopy. The frequency of this problem has not been evaluated in veterinary medicine. If a similar decrease does occur there is a real potential for the development of significant hypoxemia. The combined cardiopulmonary effects of general anesthesia, mucosal stimulation, and the hypoxemia in addition to the existing respiratory disease could result in cardiac arrhythmias.

There are two positions that have been used for bronchoscopy in small animals. Selection of either sternal or dorsal recumbency is based on preference and training. If bronchoscopic training is supervised by a physician (or those originally trained under one), the preference is usually for the animal to be dorsally recumbent because it is the position favored for intubation and rigid bronchoscopy in humans. The author prefers that animals be in sternal recumbency because that position is familiar to veterinarians, it avoids any possible gravitational influence on the airways and on cardiorespiratory function, and it is easier to maintain. To avoid confusion, endoscopic photographs (see references and supplemental reading) should be studied with the animal's position in mind.

NORMAL AND ABNORMAL BRONCHOSCOPIC FINDINGS

The differentiation (recognition) of what is normal from what is abnormal is a subjective one. Experience and practice greatly improve the clinician's ability to detect lesions at an early stage. The lung (bronchial epithelium) responds to irritation in limited ways, and therefore the abnormalities visualized by even an experienced bronchoscopist may not be specific (pathognomonic) for a specific disease. For this reason the samples obtained (culture, cytology, biopsy) are important and are usually relied on to establish the specific diagnosis.

The bronchoscopist should have a good understanding of the gross lung anatomy for the species at hand. Terminology used for canine bronchoscopy has recently been proposed (Fig. 1). Bronchoscopic findings and tinctorial changes in the respiratory mucosa are difficult to describe or depict through line drawings or black and white photography. The reader is strongly encouraged to review endobronchial anatomy (Amis and McKiernan, 1986) and consult color photographs of endoscopic findings (Stradling, 1976; Venker-van Haagen, 1979; Venker-van Haagen et al., 1985.)

Endobronchial anatomy is best described sequentially, as the bronchoscope is passed into the tracheobronchial tree. Figure 1 depicts the canine airways as encountered during bronchoscopy. This diagram and the terminology used are of great assistance in communicating the location of endobronchial lesions to others or in recording results for comparison at a subsequent bronchoscopy. They also are helpful in finding lesions on a radiograph or at surgery.

C-shaped cartilaginous rings are usually visible beneath the tracheal mucosa and into the larger bronchi. In the trachea a dorsal membrane, located between the ends of these rings, is stretched relatively tightly so that there is little if any redundancy (visible protrusion or collapse into the airway) in the normal animal. Changes in airway caliber and collapse of tracheal, bronchial, or both lumens with quiet respiration may be observed in animals with tracheobronchial collapse and bronchiectasis. These findings are greatly exaggerated during forceful respiration (e.g., coughing), and the bronchoscopist must be careful not to overdiagnose airway collapse in these animals.

The mucosa of the normal tracheobronchial tree should be light pink, although its appearance will vary depending on the intensity and proximity of the lighting being used. Harsh white highlights (a reflected glare) may be produced when the mucosa is at right angles to or close to the light source. The glistening appearance of the normal mucosa is due to the presence of a thin periciliary fluid layer (the "sol"). In a healthy animal small accumulations of mucus (clear to white and slightly opaque) may be observed on the mucosa, stranding across the lumen, or pushed up in front of the bronchoscope during bronchoscopy. A rich supply of submucosal vessels (mucosal capillaries) is usually visible within the submucosa and is especially noticable between the cartilaginous rings of the trachea.

Mucosal hemorrhage may be induced easily during endoscopy (from a forceful or rough endoscope insertion, suction, or biopsy). When it is present on initial examination it may be associated with thoracic trauma (lung contusion, bite wounds), parasitic infection (especially *Paragonimus*), airway foreign body, chronic mucosal trauma (e.g., from coughing) with severe external compression (e.g., a lobar *Blastomyces* granuloma, hilar lymphadenopathy), and (rarely) a lung tumor.

Focal or generalized changes may be observed in the tracheobronchial tree of a diseased animal, including those involving (1) lumen size (intraluminal obstruction, stricture, external compression, or bronchiectasis); (2) lumen shape (dynamic collapse); (3) mucosal abnormalities (edema, accumulations of secretions, irregularity or erosions, mucosal hyperplasia, and thickening or folding); and (4) submucosal changes (increased vascularity or hyperemia, hemorrhages, or nodule formation).

Mucosal edema is readily apparent owing to the gelatinous appearance it imparts to the epithelial surface. Edema may be accompanied by blunting of the bronchial bifurcations or "spurs" (the carina is just the first spur encountered) and some degree of loss of details of the submucosal vascular pattern. Generalized reddening of the mucosa (due to inflammatory changes, increased vascularity, and hyperemia) is a common finding in chronic respiratory diseases. Because only diseased animals typically undergo bronchoscopy, care must be exercised in interpreting the appearance of the mucosa so as not to accept the reddened mucosa as normal.

Larger accumulations and secretions of unusual color are associated with chronic irritation, infection (bacterial, parasitic, or fungal), allergies, and trauma. Stradling (1976) states that secretions are excessive if there is need to suction them from the airways during bronchoscopy, regardless of the characteristics of the mucus. He also reports that in humans the openings (dilated ducts) of hypertrophied mucus-secreting glands can be visualized in the bronchial wall of some chronic bronchitis patients.

BRONCHOSCOPIC TECHNIQUE IN SMALL ANIMALS

One of the biggest problems in bronchoscopy is learning how to manipulate the endoscope (especially the flexible endoscopes). It is mandatory that the bronchoscopist be able to direct the instrument (e.g., for biopsy and collection of cytology specimens) without undue risk to the patient (prolonged anesthetic time, excessive trauma/bleeding) or damage to the endoscope.

Although there are no commercially available bronchial casts of animals (as there are for the human bronchial tree), methods have been proposed for making tracheobronchial casts (inflated air-dried lung specimens), which serve as excellent training models. These hollow bronchial casts (as well as cadaver specimens) give neophytes the opportunity to safely develop the manual dexterity and anatomic recognition skills that are necessary to become a competent bronchoscopist. In addition, endoscopy training opportunities are available through certain veterinary schools. The clinician should pursue some form of special training prior to using bronchoscopy as a routine diagnostic tool.

Although preliminary procedures (obtaining history, physical examination, and thoracic radiography) may have established a list of differential diagnoses, it is valuable for the bronchoscopist to be thorough and perform all endoscopies using a standard method and technique. The author examines the larynx, trachea, carina, the right side, and finally the left side of the tracheobronchial tree. A

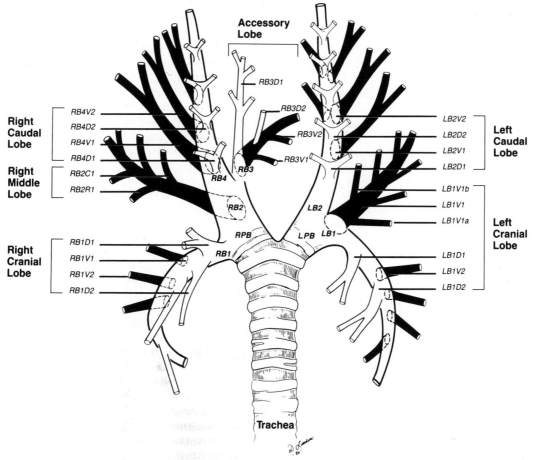

Figure 1. Artist's representation of the canine bronchial tree using a recently proposed nomenclature system. This system uses letters and numbers to identify the principal, lobar, segmental, and subsegmental bronchi by their bronchoscopic order of origination and their anatomic orientation.

Key: R, right; L, left; B, bronchus; P, principal; V, ventral; D, dorsal; C, caudal; R, rostral. Numbers indicate origination order, and lower case letters indicate origination order of subsegmental bronchi (without anatomic orientation). (From Amis, T. C., and McKiernan, B. C.: Systemic identification of endobronchial anatomy during bronchoscopy in the dog. Am. J. Vet. Res. 47:2649, 1986.)

bronchial cast model and the diagram depicted in Figure 1 are useful in localizing lesions and for recording the location (in writing) of lesions, biopsies, or photographs for future comparison and reference. One should record changes in gross anatomy, fixed and dynamic lumen size, shape abnormalities, mucosal/submucosal characteristics, and the presence of secretion accumulations.

SAMPLE PROCUREMENT AND HANDLING. When specific abnormalities are noted samples may be obtained for tests such as cytologic evaluation (via brush, curette, washing pipe, or lavage), histopathologic evaluation (via cup or crocodile biopsy forceps), and culture (from washings or tissue biopsy). The use of transbronchial biopsy techniques (using needle or forceps) has not been evaluated in veterinary medicine.

Samples obtained with endoscopic forceps are typically small. A biopsy is indicated when prolif-

erative mucosal changes are seen or when a mass lesion is visualized. When a biopsy is to be performed, multiple specimens should be taken (if feasible) to give the pathologist a greater chance to make a diagnosis. One of the biopsy samples may be gently rolled on a glass slide for cytologic evaluation prior to fixing it in formalin. The incidence of mucosal cancer is low in veterinary medicine, and therefore the diagnostic return from mucosal biopsy is relatively low or at best nonspecific.

Cytologic evaluation is of major importance. Bronchial brushings will result in better epithelial cytologic specimens, whereas washings and lavage procedures seem to collect cells that were exfoliated or loose on the surface. Bronchoalveolar lavage with the bronchoscope in a wedged position may be useful for the diagnosis of alveolointerstitial lung disease. Rebar and associates (1980) have reviewed technique and evaluation of bronchopulmonary lavage cytology in the normal dog; Hoffmann and Wellman (1986), the tracheobronchial cytology; and Venker-van Haagen (1985), the results from 228 small animal bronchoscopies (including cytology). (Also see pages 361 to 368.)

Cultures from the lower airways are helpful in establishing a specific diagnosis and selecting an appropriate antibiotic based on sensitivity results. However, samples must not be contaminated by upper respiratory tract secretions. The use of the flexible endoscope in obtaining samples for culture is controversial owing to the opportunity for sample contamination (both from the oral cavity and from an improperly cleaned endoscope channel). Guarded catheters have been developed (Microbiology Specimen Brush, Medi-Tech, Watertown, MA); these decrease the possibility of upper airway contamination of a culture sample obtained by flexible endoscopy.

COMPLICATIONS

Bronchoscopy is generally thought to be safe and to lack any serious complications. Potential complications have rarely been discussed in veterinary medicine. In human medicine a list of potentially serious complications includes those associated with anesthesia (e.g., anesthetic reaction, endotracheal tube trauma, and hypoventilation), effects of the bronchoscopic procedure itself (e.g., bronchospasm, bleeding, bacteremia, hypoxemia, and arrhythmias), and those that occur after the completion of the procedure (e.g., fever, infection, and new pulmonary infiltrates). Complications that have been mentioned in veterinary medicine are few in number and can easily be anticipated by an examination of this list and the contraindications in Table 1.

Despite the potential for complications, it is interesting to note that no serious complications have been documented in animals. However, it is imperative that *the veterinary bronchoscopist be prepared for all eventualities*. This means that he or she must have a clear understanding of patient risk factors and the limitations of the equipment and have both the knowledge and all drugs or equipment necessary to treat any complication.

References and Supplemental Reading

Amis, T. C., and McKiernan, B. C.: Systemic identification of endobronchial anatomy during bronchoscopy in the dog. Am. J. Vet. Res. 47:2649, 1986.
Hoffman, W. E., and Wellman, M. L.: Tracheobronchial cytology. *In* Kirk, R. W. (ed.): *Current Veterinary Therapy IX*. Philadelphia: W. B. Saunders, 1986, pp. 243–247.
McKiernan, B. C., and Kneller, S. K.: A simple method for the preparation of inflated air-dried lung specimens. Vet. Radiol. 24:58, 1983.
Rebar, A. H., DeNicola, D. B., and Muggenburg, B. A.: Bronchopulmonary lavage cytology in the dog: Normal findings. Vet. Pathol. 17:294, 1980.
Stradling, P. (ed.): *Diagnostic Bronchoscopy: An Introduction*, 3rd ed. New York: Churchill Livingstone, 1976.
Venker-van Haagen, A. J.: Bronchoscopy of the normal and abnormal canine. J. Am. Anim. Hosp. Assoc. 15:397, 1979.
Venker-van Haagen, A. J., Vroom, W. M., Heijn, A., and van Ooijen, P. G.: Bronchoscopy in small animal clinics: An analysis of the results of 228 bronchoscopies. J. Am. Anim. Hosp. Assoc. 21:521, 1985.
Zavala, D. C.: *Flexible Fiberoptic Bronchoscopy*. Cedar Rapids, IA: Pepco Litho Press, 1978.

CONGENITAL HEART DISEASE

MATTHEW W. MILLER, D.V.M.,
College Station, Texas

and JOHN D. BONAGURA, D.V.M.
Columbus, Ohio

The management of congenital heart disease can be a challenging and rewarding clinical experience. Dogs and cats are affected with a wide array of cardiac malformations. Although complex cardiac defects have been documented in the veterinary literature, these lesions often cause death in the immediate postnatal period. The lesions most commonly encountered in veterinary practice are relatively simple and include patent ductus arteriosus (PDA), valvular stenosis or insufficiencies, subvalvular aortic stenosis (SAS), pulmonic stenosis (PS), mitral and tricuspid dysplasia, atrioventricular septal defects (ASD, VSD), and the tetralogy of Fallot. Logical interpretation of information obtained from physical examination, thoracic radiography, and electrocardiography (ECG) will, in many cases, lead to an accurate diagnosis.

While congenital heart disease accounts for less

than 10 per cent of the clinically significant cardiovascular diseases diagnosed in small animal patients, it is the most common cause of cardiovascular disease in young animals (less than 1 year of age). Occasionally animals with congenital disease do not display clinical signs or are not diagnosed until they are mature; accordingly, congenital disease must be differentiated from the more common acquired diseases in these patients. The veterinarian should be familiar with the typical physical examination and thoracic radiographic and electrocardiographic (ECG) abnormalities encountered with the common congenital cardiac defects. Definitive diagnosis of the type and severity of congenital heart disease may require more sophisticated diagnostic techniques, including echocardiography and selective angiocardiography; therefore, pets with congenital heart disease may benefit from referral.

DIAGNOSIS

Signalment and History

The majority of animals with congenital heart disease are asymptomatic when first examined, and many clients are surprised when they are told that their pet has serious heart disease. Occasionally owners complain of the animal's exercise intolerance, fainting, respiratory distress, or stunted growth. A history of fainting should alert the clinician to the possibility of hypoxic events (right-to-left shunts), ventricular outflow tract obstruction, or paroxysmal arrhythmias. Respiratory distress may be indicative of congestive heart failure or cyanotic heart disease.

Signalment can give the clinician a great deal of valuable information. Breed and sex predilections for certain congenital malformations have been well documented (Table 1). Awareness of these genetic positions will help guide the evaluation and concentrate attention on the most common anomaly seen in that breed and help one to counsel breeders. Yet, breed predisposition alone does not permit accurate diagnosis of congenital heart disease.

Physical Examination

AUSCULTATION. The majority of pets with significant congenital heart disease have cardiac murmurs. The exceptions include some patients with outflow tract hypoplasia and right-to-left shunting and animals with polcythemia, increased blood viscosity, and a resultant reduction in murmur intensity. Auscultation, therefore, is a cornerstone of diagnosis. The most important aspect of the physical examination is determination of the point of maximal intensity (PMI) of the murmur and whether the

Table 1. *Breed and Sex Predilections for Certain Congenital Cardiac Defects*

Defect	Predilection
Patent ductus arteriosus (PDA)	Poodle, collie, Pomeranian, German shepherd, Shetland sheepdog (female:male, 2.2:1)
Pulmonic stenosis (PS)	Beagle, bulldog, fox terrier, miniature schnauzer, Chihuahua, Samoyed
Subaortic stenosis (SAS)	Newfoundland, boxer, German shepherd, German shorthaired pointer, golden retriever, Rottweiler
Ventricular septal defect (VSD)	English bulldog
Atrial septal defect (ASD)	Samoyed, boxer, Doberman pinscher
Mitral dysplasia	Great Dane, German shepherd (male > female)
Tricuspid dysplasia	Great Dane, German shepherd, Weimaraner, Labrador retriever (male > female)
Tetralogy of Fallot	Keeshond, English bulldog

Note: PDA, PS, and SAS are the most common defects seen in dogs. ASD/VSD and A-V valve dysplasias are the most common defects seen in cats.

murmur is systolic, diastolic, systolic and diastolic, or continuous (Fig. 1). Differentiating murmurs based on their shape and quality can be difficult. As a general rule, ejection murmurs are crescendo/decrescendo, whereas regurgitant murmurs are band-shaped and holosystolic. Murmurs with a high-pitched, musical quality are probably due to the vibrations of cardiac structures and are usually associated with valvular lesions. Most of the more common congenital anomalies can be grouped based on PMI of the murmur, timing during the cardiac cycle, and points of radiation. Knowing the expected PMI, as well as the characteristic patterns of radiation of murmurs, is a necessity for excluding some defects and refining the differential diagnosis.

In animals with valvular lesions, the PMI is usually located over the anatomic lesions, and the area of characteristic sound radiation often marks the resultant abnormal blood flow. The murmur of pulmonic stenosis is heard best at the ventral left base and invariably radiates to the left craniodorsal thorax (into the dilated, poststenotic main pulmonary artery). Mitral dysplasia produces a systolic murmur that radiates to the left apex, whereas the regurgitant murmur of tricuspid dysplasia is heard best over the right cardiac impulse. With congenital SAS, the murmur is heard below the aortic valve at the left third to fourth intercostal space, but the PMI of the murmur actually may be located over the dilated ascending aorta at the right base. Presumably, this is because the aortic root initially turns to the right before descending to the left. It is also common for the murmur of SAS to radiate up the neck along the carotid arteries and occasion-

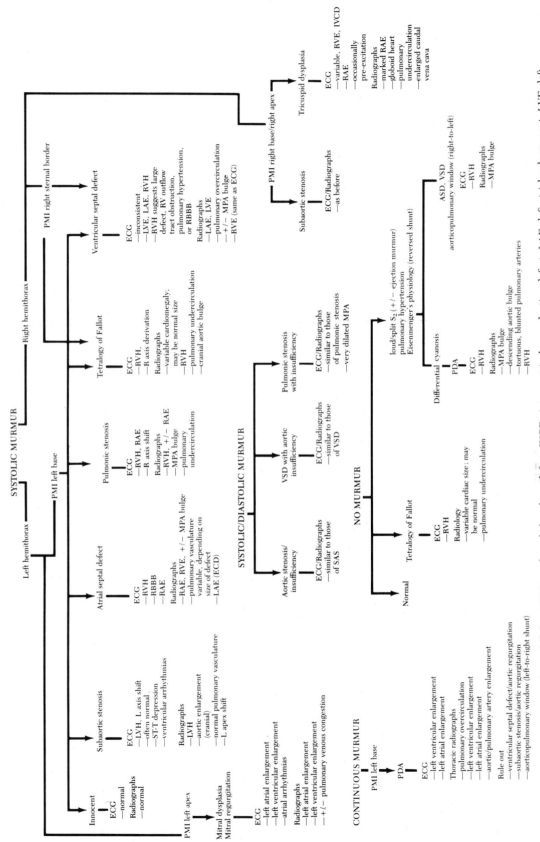

Figure 1. ASD, atrial septal defect; ECD, endocardial cushion defect; IVCD, intraventricular conduction defect; LAE, left atrial enlargement; LVE, left ventricular enlargement; LVH, left ventricular hypertrophy; MPA, main pulmonary artery; PDA, patent ductus arteriosus; PMI, point of maximal intensity; RAE, right atrial enlargement; RBBB, right bundle branch block; RV, right ventricle; RVE, right ventricular enlargement; RVH, right ventricular hypertrophy; SAS, subaortic stenosis; VSD, ventricular septal defect.

ally to be heard on the head. The murmur associated with ASD and VSD is often heard best at the left base, as the flow murmur of relative pulmonic stenosis is caused by the left-to-right shunt. In the case of an ASD, the first heart sound (S_1) is usually audible and there is splitting of S_2. A short left basilar systolic ejection murmur with a loud or split S_2 is characteristic of pulmonary hypertension associated with a reversed shunt such as a right-to-left PDA.

Systolic murmurs heard best at the *right* hemithorax are usually due to tricuspid dysplasia (or tricuspid regurgitation [TR] caused by right ventricular enlargement [RVE]), SAS, or a subcristal VSD. The murmur of SAS is usually heard well at the cranial cardiac base, whereas that of tricuspid dysplasia is heard better over the right cardiac impulse. In many animals, the murmur associated with VSD is loudest at the right sternal border. Either the murmur of PS or that of the VSD can predominate in dogs with the tetralogy of Fallot. Differentiation of the defects requires interpretation of other aspects of the physical examination as well as the results of ECG and thoracic radiographs.

The characteristic continuous murmur of a PDA is heard best high on the left base over the main pulmonary artery, peaks at the second heart sound, and has a lower frequency diastolic component. It is not uncommon to hear a systolic murmur at the left apex in animals with PDA. In some dogs this may be caused by mitral regurgitation. Systolic and diastolic (to-and-fro) murmurs, heard with aortic stenosis and insufficiency, with pulmonic stenosis and insufficiency, or with VSD with aortic insufficiency, may be difficult to differentiate from a true continuous murmur and may lead to an erroneous diagnosis of PDA.

The vast majority of congenital heart defects cause a systolic murmur; however, it is important to remember that not all animals with systolic murmurs have cardiac defects. Physiologic or innocent systolic ejection-type murmurs often are heard best over the left cardiac base. These soft murmurs will frequently disappear after the animal is 4 to 5 months of age and are of no clinical significance, except when they prompt a tentative diagnosis of congenital heart disease. Animals with innocent murmurs have normal thoracic films and electrocardiograms and, other than their murmurs, a normal cardiovascular examination. When soft systolic murmurs persist in pets older than 6 months of age, the possibility of congenital heart disease (e.g., SAS) must be considered.

MUCOUS MEMBRANES. Evaluation of the mucous membranes (MM) and capillary refill time (CRT) gives important information regarding cardiac output and oxygenation. Blanched MM and a prolonged CRT suggests cardiac failure, whereas cyanotic MM should alert the clinician to the possibility of a right-to-left shunt, severe congestive heart failure, or concurrent lung disease. The most common form of cyanotic heart disease encountered in veterinary medicine is the tetralogy of Fallot. Other forms of cyanotic heart disease are primarily intracardiac or extracardiac shunts complicated by pulmonary hypertension (Eisenmenger's physiology) or pulmonic stenosis. Both the oral and vulvar or preputial mucous membranes should routinely be evaluated to rule out the possibility of a reversed PDA with differential cyanosis (cranial membranes pink/caudal membranes blue).

VENOUS PULSES. Evaluation of the jugular vein is an important and frequently overlooked portion of the physical examination. It may be necessary to shave the hair over the jugular furrow to adequately evaluate the jugular vein for distention or abnormal pulsation. The venous pulse in the standing animal can normally be seen to extend one fourth to one third of the way up the neck. Jugular venous distention or abnormal pulsations above the level of the right atrium should alert the clinician to the possibility of elevated right-sided pressures and a right-sided heart lesion.

Accentuation of the jugular venous pulse during compression of the liver is known as the hepatojugular reflex. Pressure on the liver increases venous return to the right atrium. This increased blood volume is well tolerated by the normal right side of the heart, but in right-sided heart disease this increased blood volume may result in elevations in right atrial pressure and be manifested as changes in the character of the venous pulse.

PRECORDIAL PALPATION. Palpation of the precordium can help the clinician differentiate among certain cardiac defects. The points of the left and right cardiac impulses are the general areas of the mitral and tricuspid valve sounds, respectively. This knowledge helps orient the examiner to the location of the valve areas relative to the sternal borders and intercostal spaces. Palpable thrills generally identify the PMI of a murmur and also suggest that the lesion is of hemodynamic significance. The strength of the apical impulse can give the clinician an indication of the systolic function of the ventricles, and an intense apical impulse is suggestive of ventricular hypertrophy. If the right apical impulse is equal to or stronger than that on the left (right ventricular heave), defects that result in right ventricular hypertrophy (PS, tetralogy of Fallot, right-to-left shunts) should be suspected.

ARTERIAL PULSES. Changes in arterial pulse character are associated primarily with lesions of the left side of the heart. The arterial pulse is usually reduced in intensity and slow to rise in dogs with SAS, whereas animals with PDA or aortic regurgitation have bounding "water hammer" pulses owing to diastolic run-off of blood from the aorta. Significant right-sided lesions may also decrease arterial pulse intensity because of reduced right-sided cardiac output and a subsequent reduction in left-sided preload. Weak arterial pulses also may be a manifestation of cardiac failure, whereas pulses of variable intensity or pulse deficits suggest an arrhythmia.

Electrocardiography

Although it is prudent to examine all aspects of the ECG, when evaluating the electrocardiogram in patients with congenital heart disease, the primary abnormalities to recognize are those associated with right- or left-sided chamber enlargement/hypertrophy and alterations in the mean electrical axis (MEA). Other abnormalities encountered less frequently include ST-T segment changes (e.g., in SAS), conduction abnormalities, and arrhythmias. Chamber sizes change in response to the hemodynamic (volume or pressure) abnormalities associated with each cardiac defect.

P-wave changes associated with left atrial enlargement (P wave > 0.04 sec) are commonly seen with left-to-right intracardiac (VSD) or extracardiac (PDA) shunts and with mitral dysplasia. Although a secundum ASD results in left-to-right shunting, the left atrium decompresses into the right atrium, causing right atrial instead of left atrial enlargement. Wide and peaked P waves (P wave > 0.4 mV) are associated with ASD or tricuspid dysplasia and occasionally with PS. Atrial arrhythmias, including atrial premature contractions and atrial fibrillation, occasionally develop in patients with defects that cause atrial enlargement.

Left ventricular hypertrophy (LVH) and left ventricular enlargement (LVE) are seen with lesions causing left ventricular outflow tract obstruction and left ventricular volume overload, respectively. Electrocardiographic changes include increased R-wave amplitude (> 2.5 to 3 mV in lead II) and a left axis deviation (MEA $< 40°$). The most dramatic increases in the R-wave amplitude are usually seen with PDA. Left ventricular hypertrophy is most commonly seen with SAS and may be accompanied by a left axis shift. Lesions associated with left ventricular volume overload and subsequent enlargement include PDA, VSD, and mitral dysplasia. The mean frontal axis in these defects is usually normal.

The causes of right ventricular hypertrophy or enlargement (right axis deviation with prominent S waves in leads I, II, III, aVf, and V_2 to V_6) include PS, ASD, tetralogy of Fallot, large VSD with equilibration of intraventricular pressures, and shunts complicated by pulmonary hypertension. Because the right bundle branch is more susceptible to injury, it is not uncommon for defects affecting the right side to result in a right bundle branch block (RBBB).

Thoracic Radiography

Thoracic radiographs are frequently helpful in the diagnosis of congenital heart disease. Special attention should be directed to overall cardiac size, individual chamber size, the great vessels, and pulmonary vascularity. As a general rule, volume overload (PDA, VSD) will result in more dramatic changes in cardiac size than will pressure overload (SAS, PS, or right-to-left shunts). Changes in thoracic radiographs reflect the response of the heart and blood vessels to the underlying hemodynamic abnormality.

Volume overload leads to enlargement of the cardiac chambers or great vessels that carry the increased volume. Pulmonary overcirculation is usually indicative of a left-to-right shunt (PDA, VSD, or ASD), and differentiation of the lesions causing pulmonary overcirculation is facilitated by determining the associated chamber enlargements. Ventricular septal defect, endocardial cushion defect (in cats), and PDA force the left atrium and left ventricle to accept the increased pulmonary flow; subsequently these chambers enlarge. When there is left atrial enlargement without pulmonary overcirculation, mitral dysplasia should be considered. In the case of an ostium secundum ASD, the increased pulmonary flow returns to the left atrium, but the left atrium decompresses into the right atrium, and tends not to enlarge. Instead the right atrium and ventricle must handle the increased flow so these chambers dilate. In the case of VSD or ASD an increased amount of blood flows across the pulmonic valve. This increased flow dilates the main pulmonary artery. Turbulent blood flow across a PDA causes dilation of both the descending aorta and the pulmonary artery in the area of the communication. Thus, radiographic changes typical of a PDA include pulmonary overcirculation, elongation of the cardiac silhouette, left atrial enlargement, and dilation of the aorta ("ductus bump") and main pulmonary artery. Dysplasia of the AV valves causes volume overload of the atrium and ventricle on each side of the affected valve. Therefore, mitral dysplasia is associated with left atrial and ventricular enlargement, whereas tricuspid dysplasia causes enlargement of the right atrium and ventricle (often a globoid heart). Pulmonary undercirculation is commonly seen with tricuspid dysplasia owing to the decreased forward flow caused by the incompetent tricuspid valve.

Stenotic lesions of the ventricular outflow tracts result in pressure overloads of the respective ventricles and subsequent muscular hypertrophy. As stated previously, this hypertrophy usually does not cause the degree of cardiac enlargement that is frequently seen with lesions causing volume overload. Stenotic lesions result in turbulent blood flow distal to the point of obstruction and cause dilation of the chamber or vessel that is receiving the flow. In the case of SAS, the proximal aorta dilates and is frequently evident as a bulge at the 12 o'clock position with widening of the cranial mediastinum on the ventrodorsal (VD) radiograph, or as a loss of the cranial cardiac waist on the lateral film. If SAS is complicated by mitral insufficiency or CHF, the left atrium may be enlarged. The high-velocity turbulent flow associated with pulmonic stenosis causes dilation of the main pulmonary artery. Right ventricular hypertrophy is usually manifested as rounding of the right cardiac border and a decrease in the distance between the cardiac silhouette and the right thoracic wall on the VD film. The lateral film frequently demonstrates widening of the cardiac silhouette, increased sternal contact, and an elevation of the cardiac apex. The pulmonary vasculature varies from normal to significantly diminished in size.

Right-to-left shunting defects typically exhibit minimal cardiomegaly, which is manifested primarily as right ventricular hypertrophy. These changes are similar to those seen with PS. Dilation of the main pulmonary artery with peripheral pulmonary hypovascularity is often seen with pulmonary hypertension but is much less common with the tetralogy of Fallot. When tetralogy of Fallot is associated with pulmonary hypoplasia or atresia, the pulmonary bulge is totally absent, the left auricle is small, and there is dramatic pulmonary hypoperfusion. With reversed shunts, the peripheral pulmonary vasculature may appear normal or diminished, whereas the proximal lobar pulmonary arteries are enlarged, blunted, or tortuous.

Echocardiography

The ever-decreasing cost of ultrasound equipment has made echocardiography increasingly available. The more common echocardiographic abnormalities seen with congenital cardiac defects are listed in Table 2. Echocardiography allows the clinician to gain qualitative (valvular morphology) as well as quantitative information (chamber size, wall thickness) regarding cardiac anatomy. In certain defects (ASD, VSD) the actual anatomic abnormality may be visualized, whereas in other cases visualization of the compensatory response to the lesion may be just as informative. Saline injected into a peripheral vein acts as a contrast medium and demonstrates right-to-left shunting defects readily. Right ventricular hypertrophy and flattened septal motion suggest elevated right ventricular pressure.

The development of Doppler echocardiography and, most recently, color flow mapping has revolutionized noninvasive imaging. Doppler echocardiography uses ultrasound to detect the direction and velocity of normal and abnormal blood flow within the heart. Quantitative measurements allow *noninvasive* measurement of cardiac output, transvalvular pressure gradients, regurgitant volumes, and shunt fractions. As more experience is gained with this exciting imaging modality, the indications for invasive diagnostic procedures such as cardiac catheterization should diminish.

Cardiac Catheterization

Even though noninvasive imaging modalities are now able to quantitate the severity of some lesions, cardiac catheterization is still considered the "gold standard" by which all other diagnostic modalities are measured. When considering surgical intervention, anatomic information gained by angiography allows the surgeon to determine the feasibility of a given procedure. Pressure gradients obtained during catheterization help determine prognosis and whether surgical intervention is indicated. With the advent of percutaneous balloon valvuloplasty, cardiac catheterizations can now be therapeutic as well as diagnostic procedures. For instance, percutaneous balloon valvuloplasty should be attempted on every patient with pulmonic stenosis undergoing cardiac catheterization.

THERAPY

Congestive Heart Failure

Congestive heart failure (CHF) is a common sequela to most forms of uncorrected congenital defects. Management of CHF associated with congenital disease is similar to management of CHF caused by acquired disease. Therapy usually consists of digoxin (0.01 to 0.02 mg/kg divided b.i.d. PO) for inotropic support and control of supraventricular arrhythmias; diuretics (furosemide, 0.5 to 2.0 mg/kg s.i.d. to t.i.d. PO) to reduce sodium and fluid retention; and vasodilators (hydralazine, 0.5 to 2.0 mg/kg b.i.d. PO; captopril, 0.5 to 2.0 mg/kg t.i.d. PO). In defects with left-to-right shunting, use of arterial vasodilators (hydralazine and captopril) may reduce left-to-right shunting by reducing the pressure gradient between the systemic and pulmonary circulations. Patients with congestive heart failure must be stabilized prior to surgical intervention. Animals with cyanotic heart disease usually do not develop congestive heart failure but may be incapacitated by tissue hypoxia and hyperviscosity from polycythemia.

Arrhythmias

Atrial arrhythmias such as atrial flutter or fibrillation frequently result from defects that cause atrial

Table 2. Echocardiographic (Doppler) Features of Select Congenital Heart Defects

Defect	Echocardiographic (Doppler)
Patent ductus arteriosus (PDA)	Dilated left atrium, left ventricle, and pulmonary trunk; possible identification of PDA; turbulent flow in main pulmonary artery, with retrograde diastolic flow and increased transmitral and aortic flow velocities
Pulmonic stenosis (PS)	Right ventricular hypertrophy, right atrial and pulmonary artery enlargement, outflow tract obstruction, thickened valve leaflets, septal flattening and/or paradoxical septal motion, high-velocity flow (> 1.5 m/sec) across the pulmonic valve
Subaortic stenosis (SAS)	Left ventricular hypertrophy, dilated aorta, subvalvular narrowing, high-velocity flow (> 2.0 m/sec) across the aortic valve
Ventricular septal defect (VSD)	Variable chamber enlargement, most commonly left atrial and ventricular, possible identification of defect, right ventricular hypertrophy if pulmonary hypertension (PH) or very large defect, visualization of flow across defect, may be bidirectional, increased transmitral and PA flow velocity, right to left in the case of PH
Atrial septal defect (ASD)	Right atrial and ventricular enlargement, possible identification of defect, main pulmonary artery enlargement, flow across defect, increased velocity flow across tricuspid (diastole) and pulmonic (systole) valves
Mitral valve dysplasia	Left atrial and left ventricular enlargement, abnormal mitral valve anatomy, increased transmitral diastolic flow velocity, turbulent retrograde systolic transmitral flow
Tricuspid valve dysplasia	Right atrial and ventricular enlargement, abnormal tricuspid valve anatomy, increased transtricuspid diastolic flow velocity, turbulent retrograde systolic transtricuspid flow
Tetralogy of Fallot	Right ventricular hypertrophy, right ventricular outflow tract obstruction, identification of VSD, over-riding aorta, small left heart, contrast study indicating right-to-left shunting, septal flattening and/or paradoxical septal motion, right-to-left flow across VSD, decreased diastolic transmitral flow, possibly increased transaortic systolic flow, increased flow velocity across the pulmonic valve
Pulmonary hypertension (PH)	Right ventricular hypertrophy, right atrial enlargement, dilated main pulmonary artery, visualization of associated shunt, right-to-left shunt by Doppler or bubble study, increased flow acceleration across pulmonary valve

enlargement. Therapy consists of digoxin (0.01 to 0.02 mg/kg divided b.i.d. PO); beta-adrenergic blockers (propranolol, 0.5 to 1.0 mg/kg t.i.d. PO); calcium channel blockers (diltiazem, 0.75 to 1.25 mg/kg t.i.d. PO); or a combination of these drugs. Ventricular arrhythmias are most commonly seen with SAS and are believed to predispose to sudden death, which is common with this defect. These arrhythmias are probably due to myocardial ischemia. Therapy with beta-adrenergic blockers or calcium channel blockers at previously mentioned dosages may be used to reduce myocardial oxygen demand and might prevent episodes of tachyarrhythmias. Indications for medical therapy in animals with SAS include significant depression (> 0.3 mV) of the ST-T segment on a postexercise, "stress test" ECG, or a systolic gradient of greater than 75 mm Hg measured during cardiac catheterization or by continuous wave Doppler echocardiography. The authors most commonly use propranolol (Inderal) (0.5 to 1.0 mg/kg t.i.d. PO), nadolol (0.25 to 0.5 mg/kg b.i.d. to t.i.d. PO); or atenolol (0.2 to 0.5 mg/kg b.i.d. PO).

Surgical Correction

Definitive therapy of congenital disease involves surgical correction of the underlying defect. To date no surgical procedures are routinely done for the treatment of *subaortic stenosis* or *dysplasia of the AV valves*, and therapy is limited to medical management of CHF and associated arrhythmias. Although open heart surgery using cardiopulmonary bypass has been employed in a limited number of cases of SAS in dogs, the procedures are difficult, expensive, and fraught with complications. Ventricular apex–to-aorta valved conduit, for bypass of SAS, is not widely employed.

Ligation of *patent ductus arteriosus* is the therapy of choice for this defect and is associated with a surgical mortality of less than 5 per cent at most institutions. If ligation is performed early in life (before 6 months of age), most animals have a normal life expectancy. If ligation is not performed, about 50 per cent of affected animals with PDA will die within the first year of life.

Palliation and definitive surgical repair of *atrial septal defects* and *ventricular septal defects* has been described in the veterinary literature with varying degrees of success. Placement of a pulmonary band, resulting in supravalvular pulmonic stenosis, decreases the left-to-right shunting and has been used as a palliative therapy for VSD with some success. Indications for pulmonary banding include left-sided CHF, a left-to-right shunt of greater than 3:1 by catheterization, or pulmonary hypertension associated with increased flow (not resistance). Decreasing the left-to-right shunt fraction will decrease the likelihood of left-sided CHF and theoretically will reduce the chances of development of high-resistance pulmonary hypertension. After pulmonary hypertension and reversed shunting have developed as a result of previously left-to-right shunt, surgical correction is contraindicated.

The *tetralogy of Fallot* can be palliated with the formation of an extracardiac shunt between a systemic artery (aorta or left subclavian artery) and the pulmonary artery to increase pulmonary circulation and reduce the severity of hypoxemia. Results can be quite rewarding with improved Pa_{O_2} and activity and stabilization of the packed cell volume (PCV) for years. Reducing the degree of polycythemia to obtain a PCV between 55 and 60 per cent and therapy with propranolol (0.5 to 1.0 mg/kg b.i.d. to t.i.d. PO) may provide temporary relief in some animals.

Several procedures, including partial valvulectomy, right ventricular patch grafts, right ventricular outflow tract reconstruction (partial myectomy), and more recently pulmonary balloon valvuloplasty, have been used for the therapy of *pulmonic stenosis*. Any animal with a transpulmonary valve systolic gradient of greater than 50 mm Hg (measured during anesthesia) should undergo surgical correction. Although the vast majority of humans with congenital pulmonic stenosis respond well to pulmonary balloon valvuloplasty, in the authors' experience, less than 30 to 40 per cent of the dogs with PS will benefit significantly from this procedure. This is due to the marked difference in the type of valvular lesion seen in the dog (dysplasia) compared with the type most commonly seen in humans.

Because studies have shown that PDA, as well as many other congenital cardiac defects, including PS, SAS, and the tetralogy of Fallot, are hereditary (Patterson, 1976), animals with such defects should be neutered.

SUMMARY

Congenital heart disease is the most common cause of cardiovascular disease in animals less than 1 year of age. Most animals are asymptomatic, while some show signs, including respiratory distress and exercise intolerance, causing premature disability and death. Practicing veterinarians can frequently base a tentative diagnosis on careful physical examination, thoracic radiography, and electrocardiography. Definitive diagnosis usually requires cardiac catheterization or echocardiography. Referral is useful because a variety of management approaches are available, depending on the type and severity of the defect. A polygenetic basis has been established for cardiac defects in several breeds (Patterson, 1976), and knowledge of this helps the veterinarian counsel breeders regarding future matings.

References and Supplemental Reading

Bolton, G. R., and Liu, S. K.: Congenital heart diseases of the cat. Vet. Clin. North Am. [Small Anim. Pract.] 7:341, 1977.

Bonagura, J. D.: Congenital heart disease. *In* Bonagura, J. D. (ed.): *Cardiology. Comtemporary Issues in Small Animal Practice.* Vol. 7, New York: Churchill Livingstone, 1987.

Ettinger, S. J., and Suter, P. F.: *Canine Cardiology.* Philadelphia: W. B. Saunders, 1970.

Patterson, D. F.: Congenital defects of the cardiovascular system of dogs: Studies in comparative cardiology. Adv. Vet. Sci. Comp. Med. 20:1, 1976.

Thomas, W. P.: Congenital heart disease. *In* Kirk, R. W. (ed.): *Current Veterinary Therapy VIII.* Philadelphia: W. B. Saunders, 1983.

ACQUIRED VALVULAR HEART DISEASE IN THE DOG

JOHN R. REED, D.V.M.

Carmichael, California

Acquired valvular heart disease encompasses two distinct disorders in the dog. The first and the most common is chronic valvular degeneration. Atrioventricular (AV) valvular regurgitation of the mitral value is the most frequently encountered cardiac disorder in aging patients. In conjunction with mitral valvular degeneration, degeneration of the tricuspid valve frequently occurs. The second distinct disorder is bacterial endocarditis (BE), which occurs sporadically in the dog. This chapter will only deal with acquired valvular heart disease. Discussion of atrioventricular valvular regurgitation due to congestive cardiomyopathy and congenital valvular defects can be found elsewhere (see pp. 224–231 and 240–251). Those who would like more in-depth information are referred to the excellent review by Sisson (1987).

DEGENERATIVE MITRAL AND TRICUSPID VALVULAR DISEASE

Anatomy and Function

The histologic structures of the mitral and tricuspid valves are similar. The tissues of the tricuspid valve leaflets are normally thinner and more transparent than those of the mitral valve leaflets. There are four distinct layers that make up the valve leaflets: (1) *atrialis*, which contains endothelial cells, connective tissue, and a layer of smooth muscle; (2) *spongiosa*, which contains collagen, fibroblast, and elastic fibers; (3) *fibrosa*, a dense layer of collagen that infiltrates similar tissue in the annulus of the AV valve and central core of the chordae tendineae; and (4) the *ventricularis*, which lines the ventricular surface of the valve (it is similar to the atrialis but without the smooth muscle layer).

In the dog, there are two main mitral valvular cusps. They are identified as the larger anterior (cranioventral, septal) and the smaller posterior (craniodorsal, mural) cusps. The valve cusps are anchored to the anterior and posterior papillary muscles via chordae tendineae. The tricuspid valve really consists of only two cusps. There is a large ventral and smaller dorsal (septal) cusp with numerous secondary cusps. The chordae tendineae of the dorsal leaflet attach directly to small ridges on the interventricular septum. The ventral leaflets attach to a single small papillary muscle of the conus and numerous other papillary muscles that arise from the interventricular septum. The function of both AV valves is to prevent regurgitant volumes of blood from returning to the atria.

The proper closure of the mitral valve requires six anatomic components of mitral valve apparatus to work as one unit. The six components are the mitral leaflets, chordae tendineae, mitral annulus, papillary muscles, the left ventricular wall, and the left atrial wall. It is important to realize that failure of one or more of these structures can result in valvular incompetence. In time, one structural failure may cause the other structures to malfunction, thus leading to further mitral valvular dysfunction.

Incidence and Pathology

Various investigators have reported from 11 to 42 per cent incidence of valvular heart disease in dogs. They have noted that the prevalence of the disease clearly increases with advancing age. Detweiler and associates (1965) determined by clinical means that 10 per cent of dogs 5 to 8 years old, 20 to 25 per cent of dogs 9 to 12 years old, and 30 to 35 per cent of dogs over 13 years old exhibit murmurs. Whitney (1974) found that 58 per cent of dogs older than 9 years of age had significant valvular heart disease. All evidence suggests that male dogs are affected more frequently than female dogs (1.5:1.0) and that small breeds have a greater incidence than larger breeds. Buchanan (1979) studied the incidence of valve involvement in dogs with chronic valvular disease. He found that in 62 per cent the mitral valve alone was involved; 32.5 per cent, both the mitral and tricuspid valves; 2.5 per cent, mitral and aortic valves; 1.3 per cent, the tricuspid valve alone; and 1.3 per cent, the aortic valve alone.

The chronologic changes to the mitral and tricuspid valves were best described by Whitney (1974). The lesions that develop in the tricuspid valve are similar to but less severe than those in the mitral valve. The histologic changes in dogs with chronic valvular fibrosis are best described by the term *myxomatous degeneration*. These lesions also occur in the chordae tendineae. Type I changes consist of a few small, discrete nodules in the area of valvular apposition. In type II lesions, the nodules are larger, are more numerous, and are starting to coalesce. Type III changes are characterized by large plaquelike lesions, which are the result of coalescence of nodules. In type IV lesions, the valve cusps are contracted and grossly distorted. In type III and IV valvular lesions, regurgitation is usually present. The most prominent histologic features are degeneration of the fibrosa and thickening of the spongiosa.

Pathophysiology

The long-term effect of chronic mitral valvular regurgitation (MR) is volume overload of the left ventricle. Initially, the tendency for cardiac output to decline is compensated by the Starling mechanism (Fig. 1), by neurohumoral and renal mechanisms, and eventually by eccentric hypertrophy of the left ventricle. These compensatory mechanisms are able to maintain normal cardiac output for several months or years even when the regurgitant fraction is large. The volume of MR depends on the size of the regurgitation orifice, the pressure gradient between the left ventricle and atrium, the aortic diastolic pressure, and the duration of systole. Decompression of the left ventricle into the low-pressure left atrium results in the enlargement of the left atrium owing to increased volume and pressure. Because more than half of the left ventricular stroke volume can be regurgitated into the left atrium, the left side of the heart has to increase

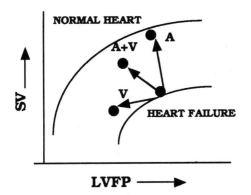

Figure 1. Frank-Starling left ventricular function curves of a normal heart and of a diseased heart. The black circle on the heart failure curve represents a patient's condition at a point in time. With the use of various types of vasodilators a particular response can be seen. SV, stroke volume; LVFP, left ventricular filling pressure; A, arterial dilator; A + V, arterial and venous dilator; V, venous dilator and/or diuretic.

its stroke work to maintain a normal forward stroke volume.

Increases in preload or afterload and decreased contractility result in ventricular dilation, which produces an increased regurgitant volume. The aforementioned compensatory mechanisms evoked in MR increase preload and afterload. A vicious cycle is established whereby MR results in ventricular dilation, which in turn leads to increasingly severe MR. An acceleration of this process is associated with declining contractility. The administration of diuretics, vasodilators, and positive inotropic drugs decreases ventricular size and thus retards the vicious cycle.

When the mean left atrial pressure rises above a threshold level, pulmonary congestion will occur, causing signs of left-sided heart failure (pulmonary edema). The left atrial pressure is dependent on the amount of regurgitant volume and the compliance of the left atrium. Severe pulmonary congestion is likely to develop when the left atrial compliance is low and the regurgitant volume is large. An example of this situation occurs with rupture of a primary chorda tendinea. When MR occurs over a long period of time, the atrium is often large, its compliance is high, and the left atrial pressure is often normal. Left atrial pressure is also dependent on myocardial contractility and the compliance of the left ventricle. When contractility decreases, pulmonary congestion occurs as a result of an increase in left atrial pressure.

The assessment of myocardial oxygen consumption and contractility in dogs with MR relative to therapeutic implications has received much attention. Myocardial oxygen consumption rises only modestly in dogs with MR. This occurs because contractility, myocardial wall tension, and heart rate

are the major determinants for oxygen consumption. Oxygen consumption is little affected by the increased work of myocardial fiber shortening, and ventricular wall tension is not likely to increase greatly when there is MR. Myocardial contractility in MR is difficult to assess without sophisticated equipment. The traditional measurements used to describe ventricular function in conditions such as cardiomyopathy (e.g., ejection fraction) are not reliable indicators in dogs with MR. In patients with MR, myocardial contractility can be accurately assessed only by methods that take into account loading conditions (preload and afterload). It is important to keep in mind that varying degrees of myocardial failure can develop from chronic MR and that myocardial failure causes a deterioration in the clinical status of the patient.

When tricuspid regurgitation (TR) develops, the right atrial pressure will start to rise. This rise depends on the size of the orifice within the valve and the severity of pulmonary hypertension. When the right atrial pressure exceeds 10 to 12 mm Hg, signs of right-sided heart failure develop (ascites and pleural effusion). TR in the dog most often results from a combination of valvular degeneration and functional dilation of the right side of the heart due to increased pulmonary vascular resistance caused by MR and left-sided heart failure. Effective cardiac output tends to decline with TR, especially when pulmonary vascular resistance is high. Under these circumstances, signs of low-output heart failure (syncope) are more common than signs of severe pulmonary congestion in dogs with advanced MR and TR.

Two peracute sequelae to chronic MR can occur. Rupture of a primary chorda tendinea is characterized by the sudden development of fulminating pulmonary edema in previously compensated patients. Ruptured chordae tendineae tend to occur in males more than in females and are frequently seen in the poodle breed. Myxomatous degenerative changes are almost always present in the offending chordae tendineae. Left atrial rupture (second sequela) is the result of endocardial splitting of the left atrium due to chronic MR. The regurgitant fraction causes jet lesions in the left atrial wall over time. The dachshund and cocker spaniel breeds seem to be predisposed to this phenomenon. When the left atrium ruptures, a hemopericardium will occur. This usually results in cardiac tamponade and severe cardiogenic shock.

Clinical Signs

The development of clinical signs due to MR results from the progressive degeneration of the valve leaflets. Mild degrees of valvular regurgitation can be tolerated for many years owing to the interaction of compensatory mechanisms mentioned previously. Most dogs with chronic valvular heart disease remain compensated throughout life and eventually die for reasons other than heart failure. Clinical signs of heart failure generally occur after 7 years of age and are represented by signs of left-sided heart failure (pulmonary congestion), right-sided heart failure (ascites), or both.

The cough is the most common and often the earliest sign of heart failure. The cough is usually dry and harsh and generally occurs during the night, during early morning hours, and after exercise. Frequently the owners state that their dogs seem restless at night, and the dogs cannot find a comfortable position in which to rest. Eventually these dogs experience orthopnea and cannot lay down. As the respiratory signs increase, tachypnea and exercise intolerance may develop. Exercise intolerance is more prevalent in dogs with advanced disease when forward output falls because of severe regurgitation. If forward output continues to fall, syncope may be observed. Syncope can also result from arrhythmias, prolonged periods of coughing, drug therapy (from hypotension), and cardiac tamponade caused by a left atrial tear.

Diagnosis

The murmurs of MR and TR are usually diagnosed during routine *physical examination*. The murmur of MR initially begins as an early to late systolic murmur that progresses to a holosystolic murmur best heard over the left apex. Frequently, the holosystolic murmur will have a musical pitch on auscultation. Sometimes auscultation will reveal a systolic click without the presence of a murmur. It has been suggested that this is an early sign of impending MR or may represent mitral valve prolapse as in humans. The author has not been able document either in the dog.

It is difficult at times to determine whether murmurs auscultated over the tricuspid valve originate from that valve or if they are referred from the diseased mitral valve. Other clinical findings that will support identification of TR are jugular distention or pulse, a precordial thrill at the right fourth or fifth intercostal space, and an auscultable difference in the frequency of the murmurs from the right to left side. The murmur may be soft or absent when severe TR occurs, and usually ascites is present under these circumstances.

Dogs with symptomatic MR are generally dyspneic, cough, and may faint. On auscultation, pulmonary crackles are common. Sinus tachycardia, premature beats, or atrial fibrillation may be heard as well. In dogs with severe TR, hepatomegaly, ascites, dependent edema, jugular pulses, and muf-

fled heart sounds due to pleural effusion may be present.

Electrocardiograms (ECGs) in dogs with chronic MR, TR, or both are frequently insensitive for chamber enlargement and quite often normal. The ECG becomes valuable when sequential recordings are performed. Left atrial enlargement (P wave > 0.04 sec) is a common finding with MR. Left ventricular enlargement (QRS > 0.06 sec, R wave > 2.5 to 3.0 mV) is frequently seen. The mean electrical axis (MEA) in MR patients is usually normal. Increased amplitude of the P waves (> 0.4 mV) is an insensitive finding for evidence for right atrial enlargement in TR patients. Evidence for right ventricular enlargement in conjunction with left ventricular enlargement is difficult to recognize because left ventricular enlargement prevents its recognition. If significant pulmonary hypertension develops, evidence of right ventricular enlargement may be present (MEA > 100°, S wave in leads I, II, III, aVF, V_2, and V_4).

Thoracic radiographs are obtained to examine the cardiac silhouette for chamber enlargement as well as to evaluate the lungs and chest cavity for evidence of either left- or right-sided heart failure. In typical cases there is usually a prominent left atrium in both radiographic views. It is difficult to distinguish between pure left ventricular enlargement and biventricular enlargement without the use of ultrasound or angiocardiography. When there is significant left-sided heart enlargement, the trachea is displaced dorsally. The carina is often compressed between the heart and the thoracic vertebrae. The left mainstem bronchus is elevated and often compressed owing to the enlarged left atrium. The left mainstem bronchi and carinal compression are responsible for a cardiogenic cough in many patients. As left-sided heart failure develops, changes in the pulmonary veins and interstitium (pulmonary edema) can be visualized. An engorged caudal vena cava, pleural effusion, and hepatomegaly indicate right-sided heart failure.

Echocardiography is useful in reflecting changes caused by volume overload of the left side of the heart. These changes include an enlarged left atrium (increased left atrial–aortic ratio), an increased left ventricular diastolic dimension, exaggerated left ventricular free-wall and septal motion, excessive mitral valve amplitudes of motion, a steep E to F slope, and a thickened anterior mitral leaflet. Assessing left ventricular function with echocardiography in MR cases is difficult and usually requires the use of more sophisticated instrumentation. Generally ventricular fractional shortening (FS) is high (> 45 per cent) owing to reduced resistance to ventricular emptying. Normal FS in cases of severe MR may signify severe myocardial failure.

A complete *blood chemistry profile* is essential in the workup of dogs with MR, TR, or both. When a patient has been receiving treatment and has been compensated for some time and then decompensates, the reason for decompensation is often found in the blood chemistry profile. Particular attention should be placed on renal and liver function, electrolyte concentrations, serum protein levels, thyroid function, and detection of anemia. Renal function is probably the most critical when treating heart disease. Hypokalemia and renal failure will enhance the likelihood of digoxin toxicity and ventricular ectopia. Drug therapy (diuretics and vasodilators) can result in renal decompensation and failure.

The *differential diagnosis* of MR and TR is important. Usually, the diagnosis of MR and TR is straightforward and can be based on the physical examination and other diagnostic tests. However, other causes of cough, dyspnea, and pulmonary crackles in a mature dog need to be evaluated (see pp. 361 and 188). MR is often heard in dogs with cardiomyopathy but usually the intensity of the murmur is less; larger breed dogs tend to be affected, and an echocardiogram will demonstrate markedly decreased FS. The chest radiograph and other diagnostic tests are used to rule out other possible diagnoses before therapy for cardiac failure is initiated. Never is a heart murmur by itself a definitive finding for diagnosis of heart failure.

Medical Management

The *goal of therapy* in any animal with heart disease is to prolong and maintain quality of life. In dogs with MR and TR, the specific objectives are to reduce the severity of the regurgitant fraction; to alleviate pulmonary congestion pleural effusion, or both; to maintain cardiac output; to control significant cardiac arrhythmias; to control or eliminate aggravating conditions; and to preserve any remaining cardiovascular reserve mechanisms. These goals should be accomplished with as few unpleasant side effects as possible. The most ideal treatment method is the surgical replacement of the diseased valve prior to irreversible myocardial damage. Unfortunately in veterinary medicine, this is not practical at this time. Medical intervention is the only available option in attempting to reduce the severity of MR and TR. The effective utilization of the numerous drugs available is contingent on knowledge of pharmacology and pharmacokinetics. The inadequate and inappropriate use of cardiac drugs is a frequent cause of treatment failure.

Sodium restriction and administration of diuretics, positive inotropic drugs, and vasodilators all have demonstrated a capacity to lessen the severity of MR and TR in various circumstances. Specific drugs within each of these groups have certain beneficial effects as well as deleterious side effects, which must be considered before therapy is initi-

ated. There is no single effective therapy for patients in various stages of valvular heart disease.

INITIAL THERAPY

Dietary sodium restriction has been recommended in class I patients (classification system developed by the New York Heart Association, class I patients have murmurs but are asymptomatic); however, the author prefers to initiate sodium restriction when congestive heart failure develops (class II or III) because low-sodium diets frequently seem to be unpalatable. The owners are advised not to give any salty treats. As the first signs of heart failure appear (class II), diuretic therapy in conjunction with further sodium restriction is instituted. The resulting reduction in fluid volume usually relieves signs of pulmonary congestion or ascites. A reduction in the regurgitant fraction may result owing to a decrease in preload and afterload. The most widely used diuretic is furosemide (1 to 4 mg/kg up to t.i.d. PO), because it is effective and well tolerated. The lowest effective dose should be used. Another useful medication at this early stage can be aminophylline (6 to 9 mg/kg t.i.d. PO). It has one major action (bronchodilator) and two minor ones (weak inotropic and diuretic). As the disease progresses (to class III or IV), aminophylline is of less value (unless there is concurrent bronchial disease) and higher and more frequent doses of furosemide are necessary. Overzealous diuretic therapy can result in a decrease in preload to the extent that cardiac output can fall (see Fig. 1). Diuretics should be used cautiously in renal disease patients and in those with low cardiac outputs.

INOTROPIC DRUGS

The use of inotropic drugs (digitalis) in dogs with MR and TR is controversial in veterinary medicine. It has been argued that myocardial contractility is normal in most dogs with MR, and therefore digoxin is not indicated. Others question the extent of inotropic effectiveness and cite the prevalence of serious toxicities. There is experimental evidence that myocardial contractility declines in dogs with MR, but it is difficult to assess myocardial contractility in clinical cases. Some investigators have chosen to initiate digoxin concurrently with diuretics at the first signs of heart failure (class II) and prior to vasodilator therapy. Others use digitalis later in the course of disease (class III or IV) when diuretics and vasodilators are no longer able to control clinical signs, or when atrial arrhythmias supervene. This author prefers to utilize diuretics initially and then use digoxin (0.01 to 0.02 mg/kg divided b.i.d.) and vasodilators in conjunction with diuretics. The author has found that giving digitalis with care and with thorough follow-up allows safe utilization of the drug.

Most practitioners agree that digoxin should be used to treat dogs with severe heart failure, atrial fibrillation, and other recurrent supraventricular arrhythmias. The negative chronotropic effect of digoxin improves ventricular filling and thus promotes a greater stroke volume. The use of intravenous positive inotropic agents other than digoxin (e.g., dobutamine or amrinone) is reserved for dogs in severe heart failure (class IV) that are not responsive to maximally tolerated doses of digoxin, diuretics, and vasodilators. There are currently two potent catecholamines available to treat severe myocardial failure. Dopamine or its close relative dobutamine (2 to 10 μg/kg/min) has to be given continuously in an infusion for 24 to 48 hours. Quite often a potent intravenous vasodilator such as nitroprusside (1 to 10 μg/kg/min) has to be given in conjunction with these inotropic agents to prevent arterial constriction and to stabilize patients with intractable heart failure. When this final effort fails, the patient usually dies or is euthanatized.

VASODILATORS

Vasodilators (Table 1) have been utilized in veterinary medicine within the last several years with much success (see *Current Veterinary Therapy IX*, p. 329–333). The short-term benefits have been well documented in experimental cases as well as in naturally occurring MR. Questions that still need to be answered concern the long-term hemodynamic effects prevalence of adverse reactions, and the relative merits (arteriolar, venous, and mixed) for each vasodilating drug. Although the choice remains an individual one, hydralazine, captopril (or enalapril), or prazosin can be considered for

long-term treatment of advanced valvular heart disease.

Hydralazine (0.5 to 3 mg/kg b.i.d. PO) is a direct-acting arteriolar dilator that has been shown to be effective in the short-term management of chronic MR in dogs. To understand the action of this drug as well as the others, one must understand the anatomy and physiology of MR. Because the mitral regurgitation orifice and the root of the aorta are parallel, the ratio of forward blood flow to regurgitant flow depends on the ratio of aortic impedance to regurgitant impedance. An increase in systemic arteriolar resistance (vasoconstriction) results in diminution of forward flow and causes regurgitant flow to increase. This is exactly what happens in heart failure patients (i.e., the systemic vascular resistance goes up [increased afterload]). The administration of an arteriolar dilator decreases the volume of regurgitant flow independent of any change in the mitral regurgitation orifice by decreasing the diastolic blood pressure and the systemic vascular resistance. In conjunction with a decrease in systemic vascular resistance (decreased afterload), there is an increase in stroke volume and venous pressures often decline (see Fig. 1). However, the venous pressure and preload may not always decrease significantly with the use of a pure arteriolar dilator. The problems that have been encountered with the use of hydralazine include a variable dose requirement, development of tolerance with long-term use, and adverse side effects, including hypotension, reflex tachycardia, sodium retention, and gastrointestinal signs.

Nitroglycerin and *isosorbide dinitrate* are direct-acting venodilators (see Table 1). Both agents increase systemic venous capacitance (decrease preload) and effectively lower pulmonary venous pressure, thus reducing pulmonary congestion. The regurgitant volume may decrease as a result of decreased venous return, lower left ventricular filling pressures, and reduced size of the left ventricle

Table 1. *Site of Action and Hemodynamic Effects of Vasodilator Agents in Congestive Heart Failure*

Drug	Site		Hemodynamic Effects				
	Arterial	Venous	HR	AP	CO	LVFP	SVR
Parenteral							
Nitroprusside	+ + +	+ +	NC, ↑	NC, ↓	NC, ↑	↓	↓
Nitroglycerin	+	+ + +	NC, ↑, ↓	NC, ↓	NC, ↑, ↓	↓	↓
Phentolamine	+ + + +	0	↑	↓	↑	↓	↓
Nonparenteral							
Nitroglycerin ointment 2% (Nitrol, Nitro-Bid)	+	+ + +	NC, ↑, ↓	NC, ↓	NC, ↑, ↓	↓	NC, ↓
Hydralazine	+ + + +	0	NC, ↑	NC, ↓	↑	NC, ↓	↓
Prazosin	+ +	+ +	NC, ↑	NC, ↓	↑	↓	↓
Captopril	+ +	+ +	NC, ↑	NC, ↓	↑	↓	↓

HR, heart rate; AP, arterial pressure; CO, cardiac output; LVFP, left ventricular filling pressure; SVR, systemic vascular resistance; + to + + + +, degree of vasodilation: + = weak, + + + + = strong; NC, no change; ↑, increase; ↓, decrease.

and of the mitral regurgitation orifice. Effective cardiac output usually increases modestly but may decline if adequate ventricular filling pressures are not maintained. These drugs, in conjunction with diuretics, could actually decrease stroke volume. They are often combined with hydralazine to relieve persistent pulmonary edema. Their use in veterinary medicine has not been critically evaluated. In humans, they have sustained actions and few side effects. The author has not found these drugs to be consistently effective in dogs, although others have reported success with their use.

Nitroprusside is an extremely potent arterial and venous vasodilator that can only be given intravenously. Nitroprusside (1 to 10 μg/kg/min) is used in refractory cases of heart failure or with acute life-threatening MR due to ruptured chordae tendineae. Hypotension is by far the most serious side effect, but this can be reversed within 10 minutes after discontinuation of the drug.

Prazosin and captopril are both arteriolar and venous vasodilators in equal proportions. *Prazosin* (1 to 2 mg b.i.d. to t.i.d. PO) is an alpha-adrenergic blocking agent. Adverse reactions to prazosin in humans are minimal, and the dosages are more constant than for hydralazine. The one main criticism of this agent in humans concerns its effectiveness over a long theraputic period. Long-term studies of its usefulness in canine MR cases have not been performed. *Captopril* (0.5 to 2 mg/kg t.i.d., PO) is an angiotensin-converting enzyme inhibitor. It prevents the conversion of angiotensin I to angiotensin II. This causes an immediate reduction in systemic arteriolar resistance and a slight degree of venodilation. Because of the conversion block, aldosterone and angiotensin II levels usually decline and renal blood flow increases. This results in a marked natriuresis. In humans, captopril appears to offer sustained long-term hemodynamic improvement without severe side effects. Hypotension has been seen especially in hyponatremic patients. Renal complications have been reported in humans, and the author has noted this adverse effect in dogs. The blood urea nitrogen, serum creatinine levels, or both should be monitored in patients receiving captopril. Anorexia is another adverse effect that may persist even at lower dosages. The author prefers the use of captopril over the above named vasodilators because of the clinical results.

OTHER THERAPY

Additional therapeutic measures should be considered in selected individuals. Exercise should be curtailed as signs of heart failure progress. In an acute heart failure crisis, oxygen and bronchodilator therapy are beneficial. Although used in some hospitals, morphine is not used by the author to reduce anxiety in an acute episode of fulminating heart failure because it can depress the patient's respiration. Cough suppressants are often needed in the chronically medicated MR patient owing to carinal and caudal airway compression. Hycodan (2.5 to 5 mg/dose) is the author's choice for a cough suppressant. The lowest possible dosage should be used to control the cough.

When congestive heart failure develops in a MR patient as a result of ruptured chordae tendineae, therapeutic measures are often futile. The prognosis is grave, and death usually results. Left atrial tears are a consequence of endocardial splitting as explained previously. A left atrial tear results in a hemopericardium, which can cause cardiac tamponade and sudden death. The triad of cardiac tamponade findings is jugular distention, muffled heart sounds, and a decreased arterial pulse. Immediate high-volume intravenous fluid therapy is essential when cardiogenic shock is present. Pericardiocentesis is also recommended to reduce the intracardiac diastolic pressures, which will then allow cardiac filling. A sequela to long-term TR is a nonresponsive ascites. Diuretics and vasodilators such as captopril (Capoten, Squibb) given at maximum dosages may not be able to relieve the ascitic fluid. Periodic abdominocentesis may be the only means to reduce the ascitic fluid. Injectable furosemide may be more effective than oral diuretics if there is intestinal congestion with drug malabsorption. Sustained cardiac arrhythmias may develop, and management of these problems is described on pages 271–278 and 278–286.

BACTERIAL ENDOCARDITIS

Bacterial endocarditis (BE) can be a life-threatening disorder and can cause a variety of serious cardiac and systemic complications. Bacterial infections of the heart valves or mural endocardium can be disguised by the manifestation of disease in other organ systems. Because of the difficulty of recognizing clinical cases, the prevalence of endocarditis in the dog is unknown. The incidence of endocarditis in necropsied dogs has been reported to be as low as 0.06 per cent or as high as 6.6 per cent. Medium to large breed dogs over 4 years of age are the most frequently affected. The German shepherd breed is at risk of acquiring BE. No relationship between BE and myxomatous degeneration of the heart valves has been found in the dog. Endocarditis has been reported in association with a variety of congenital defects, especially subaortic stenosis.

Pathology and Pathogenesis

The lesion of BE in the dog is usually located on the aortic, the mitral, or both valves. Right-sided valvular involvement is rare. The pathologic findings vary with the duration and the virulence of the infecting organism. There are two different types of infection (acute ulcerative and chronic or subacute). In acute ulcerative cases, destruction of valvular tissue proceeds rapidly. Necrosis of the valve stroma occurs. Above this lesion, large numbers of bacteria and neutrophils are observed in a platelet-fibrin thrombus. In subacute infections, the underlying valve cusp reveals some necrosis but also shows evidence of attempted repair. Valve dysfunction occurs most commonly owing to necrosis, perforation, or prolapse. Chordae tendineae, if involved in the infective process, can rupture. Left-sided heart failure usually occurs when either the aortic or mitral valvular leaflets are involved. Stenosis of the affected valves can occur, but it is less common.

Systemic metastatic infections are common owing to the central location of the infection and the friable structure of the vegetation. Abscess formation can occur either at the site within the heart or systemically through the metastatic spread of the infective emboli. The kidney and spleen are the most common sites of embolization at necropsy. Other organs, including the heart, can be affected as well. Emboli can vary in size and can be sterile or infective. The consequences of arterial embolization depend on the organ affected and the degree of obstruction. Infections in areas away from the heart can be primary or secondary (caused by infective emboli). Thus the significance of urinary tract infections, discospondylitis, and septic arthritis is uncertain because its origin is unknown (i.e., cause or effect?).

Streptococcus, Staphylococcus, and *Corynebacterium* species and *Pseudomonas aeroginosa, Escherichia coli, Erysipelothrix rhusiopathiae,* and *Aerobacter aerogenes* are the most commonly reported isolates in dogs with BE. *Streptococcus* has historically been the primary agent in reported cases. However, recent studies suggest that more variable causative agents are involved. As in human patients, it appears that, with the changing spectrum of antibiotics, new bacterial agents will become predominant as causes of BE.

Transient or persistent bacteremia is an absolute requirement for the establishment of BE. Bacteremia can result from an active infection anywhere on or in the body. Certain bacteria (*Streptococcus* and *Pseudomonas* species) are more able to adhere to the surface of the valve leaflets than are other bacteria. Pre-existing acquired cardiac lesions are not thought to be necessary for the establishment of these infections. The course of acute ulcerative BE is often short, and clinical signs of sepsis may be severe. In subacute BE, the resulting infection is often less fulminating. The bacteria involved are usually part of the indigenous flora and may gain access to the circulation as a result of trauma,

surgery, and urogenital gastrointestinal, or dental manipulation. A previously damaged valve or mural lesion can facilitate infection. In both forms of endocarditis there may be neither physical or historical evidence of a previous infection nor pre-existing cardiac abnormality.

Clinical Signs

Bacterial endocarditis can manifest clinically in many different ways and involve many different organ systems. The early signs often suggest systemic infection rather than cardiovascular disease. Anorexia, fever, shaking, weight loss, weakness, lethargy, and shifting leg lameness are among the most frequent owner complaints. Vomiting, diarrhea, seizures, hemi- or paraparesis, visual disturbances, and hematuria have also been reported. In some patients there is a history of recent surgery, dental manipulation, or the use of immunosuppressive drugs. A persistent recurrent fever is common. Cardiac signs may be silent and may occur singly or, more commonly, together with central nervous system (including the eyes), renal, orthopedic, and peripheral disorders. Pulmonary edema, dyspnea, tachypnea, and other signs of heart failure are usually present when the aortic valve is involved, rather than with isolated mitral valve disease.

Diagnosis

A thorough *physical examination* is extremely important in bacterial endocarditis cases. The findings of a heart murmur, evidence of embolization to other organ sites, and a fever are highly suggestive of the diagnosis of BE. BE is rarely diagnosed this easily, however. A common finding in most dogs with BE is a persistent or recurrent fever. Fever also is more commonly found in dogs when the mitral valve is affected rather than the aortic valve. Significant systolic murmurs are frequently auscultated in dogs with endocarditis of either the mitral or the aortic valve. Physiologic murmurs, caused by fever, are usually shorter in duration and of a lower intensity of sound than significant pathologic murmurs and therefore should not be misinterpreted. The murmur of MR is common in older, smaller breed dogs and should not be over-interpreted as a murmur due to endocarditis. The development of a diastolic murmur in conjunction with a bounding arterial pulse strongly suggests BE involvement of the aortic valve. A variety of heart arrhythmias due to heart failure, myocarditis, myocardial infarction (embolization), and destruction of the conduction system by a mural lesion may be auscultated. Gallop sounds can commonly be heard in dogs with signs of heart failure.

As alluded to above, signs of secondary organ embolization need to be looked for aggressively. Retinal emboli, hemorrhages, and hyphema are some of the ocular manifestations of BE. Epistaxis and petechiation of the skin and mucous membranes are noted infrequently. Pain, pallor, and the lack of an arterial pulse are indicative of arterial obstruction. Joint pain and stiffness may be due to immune complex disease or to septic arthritis. Thoracolumbar pain and abdominal pain may be present when the kidneys or other abdominal organs are involved. A variety of neurologic deficits may also be seen. BE can mimic immunologic disease and will be exacerbated by corticosteroid therapy.

The *ECG* and *chest radiographs* may be normal in dogs with BE. In 50 to 75 per cent of BE cases there will be arrhythmias, conduction disturbances, or both. Left-sided cardiac enlargement patterns frequently occur and are associated with advancing cardiac disease. Evidence of BE on chest radiographs is rare. There may be evidence of cardiac enlargement and signs of impending heart failure on survey radiographs. Occasionally, presence of a pulmonary infarction or bone infection may give the investigator a clue to the diagnosis of BE. Angiocardiography, Doppler echocardiography, and intracardiac pressure studies can assess the severity of valvular involvement in some cases.

Laboratory analysis will reveal a mild normocytic normochromic anemia in 60 per cent of cases. A left shift in the white blood cell count does not occur on a regular basis. Neutrophilia, monocytosis, or both occur 80 per cent of the time. When the kidneys are involved, the blood urea nitrogen is commonly abnormal. In fact, this may be the only initial abnormality in a complete workup. Often the elevation in the blood urea nitrogen reflects embolization and infarction of the kidneys. The urinalysis may be normal or reveal pyuria, hematuria, or proteinuria due to pyelonephritis, renal infarction, or glomerulonephritis. Urine cultures are often negative and should never be substituted for a series of blood cultures. Joint fluid analysis may reveal a septic or nonseptic inflammatory response. Results of autoimmune tests (Coombs', antinuclear antibody, and rheumatoid factor) may be positive in dogs with BE. When performed correctly blood cultures will be 75 per cent accurate. One of the most common reasons for a negative culture in positive BE is recent antibiotic therapy. Ideally, three to four samples of blood should be collected longer than 1 hour apart and within 24 hours. Aerobic and anaerobic cultures should always be done.

Echocardiography is not a substitute for properly performed blood cultures but often allows a diagnosis in animals in which the blood cultures have been negative. Lesions as small as 2 mm may be visualized via echocardiography but may be con-fused with those caused by degenerative valvular disease. Cardiac dilation, flail leaflets, and ruptured chordae tendineae may also be visualized. Aortic valve vegetations are usually readily imaged and easily identified. On the other hand, mitral valvular lesions may be difficult to differentiate from myxomatous changes. Two-dimensional echocardiography is more sensitive in the detection of involvement of vegetative lesions and flail leaflets than M-mode echocardiography. Determination of systolic-diastolic dimensions and other indices of left ventricular function by M-mode and Doppler echocardiography are valuable in the initial and progressive follow-up studies during therapy. By using echocardiography and serial studies, a prognostic tool is developed.

Medical Management

Management and *prevention* of BE initially requires the proper diagnosis. A definitive diagnosis requires a positive blood culture and evidence of cardiac involvement (progressive new murmur or echocardiographic findings). After the diagnosis has been made, management can attempt to eradicate the infection. Therapy must be aggressive, intense, and closely monitored. An organism must be identified via blood cultures and antimicrobial sensitivity must be determined for successful results. The parenteral administration of bactericidal doses of drugs for up to 4 to 6 weeks is recommended in humans. In the dog it is unrealistic to consider intravenous therapy for this period of time. The administration of IV antibiotics for 7 to 14 days is not unrealistic and is followed by appropriate oral antibiotics for another 4 weeks. Antibiotics (IV and PO) should be given every 4 to 6 hours. In culture-negative endocarditis cases or when results are pending in acute BE, an aminoglycoside and a penicillin-type antibiotic may be used. Frequent daily examinations should be performed to determine changes in heart sounds, cardiac rhythm, arterial pulse pressure, and any systemic complications. If recurrent fevers are persistent during antibiotic therapy, blood cultures using an antibiotic removal system should be attempted to determine the efficacy of the antibiotic in use. Blood cultures should be attempted after the completion of therapy to ensure the organism has been successfully eliminated.

One should determine the probable portal of entry of the infection. All extracardiac infections should be eliminated even if surgery is needed for total ablation. Concurrent conditions that may lead to BE in dogs include abscesses, periodontal disease, prostatitis, osteomyelitis, urinary tract infections, and pneumonia. Common cardiac disturbances that may have to be treated are congestive heart failure and arrhythmias. Congestive heart failure is the most common cause of death in dogs with BE, especially if the aortic valve is involved. Because valve replacement is not a choice in veterinary medicine, the administration of digitalis, diuretics, and vasodilators is indicated when signs of heart failure are present. Antiarrhythmic therapy is given when serious tachyarrhythmias occur. A pacemaker may be indicated if third-degree heart block results from the infection.

The *prognosis* of BE depends on the virulence of the bacterial organism, the hemodynamic consequence to valvular damage, the presence of heart failure, and the degree of involvement of extracardiac organs such as the kidneys. Prevention of BE in veterinary medicine is not well documented. Potentially when there is dental or urogenital ma-

nipulation bacteremia can occur. When there is pre-existing heart disease and dental manipulation is going to occur, use of prophylactic antibiotics should be considered.

References and Supplemental Reading

Buchanan, J. W.: Valvular disease (endocardiosis in dogs). Adv. Vet. Sci. Comp. Med. 21:75, 1979.

Detweiler, D. K., Lunginbuhl, H., Buchanan, J. W., et al.: The natural history of acquired cardiac disability in the dog. Ann. N.Y. Acad. Sci. 147:318, 1965.

Keene, B. W., and Bonagura, J. D.: Valvular heart disease. *In* Kirk R. W. (ed.): *Current Veterinary Therapy VIII.* Philadelphia: W. B. Saunders, 1983, pp. 311–320.

Sisson, D.: Acquired valvular heart disease in dogs and cats. *In* Bonagura, J. D. (ed.): *Cardiology. Contemporary Issues in Small Animal Practice.* Vol. 7. New York: Churchill Livingstone, 1987, pp. 59–116.

Whitney, J. C.: Observations on the effect of age on the severity of heart valve lesions in the dog. J. Small Anim. Pract. 15:511, 1974.

CANINE CARDIOMYOPATHY

BRUCE W. KEENE, D.V.M.
Madison, Wisconsin

The term cardiomyopathy refers to diseases of the heart muscle that occur in the absence of significant malformation or disease of the heart valves or vasculature. Cardiomyopathies have been categorized into three major groups by the World Health Organization as dilated, hypertrophic, or restrictive based on the predominant structural and functional abnormalities observed. Both dilated and hypertrophic cardiomyopathies have been reported in dogs, with the dilated form being far more common. In addition to this classification, these diseases may also be divided into primary (idiopathic), accounting for the majority of cases in which no specific cause can be identified, and secondary cardiomyopathies known to be caused by some infectious, inflammatory, toxic, or metabolic insult to the myocardium. The hallmark of dilated cardiomyopathy (DCM) is dilation of the ventricles, with some increase in myocardial mass (hypertrophy) and loss of contractile function. Hypertrophic cardiomyopathy (HCM) is characterized by tremendously increased myocardial mass, accompanied by either normal or more often decreased ventricular cavity size and abnormal diastolic function. Restrictive cardiomyopathy (RCM) has not been specifically reported in dogs but refers to diseases that restrict the normal diastolic filling of the ventricles by reason of myocardial or endocardial disease that

effectively stiffens the ventricle without causing massive myocardial hypertrophy.

This classification system supplies convenient diagnostic labels and provides a therapeutically useful pathophysiologic grouping of what are probably several etiologically distinct diseases within each category. With a few exceptions (for example, the recent discovery of taurine deficiency as a major cause of dilated cardiomyopathy in cats), the causes of cardiomyopathy remain unknown. Treatment of these diseases has therefore generally been designed to adjust the mechanical function of the heart, peripheral circulation, or both to compensate as long as possible for the malfunctioning heart muscle. Although this kind of therapeutic intervention may ameliorate the clinical signs of heart failure for variable periods of time, it is not usually effective in altering the ongoing pathologic muscle changes that cause these diseases. As more is learned about the heart muscle and the cellular events surrounding the onset and progression of cardiomyopathy, treatment of this group of diseases may include specific measures designed to reverse or at least halt the progression of muscle damage and the subsequent geometric and functional changes that eventually lead to heart failure and death. This article will provide an update on the diagnosis and treatment of the more commonly recognized forms of canine cardiomyopathy.

DILATED CARDIOMYOPATHY

Dilated cardiomyopathy is a syndrome characterized by progressive ventricular dilation and loss of myocardial contractile function in the absence of valvular or vascular heart disease. DCM occurs in a wide variety of mammalian and avian species, the first report in dogs occurring in 1970. Although there are no published studies examining the incidence of DCM in dogs, the incidence in the author's practice appears to be increasing. This increase may be the result of genetic selection and line breeding in specific geographic areas and breeds or may be artifactual, possibly resulting from increased disease awareness and recognition by veterinarians, breeders, and dog owners. Regardless of the cause, canine DCM is clearly an important clinical problem, accounting for a substantial percentage of canine morbidity and mortality from cardiac causes.

Preliminary studies in the author's laboratory have produced biochemical evidence that canine DCM is probably not a single disease, but rather the result of a variety of different pathologic processes or defects in myocardial metabolism. The situation may in fact have some parallels to that found with "end-stage" kidney or liver disease, in which a variety of insults may lead to chronic, end-stage organ failure. Evidence for this hypothesis includes the results of a pilot study in which three of four dogs with severe heart failure caused by DCM were shown to have depressed myocardial adenosine triphosphate (ATP) concentrations compared with normal dogs, whereas one dog with DCM (a cocker spaniel) did not (Keene et al., 1986). Myocardial L-carnitine deficiency was also demonstrated in association with DCM in some dogs (35 per cent of a series of 20 consecutive cases) but not others, and there is evidence to suggest that different metabolic causes of DCM exist even among dogs known to be carnitine deficient (Keene et al., 1988b). Some dogs with dilated cardiomyopathy appear to have a generalized form of metabolic muscle disease (muscular dystrophy), whereas others appear to have only myocardial involvement.

Although DCM has been recognized in many breeds, it is infrequently seen in dogs weighing less than 15 kg. Distinct clinical forms and features of DCM have been recognized and described in some breeds, including Doberman pinschers, boxers, English cocker spaniels, and giant breed dogs. Despite the recognized differences in clinical presentation, prognosis, and possibly even biochemical characteristics of the myocardium and skeletal muscle among the breeds affected, DCM occurs most often in relatively young to middle-aged male dogs. Detailed descriptions of the typical clinical and pathologic findings of DCM in specific breeds are available (Harpster, 1983; Calvert et al., 1982; Staaden, 1981). The following sections provide a brief review of the clinical characteristics of DCM in boxers and Doberman pinschers, breeds in which the clinical characteristics are most distinctive and the disease takes its highest toll.

BOXER CARDIOMYOPATHY

As in other forms of DCM, boxer cardiomyopathy occurs more frequently in male dogs. The hallmark of this form of DCM is the presence of ventricular arrhythmias, often having a left bundle branch block pattern electrocardiographically. Although ventricular arrhythmias in boxer cardiomyopathy may occur in any pattern, paroxysmal or sustained ventricular tachycardia is a common finding. Harpster's (1983) report of the disease, categorized affected dogs as follows:

1. Asymptomatic animals without evidence of myocardial failure whose ventricular arrhythmia is noticed on auscultation. These animals have a guarded prognosis but often survive 2 years or longer with antiarrhythmic therapy.

2. Animals that have a history of episodic weakness or syncope related to episodes of sustained ventricular tachycardia but without evidence of heart failure. These animals have a more guarded prognosis but may survive for a year or more if effective therapy can be found.

3. Animals in heart failure with or without atrial fibrillation at the time of presentation. These animals also frequently have ventricular arrhythmias and have a poor prognosis, with most dying within 3 months of presentation.

It is important to remember that disease in animals in either of the first two categories may progress to heart failure at any time, and that dogs in all three categories are predisposed to sudden death. The factors influencing the rate of progression of the disease remain unknown. Although treatment is strongly recommended, the efficacy of antiarrhythmic therapy in prolonging the life of these animals is also unknown at this time.

There appear to be significant geographic (or possibly familial) differences in the distribution and clinical characteristics of boxer cardiomyopathy. In the author's practice in the upper Midwest, the incidence of boxers in heart failure with atrial fibrillation is substantially higher than in Harpster's report. Although not definitively proven at this time, biochemical investigations performed on endomyocardial biopsy specimens from several boxers in heart failure caused by DCM indicate that myocardial carnitine deficiency is a frequent finding in these animals. Preliminary (uncontrolled) therapeutic trials suggest that L-carnitine supplementation (2 gm b.i.d.) provides a useful adjunct to and may even replace conventional therapy in some of these dogs (Keene et al., 1988c).

DOBERMAN CARDIOMYOPATHY

Several clinical characteristics appear to distinguish DCM in Doberman pinschers from that in other large breed dogs. As in other breeds, male are much more commonly affected than females. In general, however, Dobermans have ventricular arrhythmias more frequently, and they have an even poorer prognosis than other dogs with severe DCM. They often exhibit extremely poor systolic myocardial function as evidenced by severely depressed echocardiographic indices of contractility (prolonged pre-ejection periods and low left ventricular fractional shortening). These dogs frequently have an acute onset of dyspnea, orthopnea, or a soft cough sometimes productive of blood-tinged froth or sputum.

Despite poor myocardial contractility and echocardiographically demonstrable left ventricular dilation, the heart shadow may not appear to be grossly enlarged radiographically, although generalized alveolar pulmonary edema is common. In the author's clinical experience, the truly life-threatening severity of the pulmonary edema in these patients is often belied by the patient's seemingly moderate signs of respiratory distress, making high-quality radiographs essential in the workup of Doberman DCM. If these animals are stressed (even with minor exertion), however, clinical signs can worsen dramatically. Despite their seemingly good condition at the time of presentation and the clinician's and owner's best efforts, affected animals frequently deteriorate rapidly. Many Dobermans with DCM suffer anorexia and progressive weight loss, and some seem to balance on an almost impossibly fine line between clinical dehydration, pre-renal azotemia, and other signs of low cardiac output (depressed mixed venous oxygen tension, lethargy, or weakness) and signs of congestive heart failure (pulmonary edema, pleural effusion, or ascites). These problems (especially persistent anorexia and weight loss) represent the most frustrating aspects of the long-term medical management of Doberman DCM for both owners and veterinarians. Sudden death, presumably caused by sustained ventricular arrhythmias that degenerate into ventricular fibrillation, is observed all too frequently in these patients. This fatal complication can arise at any time, often when the animal appears to be doing well at home. The efficacy of antiarrhythmic drugs in preventing sudden death is an active area of investigation, although no hard data are currently available to guide drug selection.

Diagnosis

In establishing a clinical data base for any animal suspected of having heart disease, a thorough history and physical examination are always indicated. In addition, thoracic radiography, electrocardiography, and clinical laboratory tests are necessary to obtain an accurate and specific diagnosis in most cases. This data base is then expanded as needed to include specialized cardiovascular examinations such as echocardiography and cardiac catheterization, angiography, and endomyocardial biopsy. The following sections will provide a brief summary of the pertinent findings and usefulness of these tests in the diagnosis of canine DCM.

HISTORY AND SIGNALMENT

Because of strong breed and gender predispositions, the signalment in combination with a history suggesting the presence of heart disease is a valuable tool in the diagnosis of canine DCM. Although some clinical signs and findings are more typical of some breeds than others, the onset of DCM is generally characterized by manifestations of heart failure. These signs usually include some combination of weakness, weight loss, anorexia, lethargy, exercise intolerance, dyspnea, a soft cough, syncope, or ascites. Not all of these signs are likely to be present in any individual, and the alert clinician will occasionally find auscultatory evidence of underlying DCM (atrial fibrillation, ventricular premature contractions [VPCs], or a gallop sound) in an otherwise asymptomatic patient. The progression of clinical signs and weight loss may be astonishingly rapid, especially in Doberman pinschers and boxers, when signs of heart failure are present.

PHYSICAL EXAMINATION

Many of the physical examination findings in DCM depend largely on the clinical stage of heart failure at presentation. Findings such as respiratory distress; auscultation of inspiratory crackles; dullness to thoracic percussion, suggesting pleural effusion; and pale, cold mucous membranes, suggesting peripheral vasoconstriction, are important in assessing the severity of congestive heart failure. The physical diagnosis of DCM, however, is usually based on the signalment and cardiac auscultatory findings. In predisposed breeds, physical examination findings that suggest the presence of DCM include the rapid, irregular, or "chaotic" heart sounds and frequent peripheral arterial pulse deficits of atrial fibrillation; the presence of extrasystoles (sometimes described as "dropped beats"), with corresponding arterial pulse deficits often caused by ventricular premature contractions; or the presence of a gallop sound. Gallop sounds are the auscultatory manifestations of excessive ventricular stiffness and are usually associated with frank or impending heart failure in the dog. Gallop sounds are transient sounds that occur during diastole and are generally heard best over the left apex. The third heart sound (S_3) occurs early in diastole, when a stiff, relatively noncompliant ventricle causes the sudden deceleration of blood during the period of rapid ventricular filling. Because of its timing, S_3 can occur during sinus rhythm or atrial fibrillation. The fourth heart sound (S_4) is a late diastolic sound produced after the contraction of the atria into an excessively stiff ventricle. Sometimes, a summation gallop (S_3 and S_4 together) is produced if both sounds are present during sinus tachycardia. Although most dogs with DCM will have at least one of these auscultatory findings, in any given patient some, all, or occasionally none may be present.

Of the typical physical findings, gallop sounds are the most elusive and difficult to recognize. Because gallop sounds are often soft, transient (short duration), low-frequency heart sounds, it is important that auscultation be performed in a quiet environment using the bell of the stethoscope as well as the diaphragm. When lightly applied to the chest wall, the stethoscope's bell maximizes the transmission of low-frequency sounds and thus optimizes the clinician's ability to recognize gallops. Heart murmurs are usually not prominent features of DCM, although soft murmurs of mitral or tricuspid regurgitation may be present when papillary muscle dysfunction or alterations in ventricular geometry are severe enough to produce (usually mild) atrioventricular (AV) valve regurgitation. Weight loss can be dramatic, and many owners relate a history of rapid muscle wasting just prior to presentation. It is unclear at the present time whether the loss of muscle mass typical of severe DCM is the result of "cardiac cachexia" or of specific metabolic defects affecting skeletal as well as cardiac muscle.

THORACIC RADIOGRAPHY

The radiographic hallmark of DCM is generalized cardiomegaly, although the radiographic findings are highly dependent on the severity of the disease as well as the chest conformation and hydration of the patient. Cardiomegaly may be so severe in some patients as to suggest the presence of pericardial effusion. In deep-chested breeds (especially Doberman pinschers), however, minimal or even undetectable cardiomegaly or primarily left atrial enlargement may be evident on plain radiographic studies. Likewise, patients that have undergone extensive diuresis and volume contraction may show minimal cardiomegaly. Often, the consequences of myocardial failure (i.e., pulmonary edema, pleural effusion, or both) partially obscure the heart shadow, making radiographic diagnosis of cardiac changes more difficult. Pulmonary edema is char-

acterized by increased pulmonary interstitial and alveolar densities, especially in the hilar or dorsocaudal lung fields, although they may be generalized in severe cases. Enlargement of the pulmonary vein (as compared with the pulmonary artery to the same lung lobe) is an important adjunct in the diagnosis of cardiogenic pulmonary edema and is usually evident in dogs with edema as a result of DCM. Pleural effusion, ascites, or both may be seen in dogs with right-sided heart failure due to DCM, and these patients are expected to demonstrate distention of the caudal vena cava, hepatomegaly, or jugular venous distention or abnormal jugular vein pulsations—signs of elevated right-heart filling pressures.

ELECTROCARDIOGRAPHY

Electrocardiography (ECG) is a useful adjunct in the diagnosis of canine DCM. It often confirms the presence of atrial fibrillation or ventricular ectopia, which might be suspected on auscultation. Even in the presence of sinus rhythm, the ECG may indicate the presence of left ventricular enlargement ($R_{II} > 3.0$ mV) or myocardial disease (QRS complexes > 0.06 sec in duration with a slurred or "sloppy" R-wave descent). Dogs in sinus rhythm may also display ECG evidence of left atrial enlargement ($P_{II} > 0.05$ sec in duration, often "notched"). In addition to its central role in diagnosis, the ECG is also used extensively in the long-term management of DCM to monitor the progress of antiarrhythmic therapy or to facilitate the rapid diagnosis of new arrhythmias that may arise.

CLINICAL LABORATORY TESTS

No specific clinical laboratory tests exist for the diagnosis of DCM, although it is important to screen DCM patients for common systemic sequelae of cardiac disease. Azotemia caused by decreased renal perfusion, mild elevations in serum liver enzyme levels resulting from chronic hepatic congestion, and mild hypoproteinemia and anemia are common findings and may influence therapeutic decisions or require dosage adjustments of some cardiac drugs. Routine clinical laboratory tests (i.e., complete blood count automated biochemical profile, and urinalysis) are also useful in screening for intercurrent diseases that may affect the management or prognosis of DCM. For example, hypercholesterolemia may be an indication of hypothyroidism, the correction of which may significantly improve the symptoms of DCM in some dogs.

ECHOCARDIOGRAPHY

Echocardiography has become the "gold standard" for the diagnosis of DCM in veterinary medicine. In the hands of a well-trained, experienced operator, two-dimensional or M-mode echocardiography supplies accurate, noninvasive measurements of cardiac dimensions and function. Echocardiography allows the reliable differentiation of cardiomegaly resulting from pericardial effusion from that caused by DCM. Echocardiography is especially useful in determining the cause of heart failure in breeds predisposed to both chronic valvular heart disease and DCM (e.g., Afghan hound, English and other cocker spaniels). In addition to its proven initial diagnostic utility, Doppler echocardiography may provide a reasonably effective means of quantitating the response to drug therapy in intensive care settings and of monitoring the long-term success or failure of treatment.

ENDOMYOCARDIAL BIOPSY

While still considered an investigational technique, endomyocardial biopsy can be performed safely and effectively in animals with DCM (Keene et al., 1988a). This technique provides a reliable means of tissue acquisition for metabolic, biochemical, histologic, or ultrastructural investigation of heart muscle. The clinical utility of endomyocardial biopsy is unclear at the present time. In a pilot study of 20 consecutive dogs with a clinical and echocardiographic diagnosis of DCM, results of endomyocardial biopsy directly influenced the therapy of nine of these patients. Seven of the latter dogs were shown to have myocardial carnitine deficiency and subsequently underwent L-carnitine supplementation. Biopsy of the other two dogs identified hemangiosarcoma infiltrating the ventricle in one and demonstrated changes compatible with doxorubicin toxicity in the other. Further studies are needed to determine whether endomyocardial biopsy deserves a role in the routine evaluation of dogs with DCM.

Therapy of Primary Dilated Cardiomyopathy

HEMODYNAMIC ASSESSMENT AND PATIENT MONITORING

As previously discussed, unless a specific etiologic or metabolic association with DCM can be established, therapy is generally directed at alleviating the patient's clinical signs of heart failure. Accurate initial assessment of the patient's hemodynamic status is essential in choosing appropriate therapy in DCM. A wide and ever-increasing variety of drugs are available to regulate the heart rate and rhythm, increase contractility (the intrinsic ability of the myocardium to contract), and regulate the blood volume as well as the peripheral venous and arterial tone to influence both preload (the amount of "stretch" on the muscle fibers just prior to contraction) and afterload (the force acting on the myocardium that resists ejection after the onset of shortening). Repeated clinical assessment and some form of hemodynamic monitoring are necessary for the clinician to make informed decisions regarding heart failure therapy in canine DCM. The initial assessment of the patient's hemodynamic status should include some determination of the heart rate and rhythm as well as a measurement of cardiac preload. If possible, a quantitative or semiquantitative indicator of afterload, contractility, and cardiac output should also be examined before deciding on a therapeutic strategy. However, when the clinical signs of heart failure are severe, the pretherapy assessment must be abbreviated.

In animals with acute, fulminating cardiogenic pulmonary edema, administration of intravenous or intramuscular furosemide (2 mg/kg), combined with subcutaneous morphine (starting dose 0.1 to 0.2 mg/kg), an oxygen-enriched (40 per cent O_2) atmosphere, and a 5-mg transdermal nitroglycerin patch (available from several manufacturers) may be life-saving until the animal is stable enough to withstand the stress of more thorough examination.

The heart rate and rhythm are easily and reliably monitored electrocardiographically. Indicators of venous pressure and preload may be direct (e.g., pulmonary capillary wedge pressure for left ventricular preload, central venous pressure for right) or indirect (e.g., radiographic evidence of pulmonary venous distention and pulmonary edema; crackles on thoracic auscultation for the left ventricle; and jugular venous distention, pleural or peritoneal effusion and distention of the caudal vena cava and liver, or both for the right). Afterload is difficult to measure and is often roughly estimated by measuring only one of its determinants, the arterial blood pressure. Arterial blood pressure can be determined either by direct arterial catheterization or by noninvasive Doppler or oscillometric methods. Because afterload depends on the ventricular diameter and wall thickness as well as the arterial blood pressure (larger diameters and thinner ventricular walls increase the wall tension, a more accurate reflection of afterload), it is possible that the blood pressure may be normal or even decreased when ventricular afterload is elevated. Contractility is also difficult to quantitate, with echocardiographic indices being the most commonly used measure of contractility in clinical veterinary practice. Of the various echocardiographic indices available, the pre-ejection period and left ventricular fractional shortening (FS) are probably the most frequently reported but aortic blood acceleration, measured by Doppler echocardiography, may be most sensitive (Table 1).

Cardiac output (the net effect of alterations in heart rate and rhythm, preload, afterload, and con-

Table 1. *Normal Values for Commonly Used Quantitative Indices of Preload, Afterload, and Contractility in the Dog, and Directional Changes Expected with Untreated DCM*

Cardiac Variable	Measurement	Normal Value	DCM Value
RV preload	CVP	0–6 mm Hg	•/+
LV preload	PCWP	5–15 mm Hg	•/+
LV afterload/(tension)	MAP	80–100 mm Hg	•/−/+
LV contractility	PEP	45–55 msec	/+
	FS	28–50%	−
Cardiac output	CI	4–5 L/min/m²	•/−
	pV$_{O_2}$	>30 mm Hg	•/−

RV, right ventricle; LV, left ventricle; CVP, central venous pressure; PCWP, pulmonary capillary wedge pressure; MAP, mean arterial pressure; PEP, pre-ejection period; FS, fractional shortening; CI, cardiac index; PV$_{O_2}$, free-flowing jugular venous oxygen tension, • indicates that normal values can be expected with DCM, + indicates values above the normal range are expected, and − indicates that values below the normal range are expected.

tractility) is also a useful measurement in the management of heart failure caused by DCM. Cardiac output can be determined directly via a thermistor-tipped thermodilution catheter placed in the pulmonary artery. Unfortunately, the required equipment is expensive and the placement and maintenance of these catheters requires a substantial time commitment and highly skilled nursing care. Because of these factors, measurement of cardiac output is generally too expensive to be practical in most veterinary settings. Directional changes in cardiac output may be relatively easily monitored by measuring the free-flowing jugular venous oxygen tension (see *Current Veterinary Therapy VIII*, pp. 283–284). Increases in cardiac output are theoretically accompanied by commensurate increases in venous oxygen tension. Clinically, the patient's general attitude, mucous membrane color and refill time, and renal function status provide useful indicators of cardiac output. Normal values for the hemodynamic indices useful in the management of DCM are summarized in Table 1.

PHARMACOTHERAPY OF HEART FAILURE IN DCM

The medical therapy of heart failure in DCM is designed to pharmacologically manipulate the heart rate and rhythm, preload, afterload, and contractility to support the failing myocardium. The goal of therapy should be to provide adequate cardiac output for a relatively quiet life style, while minimizing myocardial oxygen demand (reducing the tendency toward arrhythmia, sudden death, and hypertrophy) and abnormal fluid accumulations. Client education and communication is important in all phases of treatment. Unrealistic expectations of a rapid recovery and return to former levels of athletic performance and vigor are a common but usually avoidable cause of client dissatisfaction. The benefits of cage rest, especially in the initial treatment of canine DCM, cannot be overemphasized.

Because reduced cardiac contractility is the pathophysiologic hallmark of canine DCM, and most dogs with DCM are in atrial fibrillation with a rapid ventricular response (> 160/min), digitalization remains the backbone of therapy. Although both digoxin and digitoxin are available, digoxin's more convenient formulation for the size of most dogs with DCM make it the most frequently prescribed digitalis glycoside in these patients. If heart failure is not immediately life threatening, and the ventricular response to atrial fibrillation is less than 220 to 230 beats per minute, slow oral digitalization is begun with maintenance doses of digoxin (0.01 to 0.015 mg/kg divided b.i.d., not to exceed 0.5 mg/dog/day unless serum digoxin levels are shown to be inadequate). Doberman pinschers with DCM appear to be especially prone to digitalis intoxication, and digitalization is often accomplished with 0.375 mg of digoxin divided into two doses daily. Near–steady state plasma concentrations of digoxin are reached approximately 3 to 5 days after the initiation of therapy. Serum creatinine levels, urea nitrogen concentrations, or both should be measured at the outset of therapy. Because digoxin is excreted primarily by the kidney in the dog, even marginally reduced renal function is often accompanied by significant prolongations of the half-life of the drug. If ventricular premature complexes complicate heart failure in DCM, digoxin must be administered with extra caution because of its propensity to exacerbate ventricular arrhythmias. In these cases, frequent or continuous ECG monitoring is essential, and concurrent initiation of specific ventricular antiarrhythmic therapy may be indicated.

In the author's practice, serum concentrations of digoxin are routinely checked 4 to 7 days after digoxin administration is begun. The serum sample should be drawn 8 to 10 hours after the previous dose, and therapeutic levels are considered to be 0.8 to 2.0 ng/ml. Although digoxin serum levels do not provide an absolute indicator of appropriate digitalization (occasionally dogs will tolerate higher levels without signs of toxicity or conversely show signs of toxicity when their serum concentrations are within this range), when combined with the clinical response, they provide a useful framework for dosage adjustment. Ideally, digitalization should substantially slow the heart rate, decreasing the significance of the absent atrial contribution to cardiac output and reducing myocardial oxygen demand. Conversion to sinus rhythm occurs infrequently and is not a realistic goal in patients whose atrial fibrillation is associated with significant atrial enlargement.

Often, digoxin alone will fail to decrease the resting heart rate to an acceptable range (80 to 150/min), and either a beta-blocker or a calcium antagonist must be added (see pp. 271–278).* Because all of these drugs have potentially significant negative inotropic effects in the setting of heart failure, digitalization should be accomplished before these drugs are used. The best studied drug for this purpose is propranolol, a nonspecific beta-adrenergic blocker. Propranolol (Inderal, Ayerst) is started orally at low doses (5 to 10 mg/dog t.i.d.) and increased over a period of days, titrating the dose in 5 to 10-mg increments to obtain a heart rate in the target range. Most large breed dogs in atrial fibrillation eventually require 10 to 50 mg t.i.d. Atenolol (Tenormin, Stuart), a relatively specific beta₁-receptor blocker, is being used with increasing frequency for this purpose. In the author's experience, atenolol has a more potent and predictable negative chronotropic effect, but caution is urged as some dogs become weak and exacerbations of heart failure have been observed. The currently recommended dose of atenolol is 12.5 mg (1/4 of a 50-mg tablet) b.i.d.

Calcium channel blocking drugs are being used with increasing frequency in the management of supraventricular arrhythmias (see *Current Veterinary Therapy IX*, p. 340). Although verapamil is effective in rapidly decreasing the ventricular response to atrial fibrillation, its potent negative inotropic effect poses a real danger in the setting of heart failure. Recently, oral diltiazem (Cardizem, Marion) has been advocated in the long-term management of atrial fibrillation (Hamlin, 1988). Diltiazem has theoretic advantages over verapamil (diltiazem is a less potent negative inotrope) and the beta-blockers (diltiazem is a vasodilator, circumventing the increased peripheral vascular resistance that accompanies beta-adrenergic receptor blockade). Diltiazem has been used successfully to decrease the ventricular response to atrial fibrillation at dosages of 0.5 to 1.25 mg/kg t.i.d., therapy being initiated at the low end of the dosage range and gradually increased to effect.

When ventricular arrhythmias represent a serious clinical problem in DCM (e.g., in most boxers, many Doberman pinschers, and other dogs in which frequent bouts of sustained or nonsustained ventricular tachycardia or frequent, hemodynamically significant ventricular premature beats complicate the presentation), specific ventricular antiarrhythmic therapy is indicated. Such therapy is directed at minimizing the hemodynamic impact of the ventricular arrhythmia and preventing sudden death. Many antiarrhythmic drugs and drug combinations are available and have been used in canine DCM.

Because most of these patients are or potentially will be given digitalis, quinidine is generally avoided because of the quinidine-digoxin interaction that significantly prolongs the half-life of digoxin. Sustained ventricular tachycardia in the hemodynamically compromised dog with DCM is best managed with intravenous lidocaine. Intravenous boluses of 2 mg/kg may be given up to three times in a 5-minute period under constant ECG monitoring to achieve conversion to sinus rhythm. Intravenous diazepam (Valium) (5 mg) should be available if the bolus is repeated a third time to treat the neurologic manifestations (seizures, excitement) of lidocaine toxicity should they occur. If conversion to sinus rhythm occurs, a continuous infusion of lidocaine is administered at a dose of 50 μg/kg/min. Oral therapy with tocainide (Tonocard, Merck) has been successful in the long-term therapy of many lidocaine-responsive patients at doses of approximately 15 mg/kg t.i.d.; however, this drug is expensive compared with those used more commonly in veterinary medicine. The sustained release formulation of oral procainamide (Procan SR, Parke-Davis) is also useful in the long-term management of some patients at dosages of 15 to 20 mg/kg t.i.d. (or 10 to 15 mg/kg q.i.d.). If conversion of sustained ventricular tachycardia to sinus rhythm does not occur following intravenous lidocaine administration, several therapeutic options exist. Procainamide (Pronestyl, E. R. Squibb & Sons Inc.) may be administered at a dose of 2 mg/kg in a slow intravenous bolus over 3 to 5 minutes. These boluses may be repeated up to a dose of 15 mg/kg over a 20 to 30-minute period. Conversion to sinus rhythm should be followed with oral Procan SR as outlined above. Other ventricular antiarrhythmic drugs and combinations (e.g., addition of a beta-blocker or amiodarone) should be administered after consultation with a veterinary cardiologist familiar with the case, as their use in inappropriate situations may involve substantial risk to the patient.

In the author's practice, 24-hour ECG monitoring (Holter) is helpful in drug selection. This technique is used to establish the baseline frequency of ventricular depolarizations 24 hours before antiarrhythmic medication is begun. The characteristics of the arrhythmia (e.g., number and rate of premature depolarizations; number, rate, and duration of paroxysms of nonsustained and sustained episodes of tachycardia) are quantitated and compared with results obtained following administration of a specific antiarrhythmic drug. Preliminary results from these and similar studies suggest that the response to antiarrhythmic therapy is far from uniform, with some animals actually experiencing exacerbations of their arrhythmia on some antiarrhythmic drugs (Hamlin, 1987).

If cardiogenic shock is present (e.g., in many Doberman Pinschers) and cardiac output and con-

---

Editor's Note: The optimum heart rate for dilated failing ventricles has yet to be determined.

tractility appear to be severely depressed, more potent inotropic support than digoxin is indicated. Both catecholamines (dobutamine, dopamine) and bipyridine derivatives (amrinone, milrinone) are available for this purpose. All of these drugs share the disadvantage that they can only be administered by carefully monitored continuous intravenous infusion. All are potentially arrhythmogenic, and the cost associated with their use may be substantial (especially with dobutamine and amrinone). If atrial fibrillation is present, digoxin is administered intravenously (0.01 mg/kg in two divided doses 2 hours apart). Following digitalization, a constant intravenous infusion of dobutamine (Dobutrex, Eli Lilly and Company; 2 to 10 μg/kg/min) or dopamine (Intropin, American Critical Care; 1 to 10 μg/kg/min) may dramatically improve cardiac output and signs of heart failure. These drugs may cause tachycardia, exacerbations of supraventricular or ventricular ectopy, or both. They should ideally be used in conjunction with continuous or at least regular ECG monitoring or careful cardiac auscultation. Drip rates should be halved or stopped temporarily if significant increases in the heart rate (> 20 per cent) or arrhythmia frequency occurs. Although dobutamine has several theoretic advantages over dopamine (less arrhythmogenic, less vasoconstriction at higher doses), dopamine is significantly cheaper, which may influence drug selection in some cases. Amrinone (Inocor, Winthrop-Breon) has potent vasodilator as well as inotropic effects. In the dog, therapy is initiated with a slow 0.75 mg/kg bolus administered over 2 to 3 minutes, followed by a constant infusion of 5 to 10 μg/kg/min, depending on the response to therapy. Amrinone is expensive and has not been used extensively in veterinary medicine. Its use should be limited to well-monitored situations in which heart failure has been unresponsive to more conventional therapy. Milrinone, a close chemical relative of amrinone, can be administered orally and has been shown to be useful in the management of heart failure in dogs at dosages of 0.5 to 1.0 mg/kg b.i.d. This compound is only available for investigational use in the United States at this writing, and more clinical experience with the drug is needed before general recommendations can be made about its place in the pharmacotherapy of canine DCM. A more extensive review of positive inotropic drug therapy is available in *Current Veterinary Therapy IX* (pp. 323–328).

Dogs with congestive heart failure as a result of DCM require preload restriction to eliminate the accumulation of unwanted fluid within the lung (pulmonary edema) or body cavities (ascites or pleural effusion), in addition to positive inotropic support. Reductions in cardiac preload may be accomplished by salt-restricted diets (e.g., h/d, Hill's Pet Products), diuretics, or venodilators. If failure is severe, some combination or even all of these therapeutic modalities may be necessary. Moderate salt restriction (such as the use of a commercial low-salt diet) is useful in most cases. In addition, furosemide (Lasix, Hoechst) is usually administered. The smallest effective dosage of furosemide is generally used for long-term therapy to minimize the adverse effects of excessive preload restriction, including signs of lethargy and prerenal azotemia that may result from decreased cardiac output. This generally results in furosemide doses in the range of 1 to 4 mg/kg administered one to three times daily. Additional preload restriction can be attained with the use of a venodilator such as nitroglycerin. The author is currently using several transdermal nitroglycerin delivery systems marketed for human use. In carefully monitored clinical situations, application of a 5-mg patch to the shaved skin of dogs in heart failure caused by DCM results in prompt (within 20 minutes) reductions in both central venous and pulmonary capillary wedge pressures. Because of recent evidence in humans that intermittent application of nitroglycerin results in a better and more sustained therapeutic response, current recommendations are that these patches be applied for 12 of every 24 hours if long-term home use is contemplated. Ideally, preload should be "optimized" to levels that support cardiac output without resulting in fluid accumulation. Significant individual variation in these optimal levels occurs, depending on the rate at which cardiac filling pressures were elevated, and the degree of subsequent lymphatic adaptation, protein loss, and other hemodynamic compensations and consequences known to occur as a result of chronic heart failure. The goal of preload reduction by any of the above methods should be to maintain the central venous pressure (CVP) at approximately 5 to 10 cm H_2O, and the pulmonary capillary wedge pressure between 12 and 18 mm Hg. If these indices are unavailable, the serum creatinine level, packed cell volume (PCV), total protein, body weight, and radiographic size of the pulmonary vessels should be monitored to ensure that the removal of abnormal fluid accumulations is not accomplished at the expense of excessive volume contraction and clinically significant reductions in cardiac output.

Afterload reduction is often indicated in the management of heart failure caused by canine DCM and may be accomplished with a number of arterial dilating drugs. Among the drugs available for this purpose, those that act by inhibiting the angiotensin-converting enzyme (ACE) appear to have significant advantages. These drugs dilate both arteries and veins by inhibiting the formation of angiotensin II. They have the added benefit in the treatment of heart failure of reducing sodium and subsequently fluid retention by secondarily reducing circulating aldosterone concentrations. Captopril (Capoten, E. R. Squibb & Sons Inc.) is the prototype drug of this class and the one most commonly used in most veterinary practices. Dosages of 0.25 to 0.5 mg/kg t.i.d. are recommended initially, with gradual increases possible up to 2 mg/kg t.i.d.. Dosages greater than 2 mg/kg t.i.d. should be avoided because renal failure has been observed in some dogs when this dosage was exceeded. Signs of gastrointestinal upset (anorexia, diarrhea, and vomiting) are not infrequent and occasionally require discontinuation of therapy if they do not resolve following dosage reduction.

Hydralazine (Apresoline, Ciba Pharmaceutical Company) is another afterload-reducing drug potentially useful in the management of heart failure due to canine DCM. As a direct-acting arterial dilator, hydralazine must be used with caution in hypotension, and some method of measuring arterial blood pressure is helpful in dosage titration. Hydralazine therapy is initiated at 0.5 to 1 mg/kg b.i.d. and gradually titrated upward to a maximum dosage of 3 mg/kg b.i.d. based on the clinical and hemodynamic response. Ideally, the mean arterial pressure should remain 70 mm Hg or greater, and the central venous oxygen tension should rise to greater than 30 mm Hg. Because of the theoretic advantages of captopril, as well as hydralazine's potent hypotensive effect and the dosage titration required to obtain the optimal dosage, hydralazine is not usually the first-choice vasodilator in the management of heart failure in dogs with DCM. In dogs that cannot tolerate captopril, or in which a maximal dose of captopril fails to adequately increase cardiac output, hydralazine may be substituted. The author has had success in a limited number of cases utilizing hydralazine and captopril in combination. These few patients had refractory heart failure and had an inadequate response to captopril. The addition of 0.5 to 1 mg/kg of hydralazine in these patients provided subjective improvement in their attitude as well as objective improvement in peripheral venous oxygen tension.

Sodium nitroprusside, a direct-acting arterial and venous dilator, has been used by the author in combination with dobutamine in several cases of severe, end-stage heart failure due to DCM. Nitroprusside (Nipride, Hoffmann-LaRoche) has an extremely short duration of action and must be administered by constant intravenous infusion. It is an extremely potent hypotensive agent and should only be used when a reliable means of arterial blood pressure monitoring is available. The initial dosage of 1 μg/kg/min is gradually increased to titrate the mean arterial blood pressure to approximately 70 mm Hg. Preliminary results indicate that tolerance to the action of sodium nitroprusside develops rapidly in the dog, and careful monitoring and dosage adjustment is necessary to maintain the therapeutic effect. At the present time, the author considers the use of sodium nitroprusside to be an effective

(temporary) emergency measure in patients that are refractory to conventional therapy, including intravenous inotropic support. Sodium nitroprusside therapy has not been continued beyond 48 hours in the author's practice, and prolonged therapy is not recommended. A more extensive review of vasodilator therapy can be found in *Current Veterinary Therapy IX* (pp. 329–339).

The choice of therapy for heart failure caused by DCM is complex, depending on the nature and severity of clinical signs, the owner's involvement with and commitment to the pet, and the availability of sophisticated monitoring techniques. A dog with an acute onset of life-threatening cardiogenic pulmonary edema (such as occurs in many Doberman pinschers) may require intravenous diuretics, inotropic agents, vasodilators, and extensive (often invasive) patient monitoring to survive even a few days. In contrast, an asymptomatic giant breed dog (e.g., an Irish wolfhound found to have atrial fibrillation with a slow ventricular response) may not require any medication unless the underlying cause of DCM can be identified (e.g., via endomyocardial biopsy) and corrected. Accordingly, the overall prognosis of DCM in the dog is influenced by the global ventricular function, breed, cardiac rhythm, and underlying cause, as well as therapy. Table 2 summarizes the drugs commonly used in the treatment of heart failure caused by canine DCM.

Secondary Dilated Cardiomyopathy

In addition to primary (idiopathic) canine DCM, several pathologic insults have been demonstrated both experimentally and clinically to cause myocardial damage severe enough to result in similar syndromes of contractile failure, cardiac dilation, or arrhythmia. These insults include infectious agents (e.g., parvovirus, Chagas' disease, and Lyme disease) as well as toxins (e.g., doxorubicin or cobalt). Some of these secondary cardiomyopathies may occur frequently enough to warrant serious consideration in the differential diagnosis of acquired cardiac disease in specific geographic areas or types of practice. In addition to these agents, some metabolic illnesses (e.g., renal failure, hypothyroidism, and diabetes mellitus) have been shown to depress myocardial function, causing (usually subclinical) cardiomyopathies that may contribute to concurrent heart disease in some dogs.

LYME CARDITIS

Most known causes of secondary canine DCM have been recently reviewed (see *Current Veterinary Therapy IX*) and are of limited clinical importance in all but a few specialized practices. The

Table 2. Drugs Commonly Used in Heart Failure Due to Canine DCM

Drug	Physiologic Effects	Usual Dosage/Remarks
Antiarrhythmics		
Digoxin	Slows the rate of ventricular response in atrial fibrillation	0.01–0.015 mg/kg divided b.i.d. (≤ 0.5 mg b.i.d. total) PO
	Increases cardiac contractility	Discontinue if vomiting, anorexia occur
Propranolol	Beta-Blocker	Start 5 mg/dog t.i.d. PO, titrate slowly to effect
	Slow ventricular response to atrial fibrillation	
	Negative inotrope	Initiate after digoxin
Atenolol	Same as propranolol, greatest duration of action, greater beta$_1$ specificity	12.5 mg/dog b.i.d. PO, can cause bradycardia, heart failure
		Initiate after digoxin
Diltiazem	CA antagonists	0.5–1.25 mg/kg t.i.d. PO
	Slows ventricular response to atrial fibrillation	Can cause bradycardia, heart failure, hypotension
	Negative inotrope	
Lidocaine	Ventricular antiarrhythmic	2–6 mg/kg IV bolus, 50 µg/kg/min IV infusion
Procainamide	Ventricular antiarrhythmic	2–15 mg/kg IV over 20 min, 15–20 mg/kg t.i.d. PO
		Use sustained release preparation
Tocainide	Ventricular antiarrhythmic	10–20 mg/kg t.i.d.
	Similar to "oral lidocaine"	
Positive Inotropes		
Digoxin	See above	See above
Dobutamine	Catecholamine	2.0–10 µg/kg/min IV
	Increases contractility	May cause tachyarrhythmia
Dopamine	Catecholamine	1.0–10 µg/kg/min IV
	Increases contractility	May cause tachyarrhythmia
Amrinone	Bipyridine derivative	0.75 mg/kg IV over 3 min
	Increases contractility	5–10 µg/kg/min infusion
	Arterial vasodilator	
Diuretics		
Furosemide	Loop diuretic	1–4 mg/kg IV, SC, PO
	Reduces preload	Administer 1–3 times daily
Vasodilators		
Nitroglycerin	Venodilator	5-mg transdermal patch
	Reduces preload	Apply 12 of 24 hours
Hydralazine	Arterial dilator	0.5–3 mg/kg b.i.d. PO
	Reduces afterload	Titrate dosage, beware of hypotension
Captopril	ACE inhibitor (see text)	0.25–2 mg/kg t.i.d. PO
	Reduces preload and afterload	Start low and titrate up
		Watch for hypotension, GI side effects
Sodium nitroprusside	Dilates arteries and veins	1–10 µg/kg/min IV
	Reduces preload and afterload	Monitor blood pressure
		Watch for hypotension

recognition of Lyme disease as a potential cause of myocarditis and DCM in the dog, however, has not been reviewed in any readily accessible source and deserves mention. Lyme disease, and subsequently Lyme carditis, is being diagnosed with increasing frequency in dogs in some geographic areas. Lyme disease is a systemic illness that can have rheumatologic, cardiac, neurologic, or dermatologic manifestations in the dog. It is caused by the spirochete *Borrelia burgdorferi*, which is transmitted to dogs primarily by the tick *Ixodes dammini* but possibly by other biting insects as well. Since the disease was originally described in the human population of Lyme, Connecticut, in 1977, the distribution of Lyme disease has been recognized to be nationwide. Endemic areas include Wisconsin and Minnesota, as well as the northeastern and western

coastal states. Lyme disease was first reported in dogs in 1984, and Levy and Duray (1988) recently described third-degree AV block (a common result of Lyme carditis in humans) in a dog with a high serum Lyme titer and pathologic findings at necropsy similar to those of human Lyme carditis (myocarditis characterized by the infiltration of plasma cells, macrophages, neutrophils, and lymphocytes, with attendant myocardial necrosis).

The author has diagnosed three cases of apparent Lyme carditis; although syncope, high-grade second- or third-degree AV block, and signs of congestive heart failure were the presenting complaints in two of these patients, one dog was referred for the evaluation of heart failure and paroxysmal ventricular tachycardia. Two of these patients had noncardiac clinical signs that suggested the possibility of

Lyme disease (fever and joint pain). All three dogs had severely depressed systolic ventricular function echocardiographically, and two of the three died suddenly despite antibiotic and antiarrhythmic therapy. One dog with high-grade second-degree AV block and congestive heart failure has recovered clinically and is doing well 3 months after presentation. Although this animal's left ventricular systolic function has improved significantly and no further episodes of syncope or respiratory distress have occurred, high-grade second-degree AV block persists (the owners declined implantation of a ventricular pacemaker).

The fatal case reported by Levy and Duray (1988), coupled with the results of other recent cases, suggests that, unlike humans, dogs with third-degree AV block caused by Lyme carditis do not routinely recover normal AV nodal function with appropriate antimicrobial therapy. Further investigation of canine Lyme carditis is needed, but it is clear that at least temporary ventricular pacing may be required in some cases. The possibility of Lyme carditis should be considered and investigated (via serum Lyme titer determination and possibly endomyocardial biopsy) in patients with unexplained ventricular arrhythmias, symptomatic AV block, or echocardiographic evidence of ventricular dysfunction. Because the disease is difficult to definitively document even at necropsy, the diagnosis is usually based on a positive serum titer and concurrent evidence of myocarditis with or without other manifestations of the disease. If acute Lyme carditis is suspected, therapy with tetracycline (25 mg/kg t.i.d.), doxycycline (5 mg/kg q.d.), or ampicillin (20 mg/kg t.i.d.) should be instituted at once and continued for 3 weeks pending results of appropriate diagnostic tests.

HYPERTROPHIC CARDIOMYOPATHY

Hypertrophic cardiomyopathy (HCM) is the term used to describe primary myocardial disease characterized by concentric hypertrophy of the left ventricle. This hypertrophy results in a markedly thickened left ventricular free wall and interventricular septum and occurs at the expense of the left ventricular lumen. The hypertrophied ventricle is less compliant than normal and fills at a higher end-diastolic pressure. During exercise, with stress (catecholamine-induced tachycardia and decreased compliance), or simply with time as the hypertrophy progresses, the ventricle may become so stiff that left ventricular filling pressures (and therefore left atrial and pulmonary venous and capillary hydrostatic pressures) reach levels high enough to precipitate pulmonary edema. Other clinical manifestations of HCM may include episodic weakness, collapse, and even sudden death. These signs are

thought to be the result of ventricular arrhythmias that commonly occur when ventricular hypertrophy outstrips the coronary blood supply, causing myocardial ischemia. Dynamic outflow tract obstruction (the result of the hypertrophied interventricular septum) may contribute to or cause episodic weakness and collapse in some dogs. The pathologic stimulus that results in HCM is unknown, and other causes of concentric ventricular hypertrophy (e.g., outflow tract obstruction, systemic hypertension, and thyrotoxicosis) must be ruled out before HCM can be diagnosed. Relatively few clinical cases of HCM have been reported in dogs, and significant age or breed predispositions have not yet been determined, although approximately 75 per cent of the reported cases have occurred in males.

Diagnosis

Physical diagnostic findings in HCM appear to be variable. Heart murmurs may theoretically result from mitral regurgitation (caused by papillary muscle dysfunction, Venturi effect, or geometric changes in the ventricle) or aortic stenosis (caused by dynamic outflow obstruction). Ventricular premature contractions may be auscultated as the only physical diagnostic clue. The frequency with which gallop sounds are heard is unknown, although their presence is an expected sequela of decreased ventricular compliance. The definitive diagnosis rests on echocardiographic findings of left ventricular concentric hypertrophy in the absence of fixed outflow tract obstruction, systemic hypertension, or unusual metabolic disturbance such as thyrotoxicosis.

Therapy

No therapeutic trials of canine HCM have been reported to date, although exercise restriction in association with beta-blockers (propranolol, 0.5 to 1 mg/kg t.i.d.; or atenolol, 12.5 mg b.i.d. in dogs > 25 kg) should theoretically be useful in decreasing the heart rate, myocardial oxygen consumption, and stress response that is thought to result in increased diastolic dysfunction, pulmonary edema, and ventricular arrhythmias in these patients. Calcium antagonists may also be useful for this purpose, although further investigation is needed before any recommendation can be made regarding the efficacy and safety of these drugs in this setting. The prognosis must be guarded because of the possibility of sudden death, but in the author's experience prolonged (1 to 3 years) symptom-free survival has been possible in the few cases in which an antemortem diagnosis has been made.

References and Supplemental Reading

Calvert, C. A., Chapman, W. L., Jr., and Toal, R. L.: Congestive cardiomyopathy in Doberman pinscher dogs. J.A.V.M.A. 181:598, 1982.

Hamlin, R. L.: Proarrhythmic effects associated with the use of quinidine, procainamide, and tocainide in dogs with ventricular ectopia. ACVIM Proceedings of the 5th Veterinary Medical Forum, 1987.

Hamlin, R. L.: The use of oral diltiazem to reduce the ventricular response to chronic atrial fibrillation in dogs. J. Am. Coll. Vet. Intern. Med. 1988 (in press).

Harpster, N. K.: Boxer cardiomyopathy. In Kirk, R. W. (ed.): Current Veterinary Therapy VII. Philadelphia: W. B. Saunders, 1983.

Keene, B. W., Kittleson, M. D., Atkins, C. E., et al.: Modification of a technique for transvenous endomyocardial biopsy in the dog. Am. J. Vet. Res. 1988a (in press).

Keene, B. W., Kittleson, M. D., Rush, J. E., and Shug, A. L.: Frequency of myocardial carnitine deficiency associated with spontaneous canine dilated cardiomyopathy. ACVIM Proceedings of the 6th Veterinary Medical Forum, 1988b.

Keene, B. W., Panciera, D. L., Atkins, C. E., et al.: Myocardial carnitine deficiency associated with spontaneously occurring dilated cardiomyopathy in a family of dogs. 1988c (in preparation).

Keene, B. W., Panciera, D. L., Regitz, V., et al.: Carnitine-linked defects of myocardial metabolism in canine dilated cardiomyopathy. ACVIM Proceedings of the 4th Veterinary Medical Forum, Vol. II, 1986, pp. 14–55.

Levy, S. A., and Duray, P. H.: Complete heart block in a dog seropositive for Borrelia burgdorferi: A similarity to human Lyme carditis. J. Am. Coll. Vet. Intern. Med. 2:145, 1988.

Staaden, R. V.: Cardiomyopathy of English cocker spaniels. J.A.V.M.A. 178:1289, 1981.

CARDIOMYOPATHY IN THE CAT AND ITS RELATION TO TAURINE DEFICIENCY

PAUL D. PION, D.V.M.,
MARK D. KITTLESON, D.V.M., Ph.D.,
and QUINTON R. ROGERS, Ph.D.
Davis, California

Cardiomyopathy describes a group of diseases that directly affect the myocardium. By definition, this excludes acquired and congenital conditions that may secondarily affect the myocardium and whose pathophysiologic origins primarily involve the structure or function of other cardiac components.

Cardiomyopathies have been morphologically and functionally classified as dilated, hypertrophic, and restrictive. In humans, hypertrophic cardiomyopathy (HCM) has also been called idiopathic hypertrophic subaortic stenosis and asymmetric septal hypertrophy. Restrictive cardiomyopathy has also been called infiltrative cardiomyopathy. Dilated cardiomyopathy (DCM) has also been referred to in the literature as congestive, dilatative, and dilatation cardiomyopathy. The term dilated cardiomyopathy is preferred by the World Health Organization and will be used in this article. Because dilated refers to the ventricular cavities and the disease process actually occurs within the myocardium and produces myocardial failure and secondary eccentric hypertrophy, the authors prefer the term primary myocardial failure.

CARDIOMYOPATHY IN THE CAT

In the cat, two forms of primary myocardial disease are well defined—hypertrophic and dilated cardiomyopathies. Two other forms of cardiomyopathy, restrictive and excessive moderator band types, have been described, but because criteria for diagnosis of these conditions are poorly defined in cats, diagnosis of these conditions is difficult at best (see Current Veterinary Therapy IX, p. 380, for more details). It is probable that different clinicians assign these diagnoses to different patient populations.

Both dilated and hypertrophic cardiomyopathy are classified as primary diseases of the myocardium. Beyond this common classification, there are few similarities between the functional, structural, and etiologic characteristics of these disease entities. A more detailed description of the diagnosis and treatment of primary myocardial disease in cats is available (Fox, 1983; Harpster, 1986). The primary purpose of this article is to discuss dilated cardiomyopathy (DCM) and its relation to taurine deficiency. Features of feline hypertrophic cardiomyopathy (HCM) will also be presented to emphasize the similarities and differences between the pathophysiology and clinical management of these conditions.

Clinical Presentation of Myocardial Diseases in the Cat

Hypertrophic and dilated cardiomyopathies cannot be definitively differentiated from other forms of congenital or acquired feline heart disease on the basis of physical, laboratory, or radiographic evaluations alone, as there are no unique historical, clinical, radiographic, or hematologic characteristics that distinguish one form of cardiomyopathy from another. Echocardiography is the best definitive means of differentiating hypertrophic and dilated cardiomyopathy in cats (see pp. 201–218). Thus, after performing initial diagnostic studies and providing supportive measures common to the management of any form of cardiac insufficiency, it is recommended that the clinician perform, or refer the patient for, ultrasound examination.

Physical examination may demonstrate a systolic murmur, usually localized over the sternum, and an audible third or fourth heart sound (gallop). Pulmonary congestion and pulmonary edema are more common in cats with hypertrophic cardiomyopathy than in cats with dilated cardiomyopathy. However, the presence of pulmonary edema is not sufficient evidence for differentiating hypertrophic cardiomyopathy from other forms of feline heart disease. Pleural effusion and pulmonary edema may be associated with either dilated or hypertrophic cardiomyopathy. Ascites is an uncommon clinical sign in all forms of feline heart disease other than pure right-sided heart disease (e.g., tricuspid regurgitation, heartworm disease). Noncardiogenic diseases (e.g., feline infectious peritonitis, cirrhosis, and neoplasia) are the usual diagnoses underlying abdominal effusion in cats.

As a result of the cat's generally sedentary tendency, exercise intolerance and fatigue, commonly associated with cardiac insufficiency in other species, are rarely reported in cats with cardiomyopathy. It is common for owners of cats with cardiomyopathy (dilated or hypertrophic) to report that the patient appeared normal the previous day and suddenly became severely dyspneic.

Cats with cardiomyopathy may also have nonspecific signs (lethargy, dehydration, and hypothermia) that are suggestive of renal failure or other metabolic diseases. In these patients, careful physical examination often reveals abnormal cardiac sounds or rhythm, which should stimulate an attempt to rule out a coincident or primary cardiac disorder. The greatest risk to such patients is injudicious administration of fluids, leading to respiratory failure caused by pleural effusion or pulmonary edema.

Two relatively common presentations that may cause confusion are posterior paralysis and chylothorax. Posterior paralysis resulting from aortic thromboemboli may lead the clinician toward an unrewarding investigation of the neuromuscular system. Necropsy data indicate that aortic thromboembolism is more commonly associated with hypertrophic than dilated cardiomyopathy in cats. Chylothorax in cats has historically been considered to be most commonly associated with traumatic or neoplastic causes and not with cardiac disease. In this situation, chylothorax has been considered to require surgery. Recent review by Tonachini and colleagues at the University of California, Davis, has shown that congestive heart failure (caused by tricuspid dysplasia; hypertrophic, restrictive, or dilated cardiomyopathy; and hyperthyroidism) is a common cause of chylothorax in cats (also see *Current Veterinary Therapy IX*, p. 298). Treatment directed at alleviating signs of congestive heart failure (CHF) results in resolution of the chylothorax in most patients with underlying cardiac disease.

HYPERTROPHIC CARDIOMYOPATHY

Etiology and Pathophysiology

Hypertrophic cardiomyopathy is primarily a diastolic disorder, the result of an abnormally thickened, stiff left ventricular myocardium that has normal or near-normal systolic myocardial function but a decreased ability to accept diastolic flow from the left atrium. This diastolic dysfunction (decreased compliance), which results in the need for a greater pressure to fill the left ventricle, is worsened by ischemia and tachycardia. Thus, left ventricular diastolic pressure increases. Since the mitral valve is open during diastole, left atrial and pulmonary venous and pulmonary capillary pressures also increase. The increase in left atrial pressure produces left atrial enlargement; the increase in pulmonary venous pressure results in pulmonary venous congestion, and the increase in pulmonary capillary pressure produces pulmonary edema. Left ventricular volume is normal or decreased. The left ventricular papillary muscles are usually greatly enlarged in relation to the volume of the ventricle, and left ventricular wall thickness is increased. The left atrium may be normal in size but is usually enlarged. The etiology of hypertrophic cardiomyopathy in cats is unknown. In humans, there is evidence suggesting that hypertrophic cardiomyopathy is heritable. The morphologic progression of the abnormal left ventricle in cats with hypertrophic cardiomyopathy is unknown. There is no known association between hypertrophic cardiomyopathy and plasma taurine concentrations.

Definitive Diagnosis

Definitive diagnosis of hypertrophic cardiomyopathy in cats may be confirmed by echocardiography, contrast angiography, or postmortem examination. Contrast angiography may carry a significant risk in compromised patients. Echocardiography (cardiac ultrasound) is a noninvasive, safe, and relatively inexpensive procedure, which has become readily available in most regions of the United States, usually in large referral and private practices.

Echocardiographic changes associated with hypertrophic cardiomyopathy in cats include symmetric and, rarely, asymmetric thickening of the interventricular septum and left ventricular free wall. The left ventricular papillary muscles are often greatly enlarged. The end-diastolic diameter may be normal or decreased. The end-systolic diameter may be normal or decreased. The decrease in the size of the left ventricular chamber may be due to abnormal thickening of the septum and left ventricular wall but more commonly is caused by excessively large papillary muscles occupying the chamber. The left atrium is usually dilated, and, occasionally, a ball thrombus may be visualized within the left atrium. Other causes of left ventricular hypertrophy, including congenital subaortic stenosis, hyperthyroid heart disease, and chronic renal disease with systemic hypertension, should be excluded.

Therapy

Hypertrophic cardiomyopathy in cats most often causes signs of pulmonary congestion and edema or aortic thromboembolism. By contrast, in humans and dogs, the most common presentation of hypertrophic cardiomyopathy is sudden death, and signs of congestive heart failure are uncommon. The incidence of sudden death in feline hypertrophic cardiomyopathy is unknown.

Therapy for CHF in cats with hypertrophic cardiomyopathy is palliative (also see *Current Veterinary Therapy IX*, p. 380, for more details). Diuretics are the most useful class of drugs for relieving signs of congestion and edema. Furosemide (0.5 to 2.2 mg/kg s.i.d to t.i.d. PO) is the most commonly prescribed diuretic for cats. Intravenous (or often intramuscular to circumvent the stress associated with restraint for venipuncture) furosemide (0.5 to 2.2 mg/kg) is indicated in severely dyspneic cats with pulmonary edema. Captopril, an angiotensin-converting enzyme inhibitor (0.5 to 1 mg/kg b.i.d.

to t.i.d. PO), is useful, in conjunction with diuretics, for treating congestive heart failure in cats. Pleurocentesis is the preferred and most rapid means of treating significant pleural effusions. Beta-adrenergic receptor blockade with propranolol (0.5 to 1.0 mg/kg b.i.d. to t.i.d. PO) has commonly been recommended to improve diastolic function in cats with hypertrophic cardiomyopathy. Calcium entry blockers such as verapamil and diltiazem have also been theorized to have potential beneficial effects in cats with hypertrophic cardiomyopathy. Both of these drugs have been shown to be beneficial in humans with hypertrophic cardiomyopathy; however, they should not be administered to cats with uncontrolled CHF. Clinical experience with these drugs suggests that furosemide and captopril are effective and safe agents for controlling signs of congestive heart failure in cats. However, the benefits of beta-adrenergic blockade with propranolol are difficult to judge. Studies characterizing the symptomatic hemodynamic effects of beta-blockers and calcium entry blockers in cats with hypertrophic cardiomyopathy are in progress (Bright and Golden, 1988). Positive inotropic agents, such as digoxin and milrinone, are generally considered to be contraindicated in feline patients with hypertrophic cardiomyopathy.

Aspirin (25 mg/kg every third day) has been recommended for prevention of intravascular thrombus formation in feline myocardial diseases. To date, there have been no controlled clinical studies of the protective effects, if any, of aspirin therapy in this patient population. In the authors' experience, aspirin at the recommended dosage is not routinely effective in preventing thrombosis in cats with myocardial disease and previous episodes of aortic thromboembolism. Harpster (1986) and others have recommended the use of warfarin (0.08 to 0.1 mg/kg once daily) as a preventive measure in cats at risk. This therapy also is untested in a controlled clinical trial, and extremely careful patient monitoring is required to prevent signs of toxicity (bleeding). Warfarin therapy is not recommended for outdoor cats that might acquire traumatic injuries.

Prognosis

In general, the prognosis for cats with hypertrophic cardiomyopathy is favorable. In many cats, with proper management, signs of congestion and edema may be controlled for a period of months to years after the initial diagnosis. Captopril appears to be an effective addition to diuretic therapy in cats with refractory pulmonary edema or pleural effusion. Systemic thromboembolism may represent the greatest risk to cats with hypertrophic cardiomyopathy. Atrial fibrillation may lead to sudden cardiac decompensation and can be treated with propranolol or diltiazem to control the heart rate (see pp. 271–278).

In older cats with hypertrophic cardiomyopathy and signs of congestive heart failure that are difficult to control with diuretics and captopril, coincident hyperthyroidism or anemia should be ruled out. Lowering circulating concentrations of thyroid hormone in cats with coincident hyperthyroidism may allow reduction of the doses of diuretics and captopril required to control signs of congestive heart failure. It is worth emphasizing that, although hyperthyroidism can occur in conjunction with hypertrophic cardiomyopathy, the heart disease caused by hyperthyroidism should be called thyrotoxic heart disease and not hypertrophic cardiomyopathy.

DILATED CARDIOMYOPATHY

Etiology and Pathophysiology

Dilated cardiomyopathy is a primary systolic myocardial disorder. The weakened myocardium is less able to provide power to maintain the function of the heart as a pump. Decreased systolic function in patients with dilated cardiomyopathy can result in signs associated with decreased cardiac output (low-output failure) or congestion/edema (backward heart failure). End-systolic left ventricular volume increases owing to the decrease in myocardial function. Left ventricular end-diastolic volume increases because of eccentric myocardial hypertrophy. The hypertrophy is thought to result from a sequence of events. Initially, the decrease in cardiac output stimulates renal retention of sodium chloride and water via several mechanisms. This results in an increased blood volume and thus venous return. The increase in venous return increases end-diastolic pressure and thus wall stress. This stretching force is thought to somehow stimulate the sarcomeres (the contractile units in the myocardium) to replicate in series. This replication results in the left ventricle's growing larger such that it accommodates a larger end-diastolic volume. The thickness of the left ventricular myocardium remains normal as long as the myocardium hypertrophies normally. In some cats with DCM, the wall apparently is unable to hypertrophy adequately, resulting in walls that are thinner than normal. However, in almost all cases, the wall is too thin for the degree of left ventricular dilation present. The papillary muscles are usually small in relation to the volume of the ventricle. The left atrium may be normal in size but is usually enlarged.

There are no specific histologic or electron microscopic lesions associated with dilated cardiomyopathy. For this reason, it has been suggested that dilated cardiomyopathy may represent a primary biochemical and not a primary structural lesion. It is now known that taurine deficiency is a common cause of dilated cardiomyopathy in cats.

Taurine

Taurine (2-aminoethanesulfonic acid) is a sulfur-containing amino acid (Fig. 1). Taurine was first isolated from ox bile in 1827. Since then, taurine has been found throughout evolutionary history, beginning with single-celled organisms. When multicellular organisms are studied, taurine is largely confined to branches of the evolutionary tree leading to animals and is seldom encountered in plants.

A major function of most essential amino acids is incorporation into proteins in specific sequences as determined by DNA sequencing in the nucleus. Taurine, however, has not been identified as a part of any protein in mammals. The majority of intracellular taurine is thought to be freely dissolved in the cytosolic fluid of cells. Other than its role in the conjugation of bile acids and the detoxification of xenobiotics via conjugation and excretion in bile, the function of taurine in mammals is not well understood.

Tissues with the highest taurine concentrations include heart, retina, central nervous system, and skeletal muscle. Taurine is also present in high concentrations in white blood cells and platelets. Taurine is the most abundant free amino acid in myocardium and retina. In cats, intracardiac taurine concentrations range between 6 and 18 mM (compare with potassium, 150 mM; and calcium, 0.0001 mM in diastole, 0.01 mM in systole). These high tissue taurine concentrations are maintained by active transport of taurine from plasma to the intracellular space that is modulated by the beta-adrenergic receptor–adenylate cyclase system.

It has been known since the mid 1970's that taurine is essential for normal retinal function in cats. Recent evidence demonstrates that taurine is essential for normal myocardial function. Despite these and many other *in vivo* and *in vitro* studies illustrating the varied and ubiquitous effects of taurine in mammals, the basis for these effects is unknown.

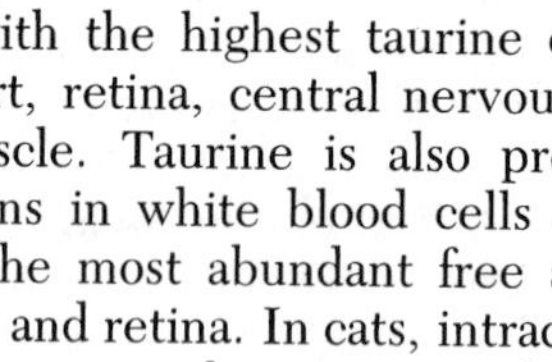

$$O = \overset{\overset{\displaystyle O}{\|}}{\underset{\underset{\displaystyle O}{|}}{S}} - CH_2CH_2\overset{\oplus}{N}H_3$$

$$\ominus$$

Taurine

Figure 1. The structure of taurine as it exists at physiologic pH. Note that (1) taurine contains a sulfonic acid group and not a carboxylic acid; (2) taurine is a β-amino acid; and (3) it is zwitterionic (carries a positive and a negative charge) a physiologic pH.

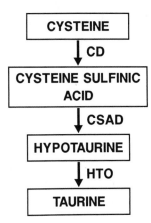

Figure 2. The primary pathway for conversion of cysteine to taurine in mammals. CD, cysteine dioxygenase; CSAD, cysteine sulfinic acid decarboxylase; HTO, hypotaurine oxidase.

Several mechanisms of action have been proposed to explain the seemingly endless list of physiologic functions altered by the presence or absence of taurine. Taurine is a small, highly charged molecule and thus is osmotically active. It is thought to be an important osmoregulatory substance in the nervous system and myocardium. Much of the available evidence supports a theory that taurine's major effects may be related to modulation of tissue calcium concentrations and availability. Inactivation of free radicals (destructive molecules with an odd number of electrons that are proposed to be involved in many forms of cellular injury) has also been proposed as a possible explanation for some of taurine's actions. In addition, taurine has metabolic effects and may interact with or be synergistic with insulin.

TAURINE AND THE CAT

Cats have a limited ability to synthesize taurine from cysteine and methionine because their tissues contain low concentrations of cysteine sulfinate acid decarboxylase (CSAD), a key enzyme in the biosynthesis of taurine (Fig. 2). However, this low synthetic ability is not unique to the cat (e.g., humans also have limited synthetic ability), and, as indicated

Table 1. *Conditions Associated with Taurine Deficiency in the Cat*

Central retinal degeneration
Degeneration of the tapedum lucidum
Reproductive failure
  Fetal resorption
  Abortion
  Stillbirths
Kitten mortality and deformities
  Abnormal hindlimb development
  Thoracic kyphosis
  Abnormal development of the cerebellum and visual cortex
Dilated cardiomyopathy

later, it is unlikely that this alone is sufficient to explain the cat's propensity for developing low plasma taurine concentrations and associated abnormalities (Table 1).

As previously stated, the best defined metabolic role of taurine in mammals is in bile acid conjugation. Mammals utilize taurine and glycine for conjugating deoxycholate to form bile acids. These systems are also utilized for conjugating other metabolites and xenobiotics. Many mammals preferentially utilize taurine for bile acid conjugation, forming taurocholic acid; however, if taurine is in low supply, glycine can be utilized so that the major bile acid produced will be glycocholate (the glycine conjugate). Cats are unable to conjugate significant amounts of their bile acids with glycine. They must utilize taurine exclusively for conjugation, and, therefore, even with dietary taurine restriction, they continue to lose taurine in the bile. It is this continued taurine loss that also predisposes the cat to development of low plasma taurine concentrations. Cats fed diets low in taurine are gradually depleted of taurine despite reabsorption of taurine (as free taurine and taurocholic acid) in the jejunum and ileum and up-regulation of renal conservation processes.

TAURINE AND THE HEART

There is a large body of literature describing *in vivo* and *in vitro* physiologic phenomena in the heart associated with alterations in intracellular and extracellular taurine concentrations. Taurine is known to have positive inotropic properties in hearts perfused with low calcium concentrations and negative inotropic effects in hearts perfused with high calcium concentrations. Myocardial taurine concentrations are increased in dogs, rabbits, and humans with disorders that result in eccentric hypertrophy of the ventricles. Taurine has been shown to have beneficial effects in rabbits and humans with valvular heart disease. These observations coupled with the high concentration of taurine normally found in the heart have led other investigators to speculate that taurine depletion might lead to a clinically significant reduction in myocardial mechanical function. However, previous investigators have been unable to demonstrate this phenomenon in acute *in vivo* studies utilizing rats and rabbits.

IDENTIFICATION OF TAURINE DEFICIENCY MYOCARDIAL FAILURE

The first cat identified as having taurine deficiency in conjunction with dilated cardiomyopathy at the University of California Veterinary Medical

Teaching Hospital had posterior paresis associated with an aortic thromboembolus (see pp. 295–302). Perfusion to the hindlimbs improved greatly during the first day of thrombolytic therapy, but unfortunately the patient died 2 days later from its heart disease. Discussion with the owner provided historical information that ultimately provided the impetus to pursue taurine deficiency as a possible cause of dilated cardiomyopathy in cats.

One year earlier, the patient had been diagnosed as having feline central retinal degeneration (FCRD). FCRD usually causes clinically insignificant vision loss but can result in blindness and is known to be caused by a deficiency of taurine. The plasma taurine concentration measured at the time was 10 nmol/ml (10 to 20 per cent of normal plasma concentrations). The veterinarian who made the diagnosis was surprised to learn that the patient had been eating a commercial cat food. Until recently, it had been generally believed that only cats eating dog food, poorly formulated home-cooked diets, or commercial diets containing less than 400 mg of taurine per kilogram of dry weight developed low plasma taurine concentrations and FCRD. This proved to be a general misconception. Several investigators have demonstrated that low plasma taurine concentrations can be detected in many cats eating a diet consisting primarily of certain commercial cat foods that contain 400 to 1500 mg of taurine per kilogram of dry diet. Feeding these same diets to cats under controlled laboratory conditions induced rapid depletion of plasma taurine concentrations.

The first evidence that appeared to confirm the hypothesis that taurine deficiency might be a cause of dilated cardiomyopathy in cats was provided by echocardiographic evaluation of 11 cats that had been eating a purified diet with marginally inadequate amounts of taurine for 4 years: three of these cats had myocardial failure. Taurine supplementation restored myocardial function to normal in these cats.

Armed with this early data, the authors began a prospective study evaluating plasma taurine concentrations in and the effects of taurine administration on cats with dilated cardiomyopathy. All patients with feline dilated cardiomyopathy diagnosed in the authors' hospital since December 1986 have had low plasma taurine concentrations. Diet histories in these cases were consistent with suspicions regarding commercial diets. The commercial diets included a wide variety of foods, including canned and dry forms formulated by almost every major manufacturer in the United States. All cats with dilated cardiomyopathy and taurine deficiency received taurine supplementation. Over 90 per cent of cats with echocardiographic evidence of myocardial failure that survived longer than 1 week after beginning taurine therapy recovered. Not only did they improve clinically, but myocardial function, as determined by echocardiography, returned to normal (Fig. 3). Prior to the identification of taurine as effective therapy for cats with taurine deficiency and dilated cardiomyopathy, most cardiologists (veterinary and human) believed that dilated cardiomyopathy in all species was, in the vast majority of cases, an irreversible disease process.

In summary, the data demonstrating that taurine deficiency is the underlying cause of feline dilated cardiomyopathy includes (1) in 100 per cent of cases observed by the authors, dilated cardiomyopathy in cats has been associated with low plasma taurine concentrations; (2) feeding cats experimental diets low in taurine has caused dilated cardiomyopathy; and (3) administering taurine to cats with dilated cardiomyopathy associated with low plasma taurine levels has resulted in normalization of the function of the heart in all surviving cases (Figs. 4 through 6).

Prior to these findings, dilated cardiomyopathy in cats had been a frustrating condition because most patients died soon after being diagnosed despite heroic therapeutic efforts. The prognosis remains guarded in the critically ill patient with signs of cardiogenic shock. However, with proper management, it is now possible to reverse the underlying myocardial failure in most cases of feline dilated cardiomyopathy associated with low plasma taurine concentrations. The majority of these patients should survive and return to function as normal healthy pets.

Definitive Diagnosis

Dilated cardiomyopathy is easy to diagnose with echocardiography, even for the novice echocardiographer. It is characterized by left ventricular chamber dilation (increased end-diastolic diameter [EDD]), increased end-systolic diameter (ESD), and decreased motion of the interventricular septum and left ventricular wall. The percentage of change in left ventricular chamber diameter from diastole to systole, or fractional shortening (FS), is defined as

$$FS = \frac{EDD - ESD}{EDD}$$

This value, an index of cardiac pump function, analogous to the angiographic ejection fraction, is decreased (to less than 35 per cent and often less than 20 per cent) in cases of dilated cardiomyopathy. The right ventricle and right atria may have normal dimensions or may appear enlarged. The left atrium usually is enlarged. Careful evaluation of the left atrium by two-dimensional echocardiography may reveal the presence of a left atrial thrombus.

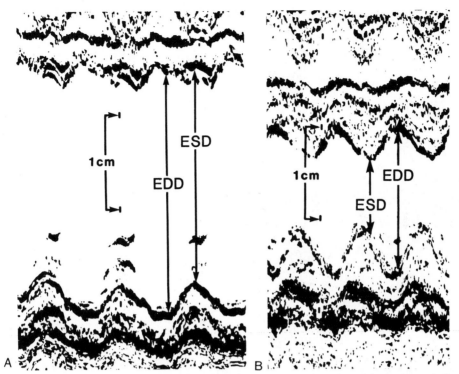

Figure 3. M-mode echocardiogram from the first cat with DCM treated with oral taurine supplementation. *A*, first examination; *B*, 10 weeks after beginning taurine therapy. The ultrasound beam is passing through (top to bottom) the right ventricular wall, right ventricular cavity, interventricular septum, left ventricular cavity (chamber with labels), and left ventricular wall. EDD, end-diastolic diameter; ESD, end-systolic diameter. (Used with permission, Pion, P. D., et al.: Myocardial failure in cats associated with low plasma taurine: A reversible cardiomyopathy. Science 237:764–768, Aug 14, 1987. Copyright 1987 AAAS.)

Nutrition

DIET HISTORY

The discovery of taurine deficiency myocardial failure serves to emphasize the importance of proper nutrition and the need for a greater understanding of the nutritional requirements of healthy and diseased companion animals. In cases of dilated cardiomyopathy associated with low plasma taurine concentrations, knowledge of the patient's dietary patterns is the best tool the practitioner has for discovering why an individual patient developed taurine deficiency–related disease. In addition, this

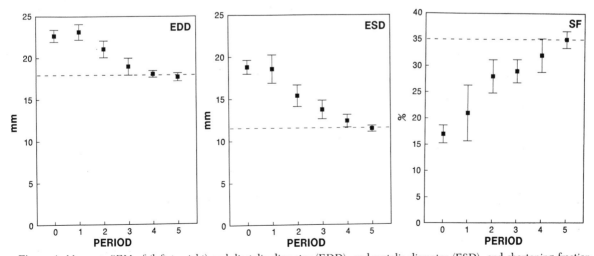

Figure 4. Mean ± SEM of (left to right) end-diastolic diameter (EDD), end-systolic diameter (ESD), and shortening fraction (SF) for 15 taurine-supplemented cats with DCM. Period 0 (P0), date of presentation; P1, 1 to 2 weeks after presentation; P2, 3 to 4 weeks; P3, 5 to 6 weeks; P4, 7 to 8 weeks; P5, 9 to 12 weeks. The horizontal dotted lines represent the upper (EDD and ESD) and lower (SF) limits of clinical normality (95 per cent confidence interval) at the time the studies were performed. (Used with permission, Pion et al. Science 237:764–768, Aug 14, 1987. Copyright 1987 AAAS.)

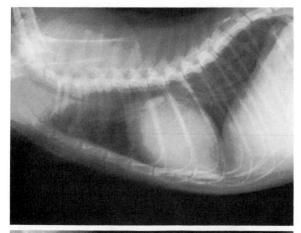

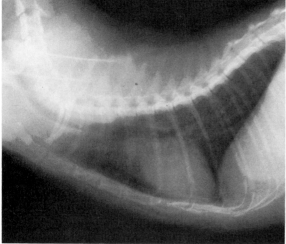

Figure 5. Thoracic radiographs (lateral projection) of a 4-year-old cat with DCM before (top) and 6 months after (bottom) beginning taurine supplementation. This cat received taurine supplementation for a total of 4 months. Altering the cat's diet to a taurine-supplemented diet then maintained adequate plasma taurine concentrations and normal myocardial function.

information serves as a guide in determining if other cats in the household are at risk. Also, correlating dietary patterns in cats with myocardial failure resulting from taurine deficiency may help identify commercial foods that do not provide adequate amounts of taurine.

Acquiring a complete diet history requires interviewing the person who is primarily responsible for feeding the patient. The aim is to define, in depth, the eating patterns of the patient. This includes the brand(s) of food, the type of food (canned, soft-moist, or dry), and the flavor(s) as well as the percentage of each food eaten. Hunting habits of other cats in the household may explain why plasma taurine concentrations are higher in some cats that are fed the same diet as the patient.

OBTAINING A SAMPLE

Many commercial laboratories offer plasma taurine analyses. However, most of these laboratories do not perform the analysis themselves. Most samples are forwarded to laboratories at research universities.

For the results of these analyses to be meaningful, precautions must be taken to avoid hemolysis or thrombosis of blood samples. Heparin is the anticoagulant of choice for collecting taurine samples. EDTA may interfere with the assay when performed by certain analytical techniques, making accurate determinations at low concentrations difficult. The ideal procedure for handling plasma taurine samples is to collect a 3-cc sample of blood from the jugular vein, using a 20- or 22-gauge needle and a preheparinized syringe. The heparinized blood should be transferred to a plastic tube or a silicone-coated glass tube (contacting glass activates platelets) and kept cool on ice. The sample should be spun immediately in a clinical centrifuge at a moderate to high speed for 10 min. As soon as the centrifuge has stopped, the plasma should be separated from the cellular pellet, making sure not to disturb the buffy coat, and the plasma should be frozen.

Taurine is a stable compound. Despite this stability, it is best to transport the sample to the laboratory frozen via overnight courier. If the sample is left at room temperature, bacteria that can utilize taurine may begin to grow in the plasma, resulting in artificially decreased plasma taurine concentrations.

INTERPRETING THE RESULTS

Plasma taurine concentrations are highly dependent on the amount of taurine in the diet and the type of diet. Canned diets generally contain meat products and therefore contain more taurine than dry diets. However, for reasons that are not fully understood, dry expanded diets require less taurine to support normal plasma taurine concentrations than do canned diets. In addition, plasma concentrations may increase after a meal and decrease during the postabsorptive period. For these reasons, normal plasma taurine concentrations are difficult to define. In the authors' experience, a plasma taurine concentration less than or equal to 20 nmol/ml in a cat with DCM is consistent with a diagnosis of taurine deficiency–induced myocardial failure in cats. The authors recommend that, if a particular diet does not support plasma taurine concentrations of at least 60 nmol/ml, the diet should be changed or supplemented with other foods that support higher plasma taurine concentrations.

Therapy

A few definitions may aid in the discussion of therapy. Heart disease is defined as any sign of

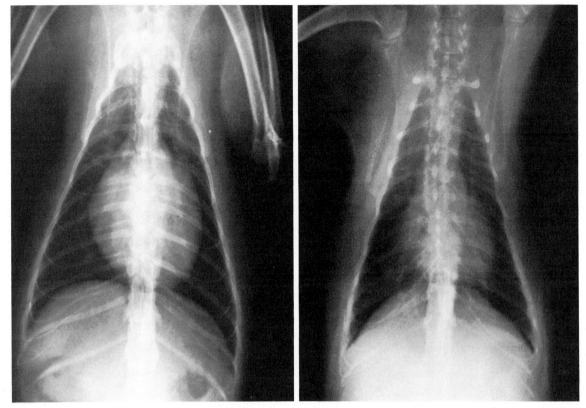

Figure 6. Thoracic radiographs (dorsoventral projection) of the same cat as in Figure 5 before (left) and 6 months after (right) beginning taurine supplementation.

cardiac dysfunction (e.g., murmur, arrhythmia, and cardiac malformation). Heart failure is a term generally describing clinical signs of congestion, such as pulmonary edema, pleural effusion, ascites, and peripheral edema, (i.e., *congestive heart failure*) or signs of low cardiac output (i.e., *low-output failure*). Most cats with DCM and congestive signs have pleural effusion that appears to be more predominant than pulmonary edema. However, the presence or absence of pleural effusion cannot be used to reliably differentiate among forms of myocardial disease. Myocardial failure is defined as a decrease in myocardial contractility. Dilated cardiomyopathy (primary myocardial failure) may occur without signs of heart failure (congestive or low output), with signs of low-output or congestive heart failure, or with signs of both congestive and low-output heart failure.

Initial management of cats with dilated cardiomyopathy is similar to that outlined earlier for hypertrophic cardiomyopathy, except that beta-blockers and calcium entry blockers are *not* indicated, whereas positive inotropic agents (digoxin, milrinone, dopamine, or dobutamine) may be indicated. Each of these points is controversial; however, a discussion of these controversies is beyond the scope of this article.

Prior to the finding that feline dilated cardiomyopathy is associated with low plasma taurine con-

centrations, therapy was palliative and based on the administration of drugs to alleviate the signs of heart failure. Positive inotropic drugs were administered to increase the heart muscle's ability to pump blood in an attempt to increase cardiac output and alleviate signs of low-output failure and to increase saluresis by increasing renal blood flow and augmenting the efficacy of diuretics. Diuretics (e.g., furosemide and hydrochlorothiazide) were utilized to increase the excretion of extracellular fluids, lower pulmonary and systemic venous pressures, and reduce signs of congestive failure. Arteriolar dilators (e.g., hydralazine) were utilized to reduce systemic vascular tone and increase cardiac output. Venodilators (e.g., nitroglycerin) were used to decrease pulmonary and systemic venous pressures, thus reducing signs of congestion and edema. Captopril, an angiotensin-converting enzyme inhibitor that inhibits the conversion of angiotensin I to angiotensin II (by converting enzyme in the lungs) and reduces circulating concentrations of angiotensin II and aldosterone, was often beneficial. The net effect of captopril's actions is reduced systemic vascular resistance and renal reabsorption of sodium chloride and water.

Many cats improved clinically after initial therapy with diuretics, vasodilators, and inotropic drugs. However, most of these cats continued to deteriorate echocardiographically and eventually died, usually within 6 months of diagnosis. With the advent of taurine therapy, definitive therapy for the myocardial failure due to taurine deficiency is possible. *Traditional heart failure therapy, including diuretics and captopril, is still required, especially during the first several weeks following diagnosis.* Whether digoxin (or other positive inotropic agents) should continue to be included in this list is unresolved. Cats treated by the authors during the past 24 months have not received positive inotropic drugs. In the absence of heart failure, taurine supplementation alone is all that is required to reverse the pathophysiologic changes described.

TAURINE AND CLINICAL MANAGEMENT OF DILATED CARDIOMYOPATHY

Many of the recommendations for managing cats with dilated cardiomyopathy outlined in this article represent the opinions of the authors, based on 2 years' experience with taurine therapy. Controlled studies have verified that taurine deficiency is a cause of dilated cardiomyopathy in cats and that taurine therapy is an effective means of managing these cats. However, the medical protocol outlined is not meant to be interpreted as the only way of managing these cases. These methods have worked in the authors' hands.

RECOMMENDED THERAPEUTIC PROTOCOL. Dilated cardiomyopathy is known to occur in almost all mammalian and avian species. The cat and possibly other obligate carnivores are the only species in which taurine deficiency myocardial failure is believed to occur. Therefore, it is unlikely that all cases of feline dilated cardiomyopathy result from taurine deficiency. However, evidence points to this as the major cause in the pet cat population. Thus, the authors recommend that *every cat with dilated cardiomyopathy should*

1. be considered taurine deficient.

2. have a plasma taurine sample submitted, prior to taurine supplementation or a dietary change, for confirmation of the diagnosis of taurine deficiency myocardial failure.

3. be treated with taurine orally *in addition to standard therapeutic modalities for the management of congestive heart failure* (e.g., pleurocentesis, furosemide, and captopril).

4. have their dietary history investigated, and all animals in the household with similar diets should have plasma taurine concentrations measured and be examined echocardiographically and treated appropriately.

TREATMENT OF THE CAT WITH TAURINE DEFICIENCY MYOCARDIAL FAILURE. Initial diagnostic procedures and therapy are identical to those described previously. These cats may be highly susceptible to stress and must be handled with minimal restraint and proper precautions before diagnostic procedures are undertaken. Most dyspneic cats tolerate pleurocentesis. Because most cats with dilated cardiomyopathy have pleural effusion and not florid pulmonary edema, this is often all that is required to stabilize these patients so that radiography and echocardiography can be safely performed.

The authors utilize the following diagnostic and treatment protocol (for the average 4–5 kg cat):

1. History (including diet history).

2. Physical examination (including fundoscopic evaluation for evidence of FCRD).

3. Pleurocentesis *prior to radiography*, if cat is dyspneic. If still dyspneic, radiography is postponed and echocardiography is attempted with minimal restraint to confirm the diagnosis. In severely dyspneic cats, all diagnostic procedures (except pleurocentesis) are postponed until cage rest (oxygen-enriched, if available) and diuretics relieve signs of congestion.

4. Radiography—to determine cardiac size and detect signs of congestive heart failure. Pleurocentesis, if pleural fluid is detected.

5. Obtain plasma for determination of plasma taurine concentration (note special handling instructions above). Baseline hemogram, serum chemistry determinations, and urinalysis, as indicated.

6. Baseline echocardiography—if unavailable, refer for evaluation and confirmation of diagnosis when stable, if possible.

7. Administration of diuretics (furosemide, 0.5 to 2.2 mg/kg equivalent to 3 to 12.5 mg s.i.d. to t.i.d.) if congestive heart failure is present.

8. Administration of captopril (0.5 to 1.0 mg/kg equivalent to 3 to 6 mg b.i.d. to t.i.d. PO) if congestive heart failure is severe or refractory to previous appropriate diuretic therapy.

9. Administration of taurine (250 to 500 mg b.i.d. PO). (Taurine is available in health food stores in 500-mg capsules.)

10. Unless the owner objects, cannot provide basic nursing care (including force feeding food and liquids), or would be unable to tolerate the animal dying at home, these cats thrive better at home. Effective client communication is important, and follow-up is essential.

11. Communication to the owner that the prognosis is guarded. Cats that are critically ill may die within hours to days of diagnosis.

The benefits of inotropic therapy in these early stages is unknown, but it is recommended by some cardiologists. Initial impressions are that minimizing stress and providing good nursing care (encouraging intake of food and water, monitoring for signs of dyspnea) are the most important factors affecting survival. The diet eaten during this initial period is not critical. Dehydration and hypothermia should be managed. The client should be advised to feed whatever the cat will eat.

RESPONSE TO TREATMENT

Most owners report clinical improvement (e.g., improved appetite, activity, respiratory patterns, and interactions with family members) within 4 to 10 days of beginning therapy. A small percentage of cats die within 7 days despite therapy. For this reason, it is important to emphasize to clients that, although the prognosis for feline dilated cardiomyopathy is much more promising than in the past, the initial prognosis must remain guarded until a clinical response is observed. After a clinical response is identified, the prognosis becomes good.

Echocardiographic improvement is usually not apparent prior to 3 to 6 weeks of taurine supplementation. By 6 weeks (or rarely up to 12 weeks after taurine therapy), an echocardiogram should demonstrate improvement in systolic function (decreased end-systolic diameter and increased fractional shortening). Radiographs should show resolution of or greatly decreased pleural effusion and a decrease in the size of the cardiac silhouette. If pleural effusion is absent or minimal, dosage of furosemide and captopril may be decreased at this time.

By 6 to 12 weeks, pleural effusion should be resolved, and furosemide and captopril may be discontinued. To be conservative, owners should be advised to continue to observe for signs of dyspnea and to return 1 week after discontinuing diuretic therapy for radiographs to confirm the resolution of pleural effusion. Echocardiographic parameters should be significantly improved in most cats by 12 to 16 weeks of taurine supplementation. However, a slower response is not cause for alarm so long as a response is observed.

When the cat's clinical and echocardiographic findings approach normal, the authors recommend adjusting the diet to one the cat will eat after discontinuing taurine supplementation. The length of time to continue taurine supplementation for optimum results is not known, but the amount prescribed can be decreased to 250 mg once daily at the time echocardiographic improvement is noted. Taurine supplementation may be discontinued by 12 to 16 weeks if echocardiographic values are near normal and the cat will eat a diet known to support "normal" plasma taurine concentrations (> 60 nmol/ml). Plasma taurine concentration is rechecked in all cats 2 to 4 weeks after discontinuing taurine supplementation to ensure that the diet fed produces adequate plasma concentrations.

Prognosis

The degree of cardiac dilation and hypomotility does not appear to correlate with clinical signs or prognosis in cats with dilated cardiomyopathy. Patients with echocardiographically severe myocardial failure (FS < 15 per cent) and a stable clinical presentation are probably less at risk of imminent death than patients with moderate myocardial failure (FS < 25 per cent) and severe dyspnea, hypothermia, dehydration, and weakness. Therefore, prognosis depends more on clinical signs and response to therapy than on the degree of myocardial failure detected by echocardiography at the time of diagnosis. Prognosis for cats with dilated cardiomyopathy, without arterial thromboembolism due to taurine deficiency, is excellent if there is survival after the first 7 to 10 days. Of the 28 cats treated with taurine by the authors, three died within the first 10 days; only one died after that time, and one cat was euthanatized because of a nonresponsive pleural effusion. Seven cats, not included in this list, died or were euthanatized within hours of presentation.

Dietary Recommendations

Prior to March 1987, most cat foods analyzed contained 1 to 15 times the National Research Council (NRC) recommendation for dietary taurine concentrations. To explain why feeding these cat foods resulted in the depletion of plasma taurine, it was hypothesized that either the recommendation was too low or cats were not absorbing or retaining all the taurine provided by the manufacturer. In actuality, both were true. Many dry foods contained 500 to 750 mg of taurine per kilogram of dry diet. Most cats fed 500 mg of taurine per kilogram of dry diet have blood concentrations of taurine that are lower than the authors' research indicates is safe. At the time the NRC recommendation was made, the evidence indicated that these blood levels were safe. In addition, even though most canned (wet) foods contained two to ten times the recommended amount of taurine (equivalent to one to five times what is now believed to be safe) some still resulted in low blood levels. This is because the taurine is, for an unknown reason, not fully absorbed or retained. Adding more taurine to these foods appears to provide enough taurine so that cats maintain adequate blood levels. Currently, it appears that dry expanded diets containing taurine concentrations of 1000 to 1200 mg/kg of dry diet will maintain normal plasma taurine concentrations, whereas taurine concentrations of 2000 to 2500 mg/kg of dry weight are necessary in canned foods to maintain normal plasma taurine concentrations in adult cats.

Most but not all of the commercial foods that had been found to cause low plasma taurine concentrations have been supplemented as of early 1988. However, there still may be unsupplemented foods in circulation on store shelves or in storage. For these reasons, it is important not to assume that food being fed is supplemented. In addition, there may be conditions (e.g., malabsorption syndromes and aminoaciduria syndromes) in which taurine depletion may occur in a cat eating normally adequate amounts of taurine. For the aforementioned reasons, it is important to determine plasma taurine concentrations in every feline patient with dilated cardiomyopathy and to correlate results with the available diet history. During this time of transition from unsupplemented to supplemented foods, it may be impossible to identify cats with dilated cardiomyopathy that have had previous taurine deficiency but who are now on a supplemented diet and have plasma taurine concentrations higher than expected for the diagnosis. Therefore, the only definitive way to rule out taurine deficiency as the cause of dilated cardiomyopathy in these cats is to demonstrate a lack of improvement in myocardial function during a 3-month period in which plasma taurine concentrations greater than 60 nmol/ml have been achieved by supplementation.

In general, it is probably most prudent to recommend a varied diet. It is convenient and has been recommended to feed dogs and cats a single type of processed food. However, common nutritional guidelines and common sense dictate that this may not be adequate. Feeding a variety of diets, all of which are marketed as being adequate, will provide a lower risk of an animal's developing a nutritional deficiency or excess than feeding only one diet.

Conclusions

Prior to the recognition of taurine deficiency myocardial failure, feline dilated cardiomyopathy was thought to be the end-stage, irreversible result of an acute or chronic insult to the myocardium. Viral, immune, and toxic etiologies were considered probable candidates in conjunction with a possible genetic predisposition.

Taurine deficiency appears to be the major cause of dilated cardiomyopathy in cats. Dilated cardiomyopathy is recognized in many species of mammals and birds, most of which are not thought to be at risk of developing taurine deficiency. Because it is likely that disease in cats shares common etiologies with that in these species, the authors believe that, although taurine deficiency is very important, it probably is not the only cause of dilated cardiomyopathy in cats.

Taurine supplementation normalizes myocardial function in cats with taurine-deficiency DCM. Because taurine-depleting diets may remain in circulation and many cats have only recently begun eating taurine-supplemented diets, it may be difficult to determine the incidence of taurine deficiency myocardial failure (a secondary cardiomyopathy) for several years. Only time and careful observation will provide information regarding the incidence of primary idiopathic dilated cardiomyopathy in cats.

References and Supplemental Reading

Bond, B. R., and Fox, P. R.: Advances in feline cardiomyopathy. Vet. Clin. North Am. [Small Anim. Pract.] 14:1021, 1984.

Bright, J. M., and Golden, A. L.: The use of calcium channel blockers in cats with hypertrophic cardiomyopathy. Proceedings of the Sixth Symposium of the American College of Veterinary Internal Medicine, Washington, D.C., 1988, p. 184.

Fox, P. R.: Feline myocardial diseases. In Kirk, R. W. (ed.): Current Veterinary Therapy VIII. Philadelpia: W. B. Saunders Co., 1983, p. 337.

Harpster, N. K.: Feline myocardial diseases. In Kirk, R. W. (ed.): Current Veterinary Therapy IX. Philadelphia: W. B. Saunders Co., 1986, p. 380.

Harpster, N. K.: The cardiovascular system. In Holzworth, J. (ed.): Diseases of the Cat. Medicine and Surgery. Vol. 1. Philadelphia: W. B. Saunders Co., 1987, p. 820.

Huxtable, R. J., and Sebring, L. A.: Cardiovascular actions of taurine. In Kuriyama, K., Huxtable, R. J., and Iwata, H.: Sulfur Amino Acids, Biochemical and Clinical Aspects (Proceedings of an International Symposium and the 5th Annual Meeting of the Japanese Research Society on Sulfur Amino Acids, August 7–10, 1982, Tokyo). New York: A. R. Liss, 1983, p. 5.

Liu, S-K.: Left ventricular false tendons associated with cardiac malfunction in 101 cats. Lab. Invest. 56:44A, 1987.

Pion, P. D., Kittleson, M. D., Rogers, Q. R., et al.: Myocardial failure in cats associated with low plasma taurine: A reversible cardiomyopathy. Science 237:764, 1987.

Tonachini, T. M. A., Breznock, E. M., and Pion, P. D.: Correlation between lipoprotein electrophoresis and triglyceride concentration in chylous and nonchylous effusions in cats (abstract). Proceedings of the Tenth Annual House Officer Seminar Day, School of Veterinary Medicine, University of California, Davis, CA, 1988.

Van Vleet, J. F., and Ferran, V. J.: Myocardial diseases of animals. Am. J. Pathol. 124:95, 1986.

CANINE AND FELINE
HEARTWORM DISEASE

THOMAS N. HRIBERNIK, D.V.M.

Baton Rouge, Louisiana

Dirofilaria immitis infection in dogs, and to a lesser extent in cats, is not uncommon throughout much of the continental United States and Hawaii. The highest incidence of infection remains in the southeastern Atlantic and Gulf Coast states. It is a completely preventable infection in the dog if appropriate protective measures are taken. The clinical abnormalities resulting from heartworm infection are varied and include exercise intolerance, respiratory signs (coughing and tachypnea), syncope, right-sided congestive heart failure, and sudden death. On the whole appropriate management of this condition is rewarding for patient, owner, and veterinarian.

A detailed account of all the various aspects of heartworm disease is beyond the scope of this article. For a more detailed discussion of the pathophysiology of heartworm disease, laboratory tests used to diagnose patent infections, and uncommon syndromes associated with canine heartworm disease, the reader is referred to the references and supplemental reading list.

CANINE HEARTWORM DISEASE

Preadulticide Evaluation

The pretreatment evaluation of the patient with confirmed heartworm infection should first, and foremost, take into account the relevant historical and physical findings of the animal in question. These will often dictate the diagnostic tests and procedures necessary prior to administration of adulticide medication. In a limited number of clinical scenarios such as the caval syndrome, the historical and physical findings may be all that are necessary and prudent in the microfilaremic patient to dictate the initial therapeutic measures.

There is currently no consensus as to what should constitute a minimum preadulticide data base. The American Heartworm Society (Otto, 1983) has suggested that, besides a thorough history and physical examination, the preadulticide evaluation include a urinalysis, complete blood count, blood urea nitrogen, and perhaps tests to assess liver function. It is also suggested that thoracic radiographs can be useful in determining the degree of pulmonary parenchymal and vascular disease present.

The decision to perform preadulticide laboratory work is often based on one or more of the following premises. Because thiacetarsamide is a potent hepatotoxin and nephrotoxin, preadulticide evidence of liver or kidney disease may preclude use in some patients. Most patients have no significant evidence of pre-existing routine biochemical test abnormalities of these organ systems. Another reason for laboratory testing is to detect underlying disorders related or unrelated to heartworm infection in patients not outwardly displaying abnormal signs or symptoms. This may enable one to identify significant abnormalities that require immediate attention or preclude adulticide therapy at least temporarily.

Laboratory testing in patients with historical or physical examination findings suggesting medical problems related or unrelated to heartworm infection definitely bears merit. This expansion of the patient's data base will often enable one to more clearly define the patient's problems. It may also result in a decision to perform additional diagnostic tests or procedures to more appropriately define potential abnormalities. In some situations, it could result in postponement of adulticide therapy.

Another reason that has been traditionally offered for performing preadulticide laboratory tests is the ability to predict which patient will have acute adverse reactions such as anorexia, vomiting, or icterus during adulticide therapy. A large retrospective study at the author's institution failed to identify any preadulticide laboratory test that would predict which patient would have reactions during adulticide therapy. While renal failure should be carefully assessed prior to any arsenical therapy, elevation of liver enzyme levels is not predictive of adverse drug reactions and does not by itself contraindicate carparsolate treatment.

It is unlikely that a consensus will ever exist regarding what should constitute a preadulticide laboratory test data base. However, it could be argued that in most young, asymptomatic dogs pretreatment laboratory tests may be unnecessary. In the final analysis, the clinician should use his or her judgment of each patient as an aid in deciding what should be included in the preadulticide laboratory test data base.

Thoracic radiographs taken prior to adulticide therapy are often beneficial. They will enable one to clinically assess the severity of pulmonary arterial and parenchymal disease. This, in turn, may alter pretreatment and preadulticide strategies and affect prognosis. Evidence of thromboembolism or eosinophilic pneumonitis dictates additional treatment (generally prednisolone, 1 mg/kg daily for 7 to 10 days) prior to adulticide therapy. Other radiographic abnormalities associated with heartworm disease may also be observed. The author believes that information gained from thoracic radiographs is of significant benefit in most patients, with the possible exception of young, asymptomatic dogs. Angiographic studies have limited utility in most cases.

The electrocardiographic (ECG) evaluation of the dog with heartworm disease is considered an optional diagnostic procedure. Although one may observe evidence of right ventricular enlargement with advanced heartworm disease, this is of little significance by itself. Patients with exercise intolerance, syncope, pulse deficits, or right-sided heart failure should have at least a lead II rhythm strip run to check for arrhythmias.

Echocardiographic evaluation is an unnecessary diagnostic procedure in most animals. In advanced heartworm disease one may note such abnormalities as right ventricular dilation, free-wall hypertrophy, abnormal septal motion, and abnormal tricuspid valve excursions. However, these findings by themselves will generally not result in alterations in therapeutic or diagnostic procedures. An exception to this limited utility may occur with the caval syndrome; the findings in this syndrome are described below.

Occult Heartworm Infection

Dogs infected with adult *D. immitis* but without demonstrable evidence of microfilaremia are said to have occult infections. The overall reported incidence of occult infections has varied from 10 to 67 per cent of the heartworm-infected canine population as a whole. Generally speaking, animals with advanced heartworm disease have the highest likelihood of being amicrofilaremic.

Occult infections can arise for a variety of reasons, although four major mechanisms are proposed. (1) Most individuals believe that immune-mediated microfilarial destruction or sequestration is the major cause of amicrofilaremic heartworm infection. (2) Prepatent infections can, on occasion, also result in significant disease. This effect is not always related to the number of developing parasites. (3) Another potential reason for an occult state is the presence of an adulticide-induced or naturally occurring unisexual infection. The former is distinctly possible in light of the relative resistance of female worms

and young adults to the parasiticidal effect of thiacetarsamide. The clinical significance of this possibility in the majority of animals treated with adulticide remains undetermined. Naturally occurring unisexual infections have been thought to be relatively uncommon and, when present, to be infrequently associated with significant clinical disease. However, it has recently been shown that a significant number of dogs with occult infections in a *D. immitis* hyperenzootic area had unisexual infections. (4) Finally, drug-induced suppression of microfilaria can also result in at least a transient amicrofilaremic state. Microfilaricides (particularly ivermectin at certain dosages) administered to dogs with adult worms can temporarily eliminate circulating microfilariae. It has not been determined whether occult states will result from the long-term administration of a low dose of ivermectin used as preventive measure in animals in which prophylaxis was begun too late to prevent maturation of developing worms.

Any dog with cardiopulmonary signs consistent with heartworm disease in which an amicrofilaremic state has been documented by a standard, acceptable technique for microfilarial detection such as the filter concentration tests or modified Knott's method should be considered a "candidate" for occult infection. In addition, in a *D. immitis*–prevalent area, any animal with a questionable, preventive administration program should be suspected of having an occult infection.

When suspicion exists for the presence of an occult infection, it becomes necessary to pursue the diagnosis with a method other than those used to detect microfilariae. Serodiagnostic tests have greatly improved the ability to do this. Earlier tests, which employed various technologies to detect host *antibody* to parasite antigen (adults or microfilariae), have been supplanted by those that detect circulating *antigens* of adult worms. The adult antigen assays utilize monoclonal antibody–based technology, which enables the detection of antigens of both male and female worms. A variety of adult antigen tests are currently available and are quite specific and sensitive for the detection of *D. immitis* infection. Most of these appear to be quite efficient in detecting infections with more than five worms. One current test is thought to be relatively effective in detecting the presence of infections with as little as one worm (Cite, AgriTech Systems, Inc., Portland, ME).

The antigen assay tests may also be used after carparsolate treatment to determine adulticide efficacy. Antigen titers have been reported to be negative by 12 weeks after adulticide administration if therapy is effective. However, most of the current tests are more inconsistent in detecting adult worm burdens of less than five. An additional future application of the adult antigen assays may reside in their potential use as a predictor of clinically significant thromboembolic disease prior to treatment. Because this will require quantitation of blood antigen levels, alterations in available assays will be needed.

Thoracic radiographs can also be used to diagnose occult infections. Radiographic abnormalities tend to be related to the adult worm burden, duration of infection, and host-parasite interactions. A number of potential radiographic findings typical of heartworm infection are possible. These may include enlargement of lobar pulmonary arteries (particularly those distributed caudally), right ventricular enlargement, increased prominence of the main pulmonary artery segment, and increased perivascular parenchymal pattern. These are the most commonly observed findings. The radiographic findings in pulmonary thromboembolism are covered below. The reader is referred to the suggested reading list for radiographic findings in dogs with allergic or eosinophilic pneumonitis.

The management of the patient with occult infection will depend to a large extent on the type of heartworm disease present. Supportive measures may be indicated prior to adulticide treatment in some cases. Occult heartworm patients should have preventive therapy initiated prior to, or concurrent with, adulticide therapy. When indicated, aspirin may be administered to dogs, as described later. Microfilaricides are obviously not necessary in the amicrofilaremic state.

Treatment

ADULTICIDE THERAPY

Thiacetarsamide remains the adulticide of choice for *D. immitis* infection. Reports in the past several years have provided enlightening information about this drug. Thiacetarsamide appears to be effective against the late fourth stage developing larvae of *D. immitis*. Its adulticide efficacy is believed to be decidedly less than originally thought. This is because young adult worms are not easily killed by the drug, plus female worms are more resistant than males to its adulticide effect. Efficacy of the drug is also related to the length of time adults are exposed to the minimum effective concentration of arsenic rather than peak blood arsenic concentrations. These findings probably account for the difficulty in totally eliminating infection in many animals.

An attempt to improve efficacy by extending the treatment period to 3 days (six injections) has been shown to result in no significant difference from that seen with the standard 2-day regimen (four injections). The 3-day regimen may also result in an increased severity of postadulticide pulmonary

embolism. Substantial improvement in efficacy has been observed when an increased dosage of thiacetarsamide is given. Preliminary reports suggest that a 20 per cent increase in dosage per injection may be indicated to improve worm kill. However, postadulticide embolism tends to be more pronounced at this dosage. Patients deemed suitable candidates for adulticide therapy are admitted to the hospital. Until additional work is published, it is recommended to use the standard dosage of 2.2 mg/kg *twice daily for 2 days* intravenously. Six- to 8-hour intervals between daily injections with overnight intervals of less than 16 hours may be more effective than longer periods of time. This suggestion is related to the effect of injection interval spacing on the postdistribution blood arsenic concentrations. Although it has been recommended not to give consecutive injections into the same peripheral vein, no consistent problems are recognized with utilization of the same vein for each injection.

It has been shown in experimental infections that aspirin will reduce or retard pulmonary arterial disease development. In addition, aspirin administration will improve postadulticide pulmonary arterial blood flow. In some animals it will improve pulmonary parenchymal disease, whereas in others it can result in a worsening of parenchymal disease. Administration of aspirin could be theoretically beneficial to all dogs undergoing adulticide therapy; however, in most dogs that are asymptomatic or have mild disease, it is doubtful whether aspirin should be given. Dogs with *advanced* clinical signs or symptoms and radiographic evidence of severe pulmonary arterial disease do appear to benefit from aspirin. The dosage of aspirin given is 5 mg/kg daily for 7 to 14 days before and for approximately 30 days after adulticide treatment. Another potential use for aspirin is in the geriatric patient that is deemed to be an unsuitable candidate for adulticide. Vomiting, melena, hemoptysis, and bleeding are reasons to stop aspirin therapy.

The major acute adverse effects of thiacetarsamide administration are anorexia, vomiting, and icterus. Approximately 15 to 30 per cent of treated animals will experience one or more of these side effects. Most of these will be noted after the first or second injection. The patient's appetite should be evaluated by feeding a portion of the daily meal prior to each injection. The dog should also be checked for evidence of icterus prior to each injection. Therapy should be suspended in any patient with evidence of profuse, protracted vomiting or icterus. Anorexia should not be used as a reason to abort adulticide treatment. However, anorexia in conjunction with vomiting may be an indication to stop therapy. If adulticide therapy is aborted for any reason, symptomatic therapy, such as intravenous fluids, should be given if necessary. These animals can be retreated in 2 to 4 weeks with the complete adulticide regimen with relative impunity.

Less common acute adverse side effects include perivascular injection of adulticide, bleeding, thromboembolism, and right-sided heart failure or an acute worsening of congestive heart failure. Any area that has received perivascular injection of thiacetarsamide should have dimethyl sulfoxide (DMSO) applied topically three to four times daily. The other aforementioned side effects are discussed on pages 131 to 134 (Calvert and Rawlings, 1986).

On completion of adulticide therapy, the dog is sent home with instructions to have severely restricted exercise for 30 days. Owners should be advised to report anorexia, lethargy, depression, coughing or increased coughing, bleeding, and breathing difficulties during this time. Patients are routinely checked at 1 week after adulticide therapy. Microfilaricide therapy is given to all microfilaria-positive patients at 3 to 4 weeks after thiacetarsamide therapy, unless they are experiencing significant complications such as thromboembolism or bleeding.

MICROFILARICIDE THERAPY

All microfilaremic dogs should undergo therapy with a microfilaricide 3 to 4 weeks after adulticide treatment. Although the only microfilaricide approved by the Food and Drug Administration (FDA) is dithiazanine iodide, ivermectin is a widely used and extremely efficacious microfilaricidal agent. FDA approval of ivermectin as a microfilaricide is not anticipated. However, it is currently the microfilaricide of choice at the author's institution, although its use is avoided in collies or mixed-breeds of suspected collie lineage.

Ivermectin will eradicate the microfilariae from most dogs within 3 weeks of administration. Dramatic declines in microfilarial counts usually occur within the first several hours after administration. This rapid kill-off may account for some of the acute adverse effects that have been observed. Additional toxicity is related to the drug's blockade of gammaaminobutyric acid in the central nervous system.

Dogs to be treated with ivermectin are admitted to the hospital in the morning. Ivermectin is administered at a dosage of 0.05 mg/kg orally. Ivermectin (Ivomec, Merck Sharp & Dohme) is most commonly diluted to a 1:10 solution with propylene glycol. This solution can be dosed orally at 1 ml/20 kg to achieve the 0.05 mg/kg dosage. During the day the animal is periodically monitored for adverse reactions (see page 141). The more common side effects include listlessness, ataxia, vomiting, diarrhea, mydriasis, and shock. Most reactions are mild, although occasionally a dog will require intravenous fluid therapy and corticosteroids. Barring any major adverse reactions, the dog is sent home with instructions to return in 3 weeks for a microfilaria concentration test. If it is negative at that time, prophylactic therapy is initiated. If microfilaremia persists, it is wise to recheck the blood 1 week later, because only 90 per cent of treated animals will be negative at 3 weeks.

Persistent microfilaremia at the end of 4 weeks can be attributed to several possibilities. Although all adults may have been killed, the occasional dog may require a second microfilaricide regimen to finally clear the microfilaremia. A second distinct possibility is that not all of the adult worms have been killed. A positive result with an adult antigen assay at 12 weeks after adulticide therapy will confirm this. Unfortunately, not all dogs with residual adult worm infection will have positive results on the occult test. In the final analysis, if direct or circumstantial evidence exists for adult worm persistence, the adulticide will need to be readministered. Because the remaining worms are likely to be resistant to the adulticide, it is best to wait a minimum of 6 months before retreating. Ivermectin can be used at a preventive dosage during the interim to prevent acquisition of additional infection.

PREVENTIVE THERAPY

The veterinary profession has two excellent preventive agents available. Diethylcarbamazine (DEC) is a time-proven product, which is available in liquid, tablets, and chewable tablets. Given at a daily dosage of approximately 6.0 to 7.0 mg/kg, it is highly efficacious against developing fourth stage larvae. It should be started prior to the appearance of mosquitoes and continued for a minimum of 60 days after the mosquito season. In subtropical regions, this means that animals continuously receive the drug. The only contraindication for DEC use is that it should not be given to microfilaremic dogs prior to adulticide and microfilaricide. However if microfilaremia is detected in a dog receiving diethylcarbamazine, it is safe to continue its use while appropriate treatment is instituted.

Ivermectin (Heartguard, Merck Sharpe & Dohme) has recently received FDA approval as a heartworm preventive. Like diethylcarbamazine, it is a highly efficacious larvicide. It may be administered with relative impunity to all breeds of dogs and to dogs with existing microfilaremia. It is given once per month at a dosage of 0.006 mg/kg. The wide safety range of the drug is readily apparent when one notes that the manufacturer markets the drug in three different dosages covering a wide weight range for each dosage.

Associated Conditions

PULMONARY THROMBOEMBOLISM

Naturally occurring and adulticide-induced pulmonary thromboembolism can result in significant morbidity, and occasional mortality, in the canine heartworm disease patient. The dead and dying adult worms cause regional arterial thrombosis, severe endothelial damage, edema and inflammation in the pulmonary interstitium and alveoli, pulmonary hypertension, increased right ventricular afterload, and ventilation-perfusion mismatching.

A number of clinical findings are possible in the thromboembolic patient. Presenting complaints most commonly reported are cough, breathing difficulty, and variable degrees of lethargy, depression, and anorexia. Hemoptysis and bleeding from other body orifices may be observed in a lesser number of animals. Physical findings are variable but often include depression, pyrexia, cough, respiratory difficulty, tachycardia, and abnormal lung sounds. Additional possible findings include evidence of right-sided heart failure, hemorrhage, and pale mucous membranes. These historical and physical findings can be observed in untreated dogs, but they are most commonly noted 5 to 21 days after adulticide treatment. Dogs with preadulticide radiographic evidence of severe pulmonary arterial enlargement and tortuosity appear to be at the greatest risk for clinically apparent postadulticide complications associated with thromboembolism.

The radiographic findings associated with both naturally occurring and adulticide-induced thromboembolism can be quite variable. As a generalization, the caudal and accessory lobes are most commonly affected. Poorly defined focal and coalescing interstitial and alveolar densities adjacent to the affected arteries are often noted.

Other diagnostic findings that may be observed in the thromboembolic patient include thrombocytopenia, neutrophilic leukocytosis, laboratory evidence of disseminated intravascular coagulation (DIC), anemia, and decreased arterial Po_2. Transtracheal aspiration sampling will reveal a microbiologically sterile inflammatory process. The cytologic findings will vary from predominantly neutrophilic to a mixed neutrophilic-mononuclear response with variable numbers of eosinophils.

Most patients with mild clinical evidence of thromboembolism can be managed on an outpatient basis. Prednisone or prednisolone is given at a dosage of 0.5 mg/kg twice daily for 5 to 7 days orally. The owners are also instructed to severely restrict the animal's exercise. Animals that have severe coughing, hemoptysis, cyanosis, or respiratory distress should be hospitalized. Corticosteroids should be given at the previously described dosage. Bronchodilators and oxygen therapy may be needed for animals with cyanosis or severe respiratory distress. Fluid therapy should be administered to animals in which it is deemed necessary. Aspirin therapy probably should be discontinued in the dog exhibiting hemoptysis or laboratory evidence of DIC.

The prognosis for most dogs with thromboembolism is good. When mortality occurs, it is generally confined to those patients with pre-existing severe pulmonary arterial disease or those with severe heart failure.

THE CAVAL SYNDROME

The caval syndrome represents an acute life-threatening form of heartworm disease associated with heavy adult worm burdens in the venae cavae and right atrium. The reason why only some dogs develop the caval syndrome is unclear. Recent experimental work has demonstrated that development of caval syndrome involves more than just the number of worms related to body weight or the severity of the worm burden. Several studies have revealed a marked predilection for the syndrome to develop in male dogs. It does appear that retrograde migration of adult worms in the venae cavae and right atrium from 5 to 17 months after infection is important. This migration results in at least a partial inflow obstruction of blood from the venae cavae to the right side of the heart, with mechanical interference to the tricuspid valve apparatus.

Pre-existing pulmonary hypertension resulting from pulmonary vascular disease has an additive effect on right ventricular dysfunction. Left ventricular preload and cardiac output may also be substantially reduced. Red blood cell hemolysis results from mechanical trauma owing to impaction on the adult worm mass, plus a fibrin meshwork if DIC is present. The hepatorenal dysfunction often observed may be caused by the combined effects of chronic passive congestion, decreased perfusion, and hemolysis.

The clinical findings of the caval syndrome are fairly characteristic. It is most commonly observed in young male dogs in which appropriate heartworm preventive measures have not been taken. The peak seasonal incidence occurs in the spring and early summer. Most dogs will have no antecedent clinical signs typical of those seen with symptomatic heartworm disease. The principal historical findings in these animals are a sudden onset of anorexia, weakness, depression, and respiratory difficulty. Physical examination findings often include pale mucous membranes, jugular vein distention and pulsation, respiratory difficulty, and a systolic murmur. Other findings include hepatosplenomegaly, abdominal distention, icterus, and abnormal lung sounds.

A number of diagnostic test abnormalities may be observed. Common laboratory findings include microfilaremia, hemoglobinemia, hemoglobinuria, regenerative anemia, red blood cell fragmentation, elevated liver enzyme levels, and elevated blood urea nitrogen. Possible additional findings include bilirubinemia, bilirubinuria, neutrophilic leukocytosis, and increased bromsulphalein (BSP) dye retention. Laboratory evidence of DIC may also be observed. Thoracic radiography will often reveal evidence of moderate to severe heartworm disease. Potential abnormal electrocardiographic findings include evidence of right ventricular enlargement, sinus tachcardia, and occasionally atrial or ventricular premature complexes. Echocardiographic evidence of echodense adult worms in the right atrium with movement into the right ventricle during diastole is considered pathognomic of the caval syndrome. Finally, an elevated central venous pressure is observed in a large number of animals.

The treatment of choice for the caval syndrome is surgical removal of the worms. The animal is restrained, and a surgically prepared lateral jugular venotomy is performed under local anesthesia. Either sterile alligator forceps (20 to 40 cm in length) or an endoscopic basket (Spiral Basket, Mill-Rose Laboratories, Mentor, OH) is passed through the venotomy site down to the level of the fourth or fifth intercostal space. One to four worms are usually removed with each retrieval attempt. The process of removal should continue until five or six successive attempts fail to retrieve worms. After the worms have been removed the jugular vein is ligated and the surgical site is closed in a routine manner.

Fluid therapy is also indicated to maintain blood pressure and tissue perfusion. Overzealous fluid delivery should be avoided, at least initially, because most animals will have high central venous pressures at the time of diagnosis and for several hours after worm removal. Concomitant central venous pressure measurement is useful to help avoid excessive fluid administration.

Approximately 15 to 40 per cent of the animals in which worms have been successfully removed will die. Those that survive should be treated with adulticide once the clinical and laboratory abnormalities have returned to normal. In most patients this takes approximately 2 to 4 weeks.

RIGHT-SIDED HEART FAILURE

Right-sided heart failure due to severe chronic heartworm disease is not an uncommon finding in endemic areas. It is the result of a protracted elevated right ventricular afterload caused by the pulmonary hypertension of severe pulmonary arterial disease. Pulmonary thromboembolism may also contribute to the development of heart failure in some dogs.

Large breed male dogs, usually 3 to 8 years of age, are most commonly affected. Presenting complaints often noted are exercise intolerance or syncope, variable degrees of anorexia and lethargy, distended abdomen, cough, weight loss, and occa-sionally respiratory distress. Physical examination will usually reveal cachexia, abdominal distention (due to hepatomegaly and ascites) and distended jugular veins with pulsations. Other possible findings include a split second heart sound, right atrioventricular (AV) valve systolic murmur, hepatomegaly, splenomegaly, abnormal lung sounds, cough, and respiratory distress. Rarely, poorly audible heart sounds may be detected in animals with significant hydrothorax or pericardial effusion. Peripheral edema is rarely noted.

Common laboratory test abnormalities noted in patients with right-sided heart failure due to heartworm disease include mild to moderate nonregenerative anemia, neutrophilic leukocytosis, eosinophilia, basophilia, mild to moderate elevations in liver enzyme levels, prerenal azotemia, prolonged BSP dye retention, and ascites classified as a modified transudative. Microfilaremia is not always evident. In this case, if doubt exists as to the diagnosis, an appropriate adult antigen assay should be performed.

Thoracic radiographic findings will not allow one to determine whether right-sided heart failure is present. However, they will invariably reveal some evidence of advanced disease such as severe right ventricular enlargement, enlarged main pulmonary artery segment, and enlarged and tortuous lobar arteries. Various pulmonary parenchymal changes may also be noted. Electrocardiographic evidence of right ventricular enlargement is a common finding in right-sided heart failure.

The pretreatment data base for right-sided heart failure patients should include hemogram, biochemical profile, complete urinalysis, lead II ECG rhythm strip, and thoracic radiographs. The finding of most of the laboratory abnormalities previously mentioned or occasional atrial or ventricular premature complexes should not deter one from contemplating adulticide therapy. Dogs with radiographic evidence of thromboembolism should receive therapy with corticosteroids for 7 to 14 days and prior to adulticide therapy.

Calvert and Rawlings (1986) have clearly shown that the most beneficial way of treating right-sided heart failure is to administer adulticide after a stabilization period. The preadulticide stabilization period consists of 7 to 14 days of cage rest, oral furosemide at a dosage of 2 to 4 mg/kg twice daily, 5 mg/kg of aspirin daily, and a low-sodium diet. At the end of this period, adulticide is administered at the previously recommended dosage and duration. This is then followed by an additional 3 to 4 weeks of cage rest, administration of diuretics and aspirin, and low-sodium diet. Dogs so treated have a markedly improved survival rate over those managed differently. It appears that, in addition to the long-term benefits of eradicating most if not all of the adults with thiacetarsamide, aspirin therapy and cage rest are major determinants of survival. It should be noted that like many others, the author does *not* use digitalis compounds (unless atrial fibriliation has developed) or vasodilator therapy.

A number of potential problems with this therapeutic regimen have become apparent. A real problem is the cost of hospitalizing these dogs for the prescribed period. A viable alternative is for the client to purchase a suitable cage and confine the animal at home. These animals should be re-evaluated at least weekly. Other problems include persistent anorexia, gastrointestinal bleeding due to the aspirin, and thromboembolism with transient intensification of the failure state and DIC. The persistent anorexia can rapidly result in hypokalemia and its attendant side effects owing to the concomitant diuretic therapy. If the animal will not eat the low-sodium diet, every effort should be made to entice it to eat (see pp. 302–307). Decreased furosemide dosage or an alternate diuretic with less kaliuretic effect (spironolactone [Aldactazide, Searle], 2 mg/kg b.i.d.) should also be considered. Aspirin administration may need to be suspended in animals with evidence of gastrointestinal bleeding. Some authors have suggested that cimetidine be used in conjunction with aspirin to avert this problem. Thromboembolism should be treated as previously mentioned. The development of DIC in most of these dogs is a harbinger of impending death in spite of supportive therapy. Despite all of these potential problems, the treatment regimen previously described remains the one of choice. The prognosis for survival in animals so treated is approximately 80 per cent.

FELINE HEARTWORM DISEASE

The cat is considered a susceptible but resistant host for *Dirofilaria immitis*. The potential for feline heartworm disease tends to parallel that of canine disease in a given area but occurs at a lower prevalence. Recognition of infection has increased over the past several years as the practicing veterinarian has become aware of associated clinical findings.

Several differences from *D. immitis* infection in the dog are apparent. The percentage of infective larvae that develop into adult worms is significantly less. Because of this, adult worm burdens are less, with a range of one to nine worms and an average of two to three. Aberrant larval migration appears to be more common, resulting in a greater possibility of ectopic worms. The patency period is quite brief, with demonstrable microfilaremia occurring in less than 20 per cent of cases. It has been generally assumed that adult worm life span was approximately 2 years as compared with approximately 5 years in the dog. However, it has recently been demonstrated that some worms may live at least 30 months. Although the pathologic findings are similar to those in the dog, pulmonary hypertension, right-sided heart failure, and particularly the caval syndrome are extremely uncommon.

Outdoor male cats of a wide age range (1 to 17 years) are most commonly affected. Although initially it was believed that infection with the feline leukemia virus was a predisposing factor for acquisition of *D. immitis* infection, this has yet to be substantiated. Infected cats may be asymptomatic or have acute or chronic medical problems. Most asymptomatic cats are never diagnosed antemortem. The most common presenting complaints are respiratory distress, coughing, anorexia, and lethargy. The respiratory distress is usually due to pulmonary thromboembolism. Other signs or symptoms observed include vomiting, weight loss, and sudden death. The vomiting can be acute or chronic and sporadic in nature. In an endemic area, *D. immitis* infection should be considered as a differential diagnosis for the chronically vomiting cat, though the reason for the emesis remains obscure. Other uncommon problems reported to occur with *D. immitis* infection include syncope, seizures, a sudden onset of blindness, chylothorax, and abdominal distention resulting from right-sided heart failure.

Physical examination findings do not always correlate with the clinical signs. In fact, in many cats no abnormalities are detected. Respiratory distress and to a lesser extent cyanosis, cough, and abnormal lung sounds are noted on occasion. Systolic heart murmurs and signs of right-sided heart failure are extremely rare.

The most common laboratory abnormalities observed are eosinophilia and mild nonregenerative anemia. On occasion, basophilia with or without a concomitant eosinophilia may be noted. Most animals (> 80 per cent) will not have microfilaremia. Except for hyperglobulinemia in some animals, results of most other routinely performed laboratory tests are normal. Transtracheal washings most commonly reveal a microbiologically sterile sample with a predominance of eosinophils, although neutrophilic or mixed neutrophilic-mononuclear cytologic findings may also be noted. Eosinophilic aspirates may develop at the time of anticipated patency or the time of arrival of L5. Increased pulmonary secretions with eosinophils may be found prior to radiographic evidence of increased pulmonary densities or enlarged caudal lobar arteries in some cats. Peripheral blood eosinophilia is not always observed in cats with eosinophilic tracheal aspirates.

One of the best ways to confirm the diagnosis is by thoracic radiography. The most consistent abnormality observed is enlarged caudal lobar arteries with ill-defined margins. Enlargement of the main pulmonary artery does occur but is not visible without contrast angiography, as it is more medial to the cardiac silhouette in the ventrodorsal (VD) view in the cat. Right ventricular hypertrophy is seldom observed. Pulmonary parenchymal changes that may be observed include perivascular densities, atelectasis, and alveolar disease. Nonselective venous angiography is seldom performed at the author's hospital, but it does enable one to more clearly visualize the previously described vascular changes as well as vascular tortuosity.

Serologic tests that have been used as an aid in the diagnosis of feline heartworm disease include enzyme-linked immunosorbent assay (ELISA) for antibodies to adults, indirect fluorescent antibody (IFA) test for antibodies to microfilaria, IFA test for antibodies to adults, and ELISA or latex agglutination (LA) for antigens to adults. Tests that utilize monoclonal antibody–based ELISA or LA technology appear to be best suited for the practicing veterinarian. They can be performed with the tests currently marketed for the dog. Unfortunately, most of these are currently inconsistent in their ability to detect adult worm burdens of less than five, and, because most cats have less than five worms, a negative test result does not eliminate the possibility of *D. immitis* infection. One adult antigen assay currently available (Cite, AgriTech Systems, Inc., Portland, ME) is purported to consistently detect adult worm burdens as low as one worm. This would obviously be a useful diagnostic test for feline heartworm disease.

As previously mentioned, eosinophilic transtracheal aspirates may be recovered in some cats without concomitant radiographic evidence of heartworm disease. This could inadvertently lead to an erroneous diagnosis of feline asthma or lungworm infection. In light of this, it seems prudent to perform an adult antigen assay in such a case if one is practicing in an area where *D. immitis* is relatively prevalent. If this test result is negative, one should treat symptomatically and radiograph the animal at a later date to see if signs of heartworm disease have developed.

Thiacetarsamide, at a dosage of 2.2 mg/kg twice a day for 2 days intravenously, has been used to kill adult heartworms. This drug has not been approved for this use in the cat. Hepatotoxicity and renal toxicity are uncommon findings. Thromboembolism is of particular concern, as it can result in sudden death, especially within the first 10 to 14 days after treatment. This risk should be carefully discussed with the owner prior to contemplating adulticide therapy. The animal with evidence of thromboembolic disease should, at the minimum, receive corticosteroids and cage rest. Animals with cyanosis will also benefit from oxygen therapy and possibly furosemide. Other supportive measures such as fluid therapy should be instituted when deemed necessary for shock.

Because microfilaremia is seldom encountered, most animals will not need to be treated with microfilaricides. However, when necessary, dithiazanine iodide and levamisole have been used successfully to eliminate microfilariae. Neither drug has received FDA approval for this use in the cat. Although preventive therapy is seldom warranted, diethylcarbamazine has been safely administered to cats.

References and Supplemental Reading

Atkins, C. E.: Caval syndrome in the dog. Semin. Vet. Med. Surg. 2:64, 1987.

Calvert, C. A., and Rawlings, C. A.: Therapy of canine heartworm disease. *In* Kirk, R. W. (ed.): *Current Veterinary Therapy IX*. Philadelphia: W. B. Saunders, 1986, pp. 406–419.

Dillon, R.: Feline heartworm disease. *In* Kirk, R. W. (ed.): *Current Veterinary Therapy IX*. Philadelphia: W. B. Saunders, 1986, pp. 420–424.

Dillon, A. R., Brawner, W. R., Grieve, R. B., et al.: The chronic effects of experimental *D. immitis* infection in cats. Semin. Vet. Med. Surg. 2:72, 1987.

Grieve, R. B.: Advances in the immunologic diagnosis of *Dirofilaria immitis* infection. Semin. Vet. Med. Surg. 2:4, 1987.

Knight, D. H.: Heartworm disease. *In* Ettinger, S. J. (ed.): *Textbook of Veterinary Internal Medicine*, 2nd ed. Philadelphia: W. B. Saunders, 1983, pp. 1097–1125.

Otto, G. F. (ed.): *Proceedings of the Heartworm Symposium, 1983*. Edwardsville, KS: Veterinary Medicine Publishing Co., 1983.

Otto, G. F. (ed.): *Proceedings of the Heartworm Symposium, 1986*. Washington, D. C.: American Heartworm Society, 1986.

Rawlings, C. A. (ed.): *Heartworm Disease in Dogs and Cats*. Philadelphia: W. B. Saunders, 1986.

ATRIAL ARRHYTHMIAS

JOHN D. BONAGURA, D.V.M.
Columbus, Ohio

Atrial tachyarrhythmias constitute some of the most common cardiac rhythm disturbances encountered in clinical practice. Abnormal electrical activation of the atria might not be troublesome were it not for the attendant rapid ventricular response to this abnormal supraventricular activity. Frequently an abnormal atrial rhythm promotes excessive ventricular rates or irregular cardiac beating. Ventricular filling is compromised by the reduction in diastolic period and by the abnormal or lost atrial contribution to filling. When superimposed on pre-existent heart disease, atrial arrhythmias can cause hypotension, decreased tissue perfusion, and syncope and may become life threatening. Previously stable pets with chronic heart disease quickly decompensate following development of atrial tachyarrhythmias. Chronic heart disease such as mitral regurgitation and cardiomyopathy may be associated with incessant atrial tachycardias, which may require lifelong medical treatment.

The purpose of this article is to review the causes, electrocardiographic recognition, and management of atrial tachyarrhythmias. For information concerning atrium-based bradyarrhythmias, such as the sick sinus syndrome and atrial standstill, the reader is referred to pages 286 to 294. Specific aspects of the clinical actions of drugs used in the management of atrial tachyarrhythmias can be found in Current Veterinary Therapy IX (pp. 346–360).

CLINICAL ASSESSMENT

Normal Atrial Activation

The atria normally are depolarized by the sino-atrial node. Atrial activation processes are orderly and are dictated by the location of the cardiac pacemaker, anatomic aspects of the atria and great veins, and functional specialized conducting pathways within the atrial muscle. The normal activation process, represented by the P wave, is well seen in leads II or aVF. The P wave is generally positive in leads I, II, aVF, and III, with the highest amplitude P wave found in lead II. In the resting dog, varying autonomic tone may generate recurrent variations in the P wave form, with the largest P waves being observed in lead II during the shortest cardiac cycles. This normal variation of sinus rhythm is termed wandering atrial pacemaker, and it should

not be confused with an atrial arrhythmia. Moreover, cardiomegaly or myocardial disease can distort the normal sinus P wave, leading to excessively tall, wide, or splintered P waves despite otherwise normal pacemaker activity. High sympathetic tone causes sinus tachycardia with prominent P waves, a rhythm that in this article will be considered a physiologic rhythm. However, because it may be confused with atrial tachycardia, sinus tachycardia will be discussed when considering the differential diagnosis of atrial tachycardia.

Identification of Atrial Tachyarrhythmias

Tachyarrhythmias generated solely within the atria include sinus tachycardia, atrial tachycardia, atrial flutter, and atrial fibrillation (Figs. 1 and 2). *Sinus tachycardia* is a normal impulse mechanism that develops at a higher than normal rate (usually > 180/min in the dog and > 240/min in the cat) owing to increased sympathetic tone. P waves are positive in leads II and aVF and atrioventricular (AV) conduction sequence is 1:1 (P:QRS) unless there is AV conduction disease. As with all supraventricular tachyarrhythmias, the QRS is of normal duration and orientation unless there is accompanying ventricular enlargement or intercurrent ventricular conduction problems such as bundle branch block.

Premature atrial complexes are impulses that arise outside of the sinoatrial (SA) node and generate early atrial muscle activation with an abnormal or ectopic P wave (P′ wave). These abnormal complexes can be envisioned as the simplest of atrial rhythm disturbances. Provided the premature impulse can be conducted to the ventricle, a premature QRS will ensue. Generally, this QRS complex appears normal in duration and orientation; however, if the bundle branches are caught "unaware" and not yet repolarized, the accompanying QRS may be abnormal. Isolated and even frequent atrial premature complexes tend to be well tolerated by the patient, but they may be harbingers of more serious atrial arrhythmias (Fig. 2).

Atrial tachycardia is an abnormal, rapid, regular activation that develops outside of the SA node and is due to abnormal impulse generation (ectopic pacemaker) or a circuit movement about the atrium (atrial re-entry). The P-wave axis may be normal or

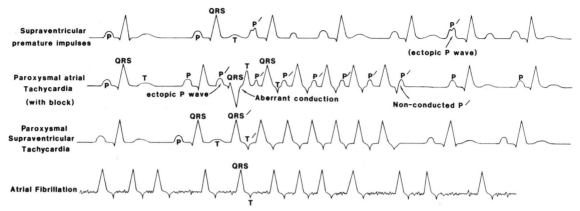

Figure 1. Common supraventricular arrhythmias. Paroxysmal atrial tachycardia may be terminated by a period of blocked P waves as increasing refractoriness of the AV node produces AV block.

altered, resulting in negative or abnormally formed P waves when compared with sinus node–generated impulses. The atrial tachycardia may be paroxysmal or sustained. Sustained atrial tachycardia in the dog usually occurs in the range of 260 to 380 atrial impulses per minute (Fig. 3). Often, P waves are blocked in the AV node because the atrial impulse formation may encroach on the refractory period of the AV nodal cells. This leads to an AV conduction sequence of greater than 1:1 (P:QRS).

Atrial flutter is an abnormal, rapid regular activation caused by circuit movement through the atria. The flutter rate is usually greater than 400/min and is characterized by saw-toothed flutter waves in the electrocardiogram (ECG) baseline. The

ventricular response is usually rapid but may be regular or irregular, depending on the pattern of AV conduction. This is an unstable rhythm in small animals and often reverts back to sinus rhythm or degenerates to atrial fibrillation.

Atrial fibrillation is a rapid, totally chaotic, and fragmented atrial activation process (Figs. 2 and 4 through 6). Although the actual atrial rate is not easily measured in the dog or cat, 500 to 600 atrial impulses may be initiated per minute. The ventricular response is invariably irregular unless there is coincident AV conduction disease with a junctional escape rhythm or unless the patient is digitalis intoxicated, exhibiting high-grade AV block of atrial impulses and development of a regular ectopic AV

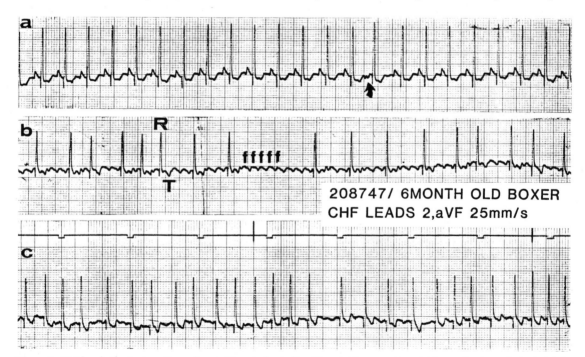

Figure 2. Atrial arrhythmias in a Boxer dog. *a*, Sinus tachycardia with a single premature atrial complex (arrow). *b*, Atrial flutter with prominent flutter waves (f) and irregular ventricular response. *c*, Atrial fibrillation with rapid, irregular ventricular response; note the absence of P waves.

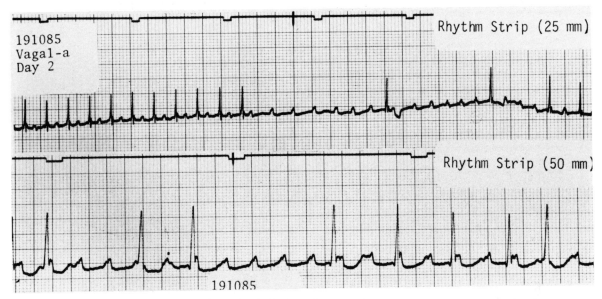

Figure 3. Probable atrial tachycardia in a dog with valvular heart disease. Following a vagal maneuver (top) multiple P waves are noted to be blocked. The bottom strip indicates the irregular ventricular response to the atrial tachycardia. Atrial rate is between 260 and 300/min.

junctional rhythm. The ventricular response in atrial fibrillation is usually rapid, except when the patient is not in heart failure, has intercurrent AV conduction disease, or has been treated with drugs that impede AV conduction.

Re-entrant supraventricular tachycardia (SVT)

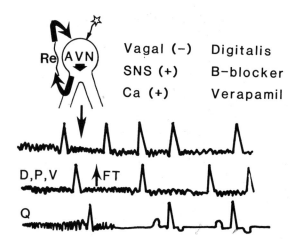

Figure 4. Role of the atrioventricular node (AVN) in supraventricular tachyarrhythmias. In re-entrant tachycardias, the impulse ascends an accessory pathway (Re) to activate the atria in a retrograde fashion. The impulse then travels down the AVN to activate the ventricles. A circuit loop is formed. Ectopic impulses (star) or atrial fibrillatory waves will be conducted to the ventricle only after crossing the AV node and bundle branches. Drugs like digitalis (D) that increase vagal tone, or beta-blockers like propranolol (P) that decrease sympathetic (SNS) tone, or agents like verapamil (V) or diltiazem that block calcium currents will impede conduction of atrial impulses. In the case of atrial fibrillation (bottom), these drugs slow the ventricular response, increasing ventricular filling time (FT). In a small subset of patients, quinidine (Q) or a calcium channel blocker can convert the patient to normal sinus rhythm.

refers to a tachyarrhythmia resulting from abnormal circuit movement that travels between the atria and ventricles using an electrical "loop." The atria, AV node, and an accessory atrioventricular pathway constitute the loop (Fig. 4). The impulse activates the atria, descends to the ventricle, and ascends back to the atrial muscle by using another atrioventricular pathway. Frequently, a premature atrial or ventricular impulse initiates the tachycardia by traversing one potential AV pathway but not the other. Re-entrant SVT is commonly observed in human patients and in some animals with ventricular pre-excitation syndromes. In the usual case of pre-excitation, the patient will have a markedly shortened P-R interval during normal sinus rhythm but a normal or long P-R interval during the re-entrant SVT. The tachycardia typically develops when the abnormal atrioventricular conduit conducts the ventricular electrical impulse up to the atria, while the AV node reciprocates by returning the impulse back down to the ventricles. In this manner, the atria and ventricles are rapidly activated in sequence, provided the critical relationship between antegrade and retrograde conduction is maintained. The P waves are normal during sinus rhythm but are negative and buried in the ST segment during SVT.

Role of Atrioventricular Conduction

Of paramount importance is an understanding of the ventricular response to atrial activation. Normally, atrioventricular conduction is 1:1, yielding a QRS complex for each P wave. However, rapid atrial activation, particularly when the atrial rate is

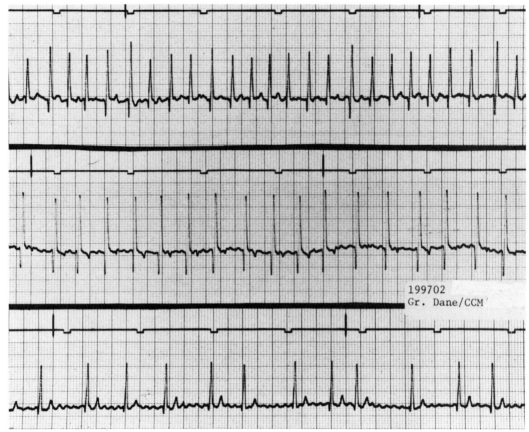

Figure 5. Effects of digoxin and propranolol on the ventricular response in atrial fibrillation. Baseline recording (top) and follow-up strips (middle and bottom). The lower strip was taken after 5 days of therapy. Paper speed, 25 mm/sec.

suddenly increased or is sustained at greater than 300 impulses per minute, often is attended by physiologic blocking of atrial impulses in the AV node (Figs. 1 through 3, 5, and 6). Owing to a variety of factors, including varying autonomic tone, the resultant ventricular rate generally tends to be rapid but erratic. This is especially true in animals with atrial fibrillation, although similar irregular responses can also be observed in some dogs with atrial tachycardia and atrial flutter. In the latter cases, the ventricular response is more likely to be regular owing to the consistent formation of atrial impulse and the development of set patterns of AV conduction (e.g., 2:1 or 3:2 ratio of P waves to QRS

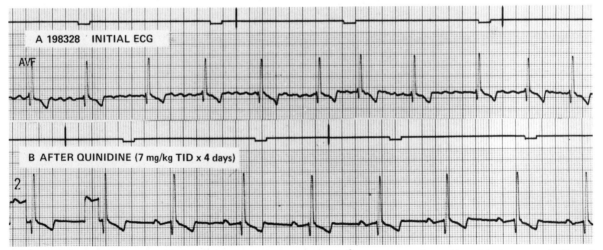

Figure 6. Conversion of atrial fibrillation (A) to normal sinus rhythm following therapy with quinidine (B). Paper speed, 50 mm/sec.

complexes). With re-entrant SVT, the atrioventricular relationship is almost always 1:1 (P/QRS) because the arrhythmia generally uses a circuit in which each end is formed by the atria or ventricles.

The clinician must appreciate factors that control depolarization and conduction of atrioventricular nodal cells. Conduction is accelerated by vagal blockade or increased sympathetic efferent traffic. The cells require calcium to attain their slow-current depolarization. Thus, if the clinician wishes to impede AV conduction, the administration of a vagomimetic drug such as digitalis, a beta-adrenergic blocker such as propranolol, or a calcium channel blocker such as verapamil will accomplish this slowing (Fig. 4). Accordingly, when a sustained atrial tachycardia is present, the ventricle may be partially protected from rapid activation by administration of one or more of these drugs. Moreover, in some cases, re-entrant SVT may be abruptly terminated by AV nodal blockade, as antegrade conduction is extinguished temporarily and the circuit is broken.

DIFFERENTIAL DIAGNOSIS

The ECG criteria for diagnosis of atrial tachyarrhythmias have not been stated conclusively for dogs and cats. Although experimental studies have generated most of these rhythm disturbances, the models and accompanying atrial rates do not always represent the naturally occurring disorder. The distinctions between sinus and atrial tachycardia, and between atrial tachycardia and atrial flutter, are not always clear. Inasmuch as there is some overlap in atrial rates with these dysrhythmias, and electrode studies are rarely done to assess the underlying electrophysiologic mechanism, the final ECG diagnosis will at times be in doubt. The following are guidelines found helpful by the author for distinguishing atrial arrhythmias.

Sinus tachycardia in the dog and cat typically develops at rates of less than 300/min, unless the animals has thyrotoxicosis; has ingested a toxin, such as caffeine or chocolate; or has been treated with atropine, glycopyrrolate, or a catecholamine. Because sympathetic tone is the cause of sinus tachycardia, AV conduction pattern is usually 1:1 (P:QRS), and vagal maneuvers do little to change the rhythm. Typical of sinus mechanisms, the P-wave configuration is positive and peaked in lead II. Many of these patients are hypotensive, and the rapid administration of fluids (40 to 75 ml/kg/hr in nonedematous patients) often leads to a dramatic decline in atrial rate. Treatment of pain, shock, or hyperthermia also may decrease the heart rate in animals with sinus tachycardia.

In patients with regular but abnormal atrial mechanisms (atrial tachycardia or atrial flutter), the atrial rate is often greater than 300/min, and the AV conduction sequence is frequently greater than 1:1 (P:QRS). *Vagal maneuvers*, including firm ocular pressure (15 to 20 seconds) or bilateral carotid massage (in the jugular furrow ventral to the mandible), are more likely to cause transient AV nodal block and unmask the atrial tachyarrhythmia (Fig. 3). In the less commonly encountered re-entrant SVT, a vagal maneuver may actually terminate the tachycardia. Vagal maneuvers can be enhanced by administering morphine (to dogs), 0.2 mg/kg intramuscularly, or by giving edrophonium chloride (Tensilon), 1 to 4 mg intravenously (atropine should be available). Similar to a vagal maneuver, drugs that impede AV conduction will increase the AV conduction ratio, or less commonly terminate a re-entrant or atrial tachyarrhythmia.

Atrial flutter and sustained atrial tachycardia may be difficult to distinguish because both produce rapid and regular atrial rates and the absence of an isoelectric shelf (saw-toothed waves) may be difficult to appreciate in some animals with atrial flutter. From a pragmatic view, the distinction between these arrhythmias is unimportant, as both are associated with heart disease and are treated similarly. By producing transient delays in ventricular activation, vagal maneuvers or therapy with AV nodal–active drugs usually unmasks P′ waves or flutter waves that might be buried in QRS-T complexes.

The diagnosis of atrial fibrillation is relatively straightforward. In the patient with a narrow QRS tachycardia, the R-R intervals should be measured with calipers. If the intervals vary in an irregular fashion, and if definitive P waves or flutter waves are not observed during the pauses, atrial fibrillation is highly probable.

CLINICAL CAUSES

The majority of sustained or recurrent atrial arrhythmias can be linked to the presence of *organic heart disease*, and the underlying cause can usually be identified by obtaining a medical and drug history, examining the heart and lungs, and obtaining routine hematologic tests. Cardiomyopathies, chronic valvular heart disease, and uncorrected congenital cardiac lesions may result in progressive atrial distention. Atrial enlargement is the most common basis for development of persistent atrial arrhythmias. Contributing factors to the development of atrial arrhythmias in animals with heart disease include high sympathetic tone, drugs such as digitalis and catecholamines, electrolyte disorders, hypoxia, ischemia, and myocardial fibrosis. Atrial arrhythmias are not uncommon in animals with cardiac neoplasia, and atrial fibrillation can develop in dogs with constrictive pericarditis or chronic pericardial diseases. Animals with accessory AV pathways (pre-excitation complexes) have the potential for development of atrial fibrillation and re-entrant SVT.

Noncardiac conditions may lead to atrial arrhythmias. Pulmonary disease, including vascular disease from heartworms, may promote atrial arrhythmias by causing cor pulmonale, hypoxia, and acid-base disturbances. Thyrotoxicosis and overtreatment with L-thyroxin frequently lead to atrial premature complexes and atrial arrhythmias. Severe anemia often causes sinus tachycardia and atrial arrhythmias. Electrocution has been associated with atrial tachycardia.

Additional *iatrogenic causes* of atrial arrhythmias include cardiac drugs, catecholamines, bronchodilator drugs, jugular catheters in the atrium, cardiac catheterization, anesthetic agents, and thoracic surgery.

DRUGS AND METHODS USED IN TREATMENT

The major treatments used to terminate or control atrial arrhythmias include vagal maneuvers and administration of digitalis, a beta-blocker, a calcium channel blocker, or quinidine. Ocular pressure or carotid massage can be attempted to assist in the diagnosis or termination of a rapid, regular (or irregular) supraventricular tachycardia. The potential merits of this diagnostic procedure have been discussed above. It should be attempted in animals with probable re-entrant SVT (see below).

Digoxin is the most frequently used drug to control the heart rate in atrial tachyarrhythmias. Rarely does it convert a sustained arrhythmia, but is slows AV conduction and decreases the rate. Usual maintenance doses are 0.01 to 0.02 mg/kg divided b.i.d. orally, or 0.015 to 0.02 mg/kg in four divided doses intravenously, as a loading dose given over 2 to 4 hours.

Beta-blocking drugs such as *propranolol* (Inderal, in dogs: 0.2 to 1.0 mg/kg q8h PO or 0.5 to 3.0 mg over 5 minutes IV; in cats: 2.5 to 5 mg q8 to 12h PO; *nadolol* (0.1 to 0.5 mg/kg q8 to 12h PO); and *atenolol* (0.1 to 0.25 mg/kg q12h PO) may either suppress abnormal atrial activity or result in slowing of the ventricular response. These are negative inotropic drugs (see *Current Veterinary Therapy IX*, p. 343) and must be used cautiously in animals with hypotension or congestive heart failure (CHF). Typically, the author begins at the low end of the dose range and gradually increases the dose with each treatment until the desired effect is attained.

Calcium channel blocking drugs such as verapamil (Isoptin, Calan) and diltiazem (Cardizem) have a potent effect on AV conduction and also have the potential to convert atrial tachyarrhythmias and re-entrant SVT to normal sinus rhythm. They are effective in controlling heart rate in atrial fibrilla-

tion, and diltiazem (0.5 to 1.25 mg/kg q6 to 8h PO) is frequently administered with digoxin to control the ventricular rate. Both drugs have the potential for significant myocardial depression and they are also vasodilators (see *Current Veterinary Therapy IX*, p. 340). Thus, as with beta-blockers, the dosage should be titrated upward, starting at a low dose and increasing the dose with each administration until the desired effect has been attained. In pets without CHF but with severe sustained supraventricular tachycardia that does not cease with a vagal maneuver, intravenous verapamil (0.05 to 0.15 mg/kg) can be given.

Quinidine and procainamide are more commonly used for ventricular arrhythmias in the dog and cat; however, they have some effect on atrial arrhythmias as well. Quinidine (6 to 8 mg/kg q6h for 24 hours IM) has been used successfully to convert acute atrial fibrillation to normal sinus rhythm in dogs as described below. Initially, the ventricular rate may increase owing to an anticholinergic-sympathomimetic effect on the AV node.

ISOLATED ATRIAL PREMATURE COMPLEXES

Drug therapy of atrial premature complexes may be unnecessary. If applicable, drugs that induce atrial arrhythmias, such as thyroxin or bronchodilators, should be reduced in dosage. In the patient that has experienced syncope but in which a repetitive atrial dysrhythmia cannot be documented, the author recommends therapy as described below for recurrent atrial tachyarrhythmias. In the dog with frequent atrial arrhythmias and CHF, oral digoxin can be prescribed. If this treatment is ineffective in reducing frequency of premature beats, a beta-blocker or diltiazem can be added. In the cat with hypertrophic cardiomyopathy or hyperthyroid heart disease, frequent atrial premature complexes can be treated with propranolol (Inderal, 2.5 mg q8h PO).

RECURRENT OR SUSTAINED ATRIAL TACHYARRHYTHMIAS

The patient with recurrent or sustained atrial tachycardia is most likely to have cardiomegaly from valvular heart disease or cardiomyopathy and is usually in congestive heart failure. A less common presentation is the patient who is not congested but has severe tachycardia, hypotension, and a relatively normal-sized heart. A third clinical presentation is the dog with asymptomatic atrial fibrillation and a slow ventricular response. Finally, there may be acute development of atrial flutter or fibrillation associated with surgery or trauma in a large-breed dog. The pet with intercurrent heart failure will be considered first.

ASSOCIATED CONGESTIVE HEART FAILURE. When heart failure is complicated by atrial tachycardia, flutter, or fibrillation, the initial treatment is administration of digitalis. Typically digoxin is administered orally. A loading dose (twice the eventual maintenance dose) is given orally for 2 days when heart failure is severe or the ventricular rate exceeds 220/min during cage rest. Alternatively, an intravenous loading dose can be given as described above. This is helpful when the clinician desires to use an intravenous infusion of dobutamine or dopamine to support myocardial failure. Other therapy for CHF is provided (pp. 231–240 and 240–251).

In the typical case, atrial tachyarrhythmias persist and do not revert to normal sinus rhythm. Moreover, most patients continue to experience tachycardia despite digitalization. Accordingly, after 24 to 48 hours of treatment with digoxin, an additional drug is added to control the ventricular rate. Although the author has had good experience using beta-blocking drugs such as propranolol, nadolol, or atenolol in some dogs (Fig. 5), these drugs have significant potential for depressing myocardial function and must be used cautiously, especially in Doberman pinscher dogs.

The drug that has become the second choice, after digoxin, to control ventricular rate is diltiazem (Cardizem), which is given as described previously and is administered long term for treatment of the atrial rhythm disorder. The ultimate dosage is titrated to the resting ventricular heart rate, of which a target rate of 120 to 160/min seems reasonable. Interestingly, some dogs convert to normal sinus rhythm following administration of either diltiazem or verapamil. Even in these cases, the drug is usually continued to maintain the rhythm.

The overall prognosis for patients with atrial fibrillation and CHF is poor, with only 30 to 35 per cent surviving more than 6 months despite drug therapy to control heart rate and clinical signs of heart failure.

ATRIAL OR SUPRAVENTRICULAR TACHYCARDIA WITHOUT CHF. Treatment of the patient with acute atrial tachycardia without congestive heart failure is centered on maintaining arterial blood pressure and either converting the tachycardia to normal sinus rhythm or slowing the ventricular response. An intravenous line should be established, and intravenous saline or lactated Ringer's solution administered to maintain blood pressure (see discussion of differential diagnosis). Vagal maneuvers should be performed. If these do not convert the tachycardia, verapamil should be administered using an initial dose of 0.05 mg/kg given over 2 to 3 minutes intravenously. This can be repeated up to a total dose of 0.15 mg/kg. If verapamil is unavailable, diltiazem can be given orally using an initial dose

of 0.5 mg/kg orally, and giving 0.25 mg/kg every hour orally up to a total dose of 1.25 to 1.5 mg/kg. If neither calcium channel blocker is available, a combination of intravenous digoxin and oral propranolol (0.25 mg/kg) can be tried.

The therapeutic end point is either conversion to sinus rhythm or marked slowing of the ventricular rate (to less than 200/min). At that time, a cardiac workup should be done. Continual oral therapy may be required to maintain sinus rhythm or a controlled ventricular rate.

ATRIAL FIBRILLATION OF ACUTE ONSET. In the large-breed dog with documented atrial fibrillation of acute onset, in which there is no significant cardiomegaly, no cardiac murmur, and no congestive heart failure, conversion to sinus rhythm can be attempted. Often these dogs have recently undergone anesthesia. Although oral quinidine can be successful in attaining conversion (Fig. 6), intramuscular administration (6 to 8 mg/kg q6h for 24 hours) is generally successful in converting most of these patients. The drug can then be discontinued, and the patient followed electrocardiographically.

ATRIAL FIBRILLATION IN THE ASYMPTOMATIC DOG. If there is no evidence of heart failure, and the ventricular rate is less than 150/min at rest, the options are (1) to attempt conversion to sinus rhythm using quinidine as described above (if this is unsuccessful diltiazem [0.75 to 1.0 mg/kg q8h PO for 3 days] can be given); (2) to administer an oral dose of digoxin (0.01 to 0.02 mg/kg divided b.i.d.) to control ventricular rate; or (3) to do nothing and follow the patient.

RE-ENTRANT SUPRAVENTRICULAR TACHYCARDIA

If re-entrant SVT is strongly suspected from evaluation of the ECG and responses to vagal maneuvers or observation of ventricular pre-excitation during normal sinus rhythm, a cardiologist should be consulted concerning potential modes of home therapy. Treatment can be directed at reduction of premature complexes, blockade of the AV node, or blockade of conduction across the accessory pathway. A calcium channel blocker, such as verapamil (0.05 to 0.15 mg/kg IV), is a reasonable first choice in the treatment of a patient with symptomatic episodes of tachycardia. Digoxin probably should be avoided because it can promote conduction down the accessory pathway. Drugs such as amiodarone or procainamide may have significant effect on the accessory pathway. There are no trials that indicate the effect of drugs in these arrhythmias.

References and Supplemental Reading

Bohn, F. K., Patterson, D. F., and Pyle, R. L.: Atrial fibrillation in dogs. Br. Vet. J. 127:485, 1971.

Bonagura, J. D., and Ware, W. W.: Atrial fibrillation in the dog: Clinical findings in 81 cases. J. Am. Anim. Hosp. Assoc. 22:111, 1986.

Hamlin, R. L.: Diltiazem for treating supraventricular arrhythmias in dogs. J. Vet. Intern. Med. (in press).

Keefe, D. L., and Kates, R. E.: Myocardial disposition and cardiac pharmacodynamics of verapamil in the dog. J. Pharmacol. Exp. Ther. 220:91, 1982.

Kittleson, M., Keene, B., Pion, P., and Woodfield, J.: Verapamil administration for the treatment of supraventricular tachycardia in the dog. J. Vet. Intern. Med. (in press).

Piepho, R. W., Blocdow, D. C., and Lacz, J. P.: Pharmacokinetics of diltiazem in selected animal species and human beings. Am. J. Cardiol. 49:525, 1982.

THERAPY FOR VENTRICULAR ARRHYTHMIAS

WENDY A. WARE, D.V.M.,
and ROBERT L. HAMLIN, D.V.M.

Columbus, Ohio

Disturbances in the heart's rhythm that originate from the ventricles are common, occurring with many diseases and metabolic abnormalities. Decisions about when and how to treat these arrhythmias depend on the severity of the rhythm disturbance as well as the patient's underlying disease process and hemodynamic state. Correct interpretation of the patient's electrocardiogram (ECG) is essential to therapeutic decision making. Rational therapy of ventricular arrhythmias also requires an understanding of the possible underlying causes of the disturbance and an appreciation for risks versus benefits of specific antiarrhythmic drugs.

Cardiac arrhythmias result from abnormal electrical impulse generation or conduction or a combination of both. Abnormal impulses can arise from specialized conducting tissues, such as Purkinje fibers, or from cells that under normal conditions do not possess automaticity, such as ischemic myocardial cells. Ectopic beats can also develop from membrane potential fluctuations, called afterdepolarizations, which are induced by the preceding impulse. Such "triggered activity" is thought to be a cause of digitalis-induced ventricular arrhythmias. Disturbances of conduction within the heart may lead to re-excitation of the atria or ventricles when the original impulse does not dissipate normally but is maintained somewhere within the ventricle and subsequently is able to "re-enter" and stimulate another depolarization.

IDENTIFICATION OF VENTRICULAR ARRHYTHMIAS

Impulses originating from a ventricular focus are usually wide and of a different configuration than the normal QRS complex. They may be mainly positive or negative. *Ventricular premature complexes* (VPCs) (or contractions, depolarizations, premature ventricular contractions [PVCs]) are ectopic impulses that occur before the next expected sinus impulse. There may be isolated VPCs (Fig. A), pairs (couplets), or runs of three or more (paroxysmal ventricular tachycardia). A bigeminal pattern occurs when each normal QRS is followed by a VPC (Fig. 1B). If all the VPCs have the same configuration they are said to be *unifocal*. If variable configurations occur (e.g., some positive, some negative) the VPCs are considered *multiform* (Fig. 1C); this may indicate multiple sites of origin and electrical instability.

Ventricular tachycardia (VT) is a rapid series of VPCs. It may be sustained (persistent) or paroxysmal (Fig. 1D). In dogs the rate of VT exceeds 100 beats/min. The R-R interval is usually regular. Nonconducted sinus P waves can often be found superimposed on or between the ventricular complexes. *Fusion complexes* may occur and represent almost synchronous ventricular activation from both an ectopic ventricular focus and a normal sinus impulse traveling down the ventricular conduction system;

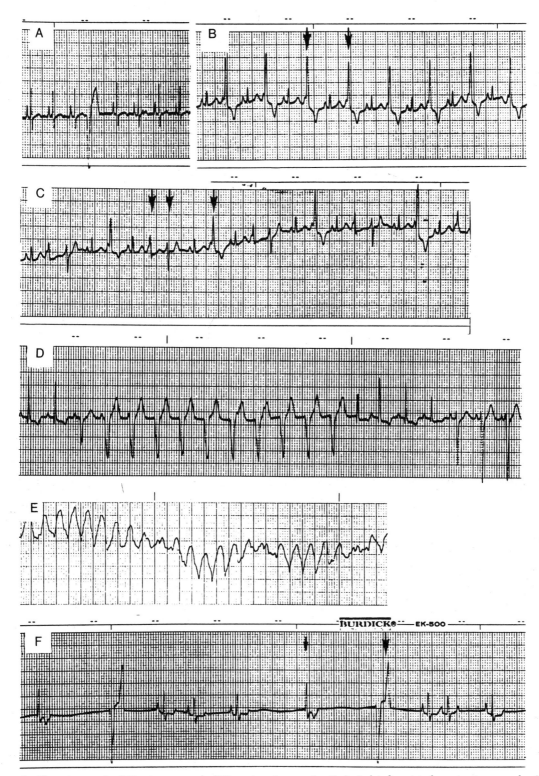

Figure 1. All tracings are lead II at paper speed of 25 mm/sec, 1 cm = 1 mV. *A*, Isolated ventricular premature complex (VPC) in a cat with hypertrophic cardiomyopathy. *B*, VPCs in a bigeminal pattern (arrows) in an older cat given a thiobarbiturate. *C*, Multiform VPCs (arrows) in the same cat as B. *D*, Paroxysmal ventricular tachycardia in a dog with metabolic acidosis, seizures, and oliguric renal failure. *E*, Polymorphic ventricular tachycardia in an older cat with dilated cardiomyopathy. Lidocaine temporarily converted this to sinus rhythm. *F*, Junctional (small arrow) and ventricular (larger arrow) escape complexes in an older dog with sinus arrest that had episodes of syncope and weakness.

thus, their configuration is a melding of the normal QRS and the VPC patterns. Ventricular tachycardia is a serious rhythm disturbance that is often associated with significant underlying heart disease. Ventricular tachycardia can lead to hypotension and congestive heart failure (CHF), as well as ventricular fibrillation.

Accelerated ventricular rhythm, also called idioventricular tachycardia, is an enhanced ventricular rhythm with a rate of about 60 to 100 beats/min in the dog. Because the rate is slower than with VT, it is usually a less serious rhythm disturbance. An accelerated ventricular rhythm may intermittently occur with sinus arrhythmia. As the sinus rate slows the accelerated ventricular rhythm becomes manifest, only to be suppressed as the sinus rate increases again. Clinically, an accelerated ventricular rhythm may have no deleterious hemodynamic effects and antiarrhythmic therapy is often not needed. However, the animal should be closely monitored, as more serious rhythm disturbances can develop. If an accelerated ventricular rhythm progresses to VT or if it causes signs of hypotension, it should be suppressed.

Ventricular tachycardia may lead to *ventricular flutter*, which is a fast, unstable ventricular rhythm. The ECG appearance is that of a sine wave, with no isoelectric shelf between complexes. Usually this rhythm progresses to *ventricular fibrillation* (VF) in which rapid, disorganized electrical activity causes ineffective contractions and cardiac arrest. Cardiopulmonary resuscitation and electrical defibrillation must then be initiated immediately. It is not known how frequently the sequence of VPCs progressing to VT to VF occurs; nor is it known yet whether frequent VPCs or VT are better predictors of impending VF and sudden death than single, sparsely occurring VPCs. It is also not known whether multiform ventricular arrhythmias are better predictors of sudden death in dogs and cats than unifocal VPCs, although the former are thought to be more serious. Other patterns of ventricular tachyarrhythmias can occur as well (Fig. 1–E), including polymorphous or multiform VT, torsade de pointes (a type of polymorphous VT), and ventricular parasystole. Information about the appearance and clinical associations of these arrhythmias can be found in the supplemental reading.

It is important to differentiate VPCs and *escape complexes*. An escape complex is one that occurs after a long pause in the dominant (usually sinus) rhythm. It is a cardiac rescue mechanism. The origin of an escape focus can be atrium, atrioventricular (AV) junction, or ventricle (Fig. 1F). If the dominant rhythm does not resume (as in persistent sinus arrest or complete AV block), the escape focus may continue to discharge at its own intrinsic rate. A ventricular escape rhythm (*idioventricular rhythm*) usually has a rate less than 40 beats/min in dogs and less than 100 beats/min in cats. As with any ventricular rhythm, the QRS complexes are wide and abnormally shaped. Animals with an idioventricular rhythm may show signs of hypotension, syncope, or congestive heart failure (CHF) owing to the slow heart rate. Anticholinergics (such as atropine or glycopyrrolate) or sympathomimetics (e.g., isoproterenol or dopamine) may increase the rate or restore AV conduction; however, ventricular pacing often is needed. Escape complexes or idioventricular (escape) rhythms should *never* be suppressed with antiarrhythmic drugs, as asystole (lack of any contractions) may result.

CAUSES OF VENTRICULAR ARRHYTHMIAS

Many diseases can affect the heart rhythm either directly by involving cardiac tissue or indirectly through neurohumoral effects. In general, automaticity or conduction can be altered by changes in local autonomic tone, ischemia, hypoxia, electrolyte imbalances (especially K^+ and Ca^{2+}), temperature, acidosis, alkalosis, drug effects, endocrine abnormalities (e.g., hyperthyroidism), and even local pressure changes (stretch). Often an arrhythmia can be abolished by correcting these abnormalities.

Disease of the central nervous system (CNS) can generate abnormal neural effects on the heart and lead to arrhythmias. Tumors, hemorrhage, seizure activity or embolization of the brain, CNS alterations from metabolic disease (e.g., hepatic or diabetic coma and uremia), and even psychologic stress may predispose to ventricular as well as supraventricular arrhythmias.

Table 1 lists many conditions that have been associated with ventricular arrhythmias. Often the distinction among cardiac, neural, and extracardiac causes of these rhythm disturbances is blurred; however, sustained or recurrent ventricular arrhythmias are more likely to develop in animals with structural cardiac lesions such as cardiomyopathy. Ventricular arrhythmias may be short lived in situations of electrolyte disturbance or drug toxicosis.

PATIENT EVALUATION AND THERAPEUTIC GUIDELINES

Ventricular tachyarrhythmias have deleterious effects on hemodynamics. These may be insignificant in patients with a normal heart; however, in the presence of underlying heart disease, rapid ventricular rates, or myocardial depression from a systemic disease, the hemodynamic impairment can be severe. The reductions in cardiac output, arterial blood pressure, and coronary perfusion that result from severe arrhythmias may lead to congestive or

Table 1. *Causes of Ventricular Tachyarrhythmias*

Cardiac
  Congestive heart failure
  *Cardiomyopathy (especially in Doberman pinschers and boxers)
  Myocarditis (infectious and noninfectious)
  Pericarditis
  *Degenerative valvular disease with myocardial fibrosis
  *Ischemia (during or following arterial hypotension of any cause, CHF, ventricular outflow obstruction, myocardial infarction)
  *Trauma
  Cardiac neoplasia
  Heartworm disease
  Congenital heart diseases
  Ventricular dilation
  Mechanical stimulation (intracardiac catheter, pacing wire)
  *Drugs (digitalis, sympathomimetics, anesthetics or tranquilizers, anticholinergics, antiarrhythmics)

Neurogenic (Autonomic Nervous System) Factors
  High sympathetic tone (pain, anxiety, fever)
  Central nervous system disease (increases in sympathetic or vagal stimulation)
  Electrical shock

Extracardiac
  Hypoxia
  Electrolyte imbalance (especially K^+)
  Acidosis/alkalosis
  Thyrotoxicosis
  Hypothermia
  Fever
  Sepsis/toxemia
  *Trauma (thoracic or abdominal)
  *Gastric dilation/volvulus
  Pulmonary disease
  Uremia
  Pancreatitis
  Pheochromocytoma
  Other endocrine diseases (diabetes mellitus, Addison's disease, hypothyroidism)

*Most common causes in the dog.

low-output heart failure or both. Clinically, poor cardiac output and hypotension may be manifest as weakness, depression, inability to exercise, syncope, dyspnea, renal failure, worsening rhythm disturbances, and, sometimes, mentation changes, seizure activity, and sudden death. Pulse deficits or an irregular, weak pulse with split heart sounds of varying intensity and regularity may be found on physical examination. Usually VT causes more severe hemodynamic compromise than isolated VPCs, with faster rates of VT being more deleterious.

Initial patient evaluation should involve a thorough history, including drugs administered; a complete physical examination, with careful attention to the cardiovascular system; identification of any concurrent disease; assessment of the animal's metabolic status; and interpretation of past and present ECGs. Careful patient monitoring, by both physical examination and ECG, is essential because cardiac arrhythmias are often not consistent and may change in response to drug therapy, prevailing autonomic

tone, baroreceptor reflexes, and variations in heart rate. A search for possible underlying causes of the arrhythmia, such as hypotension-induced ischemia, electrolyte or acid-base imbalances, or drug toxicosis, should be initiated. Other helpful measures in some circumstances include cage rest, blood transfusions, and administration of oxygen, analgesics, antibiotics, or corticosteroids, as well as specific antiarrhythmic drugs. Serum K^+ level must be maintained within the normal range for effective antiarrhythmic therapy.

The decision to use an antiarrhythmic drug is based on the type and severity of the rhythm disturbance and the degree of hemodynamic compromise. The route of drug therapy depends on patient status. The clinician's ability to correctly administer and monitor the chosen therapy, the potential for adverse drug reactions or side effects, and the potential for any detrimental drug interactions must be considered. Familiarity with the pharmacodynamic and pharmacokinetic properties of the drug to be used is wise.

Dogs with frequent VPCs (more than 20 to 30/min*), paroxysmal or sustained VT, or signs of hypotension should be treated with intravenous lidocaine (or procainamide). If this is not effective, other parenteral antiarrhythmic therapy is tried (Fig. 2, see also Table 4). Animals with more than 10 but fewer than 25 VPCs per minute often can be medicated with oral quinidine, procainamide, or tocainide. Occasional VPCs in an asymptomatic animal usually do not require therapy. Table 2 lists guidelines for initiating antiarrhythmic therapy, which, although extrapolated from the human literature, are thought to be applicable to veterinary medicine.

Antiarrhythmic therapy, even if unsuccessful in totally abolishing the arrhythmia, may be helpful by decreasing its frequency, rate, and adverse hemodynamic effects and might prevent development of ventricular fibrillation. However, it is not known whether reduction in frequency or complete abolition of an arrhythmia prolongs life in either the cat or the dog.

Antiarrhythmic Drugs

Drugs used to suppress arrhythmias have been classified according to their electrophysiologic effects on cardiac cells (Table 3). An awareness of this classification system may be helpful, although finding an effective drug is often a matter of trial and error, as it is almost impossible to determine the mechanism of an arrhythmia from the ECG alone.

Class I drugs tend to slow conduction and de-

*Editors' Note: These are guidelines, since some dogs tolerate isolated VPCs well and may not require therapy.

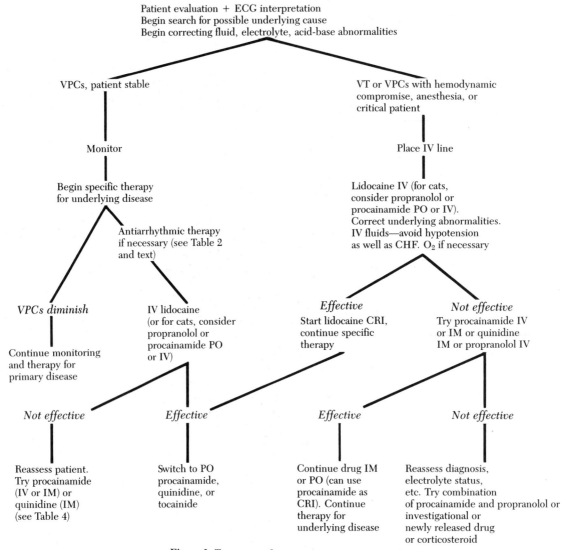

Figure 2. Treatment of ventricular tachyarrhythmias.

crease automaticity and excitability by their membrane-stabilizing effects. The "traditional" antiarrhythmic agents belong to this class. Class II drugs, the beta-adrenoceptor blocking agents, act by inhibiting catecholamine effects on the heart rather than having direct electrophysiologic effects. Some betablockers are nonselective, i.e., affect both beta$_1$- and beta$_2$- receptors (propranolol, nadolol, timolol,

Table 2. *Guidelines for Initiation of Antiarrhythmic Therapy*

1. Frequent VPCs (more than 20–30/min)
2. Repetitive VPCs (pairs, paroxysms) at rates of more than 120–130 beats/min
3. Multiform VPCs
4. R-on-T phenomenon (VPCs occurring on or close to the T wave of the preceding complex)
5. Clinical signs of low cardiac output or hypotension
6. Ventricular myocardial failure

and pindolol). Others possess relative beta$_1$ selectivity (metoprolol and atenolol). Pindolol also has weak agonist effects (intrinsic sympathomimetic activity). Class III drugs prolong the refractory period of the cardiac cell action potential without decreasing conduction velocity. They may be most effective in suppressing re-entrant arrhythmias or in preventing ventricular fibrillation. Class IV drugs, by slowing Ca^{2+} entry into myocardial cells, affect those tissues most dependent on the slow Ca^{2+} current (mainly the sinoatrial and atrioventricular nodes and ischemic tissue). Ventricular arrhythmias usually are not responsive to class IV agents. The newly proposed class V contains a drug that selectively slows the sinus node rate and has no effect on ventricular arrhythmias.

Although drugs within the same class are similar, they are not identical (e.g. lidocaine and procainamide), so that if one drug does not suppress a

Table 3. *Antiarrhythmic Drug Classification*

Class	Drug	Mechanism and ECG Effects
I		Decrease fast inward Na$^+$ current; membrane stabilizing effects (decreased conductivity, excitability, and automaticity)
IA	Quinidine Procainamide Disopyramide	Moderate decrease in conductivity, increased action potential duration; QRS and Q-T prolonged
IB	Lidocaine Tocainide Mexiletine	Little change in conductivity, decreased action potential duration; QRS and Q-T unchanged
IC	Flecainide	Marked decrease in conductivity, no change in action potential duration
II	Propranolol Atenolol Metoprolol Pindolol Nadolol Timolol	Beta-adrenergic blockade—reduce sympathetic stimulation (no direct effects on myocardium at clinical dosages)
III	Bretylium Amiodarone	Selective prolongation of action potential duration and refractory period; antiadrenergic effects; Q-T prolonged
IV	Verapamil Diltiazem	Decrease slow inward Ca^{2+} current (therefore, greatest effects on SA and AV nodes)

patient's arrhythmia another in the same class might. Alternatively, a drug from a different class might be chosen. Sometimes two drugs of different classes are used together and may have synergistic effects (e.g., propranolol and procainamide, and mexiletine plus quinidine).

Many antiarrhythmic drugs can be given intravenously. This is often desirable because the onset of action is faster and efficacy can be better assessed. However, caution must be used to avoid adverse drug effects or toxicities. For instance, some antiarrhythmic agents have negative inotropic effects that can be deleterious when they are given intravenously (Table 4). Loading doses can be used to quickly boost drug levels into the therapeutic range, especially if concurrent constant rate infusion (CRI) is being used. Loading doses increase drug blood levels; however, they do not shorten the time required to achieve steady state. Intramuscular administration of some drugs may provide a faster onset of action than oral dosing without the risks of intravenous administration, but drug absorption from this route can be variable.

Oral preparations must be used for long-term therapy. Unfortunately, bioavailability may be quite variable. Certain drugs are well absorbed into the portal circulation only to undergo extensive hepatic metabolism before reaching the systemic circulation. Drugs such as propranolol and verapamil have relatively low bioavailability because of this large first-pass effect. Drug absorption may also be adversely affected by poor gastrointestinal mucosal

blood flow from heart failure, gut hypermotility, or malabsorption syndromes. Absorption of many antiarrhythmic drugs may be enhanced by raising gastric pH.

Guidelines for dosing usually are based on prior pharmacokinetic studies, but the dosage of drug used in an individual animal should be titrated to achieve therapeutic effect without toxicity. Changes in blood flow to various organs and changes in drug protein binding can affect plasma concentration and drug elimination. Drugs such as propranolol, lidocaine, verapamil, and disopyramide are dependent on liver blood flow for their clearance. With reductions in liver blood flow (such as from low cardiac output in heart failure or administration of propranolol or cimetidine) they are not cleared as rapidly, necessitating reduction in dosage or dosing frequency. Other drugs, such as digoxin and bretylium, are cleared mainly by the kidney and need dosage adjustments for animals in renal failure. If available, measurement of plasma drug concentration is helpful.

Therapy of Frequent VPCs or VT

Lidocaine (without epinephrine) is usually the first-choice drug because it has minimal adverse hemodynamic effects (Fig. 2). For dogs, boluses of 2 to 3 mg/kg slowly intravenously repeated once or twice over 15 to 20 minutes are usually effective. Total initial doses of up to 8 mg/kg over 10 minutes can be used if necessary, but toxicity may result (see Table 4). Another method is to inject 1 ml of 2 per cent lidocaine per 5 kg of body weight. If the arrhythmia is not suppressed in 5 minutes give 1 ml/10 kg. If after another 5 minutes the arrhythmia persists and no sign of toxicity is present give 1 ml/20 kg. The latter dose may be repeated as often as necessary until conversion or signs of toxicity are noted. Alternatively, a rapid intravenous infusion of 0.8 mg/kg/min can be administered over a 10-minute period (Table 4).

If lidocaine is ineffective, procainamide or intramuscular quinidine should be tried. Quinidine is generally not given intravenously owing to its marked hypotensive effects. Propranolol is another alternative. It is recommended that propranolol be diluted to a strength of 0.1 mg/ml. This dilution can be given at 0.1 mg/min until the desired effect or maximum recommended dose is reached.

If intravenous drug use is not possible, procainamide or quinidine given intramuscularly or orally can be effective in suppressing VT. A single loading dose (14 to 20 mg/kg IM) can be tried to assess effectiveness. Results should be seen in about 2 hours. If effective, lower doses can be given every 4 to 6 hours IM or PO.

In *cats,* propranolol is said to be the drug of

Table 4. Drugs Used For Ventricular Tachyarrhythmias

Drug	Dose/Route	Therapeutic Plasma Levels*	Precautions	Side Effects/Toxicity
Lidocaine HCl	*Dog:* Initial boluses of 2–3 mg/kg slowly IV, up to 8 mg/kg/10 min; or rapid IV infusion at 0.8 mg/kg/min; if effective then 25–80 µg/kg/min CRI *Cat:* 0.25–1 mg/kg IV over 5 min	2–6 µg/ml	Caution if also using drugs that decrease liver blood flow (e.g., propranolol, cimetidine) and in CHF. Cats are exquisitely sensitive to the neurotoxic and cardiotoxic effects	Seizures (give diazepam), CNS excitation, tremors, emesis, hypotension (rare), sinus arrest, AV blocks, ventricular tachyarrhythmias, respiratory arrest
Procainamide HCl	*Dog:* 6–8 mg/kg IV over 5 min; 10–40 µg/kg/min CRI; 6–20 mg/kg q4–6h IM; 8–20 mg/kg q6h PO; Procan SR 8–20 mg/kg q6–8h *Cat:* 25–50 mg q6–8h IM or PO	3–8 µg/ml or 6–10 µg/ml	Use with caution in cats. Clearance is decreased in heart failure. Use caution with IV administration. Give on empty stomach	Weakness, hypotension, decreased myocardial contractility, vagolytic effects, GI signs (anorexia, emesis, diarrhea), agranulocytosis and lupuslike syndrome (humans), ventricular tachyarrhythmia, decreased GFR and renal function, prolongation of P-R, QRS, Q-T intervals, AV blocks
Quinidine gluconate, quinidine polygalacturonate, quinidine sulfate	*Dog:* 6–20 mg/kg q6h IM; 6–16 mg/kg q6h PO; sustained action gluconate and polygalacturonate preparations: 8–20 mg/kg q6–8h PO	2–5 µg/ml	Do not use IV. Reduce dose in liver disease, CHF, and hypoalbuminemia. Quinidine-digoxin interaction (raises serum digoxin level). Cimetidine impairs absorption and elimination of quinidine	Weakness, hypotension, decreased myocardial contractility, vagolytic effects, GI signs, cinchonism, urine retention, sinus node suppression, ventricular tachyarrhythmias, AV blocks, prolongation of P-R, QRS, Q-T intervals
Phenytoin	*Dog:* 5–10 mg/kg slowly IV (over 2–3 min); 30 mg/kg q6–8h PO	10–16 µg/ml	Used for digitalis-induced arrhythmias only. Half-life is much shorter than that of digoxin so must repeat several times a day until serum digoxin level falls. Do not use in cats	Propylene glycol diluent causes hypotension, cardiac depression, respiratory or cardiac arrest; nausea, ataxia, hepatopathy, depression, seizures, variable PO absorption
Propranolol	*Dog and Cat:* 0.02–0.06 mg/kg slowly IV; 0.2–1.0 mg/kg q8h PO	50–150 ng/ml	Strength of effect depends on prevailing sympathetic tone. Begin with low dose	Bradycardia, prolongs AV conduction, hypotension, decreased myocardial contractility, may exacerbate heart failure, bronchospasm, hypoglycemia (in diabetics), prolongs P-R interval, GI upsets, depression, dizziness
Atenolol	*Dog:* 12.5–50 mg q8–24h PO	100–200 ng/ml	As for propranolol	As for propranolol, less bronchospasm
Tocainide	*Dog:* 5–20 mg/kg q6–8h PO	4–10 µg/ml	Giving with food may decrease side effects. Reduce dose or increase dosing interval with renal disease	As for lidocaine: CNS signs, GI upsets

*Human values; thought to be similar for dog and cat.
GI, gastrointestinal; GFR, glomerular filtration rate; CNS, central nervous system; AV, atrioventricular.

choice; however, procainamide (25 to 50 mg slowly IV or IM) or lidocaine has also been used successfully in this species. Small doses of lidocaine often are effective (see Table 4) but cats are sensitive to the drug's neurotoxic effects. Occasionally quinidine has been used in cats.

Digoxin is not used in the treatment of ventricular arrhythmias unless they are caused by heart failure or accompanied by serious supraventricular arrhythmias that need suppression. Because digoxin can predipose to ventricular arrhythmias, frequent ECG monitoring is essential and simultaneous use of another antiarrhythmic drug may also be necessary and should precede administration of digoxin if frequent or repetitive VPCs are present. Phenytoin is only used for digitalis-induced ventricular arrhythmias that are refractory to lidocaine (Table 4).

In human medicine, direct-current (DC) cardioversion may be used to convert VT; however, the need for ECG-synchronized equipment and anesthesia or sedation usually precludes use of this therapy in veterinary medicine.

After successful initial therapy of VT the animal should be closely monitored for return of the rhythm disturbance, especially within the first hour. Repeated intravenous drug boluses or CRI may be needed. Small IV boluses along with CRI (or a double-infusion technique) can help maintain therapeutic plasma levels until the drug by CRI reaches steady state (4 to 6 hours for lidocaine, 12 to 22 hours for procainamide). One method of providing a constant lidocaine infusion (44 µg/kg/min) is to add 25 ml of 2 per cent lidocaine (without epinephrine) to 250 ml of 5 per cent dextrose in water. This should be infused at 0.25 ml/25 lb of body weight per minute (the 25/250/0.25 rule). The rate or concentration can be increased if needed. If necessary, IV infusions can continue for several days, although 6 hours may be sufficient. An antiarrhythmic agent given IM or PO can be started as the patient is weaned from the IV drug. If a different drug is required for IM or PO use (e.g., quinidine or procainamide following an IV lidocaine infusion), its efficacy must be monitored. For oral maintenance therapy, the choice of drug depends on the effectiveness of the parenteral drug, the species involved, any concurrent medications, adverse drug effects, drug cost, and the dosing frequency required. Sustained release preparations of quinidine or procainamide may allow t.i.d. dosing and are most commonly used; however, in dogs, the half-life of sustained release procainamide is only slightly longer than that of procainamide itself. Tocainide, although expensive, appears to be effective in many dogs that are initially responsive to lidocaine.

Animals receiving long-term antiarrhythmic therapy should be re-evaluated frequently. Most clients can be instructed in how to use a stethoscope or palpate the chest wall to count the number of "skipped" beats per minute at home. This will approximate the frequency of events of VPCs (either single or paroxysms). If the rhythm disturbance disappears the drug may be discontinued and the animal monitored several times in the following 1 to 3 days for recurrence. Unfortunately, occasional ECG recordings may not provide an accurate assessment of an arrhythmia's presence or severity because arrhythmias tend to occur sporadically. If available, 24 to 48 hour continuous ECG recordings (Holter monitor) are helpful in documenting arrhythmias and the response to therapy.

In some patients the arrhythmia cannot be totally suppressed. Consideration of the animal's clinical status, whether the drug has decreased the number of VPCs, and the daily drug dosage (whether it should be increased) can be helpful in deciding to continue or discontinue therapy or try a new drug.

Treatment of Refractory Ventricular Arrhythmias

If conventional drug therapy is ineffective, one or more of the following suggestions may be helpful:

1. Re-evaluation of the ECGs can indicate if the rhythm diagnosis is correct. As an example, supraventricular tachycardia with aberrant ventricular conduction (bundle branch block) can resemble VT.

2. Serum K^+ levels can be measured. Hypokalemia reduces the efficacy of antiarrhythmic drugs, especially the class I agents. If serum K^+ level is less than 3.0 mEq/L, KCl can be infused at 0.5 mEq/kg/hr or, if 3.0 to 3.5 mEq/L, infused at 0.25 mEq/kg/hr.

3. The possibility that drug therapy might be exacerbating the rhythm disturbance (proarrhythmic effect) should be considered; one should rule out digitalis or antiarrhythmic drug toxicity. Polymorphous VT (torsade) can result from quinidine, procainamide, or disopyramide toxicity.

4. A beta-blocking drug can be administered with a class I drug (e.g., propranolol with procainamide).

5. The dose of the conventional antiarrhythmic agent having the greatest effect might be increased or drug efficacy can be retested using IV therapy. (Can plasma concentration be measured? Have "therapeutic" levels been achieved?)

6. A newer or investigational agent can be given.

7. If the patient is tolerating the arrhythmia well, supportive care only can be continued with close monitoring. Alternatively, investigational drugs, DC cardioversion, or ventricular pacing might be available at a referral center.

References and Supplemental Reading

Adams, H. R.: New perspectives in cardiology: Pharmacodynamic classification of antiarrhythmic drugs. J.A.V.M.A. 189:525, 1986.

Bonagura, J. D., and Muir, W. W.: Antiarrhythmic therapy. *In* Tilley, L. P. (ed.): *Essentials of Canine and Feline Electrocardiography*, 2nd ed. Philadelphia: Lea & Febiger, 1985, pp. 281–316.

Mandel, W. J. (ed.): *Cardiac Arrhythmias*. Philadelphia: J.B. Lippincott, 1980.

Muir, W. W., and Sams, R.: Clinical pharmacodynamics and pharmacokinetics of beta-adrenoceptor blocking drugs in veterinary medicine. Comp. Cont. Ed. Pract. Vet. 6:156, 1984.

Novotney, M. J., and Adams, H. R.: New perspectives in cardiology: Recent advances in antiarrhythmic drug therapy. J. A. V. M. A. 189:533, 1986.

Sasyniuk, B. I.: Concept of reentry vs automaticity. Am. J. Cardiol. 54:1A, 1984.

Tilley, L. P.: Analysis of common cardiac arrhythmias. *In* Tilley, L. P. (ed.): *Essentials of Canine and Feline Electrocardiography*, 2nd ed. Philadelphia: Lea & Febiger, 1985, pp. 125–246.

BRADYARRHYTHMIAS AND CARDIAC PACING

D. DAVID SISSON, D.V.M.

Urbana, Illinois

Symptomatic bradycardia in dogs and cats most commonly results from high-grade second-degree or complete (third-degree) heart block, sick sinus syndrome, or persistent atrial standstill. Chronic, persistent bradycardia is characterized by the development of exercise intolerance, lethargy, or overt heart failure. Transient and sporadic cerebral hypoperfusion resulting from a heart rate–induced fall in cardiac output is usually manifested as episodic ataxia, weakness, syncope, or Stokes-Adams seizures. Recurrent episodes of prolonged hypotension may result in cerebral anoxia, permanent brain damage, and behavioral changes.

Most of the arrhythmias responsible for symptomatic bradycardia are easily recognized on a resting electrocardiogram (ECG) (Fig. 1). When the resting ECG is normal and an intermittent arrhythmia is suspected, a definitive diagnosis can usually be made by recording multiple resting ECGs or a continuous 24-hour ambulatory ECG. It is the responsibility of the attending veterinarian to exclude other possible causes for the observed clinical signs, such as neurologic disease or metabolic disorders. After the diagnosis of a symptomatic bradycardia is made, the primary goals of therapy are to promptly restore an adequate heart rate and then to maintain a stable cardiac rhythm. Although pharmacologic interventions can be successfully employed for the temporary management of some patients with bradyarrhythmias, reliable long-term treatment can usually be accomplished only by implantation of a permanent artificial pacemaker. Successful patient management requires careful planning and meticulous attention to detail prior to and following pacemaker implantation.

CAUSES OF SYMPTOMATIC BRADYCARDIA

Sinus Bradycardia

In dogs, sinus bradycardia is most often a normal finding or a benign manifestation of some underlying disease that is affecting the autonomic nervous system's control of the heart rate. Sinus bradycardia is an expected finding in athletic and sedated dogs. Most dogs with sinus bradycardia and a heart rate greater than 50 beats/min are asymptomatic for the arrhythmia and do not require therapy to increase the heart rate. Vague signs of lethargy in dogs with this arrhythmia are usually due to some other effect of the underlying disease rather than to low cardiac output. This fact can readily be demonstrated by performing an atropine challenge test. Following atropine administration, the heart rate usually increases dramatically, yet the animal's attitude and behavior remain unchanged. Sinus bradycardia is an uncommon arrhythmia in the cat. Most cats with sinus arrhythmia examined by the author have been critically ill with heart failure, shock, hypoxia, or some serious metabolic disorder.

Sinus bradycardia caused by hypothermia, hypothyroidism, or disturbances of serum potassium concentration is usually accompanied by historical information or clinical findings that suggest the underlying cause. Simple laboratory tests are available to confirm these diagnoses. Patients with these disorders are best managed by treating the underlying disorder. Profound sinus bradycardia that results in clinical signs can be induced in dogs and cats by a number of toxins and pharmacologic agents. Parasympathomimetic drugs, digitalis, an-

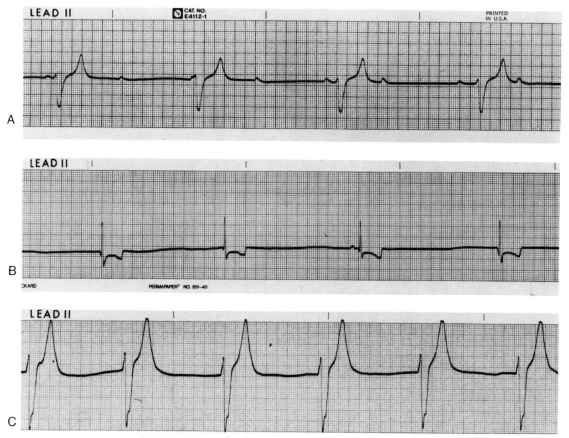

Figure 1. Representative lead II electrocardiograms are shown from three dogs with symptomatic bradycardia. *A* shows third-degree heart block and a ventricular escape rate of 40 bpm. *B* shows sinus bradycardia (or sinus arrest) and a heart rate of 50 bpm. Beats 1, 2, and 4 are junctional escape beats. Tracing *C* shows atrial standstill (no P waves) and an accelerated ventricular escape rate of 64 bpm. Paper speed, 50 cm/sec; 1 cm = 1 mV.

esthetics, xylazine, thorazine tranquilizers, and calcium channel and beta-receptor blocking drugs may all induce a pronounced sinus bradycardia. Increased intracranial pressure, meningoencephalitis, mediastinal and cervical masses, and a variety of respiratory and gastrointestinal disturbances also may cause sinus bradycardia.

The consequences of sinus bradycardia must be assessed in relation to the physical condition of the patient. Heart rates that would be well tolerated by a healthy animal may cause progressive physical deterioration in an animal with heart disease or one with a serious systemic illness. When pronounced sinus bradycardia results from a serious systemic disease and is contributing to the clinical signs, aggressive measures to increase heart rate are indicated in concert with vigorous efforts to identify and correct the underlying cause and sustain arterial blood pressure. If sinus bradycardia is suspected to be contributing to the clinical signs, trial therapy with vagolytic or adrenergic drugs is warranted. When clinical signs result from a pronounced drug-induced sinus bradycardia, an antidote specific for the drug should be administered, if available. Relevant examples include calcium salts for verapamil

intoxication and phenytoin for digitalis toxicity. It is also prudent to hasten the elimination of the offending drug and to provide general supportive therapy in accordance with the needs of the patient (e.g., administering intravenous fluids; providing a heating pad; and increasing the heart rate with atropine, adrenergic drugs such as dopamine, or a temporary pacemaker).

Heart Block

Clinically, heart block (atrioventricular block) is classified as first-degree, second-degree, and third-degree (complete) heart block. Second-degree heart block is further classified as type I when the P-R interval gradually lengthens prior to the dropped beat or beats and as type II when dropped beats are not preceded by increasing P-R intervals. The term high-grade second-degree heart block refers to the consistent blocking of two or more consecutive P waves. Occasionally, dogs or cats with intermittent high-grade second-degree or complete heart block are presented for evaluation. Many of these patients have a resting electrocardiogram characterized by first-degree heart block combined with either left or right bundle branch block. In animals suspected to have intermittent heart block, the diagnosis should be confirmed by recording the arrhythmic events on frequently repeated resting ECGs or, more reliably, by recording of a 24-hour continuous ambulatory ECG.

First-degree and type I second-degree heart block are common arrhythmias in dogs and only rarely signify intrinsic disease of the atrioventricular (AV) node or His-Purkinje system. These arrhythmias usually result from increased vagal tone and are readily abolished by exercise or atropine. It is noteworthy that electrocardiograms recorded shortly after the administration of atropine often show initial slowing of the heart rate and induction or accentuation of first- or second-degree heart block. This centrally mediated augmentation of vagal tone is a normal response to atropine and should not be interpreted as evidence of disease. In normal dogs, sinus rhythm or sinus tachycardia usually develops 10 to 20 minutes following the subcutaneous or intramuscular injection of atropine. In dogs with organic heart disease, the degree of AV block may improve or worsen.

Persistent, symptomatic high-grade second-degree and complete heart block (see Fig. 1) in dogs occur most often as idiopathic rhythm disturbances in middle-aged or older dogs. Although some of these dogs have murmurs caused by mitral or tricuspid regurgitation, few have serious valvular or myocardial dysfunction. Heart block may also develop as a sequela of bacterial endocarditis, infiltrative myocardial disease, hypertrophic cardiomyopathy, hyperkalemia, or administration of drugs that directly inhibit conduction through the AV node (e.g., digoxin and verapamil). Complete heart block has also been reported as a congenital defect of dogs. Fewer cases of symptomatic heart block have been reported in cats than in dogs. Most of these have been observed in cats with hypertrophic cardiomyopathy or in older cats, during their second decade of life. Pathologic changes in the conduction systems of cats with hypertrophic cardiomyopathy are well documented. In contrast to the situation in dogs, even low-grade heart block is an abnormal ECG finding in cats and always warrants further diagnostic evaluation and follow-up.

Animals with high-grade second-degree or complete heart block almost always exhibit signs of weakness, lethargy, and exercise intolerance. Syncope and Stokes-Adams attacks can often be historically documented. Some dogs with chronic heart block exhibit signs of congestive heart failure (CHF) that can be attributed to chronic bradycardia. In dogs with idiopathic heart block, signs of heart failure usually resolve when the heart rate is restored to the normal range. In dogs and cats with endocarditis or cardiomyopathy the prognosis is much less favorable. It is prudent, particularly when pacemaker implantation is contemplated, to thoroughly evaluate dogs with heart block by obtaining thoracic radiographs, a complete blood count, and a serum chemistry profile. Echocardiography, if available, is extremely valuable for detecting bacterial endocarditis and assessing myocardial structure and function.

Sick Sinus Syndrome

Sick sinus syndrome is a loosely defined clinical term used to describe patients that are symptomatic as a result of idiopathic sinoatrial dysfunction. The electrocardiographic findings in dogs with sick sinus syndrome include intermittent sinus arrest, sinoatrial (SA) block, sinus bradycardia, or some combination of these arrhythmias. Failure of subsidiary pacemakers to generate an adequate escape rhythm is thought to contribute to the development of clinical signs. Supraventricular tachyarrhythmias are also detected in many dogs with sick sinus syndrome. Clinical signs may result from bradycardia, tachycardia, or both.

Sick sinus syndrome has been reported in miniature schnauzers, pug dogs, dachshunds, and mixed-breed dogs. Syncope, seizures, and episodic weakness are the usual signs observed in dogs with sick sinus syndrome. The diagnosis of sick sinus syndrome is often elusive, particularly when the resting eletrocardiogram is normal and the clinical signs are infrequent. It is easy to confuse sick sinus syndrome with a seizure disorder and vice versa. Continuous ambulatory eletrocardiography often provides a diagnosis when other methods fail.

Patients with sick sinus syndrome have been segregated by some authors into two groups, those with and those without episodes of supraventricular tachycardia (SVT). Caution should be exercised when the method of treatment is based on this classification scheme. Many human patients and dogs with sick sinus syndrome without SVT based on resting electrocardiograms show a high prevalence of SVT when studied by continuous 24-hour ambulatory electrocardiography.

In the author's experience, sudden death (resulting from the arrhythmia) is extremely uncommon in dogs with this syndrome. Nonetheless, sudden death has been reported in pug dogs with sick sinus syndrome and second-degree heart block.

Atrial Standstill

Persistent atrial standstill is an uncommon rhythm disturbance in dogs and cats. P waves are not observed on the electrocardiogram, and the heart's rhythm is controlled by a junctional or ventricular escape focus. English springer spaniels with a facioscapulohumeral type of muscular dystrophy are reported to manifest this arrhythmia. Similar rhythm disturbances have been observed by the author in dogs and cats with inflammatory or infiltrative diseases of the atrial myocardium. Evidence of myocardial failure can often be detected in patients with persistent atrial standstill, either at the time of presentation or following (otherwise) successful management of the arrhythmia. For this reason, a guarded prognosis is always offered when this diagnosis is presented to the owner.

Persistent atrial standstill must be distinguished from transient atrial standstill, which is a commonly observed arrhythmia in animals with hyperkalemia due to renal failure, urinary tract obstruction, or hypoadrenocorticism. Unless death of the patient supervenes, P waves and normal sinus rhythm promptly return when blood potassium levels are returned to normal. Traditional remedies include the administration of 0.9 per cent sodium chloride, sodium bicarbonate (1 to 2 mEq/kg IV), dextrose (with or without insulin), and mineralocorticoids. If cardiac arrest appears imminent, calcium-containing solutions (10 per cent solution of $CaCl_2$, 1 ml/10 kg slowly IV) can be given intravenously to temporarily antagonize the electrogenic effects of hyperkalemia. The effects of calcium administration are short lived, but this intervention often allows the additional time required to lower blood potassium levels. Atropine (0.02 to 0.04 mg/kg IV) may increase the heart rate in animals with sinoventricular rhythm.

MEDICAL TREATMENT OF CHRONIC SYMPTOMATIC BRADYCARDIA

The only reliable method of treatment for dogs and cats with persistent atrial standstill or high-grade second-degree or complete heart block is implantation of a permanent artificial pacemaker. With rare exception, vagolytic and adrenergic drugs cannot be expected to restore and maintain sinus rhythm in patients with these arrhythmias. In an emergency, isoproterenol or dopamine, administered by constant intravenous infusion, can be used temporarily to increase the heart rate by increasing the rate of discharge of ventricular or junctional escape foci.

These drugs are often life saving when pacemaker implantation cannot be performed immediately. Unfortunately, isoproterenol and dopamine frequently induce dangerous ventricular tachyarrhythmias. Antiarrhythmic drugs should never be administered in this circumstance. Control of ventricular tachycardia in this setting is best accomplished by stopping or reducing the rate of drug administration. Orally administered isoproterenol has been recommended for the treatment of dogs with symptomatic bradycardia. Because it is not possible to maintain stable blood levels using orally administered isoproterenol, the author cannot recommend its use by this route of administration for the treatment of bradycardia due to any cause.

Vagolytic drugs, such as atropine, propantheline bromide, or isopropamide, are usually not effective remedies for dogs with heart block because they cause only a modest increase in the rate of discharge of ventricular (escape) foci. Vagolytic drugs can sometimes be used as interim therapy to accelerate the rate of discharge of junctional (escape) foci that are occasionally observed in patients with persistent atrial standstill. Test doses of atropine (0.02 to 0.04 mg/kg IM or IV) also abolish the bradyarrhythmias observed in some dogs with sick sinus syndrome. Chronic treatment with vagolytic drugs has been reported to reduce the severity of clinical signs in some dogs with sick sinus syndrome. However, the ECGs of many dogs with sick sinus syndrome do not change in response to atropine administration, and many of these dogs do not improve with trial vagolytic therapy.

Even when dogs respond to vagolytic drug therapy, the realities of owner compliance with regimens requiring the frequent long-term administration of any drug detracts from this therapeutic option. In dogs with sick sinus syndrome complicated by supraventricular tachycardia, adrenergic or vagolytic drugs given to increase the heart rate may precipitate more severe and more frequent bouts of supraventricular tachycardia. Unless a pacemaker is implanted, antiarrhythmic drugs used to suppress supraventricular tachyarrhythmias will often aggravate a pre-existing bradyarrhythmia. The limitations of medically managing dogs with sick sinus syndrome make this alternative less desirable than pacemaker implantation, particularly when the signs are frequent or severe.

PACEMAKER IMPLANTATION IN DOGS AND CATS

Equipment

Successful implantation of a permanent cardiac pacemaker requires careful planning at every stage of the procedure. An almost endless array of complications must be anticipated and guarded against. First, an equipment check should be performed. An appropriately programmed permanent pulse generator and a stimulating electrode (lead) are the essential components required to accomplish artificial cardiac pacing. The operator should ensure that the lead to be used is compatible with the pulse generator. In the event of a lapse in sterile technique, a backup pulse generator and lead should always be available. Sterile tools needed to connect the lead and pulse generator should be included in the list of necessary materials. It is also desirable to have a polypropylene mesh pouch to secure the pulse generator in position.

Most modern implantable pulse generators are lithium powered and are designed to create and detect electrical impulses in a manner described by a five-letter code. The first letter of this code indicates the chamber paced; the second letter, the chamber sensed; the third, the mode of response; and the fourth and fifth letters describe any programmable and tachyarrhythmia functions of the pulse generator (Fig. 2). Currently, only VVIPO (ventricular inhibited, demand, rate, and output programmable) and VVIMO (ventricular inhibited, demand, multiprogrammable) pulse generators are commonly implanted in domestic animals. VVI(PO or MO) pulse generators sense the electrical activity of the heart and pace the heart only if the ventricle's inherent rate falls below a predetermined rate. Pacing rates of 100 beats/min for dogs and 130 beats/min for cats are usually adequate for obtaining acceptable clinical results. It is advisable to consult with a specialist in veterinary cardiology for information regarding appropriate settings for sensitivity, refractory periods, and the output characteristics of the stimulating pulse.

The electrical current created by the pulse generator can be delivered to the heart by either epicardial or endocardial electrodes (leads). The pacing lead is also used by the pulse generator to detect the heart's inherent rhythm so that dangerous competing rhythms are avoided. Most modern permanent pacemaker leads consist of polyurethane- or silicone-coated multifilar helical coil wires. Epicardial leads are usually of unipolar design so that contact of the pulse generator to the patient's body is needed to complete the electrical circuit and to initiate pacing. Implantation of an epicardial electrode requires general anesthesia and surgical invasion of the thorax, via thoracotomy or transab-dominal approach, but offers the advantage of secure active myocardial fixation. Some epicardial leads must be sutured in place, whereas others with a corkscrewlike design can be quickly and easily screwed into place.

Permanent transvenous pacemaker implantation avoids the requirement for major surgery but requires the availability of fluoroscopy to allow accurate placement of an endocardial lead into the right ventricle. In cooperative dogs, permanent transvenous pacing can be accomplished using only local anesthesia. The author has used a variety of permanent transvenous leads and achieved good results using tined leads to obtain secure but passive fixation of the lead. Permanent transvenous leads with a retractable corkscrewlike tip that can be actively fixed to the myocardium are available but expensive. Endocardial leads may be unipolar or bipolar. When a bipolar lead system is used, pacing commences as soon as the wires from each pole of the lead are secured to the pulse generator. There is no clear consensus suggesting the superiority of either design. However, unipolar leads may be more sensitive to extraneous electrical noise and also appear to result in a higher incidence of peripheral "muscle twitching" than bipolar leads. Inasmuch as a large number of leads of different design are commercially available, interested readers are referred to the supplemental reading section for a more in-depth discussion.

Patient Preparation

In dogs and cats with high-grade heart block or atrial standstill, ventricular asystole and ventricular fibrillation are frequent sequela to the induction of anesthesia with thiobarbiturates or gas anesthetics. These arrhythmias are much less likely to develop in dogs with sick sinus syndrome, particularly if the arrhythmia is atropine responsive and the patient is

ICHD Generic Pacemaker Code

1st Letter	2nd Letter	3rd Letter	4th Letter	5th Letter
↓	↓	↓	↓	↓
Chamber Paced	Chamber Sensed	Mode of Response	Programmable Functions	Tachyarrhythmia Functions

Available Letters	
V ⟶ Ventricle	P ⟶ Rate/Output Programmable
A ⟶ Atria	M ⟶ Multiprogrammable
D ⟶ Dual Chamber	C ⟶ Multiprogrammable with Telemetry
O ⟶ Not Applicable	O ⟶ Not Applicable
T ⟶ Triggered	B ⟶ Burst
I ⟶ Inhibited	N ⟶ Normal Rate Competition
S ⟶ Single Chamber	S ⟶ Scanning
	E ⟶ External

Figure 2. The wide variety of features available on the many different pulse generators manufactured for cardiac pacing can be quickly described using a five-letter code. Letters selected from the column at the left are used to define the chamber sensed, the chamber paced, and the mode of response. Letters from the column at the right are used to describe any programmable or tachyarrhythmia functions of the pulse generator.

appropriately premedicated. Otherwise, temporary cardiac pacing initiated prior to the induction of anesthesia represents the most reliable means of preventing these often catastrophic arrhythmias. Temporary pacing is also indicated for the treatment of patients with serious but transient arrhythmias and for presurgical stabilization of seriously ill patients or those with severe CHF scheduled to receive a permanently implanted pacemaker.

Temporary pacing leads are available that can be positioned into the heart by the transvenous route or by cardiac puncture. The latter route is used only in dire emergencies. Temporary pacemaker leads are usually introduced through an indwelling large-gauge intravenous catheter that has been pre-placed in the external jugular vein. They can be advanced into position with fluoroscopic guidance or blindly until successful pacing is accomplished. It is important to note that a unipolar pulse generator intended for implantation cannot be used as an external pulse generator with a temporary bipolar pacing lead. An external pulse generator specifically designed for temporary pacing should be used with these temporary leads.

If temporary pacing is not possible, permanent pacemaker implantation can still be performed, albeit with increased risk for the patient. The selection of anesthetic agents is even more critical under these circumstances. To reduce the risk of periop-erative cardiac arrest, anesthesia should be induced with narcotics, benzodiazepines, or small doses of thiobarbiturates. For maintenance of anesthesia, low concentrations of an inhalation anesthetic can be combined with the intermittent administration of a narcotic. Preparations should be made in advance for cardiopulmonary resuscitation and electrical defibrillation, should the need arise.

Pacemaker Implantation

The attachment of an epicardial lead to the heart can be accomplished by lateral thoracotomy at the left sixth intercostal space or by using a ventral abdominal, transdiaphragmatic approach. For more detailed descriptions of these surgical approaches, see the supplemental reading section. After access to the heart is gained, the pericardium is incised near the cardiac apex to permit the operator to secure the lead to the left ventricle. Large coronary vessels should be avoided when the lead is attached to the heart. Repetitive contractions of the diaphragm are best prevented by positioning the lead as far from the phrenic nerve as possible. The author prefers epicardial leads that can be screwed into the ventricular muscle with no requirement for suturing (Fig. 3). The lead wire is then tunneled to the planned final location of the pulse generator. The lead should be sufficiently long to prevent the development of undue tension on the lead connections.

When an epicardial lead is used, the author prefers to place the pulse generator in the flank, into a pocket made by blunt dissection between the internal and external abdominal oblique muscles. The pulse generator should not be placed within the abdomen. This location often precludes noninvasive reprogramming of the pulse generator. A more superficial location of the pulse generator permits use of a reprogramming instrument without the requirement for additional surgery. Migration of the pulse generator can be prevented by placing it within a polypropylene pouch, which can be more easily secured to the surrounding musculature. Prior to connecting the epicardial lead to the pulse generator, the rate of the temporary pacemaker is decreased to avoid confusion or complications caused by competitive pacing. Before closing the surgical wounds, adequate pacing should be verified by direct observation of the heart, palpation of the arterial pulse, and recording of an electrocardiogram.

If fluoroscopy is available, permanent pacing can be more safely and more easily accomplished using an endocardial lead that is positioned into the right ventricle via the external jugular vein. The endo-cardial lead is introduced by jugular venous cut-down and secured to the vein and underlying musculature by two or more nonabsorbable sutures, being careful not to fracture the lead. To minimize the possibility of lead displacement, the electrode tip must be positioned securely in the apex of the right ventricle (Fig. 4). This requires fluoroscopic guidance. The use of tined leads also helps to prevent displacement of the lead in the early post-operative period. After the lead is adequately positioned, the pulse generator is implanted in a sub-cutaneous pocket created at the site of a separate skin incision on the dorsolateral aspect of the neck.

The main complication experienced with the transvenous technique is lead displacement in the early postoperative period (during the first 2 weeks after operation). This complication can usually be avoided by the use of tined leads, careful lead placement, and careful selection of patients. Dogs with dilated right ventricles appear to be more prone to lead displacement and should probably be paced using an epicardial lead.

Patient Aftercare and Follow-up

Implantation of a pacemaker obligates the operator to recognize and resolve complications that are likely to arise following pacemaker implantation. Pacemaker lead or pulse generator malfunction occasionally occurs. Oversensing (interpretation of P or T waves or myopotentials as QRS complexes),

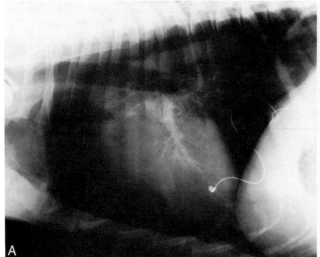

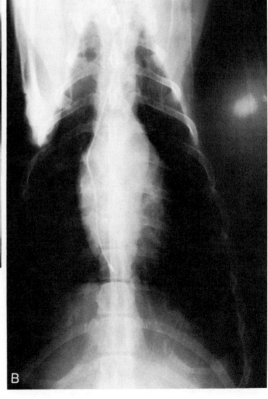

Figure 3. Proper placement of a screw-tipped epicardial pacemaker lead near the apex of the left ventricle is shown on these postoperative lateral (A) and dorsoventral (B) chest radiographs. The pulse generator was positioned in the flank of this dog.

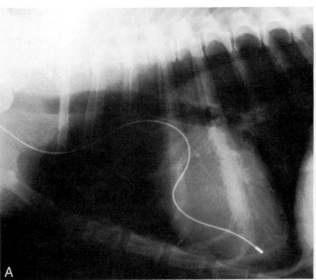

Figure 4. These postoperative lateral (A) and dorsoventral (B) chest radiographs show the desired location of a permanent unipolar endocardial pacemaker lead in the apex of the right ventricle. Lead displacement can best be avoided when tined leads are used and the lead is properly positioned.

failure to sense, and failure to pace (e.g., from fibrosis at the electrode site) are commonly encountered postoperative problems. Pacing and sensing thresholds often change over time, often within weeks of implantation, and it may be necessary to reprogram the pulse generator to resolve these problems. Lead wires may become displaced, requiring repositioning, or the lead wire may fracture and have to be replaced. Cardiac arrhythmias such as ventricular premature beats or ventricular tachycardia often develop in the early postoperative period and may require antiarrhythmic therapy. The identification of arrhythmias and pacemaker malfunction are greatly facilitated if the veterinarian is familiar with the "normal" electrocardiograms of animals with pacemakers (Figs. 5 and 6).

Bacterial infection is a constant concern in the immediate postoperative period. Regardless of the method used to accomplish permanent artificial pacing, the author administers an antibiotic (cephalexin, 20 mg/kg t.i.d.) prophylactically during and for 7 to 10 days following the procedure. Blood counts and cultures should be obtained at the first sign of a possible infection. Persistent infections often necessitate reoperation and replacement of the pulse generator and lead. Some patients receiving pacemakers will require treatment for coexisting myocardial failure (particularly those with persistent atrial standstill). Muscle twitching is another com-

monly observed problem in dogs following pacemaker implantation. Although it is not life threatening, this aggravating problem may require attention if it fails to resolve after several weeks.

Eventually, pulse generator batteries become depleted and a new pulse generator must be implanted. Most modern pulse generators signal impending battery depletion by a predetermined reduction in the pacing rate. When the pulse generator is implanted superficially, it can be easily replaced with a new pulse generator, which is simply attached to the previously implanted lead.

Recognition and successful resolution of these complications are facilitated when protocols for the care and evaluation of patients with pacemakers are developed and strictly adhered to. The brand, type, and serial number of the pulse generator as well as the programmed settings should be recorded in the patient's medical record. An electrocardiogram and thoracic radiographs should be obtained for every patient immediately after pacemaker implantation. Frequent ECGs should be obtained for several days following pacemaker implantation. Exercise should be strictly limited in dogs paced by the transvenous route, to minimize the chance of lead displacement. Exercise restriction should be continued for 2 weeks following discharge from the hospital. All patients should return for re-evaluation 10 days and 1 month following pacemaker implantation. Thoracic radio-

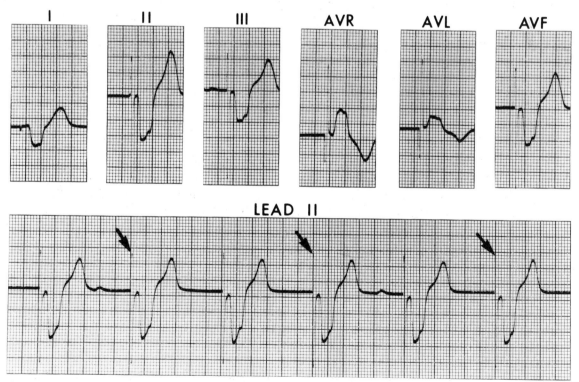

Figure 5. This ECG was recorded from a dog after pacemaker implantation for complete heart block. The pacemaker impulses (arrows) occur regularly at a rate of 100 bpm and are immediately followed by wide and bizarre QRS complexes. QRS morphologic features resemble those seen in dogs with right bundle branch block. This pattern of depolarization suggests that the heart is being paced by an epicardial lead attached to the left ventricle. Paper speed, 50 cm/sec; 1 cm = 1 mV.

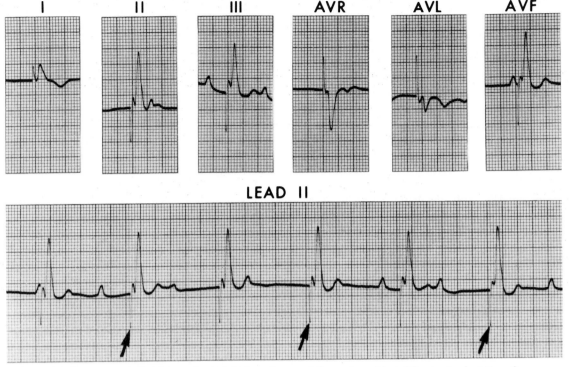

Figure 6. This ECG was recorded from a dog with high-grade second-degree heart block following implantation of a permanent transvenous pacemaker. The abnormally shaped QRS complexes that follow the pacemaker spikes (arrows) resemble those seen in dogs with left bundle branch block. Paper speed, 50 cm/sec; 1 cm = 2 mV.

graphs and electrocardiograms are repeated at the time of these visits. Thereafter, 6-month follow-up visits are recommended. With careful attention to detail, the implantation of permanent cardiac pacemakers can be a particularly rewarding procedure for the animal, the owner, and the veterinarian.

References and Supplemental Reading

Bonagura, J. D., Helphrey, M. L., and Muir M. W.: Complications associated with permanent pacemaker implantation in the dog. J.A.V.M.A. 182:149, 1983.

Fox, P. R., Matthiesen, D. T., Purse, D., et al.: Ventral abdominal, transdiaphragmatic approach for implantation of cardiac pacemakers in the dog. J.A.V.M.A. 189:1303, 1986.

Frye, R. L., Collins, J. J., DeSanctis, R. W., et al.: Guidelines for permanent cardiac pacemaker implantation, May 1984. Circulation 70:331A, 1984.

Helphrey, M. L., and Schollmeyer, M.: Pacemaker therapy. In Kirk, R. W. (ed.): Current Veterinary Therapy VIII. Philadelphia: W. B. Saunders, 1983, pp. 373–376.

Lombard, C. W., Tilley, L. P., and Yoshioka, M. M.: Pacemaker implantation in the dog. Survey and literature review. J. Am. Anim. Hosp. Assoc. 17:751, 1981.

Parsonnet, V., Furman, S., Smyth, P. D., et al.: Optimal resources for implantable cardiac pacemakers. Circulation 68:227A, 1983.

Yoshioka, M. M., Tilley, L. P., Harvey, H. J., et al.: Permanent pacemaker implantation in the dog. J. Am. Anim. Hosp. Assoc. 17:746, 1981.

THERAPY FOR FELINE AORTIC THROMBOEMBOLISM

PAUL D. PION, D.V.M.,
and MARK D. KITTLESON, D.V.M.
Davis, California

Aortic thromboembolism ("saddle thrombosis") is a common clinical entity in cats (Fig. 1). The vast majority of cats with aortic thromboemboli have an underlying cardiomyopathy (dilated, hypertrophic, or restrictive). Bacterial endocarditis with associated thromboembolism is rare in the cat. It is thought that in most cases the emboli originate in a dilated left atrium or ventricle and lodge in the distal aorta (Fig. 2). In a minority of cases it is possible to identify thrombi in the left atrium or ventricle at necropsy or by two-dimensional ultrasound examination of the heart. Aortic thromboemboli are reported to be most commonly observed in cats with hypertrophic and dilated forms of cardiomyopathy. These emboli represent a significant clinical setback because cats with hypertrophic cardiomyopathy *alone* have a good probability of long-term (months to years) functional survival.

PATHOPHYSIOLOGY OF FAILURE OF COLLATERAL VASCULARIZATION

In the cat, physical occlusion of the aorta alone does not cause ischemic damage to the peripheral nerves, muscle, and skin of the hindlimb (Fig. 3).

Imhoff (1961) clearly demonstrated that a thrombus must be present before ischemic damage occurs. Single or double ligation of the distal aorta in experimental animals produces no clinical signs; collateral circulation through epaxial and spinal arteries maintains adequate flow to the distal extremities. However, if a thrombus is produced at the site of occlusion, flow through these collateral vessels is inhibited. Vasoactive substances released by the thrombus are believed to cause vasoconstriction of the collateral vessels. Serotonin, prostaglandins, or both have been implicated as vasoactive substances. The evidence leading to this hypothesis includes the observation that administering antagonists of serotonin and prostaglandin synthesis, prior to thrombosis, prevents the inhibition of collateral circulation noted above. Administering these drugs after inhibition of collateral circulation has occurred appears to have little or no benefit in these experimental models.

CLINICAL PRESENTATION

The aortic trifurcation is the most common site for emboli to lodge (see Fig. 1), but clinical signs

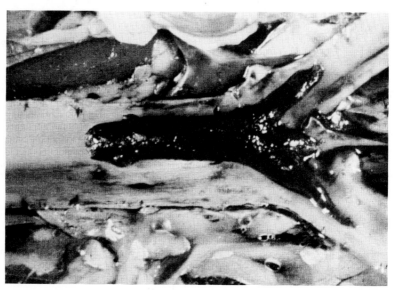

Figure 1. Postmortem photograph of a large, fresh red thromboembolus lodged at the aortic trifurcation in a cat with hypertrophic cardiomyopathy.

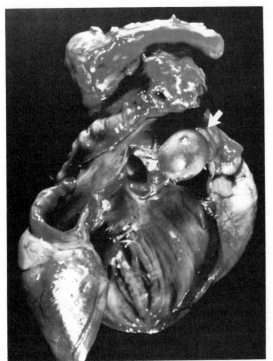

Figure 2. Postmortem photograph of a firm, partially endothelium-covered thrombus adhering to the left atrial wall in a cat with dilated cardiomyopathy.

referable to an embolus in forelimb, renal, cardiac, cerebral, mesenteric, hepatic, splenic, and ovarian arteries may be observed. Varying degrees of clinical signs result from ischemic damage to tissues distal to the occlusion. The most common clinical

signs referable to aortic thromboemboli include posterior paresis or paralysis due to ischemic myopathy and lower motor neuron ischemic sensorimotor neuropathy, cool posterior extremities, cyanotic or pale rear limb foot pads, cyanotic rear limb nail beds that do not bleed when cut back to expose the vascular ungual process, and firm, painful gastrocnemius muscles. These patients often present to veterinarians soon after the embolic episode because the onset of clinical signs is peracute and dramatic.

Although absence of arterial pulses in the affected limb or limbs is common, this sign alone should not be interpreted as pathognomonic for feline aortic thromboembolism. Palpating arterial pulses in feline patients can be difficult, especially in uncooperative or obese cats or those in pain. Typically, skeletal muscle enzyme concentrations in the serum are markedly elevated. Acute renal failure, metabolic acidosis, disseminated intravascular coagulation (DIC), and hyperkalemia may be present at the time of hospital admission. Differential diagnosis should include neuromuscular disorders such as spinal diseases (e.g., intervertebral disk extrusion, spinal abscesses, and spinal neoplasia); diabetic neuropathy; trauma; and myasthenia gravis. Imaging of the affected regional vessels by intravenous or intraarterial angiography or nuclear tracers is the definitive diagnostic procedure for thromboembolic disease but is usually unnecessary. Risks to the patient must be weighed. Stabilizing the patient is the primary consideration before attempting invasive diagnostic procedures.

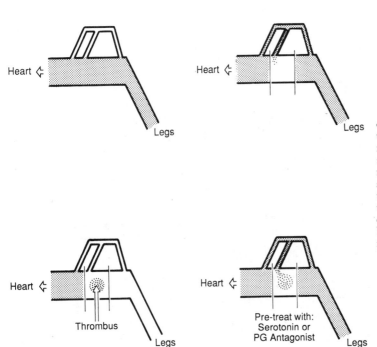

Figure 3. Pathogenesis of inhibition of collateral circulation. *Top left,* Normal circulation through abdominal aorta to pelvic limbs with minimal flow through collateral vessels. *Top right,* Ligating the infrarenal aorta results in normal flow to the periphery via collateral vessels. *Bottom left,* The presence of a thrombus in the isolated segment inhibits collateral circulation. *Bottom right,* Pretreatment with antagonists of serotonin or prostaglandins prevents the inhibition of collateral circulation when a thrombus is present.

PROGNOSIS

A guarded prognosis should be given in cases of complete aortic occlusion. Suprarenal aortic thrombosis has been associated with gastrointestinal ischemia, spinal cord dysfunction and degeneration caused by ischemia, and acute renal failure and so warrants a grave prognosis. In cases of infrarenal obstruction, given time and medical management as outlined below, some cats will regain function of the affected limb or limbs. After restoration of blood flow, whether spontaneously or as the result of therapeutic intervention, thromboembolism can recur despite prophylaxis (see following discussion of prophylaxis). Controlled clinical trials comparing therapeutic and prophylactic protocols are lacking in the veterinary literature.

If arterial occlusion is left untreated, the outcome will depend on the extent of occlusion and time to spontaneous reperfusion, via either the primary vessel or the collateral circulation. Cats may lose the affected leg because of ischemic necrosis, die of toxemia, remain paralyzed from peripheral nerve damage, or regain full or partial function of the leg. Overall, response to currently available conservative or aggressive clinical intervention often has been poor, particularly when there is associated dilated cardiomyopathy.

THERAPEUTIC OPTIONS

Surgery

Surgical removal of thromboemboli has met with mixed results. Unreliable results combined with a high anesthetic mortality in these patients have convinced most veterinary surgeons and cardiologists that surgery to remove the thrombus is not a viable alternative. This procedure is still advocated by some clinicians, particularly for suprarenal thromboembolism. The outcome of surgery is probably highly dependent on the skill of the surgeon and the anesthesiologist. Concurrent congestive heart failure (CHF) greatly increases the risk of anesthesia.

Catheter embolectomy, performed by placing a balloon-tipped (Fogarty) catheter in the affected vessel, advancing the balloon proximal to the thromboembolus, inflating the balloon, and mechanically pulling the thromboembolus free from the site of obstruction, might be effective in conjunction with medical therapies. This is the procedure of choice in humans with peripheral arterial thrombosis. However, identification, isolation, and catheterization of a collapsed unperfused artery is difficult in an animal as small as a domestic cat. Besides being technically difficult, catheter embolectomy in cats, like surgery, may be associated with the risks of

anesthesia and acute reperfusion syndrome (see below).

Medical Therapy

Medical therapy (Table 1) may include any combination of the following options:

1. Pleurocentesis and administration of diuretics and vasodilators to relieve signs of congestive heart failure from the underlying myocardial disease.

2. Anticoagulation with heparin to prevent further thrombosis. Although heparin may have thrombolytic activity, its primary therapeutic function is believed to be inhibition of thrombus formation, thereby allowing the patient's natural thrombolytic mechanisms to decrease the size of the thrombus. Heparin complexes with and activates the serine protease inhibitor antithrombin III, accelerating the neutralization of activated coagulation factors, especially factor X and thrombin (IIa). The dosage of heparin to achieve therapeutic results in cats is not well defined. Harpster (1986, p. 380) recommends an initial dosage of 220 U/kg of heparin U.S.P. IV, followed 3 hours later by a maintenance dose of 66 U/kg q.i.d. SC. In some cats the required maintenance dose may be as high as 200 U/kg q.i.d. SC. The dosage should be adjusted to maintain the activated partial thromboplastin time (aPTT) at or slightly above the normal reference range. Studies in humans conclude that this "therapeutic" aPTT should be at least 1.5 times the preheparin baseline aPTT.

In the event of hemorrhage, heparin activity may be immediately neutralized by protamine sulfate. Protamine should be administered slowly. If given minutes after administration of heparin, the dosage of protamine is 1 mg of protamine sulfate intravenously per 100 U of heparin. If 1 hour has elapsed since the last heparin dose, the protamine dose may be halved. If 2 hours have elapsed, 0.25 mg of protamine per 100 U of heparin should be administered. As explained in the discussion of prophylaxis below, excessive administration of protamine may result in a hemorrhagic condition for which there is no known therapy.

3. Vasodilation with acepromazine maleate (Prom Ace, Fort Dodge; 0.2 to 0.4 mg/kg SC t.i.d.) or

Table 1. *Therapeutic Options*

Thrombolectomy
Surgery
Catheter
Medical Treatment
Congestive heart failure therapy
Anticoagulation therapy—heparin/coumarin
Vasodilator therapy—acepromazine/hydralazine
Control of hyperkalemia and metabolic acidosis
Antiplatelet drug therapy—aspirin
Thrombolytic Therapy

hydralazine (Apresoline, Ciba; 0.5 to 0.8 mg/kg t.i.d. PO) to promote collateral blood flow. The efficacy of this therapeutic maneuver is undocumented. To avoid excessive hypotension, angiotensin-converting enzyme inhibitors should not be administered in conjunction with these agents.

4. Appropriate therapy for hyperkalemic and metabolic acidosis secondary to ischemic rhabdomyolysis and reperfusion (see following; see *Current Veterinary Therapy IX*, pp. 59 and 94). Although necessary to effectively combat these conditions, fluid therapy should be conservative and should be monitored carefully to prevent pulmonary edema in cats with underlying cardiac disease.

5. Antiplatelet therapy with aspirin to reduce further platelet activation and thrombosis (see following).

Thrombolytic Therapy

Intravascular thrombi occur in health and disease. Naturally occurring fibrinolytic agents present in all mammalian blood dissolve these thrombi. The *fibrinolytic system* (Fig. 4) is composed of plasminogen and plasminogen activators and inhibitors. Plasminogen activators are enzymes that catalyze the conversion of plasminogen to plasmin. Plasmin hydrolyzes fibrin and fibrinogen, thus dissolving existing thrombi and preventing the continued formation of intravascular thrombi.

PLASMINOGEN ACTIVATORS

The fibrinolytic agents in clinical use (streptokinase, urokinase, and tissue plasminogen activator) require adequate concentrations of circulating plasminogen, the precursor of plasmin, to be effective. Nonspecific activators of plasminogen, streptokinase and urokinase, possess little specific affinity for fibrin and therefore activate both circulating and fibrin-bound plasminogen in a relatively indiscri-

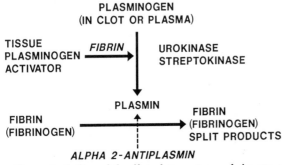

Figure 4. Outline of the fibrinolytic system and the site at which fibrinolytic agents activate fibrinolysis. Note that tissue plasminogen activator requires fibrin as a cofactor for activation of plasminogen to plasmin. Alpha₂-antiplasmin inactivates plasmin.

minant manner. Plasmin formed in circulating blood is initially neutralized rapidly by alpha₂-antiplasmin and is lost for thrombolysis. When the capacity of circulating alpha₂-antiplasmin to degrade circulating plasmin is overwhelmed, circulating plasmin concentrations rise. Plasmin, a nonspecific serine protease, degrades numerous circulating proteins, including fibrinogen, coagulation factors, plasminogen, and the administered activator itself. Degradation of circulating fibrinogen results in elevation of levels of plasma fibrin degradation products, which are in themselves potent anticoagulants. The activation of circulating plasminogen, production of fibrin degradation products, and degradation of coagulation factors give rise to what has been called a systemic fibrinolytic state, which predisposes to bleeding. These toxic effects of streptokinase and urokinase cannot be dissociated from their desired therapeutic effect. Thus, systemic use of these agents in theory involves substantial risk. However, an increasing number of studies comparing fibrin-specific and nonspecific plasminogen activators in humans with myocardial infarction cast some doubt on these theoretical disadvantages.

The utility of thrombolytic therapy with streptokinase in feline aortic thromboemboli has been investigated by Killingsworth and associates (1986). Streptokinase was administered to cats with experimentally induced aortic thromboembolism at a loading dosage of 90,000 IU intravenously over 20 to 30 min, followed by a constant-rate infusion of 45,000 IU/hr for 3 hr. The mean weight of thrombi at the aortic bifurcation of streptokinase-treated and control cats was 7.3 and 13.4 mg, respectively. Two cats had no thrombus remaining in the aorta after streptokinase administration. The reduction in mean thrombus weight was not statistically significant (p = 0.15). There was evidence of systemic fibrinolysis, but measurements of perfusion to the embolized region were unchanged. It should be noted that the thrombi in this study were isolated in a sac between ligatures and relatively isolated from the systemic vascular system. Thus, by design, these results probably underestimate the therapeutic potential of this agent in cats with aortic thromboemboli.

Streptokinase and urokinase are significantly less expensive than newer fibrinolytic agents (e.g., tissue plasminogen activator, pro-urokinase, and acylated streptokinase-plasminogen complex). Local (intra-arterial) administration of these agents provides effective thrombolysis in humans with myocardial infarction at doses below those that are usually associated with significant systemic fibrinolysis. Application of this technique to cats with aortic thromboemboli requires catheterizing the aorta (via the carotid artery) and advancing the catheter proximal to the occluding thrombus, under anesthesia. However, short-term anesthesia with a combination of ketamine and diazepam (Valium) in conjunction with local anesthesia should provide adequate immobilization and analgesia with minimal risk. Placement of a 3 or 4 French (F) 45-cm catheter (with a fixed curve at the tip) in the distal aorta without the aid of fluoroscopic guidance is not difficult. Final placement of the catheter may be confirmed by radiographic examination of the distal aortic region. This option needs further investigation in cats with aortic thromboemboli.

TISSUE PLASMINOGEN ACTIVATOR

Tissue plasminogen activator (t-PA) is an intrinsic protein present in all mammals. Recently, because of recombinant DNA techniques, it has become possible to obtain large quantities of t-PA, making its use as a therapeutic thrombolytic agent possible. Tissue plasminogen activator (Activase, Genentech) received United States Food and Drug Administration (FDA) approval in 1987. There are numerous reports of the utilization of t-PA for the lysis of thrombi as therapy for acute myocardial infarction, pulmonary thromboemboli, and peripheral vascular obstruction in humans and experimental animals.

Tissue plasminogen activator has low affinity for circulating plasminogen. Doses effective for clot lysis neither activate circulating plasminogen nor induce a systemic fibrinolytic state. Like plasminogen, t-PA hs a high affinity for fibrin within thrombi; thus, t-PA and plasminogen bind fibrin in close proximity to each other, potentiating the t-PA–catalyzed conversion of plasminogen to plasmin at the site of interest. Any plasmin that escapes into the circulation is promptly inhibited by circulating alpha$_2$-antiplasmin (Fig. 4).

TISSUE PLASMINOGEN ACTIVATOR AND THE CAT. The activity of genetically engineered t-PA in feline plasma is 90 to 100 per cent of that seen in human plasma. Early uncontrolled clinical trials by the authors with t-PA in cats with aortic thromboemboli have demonstrated acute thrombolytic efficacy (shortened time to reperfusion and ambulation) associated with the administration of t-PA at a rate of 0.25 to 1 mg/kg/hr for a total dose of 1 to 10 mg/kg IV. Forty-three per cent of cats treated survived therapy and were walking within 48 hours of presentation. Angiograms obtained after t-PA administration demonstrated resolution of the primary vascular occlusion. Thus, t-PA effectively decreased the time to reperfusion and return to function in cats with aortic thromboemboli. However, 50 per cent of the cats died during therapy, which raises major concerns regarding short-term thrombolysis or the determination of safe and effective doses of t-PA.

COMPLICATIONS OF t-PA THERAPY. Fatalities resulted from reperfusion syndrome (hyperkalemia

and metabolic acidosis) (70 per cent), congestive heart failure (15 per cent), and sudden arrhythmic death presumably due to embolization of an echocardiographically identifiable left atrial thrombus to a coronary artery (15 per cent). Deaths attributable to CHF and acute coronary thrombosis (in cats with left atrial thrombi) were expected; however, the high mortality associated with acute reperfusion was not. Reperfusion syndrome occurs when blood flow is re-established to a previously ischemic region, resulting in the release of trapped metabolic toxins into the systemic circulation. In cats treated with t-PA, death is most often due to hyperkalemia. Of the cats that died because of hyperkalemia, two also had renal arterial occlusion followed by severe hemorrhage into and around the kidney after renal blood flow was re-established. These cats died of hyperkalemia complicated by severe anemia, which could not be controlled with repeated transfusions.

RISK/BENEFIT ASSESSMENT IN CATS WITH AORTIC THROMBOEMBOLI. Is t-PA a viable therapeutic modality for veterinary medicine? Success, defined by the authors as an improvement in clinical signs associated with reperfusion within 36 hours of presentation, in 50 per cent of cases treated is a favorable outcome. The cats that successfully completed t-PA therapy exhibited signs of increasing neuromuscular function and ambulatory ability within 2 days of presentation. Although controlled studies are lacking, results of t-PA therapy contrast with those of Fox (1987), who reported an interval of 2 to 6 weeks before seeing similar signs in most cats exhibiting spontaneous resolution. These early results strongly suggest t-PA's thrombolytic efficacy in cats. It is too early to make definitive statements regarding the risks versus the benefits of this new therapy because no comparisons with placebo-treated cats were made. However, the authors' findings and those of Fox (1987) reporting return to function within 6 weeks in approximately 50 per cent of cases treated with aspirin alone raise questions regarding the benefits of early reperfusion and possible increased mortality arising from complications of t-PA therapy. At present, t-PA is too expensive, costing $2000 per 50-mg multidose vial.

PROPHYLAXIS

Feline patients with myocardial disease should be considered at risk for developing intracardiac thrombi and signs of peripheral arterial thrombosis. Therefore, preventing peripheral thrombosis is one of the most important therapeutic objectives for the veterinarian managing cats with myocardial disease.

The ideal means of preventing thrombosis is resolution of the underlying myocardial disease. This may now be feasible in cats with dilated cardiomyopathy (see pp. 251–262) but is not yet possible in cats with other forms of cardiomyopathy. The next best option is to correct the pathophysiologic alterations, either caused by or coincident with myocardial disease, which place these cats at risk. Implementing this option would require a greater understanding of the underlying clinicopathologic factors than is currently available.

The factors that predispose to the development of intracardiac thrombi in cats are not well defined. Proposed mechanisms include (1) activation of the intrinsic coagulation cascade by vascular subendothelium exposed from the trauma of turbulence in the left ventricle and as the result of "jet lesion" of mitral regurgitation in the left atrium; (2) abnormal circulatory patterns, primarily stasis of blood in the dilated left atrium, allowing platelet clumping and adhesion with activation of the intrinsic coagulation cascade; and (3) increased blood coagulability, resulting from a proposed but not well-defined underlying coagulopathy. Cat platelets are known to be "stickier" (i.e., to aggregate more readily) than those found in other species. This has been proposed as a possible explanation for why cats with myocardial disease, in the presence or absence of atrial fibrillation (a risk factor in humans), are at a higher risk for developing thrombosis than other species. In addition, recent observations by the authors suggest that the association of cardiac disease with thromboemboli may be overemphasized. Several cats treated for documented thromboemboli have had no auscultatory, radiographic, or echocardiographically demonstrable cardiac abnormalities.

It would appear that the most feasible option is to manipulate the patient's coagulation system in an attempt to alter the delicate balance between the pathways that promote clotting and those that inhibit thrombus formation to reduce the patient's thrombogenic potential. Thus, at present, antiplatelet and anticoagulant therapy provides the best means for preventing thrombi in cats with myocardial disease.

ANTIPLATELET THERAPY: ASPIRIN

Prostaglandins enhance platelet aggregation via activation of cyclic adenosine monophosphate (c-AMP). Aspirin (acetylsalicylic acid) acetylation of platelet cyclo-oxygenase prevents the formation of thromboxane A_2, a potent prostaglandinlike platelet-aggregating substance. Aspirin also inhibits cyclo-oxygenase in vascular endothelium and prevents the formation of prostacyclin, a potent prostaglandinlike compound that inhibits platelet aggregation. Thus, aspirin's action on platelets inhibits thrombotic tendencies and prolongs bleeding time, while its action on vascular endothelium inhibits prostacyclin-induced platelet inhibition, favoring local thrombosis. This paradox can be utilized therapeutically because

of the different kinetics in the two systems. The inhibition of platelet cyclo-oxygenase is irreversible, and bleeding time is restored to normal only after the production of new platelets. The inhibition of endothelial cyclo-oxygenase is reversible, and the practice of administering aspirin every third day may, in theory, allow maximal platelet inactivation (a beneficial effect) while minimizing endothelial cyclo-oxygenase inhibition and thrombotic tendencies (a detrimental effect). The dose of aspirin recommended in cats is 25 mg/kg every third day. There is no evidence that this or any other dose of aspirin is effective in preventing intracardiac or peripheral arterial thrombosis in cats with myocardial disease. Clinical impression varies among clinicians and institutions. In the authors' experience, aspirin, at the dose cited above, does not prevent recurrence of peripheral thrombosis in cats with a history of aortic thromboemboli associated with myocardial disease and previous successful medical management (whether by thrombolysis or previously described methods). Seventy-five per cent of the cats treated with t-PA by the authors have had recurrence of thrombosis despite aspirin therapy at the recommended dose of 25 mg/kg every third day.

ANTICOAGULANT THERAPY

Available anticoagulants include heparin and coumarins. As described above, heparin's anticoagulant properties are indirect, resulting from augmentation of antithrombin III activity. Antithrombin III circulates in plasma; thus heparin is an anticoagulant *in vivo* and *in vitro*. Heparin is destroyed in the gastrointestinal tract and is therefore not effective for long-term oral therapy. Heparin may be administered intravenously or subcutaneously. Repeated intramuscular injection is discouraged because local hemorrhage may result. Harpster (1986, p. 394) describes the use of long-term subcutaneous heparin administration for prevention of recurrent thromboemboli. Data are not available to evaluate the effectiveness of heparin therapy in cats.

An increase in the aPTT of 1.5 to 2 times greater than baseline may be expected when heparin is used within the normal therapeutic range. However, some studies in humans demonstrate a lack of correlation between clotting times and plasma heparin activity. The most prevalent undesirable effect of heparin overdose is bleeding. As noted above, protamine sulfate is an effective antidote for excess heparin administration. The reaction is almost instantaneous; effects of protamine last for about 2 hours. In high doses, protamine itself has anticoagulant properties that are not reversible; therefore the dosage must be carefully selected.

Coumarin anticoagulant activity is derived from

inhibition of synthesis of vitamin K–dependent clotting factors (factors II, VII, IX, and X). Coumarin derivatives exert no anticoagulant effect *in vitro*. *In vivo*, inhibitory effects on synthesis of clotting factors begin immediately. However, clotting is unaffected until already existing factor concentrations decline. Therefore, there is a delay between initial administration and effect on the prothrombin time. They are nearly always administered orally. In humans, warfarin is well absorbed from the gastrointestinal tract. The coumarins are highly bound to plasma albumin (95 to 99 per cent in humans).

Historically, oral anticoagulant therapy has been monitored with the prothrombin time (PT). This test measures the activity of factors II, VII, and X. The factor depressed most quickly and profoundly (usually factor VII) determines the prothrombin time during the initial days of therapy. Prothrombin time or partial thromboplastin time (PTT) may be used to determine adequacy of long-term oral anticoagulant dosage. The PIVKA (proteins induced by vitamin K antagonists) test is a more sensitive and specific test (see *Current Veterinary Therapy IX*, p. 513). This test was developed in Europe for monitoring human patients taking oral anticoagulant drugs. The PIVKA test detects the presence of inactive precursors of factors II, VII, IX, and X. If available, this is the assay of choice for monitoring oral anticoagulant therapy.

The anticoagulant action of warfarin-type compounds is consistent with the view that they compete with the fat-soluble vitamin K for a receptor in the liver that controls synthesis of factors II, VII, IX, and X. When the anticoagulant effect is excessive, it can be counteracted by administering vitamin K_1. However, after synthesis of factors II, VII, IX, and X is reinstituted, time must elapse before factors achieve concentrations in the plasma that will adequately reverse the bleeding tendency. If serious bleeding occurs during therapy with oral anticoagulants, it may be stopped immediately by administering fresh blood or plasma that contains the missing clotting factors. Other drugs can modify the anticoagulant actions of coumarins by altering the bioavailability of vitamin K; affecting absorption, distribution, or elimination of the coumarins; affecting synthesis or degradation of clotting factors; or altering protein binding of the coumarins. Therefore, the maintenance dose (0.06–0.1 mg/kg q 24 hr PO) should be evaluated daily during the initial titration (3 days), then every other day (2 times), and then weekly until a safe and stable dosage regimen is determined. It can take up to 1 week for new steady-state conditions to be achieved. The therapeutic effect should be re-evaluated periodically (at least once per month). Evaluation should be based upon the aPTT or PT (or preferably PIVKA, if available). In humans, frequent adjustment of the administered dose can lead to wide fluctuations in clotting test results. Some studies in humans demonstrate a lack of correlation between clotting times and the incidence of rethrombosis or bleeding. Serum warfarin concentrations have little value for predicting the anticoagulant effect of a dosage regimen in the individual patient.

In addition to its well-known effect on coagulation factors, warfarin reduces levels of protein C, a naturally occurring antithrombotic protein. Protein C has a short plasma half-life similar to that of factor VII. Therefore, in the early stages of warfarin therapy, a potential exists for a transient hypercoagulable state before other vitamin K–dependent factors (factors II, IX, and X) are affected. During this potential hypercoagulable period, in which protein C is diminished and the intrinsic clotting pathway factors are relatively unaffected, heparin should be used concurrently. Overdoses of vitamin K antagonists can have disastrous results; thus, these drugs must be used cautiously.

CONCLUSIONS

Feline aortic thromboembolism is a common and devastating clinical condition for which there is at present no effective therapy. Thrombolytic therapy with tissue plasminogen activator represents a new and promising, relatively noninvasive method for resolution of the clinical syndrome. In clinical trials in humans, tissue plasminogen activator may have advantages over previously available thrombolytic agents, which require intensive monitoring and commonly cause complications that entail large monetary and personnel costs to monitor and control. Being specific for thrombus-associated plasminogen, t-PA therapy in human patients enables more safe and effective thrombolysis without the hazards previously associated with thrombolytic therapy.

In cats with aortic thromboemboli, results of early clinical trials are promising with regard to acute thrombolytic efficacy but raise questions concerning the risks and benefits of therapy; more controlled studies are required. It is estimated that t-PA therapy for a cat with aortic thromboemboli will cost approximately $500 to $2000, including hospitalization and drug.

However, before thrombolytic therapy can be viewed as a useful therapeutic advance, the etiopathogenesis and probability of rethrombosis must be considered. There are no published controlled studies, but it is generally thought that cats have a high probability of recurrence. Finding a cure for feline myocardial diseases (cardiomyopathies) or an effective method for safely anticoagulating cats at risk would help justify the expense and personnel required for thrombolytic therapy.

Two recent developments may bring veterinary medicine closer to attaining these therapeutic goals.

First, Harpster (1986) reported successful use of warfarin sodium once daily to prevent recurrence. Second, taurine deficiency was identified as a cause of dilated cardiomyopathy in cats. Oral taurine supplementation was curative. By resolving dilated cardiomyopathy as the underlying disease, oral supplementation of taurine may prevent the recurrence of thromboemboli in cats with dilated cardiomyopathy. The use of vitamin K antagonists may reduce the incidence of recurrence in cardiac disease for which there is no cure. This type of therapy is not indicated in cases that cannot be monitored closely.

References and Supplemental Reading

Butler, H. C.: An investigation into the relationship of an aortic embolus to posterior paralysis in the cat. J. Small Anim. Pract. 12:141, 1971.

Fox, P. R.: Feline thromboembolism associated with cardiomyopathy.

Proceedings of the Fifth Annual Veterinary Medical Forum, ACVIM, San Diego, 1987, p. 714.

Greene, C. E.: Effects of aspirin and propranolol on feline platelet aggregation. Am. J. Vet. Res. 46:1820, 1985.

Harpster, N. K.: Feline myocardial diseases. In Kirk, R. W. (ed.): Current Veterinary Therapy IX. Philadelphia: W. B. Saunders, 1986, pp. 380–398.

Imhoff, R. K.: Production of aortic occlusion resembling acute aortic embolism syndrome in cats. Nature 192:979, 1961.

Killingsworth, C. R., Eyster, G. E., Adams, T., et al.: Streptokinase treatment of cats with experimentally induced aortic thrombosis. Am. J. Vet. Res. 47:1351, 1986.

Nevelsteen, A., De Clerck, F., and De Gryse, A.: Restoration of postthrombotic peripheral collateral circulation in the cat by ketanserin, a selective 5-HT$_2$-receptor antagonist. Arch. Int. Pharmacodyn. 270:268, 1984.

Pion, P. D.: Feline aortic thromboemboli and the potential utility of thrombolytic therapy with tissue plasminogen activator. Vet. Clin. North Am. 18:79, 1988.

Schaub, R. G., Gates, K. A., and Roberts, R. E.: Effect of aspirin on collateral blood flow after experimental thrombosis of the feline aorta. Am. J. Vet. Res 43:1647, 1982.

Schaub, R. G., Meyers, K. M., Sande, R. D., et al.: Inhibition of feline collateral vessel development following experimental thrombolic occlusion. Circ. Res. 39:736, 1976.

DIETARY CONSIDERATIONS IN THE TREATMENT OF HEART FAILURE

SARAH L. RALSTON, V.M.D.

Fort Collins, Colorado

Sodium restriction is not the only dietary concern in the management of dogs and cats with cardiac disease. Appropriate manipulation of dietary levels of protein, energy, sodium, and potassium may alleviate signs of edema and ascites, improve an animal's attitude, and even reduce the need for diuretic or inotropic drug therapy. The effects of chronic congestive heart disease on nutritional needs and the methods of ensuring adequate nutritional support will be stressed in this article.

NUTRITIONAL CONCERNS IN CARDIAC DISEASE

SODIUM AND WATER RETENTION. Low blood pressure and decreased renal blood flow due to valvular incompetence or a failing myocardium activate the renin-angiotensin-aldosterone system and

The author thanks Drs. Timothy Allen, Lon Lewis, Michael Hand, Mark Morris, Jr., and Wayne Wingfield for their review of this manuscript.

lead to the release of antidiuretic hormone. These cause retention of sodium and water. The clinical signs of pulmonary edema and ascites in cardiac disease are due to fluid retention. This volume expansion increases the work load on the heart, further stressing the myocardium.

CARDIAC CACHEXIA. Protein-energy malnutrition (PEM) is not uncommon in advanced cardiac disease. The severe loss of both fat and lean body mass in cardiac patients is termed cardiac cachexia. Factors that contribute to cardiac cachexia include the following:

1. Anorexia due to malaise and possible gastric compression due to ascitic fluid. Sudden changes in diet may also contribute to depressed appetite.

Table 1. *Goals of Dietary Management of Chronic Cardiac Disease*

Maintenance of lean body mass
Reduction of pulmonary edema and ascites
Maximizing immune competence and wound healing, with adequate vitamin, mineral, and protein intake
Avoidance of major electrolyte imbalances (Na$^+$, K$^+$, Cl$^-$)

2. Malabsorption due to congestion or altered splanchnic or gastrointestinal perfusion; villus atrophy caused by inadequate nutrient intake and anorexia.

3. Peripheral tissue hypoxia caused by decreased cardiac output. This, in turn, causes decreased peripheral delivery of cellular nutrients and reduced removal of cellular waste products.

4. Hypermetabolism of cardiac and respiratory tissues despite a general reduction of metabolic rates resulting from malnutrition in peripheral body tissues.

A mild (80 to 99 per cent of maintenance) reduction in food intake is adaptive to a certain degree. Reduced caloric intake and smaller meals diminish postprandial fluctuations in blood pressure and lower the overall metabolic rate. Wasting of lean muscle tissue reduces the demand for oxygen in peripheral tissues. However, prolonged, severe PEM (< 50 per cent of requirements for longer than 2 weeks) impairs immune competency and wound healing and contributes to the development of hypoalbuminemia, hypokalemia, and hypomagnesemia, which may be seen in advanced congestive heart failure (CHF).

Cardiac patients are frequently obese on presentation, but many humans rapidly lose weight while hospitalized owing to infusion of fluids containing dextrose, but lacking other essential nutrients (such as protein and fat), in a misguided attempt to preserve lean body mass. Infusion of 2.5 to 5 per cent dextrose stimulates the release of insulin, which inhibits lipolysis but permits catabolism of lean body tissue to continue at a reduced rate. Heymsfield and associates (1981) termed this "nosocomial cardiac cachexia." The primary cause for concern in these cases is the sudden loss of lean body mass without mobilization of adipose tissues. Although dogs and cats with cardiac disease are rarely hospitalized for prolonged periods of time, it is not advisable to infuse 2.5 to 5 per cent dextrose longer than necessary to initially stabilize a cardiac patient if there are no other sources of nutrients being administered to the animal.

RENAL AND HEPATIC DYSFUNCTION. Both renal and hepatic function may be compromised by reduced cardiac output. Cardiac disease is also frequently seen in older animals that have concomitant renal or hepatic disease. Some cats with chronic renal disease develop significant hypokalemia. Clinical signs of renal and hepatic disease have been reduced by the provision of low-protein diets. If renal or hepatic function or both are significantly compromised, diets containing 16 to 20 per cent high-quality protein are recommended for dogs and 18 to 28 per cent protein for cats. High-quality protein sources include eggs, chicken, and milk products.

OTHER NUTRIENT CONCERNS. Human patients with chronic cardiac failure are frequently deficient in iron, zinc, magnesium, potassium, chloride, and B vitamins. Although similar problems are not well documented in cats and dogs, B-vitamin supplementation is recommended, especially if diuretics are used. The recent discovery of a taurine-responsive cardiomyopathy in cats also warrants that attention be paid to the biologic availability of taurine fed to cats with cardiomyopathy (see pp. 251–262). Hypokalemia predisposes the patient to digitalis intoxication and to cardiac arrhythmias.

NUTRITIONAL CONCERNS WITH RELATION TO DRUG THERAPY. The inotropic drugs digoxin and digitoxin have no known direct effects on the nutritional needs of the cardiac patient. Vomiting and diarrhea, however, are drug side effects that may contribute to fluid and potassium losses.

Diuretics are frequently used in chronic cardiac failure and have a dramatic effect on the sodium and potassium needs of the animal. Thiazide diuretics and furosemide cause excretion of potassium. In the presence of high aldosterone activity as seen in chronic cardiac failure, potassium loss may be profound with diuretics. If fluid or potassium intakes are inadequate in animals receiving these drugs, the resultant volume contraction and hypokalemia may cause general weakness, azotemia, reduced glucose tolerance, altered blood pressure, and impaired urine-concentrating ability. If the dog or cat is eating maintenance amounts of a food that provide 150 to 250 mg of potassium per kilogram of body weight (0.6 to 1.5 per cent of food dry matter), further supplementation should not be necessary. In anorexic or vomiting animals, serum potassium level should be monitored in the initial stages of stabilization of a patient with these drugs.

Spironolactone and triamterene, on the other hand, are diuretics that cause some retention of potassium ions while enhancing the excretion of sodium and water. Supplemental potassium will be potentially dangerous when these two drugs are used. Sodium restriction should also not be as severe as when other loop diuretics are used. In general, sodium content of the diet should be between 0.05 and 0.5 per cent of dry matter. When using potassium-sparing diuretics it would be best not to restrict sodium content to below 0.25 per cent on a dry matter basis.

Table 2. *Reasonable Ranges of Nutrients for Cats and Dogs with Chronic Cardiac Disease**

	Cats	Dogs
kcal/kg body weight	50–80	40–60
gm protein/100 kcal	6–8	3–6
% protein (dry matter)	25–40	16–25
% Na (dry matter)	0.05–0.5	0.05–0.5
% K (dry matter)	0.8–1.5	0.8–1.5

*Use lower values for most severe cases.

Table 3. *Recipes for Homemade Diets for Dogs and Cats with Cardiac Disease*

Low-Sodium Diet for Dogs

¼ lb lean ground beef   2 cups cooked rice (no salt)
or fresh pork   2 tsp dicalcium phosphate
1 tbsp vegetable oil

Braise meat, retaining fat. Add the remaining ingredients and mix. Yield: 1 lb (0.5 kg). Give a balanced supplement that fulfills the canine minimum daily requirement for all vitamins and trace minerals.

% moisture	68	% potassium (dry matter)	1.4
% protein (dry matter)	20	% sodium (dry matter)	0.05
% fat (dry matter)	17	ME (kcal)	660/lb as fed

Restricted Mineral and Sodium Diet for Cats

1 lb regular ground beef,   1 tsp calcium carbonate
cooked   ¼ lb liver
1 cup cooked rice (no salt)   1 tsp vegetable oil or animal fat

Combine all ingredients. Yield: 1¾ lb (0.8 kg). Give a balanced supplement that fulfills the feline minimum daily requirement for all vitamins and trace minerals.

% moisture	64.0	% potassium (dry matter)	0.56
% protein (dry matter)	40	% sodium (dry matter)	0.16
% fat (dry matter)	39	ME (kcal)	940/lb as fed

Restricted Protein/Phosphorus Diet for Cats

¼ lb liver, braised   1 tsp calcium carbonate
2 large eggs, hard boiled   balanced vitamin/mineral
2 cups cooked rice (no salt)   supplement
1 tbsp vegetable oil

Mix all ingredients thoroughly. Addition of small amount of water may improve palatability (or 1 tbsp liquid, unsalted butter, or margarine).

% moisture	70	% sodium (dry matter)	0.17
% protein (dry matter)	24	% potassium (dry matter)	0.70
% fat (dry matter)	18	ME (kcal)	635/lb as fed

ME, metabolizable energy.
From Lewis, L. D., Morris, M. L., and Hand, M. L.: *Small Animal Clinical Nutrition III.* Topeka, KS: Mark Morris Associates, 1987. Modified with permission.

Vasodilators such as hydralazine and captopril are being used more frequently in patients with chronic heart failure. It is important to consider the site of action of the vasodilators, as these affect sodium and potassium balance. Captopril and enalapril are competitive inhibitors of angiotensin-converting enzyme. They reduce plasma aldosterone concentrations, which results in a dramatic increase in sodium loss, with concomitant increase in potassium retention. Potassium supplementation, potassium-sparing drugs, and low-sodium foods should not be used with these drugs. Captopril also has been shown to diminish or destroy taste sensation in humans. Some dogs become anorexic after 1 to 2 days of captopril therapy but may resume eating within 48 to 72

hours. Use of foods with strong olfactory cues may alleviate this problem.

Hydralazine is a specific arteriolar dilator, which activates the renin-angiotensin system and increases plasma aldosterone concentration. It causes moderate increases in sodium retention, with an associated enhancement of potassium loss. Food containing less than 0.1 per cent sodium and 0.8 to 1.5 per cent potassium on a dry matter basis is recommended for use with this drug.

Cachexia alters drug sensitivity by decreasing hepatic microsomal function and, if severe, by reducing plasma albumin. Drugs that are cleared through hepatic microsomal systems such as aspirin or opioids, or those that are protein bound in the plasma, such as digitoxin, should be used with caution in cachectic animals.

OBESITY AND OVERFEEDING

Obesity contributes to development and progression of chronic heart failure. The obese animal's heart has a greater mass to support. Large meals of high caloric content cause immediate increases in metabolic rate and, subsequently, in cardiac and renal output. These alterations cause reductions in perfusion in peripheral tissues and potentially loss of lean body mass. Dogs fed multiple small meals, however, have lower net energy gains than those fed similar amounts in a single meal. Small, frequent meals will be of greater benefit to the obese animal with chronic cardiac disease. This will minimize gross fluctuations in metabolic rate and, theoretically, help with weight reduction. Severe protein-energy malnutrition, however, should be avoided. If more than 10 per cent of an animal's lean body mass is lost in less than a 7- to 10-day period, the animal will have reduced resistance to bacterial infection, poor wound healing, increased incidence of decubital ulcers, and atrophy of the myocardium proportional to the reduction of lean body mass. Hypoalbuminemia and severe starvation also exacerbate the development of peripheral edema and ascites, which are common clinical problems in chronic cardiac disease. The overall goal of weight reduction in the obese cardiac patient, therefore, is slow, steady weight loss (1 to 3 per cent of total body weight per week), with adequate overall nutrition.

DIETARY MANAGEMENT OF THE CARDIAC PATIENT

Dietary goals and requirements for cats and dogs with chronic cardiac disease are presented in Tables 1 and 2. Prescription Diets such as k/d or h/d (Hill's Pet Products) may be recommended in certain

Table 4. *Nutrient Content of Human Foods That May Be Used as Treats or Substitutes in Basic Recipes*

Food	% H$_2$O	kcal /100 gm*	% Protein (dry matter)	% Calcium (dry matter)	% Phosphorus (dry matter)	% Sodium (dry matter)	% Potassium (dry matter)
Meats†							
Turkey, white meat	62	176	74	0.00	0.52	0.34	1.00
Chicken, white meat	77	107	83	0.04	0.87	0.26	1.20
Pork, fresh cooked, lean and fat	42	391	41	0.02	0.46	0.10	0.48
Lean ground beef	68	179	66	0.03	0.59	0.18	0.75
Regular ground beef	60	268	45	0.02	0.40	0.15	0.55
Lamb, broiled or roasted	61	265	38	0.02	0.36	0.18	0.65
Eggs†							
1 large (average = 50 gm)	74	163	49	0.19	0.72	0.46	0.49
1 yolk (average = 17 gm)	51	348	33	0.28	1.2	0.10	0.28
1 white (average = 33 gm)	88	51	92	0.08	0.10	1.25	0.75
Dairy products†							
Whole milk (1 cup = 244 gm)	87	65	27	0.90	0.69	0.38	1.20
Skim milk (1 cup = 244 gm)	90	59	36	1.2	1.00	0.60	1.80
Cottage cheese, creamed, un- salted (1 cup = 225 gm)	78	106	64	46	0.68	1.04	0.36
Yogurt, plain, whole milk	85	62	29	1.00	0.79	0.42	1.29
Vegetables and fruits							
Avocado‡ (California)	74	171	8	0.04	1.60	0.01	1.31
Banana‡	76	84	trace	0.33	0.08	trace	1.54
Carrots, raw, grated (1 cup = 110 gm)	88	41	8	0.33	0.33	0.42	2.83
Corn, frozen (1 cup = 165 gm)	77	79	13	0.01	0.30	trace	0.78
Whole potato, boiled‡	75	77	8	0.03	0.20	0.02	1.6
Cereals§							
Corn grits, enriched (1 cup cooked = 245 gm)‡	87	51	8	trace	0.07	trace	0.08
Farina (1 cup cooked = 245 gm)	89	43	9	0.54	0.45	trace	0.09
Oatmeal (1 cup cooked = 240 gm)	86	54	14	0.07	0.35	trace	0.50
Other grain products§							
Macaroni, cooked 8–10 min (1 cup = 140 gm)	64	110	8	0.02	0.14	trace	0.17
Egg noodles, cooked (1 cup = 160 gm)	71	125	14	0.03	0.21	trace	0.14
Other							
Butter, unsalted	16	721	trace	0.03	0.02	0.01	0.02
Corn oil (1 tbsp = 14 gm)	0	883	0	0	0	0.0	0
Molasses, blackstrap (1 tbsp = 20 gm)	24	225	0	0.89	0.10	0.01	3.84
Garlic powder (1 gm)		trace	0	trace	trace	trace	trace
Tuna fish canned in water		118	28	0.02	0.19	0.04	trace

*100 gm is roughly equivalent to 3.5 ounces.
†Palatability high for most dogs and cats.
‡Palatability high for *some* dogs and cats.
§Cooked without added salt.

Data from Lewis, L. D., Morris, M. L., and Hand, M.: *Small Animal Clinical Nutrition III.* Topeka, KS: Mark Morris Associates, 1987; and Anderson, L., Dibble, M. V., Turkki, P. R., et al.: *Nutrition in Health and Disease,* 17th ed. Philadelphia: J. B. Lippincott, 1982.

cases. Homemade recipes are avilable (Table 3). Some foods that may be used as supplements to enhance palatability are given in Table 4. Any alteration in the recipes should be made with caution and to a limited degree so that nutritional adequacy and mineral balance are maintained. Certain foods should be avoided as substitutes in the basic recipes or for use as treats (Table 5). The main goal of dietary management is to maintain lean body mass by providing adequate levels of protein, vita-

mins, and minerals in a diet that the animal will readily consume.

Dogs and cats in cardiac failure often need fewer calories per kilogram of body weight than their healthy counterparts. Normal maintenance energy requirements range from 60 to 100 kcal/kg of body weight for cats and 65 to 100 kcal/kg of body weight for dogs. One should start feeding the lower amount of calories and adjust intake according to body weight changes, taking into account fluid accumu-

Table 5. *Foods to Avoid in Diets for Dogs and Cats with Cardiac Disease*

All prepared meats (e.g., corned beef and salami)
Canned fish and vegetables, unless low salt content
Beef kidney and liver (not boiled)
All cheese, unless low in salt
All breads, unless low in salt
Dried, nonfat milk
Prepared breakfast cereals (such as cornflakes), pretzels, potato chips
Margarine or butter unless low in salt
Dog "treats"—biscuits, rawhide

lations or losses. In general, restriction of protein to 4 to 5 gm of protein per 100 kcal of metabolizable energy would be advisable in dogs. Higher levels will be required in cats: 6 gm of protein per 100 kcal is a minimum. The protein should be primarily from high-quality, highly digestible sources, such as eggs, chicken, lamb, or pork. Boiling meats will further reduce their sodium content, in that salt is leached out of the meat and into the broth during boiling. Highly digestible liquid diets (Table 6) can be used to supplement the animal's daily diet.

Most commercial dog foods contain excessive levels of sodium chloride (Table 7). Special diets (such as Prescription Diets k/d, h/d, and i/d) are formulated to have low sodium contents while meeting the other special nutritional needs of the cardiac patient. Feline Prescription Diets (h/d, k/d, and c/d) maintain plasma taurine levels in cats when given for longer than 6 months and replete plasma taurine concentrations in cats that have been depleted on experimental diets. The dietary concentration of taurine alone will not guarantee an adequate main-

tenance of plasma concentrations. To assure normal plasma taurine concentrations, it is necessary to feed diets that have been tested and found to maintain adequate plasma levels. It should also not be assumed that all commercial diets designed for geriatric animals are low in sodium content or will maintain taurine levels in cats. Sodium, potassium, and protein concentrations of any diet fed to an animal with chronic cardiac failure should be carefully checked. Reasonable ranges are given in Table 2.

The plasma concentrations of sodium, potassium, and glucose should be monitored at least once every 2 weeks until they are stable, then at 3-month intervals during the long-term dietary management of the cardiac patient. The acid-base status of the dog or cat, as well as drug therapy, may alter plasma potassium levels and should be considered when interpreting plasma potassium concentrations. Hypokalemia may be treated with KCl (e.g., salt substitute) using ½ tsp per 5 kg of body weight per day as an initial supplement added to the food.

The cat or dog in cardiac failure is frequently an older animal with fixed dietary habits. Attempts at switching the diet may be unsuccessful because the animal does not accept the new food. If the patient does not initially accept the new diet, the following should be tried:

1. Switching the diet slowly, over the course of 4 to 5 days, gradually replacing the old diet with the new.

2. Warming the new food to volatilize odors.

3. Adding flavor enhancers in *small* amounts to the new food, such as garlic, unsalted butter, tuna

Table 6. *Liquid Diet Supplements*

	kcal/ml	Protein (gm/ml)	% Sodium (dry matter)	Content of Supplement*
Ensure (Ross Lab)	1.06	0.04	0.08	Casein and soy protein, corn oil, starch
Ensure Plus (Ross Lab)	1.50	0.05	0.11	Same as above but higher in protein and vitamins
Osmolite (Ross Lab)	1.06	0.04	0.055	Medium-chain triglycerides, corn, casein and soy protein, cornstarch
Compleat B (Doyle)	1.07	0.05	0.13	Beef puree, nonfat milk, corn oil, cereal and vegetable puree, orange juice
Meritene (Doyle)	0.96	0.06	0.09	Skim milk, casein, corn oil, corn syrup, sucrose
Precision HN (Doyle)	1.05	0.04	0.10	Egg white, medium-chain triglycerides, soybean oil, maltodextrin, sucrose
Sustacal (Mead Johnson)	1.01	0.06	0.09	Casein and soy protein, soy oil, sucrose, corn syrup
Vivonex (Norwich Eaton)	1.00	0.03	0.05	Free amino acids, safflower oil, glucose, oligosaccharides
High Nitrogen Vivonex (Norwich Eaton)	1.00	0.04	0.05	Free amino acids, safflower oil, glucose, oligosaccharides
Criticare HN† (Mead Johnson)	1.06	0.04	0.06	Casein, free amino acids, safflower oil, maltodextrin, cornstarch

*All contain vitamin and mineral supplements.
†Very palatable to cats.
From *Enteral Nutrition—Ready Reference,* provided by Ross Laboratories, Columbus, OH 43216.

Table 7. *Sodium Content of Pet Foods*

Class of Food	% Sodium (dry matter)	Class of Food	% Sodium (dry matter)
Dog Foods			
Canned		*Dry*	
Ken-L-Ration	1.14	Cycle 2	0.74
Friskies Dog Food	1.03	Ken-L-Ration Biskit	0.60
Kal Kan Chunks of Beef By-Products	0.89	Gravy Train	0.56
Alpo Beef Chunks Dinner	0.86	Iams Chunks	0.54
Mighty Dog	0.58	Purina Dog Chow	0.51
Average	0.90	Gaines Meal	0.34
		Average	0.55
Semimoist		*Dietary*	
Gainesburgers	0.95	Prescription Diet k/d	0.23
Top Choice	0.81	Prescription Diet h/d (dry)	0.055
Prime	0.81	(canned)	0.090
Average	0.86	Recipe 5 (Appendix Table 3)	0.052
Cat Foods			
Canned		*Dry*	
Fancy Feast Seafood	0.89	Friskies Ocean Fish	0.89
Friskies Fish Flavor	0.86	Special Dinner Tuna & Herring	0.61
Puss-N-Boots Fish	0.83	Crave	0.60
Kal Kan Mealtime	0.79	Frish Ahoy	0.59
9-Lives Tuna	0.79	Kitten Chow	0.57
Friskies Buffet Seafood Supper	0.69	Chef's Blend	0.53
Bright Eyes Seafood Supper	0.59	Iams	0.50
Average	0.77	Tamiami	0.48
Dietary		Cat Chow Original Blend	0.47
Prescription Diet Feline c/d	0.49	9-Lives Tuna	0.37
Prescription Diet Feline k/d	0.40	Average	0.56
Prescription Diet Feline h/d	0.24	*Semimoist*	
Recipe 8 (Appendix Table 3)	0.16	9-Lives	0.74
		Happy Cat	0.65
		Tender Vittles	0.53
		Average	0.64

Modified with permission from Lewis, L., Morris, M., and Hand, M.: *Small Animal Clinical Nutrition III*. Topeka KS: Mark Morris Associates, 1987.

fish packed in water, meat variations of baby food (chicken, veal, or pork), or bouillon (which has high salt content).

4. Feeding small amounts at frequent intervals; not allowing food to remain in the cage or in the animal's bowl for more than an hour.

5. If all else fails, feeding through a nasogastric tube until the animal is stabilized nutritionally. It is important to note that none of the liquid diets listed in Table 5 contain taurine. Puréed dog or cat foods or homemade diets may be difficult to get through the relatively small-gauge nasogastric tubes but are potentially more balanced.

In general, it is better to feed a less than ideal diet than not to feed at all.

References and Supplemental Reading

Anderson, L., Dibble, M. V., Turkki, P. R., Mitchell, H. S., and Rynbergen, H. J.: *Nutrition in Health and Disease*, 17th ed. Philadelphia: J. B. Lippincott, 1982.

Blackburn, G. L., Gibbons, G. W., Bothe, A., et al.: Nutritional support in cardiac cachexia. J Thorac. Cardiovasc. Surg. 73:480, 1977.

Bonagura, J.: Current concepts in the therapy of heart disease. *In* Proceedings of AAHA 51st Annual Convention, San Francisco, 1984, p. 13.

Dudrick, S. J., and Rhoades, J. E.: Metabolism in surgical patients: Carbohydrates and fat utilization by oral and parenteral routes. *In* Sabiston, D.C. (ed.): *Davis-Christopher Textbook of Surgery, 12th ed.* Vol. 1. Philadelphia: W. B. Saunders, 1981, p. 147.

Heymsfield, S. B., Smith, J., Redd, S., and Whitworth, H. B.: Nutritional support in cardiac failure. Surg. Clin. North Am. 61:635, 1981.

Kaplan, N. M., Carnegie, A., Raskin, P., Heller, J. A., Simmons, M.: Potassium supplementation in hypertensive patients with diuretic-induced hypokalemia. N. Engl. J. Med. 312:746, 1985.

Knowlen, G. G., Kittleson, M. D., Nachreiner, R. F., and Eyster, G. E.: Comparison of plasma aldosterone concentration among clinical groups of dogs with chronic heart failure. J.A.V.M.A. 183:991, 1983.

LeBlanc, J., and Diamond, P.: Effect of meal size and frequency on postprandial thermogenesis in dogs. Am J. Physiol. 250:E144, 1986.

Lewis, L. D., Morris, M. L., and Hand, M. S.: *Small Animal Clinical Nutrition III*, Topeka, KS; Mark Morris Associates, 1987, Chapter 5.

Meguid, M. M., Collier, M. D., and Howard, L. J.: Uncomplicated and stressed starvation. Surg. Clin. North Am. 61:529, 1981.

Pion, P. D., Kittleson, M. D., Rogers, Q. R., and Morris, J. G.: Myocardial failure in cats associated with low plasma taurine: A reversible cardiomyopathy. Science 237:764, 1987.

Pittman, J. G., and Cohen, P.: The pathogenesis of cardiac cachexia. N. Engl. J. Med. 312:746, 1985.

Thomas, W. P.: Long-term therapy of chronic congestive heart failure in the dog and cat. *In* Kirk, R. W. (ed.): *Current Veterinary Therapy VII*. Philadelphia; W. B. Saunders, 1980, p. 368.

COMPLICATIONS OF CARDIOPULMONARY DRUG THERAPY

PHILIP R. FOX, D.V.M.,
New York, New York

and MARK G. PAPICH, D.V.M.
Saskatoon, Saskatchewan

A wide variety of new and emerging cardiopulmonary drugs are inundating the veterinary market. Unfamiliar products are continuously becoming available as extrapolation from human pharmacotherapy increases. Many drugs have multiple, potent actions, which are only variably predictable and often unrelated. Although these agents confer a great ability to achieve beneficial therapeutic results, they can also cause profound adverse effects, including death. Their use becomes especially complicated in animals that are critically ill or have multisystemic disorders requiring "polypharmacy." The old medical adage, *primum non nocere* (first do not harm), is well suited to today's therapeutic environment.

THERAPEUTIC STRATEGIES

The foundation of pharmacologic intervention relies on several factors: (1) an accurate diagnosis based on a complete data base; (2) a thorough understanding of the pathologic disease process; (3) realistic therapeutic end points; (4) familiarity with the mechanism of drug action; and (5) potential side effects. The clinician must understand salient pharmacokinetics, pharmacodynamics, and drug-drug interactions. Dosage adjustments are often necessary in special situations, including animals with renal failure, hepatic disease, and congestive heart failure (CHF) and cases of poor client compliance.

A constellation of clinical abnormalities is often present in animals with cardiopulmonary disease. These include tachypnea, dyspnea, auscultatory changes (e.g., abnormal lung sounds, cardiac murmurs, gallop rhythms, and arrhythmias), and coughing. Differentiating between respiratory and cardiac disease as the cause of these clinical signs may be challenging because the cardiac and pulmonary systems are closely interrelated. Congestive heart failure is often incorrectly diagnosed when heart murmurs, coughing, or abnormal lung sounds are detected without the benefit of a complete data base (e.g., chest radiograph, electrocardiogram [ECG], and clinical pathology profile). Such erroneous diagnosis may lead improperly to cardiac drug therapy when pulmonary disease is actually present. This predisposes to drug toxicities and lack of therapeutic benefit, especially in geriatric animals. Alternately, misdiagnosed pulmonary disease leads to unhelpful therapies when CHF has actually supervened. Therefore, radiographs, an ECG, and appropriate clinicopathologic tests are essential to establish whether, and to what degree, cardiac or respiratory disease is responsible for clinical signs. Therapeutic strategies may then be instituted or modified.

COMPLICATIONS OF DRUG THERAPY

Cardiopulmonary drug complications may be classified under three general categories in which much overlap exists: (1) untoward generalized, systemic effects (e.g., excessive preload reduction, hypotension, and organ underperfusion); (2) adverse drug-drug interactions; and (3) direct and indirect toxic effects on target and nontarget organs. These problems may occur with an incomplete data base, which increases the likelihood of unforeseen complications, especially in geriatric patients. Even with a complete workup, however, in veterinary medicine therapeutic regimens can rarely be designed to incorporate hemodynamic data such as blood pressure assessments.

Patients differ markedly in their responses to cardiopulmonary agents. Hemodynamic changes may also occur over the course of chronic drug therapy, which mitigates against optimal response. For example, with mitral regurgitation and low left ventricular filling pressures, vasodilators may actually lower cardiac output.

Drugs Affecting the Cardiovascular System

DELETERIOUS SYSTEMIC EFFECTS

Cardiac function may be adversely altered by certain drugs. Preload and afterload are important

308

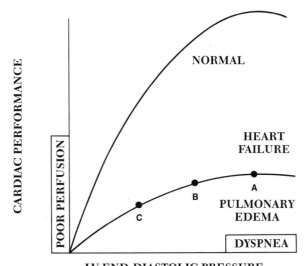

Figure 1. Effect of preload reduction on clinical signs of left-sided congestive heart failure and cardiac performance. Preload reduction from vasodilator or diuretic therapy may lower ventricular filling pressure and reduce pulmonary edema (A → B). However, overzealous use of these agents (A → C) or situations of only moderately elevated filling pressures (B → C) can result in deterioration of cardiac performance.

determinants of cardiac performance and are affected by peripheral circulatory changes. Preload may be thought of as ventricular filling pressure but is best estimated by the diastolic stretching force on the myocardium. Afterload is influenced by arterial pressure and resistance to ventricular emptying. By dilating arterioles, veins, or both, drugs with vasodilatory actions may profoundly alter cardiac loading conditions and secondarily affect cardiac performance. Blood volume reduction by diuretics ("overdiuresis") or toxic drug effects (vomiting and diarrhea) may also reduce cardiac preload. Additionally, myocardial contractility, heart rate, and rhythm may be affected by drug therapy.

Therapeutic strategies intended to correct innate neuroendocrine overcompensatory responses may themselves cause deleterious effects. For example, ventricular filling pressures may contribute to development of venous congestion and edema. Hemodynamic effects of a venous vasodilating drug (preload reducer) resemble those of a diuretic (Fig. 1) and cause a leftward shift on the ventricular function curve. When pulmonary edema is due to excessive left ventricular preload and filling pressure, preload reduction may reverse these changes and reduce pulmonary congestion (Fig. 1, A → B). However, decline of cardiac performance can result from their overzealous use (Fig. 1, A → C) or in states of normal or mildly elevated filling pressures (Fig. 1, B → C).

In heart failure, arteriolar and venous beds may be inappropriately constricted. This homeoregulatory response is intended to ensure brain and heart perfusion and maintain systemic arterial pressure at the expense of less immediately important vascular beds (skin, gut, and kidney). When congestive heart failure due to mitral valvular regurgitation is associated with increased afterload, an arteriolar dilator (e.g., hydralazine) may augment cardiac performance by reducing diastolic blood pressure and afterload, promoting greater forward stroke volume, and decreasing the mitral regurgitant fraction. However, cardiac output may be increased without resolving congestive signs in some animals (see A, Fig. 2). In contrast, when contractility is reduced but preload is normal (see B, Fig. 2), arteriolar dilating drugs may only minimally increase cardiac output but cause a detrimental decline of arterial blood pressure. This may result in hypotension and organ underperfusion.

"Balanced" vasodilators (e.g., prazosin and captopril) act on both venous and arterial beds. Patients with CHF due to elevated preload (Fig. 2A) may benefit from such agents. These drugs reduce ventricular filling pressures and augment cardiac performance with little decline in arterial blood pressure. Conversely, when preload is normal or reduced (Fig. 2B), balanced vasodilators may cause cardiac performance to remain unchanged or even decline when ventricular filling pressures and arterial blood pressure decreases.

Vasodilator therapy, by reducing preload and afterload, may potentially cause severe hypotension and organ underperfusion. This may result in myo-

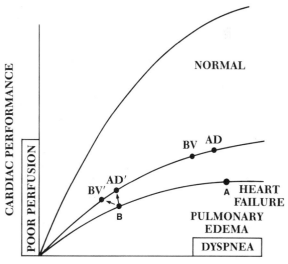

Figure 2. Effects of vasodilators on clinical signs of congestive heart failure and cardiac performance. AD, arteriolar dilator (e.g., hydralazine); BV, balanced vasodilator (e.g., captopril or prazosin). In congestive heart failure with elevated preload due to mitral valvular regurgitation, arteriolar dilators may improve cardiac performance and thereby reduce exercise intolerance and other signs of poor perfusion (A → AD). When preload is relatively normal, AD only minimally improves cardiac performance (B → AD'). Balanced vasodilators improve cardiac performance and reduce congestive signs in CHF with elevated filling pressures (A → BV) but produce less favorable effects when filling pressures are normal (B → BV').

Table 1. *Factors Affecting Pharmacokinetic Interactions*

Gastrointestinal Absorption
  Physiochemical interaction
  Gastrointestinal motility
  Bacterial flora
  Mucosal function

Distribution
  Blood flow
  Serum drug binding
  Tissue drug binding
  Active transport to site of drug action

Biotransformation
  Hepatic
  Other

Excretion
  Renal
  Biliary
  Other

Table 3. *Drugs Inhibiting Metabolism of Other Drugs*

Inducing Agent	Affected Agent
Chloramphenicol	Phenobarbital
	Phenytoin
Chlorpheniramine	Phenytoin
Cimetidine	Lidocaine
	Phenytoin
	Propranolol
	Theophylline
Metoprolol	Lidocaine
Phenylbutazone	Phenobarbital
	Phenytoin
Propranolol	Lidocaine
Sulfamethizole	Phenytoin
Trimethoprim-sulfamethoxazole	Phenytoin

cardial hypoxia and ischemia, renal dysfunction (in states of renal insufficiency), worsened hypoxia (in cases of severe, chronic cor pulmonale), and syncope.

HARMFUL DRUG-DRUG INTERACTIONS

Some drug interactions are intentionally selected for their additive or synergistic effects. Unfortunately, metabolic interactions between drugs are not always predictable, especially when absorption, distribution, binding, biotransformation, and excretion of each agent are modified by a disease process (Tables 1 through 3). Because these pharmacologic factors are poorly assessable in the clinical setting, adverse drug interactions often occur.

Drug incompatibilities can result from interactions at various sites (Tables 1, 4, and 5). For example, external drug incompatibilities may occur when drugs are mixed in the same syringe or intravenous infusion, whereby precipitation or inactivation may occur. The package insert should always be consulted regarding drug mixing, reconstitution, and administration. In contrast, internal drug incompatibilities may occur grossly (e.g., gastrointestinal protectorants altering oral digoxin ab-

Table 2. *Drugs Stimulating Metabolism of Other Drugs*

Inducing Agent	Affected Agent
Barbiturates	Digitoxin
	Phenytoin
	Oral anticoagulants
Phenylbutazone	Digitoxin
Phenytoin	Diazepam
	Digitoxin
	Glucocorticoids
	Quinidine

sorption) or at the site of drug action (e.g., beta-receptor sites on the cell membrane as with dobutamine and propranolol).

Drugs may also alter the biochemical or physiologic effects of other agents, resulting in pharmacodynamic drug interactions. For example, blocking beta-adrenergic receptor sites in congestive heart failure states may reduce beneficial effects of endogenous catecholamines, which maintain cardiac output, contractility, or pulmonary function. Diuretics, especially when administered in high doses, in combinations, or during anorexia, may cause hypokalemia. This increases susceptibility to digitalis-related arrhythmias. Hydralazine reduces total peripheral resistance, which may result in reflex tachycardia. Propranolol administration can block this reflex tachycardia, augmenting hydralazine's hypotensive effects.

Pharmacokinetic alterations may alter drug absorption, distribution, metabolism, or excretion (Tables 1 through 5). Several examples may be cited. Gastrointestinal drug absorption may be reduced by agents with a high surface area such as antacids, kaolin-pectin, sucralfate, and activated charcoal. Separating the dosing intervals may minimize these adverse interactions. However, drugs undergoing enterohepatic circulation may still interact somewhat with binding agents. Changes in gastric pH by one drug (e.g., cimetidine or antacids) may modify ionization of others. However, because most absorption occurs in the small intestine, this interaction is probably of minimal clinical importance. Gastrointestinal motility may affect absolute bioavailability by influencing rate or completeness of drug absorption. Metoclopramide increases gastric emptying. This may cause earlier and higher peak concentrations of drugs that are rapidly absorbed from the upper small intestine, such as cimetidine and some digoxin preparations. Cathartics may increase intestinal motility and decrease completeness

Table 4. *Drug Interactions or Adverse Conditions That May Occur with Digoxin*

Drugs/Condition	Possible Effects	Interventions
Antacids	Decreases GI absorption	Separate administrations
Kaolin-pectate	Decreases GI absorption	Administer digoxin at least 2 hours before kaolin-pectate
Bran	Decreases GI absorption	Separate administrations
Quinidine	Increases serum digoxin concentration	Decrease digoxin dose; monitor serum digoxin concentrations
Amiodarone	Increases serum digoxin concentration	As per quinidine
Verapamil	Increases serum digoxin concentration	As per quinidine
Diltiazem	May increase serum digoxin concentration	As per quinidine
Prazosin	May increase serum digoxin concentration acutely	As per quinidine
Spironolactone	May increase serum digoxin concentration	Monitor serum digoxin concentration
Triamterene	May increase serum digoxin concentration	As per spironolactone
Overdiuresis	Azotemia, reduced digoxin clearance	Reduce/withdraw diuretic agent; measure serum electrolytes, BUN; withdraw or modify digoxin dose
Hypokalemia	Potentiates digoxin toxicity	As per hypokalemia; judicious potassium supplementation
Hypercalcemia	Enhances patient sensitivity to digitalis; potentiates digitalis-related arrhythmias	Treat hypercalcemia; modify digoxin dose
Acid-base disturbances	May alter potassium and calcium homeostasis	Manage underlying disorder

of drug absorption. Antacids and narcotic analgesics may slow gastric emptying and potentially decrease the rate of absorption. Anticholinergics such as propantheline can slow gastrointestinal motility and increase absorption. Some phenothiazines and antihistamines (H_1-receptor blockers) have anticholinergic side effects. Bacterial flora may be modified or eliminated by certain antibiotics. Enhanced digoxin absorption by erythromycin has been reported in some humans. Drugs inducing gastrointestinal toxicity can theoretically injure the mucosa or inhibit active transport.

Disease states may also alter drug absorption, distribution, and clearance. Blood flow significantly influences uptake and clearance of drugs with high first-pass hepatic extraction such as lidocaine or propranolol. Right-sided congestive heart failure may compromise blood flow to the bowel and reduce absorption of drugs such as digoxin or furosemide. Agents interfering with hepatic uptake, drug biotransformation, intracellular binding, or biliary excretion may alter bioavailability or clearance of compounds that are highly extracted by the liver. Cimetidine, for example, may increase propranolol's plasma concentration.

Displacement of one drug from its binding site by another agent may cause toxicities. This is dependent on relative drug concentrations, binding affinities, and volume of distribution. Drugs with high binding affinities are likely to displace other drugs. Examples include digitoxin, warfarin, phenytoin, hydralazine, quinidine, salicylates, sulfon-

Table 5. *Drug Interaction That May Occur with Beta-Adrenoceptor Blocking Drugs*

Drug	Possible Effects	Interventions
Aluminum hydroxide gel	Decreases GI absorption	Separate administration; avoid this combination
Aminophylline	Potential mutual inhibition	Monitor clinical response
Barbiturates	Enhances beta-blocker metabolism	Monitor clinical response
Calcium channel blockers (e.g., verapamil)	Potentiate bradycardia; myocardial depression; hypotension; A-V block	Judicious use and close patient monitoring
Digitalis	Potentiates bradycardia	Monitor patient response
Epinephrine	Hypertension	Consider cardioselective beta-blocker; administer epinephrine cautiously
Isoproterenol, dobutamine	Mutual inhibition	Use cardioselective beta-blocker or avoid concurrent use
Lidocaine	Propranolol reduces hepatic clearance, increases lidocaine blood levels and potential for toxicity	Reduce lidocaine dose; exercise caution during administration
Phenothiazines	Additive hypotensive effects	Monitor patient response
Phenylpropanolamine	Hypertensive reaction	Avoid concurrent use
Phenytoin	Additive cardiodepression	Monitor patient response
Quinidine	Additive cardiodepression	Monitor patient response
Tubocurarine	Enhanced neuromuscular blockade	Monitor patient response
Cimetidine	Prolongs elimination half-life of propranolol by reducing hepatic clearance	Reduce dose of propranolol; monitor patient response

amides, and phenylbutazone. Volume of distribution relates the amount of drug in the body to the plasma drug concentration. If a drug has a small volume of distribution, more of the active (unbound) drug is available for delivery to sites of action. This may cause drug toxicity or altered pharmacologic response. Clinical importance of drug displacement depends on the drugs' therapeutic index (i.e., the ratio of the median toxic dose to median effective dose), their elimination rate, and the presence of other available distribution sites.

Interactions involving protein binding may be especially significant in patients with hypoalbuminemia. Low albumin levels decrease binding of phenytoin, furosemide, and digitoxin. This may reduce the total serum concentration, while their unbound active concentration remains unchanged. Hepatic cirrhosis or severe renal disease may cause dereased protein binding of digitoxin, quinidine, and phenytoin, resulting in increased fraction of unbound (free) drug.

Pharmacology of drugs metabolized and eliminated by the liver may be altered when hepatic enzyme systems are stimulated or inhibited by other drugs. Examples of agents affecting hepatic metabolism in humans are listed in Tables 2 and 3. Drugs that stimulate the metabolism of other compounds could theoretically result in subtherapeutic serum concentrations. In contrast, inhibitors of hepatic microsomal enzyme systems may delay metabolism and excretion of some agents. There is much individual variability in the metabolic capacity of this enzyme system and the degree to which it may be stimulated or inhibited. Whether resultant drug interactions are clinically important depends on the intended action of the stimulated or inhibited drug and the margin between therapeutic and toxic plasma concentrations.

Drug interactions may alter elimination of other agents through renal, biliary, or other routes. Glomerular filtration rates of some compounds are increased when they are displaced from albumin. Changes in glomerular filtration may also affect excretion of certain agents such as digoxin. Renal perfusion can be affected by vasoactive drugs such as dopamine. Tubular reabsorption of filtered drugs is decreased by diuretics, alkalinizers (for weakly acidic drugs such as salicylates), and acidifiers (for weak amines). Several drugs decrease tubular secretion of digoxin. Coadministration of digoxin and quinidine, for example, may increase the serum digoxin concentration. A similar interaction with digitoxin has not been demonstrated in dogs, however. Amiodarone, verapamil, and possibly prazosin also increase serum digoxin concentrations.

INDIVIDUAL DRUG TOXICITIES

Individual animals differ in their response to standard drug doses. Because many agents have a narrow therapeutic ratio this can result in subtherapeutic dosing or catastrophic toxicity. Toxic or adverse reactions may result from altered drug absorption in various disease states, circulatory changes associated with heart failure, altered hepatic blood flow, variations in drug metabolism and elimination, and multiple drug administration. Adverse and toxic effects of individual cardiopulmonary drugs are listed in Table 6.

Drugs Affecting the Pulmonary System

As with cardiovascular drugs, factors affecting pharmacokinetic interactions (see Table 1) or altering metabolism of other agents (see Tables 2 and 3) may result in untoward drug effects. Some specific drug-drug interactions are listed in Tables 4 and 5. Specific complications of pulmonary drug therapies are discussed below.

INDIVIDUAL DRUG TOXICITIES OF BRONCHODILATOR DRUGS

Beta-Adrenergic Drugs

Beta-adrenergic receptors are of two basic types: beta$_1$-receptors found in the heart muscle and beta$_2$-receptors in bronchial and smooth muscle. Beta-agonists stimulate bronchial smoothmuscle beta$_2$-adrenergic receptors, which relax bronchial smooth muscle. Other locations of beta$_2$-receptors are large blood vessels, pancreatic islet cells, liver, and uterine smooth muscle. Stimulation of beta$_1$-receptors leads to increases in heart rate, contractility, conduction velocity, and arrhythmias.

Beta-adrenergic drugs currently in use include isoproterenol, metaproterenol, terbutaline, albuterol, and clenbuterol. Isoproterenol is a nonspecific beta-adrenergic agonist that stimulates both beta$_1$- and beta$_2$-adrenergic receptors; the other listed drugs have a more pronounced effect on beta$_2$- than on beta$_1$-receptors. Beta$_2$-receptor–specific drugs have become popular for use in human medicine because of their lower incidence of side effects. Many are available for metered-dose inhalers, which are unfortunately impractical for small animal administration.

Anxiety, tachycardia, and occasionally more serious arrhythmias are the most common adverse effects associated with beta-adrenergic agonist administration. Isoproterenol causes adverse cardiac effects more readily than the beta$_2$-receptor–specific drugs. At high doses, the latter can also affect cardiac beta$_1$-receptors and cause a toxic response. Muscle tremors can occur at high doses as a result of beta-receptor skeletal muscle stimulation.

Table 6. *Adverse Effects of Cardiopulmonary Drugs*

Drug	Electrocardiographic Effects	Hemodynamic Effects	Other
Antiarrhythmics			
Quinidine	Increase ventricular rate in atrial fibrillation ("atropinelike" effect); depressed conduction (prolongs P-R, QRS, Q-T intervals); AV block (1st, 2nd, 3rd degree); bundle branch block; ventricular arrhythmias; "quinidine syncope"	IV administration (> 5 mg/kg in dogs) decreases stroke volume, cardiac output, contractility; standard oral doses cause milder negative inotropic effects; peripheral vasodilation	Vomiting, diarrhea; depression; toxicity potentiated by liver diseases, hypoalbuminemia, hyperkalemia
Procainamide	As per quinidine	IV rapid administration causes myocardial depression, hypotension; altered peripheral vascular resistance	Anorexia, vomiting; pyrexia; depression; autoimmune disease; decreases glomerular filtration rate, renal blood flow; toxicity potentiated by metabolic acidosis or hyperkalemia
Disopyramide	Arrhythmogenic; conduction abnormalities; "atropinelike" effect as per quinidine	Decreases contractility, stroke volume; increases heart rate, mean arterial pressure, systemic vascular resistance; aggravates CHF	Vomiting; constipation; short elimination half-life; elimination prolonged in CHF
Lidocaine	Abolishes ventricular escape rhythms; may aggravate arrhythmias	Minor	Drowsiness; ataxia; nystagmus; tremors; seizures (especially cats); respiratory depression or arrest; hypokalemia reduces antiarrhythmic effects
Tocainide	As per lidocaine	As per lidocaine	As per lidocaine
Mexilitine	As per lidocaine	As per lidocaine	As per lidocaine
Phenytoin	Minor	Minor	Depression; seizures; stimulates hepatic microsomal enzymes
Propranolol	Potentiates depression of AV conduction caused by other drugs (e.g., digitalis, quinidine, disopyramide, verapamil); bradycardia	Negative inotrope; hypotension	CNS depression; hypoglycemia; bronchospasm; reduces hepatic blood flow
Amiodarone	Bradycardia; AV block	Negative inotrope; hypotension	Altered thyroid function, hepatic enzyme abnormalities
Bretylium	Arrhythmogenic	Hypotension (infrequent)	Vomiting; ataxia; renal failure decreases clearance
Verapamil	Bradycardia; AV block potentiates depression of AV conduction caused by other drugs (e.g., digitalis, propranolol)	Negative inotrope; hypotension	Depression; may exacerbate heart failure
Diltiazem	Bradycardia; AV block	Minimal negative inotropism; mild peripheral vasodilation	Depression
Anticholinergics (e.g., atropine)	Sinus tachycardia; arrhythmogenic, especially after IV administration (transient AV block, bradycardia)	Tachycardia increases myocardial oxygen utilization	Constipation
Inotropic Agents			
Epinephrine	Arrhythmogenic; tachycardia	Positive inotrope; increases blood pressure, cardiac work, myocardial oxygen consumption; peripheral vasoconstriction	—
Isoproterenol	Arrhythmogenic; tachycardia	Positive inotrope; increases cardiac work, myocardial oxygen consumption; decreases blood pressure; hypotension	—
Dopamine	Arrhythmogenic	Positive inotrope; peripheral vasoconstriction (at 5–15 µg/kg/min); stimulates renal dopaminergic receptors (at < 2 µg/kg/min) and increases renal blood flow	Vomiting
Dobutamine	Arrhythmogenic (> 10 mg/kg/min)	Positive inotrope; minimal effect on heart rate, blood pressure (at 3–7 µg/kg/min)	Seizures (cats)
Phosphodiesterase inhibitors (e.g., amrinone)	Arrhythmogenic; tachycardia	Positive inotrope; systemic vasodilation	Poorly characterized
Digitalis glycosides	Arrhythmogenic (virtually any arrhythmia)	Positive inotrope; vasoconstriction with rapid IV bolus	Anorexia; vomiting; diarrhea; disorientation
Diuretics			
Loop diuretics (e.g., furosemide)	—	Decreases cardiac preload	Hypochloremic metabolic alkalosis; hyponatremia (rare); hypokalemia (rare in dogs, common in anorexic cats)
Thiazides	—	Decreases cardiac preload	As per loop diuretics, reduced glomerular filtration (e.g., renal insufficiency) reduces diuretic efficacy
Vasodilators			
Hydralazine, prazosin, captopril, enalapril	—	Hypotension; reduced cardiac preload; decreased stroke volume	Anorexia, vomiting; diarrhea; sinus tachycardia (especially hydralazine); acute renal failure/hyperkalemia (captopril)
Bronchodilators			
Methylxanthines (theophylline)	Tachycardia; arrhythmias	Mild positive inotrope; mild vasodilation	Mild diuretic properties; vomiting; diarrhea; drug clearance decreases with drugs that reduce hepatic metabolism; tachypnea; restlessness; tremors
Epinephrine, isoproterenol	As mentioned	As mentioned	As mentioned
Ephedrine	Arrhythmogenic	As per epinephrine	Tachyphylaxis
Terbutaline	Tachycardia; may exacerbate arrhythmias	Milder cardiac stimulation than isoproterenol	Tremors; nervousness; fatigue; vomiting

313

Anticholinergic Drugs

Although not commonly administered to small animals, anticholinergic agents can produce bronchodilating effects. These drugs include atropine, scopolamine, ipratropium bromide, and glycopyrrolate. Adverse effects are dose related and are associated with excessive parasympathetic blockade. As the dose increases, dry mouth is first observed, followed by tachycardia and miosis. At high doses, central nervous system (CNS) changes such as excitement and confusion occur. Scopolamine has a sedative effect on dogs, cats, and horses, but at high doses it can cause excitement and mania.

Homatropine and scopolamine are tertiary ammonium compounds that cross the blood-brain barrier easily, leading to central nervous system effects. Glycopyrrolate, atropine, methonitrate, and ipratropium bromide are quaternary ammonium compounds that have low lipid solubility and cross cell membranes poorly. Therefore, their CNS effects are limited. When they are administered locally in the airways, there is little systemic absorption.

Anticholinergic drugs decrease mucus production and inhibit ciliary function in the respiratory tract, which may be undesirable in an animal that has an infectious respiratory disease or chronic bronchitis. Ipratropium bromide is a recently introduced drug that was shown in experimental studies in dogs to have good bronchodilating action, minimal system effects, and no inhibition of mucociliary clearance. Unfortunately, this drug is only currently available in a metered-dose inhaler.

Methylxanthines

The methylxanthines include caffeine, theobromine, and theophylline. In dogs, theophylline toxicity has been the most thoroughly investigated.

Theophylline (aminophylline is 85 per cent theophylline) is used extensively in humans as a bronchodilator; its narrow therapeutic range requires that the dosages and plasma concentration be monitored closely. Therapeutic human plasma concentrations generally fall between 10 and 20 $\mu g/ml$. As plasma concentrations increase above 25 $\mu g/ml$, toxic reactions are common and are manifested as restlessness, tremors, cardiac arrhythmias, and convulsions.

Apparently, dogs have a higher tolerance to theophylline than people (Munsiff, 1986). In canines, increased activity (restlessness and excitement) did not correlate with theophylline plasma concentrations; convulsions did not occur at plasma concentrations as high as 111 $\mu g/ml$. Tachycardia (heart rate > 180 beats/min) was observed at dosages of 160 mg/kg and plasma concentrations of 70 $\mu g/ml$. The most common sign of theophylline toxicity is vomiting, which occurs at dosages between 80 and 160 mg/kg. For unknown reasons, dogs are most sensitive to intravenous theophylline administration. Restlessness and excitement occurred at plasma concentrations between 12 and 23 $\mu g/ml$ after an intravenous dose, but from 37 to 50 $\mu g/ml$ with oral dosages. Cardiac toxicity occurred with plasma concentrations of 16 to 23 $\mu g/ml$ after an IV dose, but at 70 $\mu g/ml$ when the drug is given orally.

Theophylline dosage recommendations in dogs is 9 mg/kg every 6 to 8 hours to maintain plasma concentrations between 10 and 20 $\mu g/ml$. Therefore, clinical toxicity is less likely using these recommended oral dosages; however, adverse effects (including anxiety and restlessness) can occur. Caution should be exercised if theophylline is administered intravenously. The intravenous administration should be given slowly, and the patient should be monitored closely for tachycardia, arrhythmias, and vomiting.

Toxicity information is currently lacking for cats. A relatively safe dose is 4 to 6 mg/kg every 12 hours orally.

The effectiveness of theophylline in small animals has been questioned. In experimental studies it has adversely affected pulmonary defense mechanisms, but the true clinical significance of this finding is not known. Theophylline continues to be a popular drug for many pulmonary conditions.

Methylxanthine toxicity is most common when errors in client dosing occur, when hepatic elimination is severely impaired, or if an intravenous dose is administered rapidly. Interference with theophylline metabolism in humans has been associated with hepatic microsomal enzyme inhibiting–drugs such as cimetidine. Drug interactions have also been noted following concurrent administration of erythromycin and quinolone and antibiotics (ciprofloxacin). Both reactions have resulted in increased plasma concentrations. Although it is possible that such interactions may occur in small animals, none have been clinically documented.

Toxic effects from methylxanthines can be diminished by enhancing their elimination. In an intoxicated animal this can be attempted by administering an intestinal adsorbent such as activated charcoal. Beta-adrenergic blocking drugs (e.g., propranolol) are the agents of choice for controlling cardiac arrhythmias. Lidocaine should be administered for refractory ventricular arrhythmias in dogs. If convulsions occur as a result of methylxanthine toxicity, they can be controlled by administering intravenous diazepam.

Antitussive Drugs

The antitussive drugs administered most commonly to dogs include codeine, hydrocodone, butorphanol, and dextromethorphan. All the drugs listed are opioids and have variable systemic opioid effects. Codeine, butorphanol, and hydrocodone can cause sedation, but usually the antitussive effects occur at dosages lower than those necessary to produce sedation. Excessive sedation indicates that the dosage should be decreased.

A possible adverse effect associated with opioid administration is constipation. Opioids inhibit intestinal propulsive movement and increase intestinal transit time. Dextromethorphan, an opioid that is contained in most over-the-counter cough preparations, has fewer side effects, and, most notably, it does not significantly affect the gastrointestinal tract at recommended dosages.

Combination Drugs

When administering antitussive agents and respiratory combination drugs, veterinarians should carefully examine the drug label to determine if all drugs contained in the formulation are safe. For example, acetaminophen is combined with codeine in over-the-counter preparations and is extremely toxic to cats. Acetaminophen has caused methemoglobinemia, hepatotoxicity, Heinz body anemia, and death. Acetaminophen toxicity, when recognized early, however, can be treated with acetylcysteine.

Anti-inflammatory Drugs

Nonsteroidal anti-inflammatory drugs (NSAIDs) such as aspirin and flunixin meglumine have been administered to decrease pulmonary reactions to endotoxic shock and heartworm disease. The most significant adverse reactions from these drugs occur in the gastrointestinal tract, and there are accounts of NSAID-induced gastrointestinal hemorrhage and ulceration in dogs. Gastrointestinal toxicity results from an inhibition of the protective influence of prostaglandins on the gastrointestinal mucosa. In dogs, reported reactions have been severe enough to cause death.

Flunixin meglumine, although shown to be efficacious in experimental models of septic shock, is a potent NSAID and should be used cautiously. Repeated administration for more than 3 to 5 days is likely to produce gastrointestinal complications.

The most common NSAID employed in small animals has been aspirin. It has been used to decrease pulmonary lesions associated with heartworm disease and heartworm adulticide treatment. The dose necessary to minimize complications of heartworm disease is considered an antiplatelet-aggregating dose, and, as such, it is lower than the usual analgesic dose. Aspirin-induced antiplatelet effects in dogs can occur with dosages as low as 3 to 20 mg/kg every 3 days. Fortunately, adverse reactions are not common with these low dosages. Cats are more sensitive to the toxic effects of aspirin than other animals owing to their decreased capacity to clear salicylates. However, at a dosage of 25 mg/kg every 2 to 3 days in cats, toxicity should not occur. Gastric mucosal irritation associated with the ingestion of aspirin can be lessened in both species by administering buffered aspirin.

References and Supplemental Reading

Bonagura, J. B., and Muir, W. W.: Antiarrhythmic therapy. In Tilley, L. P.: Essentials of Canine and Feline Electrocardiography. Philadelphia: Lea & Febiger, 1985, p. 281.

Cadwallader, D. E. (ed.): Biopharmaceutics and Drug Interactions, 3rd ed. New York: Raven Press, 1983.

Frishman, W. H.: Adverse effects, drug interactions—choosing a beta-blocker. In Frishman, W. H. (ed.): Clinical Pharmacology of the Beta-Adrenoreceptor Blocking Drugs, 2nd ed. Norwalk, CT: Appleton-Century-Crofts, 1984, p. 147.

Gross, M. J., and Skorodin, M. S.: Anticholinergic antimuscarinic bronchodilators. Am. Rev. Respir. Dis. 129:856, 1984.

Kellaway, G. S. M.: Cardiovascular iatrogenic disease and drug interactions. In Hunyor, S. N. (ed.): Cardiovascular Drug Therapy. Baltimore: Williams & Wilkins, 1987, p. 285.

McKiernan, B. C., Meff-Davis, C. A., Koritz, G. D., et al.: Pharmacokinetic studies of theophylline in dogs. J. Vet. Pharmacol. Ther. 4:103, 1981.

Muir, W. W., and Sams, R. A.: Pharmacology and pharmacokinetics of antiarrhythmic drugs. In Fox, P. R. (ed.): Canine and Feline Cardiology. New York: Churchill Livingstone, 1988, p. 309.

Munsiff, I. J.: Clinical toxicity of theophylline in dogs. Master of Science Thesis, University of Illinois, 1986.

Nelson, S., Summer, W. R., and Jakab, G. J.: Aminophylline-induced suppression of pulmonary antibacterial defenses. Am. Rev. Resp. Dis. 131:923, 1985.

Ogilvie, R. I.: Clinical pharmacokinetics of theophylline. Clin. Pharmacokinet. 3:267, 1978.

Papich, M. G.: Current concepts in pulmonary pharmacology. Semin. Vet. Med. Surg. (Small Anim.) 1:289, 1986.

Papich, M. G.: Bronchodilator therapy. In Kirk, R. W. (ed.): Current Veterinary Therapy IX. Philadelphia: W. B. Saunders, 1986, p. 278.

Petrie, J. C. (ed.): Cardiovascular and Respiratory Disease Therapy. Vol. 1. Clinically Important Adverse Drug Interactions. Amsterdam: Elsevier/North Holland Biomedical Press, 1980.

Schneeweiss, A. (ed.): Drug Therapy in Cardiovascular Diseases. Philadelphia: Lea & Febiger, 1986.

Spaulding, G. L.: The use of aminophylline and aspirin in small animal practice: Effective therapy or dangerous placebos? Semin. Vet. Med. Surg. (Small Anim.) 1:327, 1986.

Vasko, M. R., and Brater, D. C.: Drug-drug interactions. In Chernow, B., and Lake, C. R. (eds.): The Pharmacologic Approach to the Critically Ill Patient. Baltimore: Williams & Wilkins, 1983, p. 22.

Young, J. B., Leon, C. A., and Pratt, C. M.: Potentially deleterious effects of long-term vasodilator therapy in patients with heart failure. Chest 91:737, 1987.

SHOCK: PATHOPHYSIOLOGY, MONITORING, AND THERAPY

Eric R. Schertel, D.V.M., Ph.D.
and William W. Muir, D.V.M., Ph.D.
Columbus, Ohio

The dictionary defines shock as a sudden physical or mental disturbance. Traditionally, veterinary clinicians have viewed shock as a failure of the cardiovascular system due to one of several specific etiologies. These causes have included hypovolemia, heart failure, hypersensitivity reactions (anaphylaxis), bacteremia, neurologic disorders, vascular obstruction, and endocrine diseases. Although helpful for classification purposes, the categorization of shock by etiology does little to improve the clinician's understanding of the pathophysiologic process involved in the production and maintenance of shock. Furthermore, experimental studies indicate that anaphylactic and endocrine shock are primarily hypovolemic shock and that neurologic shock is caused by increases in venous capacitance. These discoveries and others focusing on the cardiovascular system have led to a functional classification of shock based on four discrete hemodynamic defects (Table 1): (1) hypovolemia, (2) heart failure, (3) obstruction to blood flow, and (4) alterations in the distribution of blood flow (distributive shock). This functional classification of shock is useful for categorizing the major components of the circulatory system regarding shock but does not provide an understanding of the physiologic responses, compensatory reactions, and pathophysiologic decompensations that can ultimately result in circulatory failure. The problem with many current views of shock, therefore, is that in real life shock frequently has several causes and that one-dimensional approaches often lead to incomplete therapy. The purpose of this article is to develop a working definition of shock; to discuss the pertinent pathophysiologic mechanisms (compensations and decompensations); to detail the pertinent signs, symptoms, and methods of monitoring patients in shock; and finally to discuss a systematic and rational approach to therapy.

DEFINITION OF SHOCK

Shock is a maldistribution of blood flow, resulting in inadequate delivery of oxygen and nutrients to tissues. Unevenly distributed capillary perfusion causes tissue ischemia, hypoxia, and acidosis, which disrupts cell function and eventually leads to cell death. Metabolic acidosis, specifically lactic acidosis, is the consequence of anaerobic metabolism and the *sine qua non* of inadequate tissue perfusion, regardless of cause.

Individual or multiple defects in various components of the circulatory system (Table 2) can be responsible for a maldistribution of blood flow. The components of the circulatory system that are involved include (1) the intravascular volume, which carries oxygen and nutrients to the tissues; (2) the blood components, particularly protein and hemoglobin, which maintain plasma oncotic pressure and carry oxygen, respectively; (3) the extravascular volume in which tissues are bathed and cellular exchange processes occur; (4) the heart, which pumps oxygenated blood to the tissues; (5) the vascular resistance vessels (arteries and arterioles), which moderate the afterload on the heart and direct the distribution of blood flow; (6) the microcirculation and capillary exchange bed, which is responsible for the exchange of oxygen, nutrients, and metabolites, (7) the venous resistance vessels, which regulate substrate filtration in capillaries; (8) shunt vessels (metarterioles), which control the flow of blood that bypasses the capillary bed; and (9) the venules and small, medium, and large veins, which collectively serve as a blood storage reservoir and regulate venous return (preload) and the "effective circulating blood volume."

When the fundamental defect in shock has been identified (maldistribution of blood flow to microcirculatory beds), an understanding of the varied hemodynamic profiles that are observed clinically and misconceptions concerning shock can begin to be appreciated. Shock is not always due to hypotension, low cardiac output, increased peripheral vascular resistance, or a combination of these hemodynamic factors. Severe hemorrhage and heart failure can result in low cardiac output and hypotension, which produces shock, but cardiac output and blood pressure may be elevated in shock patients following accidental or surgical trauma and during septicemia. As previously stated, shock is not always caused by a single, well-defined entity (e.g., hemorrhage) but generally evolves from diverse circulatory adjustments to a variety of etio-

Table 1. *Currently Accepted Classification of Shock*

Type of Shock	Primary Mechanism	Clinical Cause

Hypovolemic	Volume loss	Blood loss
		  Trauma
		  Surgery
		Plasma loss
		  Inflammation
		  Burn
		Fluid and electrolyte loss
		  Vomiting
		  Diarrhea
		  Dehydration
		  Diuresis

Cardiogenic	Heart failure	Acquired heart disease
		  Valvular insufficiency or stenosis
		  Cardiomyopathy
		  Heartworm disease
		Congenital heart disease
		  Valvular insufficiency or stenosis
		  Intracardiac defects
		Cardiac arrhythmias

Obstructive	Obstruction to blood flow	Pulmonary embolism (air) Heartworm disease Pericarditis (tamponade) Aortic emboli Intracardiac tumors Gastric dilation/displacement

Distributive
  Normal or high systemic resistance
	Increased venous capacitance (pooling)	Injury
		Surgical trauma
		Endotoxemia
		Tranquilizer, sedative, and anesthetic over-
		  dose

Low resistance	Arteriovenous shunting	Sepsis Abscess Peritonitis Pneumonia

logic events. For example, hemorrhaged dogs continue to die from shock even after the shed blood and additional fluids have been replaced. Therefore, shock should be thought of in terms of compensatory and decompensatory patterns that evolve with time. Finally, the goal of therapy should be not only to return heart rate and rhythm, blood pressure, and cardiac output to normal but also to optimize oxygen delivery to tissues.

PATHOPHYSIOLOGY

As pointed out above, a patient's response to factors that can cause shock is quite varied and is

Table 2. *Important Components of the Circulatory System*

1. Intravascular volume
2. Blood components (protein, Hb)
3. Extravascular volume
4. Heart
5. Arteries, arterioles
6. Capillary bed
7. Venous resistance vessels
8. Shunt vessels (metarterioles)
9. Venules; small, medium, and large veins

best appreciated following a complete history and thorough physical examination. The acute stress response to circulatory failure involves but may not be limited to (1) activation of the autonomic nervous system; (2) the release of epinephrine and norepinephrine from the adrenal gland; (3) the release of other hormones, including renin, angiotensin, vasopressin, and antidiuretic hormone; (4) immune system activation; (5) leukocyte release of microsomal enzymes, proteases, lipases, and oxygen free radicals; (6) activation of the arachidonic acid cascade; and (7) activation of the coagulation, complement, and kinin systems. Activation of these processes helps to protect cellular function and maintain tissue perfusion but if allowed to continue for prolonged periods or if overstimulated can result in further deterioration of cellular integrity leading to cell death, organ failure, and death.

Compensations

Sympathetic autonomic neural activity stimulation is an immediate and important defense mechanism utilized during shock. Heart rate, cardiac output, myocardial contractility, peripheral vascular resistance, and alveolar ventilation temporarily increase. Increases in peripheral vascular resistance caused by alpha-adrenergic arterial constriction reduce cutaneous, voluntary muscle, splanchnic, and renal blood flow, thereby centralizing blood volume and preferentially providing circulation to the heart, lungs, and brain.

The release of epinephrine and norepinephrine from the adrenal gland further augments cardiorespiratory stimulation and causes hyperglycemia and elevation of plasma free fatty acid concentrations, which serve as energy sources. Other hormones, including renin-angiotensin-aldosterone, glucocorticoids, glucagon, vasopressin, and antidiuretic hormone, account for exaggerated vasoconstriction of nonvital vascular beds, inotropic and chronotropic effects, salt and water retention, elevated glucose concentrations, and altered carbohydrate and lipid metabolism. Endogenous opioids (endorphins, enkephalins, and dynorphins) relieve pain and counteract the vasoconstrictor properties of other hormones, thereby helping to maintain tissue perfusion. Thyrotropin-releasing hormone acts as a physiologic opiate and antagonizes the deleterious products of arachidonic acid metabolism. Vasoactive peptides (histamine, bradykinin, and serotonin) and lysosomal enzymes are released, which increase capillary membrane permeability and cause leukocytes to accumulate at the margins of sites of inflammation and destroy cell membranes. Arachidonic acid metabolism is activated, producing biologically active cyclo-oxygenase (prostacyclin) and lipoxygenase metabolites (thromboxanes and leukotrienes), which relax or constrict various vascular beds, release lysosomal enzymes, cause platelet aggregation, and activate leukocytes. The immune system is activated to combat invading antibodies and infection. The complement cascade is activated, which facilitates phagocytosis by opsonization, lyses invading organisms, and increases capillary permeability. Oxygen free radicals are liberated; these attack cell membranes and increase capillary membrane permeability. The net result of all these mechanisms is to localize, neutralize, dilute, destroy, and remove dead and dying cells, toxins, and invading organisms. Provided the release of those substances occurs in small quantities and is appropriately timed, and tissue damage, hypoxia, ischemia, and acidosis are not extensive, these processes serve a useful purpose and protective role in preserving and maintaining organ function.

Hemorrhagic Shock

Shock caused by hemorrhage is usually categorized into four groups based on an estimation of the amount of blood loss (Table 3). Acute losses greater than 50 per cent of the total blood volume usually result in irreversible shock unless fluid and blood replacement are immediate (Table 4). Generally, acute hemorrhage produces decreases in arterial blood pressure; cardiac output; central venous pressure; the blood volume perfusing the heart, lungs, and brain (central blood volume); and oxygen delivery. Heart rate, systemic vascular resistance, and the amount of oxygen utilized by the tissue per aliquot of blood (oxygen extraction) are increased. Immediate hemodynamic compensations include tachycardia, peripheral vascular constriction, and increased myocardial contractility. Alterations in vasomotor tone caused by increases in sympathetic tone redistribute blood flow to central compartments (heart, lung, and brain) at the expense of the kidney, gut, and skin. Transcapillary refilling of plasma from interstitial and intracellular compartments may occur owing to decreases in capillary hydrostatic pressure caused by hypotension and, provided hemorrhage is not severe, results in a delayed fall in hemoglobin. Untreated severe or prolonged hemorrhagic shock, however, can lead to arteriolar vasodilation caused by local decreases in pH, persistent venulary constriction, sludging of blood, and a rapid leakage of plasma into the interstitial compartment.

Cardiogenic Shock

Acute heart failure from causes other than heart block is characterized by hypotension; elevated heart rate, central venous pressure, and oxygen extraction; and decreases in cardiac output (see Table 3). Increased sympathetic neural activity is responsible for tachycardia and increased systemic vascular resistance. Central venous pressure is often elevated. Cardiac contractility is stimulated by increases in sympathetic tone but usually deteriorates owing to the primary congenital or acquired heart disease. Blood flow is redistributed to the central compartment as in hemorrhagic shock. Activation of the renin-angiotensin-aldosterone system results in salt and water retention, hypervolemia, and edema formation.

Traumatic Shock

Traumatic shock is often complicated by hypovolemia and sepsis and therefore represents a combination of etiologic mechanisms. By itself, acute injury produces hemodynamic changes similar to those produced by stress and exercise. The demand of tissues for oxygen may be markedly increased following trauma, particularly when accompanied by sepsis. Increases in sympathetic activity increase heart rate, cardiac output, and cardiac contractility

Table 3. *Cardiorespiratory Patterns in Shock*

	Heart Rate	Arterial Blood Pressure	Central Venous Pressure	Cardiac Contractility	Cardiac Output	Peripheral Vascular Resistance	Alveolar Ventilation
Hemorrhagic shock	↑	↓	↓	↑	↓	↑	↑
Cardiogenic shock	↑ or ↓*	↓	↑	↓(↑)	↓	↑	↑
Traumatic shock	↑	↓(↑)	↓	↑	↑	↓	↑
Septic shock	↑	↓(↑)	↓	↑	— or ↑	↓	↑

↑, increase; ↓, decrease; —, no change; ( ), elevated initially by sympathetic nervous system stimulation.
*Bradyarrhythmias can cause shock.

and initially may increase arterial blood pressure, particularly if trauma is not accompanied by hemorrhage (see Table 3). Central venous pressure is decreased, as is systemic vascular resistance and oxygen extraction. Respiratory rate and alveolar ventilation are increased, producing hypocapnia and respiratory alkalosis. Traumatic shock rapidly progresses to irreversibility if hemorrhage cannot be controlled or if infection is severe.

Septic Shock

When uncomplicated by hemorrhage or trauma, early sepsis consists of tachycardia, increased cardiac contractility, normal or high cardiac output and decreases in systemic vascular resistance, and marked elevations in tissue demand for oxygen. The high cardiac output and low systemic vascular resistance characteristic of septic shock has led to the term warm shock because the patient may be warm to the touch (see Table 3). Bacteria and endotoxins, however, exert a variety of negative hemodynamic effects, depending on whether shock is produced by spontaneous infection, the infusion of live bacteria, or the injection of endotoxins. The major target organ of endotoxin in the dog is the gastrointestinal tract, particularly the liver, whereas the lung is the principal target organ in the cat. Regardless of the origin of sepsis, septic shock causes a maldistribution of blood flow that results in decreases in cerebral, renal, and coronary blood flow and the effective circulating volume. Compensatory responses include neural mechanisms that increase heart rate, myocardial contractility, and alveolar ventilation.

Septic shock frequently activates the immune and complement systems. Activation of the immune system aids in defending the animal from various antigens, whereas activation of the complement cascade initiates phagocytosis, chemotaxis, cell lysis, opsonization, and agglutination.

Decompensations

The initial physiologic response to the various etiologic factors causing shock is that of compensatory increases in cardiorespiratory function in an attempt to maintain tissue perfusion and oxygenation. However, the end result of the neurohumoral response is the uneven distribution or maldistribution of blood flow to the microcirculatory bed. Arteriolar and venular constriction in various tissue

Table 4. *Features of Increasing Degrees of Acute Hemorrhage*

Classification	Loss of Blood Volume	Blood Pressure	Signs and Symptoms	Likely Outcome
Compensated preshock	10–15%	Normal	Tachycardia Restlessness	Spontaneous recovery
Mild	15–30%	Slight fall	Tachycardia Weakness Thirst Dizziness	Usually reversible
Moderate	30–35%	70–80 mm Hg	Pallor Oliguria Lethargy	Good outcome with aggressive fluid therapy
Severe	35–40%	50–70 mm Hg	Pallor Cyanosis Collapse	Irreversible in some cases Early treatment essential
Profound	40–50%	50 mm Hg	Collapse Air hunger Anuria	

beds, including the renal, mesenteric, and pulmonic microcirculation, accounts for ischemic injury to these organs. Poor oxygen delivery results in cellular hypoxia, anaerobic metabolism, the development of lactic acidosis, and the continued release of potentially toxic substances and myocardial depressant substances. Furthermore, the net effect of continued venular constriction and arteriolar dilation (caused by release of local vasodilating factors and decreased pH) is an increase in capillary hydrostatic pressure, which forces plasma water from the capillary, thereby decreasing intravascular volume and producing hemoconcentration.

Following fluid therapy, patients with post-traumatic, postoperative, and depletional states may remain hypovolemic and have increased interstitial water, reduced intracellular water, and increased total body water. These maldistributions of water in the body fluid compartments are frequently associated with peripheral and pulmonary edema.

Continued activation of immunologic mechanisms, activation of the arachidonic acid cascade, and increases in the release of other shock mediators (histamine, kinins, bradykinin, serotonin, oxygen free radicals, and lysosomal enzymes) perpetuate the maldistribution of blood flow, loss of intravascular plasma volume, and the destruction and death of tissues. The capability of the reticuloendothelial system to destroy and clear invading microorganisms is impaired during low blood flow states. Circulating histamine and serotonin exaggerate this depression. Activation of the complement system and coagulation cascade results in the deposition of fibrin thrombi throughout the vascular system, causing further ischemia, hypoxia, and acidosis. Coagulation factors are eventually consumed, and the platelet and fibrinogen blood levels decrease. Fibrin deposition leads to activation of the fibrinolytic system. Fibrin split products are formed and hemorrhage ensues. Progressive thrombocytopenia, fibrinogen depletion, and hemorrhage characterize the syndrome of disseminated intravascular coagulation (DIC). With continued decompensation and loss of intravascular volume, the arterial blood pressure, blood flow, and oxygen delivery continue to decrease until death occurs.

MONITORING

The word monitor is derived from the Latin *monere*, meaning to warn. Clinical monitoring, therefore, should warn the clinician of changes in the patient's physiologic status. A global approach to monitoring includes a medical history and physical examination supplemented by physiologic, laboratory, and radiographic information. More often, however, monitoring focuses on methods that can be used to (1) assess physiologic imbalances created by acute hypoperfusion, hypoxia, and ischemia; (2) screen for signs of end organ dysfunction; and (3) evaluate therapy. Traditional approaches to monitoring of patients in shock have focused on simple cardiopulmonary and blood chemical values, including respiratory rate, heart rate, peripheral pulse pressure, mucous membrane color, capillary refill time, temperature, and hematocrit (Hct). Urinary output and specific gravity have been used as indirect indications of renal perfusion. Although useful as screening procedures, these indirect indices do not always provide the specific type of information required to accurately assess the patient's hemodynamic status and frequently are altered only in the later stages of shock or when the shock state is severe. Because the common denominator in shock is inadequate tissue oxygenation due to the maldistribution of microcirculatory blood flow, variables that assess tissue perfusion and oxygen transport should be monitored (Tables 5 and 6). The single most important factor that ensures adequate tissue perfusion and oxygen delivery is the effective circulating blood volume. When the effective circulating blood volume decreases, oxygen demand exceeds oxygen consumption, and anaerobic metabolism and lactic acidosis ensue.

The principal determinants of oxygen transport to tissues are arterial oxygen content and cardiac output (CO). The hemoglobin (Hb) concentration, which can be indirectly assessed from the packed cell volume (PCV), and the degree of hemoglobin saturation are the major determinants of arterial oxygen content. Over 95 per cent of the oxygen delivered to tissues is carried by hemoglobin, emphasizing the importance of transfusing packed red blood cells in anemic patients or when arterial hypoxemia is present. It should be remembered that increasing the arterial oxygen tension (Pa_{O_2}) when hemoglobin is fully saturated does little to increase the oxygen carried by blood and, therefore, minimally improves oxygen delivery.

Tissue oxygen delivery can also be enhanced by increasing the effective circulating blood volume and cardiac output. Cardiac output is determined by heart rate and stroke volume. Increases in heart rate generally increase cardiac output until rates of 180/min in the dog and 200/min in the cat are exceeded. Increases in stroke volume also increase cardiac output. The determinants of stroke volume are the venous return (preload), the impedance to the ejection of blood from the ventricle (afterload), and cardiac contractility. From this background it should be clear that noninvasive clinical assessment cannot reliably predict the direction of deviation of oxygen transport from normal and that invasive hemodynamic monitoring is necessary.

Table 5. *Useful Measured Variables for Assessing Oxygen Transport and Tissue Perfusion*

Term	Unit	Normal Range
Hemoglobin concentration (Hb)	gm/dl	12–16
Packed cell volume (PCV)	%	30–45
Arterial O_2 tension (Pa_{O_2})	mm Hg	80–100
Mixed venous O_2 tension (Pv_{O_2})	mm Hg	30–45
pH	pH	7.35–7.45
Lactic acid concentration	mmol/L	<1.0
Carbon dioxide	mm Hg	
Arterial		30–40
Venous		35–45
Temperature	°F	100–102
Heart rate	beats/min	
Dog		70–180
Cat		150–210
Central venous pressure (CVP)	mm Hg	0–3
Pulmonary artery pressure (PAP)	mm Hg	
Systolic		15–25
Diastolic		5–15
Mean		10–20
Pulmonary capillary wedge pressure (PCWP)	mm Hg	5–10
Arterial blood pressure (AP)	mm Hg	
Systolic		100–150
Diastolic		60–110
Mean		80–120
Cardiac output (CO)	ml/kg/min	150–200

Venous and Arterial Catheterization

Venous catheterization is required (1) to secure access to the venous circulation; (2) to obtain blood samples for the determination of a hemogram, blood chemical values, and mixed venous oxygen content; and (3) to administer fluids and medications. Useful information can also be obtained by utilizing catheters that can be positioned in the right atrium and pulmonary artery. Central venous pressure (CVP), measured from catheters positioned in the right atrium, provides valuable information regarding the relationship among intravascular volume, venous return, and right ventricular function. Because these factors must be considered together, central venous pressure measurements provide an important clinical guide for determining the rate of fluid administration but do not indicate the volume of fluid to be replaced. An acute, 2 cm H_2O increase in CVP during fluid administration suggests that the rate of fluid administration is too rapid. Central venous pressure measurement should not be used to predict left-sided heart pressures in critically ill patients, because of differences in the pulmonary and systemic circulations.

Pulmonary artery catheterization facilitates the sampling of true mixed venous blood samples and the direct measurement of pulmonary arterial pressures, pulmonary capillary wedge pressure, and cardiac output. Tissue oxygenation can be assessed by analysis of mixed venous blood gases and calculation of derived oxygen transport variables (see Tables 5 and 6). Pulmonary capillary wedge pressure reflects changes in left arterial pressure and

Table 6. *Useful Derived Variables for Assessing Oxygen Transport and Tissue Perfusion*

Term	Formula	Unit	Normal Range
Arterial O_2 content (Ca_{O_2})	$Ca_{O_2} = (Hb \times 1.34 \times Sa_{O_2}) + (0.003 \times Pa_{O_2})$	ml O_2/dl	16–22
Mixed venous O_2 content (Cv_{O_2})	$Cv_{O_2} = (Hb \times 1.34 \times Sv_{O_2}) + (0.003 \times Pv_{O_2})$	ml O_2/dl	12–17
Arterial-venous O_2 content difference ($Ca\text{-}v_{O_2}$)	$Ca\text{-}v_{O_2} = Ca_{O_2} - Cv_{O_2}$	ml O_2/dl	3–5
Stroke volume (SV)	$SV = \dfrac{CO}{HR}$	ml/beat	Varies with size
Systemic vascular resistance (SVR)	$SVR = \dfrac{mean\ AP - CVP}{CO} \times 80$	dyne•sec•cm^{-5}	2000–5000
Pulmonary vascular resistance (PVR)	$PVR = \dfrac{mean\ PAP - PCWP}{CO} \times 80$	dyne•sec•cm^{-5}	2000–5000
Coronary perfusion pressure (CPP)	$CPP = diastolic\ AP - PCWP$	mm Hg	60–100

can be used as an index of left ventricular filling pressure. Increases in pulmonary capillary wedge pressure suggest left ventricular failure. Finally, although arterial blood pressure can be measured noninvasively, arterial catheterization facilitates continuous blood pressure monitoring and the measurement of arterial blood gases, particularly Pa_{O_2}. Direct measurement of arterial blood pressure provides information about left ventricular contractility. A rapid rate of rise of the arterial pressure curve suggests good cardiac contractility, low impedance to blood flow, or both. A rapid fall in the arterial blood pressure suggests a decrease in systemic vascular resistance. The area under the arterial pressure curve is proportional to the stroke volume.

The adequacy of oxygen transport can be assessed by measuring mixed venous (pulmonary artery) oxygen saturation (Sv_{O_2}). Decreases in Sv_{O_2} suggest decreases in tissue oxygen supply. Abnormalities leading to a decrease in Sv_{O_2} include anemia, arterial hypoxemia, low cardiac output, and increased tissue oxygen consumption. A decrease in Sv_{O_2} in most patients with hemorrhagic, cardiogenic, or traumatic shock is generally due to reductions in cardiac output. Clinically, mixed venous oxygen content (Cv_{O_2}) and oxygen tension (Pv_{O_2}) have been used as alternatives to Sv_{O_2} to assess oxygen transport (see Table 5). These variables are dependent on Sv_{O_2} and are used to assess changes in cardiac output. A Pv_{O_2} less than 30 mm Hg is indicative of a reduction in cardiac output. When Pv_{O_2} is less than 25 mm Hg, anaerobic metabolism ensues. Therefore, low values of Pv_{O_2} suggest the severity of tissue hypoxia and herald the development of lactic acidosis.

Increasingly, indirect methods for the determination of ventilation, tissue perfusion, and oxygen transport are being utilized to assess patients during anesthesia and shock. Ventilometers quantitate respiratory rate, tidal volume, and minute volume but do not assess gas exchange. The indirect measurement of arterial blood pressure using occlusion cuffs and Korotkoff's sounds, Doppler techniques, or oscillometric methods has been advocated. Indirect techniques for the determination of arterial blood pressure require an artery that is large enough to be palpated and that is relatively superficial. The dorsal metatarsal artery in the dog or the cat is most frequently utilized for this purpose. However, regardless of accessibility, the use of indirect techniques for the measurement of arterial blood pressure is least accurate when the blood pressure is low or during vasoconstriction (i.e., during shock) and may lead to erroneous decisions regarding therapy.

New devices for measuring a variety of gas analysis variables, including transcutaneous oxygen and carbon dioxide tension, pulse oximetry, and transconjunctival oxygen tension, are available and provide quantitative information dependent on blood flow and blood oxygen content. The accuracy and utility of these devices in dogs and cats in shock has not been determined. Potentially the most useful (and most expensive) method for the serial assessment of the cardiovascular system of patients in shock is use of two-dimensional echocardiography with Doppler capabilities. These devices allow the accurate measurement of a variety of hemodynamic events indicative of myocardial function and blood flow.

Laboratory Data

The most valuable laboratory data indicate (1) the supply of oxygen to tissues and tissue oxygenation, (2) prognosis, or (3) the value of therapy. The measurement of Hb and PCV, arterial oxygen content (Ca_{O_2}), and Pa_{O_2}, Sv_{O_2}, Cv_{O_2}, and Pv_{O_2} have already been discussed. The measurement of arterial and venous pH identifies the severity of acid-base disturbances. Measurement of bicarbonate (by Oxford titrator) or total carbon dioxide (via Harleco apparatus) can provide information about acid-base status but can be misleading when the respiratory component (Pco_2) is not considered. The determination of blood lactic acid concentration indicates poor tissue perfusion and tissue oxygen deficit and serves as an excellent prognostic indicator of survival. Repeated measurements of an elevated arterial blood lactic acid concentration (> 5 mmol/L) or a progressively increasing blood lactic acid concentration are poor prognostic signs. Blood lactic acid concentrations in excess of 10 mmol/L are usually associated with a greater than 90 per cent mortality.

Other screening tests that provide additional information regarding organ function and tissue damage include determination of blood urea nitrogen (BUN), creatinine, alanine transaminase (ALT), aspartate transaminase (AST), alkaline phosphatase (ALP), lactic dehydrogenase (LDH), lipase, amylase, and serum electrolyte (Na^+, K^+, Cl^-, Ca^{2+}) levels. Measurement of blood glucose concentration yields information necessary to provide proper nutritional support. Finally, blood clotting times and platelet numbers should be evaluated to assess blood coagulability. The measurements of fibrinogen and fibrin split products suggest disturbances of blood coagulation and the fibrinolytic cascades.

Clinical-Pathophysiologic Correlations

The signs and symptoms of shock are indicative of decreases in tissue blood flow, exaggerated sympathetic autonomic responses, and circulating shock mediators. Decreases in mental alertness and coma are related to hypotension and decreases in cerebral blood flow to less than 50 per cent of normal values. Cold, pale, clammy, or dry mucous membranes reflect high sympathetic nervous system activity and reduced skin blood flow. Prolonged capillary refill time suggests poor tissue perfusion due to vasoconstriction, reduced blood volume, or both. Cyanotic mucous membranes signify the circulation of at least 5 gm of reduced hemoglobin and suggest hypoxemia. The combination of cyanosis and peripheral vasoconstriction frequently results in a pale gray coloration of the mucous membranes. Conversely, septic shock initially causes warm pink or red mucous membranes until the blood volume becomes markedly depleted. Injected (blood filled) mucous membranes combined with cyanosis result in dark red mucous membranes ($Pa_{O_2} < 60$ mm Hg, which become reddish black during marked reductions in blood flow (sludging). Tachycardia develops owing to sympathetic nervous stimulation initiated by hypoxia, ischemia, acidosis, or pain. Rapid, thready, weak pulses occur as heart rate increases, the pulse pressure (systolic and diastolic) decreases, or myocardial contractility decreases. Repeated measurements of elevations in blood lactate level (> 8 mmol/L) or a reduced venous oxygen tension (< 25 mm Hg when arterial oxygen tension is normal) indicate low cardiac output and peripheral blood flow and are poor prognostic signs. Electrocardiographic (ECG) abnormalities, including S-T–segment and T-wave changes, develop owing to reductions in myocardial blood flow, local ischemia, hypoxemia, and hyperkalemia. These changes may progress to ventricular extrasystoles and ventricular tachycardia in severe instances or following blunt thoracic and cardiac trauma. Sinus tachycardia, which progresses to sinus bradycardia or ventricular bradycardia, suggests severe cardiac hypoxemia and is a poor prognostic sign.

Reductions in renal blood flow result in marked reductions in urine output and urine sodium level and can lead to acute renal failure. Clinical signs of acute renal failure include proteinuria, hematuria, isosthenuria, and iso-osmolality with plasma. Blood urea nitrogen, creatinine, potassium, and phosphate concentrations progressively increase, while serum levels of sodium, calcium, and bicarbonate and blood pH decrease. Mentally depressed or comatose patients may be hypercapnic and hypoxemic owing to a reduced respiratory rate and hypoventilation.

Depression of liver blood flow results in decreased efficiency of protein and carbohydrate metabolism and may account for reduced detoxification capabilities and impaired coagulation. Zones of centrilobular necrosis may result in nonspecific increases in ALT, AST, ALP, and LDH. Serum bilirubin level may increase, but this is more likely to occur in patients with intravascular hemolysis and septic shock.

The initial response to stress is leukocytosis and increases in the number of circulating polymorphonuclear cells. However, low blood flow states and sludging cause intravascular aggregation of red blood cells, leukocytes, and platelets. Intravascular activation of coagulation processes results in microthrombi formation in small blood vessels, which triggers fibrinolytic mechanisms. Fibrin split products accumulate. Laboratory findings include thrombocytopenia, prolongation of prothrombin time (PT) and partial thromboplastin time (PTT), and increases in fibrinogen concentration and fibrin split products.

TREATMENT OF SHOCK

Therapeutic Goals

The basic objectives of shock therapy are to optimize the physical and functional characteristics of the cardiovascular system. The physical characteristics to be optimized are blood volume, pressure (mean arterial and atrial filling pressures), and flow (cardiac output). The single most important functional characteristic of the cardiovascular system to be optimized is oxygen delivery. The concept of "optimizing" cardiovascular function is stressed because of the common misconception that therapy should be directed at returning hemodynamic factors to normal values. Re-establishing normal values for blood volume, pressure, and flow may be adequate to resuscitate animals with mild to moderate degrees of shock but is likely to be inadequate in more severe shock, particularly when the cause of shock is one in which the metabolic demands of the patient are supranormal. Traumatic and septic shock are examples of this situation: in both of these cases normal values for volume, flow, and pressures may be found in the early compensatory stages of shock (see Table 3). However, because of the increased oxygen demand in these forms of shock, normal hemodynamic values may not be adequate to prevent deterioration of the patient. Thus, resuscitating this type of patient requires recognizing and understanding the form of shock and treating it in a manner aggressive enough to ensure that blood volume, flow, and pressure and oxygen delivery are optimal.

Fluid administration is the cornerstone of shock therapy because of the near absolute dependence of the other physical and functional characteristics of the cardiovascular system on blood volume. Cardiac output is directly dependent on blood volume (in noncardiogenic shock) through the effect of volume on venous return and cardiac filling pressures (atrial or central venous pressure). Mean arterial blood pressure is also dependent on blood volume through the influence of volume on cardiac output. Oxygen delivery is a function of cardiac output and the hemoglobin content of the blood. Thus, when guidelines (see normal ranges in Tables 5 and 6) for shock therapy (Table 7) are considered in order of temporal priority, blood volume expansion with fluids is the primary objective (except in cardiogenic shock). Ensuring adequate cardiac output, oxygen delivery, and arterial blood pressure by means other than volume expansion are the secondary issues to be addressed by shock therapy. Ancillary therapeutic measures (e.g., administration of glucocorticoids) must not supplant these basic therapeutic objectives.

Optimizing Blood Volume

Normal blood volume in the small animal patient ranges from 70 to 80 ml/kg (7 to 8 per cent) of body weight. This blood volume may not be an appropriate goal for fluid therapy in the more severe shock states because of the increased oxygen de-

mand and debt of the tissues, particularly in the late stages of shock or in septic or traumatic shock. More aggressive blood volume expansion to values between 90 and 100 ml/kg of body weight is more likely to provide optimal cardiac filling pressures and cardiac output. Because blood volume measurement is not practical and physical findings do not provide a direct estimate, blood volume must be determined by other means. Central venous pressure can be used effectively as a measure of adequate volume expansion in most forms of shock (see Table 7 for guidelines for shock therapy in order of their temporal priority). Establishing and maintaining a CVP of 5 to 12 cm H_2O will ensure optimal filling pressures to support even the highest cardiac output demands. Arterial blood pressure and pulse pressure are not necessarily good indicators of blood volume because of the intense arteriolar vasoconstriction that occurs in shock.

The choice of fluids is as important as volume expansion. Initial fluid therapy should entail admin-

Table 7. *Guidelines for Therapy of Shock Patients in Order of Temporal Priority*

Therapeutic Objectives	Therapy	Goal of Therapy	Dosage Recommendations
Blood volume	Fluids Isotonic or hypertonic crystalloids Colloids Whole blood	Central venous pressure 5–12 cm H_2O Wedge pressure 7–20 mm Hg Mean arterial blood pressure 70–120 mm Hg (systolic 100–160 mm Hg) Total protein > 4.0 gm/dl Pulse quality strong Normal skin turgor	Isotonic fluids–0.9% NaCl or LRS to effect (see Table 8) Hypertonic saline/dextran—7% NaCl or 7% NaCl in 6% dextran 70, 3–5 ml/kg *slowly* Whole blood, 20–30 ml/kg Plasma, 10–20 ml/kg Dextran 70, 10–20 ml/kg/day
Blood flow	Fluids Inotropic agents	Cardiac index 150–200 ml/min/kg Pv_{O_2} > 35 mm Hg CRT < 2 sec Bright, alert, responsive	Dopamine, 2–10 µg/kg/min Dobutamine, 2–10 µg/kg/min
Oxygen delivery/consumption	Fluids Whole blood Packed red blood cells Inspired P_{O_2} Mechanical ventilation Respiratory care	Pa_{O_2} > 70 mm Hg Pv_{O_2} > 35 mm Hg Hct > 25 Pink mucous membranes Bright, alert, responsive	Packed red blood cells, 10–20 ml/kg Inspired P_{O_2}, 40–100%

Blood pressure	Fluids
	Vasopressors
		Arterial pressure
		  Systolic 100–160 mm Hg
		  Mean 70–120 mm Hg
		  Diastolic 50–100 mm Hg
		Pulse quality strong
			Dopamine, 5–15 µg/kg/min
			Phenylephrine, 0.01–0.1 µg/kg
			Methoxamine, 0.1–0.2 µg/kg

Acid-base balance	$NaHCO_3$	pH > 7.3 and < 7.5	Sodium bicarbonate, 1–5 mEq/kg
Urine output	Fluids	1–2 ml/kg/hr	Furosemide, 2–4 mg/kg Mannitol (20%), 1–2 gm/kg
Body temperature	Warm fluids Water blanket	> 99°F and < 103°F	
Heart rate	Fluids Antiarrhythmics	70–160 beats/min	Lidocaine, 1–2 mg/kg bolus, 40–80 µg/kg/min
Sepsis	Antibiotics	Negative blood culture	Cephalothin, 20 mg/kg q6h IV Ampicillin, 20 mg/kg q6h IV Gentamicin, 2 mg/kg q8h IM
Blood glucose	Glucose Insulin	Glucose 60–120 mg/dl	Glucose 5% in maintenance fluids Glucose 50%, 0.5–2.0 gm/kg/hr Insulin (regular), 2 Units/kg q2–6h IV

CRT, capillary refill time; LRS, lactated Ringer's solution

istration of a solution with a high sodium concentration. Because of the cells' ability to maintain a low intracellular sodium concentration and the high affinity of water for sodium, isotonic fluids high in sodium (e.g., normal saline and Ringer's lactate solution) tend to stay within the extracellular space and thus in part within the vascular space. The vascular space makes up approximately 30 per cent of the extracellular fluid space. Therefore, to achieve a given degree of blood volume expansion with isotonic sodium-rich crystalloid solutions it is necessary to give three to four times this volume. Put another way, if one fourth of the blood volume (20 ml/kg) is lost to hemorrhage, approximately three to four times this amount (60 to 80 ml/kg) of isotonic fluids would be necessary to return blood volume to normal. If the crystalloid administered is low in sodium, the fluid will be further distributed within the intracellular space and the efficacy of the fluid therapy with respect to blood volume expansion will be diminished.

Hypoproteinemia and anemia are two important, life-threatening sequelae of aggressive crystalloid fluid therapy. Total protein and packed cell volume (PCV) measurements should be made prior to initiating fluid therapy and repeated during fluid therapy to prevent extreme dilution of these important blood components. Plasma proteins, specifically albumin, play an important role in maintaining vascular volume. Thus, when the total protein measurement falls below 4.0 gm/dl or albumin below 1.5 gm/dl, fluid begins to move in greater amounts from the vascular to the interstitial space because of the loss of colloid oncotic pressure. Low plasma protein concentrations can severely limit the effectiveness of subsequent efforts at blood volume expansion with crystalloids, and the edema that results can critically compromise organ function. (For the effects and treatment of hemodilution see the following discussion on optimizing oxygen delivery).

Plasma administration is probably the most effective form of colloid expansion and provides prolonged support of colloid oncotic pressure and blood volume. The half-life of canine albumin is approximately 15 days. When plasma or whole blood therapy is not available for treatment of hypoproteinemia, the synthetic colloid expanders can be used to provide the necessary oncotic pressure. Dextrans are the most commonly used synthetic colloid expander. Dextrans are high-molecular-weight polysaccharides that are marketed in low- and high-molecular-weight forms. High-molecular-weight dextran (70,000 MW; 6 per cent solution) has a much longer half-life (24 hours) than the low-molecular-weight dextran (40,000 MW; 10 per cent solution) and is preferred in shock therapy. Hydroxyethyl starch (Hetastarch; 400,000 MW; 6 per cent solution) is another form of synthetic colloid expander. It too acts to expand the blood volume

by moving fluid into and maintaining fluid within the vascular space. The dosage for each of these solutions is 10 to 20 ml/kg/day. The indications for use of these solutions in hypovolemic, hypoproteinemic states are limited. Major concerns are hypervolemia and increased blood viscosity if administration is too rapid or the dosage too high. Allergic reactions have been reported but are rare.

Hypertonic glucose and mannitol solutions can bring about blood volume expansion, but their duration of action is so limited that their use as volume expanders or colloid agents is not recommended.

An algorithm that can serve as a guideline for volume loading during emergency shock resuscitation is provided in Table 8. This or a similar organized approach should be used in the initial management of the emergency shock patient. The end points of this algorithm are establishment of an adequate pulse pressure and optimization of blood volume. Measurement of blood volume plays an important role in therapeutic monitoring during rapid volume expansion, and physical findings do not generally provide accurate information in this regard. Therefore, the authors use CVP as one of the major physiologic variables to be monitored. Because of the dominant role of volume expansion in shock therapy and the difficulty of physical detection of the degree of volume expansion, it is more important to monitor this physiologic variable than other hemodynamic variables (e.g., arterial blood pressure and cardiac output). Central venous pressure measurement does not require expensive equipment and is as easy to obtain as placement of a jugular catheter.

Optimizing Blood Pressure and Flow

Cardiac function is rarely a limiting factor in the restoration of adequate blood flow in the early stages of the types of shock discussed in this article. Adequate volume replacement generally results in the return of normal cardiac function by improving myocardial oxygen delivery through increased cardiac filling pressures, cardiac output, and coronary blood flow. Likewise, vascular function is not typically a limiting factor in restoration of blood pressure in the early stages of shock, except for the more severe forms of septic or endotoxic shock. Arterial blood pressure usually returns to normal when cardiac output is raised. Thus, as a rule, pharmacologic efforts aimed at improving cardiac function to enhance output or increasing total peripheral resistance to improve arterial pressure should never replace aggressive volume replacement.

In the more severe forms or terminal stages of shock when the heart and vasculature are unresponsive to volume replacement, inotropic and vasoac-

Table 8. *Algorithm of Fluid Therapy for Shock Patients*

Step 1.	If pulse not palpable, begin CPR and proceed to volume load, steps 2 through 5.
Step 2.	If pulse weak or barely palpable (SAP < 80 mm Hg), immediately start LRS at 60 ml/kg and run as rapidly as possible, preferably through a large-gauge central venous catheter. Obtain PCV and TP.
Step 3.	Monitor CVP at frequent intervals during infusion. Do not allow CVP to exceed 15 cm H_2O (i.e., stop fluids).
Step 4.	If PCV < 25% or TP < 3.5 gm/dl, give 10–20 ml/kg of whole blood or appropriate blood (e.g., packed cells, plasma) or synthetic colloid product (e.g., dextran).
Step 5.	Restoration of adequate pulse (SAP > 80 mm Hg) is the end-point of steps 2 to 5. If pulse still weak (SAP < 80 mm Hg) repeat steps 2 through 5. If pulse is adequate (SAP > 80 mm Hg) proceed to Step 6.
Step 6.	Obtain further history, and begin diagnostic workup. Repeat PCV and TP; treat as indicated. If no history of cardiac disease or arrhythmias, give another 30 ml/kg of fluids. If cardiac history or arrhythmias, give 5–10 ml/kg of plasma or dextran 70.
Step 7.	Fluids may be given as needed to restore circulatory integrity. Maintain CVP < 15 cm H_2O.
Step 8.	Establishing an adequate blood volume is the end-point of steps 6 to 8. This is achieved if CVP is between 5 and 12 cm H_2O and pulse is strong (SAP > 100 Hg), CRT is < 2 sec, and mucous membranes are pink. If objective is not met, repeat steps 6 through 8.
Step 9.	Finish diagnostics, evaluate for continued blood loss. If mentation depressed, evaluate for head trauma or poisoning; treat accordingly. Begin maintenance fluids.

CPR, cardiopulmonary resuscitation; SAP, systolic arterial pressure; LRS, lactate Ringer's solution; PCV, packed cell volume; TP, total protein; CVP, central venous pressure.

tive pharmacologic agents play an important role in therapeutics. In the patient with evidence of high filling pressures (i.e., central venous pressure) and poor peripheral perfusion that is unresponsive to volume therapy, the use of inotropic agents such as dopamine, dobutamine, or isoproterenol can enhance cardiac function and improve blood flow. Dopamine has positive inotropic effects and may provide some improvement in renal and splanchnic blood flows at low doses (2 to 5 μg/kg/min). At higher doses dopamine produces vasoconstriction and, commonly, tachycardia. Thus, these higher doses should be avoided unless poor cardiac function is combined with low peripheral vascular resistance (a scenario justifying its use in high doses).

Dobutamine is predominantly a beta-1 receptor agonist that acts mainly to increase myocardial contractility. Its effects on heart rate and peripheral vascular resistance are not generally significant, except at higher dosages. The use of this agent (3 to 10 μg/kg/min) in shock would be most appropriate when inadequate cardiac function is thought to contribute to poor peripheral perfusion.

Alpha-adrenergic drugs (e.g., norepinephrine, phenylephrine, and methoxamine) are not indicated in the management of most types of shock. Their use is generally reserved for low systemic resistance forms of shock (see Table 1) in which the peripheral vasculature is unresponsive and adequate blood pressure cannot be established despite aggressive efforts to expand blood volume and ensure adequate blood flow. These agents may also be used in acute, severe hemorrhage or circulatory arrest to restore blood pressure and flow until volume replacement can be instituted.

Arrhythmias are common sequelae to shock, particularly shock due to trauma. Cardiac arrhythmias can range from benign occasional premature ventricular contractions to ventricular tachyarrhythmias that markedly compromise cardiac function. Their

early detection and treatment form an important part of shock therapy. Lidocaine is generally indicated for ventricular extrasystoles or tachyarrhythmias and can be given in bolus form (1 to 2 mg/kg IV) or as a continuous infusion (40 to 80 μg/kg/min). A more thorough review of antiarrhythmic therapy is provided elsewhere (see pp. 278–286).

Arterial blood pressure can be monitored relatively well by palpation of the femoral artery. Pulse pressure should be evaluated frequently during the early phases of volume replacement to ensure a good response to fluid therapy. Direct and indirect arterial blood pressure measuring devices can be employed to assist in measurement of arterial pressure.

Urine output is also a good indicator of adequate blood flow and arterial blood pressure. Urine output should be frequently evaluated in the shock patient by either direct measurement or palpation. Efforts directed at optimizing blood volume will generally result in a return of urine output to normal. Diuretics should be used in a shock patient only after volume replacement. If urine output is less than 1 ml/kg/hr despite aggressive volume replacement, loop (furosemide) or osmotic (mannitol) diuretics can be used to improve renal blood flow and enhance urine formation. Dopamine at 2 to 3 μg/kg/min may also be effective in restoring urine output by its renal vasodilating properties.

Optimizing Oxygen Delivery

Oxygen delivery is a function of blood flow and the oxygen-carrying capacity of the blood. Establishing good blood flow by volume expansion is often enough to provide the degree of oxygen delivery to the tissues necessary to promote recovery from shock. However, when the blood loss in a patient has been significant and the oxygen requirements are heightened by trauma or sepsis, an adequate hemoglobin concentration may be the key to survival. The hematocrit or hemoglobin concentration at which whole blood or packed cell administration is warranted depends on the severity of the shock state. In patients with the excessive oxygen demands of severe septic, surgical, or traumatic shock, hematocrit levels below 30 per cent may be life threatening. A hematocrit of 20 per cent may provide acceptable oxygen-carrying capacity in less severe forms of shock.

To raise the packed cell volume from approximately 20 per cent to one of 30 to 40 per cent, 20 to 30 ml/kg of whole blood with a normal packed cell volume must be given. It is most desirable that the donor blood be from a cross-matched, A-negative donor and that it be relatively fresh (less than 1 hour old), particularly if clotting factors and platelets are needed. If an animal is a first-time recipient of blood, A-positive blood can be used, but some caution should be exercised. The patient should be monitored for urticarial reaction, vomiting, red cell lysis, icterus, and potential circulatory collapse. Preceding the blood infusion by corticosteroid treatment may help to prevent some of the problems associated with unmatched blood. In life-threatening situations of severe abdominal or thoracic hemorrhage, the shed blood can be autotransfused. This should be performed only if laboratory or surgical evaluation has eliminated the possibility of blood contamination by hollow viscus rupture.

Frequent evaluation of mucous membrane color, patient mentation, and hematocrit form the major means of monitoring oxygen delivery to the tissues of a shock patient. If blood gas analysis is available, there are numerous direct and derived cardiorespiratory values that can provide an estimate of oxygen delivery and consumption. The simplest are arterial and mixed venous partial pressures of oxygen. Arterial P_{O_2} (Pa_{O_2}) provides an estimate of pulmonary function and will determine the degree of hemoglobin saturation and oxygen content of the arterial blood. A low Pa_{O_2} (less than 70 mm Hg) on room air suggests poor pulmonary function. Increasing the concentration of inspired oxygen may help to improve the arterial P_{O_2}, but attention should also be addressed to treating possible pulmonary injuries or hypoventilation. A low mixed venous P_{O_2} (Pv_{O_2} less than 25 mm Hg) suggests inadequate oxygen delivery to the tissues, resulting in increased oxygen extraction. This should be managed by efforts to improve oxygen delivery through increasing blood flow, increasing oxygen-carrying capacity, or increasing Pa_{O_2} to improve saturation of arterial blood.

Acid-base derangements are common in shock. Poor tissue oxygen delivery results in a shift to anaerobic metabolism; metabolic acidosis is the result. If blood gas and pH meters are available, an accurate assessment of the base deficit can be obtained. The dosage of sodium bicarbonate (in milliequivalents) used to correct a given base deficit is obtained from the following formula: base deficit × 0.3 × kilograms of body weight. This formula corrects for the extracellular fluid compartment base deficit. Sodium bicarbonate should be given slowly intravenously. If blood pH cannot be measured, a clinical estimation of the malperfusion must be made. Mild, moderate, and severe malperfusion should be treated with bicarbonate dosages of 1.0, 3.0, and 5.0 mEq/kg of body weight, respectively.

Alterations in serum potassium levels are the most common form of electrolyte disturbance in shock. When metabolic acidosis is severe as a result of low cardiac output and anaerobic metabolism, hyperkalemia is a common sequela. This condition responds readily to aggressive volume expansion and improvement in the acid-base status of the patient. In fact, it is common for serum potassium levels to become low with aggressive volume replacement. Hypokalemia should be anticipated and, following the rapid phase of volume expansion, maintenance levels of potassium (10 to 15 mEq/L) should be added to subsequent fluids.

Miscellaneous Therapeutic Measures

CORTICOSTEROIDS

The use of corticosteroids for the treatment of shock has remained controversial for over four decades. The corticosteroids are believed to derive their beneficial effects from several mechanisms, including the inhibition of platelet and granulocyte aggregation, stabilization of lysosomal membranes, improved oxygen transport in peripheral tissues, inhibition of the release of vasoactive peptides, and the ability to inhibit phospholipase A_2 (a critical step in the arachidonic acid cascade). The argument over whether corticosteroids produce a beneficial effect continues because most studies do not contain controls, patients are not randomized, drug or placebo administration is not blinded, and the end point for positive drug effects is not identified. Recent studies using hemorrhage-shocked dogs, however, suggest that water-soluble dexamethasone (5 mg/kg IV) improves blood flow to the lungs, gastrointestinal tract, and kidneys and reduces cell damage as indicated by a reduction in ALP, AST, and ALT levels. Additional studies in dogs with septic shock caused by intravenous Escherichia coli injections demonstrated improved survival when gentamicin (4 mg/kg IV) and prednisolone sodium succinate (11 mg/kg IV) were administered in combination compared with dexamethasone (propylene glycol suspension, 8 mg/kg IV) and gentamicin. These experimental studies are important but do little to end the clinical questions associated with the use of steroids. Not until a well-designed prospective, randomized, and blinded clinical study is completed will the controversy surrounding steroids be ended. Most data suggest that if corticosteroids are going to be used they should be administered early and in large doses and that, although they may not produce a beneficial effect on long-term survival, the patient feels better while recovering or until death occurs.

NUTRITION

Alterations of glucose metabolism are common in shock patients. The stress involved in trauma and shock results in hormonal changes that stimulate gluconeogenesis and increased release of stored glucose. The hormones promoting the increase in blood glucose level also act to inhibit peripheral uptake and utilization of glucose, occasionally leading to hyperglycemia. On the other hand, hypoglycemia is often observed in septic shock and the late stages of other forms of shock. Neither situation is beneficial to the shock patient, particularly in light of the dramatic energy demands of shock.

Glucose solutions should be added to the fluid therapy of the shock patient. The isotonic crystalloid solution used for volume replacement can be supplemented with 5 per cent dextrose or glucose and can be given as a 50 per cent solution at a rate of 0.5 to 2.0 gm/kg/hr. If hyperglycemia develops, insulin therapy can be initiated. *Under no circumstances should insulin therapy be used without the concomitant administration of glucose.* Glucose and insulin therapy will have a tendency to drive potassium into the cells, producing hypokalemia. Therefore, potassium should be added to the fluids in quantities of 10 to 30 mEq/L.

ANTIBIOTICS

Antibiotic therapy plays an important role in both the prevention of shock and the treatment. Appropriate prophylactic and therapeutic antibiotic therapy can have a significant impact on the frequency of sepsis and shock, particularly in regard to surgically related sepsis. This is not to suggest that the other principles of aseptic surgical technique are not involved; an occasional review of both aseptic techniques and antibiotic therapy may greatly limit the occurrence of septic shock.

The prophylactic use of antibiotics in all nonseptic shock cases is not recommended. However, when shock is severe or prolonged, prophylactic antibiotics should be used to prevent the development of a septic component. The septic component is commonly the result of gastrointestinal ischemia, bacterial invasion of the intestinal submucosa, and subsequent bacteremia. Gram-positive and endotoxin-producing gram-negative bacteria are likely to invade the circulation during intestinal ischemia. Early use of broad-spectrum antibiotics can diminish the bacteremia and endotoxin release.

When sepsis is the primary cause of shock, therapeutic antibiotic use is indicated, as is culture and sensitivity testing of the source. Surgical drainage and débridement should be instituted early in therapy. The only concern that should ever delay surgical management of a septic source is stabilization of the patient. This is often difficult in the face of continuing infection. High-dose, broad-spectrum bactericidal antibiotics should be used (intravenously when possible) when culture and sensitivity are not available to guide therapy. Cephalosporins or ampicillin combined with aminoglycosides forms one good drug strategy for sepsis treatment. As always, when aminoglycosides are used, good renal blood flow should be ensured to prevent manifestation of their nephrotoxic potential.

New Therapeutic Concepts

There has been a resurgence of interest in the use of hypertonic sodium chloride solutions as an alternative form of fluid therapy for the treatment of shock. Prior to 1980, mildly hypertonic sodium chloride solutions (600 to 1800 mOsm/L) were found to be useful in the treatment of burn shock, but no real advantages had been demonstrated regarding their use in other forms of shock. In 1980, investigators demonstrated the dramatic resuscitative effects of small volumes of a hypertonic saline solution (2400 mOsm/L of NaCL; i.e., 7 per cent NaCl) used for the treatment of severe hemorrhagic shock (Velasco et al., 1980). In a canine hemorrhagic shock model with blood loss approximating 40 per cent of the blood volume, 4 ml/kg of 7 per cent sodium chloride injected as a slow intravenous bolus produced rapid, dramatic increases in cardiac output, arterial blood pressure, and splanchnic blood flow. Blood gas and acid-base status also improved rapidly, and there was 100 per cent survival in the group of dogs treated.

Since this initial study, numerous experimental studies in dogs and other species utilizing various shock models have demonstrated the potential of 7 per cent saline. Clinical reports of the use of these solutions in humans have been equally promising. The major advantages of hypertonic saline have proved to be (1) rapid restoration of circulatory function, (2) the small volume of solution necessary for initial resuscitation, (3) limited complications associated with its use, and (4) beneficial effects on hemodynamics that are not seen with isotonic solutions.

The mechanisms by which hypertonic saline exerts its resuscitative effects are not fully understood. The high sodium concentration and predominant extracellular distribution of such fluids are thought to result in an osmotic redistribution of fluid from the intracellular space to the extracellular space. The increase in vascular volume is in part responsible for the improvement in venous return and cardiac output observed but is not thought to be the sole mechanism of action. In the dog, resuscitation and the associated alterations in hemodynamics are thought to be dependent on the stimulation of a lung afferent nerve–mediated reflex that travels in the vagus. Hypertonic saline solutions are also thought to have a positive inotropic effect on the myocardium and have been suggested to cause venoconstriction, increasing venous return.

The addition of 6 per cent dextran 70 to the hypertonic saline solution has been demonstrated to potentiate and sustain the resuscitative effects of hypertonic saline. The combination of 7 per cent sodium chloride in 6 per cent dextran 70 was found in a recent human clinical study to be effective in establishing good circulatory function in trauma patients.

The available literature and the authors' clinical experience with hypertonic saline and dextran solutions suggest that the primary indications for clinical use are hemorrhagic shock, traumatic shock, surgical shock, and septic shock. These solutions should be used only as an adjunctive form of therapy directed at rapidly re-establishing good circulatory function. Their use should be followed with standard resuscitative measures, as outlined in this article, to effect clinical recovery from the signs of shock.

The dosage for 7 per cent saline or 7 per cent saline in 6 per cent dextran 70 is 3 to 5 ml/kg of body weight. These solutions should be infused intravenously through a peripheral or central vein. They should be given as a slow infusion over 3 to 5 minutes.

The contraindications for the use of hypertonic saline and dextran solutions in canine patients at this time should include hypernatremic or hyperosmotic states (e.g., moderate to severe dehydration or diabetic ketoacidosis). Seizures should also be considered a contraindication, although no reports of seizure inducement are present in the literature. Dextrans are known to diminish platelet function, and therefore the combination may not be advisable in the presence of thrombocytopenia. Cardiogenic shock is also considered to be a contraindication for their use.

Certain precautions should be exercised in the use of these solutions. The importance of slow administration must be stressed. Rapid infusion of hypertonic solutions results in reflex bradycardia, hypotension, and bronchoconstriction that, although transient, can be devastating to an animal in shock. Red blood cell lysis has not proved to be of concern, probably because of the greater resistance of red blood cells to hyper- than to hyposmotic solutions. Extravasation should be avoided, but otherwise the effects of these solutions on the veins (i.e., thrombosis and phlebitis) are not significant. Mild hypokalemia is a common finding when these solutions have been used and should be anticipated and treated as it develops. The solutions have not been studied in the presence of arrhythmias and thus caution should be used when arrhythmias are present. Re-hemorrhage has been a concern of some investigators; the rationale being that the rapid increases in blood pressure and flow may act to break down early clot formation. Certainly this potential disadvantage must be weighed against the deleterious effects of prolonging shock as a result of slower resuscitative measures.

Sodium chloride solutions of 7 per cent concentration and sodium chloride and dextran solutions are not yet available commercially. Sodium chloride solutions can be made up at 7 per cent concentration; the solution can be filtered through a 0.22-μ filter into a sterile container or autoclaved and transferred to a sterile container. If the solution is autoclaved it should still be passed through a millipore filter to ensure removal of particulates. Dextran 70 is commercially available in 6 per cent solutions, and the combination of 7 per cent sodium chloride and 6 per cent dextran 70 can be prepared by dissolving the appropriate quantity of sodium chloride in the dextran solution. Again, passing this through a millipore filter into a sterile container provides a pyrogen-free, sterile solution.

It is the opinion of the authors that hypertonic saline and dextran solutions have great potential as adjunctive therapy for shock resuscitation in the veterinary patient. However, until clinical studies are completed that further identify the indications, contraindications, and precautions regarding the administration of these solutions, caution should be exercised in their use. The authors' clinical experience suggests that these solutions can be used safely in the dog and cat by following the guidelines outlined above.

References and Supplemental Reading

Adams, H. R., and Parker J. L.: Pharmacologic management of circulatory shock: Cardiovascular drugs and corticosteroids. J.A.V.M.A. 175:86, 1979.

Clark, D. R.: Circulatory shock: Etiology and pathophysiology. J.A.V.M.A. 175:78, 1979.

Hardaway, R. M.: Cellular and metabolic effects of shock. J.A.V.M.A. 175:81, 1979.

Holcroft, J. W., Vassar, M. J., Turner, J. E., et al: 3% NaCl and 7.5% NaCl/dextran 70 in the resuscitation of severely injured patients. Ann. Surg. 206:279, 1987.

Haskins, S. C.: Shock (the pathophysiology and management of the circulatory collapse states). *In* Kirk, R. W. (ed.): *Current Veterinary Therapy VIII*. Philadelphia: W. B. Saunders, 1983, pp. 2–27.

King, E. G., and Chin, W. D. N.: Shock: An overview of pathophysiology and general treatment goals. Crit. Care Clin. 1:547, 1985.

Kramer, G. C., Perron, P. R., Lindsey, G., et al.: Small-volume resuscitation with hypertonic saline dextran solution. Surgery 100:239, 1986.

Lopes, O. U., Pontieri, V., Rocha-e-Silva, M., et al.: Hyperosmotic NaCl and severe hemorrhagic shock: Role of the innervated lung. Am. J. Physiol. 241:H883, 1981.

Ross, J. N.: Comprehensive patient management in shock. J.A.V.M.A. 175:92, 1979.

Shoemaker, W. C.: Pathophysiology of shock syndromes. *In* Shoemaker, W. C., Thompson, W. L., and Holbrook, P. R. (eds.): *Textbook of Critical Care*. Philadelphia: W. B. Saunders, 1984, pp. 52–74.

Shoemaker, W. C.: Circulatory mechanisms of shock and their mediators. Crit. Care Med. 15:787, 1987.

Shoemaker, W. C., and Czer, L. S. C.: Evaluation of the biologic importance of various hemodynamic and oxygen transport variables. Crit. Care Med. 7:424, 1979.

Shoemaker, W. C., Appel, P. L., Waxman, K., et al.: Clinical trial of survivors' cardiorespiratory patterns as therapeutic goals in critically ill postoperative patients. Crit. Care Med. 10:398, 1982.

Velasco, I. T., Pontieri, V., Rocha-e-Silva, M., et al.: Hyperosmotic NaCl and severe hemorrhagic shock. Am. J. Physiol. 239:H664, 1980.

Weil, M. H., von Planta, M., and Rackow, E. C.: Acute circulatory failure (shock). *In* Braunwald, E. (ed.): *A Textbook of Cardiovascular Medicine*, 3rd ed. Philadelphia: W. B. Saunders, 1988, pp. 561–577.

White, G. L., White, G. S., Kosanke, S. D., et al.: Therapeutic effects of prednisolone sodium succinate vs dexamethasone in dogs subjected to *E. coli* septic shock. J. Am. Anim. Hosp. Assoc. 18:1, 1982.

Younes, R. N., Aun, F., Tomida, R. M., et al.: The role of lung innervation in the hemodynamic response to hypertonic sodium chloride solutions in hemorrhagic shock. Surgery 98:900, 1985.

CARDIOPULMONARY RESUSCITATION

STEVE C. HASKINS, D.V.M.

Davis, California

Early, aggressive, and effective therapy of the patient with cardiopulmonary arrest should generate a successful long-term resuscitation rate of approximately 8 to 10 per cent. Long-term resuscitation rates in animals have been reported to be 9 per cent for dogs (Gilroy et al., 1986), and 7 (Henik et al., 1987) and 22 per cent (Gilroy et al., 1986) for cats. Forty-four per cent of 294 human patients with cardiopulmonary arrest survived the initial resuscitation in one study (Bedell et al., 1983); 14 per cent were discharged from the hospital, and 11 per cent were alive 6 months later.

The proficiency of the initial resuscitation technique and the underlying disease process determines initial survival rates. The effectiveness of the early postresuscitation monitoring and support and the severity of the underlying disease process determine early postresuscitation survival. The nature of the underlying disease process determines the long-term survival.

Cardiac arrest may be caused by any disease carried to its extreme, which directly or indirectly affects cardiovascular homeostasis. Prevention of the cardiac arrest by effective treatment of the underlying disease process is always more likely to be associated with a successful outcome than is treatment of the cardiac arrest after it has occurred. The existence of cardiac arrest must be recognized early if therapy is expected to be effective. The patient will be unconscious; there will be an absence of an auscultable heart beat or a palpable pulse; mucous membranes are often dishwater gray or blue but can be white or even normal; pupils are soon dilated; and there will be an absence of ventilatory efforts (notwithstanding agonal gasps, which should not be interpreted as true ventilation). If doubt exists as to whether a cardiac arrest exists, the resuscitation procedure should commence. It is far better to attempt resuscitation of a heart that has not truly stopped than it would be not to attempt resuscitation of a heart that truly has stopped.

Whether to resuscitate an arrested patient is a decision that must be made on the merits of each individual case and in previous agreement with the owner. Patients that have a treatable underlying disease process should be resuscitated. The resuscitation technique must be organized in advance. Necessary equipment, drugs, and supplies should be located in one place at all times, and equipment must be in working order. All available personnel should be trained to be a functional part of the resuscitation team; periodic drills should be conducted to make sure that all are well oriented to their job assignments. A cardiopulmonary resuscitation (CPR) flow sheet or check list (Table 1) should be posted to assure that essential components are not omitted from the resuscitation endeavor.

AIRWAY AND BREATHING

The airway should be secured by endotracheal intubation, and positive pressure ventilation with 100 per cent oxygen should be instituted as a first

Table 1. Cardiopulmonary Resuscitation Check List

A. Intubate endotracheally
B. Commence positive pressure ventilation (1 per 5 chest compressions)
C. Commence external chest compression (80 to 120/min)
  1. Evaluate effectiveness of the artificial circulation of blood technique. If effective, continue. If ineffective:
    a. Change the compression technique:
      Change position of animal
      Insert solid surface or sandbag underneath animal
      Change position of hands on chest
      Compress at faster or slower rate
      Compress with more or less force
      Hold the compression for longer period of time
    b. Administer epinephrine (0.1–0.2 mg/kg)
    c. Rapidly administer crystalloid fluids (40 ml/kg in the dog; 20 ml/kg in the cat)
    d. Wrap hind legs to lower abdomen tightly
    e. Wrap abdomen snugly
    f. Alternately compress abdomen and chest
    g. Simultaneously ventilate and compress chest
  2. If external technique proves ineffective after 3 to 5 min, consider a thoracotomy for internal cardiac compression
D. Drug administrations
  1. Oxygen (100%)
  2. Fluids (40 ml/kg in the dog, 20 ml/kg in the cat, per aliquot)
  3. Alpha-agonists
    a. Epinephrine (0.1–0.2 mg/kg)
    b. Norepinephrine (0.1–0.2 mg/kg)
    c. Phenylephrine (0.5–1.0 mg/kg)
    d. Metaraminol (1–5 mg/kg)
  4. Atropine (0.02–0.04 mg/kg)
  5. Sodium bicarbonate (0.5 mEq/kg after first 5 min)
E. Electrical activity of the heart
  1. None—give epinephrine (0.1–0.2 mg/kg)
  2. Chaotic—defibrillate
  3. Normal—administer fluids if cardiovascular collapse; electromechanical dissociation—catecholamine (?), dexamethasone (?)
F. Follow-up monitoring and support
  1. Cardiovascular
    a. Electrical function
    b. Mechanical function
    c. Tissue perfusion
  2. Pulmonary
    a. Nature of the breathing effort
    b. Adequacy of oxygenation
    c. Pneumothorax (?)
    d. Lung contusion (?)
  3. Cerebral
    a. Avoid hypertension, hypotension, hypoxia, hypercapnia, hyperthermia, venous outflow obstruction, head-down positioning, ketamine, inhalational anesthetics, xylazine
    b. Hyperventilate the patient until consciousness returns
    c. If consciousness is not beginning to return within 30 min from the time the heart was restarted, or the resuscitation persisted for more than 15 min, administer corticosteroids (dexamethasone, 0.5 mg/kg IV; predisolone sodium succinate, 2 mg/kg IV), mannitol (0.5/kg IV), furosemide (5 mg/kg IV)

priority. The inspired oxygen concentration should be as high as possible. One ventilation should be delivered approximately every 5 sec between external chest compressions, but twice per 15 sec if the resuscitation is being conducted by one person. Ventilation and compression should be timed so that there is essentially no pause in the provision of artificial circulation. Breathing techniques should provide for moderate hyperventilation. The respiratory alkalosis will help offset the developing metabolic acidosis, and the hyperventilation will help remove the carbon dioxide generated by the administration of sodium bicarbonate. Breathing techniques generally improve blood gas concentrations without significant effect on blood flow. Positive end-expiratory pressure, by decreasing the aortic–central venous pressure gradient, decreases cerebral and coronary blood flow. Simultaneous ventilation and chest compression (see discussion of circulation) generally increases blood flow (Rudikoff et al. 1980) but predisposes to barotrauma and pneumothorax.

CIRCULATION

Total blood flow during optimally conducted chest or heart compression techniques ranges between 20 and 40 per cent of normal (Voorhees et al., 1980). Regional blood flow is generally greater to the brain and the heart than to the viscera (Voorhees et al., 1980). Cerebral blood flow is usually higher than coronary blood flow (40 versus 20 per cent of normal) and is easiest to effect by the resuscitation technique (Voorhees et al., 1980).

Classic concepts of blood flow during CPR held that the atrioventricular (AV) valves are functional during cardiac compression and that pressure applied to the heart causes blood to move out of the ventricles and out of the chest (the *cardiac pump theory*). There is evidence for and against functional AV valves. The *thoracic pump theory* is based on the premise that the AV valves do not need to be functional and that the generalized increase in intrathoracic pressure causes the forward flow of blood. Backward flow of blood is prevented mostly by the pressure-induced collapse of the great veins in the chest and, perhaps, by upstream venous valves (Rudikoff et al., 1980). Several of the artificial circulation techniques discussed below are based on this concept.

Internal cardiac compression techniques are generally associated with better cardiac outputs (Bircher et al., 1980), but there is considerable individual variation. An immediate thoracotomy for the treatment of cardiac arrest is probably unwarranted because external chest compression works many times. If the heart can be easily started with external chest compression, the risks of an emergency thoracotomy are not warranted. If external techniques are unable to generate acceptable circulation (a second person cannot palpate a peripheral pulse with each compression; the mucous membrane color does not improve; or the pupils continue to dilate) by 3 to 5 min, an immediate thoracotomy and internal heart compression is indicated.

External chest compression should be accomplished by applying pressure directly over the heart with a force that is appropriate for the size of the patient at a rate of 80 to 120 times per min. The compression should be held for a brief period of time to maximize the elimination of blood from the heart and the chest. Time must be allowed between compressions for adequate diastolic filling of the ventricles. If the initial technique does not generate palpable pulses or an improvement in mucous membrane color, an alternate technique should be used. The compression force could be increased (Niemann, 1984) or decreased, the rate could be increased or decreased, the duration of systole could be increased, the position of the animal could be changed, the position of the hands or compressor with respect to the patient could be changed, or the compressor could be changed. Additional procedures that may help maximize the effectiveness of the artificial circulation technique include administration of fluids or alpha-agonists; application of antishock trousers, abdominal tourniquets, or abdominal wraps; intermittent abdominal compression; and simultaneous ventilation.

Cardiac arrest is a rapidly vasodilating disease process caused by tissue anoxia. The peripheral accumulation of blood volume must be replaced with exogenous fluids to maintain an effective central circulating volume. Notwithstanding pre-existing anemia or hypoproteinemia, a crystalloid fluid such as lactated Ringer's solution, should be administered rapidly intravenously in aliquots of approximately 40 ml/kg for the dog and 20 ml/kg for the cat. This bolus volume may need to be repeated periodically throughout the resuscitation endeavor in quantities sufficient to maintain an effective circulating volume. Excessive fluids predispose to fulminating pulmonary edema.

Peripheral vasoconstriction by the administration of an alpha-agonist drug (Table 2) redistributes blood to the central circulation and diminishes the loss of central blood volume into the periphery. In general, one alpha-agonist drug is as effective as another; however, epinephrine has been shown to generate the greatest arteriovenous pressure gradient and coronary and cerebral blood flow (Brillman et al., 1985; Michael et al., 1984). Isoproterenol and dobutamine cannot be recommended because of their peripheral vasodilating properties.

Antishock trousers have been reported to improve systemic blood pressure and vital organ perfusion by returning a small amount of blood from the peripheral pool to the central circulation and by preventing the runoff of central blood volume to the periphery (Bircher et al., 1980). Antishock trousers can be approximated by wrapping the hind legs and caudal abdomen with elastic bandaging material. Starting from the toes, one should wrap both hind legs and the tail and wrap up to the caudal abdomen. Care should be taken not to wrap forward on the abdomen because it will cause anterior displacement of abdominal contents and decrease ventilatory compliance. A single abdominal tourniquet can also be used to prevent the peripheral runoff of blood. Wraps and tourniquets can be removed 10 to 20 min after restarting the heart, after hemodynamic variables have had a chance to stabilize. Wraps and tourniquets should be removed slowly; rapid exposure of a precariously balanced cardiovascular system to the hypoxic vasodilated

***Table 2.** Alpha-Agonists Useful in Cardiopulmonary Resuscitation*

Drug	Receptor Activity		Dosage
	Alpha	**Beta**	
Epinephrine	+++	+++	0.1–0.2 mg/kg
Dopamine	++	+++	0.2–0.5 mg/kg
Norepinephrine	+++	+	0.1–0.2 mg/kg
Metaraminol	+++	+	1–5 mg/kg
Phenylephrine	+++	0	0.5–1 mg/kg
Methoxamine	+++	0	1–5 mg/kg

+ to +++, Relative agonist activity.

tissues caudal to the tourniquet or under the wrap may result in excessive hypotension.

A snug abdominal wrap helps splint the abdomen and decreases the posterior displacement of the diaphragm when the chest is compressed. By preventing the dissipation of the applied pressure through the abdomen, the technique enhances the generalized increase in intrathoracic pressure induced by external chest compression (Rudikoff et al., 1980; Niemann et al., 1984). Abdominal wraps reportedly improve cerebral blood flow but have little effect on myocardial blood flow (Nieman, 1984).

Intermittent abdominal compression, alternating with external chest compression, improves venous return to the chest by increasing the abdominal-thoracic venous pressure gradient. A second person compresses the abdomen between each chest compression. This increases the abdominal-thoracic pressure gradient and enhances the volume of intrathoracic blood that can be expelled during the next chest compression. The technique has been shown to improve arterial blood pressure (Yakaitis et al., 1980) and cerebral and myocardial perfusion (Niemann, 1984) but was not associated with improved survival or neurologic outcome in one study (Mateer et al., 1984).

Simultaneous ventilation and external thoracic compression have been shown to enhance the generalized increase in intrathoracic pressure (Rudikoff et al., 1980; Chandra et al., 1980) and to improve cerebral, but not myocardial, blood flow (Niemann, 1984).

Effective artificial circulation of blood must be achieved by some method until effective spontaneous electrical and mechanical rhythm has returned to the heart. If external techniques have not accomplished effective circulation within 3 to 5 min, a thoracotomy should be performed and internal cardiac compression should be conducted. A thoracotomy may also be indicated after 10 to 20 min of successful external chest compression to minimize further chest wall and lung trauma.

An elliptic strip of hair should be rapidly clipped along the line of the intended incision at the fourth or fifth intercostal space. The skin should be swabbed once with an antiseptic solution to remove hair and lose dirt, the incision should be placed midway between the ribs down to, but not through, the pleura. Pleural penetration should be accomplished with something blunt, like a finger. The incision is extended dorsally and ventrally with scissors, taking care to avoid the internal thoracic artery, which runs longitudinally about 1 cm lateral to the sternum. Small hearts can be compressed between two fingers; larger hearts, between the flats of the fingers and the palm of the hand; and still larger hearts, between the palm and the opposite chest wall.

There are additional advantages to a thoracotomy. The adequacy of diastolic filling can be assessed between each compression, and the pericardial sac can be opened to prevent pericardial tamponade during or subsequent to resuscitation. The descending aorta can be depressed with the index finger of the opposite hand, directing essential blood flow to the brain and heart. Fibrillation and flaccidity can be assessed by direct visualization.

DRUGS

The value of oxygen, fluids, and alpha-agonists in the support of the patient during CPR have been discussed earlier as part of the basic life support of artificial circulation. These therapies are also of value in the advanced life support procedures used to restart the heart. Sometimes mechanical stimulation of the heart alone by the external or internal compression technique is sufficient to restart the heart. When effective application of the basic life support procedures has not restarted the heart after 2 to 3 min, the administration of additional drugs may prove useful.

Excessive vagal tone and the lack of an idioventricular (escape) rhythm may cause and maintain asystole. Atropine may reverse this phenomenon. Low-dose atropine may cause a centrally mediated increase in vagal tone. A dose of 0.02 to 0.04 mg of atropine per kilogram of body weight is recommended. Excessive doses may predispose to ventricular fibrillation.

Catecholamines with only alpha-agonist activity (e.g., phenylephrine) or with alpha- and beta-agonist activity (e.g., epinephrine) are beneficial in CPR. Beta-agonist activity stimulates pacemaker activity and enhances contractility when the heart is beating. Both beta- and alpha-agonists are arrhythmogenic. Low starting dosages of these drugs are recommended to minimize the incidence of arrhythmias. Supplemental dosages can be increased until the desired effect is achieved. Routes of administration are described below.

Sodium bicarbonate has traditionally been recommended during CPR to combat the metabolic acidosis generated by anaerobic metabolism in hypoxic tissues. Resuscitation was more prompt and 24-hr neurologic recovery was markedly better in the group in which metabolic acidosis was prevented (Ledingham and Norman, 1962). However, sodium bicarbonate is associated with the generation of carbon dioxide (via carbonic acid) and results in hypercapnia if the patient is not well ventilated. Carbon dioxide rapidly diffuses into the intracellular compartment and into the cerebrospinal fluid (CSF). Intracellular acidosis may be associated with myocardial and central nervous system (CNS) depression (Cingolani et al., 1975; Berenyi et al.,

1975). Sodium bicarbonate may predispose to ventricular fibrillation but does not affect defibrillation. Sodium bicarbonate may or may not enhance survival rates from CPR (Weil et al., 1985). The current recommendation for sodium bicarbonate is to give none for the first 5 to 10 min and then 0.5 mEq/kg every 5 min of cardiac arrest thereafter (Standards and Guidelines, 1986).

Calcium, although classically recommended during CPR, has fallen into disfavor. Some sarcoplasmic calcium is undoubtedly necessary for muscular contraction, but excessive calcium concentrations cause sustained muscular contraction. The use of calcium during CPR may contribute to diminished coronary and cerebral blood flow following an otherwise successful resuscitation (Thompson et al., 1986) and may contribute to cell death after ischemic injury (Nayler et al., 1986). Calcium has not been shown to improve the success of the resuscitation endeavor (Yakaitis et al., 1980) and is not currently recommended in the routine management of cardiac arrest (Standards and Guidelines, 1986). If it is used, for reasons of hyperkalemia or hypocalcemia, the recommended dose is 5 to 7 mg of elemental calcium per kilogram of body weight (0.19 to 0.26 ml/kg of 10 per cent CaCl) (Standards and Guidelines, 1986).

Antiarrhythmic drugs such as lidocaine (1 to 3 mg/kg IV) or bretylium (5 to 10 mg/kg over 30 min IV) reduce the heterogeneity of ventricular refractoriness, decrease the incidence of ventricular fibrillation, and may occasionally be useful during or after CPR (Standards and Guidelines, 1986) if the ventricular arrhythmias are multiform, frequent in occurrence (> 180/min), increasing in frequency, or associated with impairment of cardiac output.

The *route of administration* of the above drugs has spurred considerable recent debate. Intracardiac (intraluminal) injections have previously been recommended; however, this route is plagued with problems such as myocardial trauma, pericardial tamponade associated with leaking puncture sites or lacerated coronary arteries, lung laceration and pneumothorax, and the possibility that an intramyocardial (intramuscular) injection of a beta-agonist drug such as epinephrine may result in refractory ventricular fibrillation. The central venous administration of these drugs is probably the best route in that it deposits the drugs close to the heart and avoids the hazards of blind cardiac puncture. Peripheral venous drug administration is associated with significant delays in the arrival of the drugs to the heart (Hedges et al., 1984) and with lower blood levels compared with the central venous route (Barsan, 1981). The intratracheal route has been advocated (Barsan, 1981; Roberts et al., 1979); however, some studies have indicated that drug uptake from the tracheal surface is sporadic, undependable, and delayed (McDonald, 1985). It is apparent that drug uptake from the tracheal surface, as well as from

any richly vascularized capillary bed (tongue, nasal cavity, conjunctival sac, or pleural space), is solely dependent on the adequacy of blood flow to the area, which, during CPR, is undependable, highly variable, and, at best, poor. It does not seem prudent to rely on such mechanisms for the uptake of drugs as important as those used during CPR. This "capillary" route should, perhaps, be relegated to those situations in which vascular access has not been secured.

ELECTRICAL ACTIVITY OF THE HEART

Electrocardiographic (ECG) monitoring during the resuscitation endeavor is important because it helps define the type of cardiac arrest and helps to guide some of the therapeutic interventions (Table 3).

Direct-current (DC) defibrillation is indicated as soon as possible when ventricular fibrillation is identified (Table 4). There is an indirect correlation between the duration of ventricular fibrillation and the success of defibrillation (Yakaitis, 1980). Early defibrillation is so important that blind defibrillation, if no ECG monitor is available, has been recommended (Standards and Guidelines, 1986). A critical quantity of energy is required to successfully defibrillate a heart and this is not affected by the prior administration of epinephrine (Yakaitis, 1980). Excessive energy can cause myocardial damage (Standards and Guidelines, 1986), and so it is prudent to start with lower settings and work up to an effective level.

If direct-current defibrillation is not available, several methods of pharmacologic defibrillation have been recommended (Table 4), but they are not as reliable as DC defibrillation.

A sharp thump to the chest may rarely restore a normal rhythm in the case of ventricular tachycardia, AV heart block, and venticular fibrillation but may also instigate ventricular fibrillation (Standards and Guidelines, 1986).

External noninvasive transthoracic, invasive transthoracic, and transvenous pacemakers may be useful if there is a problem with impulse formation or conduction but myocardial function is still preserved (Standards and Guidelines, 1986).

POSTRESUSCITATION MONITORING AND SUPPORT

Cardiovascular and pulmonary function must be monitored closely for several hours following a successful resuscitation to assure that cardiac arrest does not recur. In addition to the underlying disease process that caused the cardiac arrest, there are complications of cardiopulmonary resuscitation *per*

Table 3. *Different Types of Cardiac Arrest*

Type	Electrical Activity	Coordinated Mechanical Contraction	Visual Appearance of the Heart	Treatment
Ventricular asystole	None	No	Standstill	Beta-agonists stimulate pace-maker activity
Ventricular fibrillation	Chaotic	No	Fine to coarse myocardial rippling	Defibrillation to create simultaneous asystole
Cardiovascular collapse due to excessive vasodilation	Normal	Yes	Normal contractions	Rapid fluid administration, alpha-receptor agonists
Electromechanical dissociation	Normal	No	Standstill	Corticosteroids (?); catecholamine (?)

se that can undermine the welfare of the patient. Monitoring should include as many aspects of cardiopulmonary function as possible to attain an accurate overview of the adequacy of its performance:

1. The electrical activity of the heart (to determine whether it is beating too slowly, too fast, or too arrhythmically). Antiarrhythmic drugs should be considered if the ventricular arrhythmias become severe.

2. The mechanical activity of the heart (pulse quality, arterial blood pressure, and cardiac output).

3. The adequacy of peripheral perfusion (color, capillary refill time, urine output, and toe web temperature). Cardiotonic agents (dobutamine and dopamine) may be useful to improve myocardial performance and peripheral tissue perfusion.

4. The rate, rhythm, and nature of the breathing effort.

5. Auscultation and radiography of the thorax (to ascertain presence of a pneumothorax, a hemothorax, or lung contusion and its severity).

6. The adequacy of oxygenation (color and arterial oxygen determination).

Cardiac arrest produces cerebral hypoxia in 10 sec, depletes glucose and glycogen stores in 2 to 4 min, and depletes adenosine triphosphate (ATP) stores in 4 to 5 min. The energy-deficient cell accumulates sodium and calcium, and the cell dies. Postresuscitation cerebral failure has been attributed to

1. Global ischemia and ATP depletion, resulting

Table 4. *Defibrillation Methods*

DC Defibrillation

	Power Settings (watt-sec)	
	External	*Internal*
Small patient	100–150	10–25
Large patient	400	100–150
or		
< 7 kg	2/kg	
8–40 kg	5/kg	0.2–0.4/kg
> 40 kg	5–10/kg	

Pharmacologic Defibrillation
1. Potassium chloride (1 mEq/kg) followed by 0.2 ml 10 per cent calcium chloride/kg
2. Potassium chloride (1 mEq/kg) and acetylcholine (6 mg/kg)

in sodium and calcium accumulation. Intramitochondrial calcium accumulation prevents ATP regeneration, and sarcoplasmic calcium accumulation contributes to cell death.

2. Reperfusion injury. During ischemia, hypoxanthine is formed, which is converted to superoxide and hydroxyl radicals during reoxygenation. These free radicals, in combination with iron, cause lipoperoxidation of cellular membranes. The lipid radicals are then self-perpetuating. Initially in reperfusion failure, there are multifocal areas of "no reflow" followed by a phase of global hyperemia, delayed nonhomogeneous global hypoperfusion, and finally brain death.

3. Extracerebral derangements, such as hypotension, hypoxemia, acidemia, gut toxins absorbed through debilitated gut mucosa, an overwhelmed reticuloendothelial (RE) system, coagulopathies, activated complement and prostaglandin cascades, and other unidentified organ failures.

The most important aspect of cerebral resuscitation is to commence effective artificial circulation and to restart effective spontaneous circulation as soon as possible. Following resuscitation of spontaneous circulation, the most important aspects of cerebral resuscitation involve the physiologic management and support of the patient. One should prevent hypertension, hypotension, hypercapnia, hypoxia, hyperthermia, and excessive activity. Venous outflow obstruction and head-down positioning should be avoided. Ketamine, inhalational anesthetics, and xylazine should not be used. Hyperventilation decreased intracranial pressure but did not improve neurologic recovery in one study. It is recommended when the patient is sufficiently obtunded to tolerate endotracheal intubation. Prearrest consciousness should return within a short time after restarting the heart, although specific times cannot be given owing to variations in resuscitation effectiveness. The animal should begin to regain consciousness within 15 to 30 min. If not, or if the resuscitation exceeded 15 min, cerebral edema should be assumed. Corticosteroids may be beneficial in the support of membrane integrity and as anti-inflammatory therapy (dexamethasone, 0.5 mg/kg IV; prednisolone sodium succinate, 2 mg/kg

IV). Mannitol (0.5 gm/kg administered slowly IV) osmotically decreases cerebral edema and may scavenge toxic free radicals. Furosemide (5 mg/kg) is a weak vasodilator and redistributes blood away from the brain. Both diuretics remove fluids from the body. Additional therapies appear promising but are not routinely recommended for postresuscitation therapy at this time. Dimethylsulfoxide (0.5 to 2 gm/kg of 20 to 40 per cent solution IV) has been shown to have beneficial effects on neurologic recovery in global ischemia. Calcium antagonists have been reported to increase cerebral blood flow and to improve neurologic recovery in dogs, but results have not been uniformly favorable. Despite early promising reports, thiopental has not been found to be beneficial in cerebral resuscitation. Additional therapies that require further research include hemodilution, heparinization, induction of hypothermia, administration of free radical scavengers, administration of iron chelators, and plasma exchange or apheresis.

References and Supplemental Reading

Barsan, W. G.: Lidocaine levels during CPR: Differences after peripheral venous, central venous, and intracardiac injections. Ann. Emerg. Med. 10:73, 1981.

Bedell, S. E., Delbanco, T. L., Cook, E. F., et al.: Survival after cardiopulmonary resuscitation in the hospital. N. Engl. J. Med. 309:569, 1983.

Berenyi, K. J., Wolk, M., and Killip, T.: Cerebrospinal fluid, acidosis complicating therapy of experimental cardiopulmonary arrest. Circulation 52:319, 1975.

Bircher, N., Safar, P., and Stewart, R.: A comparison of standard, "MAST" augmented and open-chest CPR in dogs: A preliminary investigation. Crit. Care Med. 8:147, 1980.

Brillman, J. A., Sanders, A. B., Otto, C. W., et al.: Outcome of resuscitation from fibrillatory arrest using epinephrine and phenylephrine in dogs. Crit. Care Med. 13:912, 1985.

Chandra, N., Rudikoff, M., and Weisfeldt, M. L.: Simultaneous chest compression and ventilation at high airway pressure during cardiopulmonary resuscitation. Lancet 1:175, 1980.

Cingolani, H. E., Faulkner, S. L., Mattiazzi, A. R., et al.: Depression of human myocardial contractility with "respiratory" and "metabolic" acidosis. Surgery 77:427, 1975.

Gilroy, B. A., and Levine, J. F.: Survival after cardiopulmonary resuscitation in canine patients. Vet. Emerg. Crit. Care Soc. Proceedings, 1986, p. 196.

Gilroy, B. A., and Shapiro, H. M.: Survival after cardiopulmonary resuscitation in feline patients. Vet. Emerg. Crit. Care Soc. Proceedings, 1986, p. 201.

Hedges, J. R., Syverud, S. A., and Dalsey, W. C.: Central versus peripheral intravenous routes in cardiopulmonary resuscitation. Am. J. Emerg. Med. 2:385, 1984.

Henik, R. A., and Wingfield, W. E.: Cardiopulmonary arrest and resuscitation in cats. Veterinary Emergency Critical Care Society. Proceedings, 1987, p. 66.

Ledingham, I. M., and Norman, J. N.: Acid-base studies in experimental circulatory arrest. Lancet 2:967, 1962.

Mateer, J. R., Steuven, H. A., Thompson, B. M., et al.: Interposed abdominal compression CPR versus standard CPR in prehospital cardiopulmonary arrest: Preliminary results. Ann. Emerg. Med. 13:764, 1984.

McDonald, J. L.: Serum lidocaine levels during cardiopulmonary resuscitation after intravenous and endotracheal administration. Crit. Care Med. 13:914, 1985.

Michael, J. R., Niedermeyer, E., Rogers, M. C., et al.: Mechanisms by which epinephrine augments cerebral and myocardial perfusion during cardiopulmonary resuscitation in dogs. Circulation 69:822, 1984.

Nayler, W. G., and Elz, J. S.: Reperfusion injury: Laboratory artifact or clinical dilemma? Circulation 74:215, 1986.

Niemann, J. T.: Differences in cerebral and myocardial perfusion during closed-chest resuscitation. Ann. Emerg. Med. 13:849, 1984.

Niemann, J. T., Rosborough, J. P., Ung, S., et al.: Hemodynamic effects of continuous abdominal binding during cardiac arrest and resuscitation. Am. J. Cardiol. 53:269, 1984.

Ralston, S. H., Babbs, C. F., and Niebauer, M. J.: Cardiopulmonary resuscitation with interposed abdominal compression in dogs. Anesth. Analg. 61:645, 1982.

Roberts, J. R., Greenberg, M. I., Knaub, M. A., et al.: Blood levels following intravenous and endotracheal epinephrine administration. J.A.C.E.P. 8:53, 1979.

Rudikoff, M. T., Maughan, W. L., Effron, M., et al.: Mechanism of blood flow during cardiopulmonary resuscitation. Circulation 61:345, 1980.

Safar, P.: Effects of the postresuscitation syndrome on cerebral recovery from cardiac arrest. Crit. Care Med. 13:932, 1985.

Standards and guidelines for cardiopulmonary resuscitation (CPR) and emergency cardiac care (ECC). J.A.M.A. 255:2905, 1986.

Thompson, B. M., Steuven, H. S., Tonsfeldt, D. J., et al.: Calcium: Limited indications, some danger. Circulation 74:IV90, 1986.

Voorhees, W. D., Babbs, C. F., and Tacker, W. A., Jr.: Regional blood flow during cardiopulmonary resuscitation in dogs. Crit. Care Med. 8:134, 1980.

Weil, M. H., Trevino, R. P., and Rackow, E. C.: Sodium bicarbonate during CPR. Does it help or hinder? Chest 88:487, 1985.

Yakaitis, R. W., Ewy, G. A., Otto, C. W., et al.: Influence of time and therapy on ventriculation defibrillation in dogs. Crit. Care Med. 8:157, 1980.

MEDICAL MANAGEMENT OF UPPER RESPIRATORY TRACT DISEASE

SHELLY VADEN, D.V.M.,
and RICHARD B. FORD, D.V.M.
Raleigh, North Carolina

The upper respiratory tract of the dog and the cat may be regarded as extending from the external nares to the first tracheal ring. This includes the following segments: nasal cavity, paranasal sinuses, oropharynx, nasopharynx, and larynx. As a principal portal of entry, the upper respiratory tract is particularly vulnerable to trauma and colonization by a wide variety of infectious agents. This, in addition to a spectrum of congenital and neoplastic diseases, accounts for the relatively high prevalence of upper respiratory tract disease encountered in companion animal practice.

The clinical signs associated with diseases of the upper respiratory tract in dogs and cats can generally be categorized according to one of the following: (1) *sneezing*, with or without *nasal discharge*; (2) *stertor*, or snorting, sometimes referred to as "reverse" sneezing; and (3) *stridor*, or wheezing. This classification of the patient's presenting problem enables the clinician to specifically define which segment of the upper respiratory tract is involved.

The diagnostic approach to evaluating patients with signs of upper respiratory tract disease is straightforward. In most patients, even those with chronic upper respiratory tract signs, following the sequence of examinations and procedures outlined for a *routine* upper respiratory tract examination (Table 1) has high diagnostic value. Special diagnostic procedures are not indicated in every patient but should be reserved for those in which the diagnosis cannot be confirmed by routine examination (Fig. 1). The discussion that follows centers on the nonsurgical management of upper respiratory tract disease in the dog and cat according to the clinical sign, i.e., sneezing/nasal discharge, stertor, or stridor, most likely to be the initial problem for which the patient is presented.

SNEEZING AND NASAL DISCHARGE

Sneezing and rhinorrhea (nasal discharge) are clinical signs referable to diseases affecting the nasal cavity and frontal sinuses. However, these signs can be manifestations of systemic diseases, such as ca-nine distemper, or diseases of the lower respiratory tract, such as bacterial pneumonia. A thorough anamnesis should be obtained for each case and should include questions concerning character of the discharge, duration of signs, and pattern of sneezing. The value of a complete systemic evaluation, including a hemogram, biochemical profile, and urinalysis cannot be overemphasized (Ford, 1988).

Sneezing can be singular or paroxysmal and may or may not be associated with a nasal discharge. Episodic runs of sneezes, one followed by another without a pause, is characteristic of paroxysmal sneezing and most often is associated with an active intranasal lesion. Nasal discharges can be categorized according to volume, frequency, location (bilateral or unilateral), and appearance. Discharges that are definitively unilateral support intranasal disease. Serous nasal discharges are most often present initially but may go unrecognized owing to the patient's continual licking of the nose. Many discharges will progress to become mucoid, purulent, mucopurulent, or serosanguinous.

Although many discharges are blood tinged, epistaxis represents actual hemorrhage that originates from the nose; the hematocrit of the discharge approaches that of the peripheral blood. Epistaxis may result from trauma, nasal neoplasia, foreign bodies, mycotic rhinosinusitis, and severe inflammation. Because epistaxis may be due to a systemic coagulation disorder, coagulation studies and platelet count should be evaluated.

Management of epistaxis includes forced cage rest and sedation, as sneezing may worsen the bleeding episodes. The vasoconstrictive effects of intranasal flushes of dilute epinephrine (1:50,000) may decrease the severity of the bleeding episode. The nasal cavity of an anesthetized animal can be packed with gauze or ice packs to diminish bleeding. If life-threatening hemorrhage persists after these efforts have failed, nasal exploratory surgery may be indicated. If a bleeding disorder is suspected, whole blood or plasma transfusions will be required for factor replacement.

Table 1. *Evaluation of the Patient with Signs Referable to the Upper Respiratory Tract*

Routine Patient Evaluation

1. Laboratory data base
   Complete blood count (CBC), biochemical profile, urinalysis, fecal, FeLV and FTLV tests (cats), cytologic evaluation of nasal discharge
2. Nasal radiographs (general anesthesia recommended)
   Lateral projection of the skull
   Dorsoventral (occlusal) projection of the nasal cavity
3. Visual examination of the oral cavity (general anesthesia required)
   Gingival sulcus (upper dental arcade, especially medial sulcus of the upper canine teeth)
   Symmetry, consistency of the hard and soft palate
   Tonsils
   Oropharynx
   Pharyngoscopy (when available) using flexible fiberoptic bronchoscope
4. Rhinoscopy (general anesthesia required)

Special Diagnostic Studies

5. Isolation of infectious agent
   Bacterial: positive culture of nasal discharge has little or no diagnostic value; bacterial infections should be considered opportunistic
   Fungal: inoculate nasal discharge or diseased tissue (preferred) onto Sabouraud's agar (see Attleberger, 1984)
   Viral (cats only): swab oropharynx, submit in appropriate virus transport media for feline herpesvirus and/or calicivirus. *Note:* special facilities may be required
6. Serology (fungal)
   Aspergillosis: complement fixation; immunodiffusion; ELISA
   Cryptococcosis: capsular antigen test
7. Computed tomography (CT) (general anesthesia required; procedure limited to referral centers with appropriate facilities). *Note:* CT is a noninvasive technique useful in determining the extent of intranasal frontal sinus disease; CT may be able to differentiate between nasal neoplasia and mycotic rhinosinusitis in some patients
8. Intranasal biopsy (general anesthesia required; coagulation screen of patients subjected to nasal biopsy is recommended, *particularly in patients with a history of spontaneous epistaxis*
   Closed aspiration of punch biopsy
   Open biopsy: nasal flap rhinotomy

Congenital Diseases

Young dogs that develop nasal discharge during the first weeks of life should be examined for congenital defects as well as infectious disease. Although congenital disorders tend to occur more frequently in purebred dogs, mixed breed dogs are also at risk. Because of the possible heritable nature of these disorders, affected animals should not be used for breeding purposes. The oral cavity should be examined for a cleft palate. Clinical findings include bilateral nasal discharge, nasal regurgitation, poor growth, aspiration pneumonia, and death. The defects can occasionally be corrected surgically.

Oropharyngeal and cricopharyngeal dysphagia can result in a nasal discharge owing to retention and regurgitation of food and water. Megaesophagus has also been associated with a nasal discharge. Diagnosis of these disorders may require fluoro-

scopic examination of the pharynx, esophagus, or both following ingestion of solids and liquids. Depending on the cause of the disorder, surgical correction may be possible.

Primary ciliary dyskinesia is a hereditary disease seen in purebred dogs that results from the inability of the mucociliary apparatus to clear mucus and debris from the respiratory tract. The syndrome is often associated with situs inversus (seen on thoracoabdominal radiographs), chronic sinusitis and bronchitis, and bronchiectasis. The diagnosis is based on the demonstration of impaired mucociliary clearance by radionuclide imaging and defective ciliary ultrastructure. Treatment consists of long-term administration of antibiotics based on bacterial culture and susceptibility results.

Mycotic Rhinosinusitis

ASPERGILLOSIS. The most common type of mycotic rhinosinusitis in the dog is caused by the ubiquitous saprophytic organism *Aspergillus flavum*. One survey found aspergillosis to account for 12 per cent of all chronic nasal discharges in the dog (Lane and Warnock, 1977). The disease in dogs, although initially localizing to the upper respiratory tract, can eventually disseminate. Aspergillosis is rare in the cat but, when seen, is most often disseminated, particularly to the intestinal tract (Ossent, 1987; Barsanti, 1984).

Historically, the most widely recommended therapy for canine and disseminated aspergillosis has been thiabendazole (20 mg/kg/day) administered orally for 6 weeks. The results of one clinical trial were discouraging, with only 26 per cent experiencing a complete cure and improvement occurring in only 43 per cent of the dogs (Harvey, 1984). Successful therapy has been reported following the administration of ketoconazole (20 mg/kg/day for 6 weeks) (Barsanti, 1984). Preliminary results of the use of topical enilconazole administered via indwelling tubes implanted into the frontal sinuses for 7 to 10 days in combination with systemic ketoconazole are promising (Sharp and Sullivan, 1986). Surgical curettage is often combined with medical management, but many dogs experience persistent nasal discharge following surgery (see pp. 1105–1108).

RHINOSPORIDIOSIS. *Rhinosporidium seeberi* is a rare cause of mycotic rhinitis in dogs; disease prevalence is highest in the southern United States. The diagnosis is made by the visualization of polypoid nodules within the nasal cavity. Cytologic examination of impression smears from the nodules will often reveal the organism. The sporangia are as large as 400 μm in diameter; have a thin, refractile wall; and contain numerous, spheric basophilic bodies. Medical management of rhinosporidiosis has proven unsuccessful. Aggressive surgical resection

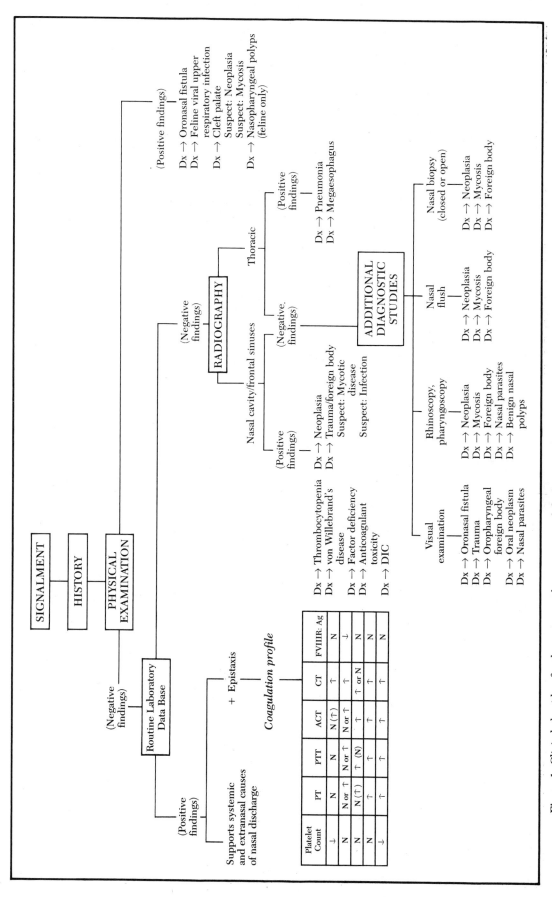

Figure 1. Clinical algorithm for the patient with sneezing, nasal discharge, or both. ACT, activated clotting time; PT, prothrombin time; PTT, partial thromboplastin time; CT, clotting time; factor VIII:Ag, factor VIII–related antigen; ↓, decreased (numbers); ↑, prolonged (time); N, normal; N (↑), usually normal, occasionally prolonged; ↑ (N), usually prolonged, occasionally normal. (Reprinted with permission from Ford. *In* Ford (ed.): *Clinical Signs and Diagnosis in Small Animals.* New York: Churchill Livingstone, 1988, p. 201.)

offers the best cure rate. Recurrence following surgery is not uncommon. Topical administration of dapsone has facilitated resolution in some human patients and at least one dog (Allison et al., 1986).

CRYPTOCOCCOSIS. *Cryptococcus neoformans* is a saprophytic fungus that commonly infects cats and infrequently infects dogs. Dogs most commonly have central nervous system or ocular manifestations of the disease, whereas nasal cryptococcosis is less common. The disease in cats is most frequently associated with the respiratory or central nervous system, although ocular and cutaneous lesions have also been reported. Feline leukemia virus (FeLV) infection may be a predisposing factor in some cats with cryptococcosis, particularly those with cutaneous infections. The average age of infected cats is 5 years, with a range of 1 to 12 years. Fifty per cent of infected cats show clinical signs referable to the nasal cavity, including sneezing, snuffling, and mucopurulent, serous, or hemorrhagic, unilateral or bilateral nasal discharge. Of the cats with upper respiratory tract disease, 70 per cent have a mass visible in the nostril or hard facial swelling. There may be an associated submandibular lymphadenopathy. Lower respiratory tract disease and fever are uncommon.

The diagnosis of cryptococcal rhinitis is confirmed by the demonstration of the thickly encapsulated, broad-based budding yeast cells in gram-stained specimens of nasal exudate. The results of fungal culture and the capsular antigen test can be used to support the diagnosis and monitor response to therapy.

Therapy for cryptococcosis involves the oral administration of ketoconazole, 10 to 15 mg/kg twice daily for up to 60 days (Legendre, 1982). The drug should be administered with food. The concomitant administration of antacids should be avoided because an acid environment is needed for drug absorption. Vomiting and diarrhea are possible side effects of treatment but can be managed simply by reducing the dose interval from twice to once daily. Subclinical increases in liver enzyme activity commonly occur during drug administration. The drug should not be discontinued unless clinical signs referable to hepatotoxicosis develop. Other therapies frequently reported include the use of 5-fluorocytosine and amphotericin B, alone or in combination. These agents are associated with a higher incidence of toxic side effects and offer no therapeutic advantage over ketoconazole. Surgical removal has been used alone or in combination with ketoconazole therapy. The majority of cats undergoing nasal surgery will have a persistence of the nasal discharge and sneezing. Therefore, surgery should be reserved for those animals not responding to medical therapy.

Nasal Neoplasia

Nasal neoplasia should be suspected in any older dog (8 to 10 years and older) with a history of nasal discharge or sneezing. There is no sex predilection for nasal neoplasia, although the incidence appears to be highest in large and dolichocephalic breeds. Nasal neoplasia accounts for 2 per cent of all tumors in dogs; 80 per cent of these are malignant. Adenocarcinoma is the most common, followed by squamous cell carcinoma and undifferentiated sarcomas. Cats most frequently have carcinomas and lymphoid tumors. The diagnosis is based on histologic examination of tissue obtained via traumatic nasal flushing and punch or aspiration biopsy. It is generally unnecessary to perform nasal exploratory procedures to obtain diagnostic tissue specimens. Computed tomography (CT) of the nasal cavity is particularly helpful in defining the extent of tumor involvement.

The median survival time without treatment is 4 months. With surgical excision alone, the survival time is reduced to 3 months. The median survival time with megavoltage therapy alone is 8.1 months (mean, 9.1 months). In some studies, surgical debulking offered no therapeutic advantage when combined with megavoltage (median survival time, 7.1 months). Although orthovoltage therapy alone resulted in a median survival time of only 4.1 months, when it was combined with surgical debulking, the median survival time increased to 8.1 months (mean, 17.5 months). Based on the mean survival times, orthovoltage and surgical debulking may provide the best results. In general, chemotherapy has not been successful in the treatment of canine nasal tumors. Dogs with adenocarcinoma usually survive longer (median survival, 12 months) than those with squamous cell carcinoma and undifferentiated sarcomas (median, 6 months) (Adams et al., 1987). Most dogs with nasal tumors die as a result of local extension and invasion of the primary tumor, or they are euthanatized. When metastasis does occur, it is most frequently to the local lymph nodes and lungs (see also pp. 399–405).

Foreign Bodies

Foreign bodies most frequently lodge in the rostral one third of the nasal cavity. The most common materials involved include grass awns, foxtails, twigs, and hay particles. Clinical signs include paroxysmal sneezing and serous to mucopurulent, fetid nasal discharge. Occasionally, sneezing will expel the foreign material, but turbinate fractures or focal osteomyelitis result in a persistent nasal discharge. The offending material, if visible on rhinoscopic examination, can often be removed with alligator forceps. Nasal flushing following the placement of gauze in the pharynx may facilitate the removal of foreign material from the nasal cavity. Because of the potential for secondary bacterial infections, it may be necessary to initiate broad-spectrum antimicrobial therapy with ampicillin, amoxicillin, cephalosporin, or chloramphenicol. Persistent nasal discharges may require surgical débridement of the nasal cavity, frontal sinuses, or both.

Dental Disease

Clinical signs of chronic rhinitis may be caused by the extension of infections originating in the maxillary teeth. This is particularly true of the incisors and canine teeth of dogs with chronic periodontal disease. Bacterial colonization of the periodontium can result in osteomyelitis of the apical bone and formation of oronasal fistulae. Paroxysms of sneezing, sometimes associated with a blood-tinged serous nasal discharge, are characteristic signs. Fistulas are easily detected by probing the gingival sulcus of the maxillary teeth. Using a periodontal probe or a male feline urinary catheter, most animals may be examined without tranquilization or anesthesia. In the anesthetized patient, saline injected into the free gingival sulcus through a catheter may actually drain from the nostril.

The most effective therapy entails extracting the affected tooth. A broad-spectrum antibiotic should be administered orally for 1 to 2 days preoperatively and 7 days postoperatively. In lieu of extraction, curettage and vigorous flushing of the alveolus combined with a 10-day course of antibiotics can be attempted. If destruction of the periodontal ligament and surrounding tissue is not extensive, the periodontium will heal and the fistula will resolve. Occasionally, the fistula will require surgical closure.

Nasopharyngeal Polyps

Nasopharyngeal polyps are benign growths that have been reported with increasing frequency in young cats; they are an uncommon disease entity in dogs. Polyps are thought to arise from the eustachian tube or middle ear and enter the pharynx via the eustachian tube. Although the etiology of these masses remains unclear, the histologic appearance suggests inflammation. Affected cats may exhibit stertorous respiration, chronic rhinitis, sinusitis, head shaking, head tilt, and otitis media. These cats may become cyanotic when stressed. Oral examination may allow for the visualization of a mass dorsal to the soft palate. Pharyngoscopy using a flexible fiberoptic bronchoscope permits visualization of the nasopharynx. Treatment involves surgical removal of the polyp. The benign nature of the mass should be confirmed by histopathologic examination of the resected tissue.

Viral and Bacterial Upper Respiratory Tract Disease

FELINE. Feline viral upper respiratory tract diseases (FVURD) most frequently result from calicivirus or herpesvirus infections; both the acute form, which occurs most often in kittens, and the chronic carrier form of adults are common. Reovirus, mycoplasma, and chlamydia have also been implicated, and leukemia virus immunosuppression may be a factor in some cases. Clinical signs include sneezing, bilateral ocular and nasal discharge, oral and corneal ulceration, salivation, depression, anorexia, fever, and dehydration. Young cats and older, debilitated cats can die from complications associated with anorexia, dehydration, and secondary bacterial infection. A presumptive diagnosis is usually based on clinical presentation but can be confirmed through viral isolation from pharyngeal swabs. In the case of mycoplasma and chlamydia infections, intracellular inclusions demonstrated on conjunctival scrapings aid in the diagnosis.

Secondary bacterial infections are typically associated with FVURD and may be persistent in some cats (Ford, 1984; August, 1984). Broad-spectrum antibiotic therapy should be instituted. Ampicillin (22 mg/kg PO q 8hr), amoxicillin (22 mg/kg PO q 8hr), cephalexin (22 mg/kg PO q 8hr), and chloramphenicol (50 mg/kg PO q 8hr) are the antibiotics most frequently recommended. If chlamydial infection is suspected, tetracycline (20 mg/kg PO q 8hr) is recommended. Tetracycline containing ophthalmic preparations should be given for 2 weeks after the disappearance of clinical signs to minimize the induction of the carrier states.

Infected cats should be isolated and kept warm and clean of ocular and nasal discharges. Copious nasal discharges can be treated with the intranasal administration of 0.25 per cent phenylephrine HCl (Neo-Synephrine), every 4 to 6 hours, or 0.025 per cent oxymethazoline (Afrin pediatric nose drops, Schering Corp., Kenilworth, NJ), q 24hr. To prevent congestive rebound, these medications should not be administered into the same nostril for more than five consecutive days. Administration of nasal decongestants to cats with thick nasal discharges is less likely to be effective. Nasal decongestants with menthol and camphor should be avoided because of their potential toxicity in cats.

Relief of nasal congestion may actually restore the sense of smell and, subsequently, restore the cat's appetite. Cats with prolonged anorexia can be given oral diazepam (0.5 mg) or oxazepam (one

Table 2. *Differential Diagnosis for Stertor*

Elongated soft palate
Pharyngeal foreign bodies
Neoplasia (pharyngeal or soft palate)
Retropharyngeal lymphadenopathy (especially multicentric lymphosarcoma)
Retropharyngeal salivary mucocele (dog)
Polyps

fourth of a 5-mg tablet) once daily as appetite stimulants. Rarely, it is necessary to initiate force feeding through a pharyngostomy or gastrostomy tube. Dehydrated and febrile cats can be given fluids by nasogastric tube or by subcutaneous or intravenous injection.

Chronic cases of bacterial sinusitis may require surgical exploration of the nasal cavities and sinuses to establish drainage or to remove inflammatory polyps. This should be considered when a thorough diagnostic evaluation fails to yield a primary diagnosis.

CANINE. Canine distemper should be suspected in young unvaccinated dogs, 3 to 6 months of age with respiratory, neurological, or gastrointestinal abnormalities. Milder respiratory forms of distemper can be seen in older dogs but are often attributed to tracheobronchitis. The diagnosis is based on a clinical suspicion, although viral isolation and serologic study may be used to support the diagnosis. Therapy is supportive and nonspecific, and owners should be made aware that neurologic signs may eventually develop. The dogs should be kept isolated, warm, and free of ocular and nasal discharges. Antibiotic therapy should be instituted to counteract secondary bacterial invasion and the immunosuppressive effects of the virus. Ampicillin, tetracycline, and chloramphenicol are effective, but tetracycline should be avoided in dogs and cats with deciduous teeth.

STERTOR

Stertorous breathing is characterized as a loud, snorting or snoring sound that originates from the nasopharynx or oropharynx. In most cases, the loudest sounds are generated during inspiration.

Table 3. *Differential Diagnoses for Stridor*

Laryngeal trauma
Brachycephalic syndrome
   Laryngeal collapse
   Eversion of the laryngeal ventricles
Laryngeal neoplasia
Laryngeal paralysis
Laryngeal inflammation
   Chronic proliferative pyogranulomatous laryngitis
Laryngeal spasm (cat)
Laryngeal edema

Because of the audible noises generated during respirations, stertor is frequently a primary presenting sign in companion animal patients with upper respiratory tract disease, particularly dogs.

Historically, the stertorous patient is described as having (1) acute, unprovoked paroxysms of respiratory distress; or (2) chronic, virtually continuous snorting. Not uncommonly, acute-onset stertor is interpreted by an owner as "severe" and justifiably prompts an emergency presentation. The owner may describe rapid, violent bursts of inspiratory effort. This physical sign, sometimes referred to as reverse sneezing, is prompted by the attempt to dislodge matter from the nasopharynx to the oropharynx and swallow the offending material. Nonetheless, acute-onset stertor may resolve spontaneously without specific treatment. Animals with additional airway compromise (e.g., collapsing bronchi) may collapse during an hypoxic episode. Death during an acute episode rarely occurs. Although animals with a history of chronic stertor may also have acute, paroxysmal episodes of respiratory distress, this is uncommon. Most animals with chronic stertor can compensate, unless the underlying cause is progressive (e.g., neoplasia), and are unlikely to be seen on an emergency basis. Chronically affected animals are more likely to be seen because of annoying, audible respirations; apparent exercise intolerance; or progressively labored breathing during periods of excitement or exercise.

Stertor is most often attributable to nasal or oral pharyngeal disorders that disrupt, or partially obstruct, air flow. None of the differential diagnoses (Table 2) can be effectively managed medically. Surgical management of these disorders is discussed in detail elsewhere in the literature and will not be reviewed here.

However, acute-onset respiratory distress characterized by stertor should be regarded as a medical emergency until proven otherwise. Even though a diagnosis has not been made, immediate supportive care is indicated when signs fail to resolve within a few minutes or when the patient's physical condition deteriorates rapidly. In most of these cases, treatment is directed at slowing the patient's respiratory rate and effort. In some cases, merely changing the patient's immediate environment is sufficient (e.g., walking outside). In others, chemical sedation (butorphanol, 0.5 to 1.0 mg/kg IV; oxymorphan, 0.05 mg/kg IV or 0.05 to 0.1 mg/kg IM) may be required. Sedation with acepromazine is not recommended. Unless anesthesia is specifically contraindicated, the clinician should be prepared to administer an ultrashort-acting or short-acting barbiturate, intubate, and administer oxygen to manage the patient. While the patient is anesthetized, a thorough visual examination of the pharynx should be performed.

STRIDOR

Stridor is characterized as a high-pitched wheezing sound that, in both dogs and cats, can usually be localized to the larynx (pp. 343–353) or the most proximal aspect of the cervical trachea (pp. 353–360). Stridor denotes partial airway obstruction, is usually associated with significant respiratory distress and, therefore, is managed as a respiratory emergency. The causes of stridor, or stridulous breathing, listed in Table 3 necessitate surgery for long-term management. The decision to delay specific surgical intervention while attempting supportive medical therapy may prove fatal for the patient.

References and Supplemental Reading

Adams, W. M., Withrow, S. J., Walshaw, R., et al.: Radiotherapy of malignant nasal tumors in 67 dogs. J.A.V.M.A. 191:311, 1987.
Allison, N., Willard, M. D., Bentinck-Smith, J., et al.: Nasal rhinosporidiosis in two dogs. J.A.V.M.A. 188:869, 1986.
Attleberger, M. H.: Laboratory diagnosis of fungal and achloric algal infections. In Greene, C. E. (ed.): Clinical Microbiology and Infectious Diseases of the Dog and Cat. Philadelphia: W. B. Saunders, 1984, pp. 129–136.
August, J. R.: Feline viral respiratory disease. Vet. Clin. North Am. [Small Anim. Pract.] 14:1159, 1984.
Barsanti, J. A.: Opportunistic fungal infections. In Greene, C. E. (ed.): Clinical Microbiology and Infectious Diseases of the Dog and Cat. Philadelphia: W. B. Saunders, 1984, pp. 728–737.
Ford, R. B.: Infectious respiratory disease. Vet. Clin. North Am. [Small Anim. Pract.] 14:985, 1984.
Ford, R. B.: Sneezing and nasal discharge. In Ford, R. B. (ed.): Clinical Signs and Diagnosis in Small Animals. New York: Churchill Livingstone, 1988, pp. 189–202.
Harvey, C. E.: Nasal aspergillosis and penicillosis in dogs: Results of treatment with thiabendazole. J.A.V.M.A. 184:48, 1984.
Lane, J. G., and Warnock, D. W.: The diagnosis of Aspergillus fumigatus infections in the nasal chambers of the dog with particular reference to the value of the double diffusion test. J. Small Anim. Pract. 18:169, 1977.
Legendre, A. M., Gomph, R., and Bone, D.: Treatment of feline cryptococcosis with ketoconazole. J.A.V.M.A. 181:1541, 1982.
Ossent, P.: Systemic aspergillosis and mucormycosis in 23 cats. Vet. Rec. 120;330, 1987.
Sharp, N. J. H., and Sullivan, M.: Treatment of canine nasal aspergillosis with systemic ketoconazole and topical enilconazole. Vet. Rec. 118:560, 1986.
Withrow, S. J., Susaneck, S. J., Macy, D. W., et al.: Aspiration and punch biopsy techniques for nasal tumors. J. Am. Anim. Hosp. Assoc. 21:551, 1985.

LARYNGEAL PARALYSIS

DENNIS N. ARON, D.V.M.
Athens, Georgia

Laryngeal paralysis, a condition in which the vocal folds cannot be properly abducted, can be either congenital or acquired. The congenital form has been reported to occur frequently in the Bouvier des Flandres, bull terrier, and Siberian husky. The onset of clinical signs occurs at 4 to 6 months of age. As an acquired disorder, laryngeal paralysis has been noted most frequently in middle-aged to older, large to giant breeds of dogs. The congenital and acquired disorder also can involve smaller breeds of dogs and cats. The clinical condition usually has an insidious onset with intermittent episodes of severe respiratory distress. In some cases, an underlying cause such as trauma, lymphosarcoma, hypothyroidism, or neuromuscular disease can be identified, but usually the cause is not determined.

ANATOMY

The larynx consists of a framework of five cartilages held together by ligaments and muscles that move on one another as a result of these muscle actions (Figs. 1 and 2). It is lined with mucous membrane that is arranged in characteristic folds. The thyroid, cricoid, and epiglottic cartilages are unpaired, whereas the arytenoid cartilages are paired.

The largest cartilage is the thyroid cartilage with its two ala that meet in the midline. The thyroid cartilage forms the lateral and ventral boundary of the larynx. The cranial cornu of the thyroid cartilage extends craniolaterally, attaching to the thyrohyoid bone of the hyoid apparatus by the hyothyroid membrane. The most caudal portion of the larynx is formed by the cricoid cartilage. It is thicker and stronger than the thyroid cartilage and resembles a signet ring. It is narrow in front, is broad behind, and forms a complete ring around the larynx caudal to the vocal folds. Caudolaterally, the cricoid articulates with the caudal cornu of the thyroid cartilage. This is a true synovial joint that permits a rocking action of the cricoid on the thyroid cartilage. The cricoid and thyroid cartilages are also connected by the cricothyroid ligament. Caudally, the cricoid cartilage is attached to the trachea. The epiglottic cartilage is a thin leaflike sheet of elastic cartilage

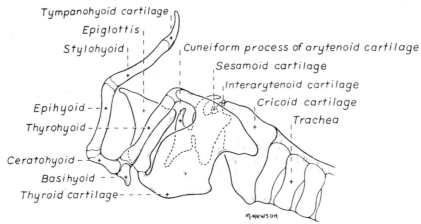

Figure 1. Laryngeal cartilages and hyoid apparatus, lateral aspect. (Reprinted with permission from Evans and Christensen (eds.): *Miller's Anatomy of the Dog*. 2nd ed. Philadelphia: W. B. Saunders, 1979, p. 520.)

that is attached to the inner surface of the cranial thyroid cartilage by its long, thin, stemlike process. The paired arytenoid cartilages form the craniodorsal extent of the larynx. They are connected to the cricoid cartilage by the cricoarytenoid joint, which is a synovial joint that allows rotation through a transverse axis and a slight sliding movement of the cartilages toward or away from each other. The interarytenoid cartilage, which lies just cranial to the cricoid lamina, attaches the two arytenoid cartilages.

The narrow passageway into the larynx is termed the rima glottidis. The boundaries of this opening are the paired arytenoid cartilages dorsally and the paired vocal folds ventrally. The vocal folds are actually mucosal folds extending from the arytenoid cartilages to the thyroid cartilage. Narrowing (adduction) and widening (abduction) of the rima glottidis is controlled by contractions of intrinsic muscles originating and inserting on the laryngeal cartilages. This muscular action regulates the functions of the larynx.

The abductors of the vocal folds and arytenoid cartilages are the paired dorsal cricoarytenoid muscles. These muscles originate from the caudal sur-

face of the cricoid cartilage and insert on the muscular processes of the arytenoid cartilages. There are three paired adductors of the glottis. They are the lateral cricoarytenoid muscle, the transverse arytenoid muscle, and, most important, the thyroarytenoid muscle. The thyroarytenoid muscle originates on the internal midline of the thyroid cartilage and inserts near the muscular process of the arytenoid cartilage. The cricothyroid muscles serve as a tensor of the vocal folds (Fig. 3).

Innervation of the larynx, both motor and sensory, is from the tenth (vagus) cranial nerve via the cranial and caudal laryngeal nerves. The cranial laryngeal nerve leaves the vagus at the level of the nodose ganglion and has two branches: the internal and the external. The internal branch provides sensory innervation to the laryngeal mucosa, whereas the external branch provides motor supply to the cricothyroid muscle. The caudal laryngeal nerve is the terminal portion of the recurrent laryngeal nerve. The recurrent laryngeal nerve originates from the vagus nerve at the thoracic inlet. The recurrent laryngeal nerve is different on the right and left sides. On the left, after leaving the vagus, it turns around the arch of the aorta; on the right,

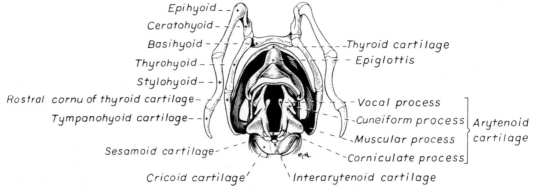

Figure 2. Laryngeal cartilages and hyoid apparatus, dorsal aspect. (Reprinted with permission from Evans and Christensen (eds.): *Miller's Anatomy of the Dog*. 2nd ed. Philadelphia: W. B. Saunders, 1979, p. 522.)

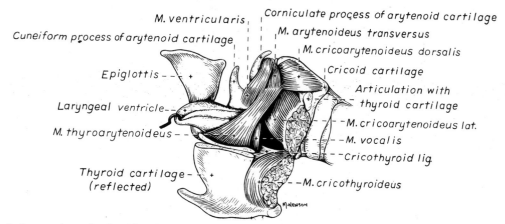

Figure 3. Laryngeal muscles, lateral aspect. (Reprinted with permission from Evans and Christensen (eds.): *Miller's Anatomy of the Dog.* 2nd ed. Philadelphia: W. B. Saunders, 1979, p. 523.)

it turns around the subclavian artery. The recurrent laryngeal nerves now course cranially to become the caudal laryngeal nerves. The caudal laryngeal nerves provide motor innervation to all intrinsic muscles of the larynx except the cricothyroid muscle.

NORMAL AND ABNORMAL FUNCTION

There are four important functions of the intrinsic laryngeal muscles: (1) The glottis is opened by rotation of the arytenoid cartilages, which are moved by the dorsal cricoarytenoid muscles. (2) The glottis is closed by the action of the thyroarytenoid and the lateral cricoarytenoid muscles, which rotate the arytenoids in a direction opposite to that which opens the glottis. This action is supplemented by that of the transverse arytenoid muscle, which approximates the arytenoids and shortens the caudal commissure. In addition, the cricothyroid muscle tenses the vocal folds and thus also may participate in glottic closure. (3) Vocal fold tension is regulated by two sets of muscles. The cricothyroid muscle tilts the cricoid cartilage backward, tensing and lengthening the vocal folds. The thyroarytenoid muscle relaxes the folds and shortens them. (4) The fourth muscle function of the larynx is that of lowering and raising the epiglottis.

The larynx serves three functions: (1) It acts as an airway, (2) it protects the lower airways; and (3) it serves as an instrument of vocalization. In the normal resting animal the glottis actively opens during inspiration and passively closes (but not completely) during expiration (Fig. 4). During strenuous activity the arytenoid cartilages and vocal folds are fixed in maximal abduction during both phases of respiration (Fig. 5). The larynx protects the airway in several ways. Most important, it effects complete and automatic closure of the glottis during swallowing; contrary to popular belief, the

epiglottis is not necessary for glottic closure or for prevention of aspiration in a properly functioning larynx. During swallowing the vocal folds are completely closed, and the epiglottis is brought over the glottis, thus deflecting the bolus of swallowed material to either side and caudally into the esophageal orifice. The other major protective function of the larynx is its role in the cough reflex, which is triggered by sensitive receptors in the larynx and the subglottic space. Stimulation of these receptors results in immediate closure of the glottis, which is followed by an explosive cough. The importance of this reflex mechanism in homeostasis cannot be overemphasized.

Most frequently laryngeal paralysis occurs because of a bilateral dysfunction of the recurrent laryngeal nerves. A dysfunction in this location results in the arytenoid cartilages and vocal folds resting in a partially open (paramedian) position. This results from the loss of the innervation of intrinsic abductor and adductor muscles of the larynx. When intrinsic muscles of the larynx cannot function with laryngeal paralysis, an inspiratory dyspnea results. This occurs because, as the intraluminal glottic pressure decreases with inspiration, the vocal folds passively move medially. This results in increased resistance to inspiratory gas flow and primary inspiratory distress. The associated laryngeal inflammation and edema can cause both an inspiratory and an expiratory component to airway obstruction. Additionally, the normal functions of deglutition and vocalization are compromised. Indeed, this abnormal function correlates well with the clinical signs of laryngeal paralysis.

SIGNALMENT AND CAUSE

At the University of Georgia Veterinary Teaching Hospital (UGVTH) 22 patients with laryngeal paralysis were diagnosed from January 1984 to February

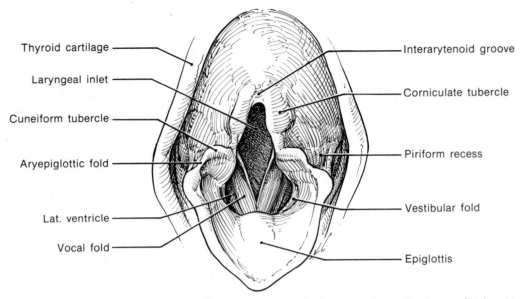

Thyroid cartilage

Laryngeal inlet

Cuneiform tubercle

Aryepiglottic fold

Lat. ventricle

Vocal fold

Interarytenoid groove

Corniculate tubercle

Piriform recess

Vestibular fold

Epiglottis

Figure 4. Normal laryngeal structures as seen during laryngoscopy. The larynx is in the resting (intermediate) position.

1987. These patients are considered to represent the recent clinical experience with laryngeal paralysis. Of these 22 patients, 5 (23 per cent) were diagnosed prior to the age of 18 months (mean, 14 months). Four different breeds of dogs and one domestic short-hair cat were represented. Included in this group were a Rottweiler, Cairn terrier, Chihuahua, and Jack Russell terrier. With three of the four dogs and the cat, no definitive cause of the laryngeal paralysis was identified. However, the laryngeal paralysis in the Cairn terrier was caused presumptively by neck wounds as a result of a dog fight.

Breed predisposition for congenital laryngeal pa-

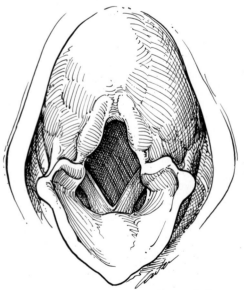

Figure 5. The same view as in Figure 4, with the arytenoid cartilages and vocal folds maxillary abducted.

ralysis has been reported to vary with the geographic location; the Siberian husky in the United States, the Bouvier des Flandres in the Netherlands, and the bull terrier in Great Britain are affected most frequently. Congenital laryngeal paralysis is not restricted to these breeds of dogs, as it has been seen in a variety of different breeds as well as in mixed breed dogs. The average age of patients at the time of treatment has been reported to be 14 months with congenital laryngeal paralysis.

In the Bouvier des Flandres breed an autosomal dominant inheritance pattern has been proved to cause the condition. On histopathologic study, wallerian degeneration of the recurrent laryngeal nerves and abnormalities of the nucleus ambiguus were noted. It has also been suggested that a hereditary predisposition to laryngeal paralysis exists in the Siberian husky. In humans, a form of laryngeal paralysis exists in the neonate or infant. Similar to the inherited condition in the Bouvier des Flandres breed, a familial form of laryngeal paralysis occurs in humans. Further, in the neonate or infant, laryngeal paralysis can have a congenital or acquired etiology, but in older children trauma is the usual cause. Table 1 lists the myriad congenital and acquired sources of laryngeal paralysis reported in children, and these conditions might also be considered in dogs and cats with laryngeal paralysis. For a significant number of children with vocal cord paralysis no apparent cause can be found (similar to the situation in the young dog and cat). It has been suggested that in these cases the recurrent laryngeal nerves have been unavoidably stretched during delivery, as with a breech presentation with twisting and stretching of the neck to deliver the head. The anatomy of the recurrent laryngeal nerves makes them vulnerable to injury

Table 1. *Congenital and Acquired Sources of Laryngeal Paralysis in Children*

Congenital
- A. Central nervous system
    1. Cerebral agenesis
    2. Hydrocephalus
    3. Encephalocele
    4. Meningomyelocele
    5. Meningocele
    6. Arnold-Chiari malformation
    7. Associated multiple congenital anomalies
- B. Peripheral nervous system
    - Congenital defect in peripheral nerve fiber at neuromuscular junction, as in myasthenia gravis
- C. Cardiovascular anomalies
    1. Cardiomegaly
        a. Ventricular septal defect
        b. Tetralogy of Fallot
    2. Abnormal great vessels
        a. Vascular ring
        b. Dilated aorta
        c. Double aortic rch
        d. Patent ductus arteriosus
        e. Transposition of the great vessels
- D. Associated with other congenital anomalies
    1. Tumors or cysts of mediastinum (bronchogenic cyst)
    2. Malformation of the tracheobronchial tree
    3. Esophageal malformation
        a. Cyst
        b. Duplication
        c. Atresia
        d. Tracheoesophageal fistula
    4. Diaphragmatic hernia
    5. Cleft palate
    6. Laryngeal anomalies
        a. Laryngeal cleft
        b. Subglottic stenosis
        c. Laryngomalacia

Acquired
- A. Trauma
    1. Birth injury
    2. Postsurgical correction of cardiovascular or esophageal anomalies
- B. Infectious
    1. Encephalitis
    2. Polyneuritis
    3. Rabies
    4. Botulism
    5. Tuberculosis
- C. Supranuclear and nuclear lesions

Partial list adapted from Dedo, D. D., and Dedo, H. H.: Neurogenic diseases of the larynx. *In* Bluestone, C. D., and Stool, S. E. (eds.): *Pediatric Otolaryngology.* Vol. 2. Philadelphia: W. B. Saunders, 1983, p. 1278.

as they course around the subclavian artery on the right and the aorta on the left. During birth the vessels provide countertraction against the nerves, thus stretching them, with subsequent paralysis.

At the UGVTH, of the 22 patients, 17 (77 per cent) were diagnosed after the age of 6 years (mean, 11 years). One domestic short-hair cat, two mixed breed dogs (both were collie mixed breeds), and nine different pure breeds of dogs were represented. There were three Labrador retrievers, three Irish setters, and two poodles. Represented one

time each were a Brittany spaniel, English springer spaniel, beagle, Doberman pinscher, Golden retriever, and Keeshond. A cause considered to be directly contributory to the laryngeal paralysis was identified in 4 of the 17 patients. These associated conditions were polyneuropathy, meningitis, cervical wounds as a result of a dog fight, and laryngeal paralysis following placement of a pharyngostomy tube for treatment of an oronasal fistula. Additionally, three of eight animals tested were diagnosed as being hypothyroid.

The vast majority of patients with acquired laryngeal paralysis have been middle-aged to older, large and giant breed dogs, with Saint Bernards and Labrador retrievers being over-represented. Acquired laryngeal paralysis has also been reported in cats. The etiology of acquired laryngeal paralysis is usually undetermined (idiopathic). However, prior to diagnosing laryngeal paralysis, certain acquired conditions need to be excluded during diagnostic workup. These include lesions involving the motor neurons anywhere along the course from the brainstem to the dorsal cricothyroid muscle, but peripheral lesions of the recurrent laryngeal nerves are responsible most of the time. Suggested causes include trauma to the cervical region or larynx, surgery or procedures in the cervical region that could have traumatized the recurrent laryngeal nerves, extrathoracic or intrathoracic masses affecting the recurrent laryngeal nerves, and generalized or specific neuropathies or myopathies that involve the innervation of intrinsic muscles of the larynx. A connection between hypothyroidism and laryngeal paralysis has been suggested because hypothyroidism has been associated with polyneuropathies and myopathies. In humans, trauma related to thyroidectomy and neoplasms causing recurrent laryngeal nerve entrapment are the primary causes of acquired laryngeal paralysis.

The congenital form of laryngeal paralysis in Bouvier des Flandres was reported to occur the majority of the time (74 per cent) in males. Other reports suggest that male dogs in general were predisposed to all forms of laryngeal paralysis, whereas one study found no sex predisposition. Of the 22 patients at the UGVTH there was found to be no sex predisposition, as exactly 11 were male and 11 were female.

In summary, laryngeal paralysis seems to occur in the dog and possibly the cat in two distinct age groups, the very young and the relatively old patient. In both groups the cause is usually undetermined. The condition appears to occur about four times more frequently in the old dog than in the young patient. The larger breeds of dogs seem to be predisposed to the syndrome in the older patient.

HISTORY AND CLINICAL SIGNS

The history and clinical signs of laryngeal paralysis were similar among the 22 patients seen at the UGVTH, whether they were young or old. The onset of clinical signs occurred between 6 and 24 weeks of age in the young patients. In the older patients the duration of clinical signs prior to presentation for diagnosis and treatment ranged from 1 day to 3 years. Ten of these 17 patients had clinical signs for more than 3 months prior to the owner's seeking veterinary help.

The most common presenting complaint was respiratory distress, while less frequently the animal had acute collapse, swallowing difficulty, hoarse bark, and noisy breathing. Besides respiratory distress, the typical history also contained early signs of change in bark and gagging or coughing while eating or drinking. More advanced signs included ptyalism, decreased exercise tolerance, exertional dyspnea, cyanosis, and syncope.

DIAGNOSIS AND MANAGEMENT

The tentative diagnosis of laryngeal paralysis is based on historical and physical findings compatible with laryngeal obstruction. The definitive diagnosis is based on direct visualization of laryngeal dysfunction, which consists of the failure of the vocal folds to abduct and collapse of the glottis on inspiration. Major errors in the initial examination for laryngeal paralysis are underestimation of distress, overzealous examination, and performance of laboratory studies that worsen the patient's condition and defeat therapeutic goals. At the UGVTH, on initial examination of the 22 patients with laryngeal paralysis, 6 required tracheostomy. This experience demonstrates that every effort should be made to keep the patient calm and to maintain a sense of security. The patient should be allowed to maintain the position that provides the most comfort and should be restrained only minimally. Fast movements that might be interpreted as threatening should be avoided. If distress is moderate to severe or likely to be exacerbated by laboratory and radiographic studies, these studies should be withheld and visualization of the oral cavity and airway should be postponed until it can be done under controlled conditions.

The definitive diagnosis of laryngeal paralysis is based on direct visualization of laryngeal dysfunction by laryngoscopy. The examination can be conducted using neuroleptanalgesia or during recovery from a light plane of thiamylal or thiopental anesthesia. Cats can be examined safely while recovering from light ketamine anesthesia. The best evaluation is accomplished when the animal is *almost awake* and beginning to vocalize. Under a deep plane of anesthesia the larynx is paralyzed, which can result in a false-positive diagnosis.

The animal is symmetrically positioned in sternal recumbency, with the neck elevated to a normal posture for examination. The tongue and epiglottis are gently depressed, while the soft palate can be elevated with a malleable retractor. Normally, the arytenoid processes should symmetrically abduct with inspiration and relax to form a relatively small glottic opening with expiration; the vocal folds can be seen to passively flutter with expiration. With laryngeal paralysis there is a failure of the arytenoid cartilages and vocal folds to abduct with collapse of the glottis on inspiration. To avoid missing the diagnosis, it is necessary to realize that, with paralysis, the vocal folds will adduct slightly with inspiration owing to pressure changes and the action of a neurologically intact cricothyroid muscle. Additionally, with paralysis, at the end of inspiration the vocal folds relax, which can appear as though they abduct. It is important to differentiate this paradoxical movement by correlating laryngeal movement with the phases of respiration. Also confusing for diagnosis is that paralysis can be unilateral or more severe on one side, making abduction and adduction asymmetric. Of the 22 patients at the UGVTH, one was noted to have total unilateral paralysis, whereas nine were noted to have bilateral paralysis but were asymmetrically affected. It is noteworthy to realize that animals with pure unilateral paralysis are uncommonly presented for diagnosis and treatment, as they are usually asymptomatic.

Radiographic evaluation of the cervical area, thorax, and other regions may become necessary to help determine a congenital or traumatic cause for the laryngeal paralysis. Skull films and dye studies of the larynx, trachea, esophagus, and cardiovascular systems may be required to document and evaluate associated defects.

Electromyography (EMG) may be employed in testing the electrical function of the laryngeal muscles. Such testing can give diagnostic as well as prognostic information for laryngeal paralysis. Electromyography may be helpful in making the diagnosis of polyneuropathy or diffuse myopathy in which laryngeal paralysis is an early component of the disease. In one study there was 100 per cent diagnostic correlation between EMG and laryngoscopy findings for laryngeal paralysis. This differs from the experience at the UGVTH. Of the 22 patients diagnosed as having laryngeal paralysis with laryngoscopy, all 22 underwent concurrent electromyography. Placement of electrodes was via the mouth to evaluate the dorsal cricoarytenoid muscle. In six patients the results of EMG of the larynx were considered normal. These normal electromyography studies may be reflective of the technique's being performed by multiple individuals possessing variable degrees of experience and expertise. Possibly some of the animals were tested prior to EMG changes in the muscles. Less likely, chronic paralysis could have led to complete atrophy and fibrosis of the dorsal cricoarytenoid muscles.

To further support the diagnosis of laryngeal paralysis an intrinsic laryngeal muscle can be sampled for histopathologic study to confirm denervation atrophy; however, this is rarely necessary. Biopsy of the dorsal cricoarytenoid muscle can be easily accomplished during arytenoid lateralization surgery. If a partial laryngectomy is performed via an oral approach, biopsy of the vocal muscle portion of the thyroarytenoid muscle can be done.

TREATMENT

The initial treatment of an animal with laryngeal paralysis is primarily symptomatic and depends largely on the amount of airway distress the patient is exhibiting. Patients with mild to moderate distress are managed primarily through avoidance of stress and provision of a cool environment. Antiedema dosages of corticosteroids can be administered to lessen airway obstruction due to inflamed edematous respiratory membranes. Administration of minimal dosages of tranquilizers, analgesics, or both helps to keep the patient calm and facilitates the examination and the administration of supplemental oxygen. If the patient progresses to severe respiratory distress, a tracheostomy may be necessary. Definitive surgical procedures to widen the rima glottidis may be necessary to help achieve patient stabilization. When possible, however, patient stabilization prior to definitive surgery or invasive diagnostic procedures requiring general anesthesia is preferred. When the condition of the patient is stabilized, the search for the cause of the paralysis may proceed; however, a diagnosis is usually not obvious in the vast majority of the patients.

At the UGVTH no treatment was performed on 6 of the 22 patients. No substantial improvement was reported in five of these patients, while one spontaneously recovered (owing to pharyngostomy tube placement). The dog diagnosed as having meningitis was treated with antibiotics only. This animal showed no improvement of the laryngeal paralysis. One dog diagnosed as being hypothyroid was treated with thyroid hormone supplementation only. This animal was reported initially to improve but underwent euthanasia 8 months after beginning treatment because of severe recurrence of clinical signs. Treatment with thyroid hormone supplementation has been reported to reverse both the clinical abnormalities and the histologic changes in humans with hypothyroid neuropathies or myopathies. Response to only thyroid hormone supplementation in dogs with laryngeal paralysis is undetermined.

Fourteen of the 22 patients at the UGVTH underwent surgical therapy for the clinical signs related to laryngeal paralysis. Generally, three different procedures were used to increase the area of the glottic lumen and to decrease upper airway resistance. These procedures were (1) partial laryngectomy (through the mouth) performed in six patients, (2) arytenoid lateralization (tie-back) performed in five patients, and (3) arytenoid lateralization with "conservative" partial laryngectomy performed in three patients.

Partial laryngectomy consists of a vocal fold resection and a partial arytenoidectomy. Before doing this procedure a tracheostomy must be performed. It has been recommended that the vocal fold resection be performed bilaterally and the partial arytenoidectomy be performed unilaterally to increase the glottic lumen by 70 to 80 per cent (Fig. 6). This procedure is accomplished with the animal in sternal recumbency; the animal's mouth is held open, with the tongue pulled rostral and ventral. The use of uterine biopsy punch to take small "bites" of the medial cartilage facilitates a clean and controlled partial arytenoidectomy and vocal fold resection. The object of this procedure is to create an adequately open glottis without removing too much tissue. Removal of too much tissue predisposes the patient to aspiration of food and liquid on deglutition. It has been recommended that the opening created with this technique should be about the size of a laryngeal lumen seen with maximum abduction in a lightly anesthetized, normal, similarly sized animal.

Of the six partial laryngectomies performed at the UGVTH only one patient had a good clinical result with this technique. Four showed minimal to no clinical improvement, and one died of aspiration pneumonia a few days after the procedure was performed. Retrospectively, with review of the surgery reports and records, the animals that showed minimal improvement probably had a conservative amount of tissue resected with their partial laryngectomy, whereas the animal that died probably had too much tissue resected. This experience points out the disadvantage of the partial laryngectomy: It is difficult to judge the amount of tissue to be resected. This is further complicated by a bloody field and swollen tissues. Not only is the animal predisposed to aspiration, but also there is an increased chance of postoperative stricture formation (webbing) when too much tissue is removed. Webbing occurs mostly at the dorsal and ventral commissures of the glottis. Webbing can be minimized if tags of the vocal folds are left ventrally and if only unilateral arytenoidectomy is performed. Partial laryngectomy has been reported to work well for those experienced in its application; however, less experienced surgeons may want to consider other methods.

Arytenoid lateralization is performed by suturing

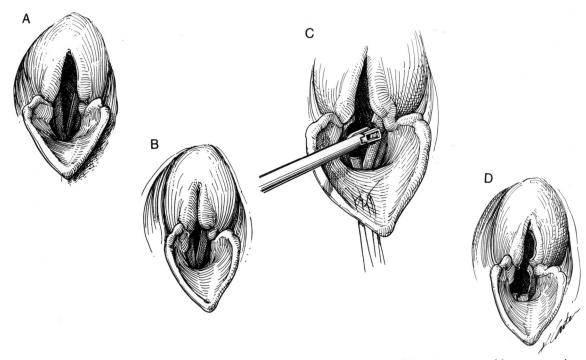

Figure 6. *A*, The larynx in a normal resting position. *B*, The appearance of a paralyzed larynx. *C*, A partial laryngectomy being performed with a uterine biopsy punch. *D*, Completed partial laryngectomy. Note the tags of ventral vocal fold, which are left to avoid webbing. (Reprinted with permission from Aron, D. N., and Crowe, D. T.: Vet. Clin. North Am. 15:891, 1985.)

the arytenoid cartilage or cartilages in an open (abducted) position, thus increasing the area of the rima glottidis. At the UGVTH this has been accomplished in two different ways. With either method, the animal is placed in dorsal or lateral recumbency. Preplacement of a tracheostomy tube is not necessary with unilateral lateralization. A lateral incision is made over the larynx and cranial trachea on the side receiving the lateralization, being careful to avoid the jugular vein and branches. Tissue plane dissection is continued to the level of the laryngotrachea. The thyroid cartilage is rotated laterally and an incision is made through the thyropharyngeal and portions of the cricopharyngeal muscles. In one technique, the cricothyroid and cricoarytenoid articulations and interarytenoid cartilage are all transected without penetrating the mucosa. The dorsal cricoarytenoid muscle is cut close to its insertion on the muscular process of the arytenoid cartilage. Then, one suture of approximately 00 size of a monofilament nonabsorbable material is passed through the muscular process of the arytenoid cartilage and the caudodorsal portion of the thyroid cartilage. The suture is placed in a mattress pattern and tied to achieve maximal abduction of the arytenoid cartilage. This position is determined by viewing the glottic lumen orally with the endotracheal tube temporarily removed. In the other technique, after the incision is made in the thyropharyngeal and portions of the cricopharyngeal muscles, a suture of 0 to 2 size is placed from the muscular

process to the cricoid cartilage without transection of the articulations (Fig. 7). The difference between these methods is the manner in which the arytenoid cartilage is abducted. In the first method described, the arytenoid cartilage is pulled into a lateral position; in the second method, the arytenoid cartilage is rotated laterally at the cricoarytenoid articulation (Fig. 8). The second method attempts to mimic the normal action of the dorsal cricoarytenoid muscle and thus requires no disarticulation. There has been no difference as far as clinical results noted between the two techniques, but the second method is technically difficult to perform in small dogs and cats, and penetration of the esophagus is a potential complication.

Of the five arytenoid lateralization procedures at the UGVTH, three were performed bilaterally and two unilaterally. A preoperative tracheostomy tube was inserted in the patients receiving a bilateral lateralization. All five patients experienced moderate to substantial improvement of clinical signs. However, the three patients that received a bilateral lateralization (performed during the same surgical episode) experienced some degree of clinical and radiographic signs of aspiration pneumonia. These three patients recovered from the pneumonia after vigorous therapy and went on to do well. It has been proposed that bilateral lateralization is necessary to resolve the clinical signs of laryngeal paralysis. Based on the author's experience and that of others, bilateral arytenoid lateralization may not be

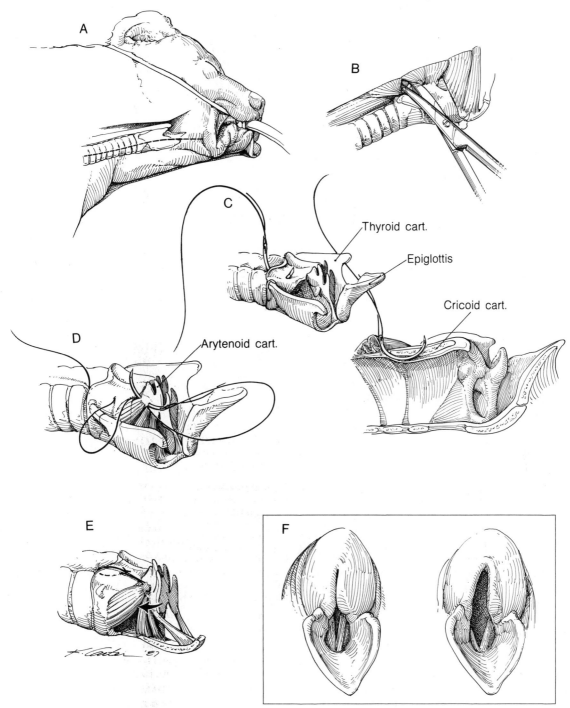

Thyroid cart.

Epiglottis

Cricoid cart.

Arytenoid cart.

Figure 7. Suture technique for palliation of laryngeal paralysis. *A*, The patient is placed in lateral recumbency with a lateral incision over the larynx and cranial trachea. *B*, Dissection is continued to the level of the laryngotrachea. An incision is made through the thyropharyngeal and portions of the cricopharyngeal muscles. A finger is passed deep to these muscles to palpate the dorsal median ridge on the cricoid cartilage and the dorsal edge of the lamina of the thyroid cartilage. A tube is passed down the esophagus to positively identify its position. *C*, Working under the thyropharyngeal and cricopharyngeal muscles, the suture needle is "walked off" the caudal edge of the cricoid cartilage and passed into the lamina of the cartilage at a lateral to medial position that is halfway between the dorsal median ridge of the cricoid cartilage and dorsal edge of the lamina of the thyroid cartilage. The needle is passed into the cartilage while not penetrating the mucosa. It is essential to avoid esophageal tissue when passing this suture. *D*, The muscular process of the arytenoid cartilage is palpated, and the suture is placed into this protuberance. *E*, The suture is tied to open the glottis. *F*, The glottic opening prior to suture placement and after suture placement. (Reprinted with permission from Aron and Crowe: Vet. Clin. North Am. 15:891, 1985.)

A

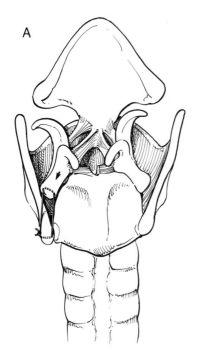

B

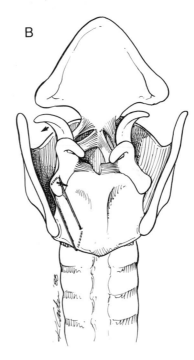

Figure 8. Two methods of accomplishing an arytenoid lateralization. *A*, The arytenoid cartilage is "pulled" into a lateral position by passing a suture from the muscular process to the caudodorsal portion of the caudal cornu of the thyroid cartilage. With this method it is necessary to transect the cricothyroid and cricoarytenoid articulations, the interarytenoid cartilage, and the dorsal cricoarytenoid muscle. *B*, The arytenoid cartilage is "rotated" into a lateral position by passing a suture from the muscular process to the cricoid cartilage. This method attempts to mimic the normal action of the dorsal cricoarytenoid muscle and requires no disarticulation.

necessary in most patients. However, if clinical signs persist, surgery on the second side can be staged 3 to 4 weeks after the initial procedure to help prevent patient morbidity associated with aspiration pneumonia. It has been suggested that a bilateral arytenoid lateralization may lead to an excess of scar tissue formation that reduces the glottic lumen to a size comparable with that achieved by unilateral arytenoid lateralization. This seems to be due to the considerable tissue manipulation required to perform the bilateral lateralization. Older patients will occasionally have calcified, fixated laryngeal cartilages. Those that have calcified laryngeal cartilages on preoperative radiographs are not good candidates for a lateralization procedure.

Recently, three patients at the UGVTH with laryngeal paralysis received an arytenoid lateralization and a "conservative" partial laryngectomy. A preoperative tracheostomy may or may not be performed. The arytenoid lateralization was achieved unilaterally, as described above. During the same surgical episode in two patients and 2 days later in one patient, a limited ventriculocordectomy (leaving ventral tags) was performed to supplement the lateralization. These three patients showed significant improvement clinically and experienced no major complications. This combination technique was attempted to achieve a "safe" maximum glottic lumen size, decrease postoperative complications, and avoid a staged second lateralization.

Other surgical techniques described in the veterinary literature for laryngeal paralysis are partial laryngectomy performed through a ventral laryngotomy incision, castellated laryngofissure and vocal fold resection, and arytenoidopexy. The author has a minimum of experience with these procedures.

POSTOPERATIVE CARE AND CONSIDERATIONS

The first 24 to 72 hours after laryngeal surgery are critical, as problems with aspiration and laryngeal edema frequently can lead to pneumonia and respiratory distress. The patient must be closely observed for this period of time and sometimes longer. During this interval only small volumes of water and soft food are offered. Water is tried after 24 hours, and, if no problems develop, a gruel of water and canned dog food is tried the second day. Evidence of gagging, retching, coughing, depression, and persistent pyrexia may require slowing the reintroduction of water and food. Radiographic views of the lungs are performed to evaluate for aspiration pneumonia, which, if present, is vigorously treated symptomatically. The animal is returned gradually over a few weeks to a more normal diet and feeding schedule.

The avoidance of respiratory distress primarily involves providing a cool environment, keeping the patient calm, and sometimes administering supplemental oxygen. Frequently, low doses of corticosteroids are given during the perioperative period to lessen airway obstruction due to inflamed edematous respiratory membranes. When needed, administration of minimal dosages of tranquilizers, analgesics, or both can help to keep the patient calm and facilitate examination of the patient and the administration of supplemental oxygen. Oxygen can be provided by an environmentally controlled oxygen cage or a nasopharyngeal catheter. If the patient progresses to severe respiratory distress, orotracheal intubation or a tracheostomy may be necessary.

Postoperative care of a tracheostomy tube, if used, requires careful monitoring and diligent cleaning of the tube and aspiration of the trachea. The tube can usually be removed 2 to 4 days after laryngeal surgery.

The owners should closely observe their animal for signs of pneumonia and respiratory difficulty for the rest of the animal's life. Problems with aspiration are forever a concern, as normal deglutition and a normal cough reflex are not re-established with the surgical procedures presented in this article. In addition, recurrence or exacerbation of clinical signs of respiratory difficulty is possible, as webbing and stricture formation can occur with the partial laryngectomy. Further, failure of the suture to hold the arytenoid cartilage in an abducted position with the lateralization procedure can result in partial or complete return of clinical signs.

References and Supplemental Reading

Aron, D. N., and Crowe, D. T.: Upper airway obstruction: General principles and selected conditions in the dog and cat. Vet. Clin. North Am. 15:891, 1985.
Dedo, D. D., and Dedo, H. H.: Neurogenic diseases of the larynx. In
Bluestone, C. D., and Stool, S. E. (eds.): *Pediatric Otolaryngology.* Vol. 2. Philadelphia; W. B. Saunders, 1983, pp. 1278–1284.
Gaber, C. E., Amis, T. C., and LeCouteur, A.: Laryngeal paralysis in dogs: A review of 23 cases. J.A.V.M.A. 186:377, 1985.
Gourley, I. M., Paul, H., and Gregory, C.: Castellated laryngofissure and vocal fold resection for the treatment of laryngeal paralysis in the dog. J.A.V.M.A. 182:1084, 1983.
Greenfield, C. L.: Canine laryngeal paralysis. Comp. Cont. Ed. Pract. Vet. 9:1011, 1987.
Hardie, E. M., Kolata, R. J., Stone, E. A., et al.: Laryngeal paralysis in three cats. J.A.V.M.A. 179:879, 1981.
Harvey, C. E., and Venker-van Haagen, A. J.: Surgical management of pharyngeal and laryngeal airway obstruction in the dog. Vet. Clin. North Am. 5:515, 1975.
Harvey, C. E.: Partial laryngectomy in the dog. I. Healing and swallowing function in normal dogs. Vet. Surg. 12:192, 1983.
Harvey, C. E.: Partial laryngectomy in the dog. II. Immediate increase in glottic area obtained compared with other laryngeal procedures. Vet. Surg. 12:197, 1983.
Harvey, H. J.: Irby, N. L., and Watrous, B. J.: Laryngeal paralysis in hypothyroid dogs. In Kirk, R. W. (ed.): *Current Veterinary Therapy VIII.* Philadelphia: W. B. Saunders, 1983, pp. 694–697.
O'Brien, J. A., and Harvey, C. E.: Diseases of the upper airway. In Ettinger, S. J. (ed.): *Textbook of Veterinary Internal Medicine.* Philadelphia: W. B. Saunders, 1975, pp. 587–598.
O'Brien, J. A., Harvey, C. E., Kelly, A. M., et al.: Neurogenic atrophy of the laryngeal muscles of the dog. J. Small Anim. Pract. 14:521, 1973.
Rosin, E., and Greenwood, K.: Bilateral arytenoid cartilage lateralization for laryngeal paralysis in the dog. J.A.V.M.A. 180:515, 1982.
Venker-van Haagen, A. J.: Laryngeal paralysis in young Bouviers. In Kirk, R. W. (ed.): *Current Veterinary Therapy VII.* Philadelphia: W. B. Saunders, 1980, pp. 290–291.
Venker-van Haagen, A. J., Hartman, W., and Goedegebuure, S. A.: Spontaneous laryngeal paralysis in young Bouviers. J. Am. Anim. Hosp. Assoc. 14:714, 1978.
Venker-van Haagen, A. J., Bourv, J., and Hartman W.: Hereditary transmission of laryngeal paralysis in Bouviers. J. Am. Anim. Hosp. Assoc. 17:75, 1981.
Wykes, P. M.: Canine laryngeal diseases. Part I. Anatomy and disease syndromes. Comp. Cont. Ed. Pract. Vet. 5:8, 1983.
Wykes, P. M.: Canine laryngeal diseases. Part II. Diagnosis and treatment. Comp. Cont. Ed. Pract. Vet. 5:108, 1983.

TRACHEAL COLLAPSE

ROGER B. FINGLAND, D.V.M.
Manhattan, Kansas

Tracheal collapse is a respiratory disease commonly diagnosed in middle-aged to aged toy and miniature breed dogs. Chihuahuas, Pomeranians, toy poodles, and Yorkshire terriers are commonly affected. Loss of intrinsic tracheal support results in dorsoventral flattening of the trachea, which is characterized clinically by a chronic cough and inspiratory or expiratory dyspnea. Dogs with tracheal collapse are frequently obese and often have concomitant pulmonary or cardiovascular abnormalities. Tracheal collapse has been reported but is rare in cats.

The trachea may be collapsed anywhere along its length. The thoracic inlet portion of the trachea is most commonly and, typically, most severely affected. Collapse of the mainstem bronchi may occur alone or in conjunction with tracheal collapse. Clinical signs associated with isolated mainstem bronchi collapse may mimic the clinical signs of tracheal collapse. Proper identification of the segment of the trachea that is collapsed is imperative for successful surgical management of the disease.

ETIOLOGY

The etiology of tracheal collapse is unknown. The condition may be acquired or congenital, although congenital tracheal collapse is rare. Several etiologies have been suggested.

TRACHEALIS MUSCLE WEAKNESS. Weakness and stretching of the trachealis muscle may allow the tracheal rings to flatten. Trachealis muscle weakness may result from a deficiency in innervation of the trachealis muscle similar to the deficient esophageal innervation observed in dogs with megaesophagus.

SMALL AIRWAYS DISEASE. Premature closure or partial obstruction of small airways results in an increase in transtracheal pressure, which may predispose to collapse, especially if there is coexistent cartilage weakness. Tracheal collapse is likely to result from primary pulmonary disease.

HEREDITARY PREDISPOSITION. Tracheal collapse has been reported to be hereditary in the Chihuahua breed (O'Brien et al., 1966).

DEMINERALIZATION OF TRACHEAL CARTILAGE. Dallman and Brown (1984) and Done and Drew (1976) have studied the histochemical properties of tracheal cartilage from dogs with tracheal collapse. They found that the hyaline cartilage was hypocellular and had a decreased glycosaminoglycan content. Soft cartilage is unable to maintain tracheal rigidity or resist changes in transtracheal pressure. Histochemical abnormalities of the tracheal cartilage may occur primarily or the changes may result from chronic deep-seated tracheitis.

SECONDARY TRACHEAL COLLAPSE. Tracheal collapse may be caused by compression from extraluminal masses such as thyroid tumors, enlarged lymph nodes, or esophageal tumors. Left atrial enlargement is a common cause of mainstem bronchi collapse. Abnormalities in the trachealis muscle or tracheal cartilage would not be expected in dogs with secondary tracheal collapse.

DIFFERENTIAL DIAGNOSIS

The differential diagnosis of tracheal collapse must include the myriad diseases that cause a chronic cough or respiratory distress in small dogs. Tonsillitis, laryngeal collapse, laryngeal paresis or paralysis, stenotic nares, eversion of the lateral ventricles, elongated soft palate, bronchitis, tracheobronchitis, chronic decompensated mitral valvular disease, hypoplastic trachea, tracheal stenosis, and tracheal neoplasia should be considered. Laryngeal paresis or paralysis and mitral valvular disease often occur concomitantly with tracheal collapse.

DIAGNOSIS

Dogs with tracheal collapse consistently have a prolonged history of cough or respiratory distress. Typically, the dog has had previous treatment for tracheobronchitis or heart failure with minimal improvement. A mild cough following exercise, stress, or leash pulling is usually the initial clinical sign.

The severity and frequency of the cough increases over months to years. Eventually, the dog coughs continuously and becomes dyspneic when excited. In the advanced stages of the disease, the dog is dyspneic and cyanotic at rest and may be syncopal. Rarely, the initial clinical sign of tracheal collapse is an acute onset of severe coughing or respiratory distress. The clinical signs of tracheal collapse are exacerbated by stress, excitement, or physical activity.

A "goose honk" cough is observed in approximately 50 per cent of dogs with tracheal collapse. The honking sound occurs when the redundant dorsal tracheal membrane vibrates or resonates as air moves through the collapsed segment. Dogs that do not have a goose honk cough frequently have a paroxysmal dry, hacking cough. Stridulous breathing without coughing is occasionally observed.

Dyspnea may occur during inspiration, with expiration, or continually throughout the respiratory cycle, depending on the segment of trachea that is collapsed. Inspiratory dyspnea occurs with cervical tracheal collapse because intratracheal pressure is decreased. Expiratory dyspnea occurs with thoracic tracheal collapse because the increased intrapleural pressure essentially compresses the flaccid thoracic trachea. Collapse of the cervical and thoracic trachea results in primarily expiratory dyspnea.

Physical examination abnormalities typically are limited to results of tracheal palpation and auscultation of the thorax. Gentle tracheal palpation usually elicits paroxysms of coughing. The prominent lateral borders of a collapsed cervical trachea may be palpable in thin dogs. Vigorous or prolonged tracheal palpation may exacerbate coughing and dyspnea and should be avoided. Thoracic auscultation often reveals a mitral regurgitant murmur and occasionally a prominent second heart sound. There may be increased bronchovesicular sounds; however, referred upper airway noise often obliterates lung sounds. The soft end-expiratory snapping together of the tracheal walls may be heard in dogs with thoracic tracheal collapse. Hepatomegaly, resulting from venous congestion due to cor pulmonale or fatty metamorphosis, may be evident on abdominal palpation.

Electrocardiographic (ECG) abnormalities are nonspecific for tracheal collapse but may include pronounced sinus arrhythmia, evidence of cor pulmonale, or (for uncertain reasons) left ventricular enlargement. A thorough cardiac workup is essential for all dogs with tracheal collapse.

Tracheal collapse is characterized by a decrease in the dorsoventral tracheal diameter on lateral cervical and thoracic radiographs. Ventrodorsal and lateral views of the cervical and thoracic trachea during maximal inspiration and expiration should be obtained. Manipulation of severely affected animals to obtain radiographs may result in life-threatening dyspnea. An appropriate-sized endotracheal tube and a supplemental oxygen supply should be available during radiographic procedures.

The cervical trachea will appear collapsed and the thoracic trachea may appear dilated on an inspiratory radiograph. The thoracic trachea will be collapsed on the expiratory radiograph, and the cervical trachea may appear dilated. Collapse may be evident on both inspiratory and expiratory views in dogs with severe tracheal collapse. Inspiratory and expiratory radiographs are essential but not diagnostic in all cases. Tangner and Hobson (1982) reported that survey radiographs were diagnostic in only 59 per cent of dogs with tracheal collapse. Airway dimensions change dramatically with respiration; consequently, survey radiographs should not be relied on to consistently provide a diagnosis.

Fluoroscopic evaluation facilitates direct visualization of abnormal tracheal dynamics during all phases of respiration and allows identification of the exact location of collapse. The entire trachea, as well as the mainstem bronchi, should be evaluated fluoroscopically in all dogs suspected of having tracheal collapse.

Tracheoscopy provides a definitive diagnosis of tracheal collapse, even in mildly affected dogs in which the diagnosis might be missed with fluoroscopy. Tracheoscopy requires general anesthesia and close attention to patient oxygenation during the procedure and must be performed judiciously. Tracheal collapse can routinely be diagnosed fluoroscopically in dogs that are candidates for surgery. Tracheoscopy is not performed if the diagnosis is evident on fluoroscopy.

GRADING SYSTEM

A grading system for tracheal collapse was devised by Tangner and Hobson (1982) to document the severity of collapse and to provide guidelines for medical versus surgical therapy. The criteria for this grading system are shown in Figure 1. Dogs with grades II through IV collapse are considered surgical candidates.

TREATMENT

Medical Management

The majority of dogs with tracheal collapse will respond to medical therapy; however, the response is often only transient or incomplete. Medical therapy is usually ineffective in dogs that are severely dyspneic, cyanotic, or syncopal. The initial therapeutic regimen should include:

ANTITUSSIVES. Hydrocodone (Hycodan, 0.25 to

Classification of Collapsed Trachea

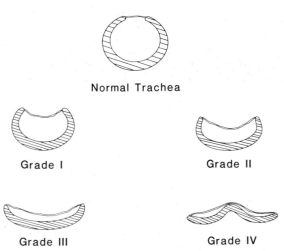

Figure 1. Grading system for collapsed trachea. (With permission from Tangner, C. H., and Hobson, H. P.: A retrospective study of 20 surgically managed cases of collapsed trachea. Vet. Surg. 11:146, 1982.)

Grade	Criteria
I	The trachea is nearly normal. The trachealis muscle is slightly pendulous, and the tracheal cartilages maintain a circular shape. The tracheal lumen is reduced approximately 25 per cent.
II	The trachealis muscle is widened and pendulous. The tracheal cartilages are partially flattened, and the tracheal lumen is reduced approximately 50 per cent.
III	The trachealis muscle is almost in contact with the dorsal surface of the tracheal cartilages. The tracheal cartilages are nearly flat, and the ends may be palpated on physical examination. The tracheal lumen is reduced approximately 75 per cent.
IV	The trachealis muscle is lying on the dorsal surface of the tracheal cartilages. The tracheal cartilages are flattened and may invert dorsally. The tracheal lumen is essentially obliterated.

0.5 mg/kg repeated every 12 hr PO) or butorphanol tartrate (Torbugesic or Torbutrol, 0.5 to 1.0 mg/kg repeated every 8 hr PO) is preferred. The response to hydrocodone in small dogs is extremely variable and may be affected by other medications such as tranquilizers and sedatives. Additionally, hydrocodone may cause constipation, necessitating the addition of stool softeners to the treatment regimen.

ANTIBIOTICS. Antibiotics should be administered based on tracheal culture and sensitivity specimens obtained via transtracheal aspiration. A broad-spectrum bactericidal antibiotic should be administered if a tracheal culture and sensitivity is unavailable. The author's preference is cefadroxil (Cefa-Tabs, 22 mg/kg repeated every 12 hr orally for 14 days). Long-term antibiotic therapy is indicated because most dogs with tracheal collapse have some degree of chronic, deep-seated bacterial tracheitis.

BRONCHODILATORS. Theophylline and its various

salts are the most commonly used bronchodilators in small animals. Dogs with thoracic tracheal collapse may especially benefit from theophylline bronchodilator therapy. Dilation of pulmonary airways decreases intrathoracic pressure during expiration, thereby decreasing tracheal narrowing. Various salts of theophylline have been formulated to increase the solubility. The most popular is theophylline ethylenediamine (aminophylline), which is 80 per cent theophylline. The dose of aminophylline is 8 to 10 mg/kg repeated every 8 hr orally. Aminophylline elixir is 20 per cent alcohol and should be used judiciously in small dogs.

Medical therapy for tracheal collapse should include exercise restriction, weight loss, and reduction in excitement and stress. The dog should wear a harness rather than a collar, and leash walking should be minimized. A cool, dry environment is beneficial. Concurrent cardiac disease should be managed appropriately.

The dog should be maintained on the initial therapeutic regimen for 2 weeks. If there has been no improvement in clinical signs after 2 weeks, the dose of antitussive should be gradually increased to the maximum recommended dose. Occasionally, a dog with tracheal collapse will respond to butorphanol but not to hydrocodone, or vice versa. A poor therapeutic response to one antitussive warrants a change to the other. Tranquilizers are indicated when excessive excitability results in paroxysms of coughing, even when antitussives are being administered. Acetylpromazine maleate (acepromazine) may be administered orally at a dose of 0.4 to 1.0 mg/kg repeated every 24 hr.

Corticosteroids should be used judiciously in the treatment of tracheal collapse. Corticosteroids seldom make the difference between long-term success and failure of medical therapy. Serious complications, including exacerbation of bacterial tracheitis or pneumonia and iatrogenic hyperadrenocorticism, may result from long-term administration of corticosteroids. Prednisone may be administered at a dose of 0.5 mg/kg repeated every 12 to 24 hr orally. Corticosteroid therapy should be discontinued if it fails to produce an improvement in clinical signs in 1 week.

Surgical management of tracheal collapse should be considered if medical therapy does not result in a substantial and sustained improvement in clinical signs after 1 month. Clinical signs often abate on medical therapy but then gradually return, even in the face of increasing dosages of drugs. This may take weeks, months, or years, but it usually does occur. It is not prudent to continue to treat the animal medically until clinical signs are so severe that the animal is no longer a functional pet. Surgery should be considered if the animal's condition deteriorates while on medical therapy.

Surgical Management

The majority of dogs with tracheal collapse managed surgically have at least some improvement in clinical signs, regardless of the severity of the disease. Mildly to moderately affected animals can be expected to have near-complete remission of clinical signs following appropriate surgical therapy. The ineffectiveness of surgery that has been previously reported likely resulted from operating on patients that were in advanced stages of the disease or from utilization of inadequate surgical techniques. Additionally, concomitant laryngeal paresis, laryngeal paralysis, or mainstem bronchi collapse is easily overlooked, and these conditions worsen the prognosis for surgical success. Surgery must be performed relatively early in the course of the disease, not when the severity of the clinical signs warrants euthanasia.

PREOPERATIVE CONSIDERATIONS

The preoperative evaluation should include a thorough physical examination, complete blood count (CBC), serum biochemical profile, ECG, inspiratory and expiratory cervical and thoracic radiographs, fluoroscopy, transtracheal aspiration for culture and sensitivity (usually done via a sterile endotracheal tube), and laryngeal examination. Cefazolin (Ancef) at a dose of 20 mg/kg should be administered intravenously at the time of induction. Minimizing stress and excitement in the immediate preoperative period is desirable.

ANESTHETIC CONSIDERATIONS

The anesthetic protocol must include provisions for rapid induction and control of the airway. Induction with an intravenous, rapidly acting agent such as thiamylal (Bio-Tal) is desirable. Mask induction should be avoided. Anesthesia should be maintained with an inhalation agent, preferably isoflurane (Aerrane.) Nitrous oxide should not be used.

The endotracheal tube should have a high-volume, low-pressure cuff that has been checked for leaks prior to insertion. Evaluation of the larynx for normal abduction of the arytenoid cartilages prior to insertion of the endotracheal tube is mandatory. The endotracheal tube should be secured to the patient in a manner that allows for repositioning of the tube intraoperatively.

SURGICAL APPROACH

CERVICAL TRACHEA. The cervical trachea is exposed from a ventral cervical midline approach. A ventral midline skin incision is made from the larynx to the manubrium. The paired sternohyoideus and sternocephalicus muscles are separated, and the left recurrent laryngeal nerve is identified. The lateral pedicles are removed from the trachea, either segmentally or in their entirety, depending on the procedure. Gentle cranial retraction on the cervical trachea facilitates placement of prostheses to the level of the first intercostal space through this approach.

THORACIC TRACHEA. The thoracic trachea may be approached through a median sternotomy or a right third intercostal space thoracotomy. Intercostal thoracotomy is preferred because this approach affords access to the thoracic trachea without major dissection, may be rapidly performed and closed, and is associated with few postoperative complications.

A right third intercostal space thoracotomy is performed, and the thoracic trachea is exposed by retracting the right costocervical vein cranially and the azygous vein caudally. The right costocervical vein may be ligated and divided to increase exposure of the cranial portion of the thoracic trachea. The right vagus nerve is retracted ventrally. The endotracheal tube should be positioned in the cervical trachea during application of prostheses to the thoracic trachea.

Placement of a thoracic drainage tube is recommended following application of prostheses to the thoracic trachea. Air may leak from around intratracheal sutures or from tears in the dorsal tracheal membrane.

SURGICAL TECHNIQUES

Surgical procedures that have been advocated for management of tracheal collapse include chondrotomy, plication of the dorsal membrane, resection and anastomosis, and application of intraluminal or extraluminal prostheses. Application of an extraluminal prosthesis has been the only surgical procedure that has resulted in repeatable, long-term success. The two most commonly used extraluminal prostheses are the total ring prosthesis and the polypropylene spiral prosthesis.

Polypropylene Spiral Prosthesis Technique

Spiral prostheses are made from the case or barrel of a polypropylene 3-ml syringe (Fig. 2A) using a rigid single-edge razor blade. A cylinder is created by removing the top and bottom of the case or barrel (Fig. 2B). A spiral cut is made at an angle of 15° from the end of the cylinder (Fig. 2C). The

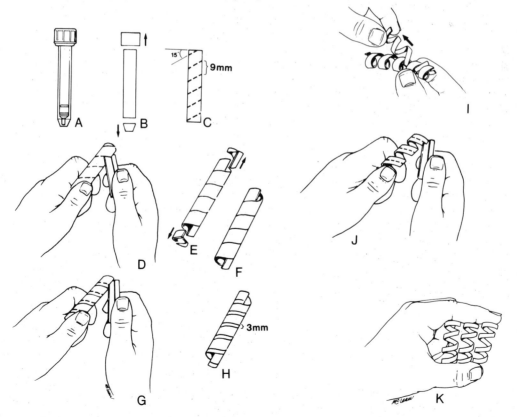

Figure 2. Technique for making polypropylene spiral prostheses from a 3-ml syringe case. See text for description. (With permission from Fingland, R. B., et al.: Surgical management of cervical and thoracic tracheal collapse in dogs using extraluminal spiral prostheses. J. Am. Anim. Hosp. Assoc. 23:163, 1987.)

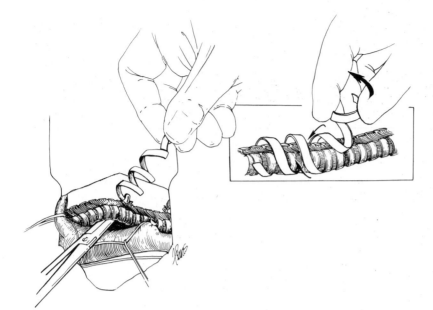

Figure 3. Application of a spiral prosthesis to the thoracic trachea. Following dissection of mediastinal fascia, a right-angle forceps is positioned medial to the trachea and one end of the prosthesis is grasped. The prosthesis is positioned on the trachea by rotating the free end (insert). Prostheses are applied to the cervical trachea in a similar manner. (Reprinted with permission from Fingland, R. B.: Tracheal collapse. *In* Bojrab, M. J. (ed.): *Current Techniques in Small Animal Surgery.* 3rd ed. Philadelphia: Lea & Febiger, in press.)

spiral cut continues down the length of the cylinder, leaving 9 mm between each cut (Fig. 2C and D). The tapered ends of the cylinder are removed (Fig. 2E and F) and a second spiral cut is made 3 mm from the first, following the same angle (Fig. 2G). The second cut divides the cylinder into a spiral with 3-mm turns and a spiral with 6-mm turns (Fig. 2H). The 3-mm spiral is removed (Fig. 2I), and the 6-mm spiral is cut in half (Fig. 2J). In this manner, three 5.5-cm-long spiral prostheses are made, each with 3-mm-wide turns separated by a 6-mm-wide space (Fig. 2K). The prostheses are gas sterilized and allowed to aerate for 24 hr before implantation.

Spiral prostheses made from the case of a 3-ml syringe are the appropriate size for the cervical trachea of most dogs weighing less than 7.5 kg. A prosthesis made from the barrel of a 3-ml syringe is the appropriate size for the thoracic trachea of dogs weighing less than 7.5 kg. Prostheses made from a 6-ml syringe barrel may be needed to support the larger cervical trachea of dogs that weigh more than 7.5 kg.

The cervical or thoracic trachea is exposed as

Figure 4. The prosthesis is sutured to the trachea with simple interrupted sutures that incorporate the prosthesis and individual cartilage rings. The sutures are tagged to facilitate rotation of the trachea for placement of additional sutures. (Reprinted with permission from Fingland *in* Bojrab (ed.): *Current Techniques in Small Animal Surgery.* 3rd ed. Philadelphia: Lea & Febiger, in press.)

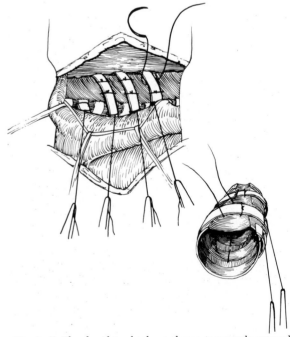

Figure 5. The dorsal tracheal membrane is securely sutured to the prosthesis. (Reprinted with permission from Fingland *in* Bojrab (ed.): *Current Techniques in Small Animal Surgery.* 3rd ed. Philadelphia: Lea & Febiger, in press.)

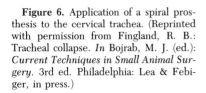

Figure 6. Application of a spiral prosthesis to the cervical trachea. (Reprinted with permission from Fingland, R. B.: Tracheal collapse. *In* Bojrab, M. J. (ed.): *Current Techniques in Small Animal Surgery.* 3rd ed. Philadelphia: Lea & Febiger, in press.)

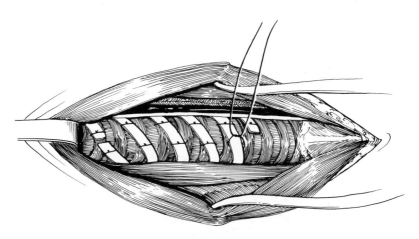

previously described. A small right-angle forceps is placed medial or dorsal to the trachea, one end of the prosthesis is grasped, and the prosthesis is directed around the trachea (Fig. 3). The prosthesis is then "turned" onto the trachea by rotating the free end (Fig. 3). The prosthesis is sutured to the trachea on the ventral, dorsal, and both lateral aspects with 4–0 polypropylene (Prolene) suture material (Fig. 4). All sutures pass through the tracheal lumen. The dorsal tracheal membrane must be securely sutured to the prosthesis (Fig. 5). The endotracheal tube should be gently manipulated within the trachea prior to closure to ensure that a suture has not been inadvertently placed through the cuff.

Spiral prostheses may be applied to the entire trachea by performing a right third intercostal space thoracotomy in conjunction with a ventral cervical midline approach (Fig. 6).

Total Ring Prosthesis Technique

Total ring prostheses are also made from the case or barrel of a polypropylene 3-ml syringe (Fig. 7). The case or barrel is cut into a 1-cm-long cylinder and a 3-mm section of the cylinder is removed, creating a C-shaped total ring prosthesis. The edges of the prosthesis are rounded and smoothed and holes are drilled to allow for passage of suture. The prostheses are gas sterilized and allowed to aerate for 24 hr before implantation.

Application of total ring prostheses begins by isolating a 1.5-cm length of trachea from the lateral pedicles, taking care to protect the left recurrent laryngeal nerve. A right-angle forceps is introduced dorsal or medial to the trachea, one end of the prosthesis is grasped, and the prosthesis is directed around the trachea (Fig. 8). The open end of the prosthesis should be positioned over the ventral

Figure 7. Technique for making total ring prostheses from a 3-ml syringe case. *A,* A 7/16 inch dowel is placed inside the syringe case for support while cutting with a pipe cutter. *B,* Holes are drilled in the total ring for sutures. *C,* A porous polypropylene total ring. (Reprinted with permission from Walker, T. L., and Hobson, H. P.: Tracheal collapse. *In* Bojrab, M. J. (ed.): *Current Techniques in Small Animal Surgery.* Philadelphia: Lea & Febiger, 1983, pp. 265–269.)

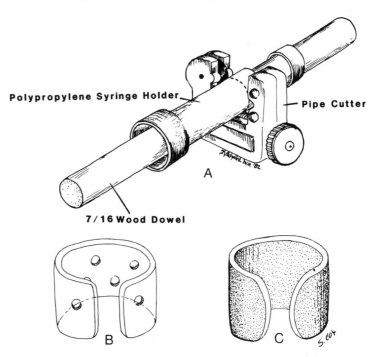

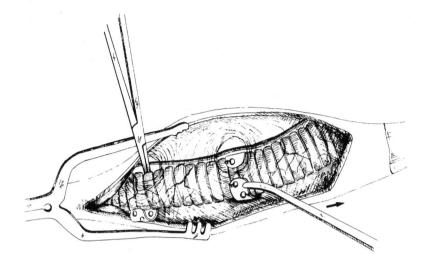

Figure 8. Application of total ring prostheses to the cervical trachea. (Reprinted with permission from Walker and Hobson *in* Bojrab (ed.): *Current Techniques in Small Animal Surgery.* Philadelphia: Lea & Febiger, 1983, pp. 265–269.)

aspect of the trachea. The prothesis is sutured to the trachea with 4–0 polypropylene (Prolene) suture material placed through the predrilled holes. Additional total ring prostheses are placed as needed, leaving approximately 1 cm between prostheses.

POSTOPERATIVE CONSIDERATIONS

The endotracheal tube is left in place with the cuff inflated until the dog has a strong swallowing reflex. The dog may be placed in a cooled, 40 per cent oxygen environment for the first few hours postoperatively. If a thoracic drainage tube was placed, it should be suctioned immediately postoperatively, hourly for 12 hr, and then as needed until pneumothorax is no longer a problem. The thoracic drainage tube should be removed 12 hr after the pneumothorax resolves.

Antibiotic therapy should be continued for 2 to 3 weeks postoperatively. Bacterial migration from the tracheal lumen through the suture tracts may lead to contamination and infection of the prostheses. Migration of tracheal mucosa over intratracheal sutures does occur, eliminating the need for long-term antibiotic therapy.

Dexamethasone (Azium) at a dose of 0.25 mg/kg should be administered intravenously immediately postoperatively and at 6 hr postoperatively to minimize tracheal mucosal swelling. Chronic or high-dose corticosteroid administration postoperatively is not indicated.

Antitussive and bronchodilator therapy is continued postoperatively as needed to control coughing. Coughing is usually severe for a period of 1 to 8 weeks postoperatively owing to tracheal irritation and mucosal swelling. Postoperative coughing must be aggressively managed because sutures may be torn out of the dorsal tracheal membrane as a result of sudden and severe changes in intratracheal pressure. The dosages of the antitussive and bronchodilator agents are gradually reduced as coughing subsides. Many dogs that have surgical correction of tracheal collapse eventually are free of clinical signs and do not require medical therapy of any type.

References and Supplemental Reading

Dallman, M. J., and Brown, E. M.: Statistical analysis of selected tracheal measurements in normal dogs and dogs with collapsed trachea. Am. J. Vet. Res. 45:1033, 1984.

Done, S. H., and Drew, R. H.: Observations on the pathology of tracheal collapse in dogs. J. Small Anim. Pract. 17:783, 1976.

Fingland, R. B.: Tracheal collapse. *In* Bojrab, M. J. (ed.): *Current Techniques in Small Animal Surgery,* 3rd ed. Philadelphia: Lea & Febiger (in press).

Fingland, R. B., DeHoff, W. D., and Birchard, S. J.: Surgical management of cervical and thoracic tracheal collapse in dogs using extraluminal spiral prostheses. J. Am. Anim. Hosp. Assoc. 23:163, 1987.

Fingland, R. B., DeHoff, W. D., and Birchard, S. J.: Surgical management of cervical and thoracic tracheal collapse in dogs using extraluminal spiral prostheses: Results in seven cases. J. Am. Anim. Hosp. Assoc. 23:173, 1987.

Hendricks, J. C., and O'Brien, J. A.: Tracheal collapse in two cats. J.A.V.M.A. 187:418, 1985.

Hobson, H. P.: Total ring prosthesis for the surgical correction of collapsed trachea. J. Am. Anim. Hosp. Assoc. 12:822, 1976.

Nelson, A. W.: Collapsing trachea. *In* Slatter, D. H. (ed.): *Textbook of Small Animal Surgery.* Philadelphia: W. B. Saunders, 1985, pp. 992–996.

O'Brien, J. A., Buchanan, J. W., and Kelly, D. F.: Tracheal collapse in the dog. J. Am. Vet. Radiol. Soc. 7:12, 1966.

Tangner, C. H., and Hobson, H. P.: A retrospective study of 20 surgically managed cases of collapsed trachea. Vet. Surg. 11:146, 1982.

Walker, T. L., and Hobson, H. P.: Trachea. *In* Bojrab, M. J. (ed.): *Current Techniques in Small Animal Surgery,* 2nd ed. Philadelphia: Lea & Febiger, 1983, pp. 265–269.

CHRONIC RESPIRATORY DISEASE IN THE DOG

JOHN D. BONAGURA, D.V.M.,
ROBERT L. HAMLIN, D.V.M.,
Columbus, Ohio

and CATHY E. GABER, D.V.M.
East Lansing, Michigan

Mature dogs are frequently afflicted with diseases of the heart, trachea, bronchial tree, and pulmonary interstitium. Although collapsing trachea, left-sided congestive heart failure (CHF), and heartworm disease can induce chronic respiratory problems in the dog, chronic bronchitis and pulmonary fibrosis are probably the most frequent causes of chronic coughing and shortness of breath in this species. Chronic bronchitis causes abnormalities of small airway function and ventilation, increased production of tracheobronchial secretions ("sputum"), and cough. Fibrosis of the lung interstitium affects pulmonary mechanics and alters ventilation-perfusion ratios in the lung, leading to chronic tachypnea. Clinical manifestations of these disorders characteristically include a long history of respiratory dysfunction; however, because initial signs of pulmonary disease may be subtle or intermittent, clients may not present their pets for evaluation until considerable disability has developed.

The clinical problems associated with small airways diseases and with pulmonary fibrosis resemble those caused by other cardiopulmonary disorders, especially chronic CHF due to mitral regurgitation. The end results of cough, cyanosis, increased lung densities, and cardiomegaly are shared by both primary cardiac and respiratory diseases. Although many cases of chronic respiratory disease can be distinguished by conducting a careful clinical examination, it is extremely difficult to attribute clinical signs to a pulmonary or cardiac origin when both conditions are present. Moreover, multiple pulmonary disorders may be diagnosed, as in cases of bronchitis, lung fibrosis, and dynamic tracheal collapse.

Little is known about the cause, prevalence, pathogenesis, or natural history of bronchitis and pulmonary interstitial disease in the dog, and a cure is rarely attained. Still, some patients benefit from symptomatic pulmonary medical therapy, and antibiotic or corticosteroid treatment reduces clinical signs markedly in some dogs. Of equal importance in the management of these cases is the assurance of a correct diagnosis and avoidance of inappropriate treatment. This article provides the authors' personal perspectives regarding identification and management of bronchitis and pulmonary fibrosis in the dog. Information detailing the clinical management of other common causes of chronic respiratory disease in the dog, including tracheal and bronchial collapse, chronic valvular disease, pneumonia, heartworm disease, and pulmonary neoplasia, can be found elsewhere in this section.

CHRONIC BRONCHITIS

Etiopathogenesis

Chronic bronchitis refers to a persistent inflammatory change in the bronchial tree that may involve lobar bronchi or the smaller airways. Chronic bronchial inflammation or irritation, regardless of cause, seems to promote the predictable responses of increased tracheobronchial secretions (sputum), cough, and progressive architectural changes in the bronchial tree with altered air flow. The morphologic changes that attend chronic bronchitis can include proliferation of goblet cells, narrowing of bronchial lumina, ectasia (or bronchiectasis) of larger airways, and alteration in the normal respiratory epithelium predisposing the airways to infection. Activation of pulmonary defense mechanisms and alteration in the cells lining the airways is anticipated and these responses have been reviewed previously (see *Current Veterinary Therapy IX*, p. 228).

The etiology of chronic bronchitis in the dog is unknown. Clearly there are cases of chronic or recurrent viral or bacterial infection that suggest an abnormality of local immunity (e.g., IgA) or in mechanical airway defense mechanisms. Chronic infection with *Bordetella bronchiseptica* should always be considered in younger dogs with lingering "kennel cough." Rare cases of bronchitis are associated with ciliary dyskinesis, and these dogs typically have recurrent bacterial sinusitis, bronchitis, and pneumonia. Environmental pollutants and hypersensitivity reactions are speculated to be causes of chronic airway irritation and injury, but it is difficult to document these etiologic factors. The relationship of chronic respiratory diseases to poor oral health is unresolved (e.g., in poodle breeds). It has been suggested that chronic or intermittent antibiotic therapy (e.g., tetracycline) combined with regular dental care may arrest or control development of chronic bronchitis in dogs, but substantive data are lacking.

Gross examination of the bronchial tree by fiberoptic bronchoscopy demonstrates hyperemia of the mucosa, mucous hypersecretion, and exudate that may plug smaller bronchi. Pathologic features of chronic bronchitis in dogs have been reviewed by Wheeldon and associates (1977) and in *Current Veterinary Therapy IX* (p. 306). Mucosal hyperemia and proliferation, with focal ulceration and squamous metaplasia, are found. The lamina propria is infiltrated by mononuclear cells and neutrophils, and the walls are edematous and may be fibrotic. It is plausible that these cells perpetuate or aggravate chronic lung disease by producing oxygen free radicals and further epithelial injury. Bronchial mucous glands and goblet cells increase in size and number. The bronchial luminal dimensions are reduced from both weakened walls and edema, contributing to decreased air flow. Mild emphysematous changes due to loss of interalveolar septae produce increased air spaces distal to terminal bronchioles. These are noted at the periphery of the lung. Although mild changes have little functional significance, severe alterations cause obstruction to flow. Bronchiectasis, pneumonia, pulmonary fibrosis, and large airways disease may be found in some cases (Fig. 1).

Pulmonary function testing in dogs with chronic bronchitis has been limited to occasional case reports; however, induced bronchitis in dogs causes chronic air flow obstruction. In addition to causing ventilation-perfusion inequalities in the lung, the small airway obstruction leads to increased work of breathing, which can be compounded by dynamic, expiratory collapse of the large airways and lead to mucus trapping peripherally. Lobar bronchi and the intrathoracic trachea may totally collapse during forced expiration or with coughing (Fig. 2). These and other factors believed to be important in the pathophysiology of chronic canine bronchitis have been reviewed (see *Current Veterinary Therapy IX*, p. 307).

The sputum obtained via tracheal or bronchial washings from affected lobes can provide insight about the type of inflammatory process (see *Current Veterinary Therapy IX*, p. 243). Normally a small number of neutrophils, alveolar macrophages, epithelial and goblet cells (more likely with bronchial brushings), and a rare lymphocyte or eosinophil are found. Cytologic findings in most dogs with chronic bronchitis are nonspecific and are characterized by a mixed inflammatory cell population dominated by the neutrophil, with reactive epithelial cells, some eosinophils, and macrophages also being present. Intracellular bacteria are found in some cases, but the majority of specimens are sterile. A mucopurulent, suppurative inflammation with intracellular bacteria is found in some affected dogs, particularly younger dogs, with chronic infective tracheobronchitis. In some patients, the tracheobronchial sputum is sterile but is characterized by an increased number of cells, predominated by the eosinophil and reactive epithelial cells. These findings are suggestive of an allergic etiology, hypersensitivity, or parasitic infection.

Clinical Findings

The typical signalment of dogs with chronic noninfective bronchitis is an adult dog of a small or medium-sized breed. Chronic infective tracheobronchitis is more common in young dogs. Regardless of etiology, a cough is the hallmark of chronic bronchitis and is usually progressive in nature. Clinical findings in dogs with chronic noninfective bronchitis include dry or productive cough (the sputum is swallowed), tachypnea, shortness of breath with exercise, and intermittent expectoration or gagging ("vomiting"). Wheezing may be evident following exertion. Small and medium-sized dog breeds are most often involved. Except in cases of persistent infective tracheobronchitis, which is more common in dogs younger than 1 year of age, the dog tends to be mature. Frequently, the pet has coughed for years prior to the owner's seeking veterinary help. The cough often is worsened with exercise and may be severe at variable times of the day. Severely affected dogs become cyanotic with exertion and may faint after coughing (cough syncope). Appetite generally is unaffected, thus, anorexia or marked depression in the dog with chronic bronchitis may suggest intercurrent respiratory tract infection or pneumonia.

The *physical examination* reveals a dog that is well fleshed, except in advanced cases, and cough is usually elicited on palpation of the trachea or during excitement. Tracheal sensitivity is a nonspecific finding and does not indicate a primary diagnosis of tracheitis, or "kennel-cough." The respiratory rate may be increased and shortness of breath may be severe, particularly in dogs with concurrent pulmonary fibrosis. The dog may appear to be "barrel chested," and some patients exhibit cyanosis with dyspnea during both inspiration and expiration.

Auscultation of the lungs is somewhat more challenging than cardiac auscultation. However, there

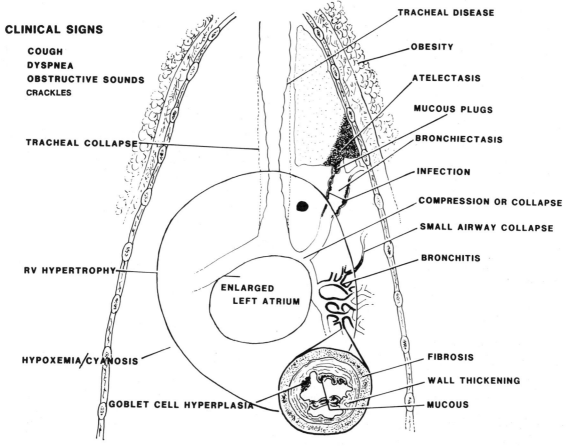

CLINICAL SIGNS

COUGH
DYSPNEA
OBSTRUCTIVE SOUNDS
CRACKLES

TRACHEAL COLLAPSE

RV HYPERTROPHY

HYPOXEMIA/CYANOSIS

GOBLET CELL HYPERPLASIA

ENLARGED LEFT ATRIUM

TRACHEAL DISEASE

OBESITY

ATELECTASIS

MUCOUS PLUGS

BRONCHIECTASIS

INFECTION

COMPRESSION OR COLLAPSE

SMALL AIRWAY COLLAPSE

BRONCHITIS

FIBROSIS

WALL THICKENING

MUCOUS

Figure 1. Important components responsible for chronic respiratory diseases in the dog. One or more of these abnormalities may be evident in a given patient. Lesions are indicated at the right and bottom; effects on the patient and clinical signs are shown at the left.

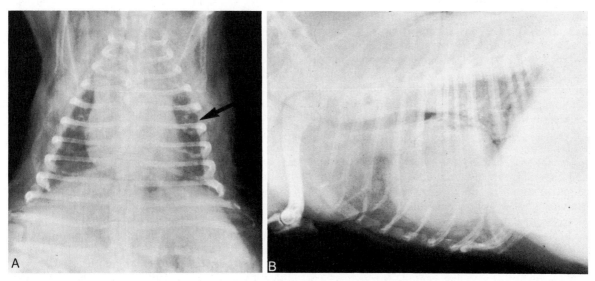

Figure 2. Thoracic radiographs from an obese dog with chronic respiratory disease. Subcutaneous and mediastinal fat are prominent. The right side of the heart appears to be enlarged. Pulmonary densities are generally increased, in part owing to an inability to attain full inspiration. *A*, The lateral borders of the lung appear to be retracted from the thoracic wall (arrow). *B*, The lateral view is expiratory and demonstrates dynamic tracheal collapse at the level of the cranial thorax.

are several simple maneuvers that can be performed to enhance the information available. First, it is important that auscultation be done while the dog is breathing deeply, as abnormal lung sounds (especially crackles) may be overlooked if the lung is not adequately expanded. To accomplish this, the mouth should be closed to prevent referral of tracheal sounds to the thorax. If necessary, the nostrils should be occluded for 10 to 15 seconds to force the dog to inspire deeply.

Auscultatory findings are quite variable and nonspecific. Some dogs have wheezing due to mucous plugging and dynamic expiratory collapse of intrathoracic airways. In advanced cases bilateral crackles will be evident during inspiration and possibly expiration. These crackles are frequently louder than those heard with pulmonary edema of CHF. A snapping sound heard over the trachea or the carina is suggestive of collapsing of the trachea or mainstem bronchus. In most cases, the heart sounds are normal, permitting the clinician to virtually eliminate valvular heart disease from the differential diagnosis.

The *thoracic radiograph* is abnormal in most cases. Typical findings include increased interstitial density with prominent peribronchial infiltrates (see Fig. 2). It may be difficult to distinguish these findings from normal aging changes of the canine thorax. Variable degrees of bronchiectasis may be evident. Aerophagia is common. Cranial and middle lung lobe consolidation or alveolar infiltrates indicate a complicating bacterial pneumonia. In some dogs, the right middle lung lobe is atelectatic from bronchial plugging and resorption of gas. The overall volume of the lung is usually normal for the breed and size of the patient; however, in some dogs there is gas trapping with pulmonary overinflation ("emphysema") causing a barrel-chested appearance. In other cases, retraction of the lung borders, typical of diffuse pulmonary fibrosis, is observed (see Fig. 2). Dynamic expiratory collapse of a lobar bronchus or the intrathoracic trachea is not uncommon. It is not surprising to find apparent cardiomegaly in dogs with chronic respiratory tract disease, but this finding should not be overinterpreted (see discussion of differential diagnosis in the following section).

Tracheobronchial cytology and culture should be done in all cases of chronic bronchitis. Sputum samples may be obtained by a transtracheal washing, via a sterile endotracheal tube, or during bronchoscopic examination. The authors prefer a transtracheal washing using either a large-bore intravenous through-the-needle catheter (Sovereign catheter, 14 or 17 gauge, 8 to 14 inches in length), or a 14-gauge intravascular cannula through which a 3.5-French (F) polyethylene urinary catheter is passed into the tracheal lumen. It is helpful to lightly sedate some patients to prevent struggling

(acepromazine, 0.1 to 0.15 mg/kg SC 30 min prior to the procedure, or diazepam, 2.5 to 5.0 mg IV 10 min prior to the procedure) and to restrain the dog in a standing or sitting position. Following tranquilization and administration of local anesthesia, most mature dogs tolerate the procedure well, and tracheobronchial secretions (sputum) are reliably obtained in this manner unless the cough is nonproductive. Intractable dogs, puppies with chronic infective tracheobronchitis, or older dogs who will undergo subsequent dental procedures can be lightly anesthetized with a thiobarbiturate or with intravenous ketamine-diazepam (Valium) combination, then intubated carefully with a *sterile* endotracheal tube. Subsequently, the tracheobronchial tree can be lavaged using a sterile male urinary catheter, which has been advanced through the endotracheal tube. Two major disadvantages of this technique are inadequate cough due to anesthesia and pooling of lavaged secretions in the endotracheal tube. Greater yield of sputum can be obtained using constant suction and a mucous trap during gentle movement of the catheter in the airways.

Bronchoscopy can be used to obtain a sample of the tracheobronchial sputum, provided a sterilized bronchoscopic port is available to obtain samples. Typical bronchoscopic features of chronic bronchitis include hyperemia and friability of the bronchial mucosa, increased quantity of mucus that must be cleared from the bronchoscope to permit further visualization, mucoid plaques, roughening of the surface, occlusion of airways with exudate and mucus, and variable degrees of airway collapse. Mucosal redundancy and polypoid structures also may be found. Bronchoscopy permits a detailed evaluation of the airways; but it is not an essential part of the workup for all cases. However, direct airway visualization is helpful in the diagnosis of focal lung disease, bronchial foreign bodies, presence of lung parasites, endobronchial tumors, and hemoptysis and in equivocal cases of tracheal or bronchial collapse.

The sputum sample is cultured aerobically for bacteria, sensitivity testing is done, and a cytofuge preparation is evaluated for abnormal cellularity. As previously mentioned, samples can be crudely classified as (1) suppurative or septic, (2) hypersensitivity reaction (eosinophilic), and (3) nonspecific inflammation or irritation. Some cases of chronic bronchitis have a superimposed bacterial infection, which may lead to an acute exacerbation of the disease. Viral isolation, though difficult to obtain, might provide insight concerning the development of these problems. Frequently nonresistant organisms like *Pasteurella* spp. are cultured, but it is difficult to assess the overall significance of this type of isolate to the bronchial disorder. Bacteria cultured from young dogs with chronic tracheobronchitis or from mature dogs with concurrent bronchiectasis or pneumonia are more likely to be significant, and these have been described (see *Current Veterinary Therapy IX*, p. 247). Following tracheal washing, and with consideration of the sputum cytology, Gram's stain results, and prior antibiotic treatment, the patient is given trimethoprim-sulfonamide, cephalexin, or another broad-spectrum antibiotic such as tetracycline pending culture results.

Other laboratory tests may be helpful in assessing the heart and lungs. The *electrocardiogram* (ECG) generally is normal in dogs with chronic bronchitis. Pronounced sinus arrhythmia (with increased heart rate during inspiration), a wandering atrial pacemaker, and peaked P waves (P pulmonale) are typical and, rarely, right axis deviation is present. Premature ventricular complexes may be observed. Some dogs have increased QRS voltages (R wave > 3.0 mV in leads II and aVF) for unexplained reasons. The *hemogram* frequently is normal, and it is emphasized that a normal white blood cell count (WBC) does *not* rule out bronchitis or respiratory infection. Neutrophilia or monocytosis may indicate bacterial pneumonia, whereas peripheral eosinophilia is found only in a small percentage of dogs with sputum compatible with "allergic bronchitis." Mild polycythemia (possibly from chronic hypoxia) may be encountered in some dogs; however, the elevation of the packed cell volume (PCV) also may be caused by inappropriate diuretic therapy and dehydration.

The *arterial blood gas analysis* is variable but most commonly demonstrates arterial hypoxemia that improves partially after oxygenation, hypocapnia, and a mixed metabolic acidosis and respiratory alkalosis. If respiratory failure (PO_2 < 60 mm Hg, increased PCO_2) ensues, the arterial carbon dioxide pressure will be increased, and artificial ventilation and vigorous medical therapy will be necessary.

PULMONARY INTERSTITIAL DISEASE

Etiopathogenesis

The causes and mechanisms for the spontaneous development of pulmonary fibrosis in the dog have not been identified. Because fibrosis is the end result of previous tissue injury, attention needs to be directed to the underlying inflammatory process in dogs with progressive interstitial disease. It is quite likely that severe, diffuse lung fibrosis in middle-aged and older dogs is preceded by multifocal alveolitis similar to that associated with chronic pulmonary fibrosis in humans and reproduced experimentally in dogs.

In human patients with interstitial lung diseases the principal lesions are found not only within the alveolar septum, but in the alveolar epithelial and endothelial cells as well. Lesions of the small airways, arteries, and veins also may be found. The pathogenesis of these lesions has been reviewed extensively (see supplemental reading), but the essential pathophysiology is believed to be injury stimulus or allergen causing alveolitis, resulting in derangement of alveolar structures, which causes loss of functional alveolocapillary units with end stage fibrosis. Effector cells, including neutrophils and mononuclear cells, are found in increased numbers in the affected tissue and in bronchoalveolar washes. Noncardiogenic pulmonary edema is found in acute cases. Fibrosis is diffuse but discrete and frequently is not adequately assessed by small transbronchoscopic biopsies. About two thirds of cases of pulmonary interstitial disease in humans are idiopathic; yet, there are over 100 known agents that can incite alveolitis and fibrosis in humans. Because many of these include inorganic and organic dusts, gases and vapors, drugs, and infectious agents, as well as chronic lung edema and chronic uremia, it is likely some dogs are exposed to similar potential risks. In animal models of pulmonary interstitial disease, alveolitis also precedes development of fibrosis.

Clinical Findings

The typical features of pulmonary fibrosis in dogs resemble those of human patients. There is usually a long and progressive history of shortness of breath. Small terrier breeds may be predisposed. Coughing can be slight or remarkably absent, except in cases of combined fibrosis with bronchitis. The most significant physical examination finding is bilateral, ventral, end-inspiratory and early-expiratory crackles that are most evident on full inspiration. In advanced cases, crackles are audible without a stethoscope. Forcing exercise usually results in tachypnea or gasping and often provokes cyanosis. If there is intercurrent bronchitis, physical findings may be similar to those previously described. Physical examination findings in dogs with pulmonary fibrosis can be quite subtle, and careful auscultation is required.

Radiography and Laboratory Studies

When considering the radiographic changes with this type of disease, it is important to realize that good film quality is essential, as several technical factors affect the amount of interstitial infiltrates that will be perceived. Expiratory films and obesity will increase overall lung density. The amount of lung density compatible with normal aging is poorly quantified. The reader is referred to *Current Vet-*

erinary Therapy IX (p. 257) for salient aspects of radiographic interpretation.

The typical patient demonstrates moderate cardiomegaly that may indicate cor pulmonale or incomplete thoracic expansion. A mild diffuse increase in interstitial lung densities is generally evident throughout the lung. Retraction of the peripheral lung edges from the ribs may be evident (see Fig. 2), and the diaphragm may be flat with poor lung expansion in some cases. In cases of concurrent bronchial disease, findings are as previously discussed.

The hemogram is almost always normal. Arterial blood gas determination is a sensitive method for verifying the presence of significant lung disease. In cases of necropsy-documented pulmonary fibrosis, arterial hypoxemia (generally in the range of 65 to 85 mm Hg) that improves when the dog is given 100 per cent oxygen by face mask and hypocapnia are found. Tracheal washes are *unlikely* to be useful if the patient is only short of breath and does not have a productive cough.

An open lung biopsy is the diagnostic method of choice to document alveolitis and lung fibrosis. However, biopsies may be difficult to perform in dogs with severe pulmonary dysfunction because of the potential anesthetic risk. Moreover, clients may not consent to this invasive procedure. When lung biopsy is not feasible, a fine-needle lung aspiration cytology is useful for identifying the cause of diffuse increases in pulmonary density related to neoplasia or infection (e.g., systemic mycosis).

The clinical experience of one of the authors (JDB) suggests that in dogs with typical historical, auscultatory, radiographic, and blood gas findings, it is likely that bronchoscopy can establish the diagnosis of alveolitis-fibrosis. Provided there is no significant bronchitis (absence of productive cough and lack of bronchial erythema and mucous hypersecretion at endoscopy), bronchoalveolar lavage can be used to obtain samples from the alveoli and to diagnose lower airway inflammation. Under direct visualization one wedges a bronchoscope in four to six bronchi and lavages each lung segment with normal saline. The lavage fluid, which is obtained from at least three different lobes, is pooled and centrifuged, and the sediment is examined by a pathologist both for cellularity and for percentage distribution of cells. Studies by Rebar and associates (1980) and Brown and coworkers (1983) have indicated that normal dogs have a predominance of alveolar macrophages and a low neutrophil count (typically less than 12 per cent). Dogs with alveolitis/ fibrosis typically have neutrophil counts exceeding 20 per cent. Again, it is emphasized that additional lung biopsy cases are needed to document this relationship and that bronchoalveolar lavage is not valuable if the dog has intercurrent bronchitis, as upper airway secretions contaminate the obtained fluid.

DIFFERENTIAL DIAGNOSIS

Diagnostic considerations in dogs with chronic respiratory signs include a variety of cardiopulmonary problems. Many dogs with chronic lung disease are overweight, whereas chronic congestive heart failure and pulmonary neoplasia often result in considerable weight loss. The absence of a cardiac murmur in a small breed dog allows chronic left-sided CHF from mitral disease to be excluded as a diagnosis. Echocardiography can identify the unusual case of dilated cardiomyopathy encountered in small breed dogs. A common error is to overestimate the heart size on the chest x-ray film in a patient with chronic bronchitis of interstitial lung disease. Possible reasons for cardiomegaly in these cases include cor pulmonale (right-sided heart enlargement from lung disease), increased intrapericardial fat, concurrent valvular disease, or inadequate pulmonary expansion, which artificially increases the cardiothoracic ratio. It is essential to integrate the results of radiography and the physical examination findings, as the absence of a cardiac murmur in small breed dogs virtually rules out valvular heart disease and congestive heart failure.

Primary respiratory conditions to be considered and ruled out include primary tracheal and bronchial collapse, pulmonary neoplasia, bacterial and fungal pneumonia, heartworm disease, bronchial foreign body, pulmonary granulomatosis and infiltrates of eosinophils, and uremic pneumonitis. This is readily accomplished by combining physical examination results with those from radiographs and hematologic tests. It is worthwhile to consult a radiologist or cardiologist in difficult-to-diagnose cases.

THERAPY

Therapy of chronic bronchitis is guided by the cytologic evaluation and culture of the tracheobronchial secretions (sputum), by the extent of radiographic changes (e.g., in pneumonia), and by response to therapy. Chronic, intermittent antibiotic or corticosteroid therapy, combined with the use of bronchodilators, administration of antitussives, and supportive care of the respiratory system form the basis for long-term therapy. Rarely is a cure obtained; however, significant improvement of clinical signs does occur in most dogs. Patients with advanced changes, including bronchiectasis or lobar atelectasis, generally respond poorly to medical therapy.

GENERAL MEASURES

There are treatments that may be helpful to dogs with chronic bronchitis regardless of cause. Obesity is a problem inasmuch as diaphragmatic function is impaired, small airways close earlier than normal, and ventilation may be impeded. Weight reduction using a diet such as Prescription Diet r/d (Hill's Pet Products) is recommended and should be accomplished over a 2 to 3 month period. If a restraint collar is worn, it should be replaced by a harness to decrease airway irritation. Environmental stresses, including house dust, vapors, chemical fumes, and tobacco smoke, should be avoided. Inhalation of humidified air, via a vaporizer or nebulizer, may liquefy secretions. The pet should be coupaged or exercised lightly following these procedures and encouraged to cough.

The use of *cough suppressants* varies on a case-by-case basis. In dogs with nonbacterial bronchitis, breaking the cough cycle is an essential part of treatment. Initial treatment with codeine derivatives (Tussinex or Hycodan, 2.5 to 5 mg q 8 to 12 hr PO) is often effective. The dosage can gradually be reduced and the lowest effective dose used. Sedation is a common side effect and may actually be beneficial if the pet develops coughing during stressful social situations. Butorphenol (Torbutrol) can also be prescribed but is less potent for reducing cough.

Bronchodilator drugs include the xanthine derivatives and the beta₂-agonists (see *Current Veterinary Therapy IX*, p. 278). Theophylline and its various salts are most commonly chosen. The authors prefer aminophylline, long-acting theophylline (Theo-Dur), or oxtriphylline (Choledyl) as initial therapy. The dosage, which must be adjusted to each patient, is usually between 6 and 10 mg/kg q 8 hr. Serum concentrations of theophylline, obtained after 1 week of therapy, can be used to guide dosage adjustment. Some dogs cannot tolerate the adverse effects, which include anxiety, restlessness, tachycardia, and emesis. The beta₂-agonist terbutaline (Brethine) can be given as an alternative agent to dogs without heart disease. The usual dose is 2.5 to 5 mg q 8 hr PO. Adverse effects are similar to those caused by the xanthines. A lower dose of terbutaline, combined with a low dose of aminophylline (2 to 5 mg/kg q 8 hr) may be used in some dogs who cannot tolerate full doses of either drug. Controlled studies supporting the use of bronchodilators are lacking; however, some dogs appear to benefit from long-term treatment, and other patients experiencing acute exacerbations of bronchitis may improve following bronchodilation. Bronchodilators also may increase the vigor of contraction of the respiratory muscles, which may be useful in dogs with chronic dyspnea.

Treatment of oral cavity infections is prudent in dogs with chronic bronchitis. As previously stated, the relationship, if any, between oral and respiratory tract infection cannot be proved but some dogs improve following dental procedures and treatment

with antibiotics. A tracheal wash can be obtained during induction of anesthesia, thereby permitting examination of tracheobronchial secretions. At that time, intravenous antibiotics (e.g., cephalothin) can be given and the dental procedures can be completed.

Anti-inflammatory therapy using prednisolone or prednisone is most effective in the dog with nonbacterial bronchitis and is most useful in the treatment of eosinophilic bronchitis (discussed below).

BACTERIAL INFECTION

Dogs with chronic bronchitis have generally received previous courses of antibiotics. In the patient with primary bacterial tracheobronchitis, or in the dog with complicating bacterial infection, a good response is obtained if the organism is susceptible to the chosen drug. In many dogs, however, antibiotic treatment causes little improvement, presumably owing to a nonbacterial cause or lack of suitable culture and sensitivity testing. Bacterial infection should be suspected in any of the following situations: (1) acute exacerbation of cough in a patient with previously stable chronic bronchitis, particularly when the cough is associated with anorexia, mucopurulent nasal discharge, or fever; (2) radiographic evidence of bronchiectasis or lobar consolidation/atelectasis; (3) recurrent signs of bronchitis in a previously documented case of bacterial tracheobronchitis; or (4) severe periodontal or dental disease, (5) leukocytosis with left shift.

Antibiotic treatment in these situations should be guided by culture of tracheobronchial secretions. As previously mentioned, following tracheal washing, cytologic study and Gram's stain should be done and the patient should be given amoxicillin, trimethoprim-sulfonamide, cephalothin or cefalexin, or another broad-spectrum antibiotic such as tetracycline pending culture results. Antibiotic treatment should continue for 2 to 3 weeks. Some dogs develop a recurrent bacterial bronchitis that responds well to antibiotic treatment until a relapse occurs. Especially in younger dogs, this may indicate a mixed infection with an unusual or resistant microorganism (e.g., mycobacterium), anatomic lesion of a bronchus, endobronchial foreign body, a lack of local immunity, or abnormal cilia. Such animals should be cultured and undergo bronchoscopy, particularly if a single lung lobe remains infiltrated or pneumonic. In dogs with bacterial bronchitis or pneumonia, breathing of humidified air or nebulization, combined with coupage of the chest, is indicated to mobilize secretions. Bronchodilators should be used to prevent reflex bronchospasm to nebulized fluid, and cough suppressants should be avoided.

When *Bordetella bronchiseptica* is cultured, the

use of gentamicin nebulization should be considered. This can be administered via an anesthetic face mask by interfacing a glass nebulizer (Devilbiss model #40) with the oxygen output line of a gas anesthetic machine. Gentamicin (2 to 6 mg/kg) is mixed with 0.5 ml of saline and placed in the nebulization pot, and 1 to 3 L/min of oxygen is used to transport the solution into the face mask. Therapy is given twice daily for 5 days. Current data indicate that gentamicin is not absorbed systemically from the lung.

EOSINOPHILIC BRONCHITIS

Presumably, bronchitis associated with eosinophilia represents a hypersensitivity reaction. For detailed discussions of these problems, see pages 369 to 376. Most dogs with "allergic" bronchitis respond well to decreasing doses of prednisone. An initial dose of 0.5 to 1 mg/kg PO q 12 hr is given for 10 to 14 days. The daily dose is then tapered over the next month. Some dogs require pulsed monthly therapy (1 week per month) or alternate-day treatment to maintain remission. The adverse effects of prednisone should be explained to the owner. Treatment with bronchodilators, cough suppressants, and antibiotics when indicated is an additional measure that can be taken. The response to treatment varies, with some pets making near-recoveries and others requiring relatively high doses of medication throughout their lives.

NONSPECIFIC CHRONIC BRONCHITIS

Treatment of most cases of bronchitis involves combinations of the aforementioned medications. Typically, antibiotics are used during exacerbations of coughing or when there is an indication of developing or recurrent infection as described above. Long-term therapy with codeine cough suppressants and xanthine bronchodilators is prescribed. Prednisone is often the most effective treatment and is given as for cases of eosinophilic bronchitis. Prednisone and cough suppressants must be discontinued if there is clinical evidence of bacterial infection.

IDIOPATHIC PULMONARY FIBROSIS

Treatment is frustrating inasmuch as the underlying cause of alveolitis is rarely determined or controlled, and therapy does not reverse pre-existent fibrosis. If the animal is exposed to dusts or fumes, these should be eliminated. Obesity, if evident, should be controlled. Because many drugs are associated with pulmonary fibrosis in humans, current medications should be scrutinized and the drug insert carefully read relative to adverse pulmonary effects. A trial course of bronchodilators using sustained-release theophylline, aminophylline, or oxtriphylline should be considered, as small airway function may be compromised and these drugs also may increase diaphragmatic contractility. The patient is treated initially with immunosuppressive doses of prednisone (1 mg/kg PO q 12 hr) for 2 weeks, and the dose is then tapered over the next month. This will not reverse the pre-existing fibrosis but may decrease ongoing alveolitis. Long-term treatment is empiric, but the authors have used pulsed prednisone (1 mg/kg q 12 hr for 1 week per month) for some cases. The benefits, if any, of cyclophosphamide have not been evaluated in the dog, but it is commonly used in humans with pulmonary fibrosis. Serial blood gas determinations and bronchoalveolar lavage cytologic studies can be used to monitor therapy and course; however, most clients refuse this type of follow-up.

References and Supplemental Reading

Brown, N. O., Noone, K. E., and Kurzman, I. D.: Alveolar lavage in dogs. Am. J. Vet. Res. 44:335, 1983.

Crystal, R. G., Bitterman, P. B., Rennard, S. I., et al.: Interstitial lung diseases of unknown cause, Parts I and II. N. Engl. J. Med. 310:154, 235, 1984.

Dungworth, D. L.: Interstitial pulmonary diseases. Adv. Vet. Sci. Comp. Med. 26:173, 1982.

Rebar, A. H., DeNicola, D. B., and Muggenberg, B. A.: Bronchopulmonary lavage cytology in the dog: Normal findings. Vet. Pathol. 17:294, 1980.

Reif, J. S., and Rhodes, W. H.: The lungs of aged dogs: A radiographic-morphologic correlation. J. Am. Vet. Radiol. Soc. 7:5, 1966.

Reynolds, H. Y.: Bronchoalveolar lavage. Am. Rev. Respir. Dis. 135:250, 1987.

Wheeldon, E. B., Pirie, H. M., Fisher, E. W., et al.: Chronic respiratory disease in the dog. J. Small Anim. Pract. 18:229, 1977.

Zinkl, J. G.: Cytology of respiratory tract disease. Semin. Vet. Med. Surg. 1:302, 1986.

PULMONARY HYPERSENSITIVITY DISORDERS

TIMOTHY BAUER, D.V.M.

Seattle, Washington

This article deals with many of the disorders of pulmonary hypersensitivity. The understanding of pulmonary immunology and its association with these disorders is poor in humans and has largely been uninvestigated in animals. It has been assumed that there are basic similarities between humans and animals; that the lungs' response to antigen-antibody interaction is similar; and that they both potentially may exhibit similar abnormal responses to extrinsic and intrinsic events.

Specific discussions of the immune mechanisms of lung injury and basic pulmonary immunology are not included in this article; the reader is referred to sections of this text that specifically deal with these phenomena. Likewise, there is considerable overlap among disorders considered to represent primary pulmonary hypersensitivities and other diseases with concomitant immunologically mediated processes. Immunologic disorders, such as systemic lupus erythematosus, rheumatoid arthritis, serologically negative immunologic polyarthritis, amyloidosis, and glomerulonephritis, may episodically have pulmonary or pleural manifestations ranging from incidental findings to the primary signs for which the client seeks medical attention. As with the primary pulmonary hypersensitivities, the mechanisms of pulmonary involvement are poorly understood. The clinician should be alerted to the presence of these problems, as they may frequently masquerade as infectious pulmonary disorders with the associated signs of fever, dyspnea, adenopathy, pulmonary infiltrates, and pleural effusion.

PULMONARY EOSINOPHILIA

Pleuropulmonary disorders affecting the pleural space, the airways, or the pulmonary parenchyma with associated circulating or tissue eosinophilia are collectively referred to as eosinophilic lung disease or pulmonary eosinophilia. These terms refer to diverse disorders that have previously been grouped together with diagnoses such as pulmonary infiltrates with eosinophilia or asthma. These classifications have led to much confusion, as they suggest the presence of blood eosinophilia, radiographically demonstrable infiltrates, or airway eosinophilia; these findings are not consistently present. The eosinophilia of these disorders varies in magnitude and may involve the blood or the pleuropulmonary structures. Although this would suggest an allergic or hypersensitivity etiology, frequently no specific mechanism can be definitely implicated. As the common feature of these disorders is the presence of tissue or blood eosinophilia, a wide variety of both intrinsic or extrinsic influences may be implicated. The subdivision of these disorders into clinical groups is of more than semantic interest, rather such division provides a framework for both recognition and guidelines for therapy. This is important, because disorders of pulmonary eosinophilia vary widely in their severity, ranging from lethal to completely benign.

It needs to be emphasized that not all patients with pulmonary involvement and eosinophilia have associated disease, i.e., the finding of blood eosinophilia may be totally unrelated. The mere presence of eosinophilia should not automatically lead to the diagnosis of pulmonary eosinophilia, as there are many noneosinophilic disorders, such as bacterial pneumonia, fungal infections, and metastatic neoplasms, that may occur in the patient with circulating eosinophilia due to an unrelated cause such as parasitism or atopy.

Transitory or Simple Pulmonary Eosinophilia (Löffler's Syndrome)

This syndrome of transient pulmonary eosinophilia is characterized by small patchy or nodular infiltrates, which may spontaneously resolve, and frequently is associated with blood eosinophilia, which is likewise transient. The diagnosis is suggested by the radiographic recognition of single or multiple infiltrates, which may resolve and migrate on serial radiographic examinations. As previously suggested, blood eosinophilia is variable, but bronchial secretions are loaded with eosinophils.

This syndrome may be observed in the absence of a known intrinsic or extrinsic agent. When a known cause is present, such as pharmacologic (drug hypersensitivity) or infectious agents, withdrawal of drugs or treatment of infections usually leads to spontaneous resolution. Little is known about the

369

pathologic sequelae of this disorder, as its course frequently is benign.

The clinical manifestations are variable with a significant number of patients being asymptomatic. This group is usually identified by radiographic evaluation during the course of medical workup for eosinophilia of unknown etiology. A dry or mildly productive cough may be the only clinical sign reported. Typically, these patients feel well, and there is no associated fever, shortness of breath, or weight loss.

If a potentially offending drug is recognized, withdrawal is advisable. Specific therapy may not be necessary, as by definition the clinical course is benign and self-limiting. If significant cough is reported, short-term corticosteroid therapy may be advisable, as these patients should respond promptly.

Chronic Eosinophilic Pneumonia or Prolonged Pulmonary Eosinophilia

This group of parenchymal disorders is distinguished from transitory pulmonary eosinophilia by both greater severity and longer duration. As with transitory pulmonary eosinophilia, there may be no known intrinsic or extrinsic cause. The author has observed two canine patients whose disease appeared following documented clostridial sepsis. Historically, some feline patients may have had cough with unremarkable radiographic evaluations, suggesting the possibility of concurrent bronchitic pulmonary eosinophilia.

Lung biopsy findings are somewhat variable, and there is some species difference, as well as differences related to chronicity. Typically, the histologic findings are the flooding of the alveoli with eosinophils, lymphocytes, and histiocytes, and there may be associated interstitial pneumonia with similar cellular elements. With chronicity, there may be proliferation of macrophages and fibrosis. Patients may have diffuse findings of bronchiolitis obliterans. If biopsy is done late in the disease course, feline patients may have fewer eosinophils and more fibrosis than their canine counterparts. Likewise, cats may have little or no eosinophilia in bronchial secretions, whereas dogs frequently have large numbers.

Radiographically, the findings are similar to those of transient pulmonary eosinophilia with single or multiple, unilateral or bilateral infiltrates. Lesions are frequently confined to the pulmonary periphery, and it is the author's impression that canine patients tend to have more frequent involvement of multiple lobes with a global distribution; infiltrates may appear more nodular than those in feline patients. Cats appear to have a predeliction for caudal lobe involvement that may have a patchy or ground glass appearance. Cats have more frequent unilateral findings. In advanced disease, there may be evidence of air trapping and increased lung volumes. Cats may develop pleural effusions and rarely pulmonary cavitation as a sequela to long-standing disease.

Clinically, patients with prolonged pulmonary eosinophilia are typically ill; there frequently are associated fever, anorexia, weight loss, and shortness of breath. Cough appears consistently in dogs but is variable in cats, and appears to be directly proportional to airway involvement. Severe hypoxemia requiring oxygen therapy appears to be unusual and is usually the result of chronic untreated disease or concurrent bacterial pneumonia.

As the underlying cause is unknown, treatment consists of corticosteroid therapy, which is usually responsible for a rapid and complete resolution of clinical signs, pulmonary infiltrates, and blood eosinophilia. Radiographic resolution may lag behind clinical resolution by 1 to 2 weeks. Patients frequently require 1 month or more of alternate-day therapy following initial "high-dose" therapy. Early withdrawal of steroids or the use of repository injections may precipitate a relapse. Frequently, patients are sicker when they relapse and may require hospitalization for high-dose, pulsed corticosteroid infusions.

Bronchitic Pulmonary Eosinophilia or Canine and Feline Asthma

This is a poorly defined broad clinical syndrome of the small airways characterized by an increased responsiveness of the tracheobronchial tree to a variety of allergens and other unrecognized agents. This presumed bronchospastic activity is reversible and episodic. Although blood eosinophilia is variable, eosinophils in bronchial secretions are a consistent finding. Airway edema and copious eosinophilic bronchial secretions may contribute to airway obstruction. These changes are responsible for the signs of cough and shortness of breath and are typically reversible, either spontaneously or with medical intervention.

The etiology of bronchitic pulmonary eosinophilia is unknown. Although the importance of an allergic etiology has been implicated, there is no comprehensive research that links specific allergens to this disorder. There are probably multiple factors potentially capable of provoking clinical signs.

Histopathologic evaluation of this disorder is infrequent. Rarely is lung biopsy indicated in this patient population; most information is obtained from postmortem examination of those few individuals that expire of their disease or that are euthanatized during acute exacerbations. Necropsy findings in these patients may not be representative of the general population. Typically, airways are found to be plugged with exudate consisting of inflammatory cells, mucus, and epithelium. Infiltration of peribronchiolar tissue with inflammatory cells may be marked by hypertrophy of bronchial smooth muscle and secretory glands.

Clinical signs may be isolated to the bronchial tree or disseminated. Although most patients, both canine and feline, have cough or shortness of breath, a significant number have associated clinical syndromes of allergic rhinitis, allergic dermatopathy, or atopy. Respiratory signs are variable and frequently change throughout the course of this disorder. Cough appears to be a consistent finding in dogs; shortness of breath may be apparent in advanced cases or when there is superimposed respiratory infection. Conversely, cats tend to have respiratory distress more frequently than their canine counterparts, and cough is a frequent but variable finding. Feline patients tend to have individual patterns to their illnesses; some have only cough without any history of dyspnea, whereas others have virtually no cough, but profound dyspnea. These findings may be referable to individual differences in the degree of bronchospasm, airway exudation, and functional airway obstruction.

The physical findings associated with bronchitic pulmonary eosinophilia are frequently striking. When crackles (rales) are auscultable, they are typically global, and they have the characteristic sound of separating Velcro. Audible ("moist") high-pitched crackling may be present during oral examination; this may be pronounced in dogs. In severely dyspneic patients with significant airway obstruction, there may be no auscultable crackles or wheezes. Bronchospasm may promote visible prolongation of expiration, and there may be increased use of accessory respiratory muscles. Changes in behavior, ranging from apparent anxiety to frantic thrashing in some cats, may be a prominent feature. Salivation and open mouth breathing with associated aerophagia and gastric distention may be present in patients *in extremis*.

Radiographic evaluation is variable and largely depends on the degree of airway obstruction or the presence of concurrent respiratory infection. Because many individuals have minimal radiographic findings, a relatively normal study does not rule out this diagnosis. In patients with significant airway obstruction, the characteristic findings of air trapping are present with hyperlucency, overinflation, and flattening of the diaphragm. Bronchial wall thickening with peribronchiolar cuffing may be evident. Dogs tend to have a higher incidence of increased interstitial density.

Laboratory examination of these patients is essential. By definition, this disorder is characterized by the presence of eosinophils in bronchial secretions. The presence of blood eosinophilia is variable; it appears to be more frequent in dogs than cats. The relative numbers of eosinophils present in respiratory secretions is variable, ranging from 20 to 90 per cent of the total white blood cells observed. The author believes that the presumptive diagnosis of bronchitic pulmonary eosinophilia must be substantiated by demonstration of eosinophils in bronchial or nasal secretions. This is of more than academic interest, as most patients will have chronic disease with episodic exacerbations. If the diagnosis is not substantiated, there is doubt regarding the appropriateness of corticosteroid therapy and expectations of permanent relief of clinical signs. As previously suggested, there are marked individual differences in severity and duration of signs. As there often is spontaneous waxing and waning of these signs without medical intervention, inappropriate therapy based on misdiagnosis may give the illusion of being palliative. As a general rule, the younger the patients are at the time of diagnosis, the more difficult they will be to manage. Cats and dogs younger than 3 years of age with significant signs tend to require both higher dosage of medication and longer duration of therapy. Likewise, those with associated allergic rhinitis or dermatitis have similar courses. It is the author's experience that these individuals become easier to manage by the time they reach middle age. Age-related disease is important to note in terms of client education and expectations. It also suggests to the veterinarian the probability of future problems; all exacerbations may not be the result of inappropriate therapy, but rather may be due to other age-related conditions.

The aggressiveness with which one provides treatment is governed by the patient's clinical signs. There is no single efficacious regimen for the chronically symptomatic patient. Therapy must be individualized, and the client must assume significant responsibility and actively participate in the animal's care. A major goal of management is client education. If long-term therapy is to be successful, clients must be well informed about the nature of their animal's disorder and the names and pharmacologic actions of their medications.

The goals of therapy depend on the patient's clinical signs and the ease with which they are palliated. A total lack of symptoms would be the best outcome, although this is not always possible. Some animals will require excessive dosage to provide total continuous resolution, which may pose more long-term liability than the disease. It may be necessary to accept a 70 to 80 per cent palliation of clinical signs of cough, with the elimination of shortness of breath, rather than producing iatrogenic Cushing's syndrome or diabetes or administering excessive medication.

Glucocorticoids act by stabilizing lysosomal membranes, decreasing levels of histamine and leukotrienes, and restoring sensitivity of smooth muscle in the small airways to endogenous or exogenous beta-agonists. There likewise is inhibition of inflammatory cell diapedesis toward the airways and a decrease in mucus production by the hypertrophied bronchial glands.

Short-acting steroids are administered orally, and the goal is to move toward alternate- or every-third-day administration. The use of repository injections, such as methylprednisolone (Depo-Medrol) or triamcinolone acetate, may pose a liability to the patient, not only in terms of adrenocortical suppression, but for exacerbation of clinical signs. It is not uncommon to see animals that have been exclusively treated with repository steroids whose clinical signs are intractable following 2 years or more of therapy. Historically, there is a typical stairstep progression of signs and of increasing dosage and frequency of administration. A similar phenomenon may be seen in patients treated with repeated high-dose, short-term oral steroids with repeated abrupt cessation of medication without tapering. This rebound phenomena may be pronounced in some patients.

OUTPATIENT THERAPY

For the definitively diagnosed patient with cough but no dyspnea, precipitating factors should be avoided. If a specific contact or inhalant irritant (e.g., litter dust) is suspected, an attempt should be made to remove it, although this is frequently impossible. Brief isolation from the home environment may be of diagnostic but rarely of long-term therapeutic value. Results of such an environmental trial must be evaluated with some caution, as most patients also have intermittent and spontaneous decreases in signs at home. Easily accomplished, but infrequently helpful, changes that can be made include (1) replace clay litter with wood shavings, newspaper, or damp sand; (2) temporarily stop application of topical insecticides, (3) replace air filters on heating or cooling systems, (4) discuss the potential effects of passive smoke inhalation, (5) remove household dust and molds, and (6) discontinue any nonessential medication, including nutritional supplements. Hyposensitization may be of potential benefit to those individuals with concurrent atopy. If results of skin testing yield a specific well-defined antigen, an attempt may be made at hyposensitization. The author's impression is that such intervention is usually unrewarding and is more capable of palliating the dermatopathy than alleviating the pulmonary manifestations.

Coexisting respiratory tract disorders must be managed, e.g., bacterial bronchitis or rhinitis. Secondary bacterial infection may coexist with ongoing bronchitic pulmonary eosinophilia, especially in newly diagnosed and untreated patients. This is a compelling reason to evaluate bronchial specimens in any undiagnosed patient (see pp. 361–368). It may be argued that treatment of the underlying disorder will result in spontaneous resolution of opportunistic infections; however, this is not always true, and concurrent specific antimicrobial therapy is advisable.

Oral dosages of prednisone are variable and range from 0.5 to 2.0 mg/kg b.i.d. given on alternate days. Therapy should be initiated twice daily and then tapered to alternate days over 2 to 3 weeks. Rapid tapering may allow exacerbation of clinical signs. Alternate- or every-third-day treatment with the lowest effective dose should continue for a minimum of 2 months, particularly for young patients. If clinical signs rapidly return following cessation of therapy, daily medication is reinstituted for 3 to 4 days, followed by the lowest previously tolerated alternate-day dosage. Attempts at complete cessation of medication have variable results.

The use of bronchodilators in the patient that is not wheezing or exhibiting dyspnea is the subject of some debate. In these patients, the use of bronchodilators will usually not substantially decrease the daily dose of prednisone required and, in the overwhelming majority of cases, has no effect on cough. The major role of bronchodilators in this patient population is to help mobilize endobronchial secretions and increase their effective clearance from the small airways.

INPATIENT MANAGEMENT

The association of dyspnea, cyanosis, and hypoxemia with bronchitic pulmonary eosinophilia is a potentially fatal condition, which necessitates aggressive treatment and supervision of definitively diagnosed patients with cough and dyspnea (status asthmaticus). A detailed physical examination and history will aid in the diagnosis of possible concomitant problems or factors that may have exacerbated clinical signs. Frequently, there is increased dry cough or wheezing for 1 day or longer. When prompted, clients may reveal that signs have been progressive over many days to weeks. Patients with truly acute onset of signs tend to require the most care. Other clues to the recognition of severe disease are profound anxiety, pulsus paradoxus, and violent use of accessory ventilatory muscles with open mouth breathing.

Adequate rehydration is important, as there are significant metabolic and respiratory water losses. In addition, adequate hydration will aid in decreasing the viscosity of endobronchial secretions and enhance clearance of this tenacious material, which is a component of airway obstruction. Pharmacologic management of the dyspneic patient includes multiple medications: beta$_1$- or beta$_2$-agents, or both;

aminophylline; and high-dose corticosteroids. Beta-adrenergic agents have different actions when inhaled; beta$_1$-agonists are cardiac stimulants, whereas beta$_2$-agonists cause bronchodilation by relaxation of bronchial smooth muscle. When given orally or parentally, beta$_2$-agonists have a longer duration of action but unfortunately lose their specificity. This has obvious implications, as the overwhelming majority of veterinary patients will not tolerate the use of medicated inhalants. Treatment appears to be best tolerated when the inhaler is attached to a mask used for anesthetic induction or oxygen delivery. The usual dosage of metaproterenol is one inhalation every 4 hr for the first 12 hr.

Epinephrine given at 0.01 ml/kg (1:1000) may be administered subcutaneously. If a beneficial effect is observed, the dosage may be repeated at 20- to 30-min intervals to a maximum dose of 0.5 ml. If the patient does not benefit from two or three doses or objectively deteriorates, one should *not* administer further doses. The excessive or inappropriate use of sympathomimetics may produce produce cardiac arrhythmia, sudden death, increased anxiety, or profuse salivation and vomiting.

Aminophylline infusions are delivered at a dosage of 2 to 5 mg/kg in 5 per cent dextrose or saline over 30 min to 1 hr. This is usually undertaken when the bronchomotor response to epinephrine or beta$_2$-drugs has not been adequate and, in combination with the above, may be more successful in reduction of the high airway resistance of this disorder. Prior to initiating therapy, one should make sure that excessive oral dosages of xanthine derivatives have not been used (8 mg/kg or more) in the previous 12 hr). Rapid, excessive, or undiluted infusions of aminophylline may lead to cardiac arrhythmias, hypotension, nausea, tremor, or acute respiratory failure. Both the beta-agonists and intravenous xanthine derivatives may acutely and adversely affect pulmonary blood flow and increase the ventilation-perfusion mismatching, thus producing further hypoxemia. When a patient receiving such medications deteriorates, it is advisable to administer oxygen if such therapy has not already been instituted.

When treating patients not *in extremis*, it is prudent to start oral bronchodilator therapy. The usual dosage is 5 to 10 mg/kg every 6 to 8 hours. However, in patients that have not previously received theophylline, one half of this dosage should be initiated arbitrarily and increased over several days in an attempt to minimize the possibility of nausea or inappetence. It may require several days or weeks to reach its maximal effect.

Corticosteroids remain the mainstay of both immediate and long-term care. The onset of action following intravenous administration is debatable, however, there appears to be a 3- to 6-hr delay until the effect may be expected. Therefore, the previously discussed drugs must provide the major therapy until the steroidal actions develop. Prednisolone sodium succinate is administered at a dosage of 2 to 4 mg/kg IV. This dose is repeated in 4 to 6 hr. Rapid infusion may be associated with vomiting, hypotension, and acute respiratory failure. These complications are most frequently observed in cats when a rapid bolus injection has been delivered.

MANAGEMENT OF REFRACTORY PATIENTS

Occasionally a previously well-managed but currently symptomatic patient, a fragile young patient, or a marginally controlled patient undergoing withdrawal of repository steroid therapy will not respond to high-dose oral prednisone. The first step in treatment is careful re-evaluation and exclusion of concurrent disorders mimicking the signs of small airways disease, e.g., respiratory infection, congestive heart failure, pulmonary vascular disease, upper airway obstruction, or other syndromes of pulmonary eosinophilia. Acute exacerbations of "asthma" or poorly controlled chronic respiratory difficulty may be treated by slow infusion, high-dose, pulsed corticosteroid therapy, using prednisolone sodium succinate. Prednisolone is infused intravenously over 4 to 6 hr at a dosage of 2 to 5 mg/kg. This is repeated several days in a row. This, in turn, is followed by several days of oral therapy at the same dosage divided twice daily. The dosage is slowly tapered over 4 to 6 weeks. During this period, use of bronchodilators is maximized, and, if aerosol therapy is tolerated, inhaled beclomethasone dipropionate is used several times daily.

Feline patients may also benefit from the limited use of progestins. Megestrol acetate, when used simultaneously with oral corticosteroids, may achieve the same effect as high-dose, pulsed prednisone. It is administered at 5 mg/day for 4 days, followed by 5 mg weekly for 4 weeks. The high-dose oral steroid therapy is tapered over the 4 weeks of progestin administration. The incidence of diabetes and mammary neoplasia does not appear to be increased in the author's patient population. However, potential adverse effects need to be related to the client prior to initiating therapy.

Intubation and positive pressure ventilation is used only as a last resort and only in patients with respiratory failure and respiratory acidosis. The incidence of pneumomediastinum and pneumothorax appears greatly increased in patients who have undergone even short-term mechanical ventilation. Arterial blood gases must be routinely monitored, and rigorous bronchial drainage should be performed. Every attempt should be made to avoid mechanical ventilatory assistance by using aggressive pharmacologic therapy as previously described.

This should be fostered by the use of supplemental environmental oxygen.

Parasitic Pulmonary Eosinophilia

This is a group of parasitic infections that evoke a similar eosinophilic response in the bronchi or the pulmonary parenchyma. They may represent aberrant migration or a normal phase of parasite development in the host. Pathologically, there are peribronchial and perivascular accumulations of eosinophils and histiocytes, as well as an interstitial pneumonitis with similar cellular elements. With chronicity, this may progress to interstitial fibrosis.

None of the agents will be discussed in depth. The parasites apparently most frequently causing pulmonary eosinophilia include *Crenosema lupus*, *Toxoplasma gondii*, *Ancylostoma caninum*, *Toxocara canis*, *T. cati*, *Dirofilaria immitis*, *Filaroides* sp., *Capilleria aerophila*, *Paragonimus kellicotti*, and *Aleurostrongylus abstrusu*. Although these parasites induce antibody production in animals, the antibodies are not protective, and serum antibody levels do not correlate with the severity of infection.

The clinical and radiographic features are variable and nonspecific. Pulmonary signs tend to predominate, with cough being the most consistently found. Dyspnea, wheezing, and weight loss may be apparent in severe cases. Systemic signs are infrequent; fever may appear and abruptly rise following specific therapy directed toward the parasite.

The diagnosis should be suspected in the following situations: (1) recent residence in endemic areas is a historical feature; (2) there is a predominance of respiratory signs; (3) significant eosinophilia is present in blood or respiratory secretions; (4) laboratory examination of feces or bronchial aspirates contains the parasite, or there is serologic evidence of infection; and (5) a clinical response is observed to specific therapy directed at the parasite. The diagnosis should always be considered in the patient with recurrent pulmonary eosinophilia.

Treatment is with the appropriate antiparasitic drugs; corticosteroids at anti-inflammatory dosages of 0.5 to 1.0 mg/kg are used concurrently to attenuate the hypersensitivity-related phenomena. Clinical signs may worsen with initial antiparasitic therapy. Death of parasites may result in liberation of increased amounts of antigen and thus a greater antigen-antibody reaction.

Pulmonary Eosinophilia Associated with Angiitis and Granulomatosis

This is a poorly understood and poorly defined group of disorders. Pathologic descriptions are few, however, the overwhelming majority of cases are observed in dogs. These disorders are characterized by widespread vasculitis, affecting not only the pulmonary circulation but also the systemic vasculature. The lesions are widely distributed throughout the body, including skin, heart, lymph nodes, spleen, alimentary organs, and kidneys. Both the parenchyma and vessels of these structures are infiltrated with plasma cells, lymphocytes, and eosinophils but with few polymorphonuclear leukocytes. Granulomas are present, often with central necrosis. The characteristic changes in the kidneys are those of glomerulonephritis. Lymph nodes undergo marked lymphocyte depletion and are replaced by a cellular infiltrate of plasma cells, histiocytes, lymphocytes, and eosinophils. There may be marked replacement with fibrous elements and amorphous eosinophilic material, and this is most noticeable in the nodes surrounding the pulmonary hilum. There is a profound circulating eosinophilia, often reaching 60 to 70 per cent of observed white blood cells. The pulmonary manifestations include pneumonitis, pulmonary nodules, and frequently consolidating lobar lesions. There is hilar adenopathy, often causing hilar compression and limited airway obstruction. Pulmonary vascular disease with thrombosis and embolism have been ubiquitous findings, with the majority of patients expiring from this aspect of their disease. Pleural effusions, which may consist entirely of eosinophils, are frequent findings. The disorder is systemic despite the predominance of pulmonary involvement. Extrapulmonary signs may develop, including dermatopathy, pericardial effusion, cardiac arrhythmias due to myocardial involvement, pancreatitis, gastric ulcer, and central nervous system involvement. Peripheral adenopathy is common.

Although this disorder has not been firmly classified and described by veterinary clinicians and pathologists, the clinical and pathologic findings would appear to be similar to those of the lymphomatoid variant of Wegner's granulomatosis described in humans. As observed in the human counterpart, two dogs with this diagnosis have died with classic multicentric lymphosarcoma. Although this disorder may resemble a reticuloendothelial neoplasm, the predominance of vasculitis and granulomatosis appears to be a distinguishing feature. The author's patients with this diagnosis had rapidly progressive disease with significant pleuropulmonary involvement.

It should be emphasized that treatment is strictly empiric. No controlled studies have been conducted in canine patients. Therapy is based on the premise that the disorder is immune mediated and, as such, therapy is twofold: (1) Corticosteroids are used for their anti-inflammatory as well as their mild immunosuppressive properties. They appear most helpful in the induction of eosinopenia. (2) Cyclophosphamide, which is assumed to have its major effect on the immune effector cells, is concurrently administered. The corticosteroids have an immediate effect, whereas the cyclophosphamide may take as long as 3 to 4 weeks to exert its effect.

Therapy is instituted with parenteral prednisone, which will usually improve the patient's status within 48 to 72 hours and decrease the dyspnea associated with the ongoing pneumonitis. This may be followed by surgical resection of the pulmonary mass lesions if they occupy the majority of a lobar segment (which they usually do). It appears fruitless to attempt surgical resection of the hilar nodes, despite their dramatic increase in size. Following healing of the surgical wound, cyclophosphamide is started at 2 mg/kg daily as a single dose, in addition to the prednisone. Routine hematologic evaluation should be obtained every 3 weeks to assure that the absolute leukocyte count remains above 3000/mm³. If leukopenia is observed, the cyclophosphamide is discontinued and the leukocyte count is allowed to return to normal. Cyclophosphamide is then restarted at one half the previous dosage. As previously stated, no controlled data are available to evaluate therapeutic regimens, but the author's limited experience would suggest that comprehensive soft tissue sarcoma chemotherapeutic protocols are of no more benefit than cyclophosphamide and prednisone alone. Owing to the consistent necropsy findings of pulmonary thrombosis and embolism, the use of anticoagulation is advisable. Any acute episode of dyspnea without obvious cause should be assumed to represent pulmonary embolism, and prompt pulmonary arteriography or perfusion scans should be performed when facilities are available. Despite aggressive care of these patients, this disorder carries a poor long-term prognosis. If the acute disorder is successfully managed, survival appears to be about 1 year. The longest survival time in the author's unpublished series is 3 years.

Pulmonary Eosinophilia Associated with Hypereosinophilic Syndrome

This rare syndrome is characterized by profound leukocytosis with eosinophilia and the diffuse infiltration of multiple organs with eosinophils. Frank eosinophilic leukemia may develop, which despite

intervention usually has a progressive, fulminant, and fatal course.

The clinical signs are similar to those of other serious disorders of pulmonary eosinophilia, including fever, weight loss, cough, dyspnea, hepatosplenomegaly, and anemia. Unlike the disorders of angiitis and granulomatosis, there is no vascular involvement or granuloma formation, and peripheral adenopathy is a variable finding. The diagnosis is suggested by the profound magnitude of the patient's illness and apparent multisystem involvement. Differentiation from other disorders is frequently aided by the presence of blast cells in the peripheral blood. If doubt exists as to the diagnosis, biopsies of lymph nodes, liver, spleen, and bone marrow should confirm the diagnosis.

Disorders Exhibiting Occasional Pulmonary Eosinophilia

A number of pulmonary and extrapulmonary disorders may be associated with blood or tissue eosinophilia. As the classification suggests, circulating or tissue eosinophilia is not a consistent finding but occurs with enough frequency to be considered in the differential diagnosis of the patient with undiagnosed pulmonary eosinophilia. Most notable examples are pulmonary lymphosarcoma, multicentric lymphosarcoma without direct pulmonary invasion, mast cell sarcoma, and syndromes of immune-mediated polyarthritis. These all may produce modest pulmonary eosinophilia. Although the primary disorder is typically recognizable, the associated syndrome of pulmonary involvement may masquerade as diffuse pulmonary spread of a neoplasm or opportunistic infection. Recognition of these syndromes will allow better care for the catastrophic disorders.

EXTRINSIC ALLERGIC ALVEOLITIS

These disorders represent a hypersensitivity pneumonitis in which the tissues of the air space are sensitized to specific antigens, and an allergic response occurs when the presensitized individual is exposed. There is documentation of these phe-

Table 1. *Allergic Agents in Humans*

Antigen	Source
Wood dust	Cedar, mahogany, oak, pine, spruce, and redwood
Actinomyces, Aspergillus sp.	Hay, grain, silage
Aureobasidium pullulans	Aerosolized contaminated fluids
Avian proteins	Avian dander and droppings
Cryptostroma corticale	Maple bark
Sitophilus granarius	Weevil-infested flour
Toluene, methylene diisacyanate, phthallic anuydride, vinyl chloride	Polyurethane and other synthetic materials

nomena in both humans and large animals, and causative agents are usually organic dusts or chemicals. Specific documentation of these maladies in small animals is infrequent. However, they are assumed to exist, as the author has evaluated numerous animals with compatible biopsy findings. A table of the known offending agents in humans are listed in Table 1.

Pathologically, both the air space and the interstitium are involved and infiltrated with a pleocellular population of plasma cells, lymphocytes, and histiocytes. Granulomas may be present, and the degree of fibrous replacement is commensurate with the chronicity of the process and the magnitude of the parenchymal destruction. Bronchiolitis obliterans is a frequent finding and may be marked.

The clinical presentation is likewise related to the chronicity and magnitude of exposure. As this is primarily a disorder of the interstitium, the early effects are those of restrictive lung disease. As the disease progresses, it takes on the features of other obstructive pulmonary disorders. Definitive diagnosis depends on serologic confirmation of antibodies to a specific extrinsic allergen, but this may be difficult to achieve with impunity. Lung biopsy coupled with the appropriate environmental history may strongly suggest the diagnosis.

Patients with acute or low-grade exposure may not be seen for evaluation, as the process may be self-limiting. Chronic or subacute disease with associated significant clinical signs should be treated with prednisone. It is important to rule out other forms of infectious interstitial lung disease, and lung biopsy is advisable. Ability to provide environmental protection also depends on specific diagnosis, making the diagnosis dependent on biopsy findings and an extensive search for the offending agent.

References and Supplemental Reading

Bauer, T.: Diseases of the lower airway; and Pulmonary parenchymal disorders. *In* Morgan, R. (ed.): *Handbook of Small Animal Practice.* New York: Churchill Livingston, New York; 1988.

Carrington, C. B., Addington, W. W., Goff, A. W., et al.: Chronic eosinophilic pneumonia. N. Engl. J. Med. 280:787, 1969.

Churg, J.: Allergic granulomatous vascular syndromes. Ann. Allergy 21:619, 1963.

Crofton, S. W., Livingstone, J. L., Oswald, N.C., et al.: Pulmonary eosinophilia. Thorax 7:1, 1952.

Liebow, A. A., and Carrington, C. B.: Hypersensitivity reactions involving the lung. Trans. Stud. Coll. Physicians Philadelphia 34:47, 1966.

Pepys, S.: Immunopathy of allergic lung disease. Clin. Allergy 3:1, 1973.

Suter, P. F., and Lord, P. F.: *Thoracic Radiography, A Text Atlas of Thoracic Diseases of the Dog and Cat.* Wettswil, Switzerland: Peter F. Suter, 1984.

Zucker-Franklin, D.: Eosinophilia of unknown etiology; a diagnostic dilemma. Hosp. Pract. 6:119, 1971.

PNEUMONIA

TODD R. TAMS, D.V.M.
West Los Angeles, California

Pneumonia refers to inflammation of the lung parenchyma due to any of a variety of causes. Often there is some degree of alveolar exudation. Pneumonitis is a term used to describe the presence of a cellular proliferation and infiltration of the alveolar septal wall, without the presence of exudation into the alveoli. These anatomic classifications share many of the same causes and may only represent different stages in the progression of the disease process.

Pneumonia may be caused by a large number of factors. Various classification schemes have been used to describe pneumonias, including etiology (e.g., bacterial, viral, mycotic, and inhalation injury), radiographic appearance, morphologic distribution, and histologic changes. Pneumonia may develop as an extension of an existing tracheobronchial disorder, from spread of a systemic disorder to the lungs, or as a primary parenchymal event.

This article presents a discussion of the important clinical features of three of the most life-threatening forms of pneumonia: acute bacterial pneumonia, aspiration pneumonia, and smoke inhalation injury. In many instances, prompt detection of respiratory compromise and rapid therapeutic intervention make the critical difference for survival.

BACTERIAL PNEUMONIA

Bacteria are among the most common causes of pneumonia in small animals. A number of predisposing factors can be involved. These include previous respiratory injury or disease (e.g., viral infections or chronic tracheobronchial disorders); debilitation; compromised immunologic status (e.g., chemotherapy- and other drug-induced immunodeficiency); endocrine-related immunodeficiency due to Cushing's syndrome, growth hormone deficiency, or diabetes mellitus; anatomic abnormalities such as cleft palate and megaesophagus; and functional defects such as the immotile cilia syndrome, a congenital defect in cilia function that affects dogs and humans. Congenital ciliary dysfunction reduces mucociliary transport, leading to chronic rhinitis, sinusitis, bronchitis, and bacterial pneumonia. Nosocomial (hospital acquired) infections commonly affect the respiratory system. Risk factors that increase the likelihood of infection include extremes of age (neonatal or geriatric patients), critical illness, chronic debilitating disease, pre-existing infection, administration of immunosuppressive drugs, and selective antimicrobial therapy. Improper preparation and maintenance of intravenous and urinary catheter sites can predispose to hematogenous spread of bacteria to the lower respiratory system in these patients. Bacterial pneumonia can also occur as a complication of other pneumonias (e.g., mycotic, allergic, or aspiration).

Clinical Findings

Clinical signs of bacterial pneumonia in the dog may include cough (often productive), fever, tachypnea, dyspnea, and nasal discharge. With progressive or severe disease, inappetence, depression, weakness, and dehydration are often present. Severely affected dogs may be orthopneic, cyanotic, or both. There may be open mouth breathing, salivation, and an apprehensive state. A pronounced foul odor coming from the mouth may be detected in patients with gangrenous pneumonia.

Bacterial pneumonia is somewhat less common in cats than in dogs. The primary clinical signs of bacterial pneumonia in cats are dyspnea; fever; inappetence; and occasionally cough, orthopnea, or both. Coughing does not seem to be as common in cats with pneumonia as it is in dogs.

Auscultation usually reveals the presence of crackles in the ventral lung regions, which may vary from fine to coarse based on the extent of involvement. Coarse crackles are bubbling or gurgling sounds, whereas fine crackles produce a cellophane-type sound. Occasionally rhonchi may be heard as slightly prolonged sounds and indicate narrowing of the airways that is most likely due to accumulation of secretions. Silent areas indicate lobar filling of exudate or a plugged bronchus. Only bronchovesicular sounds are heard in some cases of bacterial pneumonia.

Diagnosis

A diagnosis of bacterial pneumonia is suggested by a review of the history and thorough physical examination, which includes observation of the patient's breathing pattern. Diagnostic procedures that are used to confirm the presence of bacterial pneumonia and to assess extent of involvement include thoracic radiographs, complete blood count, transtracheal aspiration to obtain samples for airway cytologic study and culture and sensitivity, and arterial blood gas analysis. An elevated white blood cell (WBC) count, often with a left shift, is often seen, but the WBC count may vary from near normal to greater than $35,000/mm^3$. Monocytosis is found in some cases. A normal WBC and differential count may be seen early in the course of the disorder. Serial blood gas analyses, though not commonly used in private practice, provide sensitive indications of alteration in function of the lungs often before any changes are detected on radiographs, auscultation, and blood counts. The first change due to ventilation-perfusion abnormalities is usually a decrease in arterial partial pressure of oxygen (Pa_{O_2}), followed by a slight decrease in pH and finally by an increase in Pa_{CO_2}.

Thoracic radiographs are part of the routine data base for any patient suspected of having pneumonia. Care must be taken, however, when patients are experiencing significant respiratory distress. Initially only lateral view or lateral and dorsoventral projections are obtained if there is concern that the stress of positioning will result in decompensation of the patient's pulmonary status. The radiographic pattern can vary from pronounced alveolar pulmonary infiltrates with air bronchograms to a more mild mixed pattern of alveolar-interstitial involvement. The classic pattern of bacterial pneumonia includes fluffy alveolar opacities (the result of an exudative process that fills the alveoli and smaller airways with fluid and cells) and air bronchograms distributed particularly to ventral regions of the cranial and middle lung lobes. Both alveolar and interstitial patterns may be present simultaneously and to varying degrees. Serial radiographs should be made approximately every 48 hours during treatment and are an excellent means of monitoring response to therapy.

Airway exudate should be obtained as early as possible, preferably before antibiotic therapy, for cytologic and culture and sensitivity testing. Even though many studies have shown that the majority of organisms isolated from bacterial pneumonia patients are gram negative, the importance of isolating specific bacteria and determining sensitivity patterns should not be overlooked, especially in peracute cases and in patients that have experienced a relapse. Samples can be obtained via transtracheal wash, via bronchoscopy-guided brushings, or by passing a guarded culture swab through the larynx of a lightly anesthetized animal. Cytologic findings usually show septic, mucopurulent inflammation. Gram's stains are used to determine initial antibiotic therapy while awaiting culture and sensitivity results.

The diagnosis of bacterial pneumonia is not particularly difficult, but determining the causative mechanism may be much more troublesome. Every effort should be made to determine an underlying etiology so that future preventive measures, if indicated, can be instituted. Other diagnostic tests than those discussed above may be necessary to determine a causal relationship (e.g., biochemistry profile, feline leukemia virus [FeLV] and FIV testing in cats with pneumonia, barium contrast studies to confirm esophageal motility disorders, neurologic examination, and testing for endocrinopathies such as hypothyroidism).

Treatment

Antibiotics are the foundation of treatment for bacterial pneumonia. The initial choice of drug depends on cytology and Gram's stain results. Common bacterial isolates include *Escherichia coli*, *Klebsiella*, *Pasteurella* spp., *Pseudomonas*, *Bordetella*, and *Streptococcus*. The use of bactericidal antibiotics with a good gram-negative spectrum is recommended pending culture and sensitivity results. Trimethoprim-sulfonamide (Tribrissen, Burroughs Wellcome) is a broad-spectrum antimicrobial that is active against most gram-negative rods that are commonly isolated, except for *Klebsiella*. If the presence of *Klebsiella* is a distinct possibility, a broader-spectrum approach using a cephalosporin along with trimethoprim-sulfonamide may be best. An oxidase test can be performed 24 hr after a sample is plated, and this will help differentiate *Klebsiella* (member of Enterobacteriaceae family, which are all oxidase negative) from *Bordetella*, *Pasteurella*, and *Pseudomonas*, which are oxidase positive. A cephalosporin, trimethoprim-sulfonamide, ampicillin (amoxicillin), and potentiated amoxicillin (Clavamox, Beecham) are good choices if cocci are identified initially on cytologic study or Gram's stain. Chloramphenicol, gentamicin, kanamycin, neomycin, and tetracycline have been shown to be effective against *Bordetella bronchiseptica*. Nebulized gentamicin also may be useful in cases of chronic *Bordetella* infections. Therapy is altered based on culture and sensitivity results or lack of improvement in clinical signs by 24 to 72 hr. Radiographic improvement should be evident by 48 to 96 hr.

If moderate to severe bacterial pneumonia is present and there is marked respiratory insufficiency, aggressive antimicrobial therapy should be instituted immediately. Combination therapy using ampicillin/amoxicillin and gentamicin (2.2 mg/kg every 8 hr IV, IM, or SC in dogs and cats with normal renal function) or cephalosporins and gentamicin provides excellent broad-spectrum activity. The intravenous route should be used at the outset because of poor intramuscular absorption during hypotension. Oral administration of any antibiotic is not recommended in seriously ill patients because of low and erratic serum levels. Aminoglycosides are generally used for 5 to 10 days. Renal function and fluid balance are carefully monitored during aminoglycoside therapy (see *Current Veterinary Therapy IX*, p. 1146). Oral antibiotics are continued for 4 to 6 weeks after discharge in patients that have been hospitalized for severe pneumonia. The owner should monitor the temperature and clinical status daily. Radiographs are made every 1 to 2 weeks during the recovery phase, and an antibiotic is either continued or changed based on clinical impression of patient status and sputum culture.

Intravenous fluids are an extremely important but unfortunately often overlooked form of therapy in bacterial pneumonia patients. Because tracheobronchial secretions are about 95 per cent water, dehydration will tend to thicken secretions and lead to their retention. Retained secretions may result in further ventilation-perfusion abnormalities. Low-sodium fluids (e.g., half-strength saline or 2.5 or 5 per cent dextrose) are used if cardiac disease is also present. Lactated Ringer's solution with 5 per cent dextrose is used in patients with normal cardiac function. Glucose therapy may be important in animals with severe gram-negative infections to help maintain adequate blood glucose levels. Overhydration may result in pulmonary edema and further respiratory compromise. It may occasionally be difficult to recognize pulmonary edema radiographically in a patient that already has a radiographic pattern consistent with bacterial pneumonia.

Removal of exudate from the lungs is necessary for effective recovery. The patient should be encouraged to cough. Chest percussion (coupage) for 10 minutes followed by short leash walks should be done three to four times daily with hospitalized patients. The combination of fluid therapy, coupage, and mild exercise helps promote both cough and more effective mucociliary transport activity. Antitussive therapy of any kind is contraindicated in patients with bacterial pneumonia.

Aerosol therapy utilizing an ultrasonic-type nebulizer has proved beneficial in bacterial pneumonia cases. An ultrasonic nebulizer is capable of producing a particle size sufficiently small to be deposited in the small airways. Saline is the best nebulizing fluid; mucolytic agents should be avoided, as they are irritating. Bronchodilator therapy may prevent reflex bronchoconstriction in animals undergoing nebulization.

Bacterial pneumonia may be particularly difficult to resolve in patients that have ongoing aspiration due to megaesophagus. It is sometimes beneficial to place a gastric feeding tube in such patients (e.g., using endoscopy-guided percutaneous tube gastrostomy technique) so that no food or water is administered orally. The tube is usually left in place for 2 to 4 weeks or longer.

ASPIRATION PNEUMONIA

Aspiration pneumonia refers to the pulmonary sequelae that result from the abnormal entry of endogenous secretions or exogenous substances into the lower respiratory tract. It has two essential features: (1) compromised lower airway defense mechanisms, and (2) a pathologic event resulting from the aspiration insult.

Pulmonary complications of aspiration seldom occur in otherwise healthy animals. Intermittent aspiration of small amounts of food and liquids is common in normal animals and is usually well tolerated with no significant sequelae. The factors that determine the occurrence and extent of pulmonary complications involve primarily the frequency, volume, and character of the aspirate. In addition, the status of normal host defense mechanisms, such as reflex airway closure during swallowing, cough reflex, mucociliary transport apparatus, and pulmonary cellular defenses, is extremely important. Animals that are comatose, debilitated, or seizuring or that have swallowing dysfunction or esophageal motility abnormalities have a significantly greater potential for developing aspiration pneumonia. These conditions predispose to a breakdown of normal protective mechanisms with subsequent entry of gastric secretions, oropharyngeal secretions, and exogenous food or fluids into the tracheobronchial passages. Conditions predisposing to aspiration pneumonia are summarized in Table 1.

Pathophysiologic changes, clinical presentation, and therapeutic approach vary with the nature of the aspirated material. The term aspiration pneumonia is used only as a general description of pulmonary complications related to aspiration. Whenever possible, the character of the aspirated material should be determined. Categories of aspiration pneumonia were first delineated by Bartlett (1980). These include chemical pneumonitis, reflex airway closure, mechanical obstruction, and infection. Treatment and prognosis vary based on causative factors.

Chemical Pneumonitis

Chemical pneumonitis describes a pulmonary inflammatory reaction to any fluid that is toxic to the lower respiratory tract. Examples include gastric acid, mineral oil, animal fat, antacids, and volatile hydrocarbons such as gasoline or kerosene. Of

Table 1. *Conditions That Predispose to Aspiration*

Altered Consciousness
General anesthesia
Sedation
Seizures
Central nervous system disorders (dementia, unconsciousness)

Oropharyngeal Conditions
Cleft palate
Force feeding
Feeding too soon after local laryngeal anesthesia

Esophageal Disorders
Cricopharyngeal achalasia
Vascular ring anomaly
Esophageal stricture
Esophageal motility disorder
Megaesophagus due to any cause

Mechanical Disruption of Defense Barriers
Pharyngostomy tube, especially with placement through gastroesophageal junction or cranial to epihyoid bone
Endotracheal tube
Tracheostomy tube

Gastroesophageal Reflux

Gastric Motility Disorders
Prolonged retention of food in stomach

Persistent Vomiting Due to Any Cause

Modified from Tams, T. R.: Vet. Clin. North Am. 15:971, 1985; with permission.

these, gastric acid is most frequently encountered as a cause of chemical pneumonitis on a clinical basis.

The pH, the volume of gastric acid secretions aspirated, and the presence or absence of any particulate matter such as food in the aspirate are the most important factors in determining the severity of pulmonary reaction. If the pH of an acid inocula is less than or equal to 2.5, lung injury is consistently more severe than if a more neutralized acid inocula (pH greater than 2.5) is aspirated. If particulate matter is present, a significant reaction will occur whether the pH is less than 2.5 or more neutral, although a more severe reaction will occur with a lower-pH aspirate. The histologic response to acid aspiration is essentially a response to an acute chemical burn of the tracheobronchial tree and is characterized by atelectasis, peribronchial hemorrhage, pulmonary edema, and degeneration of the bronchial epithelium.

The presence of bile or digestive enzymes in the stomach at the time of aspiration seems to be of limited importance. In contrast, aspirates grossly contaminated with bacteria, such as those occurring in patients with bowel obstruction, are frequently associated with a fatal outcome.

CLINICAL FEATURES. The outstanding clinical feature resulting from pulmonary acid aspiration is acute tachypnea or dyspnea, which usually occurs within 2 hr of the event. Coughing and wheezing may also occur, and cyanosis may result if there is generalized pulmonary damage. Hypotension can occur as a result of an immediate reflex reaction or intravascular volume depletion with fluid accumulation in the lung. Frothy, nonpurulent sputum is expectorated in some cases.

The most characteristic physiologic feature is hypoxia. Arterial blood gas abnormalities include decreased pH and arterial partial pressure of oxygen (Pa_{O_2}) and possibly an increased Pa_{CO_2} in advanced or terminal patients. Radiographs are initially normal unless large volumes of acid have been aspirated. However, diffuse or localized alveolar infiltrates may appear and progress over the ensuing 12 to 36 hours as a result of pulmonary inflammation. Lung lobes that are dependent at the time of aspiration are most typically affected.

Aspiration of Particulate Matter

Aspiration of particulate matter causes a reaction that is more severe and prolonged than the reaction that occurs with gastric acid alone. Animals that are sedated or anesthetized when food is present in the stomach are at increased risk, as are patients that are debilitated or seizuring. Animals with cleft palate, dysphagia, vascular ring anomaly, megaesophagus, esophageal stricture, and bronchoesophageal fistula must be watched carefully for signs of aspiration. Improper pharyngostomy tube placement can also predispose to aspiration. A pharyngostomy tube should not exit cranial to the epihyoid bone and should not extend to the distal one fourth of the esophagus. Life-threatening acute respiratory distress from mechanical airway obstruction can occur at any time. Obstruction by large food particles, unless rapidly removed by coughing, endotracheal suction, or bronchoscopy, can lead to death from asphyxiation. Alternatively, severe aspiration pneumonia with secondary granulomatous reaction can occur as the result of a chronic aspiration of saliva or small amounts of food.

CLINICAL FEATURES. Unless there is significant airway obstruction, there may be minimal or no abnormal clinical signs in the first 3 to 6 hr after aspiration. This is especially true if aspiration occurs under sedation or anesthesia. However, by 6 to 8 hr there is usually an appreciable onset of dyspnea, tachypnea, and coughing. These signs should always alert the clinician to the possibility of aspiration injury. The presence of food particles or hypertonic or irritating solutions such as milk greatly exacerbates hypoxia. Severe bronchospasm with worsening airway obstruction may occur. Tachycardia, cyanosis, and shock may ensue in severe cases by 12 to 24 hr. Fever often indicates pulmonary infection.

Concurrent aspiration of bacteria-laden material is a major complicating factor. Usually organisms colonizing the oropharynx are involved. The lung damaged by aspiration provides an excellent setting for infection. Progression of infection in these cases depends not only on whether there is concurrent contamination by oropharyngeal microflora, but also on the need for ventilatory support and the use of other therapeutic agents, such as steroids or antibiotics, which might favor bacterial overgrowth. Evidence of pulmonary infection in aspiration cases may occur early or may be delayed for several days to a week, especially if early aspiration involved primarily gastric acid.

Aspiration of Inert Substances

Most nonacid or neutral substances (pH greater than 2.5) cause only transient damage to the lung. Saline, water, barium, and gastric fluid with a pH exceeding 3.0 are examples of relatively inert inocula. Limited quantities of these substances cause transient, self-limited hypoxia and, occasionally, marked hypoxia and decreased compliance. These effects most likely represent an intrinsic pulmonary reflex reaction that is independent of the chemical composition of the inoculum.

Aspiration of nontoxic fluids can also result in mechanical obstruction. If large volumes are aspirated, acute suffocation may occur (e.g., drowning). Iatrogenic cases occur during administration of barium via a stomach tube that has mistakenly been placed in the trachea. Small amounts of barium in the airways cause minimal respiratory distress. Larger volumes, however, can cause significant distress and asphyxiation, especially if there is generalized distribution.

Aspiration of Lipoid Compounds

Lipoid pneumonia is caused by chronic aspiration of exogenous lipid-containing compounds. In veterinary medicine this is almost exclusively a problem of cats in which mineral oil is used as treatment for hairballs. The tasteless and bland nature of mineral oil makes it less irritating to mucosal surfaces and therefore less likely to lead to reflex inhibition of aspiration. Residual lipid adhering to the pharyngeal mucosa may be aspirated passively with normal respiration or possibly during sleep. Gradual accumulation of lipid in the alveoli will eventually produce pathologic changes characteristic of lipoid pneumonitis. Mineral oil cannot be metabolized and remains in lung macrophages.

Most cats with mild lipoid pulmonary reactions remain asymptomatic. Moderate to severe granulomatous reaction may cause dyspnea, listlessness, and cough. Laboratory findings are usually normal. Diffuse, finely nodular densities, which could potentially be mistaken for metastatic lesions, may be seen on radiographs. Diagnosis is based on radiographic examination and clinical signs but is most supported by an accurate history. Specific questions should be advanced by the clinician regarding the possible use of mineral oil in cats that are presented for evaluation of cough or dyspnea and that have suggestive radiographic changes. Primary differential diagnosis includes neoplasia and mycotic disease. Mineral oil administration should be discontinued. If respiratory distress is significant, treatment with corticosteroids, bronchodilators, and oxygen may be necessary.

Treatment Principles

Treatment of aspiration pneumonia depends on the type and quantity of material aspirated, the degree of involvement, and the initial physical findings. If an underlying disorder is identified (e.g., megaesophagus), treatment must include management of that disorder as well as the pulmonary complications. Early recognition of conditions and clinical situations that may potentially predispose to an aspiration event may help in prevention of serious sequelae.

The three most important priorities in any aspiration patient are to identify any upper airway obstruction, to determine whether there is existent hypoxia, and to examine for signs of shock. The patient with severe respiratory compromise will be considered first. After ensuring a patent airway (using endotracheal intubation and suction, if necessary), the most important initial treatment is correction of hypoxia by administering oxygen. Patients with severe respiratory depression, comatose patients, or those that are experiencing exaggerated ventilatory effort may require continuous positive pressure ventilation. Ventilation-perfusion imbalance associated with severe aspiration pneumonia is due to perfusion of partially and completely collapsed alveoli that occurs as a result of small airway obstruction. A major advantage of continuous positive pressure ventilation is that it significantly reduces alveolar collapse and the associated ventilation-perfusion imbalance. Arterial oxygen tension and functional residual capacity are also increased significantly. Hypoxia due to ventilation-perfusion imbalance may respond poorly to the relatively low concentration of oxygen delivered by a conventional oxygen cage. Positive pressure ventilation must be initiated early in aspiration pneumonia patients when hypoxia is not corrected by supplemental oxygen (i.e., via mask or oxygen cage) or when exaggerated ventilatory effort is present. Respiratory distress from decreased lung compliance caused by alveolar collapse can lead to ventilatory failure and death. A detailed discussion of continuous pos-

itive airway pressure therapy can be found in *Current Veterinary Therapy IX* (p. 269). Several days to 1 week of continuous therapy may be required in some cases.

Patients whose respiratory capacity is not seriously compromised often respond to supplemental oxygen as administered by an oxygen cage or to short-term positive pressure oxygenation. Short-term positive pressure oxygenation can be administered to a sedated and intubated patient using manual compression of the reservoir bag of an anesthetic machine or a mechanical ventilator. For resuscitation or brief use (for a duration of time less than 12 hr), it is acceptable to use 100 per cent oxygen.

Intravenous fluid support should be initiated as early as possible. Shock requires vigorous fluid therapy. As discussed previously, fluid support is also important in treatment of bacterial pneumonia.

If a significant amount of particulate matter such as food has been aspirated with gastric or esophageal content or a foreign body has been inhaled, significant upper or lower airway obstruction may result. Bronchoscopy using flexible or rigid fiberoptic equipment can be used with accessory instrumentation to retrieve foreign material. It is important to frequently suction the oropharyngeal airway to remove accumulations of food, vomitus, and saliva that are causing obstruction or that can potentially be aspirated.

In cases of chemical pneumonitis, there is usually little opportunity to neutralize or remove the chemical insult. With acid pneumonitis, as with a flash burn, the full extent of the injury occurs within seconds to several minutes of the insult. Furthermore, aspirated acid is neutralized within minutes by tracheobronchial secretion, and adding diluents can further compromise the airways by causing mechanical obstruction. If lung or bronchial lavage is to be attempted, it must be done immediately and only sterile saline should be used.

Aspiration of small volumes of inert substances (e.g., barium) usually requires no treatment other than confining the animal and avoiding exertion. Aspiration of large volumes of nontoxic fluids, however, can cause abrupt suffocation by mechanical obstruction. If there is significant dyspnea or if asphyxiation appears imminent, immediate endotracheal intubation (using chemical restraint, if necessary) should be accomplished to maintain a patent airway. Tracheal suction and oxygen are then administered as soon as possible (positive pressure ventilation may be required). Bronchodilators may also be beneficial because bronchoconstriction is a frequent postaspiration occurrence. Emergency bronchodilation may be accomplished via parenteral isoproterenol therapy (0.01 to 0.04 μg/kg/min IV, or 0.5 ml in a nebulizer). Fluid support is required to prevent hypotension from concurrent peripheral vasodilation.

No study has documented an improved survival rate of aspiration pneumonia patients treated with corticosteroids. There appears to be no difference in arterial oxygenation, cardiac output, pulmonary artery pressure, or pathologic changes when corticosteroids are administered. Corticosteroids may interfere with the normal pulmonary defense mechanisms that act to localize and wall off foreign materials. However, if the patient is in shock, administration of steroids in conjunction with aggressive fluid support may be helpful. If steroids are used for this purpose they should not be continued beyond 24 hr after initiation of an aspiration insult.

Antibiotics are not indicated in most cases of isolated chemical pneumonitis and inert substance aspiration. These episodes are rarely associated with infection. However, aspiration of bacteria composing the normal flora of the upper airways is not uncommon in animals. Antibiotics are chosen based on guidelines presented in discussion of bacterial pneumonia. In cases of bacterial pneumonia an aggressive antimicrobial approach using cephalosporins in combination with an aminoglycoside is recommended while awaiting results of sputum culture and sensitivity testing.

Prevention

The best approach to the problem of aspiration pneumonia is to prevent its occurrence. This requires early recognition of disorders or clinical situations in which there is potential for a life-threatening aspiration event to occur. Preventive measures include ensuring that the stomach is empty before inducing general anesthesia, protecting the airways in comatose or anesthetized patients with cuffed endotracheal tubes and oropharyngeal suctioning as needed, properly placing pharyngostomy tubes, and following carefully supervised feeding regimens using elevated feeding platforms in animals with megaesophagus. Specific drug therapy can be used to maintain elevated gastric pH levels or to promote more rapid aboral gastric emptying in animals in which there is an increased likelihood that aspiration could occur (e.g., reflux esophagitis, hiatal hernia, and emergency surgery when the stomach is not empty).

If an emergency anesthetic procedure becomes necessary (e.g., cesarean section) and the stomach contains food, several options are available. Preoperative gastric emptying via administration of apomorphine or gastric lavage and aspiration through a large-bore stomach tube are effective in reducing gastric volume, but these methods are unpleasant and stressful for the patient and inappropriate in an emergency. Antacids may help to elevate gastric pH, but aspiration of food material with gastric fluid

of a more neutral pH is still quite dangerous, and colloidal antacids, if aspirated, are capable of inducing a severe pyogranulomatous pulmonary reaction.

A currently preferred alternative is to use a combination of an H_2-receptor antagonist such as cimetidine (Tagamet, SmithKline) or ranitidine (Zantac) to decrease gastric acid secretion and the gastric promotility agent metoclopramide (Reglan, Robins) to promote aboral gastric emptying. After H_2-receptor antagonist administration the gastric pH is usually greater than 3.0 within 1 hr and remains at that level for 3 to 4 hr. Cimetidine (5 mg/kg IV or IM) or ranitidine (2.0 mg/kg IM) should be administered 45 to 60 min before anesthesia in any patient in which the potential for acid aspiration is significant.

The gastric promotility drug metoclopramide is used in this situation to promote evacuation of gastric content to the small intestine. Metoclopramide also increases tone at the gastroesophageal junction, thereby reducing gastroesophageal reflux, and has central antiemetic action. To facilitate gastric evacuation, metoclopramide (0.2 to 0.4 mg/kg, maximum dose 10 mg, IM or IV) is given 30 to 45 min before anesthesia. Oral administration in a patient with a moderately full stomach would be somewhat less effective. Metoclopramide does not completely reverse gastric hypomotility caused by narcotics nor does it guarantee a completely empty stomach, but its role in reducing aspiration may be significant. Because atropine counteracts the effect of metoclopramide and reduces tone at the gastroesophageal junction, it should only be used in this situation if absolutely necessary.

SMOKE INHALATION INJURY

A majority of fire-related deaths in animals occur in the fire and most are due to carbon monoxide (CO) poisoning, not burns. Animals that survive long enough to be presented to a veterinarian may have sustained appreciable smoke or thermal damage to the respiratory tract as well as carbon monoxide intoxication. In many instances, correct emergency care makes the critical difference for survival.

Pathophysiology

Two distinct mechanisms of bronchopulmonary injury that follow smoke inhalation have been identified: carbon monoxide intoxication and smoke toxicity. Smoke toxicity is further divided into direct injury from smoke and smoke poisoning from noxious chemicals formed by the incomplete combustion of various natural and synthetic products. Although these conditions may coexist and overlap, each has distinct characteristics.

Carbon monoxide is a colorless, odorless, nonirritating gas that is produced by the incomplete combustion of carbon-containing materials. It has an affinity for hemoglobin that is 240 times greater than that of oxygen, and the resulting carboxyhemoglobin (COHb) is unable to function in oxygen transport. The resulting physiologic abnormality of carbon monoxide intoxication is inadequate tissue oxygenation. The brain is most sensitive to this oxygen deprivation. Clinical signs of carbon monoxide intoxication become evident when the COHb concentration is at 10 to 20 per cent. Early signs include shortness of breath, mild dyspnea, and confusion. At higher levels increasing irritability, nausea, vomiting, loss of coordination, and convulsions occur, and at COHb levels greater than 50 to 60 per cent respiratory failure and death may ensue. As COHb levels increase, the victim becomes disoriented and loses the desire and ability to escape.

Fortunately, thermal damage to the lower respiratory tract and pulmonary parenchyma is rare unless live steam or explosive gases are inhaled. However, mucosal burns of the mouth, nasopharynx, and pharynx may lead to upper airway obstruction any time during the first 24 hours after the burn.

Direct airway damage may be caused by inhalation of soot and other superheated particles, some of which may carry noxious particles into the lungs. Smoke poisoning results from toxic byproducts such as short-chain aldehydes, oxides of sulfur and nitrogen, and acrolein produced during burning of room furnishings, cotton clothing, plastics, and other materials. Some plastics also produce large amounts of benzene, whose anesthetic action may promote easier passage of acids and alkali into the respiratory tract. Finally, smoke poisons pulmonary alveolar macrophages. Impaired macrophage function is a likely contributing factor to the onset of bacterial pneumonia that occurs in some smoke inhalation patients.

Diagnosis

Table 2 summarizes the four stages of smoke inhalation injury. The clinician can easily recognize that an animal has been in a fire based on history provided by the presenting party and the acrid smell of smoke, which is often present on the haircoat. However, the full extent of clinical changes may not be evident for 24 to 72 hr, so careful serial examinations are required.

Careful examination of facial burns, a search for oral burns, and examination for laryngospasm are performed immediately. Hoarseness, expiratory wheeze, and carbonaceous sputum are indicators of potentially serious involvement. Inhalation injury

Table 2. Stages of Inhalation Injury

Stage I (During Smoke Inhalation)
Hypoxia, hypercapnia, acidosis
Decreased cardiac output
Hypercapnia decreasing to apnea
Bronchospasm
CO poisoning

Stage II (0 to 30 min)
Hypercapnia, mild hypoxia
Severely depressed cardiac output
Increased vascular resistance
Hyperventilation
Carboxyhemoglobinemia

Stage III (2 to 24 hr)
Increasing hypoxia
Decreasing pulmonary compliance
Altered ventilation-perfusion ratios
Clearing of CO
Mildly depressed to normal cardiac output
Pulmonary edema

Stage IV (After 24 hr)
If there is bacterial pneumonia, lung failure often occurs
If there is no bacterial pneumonia, the animal frequently recovers

From Tams, T. R., and Sherding, R. G.: Comp. Cont. Ed. Pract. Vet. 3:986, 1981; with permission.

may cause auscultable crackles or rhonchi, which may be evident on presentation or delayed until hours or days later. A cherry-red color of the skin and mucous membranes, which may result from carbon monoxide toxicity, burns, or heat from the fire, may mask cyanosis and poor perfusion from shock. The eyes are examined for evidence of conjunctivitis or corneal abrasions.

Carboxyhemoglobin determination, blood gas analysis, and thoracic radiographs are useful for better defining the initial condition of the patient and monitoring progress. Venous blood is transported on ice to a human hospital for measurement of COHb levels (reported as the percentage of saturation of hemoglobin in the carboxyhemoglobin state). High levels confirm a diagnosis of carbon monoxide toxicity and alert the clinician to the possibility of serious neurologic complications. Initial blood gas assessments may be misleading because the Pa_{O_2} can be normal in even moderately severe cases of carbon monoxide toxicity because the blood is still in tension equilibrium with alveolar gas. Thus, the Pa_{O_2} may be normal even though oxygen content is actually dangerously low.

Radiographic changes may not be evident until 16 to 24 hr after a moderate to severe inhalation injury. The most commonly seen radiographic patterns include diffuse bronchial-peribronchial densities or diffuse, patchy, interstitial infiltration representative of edema. Alveolar radiographic patterns with air bronchograms may be evident later and usually indicate bacterial pneumonia.

Transtracheal aspiration cytologic study and bronchoscopy are more sensitive means of identifying the extent of pulmonary injury. Cytologic examination reveals burned ciliated cells, strands of mucus, and soot particles in moderate to severe cases. Bronchoscopy affords a means of direct airway visualization, which may provide valuable prognostic information. Airway changes may include mucosal erythema, hemorrhage, ulceration, edema, and carbonaceous particle accumulation. The major risk of this procedure in animals is that general anesthesia is required unless a tracheostomy tube is in place.

Treatment

The mouth and larynx are examined immediately to ensure that there is a patent airway. Oropharyngeal suction or manual removal of debris may be required. If severe laryngospasm is present a tracheostomy tube should be placed before it is required as a last-minute emergency effort.

Definitive therapy for carbon monoxide poisoning is the administration of 100 per cent oxygen. The immediate goals are to reverse cerebral and myocardial hypoxia and to accelerate carbon monoxide elimination, all of which can be accomplished by a high concentration of inspired oxygen. The half-life of COHb is 4 hr when breathing room air; it is 30 min when 100 per cent oxygen is administered. Often firefighters will administer oxygen to a rescued animal at the scene.

Patients who are fairly alert at presentation usually respond to oxygen as administered in a conventional oxygen cage. If clinical signs of hypoxia (irritable or aggressive behavior, incoordination, somnolence, collapse, or convulsions) develop, the patient is sedated so that 100 per cent oxygen can be administered. Positive pressure ventilation is then performed at a rate of 8 to 12 respirations per minute for 30 to 40 min. Oxygen therapy is also beneficial for the pulmonary edema, resulting from altered alveolocapillary permeability, which may occur after smoke inhalation injury.

Intravenous fluids are indicated in hypoxic states and shock to help maintain cardiac output. Reduced perfusion aggravates tissue hypoxia; however, fluid therapy can potentiate lung edema. Dopamine (2 to 10 μg/kg/min) may be required to maintain arterial blood pressure in patients that are intolerant of fluid infusions.

The use of corticosteroids in inhalation injury is controversial. Studies using animal models have shown significant immunosuppression and decreased tracheobronchial clearance mechanisms when steroids are used. Use of steroids in patients that have sustained both smoke inhalation injury and thermal injury results in increased mortality. Because the risk of steroid use may outweigh the benefits (decreased tracheobronchial inflammation and cerebral edema associated with hypoxia), use of steroids in smoke inhalation patients is not recommended.

Studies have also failed to document the efficacy of antibiotics for late-developing bacterial pneumonia. Prophylactic antibiotics are not recommended and will only serve to select resistant bacteria. If radiographic or clinical signs of bacterial pneumonia develop, antibiotics are selected based on culture and sensitivity testing.

Bronchodilator therapy may be used to help alleviate the reflex bronchospasms caused by the effect of inhalation of soot particles on epithelial irritant receptors. Patients that frequently cough should be suspected of having this problem. Aminophylline may be beneficial at 11 mg/kg every 6 to 8 hr in the dog and 5 mg/kg every 8 to 12 hr in the cat.

Complicating Factors

Inhalation injury in conjunction with body surface burns has a poorer prognosis for survival than inhalation injury alone. The incidence of postinhalation bacterial pneumonia is increased if there are complicating factors, including surface burns or the use of tracheostomy tubes. Meticulous care of tracheostomies is of utmost importance.

References and Supplemental Reading

Bartlett, J. G.: Aspiration pneumonia. Clinical Notes on Respiratory Diseases, Spring, 1980, pp. 3–8.
Cohen, S. E.: The aspiration syndrome. Clin. Obstet. Gynecol. 9:235, 1982.
Crowe, D. T., and Downs, M. O.: Pharyngostomy complications in dogs and cats and recommended technical modifications: Experimental and clinical investigations. Vet. Surg. 15:117, 1986.
Flink, E. B., and Prasad, A. S.: Chemical agents and disease. In Sodeman, W. A., and Sodeman, T. M. (eds.): Pathologic Physiology: Mechanisms of Disease, 6th ed. Philadelphia: W. B. Saunders, 1979.
McKiernan, B. C.: Lower respiratory tract diseases. In Ettinger, S. J. (ed.): Veterinary Internal Medicine, 2nd ed. Philadelphia: W. B. Saunders, 1983.
Orton, E. C., and Wheeler, S. L.: Continuous positive airway pressure therapy for aspiration pneumonia in a dog. J.A.V.M.A. 188:1437, 1986.
Pascor, P. J.: Short-term ventilatory support. In Kirk, R. W. (ed.): Current Veterinary Therapy IX. Philadelphia: W. B. Saunders, 1986.
Schwartz, D. J., Wayne, J. W., Gibbs, C. P., et al.: The pulmonary consequences of aspiration of gastric contents at pH values greater than 2.5. Am. Rev. Respir. Dis. 121:119, 1980.
Tams, T. R., and Sherding, R. G.: Smoke inhalation injury. Comp. Cont. Ed. Pract. Vet. 3:986, 1981.
Tams, T. R.: Aspiration pneumonia and complications of inhalation of smoke and toxic gases. Vet. Clin. North Am. 15:971, 1985.
Thayer, G. W.: Infections of the respiratory system. In Greene, C. E. (ed.): Clinical Microbiology and Infectious Diseases of the Dog and Cat. Philadelphia: W. B. Saunders, 1984.
Trunkey, D. D.: Inhalation injury. Surg. Clin. North Am. 58:1133, 1978.

PULMONARY EDEMA

NEIL HARPSTER, V.M.D.

Jamaica Plain, Massachusetts

The term pulmonary edema implies the excessive accumulation of fluid within the lung. This abnormal state may occur in a wide variety of diseases; it may be a significant factor in a large number of conditions that can lead to lung injury, impairment of function, and even death, if it is allowed to progress inadequately attended.

PATHOPHYSIOLOGIC MECHANISMS

In the normal lung there is some level of transudation of intravascular fluid from the pulmonary capillaries and, perhaps, adjacent venules into the surrounding interstitial spaces. This so-called loss is minimized by normal hydrostatic and oncotic mechanisms, which work in concert to maintain fluid within the vascular compartment. The interstitial fluid that does develop is of no clinical or functional significance. It is quickly reabsorbed by pulmonary lymphatic vessels, which reside in the interstitial tissue; these transport the fluid to subsequently empty into a systemic vein. However, when pathologic states exist, normal homeostatic mechanisms, which were previously effective in the reabsorption of any interstitial fluid, are no longer adequate, and clinical signs and pulmonary dysfunction are quick to develop.

Increased Hydrostatic Pressure

Elevation of the pulmonary capillary pressure to 25 mm Hg or above results in a measurable fluid accumulation in the lung. This occurs because the normal mechanisms responsible for maintenance of lung fluid are exceeded at this level of hydrostatic pressure. These normalizing factors are substantial, as the normal left atrial, pulmonary venous, and pulmonary capillary pressures are in the range of 4 to 5 mm Hg. Nonetheless, in left-sided heart failure and other conditions (Table 1) elevation of these pressures to 25 mm Hg and above does occur and the pulmonary edema that ensues becomes a life-threatening concern.

Decreased Plasma Colloid Oncotic Pressure

Hypoproteinemia, specifically hypoalbuminemia, is the usual underlying process responsible for a

Table 1. *Pathophysiologic Mechanisms and Etiologic Factors in Pulmonary Edema*

I. Increased pulmonary capillary hydrostatic pressure
  A. Elevated left atrial pressure (LAP)
    1. Left ventricular failure
    2. Mitral stenosis
  B. Pulmonary venous pressure elevation without increased LAP
    1. Compression of left atrium
      a. Aortic body tumor
      b. Enlarged bronchial lymph node
      c. Other mediastinal masses
    2. Veno-occlusive disease
      a. Congenital stenosis
      b. Acute/chronic mediastinitis
  C. Increased pulmonary arterial pressure
    1. Acute left-to-right shunts
    2. Iatrogenic (excessive fluid administration)

II. Decreased plasma colloid oncotic pressure
  A. Hypoalbuminemia (?)
    1. Nutritional causes
    2. Hepatic disorders
    3. Protein-losing kidney, bowel, or skin disease
  B. Excessive fluid administration

III. Alterations in alveolocapillary membrane permeability
  A. Infectious agents (e.g., pneumonia, sepsis)
  B. Inhalation of irritant gases (e.g., smoke, ozone, nitrogen oxides, phosgene, carbonyl chloride, oxides of cadmium and sulfur, Teflon fumes)
  C. Aspiration of acidic gastric fluid
  D. Near-drowning
  E. Electric shock
  F. Radiation pneumonitis
  G. Disseminated intravascular coagulation
  H. Immunologic reactions (histamine, prostaglandins)
    1. Anaphylaxis
    2. Hypersensitivity pneumonitis

IV. Pulmonary lymphatic insufficiency
  A. Post lung transplant
  B. Lymphangitis carcinomatosis
  C. Silicosis (fibrosing lymphangitis)

V. Mechanisms incompletely understood
  A. High altitude
  B. Pulmonary thromboembolism
  C. Intracerebral lesions
  D. Hepatic disease
  E. Shock lung

decrease in the plasma colloid oncotic pressure. As a rule, hypoproteinemia alone does not result in clinically significant pulmonary edema but frequently does result in subcutaneous ventral edema. However, hypoproteinemia may contribute to the development of pulmonary edema when either elevated capillary hydrostatic pressure or alterations

385

in the permeability of the alveolocapillary membrane coexist. Then the lowered intravascular osmolarity will effect a more rapid movement of fluid into the interstitial space and the alveoli. These events are likely to develop during intravenous fluid administration and may occur in the absence of any definable left-sided heart abnormalities.

Alterations In Alveolocapillary Membrane Permeability

Many varied factors can be responsible for increased permeability of the pulmonary capillary and the alveolocapillary membranes, resulting in the accelerated movement of fluid from the capillary to the pulmonary interstitial space and even into the alveoli (Table 1). Some agents appear to effect a change in the size or number of pores in the pulmonary capillary membrane without causing injury to the capillary wall, and the release of histamine has been suggested as a possible mechanism (Pietra et al., 1971). Other agents have been shown to cause physical disruption of endothelial cells on electron microscopy. Proposed mechanisms for endothelial cell injury include the production of different activated and unstable oxygen derivatives (Cross and Hyde, 1978), complement activation (Craddock et al., 1977), and the release of prostaglandins (Williams and Morley, 1973). Because of the similarity of the clinical syndromes resulting in damage to the alveolocapillary membrane to that seen with respiratory distress in the neonate, these conditions in humans have been referred to as adult respiratory distress syndrome (ARDS).

Pulmonary Lymphatic Insufficiency

The pulmonary lymphatic system is responsible for most of the moment-by-moment removal of pulmonary interstitial fluid that normally accumulates over the course of a day. This system is quite extensive, with afferent vessels from the lungs coursing to the tracheobronchial lymph nodes; from there the lymph is drained via a chain of cranial mediastinal lymph nodes (Evans and Christensen, 1979). However, when there is an impairment of lymphatic function, whether the result of physical blockage or depression of physiologic pumping, drainage of fluid from interstitial spaces will be reduced. The functional capacity of the pulmonary lymphatics is felt to be the ultimate rate-limiting step in the drainage of the interstitial space.

ETIOLOGIC FACTORS

The causes of pulmonary edema are far more numerous than the pathophysiologic mechanisms previously discussed. These are outlined in Table 1, in which they are grouped according to the predominant mechanisms responsible. The differentiation among these various causes in the clinical setting is not necessarily easy, especially when the patient is in a compromised and uncooperative condition. However, patience and an organized approach will frequently yield the logical and correct conclusions.

Although the main pulmonary artery systolic pressure and the pulmonary artery wedge pressure will be elevated above normal in most causes of pulmonary edema, values in the range of 25 to 30 mm Hg should only be found when increased pulmonary capillary hydrostatic pressure is the primary abnormality (Table 1). Further identification of the cause will require additional diagnostic tests (e.g., thoracic radiography, echocardiography, and computed tomography) to separate cardiac from noncardiac lesions. When the pulmonary artery wedge pressure is consistently under 25 mm Hg in the presence of active pulmonary edema other mechanisms must be entertained.

Of all the mechanisms responsible for pulmonary edema a decrease in the plasma oncotic pressure should be easiest to define. When the serum total protein level is below 5.0 gm/dl suspicions should be raised, and serum albumin levels of less than 2.0 gm/dl (usually < 1.5 gm/dl) are confirming. It then becomes a matter of a proper search to establish the cause (see Table 1). However, in many instances hypoproteinemia alone will not result in pulmonary edema, and other contributing causes must be sought and defined. Mild elevation in the pulmonary capillary pressure frequently coexists and is responsible for the pulmonary edema in this setting.

The multifarious diseases that are responsible for altering the alveolocapillary membrane permeability are more difficult to recognize clinically. In part, this occurs because many of these conditions (see Table 1) cause other effects and injuries to the lungs beyond that affecting capillary permeability. An accurate history taking can be crucial in defining the exact cause, and this along with supportive laboratory evaluation is all-important in proper management and recovery. These conditions have been categorized as shock lung or adult respiratory distress syndrome (ARDS) in humans, meaning that a large group of etiologically diverse diseases (e.g., shock, sepsis, severe burns, uremia, blood transfusions, oxygen toxicity, aspiration, and pancreatitis) cause a similar but poorly understood effect on the alveolocapillary membrane.

Pulmonary lymphatic insufficiency is an uncommonly recognized cause of pulmonary edema. Although causes of impaired pulmonary lymphatic function have been recognized both clinically (see Table 1) and experimentally, the importance of these alone as causes of pulmonary edema has been strongly questioned (Magno and Szidon, 1976). It may be that pulmonary lymphatic insufficiency plays a role in the development of pulmonary edema only when there are other contributing factors. This combined effect may result in development of pulmonary edema at an exaggerated rate.

In addition to these well-recognized causes of pulmonary edema, there are other causes that are less well understood (see Table 1).

HIGH-ALTITUDE PULMONARY EDEMA

This syndrome occurs in various mammals with rapid exposure to altitude in excess of 2700 m (8860 ft) without a period of acclimatization. In general, it is believed to be an exaggerated vasoconstriction response of the arterioles to alveolar hypoxia. Catheterization of the pulmonary arteries reveals pulmonary hypertension, while the pulmonary artery wedge pressure remains normal. However, an exact cause for the pulmonary edema has not been identified. Theories range from transarterial leakage caused by high pressure, to inhomogeneity of arterial vasoconstriction causing local areas of overperfusion in which edema occurs, and even to transient intravascular coagulation.

NEUROGENIC PULMONARY EDEMA

Head trauma was the initial neurogenic abnormality recognized in association with pulmonary edema. Subsequently this association has also been seen with meningitis, brain tumors, encephalitis, subarachnoid hemorrhage, cerebral embolism, cerebral thrombosis, and seizures. There is general agreement that the central nervous system (CNS) lesion causes an excessive response by the sympathetic nervous system. However, beyond this initial mechanism the specific cause for the development of pulmonary edema is less clear. One current thought is that sympathetic overactivity produces shifts of blood volume from the systemic to the pulmonary circulation, with resultant elevation of the left atrial and pulmonary capillary pressures, a so-called imbalance of Starling's forces. Other theories have suggested elevated pulmonary capillary pressures due to constriction of postcapillary venous sphincters in the lungs and alterations in capillary permeability.

PULMONARY EDEMA AND PULMONARY THROMBOEMBOLISM

It seems paradoxical that a process causing interruption of blood flow to a portion of the lung should also lead to the development of pulmonary edema.

However, this observation has been made clinically in humans and has been confirmed experimentally in animals (Singer et al., 1958). The pathophysiologic mechanism by which this occurs is less clearly defined. One theory proposes the development of transarteriolar fluid leakage at the site of the microembolus owing to alterations in permeability and locally raised pressure; whereas others have considered the local release of vasoactive substances, resulting in pulmonary venoconstriction and the primary leak at the capillary bed level.

PULMONARY EDEMA AND LIVER DISEASE

Pulmonary edema has been a common complication of liver dysfunction in both an acute and a chronic setting. In the chronic situation, decreased oncotic pressure most likely plays a significant role, as the result of hypoalbuminemia. However, in acute liver disease a mechanism to explain the development of pulmonary edema is less clear. A neurologic origin has been suggested owing to the concomitant development of cerebral edema. However, as cerebral edema does not occur routinely, other less well-defined causes must also play a role.

CLINICAL MANIFESTATIONS

Fluid accumulation in the lung during the development of pulmonary edema has been depicted as occurring in four distinct phases or stages, depending on the extent of involvement of the lung tissue (Fig. 1). The earliest phase is characterized by an increase in passage of fluid and colloid from capillaries into the interstitial space; but interstitial volume does not increase, as an increase in lymphatic outflow carries away the potential surfeit. In stage 1 the passage of fluid and colloid into the interstitial compartment exceeds the functional capacity of the pulmonary lymphatic system, and fluid accumulates about the bronchioles and small vessels. As this progresses there is alveolar septal swelling owing to continued fluid accumulation (stage 2) and then the development of fluid in the alveolar angles (stage 3). Finally, alveolar filling occurs (stage 4) when alveoli reach a critical configuration at which inflation pressures can no longer maintain the existing configuration.

As might be expected, the progressive stages of pulmonary edema as explained above and depicted in Figure 1 can be related clinically to the clinical signs, physical findings, radiographic changes, and pulmonary function studies. These are summarized in Table 2. The radiographic patterns of pulmonary edema vary considerably, in some part determined by the pathophysiologic mechanism responsible. However, other factors may be equally important,

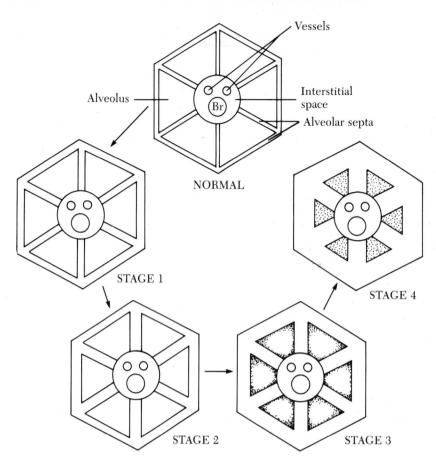

Figure 1. The progressive development of edema in the lung. Stage 1 is the development of interstitial fluid about the bronchioles and small vessels; stage 2 is alveolar septal swelling; stage 3 shows fluid accumulation in the alveolar angles; stage 4 is alveolar flooding. Br, bronchus. (Adapted from Prichard: *Edema of the Lung* 1982. Courtesy of Charles C Thomas, Publisher, Springfield, Illinois.)

such as gravitational forces in humans, particularly in pulmonary edema caused by increased pulmonary capillary pressure (West, 1970). Gravity and other poorly defined factors are responsible for the radiographic patterns seen in early left-sided heart failure in the dog, characterized by perihilar and caudal lobe pulmonary edema, which is more severe in right-sided lung lobes. This pattern of pulmonary edema is supported clinically by the presence of more pronounced crackles over the right side of the thorax.

A variety of methods have been developed for

***Table 2.** Effects of Progressive Pulmonary Edema*

Evaluation	Stage 1	Stage 2	Stage 3	Stage 4
Clinical Signs				
Cough	Absent	Present	Present	Present
Dyspnea	Absent	Absent	Present	Present
Physical Findings				
Crackles	Absent	Absent	Present	Present
Dyspnea	Absent	Absent	Present	Present
Radiographic Patterns				
Pre-edema*	Present	Present	Present	Present
Interstitial edema	Present	Present	Present	Present
Alveolar edema	Absent	Absent	Present	Present
Pulmonary Function				
Lung compliance	Increased	Increased	Increased	Increased
Airway resistance	Increased	Increased	Increased	Increased
Closing volume†	Decreased	Decreased	Decreased	Decreased
Energy of Breathing	Normal	N to Increased	Increased	Increased
Po_2	Normal	N to Decreased	Decreased	Decreased
Pco_2	Normal	N to Decreased	Decreased	Decreased

*Pre-edema suggests the presence of pulmonary vascular distention without pulmonary edema.
†See text for explanation.
N, normal.

the quantitative measurements of pulmonary edema, however, thoracic radiography remains the standard for recognition in the clinical setting. In left-sided heart failure distention and engorgement of blood vessels is the earliest recognizable radiographic finding, with lobar veins being of greater diameter than accompanying arteries. In the cat, both arteries and veins tend to be dilated. This so-called pre-edema pattern may be absent in pulmonary edema of other causes. Interstitial edema is the earliest recognizable evidence of increased lung fluid seen radiographically. Fine interstitial lines, termed Kerley's lines, are one of the earliest patterns seen in humans but are rarely recognized in animals. A perihilar haze, peribronchial cuffing, and fine increased interstitial densities are commonly noted in the dog. With progression to alveolar edema comes the loss of pulmonary lucency and the development of patchy, fluffy radiographic densities. These may be accompanied by interlobar fissure lines, suggesting the presence of mild pleural effusion.

EFFECT OF PULMONARY EDEMA ON LUNG FUNCTION

It seems logical to reason that lung function remains normal in the first two stages of pulmonary edema and becomes compromised when fluid begins to accumulate in the alveoli. Although this assumption may hold true for clinical symptoms with the patient at rest, measurable abnormalities in pulmonary function, excepting blood gases, can be recognized at earlier stages (see Table 2). These results are supported by decreased activity and reduced exercise tolerance in patients with early left-sided heart failure. Unfortunately, these more sophisticated tests for measuring pulmonary function are not readily available in clinical veterinary medicine. Nevertheless, these will be briefly discussed below.

Static Lung Compliance

The volume change per unit pressure change is known as the compliance of the lung. In the normal lung it is determined by the mixture of elastic and collagen fibers in the alveolar walls and about blood vessels. Compliance is reduced by processes that increase the accumulation of fibrous tissue in the lung and is increased with emphysema and also with age.

With pulmonary edema the lungs become stiff, i.e., less compliant. It has been reported that during acute cardiogenic pulmonary edema in humans, the average lung compliance is only 24 per cent of normal (Sharp et al., 1958). Responsible causes include the edema fluid itself, as well as the washout of alveolar surfactant as a consequence of alveolar flooding. Decreased compliance has also been demonstrated in isolated interstitial pulmonary edema, a circumstance in which alveolar surfactant content plays a minor role.

Airway Resistance

The difference in pressure between the two ends of a tube carrying air or some other gaseous medium defines the airway resistance. In the normal lung the greatest airway resistance resides in the medium-sized bronchi, whereas the small bronchioles contribute relatively little resistance (Macklin and Mead, 1967). Most of the pressure drop has been shown to occur in the airways up to approximately the tenth generation. Primary factors determining airway resistance include lung volume, tone of the bronchial smooth muscle, and density and viscosity of the gas.

In abnormal states, such as pulmonary edema, airway resistance increases. In interstitial pulmonary edema this change occurs primarily in the peripheral small airways (less than 2 mm in diameter); it is most likely the result of bronchial compression by the presence of the interstitial edema itself, but also is caused by the development of bronchial edema. Airway resistance is even further increased in acute cardiogenic edema, perhaps related to reflex bronchoconstriction, with reports of up to three times normal values (Sharp et al., 1958). In alveolar pulmonary edema additional contributions to increased airway resistance include both the accumulation of edema fluid in the airways and decreased functional lung volume.

Closing Volume

The point at which detectable numbers of small airways close during expiration is referred to as the closing volume. The end point is defined by a change in concentration of an exhaled gas that was previously inhaled. The site of closure is thought to be small airways of 1 to 2 mm, making this procedure a valuable measurement of small airway function.

In pulmonary edema, both interstitial and alveolar, the closing volume is increased. This means that small airways close earlier during expiration, owing to a combination of airway narrowing (i.e., the result of interstitial compression of airways, bronchial edema, and airway fluid) and perhaps some increase in expiratory effort.

Energy of Breathing

As expected, when increased efforts of respiration are required this ensures an increase in energy consumption. An increased work of breathing has been demonstrated in both acute and chronic heart failure. This increased energy expenditure is usually a result of increases in both elastic and viscous lung components. Respiratory arrest often develops in animals with severe, unresolved lung edema.

Blood Gas Measurement in Pulmonary Edema

Edema tends to collect heterogeneously in the lung, thereby creating significant regional variations in compliance, airways resistance, and closing volume, which result in localized air trapping, variations in ventilation, and even atelectasis. Similar changes occur in other diffuse lung disorders and effect alterations in gas exchange that have been termed ventilation-perfusion abnormalities. These findings are magnified in the presence of alveolar pulmonary edema; as gas exchange varies from normal in unaffected alveoli to negligible in alveoli flooded by pulmonary edema, while blood circulation to both these regions remains relatively normal.

Blood gas measurements commonly remain normal in the presence of interstitial pulmonary edema alone owing to the decreased perfusion of poorly ventilated and hypoxic areas. However, as alveolar pulmonary edema evolves, arterial oxygenation begins to fall (i.e., hypoxemia develops). This is usually accompanied by a fall in the carbon dioxide concentration (i.e., hypocapnia) as a result of tachypnea and hyperventilation. However, there is a subset of human patients with pulmonary edema in which hypercapnia has been documented (Avery et al., 1970). It has been postulated that this carbon dioxide retention is the result of an inability to maintain adequate minute ventilation because of extensive airway collapse and obstruction by edema fluid and froth.

MANAGEMENT

Pulmonary edema is a serious and potentially life-threatening problem, demanding prompt recognition and the immediate institution of effective measures. Theoretically, each case of pulmonary edema is quickly resolved by correction of the underlying abnormality that is responsible for its development. Unfortunately, the opportunity to accomplish this is rarely afforded, and insufficient or inappropriate treatment will hardly suffice. Perhaps of greatest importance to the clinician is an understanding of the pathophysiologic mechanism that is responsible for the pulmonary edema. This facilitates the choice of appropriate therapy.

Pulmonary edema can be an acute, life-threatening process (see below). Management depends on the pathophysiologic mechanism responsible,

and various options will be discussed. Pulmonary edema due to decreased plasma colloid oncotic pressure and that occurring as a sequela to pulmonary lymphatic insufficiency will be omitted, as the clinical significance of these mechanisms as pure causes of pulmonary edema has been strongly questioned.

Acute Cardiogenic Pulmonary Edema

This common clinical problem is seen most frequently in the dog as a result of chronic valvular heart disease and dilated cardiomyopathy and in the cat with either hypertrophic or restrictive cardiomyopathy. After the diagnosis is established, usually on the basis of physical and radiographic findings, therapy must be promptly instituted. The solution to effective management lies in prompt diagnosis, use of therapeutic agents of clinically proved efficacy, and frequent patient evaluation to ensure the desired response.

Acceptable approaches to the management of cardiogenic pulmonary edema are numerous and varied (Table 3). However, the general principles are rigid and unswerving: (1) minimize cardiac work, (2) improve oxygenation, (3) resolve pulmonary edema, and (4) enhance cardiac performance. After these goals are accomplished it remains to establish a cause for the pulmonary edema, so as to optimize long-term therapy and, thereby, reduce the chance for further episodes of this life-threatening problem.

In the majority of patients the use of oxygen, furosemide, and prazosin is usually effective in controlling the pulmonary edema and stabilizing the dog within 12 to 24 hr (see pp. 240 and 231). However, when pulmonary edema is severe it may be necessary to administer furosemide at 4.4 mg/kg every 1 to 2 hr IV for two to four doses to obtain an adequate response. Other balanced vasodilators or venodilators (see Table 3) may be as efficacious as prazosin, and personal choice and experience will guide choice of drugs. The use of aminophylline may be helpful, initially, in controlling bronchospasm, which may contribute to hypoxemia in pulmonary edema. Sedatives may also be of considerable benefit in relieving anxiety and thereby improving ventilation. It is when continued improvement in respiration and lung auscultation is not realized after a few hours, or progressive deterioration in the patient's condition continues despite the use of usually effective measures, that the use of intravenous sodium nitroprusside with or without the concomitant use of positive inotropic agents such as amrinone or dobutamine needs to be considered. Although these intravenous modalities can result in adverse effects when not used properly, with appropriate administration they are frequently life saving.

Table 3. *Summary of the Various Methods Available for the Management of Cardiogenic Pulmonary Edema*

I. Reduced cardiac work
  A. Cage rest, exercise restriction
  B. Sedation
    1. Morphine sulfate, 0.2–0.5 mg/kg IM, SC
    2. Hydrocodone bitartrate (Hycodan), 0.25–0.5 mg/kg PO
    3. Pentobarbital, 2–4 mg/kg IM or IV
  C. Arteriolar dilators
    1. Hydralazine, 0.5–1.0 mg/kg b.i.d.
    2. Sodium nitroprusside,† 1–15 μg/kg/min IV

II. Improve ventilation (oxygenation)
  A. Oxygen administration
    1. Oxygen tent or cage—50% concentration maximum for long-term use
    2. Nasal catheter
  B. Bronchodilators
    1. Aminophylline, 6–10 mg/kg q 8hr IM or *slowly* IV
    2. Isoproterenol,* 0.05–0.2 mg IM or SC
    3. Terbutaline, 0.05–0.10 mg/kg PO
  C. Sedation (see above)
  D. Improve airway patency
    1. Endotracheal tube
    2. Tracheotomy tube
  E. Ventilation (artificial)

III. Reduce venous return and excess body fluids
  A. Potent loop diuretics
    1. Furosemide (Lasix), 4.4 mg/kg IV (see text)
    2. Ethacrynic acid (Edecrin), 10 mg/kg IV
  B. Vasodilator therapy
    1. Venodilators
     a. Nitroglycerin ointment
      Dogs—⅛ inch/4.5 kg q 8hr to q 6hr cutaneously
      Cats—⅛ to ¼ inch q 8hr to q 6hr cutaneously
     b. Isosorbide dinitrate, 0.5–2.0 mg/kg q 8hr PO
     c. Sodium nitroprusside,† 1–15 μg/kg/min IV
    2. Balanced vasodilators
     a. Prazosin (Minipress), 1.0 mg/15 kg q 8hr PO
     b. Captopril (Capoten), 0.5–2.0 mg/kg q 8hr

C. Phlebotomy‡—remove 5% increments of calculated total blood volume every 30 to 60 min to effect. Do not exceed 20% of calculated blood volume.

IV. Strengthen myocardial contractility
  A. Digoxin
    1. Intravenously—0.022–0.044 mg/kg divided and given over a 1- to 2-hr period
    2. Oral
     a. Tablet, 0.009 mg/kg q 12hr
     b. Elixir, 0.008 mg/kg q 12hr
  B. Dobutamine (Dobutrex), 2.5–10 μg/kg/min IV
  C. Amrinone (Inocor), give 0.75 mg/kg bolus IV over 2 to 3 min, then infusion at 5–10 μg/kg/min

V. Management of contributing cardiac arrhythmias
  A. Supraventricular
    1. Atrial fibrillation—treat with digoxin as outlined above, IV use of digoxin may be helpful. Avoid dobutamine§
    2. Atrial or AV junctional tachycardia
     a. Try vagal maneuver to terminate
     b. Treat as outlined above, include 0.044 mg/kg digoxin given once IV
     c. Repeat vagal maneuver, if unsuccessful give antiarrhythmic drugs
      (1) Quinidine sulfate, 6–12 mg/kg q 2hr PO for no more than 4 doses
      (2) Propranolol (Inderal), 0.04–0.06 mg/kg IV over 2 to 3 min, or 0.2–1.0 mg/kg q 8hr PO
      (3) Verapamil (Isoptin), 0.05–0.3 mg/kg IV over 2 to 3 min, or 1–2 mg/kg q 8hr PO
  B. Ventricular
    1. Lidocaine
     a. IV bolus, 1–2 mg/kg
     b. IV infusion, 30–50 μg/kg/min
    2. Procainamide
     a. IV bolus, 2–4 mg/kg
     b. IV infusion, 20–75 μg/kg/min
     c. IM or PO, 12–20 mg/kg q 8hr to q 6hr

*Must be given only with great caution; will cause cardiac acceleration.
†Should be administered only with blood pressure monitoring; can result in severe hypotension.
‡Calculation of total blood volume—88 ml/kg BW.
§In atrial fibrillation dobutamine causes marked cardiac acceleration owing to increased AV conduction unless prior digitalization is accomplished and the dobutamine infusion rate is low.

After the pulmonary edema is resolved, the patient's condition will safely allow the proper diagnostic procedures to establish a definitive diagnosis. The addition of other treatment may be suggested by the results of these further studies. Cardiac arrhythmias are frequently present. These may be due to an underlying cardiac disorder or hypoxia or may be a sequela to metabolic or combined metabolic and respiratory acidosis. When severe metabolic acidosis exists, this should be treated with intravenous sodium bicarbonate. In the absence of significant acidosis the use of antiarrhythmic agents is indicated (see Table 3).

Pulmonary Edema due to Increased Capillary Permeability

Management of the pulmonary edema that occurs as a sequela to alterations in the capillary or alveolar membrane permeability or both is far more challenging than that previously discussed. First, a specific cause for the lung injury is rarely established, and the exact site and extent of the injury may be difficult to determine. Second, there is frequently injury, focal death, or both of endothelial and epithelial cells, thus creating a potential "permanent" leak until repair takes place. Lastly, therapeutic modalities that will effectively reduce capillary permeability are neither effective nor well understood.

Various mechanisms of primary injury have been proposed. These have included osmotic or cytolytic cell membrane damage, general cytotoxic change, damage caused by oxidative processes, and alterations in smooth muscle contractility resulting in increased interepithelial pore size. Thus, the solution is to find an agent or agents that will reverse or, at least, retard these changes. Unfortunately, few inroads have been made toward these ends despite extensive experimental research.

Numerous therapeutic agents have been touted as the panacea for this problem. Corticosteroids have received the most attention in this regard, based on observations that they antagonize the action of histamine and kinin, stabilize lysozymes, and interfere with the migration of phagocytes into areas of inflammation. Drugs of this family have been reported to be effective in the management of some cases of ARDS in humans. However, conclusive evidence supporting the effectiveness of these agents is lacking. Similar conclusions have been forthcoming on the use of heparin (proposed benefit in disseminated intravascular coagulation mechanisms), sympatholytic compounds (decrease in hydrostatic pressure), and superoxide dismutase (protection of phagocytosing leukocytes from the toxic effects of oxidants). On the other hand, several agents have been shown to reduce pulmonary capillary permeability, at least in isolated instances. Both antihistamines (i.e., diphenhydramine) and phosphodiesterase inhibitors (i.e., aminophylline and isoprenaline) have been shown to improve pulmonary capillary permeability in certain experimental procedures (Brigham, 1978).

The management of pulmonary edema that develops as a result of increased pulmonary capillary permeability is far less well defined and, therefore, more difficult to treat than that due to cardiogenic factors. Although the use of antihistamines and phosphodiesterase inhibitors may be tried, it is unlikely that these modalities alone will be effective and life saving. A logical, initial approach should probably begin with oxygen therapy, bronchodilators, and diuretics; the latter are given only if the patient's effective circulatory volume is adequate. (When hypovolemia exists as a complication of the patient's systemic problem, intravenous fluids and positive inotropic agents are preferred over diuretic therapy.) While the responsiveness to this therapy is being evaluated, a search for the responsible cause or causes is undertaken. However, if this approach does not quickly stabilize the patient's condition, including the normalization of blood gases, the use of positive pressure ventilation, should be considered (see *Current Veterinary Therapy IX*, p. 269). This may require the incorporation of positive end-expiratory pressure to obtain the maximum benefit. (General indications for positive pressure ventilation include (1) an arterial oxygen tension of less than 50 mm Hg with the patient breathing 100 per cent oxygen and (2) a progressive increase in the arterial CO_2 concentration.) As pulmonary infections and septicemia may be inciting causes for the development of increased pulmonary capillary permeability, cultures should be taken (i.e., blood, urine, and airway secretions) and all identified infections treated aggressively. In the absence of infection, prophylactic use of antibiotics is probably of little benefit. Finally, dexamethasone or methylprednisolone in doses given for shock for 1 to 2 days can probably be justified based on their reported benefit in ARDS in humans.

References and Supplemental Reading

Avery, W. G., Samet, P., and Sackner, M. A.: The acidosis of pulmonary edema. Am. J. Med. 48:320, 1970.

Brigham, K. L.: Lung edema due to increased vascular permeability. *In* Staub, N. C. (ed.): *Lung Water and Solute Exchange.* New York: Marcel Dekker, 1978.

Craddock, P. R., Fihe, J., Brigham, K. L., et al.: Complement and leukocyte mediated pulmonary dysfunction in hemodialysis. N. Engl. J. Med. 296:769, 1977.

Cross, C. E., and Hyde, R. W.: Treatment of pulmonary edema. *In* Staub, N. C. (ed.): *Lung Water and Solute Exchange.* New York: Marcel Dekker, 1978, p. 471.

Evans, H. E., and Christensen, G. C.: *Miller's Anatomy of the Dog,* 2nd ed. Philadelphia: W. B. Saunders, 1979, p. 542.

Macklin, P. T., and Mead, J.: Resistance of central and peripheral airways measured by a retrograde catheter. J. Appl. Physiol. 22:395, 1967.

Magno, M., and Szidon, J. P.: Hemodynamic pulmonary edema in dogs with acute and chronic lymphatic ligation. Am. J. Physiol. 231:1777, 1976.

Pietra, G., Szidon, J. P., Leventhal, M., and Fishman, A.: Histamine and interstitial pulmonary edema in the dog. Circ. Res. 29:323, 1971.

Pritchard, J. S.: *Edema of the Lung.* Springfield: Charles C Thomas, 1982.

Sharp, J. G., Griffith, G. T., Bunnell, I. L., and Green, D. G.: Ventilatory mechanics in pulmonary edema in man. J. Clin. Invest. 37:111, 1958.

Singer, D., Hesser, C., Pick, R., and Katz, L.: Diffuse bilateral pulmonary edema associated with unilobar miliary pulmonary embolism in the dog. Circ. Res. 6:4, 1958.

West, J. B.: *Ventilation Blood Flow and Gas Exchange.* Oxford: Blackwell Scientific Publication, 1970.

Williams, T. J., and Morley, J.: Prostaglandins as potentiators of increased vascular permeability in inflammation. Nature 246:215, 1973.

CHYLOTHORAX

THERESA W. FOSSUM, D.V.M.,
College Station, Texas

and STEPHEN J. BIRCHARD, D.V.M.
Columbus, Ohio

Chylothorax is the collection of chyle in the pleural space. Although diagnosed infrequently, it is a well-established clinical entity that usually presents a therapeutic challenge. Chylothorax was first described by a physician in 1633 but not until 1946 was a definitive treatment, ligation of the thoracic duct, attempted. The initial report (Patterson and Munson, 1958) of this disease in the veterinary literature described the surgical treatment of three dogs and one cat. Although the surgery has been refined since this early report, the ability to treat many animals has been hindered by a lack of understanding of the etiology of this disease.

Thoracic duct rupture, due to trauma, was once thought to be the most common cause of chylothorax in dogs and cats. Since the advent of lymphangiography, however, the thoracic duct has consistently been shown to be intact in clinical cases. Mesenteric lymphangiography is a technique in which a water-soluble contrast agent is injected into a mesenteric lymphatic to outline the thoracic duct. With this technique, dilation of the cranial mediastinal lymphatics has been repeatedly observed and is termed thoracic lymphangiectasia (Fig. 1). It is presumed that chyle leaks from these dilated, but intact, lymphatics into the pleural space. The reason why these lymphatics dilate is not known; however, thoracic lymphangiectasia and chylothorax have been produced in dogs by ligating the cranial vena cava. Thus, obstruction of thoracic duct flow is a potential cause of chylothorax. Diseases that have been reported in association with chylothorax and could obstruct the venous system where the thoracic duct enters include cranial mediastinal masses (aortic body tumor, lymphosarcoma, thymoma, and lung lobe teratoma), fungal granulomas, venous thrombi, and heartworm disease. Increased lymph flow, rather than obstruction to flow, could also result in lymphatic dilation. Increased lymph flow has been shown to occur when there is an obstruction to blood flow into or through the right side of the heart, such as in congestive heart failure (CHF). Cardiomyopathy has been reported as a cause of chylothorax in the cat; however, the pathogenesis has not been established. Despite these associations, chylothorax in most animals is termed idiopathic, because the etiology is not apparent.

A sex predisposition has not been identified with chylothorax. Afghans have a greater incidence of chylothorax than other breeds. Additionally, an abnormal termination of the thoracic duct has been described in an Afghan with chylothorax. These factors suggest a hereditary predisposition to chylothorax in this breed.

Regardless of the etiology, chylothorax is a potentially devastating disease. The basal rate of lymph flow in the thoracic duct has been estimated to be 2 ml/kg/hr. This rate varies depending on diet, being greatest following a high-fat meal. In a 30-kg dog, over a liter of chyle may be produced daily. Sixty to 70 per cent of all ingested fats are conveyed to the bloodstream by way of the thoracic duct. The thoracic duct is also the main pathway for protein transport from the capillary spaces to the venous system. Consequently, chylothorax results in both compromised respiration and debilitation because of loss of large amounts of proteins, fats, fat-soluble vitamins, and lymphocytes into the pleural cavity. Electrolyte loss would parallel that lost in a comparable volume of blood plasma. The composition of thoracic duct lymph in the dog is given in Table 1.

DIAGNOSIS

A suspicion of excess pleural fluid may be obtained from the history and physical examination. If the animal is not overtly dyspneic, thoracic radiographs will confirm the diagnosis of pleural fluid accumulation. In severely dyspneic animals it is best to remove some fluid by needle thoracentesis before taking radiographs. The most common clinical signs of chylothorax in dogs are dyspnea, coughing, weight loss, and anorexia. Muffled heart sounds, increased bronchovesicular sounds, and tachycardia are also frequently noted.

Pleural fluid may prevent adequate visualization of the structures of the thoracic cavity on radiography. In these instances ultrasonography can be used to delineate a thoracic mass or to document cardiomyopathy or heart disease and should be performed prior to removing large quantities of fluid.

393

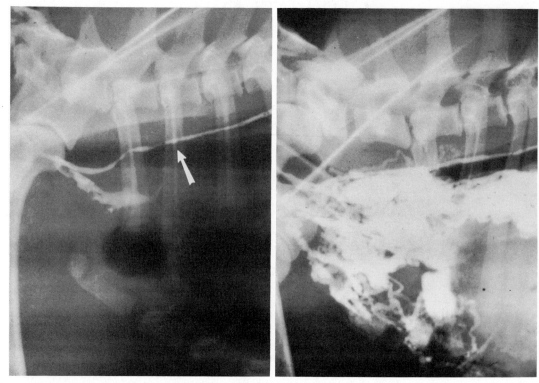

Figure 1. Lymphangiograms from a normal dog on the left (arrow points to the thoracic duct) and a dog with experimentally produced chylothorax and "thoracic lymphangiectasia" on the right.

Chylous fluid is a white or pinkish fluid in which a cream layer will form when left to stand (Fig. 2). Other characteristics of a chylous fluid are presented in Table 2. Although lymphocytes have been classically described as the predominant cell type, many chylous effusions contain more neutrophils than lymphocytes.

A simple test can be performed to determine whether a fluid is chyle, the ether clearance test. In this test, the suspect fluid is divided between two test tubes. Two drops of 10 per cent potassium hydroxide are added to each tube. A volume of water equal to that of the suspect fluid is added to the first tube and a similar quantity of ether is added to the second tube. The tubes are inverted to mix and then compared. If the fluid is chyle, the chylomicrons will be dissolved by the ether and the fluid will clear or become translucent. The tube to which water was added will simply be diluted and is used as a control. A more objective way to identify chyle is to measure the cholesterol and triglyceride content of the pleural fluid and compare with those of serum. Chylous fluid will have a higher triglyceride content than serum and a normal or low cholesterol content. The term pseudochylous fluid has been incorrectly used in the veterinary literature to define a fluid that looks like chyle but in which a rupture of the thoracic duct cannot be found, such as in cats with cardiomyopathy. True pseudochylous effusions have a high cholesterol content. Pseudochylous effusions are rare but have been reported in association with tuberculosis.

After the effusion has been identified as being chylous, every attempt should be made to define the underlying disorder before surgical therapy is undertaken. A flow chart for managing an animal with chylothorax is presented in Figure 3.

TREATMENT

Medical Management

The goal of nonoperative management of animals with chylothorax is to provide the nutritional and

Table 1. *Composition of Thoracic Duct Lymph in Dogs*

Component	Range
Total protein (gm/dl)	5.1 ± 1.0
Albumin (gm/dl)	2.9 ± 0.6
RBC (10^6/mm³)	0.002 ± 0.003
WBC (10^3/mm³)	5.7 ± 4.8
Na⁺ (mmol/L)	146.0 ± 2.0
K⁺ (mmol/L)	2.9 ± 0.3
Cl⁻ (mmol/L)	114.2 ± 2.0
LDH (IU/L)	37.4 ± 23.0
AST (IU/L)	62.2 ± 68.0

RBC, red blood cells; WBC, white blood cells; LDH, lactic dehydrogenase; AST, aspartate aminotransferase.
From Leeds, S. E., et al.: Angiology 34:769, 1983.

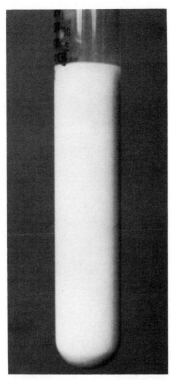

Figure 2. Typical gross appearance of a chylous effusion. Note the milky white appearance. These effusions may be blood tinged.

metabolic needs of the patient until the effusion spontaneously resolves. Animals that may have thoracic duct rupture (those with a history of trauma) and those in which an underlying disease can be identified and treated are most likely to benefit from conservative treatment. Examples of animals that may respond to medical therapy are cats with cardiomyopathy and animals with thoracic masses compressing the vena cava. Although medical management may initially control the effusion in animals with *idiopathic* chylothorax, it is the experience of the authors that eventually the effusion becomes unmanageable, necessitating surgery.

Thoracentesis and dietary management are the main components of medical therapy. Thoracentesis may be necessary initially to stabilize the patient. Daily thoracentesis enables one to quantitate the

Table 2. *Characteristics of Chylous Fluid*

Color	White to pink
Clarity	Opaque, remains opaque when centrifuged
Chylomicrons	Present
Total protein	2–6.5 gm/dl
Specific gravity	1.012–1.037
Total WBC/μl	900–16,650
Predominant cell type	Neutrophil or lymphocyte
Ether clearance test	Positive
Triglyceride content	> serum
Cholesterol content	≤ serum
Sudanophilic fat globules	Present

rate and ascertain trends in fluid formation. This is most easily accomplished by the placement of a chest tube. Strict asepsis is necessary during drainage procedures, to prevent infection.

The dietary needs of the patient can be met in a number of ways. Intravenous hyperalimentation is superior to oral alimentation in reducing the quantity of lymph flow. However, in most cases the expense and difficulty in providing intravenous hyperalimentation does not make this a viable option. A less optimum, but adequate treatment in most cases is to maintain the animal's hydration by giving a balanced electrolyte solution intravenously. The animal's caloric requirements can be met by feeding it a low-fat diet such as Prescription Diet r/d (Hill's Pet Products) or a homemade diet (Table 3). Supplementation with short- or medium-chain triglycerides is beneficial because these fats are absorbed directly into the portal system, bypassing the thoracic duct. Commercial sources of medium-chain triglycerides are available as MCT oil (Mead Johnson) (1 to 2 ml/kg/day orally) or Portagen (Mead Johnson) (1½ cups added to water to make a 1 quart mixture equals 30 cal/oz or 1 cal/ml; this solution is hypertonic and may cause vomiting or exacerbate diarrhea in dogs with gastrointestinal disease).

Although the human literature states that chyle is nonirritating, some animals with chronic chylothorax, particularly Afghans and cats, develop a severe fibrous pleuritis. This pleuritis may restrict pulmonary function, thereby complicating therapy.

Surgical Management

Surgery should be performed in those patients in which medical therapy has failed, or in patients that have no history of trauma and are likely to become debilitated if surgery is delayed.

The success of surgery depends, to a large extent, on the ability of the surgeon to identify and ligate all branches of the thoracic duct. In a majority of dogs the thoracic duct is multiple in the caudal thorax where ligation is performed. Lymphangiography is used to help identify the smaller branches of the thoracic duct, which might be difficult to visualize at surgery. This technique is easiest if intraoperative radiographic capabilities are available. Lymphangiography is particularly helpful when performed following thoracic duct ligation, to verify that no branches have been missed or to help locate those branches that were not ligated. Despite verifying complete ligation of the thoracic duct, approximately 40 per cent of dogs will have either a chylous effusion (14 per cent) or a serosanguineous effusion (28 per cent) postoperatively. Pleuroperitoneal and pleurovenous shunting can be used in these dogs to prevent respiratory distress associated

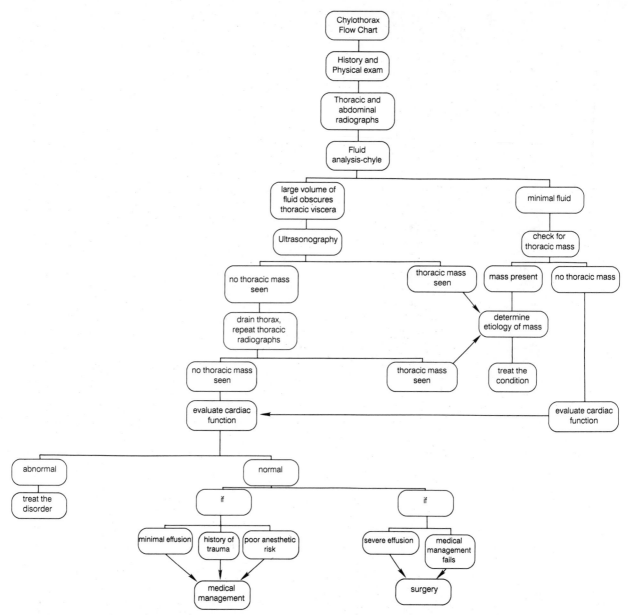

Figure 3. Flow chart for managing an animal with chylothorax. (Adapted from Fossum, T. W., and Birchard, S. J.: The surgical management of chylothorax. *In* Bojrab, M. J. (ed.): *Current Techniques in Small Animal Surgery.* 3rd ed. Philadelphia: Lea & Febiger, in press.)

with the fluid accumulation. Pleurodesis, which is an attempt to adhere the pleura of the lung and the parietal pleura of the chest wall, has been used to decrease the pleural fluid production. This technique is described on pages 405 to 408.

THORACIC DUCT LIGATION IN THE DOG

Food is withheld for 12 hr prior to surgery. The dog is fed corn oil (2 ml/kg) hourly, beginning 3 hr prior to anesthetic induction. The corn oil is absorbed by the intestinal tract and facilitates visualization of the lymphatics during lymphangiography.

PREOPERATIVE LYMPHANGIOGRAM. The right side of the chest and abdomen is clipped and prepared for aseptic surgery. A paracostal incision is made with the dog in left lateral recumbency, and the cecum is located and exteriorized. A large lymph node (mesenteric) can be palpated adjacent to the cecum. Following careful dissection of the mesentery near this lymph node, large lymphatic vessels can be visualized. Care should be taken to avoid incising these lymphatics during the dissection, because the subsequent leakage of chyle will make cannulation difficult. The use of small scissors, such as Iris scissors, will facilitate the dissection. Two 3–0 silk sutures are placed around the lymphatic and

Table 3. *Homemade Low-Fat Diet for Dogs with Chylothorax*

	Protein (gm)	Calories	Fat (gm)
1 cup of boiled rice, or potato, or oatmeal, or pasta*	5	200	2
15 ml of MCT oil	—	115	14
1 cup of low-fat (2%) cottage cheese†	35	200	4–5
1 vitamin/mineral tablet and ½ tsp. calcium carbonate (e.g., Tums)			
Total	40	515	20

*Equal amounts of baked potato or pasta may be substituted as a carbohydrate source.

†Skinned, boiled chicken breast or water-packed tuna may be substituted as a protein source; use water-packed tuna for cats.

Diet contains approximately 515 kcal, 40 gm of protein, and 6 gm of non-MCT fat. This would meet the daily needs of a 12- to 15-lb dog.

a 20- or 22-gauge over-the-needle catheter (Surflo, Burrows Co., Wheeling, IL) is placed in the lymphatic (Fig. 4). An extension tubing filled with heparinized saline is placed on the catheter. The silk sutures are tied around the catheter and looped over the extension tubing hub to secure the catheter in place. An additional suture may be placed around the extension tubing and through a segment of intestine to prevent dislodgement of the catheter. A three-way stopcock is attached to the end of the extension tubing. Moistened laparotomy pads are placed over the exteriorized intestine. Diatrezoate meglumine and diatrezoate sodium (Renovist, ER, Squibb and Sons) contrast agents (1 ml/kg diluted with 0.5 ml/kg of saline) are injected into the mesenteric catheter, and a lateral thoracic radiograph is taken while the last milliliter is being injected. The injection may be repeated while a

ventrodorsal (VD) view is taken. This preligation lymphangiogram will help determine the location of the thoracic duct and the number of branches that need to be ligated.

LIGATION OF THE THORACIC DUCT. The thoracic duct is approached via a right tenth space intercostal thoracotomy. The caudal aspect of the canine thoracic duct is located to the right of midline, just dorsal to the aorta and ventral to the azygous vein (Fig. 5). A small volume (2 to 4 ml) of methylene blue solution (U.S.P. 1 per cent, American Quinine, Shirley, NY) may be injected into the mesenteric lymphatic catheter or mesenteric lymph nodes if better visualization of the thoracic duct is needed. The mediastinum dorsal to the aorta is bluntly dissected, taking care not to incise the thoracic duct or any of its branches. The thoracic duct is identified and ligated with silk sutures. Placing a hemostatic clip on the thoracic duct gives the surgeon a radiographic marker, which, on the postoperative lymphangiogram, can be used to help locate additional branches of the thoracic duct that need to be ligated. Long-handled, right-angle forceps aid dissection and ligation of the duct.

POSTOPERATIVE LYMPHANGIOGRAM. The lymphangiogram is repeated following ligation of the duct. Often, even the caudal portion of the thoracic duct (distal to the ligature) will not fill with dye after the duct has been completely ligated. When all branches of the thoracic duct have been occluded, the mesenteric catheter is removed, and both incisions are closed routinely.

THORACIC DUCT LIGATION IN THE CAT

A similar procedure can be performed in the cat with chylothorax, except the thoracic duct is ap-

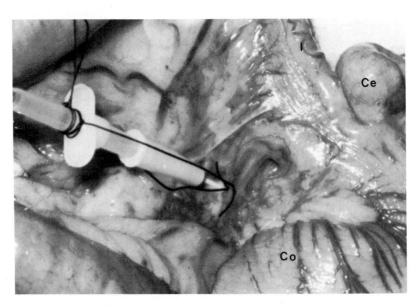

Figure 4. Placement of an over-the-needle catheter in a mesenteric lymphatic. Silk sutures are tied around the catheter and looped over the extension tubing hub to secure the catheter in place. I, ileum; Ce, cecum; Co, colon.

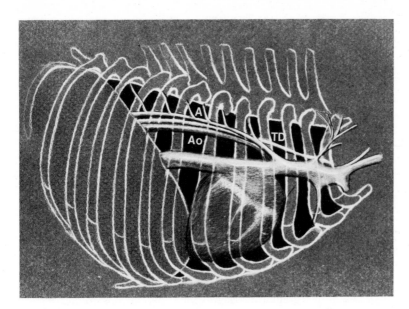

Figure 5. Diagram showing relationship of the thoracic duct to the aorta and azygous vein. Ao, aorta; A, azygous vein; TD, thoracic duct.

proached from the left side of the thorax rather than from the right side as in the dog. Placement of a catheter in a mesenteric lymphatic is more difficult in the cat owing to the large amount of mesenteric fat and the small lymphatic vessel size of most cats. However, usually a lumbar lymphatic, near the cisterna chyli, can be located and cannulated. The cisterna is found surrounding the aorta, just caudal to the diaphragm. If catheterization of an abdominal lymphatic is not possible, injection of 1 ml of methylene blue solution in a mesenteric lymph node may afford adequate visualization of the thoracic duct. Care should be taken to differentiate the more dorsally located sympathetic trunk from the thoracic duct in cats.

POSTOPERATIVE CARE

A thoracic drain should be maintained until pleural effusion stops. Up to 2.2 ml/kg of pleural fluid may be produced daily as a result of irritation caused by the presence of a thoracic drain. A record of the character and quantity of effusion should be kept. The diet may be returned to normal after the effusion stops. Chylous fluid is commonly removed from the thorax for 3 to 5 days following surgery.

If pleural effusion continues for longer than 3 to 5 days postoperatively, the character of the fluid should be assessed. This is best done by measuring the cholesterol and triglyceride content of the pleural fluid and comparing these values with similar measurements of the serum. Postoperative pleural fluid may be either chylous or serosanguineous. Chylous fluid production following ligation of the thoracic duct is more likely to occur in Afghans than in other breeds. In one study, only one of four Afghans with chylothorax responded to

thoracic duct ligation with complete resolution of the pleural effusion. Management of either type of effusion may require repeating the lymphangiogram and thoracic duct ligation, placing a pleuroperitoneal or pleurovenous shunt, or possibly pleurodesis.

PLEUROPERITONEAL SHUNTS

Pleuroperitoneal shunts were first developed for use in human neonates with chylothorax. The rationale for use of these shunts is to divert the pleural fluid into the abdomen where it can be absorbed, thereby relieving the respiratory distress. The shunt catheter (double-valve Denver peritoneal-venous shunt, Denver Biomaterials, Inc., Evergreen, CO) consists of a bivalved pump chamber, a 27-cm fenestrated (afferent) catheter, and a 66-cm heparin-impregnated efferent catheter. A Hakim-Cordis ventricular-peritoneal shunt (Cordis Corp., Miami, FL) may also be used. Under general anesthesia, the left or right hemithorax is prepared for aseptic surgery. A vertical skin incision is made over the middle of the fifth, sixth, or seventh ribs. A purse-string suture is placed in the skin at this site. Fenestrations are placed in the venous (efferent) end of the shunt catheter, and the catheter is bluntly inserted into the pleural space. A tunnel is created by blunt dissection under the external abdominal oblique muscle, and the pump chamber is pulled through the tunnel. The efferent end of the catheter is then placed into the abdominal cavity through a preplaced pursestring suture, and the incision is located just caudal to the costal arch. The shunt must be placed with the pump chamber directly overlying a rib so that the chamber can be effectively compressed. Pleuroperitoneal shunting has been successfully performed following thoracic duct ligation in a dog and cat with chylothorax.

PLEUROVENOUS SHUNTS

The placement of a pleurovenous shunt has been reported as an adjunctive procedure to surgery in dogs with chylothorax. The technique is similar to the placement of a pleuroperitoneal shunt, except that the efferent arm is placed into the caudal vena cava or azygous vein and the afferent arm is placed into the pleural cavity. The pump chamber is positioned over the lateral surface of a rib so that the venous end extends dorsally and the fenestrated end extends ventrally. The double-valve Denver shunt and the LeVeen shunt have both been used extensively in humans as peritoneovenous shunts to treat refractory ascites. Complications associated with use of peritoneovenous shunts in humans have included sepsis, shunt obstruction, peritonitis, congestive heart failure, abdominal abscess formation, gastrointestinal bleeding, pneumonia, and encephalopathy. The most common complication in children with chylous ascites is shunt obstruction due to the viscosity of the chyle. Pleurovenous shunting appears to be an attractive adjunct to the management of dogs with chylothorax. However, until additional studies are performed defining its efficacy and complication rate, the routine use of this procedure as a primary therapy cannot be recommended. At this time, pleurovenous shunting appears most appropriate for use in the management of animals with persistent pleural effusion following thoracic duct ligation.

References and Supplemental Reading

Azizkhan, R. G., Canfield, J., Alford, B. A., et al.: Pleuroperitoneal shunts in the management of neonatal chylothorax. J. Pediatr. Surg. 18:842, 1983.

Birchard, S. J., Smeak, D. D., and Fossum, T. W.: Results of thoracic duct ligation in 15 dogs with chylothorax. J.A.V.M.A. 193:68, 1988.

Fossum, T. W., and Birchard, S. J.: Lymphangiographic evaluation of experimental chylothorax after ligation of the cranial vena cava in dogs. Am. J. Vet. Res. 47:967, 1986.

Fossum, T. W., Birchard, S. J., and Jacobs, R. M.: Chylothorax in 34 dogs. J.A.V.M.A. 188:1315, 1986.

Fossum, T. W., Jacobs, R. M., and Birchard, S. J.: Evaluation of cholesterol and triglyceride concentrations in differentiating chylous and nonchylous pleural effusions in dogs and cats. J.A.V.M.A. 188:59, 1986.

Kagan, K. G., and Breznock, E. M.: Variations in the canine thoracic duct system and the effects of surgical occlusion demonstrated by rapid aqueous lymphography, using an intestinal lymphatic trunk. Am. J. Vet. Res. 40:948, 1979.

Patterson, D. F., and Munson, T. O.: Traumatic chylothorax in small animals treated by ligation of the thoracic duct. J.A.V.M.A. 133:452, 1958.

Smeak, D. D., Gallagher, L., Birchard, S. J., et al.: Management of intractable pleural effusion in a dog with pleuroperitoneal shunt. Vet. Surg. 12:212, 1987.

Smith, R. E., Nostrant, T. T., Eckhausen, F. E., et al.: Patient selection and survival after peritoneovenous shunting for nonmalignant ascites. Am. J. Gastroenterol. 79:659, 1984.

Willauer, C. C., and Breznock, E. M.: Pleurovenous shunting technique for treatment of chylothorax in three dogs. J.A.V.M.A. 191:1106, 1987.

RESPIRATORY NEOPLASIA

MARCIA CAROTHERS, D.V.M.,
and C. GUILLERMO COUTO, D.V.M.
Columbus, Ohio

Neoplasms of the respiratory tract are relatively rare in small animals, composing between 4 and 5 per cent of all neoplasms in the dog and cat (Priester and McKay, 1980). Because over 80 per cent of the respiratory tract neoplasms are malignant, tumors of this organ system should be regarded as malignant until proven otherwise (Madewell et al., 1976). In addition to the large number of histologic tumor types affecting the respiratory tract, lower respiratory organs (i.e., lungs) are common sites of metastatic neoplasia.

NEOPLASMS OF THE NASAL PASSAGES AND PARANASAL SINUSES

Neoplasms of the nasal cavity appear to be more common in dogs (1 to 2 per cent of all neoplasms) than in cats (approximately 1 per cent) and constitute approximately 75 per cent of all respiratory tract tumors. Approximately 80 per cent of primary nasal neoplasms are malignant, and their biologic behavior is characterized mainly by local invasion of the surrounding tissues. Distant metastases are uncommon at the time of diagnosis (i.e., less than 10 per cent of cases), but may occur late in the course of the disease. Common sites of metastases include the regional lymph nodes, lung, and brain. Paraneoplastic syndromes associated with nasal neoplasms are rare and include hypercalcemia (associated with an adenocarcinoma [Wilson and Bronstad, 1983]) and polycythemia (associated with a fibrosarcoma [Couto 1988]). Benign nasal tumors are exceedingly rare, although inflammatory polyps are relatively common in cats.

Nasal tumors are more common in older animals. Although there is no sex predilection in the dog, male cats appear to be at higher risk than females (2:1). In dogs, medium to large breeds are more predisposed to developing nasal neoplasms than small breeds. Nasal neoplams are more common in dolichocephalic breeds than in brachycephalic breeds; this is thought to occur because a longer nasal cavity results in entrapment of more potentially carcinogenic substances. Dog breeds reported to be at increased risk for tumors of the nasal passages and frontal sinuses include the Airedale terrier, bassett hound, Old English sheepdog, Scottish terrier, collie, Shetland sheepdog, German shepherd dog, Keeshond, and German short-hair pointer.

From the histopathologic standpoint, epithelial tumors are more common than mesenchymal tumors, representing 70 per cent of all nasal neoplasms. Nasal neoplasms are more likely to originate from the caudal two thirds of the nasal cavity and often invade the paranasal sinuses. Primary paranasal sinus tumors appear to be more common in dogs than in cats (Madewell et al., 1976). Because the caudal two thirds of the nasal passages are lined with secretory epithelium, while only the rostral one third is lined with squamous epithelium, adenocarcinomas are more common than squamous cell carcinomas. Other tumor types in dogs include undifferentiated carcinomas, chondrosarcomas, fibrosarcomas, lymphomas, osteosarcomas, and transmissible venereal tumors. In cats, squamous cell carcinomas are the most common nasal tumor, followed by adenocarcinomas and lymphomas. Table 1 presents the prevalence of different nasal tumor types in dogs and cats.

Clinical signs in dogs and cats with early nasal or paranasal neoplasia can be uni- or bilateral and include epistaxis; serous, serohemorrhagic, or mucopurulent nasal or ocular discharge or both; sneezing; reverse sneezing; and snoring. Patients with more advanced disease may exhibit facial deformity in the nasal or frontal regions or both; uni- or bilateral exophthalmos; and signs such as blindness, seizures, or behavioral changes. The latter result from direct central nervous system (CNS) invasion by the tumor through the cribriform plate. The duration of clinical signs may vary from weeks to months (average, 3 to 4 months).

Table 1. *Prevalence of Nasal Neoplasms in Dogs and Cats*

Species and Cell Type	Number of Tumors
Canine (N = 193)	
Adenocarcinoma	50
Carcinoma (not otherwise specified)	31
Chondrosarcoma	21
Squamous cell carcinoma	18
Fibrosarcoma	17
Adenoma	7
Mastocytoma	7
Fibropapilloma	7
Osteosarcoma	4
Myoepithelial tumor	4
Squamous cell papilloma	3
Sarcoma (undifferentiated)	3
Mucinous carcinoma	2
Fibroma	2
Chondroma	2
Transmissible venereal tumor	2
Histiocytoma	2
Melanoma	2
Transitional cell carcinoma	1
Basal cell carcinoma	1
Basosquamous carcinoma	1
Lymphoma	1
Reticulum cell sarcoma	1
Myeloma	1
Hemangiosarcoma	1
Myxosarcoma	1
Myxoma	1
Feline (N = 34)	
Squamous cell carcinoma	15
Adenocarcinoma	9
Lymphoma	2
Reticulum cell sarcoma	1
Fibropapilloma	1
Adenoma	1
Carcinoma (not otherwise specified)	1
Fibrosarcoma	1
Fibroma	1
Sarcoma (not otherwise specified)	1
Sympaticoblastoma	1

Adapted from Madewell, B. R., et al.: Am. J. Vet. Res. 37:851, 1976.

Physical examination in these patients usually reveals the presence of one or more of the findings discussed above. In addition, a thorough evaluation of the oropharyngeal region may reveal the presence of lesions in the hard palate; these lesions result from the invasion of the hard palate by neoplastic cells, thus causing lysis of the palatine bone, and are characterized as "soft spots" on palpation of the palate.

Plain radiographs (occlusal dorsoventral, open mouth ventrodorsal, lateral, ventrodorsal, and frontal sinus views) are beneficial in determining the extent of the disease. Abnormalities in dogs and cats with nasal neoplasms include loss of trabecular pattern or increased soft tissue density (or both) in the nasal passages, septal destruction, soft tissue swelling, facial bone destruction, frontal sinus opac-

Table 2. *Response to Therapy in Nasal Neoplasms in Dogs*

Dogs (n)	Type of Radiation	Surgery	Survival Time (Median/Mean)	Reference
10	Orthovoltage & cesium teletherapy (10 fractions × dose = 41 Gy)	None	10/4.1 months	Adams et al., 1987
14	Orthovoltage & cesium teletherapy (10 fractions × dose = 40 Gy)	Aggressive cytoreductive curettage	17.5/8.1 months	Adams et al., 1987
16	Megavoltage (cobalt or linear accelerator) (10 fractions × dose = 44 Gy)	None	9.1/8.1 months	Adams et al., 1987
10	Megavolatage (cobalt or linear accelerator) (10 fractions × dose = 44 Gy)	Aggressive cytoreductive curettage	10.1/7.1 months	Adams et al., 1987
17	Orthovoltage (5 fractions × dose = 44 Gy)	Cytoreductive curettage	19.9/15.2 months	Adams et al., 1987
3	Orthovoltage (× dose = 45 Gy)	None	29/37 months	Thrall and Harvey, 1983
4	Orthovoltage (× dose = 47 Gy)	Cytoreduction (no curettage)	12/9.5 months	Thrall and Harvey, 1983
14	Orthovoltage (× dose = 44 Gy) (3 also had chemotherapy)	Cytoreductive curettage	30.1/23.5 months	Thrall and Harvey, 1983
4	None	Cytoreduction and resection	12/5 months	Madewell et al., 1976
15	Orthovoltage (× dose = 36 Gy); cobalt (× dose = 40 Gy)	Cytoreduction and resection	5.3/5 months	Madewell et al., 1976

ification, and periosteal bone formation. Contrast rhinograms may reveal the presence of a space-occupying mass. Nasal tumors may result in radiographic changes similar to those of non-neoplastic disorders such as chronic rhinitis (e.g., mycotic infection). However, most neoplasms tend to originate in the posterior region of the nasal cavity and progress rostrally, causing severe disruption of the normal architecture, whereas mycotic diseases (e.g., aspergillosis/penicillosis) usually involve the middle nasal cavity and progress rostrally with less bony changes. Regardless of these features, a diagnosis of nasal neoplasia cannot be based on radiographs alone and must be confirmed by cytologic or histopathologic studies. Other imaging techniques that may be useful in diagnosing and evaluating the extent of nasal neoplasms include computed tomography and magnetic resonance imaging.

Techniques utilized to confirm a diagnosis of nasal neoplasia include noninvasive procedures such as cytologic evaluation of nasal flushes; rhinoscopy swabs or tissue impressions; and histopathologic evaluation of through-the-nares needle biopsy (e.g., using Tru-Cut disposable biopsy needle, Travenol Laboratories Inc.), core biopsy (e.g., polypropylene tubes or catheters), or rhinoscopy biopsy specimens. A surgical rhinotomy is a more invasive procedure but allows examination of the nasal cavity, as well as providing larger tissue specimens for histopathologic evaluation and culture. Birchard (1988) employed a simplified method for rhinotomy. Withrow and associates (1985) described a technique using the protective sheath of an intravenous catheter (Sovereign indwelling catheter feline needle gauge, Monoject, Division of Sherwood Medical) to obtain a core biopsy of nasal tissue. This approach yielded a positive diagnosis in 29 of 30 cases (97 per cent).

Love and colleagues (1987) also report a catheter technique using a 6- or 8-French Foley catheter through the nares. Fifteen of 23 cases (65 per cent) were diagnosed via catheter biopsies. In the authors' experience, noninvasive techniques yield definitive diagnoses in less than 60 per cent of cases. These false-negative results probably occur because chronic nasal disorders, regardless of whether they are neoplastic or inflammatory, result in reactive inflammation surrounding the mass. Therefore, noninvasive procedures usually yield samples from the peripheral reactive tissue, rather than from the mass itself. The following protocol is recommended to evaluate dogs and cats with chronic nasal disorders: obtain plain nasal radiographs under general anesthesia; if the radiographic changes are compatible with neoplasia or chronic inflammation, perform an exploratory rhinotomy; and obtain samples for cytologic and histopathologic study and bacterial and fungal cultures. With this approach, a diagnosis can usually be obtained in approximately 85 per cent of cases.

Therapeutic modalities utilized in the treatment of nasal neoplasms include surgery, radiation therapy, chemotherapy, and immunotherapy, either singly or in combination. Although little information is available concerning the therapy of feline nasal neoplasms, Straw and coworkers (1986) reported a mean survival time of approximately 19 months in six cats treated with radiation alone (5 cats) and with radiation and chemotherapy (one cat). Surgical cytoreduction was not performed in these cats. Several reports have compared the various therapies in the dog (see Table 2). Untreated dogs with nasal neoplasms survive approximately 3 to 5 months. Survival times with surgery alone are similar to those of untreated dogs. Although radiation therapy alone improves survival, the longest survival times are seen in dogs treated with a combination of surgical cytoreduction followed by radiation therapy. Complications with this therapy are minimal but may include recurrent nasal discharge, epistaxis, sneezing, moist desquamation of the skin at the irradiation site, conjunctivitis, keratitis, keratoconjunctivitis sicca (KCS), uveitis, and cataracts. Roberts and colleagues (1987) reported ophthalmic complications following megavoltage irradiation of nasal and paranasal tumors in 29 dogs. Severe complications (severe conjunctivitis, keratitis, cataracts, and KCS) occurred in approximately 58 per cent of the dogs. These complications developed acutely (within days) or late (within months) in the course of radiation therapy. Surgical therapy (conjunctival flaps, corneal-scleral transpositions) or topical ophthalmic therapy with corticosteroids, parasympathomimetics, or ocular emollients or a combination of these generally resulted in resolution of the problem in acute disease; however, chronic changes may persist and affect the quality of health.

Chemotherapy has been used to treat limited numbers of patients with nasal neoplasia. Transmissible venereal tumors (TVT) are generally responsive to single agent chemotherapy using vincristine (Oncovin, Eli Lilly) at 0.5 mg/m² of body surface area once a week intravenously; the response rate is over 80 per cent. Multiple-agent chemotherapy was used by the authors to treat four dogs with nasal adenocarcinomas, in which anesthesia for radiation therapy posed a significant risk. Three of the dogs were treated with VAC protocol and the fourth dog with FAC protocol (see Table 3). Two of the VAC-treated dogs showed progressive disease, and the third sustained complete remission (survival time, 157 days). The dog treated with FAC experienced complete resolution of the respiratory signs within 2 weeks of initiating therapy. Only the dog treated with FAC had surgical debulking of the mass prior to chemotherapy.

Prognostic factors in dogs with primary nasal neoplasia include mainly histologic type and tumor stage (see Table 4) at the time of treatment. Dogs with adenocarcinomas and sarcomas have longer median survival times than those with undifferentiated carcinomas or squamous cell carcinomas (10 months versus 5 months [Adams et al., 1987]). Dogs with larger and more extensive tumors (stages 2 and 3) have shorter survival times. Therapeutic failures in dogs treated with radiotherapy may be related to underestimating the tumor extent and subsequently the field of irradiation. Computed tomography may be useful in demonstrating tumor invasion and help in determining appropriate fields for radiotherapy, thus improving survival time.

NEOPLASMS OF THE LARYNX AND TRACHEA

Laryngeal neoplasms are uncommon in the dog and cat. These tumors occur in middle-aged to older animals (5 to 15 years), with the exception of oncocytomas, which occur in young to middle-aged dogs (2 to 8 years). Males appear to be more at risk than females in both dogs and cats.

Clinical signs associated with laryngeal tumors include noisy respiration, stridor, loss of bark or purr, exertional dyspnea, cough, palpable laryngeal enlargement, and cyanosis. Diagnosis is usually made by radiographic evidence of laryngeal distortion, increased soft tissue density of the larynx, or decreased laryngeal air space; laryngoscopic evaluation; and biopsy.

Although Wheeldon and coworkers (1982) found that squamous cell carcinomas were more common than other laryngeal neoplasms in the dog, Saik and

Table 3. VAC and FAC Protocol

Drug	Dose and Route	Time (1 cycle = 21 days)
VAC		
Vincristine (Oncovin, Eli Lilly)	0.7 mg/m² IV	Day 8 and 15
Doxorubicin (Adriamycin, Adria Labs)	30 mg/m² IV	Day 1
Cyclophosphamide (Cytoxan, Mead Johnson)	100 to 200 mg/m² IV	Day 1
FAC		
5-Fluorouracil (5-FU, Roche)	150 to 250 mg/m² IV	Day 8 and 15
Doxorubicin (Adriamycin, Adria Labs)	30 mg/m² IV	Day 1
Cyclophosphamide (Cytoxan, Mead Johnson)	100 to 200 mg/m² IV	Day 1

IV, intravenous injection.

Treatment consists of 4 to 8 cycles. Because of bone marrow suppression, prophylactic antibiotics (trimethoprim-sulfonamide combination at 15 mg/lb divided b.i.d.) are given throughout the chemotherapy.

Table 4. Tumor Staging: Nasal Neoplasms

Stage 1	Ipsilateral tumor
	No or minimal involvement
Stage 2	Bilateral tumor
	Moderate bone destruction
Stage 3	Extensive tumor with extranasal extension

Adapted from Adams, W. M., et al.: J.A.V.M.A. 191:311, 1987.

associates (1986) found that the prevalence of different histologic types of neoplasms was similar. Other tumor types include osteosarcoma, melanoma, mast cell tumor, adenocarcinoma, chondrosarcoma, undifferentiated carcinoma, lipoma, myxochondroma, and oncocytoma. The larynx has been a metastatic site for a thyroid carcinoma (Wheeldon et al., 1982) and a pharyngeal rhabdomyosarcoma (Ladds, 1971). In the dog, oncocytomas appear to be the second most common tumor. Oncocytes are epithelial cells present in endocrine and exocrine glands and within seromucinous glands of the upper airway and digestive tract of humans. Morphologically, oncocytes are characterized by eosinophilic cytoplasm with abundant granules (mitochondria). These neoplasms appear to have a benign biologic behavior (i.e., well encapsulated, slow growing, and rare to metastasize) (Mays, 1984). Lymphomas constitute the most common laryngeal neoplasm in the cat, followed by squamous cell carcinoma and adenocarcinoma (Saik et al., 1986).

Surgical excision constitutes the mainstay of therapy in laryngeal neoplasm. Chemo- and radiotherapy can be used in selected tumor types (e.g., lymphoma) when surgical excision is incomplete. The prognosis for most laryngeal tumors (except oncocytomas) is guarded.

Tracheal neoplasms are rare in both the dog and cat. Clinical signs of obstructive upper airway disease include cough, stridor, progressive dyspnea, exercise intolerance, panting, cyanosis, and possible collapse. Radiographs of the cervical and thoracic trachea may reveal decreased tracheal lumen or a soft tissue density within the tracheal lumen. Irregularity of the mass may be indicative of a malignant neoplasm. Diagnosis is based on biopsy specimens obtained via bronchoscopy or surgical excision.

Tracheal tumor types reported in the dog include osteosarcomas, chondrosarcomas, leiomyomas, mast cell tumors, chondromas, and osteomas. Adenocarcinomas, lymphomas, and squamous cell carcinomas have been reported in the cat.

Therapy of tracheal tumors is mostly limited to surgical excision; radio- and chemotherapy can also be used for selected tumor types. Complete excision usually results in prolonged survival or cure, except for cases of systemic neoplasia affecting the trachea (e.g., lymphoma).

PULMONARY NEOPLASIA

Although lung neoplasms are the second most common neoplasm in humans, primary pulmonary neoplasms are uncommon in the dog and cat, representing approximately 1.2 and 0.5 per cent of all neoplasms, respectively (Moulton, 1978; Stunzi, 1974). Although the etiology of primary pulmonary neoplasms is not known, experimental induction by chemicals (e.g., cigarette smoke and nitrosoamines) and radiation have been reported in the dog (Theilen and Madewell, 1979). A fibrosarcoma has been associated with aberrant migration of *Spirocera lupi* through the lung parenchyma in a dog (Stephens et al., 1983).

Primary pulmonary neoplasms typically occur in older animals, except for lymphomatoid granulomatosis, which occurs in young dogs (1 to 4 years). There appears to be no sex predilection in animals with primary pulmonary neoplasms. Although most studies do not recognize a breed predilection, Brodey and Craig (1965) reported that boxers may be at a higher risk for pulmonary neoplasms.

Clinical signs may vary depending on the tumor size and tumor doubling time. Cough, dyspnea, tachypnea, and decreased exercise tolerance are the most common signs. Others include fever, weight loss, dysphagia, hemoptysis, wheezing, and anorexia. Physical examination may reveal decreased or increased bronchovesicular sounds. Paraneoplastic syndromes associated with pulmonary neoplams include hypertrophic osteopathy (Brodey and Craig, 1965), neuromyopathy and paraplegia (Sorjonen et al., 1982) and neutrophilic leukocytosis (Chinn et al., 1985).

Plain thoracic radiographs constitute a useful diagnostic aid. Suter and associates (1974) described five radiographic patterns in dogs and cats with lung neoplasms. A solitary nodule is the most common, followed by circumscribed multiple nodules, interstitial disseminated reticulonodular pattern, mixed disseminated alveolar interstitial pattern, and homogeneous lobar consolidation. Koblik (1986) also described pulmonary calcification (generally associated with adenocarcinomas) and cavitation of masses (usually associated with solitary adenocarcinomas) in feline primary pulmonary neoplasms. Moulton and colleagues (1981) reported that the right side and diaphragmatic lung lobe are the most common locations for primary pulmonary neoplasms. The most common radiographic pattern seen in dogs and cats with metastatic neoplasms is that of circumscribed multiple nodules. Other radiographic changes may include pleural effusion, pleural thickening, thoracic lymphadenopathy, and hypertrophic osteopathy. Evaluating both right and left lateral thoracic views increases the tumor detection rate. Approximately 11 per cent of pulmonary neoplasms are missed on survey thoracic radiographs. This failure to detect the neoplasm may be due to the presence of small lesions (less than 5 to 10 mm), the lack of tumor contrast with pulmonary parenchyma, the occurrence of the tumor in a hidden location (such as the paraspinal recesses or subpleural space), the presence of pleural effusion, or atelectasis of one or more lung lobes (Suter et al., 1974).

Other diagnostic procedures in dogs and cats with pulmonary neoplasia include percutaneous fine-needle aspiration or needle biopsy for cytologic or histopathologic study; cytologic evaluation of tracheal washes or pleural fluid samples obtained by thoracentesis; bronchoscopy; and exploratory thoracotomy for biopsy.

Adenocarcinomas constitute by far the most common histologic type of primary lung neoplasm in the dog and cat. This type may be further classified as differentiated or undifferentiated. Other primary lung carcinomas include squamous cell carcinoma, bronchial gland carcinoma, and alveolar carcinoma (anaplastic–small cell and large cell and adenomatous). The biologic behavior of carcinomas appears to correlate well with histologic type. Usually, only 50 per cent of the adenocarcinomas have metastasized at the time of diagnosis, compared with 90 and 100 per cent of anaplastic/anaplastic mixed and squamous cell/squamous cell mixed, respectively (Brodey and Craig, 1965). Sites of metastases include bronchial lymph nodes, pulmonary parenchyma, pleura, pericardium, bone, and brain.

Primary mesenchymal neoplasms of the lungs are uncommon. Lymphoma, fibrosarcoma, and fibromyxosarcoma have been reported in dogs and cats. A lymphoreticular neoplasm, lymphomatoid granulomatosis, has been described in young to middle aged dogs. Histologically, the cellular infiltrate contains large reticular or plasmacytoid cells, eosinophils, plasma cells, and lymphocytes. Bronchial and hilar lymph nodes are often involved, and a peripheral basophilia may be present (Lucke et al., 1979).

Surgery (lobectomy) has been the usual mode of therapy for solitary lung tumors. Although the limited number of cases reported in the literature that were treated with surgery alone had poor survival times (2 months or less), Mehlhaff and associates (1984) reported a mean survival time of 13 months in 15 cases of primary pulmonary neoplasms. Nine dogs had recurrence of the neoplasm 1 to 12 months after surgical removal of the primary tumor. Adjuvant postoperative chemotherapy using cyclophosphamide (Cytoxan, Mead Johnson), vincristine (Oncovin, Eli Lilly), and methotrexate (Lederle); vindesine (vindesine sulfate, Eli Lilly) alone; or vindesine and cisplatin (Platinol, Bristol Laboratories) was instituted in five of these dogs. Only the two dogs treated with cisplatin and vindesine showed clinical improvement (Mehlhaff et al.,

1984). Of 210 dogs with primary lung neoplasms evaluated in a multi-institutional study, 76 had therapeutic thoracotomies. Median survival time was 120 days. Factors that decreased survival time were large tumor burden, thoracic lymph node involvement, and other metastases (Ogilvie et al., 1987).

Chemotherapy has been used to treat lymphomatoid granulomatosis. This neoplasm appears to be responsive to multiple-agent therapy using prednisone and cyclophosphamide or prednisone, cyclophosphamide, and vincristine (Postorino et al., 1987).

Lung metastases are common with many neoplasms, including mammary carcinomas, osteosarcomas, thyroid carcinomas, melanomas, and transitional cell carcinomas. Neoplastic cells of the primary tumor may form emboli, which spread via lymphatic or blood vessels. The capillary network of the lungs traps these emboli, and the neoplastic cells may proliferate and form nodules. The primary neoplasm is usually identified on physical examination, radiographic studies, or exploratory surgery. Distant metastases indicate a poor prognosis for long-term survival. The authors have treated metastatic lung neoplasms (i.e., hemangiosarcomas, thyroid carcinomas, squamous cell carcinomas, and mammary adenocarcinomas) with VAC. Complete and partial responses have been seen in dogs with hemangiosarcomas, nonmammary carcinomas, and some undifferentiated sarcomas for 6 to 12 months. Metastatic mammary carcinomas and squamous cell carcinomas have been progressive despite chemotherapy with VAC. Cisplatin has been used to treat metastatic osteosarcomas, with no response.

References and Supplemental Reading

Adams, W. M., Withrow, S. J., and Walshaw, R.: Radiotherapy of malignant nasal tumors in 67 dogs. J.A.V.M.A. 191:311, 1987.

Birchard, S. J.: A simplified method for rhinotomy and temporary rhinostomy in dogs and cats. J. Am. Anim. Hosp. Assoc. 24:69, 1988.

Brodey, R. S., and Craig, P. H.: Primary pulmonary neoplasms in the dog: A review of 29 cases. J.A.V.M.A. 147:1628, 1965.

Chinn, D. R., Myers, R. K., and Matthews, J. A.: Neutrophilic leukocytosis associated with metastatic fibrosarcoma in a dog. J.A.V.M.A. 186:806, 1985.

Couto, C. G., Boudrieau, R., and Zanjani, E.: Tumor-associated erythrocytosis in a dog with nasal fibrosarcoma. J. Vet. Intern. Med. (in press).

Engle, G. C., and Brodey, R. S.: A retrospective study of 395 feline neoplasms. J.A.V.M.A. 155:21, 1969.

Harvey, H. J., and Sykes, G.: Tracheal mast cell tumor in a dog. J.A.V.M.A. 180:1097, 1982.

Koblik, P. D.: Radiographic appearance of primary lung tumors in cats, a review of 41 cases. Vet. Radiol. 27:66, 1986.

Ladds, P. W., and Webster, D. R.: Pharyngeal rhabdomyosarcoma in a dog. Vet. Pathol. 8:256, 1971.

Love, S., Barr, A., and Lucke, V. M.: A catheter technique for biopsy of dogs with chronic nasal disease. J. Small Anim. Pract. 28:417, 1987.

Lucke, V. M., Kelly, G. A., Harrington, G. A.: et al.: A lymphomatoid granulomatosis of the lungs in young dogs. Vet. Pathol. 16:405, 1979.

Madewell, B. R., Priester, W. A., Gillette, E. L., et al.: Neoplasms of the nasal passages and paranasal sinuses in domesticated animals as reported by 13 veterinary colleges. Am. J. Vet. Res. 37:851, 1976.

Mays, M. B. C.: Laryngeal oncocytoma in two dogs. J.A.V.M.A. 185:677, 1984.

Mehlhaff, C. J., and Mooney, S.: Primary pulmonary neoplasia in the dog and cat. Vet. Clin. North Am. 15:1061, 1985.

Mehlhaff, C. J., Leifer, C. E., and Patnaik, A. K.: Surgical treatment of primary pulmonary neoplasia in 15 dogs. J. Am. Anim. Hosp. Assoc. 20:799, 1984.

Moulton, J. E.: Tumors of the respiratory system. In Moulton, J. E.: Tumors in Domestic Animals. Berkeley: University of California Press, 1978, pp. 205–239.

Moulton, J. E., von Tscharner, C., and Schneider, R.: Classification of lung carcinomas in the dog and cat. Vet. Pathol. 18:513, 1981.

Neer, T. M., and Zeman, D.: Tracheal adenocarcinoma in a cat and review of the literature. J. Am. Anim. Hosp. Assoc. 23:377, 1987.

Ogilvie, G. K., Weigel, W. M., and Haschek, W. M.: Canine primary lung tumors: Clinical evaluation of 210 cases (abstract). Veterinary Cancer Society. 7th Annual Conference, 1987.

Postorino, N. C., Wheeler, S. L., and Park, R. D.: Canine pulmonary lymphomatoid granulomatosis (abstract). UCS 7th Annual Conference, 1987.

Priester, W. A., and McKay, F.W.: The occurrence of tumors in domestic animals. Natl. Cancer Inst. Monogr. 54:1, 1980.

Roberts, S. M., Lavach, J. D., Severin, G. A., et al.: Ophthalmic complications following megavoltage irradiation of the nasal and paranasal cavities in dogs. J.A.V.M.A. 190:43, 1987.

Saik, J. E., Toll, S. L., and Diters, R. W.: Canine and feline laryngeal neoplasia: A 10-year survey, J. Am. Anim. Hosp. Assoc. 23:359, 1986.

Sorjonen, D. C., Braund, K. G., and Hoff, G. J.: Paraplegia and subclinical neuromyopathy associated with a primary lung tumor in a dog. J.A.V.M.A. 180:1209, 1982.

Stephens, L. C., Gleiser, C. A., and Jardine, J. H.: Primary pulmonary fibrosarcoma associated with Spirocerca lupi infection in a dog with hypertrophic pulmonary osteoarthropathy. J.A.V.M.A. 182:496, 1983.

Straw, R. C., Withrow, S. J., Gillette, E. L., et al.: Use of radiotherapy for the treatment of intranasal tumors in cats: Six cases (1980–1985). J.A.V.M.A. 189:927, 1986.

Stunzi, H., Herd, K. W., and Nielson, S. W.: Tumors of the lungs. Bull. WHO 50:9, 1974.

Sullivan, M., Lee, R., and Skae, C. A.: The radiological features of sixty cases of intra-nasal neoplasia in the dog. J. Small Anim. Pract. 28:575, 1987.

Suter, P. F., Carrig, C. B., and O'Brien, T. R.: Radiographic recognition of primary and metastatic pulmonary neoplasms of dogs and cats. J. Am. Vet. Radiol. Soc. 15:3, 1974.

Theilen, G. H., and Madewell, B. R.: Tumors of the respiratory tract and thorax. In Theilen, G. H., and Madewell, B. R. (eds.): Veterinary Cancer Medicine. Philadelphia: Lea & Febiger, 1979, pp. 332–356.

Thrall, D. E., and Harvey, C. E.: Radiotherapy of malignant nasal tumors in 21 dogs. J.A.V.M.A. 183:663, 1983.

Wheeldon, E. B., and Amis, T. C.: Laryngeal carcinoma in a cat. J.A.V.M.A. 186:80, 1985.

Wheeldon, E. B., Suter, P. F., and Jenkins, T.: Neoplasia of the larynx in the dog. J.A.V.M.A. 180:642, 1982.

Wilson, R. B., and Bronstad, D. C.: Hypercalcemia associated with nasal adenocarcinoma in a dog. J.A.V.M.A. 182:1246, 1983.

Withrow, S. J., Susaneck, S. J., and Macy, D. W.: Aspiration and punch biopsy techniques for nasal tumors. J. Am. Anim. Hosp. Assoc. 21:551, 1985.

PLEURODESIS

STEPHEN J. BIRCHARD, D.V.M.,
Columbus, Ohio

THERESA W. FOSSUM, D.V.M.,
College Station, Texas

and LAURA GALLAGHER, D.V.M.
Sydney, Australia

Pleurodesis is a method of treating chronic pleural effusions or spontaneous pneumothorax. An irritant is instilled into the pleural space, causing acute inflammation of the pleural membranes with the subsequent development of diffuse adhesions between the visceral and parietal pleurae. These adhesions obliterate the pleural space, preventing further accumulation of fluid or air. Pleural sclerosis and pleural symphysis are synonyms for pleurodesis. The technique has been used in animals (Laing and Norris, 1986) and humans (Austin and Flye, 1979) for a variety of pleural diseases. As little has been written on this subject in the veterinary literature, most of the information presented in this chapter is based upon studies in humans or experimental animals.

MECHANISM OF ACTION

The mechanism by which sclerosing agents cause diffuse adhesions is not well known. In normal animals, intrapleural instillation of tetracycline solutions causes an acute exudative pleural effusion, which stops by 120 hr. Histologically, the mesothelial cells of the pleural membranes are destroyed by sclerosing agents and subsequently replaced by fibroblasts, which produce collagen. Dense adhesions are formed with resultant pleurodesis.

The pH of the sclerosing agent may be an important factor in its effectiveness (Sahn and Potts, 1978). Agents with the lowest or highest pH appear to be most effective in causing pleural adhesions because they induce more inflammation and damage to the pleural surfaces than solutions with neutral pH. The importance of pH in pleurodesis has been questioned, however, as tetracycline is more effective in creating pleural adhesions than a saline solution with the same pH (Zaloznik et al., 1983).

Most authors agree that thoracic drainage is an important part of the pleurodesis procedure (Austin and Flye, 1979). Prior to infusion of the agent, the pleural space should be completely evacuated using a thoracostomy tube. Besides providing palliative relief of the patient's respiratory symptoms, thoracic drainage improves contact between the visceral and parietal pleurae and prevents dilution of the agent. After pleurodesis, thoracic drainage should be continued for 3 to 4 days or until pleural effusion stops to encourage pleural contact and subsequent adhesions. Continuous suction drainage should be considered in these patients.

INDICATIONS

The most common indication for pleurodesis in humans is effusion due to malignancy such as neoplasms of the lung, breast, and lymphoma (Austin and Flye, 1979). Pleurodesis is used as palliative therapy to stop the effusion and allow relief of the respiratory compromise. Chemotherapeutic agents have been used for pleurodesis and possible reduction of the tumor mass. The most important effect of the agents is probably the pleurodesis. In fact, tetracycline pleurodesis is currently believed by many to be superior to chemotherapeutic agents for malignant effusions, even though the tetracycline has no effect on the tumor itself (Austin and Flye, 1979). Pleurodesis agents in general have reportedly been 80 to 100 per cent effective in stopping malignant effusions in humans (Austin and Flye, 1979).

Pleurodesis has been used to treat chylothorax in both humans and animals. Although thoracic duct ligation for traumatic chylothorax in humans is sometimes effective, pleurodesis for chylothorax due to malignancy (Light, 1983) or lymphangiomyomatosis (benign proliferation of smooth muscle in lungs and other organs) is recommended by some investigators. Results of pleurodesis for chylothorax in humans have been poor. Surgical therapy for chylothorax (ligation of the thoracic duct) has been effective in some dogs and cats. However, pleurodesis should be considered for those animals with persistent effusion following duct ligation. The au-

thors have attempted tetracycline pleurodesis for chylothorax in a limited series of animals with inconsistent results. Tetracycline infusion was used in three dogs with persistent nonchylous pleural effusion after thoracic duct ligation. The rate of pleural fluid production in all three animals decreased but did not stop completely. Two dogs and one cat with chylothorax underwent pleurodesis with tetracycline, with resolution of the pleural effusion in one of the dogs but recurrence in the other two animals. Postmortem examination of the dog with recurrence revealed only partial adhesion of the visceral to parietal pleura. Standardization of the dose and technique of tetracycline pleurodesis may improve its effectiveness.

Pneumothorax is another common indication for pleurodesis in humans (Macoviak et al., 1982). Traumatic pneumothorax frequently is self-limiting and requires only conservative therapy. Spontaneous pneumothorax, such as with ruptured emphysematous bullae, often requires surgery. Pleurodesis provides an alternate method of treating persistent or recurrent pneumothorax. Pneumothorax did not recur after pleurodesis in all 50 people treated in one study (Wied et al., 1983). The authors did not recommend pleurodesis if emphysematous bullae exceeded 2 cm in diameter. Pleurodesis was effective in sealing active experimentally induced air leaks in rabbits (Macoviak et al., 1982). Pleurodesis could be considered for dogs and cats with persistent pneumothorax, especially in those patients that are poor surgical risks.

SCLEROSING AGENTS

A variety of agents have been used to induce pleurodesis. These agents share a common characteristic of being irritating to the pleural surfaces.

TETRACYCLINE

Tetracycline solution (Achromycin) has been repeatedly shown to be a safe and effective pleurodesis agent in animals and humans (Laing and Norris, 1986; Zaloznik et al., 1983; Wied et al., 1983). Experimental studies in rabbits comparing tetracycline with other sclerosing agents have shown tetracycline to be more effective than other agents in producing diffuse pleural adhesions (Sahn and Good, 1981). The effectiveness of tetracycline appears to be dose related. Three dosages of intrapleural tetracycline were used (7, 20, and 35 mg/kg) with only the highest dose resulting in greater than 75 per cent obliteration of the pleural space by adhesions (Sahn and Good, 1981).

Clinical studies in humans have also shown tetracycline to be more effective than other agents

(Wied et al., 1983). Tetracycline has been an effective treatment for malignant effusions and spontaneous pneumothorax. The recommended dose of tetracycline in adult humans is 500 mg diluted in 10 to 75 ml of normal saline per hemithorax (Zaloznik et al., 1983; Wied et al., 1983). Two dogs with pleural effusion were treated with intrapleural tetracycline (oxytetracycline) (Laing and Norris, 1986). One dog had pleural effusion caused by an aortic body chemodectoma, the other developed chylothorax after lung lobectomy. Both dogs were treated with 20 mg/kg of tetracycline diluted in 50 ml of normal saline. Although the treatment was effective in providing temporary resolution of the pleural effusions, significant pleurodesis was not found on postmortem examination. Further experimental and clinical studies in animals are needed to evaluate tetracycline as a pleurodesis agent in veterinary patients.

Intrapleural tetracycline is associated with few complications. Fever and pleural pain resulting from intrapleural tetracycline have been inconsistently reported (Zaloznik et al., 1983; Macoviak et al., 1982). Some researchers recommend adding lidocaine (15 ml of 1 per cent lidocaine solution added to 35 ml of tetracycline in normal saline solution for an adult human) to prevent pleural pain (Wallach, 1978). The tetracycline-lidocaine mixture was shown to be an effective sclerosing agent in both experimental animals and humans.

Technique is reportedly critical to the success of tetracycline pleurodesis in humans. The following protocol has been recommended for human patients: (1) complete drainage of the pleural space with a thoracic drain tube (verified by thoracic radiographs), (2) instillation of 15 to 20 mg/kg of tetracycline diluted in 75 ml of sterile water, (3) instillation of 200 ml of air to ensure contact of the solution with the pleural surfaces, (4) rotation of the patient to several different positions to distribute the solution, (5) drainage of the pleural space 2 hr later, and (6) removal of the chest tube when drainage is less than 150 ml/24 hr. This technique is 80 per cent effective in treating pleural effusions.

A higher dose of intrapleural tetracycline in dogs may be warranted because the reported dose (20 mg/kg) was not completely effective in producing pleurodesis. Parenteral tetracycline has been shown to cause renal toxicity in dogs at a dose of 40 mg/kg when administered twice a day for 14 days. The same dose given for 7 days caused only minor renal changes. Although close monitoring of renal function would be advisable, a single intrapleural dose of 35 mg/kg in dogs is probably safe.

Quinacrine

Quinacrine (Atabrine), an antimalarial drug, has been used extensively in humans as a sclerosing agent, primarily for neoplastic effusions (Rochlin et al., 1964). Response rates range from 63 to 100 per cent. Dosages of intrapleural quinacrine vary greatly. From 90 mg to 800 mg of the drug have been used in humans. Most investigators have used 100 to 200 mg of quinacrine diluted in 20 to 30 ml of normal saline.

Side effects of quinacrine pleurodesis are more numerous than with tetracycline. Pleural pain, fever, nausea, hallucinations, hypotension, and convulsions have been reported after quinacrine infusion. Significantly more patients had fever and pleuritic pain after quinacrine administration compared with those receiving tetracycline.

Chemotherapeutic Agents

Many antineoplastic drugs have been used to induce pleurodesis. Nitrogen mustard, bleomycin, 25-fluorouracil, doxorubicin (Adriamycin), and thiotepa have been used in humans with malignant effusions. Bleomycin is the most effective chemotherapeutic pleurodesing agent in humans with malignant effusions. Dosages of bleomycin range from 30 to 180 mg per instillation. Bleomycin was less effective than tetracycline in a study using experimental animals (Sahn and Good, 1981).

OTHER METHODS OF PLEURODESIS

Talc has been widely used as a sclerosing agent in humans. Talc causes an intense reactive pleuritis and therefore is an effective sclerosing agent. The talc is instilled into the pleural space either by insufflation or by injection of talc suspended in normal saline. From 1 to 5 gm of talc have been used. Two chest tubes were placed in the patients in one study and talc was insufflated through one tube until seen exiting the second. However, morbidity and mortality rates are higher with talc than with other agents (Hausheer and Yarbro, 1985). It

Table 1. *Protocol for Tetracycline Pleurodesis**

1. Place bilateral thoracic drain tubes under general anesthesia and completely evacuate the pleural space.
2. Mix 20–35 mg/kg of tetracycline hydrochloride in 25 to 50 ml of saline and administer one half of the mixture in one thoracic tube and one half in the other.
3. Position the patient in right lateral recumbency, left lateral recumbency, sternal, and then dorsal recumbency (15 min for each position).
4. Aspirate both thoracic drainage tubes every 30 min or use continuous suction for 12–24 hr. Increase interval between aspirates as fluid production decreases.
5. Pull drainage tubes when fluid production stops or is minimal (2–3 ml/kg/day).

*This is the protocol used by the authors but is not a well-established method and should be considered experimental.

is therefore recommended only for low-risk patients after other sclerosing agents have failed.

Pleurectomy (excision of the parietal pleura) is a surgical method of inducing pleurodesis (Hausheer and Yarbro, 1985). Pleurectomy is associated with a high rate of morbidity (hemorrhage and air leaks) and mortality. As with talc pleurodesis, pleurectomy is reserved for low-risk patients that have failed to respond to other forms of pleurodesis.

CONCLUSIONS

Tetracycline appears to be the drug of choice for pleurodesis in humans and experimental animals. It is safe, is effective, and can be used for a variety of pleural diseases. Addition of lidocaine to the tetracycline solution reduces pleuritic pain without reducing effectiveness. Inadequate data are presently available to recommend a dose of tetracycline for small animals. The authors have used a dosage range of 20 to 35 mg/kg in a small number of animals. The procedure used is outlined in Table 1. Controlled studies are needed to establish an effective and safe dose.

Thoracic tube drainage is a mandatory adjunct to the infusion of a pleurodesis agent. Bilateral chest tubes should be used in animals with bilateral effusion or pneumothorax. The pleural space must be evacuated as completely as possible before and after infusion of the sclerosing agent to establish contact between the pleural surfaces.

References and Supplemental Reading

Austin, E. H., and Flye, M. W.: The treatment of recurrent malignant pleural effusion. Ann. Thorac. Surg. 28:190, 1979.

Hausheer, F. H., and Yarbro, J. W.: Diagnosis and treatment of malignant pleural effusion. Semin. Oncol. 12:54, 1985.

Laing, E. J., and Norris, A. M.: Pleurodesis as a treatment for pleural effusion in the dog. J. Am. Anim. Hosp. Assoc. 22:193, 1986.

Light, R. W.: *Pleural Diseases*. Philadelphia: Lea & Febiger, 1983, pp. 209–219.

Macoviak, J. A., Stephenson, L. W., Ochs, R., and Edmunds, L. H.: Tetracycline pleurodesis during active pulmonary-pleural air leak for prevention of recurrent pneumothorax. Chest 81:78, 1982.

Rochlin, D. B., Smart, C. R., Wagner, D. E., et al.: The control of recurrent malignant effusions using quinacrine hydrochloride. Surg. Gynecol. Obstet. 118:991, 1964.

Sahn, S. A., and Good, J. T.: The effect of common sclerosing agents on the rabbit pleural space. Am. Rev. Respir. Dis. 124:65, 1981.

Sahn, S. A., and Potts, D. E.: The effect of tetracycline on rabbit pleura. Am. Rev. Respir. Dis. 117:493, 1978.

Wallach, H. W.: Intrapleural therapy with tetracycline and lidocaine for malignant pleural effusions. Chest 73:246, 1978.

Wied, U., Halkier, E., Hoeier-Madsen, K., et al.: Tetracycline versus silver nitrate pleurodesis in spontaneous pneumothorax. J. Thorac. Cardiovasc. Surg. 86:591, 1983.

Zaloznik, A. J., Oswald, S. G., and Langin, M.: Intrapleural tetracycline in malignant pleural effusions: A randomized study. Cancer 51:752, 1983.

Section

4

HEMATOLOGY, ONCOLOGY, AND IMMUNOLOGY

BRUCE R. MADEWELL, V.M.D.

Consulting Editor

Sample Preparation for the Laboratory...................................410
Parasitic Blood Diseases of Dogs and Cats...............................419
Feline Anemia..425
Hereditary Disorders of Canine Erythrocytes............................429
Diagnostic Approach to the Bleeding Patient............................436
Factor VIII (Hemophilia A) and Factor IX (Hemophilia B)
    Deficiencies in Small Animals......................................442
Von Willebrand's Disease in Dogs.......................................446
Disseminated Intravascular Coagulation.................................451
Disorders of Platelets...457
Cytochemistry of Canine and Feline Leukocytes and Leukemias...........465
Acute Phase Proteins...468
Antineoplastic Agents in Cancer Therapy................................472
Special Considerations in Drug Preparation and Administration..........475
Chemotherapy of Lymphoma and Leukemia..................................482
Chemotherapy of Solid Tumors...489
Chemotherapy-induced Myelosuppression..................................494
Cisplatin Chemotherapy...497
Radiation Therapy..502
Biological Response Modifiers..507
Cyclosporine...513
Bone Marrow Transplantation..515
Congenital and Acquired Neutrophil Function Abnormalities in the
    Dog..521
The Risk of Transmission of FeLV from Latently Infected Cats...........526
Feline Immunodeficiency Virus Infection................................530
Feline Lymphoid Hyperplasia..535
Acute Hypersensitivity Reactions.......................................537
Immune-mediated Nonerosive Arthritis in the Dog........................543

SAMPLE PREPARATION FOR THE LABORATORY

BRUCE R. MADEWELL, V.M.D.

Davis, California

The diagnostic process involves the triad of patient history, physical examination, and laboratory study. Laboratory confirmation of suspected clinical findings generally involves routine sampling methods such as use of ethylenediaminetetra-acetic acid, (EDTA)–anticoagulated blood for the hemogram or formalin-fixed tissue for histopathologic study. Increasing awareness of disease processes has resulted in clinical application of newly developed, sophisticated, sensitive testing methods, often allowing definitive diagnoses to be established. The demand for precise diagnostic methods has added to the responsibilities of the clinician—the veterinarian must know not only what tests are available routinely or by special order, but also *how* to collect the appropriate samples. (An adequately prepared sample may be crucial for the diagnosis of a life-threatening disorder in an important clinical case.) This article provides guidelines for preparation of samples for hematology, oncology, and immunology laboratories. For the routinely performed laboratory determinations, normal values derived from study of clinically healthy animals are provided in the appendices. For other determinations, however, universally accepted normal values have not yet been established, and the reader will need to consult with the individual laboratory to determine the normal range of values. Further, in some instances, the veterinarian will be requested to submit a paired, control sample from a clinically healthy animal in addition to the test sample.

ONCOLOGY

The mainstay of cancer diagnosis is biopsy; samples are collected by aspiration or imprint for cytologic methods, or scalpel-derived specimens are procured for histologic study. However, even these seemingly routine maneuvers are complex when viewed in terms of the myriad diagnostic methods that can be employed.

EXFOLIATIVE CYTOLOGY. Routine cytologic observations are done using air-dried or wet-fixed specimens. For air-dried specimens destined for Romanowsky's staining (Wright's, Giemsa, Leishman's, May-Grünwald), thin smears are made on glass slides and dried rapidly. The morphologic characteristics of exfoliated cells are extremely sensitive to degeneration and fixation artifacts. Rapid specimen drying is most important to ensure that cells dry adhered to and flattened on the slide, rather than rounding up, as occurs when thick smears are allowed to dry slowly. Superb nuclear detail can be achieved using Papanicolaou's staining methods. For Papanicolaou preparations, thin smears are fixed (wet) immediately in 100 per cent methanol or 95 per cent ethanol (the addition of 3 per cent glacial acetic acid increases the nucleoprotein-fixing properties), or using a commercial spray fixative. Most commercial fixatives contain polyethylene glycol in ethyl alcohol—the alcohol fixes the smear, while the polyethylene glycol provides a waxlike coat to prevent evaporation. Cytologic preparations may also be examined using enzyme cytochemical or immunocytochemical methods; cytochemical methods applicable to hemopoietic cells are discussed elsewhere in this volume (see p. 465), and some immunohisto(cyto)chemical methods are listed below.

HISTOLOGY. Tissue fixatives for histologic study include aldehydes (formaldehyde, glutaraldehyde), oxidizing agents (osmium tetroxide, potassium permanganate), protein-denaturing agents (acetic acid, methyl alcohol, ethyl alcohol), cross-linking agents (carbodiimides), and others (mercuric chloride, picric acid). The most widely used fixative for histopathology is formaldehyde; the commercial solution commonly contains 35 to 40 per cent gas by weight (formalin) and is prepared to 10 per cent for tissue fixation, commonly buffered with phosphate to pH 7.0. Specimens for fixation should be less than 0.5 cm in thickness and, if possible, should include margins between normal and abnormal tissues. Larger specimens should be "bread loaf" sliced to allow for adequate fixation, and the volume of fixative used should be ten times the volume of the tissue being prepared.

The hematoxylin and eosin stain is the most widely used tissue stain; the hematoxylin component stains the cell nuclei blue-black with good intranuclear detail, whereas the eosin stains cell cytoplasm and most connective tissue fibers in varying shades and intensities of pink, orange, and red. Other special stains are commonly employed (Table 1). Although many of the histologic staining methods

410

Table 1. Common Histologic Stains

Stain	Use
Toluidine blue	Demonstrates mast cells by the metachromatic staining of granules
Periodic–acid Schiff (PAS)	Stains mucin, colloid, reticulin, basement membranes, and cytoplasmic glycogen (also fungal elements)
Trichrome	Differentiates muscle and connective tissue
Fontana-Masson	Demonstrates melanin, melanin precursors, and other reducing substances (APUD cells)
Methyl green-pyronine	Identifies cells rich in RNA (e.g., plasma cells) or viral inclusion bodies
Feulgen reaction	Identifies DNA (e.g., viral inclusion bodies)
Sudan black B, oil red O	Demonstrates reticular fiber histoskeleton (e.g., glandular arrangement)

APUD, amine precursor uptake and decarboxylation.

Table 2. General Categories of Immunologic Tumor Markers

1. Products of viral genome in virus-induced neoplasms
2. Lineage-specific antigens
3. Differentiation stage–specific antigens
4. Embryonic or fetal antigens
5. Division or associated antigens
6. Antigens unique to specific tumors (i.e., immunoglobulin products of plasma cell tumors)
7. Tumor-specific or tumor-associated antigens

Modified from Evans, R. J.: Cytology in diagnosis and assessment of neoplastic conditions. *In* Gorman, N. T. (ed.): *Oncology.* New York: Churchill-Livingstone, 1986, p. 25.

used to demonstrate cellular or tissue constituents can be applied to formalin-fixed specimens, special staining methods such as those used to demonstrate enzyme activities require other fixation methods or cryostat-prepared specimens. It is prudent to check with the commercial laboratory before collecting a specimen if special studies will be required. There are a plethora of stains and staining methods used to identify connective tissues and their cells, the proteins and nucleic acids, amyloid, carbohydrates,

lipids, pigments, minerals, cytoplasmic granules and organelles, and microorganisms. The reader is referred to any standard textbook of histologic methods for details.

IMMUNOHISTO(CYTO)CHEMISTRY. Immunohisto-(cyto)chemical methods are based on recognition of tumor markers. Immunohistochemical methods utilize a tracer, which attaches to a specific antigen in the tissue section, and an enzyme histochemical reaction, which utilizes the tracer for light or electron microscopy. Some examples of immunologic tumor markers, using polyclonal or monoclonal antibodies for their identifications, are listed in Table 2.

Immunohistochemical localization of immune markers by immunoperoxidase, avidin-biotin techniques, or immunofluorescent methods is optimally performed on cryostat sections, but good results are also achieved using paraffin-embedded tissues after fixation in absolute alcohol for 36 to 48 hr. Fixation of tissues in formalin, Zenker's, Bouin's, or B-5 fixative will generally reduce sensitivity of staining, as will the paraffin embedding process. For some

Table 3. Antigens That Can Be Used as Soft Tissue Markers

Antigen	Use
Cytoskeletal Elements	
Keratin	Marker for epithelial/myoepithelial cells
Vimentin	Marker for mesenchymal differentiation
Desmin	Marker for muscle differentiation
Actin	Present in many cell types
Myosin	Strongest reactivity in muscle
Laminin	Basal lamina of smooth muscle and Schwann's cells
GFAP*	Marker for astrocytes and ependymal cells
Neurofilaments	Marker for neural cells
Proteins	
Fibronectin	Mesenchymal marker; present in fibrohistiocytes and synovium
Factor VIII rag	Specific for endothelial cells
Myoglobin	Specific for skeletal muscle
Myelin basic protein	Peripheral nerve marker
S-100 protein	Marker for peripheral nerve, Langerhans' cells, melanocytes, granular cells, and monocytes/macrophages
Alpha$_1$-antitrypsin	Histiocyte marker
Alpha$_1$-antichymotrypsin	Histiocyte marker
Enzymes	
Lysozyme	Histiocyte marker
Acid phosphatase	Markers for osseous and chondroid tissues
Alkaline phosphatase	

*GFAP, glial fibrillary acidic proteins.

Table 4. *Fixatives for Electron Microscopy*

Fixative	Buffer	Duration	Postfixation
1. 2.5% glutaraldehyde 2. Karnovsky's (modified): 2% para-formaldehyde, 2.5% glutaralde-hyde	0.05–0.1 M phosphate or caco-dylate	Hours to weeks	1% osmium tetroxide

Table 5. *Routinely Used Anticoagulants*

Anticoagulant	Content	Amount Used (ml) per ml of Blood	Clinical Use
EDTA	Potassium salt of ethylenediaminetetra-acetate, 1.00 gm; 0.07% saline solution; 100 ml	0.10	Efficient and complete anticoagulation; best for platelet counts
Oxalates	Ammonium oxalate, 1.20 gm; potassium oxalate, 0.80 gm; distilled water, 100 ml	0.10 (1 mg/ml in dry form)	Good cellular morphology; not used for platelet counts
Sodium citrate	Trisodium citrate, 3.80 gm; distilled water, 100 ml	0.15	Coagulation tests
ACD solution	Trisodium citrate, 2.20 gm; citric acid, 0.80 gm; dextrose, 2.45 gm	0.15	Blood banking
CPD solution	Citric acid, 0.32 gm; trisodium citrate, 2.63 gm; NaH_2PO_4, 0.22 gm; dextrose, 2.55 gm	0.14	Blood banking
Heparin	Stock	Wet syringe & needle for 5-ml specimen	Osmotic fragility test
Sodium fluoride	—	2.5 mg/ml	Glucose preservation
Defibrination	Glass beads, 3–4 mm	20 beads/25 ml blood	Defibrinated serum

immunohistochemical determinations, however, formalin-fixed, paraffin-embedded tissues provide satisfactory results. To procure specimens for frozen section, small pieces of tissue are frozen immediately in liquid nitrogen. Cryostat sections can be stored at −70°C or air-dried and fixed in acetone-methanol.

Immunohistochemistry provides the diagnostic histopathologist with a tool for studying tissue structure and function. For example, the undifferentiated soft tissue sarcomas often can be characterized as to their histogenesis or stage of differentiation by immunoenzyme labeling of cell products. Some of the antigens that can be used as soft tissue markers are listed in Table 3. Also included are the intermediate filament proteins, the components of the cytoskeleton that are 10 to 12 nm in diameter. These filaments are specific for tissue types, and, generally, the cell-type–specific expression of intermediate filaments is also maintained in tumor cells,

Table 6. *Causes of Hemolysis*

1. Improperly cleaned glassware, needles, or syringes
2. Use of wet needles, syringes, or glassware
3. Collecting the sample with too much pressure
4. Ejecting blood too rapidly from syringe into container
5. Placing sample in chilled glassware
6. Vigorous shaking of blood rather than slow mixing of whole blood with the chemical fixatives
7. Temperature extremes

thus allowing determination of the histogenesis of undifferentiated or anaplastic tumors.

ULTRASTRUCTURE. The electron microscope may be useful for determining the diagnosis and histogenesis of controversial neoplasms, and it is useful in distinguishing broadly among sarcoma, melanoma, and carcinoma by revealing specific structures, such as desmosomes or melanosomes.

Fixation is the most important single procedure in the whole sequence of processes involved in biologic electron microscopy—the ideal is to preserve every detail of cellular ultrastructure as it was in life the instant before the specimen was collected. Fixation must be rapid and certain. For optimal ultrastructural preservation, tissues should be fixed within seconds of removal. Tissues are carefully sliced into small cubes generally not exceeding 1 to 2 mm in thickness and placed immediately in an appropriate fixative.

Two-stage fixation procedures using glutaraldehyde buffered with phosphate or cacodylate followed by osmium tetroxide are almost universally used. Two per cent glutaraldehyde in a 0.05 to 0.1 M phosphate buffer at pH 7.2 is a superior fixative for ultrastructural detail, but it slowly penetrates into tissues, which may allow the center of thick specimens to autolyze. Glutaraldehyde fixation is optimized when the fixative is stored at 4°C or prepared fresh, the pH is adjusted, and it is allowed to warm to room temperature immediately before

Table 7. *Staining of Blood Smears*

Stain	Clinical Use
Wright's	Erythrocytes stain pink; leukocyte nuclei, blue. Nuclei and basophilic cytoplasmic components stain blue; neutrophil granules, lilac; eosinophil granules, orange; mast cell granules, deep blue-violet; nucleoli, blue-violet. Mature monocyte cytoplasm stains pale gray-blue; neutrophilic cytoplasm is pale pink
Giemsa	
May-Grünwald–Giemsa	
Wright-Leishman	
Alkaline phosphatase	Stains granules of neoplastic granulocyte precursors
Acid phosphatase	Demonstrates lymphoblasts of T-cell origin in some species
Periodic acid–Schiff (PAS)	Stains cells of granulocyte series from myelocytes on; some lymphocytes show positive granules. Megakaryocytes and platelets are positive
Peroxidase	Stains myeloid cells from promyelocytes onward; monocytes may stain weakly

the tissue is introduced. After 1 or 2 hr at room temperature, the tissue-fixative specimen is again cooled to 4°C, the total primary fixation time being 1 to 3 hr to overnight. Commercial formaldehyde as used routinely in histologic preparations is a poor fixative for ultrastructural studies because its methanol content may act as a coagulative fixative and protein denaturant. Karnovsky's fixative, a combination of paraformaldehyde and glutaraldehyde, combines the rapid fixation advantage of formaldehyde and the fixation potency of glutaraldehyde. The author uses a modification of Karnovsky's fixative (Table 4). With Karnovsky's fixative, tissue specimens can be stored for days or even weeks and refrigerated in the primary fixative before additional sample manipulation. This method may prove satisfactory to temporarily store a sample until the results of routine histopathologic evaluation are available, the decision to proceed with electron microscopic determinations being based on those findings.

CELL CULTURE. Cell culture has been used complementary to histopathologic study to allow identification of undifferentiated tumors or to distinguish benign from malignant tumors. For example, poorly differentiated malignant melanoma may express premelanosomes in culture, allowing a diagnosis to be established. Further, if a karyotype is desired, such as might be used to identify a canine transmissible venereal tumor, a tumor explant will be required. Cell culture methods are generally not within the scope of clinical practice, but sample collection for transport to an appropriate laboratory is feasible. Tissue specimens are collected using

surgical aseptic methods, and small fragments are placed immediately in transport medium. Although many transport-type (balanced salt) mediums are available, the author routinely uses sterile Hank's basic salt solution, which is designed to equilibrate with air and contains antibiotics (penicillin, streptomycin) and 2 per cent bovine fetal serum. Care must be taken to collect viable tissue representative of the neoplasm, i.e., one should avoid sampling the center of the lesion, which may contain hypoxic or nonviable cells, or the periphery, which may be composed primarily of a connective tissue capsule or inflammatory cells. After transportation to the laboratory, disaggregation of tissues to yield single cells or small groups of cells permits rapid initiation of primary cultures. Purely physical methods of disaggregation of cells may be appropriate for some tissues, whereas chemical or enzymatic methods of freeing cells from the stroma and from each other are required for other specimens. These methods include gentle mincing of tissue fragments with scissors or scalpel, teasing the tissues apart, passing the specimen through a wire mesh, or trypsinization. Rarely are explant cultures successful unless chemically defined media are supplemented with serum. Fetal bovine serum, 10 to 20 per cent by volume, is commonly used.

HEMATOLOGY

Anticoagulants are used for hematologic methods; the commonly used anticoagulants are listed in Table 5.

Table 8. *Some Laboratory Studies of Disturbances of Iron Metabolism*

Test	Method of Sample Collection	Interpretation or Clinical Utility
Blood/bone marrow iron stains	Air-dried smears of blood or marrow for Prussian blue reaction	Prussian blue reaction detects nonheme iron (i.e., ferritin and hemosiderin iron) in red blood cells, marrow, and urine. Iron appears as blue granules usually < 1 μm in diameter
Total serum iron	Serum from clotted blood collected into glassware washed with dilute HCl. Avoid hemolysis	Indirect indicators of body iron stores. Perturbations seen in conditions such as inflammation, malignancy, liver disease, iron therapy, and malnutrition
Total iron-binding capacity		
% saturation of transferrin		
Ferrokinetic determinations	In usual ferrokinetic studies, transferrin is labeled with radioactive iron (^{59}Fe)	Allows measurement of the rate of erythropoiesis; allows discrimination between effective and ineffective erythropoiesis

Table 9. Laboratory Evaluation of Erythrocyte Defects or Abnormalities

Test	Sampling Method	Interpretation or Clinical Utility
Osmotic fragility	Heparinized or defibrinated blood	Usual method of measuring the surface-volume ratio of erythrocytes
Erythrocyte volume distribution	EDTA-anticoagulated blood	Allows recognition of disturbances of erythrocyte production that result in altered cell size; also allows assessment of chronicity and severity of problem
Erythrocyte sedimentation rate (ESR)	EDTA-anticoagulated blood	Increased rate in diseases associated with tissue necrosis and degeneration; influenced by many nonspecific variables
Reticulocyte staining	Apply a drop of 0.5% NMB in physiologic saline solution and glass coverslip to an air-dried blood film and examine immediately	Valuable tool for appraising the rate of effective erythropoiesis
Heinz body staining	Equal drops of whole blood and NMB	Unstable hemoglobins (Heinz bodies) are small, deep-purplish inclusions at cell margin. They may be result of oxidative drugs, unstable hemoglobins, or splenectomy
Canine distemper inclusions	Routine Romanowsky-stained blood film, or apply NMB to dry unfixed blood film	Inclusions appear in reticulocytes, pale blue or red, varying in size and location
Erythrocyte parasites		
Babesia canis, B. gibsoni, feline babesias	Thin air-dried blood smear stained with Romanowsky's stain. Best to use microcapillary blood	*B. canis* organisms (2.4–5.0 μm) appear as large piriform bodies and may show multiple invasion of single cells. Organism size varies with species
Haemobartonella canis, H. felis	Thin air-dried blood smear stained with Giemsa	Organisms appear as basophilic coccoid, rod, or ring forms
Trypanosoma cruzi	Thin air-dried blood smear stained with Giemsa	Protozoan parasite is 16–20 μm in length and is spindle shaped and flagellated
Cytauxzoon	Thin air-dried blood smear stained with Giemsa.	Parasite appears as ring-form (1.0–1.5 μm in diameter) piroplasms in its erythrocyte phase
Toxoplasma gondii	Thin air-dried blood smear stained with Giemsa	Rarely, tachyzoites may be found in blood. Tachyzoites are crescent-shaped bodies with paracentral nuclei and measure 4–6 μm × 2–3 μm
Erythrocyte enzymes	Collect blood into EDTA, ACD, or heparin; enzymes are stable for 1 week when anticoagulated blood is stored at 4°C	To detect deficiencies in G-6-PD, pyruvate kinase, or other erythrocyte enzymes
Separation of hemoglobins	Oxalate- or EDTA-anticoagulated blood; wash erythrocytes 3 times in NaCl solution (0.85 g/100 ml) prior to preparation of hemolysate and electrophoresis on cellulose acetate	Allows quantitation of hemoglobin A and hemoglobin B in dog and cat in suspected hemoglobin disorders
Serum haptoglobin	Oxalate- or EDTA-anticoagulated blood	Increased values in patients with obstructive biliary disease, inflammations, neoplasms; decreased in hemoglobinemia and parenchymatous liver disease
Hemoglobin vs. myoglobin in urine	Fresh urine	Electrophoresis allows distinction between hemoglobinuria and myoglobinuria. Or, hemoglobin can be precipitated from urine (2.8 gm of NH_2SO_4 to 5 ml of urine) and retested with a commercial urine dipstick, a positive reading confirming myoglobin
Quantitative methemoglobin in serum	EDTA-anticoagulated blood	Various chemical compounds or therapeutic agents can cause methemoglobinemia (e.g., nitrites, aromatic amino and nitro compounds)
Serum erythropoietin	Serum	Useful in distinguishing primary from secondary polycythemias; high levels observed in aplastic anemia and pure red blood cell aplasia
Erythrocyte survival measurements	Usual method involves labeling erythrocytes with radioactive sodium chromate (^{51}Cr)	Allows measurement of erythrocyte life span

NMB, new methylene blue; ACD, acid-citrate-dextrose; G-6-PD, glucose-6-phosphate dehydrogenase.

Table 10. Leukocyte Studies

Test	Sample	Interpretation or Clinical Utility
Methyl green-pyronine stain	Air-dried smears of blood or marrow	Measure of ribonucleoprotein content of leukocytes
Serum lysozyme (muramidase) activity	Serum	May serve as reflection of macrophage activity in animals with cancer or chronic inflammatory disease. Serum lysozyme levels are increased in myeloproliferative diseases
Lupus erythematosus (LE) cell phenomenon	Collect 7–10 ml of whole blood in glass tube and allow to clot; sample is processed through wire mesh	LE cells are neutrophils showing a homogeneous, smooth, lavender inclusion. LE phenomenon is seen in animals with lupus erythematosus, but also other collagen diseases and some drug reactions
Neutrophil Function		
Bactericidal assay	Heparinized blood from which neutrophils are separated by gradient contrifugation from test animal and healthy control	*In vitro* test to measure the end product of neutrophil function—ability to kill bacteria
Nitroblue tetrazolium (NBT) test	Heparinized blood from test animal and healthy control	Estimates phagocytic function of neutrophils and provides some information on neutrophil metabolic function
Neutrophil chemotaxis	Heparinized blood from test animal and healthy control	Used to detect defects of neutrophil migration by observing directional migration in response to a gradient of chemoattractant
Chemiluminescence	Heparinized blood from test animal and healthy control	Measures the ability of neutrophil population to generate a respiratory burst accompanied by the release of photons of lights
Cellular Inclusions in Circulating Blood Leukocytes		
Feline infectious peritonitis	Routine air-dried, thin smears of peripheral blood, lymph nodes, or bone marrow, stained with Romanowsky's stain	Inclusions occasionally seen in neutrophils
Canine ehrlichiosis		Neutrophils or lymphocytes
Histoplasmosis		Monocytes and tissue macrophages
Leishmaniasis		Monocytes and tissue macrophages
Hepatozoonosis		Neutrophils and monocytes
Canine distemper		Lymphocytes, neutrophils, or erythrocytes
Toxoplasmosis		Monocytes (or erythrocytes) or free in blood

Blood collected for anticoagulation studies must be mixed immediately with proper additives. Oxalates, citrates, and EDTA-based anticoagulants remove calcium from the blood by forming insoluble or un-ionized calcium salts; heparin inactivates thrombin and thromboplastin; and defibrination removes fibrinogen converted to fibrin. Dipotassium or disodium salts of EDTA are popular anticoagulants because they neither interfere with normal staining characteristics of cells nor alter cell size, and samples may be stored in the refrigerator overnight. Oxalates produce the least cell distortion, but cells must be examined within an hour or leukocyte distortion occurs, and oxalates are not recommended for platelet counts. Heparin anticoagulation is best for osmotic fragility tests because it does not alter cell size. It may, however, influence leukocyte staining, is effective for only 10 to 12 hr, and is the most expensive of the anticoagulants. Defibrination allows serum preparation from whole blood. To defibrinate, fresh whole blood is collected into an Erlenmeyer flask containing glass beads. The specimen is then gently swirled until the fibrin precipitates around the glass beads, generally within 10 to 15 min.

Hemolysis in collected samples may be the result of an improperly collected specimen; common causes of hemolysis are listed in Table 6.

When blood samples are collected for cellular morphologic evaluation, it is advised that blood films be prepared as soon as possible after collection of the specimen. Most routinely used stains for blood smears in veterinary medicine are of the Romanowsky type, incorporating basic and acidic aniline dyes, which bring out the contrasting colors of red and blue. Some stains used for hematologic examinations are listed in Table 7. Romanowsky's stains are also commonly employed for bone marrow evaluations. The main attribute of Wright's stain is that it produces a broad spectrum of hues, whereas the Giemsa stain is especially good for nuclear and cytoplasmic detail and provides better definition of the hematopoietic cells. Giemsa stain is an aqueous solution, and smears must be fixed in 100 per cent methanol prior to staining. Some methods incorporate two stains to combine the advantages of each (e.g., Wright-Giemsa and May-Grünwald–Giemsa). May-Grünwald is a popular stain, which, when used first, results in the simultaneous alcohol fixation of the specimen. May-Grünwald, like Wright's, is a polychromatic stain that is metachromatic.

ERYTHROCYTE STUDIES. A variety of studies directed specifically at detection of erythrocyte defects or abnormalities are done, some routinely, in clinical practice. Some of these studies are aimed at assessment of iron metabolism, as an aid in

Table 11. Hemostasis Studies

Test	Sampling Method	Indications or Clinical Utility
Activated coagulation time	Draw blood into an evacuated diatomite tube, prewarmed to 37°C	Estimate of overall activity of intrinsic system of blood coagulation; prolonged only in severe deficiencies of factors in intrinsic or common pathways.
Activated partial thromboplastin time (APTT)	Venous blood is collected into a plastic syringe by clean venipuncture. Anticoagulant: 1 vol of 3.8% trisodium citrate is mixed with 9 vol of blood by gentle inversion, in a polystyrene tube. Platelet-poor plasma is achieved by centrifuging samples at 1600 g for 10 min. As for APTT, platelet-poor plasma is drawn off with siliconized or plastic pipettes, used fresh, or stored at $-70°C$	Measure of coagulant activity of extrinsic system; prolonged in deficiencies of one or more factors of XII, XI, X, IX, VIII, V, prothrombin, and fibrinogen
One-stage prothrombin time		A measure of the coagulant activity of the extrinsic system; prolonged with deficiencies of factors V, VII, X, or prothrombin, or if heparin, fibrin/fibrinogen split products are present, or if fibrinogen is low
Plasma fibrinogen concentrations	Citrated plasma or EDTA	Estimate of fibrinogen concentration in plasma
Paracoagulation test for soluble fibrin monomer	Fresh, platelet-poor citrated plasma	Detects soluble fibrin monomer in plasma as evidence of fibrinolysis
Euglobulin clot lysis time	Platelet-poor citrated plasma	Evaluates systemic fibrinolysis
Antithrombin-III	Platelet-poor citrated plasma	Measurement of the activity of a naturally occurring antithrombin. Decreased AT-III activity is observed in DIC. May be used to identify patients susceptible to thrombosis
Plasminogen	Platelet-poor citrated plasma	Decreased plasminogen activity is observed in ongoing systemic fibrinolysis or decreased synthesis
Plasminogen activator	Platelet-poor citrated plasma	May aid as a predictor of susceptibility to thrombosis
Specific factor deficiencies	Platelet-poor citrated plasma	Methodology available to detect specific deficiencies of factors V, VII, VIII, IX, X, XI, XII, and XIII
Von Willebrand factor (antigen)	Citrated plasma from patient	Measurement of factor VIII:VWF complex
PIVKA thrombotest assay	Citrated plasma	Proteins induced by vitamin K absence or antagonists are precursor proteins of factors II, VII, IX, and X. Any medical condition causing relative or absolute vitamin K deficiency causes prolongation of thrombotest assay
Fibrin/fibrinogen split products	For latex agglutination test, blood is collected into commercially available tubes containing soybean trypsin inhibitor and bovine thrombin	To detect the presence of fibrin/fibrinogen split products in serum; FDP concentration increases in DIC
Thrombin time	Citrated plasma	Measure of the rate of conversion of fibrinogen to fibrin; used as an indicator of quantitative and/or qualitative fibrinogen disorders.
Others: prekallikrein, kallikrein, kallikrein inhibitors	Citrated plasma	May be useful in monitoring disorders associated with tissue inflammation or necrosis, particularly involving the pancreas

DIC, disseminated intravascular coagulation; FDP, fibrin degradation products.

recognizing those disturbances clinically manifested frequently in companion animals (iron deficiency anemia and the anemia of chronic inflammatory diseases). Some laboratory methods useful for this assessment are listed in Table 8.

A composite of other studies aimed at detection of erythrocyte defects and abnormalities is found in Table 9. Erythrocyte volume measurements, previously purveyed by calculated Wintrobe's indices or estimated by osmotic fragility measurements, are now accurately measured with automated electronic instruments.

LEUKOCYTE STUDIES. Total blood leukocyte and differential counts are an integral component of disease investigation. Cytochemical methods for differentiation of primitive or neoplastic leukocytes are outlined elsewhere in this text (p. 465); additional leukocyte-related studies are cited in Table 10.

HEMOSTASIS STUDIES. Hemostasis is achieved by vascular factors, platelets, and the clotting mechanism. The integrity of the blood vessel wall cannot be routinely evaluated, and diagnosis of abnormal hemostasis is directed at estimation of platelet numbers and function and assessment of the coagulation mechanism. The hemostatic mechanism is evaluated by a variety of methods, some of which are outlined in Table 11. All blood samples must be collected with a minimum of trauma and blood stasis, and delay between collection and testing should be minimized. Venous blood collected from indwelling

Table 12. Evaluation of Platelet Abnormalities

Test	Sampling Method	Indications or Clinical Utility
Platelet count	Diluents include 1% ammonium oxalate, 2% disodium EDTA in saline, or commercial counting fluids	To detect thrombocytopenia or thrombocytosis
Clot retraction	Venous (0.5 ml) blood diluted 1:10 with cold buffered saline (4.5 ml) and clotted with a standardized concentration of thrombin	Clot retraction in 1–2 hr is dependent on normal platelet quantity and quality
Russell's viper venom time	Citrated platelet-rich plasma	Measure of common pathway of blood coagulation
Buccal mucosa bleeding time	Regulated length and depth of incision in upper lip mucosa	Prolonged bleeding times with qualitative and quantitative platelet defects, capillary fragility, vascular lesions, von Willebrand's disease
Platelet aggregation and release	Citrated platelet-rich plasma	Platelet aggregation disorders have been described in some collagen or connective tissue diseases, and in association with some drug administrations
Platelet retention (adhesiveness)	Citrated platelet-rich plasma	Decreased adhesiveness in association with platelet function defects or von Willebrand's disease.
Mean platelet volume	Citrated platelet-rich plasma	Provides early indication of bone marrow response to thrombocytopenia

Table 13. Immunochemical Methods

Test	Sampling Method	Indications or Clinical Utility
Serum protein electrophoresis and immunoelectrophoresis	1 ml of serum; freeze if mailing	Used for investigation of diseases in which single clone of lymphocytes or plasma cells produces a large amount of homogeneous immunoglobulin or immunoglobulin fragment
Serum viscosity	Serum; centrifuged at 3000 g for 10 min to remove particulate matter	Serum viscosity is increased in macroglobulinemia and some cases of multiple myeloma
Immunoglobulin quantitation: IgG, IgM, IgA	1 ml of serum; freeze if mailing	Used for evaluation of hypo- or hypergammaglobulinemias
Hemolytic complement (CH_{50})	1 ml of serum collected fresh	Screening test for integrity of complete complement system
C3 assay	1 ml of serum collected fresh	Reduction in C3 generally reflects total hemolytic complement activity

catheters is not suitable for coagulation studies. Samples are collected into plastic or polystyrene tubes; if glass containers are used, they must be of standardized, siliconized glass. The most commonly used anticoagulant for the collection of blood for coagulation studies is trisodium citrate.

The role of blood platelets in hemostatic disorders can be assessed quantitatively and qualitatively. Evaluation of platelet function is outlined in Table 12.

IMMUNOLOGY

Rapid advances in immunology during the last several decades have led to the widespread application of basic advances to clinical medicine. Many immunologic methods are shared with the oncology and hematology laboratories; others are unique. In that many of these methods are not done daily by many laboratories, coordination of sampling with a regional laboratory is advised.

Table 14. Examples of Tests to Detect Specific Antibody Activity

Test	Sampling Method	Indications or Clinical Utility
Rheumatoid factor	0.5 ml of serum; freeze if mailing	IgM antibody that appears early in course of rheumatoid arthritis and remains present during course of disease activity
Cold agglutinin activity	Collect 5–10 ml of blood in prewarmed (37°C) clot tube, and deliver, warmed, stat to laboratory	Often associated with infectious or neoplastic diseases, cold agglutinins are antibodies, mostly of IgM type, that react with red blood cell antigens at temperatures below 37°C
Cryoglobulins (cryoimmunoglobulins)	Same samples as cold agglutinins. Harvested serum is promptly collected and stored at 4°C	Serum proteins or protein complexes that undergo reversible precipitation at low temperatures. Cryoglobulins occur in variety of neoplastic, inflammatory, and infectious diseases

Table 15. Laboratory Evaluation of Cellular Immunity

Test	Sampling Method	Indications or Clinical Utility

Assays for T and B cells
  Lymphocytes with surface immunoglobulin (IgG)
  Lymphocytes with C3 receptors
  Lymphocytes with receptors for erythrocytes
Estimation of lymphocyte subpopulations using monoclonal antibodies
	Lymphocytes are generally collected from peripheral blood using Ficoll-Isopaque gradients.* Peripheral blood is collected in heparinized syringes (100 IU/ml blood) or into EDTA (0.1 mg/ml blood).	T- and B-cell assays may allow differentiation of benign from malignant lymphoproliferative diseases; documentation of certain immunodeficiency disorders; and distinguish benign monoclonal gammopathy from multiple myeloma
		
		Monoclonal antibodies allow categorization of lymphocyte subsets in lymphoproliferative disorders for diagnosis and prognosis purposes

Lymphocyte blast transformation; mitogen or antigen-induced transformation studies	Heparinized peripheral blood. Some lymphocyte blast transformation methods use whole blood collected into EDTA or heparin; others use Ficoll-Isopaque–separated blood lymphocytes	Test used to diagnose congenital or acquired immunologic deficiencies; to detect sensitization caused by infectious agents or in some autoimmune diseases; to monitor the effects of various immunosuppressive and immunotherapeutic manipulations
Cell migration inhibition assay	Heparinized peripheral blood from which lymphocytes are separated by Ficoll-Isopaque gradient centrifugation	Allows detection of certain lymphocyte mediators such as migration inhibitory factor (MIF). The production of MIF closely parallels the state of cellular hypersensitivity of the host
Cytotoxicity tests	Variety of cell separation methods are used, including density gradients, affinity chromatography, and adherence properties of cells	Provide assessment of (1) antibody-dependent cytotoxicity; (2) natural killer cell–mediated cytotoxity; and (3) cytotoxic T-lymphocyte mediated cytotoxicity

*To prepare Ficoll-Isopaque with a density of 1.088, mix 30 ml of 82.3% (w/v) sodium diatrozoate (Isopaque; Winthrop Laboratories, NY) with a solution of 9 gm of Ficoll (MW 40,000; Sigma Chemical Co., St. Louis, MO) in 120 ml of double-distilled water.

IMMUNOCHEMISTRY. Immunochemical studies include electrophoretic and immunoelectrophoretic methods for diagnosis of dysproteinemias; methods for immunologic quantitation of proteins in serum, urine, and other body fluids; and determinations of the role of complement in clinical disorders (Table 13).

The complete workup of an animal patient with a suspected disorder relating to the amount or nature of a specific immunoglobulin may be aimed at assessing the complications arising from these proteins. Several such tests are listed in Table 14.

CELLULAR IMMUNOLOGY. Assessment of defects in cellular immunology includes assays for T and B cells, use of lymphocyte transformation to assess clinical disorders, inhibition of cell migration as a correlate of cell-mediated immunity, and assays of phagocytic function. Several specific methods applicable to the immunology laboratory are outlined in Table 15.

DETECTION OF AUTOIMMUNE DISORDERS. Autoantibodies against many self-antigens are found naturally in the serum of normal, healthy individuals; autoantibodies against virtually all self-constituents can be elicited when appropriately immunized or stimulated. Autoimmune diseases are severe de-

Table 16. Tests for Detection of Autoimmune Disorders

Test	Sampling Method	Indications or Clinical Utility
Direct Coombs' test	1 ml of whole blood in EDTA; do not freeze	For detection of Ig or C3 on patient's erythrocytes for diagnosis of autoimmune hemolytic anemia or cold agglutinin disease
Indirect Coombs' test	1 ml of serum, freeze if mailing	Similar to above, but detects circulating autoantibody
Antinuclear antibody (ANA) test	1 ml of serum; freeze if mailing	Measures the capacity of patients with systemic lupus erythematosus (SLE) to make antibody to nucleoprotein. Some drugs will induce ANA
Pemphigus antibody	1 ml of serum; freeze if mailing	Allows detection of circulating skin/mucosal autoantibodies
Tissue biopsy for direct immunofluorescence; IgG, C3, IgM, IgA	Biopsy specimen collected in Michelle's media or use fresh tissue or snap freeze in liquid nitrogen	For diagnosis of diseases, including SLE, discoid lupus erythematosus, immune complex glomerulonephritis, pemphigus or bullous pemphigoid, immune complex vasculitis. Direct immunofluorescence detects antibody or complement fixed to tissues
Platelet factor-3 test (PF-3)	Collect 3 ml of citrated plasma; mail fresh frozen on dry ice	For diagnosis of immune-mediated thrombocytopenia

rangements of the immunologic network, or a component thereof, that are nonreversible from within the system and lead to pathologic conditions. Some tests used routinely for evaluation of autoimmune disorders are cited in Table 16.

In sum, the expanding repertoire of diagnostic services offered by commercial laboratories, hospitals, and teaching institutions has greatly enhanced the ability of clinical veterinarians to provide accurate and specific diagnoses. Care and planning in the collection of samples are responsibilities of the professionals to optimize those services.

References

Bancroft, J. D., and Stevens A.: *Theory and Practice of Histological Techniques*, 2nd ed. Edinburgh: Churchill-Livingstone, 1982.

Filipe, M. I., and Lake, B. D.: *Histochemistry in Pathology.* Edinburgh: Churchill-Livingstone, 1983, pp. 303–341.

Green, C. E.: *Clinical Microbiology and Infectious Diseases of the Dog and Cat.* Philadelphia: W. B. Saunders, 1984, p. 140.

Evans, R. J.: Cytology in diagnosis and assessment of neoplastic conditions. *In* Gorman, N. T. (ed.): *Oncology.* New York: Churchill-Livingstone, 1986, p. 25.

Hattersley, P. G.: Activated coagulation time of whole blood. J.A.M.A. 196:436, 1966.

Jergens, A. E., Turrentine, M. A., Kraus, K. H., and Johnson, G. S.: Buccal mucosal bleeding times of healthy dogs and of dogs with various pathologic states, including thrombocytopenia, uremia and von Willebrand's disease. Am. J. Vet. Res. 48:1337, 1987.

McDowell, E. M., and Trump, B. F.: Histologic fixatives suitable for diagnostic electron microscopy. Arch. Pathol. Lab. Med. 100:405, 1976.

Mitruka, B. M., and Vadehra, B. V.: *Clinical Biochemical and Hematologic Reference Values in Normal Experimental Animals.* New York: Masson Publishing, 1977, p. 38.

Vyas, G. N., Stites, D. P., and Brecher, G.: *Laboratory Diagnosis of Immunologic Disorders.* New York: Grune & Stratton, 1975.

Williams, W. J., Beutler, E., Erslev, A. J., and Rundles, R. W.: *Hematology,* 3rd ed. New York: McGraw-Hill, 1983, pp. 1601–1678.

PARASITIC BLOOD DISEASES OF DOGS AND CATS

THOMAS N. HRIBERNIK, D.V.M.,
and STEPHEN C. BARR, B.V.Sc.

Baton Rouge, Louisiana

This article concentrates entirely on the clinical aspects of the disease associated with selected blood parasites of the dog and cat. The reader interested in the proposed or confirmed pathogenetic mechanisms of disease produced by these organisms is referred to the supplemental reading.

CANINE BABESIOSIS

Canine babesiosis is a tick-transmitted, intraerythrocytic protozoal disease of wild and domestic dogs. The three species of *Babesia* known to infect dogs are *B. canis*, *B. gibsoni*, and *B. vogeli*. The latter species may, in fact, be a strain of *B. canis*. The principal vector tick for *B. canis* and *B. vogeli* is *Rhipicephalus sanguineus*, whereas *Haemophysalis bispinosa* is considered the predominant vector for *B. gibsoni*. Iatrogenic transmission can occur with transfusion of infected blood.

Subclinical, peracute, acute, or chronic forms of babesiosis may be seen. Peracute disease is usually seen in heavily parasitized young dogs, resulting in shock after a brief history of illness. Typical clinical findings associated with babesiosis include anorexia, depression, weakness, pale mucous membranes, splenomegaly, and pyrexia. A disruption of the premunitive state in an infected dog by such things as hard work, stress, splenectomy, the development of concurrent infections, or immunosuppressive therapy often precedes the development of these clinical abnormalities. Those animals with chronic infection often have loss of weight, intermittent fever, and appetite alterations. Terminal disease has many of the previous clinical findings plus evidence of icterus and hepatic and renal failure.

Early characteristic diagnostic findings in canine babesiosis include a regenerative anemia, hyperbilirubinemia, hemoglobinemia, bilirubinuria, and hemoglobinuria. Other possible abnormalities that may be observed are thrombocytopenia, azotemia, and metabolic acidosis. The latter two are thought to enhance clinical illness and potentially increase mortality in advanced or untreated cases.

Definitive diagnosis of babesiosis involves identification of the organism in peripheral blood smears, preferably obtained from the ventral surface of the pinna or toenail. When parasites are not observed, indirect fluorescent antibody (IFA) testing is indicated. Cross-reactivity between *B. gibsoni* and *B. canis* will not allow determination of species by the IFA test. However, a titer of greater than

1:40 is considered a positive result for the diagnosis of babesiosis.

Treatment should consist of the use of antibabesial compounds plus appropriate supportive measures if indicated. Imidocarb dipropionate (Imizol, Burroughs Wellcome), 5 mg/kg given as a single intramuscular injection, is efficacious for most infections. Because *Ehrlichia canis* infection may occur in conjunction with babesiosis, the use of this drug will serve the dual purpose of killing both organisms. Other compounds that have efficacy against canine *Babesia* include diminazene aceturate (Berenil, Farbwerke-Hoechst; Ganaseg, Squibb) and phenamidine isethionate (Lomadine, May & Baker). Diminazene aceturate is given as a single intramuscular or subcutaneous injection of a 7 per cent solution at a dosage of 3.5 mg/kg. A 5 per cent solution of Lomadine may be given at 15 mg/kg for 2 consecutive days subcutaneously. Total elimination of the parasitemia may not be desirable in endemic areas because animals will be susceptible to reinfection.

Premise spraying and a routine dipping program are the best way to avoid infection. Blood donors should be screened for disease to eliminate the possibility of iatrogenic transmission. Blood donors from endemic areas should have a splenectomy.

CANINE EHRLICHIOSIS

Canine ehrlichiosis is a tick-transmitted disease of wild or domestic Canidae caused by the rickettsial organisms *Ehrlichia canis*, *E. platys*, and *E. equi*. This discussion will focus on the various clinical aspects associated with *E. canis* infection. The primary natural reservoir for *E. canis* is the vector tick *Rhipicephalus sanguineus*. Iatrogenic transmission of infection can also occur from transfusion of infected blood. The disease has been reported throughout the United States, although it is most frequently seen in dogs from the southern states.

Clinical signs associated with acute ehrlichiosis are generally mild and often inapparent, although anorexia, transient fever, oculonasal discharges, limb and scrotal edema, lymphadenopathy, neurologic signs, and respiratory abnormalities can be observed. After this phase of infection, the disease enters a chronic phase. It is characterized by subclinical to mild signs in some dogs; others develop severe clinical signs. The subclinical aspects of chronic disease may persist for years in some animals. The severity of abnormal findings in animals with chronic disease is related in part to breed predilection (e.g., German shepherd dogs) and possibly to stress or immunosuppression. Severe chronic disease usually results in anorexia, depression, weight loss, hemorrhage, pale mucous membranes, fever, and signs of various organ systems

dysfunction or failure. Most of these animals will die despite intervention with rickettsiostatic drugs and appropriate supportive measures. It appears that the profound hypoplasia of the bone marrow cellular elements present is not readily reversible in these patients. Animals with mild chronic disease may have many of the same findings seen in the severe form. However, return to a normal clinical state is often achieved with appropriate specific and supportive therapy. This response may reflect, in part, the less severe bone marrow cytologic changes seen in mild chronic disease.

The most common hematologic abnormalities in ehrlichiosis are thrombocytopenia and nonregenerative anemia. Leukopenia is relatively uncommon, except in dogs with severe chronic disease. Megakaryocytosis, variable numbers of plasma cells, and adequate to increased numbers of erythroid and granulocytic precursors are usually found in bone marrow aspirate samples. However, profound hypocellularity and variable plasmacytosis are seen in the samples from dogs with severe chronic disease.

Hypoalbuminemia and hyperglobulinemia are the most frequently observed serum chemical abnormalities. Serum protein electrophoresis of hyperglobulinemic animals usually will reveal a polyclonal gammopathy, although a monoclonal pattern has been observed in a number of dogs. The hyperglobulinemia usually persists for 6 to 18 months after appropriate therapy. Other less frequently encountered serum chemical abnormalities include elevation of liver enzymes, total bilirubin and creatinine, or urea nitrogen levels.

A number of other abnormalities have been observed in canine ehrlichiosis. Qualitative platelet disorders are thought to be the cause of bleeding in patients with normal coagulation test results. Coagulation test findings consistent with disseminated intravascular coagulation may be found in dogs with severe chronic disease. Radiographic evidence of diffuse interstitial pulmonary radiodensities has been seen. Positive direct Coombs's reaction, weak-positive results on agar gel immunodiffusion for blastomycosis, increased release of platelet factor-3, neutrophilic pleocytosis of synovial fluid and cerebrospinal fluid characterized by mild protein elevation, and mononuclear pleocytosis have also been observed in some dogs with canine ehrlichiosis.

The diagnosis of infection is usually made by an indirect fluorescent antibody technique, which is sensitive and specific for *E. canis*. Finding characteristic intraleukocytic morulae in peripheral blood smears is diagnostic but is an uncommon occurrence. A simplified cell culture technique has been developed that enhances the chance of demonstrating *E. canis* in peripheral blood samples.

Oral tetracycline given at a dosage of 22 mg/kg, repeated every 8 hr for 14 days has been considered the specific treatment of choice. Doxycycline (Vibramycin, Roerig) given orally at 10 mg/kg daily for 10 to 14 days appears to be equiefficacious. An intramuscular injection of imidocarb dipropionate (Imizol, Burroughs Wellcome) at a dosage of 5 mg/kg, repeated after a 2-week interval may be more effective in eradicating the organism from the animal. In addition, some dogs may need supportive measures, such as blood transfusions and intravenous fluid therapy. The overall response to therapy in most dogs is usually quite rapid, with marked improvement in clinical abnormalities within 24 to 48 hr. Therapy for severe chronic ehrlichiosis often includes antirickettsial drugs, blood transfusions, intravenous fluid therapy, and parenteral bactericidal antibiotics. The prognosis for these animals is extremely poor in spite of appropriate therapy. An inability to properly control sepsis and hemorrhage in severe chronic disease often leads to death.

Prevention of ehrlichiosis has been accomplished by administration of oral tetracycline at a dosage of 6.6 mg/kg daily or by injecting repository oxytetracycline at a dosage of 200 mg twice weekly for up to 1 to 2 yr. Tick control, in the form of premise spraying and dipping animals, should be encouraged. Lastly, prevention of iatrogenic transmission is accomplished by routine serologic screening of blood donors.

CANINE HEPATOZOONOSIS

Canine hepatozoonosis is caused by the protozoan *Hepatozoon canis*. The disease currently is geographically limited to the Texas Gulf coast and southern Louisiana. Transmission of the parasite occurs via ingestion of infected *Rhipicephalus sanguineus* ticks.

Clinical signs most commonly associated with hepatozoonosis include anorexia, weight loss, muscular hyperesthesia, gait abnormalities, pyrexia unresponsive to antibiotics, bloody diarrhea, and oculonasal discharges. The disease course can often be prolonged, with periods of abatement of signs being possible. Diagnostic findings commonly observed include neutrophilic leukocytosis, mild nonregenerative anemia, hypoglycemia, and radiographic evidence of periosteal bone proliferation, particularly of the spine, pelvis, and extremities. The low blood glucose concentration is considered an artifact related to the extreme neutrophilia often observed concomitantly. Normal glucose values have been observed in such patients if blood is collected directly into sodium fluoride anticoagulant.

The definitive diagnosis of canine hepatozoonosis is made by finding the characteristic gametocytes in the neutrophils or monocytes of Giemsa-stained peripheral blood smears. Blood smears should be made shortly after collection because the gametocytes appear to rapidly leave the cell, leaving a nonstaining capsule, which may be overlooked. Several thousand leukocytes may need to be examined prior to finding gametocytes. An excellent alternative diagnostic method is muscle biopsy examination for characteristic macroschizonts and microschizonts.

Although several antiprotozoal drugs have been reported to reduce circulating parasitemia in treated dogs, there is currently no therapeutic agent known to effectively cause an improvement in the clinical outcome of the infection. Administration of nonsteroidal anti-inflammatory drugs is indicated as palliative therapy. The clinical course of the disease tends to be characterized by remissions and exacerbations. Environmental control measures for ticks plus routine dipping of dogs is indicated to limit the spread of disease.

CANINE ROCKY MOUNTAIN SPOTTED FEVER

Canine Rocky Mountain spotted fever (CRMSF) is caused by infection with the tick-transmitted rickettsial agent *Rickettsia rickettsii*. *Dermacentor variabilis* and *D. andersoni* are the principal vector ticks. Most reported cases have been in the southeastern United States, with sporadic occurrences being noted in a number of other geographic areas.

There is a marked variation in clinical presentations possible in infected dogs. Some dogs with sustained high antibody titers to the agent fail to develop clinical illness, whereas some purebred dogs, such as the Siberian husky, may develop severe disease. Unlike canine ehrlichiosis, clinical illness associated with CRMSF has a strict seasonal occurrence—spring through early fall. The clinical findings observed with CRMSF are the result of the severe endothelial damage and subsequent pathologic events. In general, the duration of illness is 2 weeks or less. A constellation of abnormal clinical findings is possible, with fever, anorexia, and depression commonly observed. The history usually includes exposure to vector ticks. Animals may have scleral injection, lymphadenopathy, mucopurulent oculonasal discharges, cough, respiratory difficulty, diarrhea, vomiting, facial or extremity edema or both, joint or muscle pain or both, abdominal tenderness, and occasionally weight loss. The endothelial damage incurred can result in epistaxis, petechial to ecchymotic hemorrhage, melena, hematuria, and retinal hemorrhage. Neurologic abnormalities commonly observed with CRMSF include altered mental status, vestibular dysfunction, hyperesthesia, ataxia, and seizures. In the terminal stages of disease, signs reflecting cardiovascular collapse and renal failure may be noted.

The most consistent hematologic finding associated with CRMSF is thrombocytopenia. However, platelet counts tend to be higher than in those dogs with thrombocytopenia associated with canine ehrlichiosis. White blood cell findings vary from leukopenia early in the disease to a leukocytosis of variable magnitude. The latter appears to vary according to the duration and severity of signs prior to diagnosis. A mild nonregenerative anemia may also occur.

A number of diagnostic test abnormalities may be noted, though they are generally mild. Possible serum biochemical abnormalities include hypoproteinemia, hypoalbuminemia, elevated liver enzyme levels, elevated urea nitrogen and creatinine concentration, and decreased calcium and sodium values. Elevated creatine kinase levels may be observed in dogs with evidence of muscle pain. A mild increase in protein level and increased white blood cell numbers (predominantly neutrophils) may be present in synovial and cerebrospinal fluid analysis. Thoracic radiographs will often reveal a diffuse pulmonary interstitial density. Coagulation testing may reveal abnormalities consistent with disseminated intravascular coagulation in some animals.

Canine Rocky Mountain spotted fever should be suspected in a dog with a history of tick infestation, fever, or any of the previously described clinical presentations during the appropriate seasons. Confirmation of infection is most routinely made by indirect fluorescent antibody testing. Samples for serology should be taken when CRMSF is suspected and 2 to 3 weeks later. A fourfold or greater increase in antibody titer confirms the diagnosis. Interpretation of results may be complicated by cross-reaction with other spotted fever group *Rickettsiae* and continued tick exposure. An alternative to serologic confirmation is direct immunofluorescent antibody testing for the organism in tissue biopsies, particularly from areas of hemorrhage.

Treatment of CRMSF entails both specific and supportive measures. Oral tetracyclines (22 mg/kg every 8 hr) and chloramphenicol (15 to 20 mg/kg every 8 hr given for 14 days) are equally effective rickettsiostatic drugs. Improvement in clinical abnormalities is usually noted within 48 hours. An exception to this response appears to be those animals exhibiting neurologic abnormalities or organ failure as a result of vascular damage. Supportive measures may be indicated for dogs with shock, coagulopathies, or organ failure. Intravenous fluid therapy must be administered with caution owing to the widespread vasculitis present. The prognosis is good if the diagnosis is not delayed and if appropriate therapeutic measures are instituted. Dogs that have recovered from infection are immune to reinfection for at least 6 to 12 months.

Prevention of CRMSF centers on avoidance of tick-infested areas and tick removal. Ticks manually removed should not be crushed or squeezed with bare hands because of the human health hazard associated with exposure to tick hemolymph. In addition, blood from infected dogs should be handled with caution by humans.

CANINE TRYPANOSOMIASIS

Canine trypanosomiasis results from infection with the flagellated protozoan *Trypanosoma cruzi*. It is a disease recognized primarily in Texas, although sporadic cases have been observed in Louisiana, Oklahoma, Indiana, and South Carolina. A wide range of mammals are reservoir hosts, but the principal ones are raccoons and opossums. *T. cruzi* infection is transmitted by arthropod vectors belonging to the Reduviidae family. The most common mode of transmission results from deposition of infected Reduviidae feces on bite wounds inflicted by the arthropod. Infection may also result from ingestion of contaminated meat, infected Reduviidae, or its feces or ingestion of infected milk.

Most cases of disease have been seen in dogs 2 to 18 months of age. Signs of myocardial dysfunction are noted most commonly, with rapid deterioration leading to death. Common clinical findings include weight loss, diarrhea, ascites, tachycardia, lymphadenopathy, and pale mucous membranes. Some animals will be asymptomatic prior to sudden death. Recent studies have revealed that young dogs (< 12 weeks of age) are more susceptible to the development of acute myocarditis when infected with pathogenic isolates. Clinical findings in these animals may include depression, anorexia, weight loss, vomiting, diarrhea, ascites, evidence of jugular pulses, pale mucous membranes, and abnormal heart rates and rhythms. Animals so affected usually die within 5 days or make an apparent recovery. Surviving dogs will develop a dilated cardiomyopathy up to 8 months after the onset of acute disease signs. Signs of biventricular heart failure with rapid, irregular heart rhythms are commonly observed in these animals. Except for the age of onset, these dogs have findings similar to those of canine idiopathic dilated cardiomyopathy. Death usually results from ventricular arrhythmias.

A definitive diagnosis can be made by demonstrating flagellates in peripheral blood smears, buffy coat smears, or culture in a specific medium (liver infusion tryptose). Parasitemias peak during the acute myocardial disease (2 to 3 weeks after infection), but are usually negative 2 weeks later. Dogs that develop dilated cardiomyopathy are aparasitemic. Mild creatine kinase and alanine transferase elevations coincide with acute myocarditis and represent the only specific clinicopathologic findings. In aparasitemic cases, diagnosis depends on positive serologic findings in association with clinical disease. The IFA, complement fixation, and direct hemagglutination tests are the most commonly used.

Typical postmortem findings include a necrotizing granulomatous myocarditis, which is often more severe in the right ventricle than the left. Chronic cardiomyopathy is typified by bilateral ventricular dilation. Multifocal mononuclear cell infiltrates and fibrosis are seen in chronic disease. Amastigote cysts within myofibrils are common in acute disease but are rarely found in chronic cardiomyopathy.

Treatment during acute myocarditis using an investigatory antiprotozoal drug (Bayer 2502 or Lampit, Bayer A-G Leverkusen, Bayerwerk, West Germany) in association with a 2-week course of anti-inflammatory doses of corticosteroids has been shown to improve survival. Lampit is given at 30 mg/kg/day for up to 5 months and is associated with severe side effects, including emesis and anorexia. Dilated cardiomyopathy may still develop and requires supportive therapy.

A thorough search of the dog's environment for vectors should be made. Treatment of the area with residual insecticides such as benzene hexachloride with repeated applications at monthly intervals will markedly reduce infestation. Owners and veterinarians should be aware of the zoonotic potential of discharges and blood from infected animals and handle these accordingly.

CANINE SALMON POISONING DISEASE

Salmon poisoning disease is a potentially highly fatal, trematode-transmitted rickettsial disease of wild and domestic Canidae. It appears to be geographically limited to the northwestern continental United States. The etiologic agent, *Neorickettsia helminthoeca*, utilizes as a vector the trematode *Nanophyetus salmonicola*.

Snails, fish, mammals, or birds are required for completion of the trematode life. Canidae infection is most commonly acquired through ingestion of metacercariae-infected freshwater or ocean salmonid fish. Less common means of reported transmission include ingestion of helminth-infected snail livers, helminth eggs, or adult flukes and parenteral injection of infected tissues and blood. The incubation period after ingestion of infected fish is usually 5 to 7 days.

Abnormal clinical findings associated with this disease include an initial pyrexia followed by a return to normal or hypothermic state, anorexia, depression, weakness, diarrhea, vomiting, weight loss, serous to mucopurulent nasal discharges, and lymphadenopathy. Failure to diagnose and treat the disorder often results in death within 7 to 10 days after the initial clinical findings of anorexia and fever. A suspicion of salmon poisoning disease can be made by noting the above clinical findings in conjunction with the finding of eggs of *N. salminocola* in feces. Confirmation can be obtained by demonstrating typical intracytoplasmic rickettsial bodies from an enlarged lymph node.

Therapy for salmon poisoning disease includes both specific and supportive measures. Specific drugs that have been recommended for *N. helminthoeca* include oral or parenteral penicillin, sulfonamides, chloramphenicol, chlortetracycline, or oxytetracycline. The parenteral route should be utilized, at least initially, in animals with severe vomiting. One suggested dosage schedule for oxytetracycline is 7 mg/kg given every 12 hr for a minimum of 3 days intravenously, followed by administration at the same dosage and interval for 14 to 21 days orally. Supportive measures include intravenous fluid therapy, appropriate hygiene, exogenous source of heat in hypothermic animals, and whole blood transfusions if severe anemia results from hemorrhagic diarrhea.

Preventive measures center around feeding only thoroughly cooked fish or fish that has been frozen for at least 24 hr, isolation of infected dogs, and sterilization of equipment used with infected dogs.

FELINE CYTAUXZOONOSIS

Feline cytauxzoonosis is an invariably fatal hematoprotozoal disease caused by *Cytauxzoan felis*. The mode of natural transmission remains speculative, although tick transmission is suspected. Clinical findings attributed to infection include anorexia, lethargy, depression, dehydration, respiratory distress, pyrexia, icterus, and pale mucous membranes.

Definitive antemortem diagnosis is made by observing the characteristic ring-form piroplasms in erythrocytes with Wright- or Giemsa-stained peripheral blood smears. Although fluid therapy and antibiotic administration may prolong the course of antemortem illness, it appears that cats with cytauxzoonosis invariably die.

Prevention of disease centers on indoor confinement of cats and appropriate ectoparasite control measures in tick-infested areas where cytauxzoonosis has been observed.

FELINE HAEMOBARTONELLOSIS

Feline haemobartonellosis results from infection by the rickettsial erythroparasite *Haemobartonella felis*. The mode of natural transmission is not known, although arthropod vectors have been suspected. Infection has been observed to be transmitted from clinically affected queens to their newborns in the absence of arthropod vectors.

Iatrogenic transmission is known to occur with transfusion of infected blood.

Cats of any age or sex may develop clinical disease associated with *H. felis* infection. However, it is recognized most frequently in young adult male cats. Clinical findings attributed to infection are usually related to the severity and rapidity of hemolysis, plus the presence or absence of significant concurrent disorders. Common clinical findings include anorexia, depression to moribund states, lethargy, and evidence of pale mucous membranes. Splenomegaly and icterus may also be observed in some animals. Some cats have a sudden onset of these findings, whereas those with chronic haemobartonellosis may only have a history of chronic weight loss and pale mucous membranes. It is not uncommon to see *H. felis* in peripheral blood smears of animals with concurrent problems such as infection with the feline leukemia virus. In these animals, the organism may or may not be causing clinical illness routinely associated with haemobartonellosis.

The most common diagnostic finding observed during acute disease is evidence of a regenerative anemia. Neutrophilic leukocytosis, erythrophagocytosis by mononuclear cells, monocytosis, autoagglutination of red blood cells, positive direct Coombs' test result, increased erythrocyte fragility, hyperbilirubinemia, and bilirubinuria are also seen in a number of patients. Confirmation of infection is made most commonly by demonstration of the erythroparasite in thin blood smears stained with Romanowsky-type stains. Because of the extreme cyclic nature of the parasitemia, examination of blood smears obtained on several consecutive days may be necessary to confirm the diagnosis. Treatment with tetracyclines generally results in failure to demonstrate the organisms. The detection of organisms without evidence of erythroid regeneration should alert one to the need to look for another disorder that is causing the animal's problems. It has been suggested that all cats with haemobartonellosis be checked for the presence of the feline leukemia virus.

Affected cats should be treated with oral tetracyclines, 20 mg/kg repeated every 8 hr for 21 days. Blood transfusions may be necessary in some animals. The concomitant use of immunosuppressive doses of corticosteroids has been advocated by some individuals. In addition to these specific and supportive measures, one should attempt to correct when possible any significant concurrent disorders.

References and Supplemental Reading

Canine Babesiosis
Breitschwerdt, E. B.: Babesiosis. *In* Greene, C. E. (ed.): *Clinical Microbiology and Infectious Diseases of the Dog and Cat.* Philadelphia: W. B. Saunders, 1984, p. 796.
Breitschwerdt, E. B.: Canine babesiosis. Proceedings of the Fourth Annual Veterinary Medical Forum, Washington, D. C., 1986, pp. 5–65.

Canine Ehrlichiosis
Greene, C. E., and Harvey, J. W.: Canine ehrlichiosis. *In* Greene, C. E. (ed.): *Clinical Microbiology and Infectious Diseases of the Dog and Cat.* Philadelphia: W. B. Saunders, 1984, p. 545.
Breitschwerdt, E. B.: Canine ehrlichiosis. Proceedings of the Fourth Annual Veterinary Medical Forum, Washington, D. C., 1986, pp. 5–57.
Kuehn, N. F., and Gaunt, S. D.: Clinical and hematologic findings in canine ehrlichiosis. J.A.V.M.A. 186:355, 1985.
Codner, E. C., Roberts, R. E., and Ainsworth, A. G.: Atypical findings in 16 cases of canine ehrlichiosis. J.A.V.M.A. 186:166, 1985.

Canine Hepatozoonosis
Craig, T. M.: Hepatozoonosis. *In* Greene, C. E. (ed.): *Clinical Microbiology and Infectious Diseases of the Dog and Cat.* Philadelphia: W. B. Saunders, 1984, p. 771.

Canine Rocky Mountain Spotted Fever
Greene, C. E., and Philip, R. N.: Rocky Mountain spotted fever. *In* Greene, C. E. (ed.): *Clinical Microbiology and Infectious Diseases of the Dog and Cat.* Philadelphia: W. B. Saunders, 1984, p. 562.
Breitschwerdt, E. B.: Rocky Mountain spotted fever. Proceedings of the Fourth Annual Veterinary Medical Forum, Washington, D.C., 1986, pp. 5–61.
Greene, C. E., Burgdorfer, W., Cavagnolo, R., et al.: Rocky Mountain spotted fever and its differentiation from canine ehrlichiosis. J.A.V.M.A. 186:465, 1985.

Canine Salmon Poisoning Disease
Gorham, J. R., and Foreyt, W. J.: Salmon poisoning disease. *In* Greene, C. E. (ed.): *Clinical Microbiology and Infectious Diseases of the Dog and Cat.* Philadelphia: W. B. Saunders, 1984, p. 538.

Canine Trypanosomiasis
Williams, G. D., Adams, G. L., Yaeger, R. G., et al.: Naturally occurring trypanosomiasis (Chagas' disease) in dogs. J.A.V.M.A. 171:171, 1977.
Barr, S. C., Holmes, R. A., Dennis, V. A., et al.: Experimental infections in dogs with North American isolates of *Trypanosoma cruzi.* Proceedings; World Association for the Advancement of Veterinary Parasitology, Montreal, Canada, August, 1987.

Cytauxzoonosis
Kier, A. B.: Cytauxzoonosis. *In* Greene, C. E. (ed.): *Clinical Microbiology and Infectious Diseases of the Dog and Cat.* Philadelphia: W. B. Saunders, 1984, p. 791.

Feline Haemobartonellosis
Harvey, J. W.: Hemobartonellosis. *In* Greene, C. E. (ed.): *Clinical Microbiology and Infectious Diseases of the Dog and Cat.* Philadelphia: W. B. Saunders, 1984, p. 576.

FELINE ANEMIA

GARY J. KOCIBA, D.V.M.
Columbus, Ohio

Anemia is a common clinical sign associated with a variety of diseases. A thorough clinical and laboratory evaluation is vital for diagnosis of the specific cause and selection of the most appropriate treatment. A standard approach to anemia facilitates rapid classification of the abnormality and provides valuable clues regarding the underlying cause. In the present approach, results of a few selected tests on blood are used to classify the anemia as regenerative or nonregenerative. The history, the clinical findings, and the results of specific follow-up tests are used to diagnose the underlying defect that is the cause of the anemia.

CLINICAL SIGNS

A large percentage of anemias in cats are of insidious onset. The affected cat compensates for the decreased oxygenation of tissues by restriction of physical activity. Exercise intolerance is present but rarely is noted by the owner. Anorexia and lethargy are often present. Sometimes pallor of the mucous membranes or unpigmented skin of the ears or nose is detected. When the anemia is severe, rapid respiration, dyspnea, increased heart rate, cardiac enlargement, and systolic murmurs related to decreased blood viscosity are observed. The signs of anemia are marked in cats with anemia of acute onset.

Physical examination should be directed at detection of primary diseases and other signs that provide evidence of the nature of the pathologic mechanisms. The animal should be checked for splenomegaly, and the skin and mucous membranes should be examined for evidence of jaundice. When practical, the urine should be examined for hemoglobin or blood. The history may be useful in eliciting information regarding the approximate onset of the signs of anemia and previous diseases that may be involved.

LABORATORY TESTS

Blood should be collected for a hemogram and reticulocyte count prior to any treatment. In cats with severe anemia, extreme caution should be exercised to minimize the possibility of cardiovascular failure induced by the stress of restraint and collection techniques. Ideally, the hemogram will include the packed cell volume (PCV), hemoglobin concentration, erythrocyte concentration, mean corpuscular volume (MCV), mean corpuscular hemoglobin concentration (MCHC), leukocyte concentration, absolute leukocyte differential count, estimate of platelet concentration, and evaluation of red blood cell morphology. At the minimum, the PCV and a detailed evaluation of a stained blood film are required.

CLASSIFICATION

The initial classification of anemias is based on whether evidence of a bone marrow erythroid regenerative response is present. The most helpful criteria for a regenerative anemia are increased reticulocytes and polychromasia of red blood cells (RBCs). Reticulocytes are immature erythrocytes with residual RNA, which can be precipitated as either coarse basophilic aggregates or punctate bodies when unfixed cells are exposed to vital stains such as new methylene blue. The reticulocytes are quantified as a percentage of all erythrocytes. The percentage can be converted to an absolute concentration per microliter of blood by multiplying the percentage of reticulocytes by the RBC concentration per microliter of blood. A reticulocyte concentration of greater than 50,000 aggregate reticulocytes per microliter of blood in a cat is evidence of a regenerative anemia.

Punctate reticulocyte concentrations are more difficult to interpret because they vary from about 1 to 10 per cent (60,000 to 600,000/μl) in normal cats and increase to high levels, which persist for rather long periods after an erythroid regenerative response. Following acute blood·loss, punctate reticulocyte levels peak at 10 to 14 days and then gradually subside. In contrast to aggregate reticulocytes, punctate reticulocytes persist in the blood of cats with nonregenerative anemia for up to 4 weeks. Although nucleated red blood cells sometimes are found in the circulating blood of cats with regenerative anemia, their presence is not specific. Cats with a variety of myeloproliferative diseases have extramedullary hematopoiesis in the liver and spleen. The cells in extramedullary sites are not subject to the same control mechanisms that operate within the bone marrow to retain erythrocytes until enucleation is complete.

If only a reticulocyte percentage and packed cell volume is available, the reticulocyte percentage should be corrected for the fact that in anemia the reticulocytes are being mixed with a smaller pool of RBCs in the circulation. The following formula can be used:

$$\text{Reticulocytes (corrected)} = \text{reticulocyte count (\%)} \times \frac{\text{PCV of patient}}{37}$$

A corrected reticulocyte count above 1.0 per cent is evidence of regeneration.

Anemia with a reticulocyte count of less than 50,000/μl or a corrected reticulocyte percentage of less than 1.0 is classified as nonregenerative. One exception to these criteria is acute blood loss anemia. Two to 4 days may elapse before sufficient reticulocytes are produced to make the regenerative response apparent in the peripheral blood.

The mean corpuscular volume is an estimate of the volume of individual red blood cells. When determined using modern blood counters properly calibrated for feline blood, the MCV can provide useful data for subclassification of anemias. The MCV of normal feline red blood cells should fall within the range of 37 to 49 fl. Cells smaller than 37 fl are classified as microcytic, and those greater than 49 fl are classified as macrocytic. Variations in MCV reflect nutritional or metabolic differences in developing red blood cells in the bone marrow, providing useful clues regarding pathogenesis.

Regenerative Anemia

Regenerative anemias are characterized by reticulocytosis (>50,000/μl). Polychromasia is readily detected on blood films. The red blood cells generally are macrocytic, and the MCHC is decreased. These changes reflect the increased number of reticulocytes, which have larger size and an incomplete component of hemoglobin.

The regenerative anemias are subdivided into those related to hemorrhage and those related to hemolysis.

External hemorrhage generally does not present a diagnostic problem. Initially, the decrease in red blood cell values is not dramatic, but, as the blood volume is restored over 24 to 48 hr by expansion of the plasma compartment, the expected decrease in PCV, hemoglobin, red blood cell count, and plasma protein concentration occurs. Occasionally the amount of blood loss from a surgical procedure is underestimated (especially with urethrostomy) but becomes apparent following rehydration over the day following surgery. Severe internal bleeding is unusual but occasionally occurs as the complication of a malignant neoplasm. Much of the blood can be effectively reabsorbed from the body cavities but hemorrhage in other sites can lead to increased serum bilirubin level and mild icterus as the hemoglobin from trapped red blood cells is catabolized. In kittens, severe flea infestation can cause life-threatening anemia. When blood loss is suspected but no obvious cause is apparent, chronic blood loss from gastrointestinal lesions or parasites should be suspected. Iron deficiency rarely occurs in cats with blood loss. The anemia is microcytic and hypochromic in advanced iron deficiency. Iron deficiency sometimes occurs in young kittens at about 4 to 6 weeks of age. The abnormality appears to be related to minimal iron stores, low availability of iron in milk, and expanding blood volume associated with rapid growth. The anemia can be severe, but the MCV remains in the normal range owing to heterogeneity of the RBC population. A subset of microcytic RBCs may be present but are obscured by a wide variance in red blood cell size related to macrocytic erythrocytes, which are normal in neonatal kittens. The defect is corrected rapidly after consumption of solid food alleviates the deficiency of iron.

The erythroid regenerative response usually is more dramatic in hemolytic anemia, in part because heme enhances erythropoiesis. Hemolytic mechanisms should be suspected in intense regenerative anemias accompanied by increased serum bilirubin levels, icterus, or splenomegaly. One of the early steps in determining the cause should be examination of a blood film for Heinz bodies, blood parasites, or autoagglutination.

Heinz bodies are large refractile inclusions that represent precipitates of denatured hemoglobin formed by exposure to oxidant drugs or other chemicals. The intracellular inclusions are recognized as nonstaining bodies that often cause irregular bulges in the erythrocyte membrane. Heinz bodies are much easier to see after staining with new methylene blue. They may be found in the blood of some clinically normal cats, but, when they are found in a large percentage of cells in a cat with regenerative anemia, they should be interpreted as a likely cause of hemolysis. One of the most common causes of Heinz-body anemia is acetaminophen toxicosis because of the inefficient metabolism and excretion of this drug in cats. The signs of acetaminophen toxicity include vomiting, salivation, lethargy, brown mucous membranes, and edema of the face and paws. The blood is brown because of the drug-induced formation of methemoglobin. Anoxia is related to the interference with oxygen transport.

Haemobartonella felis parasites are detected as

basophilic coccoid bodies on the surface of erythrocyte membranes or as rod-shaped bodies on the periphery of the cells. In instances where only a few organisms are present, it may be difficult to distinguish the organisms from precipitated stain or other debris. In anemia associated with *H. felis* infection, the number of parasites fluctuates quite widely, but the organisms should be readily detected on the erythrocytes. One should be confident about the identification of *Haemobartonella* organisms before making the diagnosis of haemobartonellosis in cats without erythroid regeneration. *Haemobartonella* infection has been associated with feline leukemia virus (FeLV) infection, which should lead one to test all cats with haemobartonellosis for FeLV. It has been suggested that FeLV predisposes to haemobartonellosis, but the alternative explanation that parasite-mediated immunosuppression increases the risk for FeLV infection has not been excluded. Autoagglutination sometimes occurs in association with haemobartonellosis, and the red blood cells usually are positive in the direct Coombs' test during the acute phase of the disease prior to treatment.

Cytauxzoonosis is a fatal disease characterized by hemolysis associated with protozoan infection of red blood cells. The disease is most common in cats in the lower Midwest and southern parts of the United States, but the disease has been recognized in other areas. Lethargy, fever, pale mucous membranes, and icterus are common clinical findings. Intraerythrocytic, ring-shaped parasites consisting of a dense, basophilic-to-magenta nucleus eccentrically located in a light-blue–staining ring 1 to 2 μm in diameter are found in less than 1 per cent to 25 per cent of the cells. Large schizonts can be detected in macrophages of many organs, including the spleen, liver, lung, and lymph nodes. No effective treatment has been described.

Immune-mediated hemolysis should be suspected in anemia with intense regeneration but no evidence of blood parasites or Heinz bodies. Spherocytes are difficult to identify in feline blood films because of the small size and normal, more spheric morphology of feline erythrocytes. A direct Coombs' test or osmotic fragility test may be used for identification of red blood cell abnormalities induced by immunoglobulins. Cats with immune-mediated hemolysis should be checked for feline leukemia virus, which is one of the most common causes. Propylthiouracil used for the treatment of hyperthyroidism is one of the major causes of drug-induced, immune-mediated hemolysis.

Lead poisoning can cause a mild hemolytic anemia in cats. The hematologic features include basophilic stippling and numerous nucleated red blood cells in the circulation. This is a rare disease in the cat because of discriminating eating habits, but the licking and grooming habits of the cat occasionally have led to ingestion of lead contaminants from the environment.

Nonregenerative Anemia

Decreased production of erythrocytes accounts for the majority of feline anemias. Feline leukemia virus infection is associated with about 70 per cent of all nonregenerative anemias. The anemia usually has a gradual onset, with clinical signs of the anemia not apparent until the PCV is low. One distinctive laboratory feature of FeLV-associated anemia is macrocytosis. Any cat with nonregenerative anemia and an MCV of 50 fl or greater should be evaluated for FeLV infection. The mechanism of the macrocytosis is unknown but could reflect a transient erythroid regenerative response in the early stages of the disease. The erythrocytes are normochromic, and no other remarkable abnormalities are seen. The bone marrow is of normal cellularity or slightly decreased with a markedly increased myeloid-erythroid (M/E) ratio related to a paucity of erythroid precursors. In a small percentage of cats, the marrow is hypercellular with evidence of dysmyelopoiesis. Usually the anemia gets progressively more severe and is fatal unless transfusions are administered to prolong life. Serum iron concentration is normal. Serum erythropoietin levels are markedly increased. The anemia appears to be related to defective proliferation of erythroid precursors either as a consequence of direct injury of erythroid progenitors or as a result of a defect in the microenvironment within the marrow. No effective treatment is known at this time. The anemia reverses itself in cats that are fortunate enough to clear the virus.

The anemia of chronic disease is a secondary manifestation of inflammatory or neoplastic diseases. It is a normocytic, normochromic anemia that is characterized by a decreased erythrocyte survival and usually a moderate erythroid hypoplasia. The marrow retains some responsiveness to erythropoietin, but the erythropoietin levels are not proportionate to the degree of anemia. Serum iron levels are decreased, but iron stores are normal to increased. This anemia can be more severe in cats than in some other species, probably reflecting the relatively short life span of erythrocytes in the cat (about 75 days). The disease is completely secondary to the inflammatory or neoplastic lesion and will resolve if the primary disease is treated successfully.

Nonregenerative anemia occasionally occurs as a component of aplastic anemia in the cat. Evidence of this syndrome includes the simultaneous occurrence of neutropenia, thrombocytopenia, and nonregenerative anemia. Generalized aplasia of the marrow may be a consequence of feline leukemia virus infection. If test results for feline leukemia are negative, then drug or other chemical exposure should be explored as possible etiologic factors. In most instances, an etiologic agent cannot be identified in aplastic anemia not associated with FeLV infection. Chloromycetin therapy does suppress hematopoiesis in the cat, but the suppression is related to direct injury to precursors in the bone marrow and is rapidly reversible after cessation of therapy. Only limited information is available regarding estrogen effects on feline bone marrow, but cats appear to be more resistant to estrogen myelotoxicity than dogs.

Chronic renal disease can cause nonregenerative anemia. Deficient production of erythropoietin by the diseased kidneys results in mild anemia. This defect may be accentuated by a shortened erythrocyte survival time, but usually the anemia is not severe enough to be of major clinical concern.

Hypothyroidism is accompanied by mild anemia. The anemia is a reflection of the decreased oxygen requirements associated with the lowering of the basal metabolic rate.

BONE MARROW BIOPSY

In most regenerative anemias, bone marrow biopsy is not necessary because the reticulocytosis provides evidence of functional hematopoiesis. In non-regenerative anemia of unknown cause, biopsy is a useful diagnostic procedure. Concurrent granulocytopenia or thrombocytopenia with anemia suggests primary disease of the bone marrow. Specific concerns to be addressed in the marrow sample are the presence of leukemic cells, myelofibrosis, or a disordered maturation sequence of erythroid cells. In the anemia of chronic disease, the findings in the bone marrow often include moderate erythroid hypoplasia with granulocytic hyperplasia and normal or increased amounts of hemosiderin. A core biopsy should be performed when attempts at aspiration biopsy do not yield cellular samples, because in some instances hypercellular bone marrows may be difficult to aspirate.

TREATMENT

Many of the treatments for anemic cats are supportive. In blood loss anemia, the primary concern should be to arrest the bleeding. In acute blood loss, one should be aware that the packed cell volume and other erythroid values may not reflect the decreased red blood cell mass until the blood volume is restored by shift of extracellular fluid to the vascular compartment over a period of 12 to 36 hours. The amount of blood loss from flea infestation should not be underestimated, particularly in kittens.

Because of uncertainties regarding the compatibility of many feline blood transfusions, transfusion should not be considered until the anemia is quite severe (PCV < 15%). Most cats with nonregenerative anemia of insidious onset can tolerate anemia down to a PCV of 10% if stressful conditions are avoided. Ideally, blood typing would be used to match donor and recipient red cells. Three blood groups occur in cats, with group A being the most common (73 to 97 per cent of cats). The incidence of group B in cats ranged from 3 to 26 per cent in various studies of cats in different parts of the world. Group AB is rare and occurs in less than 1 per cent of cats. Cats of blood group B often have anti-A antibody titers, which are sometimes high, posing a risk for blood transfusion reactions even in previously untransfused cats. Life-threatening transfusion reactions have been reported in cats of group B given group A blood in Australia. Because of this risk, it is recommended that crossmatching be performed whenever practical. The author and others in the United States have transfused large numbers of cats with unmatched blood without severe shock-like transfusion reactions. Donor cats should be screened for blood parasites and feline leukemia virus prior to use. Ten milliliters of blood per kilogram can be collected from a healthy donor at 2-week intervals. In an emergency, blood can be collected at much shorter intervals, but this should not be a regular practice because of the risk of iron deficiency. Blood for immediate transfusion can be collected from the jugular veins into large syringes with 5 to 20 units of heparin per milliliter of blood. Anesthesia of the donor does not pose a risk for the recipient. If the blood is to be stored, it should be collected in acid-citrate-dextrose (ACD) or citrate-phosphate-dextrose (CPD) anticoagulant solution. If the anemia is severe enough to require transfusion, blood should be administered at a dosage of 15 to 30 ml/kg. The transfusion should be given slowly with monitoring for signs of transfusion reactions. Severe bradycardia, apnea, and hypotension are signs of a transfusion reaction related to incompatible blood. Vomiting occurs in some cats during transfusions infused at high flow rates. Slowing the rate of infusions usually is effective. Febrile episodes are common during the first 24 hr after a transfusion.

If extreme difficulty is encountered in placing an intravenous catheter, blood may be administered by slow infusion through a needle placed in the intramedullary space of the femur.

Haemobartonellosis can be effectively treated with oxytetracycline at a dosage of 20 mg/kg t.i.d. PO for 2 weeks. The organisms usually disappear rapidly after initiation of treatment.

In Heinz-body anemia, if a drug or chemical is incriminated, the exposure should be eliminated. The Heinz bodies will be gradually cleared over a period of days to a week and the regenerative response ensures rapid correction of the anemia. Transfusion may be necessary in severe poisoning. If severe methemoglobinemia is present, as evidenced by chocolate brown discoloration of the blood and red-brown mucous membranes, treatment with reducing agents is recommended. N-acetylcysteine (Mucomyst, Mead Johnson) should be given orally as a 5 per cent solution at a 140 mg/kg loading dose followed by three to five treatments at 4-hr intervals at 70 mg/kg.

Immune-mediated hemolytic anemia is responsive to immunosuppressive drugs. Prednisone at a dosage of 2 mg/kg/day has been effective in a limited number of cases. As the anemia resolves, the dosage should be decreased to the minimum necessary to control the disease, preferably on a less than daily basis. A large percentage of cats with Coombs'-positive anemia are positive for feline leukemia virus. The increased risk of giving immunosuppressive drugs, which may alter defense mechanisms against feline leukemia virus and other agents, must be carefully considered when deciding on appropriate therapy for these patients.

Iron deficiency can be treated by elimination of the cause of the blood loss and oral supplementation with 50 to 100 mg of ferrous sulfate daily to an adult cat. The iron deficiency of kittens is rapidly corrected when solid food consumption begins. Intramuscular injection of iron-dextran is effective, but the drug induces local irritation at the injection site.

No effective specific therapy has been found for cats with FeLV-associated erythroid aplasia. Transfusions are effective in prolonging life, but the transfusion interval becomes shorter with repeated transfusions unless blood typing is used to match donor and recipient. The objective is to support the cat with the long-term hope that the cat eventually will control the virus. In the rare instances in which cats have reverted to an FeLV-negative state, the anemia has resolved.

As for the anemia of chronic disease, no specific treatment is indicated. Therapy should be directed at reversal of the primary disease. Complete recovery can be expected with effective treatment of the primary disease.

Insufficient evidence is available to allow specific recommendations regarding the treatment of idiopathic aplastic anemia in cats. Anabolic steroids such as nandrolone decanoate (1 to 2 mg/kg once per week) or oxymetholone may increase the packed cell volume slightly in some instances but are not likely to alter the course of the disease. Cats on anabolic steroids should be monitored for the development of liver necrosis or liver dysfunction as complications.

References and Supplemental Reading

Auer, L., and Bell, K.: Transfusion reactions in cats due to AB blood group incompatibility. Res. Vet. Sci. 35:145, 1983.
Cotter, S. M.: Anemia associated with feline leukemia virus infection. J.A.V.M.A. 175:1191, 1979.
Cotter, S. M., and Holzworth, J.: Disorders of the hematopoietic system. In Holzworth, J. (ed.): Diseases of the Cat. Philadelphia: W. B. Saunders, 1987, pp. 755–768.
Harvey, J. W., and Gaskin, J. M.: Experimental feline haemobartonellosis. J. Am. Anim. Hosp. Assoc. 13:28, 1977.
Weiser, M. G.: Correlative approach to anemia in dogs and cats. J. Am. Anim. Hosp. Assoc. 17:286, 1981.
Weiser, M. G., and Kociba, G. J.: Erythrocyte macrocytosis in feline leukemia virus–associated anemia. Vet. Pathol. 20:687, 1983.
Weiser, M. G., and Kociba, G. J.: Sequential changes in erythrocyte volume distribution and macrocytosis associated with iron deficiency in kittens. Vet. Pathol. 20:1, 1983.

HEREDITARY DISORDERS OF CANINE ERYTHROCYTES

URS GIGER, Dr. MED. VET.
Philadelphia, Pennsylvania

CANINE ERYTHROCYTES

Canine erythrocytes are biconcave disks with a mean diameter of 7 μm, a thickness of 2 μm, and a volume of 68 fl. These characteristics allow easy deformability through the microvasculature and provide a large surface area–to-volume ratio for delivery of oxygen. Reticulocytes are released from the bone marrow and complete their maturation in the spleen. The normal life span of canine erythrocytes is about 100 to 120 days, and the so-called apparent half-life (T1/2) of chromium-51–labeled cells from various breeds is about 20 to 29 days.

Devoid of a nucleus and mitochondria, erythro-

Supported in part by NIH grants DK 37602 and RR02512.

cytes have a limited and specialized metabolism (Fig. 1), which enables them to survive in circulation and to adequately transport oxygen. Energy is generated almost exclusively through anaerobic glycolysis (Embden-Meyerhof pathway), a process that also plays an essential role in the other three ancillary pathways. The hexose-monophosphate shunt reduces pyridine nucleotides and glutathione used for the degradation of environmental oxidants and, thereby, prevents membrane damage, globin denaturation, and Heinz body formation. The methemoglobin or cytochrome b_5 reductase system converts heme iron from the ferric form (methemoglobin) to the ferrous form. Methemoglobin cannot combine reversibly with oxygen. The Leubering-Rapoport pathway is responsible for the synthesis of 2,3-diphosphoglycerate (DPG), which influences the oxygen affinity of canine (but not feline) hemoglobin. A genetic polymorphism of various erythrocyte enzymes has been observed in the dog.

The erythrocyte membrane consists of a lipid bilayer, affixed to a membrane cytoskeleton, which determines cell shape and deformability. Various transmembrane glycoproteins function as receptors or transporters. Some glycolipids are assumed to determine the 13 recognized dog erythrocyte antigens (DEAs); of these, DEA 1.1, DEA 1.2, and DEA 7 are of clinical importance. Owing to proteolysis, canine (as well as feline) erythrocytes lose their Na-K-ATPase during late maturation in the bone marrow, with the exception of erythrocytes from Akitas and some mongrel dogs in Japan (Inaba and Maede, 1986). Thus, canine erythrocytes have high-sodium and low-potassium concentrations similar to those of serum electrolytes. Consequently, hyperkalemia generally does not occur following intravascular hemolysis unless immature (stress) reticulocytes or erythrocytes from some Japanese dogs are lysed. In fact, because Akitas' erythrocytes are "leaky" *in vitro*, pseudohyperkalemia has been observed in serum that has not been separated immediately from its clot (Degen, 1987). Finally, canine erythrocytes have been noted to be uniquely fragile under alkaline conditions, compared with erythrocytes of other species, presumably owing to a facilitated calcium entry under these conditions.

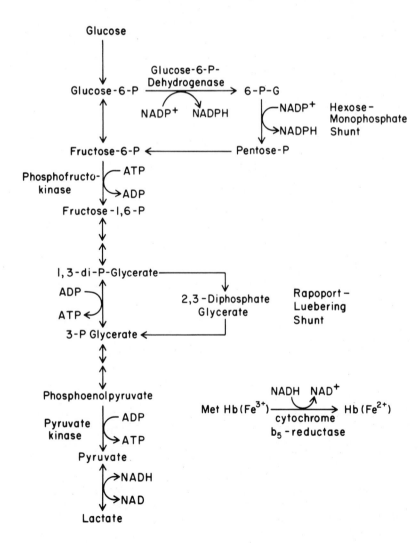

Figure 1. Embden-Meyerhof pathway and ancillary erythrocyte enzyme systems.

This pH sensitivity may explain the tendency of canine red blood cells to lyse in uncapped tubes in the laboratory. Dogs have embryonic, but no fetal, hemoglobin (Hb) and have only one adult hemoglobin (HbB) with the exception of some Japanese breeds, which have two hemoglobins (HbA and B) (Agar and Board, 1983; Harvey, 1989). An HbB polymorphism has recently been recognized in European dogs (Braend, 1988).

TYPES OF HEREDITARY DISORDERS

Several inherited erythrocyte defects have been recognized in various breeds of dog (Kaneko, 1987; Smith, 1981). Although the clinically significant erythrocyte abnormalities will be described in more detail, Table 1 provides a summary of the various defects identified in dogs. Although the degree of characterization is varied, many seem to be analogues of hereditary erythrocyte disorders in humans. The defects have been classified into four groups according to their functional and structural abnormalities: (1) hemoglobinopathies, (2) cytosolic enzyme deficiencies, (3) membrane and related abnormalities, and (4) production and maturation defects.

In contrast to the common occurrence of thalassemias and sickle cell anemias in humans, *no hemoglobinopathies* of clinical significance have been discovered in dogs. One electrophoretically abnormal hemoglobin has been seen in a dog that exhibited exercise intolerance but no anemia.

Two important cytosolic enzyme deficiencies are the classic pyruvate kinase (PK) deficiency seen in basenjis and the recently discovered phosphofructokinase (PFK) deficiency observed in English springer spaniels. Although glucose-6-phosphate dehydrogenase deficiency is the most common enzyme defect in humans, screening of over 3000 dogs revealed only one healthy Weimaraner to have a partial enzyme deficiency of this sort (Smith et al., 1976). Isolated cases of methemoglobinemia associated with cytochrome b_5 reductase deficiency were found among dogs of various breeds, including a borzoi, a Chihuahua, a cockapoo, an English setter, a poodle, a toy Eskimo, and terrier-mix dog (Atkins et al., 1981). Defects of heme synthesis known as porphyrias have been reported in cats but not in dogs.

Elliptocytosis and microcytosis due to a deficiency of the cytoskeleton protein band 4.1, which strengthens the interaction between spectrin and actin in the cytoskeleton, has been described in an inbred, nonanemic dog (Smith et al., 1983). Other presumed membrane abnormalities include stomatocytosis (Fletch et al., 1975; Giger et al., 1988a) and familial microcytosis and nonspherocytic anemia (Randolph et al., 1986, Maggio-Price et al., 1988),

as well as the production of erythrocytes with increased osmotic fragility (Rand and O'Brien, 1987) or high potassium content.

The hereditary production and nuclear maturation abnormalities of erythroid cells, including cyclic hematopoiesis of gray collies (Jones, 1983) and the recently discovered selective cobalamin (vitamin B_{12}) malabsorption of giant schnauzers, are reflected not only in erythrocyte abnormalities but also in changes in other bone marrow–derived cells. Familial macrocytosis of poodles is a presumed maturation defect and can be associated with leukopenia, neutrophil hypersegmentation, and thrombocytopenia but not anemia (Schalm, 1976).

Although overall, inherited erythrocyte defects are rare in dogs, a particular blood disorder may occur relatively frequently within a family and occasionally within an entire breed if the mutant genes involved reach a high frequency. The mode of inheritance has not been elucidated for all erythrocyte defects, but most appear to be autosomal recessive traits. Incomplete dominant inheritance has been proposed for familial nonspherocytic hemolytic anemia in poodles. Historical information concerning parents and littermates is important for genetic counseling.

CLINICAL SIGNS

Clinical manifestations are mainly determined by the degree of shortened erythrocyte survival and erythropoietic response precipitated by the erythrocyte defect. Several erythrocyte abnormalities, such as familial microcytosis in Akitas, apparently do not affect erythrocyte durability and function and could, therefore, be considered as nondiseases. The degree of hemolysis of some disorders is well compensated by an increased production of erythroid cells, and therefore no clinical signs are present. Finally, because these disorders are chronic, affected animals are usually well adapted to a mild hemolytic anemia and show no overt signs. Beagles with mild hemolytic anemia of unknown cause are an example.

Typical signs of anemia, including lethargy, exercise intolerance, pallor, and tachycardia, are commonly observed with these disorders but may not begin until the animal is several months of age. Certain environmental conditions and other diseases may exaggerate these features, as is best exemplified in canine PFK deficiency. Hepatosplenomegaly may result from severe extravascular hemolysis and extramedullary hematopoiesis. Intermittent icterus and dark pigmenturia indicate massive hemolysis. Persistent cyanosis without anemia may be observed in dogs with marked methemoglobinemia. Defects in hematopoiesis may cause leukocyte and platelet abnormalities and may there-

Table 1. Canine Inherited Erythrocyte Defects

Defects	Breed	Inheritance	PCV % (Range)	Reticulocyte % (Corrected)	Erythrocyte T½ (d)	Erythrocyte Morphology	Specific Tests	Clinical Features
Cytosolic Enzyme Deficiencies								
Pyruvate kinase (PK) deficiency	Basenjis / Beagles / West Highland white	AR / U / AR	11–25	10–45	4–9	Polychromasia, echinocytes	Abnormal PK kinetic & stability and glycolytic intermediates	Hemolytic anemia, myelofibrosis, osteosclerosis
Phosphofructokinase (PFK) deficiency	English springer spaniels	AR	11–48	5–23	4	Polychromasia	PFK activity, 8–22%	Inducible hemolytic crises, mild myopathy, pigmenturia
Glucose-6-phosphate dehydrogenase (GPD) deficiency	Weimaraner	U	N	N	U	Unremarkable	GPD activity, 40%	None
Cytochrome b_5 reductase (Cb_5R) deficiency	5 isolated cases	U	High N	N	U	Unremarkable	Cb_5R activity, 10–30% Methemoglobin > 10%	Cyanosis, no anemia, exercise intolerance
Membrane and Other Abnormalities								
Elliptocytosis (band 4.1 deficiency)	Mixed-breed dog	AR	34	2	16–23	Elliptocytes	Membrane protein electrophoresis	None
Stomatocytosis	Alaskan Malamutes / Miniature schnauzer	AR / U	N / N	3–7 / 3–7	6–18 / 10	Stomatocytes, polychromasia	Stomatocytes, increased osmotic fragility	Chondrodysplasia in malamutes, none in schnauzers
Increased osmotic fragility	English springer spaniel, mixed breed	U	N	2–5	U	Polychromasia, poikilocytosis	Increased osmotic fragility, unknown	Exercise-induced hyperthermia
High potassium erythrocytes	Akitas / Japanese mongrels	U / U	N / N	N / N	U / 14	Unremarkable	Increased erythrocyte and serum potassium	None: Pseudohyperkalemia
Familial nonspherocytic anemia	Poodles	ID	10–25	6–28	7–10	Polychromasia	Unknown	Hemolytic anemia, osteosclerosis
Nonspherocytic hemolytic disorders	Beagles	AR	29–42	8–23	7–15	Polychromasia	Calcium ATPase pump (?)	None, mild anemia
Familial microcytosis	Akitas	U	N	N	U	Microcytosis	Erythrocyte indices	None
Production and Maturation Defects								
Cyclic hematopoiesis	Gray collie	AR	N	0–8	N	Intermittent cytopenias	Serial complete blood cell counts	None related to erythrocytes, recurrent infection, bleeding
Selective cobalamin malabsorption	Giant schnauzers	AR	20–31	0	U	Nonregenerative megaloblasts, hypersegmented neutrophils	Low serum cobalamin (B_{12}), urinary organic acids	Cachexia, dementia, responsive to parenteral B_{12}
Familial macrocytosis and dyshematopoiesis	Poodles (miniature and toy)	U	N	N	U	Macrocytes, hypersegmented neutrophils	Macrocytosis, normal osmotic fragility	None, gingivitis

Data collected from references and author's unpublished observations.
N, normal; U, unknown; AR, autosomal recessive; ID, incomplete dominance.

fore be associated with recurrent infection and bleeding.

Erythrocyte defects may be a part of a multisystemic syndrome that is due to the pleitropic effects of a single mutant gene. In the collie, cyclic hematopoiesis and an unusual silver-gray coat color pattern are apparently produced by the same mutant gene in homozygous states. In the chondrodysplasia/anemia syndrome of Alaskan malamutes, skeletal abnormalities and mild anemia with stomatocytosis are related abnormalities. Dogs with PFK deficiency also have mild exertional myopathy. PK-deficient dogs and poodles with nonspherocytic hemolytic anemia develop an unexplained terminal myelofibrosis and osteosclerosis usually before 3 years of age. Cobalamin-deficient giant schnauzers fail to thrive and are cachectic.

LABORATORY DIAGNOSIS

Although the breed of dog involved, the pleiotropic and multisystemic effects observed, and the presence of anemia may provide potential clues to an inherited erythrocyte defect, a full laboratory evaluation is essential to validate the diagnosis or to discover new inherited disorders. In fact, in a few breeds, more than one erythrocyte disorder has been recognized. Hematologic laboratory tests can be divided into routine procedures, which detect a hematologic abnormality as well as rule out acquired causes, and special studies that define the nature of an intrinsic erythrocyte defect.

The routine complete blood count, including a reticulocyte count, determines the severity of the anemia and associated bone marrow response. The erythrocyte indices provide information on average erythrocyte changes, such as macro- and microcytosis, whereas examination of a peripheral blood smear may reveal immature or abnormal cells such as elliptocytes and stomatocytes (Fig. 2). Many erythrocyte defects, however, cause no changes in cell shape and are historically called nonspherocytic hemolytic anemias. The degree of reticulocytosis and erythroid hyperplasia of the bone marrow is often marked and is usually proportional to the shortened survival of the abnormal erythrocytes. The apparent half-life of erythrocytes is determined by radiolabeling erythrocytes. Signs of hemolysis may be mild but include bilirubinemia and bilirubinuria, low serum haptoglobin level, and occasionally overt hemoglobinemia and hemoglobinuria, as in PFK-deficient dogs. Some defective erythrocytes appear extremely fragile *in vitro*, resulting in artifactual lysis in blood tubes. A negative Coombs' test result and *Babesia* titer, as well as the lack of evidence of any other infection or exposure to a toxin in the face of persistent erythrocyte abnor-

malities, further support the presence of an inherited erythrocyte defect.

If a particular erythrocyte defect is suspected on the basis of signalment, physical findings, and routine test results, one specific laboratory test (e.g., an enzyme activity test) may be ordered to confirm the diagnosis. Sometimes a battery of tests in a specialized laboratory may have to be performed to reach a diagnosis. In the osmotic fragility test, erythrocytes with a membrane defect are commonly found to be more fragile at reduced osmotic conditions (Fig. 3). Membrane protein electrophoresis and ion transport studies can further characterize these abnormalities. Cytosolic enzyme deficiencies are identified by demonstrating a decrease in the activity of an enzyme, an absence of immunologic cross-reacting material, abnormal enzyme kinetics, accumulation of enzyme substrates, and lack of products. For instance, erythrocyte DPG concentration is decreased in PFK deficiency and increased in PK deficiency, as well as in other erythrocyte defects with a large number of reticulocytes and young erythrocytes. Changes in DPG also cause shifts in the hemoglobin-oxygen dissociation curve (Fig. 4). Finally, shape abnormalities of the hemoglobin-oxygen dissociation curve and abnormal electrophoretic migration of hemoglobin may identify a new hemoglobinopathy.

THERAPY AND PREVENTION

Hereditary erythrocyte defects are lifelong conditions. Fortunately, most erythrocyte defects are well compensated for and cause no or only minimal clinical signs. Therefore, they require no treatment and allow the animal to have a normal life expectancy. Splenectomy of animals with various disorders does not significantly alter the degree of hemolysis. Life-threatening hemolytic crises in PFK-deficient dogs can, however, be prevented by avoiding situations that induce hyperventilation or by administering acetazolamide prior to an expected episode. Unfortunately, disorders that have multisystemic or pleiotropic effects may cause death at an early age. PK-deficient dogs and poodles with hemolytic anemia die before 4 years of age because the bone marrow gets replaced by osteosclerosis. Overwhelming infections and amyloidosis cause death in collies that have cyclic hematopoiesis. Giant schnauzers with selective cobalamin malabsorption become extremely cachectic and lethargic, but they completely respond to parenteral cobalamin administration. Experimentally, allotransplantation of bone marrow has been shown to cure PK-deficient basenjis and collies with cyclic hematopoiesis if performed at a young age. Furthermore, lithium carbonate has been found to moderate the fluctuation of blood cell counts in collies.

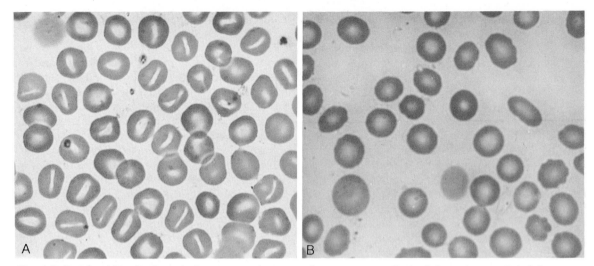

Figure 2. Peripheral blood smears. *A,* A miniature schnauzer with stomatocytosis. *B,* A cobalamin (vitamin B₁₂)–deficient giant schnauzer with anisocytosis and poikilocytosis.

Prevention is the best—and often the only—approach to a genetic erythrocyte defect. Clearly, affected animals should not be used for breeding. Because most erythrocyte disorders have an autosomal recessive pattern of inheritance, sire and dam are obligate heterozygotes (carriers) and should not be bred either. A search for and examination of littermates may reveal other affected animals that have as yet unexplained signs or that are carriers. It is possible to detect carriers of PK and PFK deficiency as well as elliptocytosis through laboratory tests.

SPECIFIC DISORDERS

Phosphofructokinase Deficiency

PFK deficiency (Giger et al., 1985, 1986, Giger and Harvey, 1987) occurs in English springer span-

iels of show and field trial lines. The disorder is characterized by chronic hemolysis with hemolytic crises and mild myopathy. Sporadic dark pigmenturia due to severe bilirubinuria is a key clinical sign and commonly develops following episodes of hyperventilation induced by extensive exercise, excessive barking, and high temperature. During these crises, affected dogs may become severely anemic or icteric. Transient hemoglobinemia and hemoglobinuria indicate massive intravascular hemolysis. These dramatic changes associated with fever, lethargy, and anorexia usually resolve within days. A marked bilirubinuria and reticulocytosis despite a normal hematocrit and hepatosplenomegaly are persistent. Still, affected dogs have a relatively normal life expectancy; however, situations

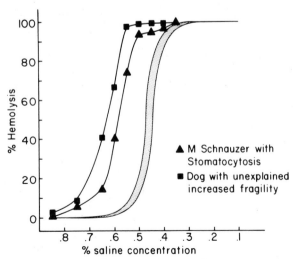

Figure 3. Increased osmotic fragility of defective canine erythrocytes. (Shaded area represents normal range.)

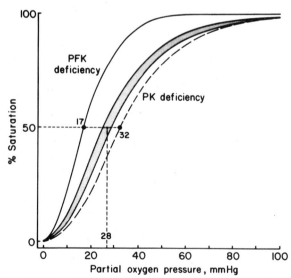

Figure 4. Hemoglobin-oxygen dissociation curves of phosphofructokinase (PFK)–deficient and pyruvatekinase (PK)–deficient canine erythrocytes. (Shaded area represents normal range.)

that can induce hemolytic crises should be avoided. Acetazolamide administration prior to an expected episode can prevent a crisis (Giger, 1987).

Erythrocyte PFK activity is severely decreased in all affected dogs (to 8 to 22 per cent of control) owing to a complete lack of muscle-type PFK. The resulting low erythrocyte DPG concentration causes increased hemoglobin-oxygen affinity (Fig. 4) and increased alkaline fragility. The alkalemia associated with hyperventilation causes hemolytic crises in PFK-deficient dogs. Since affected dogs totally lack PFK activity in muscle, they have mild metabolic myopathy, characterized by exercise intolerance. On rare occasions, they also exhibit muscle cramps and mild to moderately elevated serum creatine kinase activity (Giger et al., 1988b, 1989).

PFK deficiency in English springer spaniels has an autosomal recessive pattern of inheritance. Heterozygotes or carriers are clinically normal but have approximately half-normal PFK activity in erythrocytes and muscle.

Pyruvate Kinase Deficiency

PK deficiency (Searcy et al., 1979) in basenjis, inherited as an autosomal recessive trait, causes a severe hemolytic anemia (PCV of 12 to 26 per cent). Affected animals show clinical signs at several months of age, including exercise intolerance, retarded growth, pale mucous membranes, tachycardia, and hepatosplenomegaly. The anemia is highly regenerative, with numerous circulating metarubricytes and reticulocyte counts reaching 70 per cent; but as the dogs age, the response declines. An unexplained progressing osteomyelosclerosis of the bone marrow and generalized hemosiderosis develop, causing death usually before 4 years of age.

Erythrocytes of affected basenjis completely lack the adult erythrocyte isozyme form of PK. Instead, they express a fetal PK form that is also present in spleen and white blood cells. Affected dogs' erythrocyte PK shows abnormal enzyme kinetics and decreased stability *in vitro*. Thus, despite high PK activity in erythrocyte homogenates from affected dogs, the enzyme appears unstable and malfunctions *in vivo* as shown by the shortened erythrocyte survival and abnormal erythrocyte metabolite pattern. The blood levels of pyruvate and lactate, products of the PK reaction, are low, whereas all the other glycolytic intermediates are high in erythrocytes. The high DPG levels decrease hemoglobin-oxygen affinity (Fig. 4), which may aid in the toleration of a low hematocrit. Heterozygous basenjis or carriers are clinically normal but have half-normal erythrocyte PK activity. PK deficiency has also been reported in two beagles (Prasse et al., 1975) and recently in a West Highland white terrier (Giger and Chapman, unpublished) with similar clinical and hematologic features.

Nonspherocytic Hemolytic Anemia

Related black miniature poodles have been described as having a nonspherocytic hemolytic anemia with clinical manifestations comparable with those in PK deficiency (Randolph et al., 1983). Affected dogs have a severe macrocytic-hypochromic anemia (PCV of 10 to 26 per cent), with marked reticulocytosis and hepatosplenomegaly. They develop terminal osteomyelosclerosis before 2 years of age. The cause of this erythrocyte disorder remains unknown despite extensive studies, but a labile or kinetically abnormal PK enzyme as seen in basenjis has not been ruled out.

Selective Cobalamin Malabsorption

After binding to gastric and pancreatic intrinsic factor, dietary vitamin B_{12} (cobalamin) is specifically absorbed in the ileum. Cobalamin is an essential coenzyme in the intermediary metabolism and is required in nucleic acid synthesis for hematopoiesis and other cell growth. In humans, acquired and inherited vitamin B_{12} deficiencies are characterized by hematologic and metabolic abnormalities.

A selective cobalamin malabsorption (Fyfe et al., 1987, 1989) with an autosomal recessive mode of inheritance occurs in giant schnauzers. At 3 months of age, affected dogs fail to thrive, appear lethargic, are inappetent, and become severely cachectic. They have a moderate nonregenerative anemia with marked anisocytosis, occasional megaloblasts, and moderate poikilocytosis (see Fig. 1), as well as a neutropenia with occasional hypersegmented neutrophils. Macrocytic anemia, a typical feature of cobalamin deficiency in humans, has not been evident in dogs, although a nuclear-to-cytoplasmatic asynchrony of bone marrow cells has been seen in affected dogs.

Serum vitamin B_{12} levels are low, and urine samples contain large amounts of methylmalonic acid, an organic acid that accumulates in cobalamin-deficient patients. Gastrointestinal studies have demonstrated selective malabsorption of orally administered vitamin B_{12}, even in the presence of porcine intrinsic factor, suggesting an ileal enterocyte defect. Parenteral, but not oral, administration of vitamin B_{12} reverses all hematologic and clinical features. This disorder in dogs appears to be similar to inherited juvenile cobalamin malabsorption known as Imerslund-Gräsbeck syndrome in humans.

CONCLUSION

With the recent discovery of a number of new erythrocyte defects in various canine breeds, inherited erythrocyte disorders in dogs as a group have become important in clinical veterinary practice. Some of these hematologic disorders cause serious clinical signs or are associated with nonhematologic features, whereas others are well compensated or are simply a hematologic curiosity without clinical signs. A definitive diagnosis of an inherited erythrocyte defect requires special laboratory tests. The prognosis is variable, and only a few effective therapeutic options are available for some defects. Carrier detection is possible for certain disorders and should be used in breeding programs to limit the frequency of these genetic disorders.

References and Supplemental Reading

Agar, N. S., and Board, P. G. (eds.): *Red Blood Cells of Domestic Animals.* Amsterdam: Elsevier/North Holland, 1983.

Atkins, C. E., Kaneko, J. J., and Cougdon, L. L.: Methemoglobinemia. J. Am. Anim. Hosp. Assoc. 17:829, 1981.

Braend, M.: Hemoglobin polymorphism in the domestic dog. J. Hered. 79:211, 1988.

Degen, M.: Pseudohyperkalemia in Akitas. J.A.V.M.A. 290:541, 1987.

Fletch, S. M., Pinkerton, P. H., and Brueckner, P. J.: The Alaskan malamute chondrodysplasia (dwarfism-anemia) syndrome: A review. J. Am. Anim. Hosp. Assoc. 11:353, 1975.

Fyfe, J. C., Giger, U., Jezyk, P. F., et al.: Inherited selective cobalamin malabsorption: A canine model. Blood 70:46a, 1987.

Fyfe, J. C., Jezyk, P. F., Giger, U., et al.: Inherited selective malabsorption of vitamin B12 in giant schnauzers. J. Am. Anim. Hosp. Assoc. 1989 (in press).

Giger, U.: Survival of phosphofructokinase-deficient erythrocytes in a canine model. Blood 70:52a, 1987.

Giger, U., and Harvey, J. W.: Hemolysis caused by phosphofructokinase deficiency in English springer spaniels: Seven cases (1983–1986). J.A.V.M.A. 191:453, 1987.

Giger, U., Amador, A., Meyers-Wallen, V., et al.: Stomatocytosis in miniature schnauzers. ACVIM Proceedings, 1988a, p. 754.

Giger, U., Argov, Z., Schnall, M., et al.: Metabolic myopathy in canine muscle-type phosphofructokinase deficiency studied by P-NMR. Muscle and Nerve 1989 (in press).

Giger, U., Harvey, J. W., Yamaguchi, R. A., et al.: Inherited phosphofructokinase deficiency in dogs with hyperventilation-induced hemolysis: Increased in vitro and in vivo alkaline fragility of erythrocytes. Blood 65:345, 1985.

Giger, U., Kelly, A. M., and Teno, P. S.: Biochemical studies of canine muscle phosphofructokinase deficiency. Enzyme 40:25, 1988b.

Giger, U., Reilly, M. P., Asakura, T., et al.: Autosomal recessive inherited phosphofructokinase deficiency in English springer spaniel dogs. Anim. Genet. 17:15, 1986.

Harvey, J. W.: Erythrocyte metabolism. *In* Kaneko, J. J. (ed.): *Clinical Biochemistry of Domestic Animals,* 4th ed. New York: Academic Press, 1989 (in press).

Inaba, M., and Maede, Y.: Na, K-ATPase in dog red cells. J. Biol. Chem. 261:16099, 1986.

Jones, J. B.: Cyclic hematopoiesis: Animal models. Exp. Hematol. 11:571, 1983.

Kaneko, J. J.: Animal models of inherited hematologic disease. Clin. Chim. Acta 165:1, 1987.

Maggio-Price, L., Emerson, C. L., Hinds, T. R., et al.: Inherited nonspherocytic hemolytic anemia in beagle dogs. Am. J. Vet. Res. 49:1020, 1988.

Prasse, K. W., Crouser, D., Beutler, E., et al.: Pyruvate kinase deficiency anemia with terminal myelofibrosis and osteosclerosis in a beagle dog. J.A.V.M.A. 166:1170, 1975.

Rand, J. S., and O'Brien, P. J.: Exercise-induced malignant hyperthermia in an English springer spaniel. J.A.V.M.A. 190:1013, 1987.

Randolph, J. F., Center, S. A., Kalfelz, F. A., et al.: Familial nonspherocytic hemolytic anemia in poodles. Am. J. Vet. Res. 47:687, 1986.

Schalm, O. W.: Erythrocyte macrocytosis in miniature and toy poodles. Canine Pract. December, 1976, p. 55.

Searcy, G. P., Tasker, J. B., and Miller, D. R.: Animal model: pyruvate kinase deficiency in dogs. Am. J. Pathol. 94:689, 1979.

Smith, J. E.: Animal models of human erythrocyte metabolic abnormalities. Clin. Hem. 10:239, 1981.

Smith, J. E., Ryer, K., and Wallace, L.: Glucose-6-phosphate dehydrogenase deficiency in a dog. Enzyme 6:21, 1976.

Smith, J. E., Moore, K., Arens, M., et al.: Hereditary elliptocytosis with protein band 4.1 deficiency in the dog. Blood 61:373, 1983.

DIAGNOSTIC APPROACH TO THE BLEEDING PATIENT

I. B. JOHNSTONE, D.V.M.

Guelph, Ontario, Canada

Patients with clinically significant bleeding are commonly encountered in veterinary practice. Three questions face the veterinarian confronted with such a patient. Is the bleeding due to local factors, or does the patient have a systemic hemostatic abnormality? If a systemic disorder does exist, what is the nature of the defect? Is the defect of an inherited or acquired nature? The answers to these critical questions may be developed with a detailed patient history, a thorough clinical examination, and appropriate laboratory testing.

Recurring epistaxis may result from a nasal infection, neoplasm, or trauma, or it may be a reflection of a systemic bleeding disorder such as von Willebrand's disease (VWD) or thrombocytopenia. Likewise, hemarthrosis may be the result of a traumatic insult, or it may be a reflection of spontaneous bleeding in a dog with a severe coagulopathy such as factor VIII deficiency (hemophilia A). A generalized hemostatic defect is more likely if there is evidence of bleeding from multiple sites, if the bleeding is disproportionally severe considering the degree of tissue damage, or if both occur.

Characterization of a generalized hemostatic defect is critical to a logical therapeutic approach. Hemostatic abnormalities may result from vascular defects, quantitative or qualitative platelet defects or both, quantitative or qualitative deficiencies or both in one or more of the coagulation proteins, or combinations of these. The clinical expression of the bleeding may be helpful in differentiating between vascular/platelet and coagulation abnormalities. However, laboratory testing is usually required to determine the exact nature (and severity) of the problem.

The third question relates to whether the abnormality was acquired or was inherited from one or both parents. An answer to this question is critical, particularly with respect to prognosis. A thorough review of the patient's history and that of closely related family members may not only help to establish the hereditary nature of the condition but may also decrease the number of diagnostic possibilities because of differences in genetic transmission patterns.

CLINICAL ASSESSMENT

Patient's History

The importance of a detailed history in evaluating a patient with a suspected bleeding disorder cannot be overemphasized. The medical history is probably the most important factor in assessing whether or not a patient has a systemic abnormality. A detailed history is particularly important in a patient with a mild bleeding disorder such as von Willebrand's disease, in which results of hemostatic screening tests may be normal.

Severe expressions of hereditary hemostatic abnormalities are usually expressed clinically early in life. However, milder forms may not be recognized early unless they occur in a breed that undergoes cosmetic surgery in the early postnatal period. An attempt should be made to identify the time of apparent onset of bleeding problems and the frequency with which subsequent bleeding episodes have occurred. A history of repeated episodes of bleeding suggests the probability of an inherited abnormality. Acquired hemostatic abnormalities are more often recognized in mature animals, and there is less likely to be a history of previous bleeding episodes. One may be able to date the onset of defective hemostasis with the development of some other disease process. It is often difficult, however, to differentiate between a mild inherited hemostatic defect such as VWD and a newly acquired hemostatic disorder.

Whether bleeding episodes occurred spontaneously or required some stress such as injury or surgery to make the increased bleeding tendency apparent clinically should be ascertained. It is useful to compare the patient's response to challenges of the hemostatic mechanism with anticipated responses in normal patients to the same challenges. Reference to specific surgical procedures, such as cosmetic otoplasty and neutering, is particularly useful in this respect. Some inherited coagulopathies such as factor VIII deficiency (hemophilia A) and factor IX deficiency (hemophilia B), and many acquired disorders (disseminated intravascular coagulation [DIC], thrombocytopenia, and warfarin toxicity) produce spontaneous bleeding, whereas milder forms of these diseases and other conditions, such as VWD and factor VII deficiency, more commonly require surgery or other forms of traumatic injury to make the hemostatic impairment clinically apparent.

The assessment of response to trauma may not only strengthen the possibility of a patient's having a systemic hemostatic disorder, but it may make it possible to date its onset. If a patient has tolerated a major surgical procedure without excessive blood loss it is unlikely that it has a severe inherited bleeding disorder. The nature of the surgery (degree of hemostatic challenge) and the degree of severity of any hemostatic defect significantly influence the history pertaining to surgically induced bleeding. If it is determined that bleeding was abnormal, attempts should be made at determining how long bleeding persisted, what treatment was required, and how the patient responded.

The history should include details of previous illnesses and past and present drug treatments. Many systemic diseases can compromise hemostasis and can precipitate clinical bleeding in patients with an already compromised hemostatic response. Past bleeding episodes may have been associated with another illness. Numerous drugs can also compromise hemostasis. Questioning on the use of drugs must be specific, as owners frequently fail to equate common proprietary medications with the term drug. Nonsteroidal anti-inflammatory drugs such as aspirin are known to suppress the hemostatic response through inhibition of platelet function. The use of such drugs in a patient with an already compromised hemostatic mechanism (e.g., mild von Willebrand's disease) is potentially dangerous. Acetaminophen, digitalis, and chlorpromazine are other commonly used veterinary drugs that can suppress hemostatic activity. Live-virus vaccines may suppress the hemostatic response for 3 to 10 days after vaccination. Any association between time of vaccination and onset of bleeding should be noted. Specific questions relating to environment and habits of the patient (whether the animal is a farm or house dog, or is free roaming or closely supervised) should be determined to assess the probability of exposure to toxic agents capable of inducing bleeding. Warfarin and some of the newer warfarinlike drugs (e.g., diphacinone and brodificoum) used in rodenticides are potent inhibitors of hemostasis, as are some of the chemicals derived from poisonous plants and from snake venoms.

Whenever possible, information should be obtained concerning closely related family members (parents and littermates). A positive family history can be of great diagnostic importance, but a negative family history does not rule out the possibility of a heritable defect. A common cause of a negative family history in a patient with a genetic hemostatic deficiency is the failure to recognize affected family members. This is particularly true of clinically mild bleeding disorders, such as VWD or factor VII deficiency, or of recessive traits if many genetically affected animals (heterozygotes) are totally asymptomatic. When a positive family history does exist, the pattern of inheritance may give a clue to the nature of the abnormality. Sex-linked recessive bleeding disorders such as factor VIII and factor IX deficiencies occur almost exclusively in the male (although a female hemophiliac is theoretically possible from an affected male–carrier female breeding). A history of bleeding in female relatives suggests an autosomal transmission pattern of inheritance.

Physical Examination

The nature of the bleeding can be extremely important in making a diagnosis. The distribution, extent, and nature of current bleeding manifestations should be noted and recorded. A careful examination of the skin, mucous membranes, and joints in particular should be carried out.

Platelet or vascular defects or both are frequently characterized by multiple small bruises and purpura with spontaneous bleeding from mucosal surfaces. Epistaxis, gingival bleeding, hematuria, and melena are common clinical manifestations of the increased bleeding tendency associated with severe thrombocytopenia or qualitative platelet defects. Platelet and vascular abnormalities are difficult to differentiate by clinical examination alone. Coagulation abnormalities are most commonly characterized by single and larger bruises with bleeding into subcutaneous or muscle tissues and frequently bleeding into joints. Petechial hemorrhages are rarely seen with coagulopathies. Acquired abnormalities such as diphacinone toxicity and disseminated intravascular coagulation often defy this classification because of the multiple hemostatic abnormalities present. Likewise, von Willebrand's disease defies classification because of the spectrum of degrees of severity. In its milder form VWD tends to have the characteristics of a platelet disorder, whereas in its more severe form it shows features more typical of a coagulopathy (hemarthrosis and subcutaneous hematomas). One should ask the owner to be specific

in assessing the occurrence, location, and severity of bleeding. A history of recurring shifting lameness could be indicative of recurring hemarthrosis, although the owner never actually saw any bleeding. A red skin rash might have been purpura associated with thrombocytopenia but might not be recognized as bleeding by the owner.

The age, sex, and breed of the patient should be noted. As previously mentioned, severe inherited abnormalities are usually recognized within the first 6 months of life, depending on the size, breed, and habits of the patient (how prone to trauma or stress on weight-bearing surfaces and whether or not exposed to postpartum cosmetic surgery). Acquired bleeding disorders are more commonly recognized in mature or aged patients.

Inherited hemostatic disorders may have either autosomal or sex-linked transmission patterns. Sex-linked traits such as factor VIII and factor IX deficiencies are primarily restricted to the male of the species. Most other inherited hemostatic defects are autosomal traits and therefore occur with equal frequency in males and females. Acquired disorders can occur in either sex, although some are found more commonly in one sex than another (e.g., idiopathic thrombocytopenic purpura in female dogs).

Acquired disorders can occur in any breed, but some breeds appear to be more prone to certain types of abnormalities. Idiopathic thrombocytopenic purpura (ITP) is a particularly common problem in poodles and Old English sheepdogs. Inherited bleeding abnormalities show a much greater breed predilection with a high frequency of occurrence in certain breeds because of intensive inbreeding. VWD is an extremely common disorder in Doberman pinschers but also occurs in many other breeds. Factor IX deficiency is a well-defined entity in Scottish terriers, cairn terriers, and Alaskan malamutes but also occurs in other breeds and in cats. Because of the particular occurrence of certain genetic bleeding disorders in certain breeds of dogs and cats, knowing the breed may be useful in predicting the probability of a particular hemostatic defect.

Some systemic diseases can impair the hemostatic response to the degree that evidence of clinical bleeding can occur in otherwise healthy patients. Probably more important, milder expressions of these diseases may induce clinical bleeding in patients with already compromised hemostasis. It is important, therefore, that a thorough examination be carried out to identify, or evaluate the status of, concomitant disease processes. Liver disease can produce a variety of hemostatic abnormalities, including thrombocytopenia, thrombopathia, multiple clotting factor deficiencies, and fibrinolytic excesses. Thrombopathias have also been reported in association with renal disease, myeloproliferative diseases, and some types of malignancies. Hypothyroidism, a particularly common problem in Doberman pinschers, can increase the clinical severity of VWD.

LABORATORY ASSESSMENT OF HEMOSTASIS

General Considerations

The hemostatic mechanism is so complex that there are numerous ways in which it may become inadequate or fail completely. Although routine presurgical screening of all surgical candidates is desirable, it is usually impractical. Hemostatic testing is usually only conducted on patients when there is suspicion of a bleeding abnormality.

The importance of the history and physical examination cannot be overemphasized. Laboratory tests alone can sometimes be misleading. Patients with mild bleeding disorders such as VWD may bleed clinically but have normal screening tests. Conversely, deficiencies of some clotting factors (e.g., factor XII, prekallikrein deficiency) produce abnormal test results but little or no clinical bleeding. Laboratory tests can be divided into two general categories: screening tests, which evaluate the overall activity of the hemostatic mechanism (vascular, platelet, coagulation, and fibrinolytic responses) and specific tests, which evaluate components of these responses. Severe hemostatic abnormalities can usually be detected by a carefully selected group of screening tests. The sensitivity of these tests may be insufficient, however, to detect milder hemostatic disorders. There is no totally reliable hemostatic screening test or tests. Screening tests are useful only if carefully performed; they must be interpreted in conjunction with history and physical findings and with their limitations in mind. Specific tests are usually required to identify the precise nature of the hemostatic defect or defects. These tests are usually less readily available and much more costly to perform. The selection of specific tests is primarily based on the results of the more crude screening tests.

Testing is best done by a laboratory experienced in performing tests on the animal species in question because there can be major differences in the techniques used for animal and human testing. Proper collection and handling of blood samples is absolutely critical for reliable results. A poor venipuncture may result in the introduction of tissue thromboplastin into the blood sample, with subsequent activation of clotting factors or platelets. The test results obtained with such blood samples will be erroneous and often misleading. Removal of blood from the circulation always results in some degree of activation. The handling of the blood should be such that activation is minimized. The use of either siliconized glass or plastic syringes and tubes reduces the degree of surface activation of platelets and clotting proteins and is therefore recommended over the use of plain glass containers. Sodium citrate is the preferred anticoagulant for the preparation of plasma for coagulation testing and for specific testing of platelet function.

Careful sample handling is particularly critical for specific hemostatic tests because some clotting proteins are quite unstable and are easily depleted or activated. Advice should be sought from the testing facility as to precautions necessary in obtaining and submitting samples. For platelet function testing, it is usually necessary to refer the patient, as platelets deteriorate quickly when removed from the circulation and therefore must be tested immediately. Bowie and Owen (1984) suggested that "when tests for hemostasis are performed, the patients are the best containers for their blood samples."

If possible, species-specific normal control blood samples should be handled and tested under the same conditions as the patient's samples. Test results (e.g., normal clotting times) may vary from one laboratory to another owing to differences in reagents, equipment, and techniques. Test results must therefore be interpreted in light of expected normal values for that testing facility.

Hemostatic Screening Tests

PLATELET COUNT/BLOOD FILM EXAMINATION. Examination of a stained blood film allows for a quick semiquantitative assessment of platelet number, as well as a subjective evaluation of platelet morphology (e.g., size, degree of granulation, and presence of "shift" platelets). In addition, a quick subjective assessment of other blood cell types can be made. When platelet numbers seem abnormal, an actual count should be done to quantify the degree of deficiency or excess. Ethylenediaminetetra-acetic acid (EDTA)–anticoagulated blood minimizes platelet clumping; EDTA provides a suitable medium for counting platelets.

The most common cause of bleeding in dogs and cats is thrombocytopenia. At platelet counts of greater than $50,000/\mu l$, spontaneous bleeding is rare, but patients may bleed following injury or surgery. At platelet counts of less than $10,000/\mu l$, spontaneous bleeding is usually pronounced. Severe spontaneous bleeding in a patient with a platelet count in excess of $50,000/\mu l$ suggests the presence of some additional abnormality, possibly a functional platelet disorder. High platelet counts occur in certain types of myeloproliferative disorders and malignancies and may result in an increased bleeding tendency, probably because of a qualitative platelet defect. Thrombocytosis may be a normal event following exercise, surgery, or the administration of drugs such as adrenalin and vincristine.

BLEEDING TIME. The skin bleeding time measures the time from infliction of a small "standardized" injury to the moment of cessation of bleeding. Although probably one of the truer reflections of *in vivo* hemostasis, the bleeding time test is notorious for its lack of reproducibility and difficulty in standardization. Commercial bleeding time templates are available to induce standardized injuries; however, differences in depth and direction of the incision, location of the injury, thickness of the skin, and other factors account for considerable variability even within healthy animals. The end point (when bleeding actually stops) is sometimes difficult to identify.

The skin bleeding time is primarily a screening test for vascular or platelet disorders or both, because it measures the formation of the initial hemostatic plug. The skin bleeding time can be markedly affected by drugs such as aspirin. Patients with coagulopathies (e.g., factor VIII deficiency) may have a normal skin bleeding time but frequently "rebleed" from the injury site.

A modification of the skin bleeding time, the cuticle bleeding time, has been described by Giles and associates (1982). This technique involves severing a toenail through the cuticle under light anesthesia and determining the time to cessation of bleeding. This procedure may be a useful presurgical screening test for hemostatic deficiencies; however, it appears that the technique does not readily differentiate between platelet/vascular and coagulation abnormalities. More recently, a buccal mucosal bleeding time technique was described by Jergens and coworkers (1987).

CLOT RETRACTION (CR). When blood clots, the clot will retract owing to contraction of platelet thrombosthenin (the contractile protein of platelets). Clot retraction is therefore a useful screening test for platelet function if adequate numbers of platelets are present in the blood. Many different techniques have been described, although the diluted whole blood techniques are generally considered to be the most sensitive. The major disadvantage of the CR test is the degree of subjectivity in interpreting whether retraction is normal. It is a simple test and is often abnormal in qualitative platelet disorders.

WHOLE BLOOD CLOTTING TIME (WBCT). The WBCT is a simple screening test for the intrinsic coagulation pathway. The test is practical for the small veterinary laboratory because of its simplicity. Freshly drawn blood is placed in a glass tube, and the clotting time is determined. The major disadvantages of the WBCT are that it lacks sensitivity (i.e., the WBCT is significantly prolonged only if a clotting factor such as factor VIII is reduced to < 5 per cent of normal) and that the test is influenced by other variables, including volume of blood, size of tube, temperature, hematocrit of the blood, and concentration of blood platelets. The WBCT is prolonged with severe deficiencies of one or more intrinsic clotting factors (hemophilia, warfarin toxicity, and others).

A modification of the WBCT called the activated clotting time (ACT) test involves the use of commercial tubes containing a chemical activator. In this test, maximum activation of the intrinsic pathway is facilitated by the chemical activator. The ACT is also a potentially valuable in-office screening test for severe intrinsic abnormalities.

PARTIAL THROMBOPLASTIN TIME (PTT). The PTT is probably the most commonly used screening test for the intrinsic coagulation pathway. Plasma is activated under controlled conditions in the presence of phospholipid, and clotting is initiated by the addition of calcium. Deficiencies, abnormalities, or inhibitors of any of the intrinsic clotting factors will prolong the PTT.

Because the PTT measures the combined activities of factors XII, XI, IX, VIII, X, V, II, and I, test results may be falsely normal owing to concomitant increases and decreases in different clotting factors. The PTT is sensitive to levels of about 20 to 25 per cent of factor VIII (or IX). This sensitivity is such that a mild deficiency of a single factor may give a normal or only slightly prolonged PTT value. PTT times are prolonged in hemophilia A (factor VIII deficiency) or hemophilia B (factor IX deficiency) but are frequently normal in VWD because the factor VIII activity is often within normal limits or only slightly decreased in this disease. A prolongation (or shortening) of greater than 20 to 25 per cent of the normal control time should be considered abnormal.

PROTHROMBIN TIME (PT). The PT is the principal test for evaluating the extrinsic coagulation pathway and is prolonged by deficiencies of factors V, VII, X, II, or I or by the presence of inhibitors against one or more of these proteins. Plasma is incubated with tissue thromboplastin, and clotting is initiated by the addition of calcium. The PT is most sensitive to factor VII deficiency and least sensitive to prothrombin or fibrinogen abnormalities. The PT is prolonged in warfarin-type (vitamin K antagonist) toxicity, because three of the four factors affected are factors of the extrinsic pathway (factors II, VII, and X). Like the PTT, the PT test times vary from one laboratory to another, depending on the type of thromboplastin used. PT values are therefore reported as patient's time compared with normal control values for that laboratory. As for the PTT, a prolongation (or shortening) of greater than 20 to 25 per cent of the normal control time is generally considered abnormal.

THROMBIN CLOTTING TIME (TCT). The TCT is a simple procedure that involves the addition of thrombin to plasma with the determination of the clotting time. The test measures the last step in coagulation (the conversion of fibrinogen to fibrin). The TCT is primarily influenced by the concentration of the substrate fibrinogen and by the presence of substances that inhibit the action of thrombin on fibrinogen, such as heparin or heparinlike anticoagulants, fibrin/fibrinogen degradation products, and abnormal serum proteins (e.g., in multiple myeloma).

CLOT LYSIS AND FIBRIN/FIBRINOGEN DEGRADATION PRODUCTS (FDP). Premature lysis of a blood clot suggests hyperactivity of the fibrinolytic system. Subjective evaluation of the degree of lysis in a blood clot incubated at 37°C for 24 hr (comparing patient with normal control) may be a useful screening test for excessive fibrinolysis.

Probably a more sensitive indicator of excessive fibrinolysis is the measurement of FDP, the end product of fibrinolysis. Commercial kits containing latex particles coated with anti-FDP antibodies provide the veterinarian with a rapid and simple technique for determining whether serum FDP levels are within normal limits. Disseminated intravascular coagulation (with secondary fibrinolysis) is one of the more common causes of elevated serum FDP levels.

Specific Hemostatic Tests

Depending on the results of clinical assessment and hemostatic screening tests, specific clotting factor assays or other specialized procedures may be indicated. Invariably, such testing requires the service of a laboratory experienced in hemostatic testing on nonhuman species. When such testing is contemplated, discussions should take place between clinician and testing facility with respect to proper procedures. Specific clotting factor assays can be performed on carefully prepared and submitted plasma samples. Platelet studies, however, require referral of the patient, as platelets must be tested within a few hours of isolation from the patient.

Many clotting factor assays operate on the principle that normal plasma will correct the abnormal clotting time of congenitally factor-deficient plasma. Factor VIII assays compare the ability of normal and patient's plasma to correct the abnormal clotting time of factor VIII–deficient plasma. In a dog with factor VIII deficiency, there is little or no correction with the patient's plasma. An alternative approach to factor analysis may be the use of reagents that activate the clotting sequence at a particular point, so that a prolonged clotting time must indicate a defect at or subsequent to that point in the sequence. Fibrinogen is commonly measured by this technique. The venom of the Taipan snake (*Oxyuranus scutellatus*) can convert prothrombin to thrombin without the participation of other clotting factors and can be used to quantitate prothrombin levels in plasma.

The development of chromogenic assay techniques for various clotting factors has moved the quantitation of specific clotting factors from the coagulation-specific laboratory to any laboratory equipped with spectrophotometer. Chromogenic assay techniques are also available for quantitating specific anticoagulant factors such as antithrombin-III (AT-III). Measurements of plasma AT-III activity have potential value in the diagnosis of DIC. Von Willebrand factor antigen (VWF:Ag) is a specific protein required for platelet adhesion, which is deficient in von Willebrand's disease. Plasma levels of VWF:Ag can be measured by using an electroimmunoassay, in which plasma antigen migrates through an agarose gel containing specific antibody and precipitation rockets form. The height of the antigen-antibody precipitation rocket is proportional to the antigen concentration. VWF:Ag has also been quantitated using a specific snake venom extract (venom coagglutinin). This extract causes the clumping of formalin-fixed platelets, but only in the presence of VWF:Ag. Therefore, plasma from dogs with VWD causes subnormal clumping of platelets *in vitro*.

Platelet function is most commonly evaluated by aggregometry. Platelets are isolated from the patient (and from normal control animals of the same species) and tested *in vitro* for their ability to aggregate in response to specific aggregating agents such as adenosine diphosphate (ADP), collagen, thrombin, arachidonic acid, adrenalin, and platelet aggregating factor (PAF). Inherited platelet function disorders have been described. Liver disease, neoplasia, and drug therapy are common causes of acquired functional defects.

The detection of antiplatelet antibody has diagnostic value in differentiating immune-mediated and nonimmune-mediated thrombocytopenias. The platelet factor-3 (PF-3) test has been used to detect serum antiplatelet activity. Immunoinjury to platelets increases the availability of platelet membrane–bound PF-3, a catalyst in blood clotting. Significant shortening of the clotting time of platelet-rich plasma (in the presence of heat-inactivated serum) indicates the presence of serum-associated antiplatelet antibody. It is now recognized that increased platelet-associated antibody is a more consistent finding in immune-mediated platelet disease. Enzyme-linked immunosorbent assays (ELISA) are now being developed to detect both serum-associated and platelet-associated antiplatelet antibody.

References and Supplemental Reading

Ainsworth, D. M., Dodds, W. J., and Brown, C. H.: Deficiency of the contact phase of intrinsic coagulation in a horse. J.A.V.M.A. 187:71, 1985.

Bowie, E. J. W.: Von Willebrand's disease: State of the art. Scand. J. Haematol. 33:431, 1984.

Bowie, E. J. W., and Owen, C. A.: The clinical and laboratory diagnosis of hemorrhagic disorders. *In* Ratnoff, O. D. and Forbes, C. D. (eds.): *Disorders of Hemostasis*. Orlando: Grune & Stratton, 1984.

Campbell, K. L., George, J. W., and Greene, C. E. Application of the enzyme-linked immunosorbent assay for the detection of platelet antibodies in dogs. Am. J. Vet. Res. 45:2561, 1984.

Chinn, D. R., Dodds, W. J., and Selcer, B. A.: Prekallikrein deficiency in a dog. J.A.V.M.A. 88:68, 1986.

Davenport, D. J., Breitschkwerdt, E. B., and Carakostas, M. C.: Platelet disorders in the dog and cat part I: Physiology and pathogenesis. Comp. Cont. Ed. Pract. Vet. 4:762, 1982.

Day, H. J., and Rao, A. K.: Evaluation of platelet function. Semin. Hematol. 23:89, 1986.

Dodds, W. J.: Inherited bleeding disorders. Canine Pract. 5:49, 1978.

Dodds, W. J.: Von Willebrand's disease in dogs. Mod. Vet. Pract. 65:681, 1984.

Drazner, F. H.: Clinical implications of disseminated intravascular coagulation. Comp. Cont. Ed. Pract. Vet. 4:974, 1982.

Feldman, B. F.: Disseminated intravascular coagulation. Comp. Cont. Ed. Pract. Vet. 3:46, 1981.

Feldman, B. F.: Differential diagnosis in thrombocytopenia. Calif. Vet. 37:8, 1983.

Giles, A. R., Tinlin, S., and Greenwood, R.: A canine model of hemophilic (factor VIII:C deficiency) bleeding. Blood 60:1135, 1982.

Green, R. A., and Kabel, A. L.: Hypercoagulable state in three dogs with nephrotic syndrome: Role of acquired antithrombin III deficiency. J.A.V.M.A. 181:914, 1982.

Hamilton, H., Olson, P. N., and Jonas, L.: Von Willebrand's disease manifested by hemorrhage from the reproductive tract: Two case reports. J. Am. Anim. Hosp. Assoc. 21:637, 1985.

Ingram, G. I. C., Brozovic, M., and Slater, N. G. P.: Investigation of bleeding disorders. *In* Ingram, G. I. C., et al. (eds.): *Bleeding Disorders: Investigation and Management*, 2nd ed. Oxford: Blackwell Scientific Publications, 1982.

Jain, H. C., and Kono, C. S.: The platelet factor-3 test for detection of canine antiplatelet antibody. Vet. Clin. Pathol. 9:10, 1980.

Jergens, A. E., Turrentine, M. A., Kraus, K. H., et al.: Buccal mucosa bleeding times of healthy dogs and of dogs in various pathologic states, including thrombocytopenia, uremia, and von Willebrand's disease. Am. J. Vet. Res. 48:1337, 1987.

Johnson, G. S., Schlink, G. T., Fallon, R. K., et al.: Hemorrhage from the cosmetic otoplasty of Doberman pinschers with von Willebrand's disease. Am. J. Vet. Res. 46:1335, 1985.

Johnson, G. S., Turrentine, M. A., and Tomlinson, J. L.: Detection of von Willebrand's disease in dogs with a rapid qualitative test, based on venom-coagglutinin–induced platelet agglutination. Vet. Clin. Pathol. 14:11, 1985.

Johnstone, I. B.: Inherited defects of hemostasis. Comp. Cont. Ed. Pract. Vet. 4:483, 1982.

Johnstone, I. B.: Canine von Willebrand's disease: A common inherited bleeding disorder in Doberman pinscher dogs. Can. Vet. J. 27:315, 1986.

Johnstone, I. B., and Crane, S.: Haemostatic abnormalities in horses with colic—their prognostic value. Equine Vet. J. 18:271, 1986.

Johnstone, I. B., and Norris, A. M.: A moderately severe expression of classical hemophilia in a family of German shepherd dogs. Can. Vet. J. 25:191, 1984.

Randolph, J. F., Centen, S. A., and Dodds, W. J.: Factor XII deficiency and von Willebrand's disease in a family of miniature poodle dogs. Cornell Vet. 76:3, 1986.

Rosen, S., Andersson, M., Blomback, M., et al.: Clinical application of a chromogenic substrate method for determination of factor VIII activity. Thromb. Haemost. 54:818, 1985.

Schulman, A., Lusk, R., Lippincott, C. L., et al.: Diphacinone induced coagulopathy in the dog. J.A.V.M.A. 188:402, 1986.

Sirridge, M. S.: *Laboratory Evaluation of Hemostasis*, 2nd ed. Philadelphia: Lea & Febiger, 1974.

Williams, D. A., and Maggio-Price, L.: Canine idiopathic thrombocytopenia: Clinical observations and long-term follow-up in 54 cases. J.A.V.M.A. 185:660, 1984.

FACTOR VIII (HEMOPHILIA A) AND FACTOR IX (HEMOPHILIA B) DEFICIENCIES IN SMALL ANIMALS

JENS M. FOGH, D.V.M.

Gentofte, Denmark

The coagulation factors VIII and IX play a vital role in the intrinsic coagulation cascade. The end result of this cascade is a conversion of fibrinogen to a soluble fibrin monomer, which, in turn, with factor XIII and calcium, becomes fully converted to an insoluble fibrin clot. Inherited deficiencies of coagulation factor VIII (hemophilia A) and coagulation factor IX (hemophilia B, Christmas disease) result in varying degrees of hemorrhagic diathesis in small animals. This article reviews the current knowledge of hemophilia A and B with regard to small animals. The data are summarized for quick review in Table 1.

ETIOLOGY

Factor VIII functions in the middle of the intrinsic coagulation cascade and acts as a cofactor for factor X activation by factor IXa in the presence of calcium and phospholipid. Factor VIII is a large plasma glycoprotein that circulates tightly associated with the far more abundant von Willebrand factor (vWF).

Table 1. *Diagnosis, Distribution, and Therapy of Hemophilia A and B*

	Factor VIII Deficiency	Factor IX Deficiency
Screening Tests		
BT	N	N
APTT	I	I
PT	N	N
Coagulation activity*	0–25%	< 1%
Corrected by serum	No	Yes
Clinical symptoms	Hematomas, hemarthrosis, mild to severe bleeding episodes	Epistaxis, subcutaneous and joint hemorrhages, mild in small and severe in large breeds
Breeds	Many breeds of dogs, mongrels, cats	Many breeds of dogs, mongrels, cats
Inheritance	X-linked recessive	X-linked recessive
Therapy	Transfusion of fresh blood, fresh/frozen plasma, cryoprecipitate, DDAVP	Transfusion of fresh blood, fresh/frozen plasma/serum, cryoprecipitate

*% of normal (100%).

BT, bleeding time; APTT, activated partial thromboplastin time; PT, prothrombin time; N, normal; I, increased; DDAVP, deamino-D-arginine-vasopressin.

Factor VIII has a half-life of 6 to 14 hr *in vivo.* Factor VIII is itself activated by cleavage into proteins of 90,000 (heavy chain) and 80,000 (light chain) daltons, which are responsible for factor VIII activity. Factor VIII has been reported to be synthesized in endothelial cells and to be found in many different organs of the body.

Factor IX requires vitamin K for its synthesis, which occurs in the liver. In the intrinsic coagulation pathway, factor IX is converted to factor IXa after cleavage by factor XIa. Factor IXa then converts factor X to factor Xa in the presence of factor VIII, phospholipid, and calcium. Factor IX is a glycoprotein of 60,000 daltons, is present in both serum and plasma, and has an *in vivo* half-life of 18 to 36 hr.

INHERITANCE

Both hemophilia A and hemophilia B have a sex-chromosome–linked, recessive inheritance, which results in the diseases being reported in male dogs only. The mode of inheritance results in the following: (1) the deficiency cannot be transmitted from a hemophilic male to its male offspring; (2) the deficiency is transmitted from a hemophilic male to all female offspring, who are thereby obligate heterozygotes (carriers); (3) there is a 50 per cent probability that male offspring of an obligate heterozygote

female are hemophilic; (4) there is a 50 per cent probability that female offspring of an obligate heterozygote female are obligate heterozygotes.

BREEDS AFFECTED

Hemophilia A is the most commonly recognized congenital coagulation disorder and has been reported in most breeds of dogs and mongrels, as well as in domestic cats. One individual affected animal or carrier animal may have a dominating influence in particular breeds, if breeding stock is restricted, or in breeds in which a particular show winner is used extensively.

Hemophilia B has been reported in a number of breeds of dogs and mongrels, as well as in domestic cats. Hemophilia B has also been reported in conjunction with hemophilia A (hemophilia AB) in a family of bulldogs. It has been shown that the loci for hemophilia A and B are far apart on the X chromosome in dogs, and this distance permits free recombination by crossing over.

CLINICAL SYMPTOMS

Dogs and cats with hemophilia A or hemophilia B have normal bleeding times, as they are able to form the initial hemostatic plug. However, this plug is unstable and the secondary plug formed is defective.

Hemophilia A can exhibit severe, moderate, or mild symptoms, which cannot in all cases be attributed to the animal's factor VIII level, but can be a result of complicating factors such as thrombocytopenia (see discussion of prophylaxis).

Obligate heterozygotes have factor VIII levels of approximately 30 to 60 per cent of normal, are healthy, and exhibit no clinical symptoms.

Young animals with hemophilia A can exhibit prolonged bleeding from the umbilical cord and prolonged bleeding at teething. The most common clinical signs observed in dogs are hematomas on the body surface or in body cavities and hemarthrosis with periodic lameness. A problem encountered in hemophilic dogs as well as in cats is prolonged bleeding following surgery, which can be fatal. However, cats do not seem to be as commonly or severely affected with hemophilia A as dogs.

Hemophilia B resembles hemophilia A with regard to clinical expression in dogs and cats. Obligate heterozygotes do not exhibit any clinical symptoms. The female carriers have factor IX levels of approximately 30 to 60 per cent of normal. Bleeding tendencies in the affected animals are characterized as mild to moderate, being more severe in larger breeds. The most common signs observed are epistaxis, subcutaneous hemorrhages, hemarthroses, and severe bleeding episodes after surgery.

DIAGNOSIS

Venipuncture is performed with the utmost care to avoid tissue lesions, and the blood samples are collected in tubes containing sodium citrate (3.8 per cent), nine volumes of blood to one volume of sodium citrate. The samples are centrifuged at 2000 g for 10 min at 4°C, and the plasma fraction is aspirated from the tube and stored at below −70°C until tested.

Because factor IX is present in serum as well as plasma, the test sample for factor IX assay can also be prepared without using a stabilizer. In all tests for factor VIII or factor IX, a pool of normal dogs are used as a standard. To perform a preliminary screening for a deficiency in the intrinsic coagulation pathway, the samples are tested for activated partial thromboplastin time (APTT) and prothrombin time (PT). A prolonged APTT and a normal PT are indicative of a deficiency in the intrinsic coagulation pathway.

Owing to the similarity in clinical symptoms of hemophilia A and B and their location in the intrinsic coagulation pathway, a further differential diagnosis can only be based on specific factor VIII or factor IX assays. Animals deficient in factor VIII have factor VIII levels of approximately 0 to 25 per cent of normal, whereas animals deficient in factor IX have levels of less than 1 per cent of normal.

Factor VIII or factor IX activity can be measured in biologic assays using canine or feline factor VIII– or factor IX–deficient plasma as the test substrate. Factor VIII activity can also be quantitated using a Coatest kit (Habiuitrum), in which the activity is measured using a chromogenic substrate.

In plasma, factor VIII is noncovalently bound to von Willebrand factor (vWF). To differentiate between a diagnosis of hemophilia A and von Willebrand's disease, the samples can be screened for von Willebrand factor antigen (vWF:Ag) using an electroimmunoassay with rabbit-derived canine antibodies. A reduced factor VIII activity but normal vWF:Ag level is indicative of hemophilia A.

THERAPY

Specific Treatment

The treatment of dogs and cats with hemophilia A or B is achieved by providing the missing factor (i.e., factor VIII or factor IX). To limit the extent of the damage from hemorrhagic diathesis, it is important to treat the disorder immediately.

Hemophilia A and B can be alleviated by admin-

Table 2. *DDAVP-Induced Factor VIII Increase in Dogs Deficient in Factor VIII*

Time (min)	Dog 1, % Factor VIII*	Dog 2, % Factor VIII*
0	28	35
10	38	66
30	64	—
60	85	96
120	—	56
180	38	37

*% of normal (100%).
From author's unpublished data.

istering stabilized fresh normal whole blood at the rate of 4 to 6 ml/min to a total of 10 to 15 ml/kg of body weight. This will raise the factor VIII or factor IX levels by approximately 10 per cent for a period of about 12 to 24 hr. This increase in activity can also be achieved by administering 5 to 8 ml of plasma per kilogram of body weight. The use of fresh or fresh-frozen normal plasma reduces the risk of sensitizing the recipient. The plasma dose can be given two to three times daily for 3 days. Optimal treatment of hemophilic dogs or cats can be achieved by using cryoprecipitate. Factor IX deficiency can also be alleviated by administration of fresh normal serum, because serum contains factor IX activity.

Deamino-D-arginine-vasopressin (DDAVP), a synthetic derivative of vasopressin, can be used to treat bleeding episodes in patients with mild and moderate forms of hemophilia A. DDAVP can be administered subcutaneously (0.4 µg/kg diluted in 10 ml of saline) or intravenously (0.4 µg/kg diluted in 100 ml of saline infused over a period of 30 min). The therapeutic effect of DDAVP (0.4 µg/kg) normalizes bleeding times within 10 to 20 min, and the effect lasts for at least 1 to 2 hours (Table 2).

Symptomatic and Supportive Care

Gingival hemorrhages and other local bleeding episodes can be arrested by cauterization, administration of protein-precipitating agents, or local hemostatics. Hematomas and other physical complications can often be eased with the aid of rest and supportive bandages.

Prophylaxis

Preventive measures include the following considerations:

1. To prevent gingival injury and lesions of the digestive tract that can result in prolonged and possible fatal hemorrhage, bone or hard biscuit feeding should be avoided.

2. Painful hemarthrosis of the joints can be

Table 3. *Medications That Affect Thrombocytes*

Antihistamines
Anti-inflammatory drugs
Aspirin
Estrogens
Local anesthetics
Nitrofurans
Penicillin
Phenothiazine
Phenylbutazone
Plasma expanders
Promazine tranquilizers
Sulfonamides

caused by overexertion, hard training, or exercise and should be avoided.

3. Thrombocytopenia caused by certain medicines or vaccination with live vaccines can induce life-threatening complications for the hemophilic dog or cat (Table 3); caution in the use of any medications or drugs in hemophilic animals is advised.

4. Medication should only be given orally, intravenously, or subcutaneously if necessary; intramuscular injections can result in muscle hematomas.

MODEL FOR GENETIC RATIONALIZATION

To implement a rational elimination of the causative gene for hemophilia A or B from the population, it is necessary to set up a screening system to reliably detect and diagnose all suspected male hemophiliacs and female carriers.

For a period of 6 years, German shepherd dogs in Denmark that are suspect for hemophilia A or carrier status have been screened. The X-linked causative gene for hemophilia A in the Danish German shepherd population has been shown to be transmitted via a common ancestor, the German

Table 4. *Elimination Program*

The following rules apply to the tested dogs:

1. All suspect male dogs must submit to a factor VIII activity screening test (normal dogs 100% ±2 SD).
2. All female dogs sired by a hemophilic male are obligate heterozygotes and are disqualified as breeding bitches.
3. All pedigree-suspect female dogs siring a male hemophilic pup are obligate heterozygotes and are disqualified as breeding bitches.
4. All pedigree-suspect female dogs with a factor VIII activity value < 75% (normal females 100% ±2 SD) are obligate heterozygotes and are disqualified as breeding bitches.
5. All pedigree-suspect female dogs with a factor VIII activity value ≥ 75% (normal females 100% ±2 SD) are designated normal and qualify as possible breeding bitches.
6. All pedigree-suspect male and female dogs that do not submit to a factor VIII activity screening test are automatically disqualified as possible breeding dogs.

(From Fogh, J. M.: A study of hemophilia A in German shepherd dogs in Denmark. Vet. Clin. North Am. [Small Anim. Pract.] 18:252, 1988.)

stud dog Canto von der Wienerau, who lived from 1968 to 1973. In cooperation with the German Shepherd Club of Denmark and the Danish Kennel Club (DKK), the author has initiated an elimination program, which is based on pedigree information and evaluated factor VIII activity (Table 4). The hemophilic male dogs often reveal themselves clinically and are easily diagnosed using APTT and PT tests and specific factor VIII tests. To classify female carriers, a limit value of 75 per cent of normal factor VIII activity was chosen (normal distribution constructed from research data curve), below which the females were diagnosed as carriers. The limit was chosen to minimize the risk of diagnosing a carrier as normal. This program to date has tested over 200 suspect German shepherd dogs, resulting in the diagnosis of approximately 50 hemophilic males and 50 obligate heterozygote females.

References and Supplemental Reading

Benson, R. E., Jones, D. W., and Dodds, W. J.: A practical technique for preparation of antiserum to canine factor VIII–related antigen. Vet. Immunol. Immunopathol. 7:337, 1984.
Cambell, K. L., Green, C. E., and Dodds, W. J.: Factor IX deficiency (hemophilia B) in a Scottish terrier. J.A.V.M.A. 182:170, 1983.
Cotter, S. M., Brenner, R. M., and Dodds, W. J.: Hemophilia A in three unrelated cats. J.A.V.M.A. 172:166, 1978.
Davis, D. C., and Slappendel, R. J.: Evaluation of DDAVP on the release of F VIII in normal dogs and in a dog with hemophilia A. Proceedings of the American College of Veterinary Internal Medicine, 1984, p. 51.
Dodds, W. J.: The diagnosis, management and treatment of bleeding disorders. Modern Veterinary Practice 58:680, 1977.
Dodds, W. J.: Inherited bleeding disorders. Canine Pract. 5:49, 1978.
Dodds, W. J.: Hemostasis and coagulation. In Kaneko, J. J. (ed.): Clinical Biochemistry of Domestic Animals, 3rd ed. New York: Academic Press, 1980, p. 671.
Fogh, J. M.: A study of hemophilia A in German shepherd dogs in Denmark. Vet. Clin. North Am. [Small Anim. Pract.] 18:245, 1988.
Fogh, J. M., and Fogh, I. T.: Inherited coagulation disorders. Vet. Clin. North Am. [Small. Anim. Pract.] 18:231, 1988.
Fogh, J. M., Nygaard, L., Andresen, E., et al.: Hemophilia in dogs, with special reference to hemophilia A among German shepherd dogs in Denmark. I. Pathophysiology, laboratory tests and genetics. Nord. Vet. Med. 36:235, 1984.
Fogh, J. M., Nygaard, L., Andresen, E., et al.: Hemophilia in dogs, with special reference to hemophilia A among German shepherd dogs in Denmark. II. Clinical study, therapy and prophylaxis. Nord. Vet. Med. 36:241, 1984.
Kohler, M., Hellstern, P., Miyashita, C., et al.: Comparative study of intranasal, subcutaneous and intravenous administration of deamino-D-arginine vasopressin (DDAVP). Thromb. Haemost. 55:108, 1986.
Littlewood, J. D., Matic, S. E., and Smith, N.: Factor IX deficiency (haemophilia B, Christmas disease) in a crossbred dog. Vet. Rec. 118:400, 1986.
Lewis, J. H., Spero, J. A., and Hasiba, U.: A hemophiliac dog colony: Genetic studies and coagulation findings in hemophiliac and normal dogs. Comp. Biochem. Physiol. 75A:147, 1983.
Mertens, K., Van Wijngaarden, A., and Bertina, R. M.: The role of factor VIII in the activation of human blood coagulation factor X by activated factor IX. Thromb. Haemost. 54:654, 1985.
Prowse, C., Hornsey, V., McKay, G., et al.: Room temperature, microtray chromogenic assay of factor VIII:C. Vox Sang. 50:21, 1986.
Rebar, A. H., and Boon, G. D.: An approach to the diagnosis of bleeding disorders in the dog. J. Am. Anim. Hosp. Assoc. 17:227, 1981.
Rosen S.: A chromogenic assay for coagulation factor VIII. Thromb. Haemost. 50:A0329, 1983.
Slappendel, R. J.: Hemophilia A and hemophilia B in a family of French bulldogs. Tijdschr. Diergeneesk. 100:20, 1975.
Spurling, N. W.: Hereditary disorders of hemostasis in dogs: A critical review of the literature. Vet. Bull. 50:151, 1980.

Thomsen, A. V., Holtet, L., Nilsson, I. M., et al.: Hæmofili hos schæferhunde i Norge. Norsk Vet. 96:6, 1984.

van Dieijen, G., van Rijn, J. L. M., Govers-Riemslag, J. W. D., et al.: Assembly of the intrinsic factor X activity complex—interactions between factor IX a, factor VIII a and phospholipid. Thromb. Haemost. 53:396, 1985.

Vehar, G. A., Keyt, B., Eaton, P., et al.: Structure of human factor VIII. Nature 312:337, 1984.

Verlander, J. M., Gaman, N. T., and Dodds, W. J.: Factor IX deficiency

(hemophilia B) in a litter of Labrador retrievers. J.A.V.M.A. 185:83, 1984.

Vilhardt, H., Tomislav, B., Falch, J., et al.: Plasma concentrations of factor VIII after administration of DDAVP to conscious dogs. Thromb. Res. 47:585, 1987.

Wion, K. L., Kelly, D., Summerfield, J. A., et al.: Distribution of factor VIII mRNA and antigen in human liver and other tissues. Nature 317:726, 1985.

VON WILLEBRAND'S DISEASE IN DOGS

KARL H. KRAUS, D.V.M.,
and GARY S. JOHNSON, D.V.M.

Columbia, Missouri

Canine von Willebrand's disease is a group of related bleeding disorders that are caused by a deficiency of the protein von Willebrand factor (VWF). The diagnosis of canine von Willebrand's disease is usually made because of below-normal concentrations of von Willebrand factor antigen (VWF:Ag) in the plasma. This laboratory result is commonly encountered and has supported the diagnosis of von Willebrand's disease in mongrels and purebred dogs of at least 54 breeds (Table 1). In many of these breeds, the disease is rare or the prevalence has not been determined; however, in other breeds such as the Doberman pinscher and Airedale terrier, the prevalence of animals with abnormal laboratory findings may approach or exceed 50 per cent. Considering the large number of dogs with von Willebrand's disease, the incidence of bleeding crises is surprisingly low, suggesting that the most common forms of the disease are mild and often remain subclinical. Nonetheless, moderate to severe forms of von Willebrand's disease exist; at times, even certain of the milder forms can contribute to fatal or life-threatening hemorrhage.

VON WILLEBRAND FACTOR

The individual molecules of von Willebrand factor are polymeric, composed of 1 to 20 or more identical fibrous protomers covalently attached end to end to form a flexible string. The molecular weight of the protomer building block is slightly over 0.5 million, so the largest von Willebrand factor multimers have molecular weights of several million (Girma et al., 1987).

Von Willebrand factor participates in primary hemostasis by facilitating the adhesion of platelets to subendothelial collagen, which is exposed in injured blood vessel walls. Additional platelets stick to and accumulate on the adhering platelets, forming a growing platelet mass that eventually blocks hemorrhage by plugging vascular faults. Concurrent coagulation produces fibrin strands, which reinforce

Table 1. *Breeds of Dogs with von Willebrand's Disease*

Afghan hound	English springer	MANCHESTER
AIREDALE TER-	spaniel	TERRIER—TOY
RIER	Fox terrier—	MINIATURE
Akita	smooth	SCHNAUZER
Alaskan malamute	Fox terrier—wire	Papillon
American cocker	GERMAN SHEP-	PEMBROKE
spaniel	HERD DOG	WELSH CORGI
BASSET HOUND	German Short-	Poodle—miniature
Bearded collie	haired pointer	POODLE—STAN-
Bernese mountain	GOLDEN RE-	DARD
dog	TRIEVER	ROTTWEILER
Bichon Frise	Great Dane	Samoyed
Boxer	Great Pyrenees	SCOTTISH TER-
Cairn terrier	Greyhound	RIER
Chesapeake Bay	Irish setter	SHETLAND
retriever	Irish wolfhound	SHEEPDOG
Collie—rough	Italian greyhound	Shi Tzu
DACHSHUND—	KEESHOUND	Siberian husky
STANDARD	Kerry blue terrier	Soft-coated Wheaten
DACHSHUND—	Kuvasz	terrier
TOY	Labrador retriever	Tibetan terrier
DOBERMAN	Lakeland terrier	Vizsla
PINSCHER	Lhasa Apso	Whippet
English cocker	MANCHESTER	Yorkshire terrier
spaniel	TERRIER—	
English setter	STANDARD	

List obtained from Dr. W. Jean Dodds, New York State Department of Health, Albany.

Capitalized breeds are known to have a prevalence of von Willebrand's disease of 15% or greater.

the platelet plugs. In addition to its well-documented role in platelet-collagen adhesion, von Willebrand factor may participate in the platelet-platelet cohesions. In humans, von Willebrand factor also stabilizes coagulation factor VIII. Thus, many human patients with von Willebrand's disease have a hemophilialike coagulopathy, as well as deficient primary hemostasis. Compared with the human clotting factor, canine factor VIII appears to be much less dependent on von Willebrand factor for stabilization, so coagulation assays, such as the activated partial thromboplastin time (APTT), are not reliable indicators of canine von Willebrand's disease.

In most mammals, extracellular von Willebrand factor occurs in the plasma and throughout the vascular subendothelium. Intracellular VWF has been found in endothelial cells, megakaryocytes, and platelets. Endothelial cells and megakaryocytes are able to synthesize VWF; endothelial cells are considered to be the most important source of plasma and subendothelial VWF, whereas the VWF in platelets was provided by their megakaryocyte precursors. There is evidence that plasma, platelet, and subendothelial von Willebrand factor all participate in hemostasis; however, the relative importance of each pool has not been established. The existence of VWF in canine platelets has been questioned; however, low levels of von Willebrand factor have been detected in lysates of thoroughly washed platelets from normal dogs (Parker et al., 1988).

Laboratory and Clinical Assessment

The most frequently used laboratory procedure for determining plasma von Willebrand factor levels is an antigenic assay, the electroimmunoassay (also called the Laurell assay or rocket electrophoresis). The appropriate sample for this assay is citrated plasma, which can be obtained from blood collected into syringes containing one-ninth volume of 3.8 per cent (0.13 mol) trisodium citrate. The assay is usually performed at regional veterinary reference laboratories. If possible, samples should be shipped in a frozen state (over dry ice) to avoid possible artifactual changes that could invalidate the results. In the human and veterinary medical literature, the value measured by the electroimmunoassay for von Willebrand factor has traditionally been referred to as factor VIII–related antigen (VIIIR:Ag). Most technical journals now use the phrase von Willebrand factor antigen (VWF:Ag) instead of the outmoded terminology. Von Willebrand factor antigen levels are reported in comparison with those in pooled citrated plasma from several normal dogs. The antigen concentrations in the standard plasma pools are traditionally defined as 100 per cent or 1

U/ml. Normal dogs have baseline plasma VWF:Ag concentrations between 48 and 168 per cent (Johnson et al., 1988). Inflammatory diseases and certain stressful physiologic states, such as parturition, produce marked increases in plasma concentrations of VWF:Ag in normal dogs. A similar stress-related baseline shift occurring in a dog with von Willebrand's disease could result in a false interpretation that the dog is normal.

The platelet-associated biologic activity of von Willebrand factor can be estimated by platelet agglutination assays. In these tests the sample is stirred with washed platelets and an inducing agent is added to initiate von Willebrand factor–dependent platelet agglutination. Agglutination rates can be monitored with a platelet aggregometer and are thought to reflect the biologic activity of von Willebrand factor in the sample. The inducing agent usually used to measure VWF in human plasma is the antibiotic ristocetin; thus, the measured activity is called ristocetin cofactor activity. The ristocetin cofactor assay does not work well with canine VWF, so a snake venom protein (called either botrocetin or coagglutinin) is used instead of ristocetin to measure botrocetin cofactor activity in canine samples. As with the von Willebrand factor antigen assays, botrocetin cofactor activities are determined in comparison with standard canine plasma pools considered to contain a botrocetin cofactor activity of 100 per cent or 1 U/ml. In most canine plasma samples, there is close agreement between the VWF:Ag concentration and the botrocetin cofactor activity (Johnson et al., 1988). Notable exceptions, however, have been found in association with type II canine von Willebrand's disease or after the administration of desmopressin acetate (deamino-D-arginine-vasopressin, DDAVP, USV Laboratories, Tarrytown, NY) to dogs (see below).

The multimeric composition of von Willebrand factor can be evaluated with an electrophoretic procedure called multimeric analysis. With this technique, canine von Willebrand factor multimers have been separated into an array of bands arranged according to their molecular weights (Kraus et al., 1987).

Determination of the bleeding time (i.e., the duration of hemorrhage from small standardized incisions severing only microscopic blood vessels) is the most reliable means of assessing the severity of an insufficiency in primary hemostasis. Prolonged skin bleeding times are considered a hallmark of clinically significant human von Willebrand's disease. Because of species differences in anatomy and physiology, skin bleeding times have not been useful for assessing the severity of von Willebrand's disease in dogs. Measurement of bleeding times with incisions in the buccal mucosa, instead of the skin, has greatly improved the utility of bleeding time determinations in canine patients (Jergens et al., 1987).

For determination of the buccal mucosa bleeding time, the patient is restrained in lateral recumbency with the upper lip folded back and secured with a gauze strip tied tightly enough to partially block the venous return of blood (Fig. 1). At time zero, two 6-mm long by 1-mm deep incisions are made in the buccal mucosa with a commercially available, disposable, spring-loaded blade in a plastic cassette (Simplate-II, Organon Teknika, Durham, NC). A stopwatch is started when the incisions are made. Shed blood is absorbed at 2- to 5-sec intervals with circles of filter paper, placed within 2 mm of the incision sites with care to avoid disturbance of the forming platelet plugs. End points are reached as soon as the filter paper fails to acquire a red crescent from blood. Mean buccal mucosa bleeding times shorter than 4 min are considered normal. Prolonged buccal mucosa bleeding times are not specific for von Willebrand's disease and have also been found in dogs with thrombocytopenia, uremia, ehrlichiosis, and afibrinogenemia.

CLASSIFICATION OF VON WILLEBRAND'S DISEASE

Because of the complexity of the von Willebrand factor molecule, it could be anticipated that several different genetic mutations would result in distinct von Willebrand factor deficiencies and produce heterogeneity among von Willebrand's disease kindreds. At least 21 apparently distinct forms of human von Willebrand's disease have been described (Ruggeri and Zimmerman, 1987). Analysis of the multimeric composition of von Willebrand factor in the plasma of human von Willebrand's disease patients has provided criteria for categoriza-

Table 2. *Defining Characteristics of Major Types of von Willebrand's Disease*

Type	Characteristic Multimeric Pattern of Plasma von Willebrand Factor	Canine Breeds Involved*
Type I	Full spectrum of multimer sizes detectable (usually in subnormal concentrations)	Airedale terrier, Doberman pinscher, Pembroke Welsh corgi, Shetland sheepdog
Type II	Smaller multimers readily detectable, larger multimers missing	German short-haired pointer
Type III	All multimers absent (or present in only trace amounts)	Chesapeake Bay retrievers, Scottish terriers

*Only those breeds whose classification is confirmed by multimeric analysis are listed.

tion of the individual forms (or subtypes) of human von Willebrand's disease into three major types (Table 2).

The criteria outlined in Table 2 can be used to define the main types of von Willebrand's disease in dogs as well as in humans (Fig. 2). So far, type I canine von Willebrand's disease has been confirmed by multimeric analysis in Doberman pinschers, Airedale terriers, Pembroke Welsh corgis, and Shetland sheepdogs (Johnson et al., 1989; McCarroll et al., 1987). Indirect evidence suggests that the forms of von Willebrand's disease occurring in many other breeds listed in Table 1 belong in the type I category, even though multimeric studies have not yet been reported in these breeds. Besides being the most common type of the disease, type I canine von Willebrand's disease is also the mildest. Nonetheless, laboratory findings are sometimes extreme

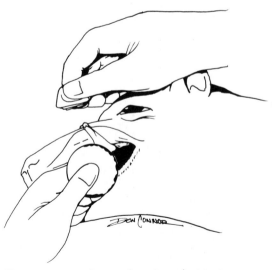

Figure 1. Dog undergoing buccal mucosa bleeding time determination. Sketch shows incision sites and position of gauze strip.

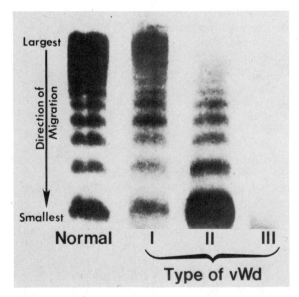

Figure 2. Multimeric analysis of plasma from a normal dog (left lane), an Airedale terrier with type In (I), a German short-hair pointer with type II von Willebrand's disease (II), and a Chesapeake Bay retriever with type III von Willebrand's disease (III).

(plasma VWF:Ag concentrations as low as 4 per cent in some Doberman pinschers), and life-threatening bleeding episodes are encountered occasionally with the type I disease.

Preliminary evidence suggests the existence of subtypes of type I canine von Willebrand's disease. For instance, multimeric analysis of plasma samples from many Doberman pinschers with von Willebrand's disease reveals a relative scarcity of the highest-molecular-weight von Willebrand factor multimers. In contrast, the various multimer sizes in plasma samples from Airedale terriers with von Willebrand's disease appear to be present in the same relative proportions as those in normal canine plasma. Most Doberman pinschers with von Willebrand's disease have prolonged buccal mucosa bleeding times, and several incidents of abnormal bleeding by affected members of this breed have been reported (Johnson et al., 1988). Most Airedale terriers with subnormal plasma levels of von Willebrand factor antigen have normal buccal mucosa bleeding times; as yet, no accounts of abnormal bleeding by Airedale terriers attributable to von Willebrand's disease have been documented.

Type II von Willebrand's disease has occurred in a family of German short-haired pointers (Johnson et al., 1989). This form of the disease was severe in puppies and young adults, but the severity appeared to lessen with age. Plasma von Willebrand factor antigen levels were less than 20 per cent in young dogs. By 3 years of age, however, the antigen level in one affected individual increased to a low normal concentration (65 per cent). Botrocetin cofactor activities were undetectable or much lower than the von Willebrand factor antigen levels in the same sample. Buccal mucosa bleeding times were markedly prolonged and often exceeded 20 min in younger dogs. In the German short-haired pointers, type II von Willebrand's disease appeared to be a recessive trait.

The most severe form of von Willebrand's disease in dogs is type III. Type III von Willebrand's disease is relatively common in Scottish terriers and has occurred in a family of Chesapeake Bay retrievers. Clinically, the disease is recessive, although heterozygous asymptomatic carriers can be detected because of their subnormal but detectable plasma von Willebrand factor antigen levels. Homozygotes lack any detectable von Willebrand factor in their plasma. They have markedly prolonged bleeding times and in most cases are afflicted with repeated hemorrhagic problems.

TREATMENT

There is currently no cure for von Willebrand's disease. Veterinarians must frequently devise management procedures in response to hemorrhagic crises or anticipated hemorrhagic crises in patients with von Willebrand's disease who are scheduled for surgery. Replacement therapy with blood or blood products has been the traditional mainstay for treating canine patients with von Willebrand's disease. Cryoprecipitate, a blood fraction rich in cold-precipitable proteins (including von Willebrand factor), is the preferred therapeutic agent for patients with normal packed cell volumes because high doses can be administered quickly by intravenous infusion without the problem of volume overload. Canine cryoprecipitate, however, is not generally available, so citrated plasma (fresh or fresh frozen and thawed) is used more commonly. When the packed cell volume has dropped acutely because of massive hemorrhage or when no centrifugation facilities for plasma preparation are available, citrated fresh whole blood may be used. At least one unit of blood or plasma should be administered for every 20 kg of body weight. In some cases, clinical benefits appear to result from lower doses. In other instances, transfusion of plasma equaling or exceeding the recommended 0.05 blood units per kilogram has failed to normalize hemostasis, perhaps because transfusion can replenish the plasma pool with von Willebrand factor but does not supply von Willebrand factor to the platelets and the subendothelium. Of course, steps should be taken to ensure that the donors have normal plasma levels of von Willebrand factor. To avoid immune sensitization of canine patients with von Willebrand's disease that may need transfusion therapy on several occasions during their lifetimes, blood donors negative for erythrocyte antigens DEA 1.1, DEA 1.2, and DEA 7 should be used whenever possible. Transfusion products with extra-high von Willebrand factor activity can be obtained from blood donor dogs pretreated with DDAVP, which stimulates endothelial cells to transfer their stores of von Willebrand factor into the blood plasma (Turrentine et al., 1988). For this purpose, the recommended dose is 1 μg of DDAVP per kilogram of body weight. Thirty minutes before the blood is to be drawn, the DDAVP should be administered by subcutaneous injection into a region relatively free of adipose tissue, such as the ventral thorax. DDAVP is available in an intranasal preparation, which is as effective injected subcutaneously as the more expensive product packaged for injection.

Direct administration of DDAVP to human patients with certain forms of von Willebrand's disease has become a commonly used alternative to transfusion therapy (Richardson and Robinson, 1985; Ruggeri and Zimmerman, 1987). Preliminary evidence suggests that DDAVP can also be effective when administered to certain dogs with von Willebrand's disease. For instance, in a study of 13 Doberman pinschers with von Willebrand's disease, the buccal mucosa bleeding time decreased from a baseline mean of 11.9 min to mean of 6.7 min, 30 min after they received a subcutaneous injection of 1 μg/kg of DDAVP. Surprisingly, the mean increase in plasma von Willebrand factor antigen was only 3 per cent; however, the mean botrocetin cofactor activity increased from 22 to 34 per cent (Fig. 3). The apparent discrepancy between the von Willebrand factor antigen response and the botrocetin cofactor response can be explained by the changed multimeric patterns found after DDAVP treatment. The disproportionately large increase in the density of slower migrating bands demonstrated that it was primarily the larger multimers of von Willebrand factor that were released into the blood in response to DDAVP (Fig. 4). The von Willebrand factor antigen concentration is affected primarily by the concentration of the smaller multimers, whereas the larger multimers are the major determinant of the botrocetin cofactor activity. The larger multimers are also thought to be particularly effective in hemostasis, which is consistent with the marked decrease in buccal mucosa bleeding times produced with DDAVP.

Although most Doberman pinschers with von Willebrand's disease appear to benefit from DDAVP treatment, certain affected individuals in this breed have repeatedly failed to exhibit a von Willebrand factor response to the drug. Furthermore, the efficacy of DDAVP treatment for von Willebrand's disease in other breeds has as yet not been demonstrated. Direct administration of this drug does not help dogs with type III von Willebrand's disease because they have no stored endothelial von Willebrand factor to secrete into their blood. Preliminary experiments indicate that the botrocetin cofac-

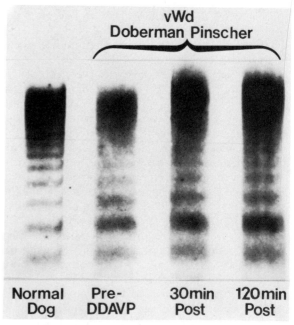

Figure 4. Multimeric analysis of von Willebrand factor in plasma from a normal dog (left lane) and plasma from a Doberman pinscher with von Willebrand's disease (vWd) drawn immediately before (pre-DDAVP) and 30 and 120 minutes after subcutaneous treatment with DDAVP (1 μg/kg).

tor activity and buccal mucosa bleeding times of German short-haired pointers with type II von Willebrand's disease do not change substantially after DDAVP administration. On the other hand, most untreated Airedale terriers with von Willebrand's disease have normal hemostasis even during surgery and therefore do not require DDAVP.

To avoid excess hemorrhage during surgery, it is suggested that dogs with type I von Willebrand's disease and prolonged buccal mucosa bleeding times be injected subcutaneously with DDAVP (1 μg/kg 20 min before induction of anesthesia). The buccal mucosa bleeding time should be remeasured immediately before induction of anesthesia to determine if the DDAVP has been effective. If there is no substantial normalization of the buccal mucosa bleeding time, the surgery should be delayed until the patient has received transfusion therapy. When necessary, frozen plasma can be rapidly thawed in a microwave oven with repeated 10-sec bursts of irradiation interrupted by manual mixing to avoid localized heat denaturation of the plasma proteins (Hurst, 1987).

References and Supplemental Reading

Dodds, W. J.: Bleeding disorders. *In* Morgan, R. V. (ed.): *Handbook of Small Animal Practice.* New York: Churchill Livingstone, 1988, pp. 773–785.

Girma, J. P., Meyer, D., Verweij, C. L., et al.: Structure-function relationship of human von Willebrand factor. Blood 70:605, 1987.

Hurst, T. S., Turrentine, M. A., and Johnson G. S.: Evaluation of

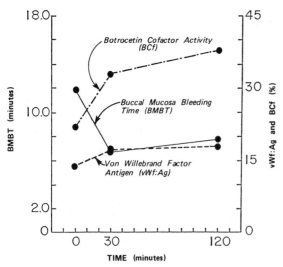

Figure 3. Mean buccal mucosa bleeding times, plasma von Willebrand factor antigen concentrations, and plasma botrocetin cofactor activities of 13 Doberman pinschers with von Willebrand's disease, immediately before (0 minutes) and 30 and 120 minutes after treatment with subcutaneously administered DDAVP (1 μg/kg).

microwave-thawed canine plasma for transfusion. J.A.V.M.A. 190:776, 1987.

Jergens, A. E., Turrentine, M. A., Kraus, K. H., et al.: Buccal mucosa bleeding times of healthy dogs and of dogs in various pathologic states, including thrombocytopenia, uremia, and von Willebrand's disease. Am. J. Vet. Res. 48:1337, 1987.

Johnson, G. S., Turrentine, M. A., and Kraus, K. H.: Canine von Willebrand's disease: a heterogeneous group of bleeding disorders. Vet. Clin. North Am. [Small Anim. Pract.] 18:195, 1988a.

Johnson, G. S., Turrentine, M. A., and Dodds, W. J.: Von Willebrand's disease in a German shorthaired pointer resembles type II human von Willebrand's disease. Am. J. Vet. Res. (in press, 1989).

Kraus, K. H., Turrentine, M. A., and Johnson, G. S.: Multimeric analysis of von Willebrand factor before and after desmopressin acetate (DDAVP) administration intravenously and subcutaneously in male beagle dogs. Am. J. Vet. Res. 48:1376, 1987.

McCarroll, D. R., Lothrop, S. A., Dolan, M. C., et al.: Canine von Willebrand factor expresses a multimeric composition similar to human von Willebrand factor. Exp. Hematol. 15:1060, 1987.

Parker, M. T., Turrentine, M. A., and Johnson, G. S.: Von Willebrand factor in the lysates of washed platelets from normal dogs and dogs with von Willebrand's disease Am. J. Vet. Res. 1989 (in press).

Richardson, D. W., and Robinson, A. G.: Desmopressin. Ann. Intern. Med. 103:228, 1985.

Ruggeri, Z. M., and Zimmerman, T. S.: Von Willebrand factor and von Willebrand's disease. Blood 70:895, 1987.

Turrentine, M. A., Kraus, K. H., and Johnson, G. S.: Plasma from donor dogs pretreated with DDAVP, transfused into a German shorthair pointer with type II von Willebrand's disease. Vet. Clin. North Am. [Small Anim. Pract.] 18:275, 1988.

DISSEMINATED INTRAVASCULAR COAGULATION

ROBBERT J. SLAPPENDEL, D.V.M.

Utrecht, The Netherlands

Disseminated intravascular coagulation (DIC) is a paradoxic clinicopathologic condition in which hypercoagulability may result in a bleeding tendency and in which a hemorrhagic diathesis and thrombosis may even occur in concert. DIC is an intermediary mechanism of disease, as well as a secondary pathologic state. This means that DIC is not a disease in itself but is always induced by some other pathologic condition or disease. Its pathologic effects not only may complicate the primary disease but may even dominate the clinical picture and become a significant factor in prognosis.

Diseases and conditions that have been reported in association with DIC in companion animals are presented in Table 1. Even though the prognosis is poor for the majority of these diseases, the outcome is not necessarily fatal in all cases if adequate therapy is instituted. For the correct diagnosis and treatment of DIC, understanding of its pathogenesis is indispensable.

PATHOGENESIS

The organization of the hemostatic mechanisms is such that injury to the vessel wall evokes a series of well-balanced responses that lead to the deposition of a hemostatic plug at the site of the injury while preventing extension of the plug beyond the local site. This is accomplished by a number of delicate interacting regulatory systems that either amplify or counteract each other. These regulatory systems include components of the blood vessel wall, blood platelets, activators and inhibitors of platelet aggregation, blood-clotting proteins, physiologic anticoagulants, fibrinolytic enzymes, and inhibitors of fibrinolysis. Following their activation in the hemostatic process, platelets as well as clotting factors and other enzymes are degraded at the site of hemostasis and eventually destroyed. Thrombi that have developed in response to local injury are gradually broken down by fibrinolysis and the reticuloendothelial system (RES), in close harmony with tissue repair. If activated clotting proteins escape into the circulation, they are efficiently eliminated by the RES and the liver. In most pathophysiologic situations, increased production readily substitutes for components that are consumed during hemostatic events.

Unlike the relatively scanty and localized activation of the hemostatic mechanisms that occurs in most types of physical injury, DIC is associated with excessive pathologic triggering of hemostasis in major parts of the vascular bed. This may result from the exposure of the blood to proteolytic enzymes or large activating surfaces or be caused by the massive entry of thromboplastic materials into the circulation.

DIC-inducing proteolytic enzymes include snake venoms, trypsin, and enzymes released from damaged leukocytes. *Activating surfaces* include damaged vascular endothelium, immune complexes, and circulating particles such as bacteria and viruses. *Thromboplastic substances* may be released from intensely necrotic tissues or damaged blood

Table 1. *Diseases and Conditions Associated with DIC in Small Animals*

Neoplasia
Metastasized thyroid carcinoma
Metastasized mammary carcinoma
Hemangiosarcoma
Lymphatic leukemia
Myeloproliferative disease

Infectious Diseases
Bacterial sepsis
Leptospirosis
Canine infectious hepatitis
Feline infectious peritonitis
Babesiosis
Dirofilariasis

Inflammatory Conditions
Suppurative bronchopneumonia
Suppurative dermatitis
Chronic active hepatitis
Acute necrotizing pancreatitis
Hemorrhagic gastroenteritis

Miscellaneous Conditions
Shock
Heat stroke
Venomous snake bite
Hepatic cirrhosis
Aflatoxicosis
Autoimmune hemolytic anemia
Cold agglutinin disease
Gastric dilation—volvulus
Congestive heart failure
Valvular fibrosis
Diaphragmatic hernia
Following extensive surgery
Hematoma of the stifle
Renal amyloidosis
Idiopathic

From Slappendel, R. J.: Vet. Clin. North Am. [Small Anim. Pract.] 18:171, 1988.

cells or may be secreted by malignant tumors. The subsequent activation of the clotting cascades induces the generation of thrombin. Thrombin converts fibrinogen into fibrin, which may be trapped in the microcirculation, and causes widespread aggregation of platelets. This may result in thrombosis of capillaries, arterioles, and venules and infarcts in many organs.

Yet microthrombosis is not a consistent event in DIC. Through the action of thrombin, fibrinogen is at first degraded to small fibrinopeptides and soluble fibrin monomers (FMs). When secondary conditions such as circulation and RES function are normal, FMs may be rapidly eliminated from the blood, even when present in high concentrations; hence, polymerization of FM to fibrin may not occur.

Clot formation may still be minimal or absent, even when fibrin polymerization does occur. Surfaces and substances that activate the intrinsic or extrinsic pathways of coagulation in DIC, as in physiologic hemostasis, also trigger the fibrinolytic system. Physiologic fibrinolysis causes slow breakdown of fibrin; the secondary systemic fibrinolysis

that occurs in DIC may rapidly dissolve small fibrin clots and may even prevent their generation by dissolving fibrin the moment it forms.

Usually hemorrhage rather than manifestations of microthrombosis attracts the attention of the clinician in patients with DIC. Systemic fibrinolysis digests not only fibrin but also fibrinogen and even other clotting proteins. Fibrinolysis and the consumption of coagulation factors and platelets in the ongoing clotting process may eventually result in thrombocytopenia and clotting factor deficiencies, hence in a hemorrhagic diathesis. The circulating fibrin/fibrinogen degradation products (FDPs), which inhibit thrombin and interfere with fibrin polymerization, may contribute to the development of the bleeding tendency.

Whether or not the hypercoagulable state of DIC results in thrombosis, a bleeding tendency, or both depends on how the various balances of hemostasis are disturbed (Fig. 1). The type of trigger itself affects the various equilibria in various ways, but the general condition of the patient and the nature of the underlying disease are just as important.

Endotoxin, for example, triggers intravascular coagulation by releasing thromboplastic material from leukocytes and aggregating agents from platelets but also blocks the RES and inhibits fibrinolysis. Endotoxin-induced DIC is therefore mostly characterized by manifestations of microthrombosis. In contrast, when DIC is induced by some types of viper venom, the plasma fibrinogen is converted to unstable fibrin strands, which are rapidly removed from the circulation by fibrinolysis and phagocytosis. Hence, defective coagulation rather than thrombosis develops in this situation.

Fibrin generation and thrombus formation will also occur more readily as DIC is more intensely stimulated. Fibrinolysis and the RES have less opportunity to dissolve the microclots in fulminant acute DIC than in low-grade chronic DIC.

Independent of whether or not thrombosis occurs, a bleeding tendency develops the more readily as the consumption of clotting factors, fibrinolytic enzymes, and thrombocytes exceeds their production. Production may be hampered by bone marrow failure and liver disease. Consumption is favored by any condition that promotes the DIC process, including paralysis of the RES, low plasma antithrombin-III (AT-III) concentrations, acidosis, anoxia, anoxemia, stasis, and shock.

Paralysis of the RES, as may occur from endotoxinemia or immunosuppression, inhibits the removal of particulate matter, activated clotting enzymes, and FM, thus allowing for continuous generation of fibrin. It also inhibits the removal of FDPs and microthrombi.

Antithrombin-III is the principal physiologic anticoagulant, which acts against all proteolytic clotting factors of the intrinsic pathway. It is produced by

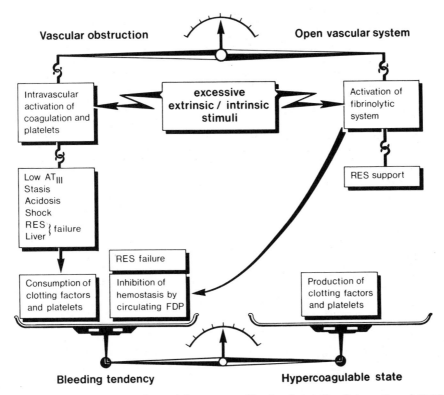

Figure 1. Pathogenesis of DIC. (From Slappendel, R. J.: Vet. Clin. North Am. [Small Anim. Pract.] 18:173, 1988.)

the liver, and it is essential for the action of heparin, both endogenous and exogenous. Low AT-III concentrations enhance clotting and thus DIC. AT-III may be reduced in patients with liver disease, nephrotic syndrome, and hereditary AT-III deficiency, and following L-asparaginase therapy or prolonged heparin administration. AT-III is consumed during the coagulation process; hence AT-III deficiency may also result from DIC itself.

Metabolic and respiratory acidosis enhance DIC because low pH inhibits heparin and its cofactor AT-III.

Anoxia and anoxemia enhance DIC because they result in anaerobic glycolysis and hence acidosis.

Stasis prevents the removal of activated clotting enzymes and debris and the supply of AT-III and heparin. It also causes local anoxemia and hypercapnia and hence acidosis. Stasis may ultimately damage the endothelium, which provides new surfaces for contact activation, and may cause necrosis of other tissues and hence *de novo* release of thromboplastic substances.

Shock enhances DIC, because most of the previously mentioned DIC-promoting conditions are present in patients with shock. Indeed, DIC is often associated with hypotension and shock. Not only may shock easily induce DIC, but DIC may also result in shock. Obstruction of significant parts of the microcirculation and hypovolemia from blood loss may be involved in the induction of shock by DIC. In addition, severe vasomotor reactions can

be induced by interactions of the activated clotting and fibrinolytic systems and the kallikrein-kinin system and by the release of vasoactive agents from triggered thrombocytes.

DIC is often associated with hemolysis. Thrombi that are generated in the lumina of small blood vessels of patients with DIC may be abnormally loose and remain permeable, probably because thrombocytopenia impedes blood clot retraction. Red blood cells that are forced through these clots by blood pressure may fold themselves around the thin fibrin strands and thereby be cut into fragments. The membranes of these fragments reseal and the remaining "fragmentocyte" or "schistocyte" may continue to circulate in the blood for some time. Wholesale fragmentation of red blood cells results in frank hemolysis, as has been described in human patients with DIC-associated diseases such as the hemolytic-uremic syndrome and thrombotic thrombocytopenic purpura.

Blood smears from dogs with DIC may contain few fragmentocytes. Yet the association of DIC and frank hemolysis rarely indicates DIC-induced hemolysis, but rather hemolysis-induced DIC. The red blood cells that are damaged in hemolytic patients release thromboplastic materials and hence promote DIC. In addition, acute hemolysis readily causes hepatic necrosis. This stimulates DIC even more, as liver cells are rich in thromboplastic materials and clotting enzymes. Hemolysis thereby induces a hypercoagulable state, which may easily turn into frank DIC with conditions such as stasis, acidosis, or shock. Thus DIC, shock, and hemolytic anemia may operate in concert to constitute a series of pathogenetic vicious circles (Fig. 2).

CLINICAL FEATURES

The consumption of platelets and clotting factors plus the antihemostatic properties of FDPs creates a potential bleeding tendency, which may be occult except for the results of laboratory tests or may result in frank hemorrhages. The latter may be petechiae, ecchymoses, epistaxis, melena, hematuria, intraocular bleedings, or accumulation of free blood in the abdomen or the thorax. Prolonged bleeding from venipuncture sites or following surgery or other trauma may also focus attention on the presence of DIC. Sometimes, the only clinically appreciable sign of DIC consists of persistent bleeding from a minor defect in the skin or mucosa, caused by some trivial, often unnoticed trauma.

Fibrin deposits trapped in the microcirculation may block capillary flow in an organ, with resulting ischemic tissue damage and clinical evidence of organ dysfunction. Clinical signs are mainly related to abnormal functioning of the kidneys, the liver, the gastrointestinal tract, the lungs, or the central nervous system. The kidney is particularly vulnerable to ischemic damage. Lesions may vary in severity from reversible tubular necrosis to complete irreversible bilateral cortical necrosis. The latter should be suspected whenever intravenous fluid therapy increases central venous pressure without restoring urine flow in a dog with DIC, anuria, and shock (Fig. 3).

LABORATORY DIAGNOSIS

With the pathogenesis of DIC in mind (see Fig. 1), its laboratory features are quite understandable. In patients with fulminant manifestations of the syndrome, the preliminary clinical diagnosis can usually be confirmed simply by the combination of thrombocytopenia and grossly abnormal blood clot formation and lysis.

In less severe DIC, the diagnosis may be much more difficult. Depending on which components of the hemostatic and fibrinolytic systems are depleted and depending on the way in which the various equilibria are disturbed, results of laboratory tests may vary from disease to disease, from patient to patient, and from moment to moment. No generally available tests are diagnostic by themselves, and correct interpretation of the results of a number of tests is required.

The following combination of relatively simple tests is recommended:

INSPECTION OF A STAINED BLOOD SMEAR. The detection of fragmentocytes supports a preliminary clinical diagnosis of DIC. However, fragmentocytes may be rare or absent, even in cases of fulminant DIC. Moreover, fragmentocytes must be distinguished from other causes of abnormal red blood cell morphology and may be present in a number of conditions not associated with DIC.

The inspection of a stained blood smear is also an appropriate method to detect severe thrombocytopenia, provided the blood is properly collected in ethylenediaminetetra-acetic acid (EDTA) by clean venipuncture.

PLATELET COUNT. Thrombocytopenia is present in many conditions that are not associated with DIC, but it is difficult to entertain a diagnosis of DIC in the presence of a (persistently) normal platelet count.

OBSERVATION OF BLOOD CLOT FORMATION AND LYSIS IN A GLASS TUBE. In fulminant DIC, the blood may fail to clot or a small piece of fibrin may appear in the clotting tube. If the tube is agitated the fibrin may be dislodged and lost among the red blood cells, giving an erroneous impression that fibrinolysis has taken place. If there is doubt concerning the size of the clot, the contents should be poured gently into a Petri's dish so that the clot may be more readily observed. In the absence of fibrinolysis a normal clot will not dissolve within 1 hr. This test can easily be performed, but the result will only be positive in case of severe depletion of clotting factors, strong fibrinolytic activity, or both.

PLASMA FIBRINOGEN ASSAY. Plasma fibrinogen is usually low in DIC but may be normal or even high from compensatory overproduction in low-grade chronic DIC. High fibrinogen concentrations may also be expected in patients in which DIC is preceded by inflammatory conditions, because inflammation increases fibrinogen production. Apart from DIC, low plasma fibrinogen level may indicate liver disease, subacute blood loss, and hereditary hypofibrinogenemia.

In patients suspected of having DIC, plasma fibrinogen is most appropriately assayed by clotting techniques. Assays based on the heating of plasma or on chemical methods precipitate soluble FMs and FDPs in addition to fibrinogen and may therefore overestimate the fibrinogen concentration. In patients treated with heparin, neutralizing protamine sulfate should be added to the sample before testing.

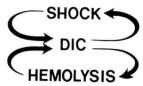

Figure 2. Pathogenetic relation among DIC, shock, and hemolysis.

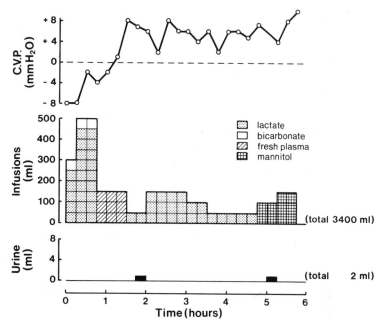

Figure 3. Fluid therapy in a dog with heat stroke, shock, and DIC. Note persistent anuria despite normal and even high central venous pressure (CVP).

FIBRIN DEGRADATION PRODUCT TEST. A commercial test kit (Thrombo-Wellco kit, Wellcome Reagents Ltd.) containing latex particles coated with rabbit antihuman FDP antiserum provides an easy and rapid agglutination technique for semiquantitative assay of serum FDP in dogs. For the exact test procedure, the reader is referred to the instruction booklet provided with the test kit. An FDP concentration of 10 μg/ml or more is considered evidence of increased fibrinolytic activity, but FDP may also be slightly increased in liver disease and in patients with internal bleeding or hematomas. Slight increases of FDP that are not associated with one of these conditions or with additional laboratory findings of DIC most probably indicate "silent" or "compensated" DIC. Close observation and careful follow-up of these patients is mandatory.

A negative test result does not rule out DIC, especially not in patients with low-grade DIC or those with low plasma fibrinogen concentrations. In those patients, soluble FM is generated in relatively small amounts, which may be cleared from the circulating blood by the RES before fibrinolytic degradation can occur. In addition, FDP fragments may complex with fibrinogen or FMs that retain thrombin-binding sites; hence these FDPs are removed during the preparation of serum for the test.

TESTS FOR FIBRIN MONOMERS. Soluble FM can be demonstrated in the plasma by the protamine gelation test, which is performed by adding 0.05 ml of protamine sulfate (10 gm/L) to 0.5 ml of citrated test plasma. If soluble FM is present in sufficient amounts, a feathery fibrin network or fine fibrin threads will form within 5 min. (The presence of amorphous material only is considered a negative result by some investigators [Dacie and Lewis,

1984].) Positive results may be obtained in many disorders in which the occurrence of DIC is uncertain. False-negative test results may also frequently be obtained, even in dogs with fulminant DIC.

A more sensitive and rather simple method to demonstrate soluble FM is the use of a commercially obtainable FM agglutination test (FM-test, Boehringer-Mannheim GmbH, Mannheim, West Germany). The FM reagent consists of a suspension of human red blood cells coated with FM from human fibrinogen. The FM test result is negative in normal dogs and almost always positive in those with DIC. As with the protamine sulfate test, positive results may be obtained in situations in which the presence of DIC is equivocal. Incorrect test results may easily be obtained if the blood has not been drawn carefully, as this may cause thrombin generation, hence FM formation *in vitro*.

CLOTTING STUDIES. The activated partial thromboplastin time (APTT), the prothrombin time (PT), and the thrombin time (TT) are prolonged in the great majority of patients with clinically evident DIC. The APTT is the most sensitive, the TT the most specific, of the three tests. APTT is prolonged when factor V or factor VIII is less than 15 to 20 per cent of normal, when prothrombin is less than 10 per cent, or when fibrinogen is less than 90 mg/100 ml. TT is prolonged when thrombin is inhibited by FDP (or heparin!) but also when plasma fibrinogen level is low. A Reptilase test (Boehringer-Mannheim GmbH, Mannheim, West Germany) rather than a TT should be performed to follow the course of DIC in patients treated with heparin. Unlike thrombin, Reptilase is not inhibited by heparin.

ANTITHROMBIN-III ASSAY. AT-III assays are not

yet available for use in veterinary practice but can be performed in any routine clinical chemistry laboratory. Low plasma AT-III concentration is a common finding in DIC and a rather specific diagnostic criterion, provided the patient is not under treatment with heparin and plasma albumin level is normal. Prolonged heparin administration reduces circulating AT-III, and reduced production or loss of albumin is usually associated with reduced production or loss of AT-III.

THERAPY

The most important and universally accepted principle in the treatment of patients with DIC is the prompt identification and elimination of the underlying trigger mechanisms. As long as the initiating cause has not been removed, the treatment of DIC will at best be only temporarily effective. If the primary disease that causes DIC cannot be cured, it is rarely warranted or even possible to keep the diseased animal alive. However, the diagnosing of the underlying disease or the fruition of a specific therapy may take time. Meanwhile DIC must be combated as well as possible to limit its deleterious consequences. In some instances, removal of the trigger *per se* may even be insufficient to stop progression of DIC, as DIC may sustain itself, especially when associated with shock.

Thus the first measure to be taken in patients with DIC is prompt and energetic combating of all unfavorable conditions that may promote DIC. This means the correction of acid-base imbalance, hypovolemia, dehydration, and shock. In addition, measures may be necessary to relieve respiratory and circulatory problems and to prevent or eradicate secondary infections.

Often no specific therapy other than supportive measures need be instituted when the trigger is minor, as in some acute postsurgical hemorrhagic episodes. In the event of severe DIC-induced bleeding, the transfusion of blood, fresh or fresh-frozen plasma, or platelet concentrates may be indicated.

Plasma expands intravascular volume and substitutes for depleted clotting factors and AT-III. Fresh whole blood also replaces lost red blood cells in patients with acute blood loss or anemia. The effect of a blood transfusion on the platelet count is usually minimal. The administration of platelet concentrates is much more effective in that respect and should be considered when thrombocytopenia seems to contribute significantly to the bleeding tendency. Plasma rather than whole blood should be given to normovolemic nonanemic patients, as plasma proteins are thereby substituted in lower volume loads. Moreover, this eliminates problems associated with

blood group incompatibility and hence possible hemolysis that might promote DIC. There is no need to fear that treatment with blood or plasma will otherwise exacerbate rather than cure DIC.

To enhance the effect of the transfused AT-III, the donor blood or plasma is incubated with heparin before transfusion (see below).

There is some controversy about the efficacy of heparin in treating DIC. Favorable, even dramatic effects, as well as disappointing results, have been documented, but objective evaluation of therapy in spontaneous DIC is hardly possible. Heparin exerts its maximal anticoagulant effect by combining with AT-III. The heparin-antithrombin complex inhibits a number of proteolytic enzymes, including plasmin and many clotting factors. It can rapidly neutralize free thrombin and retard or stop its further formation. To exert maximal effect, heparin should be administered in a dose that prolongs APTT by 1.5 to 2.0 times. This mostly suppresses hemostatic system activity in DIC. However, the regulation of the dose and prevention of hemorrhage is difficult even with frequent 24-hr monitoring of APTT, which is absolutely mandatory. The activated clotting time (ACT) test has also been promoted because it is easier to perform, but this test is inaccurate in DIC. Actually, the safest and most reliable way to monitor heparin therapy is the frequent determination of the plasma heparin concentration by a specific assay. This can hardly ever be realized in veterinary practice.

Good therapeutic responses have been documented with reduced dosages of heparin and even with minimal dosage regimens that do not significantly prolong the coagulation time. A minimal dosage regimen is effected by the administration of 5 to 10 IU/kg/hr by continuous intravenous drip or 75 IU/kg every 8 hr by the subcutaneous route (*not* 5 to 10 IU/kg SC, as probably erroneously recommended in some veterinary publications). Monitoring by APTT or other test is not necessary and the risk of inducing bleedings is almost negligible, although heparin may sometimes induce thrombocytopenia.

The effect of heparin is highly dependent on AT-III, which is often depleted in patients with DIC. Therefore, the transfusion of heparinized fresh blood or plasma is the best way to start heparin therapy after pH has been corrected and tissue perfusion restored as well as possible. The addition of a single relatively high dose of heparin to the blood or plasma (i.e., 75 IU/kg of body weight) may arrest the ongoing clotting process yet hardly contribute to the bleeding tendency, as heparin is rapidly eliminated from the circulation. Subsequently, administration of minidoses of heparin may sustain normalized hemostasis.

Once started, administration of heparin should be continued without interruption at regular intervals until DIC has completely disappeared. Waning levels of anticoagulant may otherwise cause rebound effects that intensify the clotting process. Anticoagulants other than heparin are not appropriate for the treatment of DIC.

Antiplatelet drugs such as aspirin are not an established therapy for DIC in human medicine but have been proposed for the treatment of DIC in dogs. In most DIC-associated diseases, platelet aggregation seems to be secondary to thrombin generation, which is not inhibited by aspirin. It is conceivable, however, that the administration of low doses of aspirin (10 mg/kg every other day) might be beneficial in patients in which DIC is primarily triggered by severe endothelial lesions, as in generalized vasculitis or heartworm disease.

In the author's opinion, platelet-inhibiting drugs should never be given to heparinized patients nor to patients in which DIC is associated with severe hypocoagulability. Elimination of platelet function deprives such patients of their last potential to arrest bleedings.

The long-term administration of corticosteroids blocks RES function and hence promotes DIC. Thus corticosteroids should be used only when essential for the treatment of the underlying disease, as in chronic active hepatitis or allergic vasculitis. A single intravenous injection of a high dose of corticosteroid in conjunction with other therapeutic measures, as has been propagated for the correction of shock, is not contraindicated in case of DIC.

References and Supplemental Reading

Abe, T., and Yamanaka, M. (eds.): Disseminated intravascular coagulation. Bibl. Haematol. 49, 1983.

Dacie, J. V., and Lewis, S. M.: *Practical Haematology*, 6th ed., Edinburgh: Churchill Livingstone, 1984.

Feldman, B. F., Carroll, E. J., and Jain, N. C.: Coagulation and its disorders. In Jain, N. C. (ed.): *Schalm's Veterinary Hematology*, 4th ed. Philadelphia: Lea & Febiger, 1986, pp. 388–430.

Slappendel, R. J. Disseminated intravascular coagulation. Vet. Clin. North Am. [Small Anim. Pract.] 18:169, 1988.

Wintrobe, M. M.: *Hematology*, 8th ed. Philadelphia: Lea & Febiger, 1981.

DISORDERS OF PLATELETS

BERNARD F. FELDMAN, D.V.M.
Davis, California

An adequate number of normally functioning platelets is essential not only to arrest hemorrhage after obvious vascular injury but also to prevent the leakage of red blood cells from apparently uninjured vessels. Failure of these two aspects of hemostasis is expressed, respectively, by a prolonged bleeding time and spontaneous appearance of purpuric lesions. These hallmarks of platelet disorders are also observed with various vasculitides. Purpura indicates extravasation of red blood cells from blood vessels into the skin and subcutaneous tissues. Petechiae are small pinpoint purpuric lesions, and ecchymoses are larger and usually deeper purpuric lesions. Disorders of both platelet numbers and function are relatively common. It is conventional and convenient to consider these under the general topics of thrombocytopenia, thrombocytosis, and abnormalities of function (see below). It must be emphasized that such a classification is not exclusive: in many disorders involving platelet number, both hereditary and acquired, the platelets are also functionally defective. For example, in uremia as well as in thrombocythemia, hemorrhage may be attributable to both types of abnormality.

The most common signs of hemorrhage in platelet disorders are spontaneous skin and mucous membrane petechiae and ecchymoses, epistaxis, and multiple small subcutaneous bruises. These types of lesions are seen at flexures and pressure points and in relation to scratch marks. Large spreading hematomas are extremely rare, and hemarthroses almost never occur. Conjunctival and retinal hemorrhages are also rare. Bleeding from superficial cuts and grazes tends to be mild but prolonged. This is evaluated in a semiquantitative manner by the bleeding time. In severe cases bleeding is apt to occur from venipuncture and injection sites.

PHYSIOLOGY

Effective hemostasis depends on the normal functioning of its vascular, platelet, and coagulation components. Vascular injury is followed by reflex and humorally stimulated vascular contraction. As a consequence of vascular injury, platelets exposed to subendothelial tissues are stimulated to undergo a series of release reactions, leading to the formation

Table 1. *Sequence of Hemostasis*

1. Endothelial injury resulting in vascular constriction
2. Platelet adhesion to the subendothelium
3. Platelet production of thromboxane A_2 and adenosine diphosphate release (this reaction is modulated by endothelial prostacyclin [PGI_2] production)
4. Platelet aggregation at the site of injury
5. Hemostatic plug formation
6. Stabilization of the hemostatic plug by fibrin (coagulation cascade activity)
7. Fibrinolysis

of a primary platelet plug. Activation of the coagulation cascade, a sequence of enzymatic reactions, results in fibrin formation and stabilization of the platelet plug (Table 1).

Platelets undergo three basic reactions: adherence, secretion (or release), and aggregation. Platelets represent cytoplasmic fragments of megakaryocytes. They are enclosed in a lipid bilayer cell membrane that is punctuated by a series of invaginations. These produce the open canalicular system, which increases the platelet surface area for uptake and release of substances that participate in platelet reactions. Beneath the cell membrane are filamentous structures providing support and possessing contractile properties important for platelet shape change and secretion. The cell membrane contains various functionally important receptors and phospholipids. A specific glycoprotein, GPI_b, serves as a receptor for von Willebrand factor (VWF), which mediates adherence. Another glycoprotein, $GPII_bIII_a$, mediates platelet aggregation.

The platelet cytosol contains two important types of granules, alpha- and delta- (or dense body) granules. The alpha-granules contain platelet-specific proteins, including platelet factor-4 (heparin-neutralizing factor), platelet-derived growth factor, beta-thromboglobulin, and coagulation factor V and fibrinogen. The delta-granules are storage granules for adenosine diphosphate (ADP), adenosine triphosphate (ATP), serotonin, and calcium.

Platelet adherence to collagen is mediated by VWF and other proteins, including fibronectin and fibrin. Blood flow and shear stress also determine the degree of *in vivo* adherence. There is evidence that arachidonic acid from the platelet membrane is activated, initiating prostaglandin formation. Thromboxane A_2 (TxA_2) is generated via prostaglandin metabolism and transports calcium from the delta-granules via the tubular system to the actin-myosin complex of platelets; consequently, platelets undergo a shape change and release their granular contents. Following release the platelets expose the $GPII_bIII_a$ complex, which mediates aggregation (recruitment) of other platelets. The simultaneous activation of a normally functional coagulation cascade is required to strengthen the primary platelet plug. Otherwise, hemostasis is likely to break down and bleeding may occur.

THROMBOCYTOPENIA (Table 2)

Deficient or Ineffective Thrombopoiesis

HYPOPLASIA OF MEGAKARYOCYTES

Thrombocytopenia as the result of inadequate platelet production can usually be attributed to toxic agents that cause decrease in thrombopoiesis, as well as overall hematopoiesis. Chemotherapeutic agents are the most common cause of this form of thrombocytopenia, but other drugs certainly can precipitate megakaryocytic hypoplasia (Table 3). Therapy includes removing the offending drug and supportive care.

Bone marrow infiltration (myelophthisis) by various neoplasms can lead to thrombocytopenia by interfering with thrombopoiesis. Hematologic neoplasia typically involves the bone marrow, and many forms of neoplasia can metastasize to the bone marrow. Granulomatous infectious diseases also can invade the bone marrow. Thrombocytopenia is also

Table 2. *Classification of Thrombocytopenia by Pathogenesis*

I. Defective platelet production
   A. Aplasia or hypoplasia of megakaryocytes
      1. Genetic
         a. Fanconi's anemia
         b. Pure megakaryocytic aplasia
      2. Acquired
         a. Chemical or physical agents
         b. Aplastic pancytopenia
         c. Viral infections (including feline leukemia virus)
   B. Dysthrombopoiesis
      1. Vitamin B_{12} or folate deficiency (*rare*)
      2. Myeloproliferative disorders
      3. Secondary to malignant infiltration of bone marrow
      4. Uremia
   C. Disorders of thrombopoietic control mechanisms
      1. Thrombopoietin deficiency
      2. Cyclic thrombopoiesis
II. Diminished platelet survival
   A. Immune mechanisms
      1. Antibodies
         a. Idiopathic
         b. Drug-induced
         c. Associated with immune-mediated hemolytic anemia
         d. Systemic lupus erythematosus
         e. Lymphoid neoplasia
      2. Miscellaneous
         a. Hypersensitivity reactions to vaccines, foods, and so on
         b. Acute postinfective thrombocytopenia
   B. Excessive platelet consumption
      1. Disseminated intravascular coagulation
      2. Microangiopathic processes (e.g., hemolytic-uremic syndrome)
      3. Thrombotic thrombocytopenic purpura
      4. Acute infections
III. Loss of platelets from the systemic circulation
   A. Redistribution (splenomegaly)
   B. Loss from the body due to hemorrhage (mild thrombocytopenia)

Table 3. *Thrombocytopenia Due to Drugs*

1. Bone marrow suppression
   a. Predictable and dose-related
      Cytotoxic drugs
      Estrogens
      Heparin
      Phenylbutazone
      Gold compounds
      Organic arsenicals
      Chloramphenicol
      Streptomycin
      Dilantin
   b. Occasional
      Sulfonamides
      Phenobarbital
      Primidone
2. Immune mechanisms
   Arsenicals
   Sulfonamides
   Chlorthiazides
   Digitoxin
   Quinine, quinidine

observed as part of aplastic pancytopenic disorders resulting from stem cell defects, humoral immune suppression of thrombopoiesis, or a defective bone marrow microenvironment. Therapy must be directed toward the primary inciting problem.

INEFFECTIVE THROMBOPOIESIS

Abnormalities of thrombopoiesis are encountered in myeloproliferative or myelodysplastic (preleukemic) disorders and rarely can result from vitamin B_{12} or folate deficiency, deficiencies also associated with chemotherapeutic agents. The diagnosis of ineffective thrombopoiesis is based on bone marrow examination. In a well-prepared aspirate an average of at least 2 megakaryocytes per low-power field in an area of adequate bone marrow spicules will indicate adequate megakaryocytopoiesis. In the presence of ineffective platelet production the megakaryocyte number may be increased. However, the morphologic findings may be abnormal, with smaller cells, decreased nuclear lobes, and nuclear and cytoplasmic asynchrony (Table 4).

Therapy for active bleeding in these thrombocytopenic states or prophylactic therapy when the risk of hemorrhage is high involves platelet transfusion. When a unit of whole, anticoagulated blood is centrifuged at low speed (170×9 g; it is critical that plasma be removed at 1-min intervals from 1 to 5 min), the smaller platelets remain in the plasma fraction, which can be transferred as platelet-rich plasma. A 250-ml unit of blood, when fractionated into platelet-rich plasma, can increase the platelet count by 5000 to 10,000 platelets per microliter in the average-sized dog.

Thrombocytopenia Due to Accelerated Destruction or Abnormal Distribution of Platelets

Accelerated destruction of platelets is a common cause of thrombocytopenia. In this situation megakaryocytes are increased, as is platelet production, but platelet survival is reduced. Circulating platelets tend to be larger and younger in age. Younger platelets are more hemostatically effective.

IMMUNOLOGIC THROMBOCYTOPENIA

Immunologic thrombocytopenia can be caused by exposure to antibodies or immune complexes. Antibodies alter the platelet membrane, which is recognized as abnormal. Platelet destruction by the mononuclear phagocyte system results. Platelet antibodies are either autoantibodies, which occur in autoimmune diseases, or isoantibodies, which occur in sensitization to foreign antigens. Drug-induced platelet antibodies are not primarily directed against platelet membranes. The platelet behaves as an innocent bystander and is sensitized by the attachment of the drug-carrier protein complex to its membrane. This complex then stimulates antibody production. Immune complexes can also cause thrombocytopenia by attaching to the platelet membrane, resulting in platelet destruction by the mononuclear phagocyte system.

The most common form of immunologic thrombocytopenia is idiopathic. Idiopathic thrombocytopenia appears to be caused by platelet antibody. Sensitized platelets are removed by macrophages primarily in the spleen. The spleen is also the major source of antibody-producing cells. Most of these patients have increased bone marrow megakaryocyte activity. Idiopathic thrombocytopenia can be acute or chronic (Table 5). Severe bleeding and splenomegaly rarely occur.

Ehrlichia canis and *E. platys* are rickettsial organisms. *E. canis* morulae can be found in monocytes and cause thrombocytopenia, pancytopenia, or both. The vector is the *Rhipicephalus sanguineus*

Table 4. *Causes of Isolated Thrombocytopenia*

Megakaryocytic hypoplasia
   Idiopathic
   Drug-related
   Systemic lupus erythematosus
Platelet destruction, utilization, or loss
   Immunologic
      Drug-related
      Idiopathic
      Systemic lupus erythematosus
      Post-transfusion (*rare*)
   Non-antibody-mediated
      Infections
      Hemolytic-uremic syndrome
      Intravascular coagulation
Splenic pooling

Table 5. *Clinical Features of Canine Immune-Mediated Thrombocytopenia*

Age	Generally older than 18 months
Sex predilection	Females slightly more than males
Presentation	Varies but may be acute
Type of bleeding	Petechiae, ecchymoses, epistaxis
Location	Mucous membranes, flexion areas, pressure areas, abdomen
Onset of bleeding	Insidious but may be acute
Serious bleeding	Uncommon
Severe anemia	Rare
Preceding illness	Common in acute, uncommon in chronic
Palpable spleen	Rare
Platelet count at onset	Usually less than 20,000–30,000
Clinical course	Weeks in acute form; years (lifetime in chronic form)

tick. *Ehrlichia* morulae found in neutrophils and eosinophils are associated with *E. equi* and cause transient and mild canine disease. *E. platys* is found in platelets and causes thrombocytopenia. Thrombocytopenia and cell line deficits are generally considered to result from immunologic dysfunction, though specific bone marrow depression has not been completely ruled out. Specific diagnosis is accomplished with serologic evaluation. The organisms are sensitive to tetracycline therapy.

DIAGNOSIS (Table 6). Bleeding associated with immunologic thrombocytopenia rarely is severe. In fact, severe anemia associated with thrombocytopenia suggests a second disorder such as immune-mediated hemolysis. Hemorrhage alone almost never accounts for clinically significant thrombocytopenia, and clinically significant thrombocytopenia rarely occurs above 30,000 platelets per microliter. Platelet counts less than this number invariably indicate a bone marrow production defect (this almost always occurs as a multiple cytopenia or pancytopenia) or increased platelet destruction. Bone marrow aspiration biopsy is always indicated

and is rarely associated with more than mild bleeding at the aspiration site.

Immunologic thrombocytopenia is indicated by the platelet factor-3 (PF-3) test or the antimegakaryocytic antibody test. The PF-3 test utilizes the patient's citrated plasma, which is mixed with washed platelets from a normal donor. Patient antibody activity against platelet membrane antigens releases PF-3, catalyzing the coagulation cascade. A shortening of the activated partial thromboplastin time (APTT) is an indication of antibody-induced PF-3 release.

Antimegakaryocytic antibody testing is accomplished on the patient's bone marrow smear. The smear is exposed to a fluorescent antibody produced against species-specific immunoglobulins. Fluorescence of megakaryocytes indicates a positive reaction.

THERAPY. Glucocorticoids are indicated initially in immunologic thrombocytopenia, but definitive responses are uncommon. There is no physiologic reason for using one form of glucocorticoid over another. Prednisone is usually given at doses of 1 to 2 mg/kg/day in the mornings. The lower dosage is preferred. Combination immunosuppressive therapy includes such agents as azathioprine and cyclophosphamide. Although azathioprine may take 3 to 4 days to become effective, it is the preferred immunosuppressive agent because of the relative infrequency of side effects and the temporal indication of its success. In combination with prednisone, it is administered and tapered at the same dosage as prednisone. Prednisone and cyclophosphamide have also been used with a modicum of success. Persistent cyclophosphamide therapy carries the risks of severe bone marrow depression and acute and sometimes uncontrollable hemorrhagic cystitis. Cyclophosphamide can be administered at 50 mg/m² of body surface area (1.5 mg/kg for dogs heavier than 25 kg, 2 mg/kg for dogs weighing 5 to

Table 6. *Tests Associated with Platelets*

Test	Factors Involved	Comments
Clot retraction	Platelet aggregability and coagulant activity	Nonspecific and insensitive test of platelet numbers and function
Buffy coat	Leukocytes, platelets	Uppermost cream-colored area represents platelets
Blood smear	All blood cells	12–24 platelets/oil immersion field is normal
Bone marrow	Megakaryocytes	Examination of megakaryocyte number and morphology
Buccal mucosal bleeding time	Vascular integrity, platelet count, platelet function	Screening test of platelet numbers and function, vascular integrity
Platelet aggregometry	Platelet function	Various platelet agonists used to stimulate *in vitro* aggregation (requires *fresh* blood)
Platelet adhesion	Von Willebrand factor	Nonspecific test of platelet adhesion and von Willebrand factor
Platelet factor-3 (PF-3) test	Platelet phospholipid	Indicator of immune-induced platelet injury and PF-3 release
Antimegakaryocytic antibody test	Bone marrow megakaryocytes	Direct or indirect test of immunoglobulin on megakaryocytes

25 kg, and 2.5 mg/kg for dogs weighing less than 5 kg) and is given once daily for 4 days of each week of therapy until a clinical response is achieved (1 to 4 weeks). Therapy should be continued, though with tapering doses, for at least 3 months. Many patients with acute disease will respond quickly, whereas chronic or insidious immunologic thrombocytopenic patients may require a lifetime of intermittent therapy. Depression of white blood cell counts to less than 5000/μl requires temporary cessation of azathioprine or cyclophosphamide.

Vincristine is never indicated as a first drug choice. It is indicated only when other forms of therapy have not been successful and only when bone marrow aspiration indicates adequate megakaryocytopoiesis. Vincristine is used at 0.02 mg/kg intravenously once a week and is discontinued when the platelet count returns to and remains at a satisfactory concentration. Vincristine often dramatically, but transiently, increases the platelet count. It is a mitotic spindle poison, interferes with phagocytosis, and seems to have an *in vivo* stimulatory effect on thrombopoiesis.

Danazol, an attenuated androgen, has shown promise of being effective in controlling the immune-mediated and idiopathic thrombocytopenias. The drug is given at a dosage of 75 mg/kg q12h PO in combination with immunosuppressive doses of prednisone.

Splenectomy is generally thought to be of value when all other forms of therapy have failed. Whereas splenectomy may not return the platelet count to normal, it has been associated with more rapid remissions in patients that have relapsed. Splenectomy has been more successful with immune-mediated hemolytic anemia.

Success is indicated when the platelet count remains over 75,000/μl. Increasing dosages or persistent high-dose therapy in an attempt to return the platelet count to some predetermined "normal" range is contraindicated and often futile. Many patients with chronic, immune-mediated thrombocytopenia will never have more than transiently "normal" platelet counts. The therapeutic question becomes one of which is more important, the platelet count or the patient's physical well being. Physical well being and client satisfaction are often achieved at lower than normal platelet counts.

NONIMMUNOLOGIC THROMBOCYTOPENIA

Thrombocytopenia is occasionally associated with certain types of systemic infections. The pathophysiology is multifactorial and includes direct effects of bacteria on platelets and indirect effects on platelets by means of immune reactions and vascular damage.

Activation and consumption of platelets in disseminated intravascular coagulation (DIC) is secondary to the activation of coagulation and formation of thrombin and intravascular fibrin thrombi on which platelets are consumed.

In a similar syndrome, thrombotic thrombocytopenic purpura (TTP), platelets are aggregated by an unknown stimulus and are consumed directly, resulting in intravascular platelet thrombi that behave in the same manner as intravascular fibrin thrombi and predispose to further thrombocytopenia. The TTP syndrome is complex. Evidence suggests that either a platelet-aggregating factor may be present or there is a deficiency in vascular prostaglandin I$_2$ (prostacyclin) production. Another possibility is an abnormal VWF. The clinical presentation of TTP includes thrombocytopenia, hemolytic anemia, transient neurologic abnormalities, fever, and renal failure. Hemolytic-uremic syndrome has a similar pathophysiology but primarily affects the kidneys.

Under normal circumstances the spleen contains approximately one third of the total platelet mass. In the presence of splenomegaly a larger percentage of platelets may be sequestered in the spleen, leading to a condition called hypersplenism. Hypersplenism occurs when there is diffuse hepatic disease and has been described in hepatic lymphoma. Platelets not only are sequestered in this condition but also show reduction in survival. All three cell lines may be involved, and occasionally splenectomy is necessary to reverse the developing cytopenias.

INCREASED PLATELET NUMBERS

An elevated platelet count, a count beyond the reference interval, can result from various clinical disorders and is referred to as reactive thrombocytosis (Table 7). In reactive thrombocytosis, results of tests of platelet function including bleeding time and measurements of platelet adhesion and aggregation (see Table 6) are generally normal, and patients do not have clinical hemorrhage or thrombosis.

In contrast, the platelet count can be autonomously elevated in myeloproliferative disorders. In myeloproliferative disorders results of platelet function tests are frequently abnormal and there is some tendency toward hemorrhage and thrombosis. There does not seem to be a correlation between platelet number and clinical manifestations. However, poorly functioning platelets predispose to hemorrhage and paradoxically to thrombosis. Neither the platelet number nor the platelet function measurements predict the degree of thrombosis or hemorrhage.

Clinically, the hemorrhagic signs include mucosal and particularly gastrointestinal bleeding, hematomas, and ecchymoses. Splenic, portal, and mesen-

Table 7. *Increased Platelet Counts*

Reactive thrombocytosis
  Exercise
  After acute hemorrhage
  Iron deficiency (late iron deficiency may result in thrombocy-
    topenia)
  Rebound: recovery from thrombocytopenia
Myeloproliferative disorders
  Essential thrombocythemia (thrombocytosis is predominant
    feature)
  Myelofibrosis (thrombocytosis is accompanying feature)
  Myeloid metaplasia (thrombocytosis is accompanying feature)
  Chronic myelocytic leukemia (thrombocytosis is accompany-
    ing feature)
Associated with spleen
  After splenectomy
  Splenic dysfunction
Miscellaneous
  Various neoplasias
  Chronic inflammatory gastrointestinal disorders
  Acute and chronic infections
  Vinca alkaloids
  Corticosteroids

teric vein thromboses have been reported without pulmonary embolism.

In thrombocythemia, defective platelet function appears to be the main problem. Chemotherapy may depress the more dysplastic megakaryocytic clones and allow the more normally differentiating clones to deliver platelets. Alkylating agents such as melphalan (in increasing doses from 1.5 to 4.0 mg/m² of body surface area given daily for 7 to 10 days PO; no medication for 2 to 3 weeks) should be administered cautiously in an attempt to reduce platelet numbers. Alternatively, hydroxyurea at a dose of 590 mg/m² of body surface area daily for 3 days PO has been used successfully in dogs. This drug may cause severe and intractable megaloblastic anemia. Two-week cycles, on therapy and off therapy, will minimize this complication. Intravenous administration of radioactive phosphorus to a total of 9.8 μCi/m² body surface area may also be used. An ultralow aspirin dosage (0.5 mg/kg q12h) has proved to be most effective in inhibiting platelet aggregation if thrombosis is suspected of becoming a potentially complicating factor. Considering the number of patients with hemorrhagic diatheses, rather than thrombosis, the use of aspirin or other nonsteroidal anti-inflammatory agent requires some thought.

PLATELET DYSFUNCTION

The buccal mucosa bleeding time test is a useful screening procedure for the adequacy of platelet function, though it can also be prolonged with vascular disorders. The bleeding time is not prolonged until the platelet count falls below 75,000/μl. Practically, a prolonged buccal mucosa bleeding time, which accompanies a normal or near-normal platelet count, is the first laboratory indication of platelet dysfunction. The bleeding time measures a complex set of platelet reactions, including adhesion and release and also aggregation. A prolonged bleeding time due to platelet dysfunction can be either inherited or acquired. Inherited disorders are uncommon but by no means rare. Acquired disorders, especially those due to drugs, are commonly encountered but often are not recognized because bleeding time determinations are not routine.

Inherited Disorders of Platelet Function (Table 8)

VON WILLEBRAND'S DISEASE

Von Willebrand's disease (VWD) is a hemorrhagic disorder caused by deficiency of von Willebrand factor (VWF), a plasma protein required for normal platelet adhesion. The disease is considered to be the most common heritable bleeding disorder of dogs and has been observed in cats (see also p. 446).

At least two cell types, endothelial cells and megakaryocytes, are able to synthesize VWF. Platelets have VWF sequestered within and adsorbed to outer membranes. This represents a substantial proportion of total VWF. Von Willebrand factor is necessary for the normal adhesion of platelets to exposed subendothelium of injured blood vessels. A secondary function is to stabilize factor VIII (hemophilia factor, hemophilia A factor, factor VIII:C). The combination of VWF and factor VIII:C is known as the factor VIII complex.

The laboratory evaluation of VWF usually depends on immune reactions between von Willebrand factor (the antigen, denoted VWF:Ag) and antibody to the antigen. For convenience the amount of VWF:Ag is reported as a percentage compared with a standard curve determined from pooled plasma arbitrarily assigned a value of 100 per cent. VWF:Ag concentrations of less than 60 per cent are considered to be abnormally low, although, in general, there is little correlation between the VWF:Ag concentration and bleeding tendencies. Some patients with modest decreases

Table 8. *Hereditary Platelet Disorders*

Disorder	Defect
Canine	
Von Willebrand's disease	Membrane defect—defect in adhesion
Canine thrombasthenic thrombopathia	Primary aggregation defect
Canine hereditary thrombopathia	Intrinsic signal transduction defect (aggregation defect)
Feline	
Chédiak-Higashi syndrome	Deficient release reaction

exhibit a bleeding tendency (von Willebrand's disease), and others with severe deficiencies do not exhibit bleeding tendencies (von Willebrand's trait).

The buccal mucosa bleeding time test is the best screening measure for hemorrhagic tendency in VWD (normal, 1.7 to 4.2 min). Many dogs with VWD are prone to mucosal or cutaneous hemorrhage, epistaxis, and hemorrhagic complications associated with surgical procedures.

Diseases associated with VWD include hypothyroidism, panosteitis, aplastic pancytopenia, and numerous neonatal problems, including fading puppy syndrome and exaggerated response to parvoviral disease.

The medical management of VWD includes transfusion therapy with whole blood, fresh or fresh-frozen plasma, or cryoprecipitate that contains concentrated factor VIII complex, fibronectin, and fibrinogen. Treatment with thyroid medications at the same dosage used for hypothyroid patients (even in euthyroid patients) will be successful in some patients, though tachyphylaxis may occur. The use of deamino-D-arginine-vasopressin (DDAVP) has also been successful in some canine patients when given daily for 3 to 4 days only. Bleeding VWD patients are given 1 μg/kg subcutaneously. Donor plasma VWF may be increased by injecting the donor with DDAVP at the dosage above, 30 min before obtaining the donor unit.

CANINE THROMBASTHENIC THROMBOPATHIA

Canine thrombasthenic thrombopathia is an autosomally inherited disorder occurring in otterhounds. Platelets from affected dogs fail to aggregate in response to physiologic stimuli and do not support clot retraction. These features are similar to Glanzmann's thrombasthenia and Bernard-Soulier syndrome in humans. Clinical signs are associated with mucosal bleeding and are exacerbated by stress. Platelets may be reduced or normal in number and exhibit deficits in both adhesion and aggregation.

CANINE THROMBOPATHIA

Canine thrombopathia is an autosomal defect of basset hounds attributable to abnormal cyclic adenosine monophosphate (c-AMP) metabolism. Platelets have increased intracellular c-AMP, which results in deficient ADP storage or secretion and platelet aggregation. In fact, most platelet agonists fail to aggregate these platelets, the notable exception being thrombin. Clot retraction is supported in contrast to the situation in canine thrombasthenic thrombopathia. Clinical signs are similar to those of this latter disease. Hematomas of the ears are

common. It should be noted that VWD is also commonly observed in basset hounds, and owners often ask their veterinarians to test for "that basset hound bleeding disorder."

Acquired Disorders of Platelet Function (Table 9)

These disorders are associated with the following diseases:

UREMIA. The major cause of bleeding associated with uremia is platelet dysfunction, but the cause is multifactorial. Bleeding associated with uremia includes epistaxis and bleeding into fascial planes, body cavities, and the gastrointestinal tract. Bleeding times are often prolonged, as are platelet aggregation studies. The biochemical abnormalities are consistent with deficiencies of thromboxane production due to functional cyclo-oxygenase deficiency resulting from the accumulation of several uremic metabolites, including urea, guanidinosuccinic acid, phenol, phenolic acids, and "middle molecules."

DYSPROTEINEMIA. Prolongation of bleeding time, decreased platelet adhesion, and aggregation are associated with myeloma. When immunoglobulin concentrations return to normal, platelet function returns.

HEPATIC DISEASE. The effects of hepatic disease are multifactorial. Severe diffuse liver disease often results in hypersplenism owing to shunting of hepatic blood to splenic vessels, resulting in thrombocytopenia. Diffuse liver disease is associated with defective coagulation protein synthesis and also with defective clearance of fibrin/fibrinogen degradation products, which interfere with platelet function.

MYELOPROLIFERATIVE DISEASE. Myeloproliferative disorders are associated with mucosal hemorrhage and hematomas, prolonged bleeding time, and biochemical defects indicating deficits in platelet granular storage of ADP.

Table 9. *Underlying Conditions in Acquired Platelet Dysfunction*

Myeloproliferative syndrome
  Thrombocythemia
  Chronic myelogenous leukemia
  Myelofibrosis
Chronic renal disease with uremia
Cardiomyopathy
Macroglobulinemia
Myeloma
Drugs (see Table 10)
Diseases associated with platelet hyperaggregability
  Nephrotic syndrome
  Hyperadrenocorticism
  Diabetes mellitus
Systemic lupus erythematosus
Hepatic disease
Hypothyroidism
Disseminated intravascular coagulation—fibrin degradation
  product interference

PANCREATITIS. Platelet aggregation in the presence of arachidonic acid, ADP, and collagen is decreased. Platelet dysfunction in pancreatitis is thought to be the result of fibrin/fibrinogen degradation products interfering with platelet function and "platelet exhaustion."

EHRLICHIOSIS. Experimental canine ehrlichiosis results in modest thrombocytopenia and significant decreases in mean platelet adhesiveness. There was no correlation between platelet numbers and adhesiveness in dogs with reduced complement levels. There was a correlation between platelet numbers and platelet adhesiveness in dogs with normal complement concentrations, and dogs with normal complement concentrations had more severe thrombocytopenia.

DRUG-INDUCED PLATELET DYSFUNCTION. The more common cause of prolonged bleeding time due to platelet dysfunction results from an acquired defect, most often caused by drugs (Table 10). Acquired disorders of platelet function affect the platelet reactions of adhesion, release, and aggregation. Frequently, acquired disorders interfere with more than one of these reactions, whereas congenital defects are more restricted in their pathophysiology. It is critical to have knowledge about drug-platelet interactions, in that they may seriously complicate the course of disease in patients already compromised with thrombocytopenia or hereditary or acquired thrombocytopathy.

ASPIRIN AND OTHER NONSTEROIDAL ANTI-INFLAMMATORY AGENTS. Aspirin irreversibly acetylates and inactivates the enzyme cyclo-oxygenase, preventing the generation of prostaglandin intermediates and TxA_2. The effect, which renders the platelet nonfunctional for its life span, occurs only with acetylsalicylic acid and not with nonacetylated forms of aspirin. These platelets no longer undergo release, bleeding time is prolonged, and aggregation is poor to absent. It may take 7 to 10 days for production of new platelets to normalize the bleeding time. Because aspirin also affects cyclo-oxygenase in endothelial cells, it interferes with endothelial cell antiaggregatory prostacyclin production. The inhibitory effect on endothelial cells requires higher doses of aspirin, and the effect is short because endothelial cells can regenerate prostacyclin.

Other nonsteroidal anti-inflammatory drugs cause similar cyclo-oxygenase defects, but the effects are reversible and last only as long as the drug is in circulation.

OTHER DRUGS. Low-molecular-weight dextran is readily cleared from the circulation, but the higher-molecular-weight forms may persist in the circulation for days, interfering with platelet surface reactions, including adhesion and aggregation. The bleeding time will be prolonged.

A number of antibiotics, including penicillin and trimethoprim-sulfonamide, have been shown to interfere with platelet aggregation and prolong bleeding times.

Modified live-virus vaccines have been associated with both thrombocytopenia and thrombocytopathy. Disorders occur within 1 to 3 weeks subsequent to the vaccination.

Table 10. *Drugs That Interfere with Platelet Function*

Class	Examples
Antibiotics	Penicillin and derivatives, nitrofurantoin, sulfonamides
Antihistamines, antitussives	Diphenhydramine and others, glyceryl guaiacolate
Anti-inflammatory agents	Aspirin and other nonsteroidal anti-inflammatory agents, corticosteroids, gold salts
Antithrombotic agents	Heparin, dextran
Cardiovascular drugs	Digoxin, digitoxin, hydralazine
Diuretics	Furosemide
Prostaglandins	Prostaglandin E, PGD_2, PGI_2
Sympathetic blocking agents	Alpha-blockers (e.g., phentolamine), beta-blockers (e.g., propranolol)
Tranquilizers	Phenothiazines, diazepam
Vaccines	Modified live-virus vaccines
Volume expanders	Dextran
Xanthine derivatives	Theophylline, caffeine, dipyrimadole

References and Supplemental Reading

Catalfamo, J. L., and Dodds, W. J.: Inherited and acquired thrombopathias. Vet. Clin. North Am. [Small Anim. Pract.] 18:185, 1988.

Davenport, D. J., Breitschwerdt, E. B., Carakostos, M. C., et al.: Platelet disorders in the dog and cat. Part I. Physiology and pathogenesis. Comp. Cont. Ed. Pract. Vet. 4:762, 1982.

Davenport, D. J., Breitschwerdt, E. B., Carakostos, M. C., et al.: Platelet disorders in the dog and cat. Part II. Diagnosis and management. Comp. Cont. Ed. Pract. Vet. 4:788, 1982.

Handagama, P., Feldman, B. F., et al.: Mean platelet volume artifacts: The effects of anticoagulants and temperature on canine platelets. Vet. Clin. Pathol. 15:13, 17, 1986.

Handagama, P., and Feldman, B. F.: Immune-mediated thrombocytopenia in the dog. Canine Pract. 12:25, 1985.

Handagama, P., and Feldman, B. F.: Drug-induced thrombocytopenia. Vet. Res. Commun. 10:1, 1986.

Jergens, A. E., Turrentine, M. A., Kraus, K. H., et al.: Buccal mucosal bleeding time of healthy dogs and dogs in various pathologic states including thrombocytopenia, uremia, and von Willebrand's disease. Am. J. Vet. Res. 48:1337, 1987.

Johnson, G. S., Turrentine, M. A., Kraus, K. H., et al.: Canine von Willebrand's disease. Vet. Clin. North Am. [Small Anim. Pract.] 18:195, 1988.

Thomason, K. J., and Feldman, B. F.: Immune-mediated thrombocytopenia: Diagnosis and treatment. Comp. Cont. Ed. Pract. Vet. 7:569, 1985.

CYTOCHEMISTRY OF CANINE AND FELINE LEUKOCYTES AND LEUKEMIAS

N. C. JAIN, M.V.Sc.

Davis, California

Cytochemical characteristics of leukocytes are being increasingly utilized in cytologic diagnosis of leukemias, particularly undifferentiated and acute (blast cell) leukemias in which cell morphology in Romanowsky-stained blood and bone marrow smears is not distinctive. Enzyme cytochemistry delineates specific cellular features that may be used to differentiate acute lymphocytic leukemia (ALL) from acute myelogenous leukemia (AML) and to subclassify AML. Considerable information on human cytochemistry is available (Bennett, 1982), and similar observations are being made on various animal species (Jain, 1986). The following is a brief discussion of normal cytochemical characteristics of blood and bone marrow leukocytes of the dog and cat and their application to diagnosis of leukemias in these animal species. The interested reader is referred to the supplemental reading for further details.

CYTOCHEMISTRY OF NORMAL BLOOD AND BONE MARROW CELLS

Table 1 lists observations on common cytochemical reactions of blood and bone marrow cells of the dog and cat. Specific comments about these and some other cytochemical reactions in various animal species and humans are briefly mentioned below. Techniques for staining blood and bone marrow smears for these cytochemical reactions can be found elsewhere (Jain, 1986).

Peroxidase (PO) activity is seen in neutrophils of all species and in eosinophils of most species. A few PO-positive granules may be seen in monocytes of some species. Lymphocytes in all species and eosinophils and basophils of the cat are PO negative. Although platelets and megakaryocytes in blood and bone marrow appear PO negative by light microscopy, a PO-like activity has been demonstrated in these cells in humans by electron microscopy.

Sudanophilic granules are present in neutrophils of various species and in eosinophils of all animals but the cat. Monocytes may stain negatively or have a few sudanophilic granules. Sudanophilia and PO positivity are found together in neutrophils, eosinophils, and monocytes of most species, although in the granulocytic precursors sudanophilia may manifest prior to the PO positivity. Lymphocytes are Sudan negative.

Mature neutrophils of the dog and cat are normally deficient in alkaline phosphatase (ALP) activity in contrast to the neutrophils of other common domestic animal species and humans. Eosinophils and basophils may reveal some ALP activity, but monocytes and lymphocytes are uniformly ALP negative. Hence, in the dog and cat, a careful differentiation of eosinophils and basophils is essential to avoid confusing them with ALP-positive neutrophils. Some myeloid precursors (5 to 10 per cent) in normal canine and feline bone marrow smears may show ALP activity, but the enzyme activity decreases with cell maturation so as to be absent in neutrophilic metamyelocytes through segmenters.

Leukocyte esterases differ with regard to their substrate specificities, pH optima, sensitivity to inhibitors, and pattern of cytoplasmic distribution. Monocytes contain two substrate specific esterases, viz., alpha-naphthyl acetate esterase (ANAE), which is demonstrated by using alpha-naphthyl acetate as a substrate, and alpha-naphthyl butyrate esterase (ANBE), which is demonstrated by using alpha-naphthyl butyrate as a substrate. Both of these enzymes are also referred to as nonspecific esterases (NSEs), and the NBE has also been referred to as lipase.

Nonspecific esterases are characteristically found in monocytes, macrophages, megakaryocytes, and platelets. Eosinophils, basophils, and lymphocytes may stain negatively or show some positive reaction, whereas neutrophils are generally negative. The pattern of NSE staining reaction has been used to differentiate monocytes and lymphocytes and to characterize certain subpopulations of human lymphocytes, although observations vary with regard to the latter. Lymphocytes generally show NSE activity as a coarse granular or spotlike staining with focal, circular, or semicircular distribution, whereas monocytes and their precursors usually have a diffuse localized staining. The esterase activity in monocytes is inhibited by sodium fluoride, whereas that in lymphocytes is not.

Neutrophils contain one substrate-specific esterase demonstrable by using naphthol AS-D chloroacetate and is referred to as chloroacetate esterase

Table 1. Cytochemical Reactions of Normal Canine and Feline Blood and Bone Marrow Cells

Cell Type	Peroxidase	Sudanophilia	Alkaline Phosphatase	Nonspecific Esterase	Chloroacetate Esterase	PAS Reaction
Unclassified cells	−	−	+	−	−	−
Myeloblasts	−	−	−	−	−	−
Promyelocytes	+	+	+†	−	+	±
Neutrophilic						
Myelocytes	+	+	+†	−	+	±
Metamyelocytes	+	+	−	−	+	±
Bands	+	+	−	−	+	+
Segmenters	+	+	−	−	+	+
Eosinophils						
Immature cells	±*	±*	+	−	+	±
Mature cells	±*	±*	±	−	±§	±
Basophils						
Immature cells	−	−	−	−	+	+
Mature cells	−	−	±	−	+	+
Lymphocytes	−	−	−	±‡	−	±
Monocytes	±	±	−	+	−	±
Macrophages	−	−	−	+	−	±
Erythroid cells	−	−	−	−	−	−
Megakaryocytes	−	−	−	±	−	±
Platelets	−	−	−	±	±	±

−, negative; +, positive; ±, positive or negative reaction.
*Positive in the dog and negative in the cat.
†Cells difficult to identify.
‡Resistant to inhibition by NaF.
§Negative in the dog and positive or negative in the cat.

(CAE). The CAE staining pattern in neutrophils parallels that of sudanophilia and peroxidase reaction. Eosinophils are CAE negative, but mast cells and feline basophils show strong CAE activity.

The periodic acid–Schiff (PAS) staining technique is used to demonstrate glycogen in leukocytes. Neutrophils show PAS positivity generally as fine granularity and occasionally as a few large coarse granules. Lymphocytes, monocytes, and eosinophils may either stain negatively or show a faint diffuse to granular staining. Platelets contain small PAS-positive granules, and megakaryocytes reveal a diffuse PAS-positive reaction. Staining intensity of myeloid cells increases with cell maturation, with the myeloblast being PAS negative, the promyelocyte and myelocyte being weakly positive, and the mature neutrophil being highly PAS positive.

CYTOCHEMICAL MARKERS OF LEUKEMIAS

Table 2 lists cytochemical criteria commonly used in classification of leukemias. Absence of peroxidase staining in lymphoid cells is utilized as a feature for differentiation of ALL from AML. Myeloblasts are normally PO negative, but in AML a proportion may reveal some PO activity. In some human patients with myelogenous leukemias, particularly during blast crisis of chronic myelogenous leukemia (CML), and in some cases of monoblastic leukemias, PO activity can be demonstrated only by electron microscopy. Peroxidase activity may be decreased in preleukemic syndromes, and it may even be absent in some neutrophils of patients with myelogenous leukemia and in neutrophils with toxic gran-

ulation. A reduction in or absence of PO activity may be seen in neutrophils of dogs with myelogenous leukemia and leukocytoses from other causes. Because of PO-negative staining on light microscopy, leukemic myeloblasts may resemble lymphoblasts, but PO activity in such blast cells can be demonstrated by electron microscopy.

Cytochemical staining of leukocytic ALP in humans has been used to differentiate CML from leukemoid reactions associated with nonmalignant causes. ALP activity is generally markedly decreased or absent in the former, whereas it is normal or remarkably increased in the latter. However, ALP activity is often increased in CML patients in blast crisis and during bacterial infection, pregnancy, and remission following treatment. Myelogenous leukemia occurs in the dog and cat. Neutrophils in these two species normally lack ALP activity and stain negatively also in patients with reactive leukocytosis accompanied by left shift from nonmalignant causes. In contrast, some to many ALP-positive mature and immature neutrophils may be found in blood of dogs and cats with myelogenous and myelomonocytic leukemias. Bone marrow smears of such patients usually contain an increased number of ALP-positive immature neutrophils, including blast cells. These findings indicate that staining blood and bone marrow smears of canine and feline patients for ALP activity is valuable in differential diagnosis of AML, although rare instances of ALP-negative AML may be encountered in both species.

Clinical application of NSE and CAE has been in differential diagnosis of AML, acute myelomonocytic leukemia (AMMOL), and acute monoblastic leu-

Table 2. Cytochemical Reactions in Canine and Feline Leukemias

Cytochemical Marker	Lymphocytic Leukemia	Myelogenous Leukemia	Monocytic Leukemia	Myelomonocytic Leukemia
Peroxidase	−	+	− ‡	+
Sudanophilia	−	+	− ‡	+
Alkaline phosphatase	−	+ †	−	+
Nonspecific esterase	− *	−	+	+
Chloroacetate esterase	−	+	−	+
PAS reaction	±	±	±	±

−, negative; +, positive; ±, positive or negative reaction.
*Occasionally + but resistant to inhibition by NaF.
†Rarely negative.
‡Sometimes weak +.

kemia (AMOL). The presence of blasts or immature cells reactive for NSE, either ANAE or ANBE, is considered suggestive of monocytic involvement, whereas the presence of CAE-positive cells suggests neutrophilic involvement, and a combination of both enzyme markers is indicative of myelomonocytic leukemia. In comparison with PO activity and sudanophilia, CAE activity is considered to be more specific for neutrophils. Species differences should be given consideration in this respect, for a weak CAE activity may be found in equine and ruminant monocytes.

The pattern of cytoplasmic PAS reactivity has been utilized to characterize acute leukemias in humans. Coarse granular or blocklike staining has been observed in a variable number of lymphocytes and lymphoblasts in ALL, whereas leukemic myeloblasts and monocytes have been found to give a diffuse, fine-dust-like PAS-positive reaction. PAS positivity has been detected in erythroid precursors in patients with erythroleukemia. PAS positivity has not been seen in erythroid precursors in feline patients with erythemic myelosis and erythroleukemia and in lymphocytes in canine and feline cases of acute and chronic lymphocytic leukemias.

In summary, myeloid leukemias can be distinguished from lymphocytic leukemias based on reactivity for ALP, PO, esterases, and Sudan black B (see Table 2). Neutrophils and their precursors stain for PO and CAE and exhibit sudanophilia, forming the basis for recognition of myeloid leukemia. In the dog and cat, increased neutrophil ALP may be considered predictive of myeloid leukemia because it is usually increased during myelogenous and myelomonocytic leukemias but not in leukemoid reactions. Monocytes and their morphologically recognizable precursors are identified by strong diffuse cytoplasmic reactivity for ANAE or ANBE, weak or no PO activity, variable sudanophilia, and absence of ALP and CAE reactions. Diagnosis of myelomonocytic leukemia entails finding enzymatic markers of both cell lineages. Lymphocytes and lymphoblasts are uniformly negative or exhibit little reaction for these cytochemical markers, except NSE. NSE activity in lymphoid cells varies with their

subclass and is resistant to inhibition by sodium fluoride; the pattern of staining is often distinctive (focal or coarsely granular) compared with that in monocytes (diffuse cytoplasmic staining). Azurophilic cytoplasmic granules in leukemic blast cells are generally considered indicative of a myeloid differentiation, but occasionally they may also be found in lymphoid cells, particularly natural killer (NK) cells. Such granular lymphoid cells give negative reactions for PO and CAE and are not sudanophilic.

Several other cytochemical markers of leukocytes have been studied in humans for characterization of leukemias, but their diagnostic significance remains relatively less defined. Enzyme markers such as acid phosphatase, terminal deoxynucleotidyl transferase, 5′-nucleotidase (5′-NP), adenosine deaminase (ADA), beta-glucuronidase, and purine nucleoside phosphorylase have been used to characterize lymphoid malignancies. The 5′-NP and ADA have also been used to investigate primary immune deficiencies. The diagnostic significance of elevations in serum lysozyme concentrations in AMOL and AML has been investigated in humans and some animal species. Acetylcholinesterase is a specific marker of megakaryocytes in the dog and cat.

It should be realized that, although certain specific cytochemical properties have been delineated for various hematopoietic cells and their malignancies, leukemogenesis may induce cytochemical heterogeneity, making it difficult to consistently predict the proper cell lineage. For example, PO-deficient neutrophils may be found in myelogenous leukemia and a subnormal number of NSE-positive monocytes may be seen in monocytic leukemia. It is because of such singular observations that a cytochemical profile is developed using multiple cytochemical criteria, and newer cell markers are constantly sought for differential diagnosis of hematopoietic malignancies. It is emphasized that a specific cytochemical finding is seldom suggestive of a neoplastic process *per se*; most often it discriminates only the cell lineage and to a certain extent cell maturity. In view of the lack of specific morphologic and positive cytochemical criteria for precise identification of lymphoid cells, immunologic markers are being increasingly used in diagnosis of lymphoma and lymphocytic leukemias in humans. Development of similar reagents in veterinary medicine is forthcoming.

References and Supplemental Reading

Bennett, J. M.: Leukemia morphology and cytochemistry. *In* Gunz, F. W., and Henderson, E. S. (eds.): *Leukemia*, 4th ed. Orlando: Grune & Stratton, 1982, pp. 463–486.

Facklam, N. R., and Kociba, G. J.: Cytochemical characterization of leukemic cells from 20 dogs. Vet. Pathol. 22:363, 1985.
Grindem, C. B., Stevens, J. B., and Perman, V.: Cytochemical reactions in cells from leukemic cats. Vet. Clin. Pathol. 14:6, 1985a.
Grindem, C. B., Stevens, J. B., and Perman, V.: Cytochemical reactions in cells from leukemic dogs. Vet. Pathol. 23:103, 1985b.
Jain, N. C.: *Schalm's Veterinary Hematology*, 4th ed. Philadelphia: Lea & Febiger, 1986, pp. 909–939.
Jain, N. C., Madewell, B. R., Weller, R. E., et al.: Clinical-pathological findings and cytochemical characterization of myelomonocytic leukaemia in 5 dogs. J. Comp. Pathol. 91:17, 1981.
Sun, T., Li C-Y., and Yam, L. T.: *Atlas of Cytochemistry and Immunochemistry of Hematologic Neoplasms*. Chicago: American Society of Clinical Pathologists Press, 1985.
Tsujimoto, H., Hasegawa, A., and Tomoda, I.: A cytochemical study on feline blood cells. Jpn. J. Vet. Sci. 45:373, 1983.

ACUTE PHASE PROTEINS

N. C. JAIN, M.V.Sc.
Davis, California

Acute phase (AP) proteins are plasma proteins whose synthesis is rapidly and markedly increased in response to tissue injury. Most of the AP proteins are glycoproteins, and almost all are produced by the liver parenchymal cells. They vary markedly in carbohydrate content and electrophoretic mobility. Acute phase proteins include a variety of functionally diverse plasma proteins normally present in blood in small quantity and some detectable in blood in appreciable amounts only after a response to injury. Principal AP proteins and some of their characteristics are listed in Table 1. Other AP proteins include ferritin, certain proteases, and complement components such as C3. AP proteins are investigated in clinical situations because they are believed to be a better indicator of systemic response to inflammatory processes and infections than are some of the other variables, such as fever, increased erythrocyte sedimentation rate, and leukocytosis associated with neutrophilia. Most of the literature on AP proteins concerns studies on humans and laboratory animals (see reviews by Engler and Mege, 1986; Fischer and Gill, 1975; Koj, 1985; Schreiber, 1987), whereas observations on common domestic animals are meager.

CHANGES IN ACUTE PHASE PROTEINS

The magnitude of change in the plasma concentrations of AP proteins varies with the type of injury and the extent of tissue damage. Minor inflammatory conditions may cause only a small increase, whereas marked increases may be seen in severe inflammatory conditions. The response of individual proteins differs greatly and prominent species variability exists in such a response (Koj, 1985). For example, in humans concentrations of C-reactive protein (CRP) and serum amyloid A (SAA) may increase by 20- to 1000-fold; alpha$_1$-antichymotrypsin (ACh), alpha$_1$-antitrypsin (AT), alpha$_1$-acid glycoprotein (AGP), fibrinogen, and haptoglobin may increase by two- to fivefold; and ceruloplasmin may increase by only 30 to 60 per cent. Marked increases are seen in CRP and SAA in humans, whereas such elevations occur in mice only in SAA, in rabbits in CRP, and in rats in AGP and alpha$_2$-macroglobulin (MG). In addition, plasma concentration of another acute phase protein, alpha$_1$-acute phase protein, increases in rats by 10- to 20-fold (Engler and Mege, 1986). Concentrations of some plasma proteins (such as albumin and transferrin) may decrease within hours of an acute inflammatory episode owing to leakage in tissues from increased vascular permeability. These proteins have been referred to as "negative" acute phase reactants.

In general, the synthesis of AP proteins is stimulated within 6 to 8 hr after an injury, and peak levels are attained within 2 to 5 days. For example, after uncomplicated surgery (i.e., surgery without infection) in humans, increased synthesis of CRP and ACh was evident within 8 hr and maximal values were apparent within 2 days. Rise in fibrinogen, haptoglobin, AGP, and AT levels was seen by 24 hr, with peak values within 3 to 5 days (Aronsen et al., 1972). Ceruloplasmin showed a delayed response, whereas MG did not change significantly. Transferrin diminished initially and then showed a delayed increase. During convales-

Table 1. Characteristics of Acute Phase Proteins

Protein	Electrophoretic Mobility	Molecular Weight	Normal Serum Content (mg/dl)	Half-life (days)	Biologic Function
C-reactive protein	Alpha$_1$-globulin	110,000	< 0.8	< 2.0	Regulation of inflammatory process and microbial defense
Alpha$_1$-acid glycoprotein (orosomucoid)	Alpha$_1$-globulin	39,500	55–140	5.2	Modulation of hemostasis, binds drugs
Alpha$_1$-antitrypsin	Alpha$_1$-globulin	54,000	180–260	3.9	Protease inhibition
Alpha$_1$-antichymotrypsin	Alpha$_1$-globulin	68,000	30–60	—	Protease inhibition
Serum amyloid A	Alpha$_1$-globulin	11,000	< 2.0	—	Amyloid precursor
Ceruloplasmin	Alpha$_2$-globulin	151,000	15–60	4.25	Copper carrier, oxidase activity
Haptoglobin	Alpha$_2$-globulin	80,000–160,000	83–267	3.5	Binds free hemoglobin
Alpha$_2$-macroglobulin	Alpha$_2$-globulin	820,000	150–350	—	Protease inhibition, macroglobulin transport of hormones
Fibrinogen	Beta-globulin	341,000	200–450	3.2	Coagulation
Transferrin	Beta-globulin	76,000	200–400	8.7	Transport of iron
Hemopexin	Beta-globulin	57,000	50–115	—	Binds oxidized heme

Data compiled from human literature (Fischer and Gill, 1975; Koj, 1985; Ritzmann and Finney, 1983).

cence some AP proteins such as CRP and AGP decline to normal levels rapidly within 1 week, whereas others such as fibrinogen, AT, haptoglobin, and ceruloplasmin may take 2 to 3 weeks to attain normal levels. Persistent elevations of AP proteins may be seen in chronic inflammatory conditions, but values observed are usually lower than those attained during acute inflammatory conditions (Sipe, 1985b). Recurrent acute inflammatory episodes may be associated with progressively lower responses in AP proteins, as reported for changes in CRP concentrations in rabbits given repeated intramuscular injections of turpentine (Macintyre et al., 1982). It should be noted that conditions influencing the catabolism, extravascular leakage, and tissue deposition of a particular AP protein may influence its peak and persistent serum concentration. For example, disseminated intravascular coagulation (DIC) and fibrinolysis may diminish fibrinogen concentration, and intravascular hemolysis may reduce the concentration of haptoglobin and hemopexin in face of an acute phase response.

CONDITIONS ASSOCIATED WITH INCREASES IN ACUTE PHASE PROTEINS

Increased production of AP proteins in response to various forms of tissue injury has been demonstrated in humans and laboratory animals, and their clinical significance has been evaluated in studies on humans (Fischer and Gill, 1975; Morley and Kushner, 1982). Conditions commonly associated with elevations of AP proteins are listed in Table 2. Levels of some AP proteins (fibrinogen, ceruloplasmin, and AT) may increase during gestation. The concentrations of AP proteins and their responses have been found to differ in the human neonate as compared with the adult.

In general, the increase in AP proteins is a nonspecific response to injury in that there is no disease specificity. Different AP proteins vary in their response to tissue damage, with some being more sensitive (CRP and SAA) indicators than the others (AGP and ceruloplasmin). Hence, measurement of several AP proteins or a serum protein profile (e.g., a panel consisting of CRP, AGP, AT, and haptoglobin determinations) may be more meaningful than making observations on a single protein. C-reactive protein, AGP, AT, and haptoglobin increase markedly in bacterial infections, whereas viral infections result in small increases in CRP and AG and moderate increases in AT and haptoglobin (Fischer and Gill, 1975). Determination of AP proteins is particularly important when total and differential leukocyte counts may not reflect the underlying disease process, as in neutropenic patients with bone marrow suppression, in surgical cases with septic complications, and in cattle with chronic inflammatory conditions. Sequential changes in various AP proteins may be of prognostic value and may be useful to monitor convalescence and evaluate therapeutic responses. Antimicrobial and corticosteroid therapy decrease CRP concentrations in humans by suppressing the inflammatory response (Laurent, 1982), although considerable species variations occur in hormonal influences on responses to AP proteins (Koj, 1985). Nonsteroidal anti-inflammatory drugs generally do not influence the response of AP proteins (Laurent et al., 1984).

REGULATION OF SYNTHESIS

Available evidence indicates that mediators originating from the site of injury are transported to the liver to stimulate the hepatocytes to synthesize and release various AP proteins (Fig. 1). The chief

Table 2. *Conditions Associated with Increases in Acute Phase Proteins*

Acute and chronic inflammatory conditions
Bacterial infections
Endotoxemia
Surgeries
Trauma
Burns
Malignancies
Myocardial infarction
Neonatal infections
Organ transplantations
Viral infections
Certain parasitic infections
Pregnancy

cytokine implicated in such a systemic response to injury is interleukin-1 (IL-1) produced by macrophages responding to products of tissue damage and bacterial infection (Mortensen, 1986; Sipe, 1985a). Another protein, a monokine called hepatocyte-stimulating factor (HSF), produced by activated blood monocytes, has been shown to stimulate fibrinogen synthesis by hepatocytes (Sipe, 1985b). The inter-relationship of IL-1 and HSF and their mechanisms of action remain to be elucidated. IL-1 is a family of low-molecular-weight (12,000 to 16,000) polypeptides exhibiting a broad range of activities on the immune system and other body tissues. Its production is induced under a variety of conditions associated with induction of AP responses. Mononuclear phagocytes *in vitro* begin to synthesize IL-1 within an hour in response to such stimuli.

QUANTITATION OF ACUTE PHASE PROTEINS

Acute phase proteins in serum or plasma can be rapidly and accurately quantitated using radial immunodiffusion (RID), electroimmunodiffusion (EID), and nephelometric techniques. Semiquantitative estimation of CRP can be done using a less sensitive latex agglutination test. Fibrinogen concentration can be rapidly estimated using a refractometer. Acute phase proteins can also be measured in other body fluids such as cerebrospinal fluid and synovial fluid to detect localized responses to inflammatory and infectious processes such as meningitis and arthritis, respectively.

OBSERVATIONS ON ACUTE PHASE PROTEINS IN VETERINARY MEDICINE

Fibrinogen has been investigated in greater detail than any other AP protein. The following are broad normal values of plasma fibrinogen (mg/dl): cats, 50 to 300; dogs, horses, sheep, and pigs, 100 to 500; cattle, 300 to 700; and goats, 100 to 400 (Jain, 1986). Marked increases in fibrinogen concentrations are seen in inflammatory conditions, trauma, and neoplastic conditions. When both total plasma protein and fibrinogen concentrations are elevated, a total plasma protein–fibrinogen ratio is determined to differentiate AP responses in fibrinogen (ratio < 10:1) from increases in fibrinogen due to dehydration (ratio > 15:1).

Serum concentration of CRP in dogs is normally

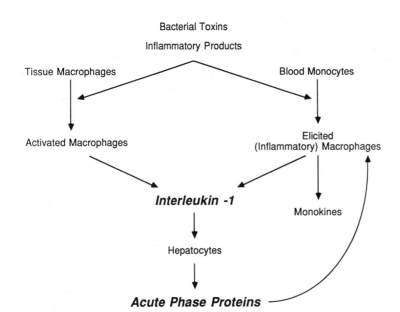

Figure 1. Cellular and molecular mechanisms involved in synthesis of acute phase proteins. (Modified from Mortensen *in* Bienvenu et al. (eds.): *Marker Proteins in Inflammation.* Vol. 3. Berlin: Walter de Gruyter & Co, 1986.)

less than 0.5 mg/dl, but it increases significantly within 4 hr of major surgery (Caspi et al., 1984). Canine CRP does not cross-react with human CRP.

Haptoglobin concentrations have been found to increase in cattle with infections, severe inflammatory conditions such as mastitis, pyometra and traumatic reticulitis, and abortions; in horses with infections; in sheep and goats with turpentine-induced inflammatory process; and in cats with abscesses, feline infectious peritonitis, and upper respiratory tract infections (Jain, 1986). Haptoglobin concentrations in cats increased following splenectomy and decreased after hemolysis associated with haemobartonellosis.

Prednisone administration in dogs induced increases in serum haptoglobin concentrations within 24 hr with a peak on the third day, and dogs with inflammatory diseases exhibited marked elevations in serum haptoglobin concentrations (Harvey and West, 1987). Changes in haptoglobin concentrations correlated highly with elevations in serum $alpha_2$-globulin levels in those dogs.

Serum ferritin and ceruloplasmin levels increased in Shetland ponies in response to turpentine-induced localized inflammation. Peak values were observed on the fifth or sixth day, and then a decline was seen, but values remained elevated for 1 to 3 weeks (Smith and Cipriano, 1987).

It is obvious from the above that AP proteins have not received much attention in veterinary medicine. Their investigations in food and pet animal populations are expected to expand as specific reagents become available for immunologic assays of AP proteins in different species. Quantitation of AP proteins in clinical veterinary medicine is encouraged, particularly to evaluate systemic responses to inflammatory and infectious conditions.

References and Supplemental Reading

Aronsen, K. F., Ekelund, G., Kindmark, C. O., et al.: Sequential changes of plasma proteins after surgical trauma. Scand. J. Clin. Lab. Invest. 29(Suppl.):127, 1972.

Caspi, D., Baltz, M. L., Snel, F., et al.: Isolation and characterization of C reactive protein from the dog. Immunology 53:307, 1984.

Engler, R., and Mege, F.: Biochemical characteristics of acute phase proteins in the rat. In Bienvenu, J., et al. (eds.): Marker Proteins in Inflammation. Vol. 3. Berlin: Walter de Gruyter & Co., 1986, pp. 231–241.

Fischer, C. L., and Gill, C. W.: Acute phase proteins. In Ritzmann, S. E., and Daniels, J. C. (eds.): Serum Protein Abnormalities. Diagnostic and Clinical Aspects. Boston: Little Brown, 1975, pp. 331–350.

Harvey, J. W., and West, C. L.: Prednisone-induced increases in serum alpha₂-globulin and haptoglobin concentrations in dogs. Vet Pathol. 24:90, 1987.

Jain, N. C.: Schalm's Veterinary Hematology, 4th ed. Philadelphia: Lea & Febiger, 1986, pp. 104, 127, 141, 179, 209, 226, 240, 947–950, 960–962.

Koj, A.: Liver response to inflammation and synthesis of acute phase plasma proteins. In Gordon, A. H., and Koj, A. (eds.): The Acute Phase Response to Injury and Infection. New York: Elsevier, 1985, pp. 139–246.

Laurent, P.: Clinical usefulness of C-reactive protein measurement. In Allen, R. C., et al. (eds.): Marker Proteins in Inflammation. Berlin: Walter de Gruyter & Co., 1982, pp. 69–88.

Laurent, P., Delvil, A., Bienvenu, J., et al.: Effect of nonsteroidal anti-inflammatory drug (niflumique acide) on acute phase protein response. In Arnaud, P., Bienvenu, J., and Laurent, P. (eds.): Marker Proteins in Inflammation, Vol. 2. Berlin: Walter de Gruyter & Co., 1984, pp. 71–74.

Macintyre, S. S., Schultz, D., Kushner, I.: Biosynthesis of C-reactive protein. Ann. N.Y. Acad. Sci. 389:76, 1982.

Morley, J. J., and Kushner, I.: Serum C-reactive protein levels in disease. Ann. N.Y. Acad. Sci. 389:406, 1982.

Mortensen, R. F.: Mechanisms of induction of synthesis of serum amyloid P-component (SAP) by mouse hepatocytes in culture. In Bienvenu, J., et al. (eds.): Marker Proteins in Inflammation. Vol. 3. Berlin: Walter de Gruyter & Co., 1986, pp. 105–115.

Ritzmann, S. E., and Finney, M. A.: Proteins—synopsis of characteristics and properties. In Ritzmann, S. E., and Killingsworth, L. M. (eds.): Proteins in Body Fluids, Amino Acids, and Tumor Markers. Diagnostic and Clinical Aspects. New York: Alan R. Liss, 1983, pp. 415–455.

Schreiber, G.: Synthesis, processing, and secretion of plasma proteins by the liver and other organs and their regulation. In Putnam, F. W. (ed.): The Plasma Proteins. Structure, Function, and Genetic Control, 2nd ed. Vol. V. Orlando: Academic Press, 1987, pp. 293–363.

Sipe, J. D.: Interleukin 1 as a key factor in the acute phase response. In Gordon, A. H., and Koj, A. (eds.): The Acute Phase Response to Injury and Inflammation. New York: Elsevier, 1985a, pp. 23–35.

Sipe, J. D.: Interleukin 1 target cells and induced metabolic changes. In Gordon, A. H., and Koj, A. (eds.): The Acute Phase Response to Injury and Inflammation. New York: Elsevier, 1985b, pp. 51–68.

Smith, J. E., and Cipriano, J. E.: Inflammation-induced changes in serum iron analytes and ceruloplasmin of Shetland ponies. Vet. Pathol. 24:354, 1987.

ANTINEOPLASTIC AGENTS IN CANCER THERAPY

JAMES P. THOMPSON, D.V.M.

Gainesville, Florida

The recommendation to treat a patient with chemotherapy should be based on the likelihood that treatment will lead to cure, relief of pain or discomfort caused by the neoplastic disease, or prolongation of quality life. Anticancer chemotherapy should not be recommended unless one of these objectives can be met.

The use of anticancer drugs should be approached with caution, but they are not necessarily more dangerous than other commonly used medications such as insulin, digitalis, anesthetic agents, and carparsolate. However, the primary care clinician should have an understanding of (1) what constitutes a safe dose, (2) the best way to administer the agent, (3) the time course of life-threatening toxicity, (4) how the agent is cleared from the body, and (5) necessary dosage adjustments based on organ failure.

The antineoplastic agents have been commonly classified into six major categories: alkylating agents, antimetabolites, plant alkaloids, antitumor antibiotics, hormonal agents, and miscellaneous agents. This article will discuss the antineoplastic agents used in veterinary cancer medicine. For dosage regimens and expected toxicities, see the table on antineoplastic agents in the Appendix (p. 1367). Recommendations regarding dosage adjustments based on abnormalities in organ systems are presented in Table 1.

ANTINEOPLASTIC DRUGS

Alkylating Agents

The alkylating agents all are cell cycle nonspecific and their modes of action are similar; the major differences in activity between different alkylating agents rest not in biochemical mechanisms of action, but rather in the extent of drug absorption, rate of drug metabolism, and tissue affinity of the various agents. These drugs have been termed alkylating agents because their reactive chemical structure consists of an alkyl group (RCH_2CH_2+). The drugs are considered unifunctional or bifunctional, based on whether one or two separate alkyl groups exist, respectively. All alkylating agents establish covalent bonds with a variety of intracellular molecules, but evidence suggests that the alkylation of DNA bases produces the most extensive cytotoxic effects. The alkylating agents generally bind to the DNA base guanine and are capable of creating intra- and interstrand covalent cross-links in the DNA double helix. The net result is a disruption of normal DNA

Table 1. *Modification of Drug Dosages Based on Clinocopathologic Data*

Clinicopathologic Test Results	Drugs Requiring Dose Modification	Suggested Modification	
Hyperbilirubinemia	Doxorubicin Vincristine Vinblastine	*Bilirubin* >1.5 mg/dl > 3.0 mg/dl	*Decrease Dose* 50% 75%
Creatinemia	Methotrexate Cisplatin Bleomycin Hydroxyurea Cytoxan Triethylenethiophosphoramide	Decrease dose in proportion to decrease in creatinine clearance	
Neutropenia, thrombocytopenia, or both	Most drugs *Note:* Steroids, asparaginase, and bleomycin may be used with caution despite bone marrow suppression. Vincristine may be used in cases of thrombocytopenia without concurrent neutropenia	*Neutrophils* < 4000/μl < 2000/μl < 1000/μl	*Decrease Dose* 25% Discontinue Discontinue and add antibiotics
		Thrombocytes 80,000–150,000/ μl < 80,000/μl	*Decrease Dose* 25% Discontinue

472

synthesis and the inhibition of messenger RNA (mRNA) synthesis; the decreased mRNA synthesis produces a concurrent decrease in protein synthesis.

The alkylating agents generally cause leukopenia, thrombocytopenia, and anemia, with the nadir of leukocyte counts observed 7 to 14 days following treatment and recovery noted in an additional 7 to 14 days. Cyclophosphamide has been shown to induce a sterile form of hemorrhagic cystitis and has been associated with the development of transitional cell carcinoma of the bladder. Busulfan, cyclophosphamide, and chlorambucil have been associated with a rare form of bronchopulmonary dysplasia, leading to pulmonary fibrosis; cisplatin chemotherapy can cause nephrotoxicity. The mechanism of permanent tumor cell resistance to these particular agents is considered to be directly related to increased repair of drug-induced DNA damage (Table 2).

Because the mode of action of the alkylating agents is similar, tumor cells resistant to one agent generally are resistant to all of the various alkylating agents. It should be noted that tumor cell resistance to antineoplastic drugs is either temporary or permanent (Table 2). Temporary tumor cell resistance is related to either an inability of the drug to be delivered to the tumor bed or a lack of active tumor cell division. Permanent tumor cell resistance is the result of tumor cell adaptation and avoidance of the biochemical mechanisms leading to tumor cell death by the antineoplastic agents.

Antimetabolites

The antimetabolites all are considered cell cycle specific and affect the cell cycle in the DNA synthesis phase (S-phase specific). The antimetabolites are structurally quite similar to purine bases, to pyrimidine bases, or to folic acid. These antimetabolite molecules inhibit normal DNA synthesis through "feedback" inhibition or through competitive inhibition of specific enzymes needed to produce the DNA bases. Regardless of which mechanism of enzyme inhibition is utilized, the antimetabolites interfere with intracellular enzymes vital for the maintenance of cellular integrity. Toxicities induced by the antimetabolites generally include bone marrow suppression, gastroenteritis, and hepatotoxicity. Fluorouracil, a pyrimidine base analogue, has been demonstrated to induce cerebellar ataxia in dogs and severe neurotoxicity and death in cats. Fluorouracil is contraindicated in cats because of the severe side effects. Tumor cell resistance to these agents may be through decreased cell uptake of the drug, decreased cell activation of the drug, increased cell inactivation of the agent, increased quantities of cellular enzymes that effectively compete with the antimetabolites, altered cellular enzyme activity, or the utilization of an alternative metabolic pathway to produce required DNA bases.

Table 2. *Tumor Cell Resistance to Antineoplastic Agents*

Drug Resistance	Mechanism	Example
Temporary	Inability to enter affected body compartment	Blood-brain barrier
	Inability to diffuse into tumor mass	Tumor too large with poor blood supply
	Inability to interact with vital cell functions	Tumor cells resting in G_0-phase
Permanent	Decreased cell uptake	Methotrexate
	Increased excretion from cell	Doxorubicin
		Vincristine
		Vinblastine
		Dactinomycin
	Decreased drug activation	Mercaptopurine
		Thioguanine
		Fluorouracil
	Increased drug inactivation	Cytosine arabinoside
	Increased drug targets	Methotrexate
	Altered drug targets	Methotrexate
		Vincristine
	Decreased metabolic product required	Asparaginase
	Increased alternate pathway utilization	Antimetabolites
	Repair of drug-induced lesions	Alkylating agents
	Pleiotropic resistance	Doxorubicin
		Vinca alkaloids
		Dactinomycin

Modified from DeVita, V. T., Jr.: Principles of chemotherapy. *In* DeVita, V. T., Jr., Hellman, S., and Rosenberg, S. A. (eds.): *Cancer, Principles and Practice of Oncology*, Philadelphia: J. B. Lippincott, 1985, p. 266.

Plant Alkaloids

Vincristine and vinblastine are natural alkaloids extracted from the periwinkle plant, *Vinca rosea* L. The exact mode of action of these agents is not well understood, but they appear to bind cytoplasmic microtubular proteins and inhibit the formation of the mitotic spindle apparatus. As a result, the agents arrest cellular division in metaphase and are classified as M-phase specific. Vincristine and vinblastine may cause gastroenteritis, lymphoid depletion, decreased spermatogenesis, anemia, and leukopenia; they may lead to elevations in serum aspartate aminotransferase, alkaline phosphatase, and lactate dehydrogenase activities. Alopecia, stomatitis, constipation, and peripheral neuropathy have also been observed. The neurotoxicity caused by the plant alkaloids is limited to the peripheral nerves, as these agents do not cross the blood-brain barrier.

The mechanism of the neurotoxicity appears to be impairment of axoplasm transport and is manifested by decreased sensory and motor nerve function. The neurotoxicity is not considered permanent and should reverse with discontinuation of the drug. The plant alkaloids are potent vesicants and, if extravasated during infusion, will result in cellulitis and potentially in tissue sloughing. Unlike the alkylating agents, resistance to one plant alkaloid does not imply resistance to another. Tumor cell resistance to the plant alkaloids appears to be the result of increased excretion from the tumor cell or altered intracellular targets affected by these agents.

Antitumor Antibiotics

The anticancer antibiotics are cell cycle nonspecific and are each natural products of soil fungi. They exert their major antitumor effect by forming complexes with DNA and inhibiting DNA synthesis, transcription of mRNA, and subsequent protein synthesis; drug interactions with DNA may be through intercalation between DNA base pairs or through noncovalent binding. The most commonly used antitumor antibiotic is doxorubicin, and it is a product of the fungus *Streptomyces peucetius*. Bone marrow suppression is the major toxic effect; however, alopecia, gastroenteritis, and stomatitis are frequent. Doxorubicin is a vesicant and also causes a dose-dependent cardiotoxicity characterized by a dilated form of cardiomyopathy nonresponsive to digitalis. The pathogenesis of the cardiomyopathy induced by doxorubicin is controversial. Another toxicity associated with doxorubicin is urticaria, pruritus, and collapse at the time of drug administration. Premedication with antihistamines has been recommended because serum histamine concentrations have been reported to be elevated following drug injection, but whether pretreatment with antihistamines is truely beneficial is currently unresolved. Tumor resistance to the antitumor antibiotics appears related to increased drug excretion from the neoplastic cells.

Hormonal Agents

Prednisone and prednisolone are the most frequently used hormones in the management of neoplastic diseases and are cell cycle nonspecific. Steroids function in the management of neoplasia to reduce tumor volume and to manage secondary complications of malignant disease, which may include immune-mediated hemolytic anemia, immune-mediated thrombocytopenia, and hypercalcemia. The glucocorticoid activity of prednisone and prednisolone is responsibile for the direct inhibition of tumor growth. A major advantage is the lack of

or minimal bone marrow–suppressive actions induced by these drugs. Although lymphocytes are sensitive to glucocorticoids and may undergo lymphocytolysis, lymphoreticular neoplasms quickly become resistant to glucocorticoids; the resistance is manifested by extensive cross-resistance to other glucocorticoid agents. Steroids have also been implicated in inducing pleiotropic drug resistance in tumor cells. Because of this phenomenon, it is currently not considered wise to recommend treatment with only steroids for several weeks while pet owners decide whether they wish their pet to be treated with combination chemotherapy.

Miscellaneous Agents

Of the miscellaneous agents, asparaginase is the most widely used. This antineoplastic agent is G_1-phase specific; it is an enzyme preparation extracted from bacteria. The antineoplastic activity is secondary to the depletion of extracellular asparagine stores following enzyme injection. The decrease in serum asparagine concentration leads to death of tumor cells that lack the cytoplasmic enzymes necessary to synthesize asparagine. Asparaginase has no effect on normal tissue cells owing to the abundance of cytoplasmic enzymes capable of synthesizing asparagine. Because asparaginase is a foreign protein, repeated injections of this preparation can lead to signs of immediate hypersensitivity; these signs include urticaria, vomiting, diarrhea, dyspnea, hypotension, pruritus, and collapse. In addition, hemorrhagic pancreatitis has been observed in the dog. Resistance to asparaginase is due to a decreased requirement of the tumor cells for asparagine.

THERAPY FOR EXTRAVASATION OF ANTINEOPLASTIC AGENTS

Extravasation of antineoplastic agents is not uncommon. Fortunately, there are no significant irritating effects with most chemotherapeutic agents. Extravasation of doxorubicin, dactinomycin, plicamycin, vincristine, vinblastine, and mechlorethamine can, however, lead to catastrophic subcutaneous damage. The chemotherapeutic agents that do not bind DNA (vincristine, vinblastine, and mechlorethamine) usually cause immediate irritation similar to a burn but typically are quickly inactivated, and normal healing generally occurs. Chemotherapeutic agents that bind DNA (doxorubicin, dactinomycin, and plicamycin) also cause immediate tissue damage, consisting of pain, erythema, and edema; but because these agents tenaciously bind DNA, they remain in the tissues for up to 5 months and contribute to long-standing injury. The severity of tissue damage is related to the dose of the drug extravasated into the subcutaneous tissue. Should extravasation occur, the injection should be stopped immediately, and one should attempt to withdraw 3 to 5 ml of blood while the needle remains in place; the needle should not be removed until efforts to withdraw blood and drug have been made. A 27-gauge needle and syringe are used to aspirate and withdraw as much of the subcutaneous bleb as possible. Following these manipulations, ice should be applied to the area for approximately 30 min and then for 15 min four times daily for the next 2 days; the instillation of approximately 5 ml of 8.4 per cent sodium bicarbonate (doxorubicin, vincristine, and vinblastine) or 5 ml of 10 per cent sodium thiosulfate (dactinomycin) into the extravasation site has been recommended by some investigators, but clinical data to support this practice are lacking. Close monitoring of the area is indicated. A surgical consultation should be obtained if pain, erythema, and edema persist; one should not wait for ulceration to occur.

References and Supplemental Reading

Boyd, J. R. (ed.): *Facts and Comparisons*. Philadelphia: J. B. Lippincott, 1985. (Updated monthly.)

Crow, S. E., Theilen, G. H., Madewell, B. R., et al.: Cyclophosphamide-induced cystitis in the dog and cat. J.A.V.M.A. 171:259, 1977.

DeVita, V. T., Jr., Hellman, S., and Rosenberg, S. A. (eds.): *Cancer: Principles and Practice of Oncology*. Philadelphia: J. B. Lippincott, 1985.

Hansen, J. F., and Carpenter, R. H.: Fatal acute systemic anaphylaxis and hemorrhagic pancreatitis following asparaginase treatment in a dog. J. Am. Anim. Hosp. Assoc. 19:977, 1983.

Harvey, H. J., MacEwen, E. G., and Hayes, A. A.: Neurotoxicosis associated with the use of 5-fluorouracil in five dogs and one cat. J.A.V.M.A. 171:277, 1977.

Ignoffo, R. J., and Friedman, M. A.: Therapy of local toxicities caused by extravasation of cancer chemotherapeutic drugs. Cancer Treat. Rev. 7:17, 1980.

Loar, A. S., and Susaneck, S. J.: Doxorubicin-induced cardiotoxicity in five dogs. Semin. Vet. Med. Surg. (Small Anim.) 1:68, 1986.

Rudolph, R., and Larson, D. L.: Etiology and treatment of chemotherapeutic agent extravasation injuries: A review. J. Clin. Oncol. 5:1116, 1987.

Theilen, G. H., and Madewell, B. R. (eds.): *Veterinary Cancer Medicine*. Philadelphia: Lea & Febiger, 1987.

Weller, R. E., Wolf, A. M., and Oyejide, A.: Transitional cell carcinoma of the bladder associated with cyclophosphamide therapy. J. Am. Anim. Hosp. Assoc. 15:733, 1979.

For dosages and more information on the drugs mentioned in this article, see the table "Antineoplastic Agents in Cancer Therapy" in the appendix.

SPECIAL CONSIDERATIONS IN DRUG PREPARATION AND ADMINISTRATION

BRUCE R. MADEWELL V.M.D.,
and ERIC R. SIMONSON, A.H.T.

Davis, California

The purpose of anticancer chemotherapy in clinical practice is to provide palliation for those animals with widespread or advanced neoplastic disease. In some instances, chemotherapeutic agents are used as adjuvants, usually in combination with surgery or radiotherapy, with the aim of preventing recurrence or decreasing the likelihood of regional or systemic spread. For some neoplasms, there is incontrovertible evidence that chemotherapy is indeed useful for prolonging disease-free intervals or effectively prolonging survival; but despite the application of anticancer chemotherapy to clinical practice for over one decade, many drug applications must still be considered investigational. Thus, it is of paramount importance that the owner of the cancer-bearing pet understand from the onset that the goal of therapy may not be cure, and that all of the consequences of the drug regimen itself have yet to be fully realized.

A major consideration to the veterinarian administering the chemotherapeutic agent is that the majority of the commercially available anticancer

Table 1. *Commercially Available Chemotherapeutic Agents*

Agent	How Supplied	Reconstitution	Stability	Administration	Acute Toxicity	Personnel Hazards
Alkylating Agents						
Chlorambucil (Leukeran, Burroughs Wellcome)	2-mg sugar-coated tablet	None	Short shelf life	Oral	Nausea and vomiting with large single dose.	None reported unless dose reduction is attempted by cutting tablets. Wear gloves and mask if attempted
Cyclophosphamide (Cytoxan, Mead Johnson) (endoxan)	25- and 50-mg tablets. 100-, 200-, 500-mg vials	Sterile water for injection, USP. Paraben-preserved bacteriostatic water for injection, USP. Agitate to dissolve completely	Solution stable for 24 hr at room temperature, or 6 days under refrigeration	Solution may be given as an IV bolus or diluted in 5% dextrose in water, USP, or 0.9% sodium chloride, USP for infusion	Nausea and vomiting have been reported when used as an infusion	Wear gloves when handling tablets or infusing.
Dacarbazine (DTIC-Dome, Miles)	100- and 200-mg vials	Sterile water for injection, USP	Solution stable for 8 hr at room temperature, or 72 hr when refrigerated. Light sensitive	IV push or diluted in 5% dextrose in water, USP	Vesicant, nausea and vomiting. Burning sensation when injected. Anaphylaxis has been reported in some patients	Wear gloves
Melphalan (Alkeran, Burroughs Wellcome)	2-mg tablets	None	See manufacturer's recommendations	Oral	Rare cases of nausea and vomiting	None reported
Antimetabolites						
Methotrexate	2.5-mg tablets, 5–50 mg vials, 20-mg vials preservative free	5-mg vials with sterile water for injection, USP. 20-mg vials with preservative-free NaCl, USP	Tablets and intact vials are stable at room temperature for 2 yr	Oral, IV, intrathecal, intra-arterial. Use preservative-free preparation for intrathecal use	Nausea and vomiting CNS reactions after intrathecal administration	Wear gloves
Cytosine arabinoside (Cytosar-U, Upjohn)	100- and 500-mg vials	Reconstitute with accompanying diluent. For intrathecal use, reconstitute with 5% dextrose in water	Refrigerate lyophylized drug. Solution stable for 48 hr at room temperature, or 7 days when refrigerated	IV, subcutaneous, intrathecal. Infuse solution with 0.9% NaCl, USP, or 5% dextrose in water	Rare nausea and vomiting	Wear gloves

Drug	Packaging	Reconstitution	Stability	Administration	Side Effects/Comments	Precautions
5-Fluorouracil (5-FU) (Adrucil, Adria; Efudex, Roche)	10-ml ampules containing 500-mg Efudex solution; also Efudex cream	None required	Discard unused solution. Light sensitive	IV, intralesional, topical	Pain at injection site. Not a vesicant, but if extravasated will cause localized pain and erythema. Not recommended in cats	Wear gloves
Antibiotics						
Bleomycin sulfate (Blenoxane, Bristol-Myers)	15-unit ampules	Sterile water for injection, USP, or 0.9% NaCl, USP, or 5% dextrose in water	7 days under refrigeration	IM, IV, SC	Nausea and vomiting, anaphylaxis. Pain at injection site. Skin reactions include rash, striae, erythema	Wear gloves
Doxorubicin hydrochloride (Adriamycin, Adria Labs)	10- and 50-mg vials	0.9% NaCl, USP	24 hr at room temperature, or 48 hr under refrigeration. Forms a precipitate if mixed with heparin or 5-FU	IV, dilute with 0.9% NaCl, USP, or 5% dextrose in water. Can be given as slow bolus or IV drip. Requires premedication with diphenhydramine and dexamethasone sodium phosphate. Refer to specific protocols	Severe vesicant; anaphylaxis. Life-threatening arrhythmias may occur during infusion and for several hours after therapy. Congestive heart failure. Dose-related irreversible cardiomyopathy. Rare hypertensive crisis following infusion	Carcinogenic to handle. Wear gloves. Should be reconstituted in a class II biologic safety cabinet
Plant Alkaloids						
Vinblastine sulfate (Velban, Eli Lilly)	10-mg vials	Add 10 ml NaCl, USP.	30 days under refrigeration when reconstituted	IV; IV push or infused in 0.9% NaCl, USP, or 5% dextrose in water	Vesicant. Rare nausea and vomiting have been reported. Neurotoxic	Wear gloves
Vincristine sulfate (Oncovin, Eli Lilly)	1- and 5-mg vials	None required	See manufacturer's recommendations	IV push	Vesicant. Tissue necrosis and sloughing may occur if extravasated. Neurotoxic	Wear gloves
VP16-213 (etoposide)	5-ml multiple dose vials; 100-mg capsules	None required	Ampules stable for 3.5 yr at room temperature. 15 days under refrigeration when reconstituted. Stability of drug when reconstituted is concentration dependent	IV infusion with 0.9% NaCl. Forms a precipitate in 0.9% NaCl, over time. Infusion rate varies in relation to volume of diluent and amount of drug. Requires premedication of diphenhydramine and dexamethasone sodium phosphate	Vesicant. Hypersensitivity reaction. Hypotension can occur when given too rapidly	Wear gloves

Table continued on following page

Table 1. *Commercially Available Chemotherapeutic Agents Continued*

Agent	How Supplied	Reconstitution	Stability	Administration	Acute Toxicity	Personnel Hazards
Miscellaneous Agents						
L-Asparaginase (Elspar, Merck, Sharp & Dohme)	10,000-unit vials	Preservative free sterile water, USP, or 0.9% NaCl, USP	Reconstituted solution stable for 8 hr under refrigeration	Subcutaneous, intraperitoneal, IV, IM. Requires premedication with diphenhydramine and dexamethasone sodium phosphate	Pain on injection. Anaphylaxis. Hypersensitivity reactions may increase with successive treatments	Wear gloves
Bacille Calmette-Guérin (BCG)	Freeze dried live *Mycobacterium bovis*	Sterile water for injection, USP	Reconstituted solution should be used immediately. Light sensitive	Scarification, intralesional, intradermal, intrapleural	Rare anaphylaxis; flulike syndrome	Wear gloves. Contact may result in conversion to tuberculin reactivity
Cisplatin (DDP, Platinol, Bristol-Myers)	10- and 50-mg vials	Sterile water for injection, USP	Stable for 20 hr at room temperature when reconstituted. Do not refrigerate after reconstitution. Forms a precipitate when in contact with aluminum. Light sensitive	IV and intralesional. Pretreat with 0.9% NaCl, USP, for diuresis to include mannitol or furosemide. Posttherapy diuresis with 0.9% NaCl, USP. Refer to specific protocols. Antiemetics are required	Nausea and vomiting in almost all cases. May increase with subsequent infusions. Tinnitus, hearing loss	Wear gloves
Hormones						
Diethylstilbestrol	0.1-, 0.25-, 0.5-, 1-, 5-mg tablets	None required	See manufacturer's insert	Oral	None reported	None reported
Prednisone (Deltasone, Upjohn; Meticorten, Schering; Orasone, Reid-Rowell)	1-, 2.5-, 5-, 10-, 20-, 50-mg tablets	None required	See manufacturer's insert	Oral	None reported	None reported

drugs are not licensed for use in domestic animals. Therefore, the consequences of drug reactions, be they favorable or otherwise, are the responsibility of the veterinarian administering that product, i.e., there is no liability on the part of the drug manufacturer. To that end, one should inform the owner as explicitly as possible that the agent or agents to be administered, although approved for use in human patients with similar neoplasms, are not specifically approved for use in animals. Further discussion is aimed at informing the animal owner of the goals of therapy and also the possible adverse reactions that may be attributed to the anticancer drug *per se*. Documentation of the owner's informed consent can occur at several levels. A statement might be made in the record that such a discussion had occurred, and perhaps the owner might even sign the record confirming that the discussion had transpired. Another level of documentation is to provide an informed consent form, stating the extralabel use of the agent to be used, the possible consequences of the treatment regimen to be employed, the veterinarian's responsibility in managing an adverse reaction should it occur, and the owner's responsibilities in the treatment program. A copy of that form then becomes an integral part of the medical record, which may be updated as the treatment regimen changes. Simply stating possible adverse reactions of therapy to an owner of an animal with cancer may not be adequate; the owner is often emotionally preoccupied with other facets of the situation and may simply forget that such a discussion had ever occurred.

DRUG HANDLING

Since the introduction of modern cancer chemotherapeutic drugs, there have been a number of reports of second malignancies following their use. As the carcinogenic and teratogenic properties of the chemotherapeutic agents have been documented over the last several years, there has been increasing concern regarding the potential hazards of preparing and administering chemotherapy. Although the degree of risk involved in the handling of most of these agents is unknown, it seems prudent to exercise caution when handling potentially toxic drugs. Dangerous exposures to cytotoxic drugs may occur in a variety of ways, such as the inhalation of drug dusts or droplets, direct skin or eye contact, or the inadvertent ingestion of drug that may have contaminated foodstuffs. Several variables influence the occupational hazard of individual agents: those variables include the chemical properties of the drug (e.g., alkylating agents are particularly hazardous); the individual's susceptibility to the drug's toxic effects; cofactors such as dietary or social factors; the number and magnitude of cumulative

exposures; and the type of exposure, such as skin contact or inhalation. Only the last two of these variables can be controlled to any degree in the workplace.

Strict attention to detail in drug handling is of paramount importance, and only personnel with adequate training should prepare and administer antineoplastic agents. Pregnant women or those likely to become pregnant should not handle these agents. Eating, drinking, smoking, and food storage are not permitted in the working area. The following guidelines have been recommended as precautionary measures for personnel involved in drug preparation and administration. For drug preparation, latex gloves are used (polyvinyl gloves may not provide adequate protection for some vesicant agents). A gown and protective eyewear are advised, particularly when handling irritating drugs such as vinblastine or cyclophosphamide. A vertical air flow hood may be required in some institutions, and the Division of Safety of the National Institutes of Health recommends the use of a class II laminar air flow biologic safety cabinet for these drug preparations. Care should be taken to vent vials to reduce pressure and the possibility of spraying the drug solution. Several filter apparatuses are available commercially to prevent such aerosolization, and the introduction of prediluted antineoplastic agents in partially filled bottles and premixed drug systems minimizes the possibility of drug aerosols. The latter contained systems also provide for waste removal. The United States Department of Health and Human Services recommends that an alcohol pad be wrapped around the needle when drawing contents from the drug-containing vial, while ejecting air bubbles from the syringe, or when breaking an ampule. Unused material should be disposed of in a leak-proof, puncture-proof container. Hands should be thoroughly washed after removing gloves. Guidelines for handling drug spills should be clearly defined.

When administering the chemotherapeutic agents, gloves should be worn with potentially vesicant, carcinogenic, and mutagenic drugs. A sterile alcohol pad is used for the absorption of any drug inadvertently discharged while infusing or withdrawing the needle. If skin contact does occur, the area is washed thoroughly with soap and water; if eye contact has occurred, one should rinse thoroughly and consult an ophthalmologist. All equipment used in the drug administration should be disposed of in a polyethylene bag and sealed within a puncture-resistant container. The container should bear a caution label and be designated as hazardous waste or toxic material for incineration. In general, urine and feces from patients treated with antineoplastic agents are handled carefully but in the usual manner. For those agents removed rapidly by the kidneys (such as cisplatin), collection of urine in metabolic cage containers during the animal's hospitalization is advised to prevent aerosolizing the drug during cleaning procedures.

DRUG ADMINISTRATION

The first consideration in delivery of chemotherapy is to determine that all necessary analyses have been determined as outlined in the treatment protocol (see pages 482, 489, and 497 and previous editions of *Current Veterinary Therapy* for model cancer chemotherapy protocols). The second is to examine the drug presciption to ascertain that it is in accordance with the treatment protocol; this step is most important to be absolutely certain that a drug overdose does not occur. When intravenous chemotherapy is to be used, the necessary equipment as well as emergency drugs must be on hand in case of an adverse reaction or inadvertent drug extravasation.

It is prudent to use jugular veins for blood sampling, thus leaving the large peripheral veins for drug delivery. Small-gauge butterfly needles may be adequate for delivery of a drug to be given over a short period of time. Small-gauge Teflon catheters may be preferred for longer infusions. It is good practice to consult a colleague if two or three unsuccessful attempts are made to insert a catheter. For intravenous bolus injection, the drug is injected directly or through the port of an infusion tubing. One should test the vein with saline solution; administer the drug with slow, even pressure on the syringe plunger; and check blood return with every 3 to 4 ml of the drug given. After the injection is completed, the vein is flushed with at least 20 ml of normal saline. For the infusion of drugs by continuous drip, one should check the running infusion every 2 to 3 min and conclude treatment with the flushing of saline. For long-running infusions, the cannula and tubing must be changed every 48 to 72 hr. At the conclusion of treatment, the medications given, injection site, time, dose, and any unusual reaction are documented in the record. Equipment disposal is performed according to the institution's policies.

There are several specific considerations when administering certain drugs:

Painful Infusions

The administration of some chemotherapeutic agents may cause pain. This occurs particularly with the administration of dacarbazine and, to a lesser extent, cytosine arabinoside. Other antineoplastic agents commonly associated with irritant activity are bleomycin, etoposide, L-asparaginase, and 5-fluorouracil. Reduction of the flow rate, dilution of drug in a larger volume of saline, or the use of 1 ml of 1 per cent lidocaine may provide relief.

Extravasation of Drug

The extravasation of vesicant drugs may be a disastrous complication of drug treatment. Fortunately, this complication is preventable in most cases with good technique, although local tissue reactions account for 2 to 5 per cent of all adverse reactions from antineoplastic agents in human practice. Any of the anticancer drugs are capable of inducing tissue damage when infiltrated locally outside the vein; severely vesicant drugs include doxorubicin, vinblastine, and vincristine. The onset and intensity of local reactions range considerably from hours to weeks and from minor skin or venous discoloration to severe local necrosis of the dermis and underlying structures. The treatment of infiltrations of vesicant drugs is controversial, and most remedies are based on anecdotal data. Common policies recommend the use of warm, moist soaks for drug-related tissue or vein irritations. The rationale is to enhance local circulation to remove the drug. Other recommendations include the local injection of various agents such as hydrocortisone (50 to 200 mg). The local injection of hyaluronidase and the application of heat has been proposed to reduce the morbidity of extravasation of the vinca alkaloids, and sodium bicarbonate is advised for doxorubicin extravasation. Some recommend the local application of cold compresses to limit the diffusion of the vesicant drug. Some authorities suggest removal of the needle, whereas others recommend that the needle be left in place for injection of agents such as hydrocortisone. When drug extravasation is thought to have occurred, it seems wise to try to aspirate as much of the infiltrated agent as possible by using a 25-gauge needle.

Acute Drug Reactions

Although idiosyncratic hypersensitivity responses have been recognized most frequently with L-asparaginase administration, all drugs possess the potential to cause these responses. The risk increases if the drug had been previously used in that patient. In human practice, the overall mortality rate from anaphylaxis is estimated to be as high as 1 per cent in patients receiving chemotherapy. Among the chemotherapeutic agents used rather commonly in veterinary oncologic practice that have some risk for the development of acute hypersensitivity reactions are L-asparaginase, cisplatin, and doxorubicin; the epipodophyllotoxin drugs (VP-16 or etoposide) have also been reported to cause acute hypersensitivity reactions. In the event of a hypersensitivity reaction, it is advised to stop the flow of drug but keep the intravenous line open with saline. One should give dexamethasone sodium phosphate (intravenously at a dose of 0.25 mg per kilogram of body weight), or epinephrine (0.1 to 0.5 ml diluted 1:1000 IM), or both, and monitor vital signs carefully. An antihistamine, such as diphenhydramine (1.0 to 2.0 mg/kg IM or by slow IV injection), may also be of value.

For animals with a prior history of drug-induced acute hypersensitivity reaction, precautionary measures prior to treatment include test dosing and anithistamine or steroid pretreatment.

Vomiting and Antiemetic Therapy

Vomiting and possible nausea are commonly encountered complications of cancer chemotherapy associated with the use of some agents in animals. Chemotherapy-associated vomiting may result from stimulation of the central nervous system or by means of toxicity to the mucosal lining of the gastrointestinal tract. Acute-onset vomiting occurs within 12 to 24 hr of treatment and is usually self-limiting. Delayed-onset vomiting occurs 24 hr or more after treatment; the mechanism for delay is not clear but may involve protein or tissue binding of the drug, followed by slow release. Anticipatory nausea and vomiting, presumably less important in animals, is a conditioned response arising from fear and anxiety and perhaps triggered by a combination of external and internal sensory stimuli.

Virtually every class of chemotherapeutic agent can give rise to nausea and vomiting at one time or another, and the manifestations of this response are variable from patient to patient. Vomiting may be a relatively minor inconvenience in the administration of drug or may be so severe as to pose a dose-limiting toxicity. A number of well-conducted studies in human oncologic practice have assessed the efficacy of a variety of antiemetic compounds, although the best agents or combinations of agents have yet to be defined. The agents most often used include the phenothiazines, glucocorticoids, butorphanol, butyrophenones, and the cannabinoids. Some of these agents have been applied to veterinary clinical practice, and there are now some data regarding their effectiveness.

The phenothiazines are probably the most widely used antiemetics, and prochlorperazine and chlorpromazine are the most commonly used; they presumably exert their effect by blocking dopamine receptors in the chemoreceptor trigger zone (CTZ) and perhaps by reducing intestinal spasms. These drugs are generally well tolerated and exert a mild sedative effect as well.

Metoclopramide is a substituted benzamide with significant antiemetic activity; it is thought to exert its antiemetic activity by dopamine receptor blockade in the CTZ and the upper gastrointestinal tract.

Corticosteroids may have a role in the treatment of chemotherapy-induced emesis, although this is controversial. The mechanism for this activity is unknown but is thought to be related to inhibition of prostaglandin synthesis. Butorphanol, a member of the phenanthrene series, has been useful in the prevention of cisplatin-associated emesis in the dog when used at a dosage of 0.4 mg/kg, given intramuscularly, at the beginning and end of a 3-hr cisplatin infusion. The butyrophenone tranquilizers haloperidol and droperidol as well as the cannabinoid drugs, have been tested and found effective in some human patients when used alone or in combination with other antiemetics. Indeed, the cannabinoid agents may be useful in a variety of settings when patients have become refractory to other conventional antiemetics. There is no information as to the use or the effectiveness of these agents in animals.

DRUG PROPERTIES

Table 1 relates the stability of some of the more routinely used chemotherapeutic agents in veterinary practice as well as some other special considerations in the use of these products. It includes guidelines for reconstitution, routes of administration, acute toxic reactions, and personnel hazards. In that there are some variations in products between manufacturers and that products are changing as they are improved, it is advised that the package insert be consulted in each instance before the drug is prepared for administration.

References and Supplemental Reading

Becker, T. M.: Cancer chemotherapy—a manual for nurses. Boston: Little, Brown, 1981, p. 29.

Cancer chemotherapy. *In The Medical Letter.* New Rochelle, NY: The Medical Letter, Inc., 1985, pp. 13–20.

deBroe, M. E., and Wedeen, R. P.: Prevention of cisplatin nephrotoxicity. Eur. J. Cancer. Clin. Oncol. 22:1029, 1986.

Dorr, R. T., and Fritz, W. L.: Complications and toxicities of cancer chemotherapy. *In Dorr and Fritz: Cancer Chemotherapy Handbook.* New York: Elsevier, 1980, pp. 101–115.

Dorr, R. T., and Alberts, D. S.: Vinca alkaloid skin toxicity: Antidote and drug disposition studies in the mouse. J. Natl. Cancer Inst. 74:113, 1985.

Fiore, J. J., and Gralla, R. J.: Pharmacologic treatment of chemotherapy-induced nausea and vomiting. Cancer Invest. 2:351, 1984.

Gralla, R. J.: Antiemetic therapy and cancer chemotherapy. *In Hellmann, K., and Carter, S. K.: Fundamentals of Cancer Chemotherapy.* New York: McGraw-Hill, 1987, pp 387–396.

Hannah, H. W.: The veterinarian's civil liability in the use of drugs. J.A.V.M.A. 191:1062, 1987.

Hutson, C.: Anti-emetic effect of butorphanol in management of cisplatin-induced vomiting in the dog. Veterinary Cancer Society, Proceedings, 7th Annual Conference, Madison, WI, 1987, p. 23.

Ignoffo, R. J., and Friedman, M. A.: Therapy of local toxicities caused by extravasation of cancer chemotherapeutic agents. Cancer Treat. Rev. 7:17, 1980.

Kastrup, E. K. (ed.): *Drug Facts and Comparisons*. Philadelphia: J. B. Lippincott, 1987, p. 950.

Macy, D. W.: Chemotherapeutic agents available for cancer treatment. *In* Kirk, R. W. (ed.): *Current Veterinary Therapy IX*. Philadelphia: W. B. Saunders, 1986, pp. 467–470.

Madewell, B. R.: Adverse affects of chemotherapy. *In* Kirk, R. W. (ed.): *Current Veterinary Therapy VIII*. Philadelphia: W. B. Saunders, 1983, pp. 419–422.

Rieche, K.: Carcinogenicity of antineoplastics agents in man. Cancer Treat. Rev. 11:39, 1984.

Tish Knobf, M. K., Fischer, D. S., and Welch-McCaffrey, D.: Extravasation and cutaneous reactions. *In* Tish Knobf, M. K., et al. (eds.): *Cancer Chemotherapy—Treatment and Care*. Boston: GK Hall, 1984, pp. 327–335.

Yarbro, C. H.: The role of the oncology nurse in cancer chemotherapy practice. *In* Hellman, K., and Carter, S. K. (eds.): *Fundamentals of Cancer Chemotherapy*, New York: McGraw-Hill, 1987, pp. 379–386.

CHEMOTHERAPY OF LYMPHOMA AND LEUKEMIA

ROBERT E. MATUS, D.V.M.

New York, New York

Lymphoma and lymphoid leukemia are the most common hematopoietic malignancies in the dog and cat. All veterinarians involved in small animal practice should have some knowledge of current treatment recommendations and conventional chemotherapy protocols, which may be offered to the owner of a pet with lymphoproliferative malignancy. Evaluation by a referral or consulting oncologist who has advanced training and experience in the treatment of cancer can be of considerable value in most cases. Prognosis for both response to treatment and probability for long-term survival are the major variables in the decision to accept the possible inconvenience of treatment schedules and the costs of chemotherapy. Knowledge and understanding of the clinical stage of disease, related hematologic and biochemical abnormalities, and performance status of the animal all contribute to the decision to recommend chemotherapy.

CLINICAL EVALUATION

In the dog, lymphoma most commonly causes a painless, generalized lymphadenopathy. Diarrhea, vomiting, and marked weight loss with lethargy and inappetence are commonly associated with intestinal involvement of lymphoma. Hypercalcemia and related alterations in renal function may cause polydipsia and polyuria. Findings on physical examination might include mucous membrane pallor, enlargement of the liver and spleen, and fever. Elevations in temperature greater than 103°F (39.4°C) may be due to concurrent infection. Cutaneous lesions that resemble plaquelike raised proliferative masses or diffuse ulcerated areas with erythema might indicate skin involvement. Labored breathing, dyspnea, and muffled heart sounds are suggestive of either the presence of pleural effusion or an anterior mediastinal mass caused by thymic or lymph node enlargement. The presence of petechia, ecchymosis, retinal hemorrhages, or hyphema are indicative of either thrombocytopenia or a coagulopathy associated with the disease process (Leifer and Matus, 1986a).

In the cat, lymphoma less often causes a generalized lymphadenopathy. More commonly the disease is associated with an anterior mediastinal mass, gastrointestinal involvement, or kidney infiltration by malignant lymphocytes. Clinical signs are often nonspecific in the early stages of the disease process. With progressive lymphoma, more specific signs related to organ involvement may be seen, as previously mentioned for the dog. Although lymphoma in the cat is caused by the feline leukemia virus (FeLV), viremia, determined by either the indirect fluorescent antibody (IFA) test or enzyme-linked immunosorbent assay (ELISA) method for demonstration of viral antigen, is not always detected. In general, the younger cat with lymphoma is more likely to be FeLV positive than the older cat with lymphoma if there is no recent history of exposure (Mooney and Hayes, 1986).

Lymphoid leukemia generally causes nonspecific clinical signs in both dogs and cats. Lethargy and inappetence are commonly reported. Weight loss, diarrhea and vomiting, and dehydration may be observed with progressive disease. Bleeding episodes such as epistaxis, hyphema, or the occurrence of petechia and ecchymotic bruising are due to thrombocytopenia and generally reflect progressive marrow involvement with decreased numbers of normal precursor cells. Fever and concurrent infection may be due to insufficient production of gran-

Table 1. Clinical Stage of Disease in Lymphoma

Stage	Canine*	Feline†
I	Involvement of single node or lymphoid tissue in single organ	Single tumor (extranodal) or anatomic area (nodal). Includes primary thoracic tumors
II	Regional involvement of many lymph nodes or without involvement of the tonsils	Single tumor with regional lymph node involvement Two or more nodal areas on same side of diaphragm Two single tumors with or without regional lymph node involvement on same side of diaphragm Resectable primary GI tract tumor, with or without involvement of associated mesenteric nodes
III	Generalized lymph node enlargement	Two single tumors on opposite sides of diaphragm Two or more nodal areas above and below diaphragm All extensive primary unresectable intra-abdominal disease All paraspinal or epidural tumors, regardless of other tumor site or sites
IV	Involvement of liver, spleen, or both, with or without generalized lymph node involvement	Stages I–III with involvement of liver, spleen, or both
V	Involvement of blood, bone marrow, or other organs	Stages I–IV with initial involvement of CNS, bone marrow, or both

*TNM Classification of Tumors in Domestic Animals. Geneva: World Health Organization, 1980, pp. 46–47.
†Mooney, S. C., et al.: Treatment and prognostic factors in feline lymphoma: 103 cases (1977–1981). J.A.V.M.A. 1989 (in press).

ulocytes and decreased immunoglobulin synthesis by normal lymphocytes. Occasionally, syndromes related to abnormal immunoglobulin production such as hemolytic anemia, immune-mediated thrombocytopenia, or monoclonal gammopathy and hyperviscosity with hemorrhage or central nervous system abnormalities may occur (Leifer and Matus, 1985).

Compared with lymphoma, acute lymphoblastic leukemia (ALL) is generally associated with more rapidly progressive clinical signs. In the author's experience, cats with acute lymphoblastic leukemia are usually young and FeLV positive. In the dog, both young and old age groups appear to be equally affected. Physical findings commonly include mucous membrane pallor, marked splenomegaly, and hepatomegaly. Lymphadenopathy is present in about half of the dogs and perhaps one third of the cats and is generally less impressive compared with the marked lymphadenopathy seen in lymphoma.

Chronic lymphocytic leukemia (CLL) is a slower, more insidious disease. A protracted history of nonspecific changes in physical activity and appetite may be the only clinical signs observed. It is not unusual to diagnose chronic lymphocytic leukemia in an asymptomatic older dog in which a complete blood count, performed as part of a routine geriatric examination, reveals a mature lymphocytosis. Physical findings can include mild to moderate mucous membrane pallor, splenomegaly, hepatomegaly, and lymphadenopathy. Chronic lymphocytic leukemia is uncommon in the cat, and the few cats followed by the author have been older than 10 yr and FeLV negative.

CLINICAL STAGE OF DISEASE

Clinical evaluation should include a complete hematologic and biochemical profile and urinalysis.

Radiographic and ultrasound studies of the chest and abdomen may be performed to assess internal lymphadenopathy and organ enlargement. Coagulation profiles and specialized radiographic studies, such as gastrointestinal contrast series or intravenous pyelograms, should be performed based on initial physical and laboratory findings. An FeLV test should be done in the cat. A bone marrow aspiration biopsy should be performed in all animals undergoing evaluation.

Based on results of these studies, clinical stage of disease can be assessed. In the dog, clinical staging for lymphoma is usually described by the World Health Organization (WHO) system. A proposed clinical staging system for lymphoma in the cat may actually provide a better clinical assessment of disease than does the currently accepted WHO classification for lymphoma. These two staging systems are compared in Table 1. Syndromes of anemia, azotemia, and hypercalcemia play no role in the determination of clinical stage of disease yet may have a profound effect on response to treatment and prognosis. Marked anemia may occur in over 20 per cent of all dogs evaluated for lymphoma. In the cat, anemia is more often observed in cats that are FeLV positive; however, bone marrow involvement of lymphoma does not appear to be dependent on concurrent FeLV infection. The prevalence of azotemia is unknown but is higher in cats with renal lymphoma and in those animals that are hypercalcemic. Hypercalcemia may occur in 10 to 15 per cent of dogs with lymphoma. Hypercalcemia is uncommon in the cat with lymphoma and is often associated with active FeLV infection and advanced clinical stage of disease. Neither staging system allows for differentiation of the dog or cat with leukemia from those with stage V lymphoma based on bone marrow involvement. Table 2 summarizes

Table 2. Lymphoma and Leukemia in Dogs and Cats

	ALL	CLL	Stage V Lymphoma
Clinical signs	Short duration with rapid progression	Protracted slowly progressive to asymptomatic	Moderate duration with marked progression. Prolonged clinical illness
Lymph node	Mild enlargement	Mild enlargement	Moderate to massive enlargement
Spleen	Massive enlargement	Moderate enlargement	Moderate enlargement with hepatomegaly
Anemia	Marked to moderate	Mild to moderate	Moderate
Total white blood cell count	Variable, extreme leukocytosis to leukopenia	Usually increased	Normal to increased
Total lymphocyte	Usually increased	Increased	Normal to increased
Lymphocyte morphology	Blast cells observed	Normal to mild atypia	Moderate atypia
Bone marrow	Marked infiltration with lymphoblasts and atypical lymphocytes	Marked infiltration with predominately normal to mildly atypical lymphocytes	Mild to moderate infiltration with atypical lymphocytes

the differences in clinical signs and physical and hematologic findings in stage V lymphoma, acute lymphoblastic leukemia, and chronic lymphocytic leukemia.

DIAGNOSIS

Ideally, the diagnosis of lymphoma should be based on the histologic examination of a tissue biopsy. However, the diagnosis of lymphoma may be confirmed by cytologic demonstration of malignant lymphoid cell infiltration in specimens aspirated from liver, kidney, and pleural effusion associated with an anterior mediastinal mass. Cytologic evaluation of lymph node and splenic aspiration biopsy specimens is of limited value in the definitive diagnosis of lymphoma: although cytologic examination may be suggestive of or compatible with a diagnosis of lymphoma, most pathologists recommend histopathologic examination of tissue to substantiate the diagnosis.

As a general screening procedure for dogs with lymphadenopathy without other clinical signs, cytologic examination of fine-needle aspiration biopsy specimens may help to convince the reluctant owner to permit further evaluation. In the cat with generalized lymphadenopathy, cytologic evaluation does not help differentiate lymphoma from extreme lymphoid hyperplasia. Lymphoid hyperplasia in the cat is not uncommon, and clinical differentiation from lymphoma is important because spontaneous regression may be seen in cats with hyperplasia (Mooney et al., 1987a).

The diagnosis of lymphoid leukemia is based on cytologic evaluation of bone marrow aspirates. Leukocytosis and lymphocytosis are not always present in leukemia and, although lymphocytosis may occur, it is not diagnostic of leukemia. Approximately 20 per cent of all cases of lymphoma in the dog and the cat are associated with lymphocytosis and lymphoid cell atypia. Bone marrow infiltration of atypical lymphocytes may occur with lymphoma, but

the degree of infiltration is usually not as severe as in leukemia. In stage V lymphoma, infiltration is usually not greater than 25 per cent, whereas in leukemia, marrow infiltration often approaches total replacement by the malignant cell line. Bone marrow involvement, characterized by atypia rather than blast transformation, commonly occurs with anterior mediastinal lymphoma in the dog and is often associated with hypercalcemia. Cytologic examination of bone marrow aspirates is important because dogs and cats with leukemia and stage V lymphoma may exhibit lymphadenopathy, splenomegaly, and hepatomegaly.

When a diagnosis of lymphoid leukemia is made, it is important to establish whether the morphology of the cells is lymphoblastic, lymphocytic, or intermediate. The intermediate cell form is moderately well differentiated, yet obviously atypical, and may make the diagnosis of chronic lymphocytic leukemia versus acute lymphoblastic leukemia difficult. In this case, one must rely on differences in clinical evaluation, as previously mentioned, in establishing a definitive diagnosis.

In some instances the pathologist may not be able to establish a diagnosis of lymphoid versus nonlymphoid cell type in acute leukemia owing to extreme undifferentiated morphology of the cells. The diagnosis of the type of leukemia must then be based on the use of enzymatic cytochemical staining patterns of the malignant cell line. Unfortunately, these specialized diagnostic stains are not routinely available. However, the diagnosis of lymphoid versus nonlymphoid leukemia can often be achieved by the skilled pathologist with careful evaluation of standard Wright- or Giemsa-stained slides of blood and bone marrow.

Chemotherapy and Prognosis for Lymphoma

Chemotherapy protocols are effective in the treatment of lymphoma in the dog and the cat. The foundation of treatment regimens includes vincristine (cell cycle specific, mitotic spindle inhibition), cyclophosphamide (cell cycle nonspecific, bifunctional alkylation), and prednisone (cell cycle non-specific, lymphocytolytic). The additional drug combination of asparaginase (cell cycle nonspecific, nutrient depletion of asparagine in malignant lymphocytes) and doxorubicin (cell cycle nonspecific, inhibition of DNA synthesis and replication) is incorporated during an intensive induction treatment period. Methotrexate (cell cycle specific, folate inhibition, altered thymidine synthesis) is added to the treatment protocol during a prolonged maintenance phase of chemotherapy. Table 3 illustrates the current treatment protocol for lymphoma in the dog and the cat. This regimen utilizes the combined cyclic administration of drugs based on a weekly period of induction, followed by prolonged maintenance at bi- and tri-weekly intervals.

Body surface area (BSA) is used to calculate dosage for the majority of drugs administered in the dog. Administration based on body surface area estimates distribution, metabolism, and elimination of drug better than does use of body weight alone. Body surface area is determined by the following formula: $k \times w^{2/3}$ (kg)/10^4, in which k represents the relationship of body length to body weight. In the dog this constant is 10.1, and in the cat k is 10.0. It may not be entirely appropriate to determine drug dosage in the cat based on tables of BSA for the dog. Additionally, it may be necessary to determine dosage of chemotherapeutic drugs based on body weight rather than body surface area in both the dog and the cat if either the activity or the side effects are independent of basal metabolic rate. The use of body weight rather than body surface area allows for better clinical manipulation of drug

dosage in the cat owing to the small quantities of drug administered in each treatment. Even in the dog it is preferable to establish the dose of methotrexate based on body weight rather than body surface area, as small changes in dosage greatly alter the severity of gastrointestinal toxicity. Asparaginase also is administered based on body weight and is limited to a maximum total dose of 10,000 IU in the attempt to prevent potential acute hepatic toxicity and drug-induced pancreatitis.

Chemotherapy is administered once a week for 6 weeks, biweekly for 12 months, and then triweekly and monthly for 6-month periods. Thus the total treatment period would be 2 years for animals that achieve and maintain complete remission. In the cat, the treatment interval is extended to every 10 days for eight treatments following the 6-week period of induction chemotherapy and then to 2-week intervals. If owners cannot bring the cat for treatment every 10 days, the interval is extended to 2 weeks for 12 months as in the dog. Maintenance chemotherapy is then the same in both dogs and cats. There is some controversy over the necessity of prolonged maintenance treatment. In the author's experience, the maintenance period with extended treatment intervals is warranted, based on observed differences in relapse and survival rates following induction chemotherapy without a maintenance protocol.

Based on results of previous studies using cyclic combination chemotherapy without doxorubicin in the dog and cat, at least an 80 per cent rate of remission is expected. Overall median survival times of 10 months in the dog and 7 months in the cat were demonstrated using this protocol. Long-term survival of 12 months or longer was observed

Table 3. Chemotherapy Protocol for Lymphoma

Week	Drug	Canine Dose	Feline Dose
1	Vincristine	0.7 mg/m² IV	0.025 mg/kg IV
	Asparaginase	400 IU/kg, IP*	Same
	Prednisone	30 mg/m² PO, OD	5 mg b.i.d. PO
2	Cyclophosphamide	200 mg/m² IV†	10 mg/kg IV
	Prednisone	20 mg/m² PO, OD	5 mg b.i.d. PO
3	Doxorubicin	30 mg/m² IV	20 mg/m² IV
	Prednisone	10 mg/m² PO, OD	5 mg b.i.d. PO
4–6	As weeks 1–3 above but discontinue:	Asparaginase and prednisone	Asparaginase
8	Vincristine	0.7 mg/m² IV	0.025 mg/kg IV
	Prednisone	None	5 mg b.i.d. PO
10	Cyclophosphamide	200 mg/m² IV	10 mg/kg IV
	Prednisone	None	5 mg b.i.d. PO
12	Vincristine	0.7 mg/m² IV	0.025 mg/kg IV
	Prednisone	None	5 mg b.i.d. PO
14‡	Methotrexate	0.5 mg/kg IV§	0.8 mg/kg IV
	Prednisone	None	5 mg b.i.d. PO

IP, intraperitoneal; OD, once a day.
*Maximum dose is 10,000 IU.
†Maximum dose is 250 mg.
‡Protocol is continued in sequence biweekly as described for weeks 8–14 for 12 months, triweekly for 6 months, and then monthly for 6 months.
§Maximum dose is 25 mg.

in more than 30 per cent of all animals treated. However, only 10 to 15 per cent lived more than 2 years (MacEwen et al., 1981, 1987; Mooney et al., 1989).

Incorporation of doxorubicin with cyclic combination chemotherapy treatment in the dog accounted for an increase in overall median survival time to longer than 12 months, and approximately 25 per cent of the dogs lived 2 years or longer. However, a 20 to 30 per cent incidence of doxorubicin-induced cardiac abnormalities in these dogs was observed. Conduction disturbances, arrhythmias, and decreased myocardial contractility occurred following an average cumulative dose of 120 mg/m^2, and 5 to 10 per cent of all dogs treated developed drug-induced congestive heart failure. The total cumulative dose of doxorubicin administered in this protocol was 180 mg/m^2 (Donaldson-Atwood Cancer Clinic, 1988, unpublished data).

In the author's current protocol, doxorubicin is given for two treatments during the 6-week period of intensive induction chemotherapy. Thus the total cumulative dose is only 60 mg/m^2. Recently, doxorubicin has been used during induction chemotherapy in the cat. The dosage is decreased to 20 mg/m^2, allowing for a total cumulative dose of 40 mg/m^2. This dosage of doxorubicin causes only mild anorexia in the cat and has not been associated with cardiac toxicity or nephrotoxicity.

Prednisone is given for only the first 3 weeks of the chemotherapy protocol in the dog. In the cat, prednisone is continued for the entire course of treatment. In the author's experience the cat tolerates daily prednisone better than the dog. Side effects such as muscle wasting, hair loss, and iatrogenic hyper- or hypoadrenocorticism have not been frequently observed in the cat, and secondary development of diabetes mellitus is uncommon.

In clinical practice, alternative protocols must be considered for those animals that either fail to respond to chemotherapy or relapse following initial response. The author routinely reinduces dogs and cats that relapse by administering the combination of vincristine, asparaginase, and prednisone, followed by cyclophosphamide (week 2), vincristine (week 3), methotrexate (week 4), and vincristine (week 5). The treatment interval is then extended to every 2 weeks. In the dog prednisone is administered in a tapered dosage of 30 mg/m^2 initially, once a day for 1 week, then 20 mg/m^2, once a day for 1 week, and then continuously at this dosage every other day. In the cat, prednisone is simply continued at 5 mg twice a day. Approximately half of the dogs and a third of the cats so treated achieve a second remission. Those animals that do not respond are treated with asparaginase a third time and are then given chlorambucil (a cell cycle nonspecific, slow-acting, alkylating agent) at a dosage of 0.1 to 0.2 mg/kg PO daily, in combination with

biweekly cyclic chemotherapy. In the cat chlorambucil is more easily given as a 2-mg total dose every other day to eliminate dividing the coated tablet. Following complete failure to these procedures, doxorubicin is administered at the previously mentioned treatment dosages once every 3 weeks.

A dog that has relapsed with moderate generalized lymphadenopathy may survive for several months on biweekly chemotherapy plus prednisone and chlorambucil despite lack of regression in lymph node size. The decision to administer doxorubicin will depend on the physical status of the dog and the progression rate of lymphoma. Some investigators suggest that the use of doxorubicin alone may achieve equivalent response and survival rates compared with protocols using vincristine, cyclophosphamide, and prednisone, However, in the author's experience, cyclic combination chemotherapy incorporating doxorubicin is associated with a higher response rate and more long-term survivors.

In some instances the treatment protocol should be changed, even if a complete response has been achieved. Cyclophosphamide causes a chemically induced inflammatory cystitis, which appears to be independent of previous drug tolerance or cumulative dose. It occurs more commonly in the dog than in the cat. If drug-induced cystitis occurs, chlorambucil should be substituted at a dosage of 1.4 mg/kg, divided into two equal doses and given orally. Approximately 20 per cent of all dogs treated with methotrexate show some gastrointestinal toxicity from a dosage of 0.5 mg/kg IV. If severe anorexia, vomiting, or diarrhea occurs, cytosine arabinoside should be substituted at a dosage of 600 mg/m^2, administered subcutaneously in divided doses once a day for 2 days. Cats seem to tolerate a dosage of 0.8 mg/kg of methotrexate extremely well; there are only occasional reports of moderate anorexia, vomiting, and diarrhea.

During maintenance treatment, cats with renal lymphoma receive cytosine arabinoside, instead of cyclophosphamide, at a dosage of 30 mg/kg divided in two doses and administered subcutaneously once a day for 2 days. A high prevalence of central nervous system metastases was noted in cats following apparent remission of renal lymphoma using cyclic combination chemotherapy without cytosine arabinoside. Since incorporating this change, central nervous system metastasis has not been observed in any of the cats treated. Drug levels approaching 30 to 40 per cent of serum concentration may be achieved in the central nervous system (Mooney et al., 1987b).

Determination of *prognosis* in the individual dog or cat with lymphoma can be difficult. Prognosis is favorably affected by early diagnosis and the initiation of treatment. Individual response to chemotherapy is the best prognostic indicator. Animals that achieve a complete response live much longer than those that show only partial or no response.

The following guidelines reflect the clinical observations made by using cyclic combination chemotherapy. In the dog and the cat, clinical stage of disease can affect response and survival. In the cat, FeLV status is important to long-term survival but not to initial response to chemotherapy. Biochemical abnormalities related to lymphoma may affect prognosis in both the dog and the cat.

In the dog, clinical stage of disease is associated with prognosis following chemotherapy only in stage I or II disease. The prognostic value of the stage III to V classification is not reliable, as the WHO system does not take into account the total tumor burden: no criteria are set for degree of lymphadenopathy, hepatosplenomegaly, or degree of bone marrow infiltration by malignant lymphocytes. All dogs with any bone marrow involvement are classified as having stage V disease regardless of concurrent tumor burden (MacEwen et al., 1987).

Cats with clinical stage I or II disease, as determined by the proposed staging system (Mooney et al., 1989), survive longer than cats with clinical stage III to V disease. FeLV-positive cats with stage I or II disease do not survive as long as FeLV-negative cats with stage I or II disease following complete response to chemotherapy (Mooney et al., 1989).

Dogs with hypercalcemia generally do not survive as long as dogs with serum calcium concentrations of less than 12 mg/100 ml. However, if appropriate fluid and blood product support are provided to prevent acute renal failure, hypercoagulability, and thrombosis during initial treatment, response to chemotherapy and survival may equal those of dogs that are not hypercalcemic. In the cat, hypercalcemia is rare and may be related to tumor burden. Hypercalcemia is seen more often in cats that are FeLV positive. In the few cases treated by the author, response to chemotherapy has been poor and long-term survival was not achieved.

Azotemia due to any cause may be a predisposing factor to the development of acute renal failure during initial treatment in dogs and cats with lymphoma. Rapid reduction in tumor volume may cause acute kidney failure in the compromised animal with renal insufficiency unless adequate fluid administration is given during the initial chemotherapy treatment. This is especially true in the cat with renal lymphoma.

Histologic grade of malignancy has not yet been proved to reliably predict biologic behavior or prognosis with respect to response and survival following chemotherapy. Studies involving morphologic and immunophenotypic classification are currently ongoing. Perhaps a more definitive prediction of response will ultimately be possible for dogs and cats with lymphoma based on differences in histologic classification.

CHEMOTHERAPY AND PROGNOSIS OF ACUTE LYMPHOBLASTIC LEUKEMIA

Results of chemotherapy of acute leukemia in the dog and cat have been disappointing. Remission rates are less than 50 per cent, and survival for longer than 6 months is not often achieved. In the dog, response to treatment has been associated with a median survival time of only 5 months, and less than 10 per cent of all dogs treated live a year or longer. Response rates and survival times are similar in the cat. Treatment of acute lymphoblastic leukemia will probably require intensive blood product support in addition to chemotherapy. Although individual animals may respond to chemotherapy and achieve long-term survival, the prognosis is poor. Death due to hemorrhage or infection is probable. Table 4 summarizes the chemotherapy protocol utilized in the treatment of acute lymphoblastic leukemia in the dog and the cat (Matus et al., 1983).

Supportive blood product administration in the treatment of acute leukemia is perhaps as important as chemotherapy. Severe thrombocytopenia, leukopenia, and anemia may result from either chemotherapy or the disease process itself. Repeated transfusion of whole blood, packed red blood cells, fresh frozen plasma, and, if available, platelet-rich plasma should be administered, as dictated by the determination of complete blood counts, differential examination, and platelet counts. Broad-spectrum antibiotics should be prescribed if indicated by clinical signs of infection, such as fever and leukopenia. Any potential infection must be aggressively treated to avoid the occurrence of sepsis and probable death. Treatment for acute lymphoblastic leukemia is probably better performed at a practice or institution where clinical support services include a reliable source of blood products, an intensive care unit, and emergency services available on a 24-hr basis.

PROGNOSIS AND INDICATIONS FOR TREATMENT OF CHRONIC LYMPHOCYTIC LEUKEMIA

Chronic lymphocytic leukemia has a more favorable prognosis than acute lymphoblastic leukemia or lymphoma. In the dog, treatment of chronic leukemia is controversial. Should the asymptomatic dog with a high lymphocyte count be treated with chemotherapy or should only those dogs with clinical signs of disease be treated? In the author's experience, treatment of the asymptomatic dog does not enhance the probability for long-term survival. Treatment is recommended when there is greater than mild lymphadenopathy, marked splenomegaly with hypersplenism, anemia, thrombocytopenia or elevated white blood cell and lymphocyte counts

Table 4. *Chemotherapy for Acute Lymphoblastic Leukemia*

Week	Drug	Canine Dose	Feline Dose
1, 2	Vincristine	0.7 mg/m² IV	0.025 mg/kg IV
	Prednisone	30 mg/m² PO, OD	5 mg b.i.d. PO
3	Asparaginase	400 IU/kg IP	400 IU/kg IP
	Prednisone	20 mg/m² PO, OD	5 mg b.i.d. PO
4, 6	Vincristine	As above	As above
	Prednisone	20 mg/m² PO, qOD	As above
7	Asparaginase	As above	As above
	Prednisone	As above	As above
8–10	Chlorambucil	0.1–0.2 mg/kg PO, OD	2 mg qOD
8–12	Prednisone	As above	As above
12–52	Cyclic combination chemotherapy protocol	See Table 3	See Table 3

IP, intraperitoneal; OD, once a day; qOD, every other day.

associated with clinical signs such as listlessness, and anorexia. In the cat, chronic lymphocytic leukemia is uncommon, and the few cats followed and treated seem to exhibit similar behavior. The asymptomatic animal may survive for months to years without treatment. However, more commonly, the disease will progress and treatment will be required at some point following diagnosis. In 22 dogs followed, the median survival time was over 17 months (Leifer and Matus, 1986b).

The recommended treatment protocol includes the administration of chlorambucil and prednisone at the following dosages:

1. Chlorambucil, 0.2 mg/kg daily for 10 days PO, then 0.1 mg/kg daily on a continuous basis PO. In the cat this dosage is more conveniently given as a 2-mg total dose every other day for 10 days and then every fourth day continuously.

2. Prednisone is administered in a tapered manner for the first 3 weeks of treatment in the dog at a dosage of 30 mg/m², then 20 mg/m², then 10 mg/m², PO, daily per week for a 3-week period. In the cat prednisone is administered at the dose of 5 mg b.i.d. PO, continuously throughout the treatment period.

3. Vincristine, 0.7 mg/m² IV, may be administered to the dog with marked splenomegaly, lymphadenopathy, or lymphocyte counts greater than 50,000/μl to more rapidly reduce tumor burden and alleviate clinical signs of disease. Vincristine has not been used in the few cats treated by the author.

Treatment is continued until the white blood cell count is normal or until anemia, splenomegaly, and lymphadenopathy are resolved. As in the case of acute lymphoblastic leukemia, supportive blood product administration is indicated in the face of severe anemia and thrombocytopenia. Antibiotics

should be administered if clinical signs of infection occur. The dog or cat with chronic lymphocytic leukemia may be more prone to develop infection owing to lack of normal immunoglobulin synthesis and altered cell-mediated immunity. Additionally, altered immunoglobulin synthesis causing hemolytic anemia, monoclonal gammopathy with hyperviscosity syndrome, or light-chain (Bence Jones) proteinuria may influence both initial response to treatment and long-term survival. Chronic lymphocytic leukemia may cause a variety of clinical signs, ranging from an uncomplicated lymphocytosis to severe organ dysfunction and immunologic alterations associated with abnormal lymphocyte function. The prognosis for the individual dog or cat is extremely variable.

References and Supplemental Reading

Leifer, C. E., and Matus, R. E.: Lymphoid leukemia in the dog. Vet. Clin. North Am. 15:723, 1985.

Leifer, C. E., and Matus, R. E.: Canine lymphoma: clinical considerations. Semin. Vet. Med. Surg. 1:43, 1986a.

Leifer, C. E., and Matus R. E.: Chronic lymphocytic leukemia in the dog: 22 cases (1974–1984). J.A.V.M.A. 189:214, 1986b.

MacEwen, E. G., Brown N. O., Patnaik, A. K., et al.: Cyclic combination chemotherapy of canine lymphosarcoma. J.A.V.M.A 178:1178, 1981.

MacEwen, E. G., Hayes, A. A., Matus, R. E., et al.: Evaluation of some prognostic factors for advanced multicentric lymphosarcoma in the dog: 147 cases (1978–1981). J.A.V.M.A. 190:564, 1987.

Matus, R. E., Leifer, C. E., and MacEwen, E. G.,: Acute lymphoblastic leukemia in the dog: A review of 30 cases. J.A.V.M.A. 183:859, 1983.

Mooney, S. C., and Hayes, A. A.: Lymphoma in the cat: An approach to diagnosis and management. Semin. Vet. Med. Surg. 1:51, 1986.

Mooney, S. C., Patnaik, A. K., Hayes, A. A., et al.: Generalized lymphadenopathy resembling lymphoma in cats: Six cases (1972–1976). J.A.V.M.A. 190:897, 1987a.

Mooney, S. C., Hayes, A. A., Matus, R. E., et al.: Renal lymphoma in 28 cats. J.A.V.M.A. 191:1473, 1987b.

Mooney S. C., Hayes, A. A., MacEwen, E. G., et al.: Treatment and prognostic factors in feline lymphoma: 103 cases (1977–1981). J.A.V.M.A. 1989 (in press).

CHEMOTHERAPY OF SOLID TUMORS

STUART C. HELFAND, D.V.M.

Philadelphia, Pennsylvania

The soft tissue tumors represent a diverse group of malignancies that can arise from any extraskeletal site in the body. They are usually classified by the tissue of origin, with tumors derived from mesodermal tissues collectively known as sarcomas. Those tumors derived from epithelium are referred to as carcinomas. This article describes the current status of the use of chemotherapy in the management of (soft tissue) sarcomas and carcinomas of small animals. Excluded from current consideration are tumors derived from hematopoietic and lymphoid organs, which are described elsewhere (see p. 482). In addition, intraoral and most intranasal tumors are omitted from this discussion because they are best treated by combinations of surgery and radiotherapy.

Chemotherapeutic approaches to the management of soft tissue tumors are usually considered second line, as surgery is the mainstay of treatment of these malignancies in veterinary medicine. Soft tissue tumors have the best chance for cure when surgery consists of wide local excision, radical local excision (e.g., chest wall reconstruction), or amputation. If this type of surgery is impractical, such as when a tumor lies in close proximity to vital structures, it has become more widely practiced to investigate chemotherapeutic alternatives. Data documenting chemotherapy responsiveness of soft tissue tumors in veterinary medicine are sparse, but the pursuit of this information is an active area of clinical research in several veterinary centers in the United States. In the area of chemotherapeutics, treatment advances for solid tumors in small animals have been painstakingly slow to appear. This is especially frustrating in light of the successes enjoyed with anticancer drugs for the treatment of some lymphoproliferative and hematopoietic malignancies.

There are several lines of evidence, although somewhat anecdotal, that chemotherapy for these tumors can be a worthwhile form of treatment. These include veterinary case reports documenting remissions of soft tissue tumors following treatment with anticancer drugs, clinical impressions of extended survival in treated animals when compared with the historical survival times of untreated animals, and the extensive human literature documenting chemoresponsiveness of many soft tissue tumors in humans. The well-established role of chemotherapy for palliation of soft tissue tumors in humans provides the greatest motivation to pursue chemotherapeutic intervention in animals. This is because both the tumors and the anticancer drugs employed in veterinary medicine are quite similar to their counterparts in human oncology.

The process of collecting veterinary data about chemotherapy for soft tissue tumors has been slow because of the enormous heterogeneity of this group of neoplasms. Many of the tumors are only infrequently encountered, making it difficult to accrue a large number of animals for study. The tumors are not confined to unique anatomic sites and their biologic behavior (and prognosis) may differ by site, further complicating the process of clinical research. Extensive surgical or radiation therapy in individual animals prior to initiating their chemotherapy adds to the complexity of identifying comparably treated animals. The advanced clinical stage of many animals with soft tissue tumors limits their life expectancy, making long-term follow-up after chemotherapy impossible.

The clinical indications for chemotherapy will differ among patients. These include (1) the sole form of (palliative) treatment for a nonresectable tumor, (2) adjuvant to radiotherapy or surgery or both for local control, (3) use in delaying or preventing development of metastatic disease, (4) palliative treatment for a disseminated tumor, (5) "rescue" relapses following radiation or surgical failures. It is advisable for the clinician to carefully consider the objectives of chemotherapy usage in each case. This is necessary so that a realistic assessment of each animal's prognosis, with anticancer drug treatment, may be given to the client.

When devising a chemotherapeutic protocol for a soft tissue tumor patient, the clinician needs to decide if a single agent or combinations of drugs are to be used. Knowledge of the drug's action, toxicities, drug interactions, rate of tumor growth, degree of cellular differentiation, and previous responses of this tumor type to chemotherapy is helpful in selecting compounds. Drugs chosen in combination protocols should have shown antitumor activity as single agents. Maximal doses should be given, and combinations of drugs without overlapping toxicities best allow this to be done. Adverse effects of the anticancer drugs have been described (see *Current Veterinary Therapy VIII*, pp. 419–423). In general, intermittent treatments with higher doses of drugs, especially alkylating agents, are preferable to more frequent administration of lower doses. However, antimetabolites show increased efficacy when given at more frequent intervals. Combination chemotherapy has the advantages of obtaining drug synergism and delaying the development of drug resistance. It is generally considered more efficacious than single-agent treatment. Veterinary oncologists have followed these principles, and the result has been the development and testing of combination chemotherapy protocols in animals with soft tissue tumors. Veterinarians have the additional considerations of drug costs, practicality of drug administration to pet animals, and the commitment of the pet owner to this modality of therapy.

DOXORUBICIN PROTOCOLS

Doxorubicin (Adriamycin, Adria Labs) has shown the widest range of antitumor activity of any single agent. Its importance in human oncology is firmly established both as a single agent and in combination protocols. Clinical response rates of doxorubicin-treated people have varied widely, in part owing to differences in doses, treatment schedules, tumor type, and stage of disease. In humans, doxorubicin has shown an increase in antitumor response as the dose is increased. It is a cell cycle–nonspecific compound, and drugs with activity that is independent of the cell cycle frequently demonstrate this property. For this reason, it is advisable to administer the maximal dose that does not produce unacceptable toxicity. The question of acceptable toxicity is not always clear cut, however, and veterinarians must routinely deal with the ethical concerns associated with the development of toxic signs in treated pet animals. The currently recommended dose of doxorubicin in the dog is 30 mg/m² every 3 weeks; whereas in the cat, 20 to 25 mg/m² is given every 3 to 5 weeks (Table 1). Even at these dosages, some animals will become ill and require supportive care.

As a single agent, doxorubicin has shown activity against a variety of carcinomas and sarcomas encountered in veterinary practice. In most instances, however, the responses are only minimal or partial (i.e., 25 to 50 per cent tumor reduction) and of insignificant duration. At the Veterinary Hospital of the University of Pennsylvania (VHUP), doxorubicin is used as a single agent primarily in the treatment of nonresectable carcinoma of the thyroid gland in dogs. For this purpose, doxorubicin induced partial remission in 30 per cent of dogs with advanced (stage III and IV) disease. The median

Table 1. Chemotherapeutics

Doxorubicin (Adriamycin, Adria Labs)	Dogs: 30 mg/m² IV every 3 weeks Cats: 20–25 mg/m² IV every 21–35 days*
AC	
Doxorubicin	Dogs: 30 mg/m² IV, day 1 Cats: 20–25 mg/m² IV, day 1
Cyclophosphamide (Cytoxan, Bristol-Myers)	50–100 mg/m² per os, days 3–6
Cycle repeats on day 22 in dogs and day 22 or 36 in cats*	
VAC	
Doxorubicin	30 mg/m² IV, day 1
Cyclophosphamide	100–150 mg/m² IV day 1, or 50 mg/m² per os, days 3–6
Vincristine (Oncovin, Eli Lilly)	0.7 mg/m² IV, days 8 & 15
Cycle repeats on day 22	
ADIC (Dogs)	
Doxorubicin	30 mg/m² IV, day 1
Dacarbazine (DTIC-Dome, Miles)	200 mg/m² IV, days 1–5
Cycle repeats on day 22	
Cisplatin† (Platinol, Bristol-Myers)	60 mg/m² IV every 3 weeks (rigorous diuresis necessary)
BAC	
Doxorubicin	Dogs: 30 mg/m² IV, day 1 Cats: 20–25 mg/m² IV, day 1
Cyclophosphamide	50–100 mg/m² per os, days 3–6
Bleomycin (Blenoxane, Bristol-Myers)	10 units/m² SC days 1, 8, & 15
Cycle repeats on day 22 in dogs and day 22 or 36 in cats*	
Melphalan (Alkeran, Burroughs Wellcome)	Dogs: 7 mg/m² per os days 1–5 every 3 weeks
5-Fluorouracil† (Fluorouracil, Roche Labs)	Dogs: 150 mg/m² IV once per week
FC†	
5-Fluorouracil	150 mg/m² IV, day 1
Cyclophosphamide	50–100 mg/m² per os, days 1–4
Cycle is repeated for 24 weeks, skipping weeks 6, 12, 18, & 24	
FAC†	
Doxorubicin	30 mg/m² IV, day 1
Cyclophosphamide	100–150 mg/m² IV day 1, or 50 mg/m² per os, days 3–6
5-Fluorouracil	150 mg/m² IV, days 1, 8, & 15
Cycle repeats on day 22	

*If toxicity is mild, repeat cycle at 21 days, otherwise 35 days.
†*Do not use in cats.*

survival time of dogs receiving it for thyroid carcinoma at VHUP was 9 months in an earlier analysis.

In an efficacy study conducted in multiple institutions, the initial response to treatment with doxorubicin was evaluated in a large number of dogs. Any response to doxorubicin was determined at the end of 9 weeks, after the completion of two cycles of chemotherapy. Thirty-one per cent of animals with a variety of nonlymphoid, soft tissue tumors showed a reduction in their tumor size, indicating a broad spectrum of activity for doxorubicin in canine malignancies. Fibrosarcomas were extremely resistant, as only 1 dog of 14 with this malignancy showed a response. It is unknown whether this initial reduction in tumor size actually implies improvement in survival, because studies aimed at answering this question are lacking. Nonetheless, doxorubicin is a reasonable choice of treatment for dogs with soft tissue malignancies, as tumor palliation and improvement in the animal's quality of life are likely in some animals.

More often, doxorubicin is combined with other anticancer drugs for solid tumor therapy. The rationale for this approach is based on the demonstrated synergism of doxorubicin with several individual compounds, including cyclophosphamide (Cytoxan, Bristol-Myers), cisplatin (Platinol, Bristol-Myers), and bleomycin (Blenoxane, Bristol-Myers), in experimental animals.

At VHUP, the combination protocol of doxorubicin and cyclophosphamide (Table 1) has been used for palliation of a variety of tumors in dogs and cats. The clinical settings have varied widely, including both adjuvant and nonadjuvant usages in animals with advanced-stage disease. Analysis of the treatment results of more than 30 dogs indicated partial remission of fibrosarcoma, hemangiosarcoma, undifferentiated sarcoma, transitional cell carcinoma, prostatic carcinoma, and thyroid carcinoma. The duration of the clinical response in these dogs ranged from 2 to 12 months. There was no tumor response in a small number of dogs treated for mast cell tumor, hemangiopericytoma, anaplastic carcinoma, and mammary carcinoma.

Doxorubicin and cyclophosphamide have been used together at VHUP for control of several feline malignancies (Table 1). In general, this protocol has been more commonly employed in an adjuvant setting rather than as the sole form of tumor control. Many cats will develop inappetence of varying degrees during the first several days of this protocol. Most animals will be eating well within 5 days, however. Following excision of mammary carcinoma in cats, it is routine to administer four cycles of doxorubicin and cyclophosphamide at the author's hospital. This recommendation is based on the high metastatic rate for feline mammary carcinoma, as well as the moderate sensitivity this tumor has shown to the combination of doxorubicin and cyclophosphamide in cats. One report described a 45 per cent response rate in cats that were treated for advanced stage mammary carcinoma with this drug combination. The duration of the remissions ranged between 45 and 344 days, with 3 of 11 cats having complete remissions. Partial responses have been observed in a small number of cats that received this drug combination for salivary adenocarcinoma, fibrosarcoma, and undifferentiated sarcoma. In several cats, the reduction in tumor size enabled resection of tumors that were considered nonresectable prior to chemotherapy. There was no response in cats treated for gastric adenocarcinoma, intestinal adenocarcinoma, and osteosarcoma.

Vincristine can be added to doxorubicin and cyclophosphamide (VAC, Table 1). In human beings, this combination has been used to control a number of soft tissue sarcomas. The addition of vincristine to doxorubicin and cyclophosphamide provides a theoretic advantage over the two-drug protocol, but no clinical trials comparing this regimen to others have been conducted in dogs. Clinical responses have been observed in 26 of 34 dogs treated with the VAC protocol for a variety of tumors including hemangiosarcoma, undifferentiated sarcoma, fibrosarcoma, rhabdomyosarcoma, neurofibrosarcoma, myxosarcoma, hemangiopericytoma, and several adenocarcinomas. Small numbers of dogs with each type of tumor were treated. The survival times for dogs that responded to VAC ranged from 17 days to nearly 2 years. Only three of nine dogs with fibrosarcoma demonstrated reduction in tumor size, once again showing the extreme chemoresistance of this malignancy.

Myelosuppression is an important side effect of the VAC protocol. The median neutrophil count of 27 dogs treated with VAC was 800/μl. Rigorous hematologic monitoring is required for dogs on this protocol, as sepsis and fever almost always develop when the neutrophil count remains below 1000/μl for more than 1 or 2 days. Dogs receiving VAC at VHUP are usually placed on trimethoprim-sulfonamide prophylactically (15 mg/kg every 12 hours orally) for the first 14 days of the chemotherapy cycle. Neutropenic, febrile animals require hospitalization and are treated intravenously with an aminoglycoside, usually gentamicin, and a second-generation cephalosporin antibiotic. The neutrophil count usually rebounds within 2 to 3 days. The protocol of doxorubicin and cyclophosphamide (without vincristine) can also cause significant myelosuppression (see p. 494).

Doxorubicin is occasionally combined with dacarbazine (Table 1) for treatment of soft tissue sarcomas in humans. Although doxorubicin and cyclophosphamide are more routinely utilized in veterinary medicine, the combination of doxorubicin and dacarbazine has been therapeutic for several canine soft tissue sarcomas treated at VHUP. This protocol has also been used to treat dogs with relapsing lymphosarcoma.

CISPLATIN

Since its introduction as an antineoplastic compound, cisplatin has been widely used in human oncology. The drug has undergone toxicity and efficacy testing in several veterinary institutions in small animals. The toxicities are notable and have been described elsewhere. The compound is contraindicated in cats.

At VHUP, 26 dogs with 12 different tumor types

received 53 cycles of cisplatin. One dog achieved a complete remission of pulmonary metastases from a nasal carcinoma after two treatments with cisplatin. One other dog with an advanced intranasal adenocarcinoma experienced a partial remission after two cisplatin treatments, which rendered the tumor amenable to surgical excision and radiotherapy. One dog had a partial remission of lung metastases, which were derived from a primary limb osteosarcoma. Of the remaining 23 dogs, no animal experienced any significant antitumor effect from treatments with cisplatin. The malignancies that were resistant included tonsillar squamous cell carcinoma, prostatic carcinoma, thyroid carcinoma, thyroid carcinosarcoma, squamous cell carcinoma metastatic to bone, transitional cell carcinoma, synovial cell sarcoma, undifferentiated sarcoma, myxofibrosarcoma, intranasal chondrosarcoma, and osteosarcoma (of long and flat bones). With the exception of osteosarcoma, only one dog with each tumor type was treated.

Other investigators have observed intermittent effectiveness of cisplatin in canine solid tumors. Dramatic responses of both primary and metastatic squamous cell carcinoma were reported in two dogs treated with cisplatin. One animal experienced a complete clinical remission, lasting approximately 1.5 yr. The other dog experienced a partial remission that lasted for 3 months. Forty-one dogs with a variety of solid tumors were treated with cisplatin at Purdue University (Knapp et al., 1988). The overall response rate was 17 per cent (7 of 41 dogs responded). One dog of 11 with squamous cell carcinoma experienced a complete remission, as did one dog with an undifferentiated carcinoma in the mediastinum. Partial remissions were observed in 1 of 11 dogs with squamous cell carcinoma, one of three dogs with nasal adenocarcinoma, one dog with thyroid adenocarcinoma, and two of three dogs with metastatic osteosarcoma. Remission durations ranged from 21 to 150 days.

When determining clinical response of tumors to cisplatin, two chemotherapy treatments were given to each dog 3 weeks apart before evaluating the drug's efficacy. In most cases, clinical benefit from cisplatin was apparent within this time period in the dogs treated at the University of Pennsylvania and at Purdue University.

The role of cisplatin in the management of canine solid tumors is, as yet, undefined. It appears that as a single agent, this drug has modest efficacy in some adenocarcinomas, squamous cell carcinomas, and osteosarcomas. It is a reasonable chemotherapeutic agent to choose for tumor palliation in some dogs that have nonresectable carcinoma or metastatic osteosarcoma. In humans and experimental animal models, cisplatin has shown synergism with other chemotherapeutic agents, including doxorubicin, bleomycin, and 5-fluorouracil (Fluorouracil,

Roche Labs). Veterinary data about these drug combinations are lacking. Cisplatin is synergistic with radiotherapy and hyperthermia and is being used routinely with these modalities to treat solid tumors in dogs at a number of veterinary institutions. (For an additional discussion of cisplatin therapy in small animals, see p. 497.)

MISCELLANEOUS PROTOCOLS

Several protocols have been employed on limited numbers of animals that resulted in tumor palliation in some animals. Clinical investigations with these protocols are in an early phase of study. Controlled clinical trials are needed to firmly establish their true importance.

Cats with nonresectable squamous cell carcinoma of the tongue have been treated with the combination of doxorubicin, cyclophosphamide, and bleomycin (Table 1). One cat had a complete remission after two cycles (6 weeks), which persisted for 9 months. Partial remissions were induced in another three cats, which lasted 2 to 5 months. Only one cat of five so treated failed to show any objective improvement in its tumor. After there was reduction in the size of the lingual squamous cell carcinoma, responding cats enjoyed an improved quality of life characterized by increased appetite and weight gain. Toxicity of this protocol was no worse than that of doxorubicin and cyclophosphamide alone. The high cost of bleomycin will preclude usage of this protocol for most pet owners.

The alkylating agent melphalan (Alkeran, Burroughs Wellcome) is being investigated at VHUP in dogs following excision of anal sac (apocrine gland) adenocarcinoma (Table 1). Because anal sac adenocarcinoma has a highly metastatic behavior, adjuvant chemotherapy has a role in the management of this malignancy. One dog with an incompletely excised, metastatic sublumbar lymph node experienced a complete remission following two cycles of melphalan. Abdominal radiographs and serum calcium levels returned to normal. This dog was treated for 6 months and has remained disease free for 3 yr. Another animal, with hypercalcemia and moderately enlarged sublumbar lymph nodes containing metastases, experienced progressive disease during 6 months of melphalan treatment. Two other dogs, without signs of metastasis at the time of anal sac surgery, received melphalan for 6 months postoperatively. These dogs have remained disease free after 2 years of follow-up.

The antimetabolite 5-fluorouracil is a compound with proven efficacy for some carcinomas in human beings. In people, it has a role in the management of mammary carcinoma, hepatic and gastrointestinal malignancies, and prostatic adenocarcinoma, to name a few. This drug has been used at several veterinary institutions in combination chemotherapy protocols designed against carcinomas in the dog. To date, there have been no reports of treatment results with these protocols, although (neurologic) toxicity data have been published. *This agent is extremely dangerous in cats and should not be used in this species.* In combination protocols, 5-fluorouracil is given to dogs with cyclophosphamide (FC) and doxorubicin (FAC) (Table 1). The author has treated two dogs with FAC for prostatic adenocarcinoma. One dog went into a partial remission lasting 2 months, whereas the other animal did not respond. Two dogs with bronchogenic carcinoma were treated with FAC without benefit. Statistically significant numbers of dogs need to be treated before making conclusions about the relevance of 5-fluorouracil therapy in veterinary medicine. The protocols are presented in Table 1 for interested clinicians.

CHEMOTHERAPEUTIC GUIDELINES

Clinical response of tumors to doxorubicin-based protocols is usually detectable after two cycles. At VHUP, doxorubicin protocols are continued for at least four to six consecutive cycles. Because a total of no more than eight treatments of doxorubicin are routinely given to any animal, two to four cycles are kept in reserve for future recurrences.

It is preferable to monitor a specific tumor marker during chemotherapy to gauge the effectiveness of treatment. However, this is not always possible, especially with visceral malignancy. Periodic ultrasonography of the abdomen, with special attention to the liver and spleen, has been a useful method of following tumor response in animals with known parenchymal malignancy. At VHUP, thoracic radiographs are done every 6 to 8 weeks to follow the clinical course of pulmonary metastasis. Sublumbar lymphadenopathy can also be monitored via radiographs and ultrasonography.

Particular attention must be paid to the neutrophil count and, to a lesser degree, the platelet count in animals receiving many of these drugs. At VHUP, the neutrophil count is obtained one time 10 to 14 days after doxorubicin is given. When cyclophosphamide is combined with doxorubicin, this blood count is done one time between days 9 and 11 of the cycle. Following cisplatin administration, a neutrophil count and serum creatinine measurement are advised at day 10 of the cycle. Initially, weekly blood counts are done when 5-fluorouracil is given with cyclophosphamide. Subsequent counts are done one to two times monthly if myelosuppression is not severe.

Veterinarians who engage in chemotherapeutics must acquire a knowledge of the toxicities of these drugs. Some treated animals will require hospitalization for life-threatening, chemotherapy-induced side effects, and it is essential that those animals be recognized promptly. With an understanding of the complications of chemotherapy, there is no reason why most veterinarians cannot participate in this area of cancer medicine when presented with patients with solid tumors.

References and Supplemental Reading

Baker, L. H. (ed.): *Soft Tissue Sarcomas.* Boston: Martinus Nijhoff Publishers, 1983.
Brown, N. O.: Management of solid tumors. *In* Kirk, R. W. (ed.): *Current Veterinary Therapy VIII.* Philadelphia: W.B. Saunders, 1983, pp. 415–418.
Clemmons, R. M., Gorman, N. T., and Calderwood-Mays, M. B.: Lumbar epidural chondrosarcoma in a dog treated by excision and chemotherapy. J.A.V.M.A. 183:1006, 1983.
DeMadron, E., Helfand, S. C., and Stebbins, K. E.: Use of chemotherapy in treatment of cardiac hemangiosarcoma in a dog. J.A.V.M.A. 190:887, 1987.
Gottlieb, J. A., Baker, L. H., Quagliana, J. M., et al.: Chemotherapy of sarcomas with a combination of adriamycin and dimethyl triazeno imidazole carboxamide. Cancer 30:1632, 1972.
Gottlieb, J. A., Baker, L. H., O'Bryan, R. M., et al.: Adriamycin (NSC-123127) used alone and in combination for soft tissue and bony sarcomas. Cancer Chemother. Rep. 6:271, 1975.
Helfand, S. C.: Chemotherapy for nonresectable and metastatic soft tissue tumors. Proceedings of the 10th Annual Kal Kan Symposium, October, 1986, Kal Kan Foods, Inc, 1987, pp. 133–142.
Jeglum, K. A., deGuzman, E., and Young, K. M.: Chemotherapy of advanced mammary adenocarcinoma in 14 cats. J.A.V.M.A. 187:157, 1985.
Jeglum, K. A., and Whereat, A.: Chemotherapy of canine thyroid carcinoma. Comp. Cont. Ed. Pract. Vet. 5:96, 1983.
Knapp, D. W., Richardson, R. C., Bonney, P. L., et al.: Cisplatin therapy in forty-one dogs with malignant tumors. J. Vet. Intern. Med. 2:41, 1988.
MacEwen, E. G.: Current concepts in cancer therapy: Biologic therapy and chemotherapy. Semin. Vet. Med. Surg. 1:5, 1986.
Madewell, B. R.: Adverse effects of chemotherapy. *In* Kirk, R.W. (ed.): *Current Veterinary Therapy VIII.* Philadelphia: W.B. Saunders, 1983, pp. 419–423.
Richardson, R. C.: Solid tumors. Vet. Clin. North Am. [Small Anim. Pract.] 15:557, 1985.
Schoster, J. V., and Wyman, M.: Remission of orbital sarcoma in a dog using doxorubicin therapy. J.A.V.M.A. 172:1101, 1978.
Tilmant, L. L., Gorman, N. T., Ackerman, N., et al.: Chemotherapy of synovial cell sarcoma in a dog. J.A.V.M.A. 188:530, 1986.

CHEMOTHERAPY-INDUCED MYELOSUPPRESSION

ROBERT C. ROSENTHAL, D.V.M.

Madison, Wisconsin

With improved comprehensive veterinary care, including better vaccinations, more attention to nutritional concerns, and increased sophistication in both diagnostic techniques and medical management, pets are living longer than ever before. Cancer is in most instances a disease of the middle-aged and older animal. It is reasonable to expect that more and more pets with cancer will be presented to veterinarians and that their owners will expect treatment that is both reasonable and effective. For many years, cancer in pets was considered a surgical problem, if, indeed, any therapy was considered at all. Surgery remains a vital tool in the oncologist's approach to both diagnosis and treatment, but other therapies are gaining increased importance. Radiation therapy is available at almost every veterinary school and at some institutional and private practices as well. Chemotherapy in both primary and adjunct settings is now practiced by many veterinarians. Although there are clear benefits seen with chemotherapy for lymphosarcoma, multiple myeloma, and transmissible venereal tumors of dogs, the advantages gained by treatment with drugs for most other tumors have been more difficult to quantify. There is much to be learned about the effect of combination chemotherapy on response rates, remission times, and survival.

Two of the basic principles of combination chemotherapy are (1) to use drugs with different mechanisms of action and (2) to use drugs with different toxicities. One should always try to employ drugs with different dose-limiting toxicities so that each agent can be used in full doses. A good example of this principle is the widely used COP (cyclophosphamide, vincristine, prednisone) protocol for lymphosarcoma. The dose-limiting toxicity of the alkylating agent cyclophosphamide is myelosuppression, but the same is not true of either vincristine or prednisone. Myelosuppression is, of course, a concern with these drugs but not to the extent that it is when the myelosuppressive drug doxorubicin is substituted for prednisone in this protocol (as has been evaluated in a trial of the treatment of nonresectable and metastatic soft tissue tumors in dogs) (Helfand, 1987).

The importance of toxicity cannot be overempha-

sized. Chemotherapy is limited not by the ability to kill cancer cells, but rather by the toxicity to the host. This simple fact is complicated by the realization that most owners have had some experience with cancer and cancer therapy in either people or animals they know. The quality of their pet's life is an over-riding and reasonable concern for pet owners. That the option of euthanasia exists demands that veterinarians providing cancer care do not diminish the quality of the patient's life. There is no justification for a therapy that is worse than the disease. Dermatologic and gastrointestinal toxicities (alopecia, anorexia, vomiting, and diarrhea) are frequently of greatest concern to owners and need to be addressed with frank discussion prior to beginning therapy with drugs likely to cause such effects. To the chemotherapist, however, bone marrow toxicity and the attendant problems of infection attributable to neutropenia and the potential for the delay of further treatment are usually of greater concern. If chemotherapy is to continue to be an effective means of treatment, it will be necessary to anticipate and manage the effects of myelosuppressive drugs.

Although anticancer agents can affect all the cellular elements of the blood, the effect on granulocytes is of the greatest concern, with the effects on platelets and red blood cells usually of less importance. Granulocytes remain in the peripheral circulation for only hours; their total population turns over several times a day. Platelets remain in the circulation for days (the normal life span for canine platelets is about 5 to 6 days). Red blood cells survive longer (mean, 110 to 120 days in the dog; 70 days in the cat), and therefore are less affected by short-term effects on the marrow. It is important to recognize that both the survival of cells in the periphery and the direct effect of the drugs on the proliferating cells in the marrow determine the hematologic picture.

DEVELOPMENT OF CELLS IN THE BONE MARROW

Erythrocytes, polymorphonuclear granulocytes, monocytes, and platelets develop in the bone marrow from a population of pluripotent stem cells. The development of granulocytes provides a basis for understanding the impact of cytotoxic therapy on the total and differential white blood cell counts. Pluripotent stem cells are not differentiated and can divide essentially without limit. Each daughter cell may either remain a stem cell or differentiate into a multipotent progenitor cell, which has the capacity to give rise to a myeloblast (or other blast cell). Myeloblasts divide to form promyelocytes, which in turn divide to form myelocytes. Two or three divisions are possible at the myelocyte stage before these cells differentiate into metamyelocytes, which no longer have the capacity to divide but do undergo further maturation to band and segmented forms. The stem and progenitor cells are primitive and cannot be identified morphologically. They represent a proliferative pool with great regenerative potential. The cells in the myeloblast through the myelocyte stages represent a mitotic pool that undergoes four to five mitoses and results in as much as a 16- to 32-fold increase in cell numbers. The transit time through this mitotic pool is about 60 hr. In the storage pool, metamyelocytes develop in turn into band forms and mature segmented cells. Transit time through the storage pool ranges from 50 to 70 hr. There is a 2- to 3-day reserve of cells in this pool. Other cell lines have comparable developmental patterns. Monocytes undergo fewer divisions and have a shorter transit time than granulocytes. The transit time for red blood cells in the bone marrow has been estimated at 7 days. Platelets are produced over a 3- to 4-day period.

EFFECT OF CYTOTOXIC DRUGS

The various cytotoxic anticancer agents have been widely reviewed in this volume and elsewhere. The cycling cells of the bone marrow, those in the mitotic pool, are highly susceptible to their effects. Dose and schedule are determined by the effect on the bone marrow (or other dose-limiting tissue toxicity). The commonly used cytotoxic agents vary in their potential to suppress the bone marrow acutely or chronically. With most of these drugs as commonly used, the lethal effect seems to be on the cells of the mitotic pool and spares the total marrow destruction that would ensue if stem cells were destroyed. The nondividing cells of the maturation pool are not affected. Clinically, this is apparent as a 2- to 3-day preservation of the white blood cell count before the decrease that reflects the lack of activity in the mitotic pool. After stem and progenitor cells replenish the mitotic pool, the developmental process continues and eventually mature white blood cells return to the circulation. White blood cell counts generally recover within a week to a range that allows further treatment.

Alkylating agents, antitumor antibiotics, antimetabolites, plant alkaloids, and some of the miscellaneous agents have the potential to cause myelosuppression, but the degree and duration of the effect can vary. Cell cycle–nonspecific drugs (including the alkylating agents and doxorubicin) are likely to cause more severe myelosuppression. An understanding of the unique aspects of each drug is helpful in planning and conducting chemotherapy.

Asparaginase is essentially without myelosuppressive toxicity. Vincristine, cis-platinum, and bleomycin have relatively little myelosuppressive toxicity. The potential for myelosuppression is greater with cyclophosphamide, doxorubicin, and methotrexate, but precise responses are dose and schedule dependent. The nadir after doxorubicin therapy occurs later than that with most other drugs, and subsequent treatments should be planned 2 or 3 weeks later. The less frequently used drugs vinblastine, 5-fluorouracil, cytosine arabinoside, and nitrogen mustard are recognized as potentially quite myelosuppressive as well. Furthermore, the alkylating agents may demonstrate cumulative toxicity with prolonged use. One unique feature of cyclophosphamide is its recognized platelet sparing. As suggested above, by balancing the characteristics of the components of a protocol, the chemotherapist should be able to employ these drugs both effectively and safely.

MANAGEMENT OF CHEMOTHERAPY-INDUCED MYELOSUPPRESSION

A decrease in the white blood cell count is expected as a normal response to most cytotoxic chemotherapy. In protocols that call for the repeated use of these drugs, it is imperative that a total and differential white blood cell count be performed prior to their administration. In most instances, a complete blood count will provide additional information regarding the packed cell volume (PCV) and an assessment of platelets. It is not unusual to find a PCV in the 33 to 37 per cent range in dogs on long-term chemotherapy. This does not seem to be harmful or require treatment, but rapid decreases much below these levels should be investigated. If thrombocytopenia is noted, further therapy may need to be delayed; however, this seems to be a much less common or serious problem than granulocytopenia. Most dogs and cats receiving chemotherapy have platelet counts of greater than $50,000/\mu l$. Spontaneous hemorrhage is usually not noted until platelet counts are less than $40,000/\mu l$. Canine autologous bone marrow transplantation patients have remained free of spontaneous hemorrhage for prolonged periods with platelet counts in the 15,000 to $20,000/\mu l$ range. The thrombocytopenic bleeding patient should receive transfusions of whole blood or platelet-rich plasma. Bleeding patients with adequate platelet counts should be evaluated for other coagulopathies.

Guidelines for altering therapy by using decreased doses based on the degree of myelosuppression have been published, but it is probably better to delay therapy until treatment with full doses can be tolerated. This is especially true for solid tumors, but the concept should apply to hematologic malignancies as well. One conservative guideline states not to treat with myelosuppressive drugs if the total white blood cell count is less than 4000/μl or if the neutrophil count is less than 2500/μl. In reality, to use chemotherapeutic drugs to their fullest benefit, veterinary oncologists will frequently employ anticancer agents even when counts are somewhat below these figures, depending on several factors including the patient's history of response, the drug previously used, and the drug scheduled to be given.

Infection is a major concern in the chemotherapy-induced myelosuppressed patient. Although white blood cell counts are expected to fall below the normal range at some time following the administration of these drugs, most patients do not become infected. Antibiotics do not need to be administered routinely to cancer patients receiving chemotherapy as it is most often given now. Patients with neutrophil counts of less than 2000/μl should be monitored carefully for signs of fever or infection. The risk of infection increases with neutrophil counts below 1000/μl and rises sharply as counts fall below 500/μl. As more aggressive protocols are developed, there may be a place for prophylactic antibiotic therapy in conjunction with combinations of drugs that are expected to result in neutrophil counts of less than 1000/μl for prolonged periods. Trimethoprim-sulfonamide has been used in conjunction with an aggressive combination chemotherapy protocol using cyclophosphamide, doxorubicin, and vincristine. As a single agent, this drug appeared to reduce effectively the frequency of antibiotic-responsive febrile episodes in a patient population with a median neutrophil count of 800/μl.

In the myelosuppressed, febrile patient, a locus of infection may be difficult to identify because of the absence of the usual signs of inflammation. A diligent search should be made, however, including obtaining cultures of blood and urine. Many of the usual systemic signs of infection may be absent. The majority of infections in myelosuppressed patients involve the respiratory, alimentary, and urogenital tracts. Although many of these patients will have pneumonia, they will often lack physical signs of pulmonary congestion. Thoracic radiographs are usually helpful in demonstrating consolidation and should be considered an important part of the diagnostic workup. Erythema and pain remain important signs in localized infections, and subtle changes should be looked for carefully. A subjective assessment of the patient's status manifested by fever and malaise is likewise an important factor. The knowledge that infection is common in the seriously myelosuppressed patient and is likely to be serious should prompt the clinician to respond quickly.

The "best" antibiotic to use in this setting is the one to which the causative organism is susceptible, but there is often not enough time to await the results of culture and sensitivity testing. Most infections are caused by gram-negative bacilli, including *Pseudomonas*, *Klebsiella*, and *Escherichia*. A combination of ampicillin and gentamicin has proved helpful and economical, but certainly many other drug combinations may be as or even more useful. The use of other drugs, including ticarcillin, tobramycin, carbenicillin, amikacin, third-generation cephalosporins (e.g., ceftazidime), and fluoroquinolone antimicrobial drugs (e.g., eiprofloxacin), holds great promise in this area. Many questions remain unanswered; it is by no means clear what two- or three-drug combination might really be optimal. It is doubtful that there is an optimal combination for all cases. The role of monotherapy with newer drugs is unknown. If the expected duration of the granulocytopenia is short and granulocyte numbers do begin to rise, the chances for recovery are better than if neither of these occurs. There are currently no firm guidelines indicating at what point the antibiotic regimen might be altered in the absence of response, but it is clear that antibiotic therapy should continue until the granulocytopenia resolves.

Lithium has been considered a potentially useful agent in the prevention of chemotherapy-induced myelosuppression. Several clinical studies in human cancer patients suggest a beneficial role, but others question the conduct of these trials and the interpretation of the results. Studies in normal dogs given myelosuppressive doses of vinblastine or nitrogen mustard showed that lithium was not able to protect those dogs against chemotherapy-induced myelosuppression. Evaluation of the clinical use of lithium adjunctively in selected canine cancer patients has also failed to demonstrate a beneficial effect.

Other possible adjunctive measures include the use of anabolic steroids, aspirin or other nonsteroidal anti-inflammatory agents, granulocyte transfusions, or granulocyte-macrophage colony stimulating factors (GM-CSFs). Corticosteroids seem to have no real role here. Although such drugs increase white blood cell counts in normal animals, the mechanism involves preventing normal egress from the circulating pool and accelerated release of mature neutrophils from the storage pool rather than an effect on myelopoiesis. It is interesting to note that, in the myelosuppressed patient, granulocytes can be found in the tissues in numbers indicative of recovery before the peripheral counts rise appreciably. It seems logical, therefore, that normal egress from the circulation is a function to be maintained, not inhibited. Anabolic steroids have been used as adjunctive therapy in aplastic anemias with debatable results. They seem to have no practical role in stimulating a short-term myelopoietic response.

In the febrile neutropenic patient presumed to be septic, antipyretic drugs may be of some value. A fever that remains below 105°F is not likely to harm the patient and may inhibit the proliferation of pathogens and provide useful information regarding the likely origin of the fever and the response to therapy. Temperatures greater than 106°F, however, may be detrimental to the patient, as they are associated with brain damage, dysrhythmias, and disseminated intravascular coagulation, in addition to increasing the metabolic rate and contributing to dehydration. Administration of aspirin or other means to lower the temperature are indicated for these patients. Flunixin meglumine or corticosteroids may also be helpful if the patient has endotoxic shock, and the clinician should be certain to maintain proper hydration of the patient at all times.

Granulocyte transfusions have been shown to be of benefit in neutropenic septic human beings if the white blood cell count is expected to rise soon. Currently, technical problems limit the applicability of this approach in veterinary patients. One potential additional adjunct is the use of GM-CSF, a specific stimulator of the granulocyte-macrophage series that may become available as a product of genetic engineering. Although not likely necessary for the patient experiencing short-term myelosuppression, GM-CSF may be useful in patients expected to have long-term suppression (e.g., bone marrow transplant recipients).

SUMMARY

Veterinarians are likely to encounter more cancer patients whose owners will request therapy. Chemotherapy will be an increasingly important part of cancer treatment. Effective chemotherapy will be accompanied by some degree of myelosuppression. The ability to anticipate and react to problems associated with the myelosuppressed cancer patient will facilitate the delivery of improved patient care. The prudent and appropriate use of anticancer agents, antibiotic support, and new approaches to myelosuppressed dogs and cats should add to the veterinarian's capacity to provide a high level of care for cancer patients.

References and Supplemental Reading

Bodey, G. P.: Infections in patients with cancer. In Holland, J. F., and Frei, E., III (eds.): Cancer Medicine, 2nd ed. Philadelphia: Lea & Febiger, 1982, pp. 1339–1372.

Couto, C. G.: Toxicity of anticancer therapy. Proceedings of the 10th Annual Kal Kan Symposium, October, 1986, Kal Kan Foods, Inc., 1987, pp. 37–46.

Davis, L. E.: General care of the patient. In Davis, L. E. (ed.): Handbook of Small Animal Therapeutics. New York: Churchill Livingstone, 1985, pp. 10–19.

Helfand, S. C.: Chemotherapy for nonresectable and metastatic soft tissue tumors. Proceedings of the 10th Annual Kal Kan Symposium, October, 1986, Kal Kan Foods, Inc., 1987, pp. 133–142.

Rosenthal, R. C.: Lithium carbonate as a protectant against vinblastine-induced myelosuppression. J. Vet. Comp. Oncol. (in press).

Rosenthal, R. C.: Chemotherapy. In MacEwen, E. G., and Withrow, S. J. (eds.): Veterinary Clinical Oncology. Philadelphia: J. B. Lippincott (in press).

Schimpff, S. C.: Therapy of infection in patients with granulocytopenia. Med. Clin. North Am. 61:1101, 1977.

Sickles, E. A., Green, W. H., and Wiernik, P. H.: Clinical presentation of infection in granulocytopenic patients. Arch. Intern. Med. 135:715, 1975.

CISPLATIN CHEMOTHERAPY

WAYNE SHAPIRO, D.V.M.
Boston, Massachusetts

There are over 40 antineoplastic drugs currently available. Less than 15 of these are used routinely for the treatment of cancer in domestic animals. A relatively new drug to veterinary medicine, cisplatin (*cis*-diammine-dichloroplatinum; Platinol, Bristol-Myers), has been under careful evaluation at many veterinary centers.

While studying the growth characteristics of *Escherichia coli* in an electrical field, Rosenberg and associates (1965) discovered that cell division was inhibited when platinum electrodes were used. This effect was shown to be due to the formation of new compounds by electrolysis—the platinum diamines. The antineoplastic properties of these compounds were quickly recognized, and cisplatin was chosen for further evaluation in human clinical trials (Rozencweig et al., 1977). As a single agent or in combination chemotherapy, cisplatin was most effective for treatment of transitional cell carcinoma, head and neck squamous cell carcinoma, ovarian and testicular tumors, and osteosarcoma.

PHARMACOLOGY

Cisplatin (Fig. 1) is an inorganic complex formed by a central platinum atom surrounded by two chlorine atoms and two ammonia groups arranged in the *cis* configuration in the horizontal plane (Page et al., 1985). In fluids with a high chloride ion content (i.e., physiologic saline solution or the extracellular fluid), cisplatin remains intact and inactive. This electrically neutral form readily diffuses across cell membranes. Within a cell, the low chloride content of the intracellular fluid allows dissociation of the chloride ions, resulting in positively charged, aqueous forms of cisplatin. These active forms bind covalently to genomic DNA, especially to guanine residues, and produce inter- and intrastrand cross-links and breakage similar to the effect of bifunctional alkylating agents. This effect is considered cell cycle independent. Unrepaired damage to DNA results in death of the cell when mitosis occurs.

After intravenous administration of cisplatin to dogs, there was a biphasic clearance pattern (Litterst et al., 1976). The half-times for the rapid-phase and slow-phase clearances were less than 1 hr and nearly 5 days, respectively. Plasma levels fell by 90 per cent during the first 4 hr, and 60 to 70 per cent of the cisplatin dose was recovered in the urine. Within several hours after administration 90 per cent of the remaining serum platinum was protein bound. Tissue concentrations of platinum were measured, and those accumulations were postulated to act as reservoirs for the prolonged slow-phase clearance of platinum that resulted in easily detectable serum levels 12 days after administration.

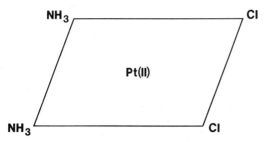

Figure 1. The structure of cisplatin (*cis*-diamminedichloroplatinum [II]).

TOXICITY

Preclinical studies with dogs, monkeys, and other laboratory animals showed the main side effects of cisplatin to be nephrotoxicity, gastrointestinal disturbances, bone marrow suppression, and ototoxicity (Schaeppi et al., 1973; Cvitkovic et al., 1977).

When used in human beings the main dose-limiting side effect of cisplatin is acute renal tubular necrosis (Rozencweig et al., 1977). This effect may be due to accumulation of cisplatin in tubular epithelial cells by active secretion, leading to uncoupling of oxidative phosphorylation, energy depletion, and necrosis. Cisplatin may also produce a heavy metal–type of toxicosis that activates the renin-angiotensin system to decrease glomerular filtration rate and renal blood flow, resulting in tubular necrosis. Pre- and posthydration with chloride-containing fluids, diuresis with furosemide and mannitol, and dosage reduction for patients with pre-existing renal compromise have greatly decreased nephrotoxicosis related to cisplatin administration. Nausea and vomiting can be so severe that human patients refuse additional cisplatin therapy, despite its proven efficacy. Antiemetic drugs decrease but do not completely eliminate this side effect. Bone marrow suppression is usually mild and not a dose-limiting problem. Tinnitus and high-frequency hearing loss may occur, but irreversible deafness is relatively rare. Additionally, seizures, peripheral neuropathies, electrolyte wasting, hyperuricemia, elevated liver enzyme values, and anaphylaxis have been described in association with cisplatin treatment.

RESULTS OF CLINICAL TRIALS

Dogs. Early clinical experience suggested that cisplatin could be used safely and effectively for treatment of canine malignancies. Two dogs treated for primary pulmonary tumors showed partial responses (PR) (> 50 per cent reduction of tumor size) for more than 4 weeks each (Melhaff et al., 1984). Two dogs were treated with cisplatin for metastatic squamous cell carcinomas (Himsel et al., 1986). One had a PR for more than 6 weeks and one had a complete response (CR) (no detectable tumor) for approximately 16 months, until a new tumor, a chemotherapy-resistant malignant lymphoma, resulted in its death. The latter dog had a mild chronic azotemia attributable to cisplatin treatment.

A number of dogs have been treated with 2 to 6 monthly infusions of cisplatin at 40 to 50 mg/m² at the University of California at Davis and the Ohio State University. One of eight dogs (12.5 per cent) with urinary tract transitional cell carcinomas had a PR of 31 weeks. Three of five dogs (60 per cent) with inoperable head and neck squamous cell carcinomas had PRs of 2, 10, and 15 weeks. Eleven dogs given cisplatin after amputation of a limb for osteosarcoma had a median survival time of 43 weeks (Shapiro et al., 1988). This was significantly longer (p < 0.003) than the median survival time of 14.5 weeks for eight dogs treated concurrently by amputation alone (Fig. 2).

For these 24 dogs toxicities attributable to cisplatin were minor. At least one episode of vomiting was recorded for 16 of 24 (66 per cent). In all cases vomiting stopped within 6 hr of the termination of cisplatin infusion. Three of 24 dogs (12.5 per cent) had single episodes of thrombocytopenia detected during cisplatin administration that were asymptomatic and resolved without incident. Gradual decreases in endogenous creatinine clearances were observed in 5 of 24 dogs (21 per cent). Whether the decreases in creatinine clearances were due to cisplatin *per se* or to concurrent disease, metastatic neoplasia, or renal insults associated with anesthesia and surgery could not be satisfactorily determined. However, most important, there were no episodes of acute renal failure or toxicosis in this series.

A low-dose cisplatin–radiotherapy combination has been developed for limb-sparing treatment of canine osteosarcoma (Withrow et al., 1986). An adaptation of this procedure has been used to treat inoperable tumors of dogs and cats (Stephens et al., 1986). Nine dogs received ten Monday-Wednesday-Friday (MWF) doses of 10 mg/m² cisplatin IV followed 2 hr later by anesthesia and a 4-Gy (400 rad) fraction of external beam radiotherapy. There were no untoward drug or radiation toxicities associated with this method in dogs.

CATS. There are data suggesting that cats are much more sensitive than dogs to cisplatin toxicosis. Ten of ten cats (100 per cent) treated with single injections of cisplatin at 40 to 60 mg/m² of body surface area developed a dose-related primary pulmonary edema (Knapp et al., 1987). Saline diuresis did not contribute to or ameliorate this effect, and renal toxicosis attributable to cisplatin administration was not found.

Four cats were treated for inoperable head and neck carcinomas with the low-dose cisplatin–radiotherapy regimen described above (Stephens et al., 1986). Two of the four cats developed malaise, fever, and anorexia during treatment but interruption of treatment for 1 week allowed completion of the ten-fraction course of cisplatin and radiotherapy without incident. The next two cats developed severe pulmonary edema acutely after the fifth and seventh cisplatin infusions, respectively. Treatment with diuretic and corticosteroid administration and enhanced oxygen atmosphere resulted in resolution of the pulmonary edema within 72 hr. During these 72 hr severe metabolic alkalosis, hypokalemia, proteinuria, isosthenuria, and hyaline casts developed, suggesting that renal damage had also occurred.

Because a cumulative pulmonary toxicity of cisplatin had not been documented in any species a study was designed by the author to determine the systemic effects of intermittent low-dose cisplatin infusions on normal cats without the complicating factors of intercurrent disease, saline and mannitol diuresis, or anesthesia and radiotherapy. This study showed that five to six cisplatin doses of 10 mg/m² IV (MWF) in normal cats quickly produces disruption of function of renal tubular epithelial cells, progressing to mild azotemia and mild pulmonary edema detectable at necropsy. Serum samples collected immediately before each cisplatin injection were assayed for total platinum concentration. These levels increased linearly through the course of treatment, suggesting that, in these cats, cisplatin accumulated in serum until levels sufficient to produce pulmonary toxicity were reached.

Six additional cats with tumors have been treated with a cisplatin dose of 7.5 mg/m² for ten treatments in combination with radiotherapy without incident. One cat with acute myelogenous leukemia was treated with two 10-mg/m² doses of cisplatin in 50 ml of normal saline solution at a 4-day interval. Two days after the second cisplatin infusion peripheral blood and bone marrow samples were free of detectable tumor cells, but after 2 more days the cat was euthanatized for hepatic failure, which necropsy showed to be due to infiltration by myeloid cells. Whether nontoxic doses of cisplatin will have significant therapeutic value in cats is still undetermined.

RECOMMENDATIONS FOR CLINICAL USE OF CISPLATIN IN DOGS

Systemic Chemotherapy

Before undertaking a course of cisplatin chemotherapy, baseline tumor measurements and thoracic

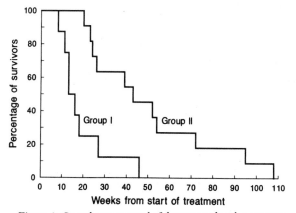

Figure 2. Cumulative survival of dogs treated with amputation alone (group I) or amputation and cisplatin (group II). (Reproduced with permission from Shapiro, W., et al.: J.A.V.M.A. 192:507, 1988.)

Table 1. Summary of Selected Cisplatin Infusion Protocols for Dogs

Step	Low Dose (MWF)*	High Dose (q 21–28 d) Short Term†	High Dose (q 21–28 d) Long Term‡
1. Prehydration with normal saline (0.9% NaCl) solution IV			
Dosage	12 ml/kg	18.3 ml/kg/hr	105 ml/m^3/hr
Duration	2–5 min	4 hr	12–18 hr
2. Mannitol (optional)			
Dosage	0.55 gm/kg		15 gm/m^2
Additional saline to make total volume	12 ml/kg		70 ml/m^2/hr
Duration	2–5 min		30 min
3. Antiemetic as needed in high-dose protocols			
4. Cisplatin			
Dosage	10 mg/m^2	40–70 mg/m^2	40–70 mg/m^2
Additional saline to make total volume	50 ml	6 ml/kg	70 ml/m^2/hr
Duration	2–5 min	20 min	6 hr
5. Posthydration (normal saline)			
Dosage	12 ml/kg	18.3 ml/kg/hr	105 ml/m^2/hr
Duration	2–5 min	2 hr	6 hr

*Stephens et al., 1986.
†Ogilvie et al., 1987.
‡Shapiro et al., 1988.

radiography are recommended for the purposes of tumor staging and monitoring responses to treatment. In addition, a hemogram, platelet count, serum biochemical and electrolyte determinations, and urinalysis should be done to monitor potential toxicosis. In the past, endogenous creatinine clearance tests were used as a sensitive method for detection of renal dysfunction, but these appear to have limited value in predicting cisplatin-induced nephrotoxicosis in dogs (Himsel et al., 1986; Shapiro et al., 1988). Dogs given high doses of cisplatin monthly should have laboratory tests repeated before each cisplatin administration and whenever toxicosis is suspected. Dogs given low doses more frequently should be monitored at weekly intervals. Tumor measurements and thoracic radiography should be performed on all dogs at monthly intervals.

Reduction of cisplatin dosage is recommended if rapid decreases in white blood cell (WBC) or platelet counts occur, if there are changes in serum electrolyte concentrations or urine specific gravity, if blood urea nitrogen (BUN) or serum creatinine levels are elevated, or if the endogenous creatinine clearance is less than 2.9 ml/min/kg (normal, 3.7 ± 0.77 ml/min/kg). Use of cisplatin is not recommended if the WBC count is less than 3200/μl; platelet count, less than 100,000/μl; or endogenous creatinine clearance, less than 1.4 ml/min/kg; or if frank uremia, electrolyte deficiency, or acid-base disturbances exist. Further, if the tumor is progressive after two full courses of therapy, additional cisplatin is not recommended.

A summary of cisplatin infusion protocols for dogs is given in Table 1. Results of clinical trials using the low-dose and the long-term, high-dose methods were discussed above. The short-term, high-dose method was evaluated after a single administration of cisplatin to clinically healthy dogs, and minimal toxicity was observed on the basis of careful laboratory and pathologic studies. Whether this method is similarly safely tolerated by geriatric, tumor-bearing animals has yet to be determined.

There are five basic steps to be followed in the use of cisplatin:

1. Prehydration with normal saline (0.9 per cent sodium chloride) solution. Hyperhydration results in dilution of the urine and hence decreases the concentration of cisplatin passing through the kidneys. In addition, the high chloride content will hold cisplatin in its inert form even within tubular epithelial cells.

2. Mannitol diuresis. This step is controversial. Hyperosmotic diuresis should further enhance urine production, thus protecting the kidneys, but adequate prehydration may be sufficient in most cases.

3. Antiemetics. Metoclopramide (Reglan, Robins), chlorpromazine (Thorazine, SmithKline Beckman), dexamethasone (Azium, Schering Corp), or a combination of these can be given as needed to decrease vomiting associated with high doses of cisplatin. A moderate amount of vomiting is to be expected and should not force discontinuation of cisplatin treatment.

4. Cisplatin infusion. Cisplatin is available as a lyophilized powder in 10-mg vials. One should not use aluminum needles or infusion sets because platinum forms a precipitate with aluminum and efficacy may be lost. Reconstitution should only be performed while wearing protective gloves and

mask and, if possible, under a vented hood. Cisplatin can be administered either intravenously or intra-arterially.

5. Posthydration. This will further protect from cisplatin-induced nephrotoxicosis.

Local Chemotherapy

Local administration of chemotherapeutic agents allows delivery of high concentrations of an antineoplastic drug to a confined area while minimizing the risk of systemic toxicosis. Because cisplatin is not highly irritating or caustic to tissues, it is ideally suited for use in local chemotherapeutic methods.

INTRACAVITARY INSTILLATION

Intracavitary instillation of cisplatin at 21- to 28-day intervals has been particularly effective in human patients for the treatment of malignant pleural effusions associated with thoracic and abdominal tumors (Lucas et al., 1985; Markman et al., 1984), and similar palliation has been noted in a limited number of animals with malignant effusions. The concurrent intravenous administration of sodium thiosulfate, an antidote to cisplatin, serves to minimize nephrotoxicosis from systemically absorbed cisplatin (Markman et al., 1985).

The following guidelines are offered for the intracavitary use of cisplatin:

1. The pretreatment tumor staging and steps for monitoring of toxicosis and handling of cisplatin as outlined for systemic administration should be followed.

2. No more than a corresponding systemic dose of cisplatin should be administered by the intracavitary route diluted to 1 mg/ml in normal saline solution.

3. Saline pre- and posthydration should be used as for systemic administration.

4. An intravenous bolus of sodium thiosulfate (2 gm/m²) should be given as the intracavitary cisplatin is instilled and an additional 6 gm/m² given in the intravenous saline over a 6-hr period.

5. After 4 hr an attempt should be made to remove all remaining intracavitary cisplatin.

INTRAVESICULAR INSTILLATION

Instillation of cisplatin directly into the urinary bladder has been effective in preventing relapse of superficial bladder tumors (Hemstreet et al., 1984; Llopis et al., 1985). Systemic toxicosis is rare, although hypersensitivity may be greater than with intravenously administered cisplatin. Concurrent saline infusions are not necessary.

There are limited data on the intravesical use of cisplatin in dogs. An appropriate dose for intravesicular instillation of cisplatin in the dog is 10 to 20 mg/m² diluted to 1 mg/ml in saline solution. The cisplatin solution should remain in the bladder for 2 hr. Intravesicular instillation can be repeated at 1- to 4-week intervals.

INTRALESIONAL CHEMOTHERAPY

Use of a purified bovine collagen (provided by Matrix Pharmaceuticals) as a vehicle for chemotherapeutic implants has been recently described (Kitchell et al., 1986). The high-molecular-weight, nonimmunogenic protein acts as a sponge or repository to slowly release drug into surrounding tissue. Cisplatin can be added to collagen at a final concentration of 3 mg/ml and injected in a gridding manner sublesionally for treatment of superficial tumors or intralesionally for mass lesions on a weekly basis. The addition of epinephrine at a final concentration of 0.25 mg/ml to the implant may further improve the local retention of drugs.

CONCLUSION

Cisplatin shows promise as an effective and relatively safe drug for the treatment of canine malignancies, especially appendicular osteosarcoma, head and neck squamous cell carcinoma, and, possibly, transitional cell carcinoma. Continued evaluation of cisplatin dosage rates and methods to protect the kidneys should improve the therapeutic index, and combinations of cisplatin and other drugs, radiotherapy, surgery, or hyperthermia will provide better methods for treatment of cancer in veterinary medicine. Until more information is available, cisplatin should only be used with extreme caution in cats.

References and Supplemental Reading

Cvitkovic, E., Spaulding, J., Bethune, V., et al.: Improvement of *cis*-diamminedichloroplatinum: Therapeutic index in an animal model. Cancer 39:1357, 1977.

Hemstreet, G. P., West, S. S., Weems, W. L., et al.: Intravesicular CDDP therapy compared with combined CDDP and external radiation in noninvasive bladder cancer. Urology 24:59, 1984.

Himsel, C. A., Richardson, R. C., and Craig, J. A.: Cisplatin chemotherapy for metastatic squamous cell carcinoma in two dogs. J.A.V.M.A. 189:1575, 1986.

Kitchell, B. E., Liskey, C., Madewell, B. R., et al.: Therapeutic drug-matrix implants for the treatment of veterinary neoplasms: A phase I–phase II study. Proceedings of the Veterinary Cancer Society Sixth Annual Conference, 1986, p. 10.

Knapp, D. W., Richardson, R. C., DeNicola, D. B., et al.: Cisplatin toxicity in cats. J. Vet. Intern. Med. 1:29, 1987.

Litterst, C. L., Gram, T. E., Dedrick, R. L., et al.: Distribution and disposition of platinum following intravenous administration of *cis*-diamminedichloroplatinum (II) to dogs. Cancer Res. 36:2340, 1976.

Llopis, B., Gallego, J., Mompo, J. A., et al.: Thiotepa vs Adriamycin vs cisplatinum in the intravesical prophylaxis of superficial bladder tumors. Eur. Urol. 11:73, 1985.

Lucas, W. E., Markman, M., and Howell, S. B.: Intraperitoneal chemotherapy for advanced ovarian cancer. Am. J. Obstet. Gynecol. 152:474, 1985.

Markman, M., Howell, S. B., and Green, M. R.: Combination intracavitary chemotherapy for malignant pleural disease. Cancer Drug Deliv. 1:333, 1984.

Markman, M., Cleary, S., and Howell, S. B.: Nephrotoxicity of high-dose intracavitary cisplatin with intravenous thiosulfate protection. Eur. J. Clin. Oncol. 21:1015, 1985.

Melhaff, C. J., Leifer, C. E., Patnaik, A. K., et al.: Surgical treatment of primary pulmonary neoplasia in 15 dogs. J. Am. Anim. Hosp. Assoc. 20:799, 1984.

Ogilvie, G. K., Kraweic, D. R., Gelberg, H. B., et al.: Evaluation of a short term saline diuresis protocol for the administration of cisplatin. Proceedings of the Fifth Annual Veterinary Medical Forum, 1987, p. 907.

Page, R., Matus, R. E., Leifer, C. E., et al.: Cisplatin, a new antineoplastic drug in veterinary medicine. J.A.V.M.A. 186:288, 1985.

Rosenberg, B., VanCamp, L., and Krigas, T.: Inhibition of cell division in Escherichia coli by electrolysis products from a platinum electrode. Nature 205:698, 1965.

Rozencweig, M., VonHoff, D. D., Slavik, M., et al.: cis-Diamminedichloroplatinum (II): A new anticancer drug. Ann. Intern. Med. 86:803, 1977.

Schaeppi, L., Heyman, I. A., Flerschman, R. W., et al.: cis-Dichlorodiammineplatinum (II): Preclinical toxicological evaluation of intravenous injection in dogs, monkeys and mice. Toxicol. Appl. Pharmacol. 25:230, 1973.

Shapiro, W., Fossum, T. W., Kitchell, B. E., et al.: Use of cisplatin for treatment of appendicular osteosarcoma in dogs. J.A.V.M.A. 192:507, 1988.

Stephens, C. H., Turrel, J. M., Theon, A. P., et al.: Low dose cisplatin as a radiation sensitizer for the treatment of advanced carcinomas and osteosarcomas in the dog and cat: A preliminary report. Proceedings of the Veterinary Cancer Society Sixth Annual Conference, 1986, p. 17.

Withrow, S. J., LaRue, S. M., Wrigley, R. H., et al.: Limb sparing treatment for canine osteosarcoma. Proceedings of the Veterinary Cancer Society Sixth Annual Conference, 1986, p. 12.

RADIATION THERAPY

SUSAN M. LaRUE, D.V.M.

Fort Collins, Colorado

Surgery remains the primary weapon against cancer in pet animals. In the past decade chemotherapy has begun to play an increasing role in small animal cancer management. Lymphosarcoma and transmissible venereal tumors are commonly treated with chemotherapeutic drugs. The use of radiation therapy has been restricted in part by its availability. Radiotherapy was occasionally presented as an option when other treatment failed.

Attitudes of veterinarians and pet owners toward cancer management have changed. There is a greater awareness of what is available for cancer treatment, and there is greater willingness by clients to invest time and money for cancer treatment for their pets. Radiation therapy is being recognized as the preferred treatment for some cancers, either alone or combined with other treatment modalities.

Although different methods of irradiation are available for cancer therapy, such as brachytherapy and systemically administered radionuclides, this article will deal exclusively with external beam irradiation or teletherapy. Three general types of teletherapy are available for the treatment of pet animals: orthovoltage; gamma-emitters, such as cobalt-60 and cesium-137; and linear accelerators. All three types of equipment produce ionizing radiation. Orthovoltage machines produce lower energy radiation (150 to 400 kVp), whereas gamma-emitters and linear accelerators produce radiation with an energy greater than 500 keV (megavoltage). Beam energy is an important factor in obtaining the desired dose distribution to the tumor, thus the treatment of tumors in certain locations may be restricted by the type of equipment available.

TYPES OF EQUIPMENT

The orthovoltage machines available at many veterinary teaching hospitals usually produce low-energy x-rays in the range of 150 to 300 kVp (Feeney and Johnston, 1983). X-rays of this energy give maximum dose to the surface being irradiated. Although this may be desirable for superficial tumors, it is impossible to give an adequate dose to deep-seated tumors without giving an excessive dose to overlying skin. Skin-related complications are more prevalent than with higher-energy external beam irradiation. Owing to the differences in absorption characteristics, low-energy x-rays are absorbed more effectively by bone than by soft tissue. Bones included in orthovoltage radiation fields may receive much higher doses than the tumor and be particularly susceptible to late complications. Despite the limitations, orthovoltage can be quite effective for certain tumors. It was recently reported that orthovoltage irradiation combined with surgery was more effective for control of nasal tumors than other radiation regimens (Adams et al., 1987).

Radioactive cobalt and cesium are the most common gamma-emitters used for teletherapy. A gamma-ray is a packet of energy identical to an x-ray except for its origin. By definition a gamma-ray originates from the disintegration of a radioactive nucleus. Cesium-137 produces 662-keV gamma-rays, whereas the energy for gamma-rays from a cobalt-60 source averages 1.25 MeV. The higher-energy gamma-rays give maximum dose below the skin and thus provide a skin-sparing effect when deep tumors are treated. For superficial tumors a "bolus" or layer of tissue density material is placed over the skin, allowing the dose to build up, resulting in maximal dose to the skin. Megavoltage radiation does not deposit excessive energy to bone-density tissues. Dosimetry techniques are well established, owing to years of use in human medicine. Cobalt machines, in particular, are versatile enough to treat tumors in a wide variety of locations.

Linear accelerators produce megavoltage x-rays that afford sparing to the superficial tissues and allow for penetration of deep-seated tumors. The maximum dose is produced below the surface. Additionally, some linear accelerators are capable of producing an electron beam. Electrons give maximal dose to superficial tissues. The dose to deeper structures drops off dramatically. This is valuable for superficial tumors and for intraoperative radiation therapy. The increased interest in cancer therapy for pet animals may lead to an increase in the availability of cobalt machines and linear accelerators.

FACTORS AFFECTING OUTCOME OF RADIATION THERAPY

Radiation is capable of destroying any tumor if the dose is high enough. However, for radiation therapy to be considered successful, there should be no loss of function or major complications associated with treatment. Therefore, the dose to the tumor is limited by the effects of that dose on normal tissues in the field. Because tumors are not necessarily more sensitive to the effects of radiation than normal tissues, a treatment regimen that spares normal tissues, yet gives a lethal dose to the tumor, should be selected.

The outcome of a tumor undergoing radiation therapy is dependent on many factors, including inherent tumor characteristics, tumor location and size, equipment available, and adequacy of treatment planning.

Tumors vary in their response to radiation. This is attributable to many factors, including the tumor doubling time, growth fraction, and tumor hypoxia. Histologic diagnosis is an important predictor of general radioresponsiveness. Therefore, biopsy and histologic evaluation should be performed on the tumor of every potential radiation therapy patient. Great heterogeneity exists within tumors of the same type; so the outcome of therapy for an individual tumor cannot be predicted, only overall probability of response of a group of tumors. In dogs, acanthomatous epulides, some brain tumors, mast cell tumors, perianal adenomas, and transmissible venereal tumors are some of the tumors that are considered radioresponsive (Thrall and Harvey, 1983; Turrel et al., 1984; Gillette, 1976; Morgan and Carlson, 1963; Thrall, 1982). Soft tissue sarcomas are generally less radioresponsive, but long-term control can be achieved (McChesney et al., 1989). Tumors such as osteosarcoma and melanoma are relatively resistant to radiation therapy alone (Banks and Morris, 1975), although combining radiation therapy with other modalities may be advantageous in these tumors (LaRue, 1989; Dewhirst et al., 1984). One method of determining the radioresponsiveness of a tumor is to establish a median tumor control dose (TCD_{50}). TCD_{50} is the dose of radiation necessary to control 50 per cent of the tumors of that type (Table 1). The TCD_{50} is useful for comparing radioresponsiveness of tumors and predicting the probability of tumor control.

Tumor location can affect the outcome of radiotherapy. For example, following treatment with radiation, rostrally located squamous cell carcinomas have a better prognosis than tonsillar squamous cell carcinomas. Whether this is due to inability to achieve adequate tumor dose to that location or to an inherent difference in biologic behavior is not fully understood (Todoroff and Brodey, 1979).

Tumor size can also affect the outcome of radiotherapy. In addition to having greater numbers of cells that must be killed, large tumors may have regions of hypoxia due to poor vascularity. Hypoxia decreases radiation sensitivity. Another complicating factor associated with large tumors is the size of the radiation field. Effects on normal tissues are exacerbated when the radiation field is large.

Appropriate treatment planning is essential for radiotherapy to be successful. The radiation therapist must be able to determine the extent of the tumor, so thorough radiographic studies, including

Table 1. *Total Radiation Doses with a 50% Probability for Tumor Control or Normal Tissue Injury in Dogs**

	Dose (Gy)
Tumors	
Mast cell tumor	36
Oral squamous cell carcinomas	39
Soft tissue sarcomas	52
Normal tissue	
Moist desquamation	38
Necrosis of bones with tumor invasion	49

*Doses were given in ten fractions over 3 weeks.

Reprinted with permission from Gillette, E. L.: Cancer therapy: Radiation and hyperthermia. Semin. Vet. Med. Surg. (Small Anim.) 1:21, 1986.

Table 2. *Radiotherapy for Clinical Patients*

Radiation as the Optimal Method of Therapy
  Acanthomatous epulis (Thrall and Harvey, 1983)
  Primary brain tumors (Turrel et al., 1984)
  Oral squamous cell (MacMillan et al., 1982; Gillette, 1982;
    Gillette et al., 1987)
  Nasal tumors* (Beck and Withrow, 1985; Bradley and
    Harvey, 1973; Norris, 1979; Thrall and Harvey, 1983;
    Adams et al., 1987).
  Fibrosarcoma* (McChesney et al., 1986)
  Hemangiopericytoma* (McChesney et al., 1986)
**Multimodality Therapy, Including Radiotherapy, as the Opti-
  mal Treatment**
  Osteosarcoma (LaRue, 1989)
  Melanoma (Dewhirst et al., 1984)
Radiation Therapy as an Alternative Method
  Mast cell tumors (Gillette, 1976)
  Perianal adenomas (Morgan and Carlson, 1963)
  Transmissible venereal tumors (Thrall, 1982)
  Lymphosarcoma (Couto et al., 1984)
Palliative Radiation Therapy
  Any metastatic spread to bone if the primary tumor is con-
    trolled

*May also require surgery for optimal results.

special studies if indicated, must be made available to the therapist. Geographic misses inevitably result in recurrence and must be avoided. Accurate histopathologic evaluation is essential, because the width of margins around the tumor is often based on tumor type.

Age of the patient is not a factor in predicting radiosensitivity or outcome of therapy. General health is an important consideration in patient selection owing to multiple anesthetic episodes and prolonged hospitalization associated with radiation therapy. The temperament of the patient must also be considered.

CASE SELECTION

Tumors in patients undergoing radiation therapy can be grouped into one of four classifications: (1) tumors for which radiation therapy is the optimal method of treatment; (2) those for which multimodality therapy, including radiotherapy, is the optimal method of treatment; (3) those for which radiation therapy offers an alternative method of treatment; and (4) tumors for which the goal is palliation (Table 2). Each of these groups will be discussed briefly.

Radiation As the Optimal Method of Therapy

Radiotherapy is the optimal method of treatment when it offers the best prognosis for tumor control and clearly offers the least chance for disabling complications. Factors to consider in making this decision are the radioresponsiveness of the tumor and the potential complications of other methods of treatment.

Acantomatous epulis, a locally infiltrative, nonmetastasizing oral tumor of periodontal origin, can be successfully treated with radiation therapy. In one study of 39 dogs with acanthomatous epulides treated with orthovoltage radiation, the epulis recurred in only three cases (Thrall and Harvey, 1983). Median survival was 37 months, and 1-yr survival was 85 per cent. Some of the dogs had surgical debulking performed prior to radiation therapy, but this was not thought to be beneficial. Although complete surgical resection can be performed on acanthomatous epulides using aggressive surgical techniques, such as partial mandibulectomies or maxillectomies, the results are not as cosmetically acceptable as in irradiated patients. The importance of obtaining a diagnostic-quality biopsy specimen and having it evaluated at a reputable histopathology laboratory cannot be overemphasized. Other types of oral tumors are treated more successfully by aggressive excision than by radiation therapy, so an accurate diagnosis is essential.

Tumor control has been achieved in primary brain tumors of various histologic types using megavoltage radiation (Turrel et al., 1984). Minimal complications and a median survival of 322 days (Turrel et al., 1984) make radiation the treatment of choice for this tumor.

Reports in the literature regarding the treatment of nasal tumors have had varying conclusions; however, the consensus appears to be that radiation therapy, either alone or in conjunction with surgery, offers the best prognosis for nasal tumors (Beck and Withrow, 1985; Bradley and Harvey, 1973; Norris, 1979; Thrall and Harvey, 1983; Adams et al., 1987).

Often radiation therapy becomes the optimal method of therapy when a tumor is located at a site where complete surgical excision of the tumor would have functionally or cosmetically unacceptable results. Depending on the situation, radiation therapy can be used alone or following surgical debulking. The surgical debulking can be planned or can result from an attempted excision in which adequate margins could not be obtained. To be most effective, debulking should remove all visible tumor, leaving only microscopic disease (Fletcher, 1979). Soft tissue sarcomas of the head and neck region and the extremities are suitable for this type of therapy. Another group of tumors that fit this category are tumors with apparent or probable metastasis to regional lymph nodes. Tumors located in the caudal third of the oral cavity metastasize early to regional lymph nodes. The regional nodes as well as the primary site usually are irradiated.

Multimodality Therapy, Including Radiotherapy, as the Optimal Treatment

This group includes many tumors that have an extremely poor prognosis with single-modality treatment regimens. Much of the ongoing work is preliminary, but encouraging results have been obtained in limb sparing for canine osteosarcoma using radiation and cisplatin prior to surgical excision and replacement with an allograft (LaRue, 1989). Radiation combined with hyperthermia is being used on dogs with melanomas (Dewhirst et al., 1984). Radiation therapy has also been combined with chemotherapeutic agents that have radiation-sensitizing properties, such as cisplatin (Bartelink et al., 1986).

Radiation Therapy as an Alternative Method

Some tumors that are successfully treated by surgery, chemotherapy, or other methods are also sensitive to radiation therapy. This group of tumors includes lymphosarcoma, transmissible venereal tumors, perianal adenomas, rectal polyps, and multiple myeloma. Although radiation therapy is not generally considered the primary treatment mode, there are instances in which radiation therapy may offer advantages. An example would be stage I or II lymphosarcoma in a dog with compromised organ function that would render chemotherapy too risky, or when rapid alleviation of signs is necessary.

Palliative Radiation Therapy

In human patients it is common to treat tumors, especially metastatic spread to bone, without intent to cure. In these cases mortality from the tumor at other locations can be predicted, and the intent of palliation is to reduce pain, thus improving the quality of life. Because short-term control, not cure, is the intent, the dosage can be reduced, limiting the complications of therapy and shortening the duration of therapy. Palliative radiation therapy has not been used commonly in veterinary medicine. This may be due to the rapid demise of many veterinary cancer patients due to growth of the primary tumor. Control of metastatic spread has not been an issue. Recent therapeutic advances have prolonged survival of many veterinary cancer patients. In the face of prolonged survival, metastatic spread to bone may result in death of the animal in spite of control of the primary tumor. Palliative therapy should be presented as an option to owners of these patients.

COMPLICATIONS OF RADIOTHERAPY

Complications of radiotherapy are classified as early or late. Early effects will occur during or shortly after radiation therapy. Early effects involve tissues that are rapidly proliferating, such as oral mucosa, intestinal epithelium, and skin. These ef-

fects are generally self-limiting, and the patient has a rapid recovery. However, they can be unpleasant for the animal and owner and, in rare instances, can result in death of the patient if not cared for properly. Late effects involve more slowly proliferating tissues, such as bone, lung, heart, kidneys, and spinal cord. When late effects occur they may be quite severe and can result in necrosis, loss of function, or even death. Treatment of late effects can be complicated and expensive. The radiation dose is usually limited by late tissue effects, and an effort is made to limit morbidity to less than 5 per cent.

In addition to early and late effects, human patients undergoing radiation therapy will often develop what is termed radiation sickness. Radiation sickness is a nausea that develops most often in head and neck cancer patients or abdominal cancer patients. The cause of this syndrome is not clear, and it does not appear to be dose related. Animal radiation patients do not develop this syndrome. Owners who have undergone radiation therapy or have known radiation therapy patients will often cite this as a reason not to use radiation therapy for their pet. They must be assured that this is not a problem.

Management of Early Effects

Management of early effects is often done by the referring veterinarian. Although medical management is straightforward, the greater burden lies in reassuring and encouraging the owner. Bringing the animal home after hospitalization for radiation therapy can be stressful for the owner. If any problems develop, even minor problems about which they have been forewarned, owners may doubt their decision to go forward with therapy. If the veterinarian understands the situation and initiates prompt and appropriate therapy, the owners' fears will be alleviated.

SKIN. Early effects to the skin are restricted to the radiation field. The severity of effect is dose related, and the patient may have a variety of lesions. Epilation is common, and several months may be required for regrowth of hair. Damage to the melanocytes may result in hypo- or hyperpigmentation of skin, alteration of coat color, or both when regrowth occurs. Dry desquamation may accompany epilation. It generally does not cause any problem or discomfort to the dog and usually is not treated. Moist desquamation occurs 3 weeks into the treatment or later, and the severity is variable. It is often associated with pruritus, and self-inflicted mutilations exacerbate the problem. The area should be cleansed with warm water. Application of petroleum-based products over the wound is contraindicated. Drying agents can be used, but no evidence of efficacy exists. Preventing self-mutilation is of paramount importance. Elizabethan collars, side braces, or padded bandages on the paws may be indicated, depending on the location of the field. Desquamation should subside in 2 to 3 weeks following therapy. If exudation is liberal, one should monitor plasma protein levels and hydration status closely.

MUCOUS MEMBRANES. Mucositis of the oral cavity, pharynx, or esophagus can occur when tumors of the head and neck region are irradiated and always occurs to some degree in patients that have received irradiation for oral tumors. The mucositis begins to develop during the second week of therapy and reaches a maximum severity in about 3 weeks. Clinical signs include increased salivation and tenderness of the mouth. The animal may become reluctant to eat or drink and thus, without treatment, can become dehydrated and debilitated. Low-salt foods are more palatable and less irritating to the oral mucosa than regular commercial diets. Hand feeding and pampering by the owner aid in maintaining caloric intake. The owners should be instructed on the specific caloric and fluid requirements of their animal and assisted in developing a diet that meets those needs. Administration of fluids, usually subcutaneously, may be necessary. If anorexia has been a problem, evaluation of electrolyte concentrations is indicated. In extreme cases the use of a nasogastric tube or gastrostomy tube for feeding is indicated. Mucositis will generally subside 2 to 3 weeks following therapy.

EYES. Effects to the eye are dose related and vary in severity. An eye that is directly in the field and receives a full dose will undergo severe early and late effects and ultimately develop end stage disease, whereas eyes at the periphery of a field may only manifest mild changes. Acute effects include blepharitis, blepharospasm, conjunctivitis, and corneal ulceration. Treatment depends on the presence or absence of corneal ulceration. If an ulcer is not present, ophthalmic preparations with steroids are indicated. The reaction should be monitored frequently by the local veterinarian, and the owners should be instructed to return the pet for re-evaluation if the appearance of the eye changes. When corneal ulceration is present it should be treated aggressively. Keratoconjunctivitis sicca can also occur following radiation. This change can be temporary or permanent. Treatment should be instituted as soon as possible to prevent corneal ulceration.

GASTROINTESTINAL TRACT. The intestinal tract may be unavoidably in the treatment field for tumors of the abdomen. Gastrointestinal signs depend on the amount and location of gut irradiated. When the pelvic region is irradiated, colitis can occur. Signs include frequent attempts to defecate; straining; and diarrhea with blood, mucus, or both.

Symptomatic therapy should be instituted. Irradiation of the stomach can result in vomition, and irradiation of the small intestine can result in small bowel diarrhea. Again, symptomatic therapy is indicated. These effects usually occur during treatment. If severe, radiation therapy is interrupted. Recovery occurs within a few days if gastrointestinal signs are caused by radiation injury.

Management of Late Effects

Late effects of irradiation are rare, but when they do occur can be quite severe, are expensive to treat, and can result in loss of function or death. Late effects occur from a few months to years after radiation therapy, and the occurrence is not readily predictable. Severity of acute effects does not correlate with the development of late effects.

OSTEORADIONECROSIS. Bone included in the radiation field will undergo cellular death and resulting osteopenia. The acellular bone is replaced by viable bone over a period of years. In most cases structural support is still provided by the bone so clinical signs are not manifested. However, if the bone is subjected to additional insult, such as infection or trauma, it is quite vulnerable. Bacterial infection of irradiated bone results in irreversible osteonecrosis. Resolution of infection will not occur without removal of involved tissues. This problem is seen most commonly when the mandible or maxilla is irradiated, owing to high levels of bacteria present in the mouth. The mandible seems particularly vulnerable, perhaps because of a limited blood supply, which also has been compromised by radiation therapy. Conservative management is most common and is the best approach. For severe cases of mandibular necrosis, partial or complete hemimandibulectomy is indicated. For maxillary necrosis aggressive debridement of the necrotic bone, followed by reconstructive surgery may alleviate the problem. Oronasal fistulas may result from maxillary osteoradionecrosis. These fistulas should not be treated in a manner comparable with treatment of fistulas in unirradiated animals. Aggressive reconstructive surgery is generally required.

Long bones included in the radiation field can also become infected, particularly if surgery involving the bone was also performed (such as a limb-sparing procedure). The resulting osteomyelitis and osteoradionecrosis may necessitate amputation. Another rare complication is fracture of the osteopenic bone. This can occur years after irradiation and is generally associated with mild trauma. The optimal method of treatment of these fractures has not been determined; however, internal fixation, particularly with compression, may offer the best prognosis for fracture healing. Aseptic technique is essential, because bacteria entering the area will promote osteoradionecrosis. Likewise, the animal must be thoroughly examined before surgery for any signs of infection. Urine obtained by cystocentesis should be evaluated and cultured if any indication of infection exists. A complete otoscopic examination should also be included in the preoperative workup. Surgery should be postponed until any infections are under control.

Treatment of late effects associated with bone can be quite frustrating because apparently simple problems can result in disaster when treatment is attempted. It is recommended that patients with these late complications be referred to a center where the surgeons are familiar with treating these disorders. If that is not logistically possible, close consultation with a surgeon experienced with late complications should be maintained throughout treatment.

OTHER LATE COMPLICATIONS. Fibrosis can occur in the muscles, subcutaneous tissue, and other soft tissue structures included in the radiation field. Radiation adjacent to or including a joint can result in loss of range of motion and joint function. Simple releasing incisions generally are not helpful. Each case must be individually evaluated for proper treatment.

Late ocular complications include cataracts, retinal atrophy, and end stage ophthalmia. Enucleation is recommended if the eye is bothersome to the animal. Late fibrosis in the intestinal wall is probably more important than early changes and can result in strictures.

References and Supplemental Reading

Adams, W. M., Withrow, S. J., Walshaw, R., et al.: Radiotherapy of malignant nasal tumors in 67 dogs. J.A.V.M.A. 191:311, 1987.

Banks, W. C., and Morris, E.: Results of radiation treatment of naturally occurring animal tumors. J.A.V.M.A. 166:1063, 1975.

Bartelink, H., Kallman, R. F., Rapacchietta, D., and Hart, G. A. M.: Therapeutic enhancement in mice by clinically relevant dose and fractionation schedules of cis-diamminedichloroplatinum (II) and irradiation. Radiother. Oncol. 6:61, 1986.

Beck, E. R., and Withrow, S. J.: Tumors of the canine nasal cavity. Vet. Clin. North Am. 6:521, 1985.

Bradley, P. A., and Harvey, C. E.: Intra-nasal tumours in the dog: An evaluation of prognosis. J. Small Anim. Pract. 14:459, 1973.

Couto, C. G., Cullen, J., Pedroia, V., and Turrel, J. M.: Central nervous system lymphosarcoma in the dog. J.A.V.M.A. 184:809, 1984.

Dewhirst, M. S., Sim, D. A., Sapareto, S., and Connor, W. G.: Importance of minimum tumor temperature in determining early and long-term responses of spontaneous canine and feline tumors to heat and radiation. Cancer Res. 44:43, 1984.

Feeney, D. A., and Johnston, G. R.: Radiation therapy: Applications and availability. In Kirk, R. W. (ed.): Current Veterinary Therapy VIII. Philadelphia: W. B. Saunders, 1983.

Fletcher, G. H.: Basic principles of the combination of irradiation and surgery. Int. J. Radiat. Oncol. Biol. Phys. 5:2091, 1979.

Gillette, E. L.: Radiation therapy of canine and feline tumors. J. Am. Anim. Hosp. Assoc. 12:359, 1976.

Gillette, E. L.: Hyperthermia effects in animals with spontaneous tumors. Natl. Cancer Inst. Monogr. 61:361, 1982.

Gillette, E. L., McChesney, S. L., Dewhirst, M. W., and Scott, R. J.: Response of canine oral carcinomas to heat and radiation. Int. J. Radiat. Oncol. Biol. Phys. 13:1861, 1987.

LaRue, S. M., Withrow, S. J., Powers, B. E., et al.: Multidisciplinary limbsparing for canine osteosarcoma. J.A.V.M.A. (submitted).

MacMillan, R., Withrow, S. J., and Gillette, E. L.: Surgery and regional irradiation for treatment of canine tonsillar squamous cell carcinoma: Retrospective review of eight cases. J. Am. Anim. Hosp. Assoc. 18:311, 1982.

McChesney, S. L., Gillette, E. L., Dewhirst, M. W., and Withrow, S. J.: Influence of WR 2721 on radiation response of canine soft tissue sarcomas. Int. J. Radiat. Oncol. Biol. Phys. 12:1957, 1986.

McChesney, S. L., Withrow, S. J., Gillette, E. L., et al.: Radiation therapy of canine soft tissue sarcomas. J.A.V.M.A. (submitted).

Morgan, J. P., and Carlson, W. D.: X-Irradiation of perianal gland neoplasms in the dog. J.A.V.M.A. 143:1227, 1963.

Norris, A. M.: Nasal neoplasms in the dog. J. Am. Anim. Hosp. Assoc. 15:231, 1979.

Thrall, D. E.: Orthovoltage radiotherapy of canine transmissible venereal tumors. Vet. Radiol. 23:217, 1982.

Thrall, D. E., and Harvey, C. E.: Radiotherapy of malignant nasal tumors in 21 dogs. J.A.V.M.A. 183:663, 1983.

Todoroff, R. J., and Brodey, R. S.: Oral and pharyngeal neoplasia in the dog: A retrospective survey of 361 cases. J.A.V.M.A. 175:567, 1979.

Turrel, J. M., Fike, J. R., LeCouteur, R. A., et al.: Radiotherapy of brain tumors in dogs. J.A.V.M.A. 184:82, 1984.

BIOLOGICAL RESPONSE MODIFIERS

CHRIS K. GRANT, PH.D., D.SC.
and GRADY H. SHELTON, D.V.M.

Seattle, Washington

In malignant disease, biological response modifiers (BRMs) are agents or approaches that alter the tumor-host relationship such that the host's antitumor response is improved, with resultant therapeutic effects. Included in this definition are molecules of either natural or synthetic origin whose mechanisms of action influence the biological responses of the recipient (Table 1). Although BRMs are primarily thought of as antitumor agents, they also have therapeutic applications in other clinical conditions,

Table 1. Examples of Biological Response Modifiers

Bacterial Agents
  Bacille Calmette-Guérin (BCG)
  Corynebacterium parvum
  Muramyl dipeptide (MDP)
  Staphylococcal protein A (SpA)
Chemical Agents
  Cimetidine
  Levamisole
  Low-dose cytotoxic drugs
Interferons
  Alpha-, beta-, gamma-IFN
Thymosins
  Thymosin fraction 5
  Alpha$_1$-thymosin
Cytokines and Lymphokines
  Interleukin-2 (IL-2)
  Tumor necrosis factor (TNF)
Monoclonal Antibodies (MAbs)
  Anti-idiotype vaccines
Bone Marrow Transplantation

including infectious, autoimmune, and immunosuppressive diseases. BRMs can modify responses in the following ways: (1) they may increase the host's defense through augmentation or restoration of effector mechanisms or mediators; (2) they may decrease the deleterious component of the host's response; (3) they may augment natural host defense by acting directly as effector mechanisms; or (4) they may increase the ability of the host to tolerate damage by cytotoxic modalities of cancer treatment.

Most disease states and particularly systemic disorders are associated with some degree of immune dysfunction or impairment, and therapy involving BRMs is intended to correct this. It is now recognized that cancer often develops in the presence of defective immunosurveillance mechanisms, is often associated with progressive immunodeficiency, and is commonly treated with chemotherapeutic agents that contribute to immunosuppression. Therefore, therapy that can either restore normal immune function or stimulate an improved immune response should be beneficial to a host with cancer or certain other systemic diseases. Recent scientific and technologic advances have so increased knowledge of biological responses, and in particular immunologic mechanisms, that manipulation of these responses for therapeutic purposes is both realistic and practical. The advent of hybridoma technology and large-scale monoclonal antibody (MAb) production has provided a powerful tool for the isolation and purification of tumor-associated antigens, cytokines, lymphokines, and other biologically active molecules. In addition, MAbs can themselves be used as therapeutic agents, as diagnostic tools (in tumor imaging), or as specific cytotoxic delivery devices when coupled with drugs or toxins. Genetic engineering, on the other hand, provides the means to produce massive quantities of highly purified, bio-

logically active proteins utilizing simple fermentation technology.

BRMs are not yet commonly used in clinical veterinary medicine, but it seems likely they will be increasingly utilized in the foreseeable future. Numerous clinical trials are in progress to evaluate the therapeutic potential of such agents in various domestic animal diseases. This article discusses some of the BRMs currently under study and indicates which agents have already demonstrated applicability in veterinary medicine.

BACTERIAL AGENTS

It has long been recognized that certain bacterial products (e.g., BCG and *Corynebacterium parvum*) possess significant immunoregulatory capabilities. Some mechanisms influenced include activation of B and T lymphocytes, natural killer cells, and macrophages; enhancement of antibody-dependent cell-mediated cytotoxicity (ADCC); interferon induction; and elaboration of tumor necrosis factor (TNF).

The attenuated live mycobacterium *bacille Calmette-Guérin* (BCG) is an extensively studied BRM. Bacterial cell wall preparations derived from BCG include free lipid and proteins, which are immunogenic, as well as a peptidoglycan-containing muramyl dipeptide, which stimulates the reticuloendothelial system (RES). Injection of BCG cell wall fractions causes activation of T lymphocytes, subsequent release of lymphokines, and attraction of macrophages and polymorphonuclear cells (PMNs), with an end result of granuloma formation. This inflammatory reaction allows for nonspecific lysis of granuloma-associated tumor cells with the subsequent release of tumor antigens. Circulating antigen can then stimulate T lymphocytes to a specific activated state to elicit further tumor destruction.

Mean tumor-free survival time of dogs with malignant mammary tumors was significantly extended when the tumors were injected with BCG cell wall preparation 4 weeks prior to surgical removal. BCG cell wall vaccines have been successfully used to treat bovine ocular squamous cell carcinoma and equine sarcoid. Ribogen (Fort Dodge), a lyophilized emulsion consisting of mycobacterial cell wall components, is approved for these veterinary uses. Ribogen is also being tested against certain canine tumors and, when administered systemically, has been shown to augment host resistance to numerous infectious diseases in laboratory animals.

Corynebacterium parvum, now classified as a *Propionibacterium*, has been studied extensively as a potential antitumor agent. *C. parvum* is known to stimulate cell-mediated immunity and to enhance both macrophage function and antibody production. The median survival time of dogs with malignant oral melanoma treated by surgery plus periodic intravenous administration of *C. parvum* exceeded that of matched dogs similarly treated by surgery alone (370 versus 228 days). The most dramatic survival improvement was found in dogs with advanced disease (median survival of 288 days versus 121 days with surgery alone), a finding that parallels results reported for human melanoma.

Immunoregulin (ImmunoVet Inc.) is a suspension of killed *Propionibacterium acnes*, which can be used as an adjunctive therapy for immunosuppressive disorders, such as feline leukemia virus (FeLV)–associated diseases, canine and feline pyoderma, and equine infectious upper respiratory tract disease. Although *P. acnes* may be beneficial for some FeLV-infected cats with non-neoplasia–associated diseases, it should not be regarded as a primary treatment modality, for it has been continually ineffective in reversing viremia in FeLV-positive cats.

Muramyl dipeptide (MDP) is a simple glycopeptide containing the bacteria-specific carbohydrate, muramic acid, and two amino acids, L-alanine and D-isoglutamine. MDP is a potent stimulator of the RES and promotes activation of tumoricidal macrophages, which nonspecifically destroy neoplastic cells. The antitumor activity of muramyl peptides can be enhanced by encapsulation in liposomes. Liposomes are produced from phospholipids and facilitate delivery of peptides to the RES, particularly in the liver, spleen, lymph nodes, and lung. Investigations are currently under way to evaluate the effectiveness of liposome-encapsulated muramyl tripeptides (which are more lipophilic and thus incorporate into liposomes better than MDPs) in preventing postoperative metastases in dogs with osteogenic sarcoma and in cats with mammary adenocarcinoma. Thus far 27 dogs with osteosarcoma have achieved significantly prolonged survival times and decreased rates of metastases when compared with dogs treated by surgery alone (MacEwen, 1987b).

Protein A (SpA) is a polypeptide cell wall component of *Staphylococcus aureus* Cowan I (SAC). SpA binds the Fc region of immunoglobulin G (IgG) and may preferentially bind IgG-associated circulating immune complexes (CICs). Tumoricidal activity has been observed in humans, dogs, and cats when plasma was perfused over SAC and then reinfused into the tumor-bearing host, a process intended to remove CICs and referred to as extracorporeal immunoadsorption (ECIA).

In one study both antitumor and antiviral responses were reported in 9 of 16 FeLV-positive cats with leukemia/lymphoma following ECIA treatments using formalin-killed, heat-stabilized SAC (Jones et al., 1984). Cats that responded (by clearance of FeLV and complete tumor regression) developed antibodies to the viral envelope glyco-

protein gp-70 and also complement-dependent cytotoxic antibodies (CDA) against virus-infected feline lymphoma cells. Antitumor and antiviral responses were also observed in FeLV-infected cats with neoplastic disease following ECIA using purified SpA, or notably after intraperitoneal injection of small quantities of purified SpA. In the latter case, marked transient elevations in circulating gamma-interferon levels preceded the appearance of CDAs.

The authors treated 11 cats with leukemia/lymphoma by ECIA using purified SpA covalently bound to silica (Prosorba, Imrè Corporation). Prior to therapy, seven cats were FeLV positive and four were FeLV negative. Five of 11 cats achieved complete tumor regressions, and three of the responder cats have now survived in excess of 1.5 years after therapy. The six cats that did not respond died of progressive disease. It was noted that responder cats had minimal tumor burden relative to nonresponders. No antiviral responses were observed in the seven FeLV-positive cats; however, latent FeLV infection was reactivated in two cats that were not viremic prior to treatment. The latter unexpected observations support the concept that previous FeLV exposure can lead to leukemia/lymphoma in the absence of overt virus production.

The mechanisms whereby SpA treatments provide therapeutic benefit are unclear. SpA is a potent lymphocyte mitogen, is an efficient activator of the complement cascade, and can potentiate some cellular immune reactions. Even when cross-linked to an inert matrix, small quantities of SpA are eluted and returned in host plasma. In addition, most commercial preparations of SpA also contain other bacterial contaminants, including enterotoxins. ECIA is currently costly and highly labor intensive and generally yields inconsistent results, except perhaps when used to treat cats with minimal tumor burden. Combination therapy that includes SpA-ECIA may prove more effective than treatment with this modality alone.

CHEMICAL AGENTS

Cimetidine is a histamine (H_2) receptor antagonist and has been reported to enhance cell-mediated immunity. Clinically beneficial results have been obtained in human patients with mucocutaneous candidiasis, herpes zoster, and herpes simplex infections. When used in combination with interferon, cimetidine has exhibited synergistic effects. Cimetidine may exert an indirect effect by preventing the release of a soluble histamine-induced factor, which in turn mediates suppressor cell activity. At this stage cimetidine would appear to be a candidate for therapeutic trials in some canine and feline immunodeficiency diseases.

Levamisole, the antihelminthic, has received considerable attention as an immunomodulatory substance. Levamisole is an imidazole derivative whose action on cyclic nucleotide phosphodiesterases causes a net increase in cyclic guanosine monophosphate (*c*-GMP) levels within lymphocytes, and this results in increased responsiveness to mitogens. The drug also causes proliferation of helper and suppressor T cells and macrophages, and it enhances delayed hypersensitivity reactions. On the other hand, levamisole has little effect on antibody production in immunocompetent hosts.

MacEwen (1987a) has evaluated levamisole as an adjunct to both surgery and chemotherapy in canine and feline mammary tumors and canine lymphosarcomas, but no significant clinical benefit was noted. However, the same investigator found that levamisole did provide some therapeutic benefit for cats with eosinophilic granuloma complex. Fourteen of 18 cats with eosinophilic granuloma responded to treatment with levamisole at an oral dose of 5 mg/kg three times weekly, and lesions completely regressed in ten of these cats after approximately 16 weeks of treatment. If, as has been suggested, feline eosinophilic granuloma lesions are due to autoantibodies against normal cat epithelial components, levamisole may exert its effect by activating suppressor cells.

It is now recognized that several classes of cytotoxic drugs (e.g., antimetabolites, antitumor antibiotics, and alkylators) given in low doses and at appropriate times can function as BRMs to augment immune defenses against tumors. Cyclophosphamide has immunomodulatory activity, in that low doses of the drug will enhance rather than depress induction of allergic contact dermatitis in guinea pigs. The ability of some cytotoxic drugs to function as BRMs, through mechanisms such as stimulation of lymphokine production or inhibition of suppressor T cells, may prove to be therapeutically significant.

INTERFERONS

Interferons (IFNs) are a family of glycoproteins produced by different cell types in response to a variety of stimuli such as B-mitogens, endotoxins, foreign nucleic acids, and neoplastic or virus-infected cells. Alpha-, beta-, and gamma-IFNs are produced by leukocytes, fibroblasts or epithelial cells, and T lymphocytes, respectively. IFNs can exert antiviral, antitumor, immunoregulatory, and cell-differentiating activities. The various subtypes of natural IFNs differ in their biochemical compositions, inciting stimuli, and functional activities. In general, alpha- and beta-IFNs have more potent antiviral activity, whereas gamma-IFNs are weak antiviral agents but have greater immunomodulatory and antitumor capabilities.

IFNs mediate antiviral and antiproliferative responses directly by acting on cell membrane receptors and indirectly by stimulating biosynthesis of a variety of mediator molecules, including prostaglandins. A complex inter-relationship exists between IFN and prostaglandins in regulating cellular functions, which, in turn, may represent a feedback mechanism to counterbalance interferon activity. IFNs enhance the cytotoxic reactivity of macrophages and natural killer cells, and they augment the differentiation or activation or both of cytotoxic T lymphocytes.

Human clinical trials have demonstrated some antitumor activity for IFN in a number of malignancies, including breast carcinoma, malignant lymphoma, multiple myeloma, malignant melanoma, Kaposi's sarcoma, renal carcinoma, chronic leukemias, bladder carcinoma, malignant gliomas, nasopharyngeal carcinoma, and hairy cell leukemia. In addition, studies have indicated a synergistic antineoplastic effect between interferon and certain chemotherapeutic agents, and clinical trials are in progress to evaluate these combined treatment modalities.

There are currently little data available on the use of interferons in veterinary medicine. Interferon was shown to be capable of inhibiting replication of FeLV in cell culture. In one report, oral administration of an IFN-containing preparation resulted in recovery of four cats from FeLV-associated nonregenerative anemia and conversion of one cat to an FeLV-negative state. Future clinical studies in veterinary medicine will be facilitated by the production of species-specific, genetically engineered interferon.

THYMOSINS

Thymic extracts often exert marked biological activity on immune cells. Similar to interferons, thymic extracts represent a family of hormonelike compounds collectively referred to as thymosins. The two most studied are thymosin fraction 5 and alpha$_2$-thymosin; however, numerous other thymic hormones or thymic peptides have been isolated, including thymic factor X, thymostimulin, beta-thymosins, thymopentin, thymulin, and thymic humoral factor.

As BRMs, thymosins function mostly as immunorestorative agents by inducing the maturation and differentiation of T lymphocytes; in addition, they can enhance immune function by stimulating lymphokine production (e.g., interferons, interleukin-2, and colony-stimulating factor). Thymosins also appear to play a role in the regulation of other important hormone systems located in the brain, such as luteinizing hormone–releasing hormone (LHRH), luteinizing hormone (LH), adrenocorticotropic hormone (ACTH), and beta-endorphin. This latter observation is relevant to the mechanisms involved in the normal aging process, in which the brain may become unable to produce and regulate certain hormones.

Thymic preparations have been used to enhance immune responses in both normal and immunodeficient animal models. Based on preliminary clinical trials, thymosins may be useful in the treatment of immunodeficiencies or immune imbalance diseases (e.g., autoimmunity, certain infectious diseases, allergies, and perhaps cancer), as well as conditions associated with neuroendocrine imbalances (e.g., reproductive problems and stress-related diseases).

CYTOKINES AND LYMPHOKINES

Many BRMs are natural cell products synthesized and secreted by various cell types in response to different specific stimuli. *Cytokines* is a general term for soluble and biologically active factors produced by cells; these factors are usually glycoproteins ranging in molecular weight from 10,000 to greater than 200,000. They are potent at very low concentrations, and they have a wide range of biologic activities, including regulation of various immune components. *Lymphokines* are soluble factors synthesized and excreted by lymphocytes in response to specific antigen or nonspecific mitogen stimulation. Lymphokines bind to specific receptor sites on lymphokine-responsive cell membranes, and as a result they stimulate the receptor cells to new activities. These responding cells may or may not be other lymphocytes. The subclass of lymphokines that activate other lymphocytes are termed interleukins. Two cytokines that have received considerable attention because of their potential clinical promise are interleukin-2 (IL-2) and tumor necrosis factor. Both have been isolated and purified, and they can be produced in large quantities by genetic engineering.

Interleukin-2, formerly T-cell growth factor, is produced by lymphocytes that have been stimulated by mitogens or by specific antigens. The primary biological activity of IL-2 is in induction and amplification of specific cytotoxic T-cell activity. In addition, IL-2 appears to play a role in restoring and enhancing B-cell activity, and it acts in concert with antibodies and cytokines, such as gamma-interferon and TNF. Exposure of lymphocytes to IL-2 *in vitro* and subsequent reinfusion can improve immune reactivity in both humans and animals that exhibit poor immune responsiveness. This finding has major implications for immunosuppressed cancer pa-

tients, as well as for patients with acquired or congenital immunodeficiency diseases.

Immunotherapy with IL-2 and with IL-2–expanded T cells has demonstrated marked antitumor effects in both animal models and human malignancies. Cytolytic T cells with nonspecific antitumor reactivity can be generated by incubation of lymphocytes in IL-2–supplemented media, and these cytotoxic cells are referred to as lymphocyte-activated killer (LAK) cells. Adoptive transfer of LAK cells in conjunction with IL-2 administration has resulted in regressions of a variety of human cancers, including renal cell carcinoma, malignant melanoma, colorectal cancer, and malignant lymphoma.

More recently it was realized that lymphocytes naturally infiltrating tumors are more likely to be tumor specific than peripheral blood lymphocytes. Adoptive immunotherapy utilizing this subpopulation of tumor-infiltrating lymphocytes (TIL) expanded in IL-2–dependent culture has caused regression of advanced pulmonary and hepatic metastases in mouse tumor models. In fact, TIL cells appear to be 50 to 100 times more potent than LAK cells.

In preliminary studies, the authors have treated 17 FeLV-infected cats (including 12 cats with lymphoma/leukemia) using high-dose human recombinant IL-2, either alone or in combination with LAK cells or with chemotherapeutic agents. Good evidence was obtained that human IL-2 does stimulate cat T cells. No antiviral effects or tumor regressions resulted from IL-2 therapy alone; however, a synergistic antitumor effect was suggested in cats treated with combinations of IL-2 and cytotoxic agents. Toxicity of IL-2 administration was dose-dependent, generally was reversible on cessation of therapy, and primarily consisted of fever, lethargy, dyspnea, and eosinophilia.

Tumor necrosis factor is a soluble oncolytic protein derived from activated macrophages found in serum of animals treated sequentially with a reticuloendothelial stimulator (e.g., BCG or *C. parvum*) and endotoxin. TNF was originally identified by its ability to induce hemorrhagic necrosis and regression in a mouse tumor model, and the effects obtained were similar to those caused by endotoxin. It is preferentially cytotoxic for neoplastic cells, and it requires the presence of specific TNF receptors on target cells to exert its action. Besides cytotoxic-cytostatic activity, TNF can activate and enhance neutrophil and eosinophil functions and can augment expression of class I and II histocompatibility antigens. Synergistic antitumor effects between TNF and gamma-IFN have been documented.

Clinical studies of TNF represent the first therapeutic attempt to utilize a toxic cellular product capable of killing tumor cells. Tumor necrosis and regression has been achieved using a spectrum of tumors growing in mice. Currently, TNF is being evaluated in human clinical trials against a variety of solid tumors and against different types of leukemias. Although results are hard to predict, this agent may be most effective when used in combination with chemotherapeutic agents or other BRMs.

MONOCLONAL ANTIBODIES

Monoclonal antibodies are secreted from hybridomas. Hybridomas are developed *in vitro* by fusing immortal, antibody nonsecreting myeloma cells with specific antibody-secreting spleen cells (generally derived from previously immunized mice). The process is carried out using large numbers of both cell types, and the specific antibody-secreting hybridomas are identified by a series of screens until the required cells are selected and cloned. By fusing antibody-producing spleen cells (B cells) with myeloma cells, a hybrid clone can be selected that will secrete high levels of specific antibody and divide indefinitely. As a result hybridoma technology provides the means to produce MAbs in virtually unlimited quantities. MAbs alone have many potential therapeutic applications (e.g., direct toxicity to tumor cells via either CDA or ADCC), but their value is greatly enhanced because they can be coupled to a variety of agents and still retain their ability to bind to antigen. As a result they can be conjugated with radioisotopes, chemotherapeutic agents, toxins, or even other BRMs, and the MAb then becomes a vehicle to specifically deliver these agents to required sites of action with minimal toxic side effects.

In humans, anti–T-cell MAbs have been used to elicit tumor regression in patients with various types of T-cell leukemia or lymphoma. MAbs have also proved beneficial in the treatment of graft-versus-host disease (GVHD) associated with bone marrow transplantation and may be useful reagents in treating certain immune deficiencies and in altering other immune responses.

Factors that may limit the efficacy of MAb therapy include (1) heterogeneity of target antigens when each MAb is epitope specific; (2) high levels of preexisting recipient antibodies to heterospecies immunoglobulins and secondary immune responses to injected MAbs; (3) high levels of circulating antigens, which bind MAbs before they reach the target site; (4) poor MAb accessibility (e.g., poor tumor vascularity); (5) nonspecific MAb uptake by the RES; and (6) antigenic modulation of tumor cells in the presence of antibody (so target cells no longer express the target antigens). Immunoconjugates, immunoglobulin fragments (i.e., F[ab']$_2$ fragments), specific tolerization to heterospecies immunoglobulins, and pools of MAbs to different tumor cell epitopes are possible solutions to these problems.

The authors have treated four FeLV-positive, leukemia- or lymphoma-bearing cats with intravenous infusions of up to 150 mg of purified MAbs specific for FeLV gp-70 (a viral envelope protein). Objective tumor regressions (> 50 per cent) were rapidly obtained in two cats; however, these regressions were transient, and all four cats eventually died of progressive disease. Anti-FeLV MAbs have also been used to treat 11 healthy FeLV-positive cats. Although circulating FeLV levels were transiently decreased, no permanent virus reversals resulted from this therapy. By 2 weeks after treatment all cats exhibited elevated levels of antibodies to mouse immunoglobulins.

It may also be possible to use MAbs to develop *anti-idiotype vaccines*. Each different MAb is directed to a specific antigen epitope. The binding of antibody to antigen is somewhat similar to a lock-and-key mechanism with one (the binding site or idiotype of the MAb) being the opposite shape to the other (the epitope of the antigen). Because the idiotype of an antibody is a novel shape to the host that develops it, the host will be immunized and then make a second antibody to it (i.e., the anti-idiotype antibody). Humoral immune responses are thus controlled by this feedback mechanism. The point is, however, that the binding site of the anti-idiotype antibody is the opposite shape to the original idiotype, and therefore, is the same shape as the original inciting epitope. It is possible to construct anti-idiotype MAbs, which can be used to vaccinate a host rather than expose the host to the pathogen directly. The host's immune response to this immunization would then resemble a positive response to the original pathogen. For example, in the authors' laboratories an anti-idiotype vaccine for FeLV infection is being developed. MAbs to FeLV are first constructed and the idiotypes of these have the opposite shape to the virus epitopes. Next anti-idiotype MAbs to the originals are developed, and these MAbs have the same shape as the virus epitopes. By immunizing cats with anti-idiotype MAbs, the production of antibodies that react directly with FeLV is induced. It is hoped that selection of the correct anti-idiotype MAbs for vaccination will result in a protective immune response.

BONE MARROW TRANSPLANTATION

The efficacy of bone marrow transplantation (BMT) has improved in recent years as a result of advances in radiotherapeutic techniques, use of more potent immunosuppressive agents, a better understanding of histocompatibility antigens, and the employment of various methods to selectively deplete T cells (to prevent GVHD). In fact, BMT is considered the treatment of choice for humans with aplastic anemia and certain forms of leukemia.

Dogs have long been used as animal models to facilitate elucidation of the principles and techniques of human BMT. BMT combined with irradiation and chemotherapy has resulted in long-term survival of 25 per cent of dogs with spontaneous malignant lymphoma. Pyruvate kinase deficiency in Basenjis and cyclic neutropenia of gray collies have also been successfully treated with BMT.

Cats would be expected to be ideal candidates for BMT because of the apparent minimal polymorphism in the feline major histocompatibility complex. Mucopolysaccharidosis VI in a cat was successfully treated by BMT. Several cats infected with FeLV have also received bone marrow transplants; although marrow engraftment was often successful, FeLV viremia consistently returned within a short period of time.

BMT promises to be a viable alternative for a variety of otherwise untreatable hematopoietic and immunodeficiency diseases in humans and animals. Despite the complexities involved, BMT is a clinically relevant technique that is within the capabilities of most veterinary medical centers.

SUMMARY

Biologic therapy has rapidly evolved to become the fourth modality of cancer treatment. There is broad potential for therapy utilizing BRMs alone, in combinations, or as adjuvants to more conventional treatments. As knowledge of immunologic mechanisms increases, so should ability to use specific biologic agents for the treatment of cancer, infectious diseases, autoimmune diseases, and immunosuppressive disorders in veterinary medicine.

References and Supplemental Reading

Appelbaum, F. R., Deeg, H. J., Storb, R., et al.: Marrow transplant studies in dogs with malignant lymphoma. Transplantation 39:499, 1985.

Engelman, R. W., Tyler, R. D., Trang, L. Q., et al.: Clinicopathologic responses in cats with feline leukemia virus–associated leukemia-lymphoma treated with staphylococcal protein A. Am. J. Pathol. 118:367, 1985.

Ford, R. B.: Biological response modifiers in the management of viral infection. Vet. Clin. North Am. [Small Anim. Pract.] 16:1191, 1986.

Harris, C. K., Beck, E. R., and Gasper, P. W.: Bone marrow transplantation in the dog. Comp. Cont. Ed. Pract. Vet. 8:337, 1986.

Jones, F. R., Grant, C. K., and Snyder, H. W.: Lymphosarcoma and persistent feline leukemia virus infection of pet cats: A system to study responses during extracorporeal treatments. J. Biol. Response Mod. 3:286, 1984.

MacEwen, E. G.: Approaches to cancer therapy using biological response modifiers. Vet. Clin. North Am. [Small Anim. Pract.] 15:667, 1985.

MacEwen, E. G.: Current immunotherapeutic approaches in small animals. In Proceedings of the 10th Annual Kal Kan Symposium for the Treatment of Small Animal Diseases. Ohio State University, Columbus, OH, Kal Kan Foods, Inc., 1987a, pp. 47–52.

MacEwen, E. G.: Personal communication, 1987b.

Oldham, R. K.: Biological response modifiers. J. Natl. Cancer Inst. 70:789, 1983.

Oldham, R. K.: Monoclonal antibodies in cancer therapy. J. Clin. Oncol. 1:582, 1983.

Rosenberg, S. A.: Adoptive immunotherapy of cancer using lymphokine activated killer cells and recombinant interleukin-2. In DeVita, V. T., Hellman, S., Rosenberg, S. A. (eds.): Important Advances in Oncology. New York; J. B. Lippincott, 1986, pp. 55–91.

Rosenberg, S. A., Spiess, P., and Lafreniere, R.: A new approach to the adoptive immunotherapy of cancer with tumor-infiltrating lymphocytes. Science 233:1318, 1986.

Torrence, P. F.: Biological Response Modifiers. New Approaches to Disease Intervention. Orlando: Academic Press, Inc., 1985.

CYCLOSPORINE

CLARE R. GREGORY, D.V.M.
Davis, California

Since its discovery in 1972 by Jean F. Borel and coworkers at the Sandoz Laboratories in Basel, Switzerland, cyclosporine has revolutionized transplantation medicine. Cyclosporine is the first potent immunosuppressive agent to act on specific T lymphocyte and T-associated B-lymphocyte responses without concomitant myelotoxicity (Fig. 1). Cyclosporine does not inhibit migration of leukocytes and has no significant effect on the viability of nonstimulated lymphocytes. This specific, reversible mechanism of action spares nonspecific host resistance and reportedly results in a lower incidence of viral and bacterial infections when compared with action of other immunosuppressive agents.

Cyclosporine has been used primarily in organ and tissue transplantation but has potential use for the treatment of several autoimmune disorders. Cases of pemphigus vulgaris, bullous pemphigoid, immune-mediated uveitis, and certain collagen vascular disorders in human patients have been successfully treated or have benefited from cyclosporine administration. Cyclosporine has been used to manage pemphigus foliaceus in a dog, immune-mediated uveitis in rats, and ocular herpes simplex keratitis in rabbits.

PHARMACOLOGIC PROPERTIES

Cyclosporine is a neutral, hydrophobic cyclic peptide composed of 11 amino acids. The drug

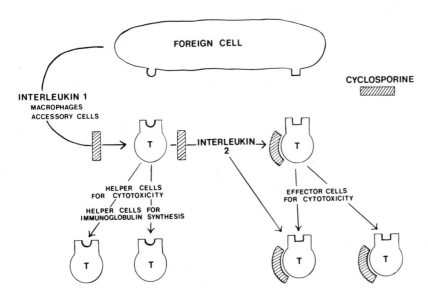

Figure 1. Activation of lymphocytes by alloantigens. Depending on the nature of the antigenic stimulation and the differentiation state of the responding T lymphocyte, cyclosporine stops interleukin 2 production by activated T helper cells, inhibits interleukin release from macrophages, and inhibits development of interleukin 2 receptors on immature alloreactive T cytotoxic cells.

undergoes hepatic metabolism and biliary excretion, with only a small amount excreted unchanged in the urine. The oral preparation, Sandimmune (Sandoz), comes in an olive oil base. After oral administration, absorption can be highly variable among individuals of the same species. Some cats, and on occasion dogs, find the oral solution highly unpalatable, resulting in profuse salivation and head shaking. These animals may receive an inadequate dose and often become unmanageable with repeated treatments. A trial of the oral solution is recommended prior to transplantation, particularly in feline patients, as the medication has to be administered for life. Inadequate or infrequent administration of cyclosporine will result in rejection of the allografted tissue or organ. Administration of the oral solution via capsules and ophthalmic cyclosporine preparations are currently being tested.

Cyclosporine is also available in a solution for intravenous adminstration. Intravenous cyclosporine is administered at a third of the recommended daily oral dose. Prior to administration, the intravenous solution is diluted in 5 per cent dextrose or 0.9 per cent saline and given over a 4- to 6-hour period. Intravenous cyclosporine is used during the perioperative period when oral administration is not possible and during periods of vomiting and malaise associated with rejection episodes or other illnesses.

Owing to the highly variable absorption of the oral solution, blood or plasma levels of cyclosporine must be monitored during therapy. This is particularly important in the transplant patient at the time of changing from intravenous to oral administration. Both high-pressure liquid chromatography and radioimmunoassay can be used to measure cyclosporine levels. Analysis of different fluids by either method will provide different results. The concentrations in whole blood are approximately twice those measured in plasma because of the

propensity of cyclosporine binding to red blood cells. Concentrations in plasma can vary greatly, depending on the temperature at which the plasma is separated from blood, requiring that conditions of collection and separation be standardized. Whole blood cyclosporine determinations appear to be more reproducible and reliable than plasma cyclosporine concentrations. High-pressure liquid chromatography can also be used to detect the individual metabolites of cyclosporine. Based on initial studies, the metabolites appear to contribute little to the immunosuppressive ability or toxicity of the parent drug.

Dosages of cyclosporine administered orally are arbitrarily divided into high dose (12 to 17 mg/kg/24 hr), moderate dose (7 to 11 mg/kg/24 hr), low dose (1.5 to 6 mg/kg/24 hr), and ultra low dose (< 1 mg/kg/24 hr). The daily dose is generally divided and administered every 12 hr. Organ allograft recipients receive high doses initially; these are reduced to moderate to low levels, depending on the immunologic tolerance of the patient to the graft, i.e., lack of rejection episodes. Alterations of dosage are also based on blood levels, *in vitro* assays of cell-mediated immunity (e.g., mitogen stimulation and mixed lymphocyte responses), and development of drug-induced side effects. Blood levels are only a qualitative indication of immunosuppression, and effects will vary among individuals. Blood levels do provide proof that a patient is able to absorb the oral solution and allow for adjustment in dose. Few guidelines exist for the selection of blood levels in veterinary patients that will allow allograft survival while minimizing toxic or lethal side effects. Whole blood levels of cyclosporine measured just prior to the next oral administration (12-hr trough level) are maintained at 400 to 600 ng/ml in renal allograft recipients. Prednisolone (0.25 to 0.5 mg/kg/24 hr) is administered in conjunction with cyclosporine.

ADVERSE EFFECTS

In human patients, cyclosporine nephrotoxicity is its major limiting factor as an immunosuppressive drug. Cyclosporine is generally not nephrotoxic in the dog and cat. Only one case of nephrotoxicity has been reported in a dog unable to metabolize cyclosporine owing to a coexisting chylous effusion. Hepatotoxicity also occurs in human patients but has not been a problem in the dog and the cat.

Despite a low risk of postimmunosuppressive infections with use of cyclosporine when compared with risk associated with other immunosuppressive agents, several studies indicate that cyclosporine can permit the development of lethal bacterial and fungal infections. In large-hospital situations, careful surveillance is necessary to identify and eliminate nosocomial sources of infection.

Other adverse reactions reported with the use of cyclosporine in dogs and cats are gastrointestinal irritation, gingival hypertrophy, and papillomatosis. One case of B-lymphocyte hyperplasia has been reported in the dog. All these effects generally abate when the dosage of cyclosporine is reduced.

Many different drug interactions have been reported with cyclosporine administration. Drugs of particular concern are those that may potentiate cyclosporine nephrotoxicity. Gentamicin, amphotericin, and melphalan are intrinsically nephrotoxic, whereas ketaconazole, erythromycin, and cimetidine depress hepatic metabolism of cyclosporine. Trimethoprim may also potentiate cyclosporine nephrotoxicity. Phenytoin and phenobarbital increase hepatic metabolism of cyclosporine and result in lower than anticipated blood levels.

CURRENT AND FUTURE APPLICATIONS

The development of cyclosporine, the evolution of estimating histocompatibility and cell-mediated immunity, and microsurgery have made renal transplantation a possible consideration for treatment of terminal renal failure in the dog and cat. Several veterinary colleges and private hospitals are currently offering renal transplantation for selected patients. The major limiting factor in the use of cyclosporine is the high cost, initially as high as $0.45/kg/day. With the development of multiple-drug immunosuppressive protocols that allow lower doses of cyclosporine to be administered, this cost could be reduced.

Cyclosporine has potential benefit in the treatment of many diseases in which T lymphocytes are involved. Areas of research that may have clinical application in the near future are the treatment of certain immune-mediated and inflammatory conditions, including atopic dermatitis, uveitis, rheumatoid arthritis, myasthenia gravis, polyradiculoneuropathy, inflammatory bowel disease, aplastic anemia, and nephrotic syndrome.

References and Supplemental Reading

Gregory, C. R., Gourley, I. M., Taylor, N. J., et al.: Experience with cyclosporin-A after renal allografting in two dogs. Vet. Surg. 15:441, 1986.

Gregory, C. R., Gourley, I. M., Taylor, N. J., et al.: Preliminary results of clinical renal allograft transplantation in the dog and cat. J. Vet. Intern. Med. 1:53, 1987.

Latimer, K. S., Rakich, P. M., Purswell, B. J., et al.: Effects of cyclosporin administration in cats. Vet. Immunol. Immunopathol. 11:161, 1986.

Page, E. H., Wexler, D. M., Guenther, L. C., et al.: Cyclosporin-A. J. Am. Acad. Dermatol. 14:785, 1986.

Rosenkrantz, W. S.: Cyclosporine therapy in a case of pemphigus foliaceus. Vet. Allergist, Summer 1984, p. 1.

White, J. V.: Cyclosporine: Prototype of a T-cell selective immunosuppressant. J.A.V.M.A. 189:566, 1986.

BONE MARROW TRANSPLANTATION

P. W. GASPER, D.V.M.
Fort Collins, Colorado

The technique of transplanting bone marrow is simple. However, management of patients who receive marrow transplants is one of the toughest medical challenges known. A marrow transplant endows the recipient with a new, lifelong source of donor origin lymphohematopoietic cells and, therefore, has the potential to cure many fatal diseases (Fig. 1). Most bone marrow transplant (BMT) techniques were developed and tested in dogs. Although some veterinary patients have received marrow

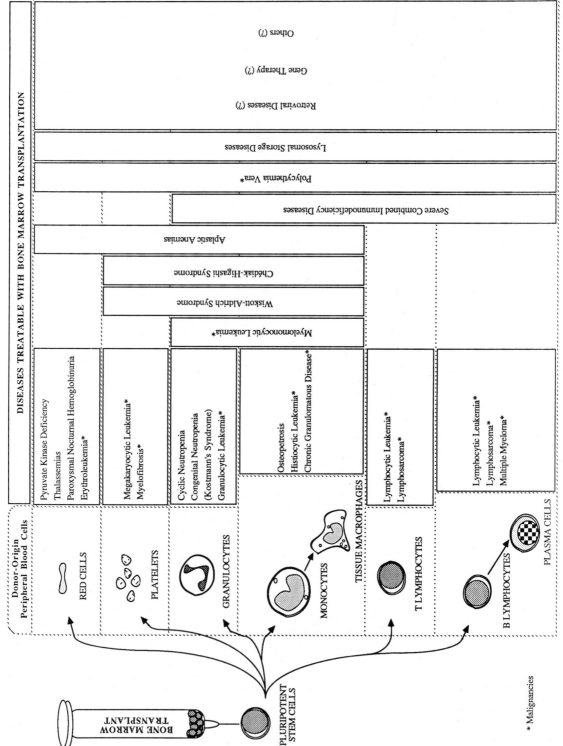

Figure 1. Diseases treatable with bone marrow transplantation.

transplants to treat their specific diseases, most BMTs of animals have been performed to obtain information to better treat humans. BMT offers hope in otherwise fatal conditions. Because there is a wealth of experience in transplanting bone marrow in dogs and increasing experience in cats, and because there is a growing understanding of and developments in immunosuppressive therapy, one can anticipate that BMT will be increasingly utilized in veterinary medicine.

Bone marrow transplantation differs from solid organ transplantation in two major ways. First, one simply infuses cells intravenously and the marrow "organ" assembles itself—pluripotent stem cells seed the recipient with a lifelong source of donor origin lymphohematopoietic cells. Second, because the transplant recipient acquires a new immune system of donor origin, marrow grafts can mount immune reactions against normal recipient tissues. This phenomenon is termed graft-versus-host disease (GVHD) and is one of the primary reasons BMT is not used more often in human and veterinary medicine.

There are different types of marrow transplants depending on the relatedness of donor to recipient and on the disease treated. Allogeneic BMTs involve donor-recipient pairing between genetically nonidentical individuals, either histocompatible or nonhistocompatible (discussed below); syngeneic BMTs are between genetically identical individuals (i.e., monozygotic twins); and autologous BMTs involve the recipient serving as its own donor. BMT therapy is indicated for two broad categories of diseases: malignant disorders and nonmalignant disorders (see Fig. 1).

Marrow transplants for malignant disorders generally follow high-dose chemotherapy or irradiation, which destroys marrow simultaneously with tumor cells. Neoplasia of any lymphohematopoietic lineage can be treated with BMT. The most common BMT-treated malignancies in humans are lymphocytic and myelogenous leukemias. The donor-recipient pairing is usually allogeneic or syngeneic, although the use of autologous BMT is an attractive and increasingly used alternative because it obviates the need for a histocompatible donor, thereby eliminating the threat of GVHD. Autologous transplantation involves removal of marrow during remission of the malignancy, elimination of residual tumor cells from the cells to be transplanted (using monoclonal antibodies coupled with complement, immunotoxins, magnetic microspheres, magnetic immunocolloids, or drug conjugates), and finally, cryopreservation of the tumor-purged marrow. When the patient relapses, it is treated with high dose total-body irradiation and chemotherapy, and frozen tumor-free marrow is thawed and seeded back into the patient.

The general objective in BMTs for nonmalignant disorders is to provide the affected individual with new marrow elements to replace malfunctioning or absent cells. These life-threatening hematologic or immunologic conditions can be either congenital or acquired. The donors are allogeneic or syngeneic and provide normal functioning marrow. The most common BMT-treated nonmalignant conditions in humans are aplastic anemias and severe combined immunodeficiency diseases. Other conditions for which BMT is indicated include inherited defects in single blood cell lineages (such as cyclic neutropenia in collies or pyruvate kinase deficiency in Basenjis) or multiple cell lineages (e.g., Chédiak-Higashi syndrome of Persian cats). The indication for BMT is less apparent in conditions such as osteopetrosis, in which one replaces defective osteoclasts, or lysosomal storage diseases (such as mucopolysaccharidosis VI of Siamese cats), in which one corrects congenitally malfunctioning or absent enzyme by installing cells that will continually manufacture and disseminate normal enzyme. In addition to peripherally circulating lymphohematopoietic cells, alveolar macrophages, Kupffer's cells, osteoclasts, dendritic cells, Langerhans' cells, and certain glial cells arise from and are continually replenished by marrow stem cells.

As transplantation techniques are perfected one can imagine additional potential indications for BMT. Retroviral infections are infections primarily of lymphohematopoietic cells and, therefore, may be treatable by BMT when coupled with other immunotherapeutic and chemotherapeutic agents to protect virus-free cells as they engraft. Molecular biologists anticipate autologous BMT as the vehicle for future gene therapy—transfecting genes into marrow stem cells in culture then seeding cells that produce the gene product back into the patient.

METHODOLOGY

The technique of bone marrow transplantation can be divided into five distinct steps (Fig. 2). First, one selects the best possible donor. Large litter sizes and relatively short gestation times of dogs and cats allow for more donor-recipient alternatives than are generally available in human medicine. After the donor is selected, the patient is prepared for its transplant. How one proceeds at this step varies with the disease being treated. Next, a cell suspension containing enough stem cells to beget a complete population of functional peripheral blood cells is infused intravenously. Hematologic engraftment occurs with donor-origin end cells appearing in the recipient's circulation within 14 to 21 days (Fig. 3). Like solid organ transplantation, one must suppress the patient's immune responses to avoid rejection of allogeneic marrow. Quick-thinking medical skills are required during the transition period between elimination of host blood cells and

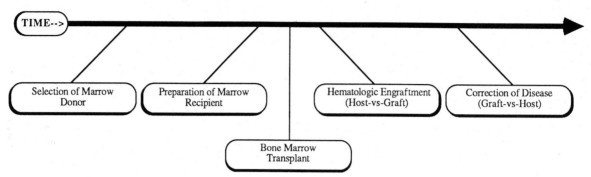

Figure 2. Sequence of events in bone marrow transplantation.

total engraftment of donor cells. As soon as donor lymphohematopoiesis can be demonstrated, the clinician may have to focus on the development and possible complications arising from graft-versus-host reactivity. The final result is a patient endowed with donor-origin immunologic and hematopoietic systems.

SELECTION OF MARROW DONOR

The dog was the first animal in which the predictive value of *in vitro* histocompatibility testing for the outcome of marrow grafts was demonstrated. The information learned in canine studies was rapidly applied to matching human donor-recipient pairs. Knowledge of the feline histocompatibility system is more sketchy than knowledge of the systems of people and dogs. Although one can

identify the usual components of the histocompatibility complex in cats, early results from performing allogeneic BMTs suggest that the cat may be more likely to accept nonsibling marrow grafts than other outbred mammals.

Histocompatibility genes are genes that control the rejection of organ grafts. The major histocompatibility complex (MHC) is a chromosomal region that contains several genes that are important in the determination of cell surface antigens. These antigens aid in the recognition of self and nonself. The major histocompatibility complex in the dog is referred to as the DLA (dog leukocyte antigen) system (similar to the human HLA system). The DLA system is composed of four loci labeled A, B, C, and D. Each locus has several alleles or determinants, which are numbered consecutively. The DLA-A, B, and C loci encode class I antigens, which are serologically defined and measured *in*

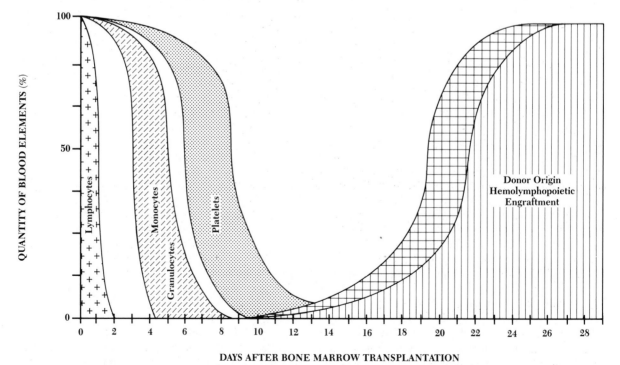

DAYS AFTER BONE MARROW TRANSPLANTATION

Figure 3. Hematologic changes following total body irradiation and bone marrow transplantation.

vitro using a microlymphocytotoxicity assay employing alloantisera originally produced by immunizing canine littermates that differed by only one allele. The DLA-D locus codes for class II antigens, which are lymphocyte defined and measured *in vitro* in the mixed leukocyte reaction (MLR). Inheritance of one DLA haplotype from each parent results in the probability that one of four littermates would be matched at all determinants of the MHC (the chances for a DLA identical donor are $1 - (3/4)^n$, where n is number of siblings). Inbred animals have an increased chance for matching at the MHC because inbreeding increases the frequency of homozygosity in polymorphic genetic systems.

The pragmatics of donor selection presently require that one respect the polymorphism of histocompatibility. Although reagents exist to identify canine and human MHC antigens, the likelihood for success of a BMT is far greater if performed between MHC-matched *siblings*, than if performed with MHC-matched nonsibling donor-recipient pairings. This indicates that present tests measure only prominent tissue differences and suggests that other histocompatibility antigens influence the outcome of transplantation. For practical reasons, one attempts to locate a sibling that is matched for the MHC and tries to suppress the inevitable remaining minor histocompatability differences by immunosuppressive therapy. Marrow grafting between DLA-matched canine littermates results in excellent probability of long-term survival.

PREPARATION OF MARROW RECIPIENT

Marrow transplant recipients are prepared for BMT in two ways. One set of procedures is performed regardless of the condition treated. The objective is to have the patient in the best possible physical condition at the commencement of the transplant. One examines the patient for potential sources of complications, including dental calculi; performs bacterial analysis and parasitologic analysis of feces; and collects baseline clinical data such as complete blood count, platelet count, and serum chemistry profile. Selective gastrointestinal decontamination has been shown to be helpful in decreasing the incidence of infections during the critical period of post-BMT immune suppression, more so than total gastrointestinal decontamination, which leaves the patient susceptible to rapid colonization of the intestine if microorganisms were inadvertently introduced.

The second set of preparations differs according to the disease treated. Here one addresses three concerns: marrow "space," host resistance to donor lymphohematopoietic stem cells, and tumor cell elimination. Table 1 illustrates how the strategy of patient conditioning varies in three representative

Table 1. *Strategy for Patient Conditioning in Representative Diseases*

	Severe Combined Immune Deficiency	Aplastic Anemia	Leukemia
Marrow "space"	No	Yes	No
Host resistance	No	Yes	Yes
Tumor cell ablation	No	No	Yes

diseases: severe combined immune deficiency (SCID), aplastic anemia (AA), and leukemia.

1. Marrow space is a conceptual rather than anatomic concern. It has been found that replication and differentiation of stem cells can proceed only if a proper microenvironment is available in the new host. Patients with aplastic anemia (AA) apparently have sufficient space in the marrow to support new hematopoiesis, whereas leukemic or severe combined immunodeficiency (SCID) patients do not.

2. Host resistance to donor cells must be blunted for the graft to seed and grow. Resistance does not occur in SCID patients, who lack a functioning immune system, whereas AA and leukemic patients must be immunosuppressed so that they will not reject the graft. If the patient has ever received blood transfusions, the potential for host resistance is increased.

3. Ablation of tumor cells is relevant when using BMT to treat patients with neoplasia. Replacement of malignant lymph or hematopoietic systems by newly transplanted systems will be of lasting usefulness only if all clonogenic leukemia cells in the host can be eliminated.

High-dose radiotherapy or chemotherapy or combinations of the two are the most commonly used conditioning regimens. Total-body irradiation (TBI) has the advantage of killing noncycling tumor cells as effectively as cycling cells; this is especially pertinent to the treatment of lymphoid malignancies. Radiation penetrates privileged sites, such as the central nervous system (CNS) and testicle, which are not accessible by most chemotherapeutic agents. Consistent and sustained engraftment of allogeneic marrow in the dog is achieved only above 12.0-gray (Gy) midline air exposure (9.0- to 10.0-Gy midline tissue) dose. Dogs grafted after radiation of 12.0 Gy usually achieve stable complete chimerism; that is, all cells analyzed in marrow, lymph nodes, and peripheral blood are determined to be of donor origin (karyotype). A dose of 300-kV x-rays is sufficient to obtain a complete radiation chimera, and the lower TBI dose is significantly less toxic; however, the lower dose may not eliminate all tumor cells nor all host stem cells, predisposing the patient to relapse of its disease or an unstable marrow graft.

Dogs conditioned with a single TBI dose of 12.0 Gy will manifest signs of gastrointestinal toxicity within 60 hr of treatment. Vomiting, diarrhea, and polydipsia are observed. Untreated dogs will die within 7 days of TBI of extreme dehydration and electrolyte loss. This can be prevented by stopping oral intake for 5 days following TBI and by aggressive fluid therapy. Currently, fractionated TBI is being used to increase the total radiation dose while decreasing the severity of acute gastrointestinal toxicity and late respiratory effects (pulmonary interstitial fibrosis). Cats conditioned with a fractionated dose of 10 Gy (five 2-Gy fractions over 3 days) show no signs of gastrointestinal toxicity; moreover, they continue to eat and drink after TBI.

Cyclophosphamide (Cy) can be substituted for TBI to condition dogs for marrow grafting. Cy-induced chimeras tend to be less than 100 per cent, resulting in persistent mixtures of host and donor lymphohemopoietic cells. Therefore, the use of Cy as the sole conditioning agent is limited to those diseases in which host cells are absent to begin with, such as AA or SCID. Trials using Cy to prepare cats for BMT have failed to identify a regimen that can be used safely.

Conditioning with a combination of agents is currently being evaluated in dogs and one can anticipate that an effective method will be derived soon. The experience in treating dogs with combinations of TBI and Cy has been negative, primarily because of overlapping toxicity. Cy-induced GI toxicity, hemorrhagic cystitis, and possibly myocardial damage have been seen in dogs. Other agents that have been and are being evaluated in combination with TBI include 6-mercaptopurine, methotrexate, silica particles, antilymphocyte serum, L-asparaginase, *Corynebacterium parvum*, glucocorticoids, and dimethylmyleran.

BONE MARROW TRANSPLANT AND HEMATOLOGIC ENGRAFTMENT

Under general anesthetic, bone marrow is collected aseptically from a histocompatible donor. In dogs, this is performed with a suction apparatus that draws marrow into a flask containing anticoagulant. Multiple aspirations of the pelvis and long bones with large-bore (15-gauge) needles yield approximately 300 ml of hemodiluted marrow. In cats, it has been found that aspiration of 3 to 4 ml of marrow from each of the donor cat's long bones (humeri, femurs, and tibias) with 18-gauge marrow biopsy needles into anticoagulant-containing syringes yields approximately 20 ml of marrow. Ordinarily, the only processing is centrifugation to remove fat and passage through a sieve screen to remove large particulate material before intravenous administration to the recipient. The transplanted marrow is a mixture of cells at various stages of development within the erythroid, myeloid, mon-

ocytic, megakaryocytic, and lymphoid lineages together with marrow stromal cells. Hematopoietic cells arise from a small population of undifferentiated self-renewing stem cells, which likely constitute the only essential part of the graft. Success of BMT is dependent on retrieving a sufficient number of hematopoietic stem cells.

Figure 3 illustrates the kinetics of TBI-induced destruction of host hematopoietic cells followed by growth of donor-origin blood cells. The decline in the cell lineages reflects their respective life spans in peripheral circulation (with the exception being lymphocytes, which are killed in interphase by irradiation). Because of the long half-life of erythrocytes, a decline in hematocrit is not usually observed. Progeny of donor stem cells generally begin to appear in the marrow and blood of the recipient between 2 and 3 weeks after transplantation. In successful BMTs, hematopoiesis appears entirely normal and persists indefinitely. The chemotherapy and TBI given in preparation for marrow transplantation cause extensive ablation of cellular and humoral immunity. All patients manifest an immunodeficiency of varying length following BMT. With time, donor-derived lymphoid cells repopulate the host, ultimately resulting in restoration of immunocompetence. Failure to engraft can be caused by unappreciated genetic disparity between the donor and recipient, inadequate immunosuppression of the recipient, abnormalities of insufficient numbers of stem cells in the graft, abnormal marrow microenvironment in the recipient, drug toxicity, or viral infections.

GRAFT-VERSUS-HOST DISEASE

Unique to marrow transplantation, graft-versus-host disease is one of the largest impediments to the routine use of BMT therapy in veterinary and human medicine. Three conditions must be met for a marrow graft to attack its new host: genetically determined histocompatibility differences between the donor and recipient; the presence of immunocompetent cells in the graft, which can recognize histocompatibility antigens of the host and mount an immunologic reaction; and inability of the host to react against or reject the graft. Two distinct forms of GVHD—acute and chronic—have been recognized. They have different onsets as well as different clinical and pathologic manifestations. Acute GVHD is characterized by inflammatory destruction of epithelial cells in the skin, liver, and gastrointestinal tract by cytotoxic lymphocytes and develops within the first 60 days after BMT. Chronic GVHD is characterized by increased collagen deposition, resulting in fibrosis, and generally appears after day 100 post-BMT; however, it can arise as early as day 70. GVHD itself seldom causes death, but it is often associated with fatal secondary infections.

Efforts are currently being directed toward preventing GVHD. Treatment of established acute GVHD poses a predicament because available methods involve the use of nonspecific immunosuppressive agents in a patient that is already profoundly immunosuppressed. Methotrexate was first developed as an agent for prophylaxis of GVHD after allogeneic BMT in dogs. Cyclosporine has been evaluated more recently. The approach has been to administer these agents to the recipient during engraftment (in the first 2 weeks after BMT) to paralyze any lymphocytes that may have been in the graft. A different preventive approach has been to deplete T cells and other lymphocytes from the donor marrow through a variety of methods, including lectin agglutination with E rosetting, elutriation, use of monoclonal antibodies and complement, or toxin-linked monoclonal antibodies. Early results from these studies are encouraging; nearly all have demonstrated a significant reduction in acute and chronic GVHD if at least a 1.5-log T-cell reduction is achieved.

SUMMARY

Marrow transplantation offers a potential cure for many conditions of dogs and cats that have heretofore been considered fatal diseases (see Fig. 1). It is a simple procedure but requires state-of-the-art patient management. Bone marrow transplantation is currently not a practical therapy for veterinary patients; however, veterinarians may be near the end of considering BMT solely an experimental procedure.

References and Supplemental Reading

Harris, C. K., Beck, E. R., and Gasper, P. W.: Bone marrow transplantation in the dog. Comp. Cont. Ed. Pract. Vet. 8:337, 1986.

Lum, L. G.: The kinetics of immune reconstitution after human marrow transplantation. Blood 69:369, 1987.

Martin, P. J., Hansen, J. A., Storb, R., and Thomas, E. D.: Human marrow transplantation: An immunological perspective. Adv. Immunol. 40:379, 1987.

Storb, R.: Critical issues in bone marrow transplantation. Transplant. Proc. 19:2774, 1987.

Vriesendorp, H. M., and Van Bekkum, D. W.: Bone marrow transplantation in the canine. In Shifrine, M., and Wilson, F. D. (eds.): The Canine As a Biomedical Research Model: Immunologic, Hematologic, and Oncological Aspects. Technical Information Center/U.S. Department of Energy publication #10191, 1980, pp. 153–202.

CONGENITAL AND ACQUIRED NEUTROPHIL FUNCTION ABNORMALITIES IN THE DOG

C. GUILLERMO COUTO, D.V.M.
Columbus, Ohio

and URS GIGER, D.M.V.
Philadelphia, Pennsylvania

The circulating blood polymorphonuclear neutrophils (PMNs) are primarily responsible for recognition and phagocytosis of relatively small particulate material, including mainly bacteria. Functional abnormalities or decreased numbers of these circulating cells can result in fulminant fatal sepsis or recurrent or chronic bacterial infections. Although a limited number of disorders associated with neutrophil function abnormalities had been suspected in the dog during the past two decades, current research has revealed an increasing number of congenital and acquired disorders affecting this cell line (Table 1).

NEUTROPHIL MORPHOLOGY AND PHYSIOLOGY

Mature neutrophils have a polymorphic segmented nucleus with clumped chromatin; in general, the nuclear lobes are irregular and filaments joining two lobes are occasionally seen. The nuclear

Table 1. *Neutrophil Function Abnormalities*

Congenital
Leukocyte adhesion protein deficiency in Irish setters
Complement (C3) deficiency in Brittany spaniels
Immunodeficiency in Weimaraners
Neutrophil bactericidal defect in Doberman pinschers
Pelger-Huët anomaly in various canine breeds
Ciliary dyskinesia in pointers

Acquired
Endocrine
Hypercorticism
Diabetes mellitus
Hypothyroidism (?)
Growth hormone deficiency (?)

Infectious
Sepsis
Protothecosis and aspergillosis
Viral diseases and vaccines

Others
Extensive burns (?)
Drugs/chemicals (?)
Cancer (?)
Immune-mediated diseases (?)
Severe cachexia (?)
Granulocytic leukemia (?)

?, Not well documented in dogs.

membrane is irregular (i.e., moth-eaten appearance), and the cytoplasm is pale gray with indistinct, diffuse, pinkish granulation (Jain, 1986).

Ultrastructurally, they contain *primary* and *secondary* (or specific) granules. The primary granules first appear in progranulocytes, are azurophilic on Romanowsky's stains, and are peroxidase positive. The secondary granules first appear in myelocytes and are peroxidase negative. Formation of primary granules ceases when secondary granules appear (Jain, 1986). Primary and secondary granules contain a wide variety of enzymatic and nonenzymatic constituents. (For a detailed review of this subject the reader is referred to Jain, 1986.)

Neutrophils originate in the bone marrow from the committed colony-forming unit granulocyte-macrophage cell (CFU-GM) as follows: CFU-GM, myeloblast, progranulocyte, myelocyte, metamyelocyte, band cell, and mature neutrophil. Neutrophils undergo three phases of development: intramedullary, intravascular, and tissue phases. In dogs, the transit from myeloblast to mature neutrophil in the intramedullary phase takes approximately 3 to 5 days. The circulating life span of canine PMNs is approximately 6 to 8 hr. Little is known about the tissue phase of canine PMNs (Jain, 1986).

The primary function of PMNs is to ingest and destroy particulate material (e.g., bacteria). In order to do so, PMNs are first attracted to the injury site (via chemotaxis, margination, adhesion, and migration), where they subsequently ingest the particle (via adhesion and phagocytosis) and kill the organism (respiratory burst). Failure in any of these steps may lead to some of the clinicopathologic features discussed above.

CLINICAL ABNORMALITIES ASSOCIATED WITH NEUTROPHIL DYSFUNCTION

Dogs with PMN disorders have frequent infections and their clinical manifestations are similar, whether the disorder results from insufficient numbers of circulating neutrophils or cell dysfunction. In most cases, infections tend to be prolonged, there is a transient response to antibiotic therapy, and recurrent infections are the rule. Most infections occur in the skin and respiratory and gastrointestinal tracts, and the organisms commonly involved include enterics and pyogenic bacteria.

If PMN adhesion and chemotactic responses are normal, affected dogs tend to develop the cardinal signs of inflammation in the affected site (i.e., swelling, redness, increased tissue temperature, pain, and abnormal function) with occasional pus formation. Marked blood leukocytosis with or without left shift is common in these patients; this neutrophilic leukocytosis may be of such magnitude (i.e., $> 100,000$ cells/μl) that it may mimic chronic myelogenous leukemia.

Bacteriologic cultures obtained from obvious sites of infection (e.g., abscesses, pneumonia, and cystitis) reliably yield pyogenic organisms such as *Staphylococcus* and *Streptococcus* or gram-negative enterics such as *Proteus*, *Pseudomonas*, and *Escherichia coli*. Blood cultures in dogs with signs of bacteremia or septicemia yield the offending organism in only approximately 20 to 30 per cent of cases.

A confirmatory diagnosis of PMN dysfunction requires *in vitro* evaluation of neutrophil function (see below). However, the signalment (i.e., young Irish setter or Weimaraner), history (e.g., recurrent febrile episodes initially responsive to antibiotics), physical examination results (e.g., multiple abscesses, suppurative lymphadenopathy, and pneumonia), underlying disease (e.g., diabetes mellitus); and laboratory findings (e.g., neutrophilia with left shift) may suggest the presence of a PMN abnormality.

LABORATORY EVALUATION OF PATIENTS WITH SUSPECTED NEUTROPHIL DYSFUNCTION

Several PMN functions can be evaluated *in vitro*. Table 2 lists PMN function tests available for dogs. The major limiting factor in performing neutrophil function tests is the need for fresh cells; the majority of these assays need to be conducted within 2 hr of collecting the samples. In addition, because the majority of these tests require sophisticated laboratory equipment, their performance is mostly limited to teaching institutions and research laboratories.

Other problems involved in interpretation of

Table 2. Laboratory Evaluation of Neutrophil Function

Adhesion	Nylon wool/glass adherence
Migration	Migration under agarose
	Boyden chamber assay
Phagocytosis	Phagocytosis of bacteria, yeast, latex, or zymosan
	Phagocytosis of opsonized particles
Oxygen metabolism	O_2 consumption
	Chemiluminescence*
	Nitroblue tetrazolium reduction test (NBT)
Microbicidal capacity	Bacterial killing assay
	Candidacidal assay

*Indirectly evaluates phagocytosis if particulate material (e.g., latex beads) is used.

PMN function assays include the following: infection may enhance neutrophil function, resulting in increased nitroblue tetrazolium (NBT) reduction or chemiluminic responses; in vitro tests may not correlate with the in vivo situation; bactericidal assays measure overall function; and functional defects may only be detected with selected bacterial species.

CLINICAL MANAGEMENT OF DOGS WITH NEUTROPHIL ABNORMALITIES

Owing to the low numbers or abnormal function of neutrophils in circulation in these patients, the pyrexia should be attributed to bacterial pyrogens until proven otherwise (if one accepts that endogenous pyrogens are produced primarily by PMNs).

Appropriate antibiotic therapy constitutes the mainstay of treatment in patients with PMN abnormalities. A trimethoprim-sulfa combination has shown beneficial effects in human patients with neutropenia and neutrophil abnormalities (e.g., chronic granulomatous disease), including eliminating or reducing the numbers of gram-negative bacteria (e.g., Enterobacteriaciae) colonizing the gastrointestinal tract; preserving the anaerobic gastrointestinal flora, thus conferring resistance to the colonization by exogenous nosocomial organisms; providing therapeutic tissue levels of both drugs; and enhancing opsonization (Pizzo, 1984).

A trimethoprim-sulfa combination (Tribrissen, Burroughs Wellcome; 15 mg/kg b.i.d. PO or SC) has proved beneficial in dogs with neutrophil abnormalities or neutropenia. On a clinical basis, it appears to reduce the frequency of sepsis, shorten the duration of septic episodes, and decrease the severity of the episodes (Couto, 1986).

Fever in a patient with neutrophil dysfunction constitutes a medical emergency. The following protocol is recommended for the management of dogs with PMN abnormalities that are febrile: The patient undergoes a thorough physical examination in search of a septic focus, an indwelling intravenous catheter is placed aseptically, and intravenous fluids are administered as required. Blood samples for complete blood count (CBC) and serum electrolyte, blood glucose, and blood urea nitrogen concentrations are obtained immediately. Two or three sets of aseptically collected blood samples are obtained for aerobic and anaerobic bacterial cultures and antimicrobial sensitivity tests at 30-min intervals. After collecting the second set of samples for blood cultures, therapy with a bactericidal antibiotic combination is instituted. A combination of gentamicin (2 mg/kg t.i.d. IV) and cephalothin (40 mg/kg t.i.d. IV), or gentamicin and ticarcillin (40 mg/kg q.i.d. IM) is recommended because most bacterial isolates in these patients are Enterobacteriaciae and staphylococci, organisms commonly susceptible to these agents (Couto, 1986).

CONGENITAL NEUTROPHIL ABNORMALITIES

At least four syndromes of congenital neutrophil abnormalities have been identified in dogs and will be briefly discussed.

Leukocyte Adhesion Protein Deficiency

A family of structurally related proteins that are variably expressed on the surface of leukocytes plays an essential role in neutrophil adhesion-related functions. They include adherence of neutrophils to endothelial cells and other substrates, neutrophil aggregation and spreading, and random migration and chemotaxis, as well as complement receptor activity binding (C3bi, an opsonic fragment of the third component of complement fixed to the surface of microorganisms during complement activation). Deficiency of leukocyte surface adhesion proteins occurs in Irish setters with recurrent bacterial infections and persistent leukocytosis (Giger et al., 1987) and explains the previously reported canine granulocytopathy syndrome (Renshaw et al., 1975).

Affected dogs have severe recurrent bacterial infections. Omphalophlebitis and gingivitis are often the first infections and might be followed by pyoderma, pododermatitis, thrombophlebitis, pneumonia, pyometra, osteomyelitis, and fatal sepsis. The associated inflammatory response and pus formation appear to be markedly impaired, and regional lymphadenopathy is commonly noted. These episodes respond poorly to appropriate antibiotic therapy, and skin wounds heal only slowly. Episodes of infection are usually associated with severe pyrexia, anorexia, and weight loss. Long-term therapy with bactericidal antibiotics is required to keep affected animals alive.

An extreme leukocytosis with white blood cell counts at times exceeding 200,000/μl is persistently present, even during apparently infection-free periods, and consists predominantly of mature neutrophilia with variable increases in other leukocyte numbers. This persistent neutrophilia with only a minimal regenerative left shift and occasional hypersegmented cells is much higher than expected for a dog with infection and could easily be confused with chronic granulocytic leukemia. Neutrophils of affected dogs are apparently incapable of egress to the infection site to kill bacteria. Myeloid hyperplasia of the bone marrow without malignant features is seen. Hyperglobulinemia (polyclonal) and moderate anemia of inflammatory disease may also be associated with severe infections.

Recent *in vitro* leukocyte function studies revealed markedly decreased neutrophil adhesion to various substrates, impaired neutrophil chemotaxis and aggregation, and minimal overall bactericidal activity, but normal neutrophil (burst) oxidative activity. The *in vitro* functions of other phagocytes and the lymphocyte blastogenesis response were also diminished. A severe deficiency of leukocyte adhesion proteins was directly shown with monoclonal antibodies (Giger et al., 1987). Functional and antibody tests of related dogs and breeding studies support an autosomal recessive mode of inheritance.

Complement Deficiency in Brittany Spaniels

A colony of Brittany spaniels with spinal muscular atrophy was found to have a genetically determined deficiency of the third component of the complement (C3) (Winkelstein et al., 1982). The components of the complement system possess opsonizing (i.e., enhanced phagocytosis of bacteria and other particles) and chemotactic activities; therefore, deficiency of any of these components may result in defective chemotaxis or phagocytosis.

Infections in the C3-deficient dogs included pneumonia, sepsis, pyometra, and infection of muscle biopsy sites. Most affected dogs had neutrophilic leukocytosis with left shift (Blum et al., 1985). Serum C3 levels detected by radial immunodiffusion and enzyme-linked immunosorbent assay (ELISA) were significantly low when compared with those of normal control dogs. *In vitro* serum opsonizing activity against pneumococci was nonexistent. In addition, serum from C3-deficient dogs was markedly deficient in chemotactic activity (Winkelstein et al., 1982).

Immunodeficiency in Weimaraners

Over 50 young Weimaraners with recurrent episodes of fever, pneumonia/pneumonitis, diarrhea,

generalized lymphadenopathy, pyoderma, polyarthritides, radiographic bone changes compatible with hypertrophic osteodystrophy, and subcutaneous abscesses were evaluated over 24 months (Couto et al., 1987). Histopathologic abnormalities in the affected dogs consisted of suppurative and pyogranulomatous lesions in various tissues. The majority of the dogs experienced significant transient clinical improvement after antibiotic therapy.

Laboratory evaluation of these dogs revealed hypogammaglobulinemia, decreased serum concentrations of immunoglobulin G (IgG) and IgM, and decreased neutrophil chemiluminescence. Further evaluation of neutrophil function is currently in progress. Healthy relatives of the affected dogs had similar laboratory findings, suggesting a familial component.

The clinicopathologic findings in these dogs were similar to the ones reported in 18 related Weimaraners (Studdert et al., 1984) and in a litter of Weimaraner pups (Woodard, 1982).

Neutrophil Defect in Doberman Pinschers

A recent report describes abnormally low NBT reduction tests in a family of Doberman pinschers, from which a young animal had chronic recurrent respiratory tract infections. Serum immunoglobulin and complement levels were normal or increased, and *in vitro* lymphocyte blastogenic responses were enhanced by the addition of autologous serum in affected dogs. Neutrophil chemotaxis and phagocytosis were normal in the dogs evaluated. Superoxide production in response to opsonized zymosan was significantly decreased (Breitschwerdt et al., 1987). The decreased NBT reduction and inability to generate superoxide in these dogs indicate that the neutrophils had a defect in their ability to metabolize oxygen.

Other Congenital Abnormalities

An abnormality in PMN migration has been described in pointers with primary ciliary dyskinesia, a disease characterized by abnormal cilia in the respiratory tract and by ineffectual mucociliary clearance (Morrison et al., 1987). Affected dogs developed recurrent chronic respiratory tract infections, and two dogs died as a consequence of viral infections (parvovirus in one dog, distemper in the other).

Neutrophilic chemotactic responses were reported to be diminished in foxhounds with Pelger-Huët anomaly, a disorder of leukocyte development characterized by failure of nuclear segmentation in eosinophils and neutrophils (Bowles et al., 1979). However, a report of a Basenji with Pelger-Huët anomaly did not disclose any abnormalities in neutrophilic chemotaxis (Latimer and Prasse, 1982).

ACQUIRED NEUTROPHIL ABNORMALITIES

Although several acquired PMN abnormalities have been described in humans, a limited number of them that are of clinical significance have been documented in dogs (see Table 1). Only neutrophil abnormalities related to diabetes mellitus and infection will be addressed.

Diabetes Mellitus

The association between diabetes mellitus and increased susceptibility to infection has been well recognized in veterinary and human medicine. A high neutrophil count in a diabetic patient suggests the presence of an infectious process. Hyperglycemic diabetics frequently develop bacterial cystitis, pyoderma, prostatitis, and pneumonia. They appear to have more serious infectious processes and also to be more prone to have unusual infections, such as gas gangrene cystitis and candidiasis. In addition, infection is the most common precipitating cause of diabetic ketoacidosis and undoubtedly impairs blood glucose control with insulin. On the other hand, tight regulation of blood glucose level decreases the frequency of secondary bacterial infections in diabetic humans and presumably dogs (Rayfield et al., 1982; Latimer and Mahaffey, 1984).

The increased propensity to infection of diabetics is thought to be caused primarily by neutrophil dysfunction. Variable and different functional abnormalities of neutrophils from humans and dogs with diabetes mellitus have been reported. Slightly decreased neutrophil adherence and migration, as well as impaired phagocytosis and oxidative burst reaction, have been thought to contribute to reduced neutrophil bacterial killing activity. In addition, media factors, such as high plasma glucose concentration, the presence of ketones, and increased osmolality have been considered to alter neutrophil functions *in vitro*. For instance, the degree of neutrophil adherence was inversely correlated with the serum glucose level (Stickle et al., 1986) but was not directly influenced by insulin *in vitro*. Thus, strict control of blood glucose in diabetic patients is desirable to ensure maintenance of normal host defense.

Infection

It is well known that severe or prolonged bacterial infections may result in significant PMN bactericidal deficiency in humans. In one study, dogs with chronic bacterial pyoderma had significantly impaired neutrophil chemotactic responses (Latimer et al., 1983). However, it was not established whether the decreased PMN migration in the affected dogs was the cause or the consequence of the pyoderma.

References and Supplemental Reading

Blum, J. R., Cork, L. C., Morris, J. M., et al.: The clinical manifestations of a genetically determined deficiency of the third component of complement in the dog. Clin. Immunol. Immunopathol. 34:304, 1985.

Bowles, C. A., Alsaker, R. D., and Wolfe, T. L.: Studies of the Pelger-Huët anomaly in foxhounds. Am. J. Pathol. 96:237, 1979.

Breitschwerdt, E. B., Brown, T. T., DeBuysscher, E. V., et al.: Rhinitis, pneumonia, and defective neutrophil function in the Doberman pinscher. Am. J. Vet. Res. 48:1054, 1987.

Couto, C. G.: Toxicity of anticancer chemotherapy. Proceedings of 10th Annual Kal Kan Symposium, Columbus, OH, 1986, Kal Kan Foods, Inc., 1987, p. 37.

Couto, C. G., Lafrado, L., Johnson, G., et al.: Immunodeficiency in young Weimaraners. ACVIM Scientific Proceedings, 1987, p. 892.

Giger, U., Boxer, L. A., Simpson, P. J., et al.: Deficiency of leukocyte surface glycoproteins Mo1, LFA-1, and LeuM5 in a dog with recurrent bacterial infections: An animal model. Blood 69:1622, 1987.

Jain, N. C.: *Schalm's Veterinary Hematology*, 4th ed. Philadelphia: Lea & Febiger, 1986.

Latimer, K. S., and Prasse, K. W.: Neutrophilic movement of a Basenji with Pelger-Huët anomaly. Am. J. Vet. Res. 43:525, 1982.

Latimer, K. S., and Mahaffey, E. A.: Neutrophil adherence and movement in poorly and well-controlled diabetic dogs. Am. J. Vet. Res. 45:1498, 1984.

Latimer, K. S., Prasse, K. W., Mahaffey, E. A., et al.: Neutrophil movement in selected canine skin diseases. Am. J. Vet. Res. 44:601, 1983.

Morrison, W. B., Frank, D. E., Roth, J. A., et al.: Assessment of neutrophil function in dogs with primary ciliary dyskinesia. J.A.V.M.A. 191:425, 1987.

Pizzo, P. A.: Granulocytopenia and cancer therapy. Past problems, current solutions, future challenges. Cancer 54:2649, 1984.

Rayfield, E. J., Ault, M. J., Keusch, G. T., et al.: Infection and diabetes: The case for glucose control. Am. J. Med. 72:439, 1982.

Renshaw, H. W., Chatburn, C., Bryan, G. M., et al.: Canine granulocytopathy syndrome: Neutrophil dysfunction in a dog with recurrent infections. J.A.V.M.A. 166:443, 1975.

Stickle, J. E., Tvedten, H. W., Schall, W. D., et al.: Adherence of neutrophils from dogs with diabetes mellitus. Am. J. Vet. Res. 47:541, 1986.

Studdert, V. P., Phillips, W. A., Studdert, M. J., et al.: Recurrent and persistent infections in related Weimaraner dogs. Austr. Vet. J. 61:261, 1984.

Winkelstein, J. A., Johnson, J. P., Swift, A. J., et al.: Genetically determined deficiency of the third component of complement in the dog: In vitro studies of the complement system and complement-mediated serum activities. J. Immunol. 129:2598, 1982.

Woodard, J. C.: Canine hypertrophic osteodystrophy, a study of the spontaneous disease in littermates. Vet. Pathol. 19:337, 1982.

THE RISK OF TRANSMISSION OF FeLV FROM LATENTLY INFECTED CATS

ANGELA M. PACITTI, B.V.M.S.

Glasgow, Scotland

Feline leukemia virus (FeLV) is ubiquitous in the cat population and is the most important single nontraumatic cause of death of adult cats (Jarrett, 1985a). FeLV-related diseases occur in cats that have persistent productive infections. The majority of cats appear to recover from the infection, but it has recently been discovered that some of these cats do not recover virologically but have a latent infection that can be reactivated. This article assesses whether latently infected cats are a risk for other cats and how they might affect the epidemiology of the disease.

The major sources of FeLV are those cats that have persistent productive infections (i.e., they are viremic and excrete virus in many bodily secretions, particularly saliva, urine, and feces). Of these, saliva is the most important source of infection for susceptible cats and usually intimate direct cat-to-cat contact, such as licking, is necessary for horizontal transmission to occur. The other mode of transmission of infection is *in utero* from mother to fetus, resulting in all kittens born to persistently viremic queens being themselves persistently viremic.

Viremic cats can readily be identified, as they have free infectious virus present in blood and saliva, which can be detected in a number of ways. The most common methods of diagnosis of viremia include detection of viral antigen in blood by enzyme-linked immunosorbent assay (ELISA) or by fixed-cell immunofluorescence on air-dried blood smears. Many ELISA kits are now available for the use of veterinarians in their own offices. However, up to 10 per cent of cats with positive ELISA test results are not viremic (Jarrett, 1985b). For this reason it is advisable to test all ELISA-positive samples for virus by either virus isolation or immunofluorescence. Such persistently viremic cats do not mount an effective antiviral immune response and are susceptible to a number of diseases, which are invariably fatal. These include immunosuppression, lymphosarcomas, leukemias, and anemias and have been previously described in detail (Hardy, 1980). The average time from first diagnosis of viremia to death is 22.6 months (Francis and Essex, 1980); therefore the prognosis for viremic cats is grave.

Fortunately, the majority of cats that are exposed to FeLV do not become persistently viremic, but appear to recover, develop virus-neutralizing antibodies (VNAs), and are resistant to reinfection. Cats that recover from infection are no more at risk of developing FeLV-associated diseases than unexposed cats and have a normal life expectancy (McClelland et al., 1980).

LATENT FeLV INFECTIONS

A third possible outcome of exposure to FeLV was discovered when viremia was induced in cats that were believed to have recovered from infection, following treatment with high and prolonged doses of corticosteroids (Post and Warren, 1980). These results were confirmed by others (Rojko et al., 1982; Pedersen et al., 1984). Such cats were said to be latently infected, and the site of the latent virus was found to be the bone marrow. Latent FeLV infections have been reviewed by Pacitti (1987). It is now recognized that many apparently recovered cats have latent infections, some of which can last for years. Several questions about these infections are considered below: What is the prevalence and duration of these infections in FeLV-positive households? Are these cats susceptible to FeLV-related diseases? Do they transmit infection to other cats, either horizontally or *in utero*?

Diagnosis

The diagnosis of latent FeLV infection requires the aspiration of bone marrow, usually from the femoral shaft or the iliac crest from which cell cultures are made. Latent virus is reactivated from the cells and is released into the culture fluid. Infectious virus can then be detected in the fluid by virus isolation (Rojko et al., 1982; Madewell and Jarrett, 1983; Pedersen et al., 1984; Pacitti and Jarrett, 1985; Pacitti, 1987); alternatively, viral antigen can be detected in the cytoplasm of the cells by immunofluorescence (Rojko et al., 1982; Pacitti, 1987). Prior to culture, neither viral antigen nor infectious virus can be detected in latently infected bone marrow cells.

A latently infected cat is therefore one that does not have a productive persistent infection (i.e., it is not viremic) but has a nonproductive persistent infection in its bone marrow cells. All such cats have VNAs and are therefore ostensibly recovered from infection (Madewell and Jarrett, 1983; Pacitti et al., 1986; Pacitti, 1987).

With the discovery of latency as a possible sequel to exposure to FeLV, it became necessary to understand the significance of these infections, particularly in multicat households.

Prevalence and Duration

When a persistently viremic cat is introduced into a household of susceptible cats, the infection rapidly spreads throughout the household, resulting in a high incidence of viremia and associated disease. The percentage of cats that develop VNAs is also high. Jarrett and associates (1978) reported that 40 per cent of cats in this situation were viremic and another 42 per cent had VNAs.

The prevalence of the latent state in an experimental closed FeLV-infected multicat household has recently been studied (Madewell and Jarrett, 1983; Pacitti and Jarrett, 1985). It was found that following the introduction of viremic cats into such a household of susceptible cats, the proportion of cats with latent infections was initially high, being 56 per cent of those cats with VNAs 9 months after initial exposure. However, the number of cats with latent infections gradually decreased, so that after 3 yr only 8 per cent of cats with VNAs still harbored latent infections (Pacitti and Jarrett, 1985; Pacitti, 1987). Cats that eliminated their latent infection were believed to have recovered completely. Therefore, although the prevalence of latent infections is initially high, they are relatively short lived, with perhaps only 10 per cent of cats with VNAs having such infections for longer than 3 yr. This state is in contrast to persistent viremia, which is lifelong.

The factors that influence whether a cat becomes viremic or develops VNAs on exposure to FeLV are the age of the cat at first exposure to the virus and the frequency and dose of exposure (Hoover et al., 1976). It is not known what influences the development of latency versus recovery, but it seems likely that similar factors may be involved. Because both recovered and latently infected cats have similar levels of VNAs (Madewell and Jarrett, 1983), it is possible that the development of latency versus recovery is associated with the number of cells in the bone marrow that become infected on initial exposure to the virus. If this were the case, and because VNAs are responsible for killing both free virus and cells that are expressing virus, it would

mean that the more cells that became infected, the greater would be the chance of the cat's becoming latently infected rather than eliminating the virus completely. If an even greater number of cells become infected, then the cat would be likely to become viremic. From the results of Pacitti and Jarrett (1986), it is clear that VNAs have at least a partial role in the control and maintenance of latent FeLV infections, although cell-mediated immunity (Rojko et al., 1982) and complement (Kraut et al., 1985) may also be involved.

Clinical Significance

The incidence of disease in latently infected cats has been studied. Pacitti (1987) followed 26 cats with latent infections for up to 4 yr, and none developed any of the diseases commonly associated with FeLV. During this time only one cat died as a result of a pyometra, which was not considered to be associated with its latent infection. These results suggest that latently infected cats are not predisposed to develop FeLV-related diseases.

The possible involvement of latent infections in the development of lymphosarcomas in nonviremic cats remains controversial: Rojko and colleagues (1982) demonstrated latent virus in two such cats, whereas Madewell and Jarrett (1983) could not detect virus in two similar cases. As mentioned above, the prognosis for viremic cats is poor. McClelland and coworkers (1980) found that 83 per cent of viremic cats were dead within 3.5 yr of exposure, compared with only 17 per cent of recovered cats and 16 per cent of unexposed cats. In retrospect, a considerable proportion of the "recovered" cats in that extensive study must have had latent infections, thus confirming that latently infected cats are not at risk from FeLV-related diseases.

Epidemiologic Significance

It is well recognized that persistently viremic cats represent the major source of infection for susceptible cats, transmitting virus both horizontally and *in utero*. It was important to determine whether or not latently infected cats represented a potential source of infection either by spontaneously reactivating their infection to become viremic, thus resulting in horizontal transmission, or by infecting kittens *in utero*.

HORIZONTAL TRANSMISSION

Pacitti (1987) housed eight latently infected cats with eight FeLV-naive tracer cats that were susceptible to infection. The cats were housed together for a period of 12 months, during which time there was no evidence of horizontal transmission of infection. This is in contrast to the situation with viremic cats in which there is evidence of horizontal transmission of infection to susceptible cats within 1 month of exposure (Jarrett et al., 1973). From the results of Pacitti (1987) it can be concluded that, unlike viremic cats, latently infected cats do not frequently transmit sufficient quantities of virus to lead to horizontal infection of susceptible cats.

PRENATAL INFECTION

Several groups of workers have examined latently infected queens for evidence of prenatal transmission of infection to their kittens. However, whether or not this situation occurs remains equivocal. Pacitti and colleagues (1986) found no evidence of either latent or active infection at birth in kittens born to eight latently infected queens. In contrast, Rojko and associates (1982) reported latent infections at birth in kittens born to two such queens. However, in the latter study the queens had been given an intraperitoneal inoculation of virus during the first week of pregnancy, so that it is unclear if the infection in the kittens resulted from true transmission from their mothers or was produced by the virus given to their mothers during pregnancy. In another report, 1 of 30 kittens born to latently infected queens was alleged to have been viremic at birth (Pedersen et al., 1984), but this claim is difficult to substantiate because the first blood samples were not taken until the kittens were 2 weeks of age. Therefore, the question of prenatal infection from latently infected queens remains controversial.

MILK TRANSMISSION

Although Pacitti and associates (1986) found no evidence of prenatal transmission of infection from latently infected queens to their kittens, these investigators did find that the kittens of four consecutive litters of one such queen became viremic at 6 to 8 weeks of age and that their viremia was persistent. At no time was virus isolated from either the blood or saliva of this queen, but virus was isolated from milk. Therefore, the cat was latently infected but was producing infectious virus in its mammary glands and was thus infecting the kittens postnatally. It appeared that the kittens were protected from infection during the first few weeks of life by passively acquired colostral antibodies. These antibody titers had dropped to undetectable levels by the time the kittens became viremic.

This particular queen had low levels of VNAs and, although infectious virus could not be isolated from blood, viral antigen was intermittently detected by ELISA. This is interesting because approximately 10 per cent of cats that are ELISA positive are not in fact viremic (Jarrett, 1985b). Because the diagnosis of latency requires a bone marrow biopsy, it would be difficult to carry out the necessary field trials to ascertain what proportion of these ELISA-positive cats have latent infections. However, it is not unreasonable to assume that at least some of these cats will have latent infections because, as has already been discussed, a considerable proportion of FeLV-exposed experimental cats have latent infections at any one time. It is possible that these cats may produce infectious virus at extramedullary sites, such as the mammary glands, which would not be detected by routine diagnostic procedures carried out on blood samples. Therefore, cats that are latently infected, are antigen positive on ELISA, and have low levels of VNAs may represent a potential source of infection for susceptible cats.

In addition, the cat mentioned above that transmitted virus in its milk subsequently experienced spontaneous reactivation of the latent infection to become persistently viremic. In this case, reactivation occurred without administration of corticosteroids but followed exposure to four litters of viremic kittens. This prolonged exposure to infection, coupled with the stress of the various manipulations that the cat received during pregnancy, may have been responsible for the reactivation of the latent infection.

If such cats were to occur in the field they would seriously complicate the control and eradication of FeLV from closed multicat households, such as breeding colonies, by the test-and-removal programs that are commonly used (Hardy et al., 1976; Weijer and Daams, 1978). These cats may be responsible for the unexplained reappearance of infection in such households, which has occasionally been reported months or even years after the virus was believed to have been eradicated.

UNRESOLVED QUESTIONS

Because the latent state of FeLV infection was discovered by the treatment of ostensibly recovered cats with corticosteroids, many veterinarians are concerned about the possibility of routine corticosteroid therapy leading to the reactivation of latent infections. The regimens of corticosteroid therapy that have been used experimentally to induce viremia in latently infected cats are listed below.

1. 1 mg of dexamethasone plus 5 mg of prednisolone daily for 21 days, except days 10, 11, and 12, when no treatment was given (Post and Warren, 1981). This resulted in two of four apparently recovered cats becoming persistently viremic.

2. 10 mg/kg of methylprednisolone twice weekly for 4 weeks, resulting in reactivation of latent virus, causing viremia in two of five latently infected cats (Rojko et al., 1982).

3. 10 mg/kg of methylprednisolone once weekly for 4 weeks, resulting in reactivation of latent virus and persistent viremia in five of 49 latently infected cats (Pedersen et al., 1984).

Although it is clear from these results that excessive doses of corticosteroids can reactivate latent virus to produce viremia in a proportion of cats, there is no evidence to suggest that the lower doses of these drugs commonly used by veterinarians for the control of inflammatory or allergic conditions have similar effects. It would certainly seem unlikely that virus can readily be reactivated in this way, because these drugs are abundantly used in practice and there have been no reports of cats suddenly becoming viremic following routine corticosteroid therapy. Similarly, there are no reports of sudden viremia in cats following therapy with megestrol acetate, either for the purposes of contraception or for the treatment of conditions such as flea-bite hypersensitivity or eosinophilic granulomas. This drug is believed to affect these latter conditions by having a corticosteroid like effect (Chastain et al., 1981).

Obviously it would be necessary to carry out the appropriate trials to prove unequivocally the effect of both corticosteroids and megestrol acetate on latent infections.

SUMMARY

The prevalence of latent FeLV infections may be initially high following exposure to the virus, but these infections are usually short lived, with only a small proportion lasting longer than 3 yr. Cats that eliminate their latent infection appear to recover completely. The majority of latently infected cats are not at risk of developing FeLV-related diseases, nor are they usually a threat to other cats. However, certain cats that have latent infections, FeLV antigen in their blood, and low levels of VNAs may produce infectious virus at extramedullary sites. These cats are rare but are a potential source of virus not only for their own kittens, but also for other susceptible cats in the household. For these reasons, it would be advisable for veterinarians to consider FeLV latency when attempting to eradicate the infection from multicat households.

References and Supplemental Reading

Chastain, C. B., Graham, C. L., and Nichols, C. E.: Adrenocortical suppression in cats given megestrol acetate. Am. J. Vet. Res. 42:2029, 1981.

Francis, D. P., and Essex, M.: Epidemiology of feline leukemia. In Hardy, W. D., Jr., Essex, M., and McClelland, A. J. (eds): Feline Leukemia Virus. New York: Elsevier/North Holland, 1980, pp. 127–131.

Hardy, W. D., Jr.: Feline leukemia virus diseases. In Hardy, W. D., Jr., Essex, M., and McClelland, A. J. (eds): Feline Leukemia Virus. New York: Elsevier/North Holland. 1981, pp. 3–31.

Hardy, W. D., Jr., McClelland, A. J., Zuckerman, E. E., et al.: Prevention of contagious spread of FeLV and the development of leukaemia in pet cats. Nature 263:362, 1976.

Hoover, E. A., Olsen, R. G., Hardy, W. D., Jr., et al.: Feline leukemia virus infection: Age-related variation in response of cats to experimental infection. J. Natl. Cancer Inst. 57:365, 1976.

Jarrett, O.: Feline leukaemia virus. In Chandler, E. A., Gaskell, C. J., and Hilbery, A. D. R. (eds.): Feline Medicine and Therapeutics. Oxford: Blackwell Scientific, 1985a, pp. 271–283.

Jarrett, O.: Feline leukaemia virus. In Pract. 7:125, 1985b.

Jarrett, O., Hardy, W. D., Jr., Golder, M. C., and Hay, D.: The frequency of occurrence of feline leukaemia virus subgroups in cats. Int. J. Cancer 21:334, 1978.

Jarrett, W., Jarrett, O., Mackey, L., et al.: Horizontal transmission of leukemia virus and leukemia in the cat. J. Natl. Cancer Inst. 51:833, 1973.

Kraut, E. H., Rojko, J. L., Olsen, R. G., and Tuomari, D. L.: Effects of cobra venom factor on latent feline leukemia virus infection. J. Virol. 54:873, 1985.

Madewell, B. R., and Jarrett, O.: Recovery of feline leukaemia virus from non-viraemic cats. Vet. Rec. 112:339, 1983.

McClelland, A. J., Hardy, W. D., Jr., and Zuckerman, E. E.: Prognosis of healthy FeLV infected cats. In Hardy, W. D., Jr., Essex, M., and McClelland, A. J. (eds.): Feline Leukemia Virus. New York: Elsevier/North Holland, 1980, pp. 122–126.

Pacitti, A. M.: Latent feline leukaemia virus infection: A review. J. Small Anim. Pract. 28:1153, 1987.

Pacitti, A. M., and Jarrett, O.: Duration of the latent state in feline leukaemia virus infections. Vet. Rec. 117:472, 1985.

Pacitti, A. M., and Jarrett, O.: Neutralising antibody controls latent FeLV infections. J. Cell. Biochem. (Suppl.) 10A:209, 1986.

Pacitti, A. M., Jarrett, O., and Hay, D.: Transmission of feline leukaemia virus in the milk of a non-viraemic cat. Vet. Rec. 118:381, 1986.

Pedersen, N. C., Meric, S. M., Ho, E. W., et al.: The clinical significance of latent feline leukemia virus infection in cats. Feline Pract. 14:32, 1984.

Post, J. E., and Warren, L.: Reactivation of latent feline leukemia virus. In Hardy, W. D., Jr., Essex, M., and McClelland, A. J. (eds.): Feline Leukemia Virus. New York: Elsevier/North Holland, 1980, pp. 151–155.

Rojko, J. L., Hoover, E. A., Quackenbush, S. L., and Olsen, R. G.: Reactivation of latent feline leukaemia virus infection. Nature 298:385, 1982.

Weijer, K., and Daams, H.: The control of lymphosarcoma/leukaemia and feline leukaemia virus. J. Small Anim. Pract. 19:631, 1978.

FELINE IMMUNODEFICIENCY VIRUS INFECTION

E. ELIZABETH SPARGER, D.V.M.,
and JANET K. YAMAMOTO, PH.D.

Davis, California

Feline immunodeficiency virus (FIV) infection in cats is a recently recognized phenomenon, and the characterization of the clinical disease associated with FIV infection in domestic cats is still incomplete. FIV was originally isolated from feline leukemia virus (FeLV)–negative cats housed in a northern California cattery. Some of these cats have an immunodeficiency syndrome similar to that reported in cats with FeLV infection and in humans with acquired immunodeficiency syndrome (AIDS). Evaluation of the clinical disease in this FIV-infected cattery and in cats experimentally inoculated with FIV and early results of a serosurvey have provided some information that should be useful in diagnosing FIV infection. Additional studies will be necessary for a thorough understanding of pathogenesis, therapy, and prevention of FIV infections.

ETIOLOGIC AGENT

FIV is a retrovirus belonging to the lentivirus subfamily. Retroviruses are single-stranded RNA viruses known to package an enzyme, reverse transcriptase, which mediates the synthesis of a DNA copy of the viral RNA and the integration of the viral DNA into the host chromosomal DNA. As a member of the lentivirus subfamily, FIV is distinguished from other known feline retroviruses, including both FeLV and the feline sarcoma virus (FSV), which are members of the oncornavirus subfamily, and the feline syncytia-forming virus (FeSFV), a member of the Spumavirinae subfamily. The lentivirus subfamily includes other lentiviruses such as maedi-visna virus (MVV) in sheep, caprine arthritis-encephalitis virus (CAEV), equine infectious anemia virus (EIAV), the bovine immunodeficiency virus (BIV), the simian immunodeficiency virus (SIV), and the human immunodeficiency virus (HIV), the causitive agent of AIDS in humans. Lentivirus infections are, in general, characterized by prolonged latency periods devoid of clinical disease, followed by induction of clinical syndromes, including encephalopathies, pulmonary disease, rheumatoidlike arthritis, anemias, benign lympho-proliferative disorders, and immunodeficiency states.

The tissue culture techniques that allowed the original isolation of HIV from infected human lymphocytes were utilized to isolate FIV from lymphocytes drawn from FIV-infected cats. Cocultivation of FIV-infected lymphocytes with T lymphocytes from healthy feline donors yielded the production of viral particles with morphologic characteristics (by electron microscopy) consistent with those of other lentiviruses and with Mg^{2+}-dependent reverse transcriptase activity also typical of lentiviruses. These observations helped to distinguish FIV from FeLV, for which morphology is consistent with type-C oncornaviruses and reverse transcriptase activity is Mn^{2+}-dependent. The morphology of FeSFV viral particles is distinctive from both FIV and FeLV particles. Using western blots of FIV proteins and antisera against various animal retroviruses, FIV proteins did not bind antiserum against HIV, EIAV, MVV, SIV, or FeSFV or with monoclonal antibodies to FeLV. These findings further substantiate FIV as a unique feline lentivirus distinct from other feline retroviruses and other animal lentiviruses.

The cytopathic effects (CPE) of FIV are similar to the CPE seen in HIV-infected human T-lymphocyte cultures. These CPE consist of ballooning degeneration, the formation of multinucleated giant cells, and increased cell death in FIV-infected lymphoid cultures characterized as predominantly T cells. Primary lymphoid cells from feline fetal thymus cultures and the FeLV-producing T-lymphoid cell line FL74 were infectable with FIV, whereas early attempts to infect various feline fibroblast cell lines were unsuccessful. Owing to the apparent T-cell tropism exhibited by this new feline retrovirus, the virus was named the feline T-lymphotropic virus. Attempts to infect primary lymphoid cells or cell lines from other species, including dog, mouse, rabbit, sheep, and humans, with FTLV were unsuccessful. Once seroepidemiologic and clinical data clearly established that FTLV was a major cause of chronic immunodeficiency states in cats, the name FTLV was changed to feline immunodeficiency virus (FIV). The successful adaptation of FIV to cultivation in a feline monolayer cell line, Crandall feline kidney (crfk) cells, has greatly facilitated study of this virus. This suggests that the trophism of FIV may not be restricted only to T cells.

DIAGNOSIS

Currently, FIV infection is diagnosed by the presence of antibody in the suspect cat. Serum is tested against FIV-infected primary lymphocytes or FIV-infected crfk cells in an indirect immunofluorescence assay. Antibody can also be measured using an ELISA test, whereby ELISA plates are coated with a preparation of purified FIV. The indirect fluorescent antibody (IFA) test and ELISA are considered screening assays. Western blot analysis allows detection of antibodies against specific viral proteins and is used as a secondary assay to clarify questionable results of either IFA or ELISA. A seropositive state has consistently been indicative of active infection in all the animal and human lentivirus infections evaluated so far. Thus, assays detecting serum antibodies have been utilized for diagnosis. A consistent characteristic of most lentiviral infections is severely limited viral expression, even in the target tissues. Extremely sensitive assays for viral antigen, therefore, are necessary for detection of virus, but such assays are rarely used for routine clinical diagnosis.

There are two situations in which a negative antibody state might be seen with active FIV infection. Increased HIV expression and high levels of circulating antigen, along with depression or absence of antibodies to viral core proteins, have been observed in end-stage AIDS. A similar phenomenon may also exist in cats in the terminal stages of FIV infection, when serum antibody is no longer detectable. In this instance, an antigen detection assay or virus isolation may be necessary for diagnosis. Second, in acute FIV infection, virus isolation may precede seroconversion by at least 1 week. Similarly, in human patients exposed to HIV, viremia may precede seroconversion by weeks. This period of viremia without seroconversion during acute HIV infection is marked by an increased expression of antigen. An ELISA for detection of serum HIV antigen has been developed for diagnosis of HIV infection in these patients. Therefore, in the clinical setting, a cat recently infected with FIV may be virus positive yet seronegative. Despite these two possible situations in which a negative antibody test result might occur in a virus-positive cat, detection of FIV antibody is, in general, a suitable approach to diagnosis. An ELISA for circulating serum FIV proteins may be available in the future for diagnosis. Another approach to diagnosis is virus isolation from the cocultivation of healthy feline lymphocytes with peripheral blood lymphocytes from the suspect cat. Tissue culture supernatant is monitored for Mg^{2+}-dependent reverse transcriptase, and the cells are tested for viral antigens by IFA. This procedure is tedious, and its use as a routine diagnostic assay is limited.

A clinical diagnosis of FIV infection involves evaluation of the case history and the presenting clinical signs. Cats with persistent viral, bacterial, or parasitic infections, which are normally self-limiting, and unexplained lymphadenopathy or hematologic abnormalities are suspected of having FIV infection. These clinical findings may also be observed in cats with immunodeficiency disorders due to FeLV infection or to other primary disorders, including malnutrition, neoplasia, and immunosuppressive drug therapy. It should be remembered that FIV infection and FeLV infection may coexist in the same cat.

PATHOGENESIS AND CLINICAL SIGNS

Information in this article concerning the clinical signs and pathogenesis associated with FIV infection is derived from preliminary studies of the northern California cattery from which FIV was originally isolated, preliminary experimental inoculation experiments, and a serosurvey of FIV infection conducted by researchers at the University of California, Davis (UCD). These studies and those being conducted at other research centers are still in progress. Thus, this presentation of the clinical picture and pathogenesis of FIV infection is incomplete. These early findings, however, do provide some guidelines for selecting likely candidates for FIV infection.

IFA and western blot analysis for detection of antibody were utilized for identifying seropositive cats in the northern California cattery. This cattery included 53 pet and feral cats, 10 of which were seropositive for FIV and all of which were FeLV negative. The 10 FIV-seropositive cats were almost entirely localized within one of four outdoor pens, which housed a total of 16 cats. The clinical findings in the seropositive group included severe suppurative and, in some cases, necrotizing gingivitis and stomatitis, chronic exudative rhinitis and conjunctivitis, suppurative otitis externa usually due to chronic *Otodectes cynotis* infection, chronic diarrhea, cachexia and emaciation, miliary eczema, pustular dermatitis, and recurrent bacterial cystitis. Similar clinical signs were observed in ten cats that died during 4 years prior to this study and that were also localized to this same pen. The evaluation of this cattery was conducted for 1 year, and during this time two more FIV-positive cats died and two previously seronegative cats within this same pen of 16 cats underwent seroconversion. These findings suggest that chronic illness associated with FIV infection may last months to years before the cat succumbs. The clinical picture observed in this cattery includes a wide range of clinical signs usually associated with chronic and persistent infectious and inflammatory disorders. The severity of the suppurative and necrotizing gingivitis, stomatitis, and otitis externa is uncommon in an immunocompetent cat and has been observed in immunodeficient cats infected with FeLV. The persistent manifestations of an upper respiratory tract infection are also consistent with an immunodeficient host, and chronic diarrhea and wasting are key findings in human AIDS. Collectively the clinical signs observed in this cattery suggested an underlying immunodeficiency disorder caused by an infectious agent.

Clinical data sent with serum samples submitted for FIV antibody assay by veterinarians from various areas of the United States indicate a broad spectrum of clinical signs similar to those in the northern California cattery (Table 1). Chronic gingivitis and stomatitis were the most frequent complaints, affecting about 30 per cent of FIV-positive cats. The second most common group of complaints were chronic diarrhea, weight loss, and chronic upper respiratory tract infections, each affecting about 23 per cent. The third most common manifestation was unexplained fever in approximately 17 per cent of the FIV-positive cats. Other reported complaints were chronic abscesses, miliary dermatitis, and chronic infections in general. Anemia has been seen in some of the cats, as have neurologic signs. Neurologic signs have been observed in less than 5 per cent of cases and included dementia, aggressive behavior, psychomotor abnormalities, and convulsions. An FeLV-negative cat with a solitary lymphoma has also been found to be seropositive for FIV. It should be noted that the clinical syndromes reported in the FIV-positive cats from the northern California cattery and in the national serosurvey probably reflect chronic FIV infection.

Table 1. *Clinical Abnormalities Observed in Cats Naturally Infected with FIV*

Clinical Abnormality	Frequency
Chronic gingivitis and stomatitis	30%
Chronic diarrhea	23%
Chronic weight loss	23%
Chronic upper respiratory tract disease	23%
Fever	17%
Chronic abscesses	12%
Miliary dermatitis	5%
Recurrent cystitis	5%
Neurologic abnormalities	<5%
Lymphoma	<1%

Data from Yamamoto, J. K., et al.: Epidemiologic and clinical aspects of feline immunodeficiency virus (FIV) infection in cats from the continental United States and Canada and possible mode of transmission. J.A.V.M.A. (accepted for publication).

Ongoing studies involving experimental inoculation of kittens with FIV have provided some insight into the acute and early stages of FIV infection (Table 2). After intraperitoneal injection with tissue culture fluid containing FIV or whole blood or plasma from FIV-infected cats, virus was isolated from peripheral blood lymphocytes from the inoculated cats as early as 3 weeks after inoculation. The kittens were seropositive for FIV approximately 2 to 4 weeks after inoculation. All inoculated kittens had a generalized peripheral lymphadenopathy of varying severity within 4 to 5 weeks after inoculation. Approximately 50 to 75 per cent of the kittens experienced neutropenia with or without fever from 5 to 9 weeks following infection. Superficial bacterial infections such as cellulitis at the site of an ear tag or pustular dermatitis on the face were occasionally observed in the inoculated kittens. The generalized peripheral lymphadenopathy lasted from 3 to 6 months, whereas neutropenia persisted for 2 to 9 weeks and fever for 3 to 14 days. The clinical findings of transient lymphadenopathy, fever, and neutropenia may be observed in the acute stages of many viral infections, including FeLV infection and HIV infection in humans. With one exception, additional clinical signs have not been observed in any of the experimentally inoculated cats for up to 16 months after inoculation. The exception involved one experimentally inoculated kitten that developed a myeloproliferative disorder and was subsequently euthanatized. This prolonged asymptomatic period of FIV infection is a consistent finding in lentivirus infections in other species including HIV infection in humans, in which the virus can remain in a latent state with no signs of clinical disease for 5 years or longer after seroconversion. The length of the latent asymptomatic period that precedes the onset of clinical disease in cats naturally infected with FIV will have to be established with additional field studies of infected cats.

Ongoing studies using experimentally inoculated cats are aimed at determining the factors that may trigger clinical disease in asymptomatic FIV-infected cats. Concurrent viral, bacterial, or parasitic infections in humans, which activate the immune system and therefore activate HIV expression, have

Table 2. *Clinical Abnormalities Observed in Cats Experimentally Infected with FIV: Acute Infection*

Clinical Abnormality	Frequency
Peripheral generalized lymphadenopathy	100%
Neutropenia	78%
Cellulitis at ear tag	66%
Fever	33%
Superficial facial pyoderma	20%

From Yamamoto, J. K., et al.: Pathogenesis of experimentally induced feline immunodeficiency virus infection in cats. Am. J. Vet. Res. 49:1246, 1988.

been considered one of the cofactors for induction of full-blown AIDS. A similar mechanism may play a role in disease induction in FIV infection. How FIV as a virus actually induces an immunodeficient state in cats is not understood at this time but is also being evaluated. Early data indicate that clinically ill, naturally infected field cats have depressed lymphocyte blastogenic responses to mitogens, but the role of FIV in the dysfunction of lymphocytes is unclear. Whether FIV infection depletes a specific T-cell population (helper T cells) necessary for a functional cellular and humoral response to various pathogens, as occurs in HIV-infected people with full-blown AIDS, is not known at this time. The identification of the mechanisms by which FIV directly or indirectly allows the development of an immunodeficient state in cats will require considerable study.

PATHOLOGY

Tissue specimens from FIV-positive field and experimental cats for histopathologic examination have been limited in number. Significant microscopic lesions have been identified in the gastrointestinal tract, lymphoid tissues, and the central nervous system. Examination of the gastrointestinal tracts from three naturally infected cats from the northern California cattery revealed a diffuse enterocolitis with enterocyte necrosis in the glands and fusion and atrophy of the villi. Two of the three cattery cats had a history of chronic diarrhea and emaciation. Similar lesions have been reported in cats infected with the feline parvovirus and FeLV. In another naturally infected cat hospitalized and euthanatized at UCD, multiple foci of subacute ulceration in the colon and pyogranulomatous transmural colitis were observed. Similar lesions were observed in an experimentally inoculated cat with a severe necrotizing typhlitis and inflammation of the cecocolic lymph nodes. This cat had been exhibiting signs of abdominal pain and was neutropenic and febrile. No etiologic agent was identified in any of the enteric biopsies evaluated, although opportunistic viral or bacterial pathogens were considered likely. It should be noted that histologic alterations of the gut were seen in all the FIV-infected cats evaluated so far.

In three of the four FIV-positive field cats mentioned above, brain tissue was examined. Choroid plexus fibrosis was observed in all three cases, and a mild lymphoplasmacytic choroiditis with a mild focal suppurative meningitis was evident in one of the three cats. The cause of these lesions has not been determined. Encephalopathies have been frequently observed in other lentivirus infections including HIV infection in humans and CAEV infection in goats.

The characterization of lymphoid tissue alterations in FIV infection has been restricted because lymph nodes from FIV-infected field cats frequently were not available. Exuberant follicular hyperplasia was consistently seen in peripheral lymph node biopsies taken from experimentally inoculated cats manifesting generalized lymphadenopathy in the acute stage of FIV infection. Lymphoid depletion was observed in the spleens taken from two FIV-infected field cats with chronic illnesses.

SEROEPIDEMIOLOGY AND TRANSMISSION

The current knowledge of the epidemiology of FIV infection in cats in the United States has been derived from a UCD study of more than 1000 cats. Serum samples drawn from cats with chronic illnesses suggestive of immunodeficiency disorders indicate that approximately 15 to 20 per cent of these cats have FIV infection. It should be remembered that this study is examining a high-risk or ill population of cats and that this figure (15 to 20 per cent) does not reflect the incidence in the general population of healthy and ill cats. FIV-infected cats have been identified from almost all regions of the United States, including Hawaii, the West Coast, the Southwest, the Southeast, the Midwest, and the East Coast. The ratio of FIV-infected males to infected females is 3:1, and the age of infected cats ranges between 5 and 10 years. No breed predisposition for FIV infection has been identified at this time. The incidence is highest in outdoor and stray cats in the United States and is lowest in inner cities. The incidence in breeding catteries has not been determined. Preliminary data so far suggest that transmission in multiple-cat households is limited. An epidemiologic study conducted in Japan and including more than 1500 chronically ill cats revealed that 30 per cent of the cats were seropositive for FIV and found the highest incidence in feral cats. The data from these epidemiologic studies indicate that incidence of FIV infection is highest in older, outdoor, male cats and suggests that a primary mode of transmission might be fighting and inoculation by bite wounds. This conclusion is further supported by experimental inoculation studies.

Specific pathogen-free cats may be housed with experimentally inoculated cats for months or even a year without becoming infected with FIV. Virus has been recovered from saliva of infected cats with difficulty and appears to be shed in limited quantities. Fighting among the cats housed together in these studies is almost nonexistent. As stated above, over a period of a year, two cats converted from seronegative to seropositive in the pen housing FIV-positive cats in the northern California cattery. Infighting among the cats in this cattery and the presence of other pathogens may facilitate transmission of FIV infection. Virus-negative female cats bred by experimentally infected male cats have remained virus negative and seronegative and have given birth to virus-negative kittens. Offspring from a naturally infected female feral cat and from two experimentally inoculated female cats have been found free of FIV infection. Colostrum or milk from these three infected queens was not examined for the presence of virus, but no infections resulted from nursing.

TREATMENT AND PREVENTION

Therapy that will completely eliminate retroviral infection in any species has not yet been identified. A number of drugs that inhibit reverse transcriptase are under study for use in human AIDS patients. A dideoxynucleoside analogue, 3'-azido-3'-deoxythymidine (AZT), is a viral reverse transcriptase inhibitor that has been approved for use in AIDS patients. Immunoenhancers that may reconstitute a depressed immune system and stimulate a host antiviral response have received some evaluation as therapeutic agents. Lymphokines such as gamma-interferon and interleukin-2 when used as single therapeutic agents have been unsuccessful. Lymphokine combinations including various interferons and interleukins may be more effective. The search for a drug that will inhibit virus replication or virus infection of target cells and will not produce devastating side effects has been frustrating. Drugs that may alter virus replication may not necessarily alter the outcome of disease. Because lentiviruses, including HIV and FIV, remain latent during early stages of infection, the virus may be inaccessible to systemic drug therapy. However, the current massive effort to identify drugs that will inhibit virus replication and extend survival time in AIDS patients will involve FIV infection in cats as an animal research model and provide antiviral therapy for cats with FIV infections and FeLV infections as well. Until such therapy is available, symptomatic therapy for the chronic illnesses in FIV-infected cats is the only treatment to be recommended. Many of these cats will initially respond to antibiotic and fluid therapy, depending on the secondary illnesses present. Eventually symptomatic therapy will be of no value, and the cat will succumb to refractory secondary infections or other terminal events that have not been well characterized.

Although transmission of FIV infection is not well understood and early studies suggest that close or casual contact alone is not a major mode of transmission, isolation of FIV-infected cats from uninfected cats is recommended. This recommendation may be revised as more is known about FIV infection and pathogenesis. Because male intact cats that are out of doors and frequently fight are at higher risk for FIV infection, neutering may be considered another mode of prevention.

Prevention in the form of a vaccine for FIV may be possible but probably will not be available for some time. Results of vaccine studies in lentivirus infections in other species, including HIV infection in humans and CAEV infection in goats, have been discouraging. The ability of these viruses to maintain a latent infection in target cells and essentially "hide" from the host's immune response has proved to be one of several obstacles to successful immunization. The immunologic characteristics of lentivirus infections are being actively studied by a number of investigators, and a more thorough understanding of the host's immune response to these viruses may aid in developing an effective vaccine.

References and Supplemental Reading

Allain, J. P., Laurian, Y., Paul, D. A., et al.: Long-term evaluation of FIV antigen and antibodies to p24 and gp 41 in patients with hemophilia. N. Engl. J. Med. 317:1114, 1987.

Haase, A. T.: Pathogenesis of lentivirus infections. Nature 322:130, 1986.

Ishida, T., Washizu, T., and Toriyabe, K., et al.: Feline immunodeficiency virus (FIV) infection in Japan. J.A.V.M.A. (accepted for publication).

Lombardo, J. M.: HIV-1 testing: An overview. A.C.P.R. 11, 1987.

Pedersen, N. C., Ho, E. W., Brown, M. L., et al.: Isolation of a T-lymphotropic virus from domestic cats with an immunodeficiency-like syndrome. Science 235:790, 1986.

Reinacher, M.: Feline leukemia virus–associated enteritis—a condition with features of feline panleucopenia. Vet. Pathol. 24:1, 1987.

Tong-Starksen, S. E., Luciw, P. A., and Peterlin, B. M.: Human immunodeficiency virus long terminal repeat responds to T-cell activation signals. Proc. Natl. Acad. Sci. USA 84:6845, 1987.

Yamamoto, J. K., Hansen, S., and Ho, E. W.: Epidemiologic and clinical aspects of feline immunodeficiency virus (FIV) infection in cats from the continental United States and Canada and possible mode of transmission. J.A.V.M.A. (accepted for publication).

Yamamoto, J. K., Sparger, E. E., Ho, E. W., et al.: Pathogenesis of experimentally induced feline immunodeficiency virus infection in cats. Am. J. Vet. Res. 49:1246, 1988.

Yarchoan, R., and Broder, S.: Development of antiretroviral therapy for the acquired immunodeficiency syndrome and related disorders. N. Engl. J. Med. 316:557, 1987.

FELINE LYMPHOID
HYPERPLASIA

SUSAN M. COTTER, D.V.M.
North Grafton, Massachusetts

Mild generalized lymphadenopathy is a common finding on physical examination of cats presented to a veterinarian for illnesses or routine visits. Because the enlargement is usually mild, it often regresses spontaneously and biopsy is not usually performed.

CAUSES OF LYMPHADENOPATHY

Lymphadenitis may occur in nodes draining a local infection, such as stomatitis, or as a consequence of generalized infection, such as pyoderma. Certain infections have a predilection to invade nodes. Some that have been described in cats are cryptococcosis, plague, listeriosis, nocardiosis, tuberculosis, and streptococcosis (group G). Mesenteric lymphadenitis has been described in cats with toxoplasmosis involving intestines or pancreas. Systemic infections may cause generalized lymphadenitis; an example is granulomatous lymphadenitis seen in feline infectious peritonitis.

Local lymphadenopathy may occur because of metastatic tumor in the area drained by the node. For example, an enlarged node behind the ear may occur with ceruminous gland carcinoma in the ear canal; an enlarged mandibular node may be found with an oral tumor; or enlarged axillary or inguinal nodes frequently occur with metastatic mammary carcinomas.

Cats infected with feline leukemia virus (FeLV) frequently have mild lymphadenopathy at some stage of their infection. Shortly after experimental infection, the virus localizes in germinal centers of lymph nodes and replicates in B lymphocytes. Transient enlargement of lymph nodes occurs in the absence of neoplastic transformation. The enlargement varies from clinically imperceptible to severe, but is typically mild. Splenomegaly and sometimes hepatomegaly may occur as well. Although cats with lymphoma may have generalized lymphadenopathy from infiltration by lymphoblasts, this form is less prevalent than in dogs.

Anemic cats, regardless of FeLV status, are prone to the development of extramedullary hematopoiesis (EMH), which is most prominent in the spleen but also occurs in lymph nodes and liver. Histologic examination of a node enlarged by EMH reveals granulocytic, erythroid, and even megakaryocytic precursors in all stages of maturation, as would be expected in a section of bone marrow. The existence of EMH associated with refractory anemia has, in the past, been interpreted as an attempt at a response to the anemia. The degree of effective hematopoiesis in extramedullary sites is too small to be beneficial. In fact, the infiltration in organs such as liver may be so extensive as to interfere with normal function.

On occasion, it may be difficult to distinguish between severe EMH and myeloproliferative malignancies. If blast cells predominate in a lymph node biopsy or aspirate, a diagnosis of malignancy may be made. Subclassification into lymphoblastic, granulocytic, or erythroid leukemia can then be made in most cases by further examination. Some cats with lymphadenopathy that are subsequently proved to have hematopoietic malignancy have lymph node biopsy specimens showing only nonspecific EMH.

Severe EMH, sometimes called myeloid metaplasia, may occur in the spleen and occasionally the lymph nodes of cats with myelofibrosis. Myelofibrosis is classified as a myeloproliferative disorder but probably represents end stage refractory anemia rather than malignancy.

The most common cause of lymphadenopathy in cats is reactive or lymphocytic hyperplasia. Because lymph nodes filter the blood for antigens, nodal enlargement may occur as a result of local or systemic stimulation. When antigenic stimulation occurs, the interaction of antigen, lymphocytes, and macrophages in the node stimulates an influx of lymphocytes from the blood. This results in an increase in the size of the perifollicular and pericortical areas, which begins within 24 hr and is most noticeable after 4 to 7 days. Within 48 hours after arrival of the antigen, hyperplasia of germinal centers occurs with an increase in blasts. This reaches a peak after 7 to 10 days.

Moore and associates (1986) reviewed the records of 132 cats that had undergone lymph node biopsies. The largest category of lesions was not associated with changes allowing a specific cause to be established; these were categorized as idiopathic. Histologically most nodes (71 per cent) with idiopathic hyperplasia were found to have either B-cell (follicular) hyperplasia or B- and T-cell (paracortical) hyperplasia. Common underlying conditions prompting biopsies were enteritis with enlarged mesenteric lymph nodes, bacterial lymphadenitis, metastatic neoplasia, and reactive hyperplasia associated with dermatitis. Allergic dermatitis, particularly the miliary type, was sometimes associated with enlarged nodes containing an infiltrate of eosinophils, as well as other reactive changes.

An additional category of hyperplasia was found in 14 biopsy specimens. These nodes grossly were firm and light tan with smooth surfaces. Nodal architecture was severely distorted, with loss of trabeculae and subcapsular, trabecular, and medullary sinuses. A cellular infiltrate consisting of histiocytes, lymphocytes, plasma cells, and immunoblasts was present throughout the nodes. Numerous prominent postcapillary venules were present. This syndrome was called distinctive peripheral lymph node hyperplasia. Cats with this condition were all domestic short-hairs of either sex, ranging in age from 5 months to 2 yr (with most under 1 yr of age). Lymphadenopathy was generalized in 12 cats, and nodes were two to three times normal size. Eight of the 14 cats were clinically normal at the time of examination, except for lymphadenopathy. The others had mild signs of fever, lethargy, or anorexia. There was no common vaccination history. Three cats had hematocrits of less than 25 per cent, three were neutropenic, and two had increased serum globulin levels. Examination of bone marrow aspirates from two of the anemic cats showed erythroid hyperplasia. Three nodes were cultured aerobically, and all were negative for bacteria. Four of nine cats tested positively for FeLV, and toxoplasma titers were negative in two cats tested.

The course of the illness was known in 11 of the 14 cats. Two were euthanatized, eight recovered within 1 month, and one developed mediastinal lymphoma 2 yr later. Some cats were not treated for their lymphadenopathy, and some received antibiotics or corticosteroids alone or in combination. Regression of lymphadenopathy did not correlate with therapy. One cat required therapy with steroids and later cyclophosphamide and vincristine intermittently over 5 yr to control massive lymphadenopathy with upper airway compromise.

In addition, a group of seven specific pathogen-free kittens inoculated with Rickard FeLV developed peripheral and visceral lymphadenopathy. Four kittens showed follicular and parafollicular hyperplasia with preservation of architecture; three had the distinctive hyperplasia. For this reason it is suspected that FeLV may play a role in the pathogenesis of the condition.

A similar syndrome was described by Mooney and associates (1987) in six young cats with generalized lymphadenopathy. Of five cats tested for FeLV, all had negative results, although two had

lived with FeLV-positive cats. Four of these cats were recovering from respiratory or urinary tract infections. Serum protein electrophoresis in five cats revealed a polyclonal gammopathy in three. The lymphadenopathy regressed without therapy in five cats that were followed over a period of 4 months.

A recently described retrovirus of cats, feline immunodeficiency virus (FIV), formerly called feline T-cell lymphotropic virus (FTLV), has been found to cause immunosuppression and lymphadenopathy associated with lymphocytic hyperplasia. The lymphadenopathy occurred in spontaneous and experimentally induced infections. Both FeLV and FIV may cause an aberrant response either to the virus itself or to concurrent infectious agents. For example, FeLV causes ineffective primary humoral antibody response to specific antigens but may cause polyclonal gammopathy.

Similar lesions have been found in humans with syndromes such as angioimmunoblastic lymphadenopathy, one of the conditions associated with retroviral immunodeficiency syndrome (AIDS). Hypergammaglobulinemia and lymphadenopathy occur simultaneously with suppressed humoral antibody response. This suppression in humans and cats may be caused primarily by loss of helper T-cell function.

APPROACH TO THE CAT WITH LYMPHADENOPATHY

Whether or not signs of illness are present, a complete history and physical examination are indicated. Environmental factors and exposure to other cats may give clues as to systemic infections that may be present. If lymphadenopathy is localized, careful search for inflammation or tumor in the area drained by that node is essential. With generalized lymphadenopathy one must consider diffuse dermatologic or systemic causes. Cats with slight generalized lymphadenopathy without signs of illness may not need to have a biopsy performed. They should have a complete blood count (CBC) and FeLV test and perhaps an FIV test as a minimum data base. The size of the nodes should be followed to see whether the nodal disease subsides or whether other signs of illness develop. If the cat is showing signs of systemic illness, a urinalysis, blood chemistry profile, and possibly tests for feline infectious peritonitis (FIP), toxoplasmosis, or other conditions may also be indicated.

Lymph node aspirates are not likely to provide a diagnosis, except in some cases of lymphadenitis in which organisms may be found (e.g., cryptococcosis) or with some metastatic neoplasms (e.g., mast cell tumors, carcinomas, and rarely melanomas). An excision biopsy is more accurate than a needle aspirate to distinguish between hyperplasia and lymphoma. This distinction may be difficult even with excision biopsies because the hyperplasia may be so severe as to destroy the nodal architecture. If a biopsy is done, part of the node may be sent for culture if the cat is febrile or if lymphadenitis is suspected.

TREATMENT

Treatment is directed toward the underlying disease if one can be found. The presence of FeLV or FIV may explain the lymphadenopathy, but if fever or other signs of illness are present, one must continue to search for a superimposed infection, because these viruses alone will not cause fever. In the asymptomatic cat mild lymphadenopathy should be monitored but not treated. If it progresses, biopsy is indicated. Only one cat in Moore and colleagues' survey (1987) had such severe hyperplasia as to require treatment because of signs of upper airway compromise. This case was an exception,

and multiple biopsies were done over a period of time to rule out lymphoma. Routine use of corticosteroids to control benign lymphadenopathy is contraindicated, as it may inhibit an immune response to an undetected agent.

References and Suggested Reading

Cotter, S. M., and Holzworth, J.: Disorders of the hematopoietic system. *In* Holzworth, J. (ed.): *Diseases of the Cat.* Philadelphia: W. B. Saunders, 1987, pp. 755–807.

Frizzeria, G., Moran, E. M., and Rappaport, H.: Angio-immunoblastic lymphadenopathy. Am. J. Med. 59:803, 1975.

Mooney, S. C., Patnaik, A. K., Hayes, A. A., and MacEwen, E. G.: Generalized lymphadenopathy resembling lymphoma in cats: Six cases (1972–1976). J.A.V.M.A. 190:897, 1987.

Moore, F. M., Emerson, W. E., Cotter, S. M., and DeLellis, R. A.: Distinctive peripheral lymph node hyperplasia of young cats. Vet. Pathol. 23:386, 1986.

Pedersen, N. C., Ho, E. W., Brown, M. L., and Yamamoto, J. K.: Isolation of a T-lymphotropic virus from domestic cats with an immunodeficiency-like syndrome. Science 235:790, 1987.

Pedersen, N. C., Theilen, G., Keane, M. A., et al.: Studies of naturally transmitted feline leukemia virus infection. Am. J. Vet. Res. 38:1523, 1977.

Yamamoto, J. K., Sparger, E., Ho, E. W., et al.: Pathogenesis of experimentally induced feline immunodeficiency virus infection in cats. Am. J. Vet. Res. 49:1246, 1988.

ACUTE HYPERSENSITIVITY REACTIONS

MELISA A. DEGEN, D.V.M.
Hermosa Beach, California

Hypersensitivity reactions are also called allergic reactions. A hypersensitivity is an exaggerated immune response that is detrimental to the host. The four major mechanisms involved in hypersensitivity reactions (types I through IV) were originally described by Gell and Coombs. Although one of these mechanisms usually predominates in an allergic reaction, most hypersensitivity reactions are a combination of two or more types.

The definition of an acute reaction is somewhat arbitrary. This discussion will be limited to reactions occurring within minutes to hours after exposure to the responsible antigen. Acute reactions may involve any of the four mechanisms but most commonly are due to type I reactions.

TYPE I REACTIONS

Type I hypersensitivity reactions are also called immediate hypersensitivity because they occur

within minutes of exposure to the allergen. They are mediated by reaginic or cytotropic antibody. Reaginic antibody is usually immunoglobulin E (IgE). Although IgE has not been found in cats, cats produce reaginic antibody and are believed to experience type I hypersensitivity reactions. The Fc fragment of reaginic antibody has the unique ability to bind to receptor sites on host basophils and mast cells. When the Fab fragment of this cytotropic antibody combines with specific antigen, the basophil or mast cell degranulates. Preformed mediators are released, and other vasoactive substances are formed *de novo*.

The mediators of type I hypersensitivity cause inflammation by affecting vascular tone and permeability, by altering the balance of the coagulation system, and by altering airway resistance and compliance. Leukotrienes C4, D4, and E4 (formerly called slow-reacting substances of anaphylaxis [SRS-A]) and histamine are believed to be the major mediators in dogs and cats. Characteristics of immediate hypersensitivity mediators are listed in Table 1.

Clinical syndromes resulting from acute type I reactions include anaphylaxis, urticaria, and angioedema. The extrinsic form of asthma in people is due to an immediate hypersensitivity reaction. Asthma in dogs is extremely rare; however, a syndrome in Basenjis and Basenji crosses has been reported, which clinically resembles human asthma. It is not yet known if feline "asthma" is a result of a type I hypersensitivity or some other mechanism.

Anaphylaxis

Anaphylaxis is a peracute systemic hypersensitivity reaction. The reaction is called anaphylactic shock if systemic hypotension is a component. Anaphylaxis is usually caused by IgE-mediated mast cell degranulation; however, certain substances such as polysaccharides, trypsinlike enzymes, bacterial and fungal cell walls, some tumor cell walls, immunoglobulin aggregates, and helminth cuticles can trigger anaphylaxis by activating the alternate complement pathway. Complement components C3a and C5a, which are generated in this pathway, are potent anaphylatoxins and are capable of degranulating mast cells and basophils.

The onset of anaphylaxis usually occurs within seconds to minutes after exposure to the initiating allergen, peaks in approximately 10 to 30 min, and subsides over a few hours. The manifestations of systemic mast cell degranulation vary among species, depending on the anatomic distribution of mast cells, the relative content of each of the mediators in the mast cells, and the reaction of the target tissues to the mast cell mediators. Urticaria, angioedema, laryngeal edema, bronchial obstruction, gastrointestinal inflammation, and shock may be components.

The organ most severely affected by anaphylaxis in dogs is the liver. Specifically, the hepatic veins are most reactive. Anaphylaxis in dogs consists of portal hypertension and splanchnic blood pooling. If the reaction is severe, decreased cardiac return and shock are the results. The clinical signs are pale, cool mucous membranes, tachycardia, vomiting, diarrhea, dyspnea, and collapse. Urticaria and angioedema also may be present.

In cats, the organs most severely affected by anaphylaxis are the respiratory tract and the intestines. The signs of anaphylaxis in cats are dyspnea, vomiting, diarrhea, and collapse. Cutaneous signs, including intense pruritus, are more common in cats than in dogs and may be the initial sign. In both cats and dogs, the presence of concomitant cutaneous signs helps support the presumption of a mast cell–mediated reaction.

Virtually any foreign substance can produce anaphylaxis. A list of allergens commonly incriminated in anaphylactic reactions in people is provided in Table 2. Blood products and other biologics, drugs, Hymenoptera (bees, yellowjackets, wasps, hornets, fire ants) venom, and foods are the main offenders.

Anaphylaxis is extremely rare. It has been estimated to occur at a rate of 0.4 cases per million population per year in people. Differential diagnoses that should be considered for anaphylactic shock include cardiogenic, endotoxic, hypovolemic, and neurogenic shock; systemic mastocytosis; anaphylactoid reactions; cardiac arrhythmias; acute airway obstruction; pulmonary thromboembolism; hypoglycemia; pheochromocytomas; vasovagal collapse; cerebrovascular disturbances; and acute toxic reactions.

Table 1. *Major Mediators of Type I Hypersensitivity Reactions*

Mediator	Formation	Actions
Histamine	P	Contraction of bronchiolar and vascular smooth muscle. Increased vascular permeability. Increased secretion of respiratory mucus. Increased prostaglandin release
Serotonin	P	Smooth muscle contraction. Increased vascular permeability
Leukotrienes C4, D4, E4 (SRS-A)	N	Bronchospasm of peripheral airways. Increased vascular permeability, hypotension
Platelet activating factor (PAF)	N	Platelet aggregation and release reactions. Neutrophil activation. Smooth muscle contraction
Eosinophilic chemotactic factor of anaphylaxis (ECF-A)	P	Recruits eosinophils
Heparin and chondroitan sulfate E	P	Anticoagulants
Prostaglandins, thromboxane	N	Various effects on smooth muscle tone and platelet aggregation
Neutrophil chemotactic factor of anaphylaxis (NCF-A)	P	Recruits neutrophils. Important in late phase reactions
Kinin-generating proteases	P	Generate kinins that cause smooth muscle contraction, increased vascular permeability, increased mucus secretion, and pain

P, preformed; N, synthesized *de novo.*

Table 2. *Substances Associated with Anaphylaxis in People*

Antibiotics—penicillin, cephalosporins, streptomycin, amphotericin B, nitrofurantoin, sulfa drugs
Foods—seafood, legumes, nuts, berries, egg white, milk, seeds
Vitamins—thiamine, folic acid
Enzymes—trypsin, chymotrypsin, chymopapain, L-asparaginase
Hymenoptera venom—bees, yellowjackets, wasps, hornets, fire ants, carpenter ants
Polypeptide hormones—oxytocin, antidiuretic hormone (ADH), adrenocorticotropic hormone (ACTH), insulin
Anticonvulsants—diazepam, barbiturates, phenytoin
Polysaccharides—dextran, iron dextran, *Acacia*
Vaccines
Toxoids
Allergy extracts
Foreign sera
Sulfobromophthalein
Protamine
Acetylcysteine
Local and systemic anesthetics

The first step in treating any allergic reaction is to stop further exposure to the allergen. Treatment of anaphylaxis also should include administration of epinephrine, antihistamines, and corticosteroids. If shock is present, intravenous fluids should be given. Epinephrine is the drug of choice in anaphylaxis because it is a potent alpha- and beta-receptor agonist. It therefore antagonizes the effect of anaphylaxis on the smooth muscles of both the vasculature and the airways, alleviating bronchoconstriction and splanchnic blood pooling. Epinephrine can be given intramuscularly at a dose of 0.01 ml/kg in a 1:1000 dilution. If the antigen was administered through an extravascular injection, an additional 0.1 to 0.2 ml of 1:1000 epinephrine should be injected locally to delay absorption of the antigen. If profound hypotension is present, intravenous administration is preferable to the intramuscular route. Epinephrine should be used in a 1:10,000 dilution for intravenous administration and given in 0.5- to 1.0-ml increments to a total of dose of 0.5 to 5.0 ml. Epinephrine administration can be repeated every 15 to 30 min as needed.

Antihistamines may be beneficial in anaphylaxis. They should never be substituted for epinephrine, however, because histamine is only one of the many mediators involved. Diphenhydramine can be used intramuscularly or by slow intravenous injection at a dose of 1.0 to 2.0 mg/kg. The role of H_2-receptor activation in anaphylaxis is uncertain. Some investigators recommend the use of an H_2-blocker such as cimetidine in addition to traditional H_1-blockers. The efficacy of this measure is unproven, however, and stimulation of the H_2-receptor on the surface of mast cells will actually inhibit degranulation.

Although the efficacy of corticosteroids in reducing shock fatalities is still controversial, they are probably helpful as adjunctive therapy in acute hypersensitivity reactions. Corticosteroids help prevent further mast cell degranulation, stabilize lysosomal and endothelial membranes, decrease complement activation, decrease neutrophil aggregation, and decrease activation of the clotting cascades and the kinin system. Water-soluble corticosteroids should be given intravenously in high doses for anaphylactic shock (prednisolone sodium succinate, 35 mg/kg, or dexamethasone sodium phosphate, 5 to 10 mg/kg).

Rapid intravenous crystalloid fluid therapy is indicated to help restore adequate blood pressure in anaphylactic shock. The volume administered depends on the patient's response to therapy but may be as high as 90 ml/kg in dogs and 60 ml/kg in cats. Additional supportive therapy should be administered as needed and may include oxygen therapy, tracheal intubation or tracheostomy, and administration of aminophylline or additional vasopressors.

Finally, anaphylaxis should be prevented when possible by taking a complete history to determine any possible hypersensitivities. Animals receiving substances, such as doxorubicin and L-asparaginase, with a high potential for producing anaphylactic-type reactions should be routinely premedicated with steroids and antihistamines.

Anaphylactoid Reactions

Anaphylactoid reactions are reactions that are mediated by systemic mast cell degranulation but that are caused by nonimmunologic mechanisms. Anaphylactoid reactions can be caused by certain drugs, such as morphine, which directly degranulate mast cells. Physical factors also can cause mast cell degranulation. An example of this mechanism is the rapid infusion of hypertonic solutions. Substances capable of causing nonimmunologic mast cell degranulation in people are listed in Table 3. Unlike anaphylaxis, anaphylactoid reactions can often be prevented by slowing the rate of administration of the responsible substance. Pretreatment with steroids may also help prevent these reactions. In one study, administration of steroids at 12 and 2 hr prior to injection of radiographic iodinated contrast media greatly decreased the incidence of ana-

Table 3. *Substances Causing Anaphylactoid Reactions in People or Animals*

Nonsteroidal anti-inflammatory agents
Sulfiting agents
Opiates
Mannitol
Dextrans
Radiographic iodinated contrast media
Curare and *d*-tubocurarine
Chymopapain
Cremophor surfactant (in alfhaxalone-alfhadolone acetate anesthetics)
Doxorubicin

phylactoid reactions to these agents. Steroids are known to generate inhibitors of contact system activators. It was hypothesized that inhibition of bradykinin production as a result of the steroids was responsible for the decreased incidence of anaphylactoid reactions. A patient having an anaphylactoid reaction will not necessarily have a similar episode on subsequent exposure to the responsible substance; however, the patient is at a higher risk. The only way to distinguish true anaphylaxis from an anaphylactoid reaction is by the demonstration of significant concentrations of allergen-specific IgE. Anaphylactoid reactions are treated similarly to anaphylactic reactions because the same mediators are responsible.

Rapid intravenous injections of many substances can cause acute cardiovascular depression, with ataxia, dyspnea, and collapse. These toxic reactions are often mistaken for anaphylactic or anaphylactoid shock. Examples of substances capable of producing this type of reaction include chloramphenicol, propylene glycol, tetracycline, meperidine, and aminoglycosides.

Urticaria and Angioedema

Angioedema and urticaria are localized forms of increased vascular permeability. They occur as a result of the same reactions that induce anaphylaxis. Urticarial lesions (hives) consist of raised, circular, well-demarcated, cutaneous areas of pruritus and inflammation. Angioedema occurs when the deeper cutaneous and subcutaneous vessels are affected. The result is a diffuse swelling. Angioedema has a predilection for the head and neck, producing erythematous, pruritic pinnae, severe chemosis, and edema of the face and neck. Laryngeal and bronchial edema may occur, causing life-threatening airway obstruction in rare cases. Some people with angioedema have swelling of the gastrointestinal mucosa as well.

As with anaphylaxis and anaphylactoid reactions, urticaria and angioedema may result from immunologic or nonimmunologic reactions. Drugs associated with urticaria and angioedema in people are the same as those associated with anaphylaxis. Pressure, friction, cold, heat, emotional stress, exercise, and malignancies also have been cited as causes in people. A recurrent form of angioedema occurs in people with an inherited deficiency of C1 inactivator. Substances that have produced hives or angioedema in companion animals include vaccines, Hymenoptera venom, insecticide sprays, foods, penicillin, xylazine, tetracycline, doxorubicin, L-asparaginase, iodinated contrast media, and vitamin K_1. A case of cold-induced urticaria has also been described in a dog.

Hives respond well to antihistamines; steroids are not needed in mild cases. However, severe cases of urticaria and cases of angioedema should be treated with subcutaneous epinephrine and corticosteroids in addition to antihistamines to prevent the development of laryngeal edema or anaphylaxis. If airway obstruction is present, tracheal intubation or tracheostomy and oxygen administration are indicated. Aminophylline is helpful if bronchial constriction is a component.

TYPE II REACTIONS

The initial event in type II hypersensitivity reactions is the binding of antibody to a cell membrane–bound antigen. This leads to antibody-dependent cell lysis, usually through complement activation. Examples of type II reactions include immune thrombocytopenia in some cats receiving propylthiouracil and immune hemolytic anemia in some dogs receiving levamisole. Type II reactions typically occur between 5 and 40 days after initial administration of the antigen. They will be immediate only if prior sensitization has occurred.

The most common example of an immediate type II reaction is an acute hemolytic transfusion reaction in a sensitized recipient. A crossmatch that results in no agglutination does not eliminate the possibility of a hemolytic reaction in a previously sensitized recipient. A crossmatch using species-specific Coombs' antisera would help identify the presence of nonagglutinating anti–red blood cell IgG antibodies, which might cause a hemolytic reaction.

TYPE III REACTIONS

Type III reactions occur when immunoglobulin binds circulating antigen to form immune complexes. The disease is favored in situations of slight antigen excess. The complexes fix complement, and this initiates an inflammatory reaction. Inflammation occurs mainly in small blood vessels in the synovium, skin, kidneys, and muscle. The damaged endothelium, in turn, releases Hageman factor. Hageman factor activates the kinin system, causing more inflammation.

Serum sickness is the prototype of a systemic immune complex disease. It was first recognized in people as a sequela to treatment with equine antiserum. Many researchers now use the term serum sickness to denote systemic immune complex disease due to any foreign antigen. Common signs of serum sickness include arthritis, fever, and lymphadenopathy. Proteinuria, urticaria, neuropathies, retinitis, myositis, cutaneous eruptions, and gastroenteritis may also be seen. An example of this reaction in dogs is the polyarthritis that develops in some Doberman pinschers treated with sulfadiazine. Glomerulonephropathy, retinitis, thrombocytopenia, polymyositis, urticaria, fever, anemia, leukopenia, and skin rashes were also reported in these dogs. Immune complex disease usually develops 10 to 20 days after initial exposure to the antigen; however, it may present as an acute reaction after as little as 1 to 2 days if prior sensitization has occurred. The signs of type III reactions are usually reversible within a few days after clearing the antigen.

TYPE IV REACTIONS

Type IV reactions are an example of cell-mediated immunity. These reactions are also referred to as delayed-type hypersensitivity reactions because the inflammation usually peaks 24 to 48 hr after exposure to the allergen. A mononuclear cell infiltrate dominates this reaction. Sensitized T lymphocytes produce lymphokines, which produce inflammation and recruit mononuclear cells to the site of antigen exposure.

The most common clinical example of delayed-type hypersensitivity is allergic contact dermatitis. Delayed hypersensitivity lesions may be seen in as little as 6 hr after exposure to the hapten in some sensitized individuals. However, most acute reactions to topical agents are irritant reactions rather than allergic reactions. The responsible agent in contact hypersensitivity reactions is usually a hapten. The hapten binds to a skin protein to form a complete allergen. Common sensitizing agents include sulfa drugs, penicillins, neomycin, bacitracin, formaldehyde, idoxuridine, para-aminobenzoic acid (PABA), thimerosol and paraben preservatives, benzocaine and related topical anesthetics, disinfectants, cresol and tar shampoos, dyes, plant resins, lanolin, rubber products, metals, and tanned leather. Animals are predisposed to sensitization by any condition that makes the skin easier to permeate. Inflamed, irritated, wet, or defatted skin is more easily sensitized. Delayed hypersensitivity reactions can be treated with cool compresses, Burow's solution, and steroids if needed. Because the sensitizing agents are bound to cutaneous proteins, it may take several days to several weeks for the reaction to subside.

FACTORS INVOLVED IN SENSITIZATION

Host Factors

The ability to mount an immune response to any antigenic determinant is partially genetic. This ability is controlled by the major histocompatibility antigens coded for by immune response genes. The type of response produced by an individual, IgE or IgG, also seems to have a strong genetic basis. Identical twins raised in different environments will have nearly identical levels of IgE antibodies to specific allergens. Several investigators have reported an increased incidence of anaphylaxis in atopic individuals; however, this finding is controversial. Most people who have had acute type I hypersensitivity reactions have no history of chronic allergies.

Pharmacogenetics is also an important factor in determining susceptibility to allergies. Pharmacogenetics is the genetically determined variation among individuals in their response to drugs. One example of this principle is seen in people with genetically slow acetylation pathways. People with this phenotypic trait have an increased risk of developing drug-induced systemic lupus after procainamide or hydralazine therapy. It may be that prolonged drug exposure due to delayed metabolism increases the risk of hypersensitization in these people or that alternate metabolic pathways lead to the production of more allergenic moieties. Acquired metabolic disorders, such as hepatic failure or renal failure, will similarly alter susceptibility to hypersensitivity reactions by influencing the processing and retention of antigens. Immunopathologic changes due to chronic infections, cyclophosphamide, or antilymphocyte serum increase the risk of sensitization. The depression of suppressor T cells in these situations permits increased IgE production and "allergic breakthrough."

The autonomic balance of the animal is another important factor. Cholinergic stimulation or alpha-adrenergic stimulation will augment mast cell degranulation. In contrast to these effects, beta-adrenergic stimulation will inhibit degranulation. It is believed that people on beta-blockers are predisposed to type I reactions and that an endogenous, partial beta-blockade is important in the pathogenesis of human asthma. These effects are mediated through the cyclic adenosine monophosphate (c-AMP) system. Generally anything that decreases the content of c-AMP or increases the content of cyclic guanosine monophosphate (c-GMP) in the mast cell will augment degranulation.

Antigen Factors

Some antigens, such as pollens and venoms, are intrinsically more allergenic. Most natural allergens have a molecular weight in the range of 10,000 to 70,000. Polymerization of smaller allergens can reduce the allergenicity while increasing the antigenicity. This generalization is not universal, and some larger allergens are potent sensitizers. Allergens must be multivalent to elicit a type I reaction, because the antigen needs to bridge adjacent IgE molecules on the mast cell to cause degranulation.

Some substances are allergenic owing to cross-reactivity with a similar compound. Penicillins and cephalosporins are often cross-reactive. Sulfa drugs can cross-react with a wide variety of compounds, including sulfonylureas, procaine derivatives, thiazides, and PABA. Allergies to many biologic and pharmacologic preparations are actually due to additives and contaminants. Most drugs are too small to be complete antigens; they function as haptens. The ability of a drug to act as a hapten is dependent on its ability to form stable, covalent bonds with host proteins. Simple complexing to plasma carrier proteins is too weak to produce an immunogenic response.

Exposure Factors

In any allergic reaction, a sensitization period of at least 5 to 7 days is required. For some foods and contact allergens, the sensitization period may be months to years. Intermittent dosage schedules are more likely to produce sensitization. Intravenous administration is more likely to tolerize and less likely to sensitize. After an individual has been sensitized, however, this route is more likely to elicit a reaction.

DIAGNOSIS

Definitive diagnosis of a hypersensitivity reaction is difficult for several reasons: (1) Diagnostic challenge with the suspected allergen is potentially dangerous and therefore contraindicated in most situations. (2) False-negative results are common because the parent compound is usually the only substance tested and the allergenic moiety is often a metabolite, impurity, or additive. (3) Demonstration of allergen-specific antibodies does not always correlate with disease: most people treated with penicillin develop antibodies to the penicilloic group but only a small percentage of these people have allergic symptoms. (4) False-positive reactions to *in vivo* tests commonly are encountered as a result of direct toxicity, irritation, or nonimmunologic histamine release by the suspected allergen.

Table 4. *Clinical Criteria Suggestive of a Hypersensitivity Reaction to a Drug*

1. The reaction occurs in only a small proportion of individuals receiving the drug.
2. The reaction occurs only after a sensitizing period of 5–7 days minimum.
3. The reaction can be elicited with small doses of the drug.
4. The reaction does not resemble the pharmacologic effects of the drug.
5. The reaction includes classic signs of a hypersensitivity reaction.

Owing to the difficulties involved in performing and interpreting these tests, a presumptive diagnosis is often made on the basis of a careful history and physical examination at the time of the reaction. The client should be questioned carefully about exposure of the patient to allergens, including drugs, biologics, over-the-counter preparations, dietary additives, chew toys, foodstuffs, bites or stings of venomous animals, insecticides, shampoos, coat conditioners, household products, or plants. A complete physical examination and history supplemented with an appropriate laboratory data base should be performed to help rule out nonimmunologic causes of reactions that resemble allergic reactions. Nonimmunologic adverse reactions to drugs, biologics, and blood products are far more common than allergic reactions, and all possibilities should be carefully considered. Hymenoptera venom contains histamine and kinins, making it difficult to distinguish between toxic and allergic reactions in some cases. Factors supporting the diagnosis of a drug allergy are listed in Table 4. These principles can be extrapolated to acute hypersensitivity reactions due to most other allergens.

The clinician may wish to perform appropriate tests to identify the specific allergen. Although none of these tests is ideal, evidence may be gained to support the presumptive diagnosis. A few of the tests commonly used to identify acute hypersensitivity reactions include intradermal allergen testing, the Prausnitz-Küstner (PK) test, passive cutaneous anaphylaxis (PCA), the Schultz-Dale technique, and the radioallergosorbent test (RAST).

An intradermal allergen test is performed by injecting a small volume (usually 0.1 ml) of diluted allergen intradermally and comparing the reaction with that from an injection of histamine (positive control) and an injection of saline (negative control). This test is used commonly in the diagnosis of canine atopy. Although the risk of inducing anaphylaxis is low, this possibility should be considered. This test produces many false-positive and false-negative results for the reasons mentioned above.

In a PK test, the patient's serum is injected into the skin of a nonallergic animal. Any IgE in the patient's serum is allowed to bind to the recipient's mast cells over a period of 24 to 48 hr. Test antigen is then injected into the same site. In a positive reaction, a wheal will be produced. In a PCA test, the recipient is injected with patient serum in a similar manner to the PK test; however, the antigen is injected intravenously along with Evans blue dye. If the reaction is positive, mast cell degranulation occurs, and increased vascular permeability is a result. Because the dye binds to albumin, it is easy to detect the extravasation of plasma, which occurs when the reaction is positive. Owing to the high binding affinity of IgE, there may be insufficient circulating IgE in the patient's serum to passively sensitize the recipient. Thus false-negative results may occur with both PK and PCA tests.

The radioallergosorbent test is an *in vitro* assay for allergen-specific IgE. The assay recently has been modified to use an enzyme marker rather than a radioactive label so this test is now more accessible. However, the level of allergen-specific IgE that corresponds to clinical disease is highly variable, and the clinical usefulness of this test is therefore limited.

References and Supplemental Reading

Auer, L. K.: Feline blood transfusion reactions. *In* Kirk, R. W. (ed.): *Current Veterinary Therapy IX*. Philadelphia: W. B. Saunders, 1986, pp. 515–520.

Davis, L. E.: Hypersensitivity reactions induced by antimicrobial drugs. J.A.V.M.A. 185:1131, 1984.

Frick, O. L.: Immediate hypersensitivity. *In* Stites, D. P., Stobo, J. D., and Wells, J. V. (eds.): *Basic and Clinical Immunology*, 6th ed. Norwalk, CT: Appleton and Lange, 1987, pp. 197–227.

Killingsworth, C. R.: Use of blood and blood components for feline and canine patients. J.A.V.M.A. 185:1452, 1984.

Reisman, R. E.: Allergy to stinging insects. *In* Patterson, R. (ed.): *Allergic Diseases*, 3rd ed. Philadelphia: J. B. Lippincott, 1985, pp. 408–417.

Terr, A. I.: Allergic diseases. *In* Stites, D. P., Stobo, J. D., and Wells, J. V. (eds.): *Basic and Clinical Immunology*, 6th ed. Norwalk, CT: Appleton and Lange, 1987, pp. 435–456.

Terr, A. I.: Anaphylaxis. Clin. Rev. Allergy 3:3, 1985.

Tizard, I.: *Veterinary Immunology, An Introduction*, 3rd ed. Philadelphia: W. B. Saunders, 1987, pp. 281–306.

Willemse, A.: Acquired cold urticaria in a dog. J. Am. Anim. Hosp. Assoc. 18:961, 1982.

IMMUNE-MEDIATED NONEROSIVE ARTHRITIS IN THE DOG

PATRICK E. HOPPER, D.V.M.

Davis, California

Arthritis is a term used to describe conditions that are inflammatory in nature and are confined to the joints. The arthritis may involve a single joint (monarticular), two to five joints (pauciarticular), or more than five joints (polyarticular), simultaneously. Inflammatory joint disease, or arthritis, in the dog is characterized by cellular infiltrates in the synovial membrane and inflammatory changes in the synovial membrane and synovial fluid. The causes of inflammatory joint disorders are diverse and are categorized as infectious (septic) and noninfectious (nonseptic). Noninfectious inflammatory joint diseases are the immune-mediated arthritides, which are subdivided into nonerosive (nondeforming) and erosive (deforming) arthritis (Table 1).

Immune-mediated nonerosive arthritis in dogs is a common articular disease and the most common manifestation of immune complex disease (type III hypersensitivity reaction). The causes are diverse and include idiopathic disease and arthritis due to chronic infectious diseases and immunologic diseases, such as systemic lupus erythematosus (SLE). Causes also include plasmacytic-lymphocytic synovitis, chronic inflammatory bowel or hepatic diseases, allergic drug reactions, and malignant neoplasms (Table 2). The immune-mediated (nonerosive) arthritides are believed to be mediated through similar immunopathologic mechanisms independent of their diverse origins. The manifestations are caused by inflammatory reactions as a result of the deposition and phagocytosis of immune complexes within the synovial membrane. Complement, neutrophils, macrophages, and macrophage kinins play an important role in the pathogenesis. Because the synovial membrane's response to inflammation is similar for both infectious and noninfectious causes, inflammatory joint disease presents a diagnostic and therapeutic challenge to veterinarians.

HISTORY AND PHYSICAL EXAMINATION

Idiopathic polyarthritis is the most common form of immune-mediated joint disease. The disease can occur at any age in both sexes, although the majority of cases occur in dogs between 2.5 and 4.5 years of age. Any breed, as well as mongrels, can be affected. An increased risk is observed in large breeds (German shepherds, Doberman pinschers), sporting breeds (collies, spaniels, retrievers, pointers), and toy breeds (terriers, poodles). Systemic lupus erythematosus has no age predilection (it has been found in dogs aged 8 months to 14 years), but

Table 1. *Classification of Canine Arthropathies*

I. Noninflammatory joint disease
  A. Degenerative joint disease
    1. Primary (osteoarthrosis, osteoarthritis)
    2. Secondary (acquired or congenital defects)
  B. Traumatic joint disease
  C. Meniscal disorders and cruciate ligament ruptures
  D. Luxations and subluxations
  E. Neuropathic arthropathies
  F. Developmental arthropathies
  G. Arthropathies due to inborn errors of metabolism
  H. Dietary arthropathies
  I. Neoplastic arthropathies
II. Inflammatory joint disease (arthritis)
  A. Infectious arthritis
    1. Bacterial arthritis
    2. Mycoplasmal arthritis
    3. Fungal arthritis
    4. Protozoal arthritis
    5. Viral arthritis
  B. Noninfectious arthritis
    1. Immunologic
      a. Erosive (deforming) arthritis
        1. Rheumatoid arthritis
        2. Polyarthritis of greyhounds
      b. Nonerosive (nondeforming) arthritis
    2. Nonimmunologic
      a. Crystal-induced arthritis
      b. Chronic hemarthrosis
        1. Hemophilia
        2. Bleeding diathesis
        3. Multiple myeloma with hyperviscosity syndrome

females and certain breeds (German shepherds, collies, Shetland sheepdogs, beagles, and poodles) may be predisposed (Drazner, 1980; Grindem and Johnson, 1983; Scott et al., 1983). In plasmacytic-lymphocytic synovitis an increased risk is observed

Table 2. *Immune-Mediated Nonerosive Arthritides*

1. Idiopathic polyarthritis
2. Arthritis associated with chronic infectious diseases
  a. Bacterial:
    Subacute bacterial endocarditis
    Diskospondylitis
    Chronic actinomyces granulomas (fox tail, grass awn migration)
    Pyometra
    Periodontitis
    Deep pyoderma
    Rocky Mountain spotted fever
    Chronic ehrlichiosis
    Chronic salmonellosis
    Lyme disease
  b. Fungal: coccidioidomycosis
  c. Parasitic: dirofilariasis
3. Arthritis associated with immunologic diseases
  a. Systemic lupus erythematosus
  b. Bullous dermatitides
4. Enteropathic/hepatopathic arthritis
  a. Chronic ulcerative colitis
  b. Chronic active hepatitis
5. Plasmacytic-lymphocytic synovitis
6. Drug-induced polyarthritis (e.g., due to trimethoprim-sulfadiazine)
7. Arthritis associated with malignant neoplasia

in large breeds, particularly German shepherds. There appears to be no age, breed, or sex predilection for the remaining nonerosive arthritides. Independent of the type of immune-mediated joint disease, the presenting clinical features are similar and include fever, anorexia, and malaise accompanied by lameness of varying degrees. The joint disease and clinical manifestations tend to be cyclic in nature. Diarrhea can be present and may precede clinical signs by a day or more. Occasionally, behavioral changes, such as aggression and increased irritability, are observed, particularly when affected dogs are approached suddenly or touched. The arthritic manifestations range from overt lameness to subtle signs of weakness. A single (monarticular, pauciarticular) or shifting (pauciarticular, polyarticular) leg lameness may be observed. Dogs with polyarticular involvement show generalized weakness or stiffness (stilted gait) and difficulty in rising and lying down, involving the hindquarters predominantly. Some affected dogs, particularly small or toy breeds, will refuse to stand, walk, or move. In these instances, joint disease is difficult to appreciate and is often overlooked.

Physical examination, including palpation and manipulation of joints, cannot eliminate diagnosis of inflammatory joint disease because pain or effusion is often not demonstrable. Idiopathic polyarthritis is often characterized by the absence of effusion. Accurate evaluation of joints by physical examination is complicated by variables such as breed variation or conformation, skin and hair coat thickness, and the presence of limited volumes of synovial fluid. Regardless of the type of immune-mediated arthritis, distal extremities, including the carpus and tarsus joints, are most commonly affected. Obvious swelling, heat, or pain in one or more of the joints is a physical finding more frequently associated with acute, febrile states. In more chronic forms, swelling and heat are often absent and only subtle signs of discomfort or joint capsule thickening are detectable. Hyperesthesia, involving the neck, back, or tail, from passive manipulation rather than from specific joint pain, is a predominant clinical feature. Additional physical findings are peripheral lymphadenopathy and fever (103 to 106°F). In severely affected dogs, the disease can be debilitating, resulting in generalized muscle atrophy and weight loss. Inflammatory joint disease should be suspected whenever joint palpation reveals abnormalities in multiple joints or whenever persistent or episodic fevers are detected, especially fevers of unknown origin.

History and physical examination alone cannot distinguish among specific immune-mediated arthritides. Joint disease is the sole manifestation in idiopathic polyarthritis. In canine SLE, polyarthritis is the most common finding (60 to 90 per cent of cases) and frequently the primary presenting complaint. The clinical features are diverse, but arthritis commonly is the sole manifestation of canine SLE, indistinct from idiopathic polyarthritis. Skin and mucocutaneous lesions are prevalent in SLE (occurring in 43 per cent of cases) but not necessarily a concurrent finding with polyarthritis. Less common physical abnormalities found in dogs with SLE include muscular (myositis), neurologic (meningitis, myelopathy), or vascular (edema) disorders (Pedersen, 1978; Grindem and Johnson, 1983; Scott et al., 1983). In plasmacytic-lymphocytic synovitis, the stifle joint is primarily affected, resulting in gonitis and leading eventually to degeneration of the cruciate ligaments and drawer motion. The arthritis that is seen in the secondary immune-mediated arthritides is most often a minor manifestation of the disease syndrome. Monarticular and pauciarticular involvement of the carpi and tarsi are the most frequent musculoskeletal findings in the secondary arthritides. In the dog, allergic drug reactions are frequently associated with cutaneous manifestations. In human beings, certain drugs (procainamide, hydralazine, sulfonamides, propranolol, and quinidine) are well recognized for inducing polyarthritis and an SLE-like syndrome (Hess, 1981). Drug-induced polyarthritis is not as well recognized in the dog. However, treatment with trimethoprim-sulfadiazine has been reported to cause polyarthritis and other immune-mediated disorders in the dog. A genetic predisposition in the Doberman pinscher breed to develop an allergic drug reaction to sulfadiazine is suspected (Giger et al., 1985; Werner and Bright, 1983). A thorough history, including previous therapy and travel, and physical examination are often helpful in recognizing infectious and other secondary immune-mediated inflammatory joint diseases.

DIFFERENTIAL DIAGNOSIS

The clinical signs manifested in the immune-mediated nonerosive arthritides are similar to and compatible with those of more common diseases such as infection and neoplasia. Occasionally arthritis is the main or only presenting clinical sign superimposed over a primary disease. Infectious arthritis presents the greatest concern because inaccurate diagnosis and subsequent therapy with a glucocorticoid hormone or immunosuppressive drug may exacerbate the infectious disease. Blood-borne infections are more likely to be associated with infectious polyarthritis than are those spread by nonhematogenous routes. Experimentally, bacteria localize rapidly in the synovial membrane and cells of the reticuloendothelial system following intravenous injection (Curtiss, 1973). Infectious arthritis can be diagnosed in any age, breed, or sex, although male dogs of large breeds (German shepherd, Great

Dane, and St. Bernard) and sporting breeds have an increased risk (Pedersen et al., 1983; Calvert, 1986). The pattern of joint involvement tends to be monarticular or pauciarticular, rather than polyarticular. Specific joints involved are most often large proximal joints (shoulder, elbow, hip, and stifle) and intervertebral disk spaces as distinguished from involvement of smaller distal joints seen in immune-mediated arthritis. Pain, heat, and distention of affected joints are frequent physical findings. Local edema of soft tissue over, and occasionally distal to, infected joints is detected. Prior joint pathologic changes, including degenerative joint disease and trauma, may be an important predisposing factor for the development of infectious arthritis. Often a source of predisposing infection can be detected. The skin, urogenital tract, oral cavity, and respiratory tract are common infection sites noted on physical examination. Other predisposing factors, such as recent glucocorticoid or immunosuppressive drug therapy, should suggest an infectious etiology.

Subacute and chronic bacteremias present the most difficulty in differentiating infectious from immune-mediated causes of arthritis. Bacteremia is most frequently associated with bacterial endocarditis and diskospondylitis (Calvert, 1986). Bacterial endocarditis and bacteremia should be considered in all dogs with unexplained fevers; lameness, especially a shifting leg lameness; cardiac abnormalities; and multisystemic involvement compatible with circulating immune complexes or embolic phenomena. In contrast, diskospondylitis often is less severe or produces no clinical signs. Clinical signs characteristic of diskospondylitis are a stilted gait and hyperesthesia of the spine. Other conditions with demonstrable hyperesthesia of the head, neck, or limbs are meningitis, polymyositis, polyneuritis, and intervertebral disk disease. Interestingly, lymphadenopathy is not a common clinical sign of bacteremia associated with most microorganisms. When lymphadenopathy, fever, and lameness are present, immune-mediated arthritis, neoplasia, and chronic infections, including rickettsial, mycotic, and spirochetal diseases, should be suspected.

Rheumatoid arthritis (RA) and immune-mediated nonerosive arthritis are similar early in the course of disease. Rheumatoid arthritis, an erosive, immune-mediated arthritis, is a rare form of joint disease, affecting dogs predominantly in small or toy breeds, with no apparent sex predilection. The age at onset of clinical signs in dogs affected by RA ranges from 2 to 8 years, while the mean age at onset occurs at approximately 4 years (Newton, 1976; Pedersen et al., 1976a; Bennett, 1987). Rheumatoid arthritis is characterized by a shifting leg lameness and generalized stiffness after rest. The joint disease tends to be polyarticular in a bilaterally symmetric fashion. Some dogs affected with RA are unable to sit or lie down without extreme discomfort or effort. If undetected, RA tends to localize in distal joints, especially the carpus and tarsus. This rare form of arthritis in the dog is progressive and episodic, with clinical signs increasing in frequency and duration. In chronic RA, continuous destruction of affected joints leads to rupture of ligaments, joint luxation, and angular deformities.

Noninflammatory arthropathies, particularly hip and elbow dysplasias, are suspected in some cases because of the signalment and the clinical signs. Further confusion comes from the dog's apparent discomfort on manipulation of the hip, which may in fact be due to movement or pressure applied to distal joints. A joint aspirate and analysis is indicated in suspected noninflammatory arthropathies, especially when the history does not include acute trauma or when signs of systemic illness are present (fever and leukocytosis).

CLINICOPATHOLOGIC FINDINGS

HEMOGRAM

Anemia and thrombocytopenia are infrequently seen in idiopathic polyarthritis. However, dogs with SLE will frequently have anemia and may have thrombocytopenia. When anemia is present in canine SLE (35 per cent of cases), a nonregenerative anemia is detected most often (80 per cent). A Coombs' test result is positive in approximately 25 per cent of the SLE cases, although autoimmune hemolytic anemia is infrequently observed (in 20 per cent of cases). Thrombocytopenia, due to an immune-mediated process, is rarely found in SLE dogs (in only 10 per cent). Circulating antiplatelet antibodies can be present and may be responsible for the decrease in platelet numbers. Leukocytosis, absolute neutrophilia, and hyperfibrinogenemia are common findings in acute febrile attacks, although the leukogram can be normal or reflect a stress response. Leukopenia is a rare finding in most dogs with polyarthritis. Most often the leukopenia seen in canine SLE patients (in 23 per cent) is due to autoantibodies directed against leukocytes. Overall, the hemogram does not differentiate between the arthritides because the changes observed are consistent with either infectious or immune-mediated disease processes.

BLOOD CHEMISTRY AND URINALYSIS

Serum chemistry profiles in idiopathic polyarthritis either are normal or show variable decreases in albumin and variable increases in globulin levels. In patients with these abnormalities, serum electrophoresis is valuable to confirm hypoalbuminemia and demonstrate elevations in alpha$_2$- and gamma-globulins. Similarly, hypoalbuminemia ($<$ 2.5 mg/dl) is a common finding in patients with SLE (vasculitis and glomerulonephritis) and secondary polyarthritis due to chronic infection (embolic or immune-mediated vasculitis and glomerulonephritis), chronic inflammatory bowel disease, or hepatic disease. In contrast to findings in idiopathic polyarthritis, blood chemistry abnormalities reflecting multisystemic involvement are suggestive of infectious processes, such as bacterial endocarditis, or multisystemic immune disorders, such as SLE.

Urine must be examined for evidence of infection and glomerulonephritis. The urine protein-creatinine ratio is helpful to evaluate the significance of proteinuria in dogs with suspected protein-losing nephropathy (Center, 1985). Proteinuria is consistent with SLE and bacteria-associated glomerulonephritis. Approximately 50 per cent of the dogs affected by SLE have proteinuria (Pedersen et al., 1976b; Drazner, 1980; Grindem and Johnson, 1983; Scott et al., 1983).

SYNOVIAL FLUID ANALYSIS

To establish the diagnosis and differentiate between inflammatory and noninflammatory joint diseases in the dog, arthrocentesis and synovial fluid analysis are essential. There are few, if any, contraindications for obtaining synovial fluid, with the exception of infected skin (moderate to severe pyoderma or lick granuloma). The complications and risks of this procedure are minimal. Trauma or hemorrhage from obtaining synovial fluid is usually minor and of no clinical significance. Iatrogenic contamination or inoculation of the joint, although a potential risk, has not been recognized and can be avoided by proper preparation of the site. Arthrocentesis and description of specific sites have been previously described and illustrated (Werner, 1979; Pedersen et al., 1983).

A single drop of synovial fluid is sufficient for gross appearance and cytologic examinations including a Gram's stain for microorganisms. Analysis is completed with an additional small amount of synovial fluid for bacterial culture (aerobic, anaerobic, and *Mycoplasma* spp.). Arthrocentesis of multiple joints is recommended because occasionally analysis of synovial fluid from a single joint may be inconclusive. An increased volume of synovial fluid can be observed in inflammatory joint diseases but can also be seen in noninflammatory arthropathies, particularly with acutely traumatized or degenerative joints. More often inflammatory joints contain only a small amount ($<$ 0.1 ml) of synovial fluid. This often confuses the clinician in diagnosing inflammatory joint disease. Normal synovial fluid is colorless, clear, viscous, and tenacious. Synovial fluid containing blood is typically associated with acute trauma, although septic arthritis and generalized bleeding diathesis also produce hemarthrosis. The occurrence of blood due to traumatic collection can usually be distinguished from that of hemarthrosis because in the former the blood is incompletely mixed with the synovial fluid. Yellow-tinged fluid is the result of previous hemorrhage with release of hemoglobin pigments into the joint fluid. If either red blood cells or white blood cells or both are in excess, an increase in turbidity is observed. Flocculation and clot formation qualify the synovial fluid as an exudate and indicate severe inflammation. The viscosity can be evaluated by observing the fluid exiting from the needle and onto a slide. A sample from a normal joint will form a long "string" between the needle and the slide. In addition, the drop on the slide should remain spheric rather than dispersing over the slide. A thin, runny consistency indicates a deficiency in polymerized hyaluronic acid or dilution from excess serum. This is a frequent finding in inflammatory disorders caused by the action of hyaluronidase, which is produced by either bacteria or inflammatory cells. Occasionally poor viscosity is observed in degenerative or acutely traumatized joints.

Often small volumes of synovial fluid are obtained, but a nucleated cell count and differential count can be accurately estimated. This can be accomplished by cytologic examination of both synovial fluid and peripheral blood smears and comparison of nucleated cell counts. Synovial smears, as with routine blood smears, are stained with Wright's or Wright-Giemsa stain. The nucleated cell count for several high-power fields is averaged for both smears. The white blood cell (WBC) count of the peripheral blood is determined and, accordingly, an estimation of the nucleated cell count in synovial fluid can be calculated.

Peripheral blood WBC count
$= 27,000/mm^3$

Average number of nucleated cells
in five fields $= 5.0$

Synovial fluid: Average number of nucleated cells
in five fields $= 12.0$

Estimated nucleated cell count
in synovial fluid $= \dfrac{27,000}{5} \times 12 = 64,800$

A clinical impression, at the least, can be obtained as to the approximate cell count in the synovial fluid, which may be normal (0 to 3 mononuclear cells and a rare neutrophil per high-power field) or elevated (mild, moderate, or severe). Samples can be submitted to a reference laboratory and synovial fluid can be placed in an ethylenediaminetetraacetic acid (EDTA) anticoagulant tube. Anticoagulants are necessary to prevent clotting, as joint aspirates from inflamed joints can have high concentrations of fibrinogen and clotting factors.

Normal synovial fluid contains a mixture of small and large mononuclear cells, including lymphocytes, histiocytes, and desquamated synovial cells (clasmatocytes) along with an occasional or rare polymorphonuclear neutrophil (Table 3). Increased numbers of mononuclear cells tend to occur following trauma and in joints with degenerative joint disease, chronic inflammation, and osteochondrosis. Neutrophils are generally absent or, if present, should account for less than 10 per cent of the nucleated cell count. An increase in the relative or absolute number of neutrophils indicates inflammation of the synovial membrane. The presence of neutrophils only indicates inflammation and has no differentiating diagnostic value for specific inflammatory arthritides. Septic arthritis has a tendency to result in more severe toxic changes in the neutrophil, although vacuolization is sometimes seen in RA and nonerosive immune-mediated arthritis. Generally, the more severely inflamed joints will contain a greater concentration of nucleated blood cells and a corresponding greater percentage of neutrophils. Red blood cells, as with neutrophils, are rare in normal synovial fluid, but numbers of such cells increase in all forms of joint disease, particularly those associated with acute trauma.

When sample volume is adequate, additional procedures include mucin clot test and determination of protein and glucose content. The mucin clot test is designed to indirectly determine the extent of polymerization of hyaluronic acid. Inflammation, as a rule, causes depolymerization of the polymer, which results in a poor clot. Protein levels are generally less than 1.0 gm/dl and increase with any form of synovitis, although excessive protein (4 to 5 gm/dl) suggests infection. The synovial fluid glucose–blood glucose ratio is generally low with all forms of immune-mediated arthritis (0.5 to 0.8) and extremely low (< 0.5) in septic arthritis (Werner, 1979).

SEROLOGIC FINDINGS

Difficulty in distinguishing immune-mediated diseases from chronic infectious diseases associated with arthritis should prompt immunologic testing. Rheumatoid factor (RF) is found in 20 per cent to as high as 70 per cent of the dogs affected with erosive, immune-mediated arthritis, depending on the sensitivity of the specific test system utilized (Pedersen et al., 1976a; Bennett, 1987). Rheumatoid factors (antibodies) will react with immune-complexed immunoglobulin G (IgG) or denatured IgG. Therefore, any disease, infectious or noninfectious, associated with immune complex production, can potentially result in low positive titers. Moreover,

Table 3. *Synovial Fluid Characteristics in Various Types of Canine Arthritis*

| Condition | Nucleated Cells/mm³ | Differential (%) | |
		Mononuclear	*Neutrophils*
Normal	250–3000	94–100	0–6
Degenerative	1000–5000	88–100	0–12
Rheumatoid arthritis	8000–38,000	20–80	20–80
Nonerosive arthritis (all types)	4400–371,000	5–85	15–95
Plasmacytic-lymphocytic synovitis	5000–20,000	60–90	10–40
Septic arthritis	40,000–267,000	1–10	90–99

Modified from Pedersen, N. C., and Pool, R.: Canine joint disease. Vet. Clin. North Am. [Small Anim. Pract.]. 8:465, 1978.

significant titers of RF have been detected in 5 per cent of the normal dog population (Newton, 1976). Dogs with SLE, idiopathic polyarthritis, or plasmacytic-lymphocytic synovitis can occasionally have low titers for RF. At present, lupus erythematosus (LE) cell preparations and fluorescent antinuclear antibody (FANA) are available to test for the presence of antinuclear antibodies. LE cells are found only in a low percentage of SLE-affected dogs and can be confused with tart cells. Thus, LE cell preparations are not routinely done owing to the limitations of the test results. Indirect FANA determination is the most specific and sensitive serologic test for SLE. Dogs with SLE occasionally have low or negative (seronegative lupus) FANA titers. Low titers of FANA can be found in a number of infectious, inflammatory, and neoplastic disorders. In the dog, subacute bacterial endocarditis with polyarthritis, resulting in the production of autoantibodies, including FANA and RF, has been documented (Bennett et al., 1978). The significance of a positive FANA finding, therefore, should be interpreted with caution and based on clinicopathologic criteria. Georgraphic location and clinical signs, in addition to polyarthritis, may require serologic testing for chronic infectious diseases, such as occult dirofilariasis, coccidioidomycosis, Lyme disease, erlichiosis, and Rocky Mountain spotted fever.

MICROBIOLOGIC FINDINGS

Synovial fluid should be cultured whenever septic arthritis is suspected or confusion between infectious and immunologic joint disease exists. In addition to routine culturing, bacteriologic studies are enhanced by utilizing broth enrichment media, such as thioglycolate. Anaerobic cultures should also be taken in suspected immunodeficient patients. A negative culture should not be interpreted as evidence that an infectious disease is not present because chronic infectious diseases are frequently associated with a sterile immune-mediated arthritis. If joint cultures are negative, isolation and identification of the organism from blood or urine should be considered diagnostic. Blood cultures are positive in 75 per cent of dogs with bacteremia, bacterial

endocarditis, or diskospondylitis. Bacteriuria and positive urine cultures are less common (35 to 45 per cent) (Calvert, 1986). Other infectious agents, such as *Borrelia burgdorferi* (Lyme disease), are difficult to culture, and at present determination of antibody titers is the most useful diagnostic test.

RADIOGRAPHIC FINDINGS

Radiographic evaluation of immune-mediated nonerosive arthritis is usually normal or limited to nonspecific signs of soft tissue swelling and joint distention. Even in chronic cases, radiographic signs are minimal: increased periarticular soft tissue due to fibrosis; periosteal bone proliferation at ligament or joint capsule attachments; and secondary degenerative joint disease. Consequently, radiographic joint surveys are often noncontributory in differentiating among the inflammatory joint diseases, including the early stages of septic or rheumatoid arthritis. However, radiographic joint surveys should not be excluded from the initial examination. Abnormal radiographic findings associated with concurrent orthopedic disease can be present. This can be confounding to the clinician, and thus inflammatory joint disease must always be suspected in patients with lameness. In septic or rheumatoid arthritis, which tend to be deforming and progressive, destructive radiographic findings may be present in initial or subsequent evaluations. In addition, sequential radiographic joint surveys during the course of treatment may be beneficial when synovial fluid analysis is normal but minor clinical signs persist.

DIAGNOSIS

Diagnosis of immune-mediated nonerosive arthritis is based on careful evaluation of the history (including disease course), clinical signs, radiologic features, and clinicopathologic findings. Arthrocentesis for analysis of synovial fluid is the single most helpful test to establish the presence, severity, and distribution of joint involvement in inflammatory joint diseases. Ideally, synovial membrane biopsies should be taken and subjected to histologic and immunofluorescence examinations to differentiate between the immune-mediated arthritides and RA. However, rheumatoid arthritis is rare, and treatment is often unrewarding. A synovial biopsy may be helpful, therefore, when clinical signs persist or worsen in spite of treatment.

The most common type of immune-mediated arthritis is idiopathic polyarthritis. Accordingly, in the diagnostic investigation, there is no evidence of a primary chronic infectious disease process; serologic abnormalities are absent; and cultures for bacteria are negative. Criteria for the diagnosis of canine SLE include positive serologic test result for either LE cells or FANA. However, absence of LE cells and FANA does not exclude the diagnosis. Histopathologic examination and immunofluorescence testing (lupus band test) of diseased skin or oral mucosa can also be of diagnostic benefit. Identification of serologic abnormalities, such as FANA, can be the sole basis for classifying this immune-mediated arthritis as SLE. The diagnosis of canine SLE is more easily made when serologic abnormalities and negative results of bacteriologic studies are coupled with multisystemic manifestations, especially joint, skin, kidney, oral mucosa, and hematopoietic abnormalities. Diagnosis of immune-mediated arthritis associated with chronic infectious diseases is dependent on finding a sterile polyarthritis and on determining an infectious agent in other parts of the body.

The overlying disease is usually apparent for the less common forms of immune-mediated arthritis. Enteropathic arthritis is suspected in the differential diagnosis by detection of inflammatory bowel disease, such as chronic ulcerative colitis or fulminating enterocolitis, concurrently with sterile arthritis. Hepatopathic arthritis is substantiated when chronic active hepatitis or cirrhosis is identified and no other cause of polyarthritis is found. The presence of any malignancy or prior drug therapy should be suspected as the cause of the sterile arthritis until proved otherwise.

Plasmacytic-lymphocytic synovitis in the dog is usually not diagnosed prior to surgical intervention for cranial cruciate ligament (CCL) rupture. Gonitis and synovial effusion usually precede CCL rupture by weeks or months. Synovial fluid analysis prior to surgery can be misleading as to the underlying cause of gonitis. The total nucleated cell count is not dramatically increased, and mononuclear cells are the predominant cell type. These findings are also consistent with those of degenerative joint disease or acute trauma. At surgery, abnormal synovium and synovial fluid are observed, but marginal erosions of subchondral bone and pannus formation usually identified with RA are absent. Histologically, the synovitis is characterized by marked diffuse plasmacyte and lymphocyte infiltrations. These histologic findings are similar to those observed in RA, but differ significantly in intensity from those found in spontaneous CCL rupture and degenerative joint disease of dogs. If these changes are not appreciated or suspected at the time of surgery and the synovitis is not controlled by drug therapy, the success of the surgical stabilization is doubtful.

It should be clear that no single clinical finding or test result is pathognomonic for any specific type of inflammatory joint disease. Most often a specific diagnosis is substantiated by elimination of other causes of polyarthritis. The many similarities shared by inflammatory joint diseases, particularly the immune-mediated forms, should stress the importance of a systematic approach and careful interpretation of all test results.

TREATMENT

The treatment of immune-mediated nonerosive arthritis is dependent on the primary disease identified. For chronic infectious diseases associated with arthritis, antibiotic selection is based on culture and antibiotic sensitivities of the isolated organism. Occasionally, rickettsial and spirochetal infections are suspected but cannot be definitively diagnosed. Under these circumstances, with the diagnosis of idiopathic polyarthritis uncertain, administration of tetracycline (rickettsial infections) or penicillin (spirochetal infections) is recommended for at least 2 weeks. If clinical signs and abnormal joint cytologic findings persist, an infectious etiology is unlikely and the diagnosis of idiopathic polyarthritis may be more certain. Idiopathic polyarthritis, SLE, and plasmacytic-lymphocytic synovitis are treated in a similar fashion with a glucocorticoid hormone or combination immunosuppressive drugs.

GLUCOCORTICOIDS. Prednisone and prednisolone are the glucocorticoid drugs of choice for induction therapy. Prednisone or prednisolone are administered orally at a dosage of 2 to 4 mg/kg or 100 mg/m^2 of body surface area (BSA) in divided dosages for 2 weeks. The highest dosage levels are recommended during the first few days until clinical signs subside, at which time the dosage can be reduced, while continuing the immunosuppressive dosage of 2 to 4 mg/kg/day (75 mg/m^2 BSA), to minimize the side effects of therapy.

At the end of the 2-week period, the dog is again evaluated. Clinical signs and physical abnormalities should have improved but may not have resolved completely. Prior hematologic abnormalities should be monitored until normality is achieved. As in the diagnosis of inflammatory joint disease, arthrocentesis and cytologic examination of synovial fluid are essential in evaluating the response to treatment. Those joints containing the most dramatic synovial fluid abnormalities can be monitored and used as reference points on subsequent examinations. Clinical signs and physical examination findings, although helpful, should not be the basis for adjusting glucocorticoid dosages or adding immunosuppressive drugs to the treatment protocol. A set schedule for reducing glucocorticoid therapy is not recommended. In spite of clinical improvement and marked reduction in absolute count or relative percentage of neutrophils, the synovial fluid may still contain increased numbers of mononuclear cells and neutrophils. Without recognition of these changes, therapy reduction may be precipitous. Two possible consequences of early reduction of treatment are recurrence of the disease and unnecessary subjection of the patient to more potent drugs or prolonged glucocorticoid therapy. Opposite assessment can occur when abnormalities in joint function persist, even though the immune disease is in remission. The most accurate method, therefore, to assess persistence of clinical signs is synovial fluid analysis. In patients with normal synovial analysis findings, comparison of serial radiographs can aid in determining the extent of joint dysfunction due to degenerative joint disease and ligamentous changes.

Treatment is modified or altered depending on whether the disease is in remission. Remission is described as the resolution of clinical abnormalities and the absence of inflammatory changes in the synovial fluid. Remission is observed within 2 to 4 weeks if prednisolone alone is to be a successful therapy. If remission has occurred, prednisolone dosage is reduced to half of the previous dosage for 2 weeks, and then to maintenance levels, approximately 1 mg/kg every other morning. Synovial volume diminishes during remission, making the obtainment of synovial fluid more difficult. If synovial fluid cannot be obtained, but the dog is clinically stable, prednisolone dosage can be safely reduced. In such cases, a hemogram can be done and evaluated for evidence of inflammation to assist in the determination of the clinical status of the patient. Any degree of inflammation in synovial fluid should be considered to indicate active disease and, therefore, medication should not be reduced or discontinued. If remission has been maintained, alternate-day therapy (1 mg/kg) should be continued for an additional 1 or 2 months and follow-up examinations extended to once a month. If complete remission has been maintained after this period of time, medication is discontinued.

Increased dosages of a glucocorticoid are not recommended if remission has not been achieved at the first 2-week re-examination. Prednisolone can be continued at the same previous dosage for 2 more weeks, or combination therapy consisting of prednisolone and cytotoxic drugs (alkylating and thiopurine agents) can be initiated. Combination therapy can also be used as the initial induction treatment, avoiding undesirable effects from high dosages of prednisolone. It may also be used when a more rapid improvement is desirable.

CYTOTOXIC AGENTS. Alkylating agents, cyclophosphamide (Cytoxin, Mead Johnson) and chlorambucil (Leukeran, Burroughs Wellcome) are the most potent immunosuppressive drugs available and, therefore, are preferred to the thiopurines. The dosage of cyclophosphamide is 50 mg/m² BSA given orally once daily on 4 consecutive days or on alternate days for a week. This would constitute one cycle of therapy. Chlorambucil is given orally at a dosage of 2 mg/m² BSA once daily. Chlorambucil may be as effective as cyclophosphamide in maintaning remission, although its efficacy in inducing remission has not been sufficiently evaluated. Thiopurines, azathioprine (Imuran, Burroughs Wellcome), and 6-mercaptopurine (6-MP) (Purinethol, Burroughs Wellcome) can be used for induction therapy, but remission may take longer than when alkylating agents are used. The thiopurines, although not as effective as the alkylating agents, are less toxic and are preferred for the few cases in which long-term therapy is necessary. The dosage for both azathioprine and 6-mercaptopurine is 50 mg/m² BSA given orally once daily. A glucocorticoid is administered simultaneously with cytotoxic drugs at the same dosage or at one half the dosage outlined previously.

Bone marrow toxicity is the most common adverse effect of the cytotoxic drugs. Bone marrow suppression with cyclophosphamide occurs after several months on therapy. At the prescribed dosage, thiopurines are infrequently associated with bone marrow suppression. Bone marrow suppression with azathioprine, if it occurs, appears in 3 to 6 weeks. Cytotoxic drugs, especially cyclophosphamide and chlorambucil, delay new hair growth in shaved areas (joints) and cause alopecia in some dogs (poodles, Kerry blue terriers). Dogs with pre-existent hepatic disease should not be given azathioprine or cyclophosphamide.

Azathioprine is cleaved by the liver to two molecules of 6-MP, the active metabolite. Cyclophosphamide requires conversion to its active metabolite by the liver, thus requiring adequate liver function also. A sterile hemorrhagic cystitis is a common sequela of chronic cyclophosphamide therapy. If cyclophosphamide is not used for longer than 3 or 4 months, the potential problems with sterile hemorrhagic cystitis are rare. In addition, observation should be directed toward early signs of cystitis (pollakiuria, stranguria, and dysuria), which often precede, by days or even weeks, the signs of hemorrhagic cystitis.

The treatment of the immune-mediated disorders, using combination immunosuppressive drugs, necessitates evaluation of complete blood cell counts, in addition to clinical signs and synovial fluid analysis. Complete blood cell counts are recommended every 2 weeks until complete remission is achieved. Occasionally, cytotoxic drugs, particularly cyclophosphamide, must be reduced or discontinued temporarily owing to bone marrow suppression, even though complete remission has not been achieved. Cytotoxic drugs are discontinued for a period of 1 week if the white blood cell count falls below 5000 cells/mm³ or if the neutrophil count falls below 2500 cells/mm³. If the WBC and neutrophil counts have improved, the cytotoxic drug should be reinstituted at one half of the original dosage.

Combined immunosuppressive therapy, at induction or highest tolerable dosage, is continued as long as there is active disease present and steady improvement is seen. The time period before remission is observed can range from 2 to 16 weeks, depending on whether alkylating agents or thiopurines are used in combination with prednisolone. The dosage for cyclophosphamide is not changed for maintenance therapy and is continued for at least 1 month following remission. However, chlorambucil, or one of the thiopurines, is given every other day at the dosage used for induction. The daily dosage of prednisolone is reduced by half during maintenance therapy until alternate-day treatment can be given (1 mg/kg). Glucocorticoids can usually be alternated with chlorambucil or thiopurines on consecutive days. If complete remission has been maintained at the end of 1 or 2 months, cytotoxic drugs are withdrawn. Prednisolone, at maintenance dosage, is continued for 2 to 3 more months. If complete remission is maintained after this time period, glucocorticoid is also withdrawn.

If abnormal joint fluid is detected or clinical signs reappear while on maintenance therapy, remission may be re-established by using combined immunosuppressive drug therapy. Abnormal joint fluid findings usually precede clinical signs and consist predominantly of mononuclear cells. Active disease or relapse is not excluded by finding fewer numbers of neutrophils than detected on initial presentation. The same cytotoxic drug previously used can be selected again for induction therapy. Therapy is adjusted, as previously described, except maintenance therapy of prednisolone and cytotoxic drugs is extended for 3 or 4 months following remission. If therapy is necessary for more than 5 months, chlorambucil, or one of the thiopurines, should be used. Neither drug is associated with sterile hemorrhagic cystitis and at alternate-day therapy is rarely associated with bone marrow suppression.

The prognosis for idiopathic polyarthritis is good. Glucocorticoid therapy alone can successfully induce remission in approximately 50 to 60 per cent of cases. Those patients not responding to glucocorticoid therapy usually respond favorably to combined immunosuppressive drug therapy. However, a small percentage (< 5 per cent) will be extremely difficult to treat. In all patients, recurrence of the disease is common (in 30 to 40 per cent of cases for a considerable period of time after drug therapy has been discontinued. Treatment for indefinite periods is necessary in about half of these patients with recurrent disease. The prognosis for SLE is variable, depending on the extent of systemic involvement. Dogs with SLE can often achieve long-term remission on alternate-day therapy of glucocorticoids, and some may achieve long-term remission on a drug-free basis. Prolonged therapy based on a positive ANA titer in a dog that has achieved remission is unsubstantiated. In human beings, SLE patients may be ANA positive and asymptomatic for long periods of time without drug therapy. The prognosis for plasmacytic-lymphocytic synovitis is favorable with proper surgical repair to stabilize the joint and with drug therapy to control the synovitis.

In conclusion, immune-mediated nonerosive arthritis occurs frequently and is not a single disease but includes a diverse group of diseases that have in common immune-mediated joint disease. Finally, arthrocentesis and joint fluid analysis are practical and essential for the diagnosis and treatment of immune-mediated arthritis.

References and Supplemental Reading

Bennett, D.: Naturally occurring models of inflammatory polyarthropathies in the domestic dog and cat. Br. J. Exp. Pathol. 40:3, 1986.

Bennett, D.: Immune-based erosive inflammatory joint disease of the dog; canine rheumatoid arthritis. J. Small Anim. Pract. 28:779, 1987.

Bennett, D., Gilbertson, E. M., and Grennen, B.: Bacterial endocarditis with polyarthritis in two dogs associated with circulating autoantibodies. J. Small Anim. Pract. 19:185, 1978.

Calvert, C. A., and Greene, C. E.: Bacteremia in dogs: Diagnosis, treatment, and prognosis. Compend. Cont. Ed. Pract. Vet. 8:179, 1986.

Center, S. A., Wilkinson, E., Smith, C. A., et al.: Twenty-four-hour urine protein/creatinine ratio in dogs with protein-losing nephropathies. J.A.V.M.A. 187:820, 1985.

Curtiss, P. H.: The pathophysiology of joint infections. Clin. Orthop. Rel. Res. 96:129, 1973.

Drazner, F. H.: Systemic lupus erythematosus in the dog. Comp. Cont. Ed. Pract. Vet. 2:243, 1980.

Giger, U., Werner, L. L., Millichamp, N. J., et al.: Sulfadiazine-induced allergy in six Doberman pinschers. J.A.V.M.A. 186:479, 1985.

Grindem, C. B., and Johnson, K. H.: Systemic lupus erythematosus, literature review and report of 42 new canine cases. J. Am. Anim. Hosp. Assoc. 19:489, 1983.

Hess, E. V. (ed.): Drug-induced lupus. Proceedings of the Kroc Foundation Conference. Arthritis Rheum. 24:979, 1981.

Newton, C. D., Lipowitz, A. J., Halliwell, R. E., et al.: Rheumatoid arthritis in dogs. J.A.V.M.A. 169:113, 1976.

Pedersen, N. C.: Synovial fluid collection and analysis. Vet. Clin. North Am. [Small Anim. Pract.] 8:495, 1978.

Pedersen, N. C., Pool, R., Castles, J. J., et al.: Noninfectious canine arthritis: Rheumatoid arthritis. J.A.V.M.A. 169:295, 1976a.

Pedersen, N. C., Weisner, K., Castles, J. J., et al.: Noninfectious canine arthritis: The inflammatory, nonerosive arthritides. J.A.V.M.A. 169:304, 1976b.

Pedersen, N. C., Pool, R. R., and Morgan, J. P.: Joint diseases of dogs and cats. In Ettinger, S. J. (ed.): Textbook of Veterinary Internal Medicine, 2nd ed. Philadelphia: W. B. Saunders, 1983, pp. 2187–2235.

Scott, D. W., Walton, D. K., Manning, T. O., et al.: Canine lupus erythematosus. I: Systemic lupus erythematosus. J. Am. Anim. Hosp. Assoc. 19:461, 1983.

Werner, L. L.: Arthrocentesis in joint fluid analysis: Diagnostic applications in joint diseases of small animals. Compend. Cont. Ed. Pract. Vet. 1:855, 1979.

Werner, L. L., and Bright, J. M.: Drug-induced immune hypersensitivity disorders in two dogs treated with trimethoprim-sulfadiazine: Case reports and drug challenge studies. J. Am. Anim. Hosp. Assoc. 19:783, 1983.

Section
5

DERMATOLOGIC
DISEASES

DANNY W. SCOTT, D.V.M.
Consulting Editor

Retinoids in Dermatology...553
Ivermectin in Small Animal Dermatology.................................560
Fatty Acid Supplements as Anti-inflammatory Agents.....................563
Nonsteroidal Anti-inflammatory Agents in the Management of
  Canine and Feline Pruritus 566
Immunomodulating Drugs in Dermatology 570
Imidazoles and Triazoles 577
Lasers in Dermatology..580
Miliary Dermatitis, Eosinophilic Granuloma Complex, and
  Symmetrical Hypotrichosis as Manifestations of Feline Allergy.........583
Fleas and Flea Control...586
RAST and ELISA Testing in Canine Atopy 592
Sex Hormone–Related Dermatoses in Dogs 595
Hormonal Replacement Therapy in Veterinary Dermatology 602
Familial Canine Dermatomyositis 606
Staphylococci and German Shepherd Pyoderma............................609
Lichenoid Dermatoses in Dogs and Cats.................................614
Dermatoses of the Nose and Footpads in Dogs and Cats..................616
Dermatoses of the Pinnae...621
Canine Cutaneous Histiocytoses...625
Feline Cutaneous Mast Cell Tumors 627
Disorders of Melanin Pigmentation in the Skin of Dogs and Cats 628
Sporotrichosis and Public Health.......................................633

RETINOIDS IN DERMATOLOGY

KENNETH W. KWOCHKA, D.V.M.

Columbus, Ohio

Over the past ten years, the retinoids have revolutionized treatment of a number of different dermatoses in human medicine. Potential uses for this exciting group of compounds in veterinary dermatology are just beginning to be explored. During the next several years, additional synthetic derivatives will become available with even greater potential efficacy for veterinary dermatoses.

The term "vitamin A" is now used not in reference to any one compound but to characterize the biologic activity of a group of compounds. The term "retinoids" refers to this entire group of compounds including retinol (vitamin A alcohol) and all the naturally occurring and synthetic derivatives. The three major naturally occurring compounds are retinol, retinal, and retinoic acid. Retinol is the most potent analogue, the main dietary source, and the main transport and storage form of vitamin A. Retinol is metabolized to retinal and retinoic acid. General functions of the retinoids include growth promotion, differentiation and maintenance of epithelial tissue, and maintenance of normal reproductive and visual functions (Peck and DiGiovanna, 1987).

The importance of vitamin A for the maintenance of normal skin was first discovered in the 1920's. Epithelial changes due to abnormal keratinization were identified in vitamin A–deficient animals. This led to the use of high doses of oral vitamin A and topical vitamin A for a number of different dermatoses involving keratinization abnormalities. The potential importance of vitamin A in chemoprevention of cancer was also realized in the 1920's, when rats being fed vitamin A–deficient diets developed carcinomas of the stomach.

Naturally occurring retinoids and their metabolites have been useful in treating various dermatoses and neoplasms for a number of years. In the last 20 years, many retinoid derivatives have been synthesized and tested to develop compounds with a better therapeutic index and less toxicity than naturally occurring retinoids. Most of this work has been done with compounds targeted at cancer treatment and prophylaxis. Ironically, the two most successful synthetic retinoids that are now commercially available are used for dermatoses and not cancer therapy or chemoprevention. Isotretinoin (Accutane, Roche), 13-*cis*-retinoic acid, is efficacious in severe recalcitrant cystic acne, Darier's disease, pityriasis rubra pilaris, and other disorders of keratinization. Etretinate (Tegison, Roche), the trimethylmethoxyphenyl analogue of retinoic acid ethyl ester, is used for psoriasis, lamellar ichthyosis and, other disorders of keratinization.

PHARMAKOKINETICS

The naturally occurring retinoids are derived from dietary precursors of animal and vegetable origin. Retinyl esters are obtained from animal fats and fish liver oils, while the beta-carotene precursor comes from yellow and green leafy vegetables. Retinyl esters are hydrolyzed in the digestive tract to retinol, which is absorbed into the mucosal cells. Beta-carotene undergoes oxidative cleavage to retinal, which is reduced to retinol in the intestinal mucosa. Retinol is then esterified, complexed with long-chain fatty acids into chylomicrons, and transported to the liver via the lymphatics and the blood. Retinol is stored in the liver as retinyl ester in Ito's cells.

When needed, retinol is released from the liver in a 1:1 ratio with serum retinol-binding protein (RBP), which is synthesized in the liver. This complex, in turn, binds to a serum prealbumin protein, termed transthyretin (TTR), which also binds thyroxine but at a different binding site.

The RBP-retinol-TTR complex circulates in the blood until RBP-retinol binds to a membrane receptor on the target cell. Retinol is translocated into the cell and binds to a specific cytosol-binding protein, called cellular retinol-binding protein (CRBP). Translocation to the nucleus is then thought to occur with another receptor protein facilitating the hormone action. Retinoic acid has its own distinct cellular binding protein (CRABP). At the molecular level, the retinoid may affect RNA synthesis, protein synthesis, post-translational glycosylation of protein, prostaglandin synthesis, labilization of membranes, and the effects of enzymes such as ornithine decarboxylase. These effects explain the ability of retinoids to affect cellular proliferation, differentiation, and surface composition. In their direct action on the cell genome, retinoids appear to be similar to steroid hormones.

MECHANISMS OF ACTION

Retinoids have a variety of biologic effects that result in their usefulness for treatment of various dermatoses and neoplasms. Vitamin A compounds have profound effects on cell proliferation and differentiation, especially of keratinizing epithelia. Vitamin A deficiency is associated with inhibition of cell proliferation and growth. However, the same effect can be seen in cultured cells when excess amounts of retinoids are added. Thus, maintenance of normal epithelia requires the correct concentration of retinoids.

Retinoids also have the ability to control malignant transformation in certain tissues. Vitamin A deficiency may lead to squamous metaplasia of a variety of epithelia, a premalignant condition. Naturally occurring retinoids have been shown to protect animals against skin papillomas and carcinomas of the skin and other organs. Retinoids suppress malignant transformation in vitro caused by chemical carcinogens, ionizing radiation, growth factors, and viruses. In most cases, retinoids interfere with the promotion phase of carcinogenesis. They appear to act better as chemopreventive agents than as therapeutic agents.

Another mechanism of the antiproliferative effects of retinoids may be their ability to block the cell cycle in the G-1 phase and thus inhibit the ornithine decarboxylase induction necessary for cell cycle progression.

Retinoids may elicit some of their effects through the immune system. They are generally thought to stimulate humoral and cellular immunity, but, depending upon the retinoid and dosage, inhibition may be observed. Some of the antitumor effects are thought to be due to the immunostimulatory effects, resulting in their use as adjuvant therapy for cancer patients.

Additional retinoid effects may result from actions on cell membranes. At lower doses, retinoids appear to stabilize cell membranes, whereas at higher doses, they have a detergentlike effect that leads to labilization of lysosomal membranes, with enzyme release and toxicity. It has been demonstrated that gap junctions increase in number in neoplastic and embryonic keratinizing epithelia in response to retinoids. This may lead to better cell-to-cell communication and better control of tissue organization and growth.

CLINICAL APPLICATIONS

Isotretinoin has revolutionized treatment of severe recalcitrant cystic acne in humans. Efficacy in cystic acne and other follicular diseases is primarily due to inhibition of sebum production, with alterations in the skin surface lipid film. In fact, isotretinoin is the most effective inhibitor of sebum production known at this time. Histologically, sebaceous glands virtually disappear during therapy, and partial sebaceous gland inhibition remains for a prolonged period even after discontinuation of therapy.

The sebaceous gland and the follicular effects of 13-cis-retinoic acid have prompted interest in this compound for use in veterinary diseases in which there are suspected or confirmed abnormalities in sebaceous gland activity or follicular keratinization such as primary idiopathic seborrhea and comedo syndromes.

Etretinate is the synthetic retinoid of value as primary or adjunctive treatment of psoriasis, a hyperproliferative epidermal disorder. Both isotretinoin and etretinate have demonstrated efficacy for disorders of keratinization including Darier's disease, lamellar ichthyosis, nonbullous congenital ichthyosiform erythroderma, and pityriasis rubra pilaris. Both drugs have been shown to be effective adjunctive therapy for chronic actinic dermatitis, nevoid basal cell carcinoma syndrome, xeroderma pigmentosum, multiple keratoacanthomas, oral leukoplakia, cutaneous metastasis of malignant melanoma, and cutaneous T-cell lymphoma.

Based on the evidence from human clinical studies, most of the interest in utilizing these drugs in veterinary dermatoses has been for their potential usefulness in suspected or confirmed disorders of keratinization, abnormalities in follicular keratinization, and abnormalities in quantitative or qualitative secretions of the sebaceous glands. Only a limited number of cases have been reported in the veterinary literature, although many clinicians have made unpublished observations over the last several months (Table 1).

Vitamin A–responsive Dermatosis in Cocker Spaniels

This condition has been described in seven cocker spaniels (Scott, 1986; Ihrke and Goldschmidt, 1983). It is a nutritionally responsive disorder and does not represent a true dietary deficiency of vitamin A. It may represent a local vitamin A deficiency, a problem with uptake in the skin, or a problem with cutaneous utilization. Clinically, the dermatosis has been characterized by refractory seborrheic skin disease, with marked follicular plugging and hyperkeratotic plaques with surface "frondlike" plugs from the follicles. These lesions were present primarily on the ventral and lateral thorax and abdomen. Histologically, the abnormalities were very distinct and dramatic, consisting of marked orthokeratotic hyperkeratosis and dilation of hair follicles, mild orthokeratotic hyperkeratosis of the epidermis, and mild, irregular epidermal hyperplasia. In humans, this pattern of extreme follicular hyperkeratosis is known as phrynoderma and is consistent with dietary deficiency of vitamin A. This finding prompted treatment of the disorder with vitamin A

Table 1. *Reports of Oral Retinoid Therapy in Veterinary Dermatology and Cutaneous Oncology*

Retinoid	Disease	Dosage	Species or Breed	No. of Animals	Result	Side Effects (No.)	Time on Retinoid*	Reference
Retinol (Vitamin A alcohol)	Vitamin A–responsive dermatosis (phrynoderma-like)	625 IU/kg every 24 hr PO	Cocker spaniel	2 Black, 2 blonde, 1 chocolate	Excellent	None	6 mo–2 yr	Scott, 1986
		800 IU/kg every 24 hr PO	Cocker spaniel Miniature schnauzer	2 Black 1	Excellent	None	1–4.5 yr	Ihrke and Gold-schmidt, 1983
		50,000 IU, total dose, every 12 hr PO for 2 mo; then every 24 hr for maintenance	Labrador retriever	1	Excellent	None	2 yr	Parker et al., 1983
	Seborrheic dermatitis (unlike phrynoderma)	800 IU/kg every 24 hr PO	Cocker spaniel Canine	4 3	Poor	None	12–16 wk	Ihrke and Gold-schmidt, 1983
Isotretinoin (13–cis-retinoic acid)	Granulomatous sebaceous adenitis	1 mg/kg every 24 hr PO	Visla Labrador retriever mix	1 1	Excellent	None	2 mo	Stewart, personal communication, 1988
	Schnauzer comedo syndrome	1 mg/kg every 24 hr PO	Miniature schnauzer	1	Excellent	None	Unknown	Scott, personal communication, 1988
		1–2 mg/kg every 24 hr PO	Miniature schnauzer	3	Excellent	None	Unknown	Breen, personal communication, 1988
	Epidermal dysplasia	1 mg/kg every 12 hr PO	West Highland white terrier	2	Poor	None	2 mo	Scott, personal communication, 1988
	Congenital lamellar ichthyosis	1 mg/kg every 12 hr PO	American pit bull terrier	1	Excellent	None	2 mo	Scott, personal communication, 1988
			West Highland white terrier	1	Excellent	None	Unknown	Miller, personal communication, 1988
	Idiopathic seborrhea	1 mg/kg every 24 hr PO	Brittany spaniel	1	Good	None	1 mo†	DeBoer, personal communication, 1988
		3 mg/kg every 24 hr PO	Cocker spaniel	5	Poor	Conjunctivitis (2), hyperactivity (1), ear pruritus (1)	2 mo	Fadok, 1986‡
			Alaskan malamute	1	Poor		2 mo	
			Pekingese-poodle cross	1	Poor		2 mo	
			Poodle	1	Excellent	Transient erythema of mucocutaneous junctions and feet	2 mo	
		1 mg/kg every 12 hr PO	Cocker spaniel	4	Poor	Conjunctivitis (2); lethargy, vomiting, abdominal distention, abdominal erythema (1); transient liver enzyme elevation (1)	5 mo	Kwochka, K.W., unpublished observations, 1984
		0.25 mg/kg every 12 hr PO	Cocker spaniel	1	Excellent	None	4 wk	Bates, 1984
	Multiple epidermal inclusion cysts	1 mg/kg every 24 hr PO	Canine	2	Subjective decrease in incidence of new lesions in one dog	None	Unknown	DeBoer, personal communication, 1988

Table continued on following page

Table 1. *Reports of Oral Retinoid Therapy in Veterinary Dermatology and Cutaneous Oncology*
Continued

Retinoid	Disease	Dosage	Species or Breed	No. of Animals	Result	Side Effects (No.)	Time on Retinoid*	Reference
	Multiple kerato-acanthomas	2 mg/kg every 24 hr PO	Norwegian elk-hound	1	Excellent	None	Unknown	Breen, personal communication, 1988
	Cutaneous epidermotrophic lymphoma	1 mg/kg every 12 hr PO	Canine	1	Poor	None	Unknown	Miller, personal communication, 1988
		1 mg/kg every 12 hr PO, and 0.25 mg/kg prednisone, every 12 hr PO for 6 wk; then every 24 hr for maintenance	Canine	1	Excellent	Anorexia, lethargy, collapse, swollen tongue§	9 mo	Rosser, personal communication, 1988
		10 mg, total dose, every 24 hr PO for 6 wk; then every 24 hr for maintenance	Feline	3	Good	Diarrhea (1)	6–18 mo	Griffin and Rosenkrantz, personal communication, 1988
	Squamous cell carcinoma and epidermal dysplasia	3 mg/kg every 24 hr PO	Feline	10	Poor	Periocular erythema (6), periocular crusting (6), epiphora (4), blepharospasm (1)	37–162 days	Evans et al., 1985
Etretinate (trimethylmethoxyphenyl analogue of retinoic acid ethyl ester)	Idiopathic seborrhea	1 mg/kg every 24 hr PO	Cocker spaniel	1	Poor	None	Unknown	Evans, personal communication, 1988

*Duration of therapy at time of writing, or time on retinoid before discontinuation of treatment.
†Died of unrelated causes after 1 month.
‡Additional clinical pathologic abnormalities included increased platelet count (1), hypertriglyceridemia (3), hypercholesterolemia (2), increased alanine aminotransferase (2).
§Not determined if related to the drug.

(retinol, various manufacturers) at a dosage of 10,000 IU every 24 hr PO. In all dogs, marked improvement was seen within 2 to 3 weeks, with complete clinical remission by 10 weeks. Follow-ups of 6 months to 4.5 years were reported, with continued remission and no obvious side effects. The retinol dosage was decreased to 5000 IU every 24 hr PO in two of the dogs, and a generic formulation was used in another patient, resulting in exacerbation of symptoms. These were quickly brought back under control with administration of initial therapy. Thus, it appears that continual treatment is needed for life.

It is important to understand that this syndrome has very distinct clinical signs and histopathology and does not represent all cases of cocker spaniel seborrhea or idiopathic seborrhea in other breeds. The follicular hyperkeratosis is much more severe than that seen in typical seborrhea. Seven dogs (four cocker spaniels) with seborrheic dermatitis but without the severe histopathologic change of follicular hyperkeratosis were treated with oral vitamin A at the same dosage for 12 to 16 weeks with no improvement. The diagnosis should be confirmed by biopsy, other causes of metabolic seborrhea should be considered, and other antiseborrheic therapy should be employed prior to the use of vitamin A. The same condition has also been seen in a miniature schnauzer that responded to the same therapy (Ihrke and Goldschmidt, 1983).

Other Seborrheic Syndromes

A 6-month-old male Labrador retriever with severe generalized crusting, small cutaneous nodules, and mild pruritus beginning at 2 months of age was reported to respond well to retinol therapy (Parker et al., 1983). The animal was on a good commercial diet and had shown no improvement with antibiotics, steroids, or shampoos. This dog did not have the hyperkeratotic plaquelike lesions reported for the cocker spaniels but did have severe parakeratotic and orthokeratotic hyperkeratosis of the follicular infundibulum (lamellated comedones) and surface epithelium on histologic examination. In addition, there were epidermal abnormalities consistent with faulty keratinization, dilated apocrine sweat glands, and hypertrophied sebaceous glands. The dog was treated with 50,000 IU of retinol every 12 hr PO, decreased to every 24 hr after 2 months. Clinical improvement was seen after 5 weeks, with complete resolution by 6 months. The dog had been normal for 2 years without signs of toxicity at the time of writing. Lowering of the dosage resulted in reappearance of lesions. Serum vitamin A and zinc levels were normal in this dog, again suggesting a vitamin A–responsive dermatosis rather than a nutritional deficiency.

Since the synthetic retinoid, isotretinoin, has demonstrated beneficial effects on sebaceous gland abnormalities and keratinization disorders in humans, it seemed logical to utilize this compound for idiopathic seborrheic syndromes in dogs. Fadok (1986) treated eight dogs with idiopathic seborrhea with isotretinoin at a dosage of 3 mg/kg every 24 hr PO for 2 months in a double-blinded, placebo-controlled, crossover study. Only one dog showed 100 per cent improvement, with relapse after discontinuation of therapy, no response to vitamin A alcohol (25,000 IU every 24 hr PO for 2 months), and improvement with readministration of isotretinoin. Three additional dogs showed less than 50 per cent improvement. Although these dogs did not have the hyperkeratotic plaquelike lesions clinically, seven of the eight had severe follicular hyperkeratosis histologically. No histologic improvement in the degree of hyperkeratosis or follicular keratosis was demonstrated after therapy, even in the one dog that responded clinically.

Four cocker spaniels with idiopathic seborrhea were treated by the author with isotretinoin at 1 mg/kg every 12 hr PO for 5 months. Only one dog showed slightly decreased scale production while on therapy. There was no improvement in post-treatment skin biopsies. Epidermal cell migration rates were also measured. While these cocker spaniels had epidermal cells proliferating at twice the rate of normal cocker spaniels, there was no improvement seen during or after therapy.

In spite of these treatment failures, other breeds and various dosages of isotretinoin should be studied. One cocker spaniel with idiopathic seborrhea was reported to respond to this drug at 0.25 mg/kg every 12 hr PO for 4 weeks (Bates, 1984). No adverse reactions were seen, and the dog did not respond to vitamin A prior to isotretinoin usage. DeBoer (personal communication, 1988) has indicated successful treatment of a Brittany spaniel with idiopathic seborrhea with isotretinoin at 1 mg/kg every 24 hr PO. Noticeable clinical response was obtained after 1 month. Unfortunately, no long-term follow-up is available, since the dog died of causes unrelated to the drug or skin disease.

Scott (personal communication, 1988) has indicated poor response using isotretinoin, 1 mg/kg every 12 hr PO, in 2 West Highland white terriers

with greasy seborrhea characterized histologically by epidermal dysplasia.

Etretinate has not been utilized extensively for idiopathic seborrhea. There is a considerable degree of excitement over this compound, since it has profound beneficial effects on a hyperproliferative epidermal disorder in humans, psoriasis. Like psoriasis, idiopathic seborrhea, at least in the cocker spaniel, is partially characterized by a hyperproliferative epidermis. Toxicity studies indicate that etretinate may be safer to use in dogs than is isotretinoin. Evans (personal communication, 1988) has reported lack of response in a male cocker spaniel with idiopathic seborrhea at a dosage of 1 mg/kg every 24 hr PO. More work will be needed to establish an optimal dose in the dog.

Localized Keratinization Abnormalities

In general, the systemic retinoids would not be considered practical for localized follicular or epidermal keratinization disorders because of their cost. However, topical 0.05 per cent tretinoin (*trans*-retinoic acid) (Retin-A, Ortho) may be useful in these cases. Chin acne in dogs and cats is most probably due to a follicular keratinization disorder, with comedo formation and secondary bacterial folliculitis. Topical tretinoin has been used successfully to manage some of these patients (Breen, personal communication, 1988). Daily application to the affected area is recommended until remission, followed by a decrease in frequency for maintenance. Benzoyl peroxide washes (OxyDex Shampoo, DVM; Pyoben Shampoo, Allerderm) have been used concurrently. Allergic or irritant cutaneous reactions may occasionally be a problem, especially in cats. Tretinoin is available in lower concentrations (0.025 per cent and 0.01 per cent) in gel formulations for these patients. Since tretinoin increases epidermal turnover rate and reduces cohesion of keratinocytes, it may be useful in other localized hyperkeratotic scaling disorders. It is reported to be effective when used concurrently with topical emollients for calluses and idiopathic nasal hyperkeratosis (Moriello, personal communication, 1988). The author has also found tretinoin useful when alternated with topical steroids in severely lichenified lesions such as those associated with acanthosis nigricans.

Lamellar Ichthyosis

This rare hereditary congenital disorder of dogs, primarily seen in terrier breeds, is characterized clinically by tightly adhering, verrucous, tannish-gray scales and feathered keratinous projections on all or large portions of the skin. Skin biopsy reveals extreme orthokeratotic hyperkeratosis, follicular keratosis and plugging, a prominent granular layer, and many mitotic figures. This disease in a West Highland white terrier (Miller, personal communication, 1988) and an American pit bull terrier (Scott, personal communication, 1988) has been successfully managed with isotretinoin, 1 mg/kg every 12 hr PO, after a period of 8 weeks. Unfortunately, follow-ups are not available, since cost of the drug precluded long-term management and at least one dog was eventually euthanized.

Schnauzer Comedo Syndrome

Schnauzer comedo syndrome is a seborrheic disorder of certain predisposed miniature schnauzers. It is characterized by multiple comedones along the back that present as follicular papular lesions. Clinical management is usually successfully achieved with topical antiseborrheic agents or the follicular flushing agent, benzoyl peroxide. However, severe refractory cases occur that do not respond to topical therapy. Also, continual topical therapy may not be practical for all clients. Four schnauzers have been managed successfully using isotretinoin at doses ranging from 1 to 2 mg/kg every 24 hr PO (Breen, Scott, personal communications, 1988). Rapid response was seen within 3 to 4 weeks. In three of these dogs, no hematologic or liver enzyme abnormalities were seen while they were on therapy. These three dogs relapsed with comedones when therapy was discontinued and were again brought into remission with isotretinoin.

Sebaceous Adenitis

Sebaceous adenitis is a dermatosis characterized by severe, localized or generalized seborrhea sicca and granulomatous inflammation with destruction of sebaceous glands. A Visla and a Labrador retriever mix with granulomatous sebaceous adenitis have recently been successfully treated with isotretinoin (Stewart, personal communication, 1988). The drug, given at 1 mg/kg every 24 hr PO, resulted in rapid clinical response over a 2-month period. Recurrence of lesions was noted when alternate day therapy was instituted in one of the dogs. No side effects of the medication have been noted.

Epidermal Inclusion Cysts

Multiple epidermal inclusion cysts can be a frustrating problem in certain individual dogs, requiring frequent use of antibiotics, surgical drainage, and surgical removal. Since these lesions are thought to result from, at least in part, occluded pilosebaceous follicles, there is some indication that retinoids may be useful in clinical management. Two dogs with multiple epidermal inclusion cysts have been treated with isotretinoin at 1 mg/kg every 24 hr PO (DeBoer, personal communication, 1988). There was no regression of existing lesions. However, one dog subjectively appeared to develop fewer new lesions while on therapy.

Cutaneous Neoplastic Disorders

There has been no work exploring the use of retinoids as chemopreventive agents in dogs and cats. However, the use of these compounds in chemotherapy has been studied in a small number of cases.

The most complete work has been done with squamous cell carcinoma and preneoplastic (epidermal dysplasia) lesions on the heads of cats (Evans et al., 1985). Ten cats with 15 lesions were treated with isotretinoin at an average dosage of 3 mg/kg every 24 hr PO, for an average of 68 days. Based upon clinical and histologic observations, only one of the 15 lesions showed partial clinical and histologic improvement.

Isotretinoin may be effective primary or adjunctive therapy for the control of mycosis fungoides in dogs and cats. One dog that presented with 12 to 15 plaque and ulcerative lesions was brought into complete clinical remission within 4 weeks with prednisone, 0.25 mg/kg every 12 hr PO, and isotretinoin, 1 mg/kg every 12 hr PO (Rosser, personal communication, 1988). This dog had no clinical or clinical pathologic signs of internal disease. After approximately 6 weeks, the dog developed lethargy, anorexia, collapse, and a swollen tongue. The animal was not presented to the clinician until 7 days after this incident, at which time it was clinically normal with normal laboratory values. Isotretinoin was reinstituted at 1 mg/kg every 24 hr PO. The dog has been in clinical remission for 9 months at the time of this writing. No prednisolone has been administered for the last 3 months.

Three cats with cutaneous epitheliotrophic lymphoma have been treated with isotretinoin at a total dose of 10 mg every 24 hr PO (Griffin and Rosenkrantz, personal communication, 1988). All cats showed a good clinical response, with a reduction in erythema and scaling and with abundant new hair growth. There was some improvement in biopsy findings, but evidence of the epitheliotrophic neoplasia remained. Although complete remission could never be achieved, the cats were able to lead more comfortable lives while on therapy. Survival time in the three cats ranged from 6 to 18 months. Diarrhea was a side effect in one of the three cats.

Although quality of life was improved while the animals were on therapy, it is not known whether isotretinoin alters the time of remission prior to the development of systemic lymphoma and death.

RETINOID TOXICITY

In humans, numerous adverse clinical conditions have been associated with retinoid usage, including cheilitis, inflammation and xerosis of the skin, pruritus, facial dermatitis, dryness of mucous membranes, epistaxis, thinning of the hair, palmoplantar desquamation, conjunctivitis, headache, ataxia, lethargy and fatigue, psychologic changes, and visual disturbances. Other abnormalities may include transient minor elevations in liver enzymes that return to normal even with continuation of therapy, hyperlipidemia, increased platelet count, hypercalcemia, arthralgias, photosensitivity, and teratogenicity. Teratogenicity is a serious problem in a high percentage of women who take isotretinoin during pregnancy. Abnormalities have included spontaneous abortions or children with birth defects including hydrocephalus, deformed external ears, and cardiac abnormalities. Chronic hypervitaminosis A has been associated with demineralization, thinning of the long bones, cortical hyperostosis, periostitis, and premature closure of the epiphyses.

In the nine dogs (Table 1) treated with retinol at dosages of 10,000 IU every 24 hr PO (cocker spaniels and a miniature schnauzer), to 50,000 IU every 24 hr PO (a Labrador retriever), for periods ranging from 6 months to 4.5 years, there have been no adverse effects reported. Retinol appears to be well-tolerated in dogs.

Of the 29 dogs treated with isotretinoin in this review (Table 1), the incidence and severity of side effects appear to be low. However, this may be somewhat misleading, since most patients have been treated only for short periods of time and clinical pathologic evaluations have not been performed in many patients. Four dogs have developed conjunctivitis, which was reversible upon discontinuation of therapy. Other clinical abnormalities seen in single cases include hyperactivity; ear pruritus; erythema of mucocutaneous junctions and feet; lethargy with vomiting, abdominal distention and erythema; and anorexia with lethargy, collapse, and a swollen tongue. All these abnormalities were reversible or transient upon discontinuation of therapy. One patient had an increased platelet count, three had hypertriglyceridemia, two had hypercholesterolemia, and three had transient elevations in alanine aminotransferase.

A higher incidence of clinical abnormalities has been seen in the 13 cats treated with isotretinoin. Six developed periocular erythema, six periocular crusting, four epiphora, one blepharospasm, and one diarrhea. Clinical pathologic evaluations were not reported.

Etretinate has not been utilized in a sufficient number of clinical cases to comment on toxicity. Toxicity studies from the manufacturer suggest that in dogs it may be less toxic than isotretinoin.

CONCLUSION

It is difficult to make definitive recommendations on the use of natural and synthetic retinoids in veterinary dermatoses, since this mode of therapy is still relatively new and small numbers of patients have been treated. From our current knowledge of the types of diseases against which retinoids have been effective in human and veterinary dermatology, it seems most rational to reserve these drugs for cases with clinical and histologic abnormalities most consistent with disorderly keratinization of either or both the surface and follicular epithelia. Other causes of clinical scaling (ectoparasitism, allergies, infections, endocrinopathies) should first be eliminated from the list of differential diagnoses.

The synthetic retinoids, etretinate and isotretinoin, may be prohibitively expensive for many clients. Therefore, other forms of therapy such as topical therapy should first be employed before considering a retinoid. Since natural vitamin A alcohol (retinol) is less expensive than the synthetics and appears to be well-tolerated in the dog, it should be considered prior to using isotretinoin or etretinate for a nonspecific epidermal scaling disorder.

Best response has been seen with phrynoderma-like vitamin A–responsive dermatosis (retinol), granulomatous sebaceous adenitis (isotretinoin), schnauzer comedo syndrome (isotretinoin), and congenital lamellar ichthyosis (isotretinoin). In cutaneous oncology, there is some indication of efficacy of isotretinoin as primary or adjunctive therapy for cutaneous epidermotrophic lymphoma in the dog and cat. Treatment should be continued for 8 to 12 weeks before a determination of efficacy is made in most keratinization disorders.

The retinoids should not be used in breeding animals because of potential teratogenicity and inhibition of spermatogenesis. While the animal is receiving therapy, blood work should be monitored, especially lipid values and liver enzymes. Radiographic evaluation for bony changes should be considered in patients being administered long-term treatment.

References and Supplemental Reading

Bates, J. R.: Treatment of idiopathic seborrhea in a dog. Mod. Vet. Pract. 65:725, 1984.

Evans, A. G., Madewell, B. R., and Stannard, A. A.: A trial of 13-cis-retinoic acid for treatment of squamous cell carcinoma and preneoplastic lesions of the head in cats. Am. J. Vet. Res. 46:2553, 1985.

Fadok, V. A.: Treatment of canine idiopathic seborrhea with isotretinoin. Am. J. Vet. Res. 47:1730, 1986.

Ihrke, P. J., and Goldschmidt, M. H.: Vitamin A–responsive dermatosis in the dog. J.A.V.M.A. 182:687, 1983.

Parker, W., Yager-Johnson, J. A., and Hardy, M. H.: Vitamin A–responsive seborrheic dermatosis in the dog: A case report. J. Am.

Anim. Hosp. Assoc. 19:548, 1983.

Peck, G. L., and DiGiovanna, J. J.: Retinoids. In Fitzpatrick, T. B., Eisen, A. Z., Wolff, K., et al. (eds.): Dermatology in General Medicine, 3rd. ed. New York: McGraw-Hill Book Co., 1987, pp. 2582–2609.

Scott, D. W.: Vitamin A–responsive dermatosis in the cocker spaniel. J. Am. Anim. Hosp. Assoc. 22:125, 1986.

IVERMECTIN IN SMALL ANIMAL DERMATOLOGY

MANON PARADIS, D.V.M.

St. Hyacinthe, Quebec

The avermectins constitute a new class of chemicals that have a novel mode of action against a broad spectrum of nematode and arthropod parasites of animals. Avermectins appear to be the most potent broad-spectrum antiparasitic agents yet discovered. Ivermectin is the 22, 23-dihydro derivative of avermectin B_1, a macrocyclic lactone produced by an actinomycete, *Streptomyces avermitilis*, which was first isolated from soil in Japan. Research on ivermectin and its precursors has been carried out since 1975. Ivermectin was selected for development because of its superior anthelmintic efficacy. In addition, ivermectin has been shown to possess a wide range of insecticidal activity. This discovery was so significant that it was used in the generic name of this new family of compounds: "anti*vermes*" and "anti*ecto* parasites," hence the generic name avermectins.

Ivermectin was introduced commercially on the international market in 1981 and was licensed in the United States in 1983. It is now used commercially in various countries for the treatment and control of endoparasites and ectoparasites. In cattle and swine, ivermectin (10 mg/ml) (Ivomec, Merck) is administered by injection. In horses, ivermectin is available in an oral paste (18.7 mg/ml) (Eqvalan, Merck). An oral drench (0.8 mg/ml) is used for sheep (Ivomec, Merck). Ivermectin is now available for use in dogs for the prevention of heartworm disease (Heartguard tablets, Merck; 68, 136, 272 μg of ivermectin).

PHARMACOLOGY

Ivermectin is believed to act on susceptible nematodes and arthropods by increasing the release and binding of gamma-aminobutyric acid (GABA) in nerve synapses in certain areas of the brain, thus blocking GABA-mediated transmission of nerve signals. This blockage results in the nonfunction of muscle cells and, for many parasites, paralysis and death.

The preparations most commonly used in dogs and cats are the bovine and the ovine dosage forms. The bovine injectable product (Ivomec, Merck) is a 1 per cent solution (10,000 μg/ml) that can be given subcutaneously or orally. It can easily be diluted with propylene glycol for accurate doses in very small animals. The oral drench for sheep (800 μg/ml) must be given orally. Syringes can be prepared and dispensed to the owner for oral administration. Ivermectin is sensitive to ultraviolet light and should be stored in the dark (or dispensed in a brown paper bag) to prolong its shelf life.

SAFETY

One major difference exists between invertebrates and mammals as regards GABA-mediated nerve synapses. In mammals, these synapses are present only in the central nervous system, whereas in many invertebrates, such nerve synapses regulate peripheral muscle activity. Thus, ivermectin, which acts only on GABA-mediated nerve synapses, should have a wide margin of safety in mammals as it does not readily cross the blood-brain barrier. In theory, there may be a risk when it is used in animals with disorders of the central nervous system. Ivermectin has no teratogenic effects in the domestic species studied.

Ivermectin appears to have a very wide safety margin in target species. At least ten times the therapeutic dose is required to produce adverse reactions related to the action of GABA. In dogs, mydriasis and tremors were seen at 5000 μg/kg, and more pronounced tremors and ataxia were recorded at 10,000 μg/kg. In beagles, the approxi-

---

Editor's Note: Extra-label use of ivermectin outlined in this article is *not approved* by the FDA for use in the United States.

mate median lethal dose (LD$_{50}$) was found to be 80,000 μg/kg (80 mg/kg).

Collies are particularly susceptible to ivermectin toxicity. Breed idiosyncrasy may be involved. One study (Pulliam et al., 1985) was designed to determine whether ivermectin was toxic in collies at doses generally not toxic in other breeds of dogs, and whether or not the collie eye anomaly (CEA) was related to ivermectin sensitivity. Because CEA involves developmental defects in several parts of the eye, including the optic disk, it may also involve a functional anomaly of the blood-brain barrier. The results of this study indicated greater penetration of ivermectin through the blood-brain barrier in this breed. Adverse reactions, often fatal, were encountered in collies receiving doses (200 to 600 μg/kg) generally not toxic in other breeds. However, no relation was established between the CEA and toxic reactions to ivermectin in this breed.

Another study (Paul et al., 1987) demonstrated that collies have a variable sensitivity to ivermectin toxicity. Approximately 50 per cent of these dogs developed signs of toxicity at doses generally not toxic in other breeds. In addition, some of the collies sensitive to toxicity showed no signs of toxicity after receiving an oral dose of 100 μg/kg but developed severe signs of toxicity with 200 μg/kg.

The results of these studies do not preclude the possibility that individual dogs other than collies could show signs of toxicity after receiving relatively low doses of ivermectin. In fact, ivermectin toxicoses have been reported in collie crosses as well as in other breeds. However, the possibility of overdose was not excluded in all of these cases. To the author's knowledge, no such toxic reactions have been reported in cats.

There is no known specific antidote for ivermectin intoxication. There is evidence that in ascarids and lobster muscle, picrotoxin blocks or reverses the effects of ivermectin (at least in vitro). However, no evidence supporting this phenomenon exists for mammals. Supportive therapy is indicated, and several dogs severely depressed and even comatose after ivermectin administration made a complete recovery following several days of treatment of symptoms.

In addition to breed idiosyncrasy encountered in collies (such idiosyncrasy most probably exists in other breeds), anaphylactoid reactions attributable to polysorbate 80, a micelle vehicle present in the equine injectable formulation, have been described in dogs. That formulation was withdrawn from the market in 1984.

Another side effect occasionally encountered with ivermectin is associated with the rapid destruction of microfilariae. Ivermectin is highly effective against the microfilariae of Dirofilaria immitis in dogs. However, adverse reactions have been recorded in up to 5 per cent of the dogs treated. Most

reactions occur within 1 to 4 hr and are usually of a mild nature. Vomiting, trembling, tachypnea, and collapse occasionally develop. When evidence of shock is present, intravenous fluid therapy and glucocorticoids are indicated. Fatalities are rare when careful observation and appropriate therapy are provided. Acute reactions are most common when microfilaria counts are relatively high. For this reason, the author suggests that dogs in endemic areas be tested for heartworm infestation prior to treatment with ivermectin if a dose of 50 μg or more is to be given.

Even at high doses, ivermectin is inactive against the adult stage of D. immitis in dogs. Thus, the use of ivermectin as an antiparasitic agent in dogs would not be expected to result in the inadvertent destruction of adult heartworms, with the attendant risk of pulmonary embolism.

CLINICAL APPLICATIONS

Ivermectin is now licensed for heartworm prevention in dogs, at a recommended dose of 5 to 7 μg/kg once a month (this preventive treatment is safe for use in collies). However, ivermectin is not approved for the treatment of microfilariae (minimum dose, 50 μg/kg) or of endoparasites and ectoparasites (minimum dose, 200 μg/kg) in dogs and cats. Attempts have been made to warn veterinarians that some dogs (particularly collies) are abnormally sensitive to ivermectin and that unfortunate consequences are possible. If, in spite of these warnings, one elects to use ivermectin developed for another species and not licensed for dermatologic purposes in dogs and cats, the following information can be used as a "guideline." *Prior to such "extra-label" usage, it is imperative that the risks and benefits be explained to the client and that the veterinarian have the owner of the animal sign a release form.*

Canine Ectoparasites

Ivermectin is generally a very effective miticide. A single subcutaneous dose of ivermectin at 200 μg/kg is curative in naturally occurring infestations with Otodectes cynotis and Sarcoptes scabiei. In severe cases of canine scabies, two treatments at a 14-day interval have been advocated. The route of administration most probably plays an important role in the number of treatments required. Ivermectin is well absorbed when administered orally or parenterally, but lower efficacy and shorter duration of action of orally administered ivermectin have been documented. A single oral dose of 200 μg/kg of ivermectin has been shown to cure cases of canine scabies. The author currently uses two subcutaneous or oral treatments, at a 2-week interval, with a dose of 300 μg/kg of ivermectin.

Recently, the efficacy of ivermectin against *Cheyletiella* infestation in dogs has been investigated. In spite of the fact that *Cheyletiella* mites do not appear to feed on blood, ivermectin proved to be very effective against *Cheyletiella yasguri* infestation in dogs. All treated animals were completely cured after one or two subcutaneous ivermectin injections of 300 μg/kg. The exact number of treatments required to cure canine cheyletiellosis has not been precisely determined. As for other mites, it most probably varies according to the dosage, route of administration, and severity of infestation. The attention paid to treating the environment is another important factor in cheyletiellosis, since adult female mites may live off their host for up to 10 days.

Little has been reported on the efficacy of ivermectin in canine demodicosis. One paper (Belot et al., 1984) described six patients with localized demodicosis that responded well after three subcutaneous injections of 400 μg/kg of ivermectin over a 2½ month period. It is difficult to assess the efficacy of this treatment, since it is known that over 90 per cent of dogs with localized demodicosis undergo spontaneous remission without any treatment. Another paper (Scott and Walton, 1985) reported the results of treatment of four dogs with amitraz-resistant chronic generalized demodicosis. A dose of 400 μg/kg was given subcutaneously weekly for a total of eight treatments. At the time of the writing of the article, one dog was apparently cured, but no significant improvement was noted in the other three dogs. Subsequently, the dog that had apparently been cured also relapsed.

The author's experience with the use of ivermectin in generalized canine demodicosis is limited to a dozen cases. Encouraging results *were not obtained*. Because of the unpredictable clinical evolution of canine demodicosis and the very limited number of patients treated, it is probably premature to finalize opinion on the efficacy or lack of efficacy of ivermectin against *Demodex canis*. At present, results have been disappointing.

Nothing has been documented on the efficacy of ivermectin against fleas. One could expect similar results and limitations as experienced with other systemic insecticides. Systemic insecticide efficacy is dependent on the flea taking a blood meal. Thus, such products have limited value for dogs (and cats) with flea-bite hypersensitivity, since the deposition of antigen in the skin will have occurred before the insecticidal effect. The other prerequisite for effective antiflea activity would be the maintenance of an appropriate blood level of ivermectin. No such studies have been conducted in dogs. The plasma half-life of ivermectin could be approximated to a few days when used orally, and up to 2 or 3 weeks when used parenterally, but these figures require documentation. Because of the unfortunate idiosyncratic reaction encountered in some dogs, one should not expect to have a canine ivermectin product marketed for uses other than heartworm prevention.

Feline Ectoparasites

Less information is available on use of ivermectin against ectoparasites in cats. Ivermectin, given as a single subcutaneous injection of 200 μg/kg, is effective against *Otodectes cynotis*. Signs of otitis externa and pruritus disappear in 2 to 3 weeks. Ivermectin is also effective against *Notoedres cati*, at the dosage of 400 μg/kg given subcutaneously.

No reports were found on the efficacy of ivermectin in the treatment of cheyletiellosis in cats, but the author has obtained excellent results with one or two subcutaneous injections of 400 μg/kg in catteries of Persian and Himalayan cats infested with *Cheyletiella* mites. No toxic reactions have been seen.

CONCLUSION

In selected cases, ivermectin has proved to be very useful in the treatment of canine and feline ectoparasitisms such as ear mite infestation, scabies, and cheyletiellosis. It is especially useful when large numbers of animals are involved (e.g., in kennels or catteries) or when standard topical treatment regimens are unsuccessful or impossible (e.g., in large dogs or long-haired animals; when owners are physically disabled; when inclement weather conditions prevail).

Because of its broad spectrum of activity, lack of known resistant parasites, ease of administration, residual duration of effect, and margin of safety in cats and most dogs, ivermectin could have great potential for use in small animals. However, because of unfortunate idiosyncratic reactions in collies, collie crosses, and, probably, other breeds, this drug will most likely never be licensed for use in dogs other than for heartworm prevention.

References and Supplemental Reading

Barragry, T. M.: A review of the pharmacology and clinical uses of ivermectin. Can. Vet. J. 28:512, 1987.

Belot J., Parent R., and Pangui, J. L.: Démodécie canine: observations cliniques à propos d'un essai de traitement par l'ivermectine. Point Vét. 16:618, 1984.

Bigler B., Waber, S., and Pfister, K.: Successful treatment of Notoedres cati infestation with ivermectin. Schweiz. Arch. Tierheilkd. 126:365, 1984.

Campbell, W. C., and Benz, G. W.: Ivermectin: A review of efficacy and safety. J. Vet. Pharmacol. Ther. 7:1. 1984.

Chauve, C., Reynauld, M. C.: Traitement parentéral de l'otocariose du chat: Efficacité de l'ivermectine. Sc. Vét. Med. Comp. 86:189, 1984.

Paradis, M.: L'ivermectin chez les petits animaux. Méd. Vét. Québec 17:113, 1987.

Paradis, M., and Villeneuve, A.: Efficacy of ivermectin against *Cheyletiella yasguri* infestation in dogs. Can. Vet. J. (in press).

Paul, A. J., Tranquilli, W. S., Seward, R. L., et al.: Clinical observations in collies given ivermectin orally. Am. J. Vet. Res. 48:684, 1987.

Pulliam, J. D., Seward, R. L., Henry, R. T., et al.: Investigating ivermectin toxicity in collies. Vet Med. 80:33, 1985.

Scheidt, V. J., Meldleau, C., Seward, R. L., et al.: An evaluation of ivermectin in the treatment of sarcoptic mange in dogs. Am. J. Vet. Res. 45:1201, 1984.

Scott, D. W., and Walton, D. K.: Experiences with the use of amitraz and ivermectin for the treatment of generalized demodicosis in dogs. J. Am. Anim. Hosp. Assoc. 21:535, 1985.

Yazwinski, T. A., Pote, L., Tilley, W., et al.: Efficacy of ivermectin against *Sarcoptes scabiei* and *Otodectes cynotis* infestation of dogs. Vet. Med. Small Anim. Clin. 76:1749, 1981.

FATTY ACID SUPPLEMENTS AS ANTI-INFLAMMATORY AGENTS

WILLIAM H. MILLER, JR., V.M.D.

Ithaca, New York

Fatty acids have been used for years to treat seborrhea associated with fatty acid deficiency. The polyunsaturated fatty acids are necessary for caloric energy and the formation and maintenance of the fluidity and function of cell membranes. The oxidative metabolism of certain fatty acids results in the formation of eicosanoids, which include the prostaglandins (PG) and leukotrienes (LT). Currently, the effects of prostaglandins and leukotrienes are being extensively studied, as these compounds play pivotal roles in immunoregulation, inflammation, and the maintenance of normal epidermal integrity. Certain nutritional supplements appear to modulate the formation of the eicosanoids and may be useful in treating a variety of dermatologic disorders.

FATTY ACID METABOLISM

Linoleic, linolenic, and arachidonic acids are essential fatty acids. The cat requires dietary sources of arachidonic acid, whereas the dog can synthesize both arachidonic and linolenic acids from linoleic acid. The metabolic pathway of the essential fatty acids is summarized in Figure 1. It is commonly believed that both the m-6 and m-3 fatty acids share the same enzyme systems and that the desaturation steps appear to be the rate-limiting points. Dihomo-gamma-linolenic, arachidonic, and eicosapentaenoic acids are further metabolized to the eicosanoids via cyclo-oxygenase and lipoxygenase pathways. Each of the three series of eicosanoids appears to have different biologic effects. The two-series is thought of as proinflammatory, whereas the one-series and the three-series may be anti-inflammatory.

Eicosapentaenoic acid (EPA), found in marine lipids, is metabolized to the three-series of eicosanoids and is a potent competitive inhibitor of arachidonic acid metabolism via a number of different mechanisms. Supplements containing EPA can have a profound effect on the cellular levels of free arachidonic acid and the two-series of eicosanoids and thus can interfere with the proinflammatory effects of these compounds.

ATOPY

In humans, atopic dermatitis is a chronically relapsing disorder of uncertain etiology. In the early part of this century, there were reports that fatty acid supplementation was of some therapeutic value, but the advent of corticosteroids lessened the interest in this line of therapy. More recently, there has been a resurgence of interest, as some individuals theorize that a defect in delta-6-desaturase function exists in atopic individuals and plays some role in the disorder. Multiple studies using evening primrose oil (EPO) (70 per cent linoleic and 9 per cent gamma-linolenic acids) were performed, and many, but not all, showed a dose-dependent improvement in symptoms. In these studies, a variety of changes in the levels of the various fatty acids and eicosanoids were detected, which suggests that dietary manipulation can alter the formation of prostaglandins and leukotrienes.

In the United Kingdom, 16 atopic dogs were treated with evening primrose oil, and ten of the dogs responded positively. There was improvement in coat quality and a lessening of seborrheic changes, but there was no change in the level of pruritus. When fish oil, an excellent source of EPA, was added (3:1, EPO:EPA), no dog showed any

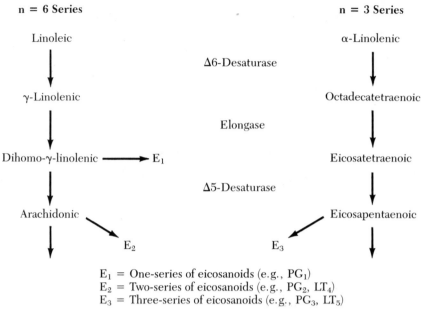

E_1 = One-series of eicosanoids (e.g., PG_1)
E_2 = Two-series of eicosanoids (e.g., PG_2, LT_4)
E_3 = Three-series of eicosanoids (e.g., PG_3, LT_5)

Figure 1. Schematic of fatty acid metabolism.

sustained change in coat quality of level of pruritus. Alterations in the levels of various fatty acids were detected, which suggests that dietary manipulation of eicosanoid formation also may be possible in dogs.

DVM Derm Caps (Dermatologics for Veterinary Medicine, Inc.) have been used by a large number of investigators for the treatment of allergic pruritus, and, although the success rates vary, this supplement can lessen or eliminate allergic pruritus. In one study of 93 allergic dogs, 17 dogs (18.3 per cent) showed an excellent response, with the pruritus being eliminated or decreasing to an insignificant level. Another 16 dogs (17.2 per cent) experienced a substantial reduction in, but not the elimination of, their pruritus. In another study, 11.1 per cent of the dogs showed an excellent response, while another 11.1 per cent showed moderate improvement.

The author has treated eight chronically atopic dogs whose symptoms could be managed only with alternate-day steroids. When DVM Derm Caps were added to the well-established steroid regimen, all dogs responded favorably in that their steroid dose was reduced by approximately 50 per cent. In no instance could the steroids be discontinued.

HYPERPROLIFERATIVE EPIDERMAL DISORDERS

In humans, the most common hyperproliferative skin disease is psoriasis. In the involved skin of these patients, the cellular content of free arachidonic acid and the two-series of eicosanoids is elevated. This suggests that arachidonic acid and its oxidative products, especially the leukotrienes, play some significant role in the pathogenesis of this disorder. Drugs that inhibit the cyclo-oxygenase pathways worsen psoriatic lesions, whereas lipoxygenase inhibitors cause improvement. In one study in which the patients were fed a diet very low in arachidonic acid but high in fish oil, 62 per cent of the individuals showed marked improvement.

Psoriasis does not occur in dogs, but canine idiopathic seborrhea does occur as a hyperplastic and hyperproliferative disorder. It is unknown what role, if any, arachidonic acid and its metabolites play in this disorder. The response of dogs with idiopathic seborrhea to 13-*cis*-retinoic acid (Accutane, Roche) a potent inhibitor of 5-lipoxygenase, has been unrewarding, which may indicate that eicosanoids are not important in dogs. Four dogs with idiopathic seborrhea were treated by the author with DVM Derm Caps, and all dogs showed a marked improvement. If this information is coupled with the improvement seen in the seborrheic signs in the atopic dogs treated with EPO, it is apparent that fatty acids play some important role in idiopathic seborrhea.

Several West Highland white terriers with epidermal dysplasia and two springer spaniels with lichenoid psoriasiform dermatitis have not responded to treatment with DVM Derm Caps. The effect of nutritional supplementation on other disorders of keratinization is unknown.

ARTHRITIS

The causes of arthritis are numerous, and, in humans, nonsteroidal anti-inflammatory drugs commonly are used for therapy. In one study of 52 people with rheumatoid arthritis, 83 per cent of the patients receiving EPO and 94 per cent of the patients taking EPO and fish oil were able to reduce by 50 per cent or more their dosages of other drugs. In the psoriasis study previously mentioned, two patients had moderately severe psoriatic arthritis in which symptoms decreased with the dietary manipulation.

The author used DVM Derm Caps to treat six atopic dogs that also had symptomatic hip dysplasia. The owners reported that while the dogs received the supplement, they showed improvement in gait, less pain, or both. One dog with an immune-mediated arthropathy showed no change with the supplement.

MISCELLANEOUS DISORDERS

The bibliography on the effectiveness of evening primrose oil with or without marine lipids is extensive and covers almost any disorder one can imagine. In humans, the tumor prostaglandin levels in more aggressive basal cell carcinomas, breast tumors, and malignant melanomas are different from those found in their less malignant counterparts. This suggests that prostaglandins may aid in the control of metastasis or invasion. In consideration of all the known and presumed anti-inflammatory and immunoregulatory effects of prostaglandins and leukotrienes, fatty acid supplements may be valuable as an adjuvant mode of therapy in many disorders.

SUMMARY

There are a large number of fatty acid supplements marketed in North America, and each might have some anti-inflammatory effects. Currently, the author is aware of three supplements, namely DVM Derm Caps, Opticoat II (Natural Animal Nutrition), and EfaVet (Efamol Ltd.), which are combinations of vegetable and marine lipids and were formulated to have anti-inflammatory effects. This article reflects the author's experiences with DVM Derm Caps as it was the first marketed. The other products may be equally or more effective.

Since this mode of anti-inflammatory therapy is new, it is best to say that these supplements have great potential. As inflammation is a very complex process, it is not surprising that fatty acid supplements can lessen but not completely eliminate symptoms. This diminution of signs should allow the clinician to decrease the dose of other, possibly harmful, medications.

References and Supplemental Reading

Belch, J. J., and Ansell, D.: Effects of evening primrose oil (Efamol) and evening primrose oil plus fish oil (Efamol Marine) in rheumatoid arthritis. Presented at Br. Soc. Rheumatol., London, November 20, 1986.

Fadok, V. A.: Nutritional therapy in veterinary dermatology. In Kirk, R. W. (ed.): Current Veterinary Therapy IX. Philadelphia: W. B. Saunders Co., 1986, pp. 591–596.

Lloyd, D.: Investigation of effects of essential fatty acid supplementation in atopic dogs. Presented at Congress of the Dermatology Study Group, Br. Soc. Vet. Dermatol., London, April 2, 1987.

Miller, W. H., Griffin, C. E., Scott, D. W., et al.: Clinical trial of DVM Derm Caps in the treatment of allergic diseases in dogs: A nonblinded study. J. Am. Anim. Hosp. Assoc. (in press).

Rola-Pleszczynski, M.: Immunoregulation by leukotrienes and other lipoxygenase metabolites. Immunol. Today 6:302, 1985.

Scott, D. W., and Buerger, R. G.: Nonsteroidal anti-inflammatory agents in the management of canine pruritus. J. Am. Anim. Hosp. Assoc. 24:425, 1988.

Vanderveen, E. E., Grekin, R. C., Swanson, N. A., et al.: Arachidonic acid metabolites in cutaneous carcinomas. Arch. Dermatol. 122:407, 1986.

Ziboh, V. A., Cohen, K. A., et al.: Effects of dietary supplementation of fish oil on neutrophil and epidermal fatty acids. Arch. Dermatol. 122:1277, 1986.

NONSTEROIDAL ANTI-INFLAMMATORY AGENTS IN THE MANAGEMENT OF CANINE AND FELINE PRURITUS

WILLIAM H. MILLER, JR., V.M.D.

Ithaca, New York

Pruritus is described as an unpleasant sensation that provokes the desire to scratch. Clinically, pruritus is the result of chemical stimulation of the nerve endings in the skin by a wide variety of compounds that include histamine, proteases, peptides, serotonin, prostaglandins, and leukotrienes. It has been stated that proteases (proteolytic enzymes) apparently are the major mediator of pruritus in dogs and cats. As some pruritic animals stop scratching when they are given a drug that has no effect on proteases, it would appear that the other mediators also are very important.

The term nonsteroidal anti-inflammatory drug (NSAID) conventionally is used to describe the compounds that inhibit prostaglandin synthesis. In the context of this article, the term is used to describe nonsteroidal drugs that have been effective in controlling pruritus in companion animals.

ANTIHISTAMINES

The effects of histamine are mediated by its binding to histamine receptors. Two types of receptors, designated H_1 and H_2, have been identified. H_1 receptor activation initiates the classic inflammatory effects of histamine, whereas H_2 activation causes gastric acid secretion, chronotropic effects on the heart, and modulation of further histamine release from mast cells and basophils. The present-day antihistamines bind to either the H_1 or the H_2 receptors, but not to both.

All antihistamines work via competitive and reversible binding of the drug to the receptor site. Through this action, the drug can only prevent the action of histamine and not reverse its effects once they are present. The actions of antihistamines appear to be extremely complicated. It has been shown that antihistamines may directly inhibit or stimulate mast cell secretion; may change the number, activity, or both of helper or suppressor T-lymphocytes; and may activate other cells, such as the eosinophil, which can alter mast cell function.

These findings may or may not have clinical applications in dogs and cats.

H_1 Antagonists

The large number of H_1 blockers fall into six different classes. As a general rule, all H_1 antagonists have antihistaminic, anticholinergic, sedative, and local anesthetic properties but vary greatly in their potency, dosage, incidence of side effects, and cost. In humans, there is a great deal of individual variability in the response to an antihistamine.

H_1 antagonists not only prevent the action of histamine but also may alter the release of histamine and other mediators from mast cells and basophils. In a study using an *in vitro* model of human allergy, it was found that H_1 antagonists could cause histamine release from basophils or could inhibit antigen-induced histamine release. The inhibitory effect was seen with low drug concentrations, while spontaneous release occurred at higher concentrations. The different classes of antihistamines showed differing patterns of release and inhibition. The phenothiazine antihistamines were the most potent inhibitors of histamine release. Of the drugs tested, diphenhydramine had the ability to cause histamine release, whereas chlorpheniramine had little power to do so. Both of these drugs would inhibit histamine release when they were used at low concentrations.

Table 1 lists examples of H_1 antihistamines used in veterinary medicine. The dosages listed are those found in standard veterinary texts or those used by the author. Some publications suggest much different and typically higher doses. If H_1 antagonists could cause or block histamine release *in vivo*, proper dosage of the various drugs would be critical. Unfortunately, there is little pharmacokinetic data for pets on which to base the dosage.

In a study in which chlorpheniramine, diphenhydramine, and hydroxyzine were given on a rotating basis to 45 allergic dogs, the pruritus in ten dogs decreased significantly with antihistamine

566

Table 1. H_1 *Antagonists for Use in Dogs*

Drug Class	Drug Name	Oral Dosage
Alkylamine	Chlorpheniramine	2–12 mg b.i.d.–t.i.d.
Ethanolamine	Diphenhydramine	2–4 mg/kg t.i.d.
	Dimenhydrinate	8 mg/kg t.i.d.
Ethylenediamine	Pyrilamine	1–2 mg/kg b.i.d.
	Tripelennamine	1–1.5 mg/kg b.i.d.
Piperazine	Hydroxyzine	2.2 mg/kg t.i.d.
	Meclizine	25 mg s.i.d.
Piperidine	Cyproheptadine	0.3–2.0 mg/kg b.i.d.
Phenothiazine	Promethazine	0.2–1.0 mg/kg b.i.d.–t.i.d.
	Trimeprazine	1–2 mg/kg t.i.d.

therapy, while another 19 dogs showed a moderate improvement. It was common for a dog to respond to one drug but not to the other two, and there was no apparent increased efficacy of one drug over the other two. This indicates, as in humans, that a dog's response to H_1 antagonists is very individualized and that a drug (or possibly several drugs) from each class of antihistamines should be used before an animal's pruritus is termed nonresponsive to antihistamines.

In nonseasonally pruritic cats, the author has had good success in managing their pruritus with chlorpheniramine at an oral dose of 2 to 4 mg given once to twice daily.

As a group, antihistamines tend to cause drowsiness, which can limit their applicability. Other reported side effects include gastrointestinal signs and an increase in pruritus. The increase in pruritus may indicate that these drugs can indeed cause histamine release *in vivo*. Acute poisoning following an overdose is characterized by central nervous system hyperexcitability, which can be fatal. Some antihistamines are teratogenic and should be avoided in pregnancy.

Many new antihistamines are being marketed, and one report suggests that terfenadine (Seldane, Merrell Dow) at an oral dose of 5 to 10 mg/kg given every 12 hr is effective in dogs, with few side effects. The expense of this drug may limit its usefulness.

H_2 Antagonists

Cimetidine (Tagamet, SmithKline) 6 to 10 mg/kg PO every 8 hr, has been widely used in pets to inhibit histamine-evoked gastric acid secretion. Since H_2 receptors are not involved in itching, cimetidine should have no place in the treatment of pruritus. As histamine acts on the H_2 receptors on basophils and mast cells to limit further histamine release, blockade of this receptor could worsen allergic pruritus. In an ongoing study of the effects of cimetidine and diphenhydramine on allergic pruritus in dogs, the condition of 1 of 15 dogs worsened with cimetidine, whereas that of one dog improved significantly.

There are reports in both humans and dogs that the combination of an H_1 antagonist with cimetidine gave better results than those seen with just the H_1 blocker. In the author's study, no dog responded better to the combination than it did to just the diphenhydramine. It would appear that cimetidine is of little or no value in treating pruritus in dogs.

TRICYCLIC ANTIDEPRESSANTS

The tricyclic antidepressants (TCA) are structurally related to the phenothiazine antipsychotic agents. All have antihistaminic, anticholinergic, and local anesthetic properties. Doxepin hydrochloride and amitriptyline hydrochloride are two TCA drugs that are the most potent antihistamines known. They both also have high anticholinergic effects. They antagonize both the H_1 and the H_2 receptors. As an H_1 antagonist, doxepin is 800 times more potent than diphenhydramine and 67 times more potent than hydroxyzine. Doxepin is six times more potent than cimetidine in blocking H_2 receptors.

Amitriptyline has been used successfully to treat behavioral disorders in dogs and cats. The drug is given PO once daily at a dose of 1 to 2 mg/kg for dogs and 5 to 10 mg for cats. Because of its strong anticholinergic effects, virtually all animals experience a dry mouth but adapt to it. There also is a low incidence of urinary retention and constipation. Hallucinations, disorientation, and hyperactivity also can be seen. This drug is contraindicated in animals with cardiac problems, a history of urinary retention, or seizures as it lowers the seizure threshold. This drug currently is being investigated as an antipruritic agent in dogs. To date, two of five dogs have shown an excellent response to amitriptyline.

ACETYLSALICYLIC ACID AND ASPIRIN SUBSTITUTES

Aspirin is the progenitor of nonsteroidal anti-inflammatory drugs and its pharmacologic actions relate to its irreversible inhibition of cyclo-oxygenase enzymes, with a subsequent reduction in prostaglandin production. Other salicylates and some of the newer aspirin substitutes only competitively inhibit this enzyme. Aspirin is a gastric irritant that causes increased gastric acid secretion, decreases gastric blood flow, and inhibits the secretion of cytoprotective mucus. Gastric irritation and blood loss are common side effects and gastric ulceration can occur. Aspirin alters prostacyclin and thromboxane formation and increases bleeding tendencies. The anti-inflammatory dose of aspirin in dogs is approximately 30 mg/kg, given every 8 hr. This dose is approximately six times higher than that required to inhibit platelet aggregation.

A reduction in pruritus was seen in only one dog in 45 receiving aspirin. As this response rate is very poor and was achieved at levels that affect clotting, aspirin is not recommended.

In human medicine, the relatively high incidence of aspirin intolerance led to the development of acetaminophen and a wide variety of prescription nonsteroidal anti-inflammatory drugs such as ibuprofen and indomethacin. Acetaminophen has no clinically significant anti-inflammatory effects, whereas such drugs as ibuprofen and indomethacin are potent cyclo-oxygenase inhibitors. In humans, there is a high incidence of adverse reactions to these newer, potent anti-inflammatory drugs. The incidence of adverse reactions to all of these newer drugs appears to be much higher in dogs and cats, and, therefore, their use is not suggested.

FATTY ACID NUTRITIONAL SUPPLEMENT

Some fatty acids appear to modulate the formation of prostaglandins and leukotrienes; they are discussed more fully on page 563.

VITAMIN E

Vitamin E is an essential fat-soluble vitamin that is necessary for the integrity and optimum function of all body cells. Vitamin E–deficient animals show multiple immunologic abnormalities and seborrheic skin disease. Vitamin E has been used as an anti-inflammatory agent to treat discoid lupus erythematosus, dermatomyositis, and acanthosis nigricans. The anti-inflammatory effects can be explained by its modulation of prostaglandin formation, enhancement of humoral and cellular immunity, stabilization of lysosomal membranes, inhibition of proteolytic enzymes, enhancement of phagocytic activity of neutrophils and macrophages, quenching of singlet oxygen, and scavenging of free radicals.

When allergic dogs were treated with 400 IU of dl-alpha-tocopherol acetate orally, twice daily, only 1 dog in 15 showed any reduction in its itching. As an antipruritic agent, vitamin E would appear to be of little value by itself.

ZINC

Zinc is a trace mineral found in all body tissues. The primary biochemical function of zinc is via its incorporation into a variety of enzyme systems, and zinc is necessary for normal immunologic reactivity. Zinc-deficient individuals show a variety of immunologic abnormalities, especially of the cell-mediated immune system.

Zinc-deficient animals typically develop seborrheic skin lesions of variable pruritus and may show signs of immunologic hyporeactivity. Adequate therapy resolves the cutaneous and immunologic abnormalities. Since the cell-mediated immune system plays a pivotal role in allergic disorders, zinc methionine (Zinpro, Zinpro Company), 1 tablet per 20 lb body weight per day was given to 15 allergic dogs. No dog showed any change in its level of pruritus, so zinc supplementation would appear to have no place in the treatment of allergic pruritus.

ANTIBIOTICS

Tetracycline and erythromycin have anti-inflammatory as well as antibacterial effects. Both inhibit neutrophil chemotaxis and random migration, and erythromycin inhibits the mitogenic response of lymphocytes. Both of these drugs have been used successfully in humans to manage autoimmune skin diseases. When 45 noninfected allergic dogs were treated with erythromycin, two dogs showed a sustained significant reduction in pruritus. An additional four dogs experienced some reduction in pruritus. The common side effect of vomiting was seen in four dogs. It is unknown whether the reduction in pruritus was due to the anti-inflammatory action of erythromycin or to a subclinical pyoderma in the dogs that was successfully managed with antibiotics. If a pruritic animal has a concurrent pyoderma, erythromycin may be the drug of choice because of its dual actions.

ORGOTEIN

Orgotein (Palosein, Coopers Animal Health, Inc.) is a copper- and zinc-containing metalloprotein that acts as an extracellular superoxide dismutase. Its anti-inflammatory effects probably occur through the stabilization of cell membranes, particularly the phagocytes. In dogs, it has been used to successfully treat orthopedic pain, a variety of ophthalmologic conditions, and acral lick dermatitis. Its use for the treatment of allergic pruritus has been suggested, but the injectable nature and expense of the product limits its potential usefulness. As it is a protein of bovine origin, anaphylaxis could occur with its repeated use.

CYTOTOXIC IMMUNOSUPPRESSANTS

Cyclophosphamide (Cytoxan, Mead Johnson) and azathioprine (Imuran, Burroughs Wellcome) are the two most common cytotoxic immunosuppressants used in veterinary dermatology. Cyclophosphamide has relatively little anti-inflammatory activity but is a potent, cell cycle–independent immunosuppressant, affecting both the humoral and the cell-mediated immune response. Azathioprine has both anti-inflammatory and immunosuppressive effects. The humoral immune system appears to be more sensitive to the effects of this drug.

Both drugs are potent agents and can cause a wide variety of side effects. In dogs, azathioprine has a low incidence of adverse effects and is widely used in the treatment of autoimmune skin diseases. It is administered at a dose of 2.2 mg/kg PO once daily or every other day. Hemograms are monitored every 1 to 2 weeks. This drug has been used successfully to control pruritus in intractable atopic dogs. Obviously, this therapy should be considered a last resort.

GOLD SALT THERAPY

Gold salt therapy (chrysotherapy) is used in the treatment of rheumatoid arthritis and certain autoimmune skin diseases in animals (refer to Scott, 1983, for a complete description). Among their effects, gold compounds can stabilize lysosomal membranes, decrease migration and phagocytic activity of macrophages and neutrophils, inhibit prostaglandin synthesis, and suppress immunoglobulin synthesis. The author is unaware of any reports in which chrysotherapy has been used to control pruritus. However, because of its anti-inflammatory effects, chrysotherapy has some potential for use in animals in whom all else has failed.

SUMMARY

Classically, pruritus in companion animals has been managed with glucocorticoid steroids. The owner-observed and medical side effects of these drugs, especially when used long term, can be unacceptable. In those instances when glucocorti-coid steroids are effective, nonsteroidal anti-inflammatory drugs should be tried to eliminate or minimize the steroid use. Since there are multiple mediators of pruritus and the various nonsteroidal drugs tend to work only on one arm of the inflammatory response, it is not unusual to find that the pruritus is lessened but not eliminated with the various drugs mentioned. Combinations of different types of drugs (e.g., an antihistamine plus a fatty acid supplement) may have an additive effect on lessening the pruritus. If one or several of the nonsteroidal drugs only lessen the pruritus, they are still of therapeutic value, as their use should lessen the dose of steroids used to control the residual pruritus.

References and Supplemental Reading

Ackerman, L.: Antihistamines in the treatment of canine allergic skin disease. Vet. Allergist, Fall 1986.

Bickers, D. R., Hazen, P. G., and Lynch, W. S.: Clinical Pharmacology of Skin Disease. New York: Churchill Livingstone, 1984, pp. 17–56.

Chastain, C. B.: Aspirin: New indications for an old drug. Comp. Small Anim. 9:165, 1987.

Denan, S. T.: A review of pruritus. J. Am. Acad. Dermatol. 14:375, 1986.

Greaves, M. W.: Pharmacology and significance of nonsteroidal anti-inflammatory drugs in the treatment of skin diseases. J. Am. Acad. Dermatol. 16:751, 1987.

Gupta, M. D., Gupta, A. K., and Ellis, C. N.: Antidepressant drugs in dermatology. Arch. Dermatol. 123:647, 1987.

Lichtenstein, L. M., and Gillespie, E.: The effects of H_1 and H_2 antihistamines on "allergic" histamine release and its inhibition by histamine. J. Pharmacol. Exp. Ther. 192:441, 1975.

Scott, D. W.: Chrysotherapy (gold therapy). In Kirk, R.W. (ed.): Current Veterinary Therapy VIII. Philadelphia: W. B. Saunders, 1983.

Scott, D. W., and Buerger, R. G.: Nonsteroidal anti-inflammatory agents in the management of canine pruritus. J. Am. Anim. Hosp. Assoc. 24:425, 1988.

Scott, D. W., and Sheffy, B. E.: Dermatosis in dogs caused by vitamin E deficiency. Comp. Anim. Pract. 1:42, 1987.

Theoharides, T. C.: Allergy and antihistamines: A new riddle. Arch. Dermatol. 122:995, 1986.

Thornfeldt, C. R., and Menkes, A. W.: Bullous pemphigoid controlled by tetracycline. J. Am. Acad. Dermatol. 16:305, 1986.

Voith, V. L.: Behavioral disorders. In Davis, L. E. (ed.): Handbook of Small Animal Therapeutics. New York: Churchill Livingstone, 1985, pp. 519–548.

IMMUNOMODULATING DRUGS
IN DERMATOLOGY

WAYNE ROSENKRANTZ, D.V.M.

Garden Grove, California

Immunomodulation refers to changing, varying, or adjusting the immune response mechanism by pharmacologic manipulation. The clinical use of immunomodulators primarily has been centered around immunosuppressive therapy in the treatment of neoplasia and autoimmune disease and in the prevention of transplant rejections. Immunostimulation is used for the treatment or prevention of infectious diseases and has received more attention recently in both human and veterinary medicine.

Immunosuppression is easier to produce than immunostimulation. Many of the immunosuppressive drugs function by affecting specific stages in the cell cycle. The response of cells to the drug varies, depending on their stage in the cell cycle. Generally, the most sensitive cells are those that are rapidly proliferating. Some of the newer immunosuppressive drugs may also function by lymphokine regulation.

Immunostimulation is a less well understood type of immunomodulation. The goal in this situation is to try to selectively influence or regulate a specific cell population or signal that will result in an enhanced immune response. It is unfortunate that the exact mechanism of action of many of the immunostimulants is unknown, and we are left with a more general type of stimulation.

Drugs that stimulate macrophage function, either directly or indirectly via lymphocyte activation, have the most potential for augmenting the host immune response. The macrophage is a key cell at the inducer and effector end of the immune response. It often functions as an antigen presenting–cell for helper and suppressor T-cells. Such interaction results in a controlled release of various lymphokines: interleukin-1 (lymphocyte-activating factor) and interleukin-2 (T-cell growth factor). These lymphokines function in clonal expansion of antigen-specific effector T-cells. Macrophage antigen presentation to B-lymphocytes results in the release of a different set of lymphokines, which direct their activities toward specific immunoglobulin production. At the effector end, the release of gamma-interferon from helper T-cells stimulates macrophage proliferation, maturation, and antimicrobial activity.

Before utilizing an immunomodulating drug,

there are some important pretreatment considerations. First, always make sure the diagnosis is correct. Using an immunosuppressant in a case of suspected pemphigus, which is actually demodicosis, could be devastating. Second, always obtain a pretreatment data base. By performing pretreatment laboratory work, a base line data base is established and may uncover a pre-existing condition that would make a specific therapy contraindicated. Lastly, prior to using immunostimulation, other underlying conditions should be ruled out or controlled (e.g., hypothyroidism, hyperadrenocorticism, demodicosis, allergies).

This article will specifically deal with some of the most current immunosuppressive agents used in the treatment of cutaneous immune-mediated diseases and related dermatoses, and the current immunostimulant agents used in the prevention or reduction of recurrent pyoderma in dogs.

CYCLOPHOSPHAMIDE

MECHANISM. Cyclophosphamide is a potent alkylating agent. Alkylating agents form covalent bonds with organic compounds, particularly nucleic acids, replacing a hydrogen atom with an alkyl group. This usually occurs at the N-7 of guanine in DNA. This results in misreading of the genetic code as well as DNA breakage and cross-linking. The main cytotoxic effects result from the alkylating reactions with nuclear DNA and cytoplasmic RNA. Cyclophosphamide has cytotoxic effects throughout the entire cell cycle but has relatively greater action against rapidly dividing cells.

PHARMACOKINETICS. Cyclophosphamide has a wide tissue distribution, being moderately lipid soluble. It is well-absorbed orally, with peak levels 1 hr after administration. Its plasma half-life is between 4 and 6.5 hr. The parent compound requires hepatic metabolism to its active forms. The initial pathway is oxidation to 4-hydroxycyclophosphamide, which equilibrates with aldophosphamide, which enters cells and is cleaved to acrolein and phosphoramide mustard. Both are highly cytotoxic.

CLINICAL USE. Cyclophosphamide has been used extensively for a wide variety of neoplasias, partic-

570

ularly lymphoreticular neoplasia. Many veterinary researchers report it to be effective in immune-mediated skin diseases. Reports in humans have included its use as a sole or combined agent in mycosis fungoides, pemphigus vulgaris, systemic lupus erythematosus, dermatomyositis, and systemic vasculitides. Cyclophosphamide (Cytoxan, Mead Johnson) is available in 25-mg or 50-mg tablets. This drug is often used as a combined therapy with prednisone as an every-other-day treatment at 1.5 mg/kg to 2.5 mg/kg. Usually, the prednisone can be reduced to an every-other-day treatment, alternating with the cyclophosphamide. The major limiting factor with this drug is its myelosuppression. During the early phases of therapy, a complete blood count (CBC) should be taken weekly. If the white blood cell count (WBC) drops to less than 4000 cells/mm³, or the platelet count drops to 120,000/mm³, therapy should be discontinued until values return to normal. The drug can be restarted at 75 per cent of the initial dose once values return to normal.

TOXICITY. The side effects are the major limiting factor for this drug's clinical use. In addition to its potent myelosuppression, the development of hemorrhagic cystitis and bladder fibrosis is a major concern. The bladder side effects are thought to be related to acrolein. The time- and dose-related administration of N-acetylcysteine and consumption of large volumes of water during therapy may help reduce this problem. Other side effects include bladder neoplasia, gastrointestinal inflammation, anorexia, depression, infertility, teratogenicity, alopecia, altered wound healing, and secondary immune depression.

CHLORAMBUCIL

MECHANISM. Chlorambucil is also an alkylating agent and functions similarly to cyclophosphamide. However, it is slower acting and the least toxic of the alkylating agents.

PHARMACOKINETICS. Chlorambucil is almost completely metabolized. Oral absorption is very good, and the plasma half-life in humans is about 1 hr.

CLINICAL USE. Chlorambucil can be used in a variety of cutaneous immune-mediated diseases. It is most commonly used in combination with prednisone, or with prednisone and azathioprine. Chlorambucil (Leukeran, Burroughs Wellcome) is available as 2-mg nonscored oral tablets. The dose is 0.1 to 0.2 mg/kg used daily or every other day. As with other myelosuppressives, the clinical response is usually not seen until 4 to 8 weeks after therapy. Monitoring is similar to that for cyclophosphamide treatment.

TOXICITY. Chlorambucil rarely causes serious clinical side effects, but myelosuppression and gastrointestinal side effects can occur. Hemorrhagic cystitis is not seen. Occasional urticarial reactions have been reported.

AZATHIOPRINE

MECHANISM. Azathioprine is an antimetabolite that is specific for cells in the S phase of the cell cycle. It is transformed to the active agent 6-mercaptopurine, which inhibits the enzymes necessary for purine synthesis, thereby interrupting DNA and RNA synthesis. Its immunosuppression comes from the inhibition of T- and B-lymphocytes. Evidence that T-lymphocytes are primarily affected is supported by marked inhibition of delayed hypersensitivity reactions, T-cell–dependent antibody synthesis, and prevention of host-versus-graft reactions. There are also theories that azathioprine decreases lymphokine production and, therefore, suppresses monocyte and macrophage function.

PHARMACOKINETICS. Azathioprine is well-absorbed orally and is almost completely metabolized. It is converted to 6-mercaptopurine by the action of glutathione or other nucleophilic agents or enzymatically. Metabolization of 6-mercaptopurine occurs by two pathways. One involves methylation of the sulfhydryl group and subsequent oxidation of the methylated derivatives. The second pathway results in the metabolism of 6-mercaptopurine to 6-thiouric acid by the enzyme xanthanine oxidase, which is present in large amounts in the liver. The plasma half-life in humans is approximately 90 min. Patients with liver disease or those on allopurinol (xanthanine oxidase inhibitor) are started on doses 25 per cent lower than normal.

CLINICAL USE. Azathioprine (Imuran, Burroughs Wellcome) is available in an injectable dosage and as 50-mg tablets. Azathioprine is preferred over 6-mercaptopurine because of its more favorable therapeutic index. Azathioprine is considered by many clinicians to be the first-choice cytotoxic drug used in cutaneous immune-mediated diseases because of its anti-inflammatory effects and lack of hemorrhagic cystitis as a side effect, compared with cyclophosphamide. Like other myelosuppressives, it has a slow onset of action, taking 4 to 6 weeks to produce clinical effects. The current dosage is 2.2 mg/kg/day, or every other day, usually used in conjunction with prednisone or added to prednisone therapy. Once the disease is in remission, the lowest possible effective dose is used, often in conjunction with prednisone. Laboratory monitoring before and during treatment is required. A CBC should be performed initially every 1 to 2 weeks, and every 1 to 2 months after a maintenance dose is established. If leukopenia, thrombocytopenia, or anemia develops, the drug should be discontinued until values return to normal; treatment should be reinstituted at one half to three fourths the original dose. If lethargy, depression, anorexia, vomiting, or diarrhea develops, a chemistry screen should be performed.

TOXICITY. The major side effects primarily relate to bone marrow toxicity. This is most obvious in cats, in which marked leukopenia and occasional deaths have occurred. For this reason, it is not generally recommended in this species. If used, the dose is 1.1 mg/kg every other day. Rarely, a severe but reversible hepatotoxicity results. Teratogenicity is also a concern, and treated animals should not be bred. Other side effects include gastrointestinal signs, skin eruptions, and, in canine patients treated long term, secondary demodicosis and dermatophytosis.

IMMUNOSUPPRESSANT DRUGS

Cyclosporine

MECHANISM. Cyclosporine is a cyclic polypeptide immunosuppressive metabolite of the fungus *Tolypocladium inflatum gams*. Cyclosporine's exact mechanism of action is still under investigation. The most current evidence suggests that it inhibits lymphocytes in the G-0 and G-1 phases and affects helper T-cells. It inhibits interleukin-2 (T-cell growth factor), resulting in blocking of proliferation of activated T-lymphocytes. It blocks gene activation and mRNA transcription by binding to calmodulin and may block the interaction of T-cell antigen receptor with the antigen. Cyclosporine also affects other lymphokines, including gamma-interferon.

PHARMACOKINETICS. Oral absorption is incomplete and variable but occurs in 3 hr, with peak levels by 5 hr. Distribution is largely outside the blood volume and highest within the fat, liver, kidney, endocrine glands, lymph nodes, spleen, and bone marrow. Elimination is primarily by biliary excretion. Plasma half-life is approximately 34 hr.

CLINICAL USE. Cyclosporine (Sandimmune, Sandoz) has been approved by the Food and Drug Administration (FDA) for use in humans for prophylaxis against organ rejection. It has also been used to treat a variety of other systemic and cutaneous disorders in humans, including psoriasis, pemphigus, bullous pemphigoid, Graves's disease, noninfectious posterior uveitis, systemic lupus erythematosus, ichthyosis, mycosis fungoides/Sézary's syndrome, epidermolysis bullosa, and allergic contact dermatitis. In the veterinary field, cyclosporine has been used successfully for organ transplantation and has had limited success in the treatment of pemphigus foliaceus. It was unsuccessful in the treatment of epitheliotropic lymphoma (Rosen-

krantz et al., 1988). Cyclosporine is available as intravenous and oral formulations. The oral form comes in a olive oil base, in a 50-ml bottle containing 100 mg/cc. The intravenous preparation is associated with a solubilizing agent (polyoxyethylated castor oil) that has caused anaphylactoid reactions in dogs and is therefore *not recommended*. The currently accepted oral dose is 20 mg/kg/day. This drug is very expensive ($200 for a bottle) and is still being used on an experimental basis. If used, the patient should be monitored closely with regular re-examinations and laboratory screening.

TOXICITY. The adverse reactions associated with cyclosporine are generally thought to be less than other immunosuppressants. The primary adverse reaction in humans is nephrotoxicity, which is usually reversible with dosage reduction. Other reported reactions in humans include hepatotoxicity, hypertension, increased incidence of Epstein-Barr infections and lymphoma, gum hyperplasia, hirsutism, nausea, tremor, and paresthesias. The current toxicity in animals is primarily gastrointestinal. Pyoderma, bacteriuria, nephrotoxicity, upper respiratory virus, gingival hyperplasia, hirsutism, and a papillomatous dermatitis with malignant features also have been reported.

Sulfones and Sulfonamides

MECHANISM. The common sulfones and sulfonamides used in veterinary medicine include dapsone and sulfasalazine. The bacteriostatic effects of these drugs relate to their ability to prevent the conversion of para-aminobenzoic acid to folic acid by bacteria. The exact mechanism of action in noninfectious diseases is not known, but it appears to relate to the drugs' potent anti-inflammatory actions. These drugs suppress nonspecific inflammation and Arthus's reactions and decrease the response of lymphocytes to phytohemagglutinin. They do not appear to have inhibitory effects on histamine, prostaglandins, serotonin, bradykinin, immune complex formation, or humoral immunity. They have mild analgesic and antipyretic properties. These drugs also have inhibitory effects on the release and function of lysosomal enzymes.

The most recently recognized mode of action of these drugs appears to be the inhibition of the neutrophil's cytotoxicity system, by interfering with the formation of iodine (I_2) from sodium iodide (NaI). When neutrophils phagocytize bacteria or immune complexes, they release hydrogen peroxide and myeloperoxidase to catalyze iodine to sodium iodide. Sulfones reduce this reaction, and this may explain their anti-inflammatory properties.

PHARMACOKINETICS. Oral absorption of dapsone is about 85 per cent of the given dose. Serum levels peak between 2 and 6 hr, with plateau levels occurring in 8 to 10 days. After being absorbed, metabolic transformations take place within the liver, with acetylation and deacetylation occurring simultaneously. Approximately 90 per cent of the dapsone is excreted via the kidneys, primarily as glucuronide. The remaining 10 per cent is recovered from the bile. When therapy has been chronic, drug levels can persist for 35 days after treatment is discontinued. The long half-life and persistence in the body relate to the high protein binding and enterohepatic recycling of the drug.

CLINICAL USE. Dapsone (Avlosulfon, Ayerst) and sulfasalazine (Azulfidine, Pharmacia) have been used to treat a variety of human diseases. In dogs, these drugs are used to treat cutaneous vasculitis, sterile neutrophilic and eosinophilic diseases, and, occasionally, pemphigus foliaceus. Other researchers have also used these drugs to treat subcorneal pustular dermatoses and dermatitis herpetiformis. The dosage for dapsone is 1 mg/kg, two to three times a day; sulfasalazine is to be given at a dose of 22 to 44 mg/kg three times a day. A clinical response should be seen within 4 to 6 weeks. Dosages should be reduced to once daily or every other day when a clinical response is seen. Unpublished reports from many researchers suggest better success treating noninfectious vasculitis and sterile neutrophilic diseases with dapsone, and poorer success treating pemphigus with dapsone. A CBC and chemistry screen should be performed every other week during the first 6 weeks of therapy and reduced in frequency after the dosage is decreased.

TOXICITY. In humans, numerous side effects have been reported, including hemolysis, methemoglobinemia, headache, fatigue, nervousness, dermatitis, gastrointestinal signs, hepatotoxicity, leukopenia, agranulocytosis, and others. In dogs, mild anemia and neutropenia, severe thrombocytopenia, hepatotoxicity, gastrointestinal signs, and skin reactions have been seen. Gastrointestinal signs can usually be eliminated by giving the drug with food. The most common side effect seen with sulfasalazine is keratoconjunctivitis sicca, which is generally nonreversible. For this reason, it is recommended to check tear production each time a blood analysis is performed.

Chrysotherapy (Gold Therapy)

MECHANISM. Both oral and parenteral gold have a variety of pharmacologic effects that can be divided into antimicrobial, anti-inflammatory, and anti-immunologic. The antimicrobial activity has been demonstrated by the drug's ability to inhibit or kill diverse micro-organisms including *Mycobacterium tuberculosis*, gram-positive and gram-negative bacteria, mycoplasma, and protozoa. The anti-inflammatory properties include reduction of lysosomal enzymes, histamine, and prostaglandins. Gold salts also have inhibitory effects on the first component of complement and can inhibit chemotaxis and phagocytosis of macrophages and neutrophils. These drugs can block the respiratory burst and subsequent release of superoxide free radicals, hydrogen peroxide, hydroxyl radicals, and singlet oxygen. Gold therapy affects both humoral and cellular immunity. It inhibits immunoglobulin synthesis, as supported by patients with pemphigus who have a decrease in serum antiepithelial antibody titers during gold therapy. Rheumatoid patients receiving long-term therapy also show significant declines in immunoglobulin levels and rheumatoid factor. The oral form of gold appears to be a more potent inhibitor of antibody production and antibody response than the parenteral forms. Chrysotherapy inhibits antigen and mitogen lymphocyte responses *in vitro*. Parenteral gold does not inhibit delayed hypersensitivity *in vivo*. In contrast, oral gold can suppress skin testing responses to dinitrochlorobenzene. The oral form appears to have additional immunomodulating effects by stimulating suppressor T-cells.

PHARMACOKINETICS. The parent forms of gold are water soluble and accumulate in a variety of tissues, especially within the bone marrow, liver, spleen, kidneys, and adrenal glands. Aurothioglucose (Solganal, Schering) is formulated in a sesame oil base and, therefore, has a low rate of absorption. The absorption with the parenteral form is complete, peaks in 4 to 6 hr, and increases to a steady state by 5 to 10 weeks. The half-life of the parenteral form is 6 days. However, with regard to therapeutic effect and toxicity, the serum half-life is of little value when compared with the biologic half-life. Most of the absorbed gold is protein bound. More than 70 per cent is excreted by the kidneys. The remainder is found in the feces. With oral gold, only 25 per cent is absorbed, and lower plasma levels result. The half-life is longer, approximately 21 days, but body retention and accumulation is much less than with parenteral gold. The oral form is also highly protein bound but is eliminated primarily through the gastrointestinal tract.

CLINICAL USE. Two parenteral compounds are available, aurothiomalate (Myochrysine, Merck Sharp & Dohme) and aurothioglucose (Solganal, Schering). Each compound is 50 per cent gold by weight. The oral form, triethylphosphine gold (Auranofin, SmithKline), is 29 per cent gold. Aurothioglucose is the parenteral form that is preferred. It is available in 10-ml vials, 50 mg/cc. The current dosage is 1 mg/kg/week intramuscularly (IM). It is recommended to use a test dose initially at 1 mg to 5 mg the first week, followed by a second test dose at 2 mg to 10 mg the second week to rule out idiosyncratic reactions. Some researchers do not use test doses, as many have not recognized idiosyncratic reactions. Clinical response should not be expected for 6 to 12 weeks. If there is no response by the 16th week the dose can be increased to 1.5 mg/kg/week. Once a clinical response is achieved, injections can be given as needed (i.e., every 2 to 8 weeks). Occasionally, the injections may be discontinued, and the disease remains in remission. This has been seen most commonly during treatment of pemphigus foliaceus in cats, making gold therapy the treatment of choice for this disease in this species. Other indications for gold therapy include feline plasma cell stomatitis and plasma cell pododermatitis, canine bullous pemphigoid, and pemphigus complex. The oral form, Auranofin, has only been available for a short time. It has been shown to be effective in human discoid lupus erythematosus and pemphigus vulgaris. The human dosage is 3 mg b.i.d. A few investigators have tried Auranofin in dogs, at a dose of 0.1 to 0.2 mg/kg/day, with limited success. As with other immunosuppressants, pretreatment baseline data should be obtained. During therapy, CBCs, chemistry screens, and urinalysis should be obtained every 2 weeks during the first 2 months of therapy, and then monthly to quarterly as the dosage of gold is reduced.

TOXICITY. Approximately one third of the human patients on gold experience complications. Most complications are of little consequence, but in 10 per cent of patients, discontinuation of the therapy is necessary. The major side effect is mucocutaneous, with rashes, oral ulcers, and pruritus the most common. Toxic epidermal necrolysis has also been reported. Other side effects seen in humans include leukopenia, eosinophilia, aplastic anemia, thrombocytopenia, proteinuria, cholestasis, enterocolitis, pulmonary interstitial fibrosis, neurologic effects, chrysiasis, and diarrhea. Side effects in cats and dogs are less common. Oral ulcerations, leukopenia, and thrombocytopenia have been reported. There is also an unpublished report of two dogs, with pemphigus foliaceus nonresponsive to azathioprine, that died of toxic epidermal necrolysis when immediately switched to aurothioglucose therapy.

Vitamin E

MECHANISM. Vitamin E has been reported to be efficacious in a variety of cutaneous disorders. The mechanism of action of vitamin E may be related to its role as an antioxidant by stabilizing cell and lysosomal membranes against damage induced by peroxides and free radicals. Vitamin E also has effects on arachidonic acid and prostaglandin metabolism and may enhance immunity and phagocytic function of neutrophils and macrophages.

PHARMACOKINETICS. Vitamin E is an oil-soluble vitamin. It is composed of four fractions: alpha, beta, gamma, and delta. The alpha fraction is the most effective therapeutically and is available in d (natural), dl (synthetic), and mixed forms. Most of the work done with vitamin E has been with d-alpha-tocopheryl acetate or succinate. Oral absorption ranges from 10 to 52 per cent. Serum levels reach a plateau after 3 weeks of oral supplementation, suggesting a type of negative feedback mechanism on absorption. Inorganic iron and mineral oil interfere with vitamin E absorption. Polyunsaturated fats and female hormones have antagonistic effects on vitamin E.

CLINICAL USE. Vitamin E has been used in a number of human dermatoses including epidermolysis bullosa, pemphigus, subcorneal pustular dermatosis, vasculitis, and discoid lupus erythematosus. Most of these cases represent small numbers and were uncontrolled and anecdotal in nature. In veterinary dermatology, vitamin E has been used to treat discoid lupus erythematosus (DLE), pemphigus erythematosus, dermatomyositis, epidermolysis bullosa, idiopathic acanthosis nigricans, and demodicosis. The current dosage of vitamin E used in DLE or pemphigus erythematosus is 400 to 600 IU twice a day. Most researchers report that only an occasional patient with DLE responds to just vitamin E therapy. However, there is one report in which 7 of 16 patients had complete recoveries (Scott and Walton, 1984). Although the majority of patients do not respond in this way, vitamin E may have a steroid-sparing effect and is still recommended. Currently, no benefit has been seen with vitamin E in the treatment of dermatomyositis. Vitamin E at a dosage of 200 IU twice a day has been reported to be effective in the treatment of idiopathic acanthosis nigricans (Scott and Walton, 1985). The success of other researchers with vitamin E in this clinical presentation is limited, and some use vitamin E as an adjunctive to antibiotics and shampoo therapy. The most recent use of vitamin E has been as a treatment for canine demodicosis. A report in which 147 of 149 dogs completely recovered while receiving vitamin E at a dose of only 200 mg five times a day was most impressive (Figuerido, 1985). In this report, plasma vitamin E levels in dogs with demodicosis were lower than those in normal controls. However, recent unpublished work indicates that normal vitamin E levels range from 4 to 28 μg/dl and that most dogs with demodicosis have normal vitamin E levels (Gilbert, 1987). This would suggest that these patients do not have vitamin E deficiencies and that the vitamin is working in some other fashion. Regardless of the disease, one should allow 30 to 40 days for a clinical response.

TOXICITY. The side effects reported with vitamin E in humans are as uncontrolled and anecdotal as the diseases that the therapy is claimed to help.

These side effects include hypertension, thrombophlebitis, fatigue, nausea, flatulence, diarrhea, myopathy, stomatitis, coagulopathy, urticaria, sore breasts, and decreased insulin requirements in diabetic patients. In laboratory animals, megadoses of vitamin E have been associated with coagulopathy, reduced thyroid function, adrenal degeneration, decreased weight gain, and infertility. An interesting side effect seen by one clinician occurred in a tricolored collie with discoid lupus erythematosus whose black coat turned white (Griffin, 1985).

Cimetidine

MECHANISM. Cimetidine is an H_2 histamine receptor antagonist (H_2 blocker) that has been used in upper gastrointestinal ulcerative disease. Experimental work in guinea pigs showed that histamine inhibited cell-mediated immunity as measured by reduced skin test reactivity, decreased production of antigen-induced lymphyokine migration–inhibiting factor, and, to a lesser degree, reduced lymphocyte proliferation response. This histamine-induced suppression could be completely blocked by H_2 receptor antagonists. Cimetidine has also been shown to restore cell-mediated immunity in patients with alopecia areata treated with dinitrochlorobenzene (DNCB) that had developed tolerance to DNCB. Peptic ulcer patients have been found to have enhanced cell-mediated immunity, by augmented response to a panel of skin test antigens. Cimetidine has also been shown to restore skin test reactivity and the production of lymphocyte migration–inhibiting factor, but not lymphocyte transformation in patients with chronic mucocutaneous candidiasis. The theory behind cimetidine's immunomodulation effects relates to the drug's ability to block H_2 receptors on suppressor T-cells that modulate lymphokine production. Therefore, cimetidine could act as an immunostimulator by reversing T-suppressor–mediated immune suppression in patients with chronic infectious diseases.

PHARMACOKINETICS. Cimetidine is rapidly absorbed after oral administration. Peak levels in humans occur within 45 to 90 min. Its half-life is approximately 2 hr. The primary route of excretion is urinary.

CLINICAL USE. The current dermatologic use of cimetidine (Tagamet, SmithKline) is in immunostimulation for canine patients with recurrent pyodermas or other chronically recurring infectious dermatoses. The recommended dosage is 3 to 4 mg/kg twice daily, used in conjunction with antibiotics until the pyoderma is cleared. Then, treatment is continued for a minimum of 12 weeks. If effective, the cimetidine will need to be continued at the same dosage for life. Individual patients have reportedly responded favorably to this protocol. This

drug has the added advantages of oral administration and low incidence of side effects. Some researchers advocate the concurrent use of an H_1 blocker, such as hydroxyzine hydrochloride, 1 mg/kg twice daily. The logic associated with this is that the use of only an H_2 blocker can inhibit the negative feedback mechanism on histamine release, resulting in increased levels of histamine and subsequent inflammation.

TOXICITY. The incidence of side effects with cimetidine is very low. In humans, long-term use has been reported to cause individual cases of gynecomastia, antiandrogenic effects, reversible alopecia and arthralgias, agranulocytosis, fever, hepatic reactions, and mental confusion.

Staphylococcal Antigens

MECHANISM. Several staphylococcal bacterial products have been used as immunostimulants in canine recurrent pyodermas. The staphylococcal cell wall is considered the major bacterial antigenic fraction. The constituents of the cell wall of *Staphylococcus aureus* are the capsule, clumping factor, proteins A and B, teichoic acid, and peptidoglycan. Of these, protein A and peptidoglycan are the most biologically active and important in immunostimulation. Autogenous and commercial bacterins include many of these antigenic fractions. Although autogenous bacterins can be made, they are often expensive and difficult to obtain and can be irritating. Staphoid A-B (Jensal Labs, Burroughs Wellcome) is a commercially available bacterin that contains mixtures of cell wall antigens and toxoids. Currently, this product has fallen out of vogue but reportedly has been used successfully. The most commonly used product is Staphage Lysate (SPL) (Delmont Labs, Swarthmore, PA). The remainder of the discussion will be centered on this product.

SPL is a bacteriologically sterile staphylococcal vaccine containing components of *S. aureus* bacteriophage and culture medium ingredients. It is not heated or treated with preservatives. It is prepared by using cultures of serologic type I and III *S. aureus* with a polyvalent *Staphylococcus* bacteriophage. Clinical benefits may be related to the stimulation of T- and B-lymphocytes and macrophage killing. SPL has been shown to stimulate lymphocyte blastogenesis in patients with staphylococcal pyoderma (Rosser, 1982).

CLINICAL USE. The indication for a bacterial antigen is an antibiotic-responsive, recurrent staphylococcal pyoderma. "Bacterial hypersensitivity" is a highly controversial area, as many pyodermas without a hypersensitivity reaction can present with target lesions, pruritus, and vasculitis. SPL should be reserved for those recurrent pyoderma patients in whom no underlying etiology can be found. Many protocols have been advocated. Some researchers are using an abbreviated protocol, giving 1 cc subcutaneously (regardless of weight) once a week for a minimum of 12 weeks. Antibiotics are used initially if there is active pyoderma. After the pyoderma has cleared following therapy with the antibiotics, the injections of bacterial antigen are tried as the sole therapy. If a good response is seen, the injections can be administered as needed, usually every 10 to 14 days. As *S. intermedius* is now known to be the primary staphylococcal species in pyodermas in the dog, future work will undoubtedly involve an SPL isolated from this species, with hopes of a more effective and specific immunostimulation.

TOXICITY. The side effects reported with SPL are limited. Reactions at the site of the injection can cause pruritus, swelling, and, on rare occasions, sloughing. Malaise, fever, vomiting, and quivering have also been reported. One researcher has commented on a case of polyarthritis that was associated with SPL injections (Griffin, 1985).

Immunoregulin

MECHANISM. Immunoregulin (Immuno Vet, Tampa, FL) is a suspension of killed *Propionibacterium acnes* (formerly *Corynebacterium parvum*). The mechanism of action appears to be a direct stimulation of macrophage activity.

CLINICAL USE. Immunoregulin has been advocated as an immunostimulant in a variety of immunosuppressive conditions. Many early reports were uncontrolled and anecdotal. Recently, an unpublished double-blinded crossover study evaluated Immunoregulin in a group of dogs in whom major underlying causes for recurrent pyoderma had been ruled out. The results of the study were that 12 of the 15 dogs (80 per cent) treated with *P. acnes* and antibiotics responded with complete remission or significant improvement of lesions after the first 12 weeks of therapy. In the group receiving placebos, only 5 of 13 dogs (38.5 per cent) exhibited such positive improvement. Several of the 12 dogs receiving placebos participated in the crossover, and 4 of 7 (57 per cent) showed complete remission. Two of the researchers who participated in this study had only one of five (20 per cent) of their patients exhibit complete remission (Griffin and Rosenkrantz, 1986).

The current protocol requires intravenous parenteral administration twice weekly during the first 2 weeks, and then weekly from the third to the twelfth week. The dosage is dependent on the patient's weight: less than 7 kg, 0.25 ml; 7 to 20 kg, 0.5 ml; 20 to 34 kg, 1.0 ml; and greater than 34 kg, 2.0 ml. The requirement of parenteral administra-tion and the expense make this form of immunostimulation less desirable in a clinical setting.

TOXICITY. The aforementioned study did not list side effects. However, some researchers have commented on mild anaphylactoid reactions after injection, including vomiting, anorexia, malaise, and fever. Extravascular injection can result in tissue inflammation and swelling.

Levamisole

MECHANISM. Levamisole, initially used for its anthelmintic effects, has been shown to have immunomodulating effects. Reportedly, levamisole affects only immunocompromised patients and has no effect on normal patients. The major effects occur through stimulation of production of lymphocytes, an increase in DNA synthesis in mitogen-stimulated lymphocytes, and an increase in the ratio of helper cells to suppressor cells. Levamisole also has been shown to stimulate phagocytosis, chemotaxis, and intracellular killing of macrophages and granulocytes. The exact mechanism of action is not entirely known but is thought to relate to modulation of lymphokines and cyclic nucleotides within the leukocytes.

CLINICAL USE. The current dermatologic use for levamisole is in immunostimulation for dogs with recurrent cutaneous infections. It has also been reported to be effective in some cases of canine systemic lupus erythematosus. Levamisole (Levasole, Pitman-Moore) is available as a 184-mg, scored bolus for worming sheep. The dosage must be closely calculated and followed, as low or high dosages are not effective and may actually further immunosuppress the patient. The recommended protocol is 2.2 mg/kg every other day, used in conjunction with antimicrobial agents until the infection is under control. If effective, the levamisole will need to be continued at the same dosage for life.

TOXICITY. Side effects are rarely seen but can include gastrointestinal disturbances, lethargy, neurotoxicity, and agranulocytosis. Periodic complete blood counts and chemistry screens are recommended to screen for toxic effects. The oral administration of levamisole makes this form of immunostimulation practical in a clinical setting. However, administration to a small dog can be difficult if the only dosage form available is the large bolus used in sheep.

References and Supplemental Reading

Ahmed, A. R., and Hambal, S. M.: Cyclophosphamide (Cytoxan): A review of relevant pharmacology and clinical uses. J. Am. Acad. Dermatol. 11:1115, 1984.

Ayres, S.: Vitamin E: An effective therapeutic agent in dermatology. *In* Epstein, E. (ed.): *Controversies in Dermatology.* Philadelphia: W. B. Saunders Co., 1984, pp. 379–385.

Fenuhel, R. L., and Chivigos, M. A.: *Immune Modulation Agents and Their Mechanisms.* New York: Marcel Dekker, 1984.

Figuerido, C.: Vitamin E serum content, erythrocyte and lymphocyte count, PCV and hemoglobin determinations in normal dogs, and dogs with scabies or demodicosis. Presentation, American Academy of Veterinary Dermatologists, Orlando, 1985.

Gilbert, P.: Unpublished studies, 1987.

Gilman, A. G., Goodman, L. S., Rall, T. W., et al.: *Goodman and Gilman's The Pharmacological Basis of Therapeutics,* 7th ed. New York: Macmillan Publishing Co., 1985.

Griffin, C. E., and Rosenkrantz, W. R.: Unpublished data on ImmunoRegulin therapy for recurrent pyoderma in dogs, 1986.

Jorizzo, J. L., Sams, M. W., Jegasothy, B. V., et al.: Cimetidine as an immunomodulator: Chronic mucocutaneous candidiasis as a model. Ann. Intern. Med. 92:192, 1980.

Long, R. E.: Potential of chrysotherapy in veterinary medicine. J.A.V.M.A. 5:539, 1984.

Muller, G. H., Kirk, R. W., and Scott, D. W.: *Small Animal Dermatology,* 3rd ed. Philadelphia: W. B. Saunders Co., 1983, pp. 163–177.

Roberts, H. J.: The Vitamin E enigma: Perspectives for physicians. *In* Epstein, E. (ed.): *Controversies in Dermatology.* Philadelphia: W. B. Saunders Co., 1984, pp. 386–395.

Rosenkrantz, W. R., Griffin, C. E., and Barr, R. J.: Cyclosporine therapy in cutaneous immune-mediated dermatoses and epitheliotropic lymphoma. Am. Anim. Hosp. Assoc. (in press).

Rosser, E.: Stophage Lysate. Presentation at the 49th Annual Meeting, Las Vegas, Nevada 1982.

Scott, D. W., and Walton, D. W.: Unusual findings in canine pemphigus erythematosus and discoid lupus erythematosus. Am. Anim. Hosp. Assoc. 20:579, 1984.

Scott, D. W., and Walton, D. W.: Clinical evaluation of oral vitamin E for the treatment of primary canine acanthosis nigricans. Am. Anim. Hosp. Assoc. 21:345, 1985.

Scott, D. W.: Sulfones and sulfonamides in canine dermatology. *In* Kirk, R. W. (ed.): *Current Veterinary Therapy IX.* Philadelphia: W. B. Saunders Co., 1986, pp. 606–609.

Stanton, M. E., and Legendre, A. M.: Effects of cyclophosphamide in dogs and cats. J.A.V.M.A. 11:1319, 1986.

Thomas, I.: Gold therapy and its indications in dermatology. J. Am. Acad. Dermatol. 16:845, 1987.

Werner, A., Wolff-Schreiner, E. C., Stinyl, G., et al.: Azathioprine in the treatment of pemphigus vulgaris. J. Am. Acad. Dermatol. 16:527, 1987.

White, J. C.: Cyclosporine: Prototype of a T-cell selective immunosuppressant. J.A.V.M.A. 5:566, 1986.

IMIDAZOLES AND TRIAZOLES

LINDA MEDLEAU, D.V.M.

Athens, Georgia

The imidazoles are one of the newest classes of antifungal agents available for the treatment of mycotic diseases. These agents are especially exciting because they offer the first broad-spectrum coverage against a wide variety of yeasts and fungi.

MECHANISM OF ACTION

The imidazoles are primarily fungistatic and may exert their effect through a number of mechanisms. Imidazoles interfere with the synthesis of ergosterol, a sterol that is necessary for fungal cell wall integrity. In the presence of imidazoles, C-14 methylsterols (ergosterol precursors) accumulate near the fungal cell wall. The lack of ergosterol, the buildup of precursor sterols, or both results in permeability changes, and fungal growth ceases. High doses of imidazoles inhibit the activity of oxidative and peroxidative enzymes that break down intracellular hydrogen peroxide. This results in the build-up of toxic peroxides, which leads to cellular degeneration and fungal cell death.

There may also be a synergistic relationship between imidazoles and leukocytes. Experimentally, when *Candida albicans* is cultured, mycelial growth occurs. If this culture is exposed to low doses of ketoconazole, only clusters of yeast cells will be seen. In mixed cultures of *Candida albicans* and leukocytes, long, branching mycelium predominate and remaining leukocytes are necrotic. However, if ketoconazole is added, many viable and motile leukocytes will be seen, and the *Candida* will be completely eradicated.

METABOLISM

Ketoconazole, the only imidazole compound that can be given orally, is dependent on an acidic environment for proper absorption from the gastrointestinal tract. Therefore, the H_2 antagonist cimetidine, antacids, or other drugs affecting gastric secretion should not be administered concurrently with ketoconazole. Ketoconazole is also lipophilic, which means that its absorption is increased if taken with a meal. Peak plasma levels occur in 1 to 2 hr. Ketoconazole is rapidly and extensively distributed throughout the body with adequate antifungal levels achieved in most tissues except testis, brain, and, probably, eye. Most of the absorbed ketoconazole is metabolized in the liver; therefore, little active drug is excreted in bile or urine. Consequently, dosages do not need to be adjusted in patients with renal failure. There may be impaired metabolism in patients with hepatic insufficiency, but the drug does not seem to accumulate (in humans). In dogs, 80 per cent of the drug is excreted within 48 hr, and 92 per cent of the drug is excreted within 1 week.

CLINICAL USE

Several topical imidazoles are available for treating localized dermatophytosis in animals (Table 1). These include clotrimazole, miconazole, and econazole. Clotrimazole can be used only topically because its gastrointestinal and neurologic side effects prevent its systemic use. Miconazole is available over the counter and by prescription for topical use and also is toxic if given systemically. Econazole is effective topically and possibly systemically. However, there is no available parental form of this drug. Topical imidazoles are applied b.i.d. to affected areas for 2 to 4 weeks, with treatment continuing 1 week beyond apparent clinical cure.

For generalized dermatophytosis in dogs and cats, systemic treatment with oral griseofulvin is usually the initial treatment of choice, since ketoconazole is not licensed for animal use. However, ketoconazole is also effective in small animal dermatophyte infections. Daily administration of ketoconazole, 10 to 20 mg/kg given once daily or divided into two daily doses, is usually effective. Giving it with food enhances its absorption. Regardless of whether ketoconazole or griseofulvin is used, systemic treatment must be continued until fungal cultures are negative or for at least 2 weeks beyond apparent clinical cure.

In humans, systemic mycoses with a fair to good response to ketoconazole therapy include blastomycosis (good), coccidioidomycosis (fair), chromomycosis (fair), histoplasmosis (good), paracoccidioidomycosis (good), and sporotrichosis (fair).

The treatment of choice for canine histoplasmosis, blastomycosis, and, possibly, coccidioidomycosis is

the combination of amphotericin B and ketoconazole. The major advantage of this regimen is that long-term amphotericin B therapy is avoided, which minimizes the possibility of renal toxicosis. Initially, both amphotericin B and ketoconazole are administered for 5 to 10 days, followed by ketoconazole alone until the disease is in remission. Amphotericin B may be administered intravenously at a dose of 0.5 mg/kg/day or 1 mg/kg every other day. Ketoconazole is given orally at a dose of 10 to 20 mg/kg that is repeated every 12 hr. Therapy should be continued at least 1 month beyond apparent clinical cure. Because ketoconazole is a fungistatic agent and therefore slow-acting, treatment may need to continue for at least 1 year.

Ketoconazole was ineffective in the treatment of experimental sporotrichosis in cats. However, ketoconazole has been used alone to successfully treat cats with cryptococcosis and histoplasmosis. In general, doses ranged from 10 mg/kg once daily in cats with cryptococcosis to 20 mg/kg b.i.d. every other day for a cat with histoplasmosis. However, successful treatment of one cat with cryptococcosis required long-term therapy with very high doses of ketoconazole (72 mg/kg/day). Surgical resection followed by therapy with ketoconazole (10 mg/kg once daily) was also used to successfully treat a cat with phaeohyphomycosis. As with dogs, long-term therapy (months) is usually needed to resolve systemic mycotic infections in cats.

Because ketoconazole has been found to inhibit adrenal corticosteroid and androgen production in humans and rats, the effectiveness of ketoconazole in treating canine hyperadrenocorticism has been studied. Cushingoid dogs were treated with ketoconazole, 15 mg/kg PO every 12 hr. A rapid decrease in plasma cortisol concentration, suppression of plasma cortisol response to synthetic adrenocorticotropic hormone (ACTH), and remission of clinical signs were seen in seven of eight dogs with pituitary-dependent hyperadrenocorticism and two of three dogs with adrenal tumors. The disadvantages of using ketoconazole to treat hyperadrenocorticism include the possibility of drug-related vomiting and the high cost of the drug.

SIDE EFFECTS

Side effects of ketoconazole administration in humans are uncommon but include nausea, vomiting, diarrhea, abdominal pain, and pruritus. Decreased libido, impotence, and gynecomastia have also been described. Potential hepatic reactions are the side effects of the greatest concern in humans. These include silent reactions (transient elevations of serum liver enzyme levels) and symptomatic reactions due to hepatitis. Hepatic reactions are presumably idiosyncratic and usually occur within

Table 1. Imidazoles and Triazoles

Generic Name	Trade Name
Topicals	
Clotrimazole	Lotrimin (Schering)
	Mycelex (Miles Pharm)
Miconazole	Micatin (Advanced Care)
	Conofite (Pitman-Moore)
	Monistat (Ortho)
Econazole	Spectrazole (Ortho)
Bifonazole	—
Oxiconazole	—
Tioconazole	—
Enilconazole	—
Terconazole	—
Systemics (oral)	
Ketoconazole	Nizoral (Janssen)
Fluconazole	—
Itraconazole	—

the first few months of therapy. Since ketoconazole has been shown to be teratogenic in laboratory animals, its use during pregnancy is not recommended.

In dogs and cats, anorexia, diarrhea, vomiting, elevated serum liver enzyme levels, and icterus have been associated with ketoconazole administration. Giving ketoconazole with food and dividing the daily dose b.i.d. to q.i.d. may help alleviate signs of anorexia or vomiting. If anorexia persists, ketoconazole therapy should be halted until the animal is eating normally and then reinstituted at a lower dosage, given on an alternate-day basis, or both. Change in coat color (lightening or graying) during ketoconazole therapy has also been observed occasionally in dogs.

In cases of accidental overdose, gastric lavage with a sodium bicarbonate solution, which increases the gastric pH, helps prevent the absorption of ingested ketoconazole.

NEWER ANTIFUNGAL AGENTS

Several newer imidazoles are undergoing clinical tests but are not yet available for general use. New topical agents include bifonazole, oxiconazole, tioconazole, and enilconazole. Tioconazole has fungicidal activity and may lead to more rapid clearing of infection than the other imidazoles. Topical enilconazole, 10 to 20 mg/kg/day for 1 to 2 weeks, has been used to successfully treat nasal aspergillosis in dogs.

Triazole antifungals are also in an investigational phase and are not yet available in the United States. Terconazole, a topical agent, may be more active against dermatophytes than are the imidazoles. Itraconazole and fluconazole are triazole drugs being developed for oral use. Itraconazole shares basic principles of activity with its predecessor compounds such as ketoconazole. Itraconazole has fungicidal or fungistatic activity against dermatophytes, yeasts, aspergilli, and various other pathogenic fungi. It appears to be among the most promising systemic agents in experimental and clinical trials. In general, the concentrations of itraconazole needed to inhibit fungal growth are many times lower than the concentrations needed with ketoconazole. Compared with other azole derivatives, itraconazole is the only drug that exerts a pronounced *in vitro* activity against a variety of *Aspergillus* species. Unlike ketoconazole, itraconazole may achieve adequate brain levels at therapeutic doses, and it also appears to have less toxic side effects. For instance, serum testosterone levels and plasma cortisol levels have not been affected in animals and human volunteers given itraconazole. Itraconazole appears to be at least as effective as ketoconazole against paracoccidioidomycosis and histoplasmosis in humans. It has shown excellent activity in sporotrichosis and chromomycosis. Itraconazole has also been used to successfully treat experimental cryptococcosis in mice, rabbits, and cats. Results in aspergilloma and aspergillosis in humans and dogs are also promising but need to be confirmed in future studies.

References and Supplemental Reading

Angarano, D. W., and Scott, D. W.: Use of ketoconazole in the treatment of dermatophytosis in a dog. J.A.V.M.A. 190:1433, 1987.
Bruyette, D. S., Feldman, E. C., and Tyrrell, J. B.: Efficacy of ketoconazole in the management of spontaneous canine hyperadrenocorticism. Proceedings, 5th Annual ACVIM meeting (abstract), 1987, p. 885.
De Keyser, H., and Van den Brande, M.: Ketoconazole in the treatment of dermatomycosis in cats and dogs. Vet. Q. 5:142, 1983.
Graybill, J. R., and Craven, P. C.: Antifungal agents used in systemic mycoses. Drugs 25:41, 1983.
Heel, R. C., Brogden, A., Carmine, P. A., et al.: Ketoconazole: A review of its therapeutic efficacy in superficial and systemic fungal infections. Drugs 23:1, 1982.
Lesher, J. L., and Smith, J. G.: Antifungal agents in dermatology. J. Am. Acad. Dermatol. 17:383, 1987.
Medleau, L., Hall, E. J., Goldschmidt, M. H., et al.: Cutaneous cryptococcosis in three cats. J.A.V.M.A. 817:169, 1985.
Noxon, J. O., Digilio, K., Schmidt, D. A., et al.: Disseminated histoplasmosis in a cat: Successful treatment with ketoconazole. J.A.V.M.A. 181:187, 1982.
Pentlarge, V. W., and Martin, R. A.: Treatment of cryptococcosis in three cats, using ketoconazole. J.A.V.M.A. 188:536, 1986.
Richardson, R. C., Jaeger, L. A., and Wigle, W.: Treatment of systemic mycoses in dogs. J.A.V.M.A. 183:335, 1983.

LASERS IN DERMATOLOGY

PATRICK T. BREEN, D.V.M.

Cincinnati, Ohio

The term LASER is an acronym. It stands for *l*ight *a*mplification by *s*timulated *e*mission of *r*adiation. This mechanism of stimulated emission was first postulated by Einstein in 1917; however, the first working laser was reportedly built by Theodore H. Maiman in 1960. Dermatologists owe a debt of gratitude to Leon Goldman, M.D., who pioneered the use of lasers in skin disease in 1962 at the University of Cincinnati College of Medicine.

Laser light is a unique form of light that is not found in nature. The three unique properties of laser light are (1) coherence (all light waves are in phase in both time and space), (2) collimation (the light waves all are traveling in nearly parallel directions with negligible divergence), and (3) monochromaticity (the light waves all are of the same wavelength). The laser wavelength is dependent on its generating medium. The active laser medium is a collection of atoms capable of undergoing stimulated emission of photons. The laser-generating chamber makes use of parallel mirrors and electric energy to produce spontaneous emission of photon light energy. The laser beam of light may be focused with lenses and mirrors into a precise spot, with high-power concentration to cut or vaporize tissue or with lower-power intensities to coagulate tissue for hemostasis. Medical lasers are not oncogenic, as are x-rays, since photonic ionization of living tissue does not occur. The carbon dioxide (CO_2) (10,600 nm infrared) laser and the argon dye (630 nm) laser are the two types of lasers of the greatest interest and application to veterinary dermatology.

THE CARBON DIOXIDE LASER

This laser has many unique properties that make it the choice for skin surgery in medicine today. The carbon dioxide laser is a pulsed energy beam created by passing high voltage across carbon dioxide gas. Nitrogen and helium are added to the carbon dioxide. The nitrogen cools and cleans the lens of the laser tube, while the helium provides a red-orange color to the beam, which otherwise would be invisible. The color provided by the helium establishes a focusing point, so the carbon dioxide beam can be visually directed to the proper point on the skin.

Advantages

The wavelength of the carbon dioxide laser (10,600 nm) is very well absorbed by water. Because skin is 70 to 90 per cent water, the laser absorption causes intercellular and extracellular vaporization of the water in living tissue. This process results in the release of steam, which is seen as a plume of smoke and is removed by a vacuum system to prevent inhalation and to reduce odor.

Of the advantages of the carbon dioxide laser, perhaps the greatest is that very little insult to skin tissue occurs beyond 500 μm from the spot receiving a well-focused beam of carbon dioxide laser light of the intensity used in cutting skin. This is a in significant contrast to, and has a definite advantage over, electrocautery or cryosurgery. Another advantage is that the heat produced by the carbon dioxide laser in the cutting mode also sterilizes the surgical area. However, studies indicate that in a defocused mode for vaporizations, some viral particles and bacterial spores can escape into the smoke plume. A high-quality vacuum system is used to remove this plume of smoke and to filter the air. In addition, when the carbon dioxide laser cuts the skin, it also seals blood vessels as small as capillaries as well as lymphatics. This is advantageous in surgery when malignant tumors or highly vascular areas, such as the oral cavity or the external ear, are involved. The carbon dioxide laser also produces a capping effect on the nerve ending, which may explain why humans who have laser surgery report little postoperative pain. This capping effect on the nerve ending could prove to be of great benefit in small animal dermatology for patients that mutilate the skin in conditions such as acral lick dermatitis.

Disadvantages

Along with the advantages of the carbon dioxide laser, some disadvantages must be considered carefully. The carbon dioxide laser light can cause damage to unprotected skin and the cornea of the eye; however, this damage is limited to the more superficial layers because of the absorption of the laser beam by the water in the tissue. Protection of the eye from the carbon dioxide laser beam may be accomplished by wearing special protective plastic eye glasses. During surgery, the laser beam should not be directed at any high-gloss surfaces, such as stainless steel tables or instruments in the surgical field. The carbon dioxide laser also causes combustion of paper products. In the surgical field, this is prevented by soaking the edges of the drapes with sterile saline solution. During oral procedures, the endotracheal tube must be protected, either by aluminum foil or by using a metal tube to prevent penetration of the tube by the laser. Overlooking this preventive measure could result in fire and potential explosion of the gas and oxygen used for anesthesia. The carbon dioxide laser beam cannot be passed over fiber optics to allow it to reach into body cavities; however, new materials such as ceramics offer promise for accomplishing this in the future.

Equipment

The design of the laser head is constantly undergoing modification. The objective is to make an instrument that feels more comparable to the scalpel, to better fit the hand and make it comfortable to the surgeon. New 20-watt carbon dioxide lasers are being made for medical dermatology. Model LS20-H (Directed Energy, Irvine, CA) is priced in a range making it economically feasible for veterinary use.

Application

The author has used the LS20-H model laser for several dermatologic surgery procedures. It has proved to be an effective mode for removing basal cell tumors and sebaceous adenomas from vascular areas. This model, used in the defocused mode, is very effective in vaporization of sebaceous adenomas on the body surface in general, with minimal blood loss and no suturing required. The animals have had little tendency to traumatize the areas postoperatively. This model has also been used, with fair success, in the management of eosinophilic granuloma in the feline. It should be noted that there is no assurance that this condition will not recur, since the etiology of the disorder is not known. Studies are under way to evaluate this further.

The following is a list of applications of the carbon dioxide laser in the Department of Laboratory Animal Medicine in the College of Medicine at the University of Cincinnati: (1) epulis of the gum and other oral tumors of the gum; (2) tumors of the skin in highly vascular areas (the ear, the tip of the tail); (3) débridement of wounds to aid in healing (includes fistular tracts of the skin); (4) granulation and hypertrophic tissue of the external ear canal; (5) eyelid margin tumors, and any other tumors when preserving the integrity of the skin is important; (6)

early acral lick dermatitis; and (7) eosinophilic granuloma lesions of the lip in the cat. This list will continue to grow with our increased understanding of the potential for this valuable tool, along with improvements in the technology. There has been a report of positive results with the use of the carbon dioxide laser in a defocused mode for reducing the scars of discoid lupus erythematosus in humans, which would have a direct application to veterinary dermatology.

THE ARGON DYE LASER: PHOTODYNAMIC THERAPY

The preferred term for the use of photosensitization to treat disease is termed photodynamic therapy (PDT). The use of light-absorbing chemicals to cause photoreactions in biologic systems is the basis for photodynamic therapy. This reaction requires oxygen and a photosensitizer, and then a light source, the argon dye laser beam. The mechanism of action to cause inactivation of a biologic system is thought mainly to be an energy transfer process from excited triplet state of the sensitizer to oxygen, producing singlet oxygen. This process causes the irreversible oxidation of some essential cellular components.

The ideal photosensitizer would be nontoxic in clinically useful doses, would be selectively retained in malignant tissue, would be activated by penetrating light (>600 nm), and would be photochemically efficient. One of the first photosensitizers used was a hematoporphyrin derivative (HPD). Recently, a more purified form, dihematophorphyrin ether (DHE), has been in use. Much of this work was pioneered by T. J. Dougherty and his colleagues at Roswell Park, Buffalo, New York.

To activate these photosensitizers, the argon ion laser pumped-dye laser system was developed. In this system, the argon laser light is used, and a red dye is pumped across the beam of light to obtain a wavelength of 630 nm. This is a visible wavelength of light, and protection of the eye with green lenses to shade out the 630 nm red light is necessary. Although other light sources can be used, the monochromatic light of the argon dye laser (630 nm) is the one that is the most effectively absorbed by malignant cells that are retaining HPD or DHE, thus resulting in their destruction.

Advantages

A distinct advantage of the wavelength of laser light produced by the argon dye laser is that it can be passed over fiber optics to affect areas within the deeper reaches of the skin tumor or inside body cavities. Pathologic studies show necrosis in tumors can vary from 3 to 10 mm in depth. The variation in necrosis depends on the type of photosensitizer, the light source, and the power settings.

The exact mechanism of action of photosensitizers in tumors and how they are retained there to cause damage when exposed to laser light is still not completely understood. In general terms, most tumors seem to have porphyrin associated with their vascular stroma (macrophages, mast cells, and possibly fibroblasts). It is theorized that the leaky vasculature of the tumor allows the porphyrin aggregates to enter the tumor interstitial fluid, where lack of lymphatic drainage results in relatively long exposure, and irreversible cell binding occurs. Porphyrin aggregates are apparently incorporated into the reticular endothelial cells by various phagocytic and pinocytic processes. Thus, the process appears to be one of both vascular and cell destruction, not unlike that seen in hyperthermia therapy. Indeed, some of the most exciting work is the combination of hyperthermia and PDT therapies to treat cancer.

Disadvantages

One point of caution when using PDT is that even normal skin will have relatively high levels of porphyrin retention (probably in macrophages), so the length and power of light exposure are critical. In humans, it is stressed that patients must avoid outdoor light for up to 60 days to prevent damage to normal skin areas. This may be of less concern in canine and feline patients; however, areas of the body where hair covering is sparce would cause concern.

Application

The use of photodynamic therapy is still considered to be experimental in both humans and animals. However, in investigations at the University of Cincinnati College of Medicine, Department of Laboratory Animal Medicine and Cincinnati Jewish Hospital, William Rogers, D.V.M., and colleagues have used the therapy to successfully treat squamous cell carcinoma of the extremities in cats and to reduce the size of tumors of the oral cavity. However, this treatment has not proved to be a total therapy. It has been necessary to accompany the PDT with conventional surgery and irradiation techniques.

A possible future application of PDT in veterinary dermatology is for the treatment of external skin cancer. A patient could receive an intravenous dose of the sensitizer as an outpatient 3 days prior to laser surgery. Then, upon admission to the hospital for the surgery, simple restraint, light tranquilization, and local anesthesia would be adequate to keep the patient comfortable during treatment of superficial problems. This would make hospitalization of the patient unnecessary. General anesthesia would be required only if fiber optic probes were needed to reach deeper into a tumor area. Another application under investigation is the administration of photosensitizers with acetone topically to external skin lesions and then the exposure of the lesions to the argon dye laser light. As the argon dye laser technology becomes more sophisticated and other possibilities are explored, PDT could replace conventional irradiation and surgical procedures for skin cancer.

SUMMARY

It is evident that laser therapy promises some significant advantages and advances for veterinary dermatology. Although the investigations are exciting and indicate that use of the laser could be a superior therapy mode, it is imperative that it be administered only by those with complete training in its use and understanding of how to select the conditions to be treated. Bear in mind quotations of two leaders in the field of laser investigation in human medicine: Dr. Isaac Kaplan admonishes, "If you do not know how to use the laser, do not try," and Dr. Leon Goldman cautions, "If you do not need the laser, do not use it."

References and Supplemental Reading

Carruth, J. A. S.: Photodynamic therapy: The state of the art. Lasers Surg. Med. 6:404, 1986.
Crane, S. W.: State of the art message: Lasers in veterinary surgery. Lasers Surg. Med. 6:427, 1986.
DeVita, V. T., Jr., Hellman, S., and Rosenberg, S. A.: *Cancer Principles and Practice of Oncology*, 2nd Ed. Philadelphia: J. B. Lippincott Co., 1985, pp. 2272–2279, 2326–2331.
Henderson, D. L., and Odom, J. C.: Laser treatment of discoid lupus. Case report. Lasers Surg. Med. 6:12–15, 44–45, 1986.
Goldman, L.: Laser dermatology, 1985. Lasers Surg. Med. 6:387, 1986.
Goldman, L. (ed.): *The Biomedical Laser: Technology and Clinical Applications*. New York: Springer-Verlag, 1981.
Gregory, R. O., and Goldman, L.: Application of photodynamic therapy in plastic surgery. Lasers Surg. Med. 6:62, 1986.
Montgomery, T. C., Sharp, J. B., Bellina, J. H., et al.: Comparative gross and histological study of the effects of scalpel, electric knife, and carbon dioxide laser on skin and uterine incisions in dogs. Lasers Surg. Med. 3:9, 1983.
Walker, P. J., Matthews, J., and Newsom, S. W. B.: Possible hazards from irradiation with the carbon dioxide laser. Lasers Surg. Med. 6:84, 1986.

MILIARY DERMATITIS, EOSINOPHILIC GRANULOMA COMPLEX, AND SYMMETRIC HYPOTRICHOSIS AS MANIFESTATIONS OF FELINE ALLERGY

GAIL A. KUNKLE, D.V.M.
Gainesville, Florida

Feline allergic diseases have not been well characterized according to clinical symptoms, tests for diagnosis, and appropriate therapy. There is wide agreement that allergies occur in this species, but theories on the pathogenesis of allergic disease in the cat have been made by extrapolation from what is known of canine and equine allergies. Immunoglobulin E (IgE), known to be of major importance in the pathomechanism of immediate hypersensitivities, has not been isolated in the cat. However, clinical and histopathologic findings have led veterinarians to presume that, like canine skin, feline skin is a major target organ for allergic disease. The role of allergens in the induction or provocation of symptoms in other organ systems of the cat (e.g., respiratory and gastrointestinal systems) have likewise not been well-defined.

FELINE ALLERGY

Allergic diseases in the cat that lead to dermatologic symptoms may occur from exposure to allergens through inhalation, ingestion, topical contact, or the bite of an ectoparasite. Contact allergy is uncommon in animals and especially in the feline species, whose hair coat (and grooming habits) protects the skin almost completely from contactant antigens and subsequent sensitization. Thus, contact allergy would be an unlikely differential diagnosis for the syndromes discussed in this article.

Feline Atopy

Feline atopy is presumed to occur by production of allergen-specific IgE after repeated exposure to inhaled antigens. Clinical signs vary from those of miliary dermatitis (with obvious inflammation of the skin) to simple hypotrichosis due to excessive grooming. It is probable that, like canine cases, some cases of feline atopy may exhibit no primary eruptions. Whereas dogs scratch and pruritus is a hallmark of atopy, cats may lick and groom the hair excessively without traumatizing the skin. Other clinical signs include lesions histologically similar to eosinophilic plaques. Any recurrent or chronic eosinophilic dermatitis should be evaluated for allergy. Historically, feline atopy is steroid responsive initially. Seasonality is variable, depending on the types of allergens to which the cat has become hypersensitive.

The diagnosis of atopy is best made by intradermal skin testing, with antigen selection being very similar to that used in defining canine atopy. Corticosteroids should be withdrawn prior to skin testing for 4 to 8 weeks, depending on prior drug use. Progestin therapy should also be withheld, but facts concerning length of withdrawal time are not known. Antihistamine drugs should be discontinued for at least 2 weeks before testing is attempted.

Many cats can be tested in the sitting position with minimal restraint, and others may be easily tested through the zippered hole of a cat bag. Experiences of several veterinary dermatologists indicate that ketamine hydrochloride does not appear to interfere with test results. The cat is clipped on the lateral thorax, and testing is done with 0.05 to 0.1 cc of each allergen intradermally. Interpretation of skin test results is somewhat more difficult in cats than dogs because cats have thinner skin and the wheals are less visible. Reactions are best determined by palpation, and the wheals may appear and fade more quickly than the recommended 15 min for dogs. Therefore, it is best not to leave the cat for any time but to carefully observe the skin test site during the 15 min following the injections. Skin reactions from tests with antigens are compared with skin reactions from saline (negative control) and histamine phosphate 1:100,000 (positive control). Glycerinated extracts should be avoided.

Therapy for feline atopy should be determined on an individual basis, according to severity of symptoms, seasonality, allergens involved, and response to treatment. Carefully consider other factors that may be contributing to the threshold of pruritus. Some cats with atopy can be successfully managed with oral antihistamine therapy. Chlorpheniramine, 2 to 4 mg/cat once or twice daily, may relieve clinical symptoms. The use of hydroxyzine in cats has resulted in more varied results, as reported by various veterinary dermatologists. Central nervous system signs (e.g., depression) may occur in cats receiving hydroxyzine.

Many cases of feline atopy can be clinically controlled with oral prednisone, 1 to 4 mg/kg every other day. Injectable glucocorticoids such as methylprednisolone acetate, 4 mg/kg, are also beneficial for relief of symptoms. In most instances, the long-acting injectables should not be repeated more frequently than every 30 days. Although side effects of steroids are not as common in the cat as in the dog, they do occur.

Hyposensitization therapy has been useful in a limited number of cases of feline allergy. A protocol similar to that recommended for dogs has been utilized. The exact duration of time necessary for response to hyposensitization has not been defined, and there are no controlled clinical studies. Anaphylaxis in cats is a rare phenomenon. It has been created experimentally, only with difficulty. It is an unlikely sequela to hyposensitization therapy.

Finally, as in any form of allergic disease, avoidance of the allergens should be attempted if feasible.

Feline Food Allergy

The immunologic mechanism of food allergy in the cat is also ill defined. However, there is no doubt that the clinical signs relative to hypersensitivities or reactions (probably immune-mediated) to foods are varied in cats and may involve the skin, the gastrointestinal tract, or the respiratory system. Cutaneous symptoms run the gamut from severe head pruritus with severe self-mutilation to miliary dermatitis to symmetric zealous grooming of the body, leading to hypotrichosis without inflammation. In addition, eosinophilic dermatitis, histologically similar to eosinophilic plaque, may also be seen in feline food allergy. Diarrhea and vomiting are not commonly seen with skin manifestations.

Feline food allergy is not usually due to a new food or a recent change in diet. The offending substance has usually been a component of the diet for some time. Unlike dogs, which usually receive the same dog food for years, cats often receive various products with different protein sources on a rotational basis. Thus, clinical signs are more likely to wax and wane. Prior response to corticosteroids, progestins, or both is quite variable in food allergy. A good initial response is, however, often transient.

The diagnosis of food allergy is made by the observation of gradual remission of signs while the animal is being fed a hypoallergenic diet. An unusual protein foodstuff such as lamb is usually chosen, and it should be fed for a minimum of 3 weeks. Strained baby food is usually preservative-free and palatable to most cats. Ingestion of other substances such as treats, houseplants, pet food of other animals, and human food remnants in dishes should be prevented for the duration of the dietary trial. Initially, if the pruritus is resulting in severe self-mutilation, oral prednisone, 2 mg/kg/day for 5 to 7 days, an Elizabethan collar, or both may be helpful in breaking the itch-scratch cycle. Long-acting steroids should not be given to the patient when assessing a trial diet. If the cat improves with the hypoallergenic diet, a challenge with the old food(s) usually results in return of clinical signs in 24 to 48 hr.

The treatment for food allergy in cats is to avoid the offending protein source. Some owners are able to find a commercial food that the cat tolerates well; other owners are forced to prepare home-cooked diets for their pets.

Generally, cats with food allergy cannot be effectively managed for long periods of time with steroids or progestins. Some cats with defined food allergy later become allergic to other foods. Some cats with food allergies have a minimum tolerance level; they can occasionally ingest the offending allergen without symptoms.

Flea-Bite Allergic Dermatitis

The immunologic sequence for development of flea allergy in cats has been extrapolated from work done in dogs. Since cats are known to get both immediate and delayed reactions to intradermal flea antigen injections, it is proposed that both type I and type IV reactions occur in the cat with flea allergy.

The clinical signs of flea-bite allergy may be miliary dermatitis, symmetric hypotrichosis, or the eosinophilic plaque form of eosinophilic granuloma complex. The lesions may be focal or generalized.

The diagnosis is made by clinical signs, history, presence of fleas or flea dirt, and positive skin test results with 1:1000 w/v Greer flea antigen. A final diagnosis is made when response to flea control results in resolution of symptoms.

The optimum treatment for flea allergy is total flea control on the pet(s) and in the environment.

In the household with several cats that are allowed to go outdoors, flea control is most difficult. There are no known safe and effective flea repellents for use on cats. Steroids may be useful in long-term management in certain cases. Hyposensitization with flea antigen was not effective in one controlled study. There is little doubt that cats may easily have a combination of problems that may lower their pruritic threshold and lead to clinical signs. This is especially true with flea-bite allergy and other skin diseases. Therefore, initially treating the obvious may allow the clinical signs to subside even if other problems exist.

MILIARY DERMATITIS

This descriptive term delineates the clinical presentation of a cat with small papules and crusts and accompanying inflammation of the skin. The etiologies are variable, but allergic disorders are frequently implicated. Cats with miliary dermatitis exhibit superficial dermatitis (usually eosinophilic) and epidermal spongiosis, crusting, and ulceration; these histologic findings are supportive of the disease origin being allergic, parasitic, or both. It is not surprising then that flea-bite allergic dermatitis is the most common cause of miliary dermatitis in cats. Other ectoparasites, allergies, and infectious causes deserve consideration as etiologies for cats that have miliary dermatitis in the absence of fleas. Once mite infestation, dermatophytosis, and bacterial pyoderma have been ruled out, any cat with chronic miliary dermatitis should receive consideration for allergy testing. Of all the cutaneous manifestations of allergy, miliary dermatitis most probably represents the classic allergic skin disease in the feline species.

EOSINOPHILIC GRANULOMA COMPLEX

The more that is written about this group of cutaneous feline lesions, the more complicated the complex becomes. The etiologies of the various forms (ulcer, plaque, and granuloma) have not been elucidated.

Eosinophilic plaque lesions (a form of eosinophilic granuloma complex) have been noted to occur in conjunction with miliary dermatitis in some cases. Focal, raised plaques with histologic features fitting the definition of eosinophilic plaque (spongiotic, superficial and/or deep perivascular or diffuse eosinophilic dermatitis) are sometimes seen in cats with flea allergy, food allergy, or atopy. Treatment of the allergy by removal of the allergen allows the plaques to resolve. Most eosinophilic plaques are intensely pruritic and are associated with blood and tissue eosinophilia. Allergies should be considered as possible etiologies in chronic or recurrent cases, but it is improbable that all eosinophilic plaques result from allergy.

The role of allergic disease in the pathogenesis of the indolent ulcer and the collagenolytic granuloma in cats is even more obscure. The common factor for the various forms of feline eosinophilic granuloma complex is not eosinophilia but simply the fact that often two forms occur on a cat at the same time. Thus, it seems reasonable to assume that these lesions may have a common pathomechanism such as hypersensitivity.

Eosinophilic dermatitis with or without abundant mast cells may be suggestive of allergy. Chronic eosinophilic plaques in the cat deserve consideration and possible investigation for an allergic etiology. Because of confusion in the histopathologic reporting of the various forms and their clinical signs, it seems best to keep an open mind regarding the etiologies of all forms.

SYMMETRIC HYPOTRICHOSIS

In cats, this condition is a common manifestation of pruritus. Whereas dogs may scratch and break the hairs with no primary cutaneous lesions in atopy, cats that are itchy or have uncomfortable cutaneous sensations may groom themselves overzealously. Cats that have self-induced hair loss may have allergies, behavior problems, or both that are responsible for the clinical signs. These animals become exquisite groomers, sometimes plucking and pulling the hair out (leaving a nice velvety skin) or sometimes licking and chewing (leading to hair breakage and a stubbly hair coat). The only way to differentiate the cat that is removing hair manually from one in which the hair is falling out is by use of an Elizabethan collar or some other mechanical device (such as a jacket).

The author believes that endocrine alopecia is rare in the cat and that most cases of symmetric hypotrichosis are cat-induced. Although some may be behavior-induced and the history may aid the diagnostician, most cats deserve the benefit of being given careful consideration for allergy as the cause of their overzealous grooming. Food allergy, atopy, and, surprisingly, even flea allergy can result in a cat with clinically normal skin but a self-inflicted "barbering."

Editor's Note: Cats with miliary dermatitis due to flea-bite allergy, atopy, or food allergy often have peripheral and tissue eosinophilia and may have prominent peripheral lymphadenopathy (lymphoid hyperplasia and eosinophilia) (Gross et al., 1986; Scott et al., 1986).

Editor's Note: It has been reported that other forms of the eosinophilic granuloma complex in addition to eosinophilic plaque also have an allergic basis (McDougal, 1986; Reedy, 1982; Scott et al., 1986).

The cat with symmetric hypotrichosis deserves a thorough search for fleas or flea dirt. Skin testing, a trial hypoallergenic diet, or a trial-response to corticosteroid therapy should be considered if the history does not immediately point to an environmental or behavioral change. Sometimes, even cats with allergy have a sudden onset of behavioral changes resulting from the discomfort in their skin.

It is unfortunate that skin biopsies do not usually help the diagnostician differentiate hypotrichotic cats with allergies from those with behavior problems and endocrinopathies. The degree of inflammation in these hypotrichotic allergic cats is usually mild to unremarkable. Having the owner keep a diary of the degree of hypotrichosis and the season, diet, and therapy may help elucidate the cause.

The treatment of cats with symmetric hypotrichosis should be directed against a defined cause. If results of skin testing are negative and a trial hypoallergenic diet is not beneficial, some cats can be treated successfully with oral prednisone.

Finally, the treatment of these cats should be approached with the owners' understanding that the various types of medical therapy (central-acting drugs as well as corticosteroids) may have more severe consequences over time than doing nothing for treatment. The author believes that drugs should be used to try to break the cycle for 60 to 90 days if an etiology cannot be determined. However, in cats in which a definite pathogenesis cannot be found, chronic drug therapy should be avoided unless the cat is thought to be in great distress.

SUMMARY

There is clinical evidence to indicate that miliary dermatitis, eosinophilic plaque, and self-induced symmetric hypotrichosis in cats may be caused by allergy. Until the immunology of the cat and the factors that influence eosinophilic migration, chemotaxis, and mast cell degranulation are better understood, practitioners and diagnosticians of dermatologic problems should keep allergic etiologies in mind as distinct possible differential diagnoses.

References and Supplemental Reading

Gross, T. L., Kwochka, K. K., and Kunkle, G. A.: Correlation of histologic and immunologic findings in cats with miliary dermatitis. J.A.V.M.A. 189:1322, 1986.
Kunkle, G. A.: Feline Dermatology. Vet. Clin. North Am. [Small Anim. Pract.] 14:1065, 1984.
McDougal, B. J.: Allergy testing and hyposensitization for three common feline dermatoses. Mod. Vet. Pract. 67:629, 1986.
Reedy, L. M.: Results of allergy testing and hyposensitization in selected feline skin diseases. J. Am. Anim. Hosp. Assoc. 18:618, 1982.
Scott, D. W., Walton, D. K., Slator, M. R., et al.: Miliary dermatitis. A feline cutaneous reaction pattern. Proceedings of the Annual Kal Kan Seminar 2:11, 1986.
Scott, D. W.: The skin. In Holzworth, W. B. (ed.): Diseases of the Cat, Vol. I. Philadelphia: W. B. Saunders Co., 1987, pp. 619–675.
White, S.: Food allergy in the cat. J.A.V.M.A. (in press).

FLEAS AND FLEA CONTROL

DIANE E. BEVIER-TOURNAY, D.V.M.
Boston, Massachusetts

A recent survey of more than 42,000 households found that members of 75.8 per cent of those households listed their veterinarian as the primary source of informed counsel on flea control for their pets. These respondents also listed flea control as the reason for visiting their veterinarian in about one third of their past years' visits to veterinary hospitals. In the southeastern United States, flea-related diseases account for over 50 per cent of dermatologic cases presented to veterinarians.

These figures make it obvious that veterinarians must be knowledgeable about and able to cope with the myriad problems fleas and flea control entail or risk their credibility and jeopardize the remaining 70 per cent of their business.

Several excellent, extensive chapters and articles devoted to flea biology, flea-related disease, flea control, and insecticides have been published in the veterinary literature. These contain valuable information for veterinarians and their staffs

(Kwochka, 1987; Kwochka and Bevier, 1987; MacDonald and Miller, 1986; Schick and Schick, 1986).

ETIOLOGY AND IMMUNOPATHOGENESIS

Ctenocephalides felis continues to be the most common flea species to parasitize dogs and cats. It is also the least host-specific flea and will infest humans. *C. felis* dies in 6 to 8 weeks without exposure to a dog or a cat, since human blood is not nutritionally complete for successful reproduction. *C. canis* is rarely isolated from dogs or cats in the United States.

Pulex irritans (human flea) is also found frequently on dogs, but seldom on cats, in certain areas of the country. In a study of 35 dogs from Georgia and Mississippi, 5831 fleas were collected and identified according to species: *P. irritans* accounted for 81.2 per cent and *C. felis* for 9.9 per cent (Kalkofen and Greenberg, 1974). *Echidnophaga gallinacea*, the poultry stick-tight flea, is common in the southeastern United States and parasitizes a great variety of hosts, including dogs and cats.

Halliwell has done numerous studies to elucidate the immunopathogenesis of flea allergy dermatitis in the dog. His studies would suggest that dermatitis rarely occurs in the absence of an allergic hypersensitivity reaction. Halliwell also demonstrated, using flea-naive dogs, that intermittent exposure to flea bites would cause the development of positive skin test reactions within 12 weeks and flea-specific immunoglobulin E (IgE) and IgG antibody development. In this same group of dogs, sequential intradermal skin testing showed that delayed and immediate hypersensitivity reactions developed in a random sequence, contrary to what the previous classic research of Feingold and Benjamini (1968) had shown in the guinea pig. Dogs showed both delayed and immediate types of reactions during the course of the 44-week study. Continual exposure of dogs to flea bites caused failure to develop hypersensitivity or delayed development of a lesser degree of hypersensitivity. Lastly, it was found that, in comparison to the general canine population, a greater percentage of dogs with allergic inhalant dermatitis are also allergic to fleas.

Histopathologic examination of skin biopsies from sequential lesions in dogs with experimental flea-bite hypersensitivity revealed that the allergic reactions to fleas probably included late-onset IgE-mediated response and cutaneous basophilic hypersensitivity in addition to the classic immediate and delayed hypersensitivities.

Work on flea saliva showed that, in addition to a low-molecular-weight hapten, allergenic compo-

nents included at least two additional allergens of greater than 20,000 dalton molecular weight.

The aforementioned findings have important implications for future therapeutic programs for flea-allergic animals based on hyposensitization, the induction of immunologic tolerance to fleas, or both.

Life Cycle

Client misconceptions regarding the life cycle of the flea are common. Failure of the veterinarian to understand and explain the rudimentary aspects of the flea life cycle to clients results in flea control failures. Appropriate use of many of the newer insecticides also requires this knowledge.

C. felis, as an adult, is a blood-feeding parasite. Mating and egg production do not occur until the newly emerged adult flea finds a host and ingests its first blood meal. The adult flea usually spends its entire life on the host unless it is removed to the environment by movement of the host itself or by the mechanical trauma of scratching.

The white, oval eggs (0.5 to 2.0 mm) are laid primarily on the host and fall off into the bedding and the surrounding environment. The female flea may lay approximately 20 to 28 eggs per day and several hundred over her life span if she has frequent blood meals. After incubation of 2 to 12 days, the eggs hatch to small, white, maggotlike larvae that feed on organic material such as skin scale, insect parts, and adult flea fecal material that falls off the host. These larvae are secretive and motile and will burrow down into carpeting or floor cracks and crevices.

Depending on environmental conditions, the larvae grow and molt twice over a period of 9 to 200 days. This occurs in 14 to 21 days in the typical indoor environment. The third instar larva forms a white cocoon, followed by pupal formation within a few days. The adult flea emerges from the cocoon after several days to several months (14 to 21 days under ideal conditions), depending on temperature and humidity. A moist, warm environment with a relative humidity of 75 to 85 per cent and a temperature of 65 to 80°F (18.3 to 26.7°C) is most favorable for rapid completion of the life cycle. The emergence of the adult from the cocoon is usually triggered by vibration caused by the pet or persons walking in the cocoon's vicinity. The entire flea life cycle may be as short as 16 to 21 days under optimal conditions or as long as a year when unfavorable conditions prevail. After hatching, the adult flea immediately searches for a host.

The flea is attracted to the host by the increase in carbon dioxide levels from the breath of the host and changes in light intensity caused by the host. The entire life span of the flea ranges from 6 to 12 months. Adult fleas in humid environments can live from 4 to 12 months without nutrition.

The percentage of fleas in each stage of development within the life cycle at any one time shows only 1 per cent adult flea population (the stage the client sees), with 99 per cent either in the "invisible" egg, larval, or pupal stages. It is critical to convince clients of the existence of this major part of the flea life cycle and of the need to eliminate it to rid their pets of the adult fleas they observe.

FLEA CONTROL STRATEGIES

Pest Control Operators (PCOs) Versus Veterinarians

This was the title of a recent article in *Pest Control Technology*. The farther we as veterinarians distance ourselves from this idea, the higher will be the quality of pet health care and client service we provide.

Our pet population is exposed to an incredible variety of cholinesterase-inhibiting pesticides (organophosphates and carbamates) through their veterinary care, PCOs, and owner-purchased retail products. The additive effects of several of these products can be deadly. Several cases of animal death have been reported in Florida and other states in which cythioate (Proban, Haver) or fenthion (Pro-Spot, Haver) was being used, and a PCO or owner unknowingly sprayed another cholinesterase inhibitor in the indoor or outdoor environment. The veterinarian, as the dispenser of the animal product, is viewed as the responsible party in providing owners with precautions, preferably written, against certain combinations of insecticide usage to prevent these tragedies and potential legal entanglements.

Dispensing flea control products to clients or recommending a PCO whose methods are known to us keeps the medical problem of fleas under our control as veterinarians. A percentage of clients want to use a PCO for convenience, whereas others prefer to be educated to control their own pest problems. The veterinarian who works with one or several PCOs in his or her area may reap the benefit of that PCO recommending professional treatment of the pet for fleas at the same time the premises are being treated.

Flea Control Programs

In the last 5 years, the field of insecticides has changed dramatically. New insecticides have entered the market while older, less effective, more toxic products are being removed. New methods of formulation have been developed that are superior to older, standard formulations (for an exhaustive review of these products and application methods, see *Current Veterinary Therapy IX*, pp. 571–590). This section will concentrate on flea control strategies for the three-pronged attack on fleas on the pet and in the indoor and outdoor environments, with a special focus on avoiding toxicoses.

Programs must be individualized, based on the number and type of animals in the environment, size of the internal environment, degree of outdoor exposure to fleas, size of the outdoor area, time of year, and family situation, such as the presence of young children.

It is difficult to do an adequate job of explaining all aspects of flea control in the examination room with a client. Videotapes and a client education handout explaining flea allergy dermatitis, the life cycle of the flea, and a flea control program are invaluable. An additional handout with blank spaces

***Table 1.** Synchronized Flea Control for Animals on Systemic Organophosphates or for "Special-need"* Households*

Day of Program	Indoor Treatment	Outdoor Treatment	Pet
1	General sanitation followed by non–cholinesterase-inhibiting surface sprays (1)† followed by adulticide-methoprene foggers (2) OR Adulticide-methoprene sprays (3) followed by pyrethroid foggers (4)	Environmental clean-up followed by insecticidal dust or spray (5) at night and watered in next day; allow to dry before pet contacts sprayed area	Dog on cythioate (6) or fenthion (7). Do not administer product on same day house or yard is treated
14	Surface spray, especially animal sleeping areas, with adulticide-methoprene spray (3) or non–cholinesterase-inhibiting sprays (1)	Same as for day 1	
30	Same as for day 14	Same as for day 1	
Maintenance	Every 8–12 weeks, repeat as for day 1	Every 14 days, as long as environmental temperature > 50° F (10° C) at night	

*Households with small children, insecticide-sensitive cats, or exotic pets.
†Numbers correspond to product listings in Table 3.

to enter which products will be utilized for an individual patient is also helpful. Some practitioners are using a reminder card system, similar to those used for vaccinations, to signal the onset of flea season, attempting to avoid heavy infestations and to prevent the skin manifestations of flea allergy dermatitis.

Synchronized flea control programs for animals on systemic organophosphates and special-need households and for animals not on systemic organophosphates are described in Tables 1 and 2. Table 3 contains available insecticide products that can be used in the appropriate area of Tables 1 and 2.

In addition to the insecticides recommended, an important aspect of indoor and outdoor flea control is sanitation. This should be completed before insecticides are dusted or sprayed or foggers are activated. Indoor sanitation physically removes flea eggs and larvae from the environment. Vacuuming removes the eggs and larvae from the carpeting and furniture. Vacuum bags should be discarded after completion. It is unsafe to recommend crushed naphthalene crystals (moth balls) in a closed vacuum bag because cyanide gas, which can be explosive, is generated. Also, flea collars placed in vacuum bags are not recommended as the insecticide may be aerosolized to toxic levels in the house through the operation of a powerful vacuum cleaner motor. Floors should be mopped, with particular attention paid to cracks and crevices where organic debris and flea eggs accumulate. With severe infestation, steam cleaning of the carpeting is highly effective in removing and killing larvae and eggs. Insecticides can be used in the water of the steam cleaning machine. Specific products are now available for this purpose where steam cleaners are rented. Carbaryl products may stain carpeting. All animal and human bedding frequented by pets must be washed and dried on the maximal heat setting to ensure flea death.

Outdoor sanitation prior to spraying includes the removal of organic debris by mowing, raking, and discarding the debris. Flea control in yards with St. Augustine or Bermuda grass is made more difficult because surface root systems of these plants provide an excellent hiding place for fleas. When spraying the outdoor environment, special attention should be given to any favorite pet sleeping areas, such as under the porch and the garage. Doghouses and automobiles should be thoroughly cleaned and treated with insecticides appropriate for indoor usage.

Even when insecticides are chosen carefully and are diligently applied by the owner, there are two potential pitfalls that might occur, especially when there is heavy flea infestation. These pitfalls will be perceived as efficacy problems by the owner and are

1. The owner fogged with an adulticide-methoprene fogger, left the house for 4 hr, returned, and still found live adult fleas.

2. The owner fogged and 1 week later started seeing live adult fleas.

Both of these problems are related to extremely heavy flea infestation of the environment. In the first situation, there was a large number of fleas in the pupal stage that were hatching at a very fast rate. When the newly hatched flea is exposed to a

Table 2. Synchronized Flea Control for Animals Not on Systemic Organophosphates

Day of Program	Indoor Treatment	Outdoor Treatment	Pet
1	General sanitation followed by organophosphate or combination surface spray (8)* followed by adulticide-methoprene foggers (2) (if using organophosphate-only spray) or methoprene foggers (if using combination sprays) OR Methoprene combination surface spray (10) followed by pyrethroid foggers (4)	Environmental clean-up followed by insecticidal dust or spray (5) at night. Can also use microencapsulated outdoor products (11)	Many choices (12): If using organophosphate in house and yard, avoid organophosphate- or carbamate-containing dips (13), sprays (14), and dusts (15). If using pyrethroids primarily in environment, these products (13, 14, 15) are acceptable
14	Surface spray, especially animal sleeping areas, with adulticide-methoprene sprays (3) or non–cholinesterase-inhibiting sprays (1)	Same as for day 1. Check label instructions on microencapsulated products, as spraying interval may be longer	
30	Same as for day 14	Same as for day 14	
Maintenance	Every 8–12 weeks, repeat as for day 1	Every 14 days for nonmicroencapsulated products as long as environmental temperatures > 50°F (10°C) at night. Check label for microencapsulated product recommendations	Product rotation recommended q 14–30 days

*Numbers correspond to product listings in Table 3.

Table 3. *Product Choices**

Trade Name	Manufacturer	Active Ingredient
1. Expar Home and Carpet Spray	CO	Permethrin
Permisyn Home and Carpet Spray	SX	Permethrin
Siphotrol Premise Spray	VK	Synergized natural pyrethrins, methoprene
Synergized natural pyrethrin sprays	Many	Synergized natural pyrethrins
2. Siphotrol Plus Fogger	VK	Permethrin, methoprene
3. Siphotrol Premise Spray	VK	Synergized natural pyrethrins, methoprene
4. Sprecto-CF Insecticide Fogger	PM	Permethrin, tetramethrin
Vet-Fog Fogger	VK	Permethrin
Mycodex Mini-Fog	BE	Allethrin, sumithrin
5. Malathion	Several	Malathion (liquid)
Vet-Kem Yard and Kennel Spray Concentrate	VK	Chlorpyrifos
Sevin	UC	Carbaryl (dust)
VIP Concentrated Yard Spray	HI	Fenvalerate
6. Proban	BV	Cythioate
7. Pro-Spot	BV	Fenthion
8. Controller House & Carpet Spray	TA	Chlorpyrifos
Mycodex Room and Carpet Accu-Spray	BE	Synergized natural pyrethrins, chlorpyrifos
Duratrol Household Flea Spray	3M	Microencapsulated chlorpyrifos
Several	Several	Malathion
Knox-Out 2 FM	PW	Microencapsulated diazinon
9. Siphotrol-10 Fogger for Fleas	VK	Methoprene
10. Siphotrol Plus II House Treatment	VK	Synergized natural pyrethrins, chlorpyrifos, methoprene
11. Duratrol Yard and Kennel Flea Spray	3M	Microencapsulated chlorpyrifos
Knox-Out 2 FM	PW	Microencapsulated diazinon

Trade Name	Manufacturer	Active Ingredient	Approach for Use in
12. *Dips*			
Adams Flea Off Dip	AD	Synergized natural pyrethrins	Dogs, cats
Expar 3.2% EC	CO	Permethrin	Dogs
Permisyn Flea and Tick Dip	SX	Permethrin	Dogs
Sprecto-D Dip	PM	Synergized natural pyrethrins, permethrin	Dogs, cats
VIP Flea Dip	HI	*d*-Limonene	Dogs, cats
Powders			
Adams Flea Off Dust II	AD	Synergized natural pyrethrins, carbaryl	Dogs, cats
Diryl Flea Powder for Dogs and Cats	PM	Synergized natural pyrethrins, carbaryl	Dogs, cats
Mycodex Powder Plus	BE	Synergized natural pyrethrins, carbaryl	Dogs, cats
Vet-Kem Flea and Tick Powder	VK	Carbaryl	Dogs, cats
Controller Flea and Tick Dust Plus	TA	Synergized natural pyrethrins, carbaryl, rotenone	Dogs, cats
13. *Dips*			
Adams Flea Off Dip	AD	Malathion	Dogs
Paramite	VK	Phosmet	Dogs
VIP Flea and Tick Dip for Dogs	HI	Chlorpyrifos	Dogs
Mycodex Chlorpyrifos Dog Dip and Sponge-On	BE	Chlorpyrifos	
Controller Flea and Tick Dip for Dogs	TA	Chlorpyrifos	Dogs
Dermaton 3	CO	Chlorfenvinphos	Dogs
14. Mycodex Flea and Tick Spray	BE	Propoxur	Dogs, cats
15. Paramite Insecticidal Dust for Dogs	VK	Phosmet	Dogs
Dermaton Dust	CO	Chlorfenvinphos	Dogs

*Numbers relate to synchronized flea control charts.

AD, Adams Division of Norden Laboratories, Miami, FL; BE, Beecham Laboratories, Bristol, TN; BV, Bayvet Division of Miles Laboratories, Shawnee, KS; CO, Coopers Animal Health, Inc., Kansas City, MO; HI, Hills Pet Chemicals, Miami, FL; 3M, 3M/Animal Care Products, St. Paul, MN; PM, Pitman-Moore, Inc., Washington Crossing, NJ; PW, Pennwalt Chemicals, Philadelphia, PA; SX, Syntex Animal Health, Inc., West Des Moines, IA; TA, TechAmerica Group, Inc., Elwood, KS; UC, Union Carbide, Danbury, CT; VK, Vet-Kem, Division of Zoecon Corp., Dallas, TX.

pyrethroid and methoprene, it is irritated and becomes very active in its dying phase. The flea will die within 2 hr after exposure. If you do nothing about this situation, all of the pupae will hatch and die within 4 to 5 days. To control the immediate problem, the client can spray the carpet with a pyrethrin spray to rapidly knock out the newly hatched adults.

The second problem also stems from a heavy flea infestation but one that is not as severe as in the first instance. In this second case, initial fogging eliminated all the adults and larvae. However, the existing pupae hatch over a period of 4 to 5 days, and the inside environment is being reinfested by an infested pet or carryover from an infested yard. This problem requires a re-evaluation of the treatment program used as well as treatment of those areas not previously treated. If the re-treatment program occurs 7 to 10 days after the initial fogging, it may be necessary to refog the house with a pyrethrin or pyrethroid fogger. It will not be necessary to re-treat the environment with methoprene.

Exotic Pets

It is difficult to find written reference to recommendations for safe flea control in households with exotic pets. Several veterinary experts involved with these groups of animals were kind enough to share their experience regarding this subject.

Although there have been numerous references to birds being more susceptible to insecticides, this does not appear to present a major medical problem for avian veterinarians. They recommend that birds be kept out of the house after flea control products are used, according to the label instructions for dogs and cats. Keeping the bird out of the house until the odor from the insecticide is gone provides extra assurance of safety. It is recommended that special attention be paid to wiping cage surfaces and making sure that food bowls are cleaned before they are used again. There was an observation that Lady Gouldian finches are more likely to exhibit insecticide side-effects than other finch species. Interestingly, in one hospital, reproduction stopped when an ultrasonic pest device was used in a bird room. The birds began laying eggs again after the device was removed. None of the veterinarians had noticed fleas on their avian patients, even on birds from households with heavy flea infestation.

It is recommended that people with snakes and other reptiles also follow label precautions listed for dogs and cats. Again, no fleas have been noticed on these species.

The usual suggestion when spraying and fogging around areas with fish tanks has been to cover the tank with a sheet of plastic and tape this completely around the sides. There is concern that the newer underground power filters that have a plastic head and tubing suck outside air into the aquarium may act as a source of intoxication to the fish. This equipment should be removed from the aquarium, along with covering the top, while spraying and fogging for fleas.

Ferrets have problems with *C. felis* from the standpoints of infestation and development of flea allergy dermatitis. Flea-allergic ferrets present with alopecia in a ring around the neck or patchy alopecia involving the entire trunk, often sparing the guard hairs, with or without a papular eruption. Some will also develop a superficial pyoderma. Ferrets can undergo intradermal skin testing with aqueous flea allergen, identical to that used in dogs and cats, and will show positive immediate hypersensitivity reaction. Flea control products safe for use in cats have been used successfully in ferrets. Flea dips appropriate for cats may be used in ferrets at one-half the recommended strength.

Alternative Flea Control Methods

Even with the advent of the newer and safer insecticides and insect growth regulators (IGRs), some owners desire alternatives to the standard pest control recommendations. These would include the application of boric acid, diatomaceous earth, and silica aerogel to indoor and outdoor environments. These products act primarily as desiccants by absorbing waxes from the insect cuticle. Because of their nature, they can cause carpet fibers to wear out quickly. Diatomaceous earth can be purchased from swimming pool supply outlets. Boric acid is again being used by some pest control operators and is found in 20 Mule Team Borax laundry detergent.

Alternative flea control methods in pets, including oral repellents such as brewer's yeast, thiamine, sulfur, and garlic as well as ultrasonic collars or boxes, have not been shown to be effective in field condition studies.

Well-controlled double-blind studies in dogs and cats to evaluate flea antigen for use in hyposensitization in cases of flea allergy dermatitis have shown no statistically significant beneficial response, although an occasional animal showed marked improvement on vaccine (Schemmer and Halliwell, 1987; Kunkle and Milcarsky, 1985; Halliwell, 1981).

The Future of Flea Control Products

Methoprene (Vet-Kem), a highly effective environmental insect growth regulator, appeared on the market in June 1988 in a spray form for topical use on animals. When used outdoors, methoprene is rapidly degraded by ultraviolet light but appears to be stabilized when combined with the hair on the animal. This product is extremely safe and has a very high median lethal dose (LD_{50}).

Fenoxycarb (Mog Corp.), another IGR that is stable in ultraviolet light and appropriate for outdoor environmental flea control, is on track for approval by the Environmental Protection Agency. It should provide an extremely safe adjunct to outdoor flea control.

Insecticides are poisons. If used improperly or without sufficient knowledge of their side effects, they can endanger humans and animals. Extra-label use of insecticides poses an increasing legal liability for the veterinarian.

Veterinarians also must be familiar with Environmental Protection Agency regulations regarding the repackaging or mixing of insecticides to minimize their potential for toxicity and environmental hazards.

References and Supplemental Reading

Feingold, B. F., Benjamini, E., and Michaeli, D.: The allergic responses to insect bites. Ann. Rev. Entomol. 13:137, 1968.

Gross, T. L., and Halliwell, R. E. W.: Lesions of experimental flea bite hypersensitivity in the dog. Vet. Pathol. 22:78, 1985.

Halliwell, R. E. W.: Hyposensitization in the treatment of flea-bite hypersensitivity: Results of a double-blind study. J. Am. Anim. Hosp. Assoc. 17:249, 1981.

Halliwell, R. E. W.: Factors in the development of flea-bite allergy. Vet. Med. Small Anim. Clin. 79:1273, 1984.

Halliwell, R. E. W.: Frank Kral Memorial Lecture in Dermatology. Phoenix, Arizona, March 22, 1987.

Halliwell, R. E. W., and Longino, S. J.: IgE and IgG antibodies to flea antigen in differing dog populations. Vet. Immunol. Immunopathol. 9:215, 1985.

Halliwell, R. E. W., and Schemmer, K. R.: The role of basophils in the immunopathogenesis of hypersensitivity to fleas (Ctenocephalides felis) in dogs. Vet. Immunol. Immunopathol. 15:203, 1987.

Kalkofen, V. P., and Greenberg, J.: Public health implications of Pulex irritans infestations of dogs. J.A.V.M.A. 165:903, 1974.

Katz, H.: PCO's versus veterinarians. Pest Control Technol. 15:34, 1987.

Kunkle, G. A., and Milcarsky, J.: Double-blind hyposensitization trial in cats. J.A.V.M.A. 186:677, 1985.

Kwochka, K. W.: Fleas and related disease. Vet. Clin. North Am. [Small Anim. Pract.] 17:1235, 1987.

Kwochka, K. W., and Bevier, D. E.: Flea dermatitis. In Nesbitt, G. H. (ed.): Contemporary Issues in Small Animal Practice, Vol. 8. New York: Churchill Livingstone, 1987, pp. 21–55.

MacDonald, J. M., and Miller, T. A.: Parasiticide therapy in small animal dermatology. In Kirk, R. W. (ed.): Current Veterinary Therapy IX. Philadelphia: W. B. Saunders Co., 1986, pp. 571–590.

Metrokotsas, M. J.: Merchandising effective parasite-control programs. Vet. Med. 7:43, 1985.

Schemmer, K. R., and Halliwell, R. E. W.: Efficacy of alum-precipitated flea antigen for hyposensitization of flea allergic dogs. Semin. Vet. Med. Surg. [Small Anim.] 2:195, 1987.

Schick, M. P., and Schick, R. O.: Understanding and implementing safe and effective flea control. J. Am. Anim. Hosp. Assoc. 22:421, 1986.

Veith, L.: Biorational Flea Control. Technical bulletin, Zoecon Corporation, 1987.

RAST AND ELISA TESTING IN CANINE ATOPY

CRAIG GRIFFIN, D.V.M.
Garden Grove, California

Veterinarians frequently are presented with patients with the chief symptom of pruritus. The differential diagnosis of pruritus is lengthy. Proper management of the patient depends on making an accurate diagnosis of all the problems contributing to the dog's pruritus. Canine atopy is one of the more common causes of chronic pruritus.

The diagnosis of canine atopy is suggested in patients with a compatible history and physical examination. A definitive diagnosis is based on positive intradermal skin tests that correlate with the historical findings together with the ruling out of other diagnoses. The intradermal skin test detects the presence of antigen-specific immunoglobulin E (IgE) fixed to dermal mast cells as well as the ability of the mast cells to release mediators following exposure to the specific antigen. It is unfortunate that intradermal skin tests are not always positive in some dogs believed to have atopy. Intradermal skin testing also requires extensive patient preparation and is subject to multiple variables that lead to false-negative or false-positive results (even when the tests are performed by experienced veterinary allergists).

The development of an accurate *in vitro* test for the diagnosis of canine atopy would be a tremendous step forward. Two laboratories have developed *in vitro* tests for the diagnosis of canine atopy. These *in vitro* tests measure allergen-specific IgE that is present in the patient's serum.

One test, offered by A & M Biosciences, Inc. (Mesa, AZ), utilizes the method referred to as the radioallergosorbent test (RAST). The test is done by using a solid-phase substrate that has a specific allergen or mixture of allergens bound to it. The allergen-bound substrate is then incubated with the patient's serum. The serum IgE specific for the allergen being tested should bind to the fixed allergen. The substrate with specific allergen and bound IgE is then washed and separated from all other serum components. The next step is to incubate the substrate-allergen-IgE complex with labeled anti–canine IgE. The labeled anti–canine IgE then binds to the allergen-specific IgE. In the RAST, the label is a radioisotope, and following incubation and repeated washing, a gamma counter determines the radioactivity of each test sample. The ratio of counts per minute is proportional to the amount of allergen-specific IgE that is present in the patient's serum.

The other test, offered by Bioproducts for Medicine, Inc. (Tempe, AZ), utilizes the method referred to as enzyme-linked immunosorbent assay (ELISA). In the ELISA, the procedures are basically similar to those of the RAST except that the anti–canine IgE is labeled with an enzyme. Following washing, the bound enzyme and anti–canine IgE complex is reacted with the enzyme substrate, and the amount of enzyme reactivity is measured. Generally, this is a colorimetric change measured by a spectrophotometer. As with the RAST, the amount of enzyme present, as determined by colorimetric analysis, correlates with the amount of allergen-specific IgE present in the patient's serum.

The major advantages of these two tests are the lack of risk and discomfort to the patient, the quantitative nature of the results, and the fact that the test can be performed on patients with widespread cutaneous inflammation or dermographism. A & M Biosciences, Inc., also claims that their RAST is unaffected by glucocorticoid therapy. This statement has not been supported by any published studies in dogs and was extrapolated from human studies. Bioproducts for Medicine, Inc., cautions veterinarians that glucocorticoid therapy may affect the test results. The tests are being marketed to veterinarians with various claims about their accuracy, reliability, and usefulness in the diagnosis and treatment of canine atopy.

The RAST was first described in 1967 (Wide et al.). Since then, the RAST and a variety of modified RASTs (Hoffman, 1980) and, later, the ELISA and fluoroallergosorbent test (FAST) have been available for use in human medicine (Seltzer et al., 1985). These tests have been shown to have value as experimental and clinical diagnostic tools in the diagnosis of IgE-mediated diseases. These *in vitro* tests have been the subject of numerous studies. Complete endorsement is still lacking, and intradermal skin testing has not been totally replaced by the simpler *in vitro* tests (Adkinson, 1981). However, in 1982 an executive committee of the American Academy of Allergy considered RAST substantially equivalent to intradermal skin testing.

In some studies, the *in vitro* tests have been found to be less sensitive, with false-negative results being a problem. In other studies, the *in vitro* tests are too sensitive, with false-positive results posing difficulties. Some researchers concluded that the intradermal skin test had more false-positive results. Several problems have been identified that help explain the conflicting data. The substrate being utilized may nonspecifically bind some IgE. The type and the number of controls utilized may vary from system to system. The type of reference curves established for different tests can affect the low and high results. Allergen quality and consistency from lot to lot may vary. The specificity of anti-IgE may vary, as different polyclonal anti-IgE antibodies and, now, monoclonal or polymonoclonal anti-IgE antibodies may be used in the test system. The binding capacity of the labeled anti-IgE can vary from lot to lot and can be affected by storage. Other serum factors have also been reported to affect *in vitro* test results. The level of blocking IgG is felt to be an important cause of false negative results. In addition, non-IgG serum blockers have been hypothesized to affect test results (Wojdani et al., 1985). Of major concern to veterinarians is a study that showed that the level of total IgE can affect test results.

In humans, Caprio and colleagues (1983) demonstrated that high serum IgE levels are associated with more false-positive RAST results. Normal dogs have serum IgE levels around 190,000 ng/ml, and atopic humans have levels of 700 ng/ml. Although there is tremendous variation, 8000 ng/ml would be very high for most normal humans. Therefore, the average dog has 20 to greater than 200 times the background of IgE found in humans. Dogs are believed to have high levels of IgE because of their exposure to internal and external parasites. This fact is just one compelling reason to require well-controlled studies and documentation of *in vitro* testing in dogs. If results from humans are to be extrapolated to dogs, these high IgE levels may lead to false-positive results.

One study by Halliwell and Kunkle (1978) on RAST testing in the dog utilized high-level IgE serum as a control for positive RASTs. The cutoff was defined so that false-positive results did not occur. With these criteria, the results of the RASTs were found to be quite variable in their correlation with the results of skin testing. The agreement between positive skin tests and RASTs was best for ragweed (82 per cent) and lowest for dandelion (12.5

per cent). There was very poor correlation with dogs that had positive Prausnitz-Küstner (P-K) tests to house dust extract. However, there was a better positive correlation (41.7 per cent) when house dust mite extract was used. The authors of this study and more recent reviews of canine atopy (Willemse, 1987) have indicated that *in vitro* tests do not replace intradermal skin testing in dogs. However, the potential value of *in vitro* tests certainly warrants further efforts and investigation.

Before canine *in vitro* diagnostic tests for the diagnosis of canine atopy can be readily accepted, certain questions need to be answered. The commercial test offered to the practitioner must be reproducible at an acceptable level. The quality control and safeguards utilized in some research studies are not always followed in commercial settings. The *in vitro* test needs to be relatively sensitive and accurate in the detection of allergen-specific IgE. The cutoff levels that are employed to determine results compatible with canine atopy need to be thoroughly explained and understood by veterinarians utilizing the test. Possibly one of the most important contributions would be the collection and publication of the effects that other chronic pruritic diseases of dogs may have on *in vitro* tests.

A study supported by a grant from the Academy of Veterinary Allergy was recently completed at the author's practice. This study was designed to evaluate the reproducibility of the two commercial test systems. Six dogs, four with atopy (intradermal skin test positive) and two normal (intradermal skin test negative), were tested. Each animal had a single blood sample taken. This was divided into ten specimens. Five specimens from each dog were submitted to each commercial laboratory. The laboratories were totally blind regarding all the samples. All possible sample pairs for each group tested by the commercial laboratory were examined. In summary, the results of this study showed that the reproducibility of Bioproducts for Medicine, Inc., was statistically better than that of A & M Bioscience, Inc., for each type of comparison made. The comparison most important to the clinician was the percentage of test pairs that changed the recommendations from treatment to nontreatment. The determination of nontreatment versus treatment was based on the laboratories' recommendations for interpretation of test results. The percentage treatment change for RAST (A & M Bioscience, Inc.) was 21.28 per cent of 672 pairs. The percentage treatment change for ELISA (Bioproducts for Medicine, Inc.) was 6.90 per cent of 840 pairs. These results showed statistically significant differences. The paired comparison T test and the two sample T test had p-values less than 0.025. The Wilcoxon signed rank test had a p-value equal to 0.0083. If the clinician decides that reproducibility regarding treatment recommendations should be greater than

95 per cent, neither laboratory is currently acceptable. If the clinician accepts 90 per cent or greater, the ELISA offered by Bioproducts for Medicine, Inc., is currently acceptable at a level of 93.1 per cent.

Some preliminary observations have also been made regarding the discriminatory ability of the two commercially available tests. Two clinically normal dogs (one owned for 2 years, the other for 10 years) had negative intradermal skin test results. In addition, these dogs had never developed pruritus, even when exposed to fleas. A & M Biosciences (RAST test) recommended treatment, with 4 of 12 allergen groups tested for one dog and 7 of 12 allergen groups tested for the second normal dog. Bioproducts for Medicine, Inc. (ELISA), would have treated both dogs for 13 of 14 allergen groups. Obviously, in clinical practice, normal dogs would not be misdiagnosed as having canine atopy because they would not be tested. One dog with dermatomyositis whose intradermal skin test result was negative would have been treated based on the RAST and ELISA results. Three dogs with scabies confirmed by skin scrapes and cured with lime sulfur dips or ivermectin were also tested by RAST and ELISA. Two of these dogs were intradermal skin tested and only positive to flea or mosquito. All three dogs would have been put on hyposensitization therapy according to both RAST and ELISA results.

Another potential problem is the question regarding the effect of glucocorticoids. Although these drugs should not directly interfere with the assay itself, they may affect the value of the test in the diagnosis of canine atopy. In a study being conducted by the author, some animals have doubled the amount of allergen-specific IgE in their serum when steroid withdrawal times used for skin testing were followed. This suggests that, again, results in humans cannot always be extrapolated to dogs. Further studies are warranted and are in progress.

Certainly, intradermal skin testing has its problems and may not be the best determinate with which to compare *in vitro* tests. Investigators and clinicians should not assume that intradermal skin testing is the most sensitive indicator of clinical allergy. Optimally, the results of *in vitro* tests and intradermal skin tests should be compared to the development of clinical hypersensitivity following exposure to an allergen. This would allow one to determine which test is most sensitive in determining clinical allergy. The results of hyposensitization based on *in vitro* testing and intradermal testing need to be evaluated and compared.

The controversy over individual allergen testing versus testing with mixtures must also be evaluated. This is necessary not just because the mixtures may theoretically lead to false-negative results or lower scores, but also because hyposensitization treatments would be much more likely to contain allergens to which the patient is not sensitive. This could be significant, since hypersensitivity can be induced in humans who are parenterally treated with allergens to which they previously did not react (Turkletaub et al., 1978).

Certainly, many questions must be answered, and much work still needs to be done before *in vitro* tests can be routinely recommended as an accurate method for the diagnosis of canine atopy. Both the *in vitro* and the *in vivo* tests have their limitations and drawbacks, which is one reason that the diagnosis and management of allergies is still a medical art.

Currently, research is being done on the effects of internal and external parasites as well as total IgE levels on the results of ELISA testing. It is hoped that this research will lead to a better understanding of allergen-specific IgE in canine atopy and the ability to discriminate between other pruritic diseases. In the meantime, the clinician should be aware of these pitfalls of *in vitro* allergy testing. A diagnosis of atopy still requires a careful history, physical examination, and elimination of other pruritic diseases.

References and Supplemental Reading

Adkinson, N. F.: The radioallergosorbent test in 1981: Limitations and refinements (editorial). J. Allergy Clin. Immunol. 67:87, 1981.

Caprio, R. E., Furth, K., Rosner, I., et al.: Predictive value of serum IgE on the correlation of RAST and intradermal testing in an atopic population. Immunol. Allergy Pract. 5:13, 1983.

Halliwell, R. E. W., and Kunkle, G. A.: The radioallergosorbent test in the diagnosis of canine atopic disease. J. Allergy Clin. Immunol. 62:236, 1978.

Hoffman, D. R.: Comparison of methods of performing the radioallergosorbent test: Phadebas, Fadal-Nalebuff, and Hoffman protocols. Ann. Allergy 45:343, 1980.

Seltzer, J. M., Halpern, G. M., and Tsay, Y. G.: Correlation of allergy test results obtained by IgE FAST, RAST, and prick-puncture methods. Ann. Allergy 54:25, 1985.

Turkletaub, P. C., Marsh, D. G., Lichtenstein, L. M., et al.: Development of long-lasting immediate hypersensitivity in nonatopic volunteers parenterally immunized with a purified grass pollen extract. J. Allergy Clin. Immunol. 61:171, 1978.

Wide, L., Bennick, H., and Johansson, S. G. O.: Diagnosis of allergy by an *in-vitro* test for allergen antibodies. Lancet 2:1105, 1967.

Willemse, T. A.: Atopic dermatitis. *In* Nesbitt, G. H. (ed.): *Contemporary Issues in Small Animal Practice: Dermatology.* New York: Churchill Livingstone, 1987, p. 57.

Wojdani, A., Etessami, S., and Cheug, G. P.: IgG is not the only inhibitor of IgE in the RAST test. Ann. Allergy 55:463, 1985.

SEX HORMONE–RELATED DERMATOSES IN DOGS

WILLIAM H. MILLER, JR., V.M.D.

Ithaca, New York

In dogs, hypothyroidism and hyperadrenocorticism are the most common causes of endocrine-related hair loss, while sex hormone and growth hormone problems are much less frequent. With the availability of good thyroid, adrenal, and growth hormone assays, the verification of disorders associated with these hormones can be relatively straightforward. In the past, the diagnosis of a sex hormone problem was made by exclusion and by response to therapy. With the availability of valid assays for testosterone, estradiol, and progesterone, the diagnosis of sex-associated dermatoses has been made easier, but by no means have all the problems been resolved. The best diagnostic tool is a strong index of suspicion based on the clinical findings. This article will describe the dermatologic problems that the author has seen caused by the sex hormones.

PHYSIOLOGY OF THE SEX STEROID

Sex hormones are produced by the adrenal glands and by the gonads. The adrenal gland of the dog produces primarily weak androgenic steroids, although some estrogens are made. Adrenal production increases after puberty. In males, adrenal androgens make up less than 10 per cent of the androgen pool. It appears that adrenal androgens have little primary effect but act as precursors for other sex steroids generated by peripheral conversion.

Gonadal function is influenced by luteinizing hormone (LH) and follicle-stimulating hormone (FSH), which are regulated by hypothalamic gonadotropin-releasing hormone (GnRH). In the classic feedback fashion, serum levels of testosterone and estradiol alter LH and FSH secretion via influencing GnRH synthesis, release, or both. The testes secrete primarily testosterone under the influence of LH. Small amounts of other androgenic steroids and estradiol also are produced. Ovarian sex hormone production is under the influence of both LH and FSH. The ovaries produce primarily estradiol and progesterone, but some androgenic steroids and weaker estrogens also are produced.

Over 90 per cent of the sex steroids are protein bound and inactive. Sex hormone–binding protein (SHBP) is found in dogs in the beta-globulin fraction. In mature dogs, the concentration of SHBP is higher in females, whereas in prepubescent dogs the levels are equal in both sexes. SHBP primarily is an androgen-binding protein, with the highest affinity for dihydrotestosterone. Other androgens, estrogens, and progesterone also will bind, but with a much lower affinity. Dihydrotestosterone, testosterone, and estradiol all compete for the same binding site, so the levels of one sex steroid can influence those of another by inhibiting binding of the latter. The concentration of SHBP is increased by estrogens and thyroid hormones, and decreased by androgens, progesterone, and growth hormone. Estrogens and progesterone are bound primarily to albumin with a weak affinity. Unbound hormones are biologically active and can be converted peripherally to other sex steroids. Androgenic steroids can be converted to more or less potent androgens or to estrogens, whereas estrogens are interconverted to more or less potent estrogens.

In mammals, an individual's hair pattern is influenced by the individual's genetic makeup and by hormones, including the sex steroids. The effects of the sex hormones are mediated through androgen, estrogen, and progesterone receptors that, in humans, vary in their concentration, depending on the sex of the individual and the part of the body examined. In humans, androgen receptors are highest in the genital skin. The concentration of estrogen and progesterone receptors are highest in the face and the breast and retroauricular area, respectively. Androgen receptors have a high affinity for androgenic steroids, but estrogens and progesterone also can bind weakly. Androgen receptors will bind all androgenic steroids, but the binding affinity varies with the hormone. The highest binding affinity is for dihydrotestosterone.

In humans, the sex hormones influence primarily the ambisexual hairs of the axillae and lower pubis and the male sexual hairs of the beard, presternal area, and upper pubic triangle. At puberty, in both sexes, the ambisexual hairs transform from vellus to terminal hairs under the influence of androgens. Since androgen levels are low in women, the concentration of androgen receptors in the ambisexual areas is higher than it is in males. Both sexes have acne-prone areas of the skin, where the sebaceous glands are more responsive to androgens. Diseases that influence sex hormone production can be manifested by changes in either or both the ambisexual and sexual hairs or by acne. In dogs, information on the distribution of cutaneous sex hormone receptors is unavailable. However, hormonal abnormalities produce patterned hair loss, and the pattern appears to vary with the different hormones. This suggests that there is a geographical variation in the concentration or activity of the sex hormone receptors in the dog's skin.

CLINICAL EVALUATION

The completely bald dog offers the clinician very few clinical clues as to the cause of the hair loss. Dogs with sex hormone problems typically start to lose hair in specific areas, and this patterned hair loss persists for long but not indefinite periods. Aside from physical changes or sexual behavior changes, most dogs with gonadal problems do not show signs of systemic disease. When examining patterned hair loss in an otherwise normal dog, the practitioner should place a sex hormone problem at or near the top of the list of differential diagnoses. Since any or all of the sex hormones may be involved in any one case, it is best to describe the problem in broad terms.

NEUTERED FEMALE DOGS

Hair loss following an ovariohysterectomy is very uncommon and has been associated with premature neutering of the animal. Because early neutering appears to be fairly common, while the development of hair loss is rare, the timing of the ovariohysterectomy probably is not critical. Although no breed predilection is referenced in the literature, most dermatology texts show photographs of boxers and dachshunds. The author's case material would support a predilection for the dachshund breed.

Affected dogs lose hair ventrally, from the chin to the vulva, in the retroauricular areas, and over the perineum. Some secondary hairs may be observed in the affected areas. The skin and the external genitalia tend to be infantile. Urinary incontinence is a rare concurrent complaint.

Caution must be used in making the diagnosis of ovariohysterectomy-associated alopecia in the dachshund, Boston terrier, and boxer breeds, because in certain lines or individuals within these breeds, a patterned, sparse coat in these areas is normal. Dogs with the patterned sparse coat have a full puppy coat and then develop their sparse coat when the adult coat comes in. Historically, if a dog from these breeds or any breed has always had a sparse coat in these areas, one may be dealing with a normal dog or one that has an endocrinopathy, and skin biopsies should be done. However, if the dog had a full adult coat and then lost hair, the diagnosis of an endocrinopathy is much more probable.

Therapy consists of observation without treatment or sex hormone replacement therapy. As the hair loss tends to stay localized to the ventrum, some owners prefer not to treat the dog.

Occasionally, an Irish setter will be presented for a poor coat, but instead of having hair loss, the dog will have a dense, dull, dry, blond-colored coat. This is a generalized phenomenon and not the blonding of the feathers seen in some dogs. This hypertrichotic condition has been associated with hypothyroidism, but some of these dogs are euthyroid or fail to respond to adequate thyroid replacement therapy.

The author has examined three of these dogs, and all were neutered females that developed the condition within 6 months after the neutering. All of these dogs developed and maintained a normal coat when they were treated with sex hormones. The author also is aware of reports in which this phenomenon has occurred in intact dogs and the animals' coats returned to normal when the dogs were neutered.

The author has not recognized a generalized truncal alopecia associated with the neutering of a female dog.

INTACT FEMALES

Sex hormone–related dermatoses in the intact bitch are uncommon and always are associated with some reproductive event or abnormality. As primary hypogonadism should not occur in the mature female, dermatologic disorders in the anestral bitch are likely to be the result of other disorders, such as hyperadrenocorticism and hypothyroidism, which affect both the skin and the ovaries. Anestral bitches should be evaluated carefully before the skin changes are attributed to an ovarian problem.

The most common sex hormone–related problem in the bitch appears to be the telogen defluxion (effluvium), or "blown coat," which occurs 1 to 2 months after whelping. During pregnancy, the number of hairs entering the telogen, or resting, phase is decreased, and the coat appears fuller. At or around parturition, the change in hormone levels causes many of the hair follicles to enter the telogen phase simultaneously, with subsequent truncal hair loss. Telogen defluxion is possible in the nonpregnant bitch, as hormone levels in the pregnant and the nonpregnant bitch are very similar. However, this phenomenon appears to be rare in the nonpregnant dog; in the author's experience, it has occurred only in bitches showing signs of pseudopregnancy. An occasional bitch will develop focal alopecia on the flank area at the time of overt pseudopregnancy. The dogs with telogen defluxion or flank alopecia will spontaneously regrow the coat in 2 to 4 months but may lose hair again if the reproductive event is repeated.

The next most easily recognized ovarian dysfunction occurs in dogs with polycystic ovaries or functioning ovarian tumors. These dogs develop alopecia of the ventrum, perineum, and flank area and have enlargement of the nipples and vulva. Some dogs lose hair over the trunk so that the entire coat is sparse. Many dogs show signs of nymphomania; blood dyscrasias are rare.

The last and vaguest syndrome involves the dog that has dermatologic changes and irregular interestral intervals, irregular estral cycles, or severe, prolonged pseudopregnancies. These dogs have no specific pattern of dermatologic change. Some will have asymptomatic perineal and ventral hair loss, some will have flank alopecia, some will have male patterned hair loss, and some will have seborrheic skin disease that is pruritic. Changes in the external genitalia may or may not be present. Although the features of a sex hormone–related problem are predominant, these dogs should be evaluated for evidence of other endocrine disorders, as they may have two intercurrent or interrelated endocrine disorders.

NEUTERED MALES

Coat changes associated with the castration of male dogs are very rare. Some develop a truncal alopecia that clinically is virtually indistinguishable from that seen in hypothyroidism. The coat color of black dogs may change to auburn. Diagnosis is by the exclusion of other appropriate endocrine disorders and the response to testosterone supplementation. Some dogs that are neutered during the winter do not regrow hair in clipped areas until the following spring, so it is advisable to postpone replacement therapy until the next shedding cycle is completed.

Occasionally, one will see a dog with no scrotal testes and an endocrine type of hair loss, and the owner will not know whether the dog was completely castrated. If the dog is showing no physical or biochemical evidence of hyperadrenocorticism but has signs of feminization, the dog should be surgically explored for a testicular tumor, as the frequency of estrogen-secreting tumors increases in cryptorchid testes. If the dog is not showing signs of feminization, the hair loss could be associated with the neutering or could be a manifestation of a bilateral cryptorchid state. As interstitial cells are relatively unaffected by higher body temperatures, testosterone production by a cryptorchid testis may be normal. Accordingly, a normal plasma testosterone level indicates the presence of abdominal testes. If the retained testes are very atrophic or if there is an estrogen-secreting tumor that has not yet feminized the dog, the testosterone levels may be very low, suggesting castration. Thus, an hCG (human chorionic gonadotropin) response test is the preferred diagnostic test to detect cryptorchid testes. A baseline sample is collected, and then 250 IU of hCG is given intravenously. A blood sample is taken 2 hr after the injection, and both blood samples are submitted for testosterone levels. A normal dog with scrotal testes will show a five- to sevenfold increase in testosterone levels after hCG administration, whereas the castrated dog will show little or no response. Dogs with cryptorchid testes will respond more like the normal dog.

INTACT MALES

In male dogs with a sex hormone problem, the testes can appear normal on palpation or show abnormalities of uniform, bilateral, testicular atrophy; unilateral or bilateral testicular neoplasia; or significant testicular dyssymmetry. The dyssymmetric and neoplastic conditions are the simplest to deal with and are discussed under testicular neoplasia.

Hypogonadism or bilateral testicular atrophy or atresia can be due to hypothalamic-pituitary defects, disorders of sex differentiation, or defects in androgen action or production. The author never has examined a mature dog with hypogonadism in which the predominant clinical signs were of a sex hormone–related dermatosis. The hypogonadism was secondary to hyperadrenocorticism, hypothyroidism, or drug administration, and other clinical signs were more evident or important. Animals with hypogonadism should have a complete medical evaluation before the clinical signs are attributed to a primary hypogonadism.

TESTICULAR NEOPLASIA

Testicular tumors are quite common in the older dog, and they may be coincidental findings or the cause of dermatologic abnormalities. The interstitial-cell tumor is the most common, followed by the seminoma, and then the Sertoli-cell tumor. Tumors can be singular or multiple and can involve one or both testes. Multiple tumor types are present in the same dog in approximately 25 per cent of the cases. The frequency of seminomas and Sertoli-cell tumors increases significantly in cryptorchid testicles.

Dermatologic signs can be seen with any type of testicular tumor, because of hormone production by the tumor or because of loss of hormones due to the replacement of normal testicular cells with neoplastic cells. Sertoli-cell tumors and seminomas can produce estrogens, while interstitial-cell tumors may produce androgens. With a functioning, unilateral neoplasm, the contralateral testicle usually is atrophic because of an interruption in the normal regulatory mechanisms.

Dogs with testicular tumors can present for hair loss, seborrhea, or both with or without signs of feminization. Feminization includes gynecomastia of all mammae, decreased libido, sexual attractiveness to other males, squamous metaplasia of the prostate, and a pendulous prepuce. Blood dyscrasias also may be seen. Coat changes typically start with hair loss in the collar area and along the ventrum and perineum. As the hair loss in these areas becomes more apparent, the dogs tend to lose the primary hairs on their trunk, while maintaining their undercoats. Dogs with estrogen-secreting tumors also tend to lose hair over the tail-head area, and the skin hyperpigments early. Dogs with testicular tumors tend to maintain their patterned hair loss for prolonged periods of time, but generalized truncal alopecia can be seen in very chronic cases.

Any dog with a patterned alopecia and a palpable testicular tumor or a cryptorchid testicle should be castrated. Dogs with testicular dyssymmetry probably have a small functioning tumor in the apparently normal testis and also should be castrated. Evidence of feminization, blood dyscrasias, or both emphasizes the need for surgery.

Not all cases are as clear-cut as those previously described. Some dogs with testicular tumors present with seborrhea or a nonpatterned hair loss, whereas other dogs with a patterned hair loss have equivocal testicular consistency. One must decide if a tumor is present or if a tumor is of functional significance. In these cases, the preputial and inguinal skin, tail gland, and anus should be examined carefully. Dogs with dermatologically significant testicular tumors often have linear preputial pigmentary changes, macular melanosis of the inguinal and perianal skin, tail gland hyperplasia, hyperplasia of the perianal glands, or some combination thereof. The preputial changes consist of a linear discoloration, either erythematous or melanotic, along the ventral surface of the prepuce, from the preputial orifice to the base of the scrotum. Both linear preputial pigmentation and macular melanosis are fairly specific indicators of testicular neoplasia, whereas tail gland and perianal gland hyperplasia is suggestive of, but not diagnostic for, a neoplasm. If any of these changes are detected, castration should be beneficial.

Castration is the treatment of choice when a testicular tumor is present. In those dogs for whom anesthesia poses an unacceptable risk, testosterone supplementation may be of some benefit, provided that the dog is not showing signs of feminization, perianal gland hyperplasia, or tail gland hyperplasia.

MALES WITH PALPABLY NORMAL TESTES

Dogs in this category can be the most troublesome to deal with, as the results of the available diagnostic tests can be normal and yet the dogs will respond to castration. In those instances in which the owner is unwilling to neuter the dog without firm evidence of a sex hormone imbalance, the condition may go undiagnosed. The author recognizes two syndromes in dogs with palpably normal testes.

The first and most common condition results in a patterned hair loss with no signs of feminization. Libido changes are not common signs, and some affected dogs have been used successfully for breeding. The patterned hair loss is identical to that described in the discussion on testicular neoplasia, namely alopecia of the collar area, ventrum, and perineum, with loss of primary but not secondary hairs over the trunk. In the Siberian husky and malamute breeds, these dogs are called "woollies," and a familial predisposition has been suggested in both of these breeds. Some dogs with black or dark-brown hairs exhibit changes in coat color to auburn or blond prior to or simultaneously with the patterned hair loss. In all dogs, the progression from the patterned alopecia to a generalized truncal alopecia is very slow.

Plasma sex hormone levels in these dogs can be within the normal ranges or can be abnormal. The author has seen hypotestosteronemia, hypoestrogenemia, hyperestrogenemia, and hyperprogesteronemia in various dogs, all with the same clinical picture. Therefore, the clinical presentation does not adequately describe which hormone(s) is at fault. Medical management of these dogs often is unrewarding even if the replacement therapy is based on the results of the sex hormone assays. Castration is the preferred method of treatment. Even dogs with hypotestosteronemia respond to castration, suggesting that peripheral hormonal interconversion, hormonal interactions, or receptor effects are more important than the level of any one individual hormone.

A very rare condition, which the author has recognized in two Pomeranians and one Golden retriever, involves the loss of hair, coupled with signs of physical or sexual aggression. Although the hair loss starts in the patterned areas previously described, there is fairly rapid progression to a truncal alopecia in which the secondary hairs may or may not be retained. These dogs all had very low baseline thyroid values but did not respond to adequate replacement therapy. All the dogs had high plasma testosterone levels, and the behavioral and coat changes responded completely to castration.

THE MALE FEMINIZING SYNDROME

The male feminizing syndrome is a rare, idiopathic condition that may be due to androgen receptor abnormalities or androgen interference by an antiandrogen. Affected dogs have normal testes, produce normal levels of testosterone and estradiol, and usually are fertile. A decreased libido or sexual attractiveness to other male dogs may be noted but is unusual.

Affected dogs have a symmetric alopecia of the perineum and inguinal areas, and the hairless areas are lichenified, hyperpigmented, and seborrheic. In chronic cases, the entire ventrum, axillary regions, and face also may be involved. Pruritus and ceruminous otitis externa are common signs. Gynecomastia is a consistent finding.

The author feels that most, if not all, dogs described as suffering from the male feminizing syndrome have a hormonal hypersensitivity rather than a sex hormone–related endocrine skin disease. This contention is supported by the early presence of pruritus and by skin biopsies that show hypersensitivity rather than endocrinelike changes. The gynecomastia seen in these dogs probably is associated with the pruritus rather than with hormonal changes. Chronically irritated nipples will enlarge in response to the irritation. When these dogs are examined early, only the caudal nipples are involved, whereas there is uniform gynecomastia in dogs feminized by a Sertoli-cell tumor. As this condition becomes more chronic, the hair loss, seborrheic changes, and pruritus progress up the ventrum, and thus, all the nipples can be enlarged in chronic cases.

In those cases in which the dog has the clinical signs previously described but is not pruritic or only becomes pruritic after all the skin changes have occurred, the diagnosis of the male feminizing syndrome rather than hormonal hypersensitivity is plausible, and the recommended therapy is castration. Before surgery, testosterone administration can be a valuable diagnostic tool. If the condition worsens, hormonal hypersensitivity is the most probable diagnosis, and castration is necessary. If improvement is noted, medical management can be continued or the animal can be neutered.

ADRENAL FEMINIZATION OR MASCULINIZATION

In dogs suffering from spontaneous hyperadrenocorticism, plasma testosterone levels tend to be decreased in males and elevated in females. In males, the decrease is associated with the inhibitory effect that cortisol has on GnRH, whereas in females, adrenal androgen production increases. Some females develop clitoral hypertrophy because of this increased androgen secretion. In the vast majority of cases, the dermatologic effects of the excessive glucocorticoid levels overshadow any changes caused by the testosterone imbalance.

Rarely, one will see cutaneous signs of a sex hormone imbalance as the first or predominant sign of hyperadrenocorticism. Dogs with black or dark brown hair will start to exhibit changes in coat color to auburn or blond, respectively. Females may develop significant clitoral hypertrophy without any other classic changes of hyperadrenocorticism. In the author's experience, these sex hormone predominating signs have uniformly occurred in dogs with adrenal neoplasia. Careful review of the history or routine blood work results will support the tentative diagnosis of hyperadrenocorticism, which can be verified by adrenal function tests.

FLANK ALOPECIA

The alopecia associated with any endocrine disorder could start in the flank area, but there are some dogs with hair loss restricted to the flank area. These dogs lose hair symmetrically over the paralumbar area, and the exposed skin can become hyperpigmented. Flank alopecia has been associated with hypothyroidism, hyposomatotropism of the mature dog, a local hyperestrogenism due to increased numbers of estradiol receptors in this area, and a generalized hyperestrogenism in the bitch with cystic ovaries or an ovarian tumor.

A more interesting and troublesome problem is flank alopecia that is seasonal. The dogs start to lose hair in the late fall or early winter and maintain the flank alopecia until spring, when the coat spontaneously regrows. The coat remains normal until the following fall when the cycle is repeated. This condition has been recognized solely in the male dog and almost exclusively in Airedale Terriers, English bulldogs, and boxers.

The affected dog responds abnormally in a growth hormone response test, but this finding does not adequately explain the clinical disease. Because of the striking breed, sex, and site predilections, a genetically influenced sex hormone imbalance caused by the interaction of multiple hormones is plausible.

The pineal gland produces melatonin and a family of chemically related hormones that have various antigonadotropic effects. Pineal hormones inhibit hypothalamic-pituitary gonadotropin release, inhibit testicular androgen production, and inhibit the effects of testosterone on the male accessory sex organs. Pineal hormone levels vary with the photoperiod and are highest during the times when darkness predominates.

Growth hormone is essential for normal growth and acts as a synergistic factor to allow testosterone to be fully effective. Androgens may enhance pituitary growth hormone secretion. In the growth hormone–deficient state, the response to testosterone is markedly diminished, and there may be an increased hypothalamic-pituitary sensitivity to pineal hormones.

The author speculates that dogs with seasonal flank alopecia have a genetically influenced, borderline growth hormone deficiency that sensitizes them to the effects of the pineal hormones. Until the pineal hormone levels increase in the fall, a photoperiod when darkness predominates, the dogs remain normal. Under the pineal influence, the dogs' androgen production decreases and, coupled with the androgen insensitivity and increase in SHBP caused by decreased growth hormone levels, results in an estrogen patterned alopecia due to a relative or absolute androgen deficiency. When spring arrives, the pineal hormones decrease, the androgen production increases, and the dog regrows its coat. Since the growth hormone deficiency will persist, the cycle will be repeated. If the growth hormone deficiency becomes more pronounced, the sensitivity to the pineal hormones may increase, resulting in an alopecia that is nonseasonal and more widespread.

The clinical diagnosis of a seasonal flank alopecia is easy, whereas laboratory confirmation is difficult. If thyroid and adrenal function tests are normal, one should suspect either or both growth hormone and sex hormone problems. Castration is of no benefit. Theoretically, androgen supplementation should cause hair regrowth, whereas antiandrogen therapy should accelerate hair loss. Since hair regrowth with any hormone can take 12 to 16 weeks, the regrowth would occur in the spring, when it naturally would have occurred. Thus, the response to therapy is unproven. Again, on a theoretical basis, androgen supplementation starting in the late summer should prevent hair loss, but this remains unproven.

HORMONAL HYPERSENSITIVITY

Hormonal hypersensitivity is a rare condition of the dog in which the animal develops an allergy to its endogenous sex hormones. The condition is virtually impossible to diagnose definitively, but the clinical syndrome is easy to recognize, at least in females.

In females, the dog starts to itch during an estral cycle and stops at the end of the cycle. Initially, the pruritus is focused over the lower back, perineum, and inguinal regions and responds poorly to glucocorticosteroid therapy. At the next cycle, the pruritus returns, usually is more intense and wider in distribution, and lasts longer. In chronic cases, the pruritus is generalized and nonseasonal, with estral intensification. Gynecomastia often accompanies the pruritus.

Hormonal hypersensitivity in males does occur, but because of its nonseasonal nature, the index of suspicion for this disorder can be low. Affected dogs show tailhead, perineal, and ventral pruritus, with secondary hair loss, hyperpigmentation, and seborrheic changes. A ceruminous otitis externa also occurs. These dogs have gynecomastia of the caudal mammae, as well as a pendulous prepuce. The testes palpate normally, and these dogs are not attractive to other males.

The diagnosis of hormonal hypersensitivity is made by the exclusion of all other appropriate differential diagnoses such as food hypersensitivity, flea-bite hypersensitivity, and atopy and by the elimination of the signs that accompany neutering. In females, testosterone often eliminates the pruritus, and the administration of repositol testosterone can be a valuable, presurgical, diagnostic test. In males, antiandrogenic compounds such as progesterone may have some applicability, but this is unproven.

SEX HORMONE–RESPONSIVE PRURITUS

Schwartzman at the University of Pennsylvania has treated allergic-looking dogs whose pruritus stops with sex hormone supplementation. Whether the elimination of the pruritus represents a correction of a sex hormone imbalance or is an effect of the sex hormones on the dog's immune system is unknown. Before a dog with idiopathic pruritus is treated with lifelong glucocorticoid steroids, sex hormone therapy might be indicated.

DIAGNOSIS AND THERAPY

Dogs with obvious tumors of the ovaries, testes, or adrenals require no further diagnostic work and should undergo surgery. The diagnostic test for the neutered dog is response to sex hormone supplementation. In the nontumorous intact dog, the absolute confirmation of the diagnosis can be difficult. Sex hormone levels should be measured, and if a definitive abnormality is detected, there is support for the diagnosis. Since there are many androgens and estrogens produced by the adrenal glands and gonads or by peripheral conversion, serum testosterone and estradiol levels can be normal. Additionally, abnormalities of the receptors or SHBP can cause sex hormone–associated hair follicle changes in the presence of normal serum sex hormone levels.

As a diagnostic test, the intact dog with normal serum sex hormone levels can be neutered or treated with sex hormones to make the dermatosis worse or better. The author prefers neutering as the method of diagnosis (and therapy), but some owners are unwilling to consent to surgery. Spironolactone, progestational compounds, ketoconazole, and cimetidine all have antiandrogenic activity. The "hypoandrogenic" dog should be made worse with this therapy, whereas the "hyperandrogenic" dog should improve. The hypoandrogenic state can be created by an absolute androgen deficiency or an estrogen excess. The hyperandrogenic state can be caused by an absolute androgen excess or an estrogen deficiency. As worsening can be detected within 1 month (whereas improvement may take 12 to 16 weeks), the author attempts to make the dog worse, with the understanding that this is a diagnostic step. The author uses megestrol acetate, 1.1 mg/kg PO s.i.d., as an antiandrogen to make hypoandrogenic dogs worse. Methyltestosterone, at the dosage described later, is used to make the hyperandrogenic dog worse. If the animal responds as anticipated, the hormone therapy is discontinued, and the dog is neutered. If the expected response is not seen, the diagnosis may be incorrect, although the dog still may respond to neutering.

Diethylstilbestrol (0.1 to 1.0 mg given daily with no therapy every third week) or methyltestosterone (1 mg/kg every other day, to a maximum dose of 30 mg) can be used for oral supplementation. The author has treated neutered female dogs with methyltestosterone instead of diethylstilbestrol, and the response has been excellent. The reason(s) for the response is unknown, but peripheral conversion to estrogens or altered sex hormone receptors in these dogs are the most probable explanation. Testosterone can cause physical and sexual aggression; either or both prostatic and perianal gland hypertrophy; epiphora; and liver changes. However, these changes are infrequent. Response to neutering or sex hormone replacement can take 12 to 16 weeks. Once a response is obtained with replacement therapy, the frequency of administration is decreased. Most dogs maintain their haircoats with once or twice weekly administration.

If no response to neutering or replacement therapy is seen, the diagnosis or therapy is incorrect. If one follows the clues offered by the skin, these nonresponsive cases should be infrequent.

References and Supplemental Reading

Chastain, C. B., and Ganjam, V. K.: *Clinical Endocrinology of Companion Animals.* Philadelphia: Lea and Febiger, 1986.

Eigenmann, J. E., Poortman, J., and Koeman, J. P.: Estrogen-induced flank alopecia in the female dog: Evidence for local rather than systemic hyperestrogenism. J. Am. Anim. Hosp. Assoc. 20:621, 1984.

Muller, G. H., Kirk, R. W., and Scott, D. W.: *Small Animal Dermatology III.* Philadelphia: W. B. Saunders Co., 1983.

Parker, F.: Skin and hormones. *In* Williams, R. H. (ed.): *Textbook of Endocrinology,* 5th ed. Philadelphia: W. B. Saunders Co., 1974, pp. 977–993.

Ponec, M. N.: Hormone receptors in the skin. *In* Fitzpatrick, T. B.,

Eisen, A. Z., Wolff, K., et al. (eds.): *Dermatology in General Medicine*, 3rd ed. New York: McGraw-Hill, 1987, pp. 367–374.

Reichlin, S.: Neuroendocrinology. *In* Wilson, J. D., and Forster, D. W. (eds.): *William's Textbook of Endocrinology*, 7th ed. Philadelphia: W. B. Saunders Co., 1985, pp. 492–567.

Sorrentino, S., Reiter, R. J., and Schalch, D. S.: Interactions of the pineal gland, blinding, and underfeeding on reproductive organ size and radioimmunoassayable growth hormone. Neuroendocrinology 7:105, 1971.

Tabei, T., Mickelson, K. E., Neuhaus, S., et al.: Sex steroid binding protein (SBP) in dog plasma. J. Steroid Biochem. 9:983, 1978.

Underwood, L. E., and Van Wyk, J. J.: Growth and reproduction. *In* Wilson, J. D., and Forster, D. W. (eds.): *William's Textbook of Endocrinology*, 7th ed. Philadelphia: W. B. Saunders Co., 1985, pp. 155–205.

Wurtman, R. J., and Cardinali, D. P.: The pineal organ. *In* Williams, R. H. (ed.): *Textbook of Endocrinology*, 5th ed. Philadelphia: W. B. Saunders Co., 1974, pp. 832–840.

HORMONAL REPLACEMENT THERAPY IN VETERINARY DERMATOLOGY

STEPHEN D. WHITE, D.V.M.

Ft. Collins, CO

Hormonal preparations that replace deficient or presumedly deficient endogenous hormones are used as therapy for several diseases in dogs and cats. These conditions commonly or exclusively affect the skin and include hypothyroidism, adult-onset hyposomatotropism, testosterone- and estrogen-responsive dermatoses, and feline symmetric alopecia (feline endocrine alopecia).

THYROID HORMONES

HORMONES. Thyroxine (T_4) and tri-iodothyronine (T_3) are the important endogenous thyroid hormones and are also the hormones used for supplementation. Both are produced in the thyroid, with T_3 also produced in the body tissues by conversion from T_4. T_4 is found in greater concentrations in the serum, but T_3 has the greater biologic potency and is considered to be the major mediator of thyroid hormone effects at the cellular level. The biologic importance of T_3 is mentioned because of rare reports of hypothyroid states with normal T_4 production but failure of conversion of T_4 to T_3. In those cases, T_3 supplementation achieved clinical euthyroidism (Rosychuck, 1982).

EFFECTS ON THE SKIN. Thyroid hormones are important for maintaining a normal rate of sebum production, keratinization, shifting telogen (resting) hair follicles to anagen (active growth phase), and maintaining a normal bacterial flora. Thus, common cutaneous signs of dogs with hypothyroidism are seborrhea, alopecia, and secondary pyodermas. While generally nonpruritic, pruritus may be present if seborrhea, pyoderma, or both are present.

DISEASE. Primary hypothyroidism, caused by idiopathic thyroiditis, atrophy, or both, is the most common form of the disease in dogs. Secondary hypothyroidism, caused by a deficiency in the thyroid-stimulating hormone (TSH) produced in the anterior pituitary, and tertiary hypothyroidism, a hypothalamic deficiency of thyrotropin-releasing factor (TRF), are rare in dogs (Chastain and Ganjam, 1986). No form of spontaneously occurring hypothyroidism has been convincingly documented in the adult cat.

DIAGNOSIS. Diagnosis is best made by the TSH-response test. Various regimens exist in the literature. The author prefers giving 1.0 IU of TSH per dog (regardless of body size) intravenously, with serum values analyzed before and 4 hr after injection. A normal response test should show at least a twofold increase in T_4 levels, with the postinjection value equal to or greater than 3.0 µg/dl. There are not much data available for interpretation of T_3 values; as a guideline, an increase of at least 30 ng/dl from baseline to postinjection value is probably normal. A normal T_4 response with a poor T_3 response may indicate a peripheral conversion problem.

Baseline T_3 and T_4 values may also be used to diagnose hypothyroidism, but many factors (e.g., episodic release of hormones from the thyroid, corticosteroids and other drugs, illness, breed, time of day) may affect these values and make them unreliable. If baseline values are used, the author believes that euthyroidism is best diagnosed when the T_4 value is equal to or greater than 3.0 µg/dl. In contrast, hypothyroidism *probably* exists when the T_4 value is less than 1.0 µg/dl (and other causes of hormone suppression, as stated previously, are ruled out). Again, T_3 values are more difficult to interpret, but levels above 90 ng/dl are probably euthyroid, whereas values below 25 ng/dl are probably hypothyroid. Values of T_3 and T_4 between these indicator values are in a gray zone, and, at least for the author, are difficult to interpret as to the presence of disease. Clinicians should be aware that different laboratories may have normal values that are somewhat different from the author's.

PREPARATIONS AND DOSAGE. Desiccated thyroid, usually produced from the thyroids of cattle, sheep, or hogs, is a nonsynthetic preparation with variable biologic activity. The exact amount of T_3 or T_4 in desiccated thyroid preparations is usually unknown. Some evidence points toward hog thyroid as being more biologically active. Desiccated thyroid also has an unreliable shelf-life. For these reasons, the author does not use this drug; however, there are anecdotal reports of dogs that cannot tolerate or absorb the synthetic preparations listed later, but do well on desiccated thyroid. The recommended dosage is 15 to 20 mg/kg q 24 hr or divided q 12 hr.

Synthetic preparations of both T_4 (sodium levothyroxine) and T_3 (sodium tri-iodothyronine) are available both as separate drugs and in combination. The T_4 preparations are the therapy of choice. Supplementing with T_4 causes a return to normal levels of both T_4 and T_3, supporting the conclusion that giving T_4 to a hypothyroid dog more closely mimics its own biology, as opposed to giving T_3, which bypasses the peripheral conversion process. The author reserves use of T_3 supplementation for proven cases of animals unable to convert T_4 to T_3.

Recommended dosages vary, but for dermatologic cases, the author prefers T_4 to be given at 0.02 mg/kg q 12 hr. For old dogs or dogs with cardiac problems, the dosage is divided in half. The T_3 dose is 4.4 mg/kg q 8 hr. Thyroid supplementation may increase insulin and digitalis requirements in dogs treated with these drugs. Thyroid supplementation may also increase the effectiveness of anticoagulant therapy. In addition, concurrent hypoadrenocorticism should be treated prior to initiation of thyroid supplementation, as the increase in metabolic rate due to thyroid hormones may precipitate a hypoadrenal crisis in a dog with untreated hypoadrenocorticism.

RESPONSE AND MONITORING. Most dogs show improvement dermatologically within 6 weeks. Improvement in other signs (mental awareness, heatseeking) is usually noted sooner. Six weeks after initiation of therapy, a blood evaluation of thyroid hormone levels 4 hr after administration of the pill is recommended. It seems that 4 hr is a good compromise regarding the biologic states of T_4 (plateau after administration is between 4 and 8 hr,

half-life is between 14 and 16 hr) and T_3 (plateau between 2 and 5 hr, half-life between 5 and 6 hr) (Rosychuck, 1982). A T_4 value of 3 μg/dl or higher and a T_3 value of 90 ng/dl or higher indicates relatively normal levels of these hormones. Persistence of clinical signs in the presence of such values should direct the clinician to investigate concurrent disease. Persistence of clinical signs *and* inadequate thyroid hormone levels suggest poor owner or patient compliance (animal is not receiving pills or is spitting them out), poor absorption (rare; possibly seen more commonly with generic synthetic preparations), inactivity of the preparation (especially if desiccated thyroid is being used), or antibodies against thyroid hormones (rare; diagnosed and treated by giving prednisone 1 mg/kg q 12 hr, continuing thyroid supplementation, and noting normal thyroid levels on testing 1 week later). If persistence of clinical signs and inadequate T_3 values are associated with adequate T_4 values while supplementing with T_4, then a peripheral conversion defect is probable and T_3 supplementation is suggested.

Thyrotoxicosis as a side effect of oversupplementation is uncommon in dogs, owing to the canine ability to catabolize and excrete thyroid hormones. Occasionally, a dog shows clinical signs such as polydipsia, polyuria, panting, weight loss without anorexia, and either or both tachycardia and nervousness. The presence of these signs should result in evaluation of T_3 and T_4 serum concentrations to confirm the diagnosis, and immediate discontinuance of the supplementation. Once the signs have abated (days to weeks), the thyroid dosage has been reviewed, and the animal has fully recovered, a lower dosage may be instituted, with the dog being monitored closely.

Thyroid hormones have also been recommended in the treatment of feline symmetric alopecia, at a dose of 0.1 to 0.3 mg T_4 per cat daily (Muller et al., 1983) or 20 to 50 μg T_3 per cat b.i.d. (Thoday, 1986). Hair regrowth occurs within 3 months. The mechanism of action is not well understood, as these cats are *not* hypothyroid. The diagnosis is made by ruling out other more common causes of feline symmetric alopecia. The author has witnessed undesirable behavior changes in cats treated with these T_4 dosages, and as "feline endocrine alopecia" seemingly affects only the skin, owners may reasonably elect to decline therapy.

It must be stressed here that the administration of thyroid hormones can force variable degrees of hair regrowth in numerous nonthyroidal diseases. Thus, the partial or complete regrowth of hair in a dog or a cat following the administration of these hormones is not synonymous with a diagnosis of hypothyroidism.

GROWTH HORMONE

HORMONE. Growth hormone (somatotropin) is produced by the anterior pituitary and acts on many peripheral tissues through another hormone, somatomedin. Immunologic cross-reactivity from species to species varies, with the canine growth hormone being closer to the porcine hormone than to the bovine or the ovine hormone.

EFFECTS ON THE SKIN. Growth hormone increases the growth of muscle and connective tissue of the body, including the skin. Lack of growth hormone induces histologic changes of orthokeratotic hyperkeratosis; follicular keratosis, dilatation, and atrophy; epidermal melanosis; sebaceous gland atrophy; thin dermis; and decreased or absent elastin fibers.

DISEASE. Two diseases resulting from growth hormone deficiency are documented in the dog. *Pituitary dwarfism*, seen most commonly in the German shepherd, is caused by a congenital pituitary cyst (cystic Rathke's pouch) or a hypoplastic anterior pituitary. Such dogs may also be deficient in thyroid and gonadal hormones, owing to the lack of pituitary production of these glands' stimulating hormones. Affected dogs are dwarves, with markedly small stature, failure of the epiphyses of the long-bones to close properly, retained puppy dentition and hair coat, and dull (cretinous) personalities. As these dogs get older, their skin often becomes seborrheic and alopecic. While supplementation with growth hormone has been reported, results have been less than satisfactory (DeBowes, 1987).

Adult onset hyposomatotropism (growth hormone–responsive dermatosis in the mature dog) is a disease most commonly seen in male Pomeranians, chow chows, miniature poodles, and keeshonds between the ages of 9 and 24 months; however, affected females, other breeds, and variable age of onset have been reported. The typical presentation is one of symmetric truncal alopecia and hyperpigmentation, although alopecia without hyperpigmentation as well as nontruncal alopecia has also been noted. Pruritus is absent unless folliculitis is concurrent. Failure of production of adequate levels of growth hormone by the anterior pituitary is believed to be the cause of this disease, but the reason for this onset of production failure is not known. One dog has been reported as recovering spontaneously (Scott and Walton, 1986).

DIAGNOSIS. Diagnosis of both pituitary dwarfism and adult-onset hyposomatotropism is based on clinical signs and the failure to respond to a clonidine (Catapres, Boehringer Ingelheim) or a xylazine (Rompun, Haver-Lockhart) response test. Both of these chemicals stimulate growth hormone release in dogs. Various protocols have been reported in the literature. The author prefers serum samples collected before and 15, 30, and 60 min after an intravenous xylazine injection of 0.3 mg/kg body weight. The serum must be frozen and shipped on dry ice to a laboratory with a validated assay for canine growth hormone. Basal growth hormone levels in normal dogs vary from 1.4 to 4.5 ng/ml. A marked (greater than five times the baseline) increase in serum growth hormone levels is seen within 30 min of xylazine administration in normal dogs, whereas pituitary dwarves and dogs with adult-onset hyposomatropism fail to respond. Baseline values alone are inadequate for diagnosis, and as the two most probable differential diagnoses (hypothyroidism and hyperadrenocorticism) may decrease baseline values, it is important for the veterinarian to rule out these diseases.

PREPARATION AND DOSAGE. There is no commercially available growth hormone for use in dogs. The recommended empiric dosage for adult-onset hyposomatotropism is 2.5 IU (for dogs weighing less than 14 kg) or 5 units (for larger dogs) administered subcutaneously every other day for a total of ten treatments. Bovine or porcine growth hormone preparations are preferred; ovine growth hormone is ineffective. Hair regrowth usually commences during therapy. While a majority of dogs do respond to therapy, dogs may also either fail to respond, have only partial hair regrowth, or regrow all their hair but redevelop alopecia at a later date. In addition, dogs may develop diabetes mellitus as a result of the gluconeogenic properties of growth hormone. The diabetes is reversible in most (but not all) dogs, provided therapy is stopped immediately. Because of possible side effects, difficulty in acquiring growth hormone, potential for spontaneous recovery, and the fact that untreated dogs with adult-onset hyposomatotropism remain healthy (if perhaps with an unpleasant appearance), the author rarely encourages treatment.

ESTROGENS

HORMONE. Estrogens are steroidal hormones produced by the ovarian follicles, Sertoli's cells of the testicles, and the zona reticularis of the adrenal cortex. At least 95 per cent of estrogens in the dog are bound primarily to albumin or sex hormone–binding globulin. Only the unbound serum estrogen enters peripheral cells to bind with hormonal receptors. Estrogens are metabolized by the liver, conjugated, and eliminated in the bile and urine. There are several estrogenic substances produced in the dog (estradiol, estrone, estriol). Most available commercial assays detect only one of these substances; thus, their ability to be utilized for diagnosis is disappointing. Reported values for blood estradiol in female dogs vary from 10 to 80 pg/ml.

EFFECTS ON THE SKIN. Administration of estrogen to various laboratory mammals and humans has resulted in a multitude of experimental data. Because the effects of hormones vary according to dosage, route of administration, and species, it is sometimes difficult to assess the relevance of such data to clinical medicine. Estrogens may increase or decrease epidermal thickness, increase pigmentation, reduce sebum production and sebaceous gland size, increase dermal ground substance, decrease subcutis thickness, and suppress anagen (growth phase) of the hair follicle.

DISEASE. Estrogen-responsive alopecia (ovarian imbalance type II) is a rare, poorly understood disease occurring in spayed female dogs. The disease has also been reported as occurring in dogs prior to first estrus, during pseudocyesis, and in conjunction with abnormal estrus cycles. Hypoestrogenism has been hypothesized but not well documented as the cause.

No age or breed predilections have been noted. Clinical signs consist of a symmetric alopecia, often starting in the perineal or genital areas, but eventually involving the trunk, ventral abdomen and thorax, neck, and pinnae. Pruritus is absent unless seborrhea develops. The dogs are usually otherwise healthy, although estrogen-responsive urinary incontinence is occasionally seen concurrently.

DIAGNOSIS. Diagnosis is based on the clinical presentation of an endocrine-type alopecia in a spayed female dog and the ruling out of other causes of alopecia, particularly hypothyroidism, hyperadrenocorticism, and adult-onset hyposomatotropism. Because of the aforementioned difficulties in assays for estrogens, such tests are rarely informative.

PREPARATION AND DOSAGE. Diethylstilbestrol (DES) is the treatment of choice. The oral preparation is preferred because of the high risk of side effects with parenteral administration. The author gives 1 mg twice weekly until hair growth is evident. Dogs weighing less than 5 kg receive 0.5 mg twice weekly. Clinical response should occur within 6 to 12 weeks. Once a good response is achieved, the dosage is lowered to the least amount necessary to maintain normal appearance.

DES is not without side effects. Bone marrow suppression (thrombocytopenia, leukopenia, anemia) is the most serious potential adverse reaction. Because this effect is not always dependent on dosage or length of therapy, it is recommended to do complete blood and platelet counts every 4 to 8 weeks initially, and then every 3 to 4 months for as long as the dog receives DES. Should blood dyscrasias be noted, DES therapy should be stopped immediately and supportive care given as needed. DES occasionally causes signs of estrus, as well as an endocrine-type alopecia and hyperpigmentation syndrome. Lowering the dosage may resolve these side effects.

Because of the side effects of DES, as well as the otherwise healthy status of these dogs, the author does not recommend treatment unless pruritus is a sign.

Combined repositol diethylstilbestrol (0.625 mg per cat) or estradiol (0.5 mg per cat) and testosterone (12.5 mg per cat) have been used to treat "feline endocrine alopecia." Overdosage of any of these sex hormones can cause severe liver disease in cats. The necessity of treating an essentially benign disease with potentially harmful drugs must be weighed by the clinician.

ANDROGENS

HORMONE. Androgens are steroidal hormones produced by the interstitial cells of the testicle, by the zona reticularis of the adrenal cortex, and, in small amounts, by the ovary. As with estrogens, there are various androgenic substances produced by the dog, and thus using blood values as diagnostics is fraught with the same problems as with the estrogens. Testosterone, the androgen with the highest serum concentrations, is bound in the blood to sex hormone–binding globulin and to albumin. Only about 2 per cent of total serum testosterone is unbound and enters peripheral cells. Most testosterone in the dog is metabolized by the liver and excreted in the bile, though some is conjugated and excreted in the urine. Normal male dogs are reported to have blood testosterone values of 1 to 7 ng/ml.

EFFECTS ON THE SKIN. Like estrogens, androgens administered to humans and animals have generated a large amount of experimental data. Androgens may increase epidermal mitosis and thickness, increase pigmentation, enlarge sebaceous glands, increase sebum production, cause thickening of the dermis, and retard anagen (though accelerated hair growth has been noted in humans).

DISEASE. Testosterone-responsive dermatosis is a rare, bilaterally symmetric alopecia usually seen in castrated male dogs. However, older dogs with normal, atrophied, cryptorchid, or neoplastic testicles have also been reported with the disease. No breed predilections are known. The etiology has been theorized but not documented as hypoandrogenism. The alopecia begins in the perineal and genital region but may eventually affect the flanks, rear legs, and ventral abdomen. The coat tends to be dry and dull, with seborrhea sicca. Pruritus and hyperpigmentation are usually absent.

DIAGNOSIS. Testosterone-responsive dermatosis is diagnosed on the basis of clinical signs and the ruling out of other more common causes of alopecia. As stated previously, blood values of androgens are not particularly helpful.

PREPARATION AND DOSAGE. Methyltestosterone, 1 mg/kg PO (up to a maximum of 30 mg total dose) every 48 hr, is the therapy of choice. A good response should be seen within 3 months, at which point the dosage should be reduced to the lowest effective maintenance dose. Methyltestosterone is expensive and may cause cholestatic liver disease and aggression. Because of these side effects, as well as the fact that these dogs are generally healthy otherwise, the author does not usually recommend therapy unless pruritus is present.

As mentioned earlier, combined repositol testosterone–diethylstilbestrol injections have been used to treat feline endocrine alopecia.

References and Supplemental Reading

Chastain, C. B., and Ganjam, V. K.: *Clinical Endocrinology of Companion Animals.* Philadelphia: Lea and Febiger, 1986, pp. 74–79, 135–150, 450–460.

Chester, D. K.: Endocrine dermatoses. *In* Nesbitt, G. H. (ed.): *Contemporary Issues in Small Animal Practice: Dermatology.* New York: Churchill Livingstone, 1987, pp. 159–187.

DeBowes, L. J.: Pituitary dwarfism in a German shepherd puppy. Compend. Contin. Ed. Pract. Vet. 9:931, 1987.

Morgan, R. V.: Blood dyscrasias associated with testicular tumors in the dog. J. Am. Anim. Hosp. Assoc. 18:970, 1982.

Muller, G. H., Kirk, R. W., and Scott, D. W.: *Small Animal Dermatology,* 3rd ed. Philadelphia: W. B. Saunders Co., 1983, pp. 492–560.

Parker, W. M., and Scott, D. W.: Growth hormone–responsive alopecia in the mature dog: A discussion of 13 cases. J. Am. Anim. Hosp. Assoc. 16:824, 1980.

Rosychuck, R. A. W.: Thyroid hormones and anti-thyroid drugs. Vet. Clin. North Am. [Small Anim. Pract.] 12:111, 1982.

Scott, D. W., and Walton, D. K.: Hyposomatotropism in the mature dog: A discussion of 22 cases. J. Am. Anim. Hosp. Assoc. 22:467, 1986.

Thoday, K. L.: Differential diagnosis of symmetric alopecia in the cat. *In* Kirk, R. W. (ed.): *Current Veterinary Therapy IX.* Philadelphia: W. B. Saunders Co., 1986, pp. 545–553.

FAMILIAL CANINE DERMATOMYOSITIS

KIRK H. HAUPT, D.V.M.,
Edmonds, Washington

and ANN M. HARGIS, D.V.M.
Pullman, Washington

Canine dermatomyositis is an inflammatory disease of the skin, muscle, and sometimes vasculature of collies and Shetland sheepdogs (Hargis et al., 1984; Haupt et al., 1985; Kunkle et al., 1985; Hargis et al., 1985). In humans, dermatomyositis is a rare disorder that is generally believed to have an immune-mediated pathogenesis. Dermatomyositis in humans and dogs has many similarities; in contrast to current information on human dermatomyositis, the canine disease has a strong genetic basis and is termed familial canine dermatomyositis.

CLINICAL FEATURES

Dermatomyositis has been documented in collies in 19 states of the United States of varied geographic locations and appears to be widespread (Kunkle et al., 1985). In collies, there is no apparent restriction to one sex, coat, or color (Kunkle et al., 1985). Dermatomyositis is less well documented in Shetland sheepdogs but appears to be a similar disease.

Several generalizations can be made about the manifestation of dermatomyositis in dogs:

1. Clinical disease occurs primarily in juvenile dogs. Adults are also affected but often with subclinical disease. In rare cases, an adult may present with dermatomyositis, lacking a history of disease as a puppy.

2. Typically, canine dermatomyositis is a clinical syndrome of dermatitis and less apparent myositis. The majority of affected dogs have dermatitis but display few overt signs of muscle disease. Moreover, muscle biopsies may fail to reveal myositis in some dogs with dermatitis. Conversely, histologic evidence of myositis has been found in a few dogs without a history of dermatitis, whose littermates had confirmed dermatomyositis (Kunkle et al., 1985; Hargis et al., 1986b).

3. For most puppies, signs of clinical disease improve spontaneously and are self-limiting. Some puppies are so mildly and briefly affected that their owners may fail to recognize a problem. Uncommonly, dogs have active and severe disease throughout life.

Skin lesions are often first observed between 2 and 6 months of age. The earliest lesions usually appear on the face, especially around the eyes and on the nose and lips; on the inner surfaces and tips of the ears; or on the tip of the tail. Subsequently, some puppies may develop lesions on the extremities and trunk, specifically over bony prominences of the elbows, stifles, carpi, tarsi, phalanges, and sternum. Early skin lesions are erythema, vesicles, pustules, papules, or small nodules that progress rapidly to crusts, ulcers, and areas of alopecia and scaling. Early, transient vesicles and ulcers may be observed on the mucocutaneous junctions of the lips and oral mucous membranes, and transient ulceration of the footpads may occur. Older lesions, found principally on the bridge of the nose and around the eyes, consist of alopecia and areas of hyperpigmentation and hypopigmentation. The dermatitis is usually nonpruritic. Peripheral lymph node enlargement may occur, especially in areas of dermatitis. Acute, transient facial swelling has been observed in a few puppies preceding onset of dermatitis (Kunkle et al., 1985).

As described by Kunkle and coworkers (1985), the clinical course and the severity of dermatitis are quite variable. Typically, skin lesions are cyclical in severity, and dermatitis lasts weeks to months. Many puppies have mild, transient lesions and heal spontaneously by 6 to 8 months of age. More severely affected puppies develop ulcers and exudative, painful lesions (often secondarily infected by *Staphylococcus*) affecting the head and extremities. These puppies usually recover by 1 year of age, although a few have scarred areas on the face. In some recovered dogs, active skin lesions recur with onset of estrus or exposure to sunlight. Uncommonly, affected dogs have a variably severe dermatitis throughout life. These dogs are usually extensively disfigured with ulcerated, crusted lesions and scars involving the head, tail, extremities, and trunk. It must be emphasized that dermatomyositis in dogs may be complicated by localized or generalized demodicosis.

Signs of muscle disease follow the onset of skin lesions and are usually minimal. Myositis may be more pronounced in puppies more severely affected by dermatitis, but not always. In Shetland sheepdogs, the severity of myositis may not correlate with the severity of dermatitis (Ihrke, 1987). Furthermore, myositis in Shetland sheepdogs on the whole seems to be less severe than myositis in collies (Hargis et al., 1985; Ihrke, 1987). The most common (and often only) sign is symmetric temporal and masseter muscle atrophy, which is easily overlooked because of the dolichocephalic shape of the head in collies and Shetland sheepdogs. Some puppies develop prehension difficulties and dysphagia manifested by difficulty in lapping water, chewing, and swallowing. A few severely affected dogs, as they mature, remain smaller than littermates and develop variably severe generalized muscle atrophy.

These dogs may exhibit a stiff gait, exercise intolerance, and generalized weakness. Severely affected dogs may have facial palsy (decreased or absent palpebral response), decreased jaw tone, and, paradoxically, hyperactive patellar reflexes. In rare instances, extensive atrophy and fibrosis of the muscles of mastication cause trismus, and uncommonly, severely affected dogs develop megaesophagus.

Other clinical findings may include conjunctivitis, infertility, and, uncommonly, transient polyarthritis. Infertility is especially evident in more severely affected males.

DIAGNOSIS

Diagnosis of canine dermatomyositis is currently based upon breed, age of onset, clinical appearance of skin lesions, cutaneous histopathology, and histologic or electromyographic evidence of myositis. Evaluation of the pedigree may reveal similarly affected dogs or a particular line of dogs in which dermatomyositis is common. Other conditions that must be ruled out include other immune-mediated skin disease, epidermolysis bullosa, pyoderma, dermatophytosis, and demodicosis. Mild forms of dermatomyositis may be confused with common dermatopathies of puppies, such as localized demodicosis and dermatophytosis.

Dermatophyte cultures, skin scrapings, and cutaneous biopsies should be performed to rule out other primary or concurrent skin conditions and to support a diagnosis of dermatomyositis. Histologically, early cutaneous lesions consist of a nonspecific, occasionally vesiculating, pustular, and ulcerative dermatitis. The inflammatory reaction is mild to severe and consists of many cell types including but not limited to neutrophils, lymphocytes, and mast cells. Basal cells may be pyknotic or vacuolated. Vasculitis is sometimes seen. Results of direct immunofluorescence testing for immunoglobulin G (IgG) and C_3 in skin have been negative. In older lesions, the epidermis is often thickened by hyperkeratosis and acanthosis. Scattered or clustered lymphocytes, macrophages, plasma cells, mast cells, and eosinophils occur in the papillary dermis or in perivascular or perifollicular areas. Dermal macrophages may contain melanin pigment. Dermal fibrosis is present, and adnexal structures may be absent or atrophic. In more severely affected dogs, lesions caused by secondary bacterial infection or demodicosis may develop.

Evaluation of the myopathy should include muscle biopsies and, when available, electromyography (EMG). Serum muscle enzymes, creatine kinase (CK), and aspartate aminotransferase (AST, SGOT), are normal. Needle EMG abnormalities include fibrillation potentials and, less frequently, positive sharp waves and bizarre high-frequency discharges. Needle EMG changes are most common in the muscles of mastication, tongue, distal extremities, laryngeal muscles, and tail (Haupt et al., 1985; Kunkle et al., 1985). Motor nerve conduction velocities are normal, but repetitive nerve stimulation studies reveal mild decremental responses in some dogs.

Histopathology of muscle is necessary to confirm dermatomyositis. Ideally, muscle biopsies should be performed approximately 2 to 3 months after onset of dermatitis and before 1 year of age, since active myositis spontaneously improves in most dogs. Myositis is more commonly found in, and is more severe in, the temporalis and masseter muscles, followed by muscles of the extremities below the elbow and stifle. With the exception of those dogs with severe atrophy and fibrosis of the muscles of mastication, the temporalis muscle is the single biopsy site of choice. Histologically, multifocal accumulations of lymphocytes, plasma cells, macrophages, and fewer neutrophils and eosinophils are present in the endomysium and perimysium. Myofibers in inflamed areas are often fragmented, vacuolated, atrophic, or regenerative. Perifascicular atrophy is occasionally seen. Both type I and type II myofibers are smaller in areas of myositis. More severely affected dogs may have vasculitis, and small nerves are occasionally incorporated in the inflammatory reaction. Results of direct immunofluorescence for IgG and C_3 have been negative.

Results of the hemogram, serum biochemical profile, and urinalysis are usually normal. The hemogram may show mild increases in neutrophil and band cells in some dogs, and a low-grade, nonregenerative anemia in severely affected dogs with chronic disease. Basal T_4 levels may be depressed in severely affected dogs, but these dogs demonstrate a euthyroid response to TSH-stimulation ("euthyroid sick syndrome"). Results of standard tests for autoimmunity, Coombs's test, lupus erythematosus (LE) cell test, antinuclear antibody (ANA) titer, and rheumatoid factor, are usually negative.

CAUSE AND PATHOGENESIS

The cause of canine dermatomyositis is unknown but may comprise a complex pathogenesis involving heredity, the immune system, and numerous other internal and external factors.

Prospective breeding studies using collies with dermatomyositis have revealed a mode of inheritance that is autosomal dominant, with variable expressivity (Hargis et al., 1984; Kunkle et al., 1985). Variable expression of dermatomyositis may, in part, be due to variation in genotype (i.e., dogs with the more severe form may be homozygous,

whereas more mildly affected dogs may be heterozygous for the gene of dermatomyositis).

Moreover, variation in the expression of dermatomyositis in different dogs suggests that more is involved in causing disease than simple inheritance. Indeed, phenotypic expression of dermatomyositis may involve an inherited immunologic defect that predisposes dogs to developing the disease. Immune complexes appear to be involved in the pathogenesis of canine dermatomyositis. Prospective studies of collies with dermatomyositis showed that (1) levels of circulating immune complexes (CICs) became elevated before or concurrent with onset of dermatitis; (2) usually, the severity of dermatomyositis correlated positively with higher levels of CICs; and (3) in more severely affected dogs, levels of CICs tended to reach a plateau or increase, whereas in mildly affected dogs the CICs tended to decrease to normal levels. In addition, histopathology has revealed lesions of vasculitis and perivasculitis, especially in dogs with severe dermatomyositis and dogs with higher levels of CICs.

Other internal and external factors may play roles in the pathogenesis of canine dermatomyositis. Distribution of lesions in peripheral parts of the body suggests that cooler temperatures in peripheral regions may be involved in lesion pathogenesis. Dermatitis is most severe on the ears, face, distal extremities, and tip of the tail. Furthermore, when muscle lesions are more generalized, only the superficial portions of muscles are involved. Distribution of cutaneous lesions over bony prominences of the extremities suggests that trauma may also have a role. Onset of estrus and exposure to sunlight have been incriminated in relapses of dermatitis in some dogs. Finally, electron microscopy has revealed structures resembling viruses within endothelial cells of muscle of some dogs, suggesting that a virus may have a role in the pathogenesis of canine dermatomyositis.

TREATMENT AND MANAGEMENT

There are few sound recommendations for effective treatment of canine dermatomyositis. Variation in severity of dermatomyositis in different dogs and the cyclic and self-limiting nature of the disease make assessing therapy difficult.

"Tincture of time" may be the affected puppy's greatest ally. Baths with hypoallergenic shampoos are beneficial. Since cutaneous trauma may play a role in causing dermatitis, measures that minimize injury are important (Ihrke, 1987). Affected puppies should not be housed on hard surfaces and should be separated from littermates and other dogs to prevent rough play. Avoidance of ultraviolet light and control of estrus (preferably by ovariohysterectomy) are other management considerations.

Treatment of dermatomyositis in humans is usually with corticosteroids, with satisfactory responses seen in the majority of patients. Corticosteroids may have a place in treating dogs more severely affected by dermatomyositis, but evidence of their effectiveness is inconclusive (Kunkle et al., 1985; Ihrke, 1987). An immunosuppressive dosage of prednisone or prednisolone, 1 to 2 mg/kg PO every 12 hr, is advised for induction of treatment. The corticosteroid dosage can be tapered, preferably to alternate-day administration, once a satisfactory response is achieved. Relapses may require reinstitution of corticosteroid therapy. Secondary staphylococcal pyodermas should be controlled with appropriate systemic antibiotics and antimicrobial baths. Identification and treatment of complicating demodicosis is essential and would negate the use of corticosteroids.

Until a practical and reliable method is found to identify minimally affected puppies and adult dogs that had mild disease as puppies but have recovered without cutaneous scarring or muscle atrophy, elimination of dermatomyositis by selective breeding will be difficult. Rigorous testing, including muscle biopsies, may fail to identify some puppies and especially adults that are genotypically but not phenotypically affected. Dogs with clinical disease should not be bred. Furthermore, all clinically normal related dogs should be removed from breeding programs, since they may be genotypically affected.

References and Supplemental Reading

Hargis, A. M., Haupt, K. H., Hegreberg, G. A., et al.: Familial canine dermatomyositis: Initial characterization of cutaneous and muscular lesions. Am. J. Pathol. 116:234, 1984.

Hargis, A. M., Haupt, K. H., Prieur, D. J., et al.: A skin disorder in three Shetland sheepdogs: Comparison with familial canine dermatomyositis of collies. Compend. Contin. Ed. Pract. Vet. 7:306, 1985.

Hargis, A. M., Prieur, D. J., Haupt, K. H., et al.: Prospective study of familial canine dermatomysitis: Correlation of the severity of dermatomyositis and circulating immune complex levels. Am. J. Pathol. 123:465, 1986.

Hargis, A. M., Prieur, D. J., Haupt, K. H., et al.: Postmortem findings in four litters of dogs with familial canine dermatomyositis. Am. J. Pathol. 123:480, 1986a.

Hargis, A. M., Prieur, D. J., Haupt, K. H., et al.: Post-mortem findings in a Shetland sheepdog with dermatomyositis. Vet. Pathol. 23:509, 1986b.

Haupt, K. H., Prieur, D. J., Moore, M. P., et al.: Familial canine dermatomyositis: Clinical, electrodiagnostic, and genetic studies. Am. J. Vet. Res. 46:1861, 1985.

Haupt, K. H., Prieur, D. J., Hargis, A. M., et al.: Familial canine dermatomyositis: Clinicopathologic, immunologic, and serologic studies. Am. J. Vet. Res. 46:1870, 1985.

Ihrke, P. J.: Personal communication, University of California, Davis, 1987.

Kunkle, G. A., Chrisman, C. L., Gross, T. L., et al.: Dermatomyositis in collie dogs. Compend. Contin. Ed. Pract. Vet. 7:185, 1985.

Mills, J. A.: Dermatomyositis. In Fitzpatrick, T. B., Eisen, A. Z., Wolff, K., et al. (eds.): Dermatology in General Medicine. New York: McGraw-Hill, 1979, pp. 1298–1304.

Winklemann, R. K.: Dermatomyositis in childhood. Clin. Rheum. Dis. 8:353, 1982.

STAPHYLOCOCCI AND GERMAN SHEPHERD PYODERMA

ROBERT G. BUERGER, D.V.M.
Baltimore, Maryland

Bacterial pyoderma in dogs is without doubt the most underdiagnosed disease in veterinary dermatology and has been the subject of several excellent reviews. The causative agent in most canine pyodermas is *Staphylococcus intermedius*, not *S. aureus*, as was thought previously. Our knowledge of staphylococcal ecology and of staphylococcal pyodermas has grown by leaps and bounds over the last several years. One particular type of deep pyoderma, German shepherd pyoderma (GSP), has been mentioned in chapters and reviews on canine pyoderma and has been the subject of several recent studies. Many practitioners who have seen individual cases are unaware that veterinary dermatologists consider GSP to be a distinct clinical syndrome and that it is the subject of ongoing research.

STAPHYLOCOCCAL ECOLOGY

Staphylococci are gram-positive aerobic or facultatively anaerobic bacteria. They can be placed in one of two groups, based on their ability to coagulate plasma *in vitro*. It was once widely believed that only coagulase-positive staphylococci were pathogenic; coagulase-negative staphylococci were considered innocuous. While it is true that coagulase-negative staphylococci have a relatively low intrinsic virulence, they have been considered by some to be opportunistic pathogens. Several studies have shown the importance of coagulase-negative staphylococci in certain infections. Many laboratories that in the past reported only the coagulase status of staphylococcal isolates are now utilizing the API Staph-Ident system (Analytab Products, Plainview, NY) to identify the species of *Staphylococcus* isolated. If only the coagulase status of the isolate is reported, one should be aware that Cox and associates (1985) have questioned the accuracy of several popular coagulase tests. *S. intermedius* is the most common coagulase-positive organism isolated from canine pyodermas (representing at least 90 per cent of all isolates), with *S. aureus* being much less common, and *S. hyicus* very rare (Medleau et al., 1986). Coagulase-negative staphylococci have been isolated less commonly (especially *S. epidermidis*, *S. xylosus*, *S. simulans*, and *S. hominis*) (Medleau et al., 1986). It is interesting that White and co-workers (1983) were able to isolate "pathogenic" coagulase-positive staphylococci from the hair coat of 18 of 20 normal dogs.

Factors that influence the virulence or pathogenicity of staphylococci are pertinent to this discussion. The effect of exotoxins and hemolysins are perhaps best known, but other factors are also important. As mentioned previously, the organisms that are able to produce the enzyme coagulase may be able to create a protective fibrin thrombus within the tissues; thus, coagulase-positive staphylococci are more likely to be pathogenic.

The ability of bacteria to adhere to the skin surface is important, as adherence and colonization are initial steps in the development of cutaneous infections. Studies in humans suggest that protein A, a component of the staphylococcal cell wall, may be responsible, at least in part, for the adherence of staphylococci to the corneocytes of atopic individuals (Cole and Silverberg, 1986). The nature of the corneocyte receptor has not been characterized. Humans with atopic dermatitis are heavily colonized with *S. aureus* on both normal and abnormal skin, and *S. aureus* is known to be an avid producer of protein A. In fact, over 90 per cent of *S. aureus* isolates produce it. It had not been known whether *S. intermedius* produced protein A. Studies by Cox and colleagues (1986) and Fehrer (1987) have shown that *S. intermedius* does indeed produce protein A and that 84.9 per cent and 4.3 per cent of canine *S. intermedius* isolates produce extracellular and cell-bound protein A, respectively. It is not yet known whether dogs with cutaneous hypersensitivity diseases have greater numbers of pathogenic staphylococci on their skin surface and whether adherence factors or adhesins such as protein A play a role in the pathogenesis of pyodermas in these individuals.

Protein A is also immunologically active. It has the ability to interact with the F_c receptor of immunoglobulin molecules, the result of which can include the activation of complement, the induction of hypersensitivity reactions, the impairment of phagocytic function, and the activation and mitogenic stimulation of lymphocytes. Fehrer (1987) has speculated that there may be a correlation between the amount of protein A produced and the type and severity of cutaneous staphylococcal infections. The severity of some pyodermas could be explained at least in part by the production of virulence factors such as protein A.

GERMAN SHEPHERD PYODERMA

German shepherd pyoderma, also referred to as German shepherd cellulitis, is a type of deep pyoderma. Middle-aged and often otherwise healthy German shepherds have a predilection for the disease. Many veterinary dermatologists recognize GSP as a unique and distinct syndrome. The dermatology service at the New York State College of Veterinary Medicine sees, on average, one case every one to two months, most on a referral basis. It is clear that many veterinarians (including veterinary dermatologists) find the diagnosis and management of this condition very frustrating.

Clinical Features

German shepherd pyoderma has been seen in German shepherd dogs of all ages but is most common in middle-aged dogs (5 to 7 years of age) of either sex, intact or neutered. The first sign noted by most owners is lumbosacral pruritus. Without a careful dermatologic examination by the attending veterinarian, cases may be misdiagnosed as flea-bite hypersensitivity (that is not to say that flea-bite hypersensitivity does not play a part in the disease process). The lesions associated with GSP are follicular papules, pustules, furuncles, carbuncles, epidermal collarettes, multifocal crusts, alopecia, erosions, ulcers, draining sinuses, hyperpigmentation, and scars. Intact lesions often appear hemorrhagic and, when ruptured, exude a thick hemopurulent exudate. Lesions may be mild and well hidden by the hair coat, especially in the early phase of the disease. The lesions typically begin over the dorsal lumbosacral area and lateral thighs, and they may be very painful. Because the pyoderma is often not recognized initially and because of the lumbosacral pruritus and concurrent flea infestation (in most cases), a tentative diagnosis of flea-bite hypersensitivity may be made. Consequently, the dog will be treated with systemic corticosteroids. There may be a transient improvement, but the improvement is not complete and is not sustained with continued corticosteroid therapy. In spite of or perhaps because of corticosteroid therapy, the lesions and the associated pruritus often increase in severity. The lesions may become generalized in untreated or mistreated cases. The head and feet tend to be affected least, but all areas are potentially susceptible.

The most frustrating clinical feature of GSP is its propensity to recur, even after appropriate therapy. However, despite the severity of the pyoderma, most dogs are otherwise well. Rectal body temperatures are usually normal. All cases have peripheral lymphadenopathy.

Diagnosis

Cytologic evaluation of the exudate from an intact lesion reveals degenerative neutrophils and macrophages with intracellular cocci. The presence of eosinophils in the exudate is variable, and their significance is unknown. Bacterial furunculosis may be associated with a tissue eosinophilia (Muller et al., 1983). Multiple scrapings and a dermatophyte culture should be performed to rule out demodicosis and dermatophytosis.

In the author's experience and as reported by Krick and Scott (1988), biopsies reveal all phases of follicular inflammation (perifolliculitis, folliculitis, and furunculosis). Biopsies from more advanced lesions reveal nodular pyogranulomatous dermatitis (often centered around free hair shafts) to diffuse dermatitis and cellulitis. Wisselink's (1985) study did not reveal follicular inflammation, and Krick and Scott (1988) have speculated that this discrepancy was perhaps due to lesion selection.

Bacterial culture and sensitivity testing should be performed to verify the infectious nature, to identify the causative organism, and to aid in selecting an appropriate antibiotic. Coagulase-positive staphylococci (usually *S. intermedius*) are the most common organisms isolated. When performing skin cultures, it is important to obtain samples from intact lesions.

Management

Approximately one half of dogs with GSP have a recurrence of disease several weeks to months after therapy is discontinued. This emphasizes the importance of eliminating all predisposing factors and the importance of appropriate antimicrobial therapy. The most common predisposing factors in GSP include flea infestation, flea-bite hypersensitivity, atopy, food hypersensitivity, and hypothyroidism.

The most common complicating factors include therapy with inappropriate antibiotics, appropriate antibiotics at inadequate doses, an inadequate duration of therapy, and the concurrent (or sole) use of systemic corticosteroids in treating the condition.

The pyoderma must be addressed directly, with both topical and systemic therapy. Clipping the affected areas is beneficial, because in many instances the hair coat has become incorporated into a thick, adherent crust that impedes the flow of exudate from the lesion and impairs the healing process. As the condition is quite painful, sedation or general anesthesia may be necessary during this procedure. Clipping greatly facilitates healing and allows for more effective topical therapy, and owners are often impressed when they see the severity of the lesions after clipping.

In the initial exudative phase, antibacterial shampoos and whirlpools are beneficial. The author uses chlorhexidine shampoo and solution (Nolvasan, Fort Dodge) most commonly. Shampoos are given every 1 to 3 days to help facilitate the removal of infectious debris. The frequency of shampoos is decreased as the recovery becomes apparent. In severely exudative cases, the author couples shampoos with whirlpools or soaks (8 to 16 oz of Nolvasan solution is added to the whirlpool or to a small tub filled with warm water). Whirlpools or soaks can be performed at home for 15 min once or twice daily by diligent owners. Once the condition is no longer exudative, the whirlpools or soaks are discontinued. Although soaks, whirlpools, and shampoos are not directly insecticidal, such intensive topical therapy, when coupled with environmental flea control and the treatment of in-contact animals, is effective in dramatically decreasing the flea population. Once the lesions are dry, and healing is under way, flea sprays are used two to three times weekly.

Systemic antibiotic therapy is necessary. Ihrke's reviews (1983; 1986) on antibacterial therapy and the treatment of canine pyodermas are pertinent to GSP. Culture and sensitivity testing invariably identifies oxacillin, amoxicillin trihydrate–potassium clavulanate (Clavamox, Beecham), and cephalexin as the most effective antibiotics. The author finds these bactericidal antibiotics most effective in treating GSP. These bactericidal antibiotics are chosen over bacteriostatic antibiotics if an immunosuppressive state (primary or secondary) is suspected, if systemic corticosteroids (especially long-acting injectables) have been administered, or if the dog had been treated unsuccessfully with other antibiotics. While trimethoprim-potentiated sulfonamides are frequently found to be effective *in vitro*, the author finds them to be largely ineffective in deep pyodermas such as GSP. Krick and Scott (1988) concur. Wisselink and associates (1985) have reported a poor clinical response of GSP to trimethoprim-potentiated sulfonamides; however, the dose employed in the study was much less than that commonly used in treating bacterial pyodermas. A list of antibiotics that should be avoided when treating all pyodermas includes tetracycline, amoxicillin, ampicillin, penicillin, and sulfonamides. A high degree of resistance to lincomycin and erythromycin has been found with only 25 per cent and 13 per cent of isolates, respectively, sensitive (Krick and Scott, 1988). One would suspect that these results were influenced by prior antibiotic use, but the researchers could not assess this possibility. Oxacillin, Clavamox, and cephalexin are the most commonly used and most effective antibiotics in the treatment of GSP. It is unfortunate that these antibiotics are not inexpensive, and expense often plays a considerable role in the management of a case. However, the author has seen misdiagnosis and mistreatment cost more than appropriate therapy.

There is no ideal duration of treatment for GSP; however, because of the depth of the infection, its severity, and the likelihood for recurrence, the author continues therapy at least 2 weeks beyond a clinical cure. This may mean a minimum of 8 to 12 weeks of therapy. Some clients are unable to determine whether the infection is eliminated. If there is doubt in the clinician's mind, an examination should be scheduled before the antibiotic is discontinued. If an infection "returns" within 1 to 2 weeks after discontinuation of an antibiotic, it is doubtful that the infection was cleared.

All dogs that are treated appropriately will exhibit remission. It is unfortunate that approximately one half will suffer relapses within weeks to months of discontinuation of therapy. A second or third course of antibiotics may achieve a long-lasting remission. In recurrent cases, it is mandatory to identify and control all predisposing factors and to examine the dog before the antibiotic is discontinued. The ability to achieve and maintain remission is directly related to the clinician's ability to identify and control predisposing factors.

How well predisposing factors are identified on the first visit is often dictated by the severity of the condition, its duration, and the wishes of the owner. The importance of a thorough physical examination cannot be stressed too strongly. The author routinely performs a hemogram, serum chemistries, a urinalysis, a fecal examination for endoparasites, and a Knott's test (if the dog is from an area where heartworm is endemic). Dogs with GSP tend to have a mild neutrophilia, and serum chemistries usually reveal only a hyperglobulinemia. Wisselink and coworkers (1985) have reported proteinuria in three dogs with GSP, but the reasons for the proteinuria were not clear. Enlarged peripheral lymph nodes (common in GSP) can be aspirated, and cytology can be performed to rule out lymphoma.

Pyodermas may occur secondary to hypothyroid-

ism, probably because of altered immune function and cutaneous physiology. A recurrent or severe pyoderma may be the only indication of hypothyroidism. The author performs the thyrotropin (TSH) (Dermathycin, Coopers Animal Health) response test, especially if the pyoderma is recurrent. In Krick and Scott's study (1988), all four dogs that had TSH response tests performed were deemed hypothyroid. If hypothyroidism is diagnosed, the dog should receive appropriate thyroid hormone supplementation.

The dog's diet should be investigated. Feed only high-quality brand-name dog food to ensure optimal nutrition.

Pruritus (occasionally severe) can be difficult to manage. Whether pruritus preceded the onset of lesions and whether it is seasonal or nonseasonal is pertinent. If pruritus precedes the lesions, it usually suggests an underlying hypersensitivity. The location of the pruritus and its seasonality should help determine the cause. In northern climates, seasonal (summer and fall) pruritus over the dorsal lumbosacral area suggests flea-bite hypersensitivity. Wisselink and colleagues (1985) found that 10 of 23 dogs with GSP that were tested with intradermal flea antigen were allergic. This test is often done during the first office visit. Even if the immediate and delayed response to flea antigen is negative, fleas probably play at least a contributing role in GSP and should be controlled. In those cases in which it is not clear whether the pruritus preceded the infection, the dog's pruritus is monitored during the initial stages of therapy. If the pruritus is associated with the pyoderma, the fleas, or both, there should be a significant improvement with appropriate antibacterial and parasiticidal therapy. If the pruritus continues despite resolution of the pyoderma and the flea infestation, then other causes of pruritus are considered (i.e., scabies, food hypersensitivity, atopy). Addressing problems such as hypersensitivities directly and specifically (e.g., with a hypoallergenic diet, hyposensitization, flea control) is important if one is to achieve and maintain remission of the pyoderma.

If more than immediate relief from pruritus is sought, it behooves the clinician to avoid corticosteroids. A worsening or a recurrence of the pyoderma may be a high price to pay for the transient improvement seen with corticosteroid use. Other therapeutic options include antihistamines, nonsteroidal anti-inflammatory drugs, and products containing cold water fish oils (see p. 566).

When one is faced with a truly recurrent pyoderma in which all predisposing factors (e.g., ectoparasites, hypersensitivities, hypothyroidism, poor nutrition) have been controlled or eliminated, one must consider the possibility of an immunologic abnormality. Investigations into primary immunodeficiencies should not take place until all concurrent conditions have been identified and corrected. Many of the tests employed to evaluate the immune system are influenced (secondarily) by concurrent diseases such as hypothyroidism and bacterial pyoderma. In the ideal situation, immunologic tests should be performed when the dog is "normal" (i.e., between bouts of pyoderma), and all nonessential drugs should be discontinued for 48 to 72 hr before the testing is to take place (certain drugs may influence the results).

The following have been employed in the evaluation of the immune system in dogs with GSP: hemograms, serum protein electrophoresis, neutrophil chemotaxis studies, neutrophil killing function studies, and direct immunofluorescence tests. Abnormalities suggestive of a compromised immune system in dogs with GSP have not been reported. Serum protein electrophoresis usually reveals hyperglobulinemia due to elevations of alpha 2, beta 1, and gamma globulins. Wisselink (1986) has reported that neutrophil chemotaxis and killing functions are normal, that results of direct immunofluorescence studies are negative, and that there are no serum immunoglobulin deficiencies in dogs with GSP. A study recently under way at the New York State College of Veterinary Medicine has evaluated a small number of dogs with GSP. The study is evaluating IgA, IgG, and IgM levels as well as *in vitro* responsiveness to B- and T-cell mitogens. So far, the study has evaluated only a small number of patients. However, the *in vitro* lymphocyte blastogenesis studies have been normal, and the only consistent abnormality has been elevated levels of serum IgG. Halliwell (1987) has shown that dogs with recurrent pyoderma have increased levels of both IgG and IgE to staphylococcal antigens and that the magnitude of the increase was directly related to the depth and the duration of the infection. The elevation of serum IgG in GSP may be due to increased levels of IgG to staphylococcal antigens. The evaluation of many more patients will be necessary for meaningful results.

The author prefers to use immunostimulants only when an immune deficiency has been identified. With available tests, the author has not identified immune deficiency as a predisposing cause of GSP. An immune deficiency was discovered in several cases through *in vitro* lymphocyte blastogenesis studies; in these cases, remission was maintained with immunostimulants (Miller, 1987). These cases lacked pruritus, which made them distinct from most cases of reported GSP. Many practitioners have used immunostimulants in cases in which an immune deficiency is suspected, but not proven, and have seen benefit. One report (Ray and Cooper, 1984) described the successful use of ImmunoRegulin (ImmunoVet, Tampa, FL) and an oral cephalosporin antibiotic in resolving a long-standing case of GSP. The author has not used ImmunoRegulin.

In humans, the use of staphylococcal bacterins for recurrent furunculosis was determined to have no significant effect (Bryant et al., 1965) (see also p. 570).

Long-term once-a-day antibiotic therapy is mentioned by Muller and coworkers (1983) as an optional treatment for recurrent pyoderma. This therapy is best avoided, but for some patients with recurrent GSP, it provides the only long-term control. One should begin this low-dose maintenance therapy only after the pyoderma has resolved and then use a narrow-spectrum antibiotic. The author most commonly uses oxacillin.

Many questions about the cause and management of GSP are as yet unanswered. Are there virulence factors, such as staphylococcal protein A, that determine the depth and severity of an infection? Do clinical and subclinical (cases that are not pruritic) hypersensitivities predispose dogs to GSP? Are allergic dogs more heavily colonized with pathogenic *S. intermedius* than normal dogs, and if so, are adhesins such as protein A involved? Why don't we see similarly severe pyodermas in allergic dogs of other breeds? Are there unidentified immune deficiencies (either qualitative or quantitative) that predispose to GSP? Given the breed predilection, are there genetic factors that are involved in the pathogenesis of GSP, and if so, what is their nature? Is there any role of so-called bacterial hypersensitivity in GSP? The author suspects that there are a number of host and bacterial factors that interact to produce the syndrome we call GSP.

References and Supplemental Reading

Bryant, R. E., Sanford, J. P., and Alcoze, T.: Treatment of recurrent furunculosis with staphylococcal bacteriophage–lysed vaccine. J.A.M.A. 194:11, 1965.

Cole, G. W., and Silverberg, N. L.: The adherence of *Staphylococcus aureus* to human corneocytes. Arch. Dermatol. 122:166, 1986.

Cox, H. U., Newman, S. S., Roy, A. F., et al.: Comparison of coagulase test methods for identification of *Staphylococcus intermedius* from dogs. Am. J. Vet. Res. 46:1522, 1985.

Cox, H. U., Schmeer, N., and Newman, S. S.: Protein A in *Staphylococcus intermedius* isolates from dogs and cats. Am. J. Vet. Res. 47:1881, 1986.

Fehrer, S. L.: Identification and quantitation of protein A on canine *Staphylococcus intermedius*. Proceedings of the Annual Members' Meeting of the American Academy of Veterinary Dermatology, and the American College of Veterinary Dermatology, 1987, p. 13.

Halliwell, R. E. W.: Levels of IgG and IgE antibody to staphylococcal antigens in normal dogs and in dogs with recurrent pyoderma. Proceedings of the Annual Members' Meeting of the American Academy of Veterinary Dermatology and the American College of Veterinary Dermatology, 1987, p. 5.

Ihrke, P. J.: The management of canine pyodermas. *In* Kirk, R. W. (ed.): *Current Veterinary Therapy VIII.* Philadelphia: W. B. Saunders Co., 1983, pp. 505–517.

Ihrke, P. J.: Antibacterial therapy in dermatology. *In* Kirk, R. W. (ed.): *Current Veterinary Therapy IX.* Philadelphia: W. B. Saunders Co., 1986, pp. 566–571.

Krick, S. A., and Scott, D. W.: Bacterial folliculitis, furunculosis, and cellulitis in the German shepherd: A retrospective analysis of 17 cases. J. Am. Anim. Hosp. Assoc., 1988 (in press).

Medleau, L., Long, R. E., Brown, J., et al.: Frequency and antimicrobial susceptibility of *Staphylococcus* species isolated from canine pyodermas. Am. J. Vet. Res. 47:229, 1986.

Miller, W. H., Jr.: Personal communication, 1987.
Muller, G. H., Kirk, R. W., and Scott, D. W.: *Small Animal Dermatology*, 3rd ed. Philadelphia: W. B. Saunders Co., 1983, pp. 197–239.
Phillips, W. E., and Williams, B. J.: Antimicrobial susceptibility patterns of canine *Staphylococcus intermedius* isolates from veterinary clinical specimens. Am. J. Vet. Res. 45:2376, 1984.
Ray, W. J., and Cooper, J. A.: Chronic deep pyoderma in a German shepherd. Canine Pract. 11:35, 1984.

White, S. D., Ihrke, P. J., Stannard, A. A., et al.: Occurrence of *Staphylococcus aureus* on the clinically normal canine hair coat. Am. J. Vet. Res. 44:332, 1983.
Wisselink, M. A.: German shepherd pyoderma: Some clinical and immunologic observations. Proc. World Small Anim. Vet. Assoc. 11:C42, 1986.
Wisselink, M. A., Willemse, A., and Koeman, J. P.: Deep pyoderma in the German shepherd dog. J. Am. Anim. Hosp. Assoc. 21:773, 1985.

LICHENOID DERMATOSES IN DOGS AND CATS

DANNY W. SCOTT, D.V.M.
Ithaca, New York

The term lichen is a noun from Greek and Latin for those symbiotic forms of plant life that are now designated lichens. "Lichen" is also the term for those dermatoses that vaguely resemble the botanical formations because they have a surface pattern of more or less closely agminated papules (agminated is an adjective meaning "gathered together in a group"). The term "lichenoid" is an English and New Latin adjective meaning "like a lichen."

In modern-day medical terminology the word "lichenoid" has two meanings: one clinical and one histopathologic. In clinical dermatology, *lichenoid skin lesions* are defined as flat-topped papules and plaques that are angular, hyperkeratotic, and grouped. In dermatohistopathology, *lichenoid tissue reactions* are characterized by hydropic degeneration of epidermal basal cells, necrotic and apoptotic keratinocytes (Civatte bodies, colloid bodies, cytoid bodies, hyaline bodies, filamentous bodies), pigmentary incontinence, and a bandlike infiltration of predominantly mononuclear cells that extends across the superficial dermis parallel to the epidermis and often obscures the dermoepidermal interface.

The etiology and pathogenesis of lichenoid dermatoses are incompletely understood. In humans, lichenoid dermatoses may be precipitated by a variety of drugs (especially antimalarials, thiazides, gold salts, phenothiazines, sulfonamides, and penicillins), tatoos, and exposure to color-film developer and are often seen in chronic graft-versus-host disease secondary to bone marrow transplantation. However, the majority of lichenoid dermatoses in humans and all of those described in dogs and cats are idiopathic.

Because lichenoid dermatoses occur frequently in human chronic graft-versus-host disease, a review of the cytologic and immunologic findings in this condition may provide relevant insight into the etiopathogenesis of all lichenoid reactions. The earliest identifiable abnormality is an increased number of epidermal Langerhans' cells (antigen-processing and antigen-presenting cells), which is followed by dermal capillary dilatation and a perivascular accumulation of lymphocytes. These early changes are then followed by a series of lymphocyte-Langerhans' cell, interlymphocyte, and lymphocyte-keratinocyte contacts and reactions which ultimately result in satellite cell necrosis of keratinocytes. Dermal lymphocytes have been shown to possess predominantly the helper/inducer T cell phenotype. Thus, an attractive current hypothesis for the etiopathogenesis of lichenoid dermatoses suggests an initial antigenic alteration ("altered self") of keratinocytes by a number of factors (drug, infectious agent, and so forth), with resultant Langerhans' cell recognition and T lymphocyte-mediated cytotoxicity.

CLINICAL FEATURES

At present, lichenoid dermatoses appear to be rare in dogs and cats. No age, breed, or sex predilections are apparent, nor have these dermatoses been clearly associated with any prior or concurrent systemic illnesses or drug administration.

Lichenoid dermatoses are characterized by the usually asymptomatic, symmetric onset of grouped, angular, flat-topped papules that develop a scaly to markedly hyperkeratotic surface. Lesions may enlarge, coalesce to form hyperkeratotic, alopecic plaques or do both. Lesions may be localized, regionalized, or generalized but are more or less bilaterally symmetric.

A *lichenoid-psoriasiform dermatosis* has been described in springer spaniels. The dermatosis began in young dogs (4 to 18 months of age) of either sex. Asymptomatic, generally symmetric, erythematous, lichenoid papules and plaques were initially noted on the pinnae, in the external ear canal, and in the inguinal region. With time, lesions became increasingly hyperkeratotic (some almost papillomatous) and spread to involve the face, ventral trunk, and perineal area. Chronic cases resembled "severe seborrhea." The exclusive occurrence of this lichenoid-psoriasiform dermatosis in springer spaniels could suggest a genetic predilection.

Lichenoid keratoses (a keratosis is a firm, elevated, circumscribed area of excessive keratin production) are occasionally seen in dogs. Generally, solitary asymptomatic lesions are seen on the pinnae of adult dogs. Lesions are well-circumscribed, erythematous and scaly to markedly hyperkeratotic plaques, or papillomas.

DIAGNOSIS

Differential diagnosis of lichenoid dermatoses includes staphylococcal folliculitis, dermatophytosis, demodicosis, and various granulomatous and neoplastic conditions. In springer spaniels, lichenoid-psoriasiform dermatosis must be differentiated from primary idiopathic seborrhea: both conditions being possibly genetically programmed in this breed. Definitive diagnosis is based on history, physical examination, laboratory rule-outs, and skin biopsy. The clinical appearance of skin lesions is characteristic. Results of carefully performed cultures are negative.

Skin biopsy reveals varying degrees of hyperkeratotic and hyperplastic lichenoid and hydropic interface dermatitis. In lichenoid-psoriasiform dermatosis in springer spaniels, in addition to the lichenoid tissue reaction, one finds a psoriasiform (regular) epidermal hyperplasia with intraepidermal microabscesses (containing eosinophils and neutrophils) and Munro's microabscesses (small, dessicated neutrophilic microabscesses within or immediately below focal areas of parakeratotic hyperkeratosis). Chronic hyperkeratotic lesions of lichenoid-psoriasiform dermatosis in springer spaniels

and solitary lichenoid keratoses frequently show papillated epidermal hyperplasia and papillomatosis.

Results of direct immunofluorescence testing may be negative or may show nonspecific focal deposition of either or both immunoglobulin and complement in the intercellular spaces of the epidermis (in areas of spongiosis) or at the basement membrane zone.

CLINICAL MANAGEMENT

In general, the prognosis for canine and feline idiopathic lichenoid dermatoses appears to be good. All patients have undergone spontaneous remission after a course of 6 months to 2 years. No form of therapy has been shown to be beneficial.

The lichenoid-psoriasiform dermatosis in springer spaniels has been characterized by a waxing and waning course for periods of 1 to 3 years. Neither spontaneous nor therapeutic remission has been reported. Various medicaments (including antibiotics, anti-inflammatory doses of glucocorticoids, oral vitamin A, levamisole, dapsone, autogenous vaccine, and antiseborrheic shampoos) have been of little or no benefit. Repeated courses of erythromycin, 11 mg/kg t.i.d. PO, were of partial benefit in one dog, and large doses of glucocorticoid, prednisolone, 2.2 mg/kg/day PO, were partially effective in another.

Lichenoid keratoses are cured with complete surgical excision.

References and Supplemental Reading

Black, M. M., and Newton, J. A.: Lichen planus. *In* Thiers, B. H., and Dobson, R. L. (eds.): *Pathogenesis of Skin Disease.* New York: Churchill Livingstone, 1986, pp. 85–95.

Buerger, R. G., and Scott, D. W.: Lichenoid dermatitis in a cat: A case report. J. Am. Anim. Hosp. Assoc. 24:55, 1988.

Mason, K. V., Halliwell, R. E. W., and McDougal, B. J.: Characterization of lichenoid-psoriasiform dermatosis of springer spaniels. J.A.V.M.A. 189:897, 1986.

Scott, D. W.: Lichenoid reactions in the skin of dogs: Clinicopathologic correlations. J. Am. Anim. Hosp. Assoc. 20:305, 1984.

Scott, D. W.: Idiopathic lichenoid dermatitis in a dog. Canine Pract. 11:22, 1984.

DERMATOSES OF THE NOSE AND THE FOOTPADS IN DOGS AND CATS

DONNA WALTON ANGARANO, D.V.M.

Auburn, Alabama

Veterinary dermatology is sometimes considered to be repetitious by those not aware of the subtle diversity present in similar-appearing diseases. However, clinical presentations affecting the nasal planum and the footpads of dogs and cats, are frequently greeted with enthusiasm by nondermatologists and dermatologists alike because of the uncommon diseases these signs may represent. Common diseases must be considered among the possible diagnoses in animals demonstrating nasal or footpad lesions, but the final diagnosis is frequently an uncommon or even rare condition.

An understanding of the diseases with a predilection for the nose and the footpads is necessary in order to establish a differential diagnosis and a subsequent diagnostic plan. The similarities among these diseases are such that diagnostic tests are usually required to establish the definitive diagnosis. Although symptomatic therapy in the absence of a definitive diagnosis may make the patient more comfortable and sometimes may reduce clinical signs, specific treatment of dermatologic diseases is preferred. In addition, the prognosis and the possible requirement of lifetime therapy must be considered, and both will vary, depending on the final diagnoses.

Hyperkeratosis, ulceration, and depigmentation are the most common clinical lesions of the nose and footpads. Table 1 lists the diseases that may affect the nasal planum, and Table 2 lists the diseases that may affect the footpads. Both sites may be affected in the same animal, but this is not always the case. Systemic signs or cutaneous lesions at other sites are present in most of these diseases.

The diagnostic workup begins with a thorough history and physical examination. It is important to establish the disease progression, including its appearance at onset and the original site(s) affected. The animal's response to previous medication may help in the consideration of certain diseases. The physical examination must include not only a dermatologic examination but also the search for other organ system abnormalities. For example, systemic lupus erythematosus, drug eruption, and some neoplastic conditions may include multi-organ system involvement in addition to dermatologic symptoms.

Likewise, nasal depigmentation with concurrent blindness or uveitis should cause one to consider the possibility of Vogt-Koyanagi-Harada syndrome.

In examining a patient with a nasal dermatopathy, it is important to observe whether the haired or nonhaired skin is affected. Demodicosis, dermatophytosis, and bacterial pyoderma tend to restrict themselves to the haired skin because of their predilection for hair follicles. Even though these common follicular diseases are unlikely to extend onto the nasal planum, skin scrapings and a culture for dermatophytes are essential parts of the dermatologic minimum data base. Cytology should also be a routine part of the early diagnostic workup for conditions affecting the nasal planum. Impression smears may be obtained from areas of ulceration in addition to pustules or vesicles. If crusts are present, they may be gently pealed off and used to make impression smears. Cytology is not always rewarding. However, the presence of acantholytic cells may suggest the diagnosis of pemphigus, or the identification of fungal organisms may cause one to consider the possibility of a deep mycotic infection.

Skin biopsies for histopathologic examination and possible immunofluorescence testing are an important part of the diagnostic workup in most patients with nasal and footpad abnormalities, because of the strong clinical similarities of the majority of these diseases. Histopathologic differentiation is difficult in some instances, and multiple samples should be submitted whenever possible to improve the likelihood of a definitive diagnosis. Direct and indirect immunofluorescence testing may support the diagnosis of an autoimmune disease. Tissue samples for direct immunofluorescence testing should be preserved and submitted in Michel's solution. Negative results of immunofluorescence tests do not eliminate the diagnosis of an autoimmune disease, nor do positive results always confirm it.

A clinical pathology data base (complete blood count [CBC], serum biochemical profile, and urinalysis) should be obtained for the majority of animals presenting with nasal or footpad abnormalities. Such a data base aids in the search for other

616

Table 1. *Dermatologic Disorders Affecting the Nasal Planum*

Disease	Clinical Lesion		
	Hyperkeratosis	*Ulcer*	*Depigmentation*
Pemphigus foliaceus	X	X	X
Pemphigus erythematosus	X	X	X
Systemic lupus erythematosus	X	X	X
Discoid lupus erythematosus	X	X	X
Mycosis fungoides	X	X	X
Deep mycoses	X	X	X
Vogt-Koyanagi-Harada syndrome	X	X	X
Contact dermatitis	X	X	X
Plastic dish syndrome	X	X	X
Idiopathic vitiligo			X
Keratinization defects	X		
Zinc-responsive dermatosis	X		
Drug eruption	X	X	X
Cold agglutinin disease	X	X	X
Necrolytic migratory erythema	X	X	
Actinic lesions (nasal solar dermatoses)	X	X	X
Neoplasia	X	X	X

organ system involvement. In addition, this information serves as baseline data prior to the initiation of therapy, which needs to be medically aggressive in some cases.

PEMPHIGUS

Pemphigus is an autoimmune disease of dogs and cats in which autoantibody is directed against a component of the epithelial cell wall. The epithelial cells lose their adhesion to each other and separate, forming vesicles or pustules. The resulting rounded-up epithelial cells are known as acantholytic cells. These are large, round, basophilic cells. The disease is limited to the integument but may have a variety of appearances. Lesions of *pemphigus foliaceus* may include ulceration, depigmentation, and crust formation on the face and nasal planum. The ears are frequently affected, as is the trunk. The footpads may be hyperkeratotic or ulcerated and may cause the patient to have difficulty in walking. In some patients, lesions are restricted to the footpads. (Pemphigus foliaceus is the author's primary consideration for dogs that are presented with painful, hyperkeratotic footpads.) Cats with pemphigus foliaceus are usually febrile and anorexic, in addition to having cutaneous signs. Paronychia is a common finding in cats. Diagnosis is determined by histopathology (subcorneal or intragranular pustular dermatitis with acantholytic cells). Supportive immunofluorescence test results include the deposition of immunoglobulin in the interepithelial cell spaces. Serologic findings are normal or negative. Therapy may include a combination of medications such as oral glucocorticoids (most cases), injectable gold salts (chrysotherapy), and other chemotherapeutic agents. Azathioprine (Imuran, Burroughs Well-

Table 2. *Dermatologic Disorders Affecting the Footpad*

Disease	Clinical Lesion		
	Hyperkeratosis	*Ulcer*	*Depigmentation*
Pemphigus foliaceus	X	X	X
Systemic lupus erythematosus	X	X	X
Discoid lupus erythematosus	X		X
Mycosis fungoides	X	X	
Deep mycoses	X	X	X
Contact dermatitis	X	X	X
Keratinization defects	X		
Zinc-responsive dermatosis	X		
Canine distemper	X		
Drug eruption	X	X	X
Toxic epidermal necrolysis	X	X	X
Vasculitis	X	X	X
Cold agglutinin disease	X	X	X
Plasma cell pododermatitis	X	X	
Necrolytic migratory erythema	X	X	
Neoplasia	X	X	X
Cutaneous horns	X		

come) and cyclophosphamide (Cytoxan, Mead Johnson) have both been used successfully. Dosage and duration of medication is variable based on the patient's response to therapy. Topical soaks and sunscreens are helpful in many instances.

Pemphigus erythematosus is similar to pemphigus foliaceus with lesions restricted to the face and ears. The two major considerations for an animal presented with ulceration and depigmentation restricted to the nasal planum are pemphigus erythematosus and discoid lupus erythematosus. As in pemphigus foliaceus, the diagnosis is determined by histopathology. Immunofluorescence testing results may be the same. However, in most cases of pemphigus erythematosus, there is the additional finding of a positive antinuclear antibody (ANA) test and immunoglobulin and/or complement deposition at the basement membrane zone. Therapy is similar to that for pemphigus foliaceus.

SYSTEMIC LUPUS ERYTHEMATOSUS

Systemic lupus erythematosus (SLE) is an autoimmune disease that may affect multiple organ systems. It has been termed "the great impersonator" because of the variety of presentations that affected patients may demonstrate. With cutaneous involvement, there is a predilection for the facial area, with ulceration and depigmentation of the nasal planum. The footpads may be hyperkeratotic or ulcerated. Ulceration at the junction of the skin and footpads, with the appearance of sloughing of the entire pad, is suggestive of SLE. Other cutaneous signs are usually present in addition to nasal and footpad lesions. Diagnosis is based on a variety of supportive findings including evidence of multisystemic involvement (i.e., anemia, thrombocytopenia, polyarthritis, glomerulonephritis), positive antinuclear antibody (ANA) test, histopathology (interface dermatitis—lichenoid, hydropic or both) and direct immunofluorescence testing (staining of basement membrane zone). A combination of glucocorticoids and chemotherapeutic agents (azathioprine or cyclophosphamide) is required therapeutically in most cases.

DISCOID LUPUS ERYTHEMATOSUS

Discoid lupus erythematosus (DLE) is the most common cause of canine nasal ulceration and depigmentation in patients in whom no other site is affected. In some patients, the muzzle and periocular area may also show depigmentation, ulceration, and crust formation. The collie appears to have a breed predilection for DLE. An uncommon finding in DLE is hyperkeratosis of the footpads. This may occur as the only clinical abnormality or in combination with facial lesions. Diagnosis is confirmed by histopathology (interface dermatitis—lichenoid) and immunofluorescence testing (staining of basement membrane zone). Results of other diagnostic tests (e.g., cytology, CBC, ANA) are negative or normal. Depending on disease severity, therapy may include sunscreens, oral glucocorticoids, and vitamin E (*dl*-alpha-tocopherol), 200 to 400 IU PO repeated every 12 hr.

MYCOSIS FUNGOIDES

Mycosis fungoides is a form of cutaneous lymphosarcoma. It is usually a disease of older dogs. Clinical signs, in particular nasal depigmentation and ulceration of the nose and mouth, may mimic signs of autoimmune dermatoses. Truncal lesions of diffuse erythema or crust formation are frequently present. The footpads may be ulcerated. The disease is limited to the integument until late in its progression. Diagnosis is based on histopathology, and treatment usually has little effect on disease progression. Systemic chemotherapeutic agents, topical nitrogen mustard (mechlorethamine hydrochloride; Mustargen, (Merck Sharp & Dohme), or both have been used. Glucocorticoids and shampoos may help relieve symptoms.

DEEP MYCOSES

Deep mycoses, in particular blastomycosis and cryptococcosis, may affect the nasal planum or footpad. It would be unlikely for both sites to be affected in one patient. Deep mycoses produce a granulomatous dermatitis that may clinically result in a nodule or an area of ulceration. Ulcerated lesions are circular and well demarcated. Other systemic signs (respiratory, ocular, or musculoskeletal) are frequently present. Fungal organisms may be seen on cytology of impression smears or aspirates. Demonstration of the organism on fungal culture or histopathology is diagnostic. Serology is helpful, especially in evaluating response to therapy. Treatment and prognosis vary depending on severity and organ system involvement. Successful treatment has been obtained with amphotericin B (Fungizone, Squibb) and ketoconazole (Nizoral, Janssen) used separately or in combination.

VOGT-KOYANAGI-HARADA SYNDROME

Vogt-Koyanagi-Harada (VKH) syndrome is a condition of unknown etiology in which cutaneous and ophthalmic signs coexist. The Akita appears to be most frequently affected with this uncommon disease. Cutaneous lesions are limited to the face (especially the nasal planum) and include depigmentation, ulceration, and crust formation. Concurrent anterior uveitis and retinal detachment may result in blindness. Diagnosis is based on the combination of ocular and cutaneous findings and histopathology (interface dermatitis—lichenoid with histiocytic cells). Results of other diagnostic tests are negative or normal. Immunosuppressive dosages of glucocorticoids are the treatment of choice.

CONTACT DERMATITIS

Contact dermatitis may result from either an irritant or an allergic reaction. *Irritant contact dermatitis*, uncommon in dogs and cats, may produce hyperkeratosis or ulceration of the footpads or nasal planum. The *plastic dish syndrome* is a form of *allergic contact dermatitis* thought to be due to a chemical in the plastic food or water bowl. Lesions of depigmentation may develop on the nasal planum in addition to erythema of the lips. This syndrome is rare. Diagnosis of contact dermatitis is based on history, reduction of signs upon removal of the offending substance, and elimination of other disease possibilities.

IDIOPATHIC VITILIGO

Idiopathic vitiligo occurs on the nasal planum and lips. The Doberman pinscher and Rottweiler are the breeds most frequently affected by this uncommon disease. Poliosis (graying of the hair) may also occur periorally, periocularly, and over the trunk. Diagnosis is by elimination of other disease possibilities. There is no treatment. A genetic basis must be considered because of apparent breed predilection.

KERATINIZATION DEFECTS

Keratinization defects of the nasal planum and footpads have been known by a variety of names including idiopathic hyperkeratosis, nasal-digital hyperkeratosis, and senile hyperkeratosis. The etiology of this condition is unknown. Any dog may be affected, but middle-aged and older spaniels, retrievers, and terriers are most often affected. Hyperkeratosis may affect the nose, the footpads, or both. Cold weather appears to aggravate the condition, and the affected nasal planum cracks and bleeds in some situations. The hyperkeratotic pads do not appear to cause discomfort to the animal. Diagnosis is based on clinical signs and elimination of other disease possibilities. Ointments (petroleum jelly or other softening agents) may be used on the nose to make the patient more comfortable.

ZINC-RESPONSIVE DERMATOSES

Zinc-responsive dermatoses have been recognized in a variety of dogs. One form is apparently genetically based, and the arctic breeds (Siberian husky, Alaskan malamute, and samoyed) have a predilection. These dogs begin to show signs at puberty and may have facial and footpad lesions. The major lesions are those of hyperkeratosis and crust formation, although in some cases erythematous plaques or focal ulcers have been seen. Dogs fed a diet deficient in zinc and high in calcium and phytates (which tie up available zinc) may develop similar signs. The lesions are more pronounced in the latter group of dogs, with signs mimicking those of the autoimmune dermatoses. Diagnosis is supported by histopathology findings of diffuse parakeratosis. Dogs occasionally are febrile and have a lymphadenopathy along with a peripheral lymphopenia. Other diagnostic test results are usually negative or normal. Therapy includes zinc supplementation in both groups of dogs. This may be accomplished with zinc sulfate, 220 mg PO repeated every 12 to 24 hr, or with zinc methionine (ZinPro), 200 to 400 mg PO once daily. Once signs have resolved and the diet has been modified, zinc supplementation is usually no longer required in the nonarctic breeds.

CANINE DISTEMPER

Canine distemper is the classic cause of canine footpad hyperkeratosis (hard pad disease). Dogs with resolving distemper may develop footpad hyperkeratosis, in which case distemper inclusion bodies are apparent on histologic examination of footpad biopsies. As a result of canine distemper vaccination, canine distemper is now one of the least probable causes of canine footpad abnormalities.

DRUG ERUPTIONS

Drug eruptions may result in a variety of cutaneous or systemic signs. Any drug is capable of producing any type of lesion. Lesions are frequently ulcerative and may appear on the nasal planum and footpad as well as in the oral cavity or on the trunk. The drug most often implicated in this uncommon condition is trimethoprim-sulfadiazine (Tribrissen, Coopers). *Toxic epidermal necrolysis* is a disease of unknown etiology but is most often associated with a drug eruption. Full-thickness epidermal necrosis results. Ulcerative lesions of the footpads have been seen in dogs with this condition. If lesions are localized, symptomatic therapy, glucocorticoids, and removal of the offending drug are usually effective. If lesions are widespread or generalized, a guarded prognosis must be considered.

VASCULITIS

Vasculitis may be idiopathic or a component of another disease process, such as systemic lupus erythematosus. Focal areas of ulceration are the most common presenting sign and are usually present on the footpads, at the ear margins, or in the mouth. Histologic examination of skin biopsies confirms the diagnosis of vasculitis; however, other diagnostic tests should be performed to consider possible underlying causes. When no underlying etiology is identified, the treatment of choice is dapsone (Avlosulfon, Ayerst) given orally in the dog at a dose of 1 mg/kg repeated every 8 hr. Following the resolution of clinical signs, the dosage is reduced. Some cases of idiopathic vasculitis may be controlled with immunosuppressive dosages of glucocorticoids.

COLD AGGLUTININ DISEASE

Cold agglutinin disease is a rare immune-mediated disorder in which animals develop IgM class autoantibodies that react with erythrocytes at temperatures below 32°C. The resulting clinical signs are similar to those observed in animals with vasculitis: focal erythema, ulceration and necrosis of the extremities. Signs develop in affected animals after exposure to cold. Diagnosis is confirmed by a positive Coombs's test performed with IgM at 4°C. Many cases are idiopathic; however, the disease has been shown to occur as a result of infectious or neoplastic conditions. Immunosuppressive dosages of glucocorticoids is the treatment of choice in patients in whom an underlying disease is not recognized.

PLASMA CELL PODODERMATITIS

Plasma cell pododermatitis is a disease of unknown etiology that has been described in cats. Multiple pads are usually involved. Early in the disease, the pads are swollen and mildly hyperkeratotic. As the disease progresses, the pads may become painful and ulcerative. Secondary bacterial or fungal infection is not uncommon at this time. Diagnosis is established by examination of skin biopsies, which reveal a diffuse plasmacytic dermatitis. A concurrent vasculitis is often observed histologically. Treatment varies with the severity of signs, as some cats will undergo spontaneous remission. In other instances, antiseptic soaks may be combined with immunosuppressive dosages of glu-

cocorticoids or with gold salt therapy (chrysotherapy).

NECROLYTIC MIGRATORY ERYTHEMA

Necrolytic migratory erythema is the name given to a rare cutaneous disease in humans associated with a glucagon-producing tumor and diabetes mellitus. The disease has been described in dogs as diabetic dermatosis. It is unfortunate that more recent canine cases have not all had concurrent diabetes mellitus. The etiology of this disease in older dogs is unknown, but most affected dogs have concurrent hepatic disease, usually cirrhosis. Animals appear to be remain compensated until late in the course of the disease, which is ultimately fatal. Cutaneous lesions are pronounced and include footpad hyperkeratosis and ulceration; erythema and ulceration of the distal extremities; and erythema, ulceration, and crust formation of the face and genital areas. Diagnosis is confirmed by histologic examination. However, the microscopic signs may be subtle, and multiple biopsies should be submitted when considering this disease. Serum biochemical profiles usually demonstrate elevation of liver enzymes. Azotemia and hyperglycemia may also be present. Dogs may show clinical improvement with symptomatic therapy and the use of glucocorticoids; however, no successful therapy is known.

ACTINIC LESIONS

Actinic or solar-induced lesions of the nasal planum are uncommon in dogs and cats. The most frequent solar-induced lesion is actinic keratosis and subsequent squamous cell carcinoma. This lesion is more often seen on the haired part of the muzzle as opposed to the nasal planum. However, most of the autoimmune dermatoses are exacerbated by ultraviolet light. In addition to worsening of the autoimmune disease, chronic sun exposure may result in transformation to squamous cell carcinoma. Sun avoidance and the use of topical sunscreens in animals with facial dermatosis is recommended.

NEOPLASTIC CONDITIONS

Neoplastic conditions, especially squamous cell carcinoma, may affect the nasal planum and footpads. Usually only one site is affected in a particular animal. Examination of skin biopsies should be diagnostic. Therapy is dependent upon the final diagnosis.

CUTANEOUS HORNS

Cutaneous horns are the name given to focal proliferations of keratin. These have been recognized in several situations, but recently they have been documented as occurring on the footpads of cats. Several reported cats with multiple cutaneous horns have had positive titers for feline leukemia virus. Cutaneous horns may be surgically excised. The base of the horn should be examined histologically, as some neoplastic conditions (squamous cell carcinoma, in particular) may result in this type of abnormal keratinization.

CONCLUSION

This article includes a brief discussion of common canine and feline diseases that affect the nasal planum or the footpad. Undoubtedly, other dermatoses are capable of affecting these same sites. One should approach the diagnostic workup of this uncommon presentation in an organized manner, obtaining first a thorough history and physical examination. A variety of diagnostic tests, including skin scrapings, fungal cultures, cytology, hematol-

ogy, serum biochemical profiles, urinalysis, serology, histopathology, and direct immunofluorescence, may be necessary in some cases before a definitive diagnosis is reached. Although symptomatic therapy may be helpful, a definitive diagnosis is preferred. This is especially important prior to the initiation of immunosuppressive therapy, which may be contraindicated in other similar-appearing diseases.

References and Supplemental Reading

Angarano, D. W.: Autoimmune dermatoses. *In* Nesbitt, G. H. (ed.): *Veterinary Medicine: Contemporary Issues in Dermatology.* New York: Churchill Livingstone, 1987, p. 79.
Center, S. A., Scott, D. W., and Scott, F. W.: Multiple cutaneous horns on the footpads of a cat. Feline Pract. 12:26, 1982.
Ihrke, P. J., Stannard, A. A., Ardans, A. A., et al.: Pemphigus foliaceus of the footpads in three dogs. J.A.V.M.A. 186:67, 1985.
Muller, G. H., Kirk, R. W., and Scott, D. W.: *Small Animal Dermatology III.* Philadelphia: W. B. Saunders Co., 1983.
Walton, D. K., Center, S. A., Scott, D. W., et al.: Ulcerative dermatosis associated with diabetes mellitus in the dog: A report of four cases. J. Am. Anim. Hosp. Assoc. 22:79, 1986.

DERMATOSES OF THE PINNAE

VICKI J. SCHEIDT, D.V.M.
Raleigh, North Carolina

Many of the common dermatologic conditions in small animals cause similar changes in the skin and tend to overlap in their clinical appearance, especially in the chronic patient. As a result, skin diseases are often confusing to the clinician and subsequently are treated symptomatically without a cause being identified. This situation can be easily avoided, provided the clinician approaches the dermatology patient systematically and integrates historical findings with the type and location of lesions.

The pinna and external ear canal are composed of a cartilaginous framework covered by skin. The dermal component of the skin is firmly attached to the pinnal cartilage and contains blood vessels, glands, and hair follicles. The cutaneous blood supply to the pinna is extensive and forms a weblike pattern over the surface of the cartilage. Because of the location of the ears on the head, the pinnae are frequently exposed to traumatic insult and vascular injury, resulting in hemorrhage, ulceration, necrosis, and scarring.

Anatomically, the pinnae are usually associated

with the external ear canal and frequently are not included as part of the routine examination of the skin unless concurrent otitis externa is present. This is ironic, since many skin diseases have some degree of pinnal involvement and may in fact begin on the pinnae before progressing to other parts of the body (Table 1). In other skin conditions, pinnal involvement may develop concurrently with lesions on other regions of the body (Table 2). This article will review the skin diseases that should be included in a differential diagnosis when the pinnae are the primary region of the body affected.

Table 1. Dermatoses of the Pinnae*

Pinnal alopecia	Allergic dermatitis
Solar dermatitis	atopy
Frostbite	food
Ear margin seborrhea	contact
Flystrike	Scabies (canine and feline)
Trauma	Otodectic mange

*Diseases that may be limited to the ear or may begin initially on the pinnae.

Table 2. *Dermatoses of the Pinnae**

Entity	History and Diagnostic Tests
Zinc-responsive dermatitis	Breed, skin biopsy, response to zinc therapy
Pemphigus foliaceus/erythematosus	Histopathology, direct immunofluorescence test
Systemic lupus erythematosus	Histopathology, ANA, lupus erythematosus, prep, direct immunofluorescence test
Juvenile cellulitis	Age, breed, negative bacterial and fungal cultures
Dermatomyositis	Age, breed, EMG, muscle and skin biopsies
Epidermolysis bullosa	Age, breed, skin biopsy
Dermatophytosis	Positive fungal culture, skin biopsy
Vasculitis	Histopathology, direct immunofluorescence
Discoid lupus erythematosus	Histopathology, direct immunofluorescence
Drug eruption	History of drug exposure, skin biopsy, response to drug withdrawal
Cold agglutinin disease	History of exposure to cold, cold Coombs's test

*Diseases that frequently affect the pinnae in addition to other areas of the body.

FROSTBITE

Frostbite is due to freezing of tissues exposed to subzero temperatures. It can affect the ear tips of dogs or cats that are confined outdoors in extremely cold weather for prolonged periods. Frostbite is a relatively uncommon problem in small animals, since most pets live indoors and are rarely exposed to prolonged cold weather.

Clinically, the tips of both ears are usually affected. Depending on the extent of exposure to the cold, the skin may initially appear pale, cold, and hypoesthetic. Once rewarming occurs, the skin becomes erythematous and painful. Scaling and dry skin are a common secondary sequelae in mild cases. However, with prolonged exposure, the ear tips become ulcerated, alopecic, and covered with hemorrhagic crusts. Necrosis and subsequent sloughing can occur in such cases. Other body areas that have poor peripheral circulation, such as the scrotum and the tip of the tail, may also be affected.

In most cases, the diagnosis can be made based on a history of exposure to subzero temperatures and clinical signs. A differential diagnosis would include cold agglutinin disease, vasculitis, systemic lupus erythematosus, burns, and dermatomyositis. A diagnostic evaluation to eliminate these causes would include a complete blood count (CBC), antinuclear antibody (ANA) test, slide autoagglutination test at room temperature, cold Coombs's test (4°C), and skin biopsy for histopathology and direct immunofluorescence. An electromyogram and muscle biopsy would eliminate dermatomyositis. Routine skin scrapings and a fungal culture are always indicated as part of the dermatologic workup.

Therapy would include removing the pet from the cold and rapid warming of the affected skin with warm water for 30 min. A petrolatum ointment or gel (Vaseline, Chesebrough-Pond, Inc.) can be used to help soften crusts and rehydrate and protect affected areas. Plastic or corrective surgery may be indicated in severe cases associated with necrosis, ulceration, and scarring. Avoidance of cold temperatures is recommended since recurrence is common.

FLYSTRIKE

Flystrike is a seasonal disease usually affecting the ears of dogs housed outside in confined areas. The stable fly, *Stomoxys calcitrans*, is the most common species incriminated. Adult flies bite the host, suck blood, and produce an erythematous papular eruption that can be extremely irritating to the animal. Affected dogs shake their head or scratch their ears, producing pinnal excoriations, exudation, and hemorrhage. Lesions are commonly confined to the tips of the ears but may also occur on the face.

The diagnosis is based on the history (summer occurrence), clinical signs, and the presence of flies. A differential diagnosis would include sarcoptic mange, otodectic mange, atopy, vasculitis, and systemic lupus erythematosus. Rarely are diagnostic tests indicated; however, multiple skin scrapings, an otoscopic examination, mineral oil preparation of an ear smear, and an intradermal skin test would aid in the elimination of other probable causes.

Therapy is directed at fly eradication. The animal should be temporarily confined indoors during the day. Insect repellents (Skin-So-Soft, Avon) or insecticidal sprays should be used on the entire body, especially concentrating on the ears, head, and neck. Topical creams or ointments containing an antibiotic, steroid, or combination (Cortisporin, Burroughs Wellcome) decrease inflammation, soften crusts, and provide protection. The source of the flies should be identified and treated with an appropriate environmental insecticide.

SOLAR DERMATITIS

Solar-induced damage to the tips of the ears is most commonly seen in white cats who are exposed to intense sunlight in areas such as California and Florida. In the early stages, diffuse alopecia, erythema, and scaling develop along the margins of the ears. Initially, the ear tips may have a slightly curled appearance. With prolonged or repeated sun exposure, the ears become edematous and ulcerated, and squamous cell carcinoma can eventually develop. Such solar changes can also occur in white-eared dogs housed outside.

The diagnosis of pinnal solar dermatitis is based on clinical signs, history of sun exposure, and histopathologic findings. A differential diagnosis would include feline and canine scabies, frostbite, trauma, pemphigus complex, systemic lupus erythematosus, and neoplastic skin diseases. The definitive diagnosis can often be made based on the histologic findings of solar-induced changes or squamous cell carcinoma.

The management of pinnal solar dermatitis includes confining the animal indoors during hours of peak sunlight and using topical sunscreens containing PABA on the ears. In cases associated with squamous cell carcinoma, radical pinnal amputation and cosmetic surgery are recommended.

PINNAL ALOPECIA

Alopecia of the pinnae has been described in several breeds of dogs, most commonly in the dachshund. The nonpruritic alopecia observed in dachshunds occurs predominantly in male dogs and begins around 1 year of age. The cause is unknown but is probably hereditary in origin. Typically, the pinnae exhibit a symmetric thinning of the hair that slowly progresses to complete baldness over several years. A similar picture is also seen in spayed, female dachshunds, associated with hypoestrogenism. In such cases, a symmetric alopecia is also noted on the ventral neck, chest, and perineum.

The diagnosis and cause of pinnal alopecia is based on the history, physical findings, and elimination of other possible causes such as ear margin seborrhea, other hereditary alopecias (i.e., color mutant alopecia), iatrogenic causes (i.e., topical medications), and endocrinopathies, particularly hypoestrogenism. In cats, hyperadrenocorticism can cause pinnal alopecia and atrophy of the skin. There is no effective therapy for cases due to a hereditary cause. Estrogen replacement therapy is recommended in female dogs with hypoestrogenism.

EAR MARGIN SEBORRHEA

Seborrheic crusting confined to the margins of the pinnae is common in breeds of dogs predisposed to primary seborrhea, such as the cocker spaniel, dachshund, and West Highland white terrier. Focal crusts that have a greasy texture are firmly attached to the skin and the base of the hair. With time, the underlying skin becomes inflamed and ulcerated. Other areas of the body, such as the axillae and groin, may also be involved.

A differential diagnosis would include zinc-responsive dermatosis, sarcoptic mange, vasculitis, systemic lupus erythematosus, dermatophytosis, and pemphigus foliaceus. The diagnosis is based on history, clinical signs, and laboratory tests. A skin biopsy may be helpful by eliminating the aforementioned causes and revealing the histologic features compatible with ear margin seborrhea (orthokeratotic or parakeratotic hyperkeratosis).

Therapy is usually directed toward the relief of symptoms and decreasing crust formation. Antiseborrheic shampoos or gels containing sulfur or benzoyl peroxide should be used to clean affected areas after the matted hair and crusts have been removed. Topical steroid creams or synthetic vitamin A gels (Retin-A, Ortho) are effective as prophylactic therapy.

SCABIES

Scabies is a common cause of intense pinnal pruritus that is usually resistant to systemic steroid therapy. Both Sarcoptes scabiei var. canis (dogs) and S. notoedres cati (cats) are host specific and extremely contagious. In dogs, lesions include alopecia, erythema, excoriations, and severe crusting along the margins of the ears. An erythematous papular eruption is often present concurrently on the elbows, ventral chest, and extremities. Feline scabies is usually confined to the ears, head, and neck. Lesions consist of multifocal to diffuse alopecia, erythema, and adherent, grayish crusts. Notoedric mange is relatively uncommon, except in certain endemic regions of the country.

The diagnosis is based on a history of acute, severe pruritus, clinical signs, and positive skin scrapings. Sarcoptes scabiei var. canis is often difficult to isolate in skin scrapings; therefore, therapeutic dipping is recommended. Notoedres cati is easily identified in skin scrapings taken from affected cats.

Therapy in dogs includes applying an insecticidal dip every 5 to 7 days for 4 to 6 weeks. Two per cent lime sulfur, lindane, or 0.025 per cent amitraz (Mitaban, Upjohn) are effective scabicides for use in dogs. Any dog having contact with an affected dog should be treated at the same time. Ivermectin has been used in resistant cases of canine scabies at a dose of 200 mcg/kg PO or SC; however, ivermectin is not approved for use in dogs at this concentration. Because of the sensitivity of cats to many insecticides, especially lindane, a 2 per cent lime sulfur solution is the treatment of choice and should be applied weekly for four to six treatments. Recently, 0.025 per cent amitraz (Mitaban), has been found to be an effective treatment for notoedric mange. However, side effects (e.g., anorexia, diarrhea) were observed in young kittens, and amitraz has not been approved for use in cats.

TRAUMA

Traumatic insult to either one or both pinnae can occasionally cause pinnal dermatitis. Trauma-related disease is more common in hunting dogs or aggressive guard dogs used for protection. It can also occur secondary to other pruritic skin diseases that involve the ears, such as sarcoptic mange, atopy, or otodectic mange. Puncture wounds, lacerations, ulcers, and crusts are usually noted along the margin of one or both pinnae, especially in long-eared dogs. Secondary bacterial infections may be present in chronic or untreated cases.

ALLERGIC DERMATITIS

Occasionally, atopy or food allergy can be localized to the pinnae or external ear canals of dogs or cats. A contact allergic dermatitis can occur on the tips of long-eared dogs, following contact with such substances as wool rugs, floor cleaners, or polishes. Allergic animals present with a history of pinnal pruritis or head shaking that may initially be seasonal (atopy) or nonseasonal (atopy, food or contact allergy), depending on the cause or course. In the early stages of atopy, the pruritus is usually responsive to systemic glucocorticoids. Both contact and dietary allergies are less responsive to systemic steroid therapy. Typically, both ears are usually involved in all three types of allergic dermatitis.

In the early stages of atopy or food allergy, the pinnae and external ear canals may appear relatively normal or mildly erythematous, with little discharge present. However, with prolonged or persistent ear scratching, the ears become excoriated and secondarily infected. In such chronic cases, edema, exudation, ulceration, and otitis externa are noted. The pinnae and external ear canals become thickened and hyperplastic. Topical glucocorticoids are of minimal benefit in alleviating the pain or pruritus in such chronic cases. In cases involving atopy, the pruritus frequently involves other areas of the body, particularly the feet, face, and groin.

The diagnosis of inhalant or food allergy is based on history, clinical signs, and initial response to systemic glucocorticoids. A differential diagnosis would include sarcoptic or notoedric mange, otodectic mange, and other causes of otitis externa (i.e., bacteria, yeast, foreign body). Diagnostic tests would include multiple skin scrapings, ear smears, mineral oil preparation of an ear swab, elimination diet, intradermal skin test, and a thorough otoscopic examination. In the early stages, ear smears commonly reveal a mild overgrowth of yeast or coccoid bacteria. However, in chronic cases, an overgrowth of gram-negative organisms associated with inflammatory cells is seen. The diagnosis of contact allergic dermatitis is based on history, clinical signs, and improvement when the offending allergen is removed.

Once the offending allergen has been identified, avoidance is the most effective form of control. This is not a feasible alternative in most cases involving inhalant allergy; therefore, hyposensitization is recommended. Medical management includes alternate-day prednisolone therapy, systemic antibiotics, and topical otic preparations containing antibiotics, steroids, or both.

OTODECTIC MANGE

Otodectic mange is a common cause of otitis externa, especially in cats. Pinnal pruritus is common in animals that are hypersensitive to the mite. Such dogs and cats present with severe head shaking and ear scratching. Alopecia, excoriations, exudation, and crusts are noted on the pinnae in conjunction with a blackish-brown discharge in the external canal. On occasion, the ear canal may appear relatively normal, with minimal discharge present. The diagnosis is based on history, physical findings, and identification of mites on ear smears or on otoscopic examination. Various therapies are available and include a thiabendazole (Tresaderm, MSD AgVet) preparation, rotenone (Canex, Pitman-Moore) and mineral oil solution, and topical pyrethrins.

CONCLUSION

There are many other skin diseases that frequently affect the pinnae in conjunction with other regions of the body (Table 2). These can often be differentiated, based on specific historical and clinical findings or laboratory tests (Table 2). Zinc-responsive dermatitis is a crusting, facial skin disease most common in artic breeds of dogs (huskies, malamutes). It is usually diagnosed based on histologic findings (severe parakeratosis and superficial perivascular dermatitis) and is response to zinc supplementation.

The immune-mediated skin diseases that commonly affect the pinnae include pemphigus foliaceus and pemphigus erythematosus, vasculitis, cold agglutinin disease, systemic and discoid lupus erythematosus, and drug eruption. As a whole, they are rare and can be diagnosed based on histopathology and immunologic tests (antinuclear antibody [ANA]; direct immunofluorescence).

Dermatophytosis can affect any haired region of the body, including the pinnae. The diagnosis is based on the clinical appearance of the lesions and positive results of fungal cultures. Juvenile cellulitis, dermatomyositis, and epidermolysis bullosa commonly involve the pinnae, in conjunction with the face and muzzle. All three are diseases of young dogs. Dermatomyositis and epidermolysis are more common in collies and Shetland sheepdogs.

In summary, pinnal dermatitis is a challenging syndrome and one that is frequently encountered alone or in association with anyone of several common skin diseases. Identifying the exact cause is based on the ability of the clinician to integrate the historical and physical findings and to formulate a complete differential diagnosis. This discussion has attempted to review a few of the possible causes of pinnal dermatitis; however, a more detailed descrip-

tion of each disease can be found in one of several references listed.

References and Supplemental Reading

Griffin, C. E.: Differential diagnoses of nasal diseases. *In* Kirk, R. W. (ed.): *Current Veterinary Therapy VIII*. Philadelphia: W. B. Saunders Co., 1982, pp. 480–484.

Halliwell, R. E. W.: Autoimmune disease in the dog. Adv. Vet. Sci. Comp. Med. 22:221, 1978.

Kunkle, G. A.: Zinc-responsive dermatoses in dogs. *In* Kirk, R. W. (ed.): *Current Veterinary Therapy VII*. Philadelphia: W. B. Saunders Co., 1980, pp. 472–476.

Kunkle, G. A., Gross, T. L., Fadok, V. A., et al.: Dermatomyositis in collie dogs. Compend. Cont. Ed. Pract. Vet. 7:185, 1985.

Muller, G. H., Kirk, R. W., and Scott, D. W.: *Small Animal Dermatology*, 3rd ed. Philadelphia: W. B. Saunders Co., 1983.

Scott, D. W.: Feline dermatology 1900–1978: A monograph. J. Am. Anim. Hosp. Assoc. 16:365, 1980.

Scott, D. W., and Schultz, R. D.: Epidermolysis bullosa simplex in the collie dog. J.A.V.M.A. 171:721, 1977.

Scott, D. W., Walton, D. K., Manning, T. O., et al.: Canine lupus erythematosus. I. Systemic lupus erythematosus. J. Am. Anim. Hosp. Assoc. 19:461, 1983.

Scott, D. W., Walton, D. K., Manning, T. O., et al.: Canine lupus erythematosus. II. Discoid lupus erythematosus. J. Am. Anim. Hosp. Assoc. 19:481, 1983.

CANINE CUTANEOUS HISTIOCYTOSES

DANNY W. SCOTT, D.V.M.

Ithaca, New York

The primary histiocytic dermatoses are a group of skin disorders in which histiocytes predominate histologically in the absence of any known proliferative stimulus (e.g., infectious agent, foreign body, metabolic product). In humans, there are numerous primary histiocytic dermatoses, all of which are uncommon to rare in occurrence. The clinical behavior (benign or malignant) of these disorders does not necessarily correlate with the cytologic appearance of the infiltrating histiocytes.

In dogs, there are four recognized primary histiocytic dermatoses: histiocytoma, malignant histiocytosis, systemic histiocytosis, and cutaneous histiocytosis. The histiocytic nature of the cells may be confirmed by electron microscopy or enzyme histochemistry. *Electron microscopy* requires the use of special fixatives (*not* formalin), and typical histiocytes are characterized by convoluted nuclei, abundant lysosomes, and cytoplasmic filopodia. *Enzyme histochemistry* is performed on frozen sections or on tissues fixed in 2 per cent paraformaldehyde, dehydrated in acetone, and embedded in glycol

methacrylate. Typical histiocytic enzyme histochemical markers include lysozyme, acid phosphatase, nonspecific esterase, and alpha-1-antitrypsin.

HISTIOCYTOMA

The histiocytoma is a common benign neoplasm of the dog. Histiocytomas characteristically affect young dogs, with about 50 per cent of the cases occurring in dogs under 2 years of age. However, old dogs may be affected. Boxers, dachshunds, cocker spaniels, Great Danes, and Shetland sheepdogs appear to be predisposed. There is no sex predilection.

Histiocytomas are usually solitary and occur most commonly on the head, pinnae, and limbs. They are usually small (less than 3 cm in diameter), firm, dome-shaped or plaquelike, well-circumscribed, dermoepidermal in location, and frequently erythematous and ulcerated. Pruritus is variable. Lesions have an initial (few days to weeks) rapid grow phase but then stabilize.

Histopathologically, histiocytomas are characterized by uniform sheets of pleomorphic histiocytic cells infiltrating the dermis and subcutis, displacing collagen fibers, and adnexae. A characteristic feature of this neoplasm is a high mitotic index. Lymphocytic infiltration and areas of neutrophilic infiltration and necrosis develop in regressing neoplasms.

Clinical management of histiocytomas may include surgical excision, cryosurgery, hyperthermia, or observation without treatment. The majority of these neoplasms undergo spontaneous regression after a few months.

MALIGNANT HISTIOCYTOSIS

Malignant histiocytosis is a rare malignant neoplasm of dogs. Malignant histiocytosis has been recognized in several breeds of dogs, with no sex predilection but with older animals typically affected. This neoplasm has also been reported in closely related Bernese Mountain Dogs, predominantly males.

Typical clinical signs of malignant histiocytosis include lethargy, weight loss, lymphadenopathy, hepatosplenomegaly, and pancytopenia. Cutaneous lesions are rarely reported and are characterized by multiple, firm, dermal to subcutaneous nodules anywhere on the body. Skin lesions may be alopecic, ulcerated, or both.

Histopathologically, malignant histiocytosis is characterized by nodular to diffuse deep dermal and subcutaneous infiltration, with cytologically atypical histiocytes exhibiting cytophagocytosis and a high mitotic index.

Malignant histiocytosis is currently a fatal disease, with no effective treatment.

SYSTEMIC HISTIOCYTOSIS

Systemic histiocytosis is a rare histologic proliferative disorder of dogs. Systemic histiocytosis has been described in closely related Bernese Mountain Dogs, 2 to 8 years of age, predominantly in males. The disorder has been recognized in other breeds, as well, with some dogs developing the disease at 4 to 5 months of age.

Clinical signs include anorexia, weight loss, respiratory stertor, and multiple cutaneous papules, plaques, nodules, and ulcers over the entire body, especially the face and the limbs. Pruritus and pain are variable. Nasal involvement may result in depigmentation.

Histopathologically, systemic histiocytosis is characterized by superficial and deep perivascular, nodular, or diffuse dermal and subcutaneous infiltrations of cytologically normal histiocytes.

The course of systemic histiocytosis may be prolonged and fluctuating, with alternating periods of exacerbation and remission, or rapidly progressive and fatal. Ultimately, most dogs are euthanized, with histiocytic infiltration of multiple organ systems, especially lungs, liver, spleen, bone marrow, and lymph nodes. Treatment with large doses of glucocorticoids and cytotoxic drugs has been generally ineffective. Anecdotal observations indicated that treatment with bovine thymosin fraction 5 may be beneficial.

CUTANEOUS HISTIOCYTOSIS

Cutaneous histiocytosis is a rare benign histiocytic proliferative disorder of dogs. Cutaneous histiocytosis does not appear to have age, breed, or sex predilections. Lesions were characterized by multiple, erythematous, dermal or subcutaneous plaques or nodules, 1 to 5 cm in diameter, anywhere on the body. Lesions often waxed and waned and appeared in new sites. Systemic involvement and lymphadenopathy were not reported.

Histopathologically, cutaneous histiocytosis is characterized by nodular to diffuse dermal or subcutaneous infiltrations of cytologically normal histiocytes.

Treatment with large doses of glucocorticoids (e.g., prednisolone, 2.2 to 4.4 mg/kg/day PO) or cytotoxic drugs has given erratic results: some dogs appearing to be cured, others requiring long-term therapy, and others showing no response.

References and Supplemental Reading

Mays, M. B. C., and Bergeron, J. A.: Cutaneous histiocytosis in dogs. J.A.V.M.A. 188:377, 1986.

Moore, P. F.: Systemic histiocytosis of Bernese Mountain Dogs. Vet. Pathol. 21:554, 1984.

Moore, P. F., and Rosin, A.: Malignant histiocytosis of Bernese Mountain Dogs. Vet. Pathol. 23:1, 1986.

Muller, G. H., Kirk, R. W., and Scott, D. W.: Small Animal Dermatology III. Philadelphia: W. B. Saunders Co., 1983.

Rosin, A., Moore, P. F., and Dubielzig, R.: Malignant histiocytosis in Bernese Mountain Dogs. J.A.V.M.A. 188:1041, 1986.

Scott, D. W., Angarano, D. K., and Suter, M. M.: Systemic histiocytosis in two dogs. Canine Pract. 14:7, 1987.

Scott, D. W., Miller, W. H., Tasker, J. B., et al.: Lymphorecticular neoplasia in a dog resembling malignant histiocytosis (histiocytic medullary reticulosis) in man. Cornell Vet. 69:176, 1979.

Wellman, M. L., Davenport, D. J., Morton, D. M., et al.: Malignant histiocytosis in four dogs. J.A.V.M.A. 187:919, 1975.

FELINE CUTANEOUS MAST CELL TUMORS

ROBERT G. BUERGER, D.V.M.

Baltimore, Maryland

Cutaneous mast cell tumors (CMCTs) account for 2 to 15 per cent of all cutaneous tumors in cats. As a relatively common tumor, one would expect CMCTs to have a clearly defined biologic behavior, but such is not the case. Although there is much controversy, the most recent studies agree that feline CMCTs are not highly malignant neoplasms.

CLINICAL AND DIAGNOSTIC CONSIDERATIONS

Cutaneous mast cell tumors seldom offer a diagnostic challenge to clinicians and pathologists. Practitioners with good cytologic skills can make a provisional diagnosis in the examination room. Lesions arise in the dermis or subcutis and are most commonly papular or nodular in appearance, and usually one to few in number. The surface may be normal, alopecic, or ulcerated. Indolent ulcerlike CMCTs have been reported on the lip. Lesions are solitary in approximately two thirds of cases. Generalized cutaneous mast cell neoplasia is rare. Most authors agree that CMCT has a predilection for older male cats, occurring especially on the head and neck. Cutaneous and visceral mast cell neoplasms are usually unrelated.

Mast cells have characteristic intracytoplasmic granules, the contents of which include many vasoactive and chemotactic substances. These granules usually stain metachromatically with toluidine blue, a feature which is an aid in cellular identification. In certain situations, the cytoplasmic granules are indistinct and can be seen only on electron microscopy. The degree of cellular differentiation and the pH at which the cells are stained are important factors in influencing the staining properties of the granules (Macy, 1986). Histiocytic mast cell tumors (the cytoplasmic granules stain poorly with toluidine blue) have been reported to be benign, self-limiting subcutaneous neoplasms of Siamese cats that are less than 4 years of age (Wilcock et al., 1986).

Once a diagnosis of CMCT has been made (either cytologically or histopathologically), the cat should be carefully re-evaluated. Particular attention should be paid to regional lymph nodes (to identify metastasis) and the alimentary tract (because of the potential for histamine-induced gastroduodenal ulceration and bleeding). Additionally, one should routinely perform a complete blood count and a buffy coat examination. Rarely, a peripheral eosinophilia, a mastocythemia, or both can be identified. In some cases, a more intensive laboratory evaluation, including a bone marrow aspirate, is recommended. However, the information obtained from such tests seldom changes the therapy or prognosis. The cats with CMCT that the author has evaluated have had one or few lesions and have been otherwise healthy. One cat was healthy and lived for 5 years without therapy after diagnoses of cutaneous mast cell neoplasia and mastocythemia.

THERAPY AND PROGNOSIS

Surgical excision is the treatment of choice and can be accomplished easily in most cases. In the author's experience, local recurrence of CMCT is rare. However, there is recurrence of CMCT at other sites in approximately one third of cases. This does not necessarily imply a malignant nature. The lesion(s) can again be surgically excised, and many cats subsequently remain lesion free. The author knows of two aged cats whose recurrent lesions were cyclic in nature (new lesions developed and regressed spontaneously).

The likelihood of metastasis from a primary cutaneous site is the subject of great controversy. Some refer to the tumor's highly malignant nature (Muller et al., 1983). Others suggest that at least some, if not most, CMCTs have a low rate of metastasis (Garner and Lingeman, 1970; Yager and Scott, 1985; Holzinger, 1973; Wilcock et al., 1986; Buerger and Scott, 1987). Visceral metastasis is extremely improbable. Four retrospective studies (Buerger and Scott, 1987; Wilcock et al., 1986; Holzinger, 1973; and Garner and Lingeman, 1970) have collectively identified 174 cats with CMCT. Of the 174 cats, only one was known to have developed visceral metastasis. Metastasis to lymph nodes or viscera has been reported in fewer than 10 per cent of cases, and metastasis is more probable if anaplasia and a high mitotic index are present (Macy, 1986).

Several studies have attempted to correlate the

histologic appearance and clinical behavior of feline CMCT (Holzinger, 1973; Wilcock et al., 1986; Buerger and Scott, 1987). In dogs with CMCT, such studies have provided useful prognostic information. However, the feline studies usually have not produced clear-cut information. The author's own study of a small number of cats with CMCT attempted to correlate the presence or degree of anaplasia to the recurrence rate. No correlation could be established, as even tumors with a high degree of anaplasia demonstrated a benign clinical behavior.

There is still much to be learned about feline CMCT, but it appears that most are not highly malignant or metastatic.

References and Supplemental Reading

Buerger, R. G., and Scott, D. W.: Cutaneous mast cell neoplasia in cats: Fourteen cases (1975–1985). J.A.V.M.A. 190:1440, 1987.

Garner, F. M., and Lingeman, C. H.: Mast cell neoplasms of the domestic cat. Pathol. Vet. 7:517, 1970.

Holzinger, E. A.: Feline cutaneous mastocytomas. Cornell Vet. 63:87, 1973.

Macy, D. W.: Canine and feline mast cell tumors. Proceedings of the 10th Annual Kal Kan Symposium, 1986, p. 101.

Muller, G. H., Kirk, R. W., and Scott, D. W.: *Small Animal Dermatology III.* Philadelphia: W. B. Saunders Co., 1983, pp. 74, 751–757.

Wilcock, B. P., Yager, J. A., and Zink, M. C.: The morphology and behavior of feline cutaneous mastocytomas. Vet. Pathol. 23:320, 1986.

Yager, J. A., and Scott, D. W.: The skin and appendages. *In* Jubb, K. V. F., Kennedy, P. C., Palmer, N. (eds.): *Pathology of Domestic Animals.* 3rd ed. Orlando, FL: Academic Press, Inc., 1985, pp. 519–520.

DISORDERS OF MELANIN PIGMENTATION IN THE SKIN OF DOGS AND CATS

ERIC GUAGUERE, D.V.M.,
Lomme, France

and ZEINEB ALHAIDARI, D.V.M.
Roquefort les Pins, France

Disorders of melanin pigmentation are very common in many canine and feline dermatoses. Their etiologic diagnosis often requires a very methodical clinicopathologic approach. A careful history and physical examination will permit the clinician to establish an inclusive differential diagnosis, which will determine the laboratory tests used. The following is an overview of the currently recognized disorders of cutaneous melanization in dogs and cats.

HYPOMELANOSIS AND AMELANOSIS

Hypomelanosis and amelanosis refer to a decrease or complete lack, respectively, of melanin. They can affect the skin (leukoderma), the hair (leukotrichia), or both and may be genetic or acquired.

The authors sincerely thank Prof. Ortonne (Pasteur Hospital, Dermatology, Nice, France) and Prof. Magnol (National Veterinary School, Lyon, France) for their active collaboration on this article.

Genetic Hypomelanosis and Amelanosis

The pathogenesis is different in the various clinical syndromes (Table 1).

ALBINISM. Albinism is an autosomal recessive disorder, described in several dog breeds. The pathogenic mechanism is a defect in the melanization of the melanosomes. In humans, recessive oculocutaneous albinism is divided into tyrosinase-negative albinism and tyrosinase-positive albinism. Albino dogs have a normal number of melanocytes, but they lack tyrosinase to produce melanin. Clinically, it is expressed by a generalized amelanosis of the skin, hair, and mucous membranes. Ocular manifestations are milder in dogs than in humans: blue eyes (rarely, pink) and slightly modified visual acuity. Ophthalmoscopic examination reveals a normal yellow tapetal fundus, but no pigment in the nontapetal fundus. The choroidal vessels are prominent against the white scleral background. Other patients may have no color in the tapetum and a bright-orange color of the fundus. Albino animals should not be used for breeding.

Table 1. *Hypothetic Pathogenetic Mechanisms in Hypomelanosis*

Mechanism	Disease
Presence of Melanocytes	
Block in melanin synthesis	Nutritional hypomelanosis
Defect or abnormality in the synthesis of melanosomes	Nutritional hypomelanosis
Defect or abnormality in melanization of melanosomes	Tyrosinase-negative albinism
Defect or abnormality of transfer of melanosomes to keratinocytes	Tyrosinase-positive albinism; some post-inflammatory hypomelanoses
Abnormal degradation of melanosomes	Chédiak-Higashi syndrome
	Canine cyclic hematopoiesis
Absence of Melanocytes	
Absence of migration of melanoblasts or their inability to survive in the skin	Waardenburg-Klein syndrome
Absence of differentiation of melanocytes	Waardenburg-Klein syndrome
Destruction of Melanocytes	Vitiligo
	Hypomelanosis secondary to physical infectious, parasitic, or autoimmune disease; senile graying of hairs; Vogt-Koyanagi-Harada syndrome

CHÉDIAK-HIGASHI SYNDROME. This disorder is an autosomal recessive syndrome, reported in humans and "blue-smoke" Persian cats. The hereditary abnormality is characterized by a generalized hypomelanosis (pigmentary dilution) and visual disorders such as photophobia and hypochromia of the irides. Increased susceptibility to infection is secondary to decreased chemotactic and bactericidal properties of leukocytes and is responsible for early death. Leukocytes, melanocytes, and many other cell types (kidney, liver) contain enlarged lysosomal granules. Gigantic melanosome complexes are also present in the phagosomes in melanocytes and keratinocytes. It is not clearly established if the complexes are synthesized as such, or result from the abnormal combination of melanosomes. Ultrastructural aspects suggest that hypomelanosis is secondary to an accelerated degradation of the melanosomes. There is no effective treatment, and affected cats should not be used as breeders.

CANINE CYCLIC HEMATOPOIESIS. Canine cyclic hematopoiesis (gray collie syndrome, cyclic neutropenia) is a lethal autosomal recessive syndrome that affects collie puppies born with a silver-gray hair coat and a light-colored nasal planum. Sometimes, some puppies present a slightly yellow pigmentation (mixture of light beige and light gray hair). At 1 week of age, affected puppies are usually smaller and weaker than their littermates. The other clinical signs start at 6 or 8 weeks of age: pyrexia, cyclic hematopoiesis, chronic diarrhea, conjunctivitis and keratitis, arthralgia, and peripheral lymphadenopathy. Early death is observed (before 6 months of age) after pulmonary and gastrointestinal disorders. The full-term cyclic neutropenia reflects the appearance of neutropenia alternating with rebounding neutrophilia (cycles at 11- to 12-day intervals). Other hematologic abnormalities are observed: microcytic normochromic anemia, reticulocytosis, increased levels of erythropoietin, and increased serum iron levels 3 to 6 days after the increase of

neutrophils. There is no effective treatment; parents and littermates should not be used as breeders. Treatment with fluids and antibiotics may keep the puppy alive longer. Lithium carbonate, 20 to 25 mg/kg daily, stabilizes the level of neutrophils but is very toxic.

WAARDENBURG-KLEIN SYNDROME. This syndrome is characterized by a hypomelanosis or amelanosis, a blue homochromia or heterochromia of the irides, and deafness. This association of genetically determined hearing loss and hypomelanosis or amelanosis has been described in humans, cats, and several genotypes of mice. Hereditary deafness and pigmentation anomalies, such as white spotting or the merling trait, are also found in many breeds of dogs: bull terrier, Sealyham terrier, collie, and Dalmatian. Abnormalities of the inner ear responsible for the deafness are as follows: reduction in the number of cochlear coils, reduction of the saccular lumen, and retraction of the tectorial membrane (cats). The pathogenic mechanism is dual: a defect in the migration of the melanoblasts or their inability to survive in the skin and a defect in the differentiation of melanoblasts into melanocytes. In cats, this syndrome is transmitted as an autosomal dominant trait with incomplete penetrance. Affected animals should not be used for breeding.

TYROSINASE DEFICIENCY IN THE CHOW CHOW. This disorder is expressed by a color change in chow chow puppies. The normally black tongue becomes pink, and portions of the hair shafts are white. The buccal mucosa also may rapidly depigment. This abnormality results from a transient tyrosinase deficiency. The melanocytes do not synthesize melanin pigments. Melanin reappears spontaneously in 2 to 4 months.

VITILIGO. Vitiligo is an autosomal dominant hypomelanosis in humans, with a variable expressivity. In humans, three pathogeneses are commonly proposed: autoimmune, neurogenic, or hereditary. Vitiligo has been described in Belgian shepherds,

German shepherds, collies, and a Siamese cat. In the United States, canine vitiligo is most commonly observed in Rottweilers and Doberman pinschers. The gradual depigmentation is more or less symmetric and appears generally before the age of 3 years and in various sites (nose, lips, oral mucosa, and eyelids). Poliosis (leukotrichia), focal or widespread, can be seen. The evolution is very unpredictable. Leukoderma, leukotrichia, or both are often permanent. In some cases, repigmentation is possible. Histologically, the condition is characterized by an absence of melanocytes in the absence of inflammation or other dermatohistopathologic abnormalities. Vitiligo must not be mistaken for discoid lupus erythematosus, chemical hypomelanosis, or syndromes resembling Vogt-Koyanagi-Harada syndrome. The psoralen–ultraviolet light (PUVA) therapy prescribed in the human disease has been tried by one of the authors on a few patients, but without satisfactory results.

Acquired Hypomelanosis

NUTRITIONAL HYPOMELANOSIS. In this condition, a copper deficiency induces a pigmentary dilution. Lenticular depigmentations have been associated with zinc deficiency. Classically, the role of proteins, vitamins, and oligoelements has been stressed in certain hypomelanoses, even though a clear relationship has not been established.

HORMONAL HYPOMELANOSIS. Hormonal hypomelanosis, especially fading of coat color, may be seen in dogs with hyperadrenocorticism, gonadal imbalances, and hypothyroidism. In humans, hormonal hypomelanosis may be seen in hyperadrenocorticism or in hypogonadism.

PHYSICAL HYPOMELANOSIS. Physical hypomelanosis (e.g., from x-rays, ultraviolet light, burns, cold, and mechanical injuries) may produce either or both leukoderma and leukotrichia by destruction of melanocytes. Such depigmentation is usually permanent.

CHEMICAL HYPOMELANOSIS. This condition can be due to various products, such as contact dihydroquinone monobenzylether used as an antioxidant in the plastic industry, or to local reactions to corticosteroids or progestational compounds injected subcutaneously. The chemical compounds can act at different levels: (1) production of free radicals that kill the melanocyte, (2) competition with tyrosinase (especially phenol derivatives), (3) interference with synthesis of melanosomes or tyrosinase by combination with the ribosomes of the melanocyte, or (4) interference with melanosome transfer by inducing an intercellular edema.

POST-INFLAMMATORY HYPOMELANOSES. These are frequent and can be secondary to a defective melanosome transfer, pigmentary incontinence, or destruction of melanocytes. In the Vogt-Koyanagi-Harada canine syndrome, a bilateral uveitis and a cutaneous depigmentation are present. The nose, lips, and eyelids are typically affected. Variable degrees of leukotrichia may also be seen. A cell-mediated immune reaction directed against melanin or against melanocytic surface receptors may be involved. Antigenic properties could be acquired secondary to a primary disease such as a viral infection. Other inflammatory dermatoses frequently characterized by depigmentation, especially of the nose and lips, include discoid lupus erythematosus, systemic lupus erythematosus, pemphigus erythematosus, and pemphigus foliaceus. In addition, focal depigmentation of the nose, lips, or both may be seen in cats, secondary to upper respiratory viral infections.

INFECTIOUS AND PARASITIC HYPOMELANOSES. These disorders are well known in humans in leprosy and various treponemal diseases. In dogs and cats, infectious depigmentations are rarely recognized but probably belong in the post-inflammatory group as concerns pathomechanism. A true parasitic hypomelanosis has been described in chronic untreated cases of canine and human leishmaniasis.

HYPOMELANOSIS ASSOCIATED WITH TUMORS. This disease is well known in humans; peritumoral halo, or Sutton's halo, has been observed around melanocytic nevi, malignant melanomas, or their metastases, and even around seborrheic keratoses. In dogs, a peritumoral halo has been seen around basal cell tumors, but the pathogenesis is unknown and clearly different from Sutton's halo. In dogs, leukoderma and leukotrichia have been observed in certain cases of leydigioma, mammary adenocarcinoma, and gastric carcinoma, without any good explanation of the pathogenic mechanism.

Dogs with epitheliotropic lymphoma (mycosis fungoides) may develop variable degrees of depigmentation of the mucocutaneous areas, nasal planum, oral mucosa, and skin.

Primary Hypomelanosis of Difficult Classification

A syndrome currently called the *Aguirre syndrome*, described in the Siamese cat, is characterized by a unilateral periocular depigmentation associated with Horner's syndrome or with corneal necrosis accompanied by uveitis and upper respiratory tract infections.

The senile graying of hairs may be a fairly localized or generalized phenomenon. The pathomechanism is not known. Melanocytes are supposed to have a genetically determined length of life, after which they begin to disappear.

HYPERMELANOSIS

Hypermelanosis refers to an increase of melanin that can affect the skin (melanoderma), hair (melanotrichia), or both and may be genetic or acquired (Table 2).

Genetic Hypermelanosis

LENTIGINES. These are uncommonly reported in dogs and cats. These brown or black macules, 1 to 5 mm in diameter, single or multiple, correspond to an increase in the melanocyte numbers in the basal layer. There is no structural epidermal change. In humans, lentigines are often associated with visceral disorders. Such an association has not been reported in dogs and cats. A hereditary profuse lentiginosis due to an autosomal dominant trait has been described in three pugs, especially involving the trunk and medial thighs. Lentigo simplex has been described in orange cats (Scott, 1987). Affected cats usually develop macular melanosis of the lips, gums, eyelids, and nose at less than 1 year of age. The macules (not true lentigines) often increase in size and number with age.

Acquired Hypermelanosis

POSTINFLAMMATORY HYPERMELANOSIS. This disorder is very common and is seen secondary to various inflammatory disorders. Physical insults include radiotherapy, friction, and intertrigo. Focal melanotrichia has been described in the gray or apricot poodle and the Siamese cat following an inflammation, an injection, or a surgical procedure. The increase in skin temperature can induce a darkening of the hair; hair color returns to normal with the next hair cycle. Histologic findings include a greater follicular melanocytic population than the epidermal melanocytic population. Common infectious causes of hyperpigmentation include chronic canine scabies, generalized canine demodicosis, dermatophytosis, and chronic pyoderma (superficial and deep bacterial infections). *Hypersensitivity disorders* such as canine atopy, chronic contact hypersensitivity, flea-bite hypersensitivity, and bacterial

hypersensitivity frequently are associated with hyperpigmentation.

The pathogenesis of post-inflammatory hypermelanosis is poorly understood. Histologic findings reveal a melanin overload in all layers of the epidermis, often the accumulation of melanocytes around superficial dermal blood vessels, and occasionally pigmentary incontinence.

ENDOCRINE HYPERMELANOSES. The pathomechanisms of these disorders are often unknown because the action of the different hormones on melanocytic activity is not well defined. The hormones generally act directly on the melanocyte, inducing a melanin overload in the basal layer without increase of the melanocyte numbers.

Hypermelanosis in Cushing's disease can be due to an increased synthesis of tyrosinase and abnormal melanosome transfer to keratinocytes. Patchy hyperpigmentation on the abdomen is very common, with other cutaneous and systemic signs. Occasionally, this hypermelanosis may be generalized.

Ovarian imbalance type I and feminization syndromes in male dogs are frequently associated with hypermelanosis, beginning in the perineal and genital regions and extending progressively to the abdomen. Hypermelanosis in hypothyroidism is inconsistent and variable in extent.

Growth hormone deficiencies (pituitary dwarfism and adult-onset hyposomatotropism) are also characterized by a generalized hyperpigmentation and a bilaterally symmetric alopecia, which spare the face and the distal extremities. Hyperpigmented alopecias of chow chows and Pomeranians, as well as keeshonds and poodles may be growth hormone–responsive if other endocrine abnormalities are ruled out.

TUMOR HYPERMELANOSES. Tumor hypermelanoses are represented by *melanomas* and *malignant acanthosis nigricans*. In dogs, melanomas are relatively frequent, benign or malignant neoplasms arising from melanocytes and melanoblasts. Cocker spaniels, boxers, Irish setters, chow chows, Scottish terriers, and poodles appear to be predisposed. The common sites are the face, trunk, feet, and scrotum.

Table 2. Hypothetic Pathogenetic Mechanisms in Hypermelanosis

Mechanism	Disease
Increase in the number of melanocytes in the basal layer	Lentigines
Normal number of melanocytes	
Increased production of normal melanosomes or production of abnormal melanosomes	
Increased synthesis of tyrosinase	Hyperadrenocorticism
Abnormal melanosome transfer to keratinocytes	Hyperadrenocorticism
Absence of degradation of melanosomes	Acanthosis nigricans
Hyperproduction of melanosomes with secondary pigmentary incontinence	Postinflammatory hypermelanoses
Unknown mechanism	Type I ovarian imbalance; feminization syndromes in male dogs; hypothyroidism; hyposomatotropism
Abnormal presence of cells able to synthesize melanin	Melanomas

Table 3. Different Causes of Canine Acanthosis Nigricans

Secondary	
Physical causes	Conformation; obesity
Parasites	Canine scabies; canine demodicosis
Bacteria	Folliculitis
Immunologic causes	Flea-bite hypersensitivity; contact hypersensitivity; atopy; food hypersensitivity
Endocrine causes	Hypothyroidism (primary or secondary); hyperadrenocorticism; hyperestrogenism; hypoandrogenism; diabetes mellitus
Neoplasia (malignant acanthosis nigricans)	Hepatic carcinoma; thyroid carcinoma; pulmonary carcinoma; ovarian and testicular neoplasms; mammary adenocarcinoma
Primary	
Idiopathic (genetic?)	Especially dachshunds

The primary tumors are plaques or nodules of variable diameter (0.5 to 2 cm for the benign melanomas; larger than 2 cm for the malignant melanomas) that may be solitary, multiple, or ulcerated. The color is usually brown or black, but some melanomas are nonpigmented. Malignant melanomas metastasize frequently and quickly to the lungs and sometimes to the kidneys, liver, and bones. The prognosis is based on the size and the microscopic appearance of the tumor (mitotic index, histologic type).

In dogs, *malignant acanthosis nigricans* has been reported rarely in association with malignant neoplasms: hepatic carcinoma, thyroid adenocarcinoma, primary pulmonary carcinoma, ovarian and testicular tumors, or mammary adenocarcinoma with pulmonary metastasis. However, a true cause-and-effect relationship has *not* been established. In humans, 20 per cent of the cases of acanthosis nigricans are associated with visceral cancer. In humans, the pathogenetic hypothesis is a glandular hypersecretion of peptides (by adenocarcinomas or endocrine disorders) that induces hyperkeratosis, epidermal growth, papillomatosis, and epidermal melanosis.

Hypermelanosis of Difficult Classification

Canine acanthosis nigricans is a cutaneous reaction pattern, characterized by symmetric axillary hypermelanosis, lichenification, seborrhea, and alopecia in association with multiple causes (Table 3). Primary idiopathic canine acanthosis nigricans has been described in many breeds, but primarily in dachshunds. The first signs often occur in dogs younger than 1 year of age. Secondary acanthosis nigricans (e.g., secondary to hypersensitivity and endocrine disorders) may occur in any breed.

Editor's Note: *Acromelanism* is normally seen in feline breeds such as Siamese, Himalayan, Balinese, and Birman. The darker-colored "points" (muzzle, pinnae, paws, tail) of these breeds are controlled by a temperature-dependent mechanism that is not completely understood. In areas where the skin temperature decreases (e.g., areas clipped for surgery), hair regrowth is typically, though temporarily, darker (melanotrichia).

References and Supplemental Reading

Cesarini, J. P., and Prunieras, M.: Systeme pigmentaire. Dermatologie 12235A10–11, EMC Paris, France, 1975.

Guaguere, E., Alhaidari, Z., and Ortonne, J. P.: Troubles de la pigmentation melanique en dermatologie des carnivores: 2. Hypomelanoses et amelanoses. Point Vet. 18:5, 1986.

Guaguere, E., Alhaidari, Z., Magnol, J. P., et al.: Troubles de la pigmentation melanique en dermatologie des carnivores: 3. Hypermelanoses. Point Vet. 18:699, 1986.

Muller, G. H., Kirk, R. W., and Scott, D. W.: *Small Animal Dermatology III.* Philadelphia: W. B. Saunders Co., 1983.

Ortonne, J. P.: Biologie du systeme mélanocytaire de la peau. Dermatologie 12235A10–11, EMC Paris, France, 1984.

Scott, D. W.: Lentigo simplex in orange cats. Compan. Anim. Pract. 1:23, 1987.

SPOROTRICHOSIS AND PUBLIC HEALTH

EDMUND J. ROSSER, JR., D.V.M.

East Lansing, Michigan

ETIOLOGY AND DISTRIBUTION

Sporotrichosis is caused by the organism *Sporothrix schenckii*. *Sporothrix* is a dimorphic fungus that exists in mycelial form at environmental temperatures (25 to 30°C) and in yeast form in body tissues (37°C). The organism can be found around the world. It prefers soil rich in decaying organic matter and has also been isolated from *Sphagnum* moss and tree bark.

PATHOGENESIS AND PUBLIC HEALTH SIGNIFICANCE

Traditionally, sporotrichosis has been associated with puncture wounds and exposure to the infectious organism from the environment. In dogs, puncture wounds from thorns and wood splinters have been incriminated; therefore, the disease is more commonly seen in hunting dogs. Cats may be similarly infected; it is also believed that puncture wounds from cat fights and direct innoculation from a contaminated claw can serve as a source of infection (Dunstan et al., 1986). In humans, environmentally contaminated puncture wounds also serve as an important source of infection. The role of human exposure to infected cats has been examined (Dunstan et al., 1986). One unique feature of feline sporotrichosis is the copious numbers of organisms found in examined tissues and exudates as well as the feces of infected cats. This is in contrast to human and canine sporotrichosis in which it is often difficult to demonstrate the presence of the organism. Exposure to an ulcerated wound or exudate of a cat with sporotrichosis is now considered an important mode of infection in humans. Therefore, owners of an infected cat, veterinarians and their assistants, and those involved in the treatment of infected cats are considered the population most at risk for contracting this disease. In many instances, the people acquiring sporotrichosis from contact with infected cats had no known injury or penetrating wound associated with development of the disease. Lesions can occur in apparently uninjured skin. Therefore, it is recommended that people handling cats *suspected* of having sporotrichosis wear gloves, remove the gloves carefully when they are done, and wash forearms, wrists, and hands with either a chlorhexidine or povidone-iodine scrub.

CLINICAL FEATURES

The three clinical forms of sporotrichosis (cutaneolymphatic, cutaneous, and disseminated) often overlap in the same patient. Thus, the more common presentations will be described. In dogs, sporotrichosis presents as a multinodular disease; some of the lesions are ulcerated, with exudation and crust formation primarily affecting the trunk and head. Nodular, draining, and crusted lesions may also be present on the distal aspects of the limbs, with cording of lymphatics proximally and regional lymphadenopathy.

In cats, lesions are most commonly observed on the distal aspects of the limbs, the head, or the tail base (Dunstan et al., 1986). Initially, the lesions are draining puncture wounds similar in appearance to fight wound abscesses or cellulitis. They occur more commonly in intact male cats that go outdoors. Subsequently, nodular lesions with ulceration, exudation, and crust formation develop. Lesions may be so deep as to expose muscle and bone. The disease may be spread when the animal licks its wounds and by normal grooming habits. Multiple lesions on the extremities, face, and ears can occur. Lymphatic involvement may not be evident clinically. However, most necropsies of cats with sporotrichosis reveal evidence of lymph node and lymphatic involvement as well as the disseminated form of the disease (involvement of multiple internal organs) via isolation of the organism from these tissues. In addition, cats and dogs may present with fever, depression, and partial or complete anorexia.

DIAGNOSIS

In addition to the more common clinical presentations of this disease, one should suspect sporotrichosis when an apparent bacterial process does not respond to systemic antibiotics. Exudates should be examined cytologically and stained for fungal organisms, which appear as round, oval, or cigar-shaped pleomorphic yeasts. A culture of the exudate and skin biopsies (one for histopathology and one for macerated tissue culture) should be submitted. In difficult cases, a fluorescent antibody test can also be performed on serum, exudate, or tissue. In feline cases, the organism is readily demonstrated by the aforementioned methods. However, in canine cases, the organism is often difficult to demonstrate, and all the aforementioned procedures may need to be performed more than once before the diagnosis of sporotrichosis is established.

TREATMENT

As previously mentioned, any exudate and tissue should be carefully handled. People handling patients (especially cats) should first be made aware of the infectious potential and should be advised to wear gloves. When the procedures are finished, the gloves should be carefully removed, and washing with a chlorhexidine or povidone-iodine scrub should be performed. The treatment of choice for dogs is KI (saturated solution of potassium iodide [SSKI]), 40 mg/kg t.i.d., with food. It should be administered for 30 days beyond apparent clinical cure. For refractory cases, ketoconazole, 5 to 30 mg/kg given once to twice daily, may be effective. The author has successfully treated one case of canine sporotrichosis with ketoconazole, 15 mg/kg b.i.d. given for 1 month beyond the apparent clinical cure. This required 3 1/2 months of treatment (see p. 578). The treatment of cats with sporotri-

chosis poses a greater challenge because of their greater sensitivity to iodides and the development of iodism. The toxic side effects of ketoconazole, especially anorexia and jaundice, are of concern in cats. The recommended feline dosage for KI (SSKI) is 20 mg/kg b.i.d. given with food, and the dosage for ketoconazole is 5 to 10 mg/kg given once to twice daily. Medical therapy should be continued for 1 month beyond apparent clinical cure, and it may be necessary to switch from one medication to the other as problems with toxicity are observed. In both dogs and cats, the use of glucocorticoids and any other immunosuppressive drugs should be avoided during or after the treatment of this disease. Immunosuppressive doses of glucocorticoids have been shown to cause a recurrence of clinical signs after the disease had apparently resolved (Raimer et al., 1983).

References and Supplemental Reading

Burke, M. J., Grauer, G. F., and Macy, D. W.: Successful treatment of cutaneolymphatic sporotrichosis in a cat with ketoconazole and sodium iodide. J. Am. Anim. Hosp. Assoc. 19:542, 1983.
Dunstan, R. W., Reiman, K. A., and Langham, R. F.: Feline sporotrichosis. J.A.V.M.A. 189:880, 1986.
Dunstan, R. W., Langham, R. F., Reimann, K. A., et al.: Feline sporotrichosis: A report of five cases with transmission to humans. J. Am. Acad. Dermatol. 15:37, 1986.
Muller, G. H., Kirk, R. W., and Scott, D. W.: Fungal diseases. In Muller, G. H., et al.: Small Animal Dermatology, 3rd ed. Philadelphia: W. B. Saunders Co., 1983.
Raimer, S. S., Ewert, A., MacDonald, E. M., et al.: Ketoconazole therapy for experimentally induced sporotrichosis infections in cats: A preliminary study. Curr. Ther. Res. 33:670, 1983.

Section

6

OPHTHALMOLOGIC DISEASES

THOMAS J. KERN, D.V.M.,
and RONALD C. RIIS, D.V.M.

Consulting Editors

Ocular Emergencies...636
Therapeutic Use of Hydrophilic Contact Lenses...........................640
Ophthalmic Usage of Nonsteroidal Anti-inflammatory Agents..............642
Sudden Blindness 644
Medical Therapy for Glaucoma 647
Uveitis 652
Ulcerative Keratitis...656
Neonatal Ophthalmic Disorders 658
Conjunctival Disorders...673
Dermatologic Disorders of the Eyelid and Periocular Region..............678
Ocular Disorders of Rabbits, Rodents, and Ferrets.......................681
The Ophthalmology Referral Patient 686
Neuro-ophthalmology 687
Adnexal Tumors of Dogs and Cats...692

OCULAR EMERGENCIES

SUSAN A. McLAUGHLIN, D.V.M.
Urbana, Illinois

Many ocular emergencies are associated with trauma: either generalized trauma, such as being hit by a car, or localized trauma, such as a cat-scratch injury. Others involve acute pain, sudden change in the appearance of the globe, or loss of vision. Prompt evaluation, accurate assessment, and appropriate therapy may make the difference between sight and blindness, or, in many cases, between saving the eye and having to enucleate it.

PROPTOSIS OF THE GLOBE

A common sequela to head trauma is proptosis of the globe (anterior displacement of the globe beyond the margins of the orbit and eyelids). This occurs more frequently and requires less severe trauma in brachycephalic animals because of the shallowness of the orbit. Proptosis in mesaticephalic and dolichocephalic animals is less common, requires greater force, and is, therefore, frequently associated with more severe injury. Although replacement of a proptosed globe is an emergency situation, the condition of the entire animal must be evaluated before proceeding. Injury to the central nervous system or cardiopulmonary system may preclude general anesthesia. In such cases, the globe is lubricated and protected until the animal is stabilized.

Evaluation of the proptosed eye should include assessment of pupil size and pupillary light reflex (PLR), damage to extraocular muscles, and corneal integrity. In addition, an attempt should be made to determine if the globe is ruptured. Establishing an accurate prognosis for vision is difficult, except when a transected optic nerve can be seen. The presence of a direct PLR in the proptosed eye or an indirect PLR from the proptosed eye to the normal eye is a favorable prognostic sign. A dilated, unresponsive pupil implies a guarded to poor prognosis for vision.

The medial rectus muscle is often ruptured, resulting in lateral strabismus, which persists after replacement of the globe. If there is extensive damage to several extraocular muscles such that the globe is hanging loosely from the orbit, the eye should be enucleated.

Corneal or scleral laceration or marked hypotony of the globe also implies a poor prognosis. In these cases, the globe frequently becomes phthisic. If there is any question about whether to enucleate the globe, it should be replaced in the orbit and the decision made later. Many eyes that appear severely damaged respond well, and most owners prefer a blind eye to enucleation.

Treatment of proptosis is not so much a case of "pushing" the globe back into the orbit as it is of "pulling" the lids out around the globe to cover and protect it until the hemorrhage and edema in the orbital tissues resolve. Under general anesthesia, or with local anesthetic infiltration if general anesthesia is contraindicated, a lateral canthotomy is performed to widen the palpebral fissure. Two or three horizontal mattress sutures of 4–0 silk are preplaced in the eyelid margins; they are tightened and tied while gentle pressure is placed on the globe. To prevent corneal injury from the suture material, sutures are placed so that they do not penetrate the full thickness of the eyelid. The eyelids should remain slightly separated at the medial canthus to allow space to apply medication. The lateral canthotomy is closed in two layers: 4–0 to 6–0 absorbable sutures in the subcutaneous tissue and 4–0 silk in the skin. Depending on the severity of the proptosis, it may be desirable to first place a third eyelid flap or to use stents with the lid sutures.

As the swelling resolves, the sutures may loosen, making it necessary to replace them to prevent trauma to the cornea. The tarsorrhaphy is maintained for 1 to 4 weeks, depending on the amount of orbital swelling present.

Postoperative care includes administration of systemic antibiotics and topical application of antibiotic and 1 per cent atropine ointments. Topical corticosteroids are not recommended. The exposure and drying of the cornea that occurs often leads to sloughing of the corneal epithelium, which cannot be recognized after the tarsorrhaphy is in place. Only after the tarsorrhaphy sutures have been removed and the cornea has been re-evaluated should use of topical steroids be considered.

Possible sequelae to proptosis include lateral strabismus, blindness, phthisis bulbi, glaucoma, keratoconjunctivitis sicca, and lagophthalmos with exposure keratitis.

EYELID LACERATION

Repair of eyelid lacerations is performed with the objective of restoring normal eyelid conformation and function. Débridement should be minimal. The vascular supply to the eyelids is such that even long, thin skin flaps and tissue that appears dry and devitalized may be salvaged in many cases. Wounds near the medial canthus should be evaluated to determine if the nasolacrimal system is involved.

The laceration is sutured in two layers, using 5–0 or 6–0 absorbable suture in a continuous pattern in the conjunctiva and 4–0 or 5–0 nonabsorbable suture in a simple interrupted pattern in the skin. The first skin suture is placed at the eyelid margin to ensure accurate apposition. Aftercare consists of topical and systemic antibiotics for 7 to 10 days. For further details, the reader is referred to a veterinary ophthalmic surgical text.

CORNEAL LACERATION

The prognosis for an eye that has sustained a corneal laceration depends on several factors: the type of trauma (sharp or blunt), the duration of the wound before repair, the length and location of the laceration, and the presence or absence of complicating factors, such as infection, uveal prolapse, lens rupture or extrusion, and vitreous prolapse (Lavach et al., 1984).

If the laceration is small, the anterior chamber has re-formed, and there is no iris prolapse, surgical repair may be unnecessary. Cat-scratch perforation of the cornea frequently occurs in this way. Treatment consists of topical application of 1 per cent atropine and antibiotics administered topically, subconjunctivally, and systemically. Aggressive antibiotic therapy is recommended if a cat-scratch injury to the cornea is suspected (even if no obvious penetration is seen) because devastating endophthalmitis may result from inoculation of organisms into the anterior chamber.

Larger, leaking lacerations require surgical repair under general anesthesia. Clotted blood and fibrin are gently removed from the surface of the cornea. If only a small amount of iris is prolapsed, it can be freed from the wound edge with a cyclodialysis spatula and replaced in the anterior chamber. Iris that appears contaminated, traumatized, or necrotic is amputated level with the corneal surface. The anterior chamber is irrigated with balanced salt solution (BSS, Alcon) to remove blood and fibrin. If the lens is ruptured or dislocated, it is removed. Vitreous in the anterior chamber should be removed. The laceration is sutured with simple interrupted sutures of 6–0 to 8–0 polygalactin (Vicryl, Ethicon). Sutures should be placed to a depth of two thirds of the corneal thickness. If the wound cannot be tightly sealed by suturing alone or if the corneal stroma is friable or necrotic, a conjunctival flap is placed over the wound after suturing. The anterior chamber is reformed with air or a combination of air and balanced salt solution. A guarded prognosis is always given because of possible lens laceration.

Postoperative care consists of topical application of 1 per cent atropine and broad-spectrum antibiotics administered topically, subconjunctivally, and systemically. Systemic nonsteroidal anti-inflammatory drugs may also be used.

CORNEAL ULCERATION

Superficial corneal ulcers with no evidence of stromal infiltrate to suggest infection can be treated by topical application of broad-spectrum antibiotic ointment or drops (neomycin-bacitracin-polymyxin B combination or chloramphenicol, b.i.d. to q.i.d.) and 1 per cent atropine ointment (b.i.d.).

Deep or melting corneal ulcers and descemetoceles require more aggressive treatment. The patient must be handled carefully to avoid placing any pressure on the eye that might cause rupture. Sedation or general anesthesia may be needed to facilitate examination and initial treatment. Samples are collected for gram staining, cytologic examination, and bacterial culture and sensitivity testing. Scrapings and swabs should be taken from the periphery of the lesion, as that is where the highest concentration of organisms is found.

Because medical therapy must be started before results of bacterial culture and sensitivity testing are available, the initial choice of antibiotic depends on the history, clinical findings, results of Gram stains, and the reported incidence and antibiotic sensitivities of various organisms. Therapy is modified, if necessary, based on the subsequent bacterial culture and sensitivity results and the clinical response. *Staphylococcus* sp. and *Streptococcus* sp. are the organisms most commonly recovered from dogs with extraocular disease (Gerding et al., 1988; Murphy et al., 1978). Beta-hemolytic streptococci can produce a slowly progressive, melting corneal ulcer. *Pseudomonas* sp. is recovered from approximately 10 per cent of dogs with extraocular disease (Gerding et al., 1988; Murphy et al., 1978). This organism produces a rapidly progressive melting corneal ulcer, which can lead to perforation and endophthalmitis in a matter of hours.

If *Pseudomonas* infection is suspected, gentamicin (Gentocin ophthalmic solution, Schering) or tobramycin (Tobrex, Alcon) drops should be applied topically every hour until signs of stromal liquefaction abate. Subconjunctival injection of 0.1 ml of gentamicin (Gentocin solution, Schering, 50 mg/ml s.i.d.) or tobramycin (Nebcin, Eli Lilly; 40 mg/ml s.i.d.) will produce therapeutic levels of drug in the cornea and is especially recommended if intensive topical therapy cannot be maintained. When gram-positive infection is suspected, topical treatment with chloramphenicol, erythromycin (Ilotycin, Dista), or a neomycin-bacitracin-polymyxin B combination is recommended along with subconjunctival injection of chloramphenicol (Chloromycetin sodium succinate, Parke-Davis) or cephalothin (Keflin, Eli Lilly). Because of the potential for endophthalmitis, a compatible antibiotic is administered parenterally at conventional doses. Atropine, 1 per cent, is also administered topically b.i.d. to provide cycloplegia.

Many deep corneal ulcers and descemetoceles benefit from some form of surgical correction or reinforcement. Small descemetoceles (1 to 2 mm in diameter) may be closed with 6–0 absorbable suture. Larger defects may be sealed with a conjunctival flap (Hakanson and Meredith, 1987) or sliding corneal graft (McLaughlin et al., 1984).

Deep corneal ulcers frequently benefit from placement of a third eyelid flap, which will provide warmth, moisture, and support to the infected cornea. Although this prevents direct observation of the cornea, the animal's condition can be assessed by observing the amount of ocular discharge and the degree of discomfort, as indicated by the presence or absence of blepharospasm. If the single-button third eyelid flap technique (Helper and Blogg, 1983) is used, the third eyelid can be lowered when direct examination of the cornea is deemed necessary. Deep corneal ulcers may also benefit from débridement of necrotic, infected stroma followed by placement of a conjunctival flap or corneal grafting.*

ACUTE GLAUCOMA

Glaucoma should be considered as one of the differential diagnoses in any case in which the owner's presenting complaint is a "red eye," "cloudy eye," or "watery eye," especially in one of the predisposed breeds. Other signs of glaucoma include dilated, unresponsive pupil; shallow anterior chamber; enlarged globe (buphthalmos); optic disk cupping; and retinal atrophy. By the time buphthalmos, optic disk cupping, or retinal atrophy is seen, the prognosis for vision is grave. Acute glaucoma rarely develops in both eyes simultaneously, so loss of vision is not a common complaint. Ocular pain is not a prominent sign unless the lens is luxated and trapped in the pupil. Anterior lens luxation should be suspected in terriers with ocular pain and a steamy, nonulcerated cornea.

Definitive diagnosis of glaucoma depends on measurement of elevated intraocular pressure. Schiøtz tonometer readings of less than 3 with a 5.5-gm weight are indicative of elevated pressure. If the tonometer reading is 0, the 10-gm weight

should be used to more accurately estimate the intraocular pressure.

Treatment should be started immediately with intravenous mannitol (1–2 gm/kg of 15 or 20 per cent solution), which reduces intraocular pressure by its action as an osmotic diuretic. Water should be withheld for 4 to 6 hr after administration of mannitol and then given in small amounts for the next 12 hr so that rehydration is gradual. Reduction in intraocular pressure as a result of mannitol administration is usually seen within 4 hr.

At the same time, treatment aimed at reducing aqueous production and increasing facility of outflow is started. A carbonic anhydrase inhibitor is given orally to reduce aqueous production (dichlorphenamide [Daranide, Merck, Sharp & Dohme], 1 to 2 mg/kg b.i.d. to t.i.d., or acetazolamide [Diamox, Lederle], 5 to 10 mg/kg b.i.d. to t.i.d.), and a miotic is applied topically to increase aqueous outflow (0.25 per cent demecarium bromide [Humorsol, Merck, Sharp & Dohme] or 0.125 per cent echothiophate iodide [Phospholine Iodide, Ayerst], every hour for 4 hr then b.i.d., or pilocarpine, 2 per cent every hour for 4 hr then q.i.d.).

If uveitis is present concurrently with glaucoma, topical or subconjunctival corticosteroids are administered after the possibility of an infectious cause of the uveitis is eliminated. If the lens is luxated anteriorly, miotics are not used and surgical removal of the lens is performed as soon as possible. If the lens is trapped in the pupil (pupillary block), one drop of 1 per cent tropicamide (Mydriacyl, Alcon) is applied and the intraocular pressure is measured in 20 to 30 min. The resulting dilation of the pupil may break the pupillary block and aid in reduction of intraocular pressure.

UVEITIS

Acute uveitis is another differential diagnosis to consider when the owner's presenting complaint is a "red eye" or "cloudy eye." One method of differentiating between uveitis and glaucoma is tonometry. The intraocular pressure will generally be lower than normal in cases of uveitis (i.e., Schiøtz tonometer readings greater than 12 with a 5.5-gm weight). Other signs of uveitis are miotic pupil, deep circumlimbal neovascularization of the cornea, iris inflammation, and aqueous flare or hypopyon.

Acute uveitis may be the result of exogenous causes (trauma and corneal ulceration) or endogenous disease (septicemia, neoplasia, and immune-mediated processes). Symptomatic treatment consists of topical application of a mydriatic-cycloplegic agent (1 per cent atropine or 10 per cent phenylephrine combined with 0.3 per cent scopolamine [Murocoll-2, Muro]) and an antibiotic-steroid combination (unless corneal ulceration is present). Sys-

---

*Editor's Note: Conjunctival flaps are preferred by some ophthalmologists.

temic or subconjunctival corticosteroid therapy should be withheld until infectious causes of uveitis have been ruled out. Specific treatment depends on determining the underlying cause of the disease.

ORBITAL CELLULITIS/ABSCESS

Orbital inflammation occurs in the dog and cat as either diffuse orbital cellulitis or an orbital abscess. The cause can be difficult to identify, but several different causes have been documented: penetrating foreign bodies entering the orbital area via the mouth, skin, or conjunctival sac; penetrating wounds, especially bite wounds; and extension of infection from diseased upper molar teeth or sinuses.

The onset of signs is usually rapid. Clinical signs include exophthalmos, chemosis, elevation of the third eyelid, exposure keratitis, pain on opening the mouth, and fever. Examination of the mouth (which may require sedation or general anesthesia) may reveal a red swelling or a draining tract behind the last upper molar.

The primary differential diagnosis for orbital cellulitis/abscess is orbital neoplasia. The clinical signs associated with orbital tumors usually develop more slowly than those associated with inflammatory orbital disease. Exophthalmos with elevation of the third eyelid is common, and the globe may be deviated depending on the location of the mass. The globe cannot be digitally repositioned in the orbit because of the presence of a space-occupying lesion. Usually there is no pain elicited by opening the mouth. Examination of the mouth may reveal intraoral extension of the tumor in the area of the last upper molar.

Treatment of orbital cellulitis/abscess consists of establishing drainage, controlling infection, and minimizing inflammation. Under anesthesia, an incision is made behind the last upper molar and a blunt probe or a closed hemostat is advanced slowly into the retrobulbar area. If purulent material is released from the retrobulbar area, specimens should be submitted for bacterial culture and sensitivity testing. The area is flushed with sterile saline, crystalline penicillin solution, or a dilute solution of povidone-iodine using a blunt needle or lacrimal cannula. Systemic antibiotics are administered postoperatively. Hot packs to reduce orbital swelling and symptomatic treatment for exposure keratitis (antibiotic ointment, artificial tears, and third eyelid flap) are applied as needed.

Improvement in clinical signs is frequently seen following this procedure, although some cases require 1 to 2 weeks to return to normal. Failure to improve or recurrence of clinical signs suggests the presence of a foreign body or neoplasia. In these cases, further diagnostic evaluation is required and orbital exploratory surgery may be necessary.

HYPHEMA

Hyphema (blood in the anterior chamber) can occur as the result of trauma, uveitis, glaucoma, retinal detachment, neoplasia, systemic disease, or clotting disorders. The results of careful historical evaluation, physical and ophthalmic examination, and appropriate laboratory tests (complete blood count and clotting profile) are considered when attempting to determine an etiology and establish a prognosis.

If a clotting disorder is the cause of the bleeding, hemorrhages are usually found elsewhere (e.g., mucous membranes of the mouth, vulva, and penis). Hyphema that is the result of trauma usually clots and begins to resolve within a few days, with complete resolution in 1 to 2 weeks. Hyphema that does not clot and persists longer than 2 to 3 weeks may be caused by retinal detachment or intraocular neoplasia.

Symptomatic therapy is aimed at treatment of the inflammation caused by the presence of blood in the anterior chamber. This includes topical application of an antibiotic-steroid agent and 1 per cent atropine for cycloplegia and mydriasis. Because hyphema may result in secondary glaucoma, intraocular pressure (IOP) should be monitored and a carbonic anhydrase inhibitor used if elevation in IOP occurs.

ACUTE VISION LOSS

Sudden loss of vision can occur as the result of optic neuritis, bilateral retinal detachment, sudden acquired retinal degeneration, bilateral hyphema or vitreous hemorrhage, or bilateral uveitis with extremely miotic pupils and severe inflammatory exudation into the anterior chamber (see also p. 644).

Diagnosis depends on a complete ophthalmic and physical examination. The reader is referred to a general ophthalmology text for treatment of the various diseases.

References and Supplemental Reading

Gerding, P. A., McLaughlin, S. A., and Troop, M. W.: Pathogenic bacteria and fungi associated with external ocular diseases in dogs: 131 cases (1981–1986). J.A.V.M.A. 193:242, 1988.

Hakanson, N. E., and Meredith, R. E.: Conjunctival pedicle grafting in the treatment of corneal ulcers in the dog and cat. J. Am. Anim. Hosp. Assoc. 23:641, 1987.

Helper, L. C., and Blogg, R.: A modified third eyelid flap procedure. J. Am. Anim. Hosp. Assoc. 19:955, 1983.

Lavach, J. D., Severin, G. A., and Roberts, S. M.: Lacerations of the equine eye: A review of 48 cases. J.A.V.M.A. 184:1243, 1984.

McLaughlin, S. A., Brightman, A. H., Brogdon, J. D., et al.: Autogenous partial thickness corneal grafting in the dog. Transactions 15th Annual Scientific Meeting, ACVO, 1984.

Murphy, J. M., Lavach, J. D., and Severin, G. A.: Survey of conjunctival flora in dogs with clinical signs of external eye disease. J.A.V.M.A. 172:66, 1978.

THERAPEUTIC USE OF HYDROPHILIC CONTACT LENSES

KOHLE HERRMANN, D.V.M.

Houston, Texas

Hydrophilic or soft contact lenses have been available since 1960. Since their introduction, hydrophilic lenses have been improved greatly and have been adapted for use in small animals. Veterinary literature is sparse with regard to the use of soft contact lenses. Most reports have described their use for treatment of indolent ulcers.

LENS CHARACTERISTICS AND ADVANTAGES

Hydrophilic contact lenses are made of polymers capable of absorbing substantial quantities of water. Most hydrophilic lenses are made of chemically cross-linked acrylic polymers; cross-linkage adds stability to the lens. These polymers swell with the use of a solvent to form a gel whose water content at saturation can vary, depending on (1) solubility of the non–cross-linked polymers, (2) number of cross-links, and (3) nature of the aqueous solution in which the gel is equilibrated. If the molecular weight of a substance is less than 500, it can enter the interstices of a hydrogel lens. Bacteria and viruses cannot penetrate intact hydrogel contact lenses. In general, the average diameter of the spaces within the lens increases directly in proportion to the water content, from approximately 38 per cent (Bausch & Lomb) to 79 per cent (American Hospital–Sauflon). The Duragel lens (Veterinary Hydrophilics, Inc., P.O. Box 616, Edgewood, MD 21040) contains 72 per cent water by weight. Lenses vary in diameter from 13.5 mm to 18 mm, with the 14.5-mm or 15.5-mm lens being the most common size used in small animal medicine.

Hydrophilic lenses, if fitted properly, relieve pain, help promote epithelial growth, and protect the epithelium from the abrasive action of the lid margins. The lenses can absorb medication and prolong contact time to the cornea.

FITTING THE LENS

The major concerns for fitting the lens are stability, curvature, and thickness. The stability is largely related to the diameter of the lens. The lens ideally should extend from limbus to limbus. The steeper lens (smaller radius of curvature) usually exhibits more adherence and stability. The weight of the lens depends on the thickness. It is more desirable to have a thin lens. Fitting the lens sometimes is done by trial and error. The lens must be fitted under the nictitating membrane to avoid loss. The hands should be thoroughly washed before handling the lens. The lens can be placed on the cornea with the fingers, or by using a cotton-tipped applicator, or by using a smooth-tipped forceps. Topical anesthetic is used before attempting to insert the lens. All the air bubbles must be removed, as they will cause the lens to be displaced. Depending on the fit of the lens and the prominence of the globe, it may be necessary to perform a temporary lateral tarsorrhaphy to keep the lens in place.

INDICATIONS

Hydrophilic contact lenses have primarily been used for the treatment of indolent ulcers. After the devitalized epithelium has been removed, a hydrophilic lens is inserted. Topical solution medications can be used after insertion. Lenses should be removed, cleaned, sterilized, and reinserted every 7 to 10 days.

Hydrophilic lenses have been beneficial in treating spastic entropion. They protect the cornea from the abrasive action of the lids while the corneal epithelium heals. If spastic entropion has not been present for a prolonged period of time, surgery may be avoided. In entropion cases requiring surgery, the corneal protection provided by soft contact lenses helps to minimize postoperative pain and complications.

Soft contact lenses can be used to maintain corneal integrity and prevent perforation of descemetoceles. This allows the veterinarian to delay emergency surgery until patient assessment is completed or referral is made.

Soft contact lenses may be beneficial in older dogs exhibiting degenerative noninfected descemetoceles by acting as bandages to help prevent rupture. Older animals may be poor anesthetic risks, and the contact lens affords the veterinarian an alternative treatment. The lenses should be removed, cleaned, sterilized, and reinserted at 4-week intervals to help prevent complications.

It is reported that active bacterial infections are a contraindication for hydrophilic lenses, although the author has used soft lenses in these disease entities with good results. The ulcer is first débrided with a razor blade or iris scissors. Next, the cornea is swabbed vigorously with povidone-iodine (Betadine Solution, Purdue-Frederick) on a sterile cotton-tipped applicator. The ulcer is then treated topically with 1 per cent gentamicin and 1 per cent atropine solutions. After being air dried for 10 to 15 min and then soaked in a gentamicin solution (50 mg/ml) for approximately 15 min, the lens is placed on the cornea. Gentamicin or another appropriate antibiotic is injected subconjunctivally. A lateral tarsorrhaphy is used to help keep the lens in place. This allows the veterinarian the opportunity to observe the cornea during the healing process, and, if complications arise, appropriate measures can be taken quickly. The soft contact lens should be cleansed, replaced, and resoaked in antibiotics every 5 to 7 days. A high-water-content lens should be used, as it will absorb more medication. A lens that is 70 per cent water would be the best.

CONTRAINDICATIONS AND COMPLICATIONS

Contraindications to hydrophilic bandage lenses are the presence of active bacterial or fungal infection and the lack of adequate follow-up capability. The animal should be kept in a clean environment so as not to get foreign material on or under the lens. If there is a blepharitis, it must be treated vigorously so a hostile environment for the bandage lens is lessened. One must make sure there is adequate tear production or the lens will dry out and be ineffective.

Complications that arise from hydrophilic lens use are discomfort, intolerance, secondary infection, and neovascularization. In humans, giant papillary conjunctivitis has also been reported as a complication. Fluorescein and epinephrine should not be used topically with a lens in place as they will discolor the lens. In animals, the most common complication is loss of the lens.

CLEANING AND DISINFECTING THE LENS

When the lenses are shipped, they have been autoclaved and are sterile. Cleaning is necessary after use to remove mucus and other deposits that accumulate on the lens surface. Both surfaces of the lens must be cleaned before disinfecting (Opticlean II, Alcon). Either heat (Boil–Soak, Alcon) or chemical disinfection (Flex Care, Alcon) can be used, but the user should not alterate between the two methods.

References and Supplemental Reading

Aquavella, J. V.: Therapeutic uses of hydrophilic contact lenses in corneal disease. *In* Leibowitz, H. M. (ed.): *Corneal Disorders, Clinical Diagnosis and Management.* Philadelphia: W. B. Saunders, 1984, pp. 652–677.

Morgan, R. V., Bachrach, J. A., and Ogilvie, G. H.: An evaluation of soft contact lens usage in the dog and cat. J. Am. Anim. Hosp. Assoc. 20:885, 1984.

Nasisse, M. P.: Canine ulcerative keratitis. Comp. Cont. Ed. Pract. Vet. 7:686, 1985.

Schmidt, G. M., Blanchard, G. L., and Keller, W. F.: The use of hydrophilic contact lenses on corneal diseases of the dog and cat: A preliminary report. J. Small Anim. Pract. 18:773, 1977.

Startup, F. G.: Corneal ulceration in the dog. J. Small Anim. Pract. 25:737, 1984.

OPHTHALMIC USAGE OF NONSTEROIDAL ANTI-INFLAMMATORY AGENTS

SHERYL GREVE KROHNE, D.V.M.
and W. A. VESTRE, D.V.M.
West Lafayette, Indiana

Nonsteroidal anti-inflammatory drugs (NSAIDs) have a different mechanism of action than corticosteroids for suppressing ocular inflammation. The NSAIDs function by irreversibly binding to and inhibiting enzymes in one branch of the arachidonic acid cascade. This enzyme inhibition blocks the formation of prostaglandins (PGs), including PGE and PGF_{2a}, which are involved in ocular inflammation. These PGs cause conjunctival hyperemia; leukocyte migration; and congestion of the iris vasculature, resulting in breakdown of the blood aqueous barrier and aqueous flare. They may cause ocular hypertension and miosis. Ocular PGs can also be responsible for vascular congestion and leakage in the posterior segment, with subsequent subretinal exudates (Bhattacherjee, 1980). PGs are proving to be important inflammatory mediators in all organ systems, accounting for the need and active search for pharmacologic inhibitors.

Efficacious usage of NSAIDs to treat ocular disease is possible when they are used alone or in combination with other drugs. Used alone, they may have 100 per cent efficacy at blocking mild inflammation if the inflammation is entirely PG mediated. More commonly, they show 35 to 80 per cent effectiveness in clinical disease that is caused by the interaction of several inflammatory intermediates. NSAIDs are able to suppress superficial ocular inflammation without markedly interfering with wound healing. They have been shown to slow corneal epithelialization and neovascularization, but, unlike corticosteroids, they do not substantially decrease corneal or scleral wound strength. Thus NSAIDs provide another treatment option when corneal or intraocular inflammation must be controlled and a corneal wound or incision is present. Frequently, NSAIDs are used in combination with corticosteroid treatments. The result is greater inflammatory suppression than if either drug is used alone. Sometimes the effect is synergistic. Corticosteroids act by decreasing arachidonic acid's availability as a substrate, thus minimizing inflammatory intermediate formation from the entire cascade. This mode of action is different from that of the PGs, accounting for the success of combined therapies (Krohne and Vestre, 1987). Many of the NSAIDs also have an analgesic effect. Their usage thus minimizes self-trauma, which may contribute to the chronicity or worsening of the ocular disease. The mechanism of action by suppression of specific inflammatory intermediates, accompanied by analgesia, makes NSAIDs invaluable in the treatment of ocular inflammation.

The NSAIDs have relatively few deleterious systemic side effects because, unlike corticosteroids, they are not long-lived circulating endogenous hormones with multiple metabolic and organ system functions. Unlike corticosteroids, they do not suppress the pituitary-adrenal axis. Their side effects are a function of their antiprostaglandin activity, which may include gastrointestinal irritation, bleeding, and ulceration. Occasionally, longer bleeding times have been documented with their usage as a result of inhibited thromboxane synthesis.

Types of ocular inflammation that can be treated successfully with NSAIDs include conjunctivitis, keratitis, anterior uveitis, chorioretinitis, and panophthalmitis (Table 1). PGs are probably involved in both neuronal and non-neuronal inflammation, therefore NSAIDs are effective to differing degrees when treating ocular inflammation induced by either of these pathways. Active inflammation with minimal structural alteration frequently responds well to NSAIDs alone, and active inflammation with minimal to severe structural alterations responds well to combination therapy with NSAIDs and corticosteroids (Bistner and Shaw, 1983).

NSAIDs are most effective when used prophylactically (e.g., presurgically) to inhibit PG formation, thus preventing much of the inflammatory reaction from developing. Without treatment, ocular inflammation can quickly intensify, causing severe and irreversible structural changes, which may interfere with vision. In cases of inflammation due to trauma, systemic disease, infection, and idiopathic causes, immediate initiation of therapy is ideal. The endogenous mechanisms that control and limit PG formation in the uvea become inoperative if the uveitis becomes severe and chronic. This breakdown in internal control is hypothesized to be

Table 1. Ocular Disease and Nonsteroidal Anti-inflammatory Treatment

Ocular Condition	Propionic Acid Derivatives	Aspirin	Phenylbutazone	Flunixin Meglumine	Indomethacin
Allergic or traumatic conjunctivitis and/or chemosis	T, S	S	S	S	S
Thermal or chemical corneal burns	T, S	S	S	S	S
Corneal graft rejections or reactions	—	—	—	—	S
Corneal neovascularization	T	—	—	—	—
Corneal ulceration	S	S, T	S	S	S, T
Scleritis or episcleritis	—	—	S	—	S
Uveitis (acute)	S, T	S	S	S	S
Recurrent uveitis	S	S	S	S	S
Blood aqueous barrier breakdown (flare, fibrin)	S, T	S	S	S, SC	S, T
Chorioretinitis	S	S	S	S	S
Endophthalmitis or panophthalmitis	S	S	S	S	S
Presurgical treatment for intraocular procedures	T, S	S	S	—	T, S
Trauma to globe (accidental or postoperative)	S, T	S	S	S	T, S

S, systemic; T, topical; SC, subconjunctival bulbar injection.

one of the mechanisms involved in the pathogenesis of recurrent uveitis. Timely NSAID usage effectively blocks the arachidonic acid cascade and reduces the possibility of recurrent uveitis. *De novo* enzyme synthesis must then take place to overcome the irreversible enzyme inhibition caused by these drugs. Although the underlying cause of the disease must be identified and treated, appropriate concurrent symptomatic anti-inflammatory therapy is critical to limit visual axis damage while a diagnostic protocol is followed to determine the underlying etiology.

TOPICAL NSAID USAGE

Superficial and anterior segment inflammatory diseases can be effectively treated with flurbiprofen (a propionic acid derivative) or indomethacin. Flurbiprofen (Ocufen, Allergan) has excellent ocular penetration and is not metabolized by the eye, allowing high ocular bioavailability. Clinical trials have shown its efficacy for treating keratitis and anterior uveitis. These drugs can be used when corneal ulceration is present but necessitate frequent re-evaluations of healing because they may delay corneal neovascularization and epithelialization. This effect is less pronounced than the delay caused by topical corticosteroids, and the topical NSAIDs (unlike corticosteroids) have not been shown to potentiate collagenase activity. Flurbiprofen prevents miosis due to anterior segment inflammation but has not consistently inhibited changes in intraocular pressure. Topical flurbiprofen may prove more effective for chronic control of recurrent uveitis than in the treatment of acute superficial disease. Topical usage of these drugs potentiates the leukotriene pathway in the conjunctiva and thus

may cause an increase in number of leukocytes in the inflamed area. Therefore, inflammatory exudate must be monitored. A dosage of one drop of ophthalmic solution is used at a frequency consistent with the degree of inflammation and chronicity of the disease. Dosage frequencies are similar to those for topical 0.1 per cent dexamethasone (Krohne and Vestre, 1987). Topical indomethacin is not yet commercially available, but it may be used topically by making a 1 per cent solution in artificial tears. Topical drug delivery of flunixin meglumine (Banamine, Schering) is possible using bulbar subconjunctival injections of 5.0 to 25.0 mg s.i.d. This treatment should be reserved for severe, acute anterior uveitis in dogs because this treatment route, although effective, causes a severe inflammatory reaction at the injection site. Flunixin meglumine is toxic to cats.

SYSTEMIC NSAID USAGE

Aspirin, flunixin meglumine, and phenylbutazone are the most frequently used systemic NSAIDs in ophthalmology. The routes and dosages are given in Table 2. The systemic route is most effective when treating uveal diseases. The therapy should be initiated at the maximum dosage indicated for the severity of the disease. Combined NSAID and corticosteroid therapy is indicated when uveal inflammation is severe and contraindications are not present. Maximum dosages of both drugs may be used initially (Krohne and Vestre, 1987). Tapering of anti-inflammatory drug dosage following acute high-dose treatment is essential to prevent ocular rebound inflammation and systemic side effects. Flunixin meglumine is an effective ocular NSAID when used initially, but this drug and high-dose

Table 2. *Systemic Nonsteroidal Anti-inflammatory Drugs*

Drug	Concentration	Dosage Regimen*	Route
Flunixin meglumine	50 mg/ml	Dog: 1.0–2.0 mg/kg once a day for maximum of 3 days	IV
	Not applicable	Cat: do not use	Not applicable
Aspirin	5 gr = 325-mg tablet; 1.25 gr (children's aspirin) = 81 mg	Dog: 10 mg/kg twice a day Cat: 1.25 gr every 48–72 hr (watch for toxicity)	PO
Phenylbutazone	200 mg/ml; 100-mg tablets; 100-mg capsules	Dog: 40 mg/kg three times a day Cat: 10–14 mg/kg twice a day	PO

*Higher doses should not be used, as an increase in efficacy does not occur and the risk of toxicity does increase.

phenylbutazone should not be used on a long-term basis because of the possibility of gastrointestinal ulceration. Initial therapy may be followed by long-term, low-dose oral aspirin or phenylbutazone treatment regimens to suppress recurrent or rebound inflammatory reactions.

References and Supplemental Reading

Bhattacherjee, P.: Prostaglandins and inflammatory reactions in the eye. Methods Find. Exp. Clin. Pharmacol. 2:17, 1980.

Bistner, S., and Shaw, D.: Intraocular inflammation. In Kirk, R. W. (ed.): *Current Veterinary Therapy VIII.* Philadelphia, W. B. Saunders, 1983, p. 582.

Brightman, A. H., Helper, L. C., and Hoffman, W. E.: Effect of aspirin on aqueous protein values in the dog. J.A.V.M.A. 178:572, 1981.

Krohne, S. D., and Vestre, W. A.: Effects of flunixin meglumine and dexamethasone on aqueous protein values after intraocular surgery in the dog. Am. J. Vet. Res. 48:420, 1986.

Krohne, S. D., and Vestre, W. A.: Ocular use of antiinflammatory drugs in companion animals. Comp. Cont. Ed. Pract. Vet. 9:1085, 1987.

Masuda, K.: Anti-inflammatory agents: Nonsteroidal anti-inflammatory drugs. In Sears, M. (ed.): *Pharmacology of the Eye.* Vol 69. New York, Springer-Verlag, 1984, p. 539.

Regnier, A., Bonnefoi, M., and Lescure, F.: Effect of lysine-acetylsalicylate and phenylbutazone premedication on the protein content of secondary aqueous humour in the dog. Res. Vet. Sci. 37:26, 1984.

Regnier, A., Whitley, R. D., Benard, P., and Bonnefoi, M.: Effect of flunixin meglumine on the breakdown of the blood-aqueous barrier following paracentesis in the canine eye. J. Ocular Pharmacol. 2:165, 1986.

SUDDEN BLINDNESS

MARJORIE H. NEADERLAND, D.V.M.

Ithaca, New York, and *Norwalk, Connecticut*

This article discusses the evaluation and treatment of canine and feline patients with sudden loss of vision, dilated pupils, and insufficient ophthalmoscopically evident disease to account for their blindness.

Obtaining a thorough history from the owner and performing a general physical, ophthalmoscopic, and neurologic examination is vital for determination of the location of a lesion causing acute blindness with dilated pupils. In addition, maze testing and careful menace testing may reveal visual field deficiencies. This should be done with one of the patient's eyes blindfolded or covered and the exposed eye stimulated from the nasal and temporal parts of each visual field. Care should be taken to prevent air currents from stimulating a corneal reflex, causing the animal to blink. Pupillary light reflexes, both direct (constriction of the pupil in the eye being tested) and consensual or indirect (constriction of the pupil in the eye not being stimulated) should be tested with a strong light source. Measurement of intraocular pressure should be performed to rule out glaucoma as the cause of blindness.

A lesion producing both blindness and pupillary deficits must be located in the portions of the visual pathway shared by the pupillary reflex pathway. Structures common to the visual and pupillary light reflex pathways include the retina, optic nerves, optic chiasm, and optic tracts.

RETINAL DISEASE

Sudden Acquired Retinal Degeneration

The syndrome of sudden acquired retinal degeneration (SARD) has also been termed silent retina syndrome and metabolic toxic retinopathy. It is characterized clinically by the sudden onset of total blindness with moderately to widely dilated pupils that are minimally responsive to light. Ophthalmoscopically, the retina appears normal, and only after the animal has been blind for a few months are fundus changes obvious. Blindness, as perceived by the owners, occurred within 24 hr to less than 4 weeks.

The "typical" SARD patient is a purebred or mixed breed dog, middle aged, and moderately overweight. Often polyuria, polydipsia, and polyphagia have been observed from about the same time that the blindness became apparent. Many of the dogs with SARD have been found to have elevated serum alkaline phosphatase, serum aspartate aminotransferase, serum cholesterol, or serum bilirubin levels. These findings may be indicative of a physiologic hyperadrenolcorticism with secondary steroid-induced hepatopathy, a response of the body to a systemic stress. Dogs from both urban and rural areas are affected. The syndrome occurs year round, with a slight increase in incidence noted in December and January.

SARD is an acute, irreversible retinal degeneration characterized histologically by a rapid loss of photoreceptor outer segments, both rods and cones, followed by a slow degeneration of the remaining retinal layers. The diagnostic test that distinguishes SARD from optic neuritis is the electroretinogram (ERG), which reveals absence of retinal function. A recordable ERG is present with optic neuritis. An unrecordable ERG performed at the onset of blindness confirms the diagnosis of SARD. It is recommended that the ERG be performed early in the diagnostic workup, because, if the ERG response is not extinguished, SARD may be ruled out and further tests are indicated to pursue the cause of the blindness.

In SARD, the rods and cones appear to be equally affected; this is in contrast to hereditary retinal degenerations in which rods and cones may be affected differentially. The clinical signs of progressive retinal atrophy (PRA), regardless of the breed affected, begin as defective night vision with progressive loss of day vision. Although the onset of blindness, as recognized by the owner, may appear to be sudden, visual loss with PRA has been gradual, with the animal adjusting to its environment but appearing to be suddenly blind in a unfamiliar setting. Ophthalmoscopically, PRA is characterized initially by peripheral retinal vascular attenuation and altered tapetal reflectivity, slowly progressing to severe vascular attenuation, tapetal hyper-reflectivity, and optic nerve atrophy. Pupillary light reflexes are often normal until late in the disease. Secondary cataract formation frequently follows PRA in some breeds.

Later in the course of SARD, when significant retinal degeneration has occurred, it may be difficult to distinguish SARD from PRA ophthalmoscopically. ERG evaluation for cone-mediated responses may prove diagnostic for PRA.

The etiologic agent of SARD has not been identified, nor have treatments been identified that have halted or reversed the progressive retinal degeneration. This syndrome is not responsive to corticosteroid administration, which also may help to distinguish it from inflammatory conditions causing similar clinical signs.

Retinal Detachment

Complete bilateral retinal detachments can be a cause of acute blindness with dilated, unresponsive pupils. Causes of retinal detachment include congenital lesions (associated with collie eye anomaly or retinal dysplasia), trauma, infections (systemic/ocular bacterial, viral, mycotic, algal), neoplasia (lymphosarcoma), immune-mediated inflammation (Vogt-Koyanagi-Harada, hyperviscosity syndromes), metabolic defects (due to renal disease [hypertension, hypoalbuminemia, hyponatremia]), toxins (ethylene glycol), or idiopathic factors. Complete detachments are often visible with a penlight. The diagnosis can otherwise be made with direct or indirect ophthalmoscopy. The detached retina appears as a veil-like structure with blood vessels, and, depending on the etiology, a variable amount of hemorrhage or exudates behind the lens.

Diagnostic evaluation to determine the nature of the underlying disease process should include general physical examination, hemogram, serum chemistry panel, and urinalysis. The presence of a retinal granulomatous process with a cellular exudate should raise suspicion of a mycotic agent. Thoracic radiography may be beneficial in the diagnosis of a mycotic or neoplastic process.

The syndrome most responsive to therapy is idiopathic serous retinal detachment, a presumed immune-mediated disease occurring in an otherwise healthy animal. In this disease, inflammation of the choroid causes serous fluid to accumulate and detach the sensory retina from the retinal pigment epithelium. Therapy for idiopathic bullous retinal detachment includes rest (with or without tranquilization) and administration of immunosuppressive levels of systemic corticosteroids (prednisone, 2.2 mg/kg s.i.d.) and diuretics (furosemide, 2.2 mg/kg s.i.d., for 1 to 2 weeks), noting response to therapy and slowly tapering the corticosteroid dose afterward. Administration of broad-spectrum antibiotics is recommended during immunosuppression. After diagnosis and treatment, detached retinas caused by systemic conditions, such as hypertension, ethylene glycol intoxication, or immune-mediated diseases, may reattach. Surgical techniques for retinal detachment include scleral diathermy, retinocryopexy, and scleral buckling. A guarded prognosis for complete return of vision should be given whatever the cause of the detachment, as the retina begins to degenerate within 12 hr of detachment. However, vision has been restored with therapy to eyes detached for as long as 6 weeks. The retina may reattach following successful treatment or spontaneously. Some degeneration is to be expected.

OPTIC NERVE, OPTIC CHIASM, AND OPTIC TRACT DISEASES

After retinal function has been established, suggesting that the lesion lies between the optic disk and the optic tracts, diagnostic tests that need to be pursued to identify the category of disease responsible for the clinical manifestations should include hemogram, serum chemistry panel, skull radiographs, and cerebrospinal fluid (CSF) examination. Brain scan with radioisotopes, computed tomography, and nuclear magnetic resonance imaging would be helpful in localizing central nervous system lesions but are not generally available.

Optic Neuritis

Optic neuritis is a nonspecific term denoting inflammation along the optic nerve, optic chiasm, or optic tracts, resulting in decreased vision. Examination of cranial nerves, postural reactions, and spinal reflexes should be performed to gain information helpful in localizing the lesion. Ophthalmoscopically, the optic disks may appear normal or may be swollen with loss of the physiologic cup, hyperemic with fuzzy edges, or hemorrhagic. This can occur unilaterally or bilaterally, total blindness occurring only in the latter. Optic neuritis may be caused by a variety of diseases, including viral infection (canine distemper and feline infectious peritonitis), mycotic infection (cryptococcosis, blastomycosis, histoplasmosis, and coccidioidomycosis), bacterial infections, protozoal disease (toxoplasmosis), algal infection (prototheca), neoplasia (meningioma, feline leukemia virus [FeLV], and lymphosarcoma), and inflammatory causes (granulomatous meningoencephalitis [GME]). Cerebrospinal fluid examination should be performed prior to institution of any therapy and should include opening pressure measurement; total and differential cell counts; protein determination (which is usually elevated in infectious, neoplastic, inflammatory, and traumatic conditions); and culture, serologic study, or fluorescent antibody titers if indicated. Cytologic trends seen in the CSF of various diseases include the following: a predominantly mononuclear population is seen with viral, protozoal, and neoplastic conditions (tumor cells rarely seen) and GME (anaplastic reticulum cells may be seen); mixed mononuclear and polymorphonuclear (PMN) populations are seen with fungal agents (organisms may be seen); predominant PMN population is seen in bacterial infections; red blood cells (RBCs), white blood cells (WBCs), and xanthochromia may be seen in trauma.

Diagnoses of systemic infectious diseases such as distemper, feline infectious peritonitis (FIP), mycoses, and toxoplasmosis should be pursued with the appropriate therapy. Prognosis for return of vision following successful treatment of the diseases depends on the extent of irreversible damage to the involved optic nerves, optic chiasm, or optic tracts.

Without evidence of an infectious agent, neoplasia, or GME, cases are classified as idiopathic. GME and idiopathic optic neuritis are treated with immunosuppressive levels of systemic corticosteroids (prednisone, 2.2 mg/kg s.i.d.). The earlier in the course of the disease that treatment is instituted, the better is the prognosis for restoration and preservation of vision. Oral corticosteroids may be continued for up to 2 weeks, and the dose is then tapered according to the clinical response to therapy. A positive response to corticosteroid therapy, at least transiently, would be compatible with GME or the inflammatory/edematous component of a neoplastic or infectious disease. If vision and pupillary light responses return, the dosage should be slowly decreased until a deterioration is seen; the dosage is then maintained at the level that preserves vision. Prognosis is guarded, and therapy may need to be continued indefinitely. If no clinical improvement is seen in response to therapy, treatment should be slowly tapered and discontinued. Prognosis for return of vision is poor. Systemic broad-spectrum antibiotics are suggested while immunosuppressive agents are in use.

Neoplasia

Neoplasia within the central nervous system (CNS) can affect the function of the visual pathway by direct destruction of the nervous tissue, compression of surrounding structures, interference with circulation, and the development of cerebral edema and disturbance of CSF circulation. Primary neoplasms such as neurofibroma, pituitary adenoma/adenocarcinoma, meningioma, and glioma; metastatic tumors; and lymphoreticular neoplasms have been reported to cause blindness. A chronic progressive course of visual deterioration would be expected.

Diagnostic measures should include those discussed above. The prognosis for most CNS tumors is grave. Immunosuppressive levels of corticosteroids may provide transient improvement of clinical signs attributable to a decrease in the inflammatory or edematous response or both of the neoplasm. Chemotherapy is problematic owing to the inability of most chemotherapeutic drugs to cross the blood brain barrier. Surgical removal of tumors causing blindness is technically difficult because of their location. Radiation therapy may be a consideration.

Trauma

Traumatic lesions, such as avulsion, hematoma, or laceration of optic nerves, optic chiasm, or optic tracts, may cause sudden blindness. A history of trauma, physical evidence of head trauma, or radiographic evidence of skull fractures would make this diagnosis. Trauma to the occipital lobes (visual cortex), not involving the optic nerves, chiasm, or optic tracts, produces cortical blindness with normal pupillary responses. Therapy for CNS trauma is directed at removal of compression and control of resultant CNS edema to prevent neuronal death and myelin degeneration. Emergency treatment with dexamethasone (2.2 mg/kg IV, repeated in 4 to 6 hr) should be instituted. Thereafter dexamethasone (0.25 mg/kg every 8 to 12 hr IV or IM) is continued. Systemic antibiotics that penetrate the blood brain barrier, such as chloramphenicol, trimethoprim, or metronidazole, should also be utilized. Prognosis for recovery of vision after avulsion or laceration of the optic nerves, optic chiasm, or optic tracts is grave. Prognosis for visual recovery from blindness due to occipital cortical trauma is guarded.

References and Supplemental Reading

Acland, G. M., and Aguirre, G. D.: Sudden acquired retinal degeneration: Clinical signs and diagnosis. Proceedings of the ACVO, 1986, pp. 58–63.

deLahunta, A.: *Veterinary Neuroanatomy and Clinical Neurology*, 2nd ed. Philadelphia: W. B. Saunders, 1983.

Moore, C. P.: Visual disturbance in the dog. Part II. Diseases of the retina and optic papilla. Comp. Cont. Ed. Pract. Vet. 6:585, 1984.

Oliver, J. E., and Lorenz, M. D.: *Handbook of Veterinary Neurologic Diagnosis*. Philadelphia: W. B. Saunders, 1983.

MEDICAL THERAPY FOR GLAUCOMA

CHARLES L. MARTIN, D.V.M.,
and DANIEL A. WARD, D.V.M.
Athens, Georgia

Intraocular pressure (IOP) is the result of a dynamic equilibrium between the production and drainage of aqueous humor. Any disruption of this delicate balance that reduces the rate of drainage below the rate of production will result in elevation of the IOP, or glaucoma. Early diagnosis and appropriate medical therapy are necessary to halt progressive retinal and optic nerve destruction and eventual blindness. This article emphasizes pharmacologic modes of emergency and maintenance therapy of glaucoma (Table 1). For discussions of the etiopathogenesis and suggested surgical interventions, the reader is directed to the appropriate reviews (Martin and Wyman, 1978; Vainisi 1973; Martin and Vestre, 1985).

The therapeutic course chosen will vary among patients depending on the history and ophthalmic presentation. The prognosis for retention of or return to functional vision is the single most important factor in deciding how rigorously to pursue glaucoma treatment.

The most intensive medical therapy is needed for the currently or recently sighted patient with elevated IOP. Optic nerve cupping and extinguished electroretinograms (if electroretinography is available) confer poor prognoses for a return to functional vision, and owners of animals with these findings should be so counseled. The animal with chronic blindness and elevated IOP will have little chance of regaining vision, so heroic medical or surgical efforts aimed at restoring vision are seldom worth the time or expense required. However, the pain associated with glaucoma, which frequently manifests as a subtle lethargy or depression, should be addressed with one of the salvage procedures mentioned below. Chronic glaucomas will sometimes result in a subnormal IOP owing to pressure atrophy of the ciliary body.

The position of the lens may play a pivotal role in predicting the likelihood of successful medical therapy. Anterior lens luxation may be associated with glaucoma as a cause or an effect; the exact relationship between the two is often difficult to ascertain. Gonioscopy is the best means of assessing this relationship. Unfortunately, an anteriorly luxated lens will preclude visualization of the iridocor-

Table 1. Medical Treatment of Glaucoma

Drug	Dose	Route	Frequency
Emergency Therapy			
Osmotic diuretics			
Mannitol	2 gm/kg	IV	One time
Glycerol	2 gm/kg	PO	
Maintenance Therapy			
Carbonic anhydrase inhibitors			
Dichlorphenamide	2 mg/kg	PO	t.i.d.
Acetazolamide	10 mg/kg	PO	b.i.d.
Ethoxzolamide	4 mg/kg	PO	b.i.d.
Methazolamide	2 mg/kg	PO	b.i.d.
Miotics			
Pilocarpine, 1%		Topically	b.i.d.
Echothiophate iodide, 0.06%		Topically	Once/day
Adrenergic agonists			
Epinephrine, 2%		Topically	b.i.d.
Dipivalyl epinephrine, 0.5%		Topically	b.i.d.
Combinations			
Pilocarpine, 2%–epinephrine, 1%		Topically	b.i.d.
Adrenergic antagonists			
Timolol maleate, 0.5%		Topically	b.i.d.
Betaxolol, 0.5%		Topically	b.i.d.

neal angle, so gonioscopy of the fellow eye must be relied on to accurately represent the angle of the affected eye. If gonioscopy demonstrates an open iridocorneal angle (i.e., if peripheral anterior synechiae or goniodysgenesis is not present), the displaced lens is probably a cause of the elevated pressure, so medical therapy alone is unlikely to effect a long-term lowering of IOP. Lens removal is indicated in these patients if they are currently or recently sighted. If gonioscopy reveals a closed iridocorneal angle, the lens displacement is probably due to scleral stretching and zonular disruption or is a decompensating factor in an eye that is predisposed to glaucoma. In these cases the prognosis is poor for normalization of IOP with only lens removal. When unable to perform gonioscopy owing to equipment limitations or bilateral luxations, one must depend on signalment and clinical experience in deciding if lens luxation is primary or secondary. Primary lens luxations are most common in the terrier breeds.

EMERGENCY MEDICAL THERAPY

The initial goal of glaucoma therapy is to reduce the intraocular pressure as rapidly, effectively, and safely as possible. In most cases this means the administration of an osmotic diuretic (Table 1). These agents serve to increase the plasma osmotic pressure, thereby extracting water from the vitreous body and lowering IOP. Mannitol is the osmotic agent of choice in small animals. It can be administered at 2 gm/kg by slow push intravenously over a 5-min period. Rapid administration may result in

vomiting. Mannitol is commonly available as a 20 or 25 per cent solution and should be kept warm to prevent crystallization. After administration oral water intake must be prohibited for 2 to 3 hr to prevent the animal from diluting the plasma space, thus negating the drug's effect. The IOP-lowering effect of mannitol begins 30 to 60 min after administration and continues for about 6 hr. Mannitol administration can be repeated but should be viewed as temporary relief of elevated IOP until maintenance medical or surgical procedures can be instituted. Continued administration results in excessive systemic dehydration and decreasing IOP-lowering effect. In addition, mannitol should not be administered within 2 to 4 hr of an anticipated cyclocryotherapy, as the resultant breakdown of the blood-eye aqueous barrier will facilitate entry of mannitol into the eye and could cause a rebound elevation of IOP.

An alternative to mannitol therapy is oral glycerol. Glycerol comes as a 20 per cent solution and should be administered at 2 gm/kg. Mixing with syrup will improve palatability and facilitate administration. Owing to wide variability in gastrointestinal absorption and relatively greater entry into the eye, glycerol may not be as effective as mannitol. However, glycerol may be indicated for patients with severe cardiac or renal insufficiency, as the retained glycerol is metabolized, but mannitol is not metabolized.

Adjunctive emergency therapy should include the administration of a carbonic anhydrase inhibitor orally. These agents lower IOP by decreasing aqueous humor production and may be initiated concurrently with mannitol administration. Mechanisms and dosages of the various carbonic anhydrase inhibitors will be covered under maintenance therapy.

MAINTENANCE THERAPY

After osmotic diuresis has been initiated, a plan for long-term IOP control should be developed. In many instances, cyclocryosurgery (Martin and Vestre, 1985) or laser ablation of the ciliary body may be the maintenance treatment of choice. In other cases, medical therapy may be effective in controlling IOP, thus obviating the need for surgery. These medical therapies serve either to facilitate outflow of aqueous or to reduce its production and may be divided pharmacologically into carbonic anhydrase inhibitors, miotics, adrenergic agonists, and adrenergic antagonists. Commonly used agents are listed in Table 2.

CARBONIC ANHYDRASE INHIBITORS

Carbonic anhydrase (CA) is an enzyme found in many secretory epithelia, including gastrointestinal, renal, and ciliary body. CA catalyzes the reaction between carbon dioxide and water to form carbonic acid, which then reacts with hydrogen ions to form bicarbonate. Although these agents are diuretics, systemic diuresis and consequent vitreal shrinkage are not responsible for their IOP-lowering effect, as evidenced by successful reduction of IOP in ne-

phrectomized animals. Carbonic anhydrase inhibitors (CAIs) reduce IOP by decreasing aqueous humor production. In various species, this effect may be the result of decreased aqueous humor bicarbonate ion concentration, local and systemic acidosis, or a combination of these.

Dichlorphenamide (Daranide, Merck, Sharp & Dohme) is a CAI that is effective in canine glaucoma and has a minimum of side effects. Given orally at 2 mg/kg, dichlorphenamide will usually have an effect on IOP within 4 hr and should be administered every 8 to 12 hr. Acetazolamide (Diamox, Lederle) is an alternative to dichlorphenamide. Dosage is 10 mg/kg q 8 to 12 hr PO. Acetazolamide is more frequently associated with side effects than dichlorphenamide but may be more readily available in some areas. Other CAIs that are used less frequently in veterinary medicine include ethoxzolamide (Cardrase, Upjohn; 4 mg/kg b.i.d.) and methazolamide (Neptazane, Lederle; 2 mg/kg b.i.d. to t.i.d.). Carbonic anhydrase inhibitor therapy may be initiated concurrently with osmotic diuresis. Potassium supplementation may be advisable in some patients with chronic usage.

Systemic side effects of the CAIs include vomiting, panting, diarrhea, and weakness. CAIs have also been linked to urolithiasis in humans. Contraindications to CAI therapy include chronic obstructive pulmonary disease, diabetes with superimposed ketosis or ketoacidosis, and hepatic insufficiency.

MIOTICS

Topical miotic therapy has been used in the treatment of glaucoma in humans and animals for many years. The primary IOP-lowering effect of these agents is due to a configurational change in the trabecular meshwork, which facilitates the outflow of aqueous humor. However, glaucoma in small animals often results from resistance to drainage owing to closure of the iridocorneal angle superficial to the trabecular meshwork region. As aqueous humor cannot proceed through the closed angle to reach the trabecular meshwork, drainage facilitation at the level of the trabecular meshwork is unlikely to greatly lower the IOP in glaucomatous animals. Miotics are unlikely to lower the IOP in cases of glaucoma due to pupillary block and iris bombé for the same reason. The greatest benefit from these drugs would probably be realized in the uncommon case of open angle glaucoma. This type of glaucoma is common in humans and has been found occasionally in the beagle. Some cases of glaucoma in the cat have also been suspected as open angle situations.

Pilocarpine (Isopto Carpine, Alcon), a direct-acting parasympathomimetic, is the most popular miotic in use today. A 2 per cent solution applied

Table 2. *Drugs Commonly Used in Glaucoma*

Drug name	Dog and Cat
Acetazolamide (Diamox, Lederle)	10 mg/kg PO q12h
Betaxolol (Betoptic, Alcon)	1 qt of 0.5% solution topically b.i.d.
Dichlorphenamide (Daranide, Merck, Sharp & Dohme)	2 mg/kg PO q8h
Dipivalyl epinephrine	1 qt of 0.5% solution topically b.i.d.
Echothiophate iodide	1 qt of 0.6% solution topically once/day
Epinephrine	1 qt of 2% solution topically b.i.d.
Ethoxzolamide (Cardrase, Upjohn)	4 mg/kg PO q12h
Glycerol	2 gm/kg PO
Mannitol	2 gm/kg IV
Methazolamide (Neptazane, Lederle)	2 mg/kg PO q8–12h
Pilocarpine (Isopto Carpine, Alcon)	1 qt of 1% solution topically b.i.d.
Pilocarpine, 2%–epinephrine, 1% (P_2E_1, Person and Covey)	1 qt topically b.i.d.
Timolol maleate (Timoptic, Merck, Sharp & Dohme)	1 qt of 0.25% or 0.5% solution topically b.i.d.

topically three to four times a day or a 4 per cent gel applied b.i.d. may be used in suspected cases of open angle glaucoma, or in closed angles if CAIs have returned the IOP to the 30 to 35 mm Hg range. Pilocarpine may aggravate an ongoing uveitis as well as potentiate pupillary block, as the miosis may enhance adhesion of the iris to the lens.

Organophosphates such as diisopropyl fluorophosphate (Floropryl, Merck, Sharp & Dohme) and echothiophate iodide (Phospholine Iodide, Ayerst) act indirectly as parasympathomimetics by inhibiting cholinesterase. Echothiophate is available as a solution (0.03, 0.06, 0.125, or 0.25 per cent). Its long duration of action (24 to 48 hrs per application) may make it more desirable than pilocarpine in cases in which topical miotics are indicated. However, the limitations to echothiophate therapy are the same as for pilocarpine. In addition, systemic organophosphate toxicity is not uncommon, especially in smaller patients.

ADRENERGIC AGONISTS

Alpha- and beta-adrenergic agonists have demonstrated limited effectiveness at reducing IOP in several species. Alpha-agonists probably enhance outflow via the trabecular meshwork and are hence subject to the same limitations in clinical veterinary ophthalmologic practice as those noted for miotics. Beta-agonists decrease aqueous humor production via stimulation of the ciliary epithelial adenylate cyclase complex. The IOP-lowering effect of both adrenergic agonists is slight and is of questionable value in small animal glaucoma, in which the pressures are frequently twice normal.

Epinephrine is the most commonly available adrenergic agonist, having alpha-agonist properties at low concentrations and beta-agonist properties at higher concentrations. A 2 per cent solution (Epitrate, Ayerst) applied twice daily is recommended. Topically applied dipivalyl epinephrine, which is converted to epinephrine in the cornea, is equally effective at much lower concentration (0.5 per cent solution, Propine, Allergan) owing to greater corneal penetrability. Both agents are locally irritating, resulting in conjunctival hyperemia, chemosis, and blepharospasm. Conjunctival and corneal pigment depositions have been associated with topical epinephrine therapy in humans. Epinephrine and pilocarpine combinations show synergism in humans and may prove more useful than either drug alone in the dog. A combination of 2 per cent pilocarpine and 1 per cent epinephrine (P_2E_1, Person and Covey) may be used twice a day.

ADRENERGIC ANTAGONISTS

The effect of alpha- and beta-blockers on IOP has received a great deal of attention in the recent clinical literature. Of the various agents shown to have an IOP-lowering effect, timolol (Timoptic, Merck, Sharp & Dohme), a nonselective beta-antagonist, has proved to be the most efficacious and reliable. The obvious contradiction of a beta-antagonist having the same effect as a beta-agonist would make one suspect that timolol's IOP-lowering action may be due to some pharmacologic property other than beta-antagonism. However, the finding that beta-blockers structurally unrelated to timolol also decrease IOP make this hypothesis unlikely. Thus, although it has been proved that beta-blockers lower IOP by decreasing aqueous humor production, the exact mechanism by which this occurs remains unresolved. Timolol, in a 0.25 or 0.5 per cent concentration, may be used two or three times per day in the dog. As some of the topically applied drug will be absorbed systemically, caution must be used in animals with cardiovascular disease. Betaxolol (Betoptic, Alcon), another beta-blocker, is less potent than timolol but may produce fewer systemic reactions. Although controlled studies in the dog are lacking, preliminary clinical evidence indicates that timolol may be more effective in lowering the IOP of the glaucomatous small animal patient than are other topical antiglaucoma drugs.

Clinical studies have demonstrated that timolol may have an additive effect when used in combination with other antiglaucoma therapies. In a series of human patients with chronic open angle glaucoma, timolol had an additive IOP-lowering effect when used in combination with pilocarpine, epinephrine, or acetazolamide. These combinations may also be useful in cases of open angle glaucoma in the dog and cat. However, as most glaucomas in small animals are of the closed angle variety, the combination of timolol and a carbonic anhydrase inhibitor may be the most clinically useful combination.

PROPHYLAXIS

Glaucoma in small animals is often a bilateral condition that initially manifests unilaterally. Owing to frequent therapeutic failures, the ability to prevent or delay the onset of glaucoma in the second eye may be the animal's only chance to maintain vision. In one study (Slater and Erb, 1986), prophylaxis delayed but did not prevent the development of glaucoma in the second eye in a series of cases of canine glaucoma that initially presented unilaterally. Unfortunately, as the cases were not classified according to the type of glaucoma or the specific therapy employed, conclusions about the reliability of prevention are ambiguous. It might be of potential benefit to recommend topical therapy in the unaffected eye as a means of assuring that the owner is observing the eye on a daily basis. This has to be weighed against the potential for developing tolerance to beta-antagonists and for some miotics to cause proliferation of trabecular structures.

SALVAGE PROCEDURES

Chronically blind eyes in which the IOP cannot be controlled by the recommended maintenance therapies are candidates for salvage procedures. Even in those chronic cases in which the IOP is successfully controlled medically, a salvage procedure may still prove beneficial in terms of reduced client expense and effort as well as decreased likelihood of long-term systemic side effects associated with carbonic anhydrase inhibitors. Evisceration and silicone prosthesis implantation is such a surgical procedure (Martin and Vestre, 1985). Cyclocryosurgery, a useful therapy in sighted eyes, may also be used to control pressures in chronic cases (Martin and Vestre, 1985). Pharmacologic ablation of the ciliary body by means of an intravitreal injection of gentamicin (Gentocin, Schering) is an easy, inexpensive, and effective method of reducing the IOP in chronically blind eyes. With the animal under narcoleptic sedation, the limbal conjunctiva is grasped with thumb forceps, and a 22-gauge needle on a 3-ml syringe is introduced 8 to 10 mm posterior to the dorsal limbus. The needle tip should be directed toward the center of the vitreous body. Following aspiration of approximately 0.5 ml of vitreous, the syringe is detached from the needle, a second syringe containing 25 mg of gentamicin is attached, and the gentamicin is injected into the vitreous. Care must be taken not to fracture the lens capsule, as intractable phacoanaphylaxis may result. This technique should *never* be used in an eye for which any hope of vision remains because the retina will be permanently destroyed by the injection. Moreover, it should not be used in eyes suspected of having tumor involvement. Approximately 20 per cent of the eyes treated with this procedure become opaque and phthisic, resulting in a cosmetically unappealing eye.

SUMMARY

Emergency glaucoma therapy should include the use of intravenous mannitol if intraocular pressures exceed 45 to 50 mm Hg. An appropriate carbonic anhydrase inhibitor should be given at the time, so that its effect will begin as that of the osmotic diuretic wanes. Carbonic anhydrase inhibitor therapy alone may be sufficient to keep the IOP below 30 mm Hg. If a CAI alone can get the pressures in the 30 to 35 mm Hg range but no lower, a topical miotic, an adrenergic agonist, or a combination of these may be added to the regimen. If CAIs are unsuccessful at lowering the IOP, topical timolol therapy may prove beneficial. *The clinician should be cautioned about spending too much time trying to medically manage a refractory case, as further ocular damage is likely to occur. Most cases of primary glaucomas are closed angle glaucomas and are usually refractory to medical maintenance therapy.*

References and Supplemental Reading

Friedland, B. R., and Maren, T. H.: Carbonic anhydrase: Pharmacology of inhibitors and treatment of glaucoma. *In* Sears, M. L. (ed.): *Pharmacology of the Eye*. New York: Springer-Verlag, 1985, pp. 279–309.

Gelatt, K. N.: The canine glaucomas. *In* Gelatt, K. N. (ed.): *Textbook of Veterinary Ophthalmology*. Philadelphia: Lea & Febiger, 1981, pp. 390–435.

Gwin, R. M.: Veterinary ophthalmic pharmacology. Part III: Pharmacologic agents that reduce intraocular pressure. *In* Gelatt, K. N. (ed.): *Textbook of Veterinary Ophthalmology*. Philadelphia: Lea & Febiger, 1981, pp. 181–205.

Martin, C. L., and Vestre, W. A.: Glaucoma. *In* Slatter, D. H. (ed.): *Textbook of Small Animal Surgery*. Philadelphia: W. B. Saunders Co., 1985, pp. 1567–1583.

Martin, C. L., and Wyman, M.: Primary glaucoma in the dog. Vet. Clin. North Am. 8:257, 1978.

Slater, M., and Erb, H.: Effects of risk factors and prophylactic treatment on primary glaucoma in the dog. J.A.V.M.A. 188:1028, 1986.

Vainisi, S. J.: The diagnosis and therapy of glaucoma. Vet. Clin. North Am. 3:453, 1973.

UVEITIS

JAMES F. SWANSON, D.V.M.

Houston, Texas

Primary and secondary inflammation of the uvea is relatively common in small animals and produces a small constellation of functionally related clinical signs. Although specific for intraocular inflammation, these clinical signs are often of little help in determining the cause of the observed disease. Uveitis may accompany many systemic illnesses. Thus, diagnosis of uveitis is often the beginning of the diagnostic challenge facing the clinician.

FUNCTIONAL ANATOMY OF THE UVEAL TRACT

The uveal tract comprises the middle or vascular tunic of the eye. It is composed of three intimately connected subunits: the iris, the ciliary body, and the choroid. The primary functions of the uveal tract in domestic animals include (1) nourishment of the lens, cornea, and outer retinal layers; (2) maintenance of a clear ocular media; (3) control of the amount of light falling on the retina; and (4) to a limited degree, accomodation for near and far vision. The iris functions as an ever-changing diaphram that regulates the amount of retinal illumination. The pigment density of the iris is variable and imparts the color to the eye. The ciliary body produces aqueous humor, which is responsible for nourishment of the avascular ocular structures. Smooth muscle within the ciliary body allows a limited degree of accommodation in domestic species. The choroid lies between the retina/retinal pigment epithelium and the sclera. Its major function is to supply oxygen and nutrients to the outer retinal layers, including the photoreceptors. The choroid also serves as a "heat sink" that dissipates heat generated as light strikes the retina and retinal pigment epithelium, a function that protects the delicate retinal tissues from thermal damage.

The clarity of aqueous humor is largely the result of the small concentration of large refractile molecules within the watery aqueous fluid. Maintanance of clear ocular media is essential for normal vision. The group of ocular structures responsible for exclusion of large molecules found within the vascular system from the ocular media is called the "blood aqueous" or "blood ocular barrier." The so-called blood ocular barrier components contained within the uveal tract are thought to be the nonpigmented epithelium of the ciliary body and iridal blood vessels. Other portions of this functional barrier are found in the retinal vessels and retinal pigment epithelium (RPE). Disruption of the blood ocular barrier always accompanies uveitis, and the resulting loss of clarity of the ocular media is one of the hallmarks of uveal inflammation.

CLINICAL SIGNS

Clinical signs of uveitis may be arbitrarily divided into acute and chronic, although remissions and exacerbations of the disease process may superimpose one set of signs on the other. Conceptually, the clinical signs of uveitis are those that might be associated with inflammation in any other organ. The eye is perhaps unique in that direct observation of the pathophysiologic processes is possible. The hallmarks of inflammation (redness, swelling, pain, and loss of function) are readily observed in uveitis.

In acute uveitis, pain is always evident to some degree and is intensified by bright light. Blepharospasm, lacrimation, and avoidance behavior in bright light are common. The eye will exhibit varying degrees of ocular redness. Hyperemia of the anterior uveal vessels causes a subtle red flush near the limbus (ciliary flush). This pattern of redness is usually accompanied or even overshadowed by the branching, diffuse redness of conjunctival hyperemia. If acute uveitis is complicated by glaucoma, an episcleral pattern may also be evident.

Swelling of the affected tissues is common, and the extent is dependent on the cause and severity. Conjunctival swelling (chemosis), corneal edema, and iridal congestion are common. Choroidal swelling occurs but is difficult to demonstrate clinically. The iris becomes swollen and may exhibit a color change. Its texture and color should be compared with those of the fellow eye.

Turbidity of the aqueous humor also occurs to a varying degree in acute uveitis. As blood ocular barrier function is compromised, large protein molecules are allowed to enter the ocular fluid, imparting a hazy character to the ocular media and partially obscuring the details of the intraocular structures. A well-focused light source* and magnification facilitate demonstration of this phenomenon. This

---

*I = slit disposable ophthalmic pocket light, Concept Inc., Clearwater, FL 33546.

may be accompanied by influx of white cells. Magnification ($> 10 \times$) is usually necessary to demonstrate these cells, unless they are present in large clumps. In severe cases red blood cells and fibrin may also be found in the anterior chamber.

Irritation accompanying uveitis may cause miosis of the pupil, although the classic pinpoint pupillary aperture is uncommon. The pupil may also be midrange in size, dilated, or misshapen, depending on intraocular pressure, lens position, and previous synechia formation.

Intraocular pressure is commonly decreased in uveitis. Aqueous formation may diminish in response to ciliary body inflammation. An assessment of intraocular pressure should always accompany evaluation of the inflamed eye, as glaucoma may be overshadowed by the signs of inflammation.

Eyes exhibiting severe panuveitis may also have inflammatory cellular infiltrate in the vitreous humor that may obscure fundus detail. Disruption of the retinal pigment epithelium in severe inflammation of the choroid (posterior uveitis) may allow fluid accumulation between the retinal photoreceptors and RPE and result in exudative retinal detachment.

Often, different clinical signs are observed in more long-standing cases of uveitis. Keratic precipitates (KPs) are accumulations of leukocytes and inflammatory debris on the corneal endothelium. KPs may have a waxy appearance and are a sign of chronicity. Small plaquelike scars may remain on the endothelium after resolution.

Iridal changes are common in chronic uveitis and include pigment changes; affected irides are usually darker brown and more homogeneous in color than normal, and fibrovascular membranes may develop on the surface of the iris and cause a dramatic color change.

The iris will often adhere to adjacent structures during the acute phase of uveitis. Adherence to the lens (posterior synechia) usually inhibits movement of the pupillary margin and, if extensive enough, may block the normal flow of aqueous humor. Occasionally the iris may become freed with resolution of inflammation, and "rests" of pigment may be noted on the anterior lens capsule. Chronic inflammation and scarring may result in narrowing of the ciliary cleft through adherence of the peripheral iris and cornea. This peripheral anterior synechia formation results in drainage angle closure and glaucoma.

Cataract formation may also be seen in chronic uveitis. Alteration of the osmotic, nutritional, and oxidative environment of the lens causes lens capsular disruption, destruction of lens fibers, and opacity. Cataract formation may also contribute to or induce intraocular inflammation.

Inflammatory membrane formation is common in severe chronic uveitis. Fibrovascular membranes may bridge and collapse the drainage angle, causing glaucoma; cyclitic membranes may form in the anterior vitreous humor; and preretinal membranes may contract and result in traction retinal detachment.

Damage to the corneal endothelium by severe or chronic inflammation reduces endothelial cell density and function. Sufficient loss of these cells allows water influx into the corneal stroma and corneal edema. If corneal stromal edema is severe, bullous keratopathy results.

Glaucoma is a particularly frustrating sequela of chronic uveitis. Annular posterior synechia formation, pupillary block, and iris bombé may occur. Scarring and closure of the iridocorneal angle are seen in both dogs and cats. Glaucoma due to uveitis may be seen more commonly in breeds exhibiting inherited malformation of the drainage angle.

Finally, destruction and scarring of the uveal tract, as well as impairment of ocular circulation and aqueous production, if severe enough, may result in shrinkage of the globe (phthisis bulbi).

ETIOLOGY

Unfortunately, the clinical signs of uveitis are usually nonspecific and often of little assistance in establishing a cause. After a diagnosis of uveitis has been made, a thorough physical examination should be performed to determine if other systemic abnormalities are present that can be correlated with the observed ocular disease. Appropriate laboratory tests as well as other more specialized diagnostic techniques may be necessary.

A great variety of infectious, autoimmune, neoplastic, and degenerative diseases have been associated with uveitis. A logical and sequential search should be undertaken to rule out treatable disease in addition to initiating symptomatic therapy. A noninclusive list of diseases associated with uveitis is found in Table 1.

Uveitis is seen in a significant number of canine lymphoma patients and is the most common secondary intraocular tumor. Severity of signs varies, but recent retrospective studies indicate that intraocular involvement is most common in widely disseminated cases and is a poor prognostic sign.

Infectious bacterial, fungal, protozoal, and viral diseases often cause iridocyclitis, chorioretinitis, or panuveitis. Sytemic fungal infections, including histoplasmosis, cryptococcosis, coccidioidomycosis, and blastomycosis usually cause visible granuloma formation that is most easily demonstrated funduscopically. There are often related systemic signs of pulmonary, gastrointestinal, lymphatic, or central nervous system dysfunction.

Brucella canis and the *Mycobacterium* sp. are

Table 1. *Systemic Diseases Associated with Uveitis in Small Animals*

Dogs	Cats
Neoplastic/inflammatory	Neoplastic
Lymphoma	Lymphosarcoma
Hemangiosarcoma	Disseminated carcinomas
Disseminated carcinomas	Infectious
Reticulosis	Systemic fungal
Infectious	*Coccidioides immitis*
Systemic fungal	*Cryptococcus neoformans*
Coccidioides immitis	*Blastomyces dermatitidis*
Cryptococcus neoformans	*Histoplasma capsulatum*
Blastomyces dermatitidis	Protozoal algal
Histoplasma capsulatum	*Toxoplasma gondii*
Rickettsial	*Prototheca* spp.
Ehrlichia canis, E. platys	Bacterial
Rickettsia rickettsii	*Mycobacterium* spp.
Protozoal algal	*Streptococcus, Staphlycoccus, E. coli* (septicemia)
Toxoplasma gondii	Viral
Leishmania donovani	Feline leukemia complex
Prototheca spp.	Feline herpesvirus
Bacterial	Feline infectious peritonitis
Brucella canis	Autoimmune
Mycobacterium spp.	Periarteritis nodosa
Streptococcus, Staphlycoccus, Escherichia coli (septicemia)	Idiopathic
Leptospira spp.	Metabolic
Viral	Type V chylomicronemia
Canine distemper	
Infectious canine hepatitis	
Canine neonatal herpesvirus	
Rabies (chorioretinitis)	
Parasitic	
Dirofilaria immitis	
Toxocara canis	
Autoimmune	
Systemic lupus erythematosus	
Uveitis/dermal depigmentation	
Necrotizing and non-necrotizing scleritis	

reported to cause anterior and posterior uveitis in dogs and cats, respectively. Clinical signs are nonspecific and include panuveitis, granulomatous chorioretinitis, and intraocular hemorrhage.

Rickettsial and protozoal parasites have been demonstrated to cause intraocular inflammation in clinical and experimental cases. Anterior uveitis, panuveitis, and chorioretinitis have been described.

Metazoan parasites, including *Dirofilaria immitis* and *Toxocara canis*, have been associated with uveitis in dogs. The mechanism is via direct invasion of the globe or by circulating immune complexes.

IMMUNOLOGIC MECHANISMS

In many instances, a causative agent cannot be conclusively demonstrated in a uveitis patient. Ocular inflammation has been shown to be a manifestation of autoallergy in both veterinary and human medicine. The exact mechanisms of hypersensitivity that result in uveitis are being explored experimentally. All classes of hypersensitivity have been suspected although only a few have been experimentally proved to cause uveitis. Anaphylactoid reactions, antibody-mediated cytotoxicity, immune complex disease, delayed-type hypersensitivity, and stimulating antibody reactions have all been incriminated either singly or in combination as a cause of uveitis. Better characterization of immune-mediated uveitis may allow development of specific blockers of the inflammatory response in the future.

TREATMENT

The therapeutic agents listed below are those employed only to suppress intraocular inflammation or to mitigate the secondary effects of uveitis. Specific agents active against particular diseases are beyond the scope of this article.

CORTICOSTEROIDS. Corticosteroids continue to be the mainstay of treatment in noninfectious uveitis. Numerous topical, injectable, and oral preparations are available, and use of a particular steroid is often based on clinical experience. Generally, topical preparations containing dexamethasone, betamethasone, or prednisolone are more effective than other glucocorticoids, and acetates penetrate intact corneal epithelium better than phosphate or alcohol derivatives. Prednisolone acetate (1 per cent) ophthalmic suspension (Ak-tate, Akorn) is effective in suppressing signs of inflammation. Oral prednisone (2.2 mg/kg s.i.d.) administration may be used to treat posterior uveitis. The dose should gradually be reduced as inflammation is controlled. Subconjunctival injections produce high concentrations within the anterior uvea. Repository preparations should be used with caution; after injection, drug release may be prolonged. Therefore, if infectious disease is discovered or develops after a repository corticosteroid is used, successful control is more difficult.

NONSTEROIDAL ANTI-INFLAMMATORY AGENTS. Nonsteroidal anti-inflammatory drugs (NSAIDs) all exert an anti-inflammatory effect by essentially the same mechanism: inhibition of prostaglandin formation. Because this action differs from that of glucocorticoids, NSAIDs may be used in addition to steroids for increased anti-inflammatory effect. Commonly used NSAIDs include aspirin, flunixin meglumine (Banamine, Schering), and phenylbutazone. Aspirin compounds should be administered with meals or in a buffered preparation. Maximum dosage in dogs should be no more than 25 mg/kg q8h orally, although considerable effect may be noted at lower dosages and administration frequencies. Flunixin meglumine is effective in controlling intraocular inflammation in dogs and may be given intravenously or intramuscularly (0.25 to 0.5 mg/kg/day) for no more than 3 consecutive days. Its use is not approved in small animals. Phenylbutazone may be administered to dogs orally or intravenously (10 to 22 mg/kg/day). Uncontrolled studies have indicated that topical 1 per cent indomethacin drops are effective in reducing intraocular inflammation, especially when combined with topical corticosteroid treatment.

NSAID use can cause severe side effects. Gastrointenstinal bleeding, hepatotoxicity, blood dyscrasias, and acute renal failure have been reported. Renal function should be monitored closely, and NSAID use should be avoided in dehydrated patients or patients with compromised renal function (see p. 53).

IMMUNOSUPPRESSIVE DRUGS. Cyclophosphamide (Cytoxan, Bristol-Myers) is a nonspecific cell cycle inhibitor that has been used extensively for the treatment of malignancies and autoimmune disorders. The drug is quite cytotoxic, and side effects include severe bone marrow suppression and hemorrhagic cystitis. Azathioprine (Imuran, Burroughs Wellcome) was first used in the mid-1960's to prevent organ transplant rejection. The drug has since been used to treat a number of autoimmune diseases. In veterinary medicine, azathioprine has been used to treat polyarthritis, autoimmune uveitis

with dermal depigmentation, and ocular fibrous histiocytoma. Systemic side effects include hepatic toxicity and severe bone marrow suppression. The patients' hematologic status should be monitored closely while under treatment. Cyclosporine (Sandimmune, Sandoz) is a cyclic polypeptide metabolite first isolated from the fungus *Tolypocladium inflatumgams* and has been shown to be a potent specific suppressor of T-lymphocyte activity. The major use of cyclosporine has been for prevention of organ transplant rejection. Sytemic administration results in generalized helper T-cell suppression and has been reported to be effective in the treatment of experimental autoimmune uveitis in animals and in several types of severe, intractable autoimmune uveitis in humans. Systemic toxicity and expense, however, limit its usefulness in veterinary medicine at this time. Research on the efficacy of topical administration for the treatment of other ocular inflammatory conditions has shown promise.

CYCLOPLEGICS. Acute uveitis is painful, and therapeutic steps should be taken to alleviate patient discomfort as much as possible. Inflammation of the ciliary musculature accompanied by ciliary spasm can be relieved by topical administration of cycloplegic agents. Topical 1 per cent atropine is the parasympatholytic drug most commonly used in veterinary medicine to combat ciliary spasm and its associated pain. However, atropine is probably overused and is associated with significant side effects. Atropine reduces aqueous outflow facility and may precipitate glaucoma in animals with narrow or malformed iridocorneal angles or in animals with drainage angles compromised by scarring or synechia formation. Decreased tear production is also associated with prolonged atropine administration. Therefore, the patient should be monitored for signs of glaucoma or tear dysfunction if atropine administration is considered. Generally, atropine should only be used often enough in acute uveitis patients to maintain pupillary dilation and should not be used at all in patients with either antecedent tear deficiency or drainage angle abnormalities. Other parasympatholytics are available that possess shorter durations of action, including tropicamide (Tropicacyl, Akorn) and homatropine (Isopto-Homatropine, Alcon), and their use may be considered.

References and Supplemental Reading

Blogg, R.: Anterior uveitis in the dog and cat. Proceedings of 5th Annual Kal Kan Symposium, 1981, pp. 17–25.
Blouin, P.: Uveitis in the dog and cat: Causes, diagnosis and treatment. Can. Vet. J. 25:315, 1984.
James, D. G., Graham, E., and Hamblin, A.: Immunology of multisystem ocular disease. Surv. Ophthalmol. 30:155, 1985.
Krohne, S. D., and Vestre, W. A.: Ocular use of antiinflammatory drugs in companion animals. Comp. Cont. Ed. Pract. Vet. 11:1085, 1987.
Martin, C. L.: Ocular infections. *In* Greene, C. E. (ed.): *Clinical*

Microbiology and Infectious Disease of the Dog and Cat. Philadelphia: W. B. Saunders, 1984, pp. 301–319.

Peiffer, R. L.: Ocular manifestations of systemic disease. *In* Gelatt, K. N. (ed.): *Textbook of Veterinary Ophthalmology.* Philadelphia: Lea & Febiger, 1981, pp. 699–723.

Schmidt, G. M., and Coulter, D. B.: Physiology of the eye. *In* Gelatt, K. N. (ed.): *Textbook of Veterinary Ophthalmology.* Philadelphia: Lea & Febiger, 1981, pp. 129–159.

White, J. V.: Cyclosporine: Prototype of a T-cell selective immunosuppressant. J.A.V.M.A. 189:566, 1986.

ULCERATIVE KERATITIS

JOAN DZIEZYC, D.V.M.

College Station, Texas

Corneal ulcers in dogs and cats are common ocular problems. Most are superficial and will heal well; however, deep ulcers are true emergencies and require correct and timely intervention to avoid the loss of the eye.

INITIAL ASSESSMENT

The first decision in assessing a corneal ulcer is to distinguish between superficial and deep ulcers. Superficial ulcers involve the loss of epithelium, with possibly a loss of superficial stroma. The area involved can be large, but superficial ulcers are shallow, causing little change in the contour of the corneal surface. Deep ulcers involve one half or more of the thickness of the corneal stroma, but are often small in area, and can resemble a small crater in the cornea. Deep ulcers can progress rapidly. In some a white or yellow cellular infiltrate may develop in the area surrounding the ulcer. In deep melting ulcers the cornea appears to be liquefying. It is probably prudent to assume that most deep ulcers are infected, although keratoconjunctivitis sicca and alkali burns can be the cause of noninfected deep ulcers.

CAUSES OF CORNEAL ULCERS

Corneal ulcers are usually the result of trauma to the corneal epithelium, although the particular type of trauma may be difficult to determine. Causes of corneal ulcers include chemical trauma such as sprays, soaps, and dips; foreign bodies, especially those lodged behind the nictitating membrane; and eyelid pathologic changes, such as entropion, ectopic cilia, lagophthalmos, and occasionally tumors. Distichiasis rarely causes ulcers; usually dogs with distichiasis are asymptomatic. Nasal folds in brachycephalic dogs occasionally cause ulceration; more commonly, pigmentary keratitis is seen nasally.

Keratoconjunctivitis sicca, especially in acute cases, causes corneal ulcers; these dogs usually have tenacious mucous discharge as well as low Schirmer's tear test values. Infectious agents, with the possible exception of feline herpesvirus, cannot adhere to an intact, healthy corneal epithelium and therefore cannot cause a corneal ulcer. Bacteria and fungi can infect an already compromised cornea and cause deepening of the ulcer.

TREATMENT OF SUPERFICIAL ULCERS

Most superficial corneal ulcers will heal in a surprisingly short time with minimal intervention. Sliding and mitosis of epithelial cells proceeds rapidly if the basement membrane is intact. The purpose of treatment is to prevent the cornea from becoming infected and to keep the animal comfortable. Topical antibiotics are used to prevent a secondary infection. They do not aid or speed healing. If a superficial ulcer does not heal within several days, reassessment of the eye should be made. It is irrational to switch antibiotics in the hopes that this will speed the healing. Antibiotic combinations (such as neomycin, polymixin, and gramicidin or bacitracin) that are not used systemically are preferable to systemic drugs, such as gentamicin, in treating a superficial corneal ulcer. In this way, development of bacterial resistance to systemically administered antibiotics is avoided. A "super" drug is not needed in these cases, as infection is not being treated. Atropine can be used topically to relieve pain.

NONHEALING SUPERFICIAL ULCERS

If a superficial ulcer does not heal within several days, a re-examination of the eye should be made. Has an ectopic cilium been missed? Is a foreign body adherent to or embedded in the nictitating membrane? Does the dog have "dry eye"? Special attention should be paid to the pattern of fluorescein dye uptake. In recurrent erosions (also known as refractory ulcers, indolent ulcers, or boxer ulcers), the area of the cornea that stains with fluorescein is larger than the visible ulcer. In these cases the epithelium surrounding the ulcer is poorly attached to the basement membrane, and fluorescein stains beneath the epithelium at the edge of the ulcer. The basement membrane in these dogs is probably abnormal and does not allow epithelial adherence to take place. Various treatments have been described, but in all cases one must keep reminding the client and oneself that the cornea *will* eventually heal. The initial treatment of choice is to debride the ulcer with a dry cotton-tipped applicator under topical anesthesia. Loose epithelium will easily peel off; normal epithelium will stay adherent to the stroma. All loose epithelium should be removed, usually leaving a defect far larger in area than the original ulcer. Subsequent treatment consists of topical administration of antibiotics three to four times a day, with atropine used topically as needed to alleviate discomfort. Re-examination should be performed in 1 to 2 weeks, at which time the ulcer (if still present) can again be debrided. Using this therapy alone, the ulcer will heal. If speedier healing is desired, other treatments include the use of a soft contact lens, conjunctival flaps, and superficial keratectomies.

FELINE HERPES KERATITIS

A unique, chronic, ulcerative keratitis caused by feline herpesvirus is seen in the cat. The virus can cause several ocular and systemic problems, but ulcerative keratitis usually is seen only in adult cats. The typical herpes ulcer is fine, branching, and superficial (known as a dendritic ulcer), but large superficial ulcers often with granulation tissue can also be seen. If the ulcer is untreated, stromal keratitis with considerable stromal infiltrates may develop. Diagnosis is probably best made by viral isolation, although indirect fluorescent antibody (IFA) test of conjunctival biopsies and identification of intranuclear inclusions on corneal scrapings or conjunctival biopsies can also be attempted. Treatment consists of using topical antiherpetic agents (idoxuridine, Stoxil, SmithKline Beckman; adenine arabinoside, Vira-A, Parke-Davis; trifluridine, Viroptic, Burroughs Wellcome) six times a day for several weeks. Trifluorothymidine (trifluridine, Viroptic, Burroughs Wellcome) has been shown to have the best *in vitro* action against feline herpesvirus and is effective *in vitro*. As in human herpetic keratitis, feline herpes keratitis can resolve without treatment and can recur, especially in times of stress.

TREATMENT OF DEEP CORNEAL ULCER

A deep corneal ulcer is presumed to be infected and should always be cultured, preferably before fluorescein staining and the application of topical anesthesia, which may inhibit bacterial growth. The ulcer is then stained with fluorescein to assess epithelial healing, if any. Descemet's membrane will not stain in a deep ulcer; the sides stain with fluorescein, but the base does not stain; this is diagnostic of a descemetocele.

After applying topical anesthetic, the ulcer can be scraped and the scraping stained with Gram's and Giemsa stains. If gram-negative rods are seen, often indicative of *Pseudomonas* infection, the author's antibiotic of choice is gentamicin. A fortified gentamicin solution is used every 1 to 2 hr. This is prepared by using 5 ml of commercially available topical gentamicin solution (Gentocin ophthalmic solution, Schering) to which 15 mg of injectable gentamicin sulfate is added (Gentocin solution, Schering). This increases the gentamicin concentration from 3 mg/ml to 6 mg/ml. Antibiotics can be changed if indicated by sensitivity results.

If gram-positive cocci are seen, indicative of *Streptococcus* or *Staphylococcus*, either penicillin or a cephalosporin can be used. For topical medication, 5 million units of sodium penicillin G can be reconstituted with 15 ml of artificial tears (concentration of 333,000 U/ml), or 500 mg of cefazolin (Ancef, SmithKline Beckman) can be reconstituted with 15 ml of artificial tears (concentration of 33 mg/ml).

Although fungal keratitis is unlikely in small animals, if fungal hyphae or yeast is seen on cytologic study, pimaricin (Natacyn, Alcon) is an excellent though expensive topical antifungal agent and should be used every 2 hr to begin treatment. A less costly alternative is miconazole (Monistat, Ortho) used as the undiluted 10 mg/ml IV preparation every 2 hr. Fungal keratitis usually requires weeks of treatment.

If the ulcer shows evidence of melting, acetylcysteine (Mucomyst, Mead Johnson) can be added to the antibiotic solution used. Using the 20 per cent solution, one part of acetylcysteine is added to three parts of the antibiotic solution to give a final concentration of 5 per cent acetylcystein. (For example, 9 ml of gentamicin solution, 3 ml of acetylcysteine 20 per cent, and 45 mg of gentamicin sulfate yields approximately a 5 per cent solution of acetylcysteine and 6 mg/ml of gentamicin.) Atropine can be used to reduce the pain of the reflex uveitis and may be needed from once to six times a day. If the pupil remains dilated, additional atropine will not be needed.

In cases of deep corneal ulcers and descemetoceles, surgical intervention may be necessary. If the ulcer is seen early in the course of the disease and epithelial growth and neovascularization have not begun, surgery is indicated. If the ulcer is seen late in the disease process, and epithelialization has occurred, and new blood vessels are near or penetrate the ulcer, surgery will probably not be necessary. If the ulcer has perforated, surgery should be performed.

A conjunctival flap is the surgical treatment of choice for deep corneal ulcers that have not perforated. Conjunctival flaps bring blood vessels to the ulcer, provide some protection and support, allow medication of the eye, and enable observation of the ulcer. Bridge flaps and pedicle flaps allow the best observation of the eye. Nictitating membrane flaps should not be used for deep ulcers, as they do not provide support or blood vessels. More important, observation of the ulcer is impossible with a nictitating membrane flap. If the ulcer worsens one must be aware of this so that reculture and change of treatment can be instituted. Nictitans flaps do not allow these options.

Corneoscleral transpositions are ideal for perforating corneal ulcers, although they require microsurgical skills. The best prognosis can be given in cases of acute perforation when the surrounding cornea is healthy. Corneoscleral transpositions allow creation of a leak-free patch of the cornea, move blood vessels closer to the ulcer, and often leave a sighted eye.

Deep ulcers usually heal first by re-epithelialization, and then corneal thickness is restored when blood vessels reach the area. When healing is finally complete, blood vessels will regress without treatment. Because there is no evidence suggesting that corticosteroids decrease the eventual size of the scar and because the possibility of recurrence of ulceration in an already compromised cornea exists, the author does not recommend their use to speed healing after epithelialization is complete.

References and Supplemental Reading

Bistner, S. I.: Ocular emergencies and trauma. *In* Slatter, D. H. (ed.): *Textbook of Small Animal Surgery.* Philadelphia: W. B. Saunders, 1985, p. 1584.

Gelatt, K. N., and Samuelson, D. A.: Recurrent corneal erosions and epithelial dystrophy in the boxer dog. J. Am. Anim. Hosp. Assoc. 18:453, 1982.

Munger, R. J.: The conjunctiva. *In* Slatter, D. H. (ed.): *Textbook of Small Animal Surgery.* Philadelphia: W. B. Saunders, 1985, p. 1469.

Munger, R. J., and Champagne, E. S.: Multiple punctate keratotomies for the treatment of recurrent erosions in dogs. Trans. Am. Coll. Vet. Ophthalmol. 18:103, 1987.

Nasisse, M. P.: Canine ulcerative keratitis. Comp. Cont. Ed. Pract. Vet. 7:686, 1985.

Parshall, C. J.: Lamellar corneal-scleral transposition. J. Am. Anim. Hosp. Assoc. 9:270, 1973.

NEONATAL OPHTHALMIC DISORDERS

MELANIE M. WILLIAMS, D.V.M.
Guelph, Ontario

The neonatal period commences at birth and continues to 4 weeks of age. Numerous ophthalmic disorders may manifest during this time period. Some disorders are present at birth, whereas others begin after birth. Most of the ocular conditions are not detectable until after the time of eyelid separation.

Puppies and kittens are born with physiologic ankyloblepharon or fusion of the superior and inferior eyelids. Lacrimal gland function and the muscular and neurologic function of the eyelids are not developed at birth. The eyelids separate between 10 and 15 days of age when these tissues have reached functional maturity.

Intraocular examination is not possible at the time of eyelid separation owing to diffuse corneal edema. Edema results from immaturity of the corneal endothelium and its associated Na^+, K^+, ATPase pump. Corneal clarity is dependent on a state of relative dehydration maintained by the endothelial pump. Corneal dehydration approaches the adult level at about 3 weeks of age. Detailed intraocular examination is not possible until between 3 and 4 weeks of age.

Neurologic visual pathways develop primarily after eyelid separation. Retinal visual stimulation and image formation are necessary for the development of the visual pathways. Absence of normal visual stimulation due to opacities or other ocular abnormalities in the neonatal and pediatric animal will result in permanent blindness due to lack of visual pathway development.

Neonatal puppies and kittens will be presented to the veterinarian because the owner/breeder has noted a physical ocular abnormality or because the animal's behavior indicates visual impairment. Retinal maturity is not reached until approximately 42 days of age; however, vision can be detected from 3 weeks of age onward in most breeds. In a visually impaired or blind neonate, the breeder will note a decreased activity level in affected pups and kittens. There will be a lack of behavioral response to light but response to auditory stimulation, marked clumsiness in comparison to littermates, and frequent collision with solid objects. Individual neonates and entire litters will be presented to the veterinarian if the breeder is concerned or uncertain about the status of the other siblings.

Neonatal or congenital ocular disorders that manifest during the neonatal period are discussed below.

EYELID ANOMALIES

Several congenital and neonatal eyelid disorders are present in the neonatal puppy and kitten. These include eyelid agenesis, entropion, and premature or delayed eyelid separation.

Eyelid Agenesis

Eyelid agenesis, also termed eyelid coloboma, represents incomplete eyelid development. The condition is more common in kittens than in puppies. The breeder/owner will notice an abnormality of the eyelid at birth or at the time of eyelid separation.

CLINICAL SIGNS. Eyelid agenesis in the dog involves the inferior temporal eyelid and may be associated with a dermoid.

In the cat, agenesis most commonly involves the superior temporal eyelid. In some instances persistent pupillary membrane, iris and optic nerve colobomas, and choroidal hypoplasia have also been present. The eyelid agenesis may cause keratitis in the superior temporal quadrant of the cornea owing to drying from exposure or from the irritation of trichiasis or entropion. Corneal ulceration, vascularization, melanosis, or granulation may be observed in this area. The domestic short-hair and Burmese cat are the most commonly affected.

ETIOLOGY. Inheritance may be a factor; however, affected domestic short-hair cats present sporadically with the disorder. The pathogenesis of eyelid agenesis may involve a failure of embryologic adhesion of the eyelid folds. Eyelid buds develop at gestational day 28 and grow over the corneal surface to meet one another and adhere together by day 32 to 33 to form the normal physiologic ankyloblepharon seen in newborn puppies and kittens.

THERAPY AND PROGNOSIS. Slight eyelid agenesis may not result in corneal disease. Mild secondary entropion may be corrected by the modified Hotz-Celsus procedure. Severe eyelid agenesis requires immediate therapy. Because tear production is not mature in the newborn, lack of eyelid protection will require administration of ocular lubricating agents and prophylactic antibiotic therapy topically. Severe cases will require eventual eyelid reconstruction. If untreated, the secondary entropion, trichiasis, and drying will produce keratitis with or without ulceration. Several blepharoplastic reconstructive procedures have been described.

Neonatal Entropion

Entropion is an inversion of the eyelid, which may cause secondary corneal disease. Entropion usually manifests during the first year of life. Neonatal entropion occurs occasionally in some breeds of dogs and with significant frequency in the Shar Pei breed. Entropion is most common in breeds selected for a wide skull or excessive facial skin with facial folds.

CLINICAL SIGNS. After eyelid separation, the lower or upper eyelid or both are seen to roll inward. The lid margin is only partially visible or may be completely obscured from view. In response to the corneal pain produced by the epidermal lid surface's contacting the cornea and conjunctiva, contraction of the retractor bulbi muscle pulls the globe deep into the bony orbit (enophthalmos). With enophthalmos, prolapse of the nictitating membrane occurs. This sequence of events may protect the cornea from further damage. If corneal epidermal contact persists, corneal vascularization, fibrosis, melanosis, or ulceration results.

Epiphora occurs as a result of hypersecretion of reflex tear from ocular pain. Blepharospasm or spastic entropion further complicates the neonatal anatomic entropion. Blepharospasm is a response to corneal pain, producing marked contraction of the orbicularis oculi muscle near the lid margin.

ETIOLOGY. Entropion is an inherited defect inasmuch as facial characteristics are passed on from parent to sibling. It represents an imbalance among three tissues, which must complement one another to produce anatomic balance. The tissues involved are the bony socket or orbit in which the eyeball sits, the globe, and the skin of the eyelids and face. Dogs selectively bred for wide skulls may develop large orbits. A normal-sized eyeball is unable to fill such an orbit, and enophthalmos results. Eyelids are not self-supporting structures; they rely on underlying tissue for their support. The bony orbital rim terminates some distance from the center of the cornea; the eyelid thereby rests on the bulbar conjunctiva and cornea of the eyeball. When these tissues are displaced caudally as in enophthalmos, the eyelids roll inward until they find tissue to rest on. Entropion is thus created. A small eyeball in an otherwise normal-sized bony orbit would have the same effect, although this is uncommon. Excessive facial skin and folds result in formation of abundant tissue, which rests against the eyelids. The redundant tissue causes an inrolling of the eyelids, and entropion results. This latter mechanism plus selection for a somewhat smaller eyeball, as in the Shar Pei compared with other breeds of comparable size and weight, produces entropion in the Shar Pei. In brachycephalic breeds shortening of the facial bones has created redundant mucosal tissue in both the throat area and the conjunctiva. The Shar Pei has much redundant conjunctiva, which adds fullness to the eyelids, further complicating the entropion.

DIAGNOSTIC TESTS. Instillation of topical ophthalmic anesthetic, at 30-sec intervals for three instillations, will anesthetize the corneal and conjunctival surfaces and eliminate the spastic component of the entropion to permit evaluation of the anatomic component. Fluorescein dye will identify corneal ulceration.

THERAPY. When possible it is advisable to delay blepharoplastic surgery until the animal has attained adult size. Only then is the permanent relationship among orbit, eyeball, and eyelid established. If neonatal correction is required to prevent corneal damage, vertical mattress tacking sutures of 4–0 silk or black braided nylon (Ethilon, Pitman-Moore) are recommended. Soft suture material is recommended in the periocular area to offset irritation, should corneal contact occur. Sutures may be left in place for 1 to 3 weeks. After suture removal, many animals will have relatively normal lid fit, with the lid margin contacting the eyeball. The procedure may be repeated if necessary. Tacking may facilitate lid growth in a slightly altered position. Fibrosis and tissue contraction along the suture track may be sufficient to roll the eyelid outward. If entropion continues to damage the corneas, blepharoplasty may be required in the young pup. A repeat procedure is likely at maturity, and overcorrection must be avoided. Palpation for adequate lateral canthal ligament support should be performed. If support is lacking, a lateral ligament will need to be fashioned from orbicularis oculi muscle.

Premature or Delayed Opening of the Eyelids

CLINICAL SIGNS. Premature eyelid separation predisposes the cornea to desiccation. Ulcerative keratopathy may result. Corneal perforation, panophthalmitis, and permanent blindness may ensue.

Delayed eyelid separation may predispose to neonatal conjunctivitis (see below).

THERAPY AND PROGNOSIS. Intensive therapy is indicated in premature eyelid separation. Therapy should include frequent ocular lubrication, such as with sterile methylcellulose ophthalmic ointment.

Topical antibiotic ointments (q6h) may be used prophylactically or if infection occurs. In the absence of infection, a surgical temporary tarsorrhaphy will be of benefit. If tear production is adequate by 2 weeks of age and if ulcerative keratopathy and infection have resolved, medication may be discontinued or a temporary tarsorrhaphy may be released.

Delayed Eyelid Separation

Delayed eyelid separation should be treated by 16 days of age. Gentle digital traction should be applied, commencing at the medial canthus. If this is not successful, one blade of a small blunt scissors should be inserted beneath the eyelid at the medial canthus. The scissors cut should be positioned along the natural line of eyelid separation. The scissors should gently be moved laterally to effect eyelid separation.

DERMOID

Dermoids represent congenital choristomas and have been referred to as congenital tumors and dermoid cysts. They are the consequence of abnormal differentiation of tissues at the ocular surface. Dermoids consist of epidermis, dermis, fat, sebaceous glands, and hair follicles.

CLINICAL SIGNS. A dermoid is frequently recognized as an abnormality by the owner at the time of eyelid separation. Dermoids occur on the cornea, conjunctiva, and eyelids. They are frequently located on the temporal cornea in the dog. In the cat they are rare (except in Burmese) and are most often located at the limbus. A dermoid may be unilateral or bilateral and single or multiple. A dermoid may be pigmented or unpigmented. Hair shafts commonly protrude from the tissue surface and project at an angle different from that of normal skin in the area. If no hair projects from the dermoid, there are usually no associated clinical signs.

The hair projecting from a dermoid may produce epiphora, discharge, blepharospasm, and keratitis. This is more likely to be significant when the dermoid is located on the eyelid, moving against the cornea and conjunctiva with ocular and eyelid movement. Dermoids on the cornea move with the globe and tend to be somewhat less irritating. The caruncle in the medial canthus of the dog may normally contain some hair follicles and should not be mistaken for a conjunctival dermoid.

THERAPY AND PROGNOSIS. Rarely, pigmentation and vascularity will increase at the dermoid border, and the dermoid itself may thicken. Dermoids tend to grow slowly if at all.

Therapy is indicated if the dermoid is causing ocular discomfort or ocular discharge or if it is considered unsightly by the owner. An eyelid dermoid is treated by surgical excision followed by primary closure of the lid defect. If the defect is too large, plastic reconstruction of the eyelid will be indicated. Conjunctival dermoids are surgically removed; and the defect is closed, using a sliding or rotational conjunctival flap or buccal mucosa graft. Corneal dermoids are removed by surgical keratectomy. The prognosis for removal without scar formation on the cornea is guarded and depends on the depth of the lesion. Some dermoids are deep and may require deep corneal resection with subsequent grafting or flapping. After healing, application of topical steroids, under close supervision, tends to discourage persistent vascularization in some cases.

NEONATAL INFECTIOUS EYE DISEASES

Neonatal puppies and kittens occasionally acquire ocular infections *in utero*, during birth, or in the neonatal period. Canine neonatal conjunctivitis (ophthalmia neonatorum), feline neonatal conjunctivitis, and feline neonatal herpesvirus infection are the major disease entities in this category.

Feline and Canine Neonatal Conjunctivitis

Neonatal conjunctivitis occurs occasionally. If recognized by the breeder/owner in the early stages, permanent ocular and visual damage may be avoided.

If the breeder is aware of the existence of such a disease and understands the clinical signs, neonatal puppies and kittens will be presented at the first noted signs of eyelid swelling or ocular discharge.

CLINICAL SIGNS. If infection occurs prior to eyelid separation, discharge accumulates beneath the eyelids, causing the eyelids to swell. A discharge may be noted at the medial canthus as the discharge is forced against the eyelids close to the time of separation. If infection occurs after eyelid separation, ocular discharge will be more obvious. Purulent discharge may cause the eyelids to stick together. Chemosis and hyperemia may be quite marked. The conjunctiva and lids are difficult to examine owing to the small size of these structures in the neonate. Puppies, kittens, and the dam and queen, respectively, should be thoroughly examined for any signs of systemic illness, as well as for vaginal or mammary gland infection.

ETIOLOGY. Genital infections in the queen or dam result in infection during the birthing or neonatal time period. Signs develop most frequently within the first 10 days of life. Bacteria or viruses in puppies and kittens, or *Chlamydia* in the cat, may be the causative agent. Neonatal chlamydial infection may occur by transmission from a carrier queen or from other cats in the household. This infection usually occurs after eyelid separation. (Neonatal herpesvirus infections are discussed separately because of the potential seriousness and frequency of this disease.)

THERAPEUTICS AND PROGNOSIS. Untreated neonatal conjunctivitis frequently results in severe keratitis, particularly if physiologic ankyloblepharon existed at the time of infection. Ulcerative keratitis and corneal perforation with permanent blindness and phthisis bulbi are common sequelae in this situation.

If the eyelids are still fused, they should be manually separated by digital traction commencing at the medial canthus. This should be accomplished without difficulty if the animal is older than 7 days of age. If the lids will not separate, a small blunt scissors blade should be inserted beneath the lid margins at the medial canthus (see p. 660). Tenacious discharge should be removed from the conjunctiva, cornea, and fornices. Culture and sensitivity testing are advisable. Cotton-tipped applicators and a warmed physiologic saline (38.5°C) flush will facilitate the removal of exudate. Warm compresses may be necessary to loosen discharge that is gluing the eyelids together. Gentle, thorough exudate removal is required to avoid creating ulcerated surfaces on the eyelids and conjunctiva. Medication should *not* be applied on top of ocular discharge, but rather after its removal.

The corneas should be stained with fluorescein to check for ulcers. Medication should initially consist of broad-spectrum antibiotics topically applied four times daily. Antibiotic selection may change when culture and sensitivity results are available. Corticosteroids are not advisable owing to the high potential for corneal ulcers. A solution consisting of artificial tears and broad-spectrum antibiotics and acetylcysteine is necessary in ulcerative conditions or when discharge is very tenacious.

Bacterial infections tend to respond well to therapy. Viral infections do not. Systemic support and therapy is indicated in systemically ill neonates.

Breeder education is important. Neonatal conjunctivitis may rapidly progress to blindness if undiagnosed or untreated, particularly if physiologic ankyloblepharon is still present. Breeders should be instructed to observe the eyelids of neonatal puppies and kittens regularly and to seek immediate veterinary care if swelling is noted. Breeders may also be instructed in digital eyelid separation prior to presentation of the neonate at the hospital.

Feline Neonatal Herpesvirus Infection

Feline herpesvirus is highly infectious but does not survive outside the body beyond 24 hr. Herpesvirus produces a variety of clinical signs including acute conjunctivitis (often associated with clinical signs of upper respiratory tract disease) and keratitis.

CLINICAL SIGNS. Signs of respiratory tract infection may or may not be present. Kittens have signs ranging from mild conjunctivitis to keratitis. Typically all siblings in the litter are affected, and the ocular disease is bilateral. A serous ocular discharge is present initially. Mucopurulence ensues with secondary bacterial contamination. If infection occurs prior to eyelid separation, discharge will accumulate behind the eyelids and produce swelling of the lids.

Occasionally herpetic keratoconjunctivitis occurs. The keratitis may be ulcerative or nonulcerative at the time of presentation. Keratitis first occurs as epithelial necrosis. The epithelium will then slough and produce an ulcer. Ulcers are initially dendritic or linear and branching. Ulcers may coalesce into large maplike or geographic ulcers. Ulcers tend to remain superficial or epithelial. Stromal involvement and perforation rarely result.

Keratoconjunctivitis sicca (KCS) may occur with herpesvirus infection. The sicca is most frequently transient but may become a chronic problem. Symblepharon may result from the severe keratoconjunctivitis.

Systemic effects of herpetic respiratory tract infection may become marked in the neonate.

ETIOLOGY. Herpesvirus is most likely to be transmitted from the queen to the kittens at the time of birth or shortly thereafter. The source of infection is often a maternal vaginal infection. A carrier animal shedding virus in the household may also be the source of infection. Cats may carry and shed herpesvirus for years. An estimated 80 per cent of infected cats may become carriers, regardless of the presence of serum neutralizing antibody. Circulating antibodies probably are of little benefit in preventing or eliminating infection. Local secretory IgA and cell-mediated immunity are probably of greater importance.

The virus is believed to become latent within local ganglia and to reactivate during times of stress. In recurrent chronic or severe forms of herpesvirus infection, concurrent feline leukemia virus (FeLV) infection should be investigated, as immunosuppression by this virus may be underlying the susceptibility to herpes.

DIAGNOSTIC TESTS. Rose bengal dye will stain necrotic corneal epithelium in herpetic keratitis, prior to the development of ulceration. Fluorescein dye will stain corneal stroma denuded of epithelium after ulceration has occurred. Schirmer's tear test will rule out hyposecretion of tears.

A complete physical examination is indicated. Numerous diagnostic tests are available, including conjunctival smears for cytologic study; serologic examination for serum neutralizing antibody and for hemagglutination inhibition for antibody; viral isolation from culture of conjunctival epithelium; and direct and indirect immunofluorescence tests on conjunctival smears.

Conjunctival cytologic results may be supportive but are rarely diagnostic for feline herpes. Serum antibody titers often demonstrate no rise in titer in recurrent disease. Paired serum samples are required, and the tests are costly. Viral harvest is beneficial in epithelial herpes infection, provided the samples are properly handled. The virus produces a cytopathic effect in culture. Viral neutralization or fluorescent antibody test will then identify the virus. These tests are lengthy and costly. Direct and indirect fluorescent antibody tests, the preferred method of laboratory diagnosis, are reliable and relatively inexpensive, and samples are easily collected.

THERAPEUTICS. In the immunocompetent animal, acute herpetic conjunctivitis is treated supportively with topical ophthalmic prophylactic antibiotics. Specific antiviral medications may or may not be required. When secondary infection is controlled, the viral infection will often resolve spontaneously in 10 to 14 days. If physiologic ankyloblepharon is present, the eyelids should be separated as previously discussed. The scissors blade should then be directed parallel to the lid margins along the line of natural eyelid separation. The scissors should gently be moved laterally to effect eyelid separation. Discharge should be removed from the eye with warm (38.5°C) physiologic saline eye flush and swabs. A topical antibiotic should then be applied every 4 to 6 hr.

Systemic therapy may be indicated in the neonate. Owing to incomplete immunity in the very young kitten, systemic viral infection and life-threatening complications are more common than in adults. Supportive systemic treatment will be required in this event.

Herpetic keratitis, whether ulcerative or nonulcerative, requires antiviral therapy. This aspect of herpes infection is difficult to manage because of its tendency to recur and viral persistence within nervous tissue. Antiviral medication must be administered frequently (q5h for ointments and q2h for solutions). Trifluridine (Viroptic, Burroughs Wellcome) is the most effective antiviral medication against feline herpesvirus. Idoxuridine (Stoxil, SmithKline Beckman) and adenine arabinoside (Vira-A, Parke-Davis) are of intermediate effect, and acycloguanosine is of little use. Prophylactic topical antibiotic should be used simultaneously. Herpes keratitis is most common in the adult cat but may be present in the neonate.

Deep corneal ulceration is best supported by a conjunctival or nictitating membrane flap. Fortunately, this is uncommon in the neonate.

Corticosteroids are contraindicated in the treatment of ocular herpes. Corticosteroids suppress the immune response and potentiate collagenase. Host immune response is required to combat herpes infection. Chronic stromal keratitis is the only indication for steroid use. This is a rare condition and is best handled by the specialist.

PROGNOSIS. Acute infections offer the best prognosis. Chronic infections become refractory. The success of therapy is dependent on the immune status of the host in addition to the efficacy of the antiviral drug. If untreated, the corneal infection may produce a scarred unsighted eye. Conjunctival infection may result in symblepharon.

An estimated 80 per cent of infected cats will become carriers and shed the virus intermittently while remaining asymptomatic. Quarantine of new additions to a cattery and vaccination are recommended.

DISORDERS OF THE NASOLACRIMAL SECRETORY AND EXCRETORY SYSTEM

The nasolacrimal system is composed of a secretory portion and an excretory portion. The secretory portion refers to the tear-producing glands, including the orbital lacrimal gland, gland of the nictitating membrane, conjunctival goblet cells, and meibomian or tarsal glands. The tear film is eliminated via the excretory portion of the nasolacrimal system. This includes the superior and inferior lacrimal puncta, and respective lacrimal canaliculi, the vestigial lacrimal sac, and the nasolacrimal canal. The tears are propelled by lid blinking toward the medial canthus, where a lacrimal lake is formed. The aqueous layer of the tear film enters the excretory system and evaporates in the nasal cavity. The mucous layer may enter the excretory system or collect at the medial canthus as "sleep." Obstruction of the excretory pathway results in tear overflow (epiphora) down the face.

Imperforate lacrimal puncta and keratoconjunctivitis sicca (dry eye) are two conditions of the nasolacrimal system that may be present in neonates.

Congenital/Neonatal Imperforate Lacrimal Punctum

Imperforate lacrimal punctum occurs occasionally in puppies and kittens.

CLINICAL SIGNS. Following eyelid separation, tears will be noted on the skin of the medial canthus. If the disorder is chronic, rust-colored tear staining of light-colored hair coat at the medial canthus will become apparent. The inferior punctum is more often imperforate, though both puncta may be affected. The disorder may be unilateral or bilateral. Atresia of the nasolacrimal canal produces similar clinical signs but is rare in small animals.

Impatency of the superior lacrimal punctum with a patent inferior punctum rarely produces clinical signs.

Imperforate puncta are most common in the toy and miniature poodle, American cocker spaniel, and Bedlington terrier.

ETIOLOGY. In puppies this usually represents a congenital malformation. In kittens it is most often due to cicatricial obstruction from herpesvirus infection.

DIAGNOSTIC TESTS. Cannulation and saline flushing of the superior punctum, if patent, will fail to produce fluid via an inferior punctum. A slight ballooning of the conjunctiva may be detectable under the pressure of the flush. This indicates that the lacrimal canaliculi are developed but the imperforate punctum is covered by a layer of conjunctiva. This is the most common finding. Fluorescein passage through the nose will be delayed on the affected side.

THERAPY AND PROGNOSIS. This ocular disorder is cosmetically unacceptable to many owners; however, it does not cause any additional ocular damage. If tear overflow is profuse (as with hypersecretion of tears from distichiasis in the American cocker spaniel), excoriation of the skin may result.

The conjunctiva over the imperforate punctum may be grasped with forceps after identification via flushing and then snipped with scissors to create a patent opening. Topical antibiotic-corticosteroid solution is applied q 4 hr for 10 to 14 days. Should the system heal closed, it should be reopened and cannulated with 0 to 2–0 monofilament nylon. The cannula should be sutured in place for 1 to 2 weeks, and topical antibiotic corticosteroid drops should be applied again q 4 hr for 2 weeks.

Neonatal Keratoconjunctivitis Sicca

Keratoconjunctivitis sicca (KCS) describes deficient tear production that results in corneal and conjunctival disease. A congenital or neonatal absence of lacrimal gland tissue or nervous stimulation may exist in puppies and kittens.

CLINICAL SIGNS. Clinical signs become apparent after eyelid separation. The disorder may produce ulcerative keratitis if the lack of aqueous tear production is complete. Partial tear production produces corneal melanosis or epidermalization in response to desiccation. Secondary extraocular infection will produce tenacious, mucopurulent discharge. This congenital disorder is seen most commonly in the pug, Pekingese, Yorkshire terrier, and Chihuahua.

DIAGNOSTIC TESTS. Schirmer's tear test values are markedly subnormal (< 10 mm/min). Rose bengal dye will diffusely stain desiccated epithelial tissue of the cornea and conjunctiva. Fluorescein dye will stain the cornea denuded of epithelium as a result of KCS.

THERAPY AND PROGNOSIS. The prognosis in congenital or neonatal dry eye is guarded. Subsequent lacrimal gland function in complete dry eye is rare. Markedly improved tear production has been observed by the author following several months of medical therapy in a puppy with congenital partial hyposecretion.

Therapy must include frequent ocular lubrication with artificial tear drops or ointments. Topical antibiotics are indicated if infection is present, and acetylcysteine may be combined with the artificial tear drops and antibiotic if the ocular discharge is tenacious and voluminous. Pilocarpine may be administered as an oral or topical preparation in an attempt to provide parasympathomimetic neurologic stimulation to the lacrimal gland. Ophthalmic formulation of a KCS solution including pilocarpine has been well described (Severin, 1979). Oral administration of ophthalmic 1 per cent pilocarpine is recommended in food twice daily, commencing with one drop twice daily for 5 days. If no clinical signs of drug toxicity occur, therapy is increased to 2 drops b.i.d. and then to 3 drops b.i.d., provided toxicity signs do not develop. Signs of adverse drug reaction include salivation, diarrhea, vomition, anorexia, and weakness.

Topical cyclosporine is presently under clinical and experimental investigation in the treatment of KCS. It may prove valuable in congenital KCS dependent on its mode of action on lacrimal tissue.

Surgical therapies include permanent partial tarsorrhaphy to decrease the area of cornea to be lubricated and nourished by the tear film. Parotid duct transposition is also feasible if salivary production is determined to be normal.

OCULAR DISORDERS AND OCULAR HYPOPIGMENTATION

Several clinical entities exist both in the neonate and in the adult that involve ocular abnormalities and ocular hypopigmentation. Three syndromes may be present in the neonate: Chédiak-Higashi syndrome; ocular dysgenesis associated with albinism and deafness; and ocular dysgenesis associated with microphthalmia, merling, and white coat color. (The latter syndrome is discussed with microphthalmia.)

Chédiak-Higashi Syndrome

Chédiak-Higashi syndrome is an inherited defect in humans and domestic animals, including cats, cattle, mink, and mice.

CLINICAL SIGNS. Affected kittens are photophobic; pale, thin irides and decreased fundic pigmentation are noted. Choroidal vessels are detectable. Fine spontaneous nystagmus is horizontal to rotatory. Bilateral cataracts vary from posterior suture line opacities to total diffuse cataract that produces leukocoria. Prolonged bleeding times and increased susceptibility to infection may exist in affected animals.

ETIOLOGY. Inheritance is suspected. Cataract is not a feature of Chédiak-Higashi syndrome in other species and may represent a separate genetic entity in the cat.

DIAGNOSTIC TESTS. In suspected cases, hair may be examined for microscopically enlarged melanin granules typical of the disorder.

THERAPY AND PROGNOSIS. No therapy exists for these genetic maldevelopments. Prolonged bleeding times may present a problem during routine surgical procedures.

Ocular Dysgenesis Associated with Albinism and Deafness

Partial hearing loss with multiple ocular dysgenesis and white hair coat has been identified in the cat and dog. Canine breeds include the collie, Dalmatian, Australian shepherd, Great Dane, and Doberman pinscher. This disorder somewhat parallels inherited Waardenburg's syndrome in humans and, excepting the auditory manifestations, resembles ocular dysgenesis (see p. 666). The breeder will note blindness, microphthalmia, or both in predominantly white-coated animals.

CLINICAL SIGNS. All affected pups have hearing deficits and a predominantly white coat or partial albinism. Multiple ocular defects are present, including a white to blue iris, irregular pupil, cortical cataract, albinotic fundus, mesodermal filtration, angle dysgenesis, and blindness. Many affected pups are also microphthalmic and have equatorial staphyloma and occasional spherophakia and lens luxation.

ETIOLOGY. Inheritance is suspected, and an association exists between the ocular-auditory abnormalities and partial or complete albinism.

PATHOLOGY AND EMBRYOLOGY. The uvea, optic nerve, and equatorial sclera are hypoplastic. The iris dilator muscle is poorly developed with anomalous vascular channels. Pigment is deficient in the uvea and retinal pigmented epithelium. Cortical cataract and coloboma are observed. The retina is variably dysplastic. The auditory system shows cochlear-saccular degeneration with severe degeneration of the organ of Corti.

THERAPY AND PROGNOSIS. Angle dysgenesis predisposes affected animals to glaucoma. Retinal detachment with hemorrhage may also occur. Breeder counseling is indicated owing to the suspected genetic association in this disorder. Selection toward albinism or marked white coat component should be discouraged.

MICROPHTHALMIA

Following eyelid separation, pups may be presented to the veterinarian with the owner's observation of no eye, a small eye, or prolapse of the nictitating membrane. Microphthalmia may be the presenting clinical sign of several ocular disorders.

ETIOLOGY. Microphthalmia has been produced by maternal vitamin A deficiency in pigs and griseofulvin administration to pregnant queens. Experimentally, microphthalmia has resulted from x-ray hypoxia; hypoglycemia; deficiencies of vitamins, including vitamin A, riboflavin, folic acid, and vitamin E; and hypervitaminosis A. In children, microphthalmia may be caused by inheritance, congenital rubella, or *Toxoplasma* infection. Numerous reports of microphthalmia in dogs exist. The microphthalmia may be associated with other minor or major ocular abnormalities and in some instances is inherited.

Microphthalmia: Anterior Cleavage Syndrome

Anterior cleavage syndrome has also been termed anterior ocular dysgenesis. The syndrome is noted in humans and dogs, including the Doberman pinscher and St. Bernard. In the Doberman the disorder is believed to be inherited as an autosomal recessive trait. It has been identified in this breed in Norway, Denmark, the United Kingdom, and the United States. Inheritance is also suspected in the St. Bernard.

CLINICAL SIGNS. At 3 weeks of age, pups have bilateral cloudy small eyes with prolapse of the nictitating membrane. Normal visual activity initially observed by the breeder between 3 and 5 weeks of age is absent. Pups demonstrate no response to a flashlight but turn their heads in response to external noise or littermate vocalizations. The head is held low, and movement is cautious and faltering. The microphthalmic globes are enophthalmic, and prolapse of the nictitating membrane results. Corneas are frequently opaque, edematous, and fibrotic with foci of melanosis. A rotatory nystagmus may be present. Some pups reportedly have narrower heads than unaffected littermates and a narrow, short palpebral fissure.

PATHOLOGY AND EMBRYOGENESIS. The cornea is abnormal, with fibrosis, vascularization, and frequent absence of corneal endothelium and Descemet's membrane. The anterior chamber, pupil, and iridocorneal angle are not formed, as the anterior uvea is continuous with the posterior cornea. Differentiation of uveal tissue into iris and ciliary body is poor to nonexistent. In the St. Bernard, a rudimentary pupil or pupillary outline occasionally exists. The eyes are aphakic or contain vestiges of abnormal cataractous lens cells within the poorly differentiated uveal tissue. The retinas are dysplastic and not attached. Optic nerve hypoplasia and internal hydrocephalus is present in some affected St. Bernard pups. Although microphthalmia is part of the syndrome, occasional unilateral megaloglobus exists in bilaterally affected St. Bernards. This is presumably due to a slightly more advanced differentiation of tissues, with congenital glaucoma resulting from the iridocorneal angle dysgenesis.

THERAPY AND PROGNOSIS. The pups are irreversibly blind. Owing to the genetic implications in this disorder, the parent stock and normal-eyed siblings should not be bred. Breeder counseling to this effect is indicated.

Microphthalmia with Cataract

Microphthalmia with cataract has been noted in the miniature schnauzer, Cavalier King Charles spaniel, Akita, and Old English sheepdog. A percentage of pups are also affected with lenticonus. Neonatal pups are not blind but may be visually impaired. The major abnormality observed by the breeder/owner will be microphthalmia at the time of eyelid separation.

CLINICAL SIGNS. Ophthalmic examination evinces cataract and microphthalmia at the time of eyelid separation. Cataracts involve the lens nucleus and perinuclear and posterior cortex. Microphakia parallels the microphthalmia in the miniature schnauzer. Lenticonus was present in the Akita, in the Old English sheepdog, in 19 per cent of affected schnauzer pups, and in 27 per cent of affected Cavaliers. Lenticonus is a deformity of the posterior lens cortex and capsule that bulges into the vitreous. Lenticonus internus is present in a small percentage of affected schnauzer lenses and represents a caudal displacement of the nucleus into the posterior lens cortex, producing a marked posterior lens protrusion or lentiglobus into the vitreal cavity.

Retinal folds were also present in the Old English sheepdog and Akita and may represent transient folds or a more permanent form of retinal pathologic change, termed retinal dysplasia. The ocular disorder presented as both unilateral and bilateral disease in the Cavalier.

ETIOLOGY. Microphthalmia with cataract is inherited as an autosomal recessive trait in the miniature schnauzer. Inheritance was suspected in the Cavalier King Charles spaniel, as many affected dogs were related.

PATHOGENESIS AND EMBRYOLOGY. Lenticonus and nuclear cataract represent an early embryologic defect. After cortical fibers are present, posterior lens capsule is no longer formed. The posterior lenticonus described has a complete, although thinned, posterior capsule, indicating that the primary defect occurred prior to day 35 of gestation. The presence of nuclear cataract further dates the defect to gestational day 25.

THERAPY AND PROGNOSIS. The cataracts may be progressive. The degree of progression seems to depend on the amount of cortical involvement. The cataracts may progress to maturity or hypermaturity between 1 and 3 years of age. Mydriatics will dilate the pupil and may provide peripheral vision around the affected nucleus and perinuclear cortex. Therapy for clinical signs of intraocular inflammation, including cycloplegics/mydriatics, topical corticosteroids, and systemic anti-inflammatory agents or antiprostaglandins, may be indicated during lens resorption. If lens resorption is complete with minimal inflammatory change, aphakic visual return may occur.

One Cavalier pup experienced bilateral posterior lens capsule rupture at 5 months of age, producing suddenly painful blind eyes. Vision is nonretrievable in this event. The lenses were predisposed to rupture in this pup owing to probable thin posterior lens capsules in the area of the lenticonus, compounded by progression of the cataracts, with resultant lens swelling.

Breeder counseling is indicated, as the defect is inherited in the miniature schnauzer and Old English sheepdog. Parental stock, normal-eyed siblings, and affected pups should not be bred. Should a repeat breeding produce similarly affected pups in the second litter, strong support exists for a genetic influence in any breed.

Microphthalmia and Ocular Dysgenesis Associated with Merling and White Coat Color

Ocular abnormalities associated with white hair coat and heterochromia irides have been noted in humans, swine, cat, dog, and cattle. Suspected inherited microphthalmia with ocular defects of the iris, ciliary body, choroid, and optic nerve occurs in humans. Ocular albinism in humans has been associated with both ocular and systemic defects. Microphthalmia with ocular dysgenesis in merle-coated animals with excessive amounts of white has been identified in the Australian shepherd, merle rough collie, and harlequin Great Dane. Investigations have been most extensive in the Australian

shepherd, accounting for the frequent reference to that breed below.

Breeders will present affected pups with small eyes with or without prolapse of the nictitating membrane at the time of eyelid separation. Behavioral abnormalities related to visual impairment or blindness will be noted in some pups.

CLINICAL SIGNS. The disorder is usually bilateral but asymmetric. Microphthalmia, microcornea, heterochromia irides, and corectopia are present in all affected pups. Cataract, equatorial staphylomas, and retinal detachments are present in a high percentage of pups; however, the degree of microphthalmia may preclude intraocular examination and identification of these clinical signs in severely affected pups.

Pups with mild microphthalmia may demonstrate no visual impairment, and the intraocular structures may be examined. In moderate microphthalmia the eyeball fills approximately one half of the palpebral fissure. Approximately half of these pups will be blind. Pups with severe microphthalmia have marked nictitating membrane prolapse and eyeballs that vary from distinct globes to irregular cystic masses. All such pups are blind, and a searching nystagmus is usually present. The microcorneas are usually irregularly shaped. Irides are usually light blue and may be transilluminated, indicating thinness. The pupil is corectopic, being oval with the long axis vertical. A poor response to topical ophthalmic mydriatics/cycloplegics is typical. Cataracts involve the anterior or posterior cortex or both. Equatorial staphylomas are often multiple and are located medially and laterally midway between the ora serrata and the optic disk. These defects occur as single or multiple small groups of excavations. The depth of the staphylomas is often difficult to evaluate with the direct ophthalmoscope. It can vary from 3 to 20 diopters. The fundus is only faintly pigmented (subalbinotic), and choroid blood vessels are prominent. The fundi are frequently atapetal. Small optic nerves or micropapilla is present in some of the more severely affected globes. Total retinal detachment may be accompanied by vitreal hemorrhage. Retinal dialysis near equatorial staphylomas may facilitate detachment.

All affected animals are blue merles, with excessive amounts of white coat accounting for 30 to 90 per cent of the total coat color.

HISTOPATHOLOGY AND EMBRYOLOGY. Retinal dysplasia is present. The staphylomas consist of thin choroid and scleral tunic cystlike formations lined with retinal tissue. Melanin deficiency may affect ocular embryogenesis. This disorder is probably related to defective prenatal development of the retinal pigmented epithelium.

ETIOLOGY. The ocular disorder is believed to be inherited in the Australian shepherd as a recessive trait with incomplete penetrance. Microphthalmia and related ocular dysgenesis occur more often in merle dogs with predominantly white coats. Merling, inherited as a dominant trait, is located at the M locus. White spotting variations are also influenced by several alleles at the S locus. Dominance of these alleles over one another may vary among breeds. Heterozygotes for merling have merle or dappled coats with occasional ocular anomalies. Homozygotes for merling have predominantly white coats and often have ocular defects, including microphthalmia. Coat color and ocular dysgenesis with microphthalmia appear to be directly related.

PROGNOSIS. No therapy exists to alter this embryologic defect. In severe microphthalmic globes, corneal vascularization and bullous keratopathy may frequently develop within the first 4 months of life. The cataract may progress to maturity by 2 to 5 years of age, producing blindness in dogs that were previously sighted.

Breeder counseling is important. Merle-coated animals are now popular; however, production of homozygotes is to be discouraged. Breeding of parents of affected offspring or affected or normal-eyed littermates is contraindicated owing to inheritance of the microphthalmia and ocular dysgenesis.

CONGENITAL/NEONATAL GLAUCOMA

CLINICAL SIGNS. Congenital glaucoma is rare in domestic animals. It has been observed in kittens with clinical signs of mydriasis, episcleral congestion, corneal edema, and blindness. It occurs sporadically in the puppy and most frequently in a unilateral, comfortable, uninflamed, buphthalmic eye that is frequently normotensive or hypotensive. An *in utero* or early neonatal intraocular pressure elevation is suspected, possibly attributable to anterior chamber filtration angle dysgenesis. The ocular tunics of the young pup are readily distensible.

DIAGNOSTIC TESTS. Tonometry is useful in determining if intraocular pressure is still elevated in congenital or neonatal glaucoma. Gonioscopy reveals structural filtration angle abnormalities in an unaffected fellow eye and in the affected eye, provided the cornea is sufficiently clear to permit visualization. Tonography evaluates the functional integrity of the aqueous humor outflow pathways.

THERAPY AND PROGNOSIS. In the canine neonate, therapy is usually not indicated for intraocular pressure lowering or comfort; however, the enlarged blind eye may be predisposed to injury or to desiccation if complete lid closure is not possible over the enlarged eyeball. Owners may also find the buphthalmic eye unsightly. Therapy may include a permanent partial tarsorrhaphy to decrease the ocular size of the palpebral fissure and to facilitate lid closure. Evisceration with an intrascleral prosthesis and enucleation are also options.

In the cat, medical or surgical therapy for glaucoma is indicated if the pressure is elevated. Cats may or may not demonstrate signs of ocular pain. Medical therapy includes carbonic anhydrase inhibitors, topical cholinergic miotic or sympathomimetic drugs, and topical beta-blockers. Surgical therapy includes cyclocryotherapy, intravitreal chemical ablation of the ciliary body epithelium, ocular evisceration with intrascleral prosthesis, and enucleation. Feline glaucoma tends to be more resistant to the therapeutic effects of antiglaucoma medical modalities and to cyclocryotherapy.

The visual prognosis in the affected eye is guarded to nil in neonatal glaucoma. Gonioscopic examination and tonometry in the normal fellow eye are indicated for prognostic value. Preventive treatment of the fellow eye is always indicated.

PERSISTENCE OF THE EMBRYONIC TUNICA VASCULOSA LENTIS

Persistent Hyperplastic Tunica Vasculosa Lentis and Persistent Hyperplastic Primary Vitreous (PHTVL/PHPV)

PHTVL/PHPV has been reported in several species, including humans and dogs. German shepherd, miniature poodle, standard schnauzer, greyhound, Labrador retriever, Irish setter, Irish wolfhound, Staffordshire bull terrier, and Doberman pinscher have been affected. The most detailed pathologic and genetic studies have involved the latter two breeds.

The breeder will note leukocoria, visual impairment, or blindness following eyelid separation.

CLINICAL SIGNS. Behavioral observation will support a visual deficit or blindness in some affected pups. Ophthalmic examination evinces the more severe expressions of PHTVL/PHPV in neonatal pups, unless the entire litter is presented for examination. The disorder may be associated with microphthalmia or persistent pupillary membrane. Doberman pups are usually affected bilaterally. Leukocoria or a white pupil is a predominant characteristic of PHTVL/PHPV. Bilateral involvement has been reported in the Labrador retriever and greyhound. Unilateral involvement was noted in the Irish setter, Irish wolfhound, miniature poodle, and German shepherd.

Ophthalmic findings range from the most mild to the most severe expression, as follows: Pigmented dots can be noted on the posterior lens capsule. A thick, white to brownish plaque on the posterior lens capsule may be found centrally and extending along the capsule halfway to the equator of the lens. The plaque occasionally grows into the lens. Abnormal lenticular shape occurs in the form of posterior lenticonus with occasional equatorial flattening of the lens. Persistence of the hyaloid artery varies from a small fibrotic remnant at the posterior polar capsule, to Bergmeister's papilla (projection of persistent hyaloid from the optic disk), to a complete hyaloid traversing from the optic disk, through the vitreal cavity, to the posterior lens capsule. An anomalous and branching vascular pathway between the optic nerve head and lens has been reported in the miniature poodle and German shepherd.

Intravitreal hemorrhage may occur from the persisting hyaloid vessels. Occasionally, intralenticular hemorrhage occurs, and calcium deposition may follow.

Cataract varies from slight to extensive at the position of the plaque (i.e., posterior lens capsule) and may extend into the posterior cortex and equatorial cortex. Anterior cortical involvement is extremely rare. The corneas, anterior chambers, and filtration angles appear unaffected. Fundic abnormalities include Bergmeister's papilla and focal retinal dysplasia.

ETIOLOGY. In the Doberman pinscher, one major autosomal gene is predominantly responsible and incomplete penetrance is suspected. There is no correlation between the ophthalmic disorder and coat color, nor is the transmission sex linked. Common ancestry was identified in all affected dogs in the Netherlands. The incidence ranged from 40 to 50 per cent of the Doberman population in that country.

Conventional karyotyping without banding failed to identify numeric or structural chromosomal aberrations.

In the Staffordshire bull terrier, 35 per cent of examined animals were affected with the bilateral disease. Most of the dogs were from one breeding line. Inheritance is suspected to be autosomal irregular dominant.

Sporadic PHPV is presumed to arise as a consequence of some intrauterine insult. Familial hereditary investigations have not been possible in the sporadic cases of the disorder in other breeds reported to date.

PATHOLOGY AND EMBRYOLOGY. The plaque on the posterior lens capsule consists of fibrous connective tissue with capillaries. Glial tissue may also be present. The fibrovascular tissue may grow into the lens. The lens capsule in the area of the plaque may be thickened, irregular, or interrupted. The persistent hyaloid vasculature consists of connective tissue and may contain a patent blood vessel and in some cases both arterial and venous vasculature. The vessel or vessels may extend from the optic disk to the posterior lens capsule.

Cortical and equatorial cataract formation is a result of the posterior capsular cataract and the invasion of fibrovascular tissue into the lens cortex.

Embryologically, a hereditary disharmony is suspected between the posterior lens capsule and tunica vasculosa lentis, with subsequent failure of regression of the hyaloid tunica vasculosa lentis.

THERAPY AND PROGNOSIS. Some affected pups will demonstrate progression of the disease, namely cataract, secondary hyphema, or retrolental hemorrhage. Progressive visual loss accompanies this change, and aggression increases simultaneously in the Doberman pinscher. These dogs become easily frightened and aggressive from fear. The Staffordshire bull terrier does not demonstrate aggression or functional visual difficulties in later life. This may represent temperament difference between breeds and less marked cataract progression in the Staffordshire bull terrier.

Animals with mild abnormalities, such as pigment spots on the posterior lens capsule, show no or only slight cataract progression.

Cataract surgery is frequently unsuccessful owing to complications from posterior segment pathologic change, including capsular opacity necessitating posterior capsular removal and hence vitrectomy, hemorrhage of patent vasculature to the posterior lens, and the necessity of extensive vitrectomy in posterior lenticonus.

Breeder counseling is essential owing to the genetic basis for this disease in the Doberman. Affected and nonaffected littermates and parent stock of the same should not be bred. The presence of persistent pupillary membrane and posterior cataract in the Doberman is strongly suggestive of a diagnosis of PHTV/PHPV and warrants detailed ophthalmic evaluation.

In other breeds, more investigation is required. Examination of parents and littermates and a repeat breeding with examination of the second litter may be indicated to investigate if the cause is genetic.

Test breeding of a promising breeding animal (Doberman) to a severely affected Doberman may be indicated in controlled circumstances. Examination of the progeny would suggest if the unknown parent is genetically clear or a carrier animal. If seven pups are produced and all littermates are examined ophthalmoscopically in detail, absence of affected pups suggests strongly that the unknown animal is genetically clear. Production of even one affected pup determines the parent to be a carrier for the ocular defect.

Persistent Pupillary Membrane

Persistence of the pupillary membrane (PPM) has been described in cattle, horses, cats, and dogs. Many canine breeds have been identified with the defect, including the American cocker spaniel, beagle, West Highland white terrier, Lakeland terrier, Chow Chow, rough collie, Labrador retriever, English springer spaniel, Pembroke Corgi, boxer, poodle, and Bedlington terrier. The Basenji breed has been described in the most detail; a high percentage of examined animals are affected, suggesting a genetic influence.

A breeder will present affected puppies with a white spot or spots on or in the eyes or blindness following eyelid separation.

CLINICAL SIGNS. Ophthalmic examination will reveal the more severe expressions of PPM in neonatal pups presented, as mildly affected pups will not demonstrate visual impairment detected by breeder observation. The ocular disorder may occur as unilateral or bilateral disease and is often asymmetric. Ocular abnormalities vary considerably from those pups with minor changes to those with major alterations. The variation of signs is as follows: a prominent minor vascular circle of the iris, which appears to project into the anterior chamber when viewed in profile under illumination; Y-shaped pigmented stumps of tissue on the iris face at the site of the minor vascular circle of the iris; small discrete white foci in the cornea with or without a tag of tissue projecting from the deep corneal surface into the anterior chamber; diffuse corneal opacities with pigmented threads or bands of tissue stretching from the inner aspect of the cornea through the anterior chamber to the minor vascular circle on the iris face; small or large pigmented or unpigmented bands or threads of tissue attaching at one or both ends to the minor vascular circle of the iris face; single or multiple focal or diffuse opacities of the anterior lens capsule centrally or paracentrally in the pupil; and pigmented foci on the anterior lens capsule. There is no definite relationship between the size of the persistent membranes and the degree of corneal damage. Pupillary shape and mobility is not altered in most instances; however, in pups with massive or multiple thicker bands of tissue coursing from the iris face to the cornea or lens, pupillary distortion may occur, most notably after pharmacologic dilation is attempted. A combination of any of these expressions may occur in one eye or in the eyes of the same animal. Persistent pupillary strands may be pigmented or unpigmented. Mydriasis assists in the identification of the threadlike PPMs that cross the pupil, as the strands become taut with pupillary dilation, and relaxed with pupillary constriction in which case they may rest over the iris face. Slit lamp biomicroscopy will isolate the corneal opacities to the inner corneal layers, namely, Descemet's membrane and endothelium. The lenticular opacities are localized to the anterior lens capsule and in some instances to the underlying anterior cortex.

In pups with minor lesions, visual impairment is not detectable. With extensive corneal or anterior lenticular opacities, vision is impaired and a searching nystagmus may be noted.

ETIOLOGY. In the Basenji, PPM is a genetic defect. There is no sex predilection and there is no correlation between the ocular defect and coat color. There is a wide range of expressivity for this defect. The inheritance is autosomal and may be recessively polygenetic with incomplete penetration. Inheritance of PPM is suspected in certain herding, working, and terrier breeds.

PATHOLOGY AND EMBRYOLOGY. Corneal opacities involve Descemet's membrane and the corneal endothelium. In many but not all instances, the endothelium is absent over the PPM area. Persistent pupillary membrane strands consist of connective tissue cells.

Anterior capsular opacities consist of fibroblasts or a thick fibrous membrane, with the underlying cortical lens fibers being disrupted and cataractous.

Embryologically, the anterior chamber is filled with primitive mesoderm, which gives rise to the anterior portion of the tunica vasculosa lentis. In normal animals, regression of this vascular tunic commences at gestational day 45 and the majority of the atrophy has occurred by postnatal days 11 to 14. Small vestiges may still be normally present at 6 weeks of age. Regression may continue to 6 months of age. Arrest of pupillary membrane regression results in persistence of these mesodermal elements.

THERAPY AND PROGNOSIS. In minor expressions of PPM, vision is not impaired.

Breeder counseling is indicated. In breeds other than the Basenji, examination of the parent stock and all siblings is indicated. A repeat breeding with detailed ophthalmic examination of all littermates may be indicated. Reproduction of PPM in the second litter is strongly suggestive of a hereditary etiology. In the Basenji breed, affected animals and their parents should not be bred. In actuality, many of the minorly affected animals are used for breeding. Such a practice will further disseminate a defective gene throughout a breed.

CONGENITAL/NEONATAL CATARACT

Cataract is any opacity of the lens or its capsule. Cataract formation may initiate during the embryologic, neonatal, or adult period. Maternal influences during pregnancy, such as infectious, toxic, or metabolic disease, may affect the developing lens. Cataract in several species has been reported to be associated with dietary amino acid deficiency, including tryptophan, histidine, phenylalanine, methionine, and arginine. Calcium deficiency in the dog and riboflavin deficiency in the cat have also been incriminated. Hand rearing versus maternal rearing increases the risk of neonatal cataract formation.

The location of the cataract within the lens indicates the time of the cataractogenic insult. At gestational day 15, induction of surface ectoderm by the optic vesicle occurs, forming a lens placode. The placode then invaginates, detaches from the surface ectoderm, and forms the primary lens fibers or adult fetal nucleus at gestational day 25. The posterior lens capsule is fully formed by gestational day 35. The fetal nucleus becomes surrounded by cortical fibers by gestational day 40. A nuclear cataract, therefore, may date cataractogenesis to the *in utero* time period. Perinuclear cortical cataract may predate cataractogenesis to gestational day 40 at the earliest and extend into the neonatal period.

The discussion below will be limited to cataract that manifests in the neonate. After eyelid separation and when neonatal corneal edema is resolving, the owner/breeder may note leukocoria or a white pupil or visual impairment in affected puppies or kittens.

Suspected Hereditary Neonatal Cataract

Inherited cataracts are common in the dog and rare in the cat. Occasionally, these cataracts will be manifested in the neonatal puppy or kitten. The breeder/owner will note leukocoria after eyelid separation. Visual impairment will be dependent on the extent of the cataractous change within the lens.

CLINICAL SIGNS. Neonatal cataracts of suspected or proved inheritance have been reported in the Old English sheepdog, golden retriever, and American cocker spaniel and in the Birman and Persian cat. Other breeds may also be affected. In all breeds except the cocker spaniel, the cataracts involved the lens nucleus routinely, with varying degrees of perinuclear cortical and cortical involvement. Leukocoria was present in all affected animals. Hypermaturity of the cataract was confirmed in the affected Persian kitten between 4 and 5 months of age. Golden retriever puppies may have associated microphthalmia and retinal folds, although these findings are not consistent. Lens resorption has sometimes followed in affected golden retrievers monitored by the author. Cataract in the cocker spaniel affected 10 per cent of animals in a particular kennel and involved the anterior subcapsular lens with variable nuclear involvement. Some of these cataracts were diffusely cortical. Occasional microphthalmia or persistent pupillary membrane was noted. Rotatory nystagmus was occasionally observed.

In the cocker spaniel and golden retriever, the cataracts tend not to progress. It should be noted that the cataracts described are not considered typical of the recessively inherited cataract commonly seen in the American cocker spaniel or the dominantly inherited posterior polar, subcapsular, nonprogressive cataract reported in the golden retriever. The cataract in the Old English sheepdog

was only occasionally noted in the young animal and was presumed to be neonatal.

Inherited cataracts that present routinely with microphthalmos are considered in discussion of microphthalmia with cataract.

ETIOLOGY. The congenital/neonatal cataract is believed to be an autosomal recessively inherited trait in the Old English sheepdog. The cataract in the cocker spaniel and golden retrievers, in the absence of other identifiable causes, was presumed to be inherited. Affected Birman kittens were littermates. Published breeding studies are not presently available to prove or disprove the suspected inheritance.

EMBRYOGENESIS. The nuclear and perinuclear cataracts date to gestational day 25 and 40, respectively. The posterior cortical and equatorial cataracts probably represent neonatal change.

THERAPY AND PROGNOSIS. Cataract surgery is not indicated for cataracts that are nonprogressive and that cause visual impairment but not blindness. Topical mydriatic/cycloplegic ophthalmic drops may provide peripheral vision in animals with nuclear and perinuclear cataract.

Lens resorption is more likely to occur in younger animals than in older animals. Resorption involves the leakage of liquefied lens protein from the capsule and eventual ventral displacement of the lens nucleus within a deflated lens capsule. Aphakic visual return may occur in animals so affected. However, intraocular reaction to the lens protein may occur. If the inflammation is mild or controlled, the prognosis for vision improves. Patients with resorbing lenses are not acceptable candidates for routine lens extraction.

If a congenital cataract is diffuse, visual stimulation of the retina may be impaired or absent. As such, central visual pathways will fail to develop and poor vision will result. The critical period for this neurologic development is during neonatal and early pediatric life.

Breeder counseling is indicated. In suspected inherited cataracts, affected animals, littermates, and parental stock should not be bred. Parent stock and littermates of affected pups should be examined ophthalmoscopically. A repeat breeding, with detailed ophthalmic examination of all siblings, may be indicated. If seven pups are produced, absence of cataract in the second litter does not support a genetic etiology for the defect in the first litter. The presence of even one affected pup in the second litter is strongly suggestive of an inherited defect.

Neonatal Nutritional Cataract

Puppies raised on artificial diets without maternal milk may develop lenticular opacities related to the artificial diet. The breeder may also notice leukocoria and visual impairment in affected pups after eyelid separation.

CLINICAL SIGNS. The anterior and posterior cortex, corticonuclear junction, and equatorial cortex are affected with cataract. The cataract is frequently irregular in density. All littermates are not clinically affected. Reports vary from 50 to 75 per cent within a given litter.

ETIOLOGY AND PATHOGENESIS. Artificial diets such as commercial milk replacements (Esbilac [Borden]), evaporated milk formulas, and goat milk formulas may be deficient in certain amino acids essential to normal lens development in neonatal canines. The nutritional cataract was first identified by Vanisi (1981) in timber wolf pups that were artificially reared. Pups started on milk replacement at 7 days of age or earlier developed more severe cataracts than those started on the diet at 12 days of age. Wolf pups started on the diet after 14 days of age did not develop cataracts. This suggests a critical time during development when the lens is more susceptible to nutritional stresses.

The addition of arginine to the artificial diet prevented the development of the cataract, suggesting that the arginine deficiency caused the disorder. Inadequate amino acid supply may result in incorrect amino acid sequence during synthesis of lens protein, producing a clinical cataract.

Protein deficiency cataract begins with intracellular lens hydration or vacuolation along the posterior Y-suture line, progressing to involve the anterior Y and subcapsular area. Widening of the sutures with granular cortical opacities, a prominent nucleocortical junction, and variable nuclear opacities is reported in other amino acid deficiencies.

PROGNOSIS AND THERAPY. After the pup is on a solid or semisolid diet or perhaps after the pup surpasses a critical age, the lens fibers develop normally. The lens continues to grow throughout life. Growth occurs peripherally, displacing older lens fibers centrally. As such, the volume of normal, clear lens cortex increases with age relative to the cataractous lens material. Cataract regression has also been noted. No therapy is indicated for the affected pups. The cataract is believed to be nutritional and not inherited and, as such, affected animals are acceptable for breeding purposes, provided the cause is confirmed historically. Affected pups will function relatively normally. The degree of visual impairment in the adult will depend on the relative amount of lens involved.

Breeders should be made aware of the existence of this type of cataract. Nutrition from an adoptive dam is preferable to an artificial diet for the lenticular health of the neonatal puppy. A supplemental supply of arginine may be protective in the neonate reared artificially. The required daily intake in the neonate is not known. Certain foods, including lean cooked lamb, are rich in arginine. The arginine content appears to vary between lots of commercial milk replacer, probably related to a variable crude protein source. Other commercial milk replacement diets may also produce nutritional deficiencies, as may various home-formulated diets.

CONGENITAL/NEONATAL DISORDERS OF THE FUNDUS

Congenital and neonatal abnormalities of the fundus may develop and produce clinical signs of ocular disease in the neonate. Visual impairment or blindness is the common complaint. For blindness to be detected in the neonate, bilateral ocular disease must be present. Congenital and developmental defects that occur during the neonatal period, but that do not result in detectable signs of ocular disease within the neonatal time frame, are excluded.

Retinal Dysplasia

Retinal dysplasia represents invaginations of the outer retinal layers with failure of proper orderly differentiation of these layers. This ocular disorder has been recognized in several breeds of dogs and occasionally in cats and may occur as a multifocal or complete and diffuse disease. Retinal detachment or nonattachment may occur, producing blindness in neonatal puppies.

Breeders will note severely affected pups to be less active than littermates and to collide frequently with objects. A high-stepping gait may also be observed.

CLINICAL SIGNS. Behavioral observation will support the presence of visual impairment or blindness.

Ophthalmic examination evinces the most severe expressions of retinal dysplasia in neonatal pups, as mildly affected pups would not demonstrate blindness. The anterior segment is clinically normal. Pupillary light reflexes may be absent or incomplete, and pupillary dilation may be present. Posterior segment examination demonstrates bilateral retinal detachment, with a retinal veil detectable immediately behind the lens. The retina remains attached at the optic disk but is frequently detached at the ora serrata. Intraocular hemorrhage may be associated with the retinal detachment. A retinal nonattachment is suspected. Affected Bedlington terriers are slightly microphthalmic with prolapse of the nictitating membrane. Microphthalmia is present in some affected Labrador retrievers and Sealyham terriers. In the latter, it may be unilateral or bilateral. A searching nystagmus may be present, indicating lack of development of neural visual pathways from congenital or neonatal blindness.

Cataracts were present in the Sealyham and in

some Bedlington terriers and Labrador retrievers, most often as focal cortical lesions, which may progress with age. Affected Labrador pups may also have skeletal deformities, resulting from retarded growth in the radius, ulna, and tibia; ununited and hypoplastic anconeal and coronoid processes; hip dysplasia; and delayed epiphyseal development.

ETIOLOGY. Common ancestry and much inbreeding exists in affected Bedlington terriers. The ocular defect is transmitted as a simple autosomal recessive trait in the Sealyham and Bedlington.

There is no association between retinal dysplasia and coat color. *In utero* or neonatal infection with feline herpesvirus and panleukopenia virus may cause retinal dysplasia or cerebellar hypoplasia in kittens.

PATHOLOGY AND EMBRYOLOGY. Invagination of the outer retinal layers forms folds or rosettes. The nuclear retinal layers are attenuated and disorganized, with photoreceptor degeneration. Retinal nonattachment and improper formation of the pars ciliaris retinae may be the underlying cause of the observed retinal detachments.

THERAPY AND PROGNOSIS. No therapy is available for this ocular defect. The affected pups are irreversibly blind. Breeder counseling is indicated because of the hereditary nature of the retinal dysplasia/detachment. Affected pups, littermates, and parents should not be bred.

Optic Nerve Hypoplasia and Aplasia

Optic nerve hypoplasia has been identified in many species, including humans, horses, dogs, cats, mice, rats, and miniature swine. Causes include genetic syndromes with multiple ocular defects and griseofulvin administration to pregnant queens, resulting in multiple ocular defects. Optic nerve hypoplasia frequently, but not always, produces blindness. Optic nerve aplasia is extremely rare and is accompanied by absence of retinal vasculature. Aplasia has been reported in the dog and cat.

Breeders will note visual deficits and abnormal behavior, such as marked clumsiness, in bilaterally affected pups when compared with unaffected littermates. Unilateral disease is noticed later in life.

CLINICAL SIGNS. Pups will demonstrate reduced pupillary light reflexes and neonatal blindness if the ophthalmic disorder is bilateral. Unilaterally affected neonates will not be identified unless the entire litter is presented for examination. Pupils will be mydriatic, and a searching nystagmus may be intermittently observed. Funduscopically, the optic nerves will appear small and poorly myelinated. There will be no signs of circumpapillary inflammation, as the disease is attributable to lack

of tissue development rather than to tissue atrophy due to inflammatory disease.

Optic nerve hypoplasia has been identified in a puppy with multiple ocular defects, including retinal dysplasialike lesions, cataract, and coloboma of the optic papilla.

Optic nerve aplasia is noted funduscopically as an absence of optic disks and retinal blood vessels.

ETIOLOGY. The defect has been suspected but not proved to be inherited in the dog or cat. A familial form in humans and an autosomal recessively inherited form in mice have been identified. In numerous species a variety of reported *in utero* insults that cause optic nerve hypoplasia is known.

PATHOLOGY AND EMBRYOLOGY. In optic nerve hypoplasia, the optic nerves are rudimentary and are composed mainly of meningeal tissue. Neural components are sparse. Retinal nerve fiber and ganglion cell layers are thin. Outer retinal layers remain normal. Optic canals are frequently small.

In optic nerve aplasia there is complete absence of an optic disk, optic nerve tissue, retinal blood vessels, ganglion cells, lamina cribrosa, optic chiasm, and optic tracts.

Optic hypoplasia and aplasia result from abnormal development at different stages of embryogenesis. Abnormal development early in embryonic life will result in lack of ganglion cell differentiation and mesodermal ingrowth through the fetal fissure and optic nerve aplasia. Abnormal development later in gestation will produce incomplete ganglion cell differentiation or early ganglion cell death and optic nerve hypoplasia.

Normal optic nerve axons may be required for bone growth and remodeling during skull development. Absence of axons may be responsible for the small optic canals observed.

THERAPY AND PROGNOSIS. There is no therapy for optic nerve hypoplasia or aplasia. Eyes with optic nerve aplasia are blind. Visual impairment of animals with optic nerve hypoplasia is determined by the degree of hypoplasia and whether one or both eyes are affected.

References and Supplemental Reading

Bistner, S. I.: *Atlas of Veterinary Ophthalmic Surgery.* Philadelphia: W. B. Saunders, 1977, pp. 120–131.

Dice, P. F.: The canine cornea. *In* Gelatt, K. N. (ed.): *Textbook of Veterinary Ophthalmology.* Philadelphia: Lea & Febiger, 1981, pp. 350–352.

Gelatt, K. N.: Pediatric ophthalmology in small animal practice. Vet. Clin. North Am. 3:3321, 1973.

Glaze, M. B., and Blanchard, G. L.: Nutritional cataracts in a Samoyed litter. J. Am. Anim. Hosp. Assoc. 18:115, 1982.

Helper, L.: The canine nictitating membrane and conjunctiva. *In* Gelatt, K. N. (ed.): *Textbook of Veterinary Ophthalmology.* Philadelphia: Lea & Febiger, 1981, p. 335.

Martin, C. L., and Chambreau, T.: Cataract production in experimentally orphaned puppies fed a commercial replacement for bitch's milk. J. Am. Anim. Hosp. Assoc. 179:175, 1981.

Nasisse, M. P.: Manifestations, diagnosis, and treatment of ocular herpesvirus infection in the cat. Comp. Cont. Vet. Med. Ed. 12:962, 1982.

Peiffer, R. L.: Feline ophthalmology. *In* Gelatt, K. N. (ed.): *Textbook of Veterinary Ophthalmology.* Philadelphia: Lea & Febiger, 1981, p. 525.

Peiffer, R. L.: The canine eyelids. *In* Gelatt, K. N. (ed.): *Textbook of Veterinary Ophthalmology.* Philadelphia: Lea & Febiger, 1981, pp. 279–280.

Severin, G. A.: *Veterinary Ophthalmology Notes,* 2nd ed. Fort Collins: Colorado State University Press, 1979, pp. 81, 94, 121–127, 137–151, and 221–242.

Vainisi, S. J., Edelhauser, H. F., Wolf, E. D., et al.: Nutritional cataracts in timber wolves. J.A.V.M.A. 179:1175, 1981.

CONJUNCTIVAL DISORDERS

CECIL P. MOORE, D.V.M.

Columbia, Missouri

SIGNS OF CONJUNCTIVAL DISEASE

Ocular signs suggesting conjunctival disease are discharge, pain, conjunctival swelling (chemosis), the presence of surface masses, and abnormal coloration (e.g., a "red eye"). These signs, alone or in combination, generally compose the owner's primary complaint in cases of conjunctival disease. A detailed examination should rule out other forms of eye disease, confirm the presence of conjunctival disease, and, if confirmed, establish the cause.

EXAMINATION PROCEDURES

Diagnostic evaluation begins with a complete physical examination followed by a detailed ophthalmic examination that includes direct examination of conjunctival surfaces using a focal light source with magnification (preferably slit lamp biomicroscope), conjunctival cultures, Schirmer's tear tests, and the instillation of vital stains. Rose bengal stain will detect areas of devitalized conjunctival epithelial cells that, when present, indicate surface drying. Fluorescein stain application establishes whether corneal ulceration is present and aids the diagnosis of nasolacrimal obstruction.

Procedures performed after instillation of topical anesthetic solution are inspection for foreign bodies, scrapings and cytologic study, and fine-needle aspiration or biopsy of surface masses. Immunofluorescence testing of cytologic specimens is indicated when the diagnostician wishes to confirm suspicions of specific conjunctival infections (e.g., with feline herpesvirus, *Chlamydia, Mycoplasma felis,* or canine distemper virus). Intraocular pressure measurements are essential in cases of apparent conjunctival disease to rule out intraocular causes of a "red eye" (e.g., glaucoma and uveitis).

CONJUNCTIVAL DISEASES AND THERAPY

Infectious Conjunctivitis

BACTERIAL CONJUNCTIVITIS. *Staphylococcus* spp. are the most frequent bacterial isolates from cases of acute conjunctivitis. Bacterial conjunctivitis is characterized by marked hyperemia and considerable mucopurulent exudate. Affected eyes usually respond to any of the triple antibiotic combinations of neomycin, bacitracin, and polymyxin B (Mycitracin, Upjohn; Trioptic-P, Beecham; Neobacimyx, Burns Biotec; Neosporin, Burroughs Wellcome), as well as chloramphenicol (Chloromycetin, Parke-Davis; Chloroptic, Allergan) or gentamicin (Gentocin, Schering).

Either antibiotic ointments or solutions may be used topically to treat bacterial conjunctivitis. Solutions are instilled every 4 to 6 hr, and ointments are administered every 6 to 8 hr. The minimum treatment period is generally 10 days. Bacterial conjunctivitis in neonates is characterized by delayed opening of the eyelids (ankyloblepharon), acute ocular swelling, and purulent discharge. Treatment consists of separating the eyelids and cleansing the eyes with saline eyewash and cotton swabs. Broad-spectrum antibiotics are applied topically for 10 days.

Conjunctival cultures and cytologic studies are indicated in unresponsive cases. Antimicrobial therapy is then dictated by results of susceptibility tests performed on bacterial isolates. Cultures should be performed only after no medication has been given for 24 hr. If bacterial cultures are negative, nonbacterial infections and noninfectious causes must be further investigated. In dogs, keratoconjunctivitis sicca (KCS) is a frequently overlooked cause of nonresponsive conjunctivitis. Especially in unilateral conjunctivitis, foreign bodies and ectopic cilia must be ruled out by meticulous examination. Chlamydial or viral infections are the most frequent causes of nonresponsive or recurring conjunctivitis in cats.

Mycoplasmal infections, caused by *Mycoplasma felis*, may manifest as severe exudative, sometimes proliferative, conjunctivitis in cats. This is a particularly troublesome disease in catteries and research colonies. Because *M. felis* may occur simultaneously with chlamydial conjunctivitis, the treatment of choice is topical tetracycline (Achromycin, Lederle) or oxytetracycline (Terramycin, Pfizer) ointment applied four times daily for 3 weeks.

CHLAMYDIAL CONJUNCTIVITIS. *Chlamydia psittaci* is the cause of a severe and frequently chronic infectious conjunctivitis of cats. Unilateral chlamydial conjunctivitis cases frequently become bilateral in 10 to 14 days. Conjunctival follicle formation characterizes chronic cases. *C. psittaci* may cause neonatal ophthalmia in kittens. Definitive diagnosis of chlamydial conjuctivitis is achieved by identifying typical intracytoplasmic inclusions within epithelial cells (in acute stages) or by a positive immunofluorescence test result on cytologic preparations.

Treatment consists of topical tetracycline ophthalmic ointment administered four times daily for 3 weeks or for a minimum of 2 weeks after abatement of clinical signs. Duration of immunity is short, and recurrences are common in colonies in which continuous re-exposure may occur.

VIRAL CONJUNCTIVITIS. Feline herpesvirus causes a serious acute viral conjunctivitis in cats of all ages. Chronic, refractory conjunctivitis or keratoconjunctivitis, including KCS and dendritic ulcers, may occur with feline herpesvirus infection. Neonatal ophthalmia and respiratory disease of kittens are also caused by this agent. Definitive diagnosis of herpes conjunctivitis is by virus isolation or by a positive result of immunofluorescence test performed on conjunctival scrapings.

Idoxuridine (IDU) (Stoxil, SmithKline Beckman; Herplex, Allergan; Dendrid, Alcon), trifluorothymidine (Viroptic, Burroughs Wellcome), and vidarabine (adenine arabinoside) (Vira-A, Parke-Davis) are drugs manufactured for human use for treating ocular herpes simplex infections. Antiviral drops are recommended every 2 hr, or ointments are recommended 5 times daily for 1 week. Acyclovir (acycloguanosine, Zovirax, Burroughs Wellcome) is a recently developed antiviral drug that appears promising for treating ocular herpes infections. Affected eyes are also treated topically with tetracycline for secondary bacterial or concurrent chlamydial infections.

FUNGAL CONJUNCTIVITIS. Although relatively uncommon, fungal conjunctivitis should be suspected in nonresponsive conjunctivitis cases with intense conjunctival hyperemia and a history of long-term topical therapy (i.e., 4 to 6 weeks or longer) with broad-spectrum antibiotic-corticosteroid combinations. Diagnosis is confirmed by cytologic examination of conjunctival scrapings or by cultures of conjunctival swabs or scrapings.

Aspergillus sp. is the most common filamentous fungus to cause ocular surface infections, and *Candida* sp. is the most common yeast isolate. To treat filamentous fungal infections, 1 per cent miconazole (Monistat, Janssen) or natamycin (Natacyn, Alcon) drops are applied to the eye six times daily for 2 weeks. When yeast infection is diagnosed, miconazole or nystatin (Mycostatin, Squibb; reconstituted to 25,000 units/ml) is used topically at the same frequency.

CONJUNCTIVITIS ASSOCIATED WITH SYSTEMIC INFECTIONS. Infectious conjunctivitis due to systemic infectious disease (e.g., canine distemper or adenovirus infections) is treated symptomatically (see discussion of symptomatic treatment). As the animal recovers from the systemic infection, the conjunctivitis usually simultaneously improves and eventually resolves.

Parasitic Conjunctivitis

Ocular thelaziasis, caused by *Thelazia californiensis*, may occur in small animals in the western regions of the United States. Affected animals may be asymptomatic or may show signs of mild conjunctivitis. Treatment consists of manual removal of the parasite or parasites after topical anesthetic administration. Topical 0.03 per cent phosphaline iodide drops daily for several days will kill any remaining parasites. *Cuterebra* larvae may grow within the conjunctiva or periocular tissues of puppies and kittens, causing a severe granulomatous conjunctivitis or blepharitis. Treatment consists of expressing or surgically removing the larvae and treating the associated inflammatory disease and secondary infections.

Trauma

Because of the rapid reparative characteristics of the conjunctiva, most lacerations and punctures heal spontaneously and do not require suturing. Broad-spectrum antibiotics are applied topically three to four times daily, and systemic antibiotics are administered for 1 week to prevent opportunistic infections. Lacerations and puncture wounds should be explored for foreign bodies and then irrigated with betadine-saline (1:9) solution.

Lacerations that are 1 cm or longer are sutured in a continuous pattern with 6–0 polygalactin 910 (Vicryl, Ethicon). After the conjunctiva is sutured, topical and systemic antibiotics are administered. Whenever conjunctival trauma is present, the remaining extraocular and intraocular structures should be carefully examined, as the orbit, eyelids, or globe may also be involved.

Traumatically induced conjunctival hemorrhage

resorbs spontaneously in 7 to 21 days, depending on the amount of blood present and the total area involved. Spontaneous hemorrhage without a history of trauma suggests a systemic clotting disorder. In cases of conjunctival or subconjunctival hemorrhage, antibiotics are applied topically to prevent secondary infection of compromised surface tissues. It is debatable whether corticosteroids are of value in treating cases of ocular surface hemorrhage.

In cases of severe conjunctival trauma, radiography should be considered for detection of radioopaque foreign bodies or for detecting possible orbital involvement (e.g., orbital fractures).

Symblepharon

As the conjunctiva heals following infectious or traumatic ulcerations, two apposing ulcerated areas may fibrose together, leaving permanent adhesions (symblepharon). Adhesions may result in reduced ocular motility, immobility of the third eyelid, and varying degrees of enophthalmos. Symblepharon may reduce or obliterate the conjunctival fornices. Scarring of the lacrimal puncta may result in persistent epiphora. Adhesions between palpebral conjunctiva and cornea may result in extensive corneal opacification. Severe neonatal conjunctivitis due to feline herpesvirus is the most common cause of conjunctival adhesions in cats. In dogs, trauma or chemical injury is the usual cause.

Treatment for symblepharon involves surgical breakdown of adhesions and postoperative antibiotic-corticosteroid ointment application. The application of petrolatum ointments to the conjunctival surfaces will discourage readhesions. Placement of a corneal-scleral protector or large soft contact lens over the surface of the globe also minimizes readhesions. A temporary tarsorrhaphy will aid in securing these overlays in position. However, surgical correction does not ensure that readhesion or permanent opacities will not result from the scarring.

Developmental Disorders

Ocular dermoids may occur on the epibulbar surface and commonly involve the lateral conjunctiva between the limbus and the lateral canthus. Dermoids are treated by surgical removal. Conjunctivectomy and possible keratectomy or eyelid reconstruction may be needed to restore ocular function. Following removal of the dermoid, the eye is treated medically with topical antibiotics for 7 to 10 days to allow the conjunctival or corneal defects to heal.

Conjunctival agenesis is uncommon and is usually associated with eyelid agenesis. If eyelid reconstruction is performed, a pedicle graft of conjunctiva should be used to line the eyelid defect.

Focal linear areas of pigmentation of the dorsolateral bulbar conjunctiva are remnants of a vestigial encircling third eyelid and are innocuous.

Immune-Mediated Conjunctivitis

Allergic conjunctivitis manifests primarily as periocular pruritus. Mild chemosis, hyperemia, and epiphora may also be noted. On cytologic examination of conjunctival scrapes from cases of suspected allergic origin, the finding of even an occasional eosinophil is highly suggestive of allergic conjunctivitis because eosinophils are normally not found. Allergic conjunctivitis is commonly associated with seasonal allergies and atopy. Plasma cells, lymphocytes, and Russell-body cells are the typical cytological findings. Intense hyperemia may be associated with delayed hypersensitivity to topically administered ophthalmic drugs. Aminoglycoside antibiotics and preservatives in ophthalmic pharmaceuticals are most likely to cause allergic reactions. Severe, acute chemosis; conjunctival hyperemia; and extensive blepharedema occur as a result of insect stings or facial snake bites. Although these acute reactions may be direct responses to vasoactive substances and exogenous toxins, some animals appear to be hypersensitive, particularly to certain insect stings.

For acute allergic conjunctivitis topical corticosteroids (e.g., 1 per cent prednisolone acetate [Pred Forte, Allergan] or 0.1 per cent dexamethasone [Maxidex, Alcon]) and systemic antihistamines and corticosteroids are indicated. Corticosteroid drops are instilled four to six times daily or ointments are administered three to four times daily as initial therapy. Frequencies should be gradually reduced to once to twice daily after 3 to 4 days, and topical drugs should be discontinued after 5 to 7 days, if possible. When chronic allergic conjunctivitis is suspected, all topical medications should be discontinued for 1 week. The possibility of a hypersensitivity to a specific topically administered drug (e.g., neomycin) may then be explored by trial readministration of individual agents.

When allergic conjunctivitis is associated with skin allergies, the offending antigen or antigens may be identified by allergy testing. If long-term therapy for allergic conjunctivitis is necessary, topical corticosteroids may be used intermittently or as needed to control local inflammation. Systemic corticosteroids are administered sparingly, preferably on an alternate-day basis. Elimination of environmental exposure and desensitization to known allergens may be possible, particularly in cases associated with systemic allergies in which allergy testing has identified specific offending allergens.

The presence of abnormal conjunctival lymphoid follicles (follicular conjunctivitis) usually results from chronic exposure and nonspecific immunologic responses to ocular surface antigens. In dogs, this nonspecific condition usually occurs in young dogs (less than 18 months of age) and is characterized by a mucoid ocular discharge and mildly inflamed conjunctiva. The discharge may be due, in part, to frictional rubbing by follicles on apposing conjunctival surfaces.

In cats, follicular conjunctivitis is usually associated with subacute or chronic stages of chlamydial infections and, therefore, affected eyes are treated with topical tetracycline. Treatment for follicular conjunctivitis in dogs consists of topical or intralesional (subconjunctival) corticosteroids. When follicles are associated with conjunctival infections in dogs, the discharge will appear mucopurulent, and antibiotic-corticosteroid combination solutions (Gentocin Durafilm, Schering; Anaprime, Syntex) or ointments (Corticosporin, Burroughs Wellcome; Ophthocort, Parke-Davis) are used topically. Solutions are instilled four times daily or ointments are applied three times daily for 2 weeks or slightly longer if needed until follicles regress. Physical abrasion of the follicles to precipitate an acute inflammatory response may be useful to resolve the follicles; however, this has rarely been needed.

Chronic superficial keratoconjunctivitis (pannus) of the dog and feline eosinophilic keratoconjunctivitis are noninfectious inflammatory diseases that may extensively involve the conjunctiva.

Tear Deficiency

Conjunctivitis caused by drying of the ocular surface (KCS) is diagnosed by a lackluster appearance of the mucosa, thick tenacious mucopurulent discharge, low Schirmer's tear test readings, and positive rose bengal stain retention. Corneal pigmentation, vascularization, or ulceration is seen concurrently with chronic conjunctivitis.

Topical treatment for KCS consists of lubricant ointments and aqueous or mucin tear replacement. Oral or topical pilocarpine is administered to stimulate tear secretion. Recently, topical 2 per cent cyclosporine in an oil vehicle has been used twice daily to successfully treat dogs with KCS. In cases in which a primary or contributing factor is identified (e.g., hypothyroidism or sulfonamide administration) the cause should be treated (or removed).

Toxic Conjunctivitis

When a toxic chemical contacts the ocular surface, the eye should be irrigated *immediately*. Ocular irrigation should be thorough and continuous for several minutes. Saline or eyewash is preferable, but, if these are not available, tap water is a satisfactory flushing solution. After irrigation, topical antibiotics are applied and the ocular surface is kept moist with artificial tears or lubricant ointments. Symptomatic treatment is indicated until healing is complete (see discussion of symptomatic treatment below).

Frictional Irritants

In cases of refractory conjunctivitis, eyelid abnormalities and foreign bodies are frequently overlooked as causes. Therefore, the need for a thorough, detailed examination is emphasized. Foreign material of plant origin (awns, weed seeds, chaff, thorn tips, bark, or leaf fragments), ectopic cilia, chalazia, and small eyelid tumors are the usual offenders. After identifying the frictional irritant, the treatment is directed removal of the irritant or surgery, if necessary, followed by topical antibiotic administration for 7 days.

Non-neoplastic Proliferative Diseases

Hyperplasia of nonpigmented conjunctival epithelium is, in most cases, associated with chronic exposure to ultraviolet light. Therefore, the anterior surface of the third eyelid and bulbar conjunctiva near the lateral limbus are the most frequently involved areas. These focal, pink, raised lesions are initially benign but have the potential to become neoplastic (e.g., squamous cell carcinoma). Surgical removal of focal lesions, avoidance of direct sunlight, and frequent re-examinations are recommended.

Conjunctival granulation tissue may appear as vascular, smooth or granular, nonpigmented areas, which occur as a secondary healing response to sizable defects following conjunctival injury or surgery. As a conjunctival wound heals, the granulation tissue usually contracts, regresses spontaneously, and is self-limiting. In cases of exuberant granulation tissue, topical corticosteroids may expedite resolution.

Acquired conjunctival melanosis may occur as a result of exposure and drying, particularly in heavily pigmented exophthalmic dogs. Although ocular lubricants and moisturizers may help, permanent correction is dependent on reducing the eyelid fissure size and improving the blink response by performing a medial permanent tarsorrhaphy.

Fibrous histiocytoma is a proliferative disorder of the subconjunctival tissues that appears as smooth, pink, focal, multifocal, or diffuse lesions that progress and enlarge until tissue protrudes from the ocular surface into the eyelid fissure area. Corneal and third eyelid involvement are common. A high prevalence of fibrous histiocytoma in collie dogs indicates a breed predisposition for this condition.

Treatment for fibrous histiocytoma consists of surgical debulking and the administration of corticosteroids topically, intralesionally, or systemically. Immunosuppressive chemotherapeutic agents (e.g., azathioprine) may be administered orally in refractory or recurring cases.

Neoplastic Diseases

Conjunctival neoplasia is uncommon and may have a variety of appearances, depending on the location and the tissue of origin. Adenomas and adenocarcinomas may arise from the meibomian glands or the gland of the third eyelid. Conjunctival involvement is usually a result of local enlargement of the tumor. Hemangiomas and hemangiosarcomas may originate from conjunctival vessels. Conjunctival hemangiosarcomas are characterized by aggressive behavior (i.e., rapid growth, local invasion, and the tendency for metastasis). The anterior surface of the third eyelid is a common site for these relatively uncommon vascular conjunctival tumors.

Viral papillomas may arise from the conjunctival surface, and squamous cell carcinomas may originate from nonpigmented conjunctival epithelium. Ocular squamous cell tumors occur more frequently in cats than in dogs. Fibrous tumors involving the conjunctiva are uncommon and usually are extensions of orbital or eyelid fibromas or fibrosarcomas. Focal pigmentation of the conjunctiva associated with a raised perilimbal lesion is indicative of benign epibulbar melanocytoma.

For solitary, resectable conjunctival tumors the treatment of choice is removal of the mass by conjunctivectomy and treatment of the site, depending on the tumor type, with cryosurgery, hyperthermia, or beta-radiation therapy. With papillomas and adenomas surgical excision alone is usually curative. For squamous cell tumors or adenocarcinomas, excision plus the ancillary therapy of topical radiation therapy (beta-application) is recommended. Epibulbar melanocytomas are generally treated with cryosurgery following local debulking. Vascular tumors are difficult to treat effectively, and hemangiosarcomas, in particular, may recur, invade locally, or metastasize.

Systemic neoplasia (e.g., lymphosarcoma) may infiltrate around the eye, causing fleshy conjunctival thickenings. With lymphosarcoma, appropriate chemotherapy usually results in regression of conjunctival lesions. Topical corticosteroids may augment systemic therapy in cases of ocular lymphosarcoma. For fibrous tumors involving the eyelids and conjunctiva, immunotherapy (e.g., intralesional bacillus Calmette-Guérin [BCG] injections) should be considered, because these tumors are difficult to treat by other modalities, and immunotherapy has been effective in treating periocular fibrous tumors in other species.

SYMPTOMATIC TREATMENT

The following empirical treatments may be beneficial while awaiting the results of diagnostic tests or while the primary cause of conjunctival disease is being treated.

1. One should remove exudates and clean the eye and periocular area. Sterile physiologic saline or an eyewash solution (e.g., Dacriose, Cooper Vision) should be used to flush the eye to remove exudates. Clipping the periocular hairs and using cotton balls moistened with saline to remove exudates is also important.

2. Secondary bacterial infections should be controlled. Broad-spectrum antibiotic ophthalmic ointments are indicated to prevent opportunistic infection of compromised conjunctival tissues. However, prolonged indiscriminate use of topical antimicrobials should be avoided, because this may encourage development of antibiotic-resistant bacterial strains and secondary fungal infections.

3. The conjunctiva must be kept moist. The lubricating properties of antibacterial ointments are generally adequate to provide continuous moistening of swollen or injured conjunctival tissues. In cases of severe chemosis in which exposure is a problem, a temporary tarsorrhaphy may be indicated until the swelling subsides. Artificial tear solutions should be applied topically four to six times daily when Schirmer's tear test values are subnormal. Topical 5 per cent sodium chloride may be useful to reduce chemosis; however, it should be used only in eyes producing adequate quantities of aqueous tears, as it will dehydrate the ocular surface.

4. Inflammation must be reduced. Anti-inflammatory drugs may be used to reduce acute swelling and to minimize discomfort and, therefore, self-trauma. Topical corticosteroids may reduce swelling and hyperemia of the conjunctiva but should not be used in the presence of a corneal ulceration. Corticosteroids are not recommended in cases of primary infectious conjunctivitis.

In dogs, nonsteroidal anti-inflammatory drugs given systemically may be beneficial in reducing chemosis, hyperemia, and associated ocular pain, particularly following ocular trauma. An initial dose of flunixin meglumine (Banamine, Schering) may be given at a dose of 0.5 to 1.0 mg/kg intravenously as a single dose. Flunixin should be given only to patients with normal renal function. As follow-up therapy, oral aspirin may be given at a dose of 10 mg/kg twice daily until signs of inflammation subside. These drugs are contraindicated if hemorrhage is the primary manifestation of the conjunctival disease.

References and Supplemental Reading

Helper, L. C.: The canine nictitating membrane and conjunctiva. *In* Gelatt, K. N. (ed.): *Textbook of Veterinary Ophthalmology*. Philadelphia: Lea & Febiger, 1981, pp. 330–342.

Lavach, J. D., Thrall, M. A., Benjamin M. M., and Severin, G. A.: Cytology of normal and inflamed conjunctivas in dogs and cats. J.A.V.M.A. 170:722, 1977.

Nasisse, M. P., Cook, C. S., Peiffer, R. L., et al.: *Feline Infectious Conjunctivitis*. Schering Continuing Education Series. Princeton: Veterinary Learning Systems, 1984.

Wyman, M.: *Manual of Small Animal Ophthalmology*. New York: Churchill Livingstone, 1986, pp. 99–123.

DERMATOLOGIC DISORDERS OF THE EYELID AND PERIOCULAR REGION

DONNA WALTON ANGARANO, D.V.M.

Auburn, Alabama

An understanding of the dermatologic diseases with a predilection for the eyelid and periocular region is helpful in establishing a list of diagnostic possibilities and a subsequent diagnostic plan. Dermatologic diseases frequently look similar and thus require more than a physical examination to establish a definitive diagnosis. Although symptomatic therapy without a definitive diagnosis will often make the patient more comfortable and sometimes reduce clinical signs, specific treatment of dermatologic diseases is obviously preferred.

Many dermatologic diseases may affect the periocular area. A list of dermatoses that are limited to, or frequently first present with, periocular involvement is presented in Table 1. Other dermatoses that are known for their periocular distribution but that are not usually limited to the periocular area are listed in Table 2.

Table 1. *Diseases That Are Limited to or May First Occur as Eyelid or Periocular Dermatoses*

Demodicosis
Dermatophytosis
Bacterial folliculitis
Facial fold pyoderma
Atopy (allergic inhalant dermatitis)
Food hypersensitivity
Zinc-responsive dermatosis
Juvenile cellulitis
Facial keratosis
Idiopathic periocular alopecia
Self-trauma due to ocular disease

Table 2. *Diseases That Affect the Eyelid or Periocular Area in Addition to Other Sites*

Pemphigus foliaceus
Pemphigus erythematosus
Systemic lupus erythematosus
Discoid lupus erythematosus
Vogt-Koyanagi-Harada syndrome (a depigmenting disease)
Canine familial dermatomyositis
Necrolytic migratory erythema

INFECTIOUS DERMATOSES

The two immediate diagnostic considerations for focal periocular alopecia or crusting are demodicosis and dermatophytosis. Skin scrapings and a fungal culture provide the minimum data base. The majority of cases of localized demodicosis will self-cure. Topical application of benzoyl peroxide (Pyoben, Allerderm; OxyDex, DVM) will be helpful in controlling secondary bacterial involvement. Miticidal products are rarely necessary. In generalized demodicosis, amitraz (Mitoban, Upjohn) is the treatment of choice. This product should be reserved for generalized cases, and, when used, strong recommendations should be made for neutering of the dog. Care should be taken to avoid ocular contact with either product. Benzoyl peroxide, because of its abrasive consistency, is particularly irritating.

A tentative diagnosis of dermatophytosis may be based on Wood's lamp examination or microscopic examination of hairs. Fungal culture offers a definitive diagnosis. Topical therapy is usually effective, and many products are available. Chlorhexidine (Nolvasan, Fort Dodge) will provide both antifungal and antibacterial activity and is helpful for the case awaiting culture confirmation. For the uncommon case in which systemic therapy is necessary, both griseofulvin (Fulvicin, Schering) and ketoconazole (Nizoral, Janssen) are effective. Chronic dermatophytosis traditionally has been treated with griseofulvin. Recently, ketoconazole has been reported to be superior to griseofulvin in the treatment of dermatophytosis in human medicine. Ketoconazole (10 to 20 mg/kg q24h) is effective, nontoxic, and less expensive than recommended effective doses of griseofulvin (50 mg/kg q24h) in veterinary medicine.

Bacterial folliculitis may also result in a focal area of periocular alopecia or crust. Other lesions are usually present and may be confined to the face or be more generalized. The bacterium most often involved is *Staphylococcus intermedius*. Therapy may consist of antibacterial shampoos or systemic antibiotics. If antibiotic therapy is pursued, the minimum duration should be 21 days. First-time infections may respond to trimethoprim-sulfadiazine or oxacillin. Chronic infections should be treated with an antibiotic selected on the basis of culture and sensitivity results.

Facial fold pyoderma is a bacterial infection that occurs in animals with anatomic folds. Many dogs, in particular the brachycephalic breeds and Shar Pei, have facial and nasal folds as a breed characteristic. Unfortunately, these folds predispose the involved skin to inflammation and secondary bacterial infection. Spastic entropion is a common sequela. Topical treatment of the pyoderma with benzoyl peroxide, chlorhexidine, or Burow's solution (Domeboro, Miles Pharmaceuticals) may be helpful; however, care must be taken to protect the eye with a lubricant prior to their use. Surgical ablation of the fold offers the only permanent cure.

Most dermatoses are capable of causing pruritus. Therefore, classically nonpruritic diseases should not automatically be ruled out of consideration because of the presence of pruritus. When any facial dermatosis begins to crust, it is common for the patient to rub or scratch the lesions. Thus, when obtaining a history, it is important to determine when the pruritus began in relation to lesion development.

ALLERGIC DERMATOSES

Hypersensitivities frequently manifest on the periocular skin. Atopy is known to result in periocular pruritus. Other areas of pruritus commonly include the ears, muzzle, distal extremities, axilla, and groin. Periocular pruritus may be intense and lead to traumatizing scratching, which results in swelling, alopecia, and crusting. Secondary bacterial infection is frequent. Atopic patients commonly have concurrent allergic conjunctivitis. The patient may, in fact, be presented for ocular disease and only by obtaining a thorough history and physical examination is the underlying diagnosis of atopy suspected.

The therapeutic options for atopy are avoidance, chemical suppression, and hyposensitization. Intradermal skin testing is the preferred diagnostic procedure to determine the allergens involved. Certain antigens may then be avoided or included in a solution for hyposensitization. Success with hyposensitization is variable, based on many factors (including the diagnostic test); however, most canine patients will benefit. Alternate-day oral corticosteroids are most commonly used for chemical suppression of atopy. Recently, the use of various antihistamines and nonsteroidal anti-inflammatory drugs has increased in popularity. Further studies are needed to evaluate the effectiveness of these chemicals.

Dietary hypersensitivity is another allergic condition in which the patient may demonstrate periocular pruritus and subsequent lesions. Unlike atopy, food allergy does not have a classic distribution pattern. Affected patients may have localized or generalized pruritus. Diagnosis is confirmed by dietary trial and provocative exposure. Therapy includes avoidance of offending antigens. Atopy and dietary hypersensitivities are frequently seen in the same patient, complicating case management.

ZINC-RESPONSIVE DERMATOSIS

A syndrome referred to as zinc-responsive dermatosis has been described, particularly in the Siberian husky and Alaskan malamute. Lesions of erythema and crusts may be present on the muzzle and distal extremities but are most pronounced on the periocular area. Lesions may or may not be pruritic. Diagnosis is confirmed by biopsy examination, and therapy involves zinc supplementation. Cases have been recognized in young, fast-growing breeds of dogs being fed large amounts of phytates or receiving high-calcium supplementation; both decrease available zinc. A similar syndrome has been reported in dogs being fed a diet that was determined to be zinc deficient.

JUVENILE CELLULITIS

Juvenile cellulitis is seen in dogs usually less than 6 months of age. It affects the facial area with edema, crusts, alopecia, erythema, and regional lymphadenopathy. The eyelids, pinnae, and periocular and muzzle regions are most typically involved. Lymph nodes may abscess and rupture. Systemic signs of fever, depression, and inappetence are frequently found. Etiology is unknown, and aggressive therapy with glucocorticoids is required after ruling out other disease possibilities. Supportive systemic antibiotics are recommended.

IDIOPATHIC DISORDERS

Idiopathic dermatoses can affect the periocular area. Periocular alopecia is prevalent in some breeds, particularly the Labrador retriever. Facial keratosis, a seborrheic, crusting dermatosis, is also idiopathic. It manifests as focal periocular lesions, unilateral or bilateral, in the older dog. Etiology is unknown, but the condition is frequently seen in conjunction with other seborrheic diseases. There is no known therapy for either condition.

SELF-TRAUMA

Although skin conditions may influence or induce ocular disease, the opposite is also true. Several ocular conditions, corneal disease in particular, may result in pain and discomfort such that the animal traumatizes itself in the periocular area. Thus, in the dog with periocular pruritus both dermatologic *and* ophthalmic possibilities must be considered.

AUTOIMMUNE DERMATOSES

There are several dermatologic conditions in which periocular or eyelid lesions are present in conjunction with other signs. Included in this group are the autoimmune dermatoses—pemphigus foliaceous, pemphigus erythematosus, and systemic (SLE) and discoid lupus erythematosus. Affected patients usually have muzzle and other cutaneous lesions of depigmentation, alopecia, ulceration, and crust formation. In SLE, there is other organ system involvement. The periocular lesions of these autoimmune diseases are prominent. Immunosuppressive therapy is usually required following a definitive diagnosis; however, therapy varies with the particular disease and its severity. Topical sunscreens are also helpful.

VOGT-KOYANAGI-HARADA SYNDROME

Vogt-Koyanagi-Harada syndrome is an uncommon syndrome that manifests as uveitis and facial depigmentation. The skin lesions may be mild, with periocular and perioral depigmentation, or they may develop into crusts, ulceration, and alopecia. Poliosis (graying of the hairs) is frequently seen and vitiligo (skin depigmentation) may also be noted. Topical and oral glucocorticoid therapy may be helpful.

DERMATOMYOSITIS

Canine familial dermatomyositis is a hereditary disease of the collie and Shetland sheepdog. The cutaneous lesions may be mild or extensive and are similar to those of the autoimmune dermatoses. The extent of muscle involvement is also variable. Lesions usually develop at less than 1 year of age. There is no known therapy, although glucocorticoids, vitamin E, and sunscreens may be beneficial. Client education is important, and these dogs should *not* be used for breeding.

NECROLYTIC MIGRATORY ERYTHEMA

Necrolytic migratory erythema is a rare condition that has been reported in dogs and humans. Affected patients are usually diabetic, and a cirrhotic liver has been found in several canine cases. All affected dogs have demonstrated severe periocular, facial, and footpad hyperkeratosis and ulceration.

NEOPLASTIC CONDITIONS

After obtaining a thorough history and physical examination, diagnostic possibilities and a diagnostic plan can be determined. Skin scrapings and a fungal culture are mandatory. Other minor diagnostic tests, such as microscopic examination of direct smears or aspirates, may be suggestive of autoimmune or neoplastic diseases. Table 3 lists neoplastic conditions that are known to affect the eyelids or periocular area. These diseases usually occur as nodular lesions; however, some, such as mycosis fungoides, may have alopecia, erythema, and crust formation. Skin biopsy and histopathologic examination are necessary to confirm the diagnosis of many eyelid or periocular dermatoses.

Symptomatic therapy may be helpful in some cases of eyelid and periocular disease. However, in cases that are unresponsive to symptomatic therapy,

Table 3. *Neoplastic Conditions That May Affect the Eyelid or Periocular Area*

Squamous cell carcinoma
Actinic keratosis
Melanoma
Sebaceous adenoma
Fibrous histiocytoma
Dermoid
Lymphosarcoma (B cell)
Mycosis fungoides

or when lesions have been present for more than 2 or 3 weeks, testing is needed to determine a definitive diagnosis. After the diagnosis has been established, specific therapy may be prescribed.

References and Supplemental Reading

Foil, C. S.: Antifungal agents in dermatology. *In* Kirk, R. W. (ed.): *Current Veterinary Therapy IX*. Philadelphia: W. B. Saunders, 1986, p. 560.

Kern, T. J., Walton, D. K., Riis, R. C., et al.: Uveitis associated with poliosis and vitiligo in 6 dogs. J.A.V.M.A. 187:408, 1985.

Kunkle, G. A., Gross, T. L., and Fadok, V.: Dermatomyositis in collie dogs. Comp. Cont. Ed. Pract. Vet. 7:185, 1985.

Muller, G. H., Kirk, R. W., and Scott, D. W.: *Small Animal Dermatology III*. Philadelphia: W. B. Saunders, 1983.

Scott, D. W.: The differential diagnosis of facial dermatitis. *In* Kirk, R. W. (ed.): *Current Veterinary Therapy VII*. Philadelphia: W. B. Saunders, 1980, p. 436.

Walton, D. K., Center, S. A., Scott, D. W., and Collins, K.: Ulcerative dermatosis associated with diabetes mellitus in the dog: A report of four cases. J. Am. Anim. Hosp. Assoc. 22:79, 1986.

OCULAR DISORDERS OF RABBITS, RODENTS, AND FERRETS

THOMAS J. KERN, D.V.M.

Ithaca, New York

Rabbits, rodents, and ferrets kept as pets experience ocular disorders similar to those that occur under laboratory conditions. Their causes include infections, genetic influences, nutritional deficiencies, congenital malformations, and environmental and management problems. Disorders that cause ocular discharge, ocular opacities, severe discomfort, or alterations in globe size are obvious and demand attention. Orbital and intraocular disorders may cause more subtle changes, which may not be detected until they have progressed to an advanced stage.

Assessment of vision in pet laboratory animals is more difficult than in dogs and cats. Most are confined to familiar quarters and may seldom venture into strange surroundings. Nocturnal species such as rats and mice may avoid bright or daylight conditions, where visual deficits would be most obvious.

Ocular examination of laboratory animals is complicated by the difficulty of using diagnostic instruments (such as ophthalmoscopes and tonometers) on small eyes. Examination of the external eye and adnexa is facilitated by use of magnification (e.g., 20-diopter [D] or 30-D indirect condensing lens, simple pocket magnifier, and head loupe). Fluorescein dye examination of the cornea and nasolacrimal excretory system is possible even in small rodents. Tonometry and Schirmer's tear test evaluation are feasible in rabbits. Exfoliative conjunctival cytologic examination is useful in all laboratory species. Topical anesthesia should be used only sparingly in these small animals, as systemic toxicity is possible. Fundus examination of rodents, rabbits, and ferrets may be performed following mydriasis by 1 per cent tropicamide (Tropicacyl, Akorn) using indirect ophthalmoscopy with a 30-D condensing lens. The pupils of pigmented rodents may be resistant to dilation owing to binding of the mydriatic agent to uveal melanin. In such animals, mydriasis may be effected by instillation of 1 drop each of 1 per cent atropine and 10 per cent phenylephrine (AK-Dilate 10 per cent, Akorn) three to four times within a 15-min period.

RABBIT

Clinically relevant anatomic features of the rabbit include (1) superior rectus muscle, normally visible through the bulbar conjunctiva; (2) only one large punctum located inferiorly at the medial canthus; (3) four glands within the orbit: lacrimal, infraorbital, harderian, and nictitating membrane glands; (4) a merangiotic fundus in which retinal vessels are present only nasal and temporal to the optic disk; (5) a myelinated optic disk with a large, deep, central depression; and (6) an extensive orbital venous plexus. Eyelid separation in rabbits occurs about 10 days after birth.

Important ocular problems in rabbits include conjunctivitis, epiphora, blepharitis, and glaucoma.

The presence of a milky aqueous discharge in a rabbit's eye free of conjunctival inflammation suggests epiphora from excessive lacrimation or inadequate tear drainage. Epiphora may result from acquired nasolacrimal duct obstruction, an occasional sequela to chronic rhinitis or conjunctivitis. Relief of the obstruction may be effected by nasolacrimal irrigation with saline injected through the single inferior punctum with a 22-gauge nasolacrimal cannula or intravenous catheter. In some rabbits with acquired stenosis, obstruction may be permanent.

The causative agent most commonly incriminated in conjunctivitis of rabbits is *Pasteurella multocida*. This organism may be present in the normal conjunctival sac or may contaminate the sac by extension from the nasal cavity through the nasolacrimal duct. *P. multocida* also causes uveitis, orbital cellulitis, rhinitis, pneumonia, otitis media and interna, subcutaneous abscesses, vulvovaginitis, pyometra, balanoposthitis, orchitis, and generalized septicemia. Conjunctivitis may accompany any of these signs or may occur alone. *P. multocida* conjunctivitis may be treated with procaine penicillin G (60,000 U/kg of body weight s.i.d. for 10 days IM), along with topical chloramphenicol ophthalmic solution or ointment (q.i.d.). Oxytetracycline (5 mg/kg of body weight b.i.d. for 10 days IM) or tetracycline (50 to 100 mg/kg in divided doses for 10 days PO) may be substituted for the penicillin G. Rabbits receiving antibiotics should be carefully monitored for the development of potentially fatal enterocolitis. If diarrhea develops during therapy, antibiotics should be discontinued and supportive therapy should be instituted. The prognosis for cure of pasteurellosis is guarded; frequently, signs of infection resolve during therapy and recur afterward.

Blepharoconjunctivitis occurs rarely in domestic rabbits; it is a result of myxomatosis, a viral disease enzootic in wild rabbits in the western United States, Europe, South America, and Australia. Infection is transmitted by mosquitoes and fleas. Subcutaneous swelling occurs in the face, in the eyelids, and around body orifices. Presumptive diagnosis is based on clinical signs and typical gross and microscopic lesions; definitive diagnosis requires virus isolation. Mortality is high, and specific therapy is unavailable. Mosquito and flea control is recommended.

Blepharitis characterized by a dry, crusty exudate overlying ulcers in the skin and mucous membrane may be caused by infection with the spirochete *Treponema cuniculi*. The vulva and prepuce are most commonly affected, but lesions may occur on the eyelids, lips, nares, and anus. The disease is transmitted venereally or by young rabbits' contact with an infected dam. Diagnosis is confirmed by identification of spirochetes on darkfield examination of material scraped from the lesions. Successful treatment may be accomplished using three injections of 42,000 U/kg of body weight of benzathine penicillin G–procaine penicillin G (Bicillin, Wyeth) given at 7-day intervals. Eradication of trepanematosis from a colony may require treatment of all rabbits.

Other noninfectious causes of conjunctivitis, blepharitis, and ocular discharge in rabbits include dust and filthy bedding, trauma, entropion, distichiasis, and trichiasis. Entropion, while uncommon, should be surgically corrected when evident. Distichia should be removed by electroepilation, simple epilation, or cryoepilation only after all other causes of irritation have been ruled out. French Rex rabbits have been reported to have deformed cilia, which cause trichiasis and secondary keratitis. Surgical removal of offending cilia or entropion repair may be necessary.

Glaucoma occurs commonly in laboratory rabbits from New Zealand white stock; this predisposition is inherited as an autosomal recessive trait with incomplete penetrance. Onset may be as early as 2 to 3 weeks after birth, but more commonly glaucoma develops at 3 to 6 months of age. Unilateral or bilateral buphthalmos, corneal opacity, and blindness should suggest the diagnosis, which should be confirmed with Schiøtz tonometry. Medical therapy is difficult; topical miotic and beta-blocking drugs may not reduce intraocular pressure enough to preserve vision, and use of oral carbonic anhydrase inhibitors is impractical, at best. Potential surgical options in pet rabbits include cyclo-cryotherapy, evisceration with silicone prosthesis implantation, and enucleation.

Clinically significant cataracts are uncommon in rabbits; chronic uveitis (e.g., associated with pasteurellosis) may cause secondary cataract formation. Heritable cataract, cyclopia, persistent hyperplastic primary vitreous, lens coloboma, and optic disk coloboma have been rarely reported.

Enucleation of the eye could result in serious hemorrhage from the orbital venous sinus; careful intraoperative hemostasis is recommended.

RAT

Clinically relevant ocular anatomic features of the rat include (1) an extensive orbital venous plexus; (2) three lacrimal glands per eye: intraorbital, extraorbital, and harderian (associated with the third eyelid); (3) transient persistence of the hyaloid artery in weanlings; (4) an extremely large spheric lens, the distortion from which causes the retina to appear to "float" in the vitreous; and (5) a holangiotic, predominantly rod retina, with radial arterioles and venules. Eyelid separation in rat pups occurs at postnatal days 12 to 16.

Common ocular problems of rats include epiphora, conjunctivitis, keratoconjunctivitis, dacryoadenitis, and retinal degeneration.

Epiphora caused by excessive lacrimation is associated with bacterial or viral conjunctivitis and ocular irritation from soiled bedding. The harderian gland of rats and mice produces porphyrin pigment, which stains periocular hair reddish brown; thus, animals with epiphora of any cause may be identified by this discoloration. Ammonia vapor from urine-soiled bedding acts directly as an ocular irritant, causing conjunctivitis and, perhaps, predisposing to secondary bacterial infection. Frequent cage cleaning with bedding replacement minimizes this environmental cause.

Bacterial and viral agents that cause subclinical and clinical upper and lower respiratory tract disease in rats may cause mild to moderate conjunctivitis. Such agents include *Streptococcus pneumoniae*, *Pasteurella pneumotropica*, *Mycoplasma pulmonis*, *Pseudomonas aeruginosa*, and Sendai virus. Bacterial culture and sensitivity testing may be indicated in individual instances, especially if multiple animals are affected or at risk. Systemic antibiotic therapy may be indicated for animals with significant signs. Recommended antibiotics include 60,000 U of procaine-benzathine penicillin G (Bicillin, Wyeth) per rat every second day for three treatments subcutaneously; 6 to 10 mg/kg of oxytetracycline s.i.d. to b.i.d. IM; 20,000 U/kg of procaine penicillin G orally s.i.d.; 15 to 20 mg/kg of tetracycline orally b.i.d. to t.i.d. PO; or 2 to 4 mg/kg of tylosin s.i.d. to b.i.d. IM.

Two related coronaviruses, sialodacryoadenitis virus (SDAV) and rat coronavirus, cause inflammation of salivary and lacrimal glands, which often results in exophthalmos, epiphora, keratoconjuctivitis, uveitis, and multifocal retinal degeneration. Sialodacryoadenitis virus infection is highly contagious and spreads rapidly by aerosol, contact, and fomite transmission. Susceptible rats of any age may become infected; when infection is enzootic within a colony, only young rats are affected. Infection lasts about 1 week, at which time rats undergo seroconversion with no carrier state. Treatment is supportive, as no specific therapy is available. Corneal opacification, anterior and posterior synechiae, secondary cataract, secondary glaucoma, and multifocal retinal degeneration, when present, are permanent.

Dacryoadenitis may follow blood sample collection from the orbital venous plexus. Though a commonly employed laboratory procedure, orbital blood collection from pet rats should be discouraged, as the resulting orbital and lacrimal gland inflammation may cause exophthalmos, keratitis, uveitis, or phthisis bulbi.

Hypovitaminosis A causes chronic keratoconjunctivitis and xerosis. Systemic therapy with vitamin A may lead to resolution of clinical signs. An adequate commercially prepared diet is preventive.

Epiphora due to nasolacrimal duct obstruction may result from malocclusion or overgrowth of the incisors. The gums and distal nasal cavity may become inflamed, with swelling causing obstruction of the duct. Corrective dentistry usually improves the condition.

Other reported causes of epiphora include stress, riboflavin or pantothenic acid deficiency, water deprivation, and lack of grooming.

Clinically significant cataracts are relatively uncommon in rats. Secondary cataracts develop following uveitis or generalized retinal degeneration. Lens opacities may occur in rodents following prolonged eyelid separation (e.g., during anesthesia) presumably as a result of temperature or osmotic changes in the anterior chamber and lens; these usually resolve with recovery from anesthesia. Hereditary cataracts occur in some strains. Nutritional cataracts develop in rats fed diets containing excessive levels of galactose, sucrose, or xylose. Duplication of this phenomenon in pet rats is unlikely.

Retinal degeneration occurs in rats as both a primary and a secondary disorder. Primary retinal degeneration is an inherited disorder in a few strains. Secondary retinal degeneration follows (1) the focal chorioretinopathy that sialodacryoadenitis virus may cause and (2) excessive light exposure (duration or intensity), especially in albino strains. The SDAV-associated retinopathy rarely causes blindness. Phototoxic retinopathy, which causes blindness, may be avoided by maintenance of approximately 12-hr light-dark cycles. In addition, cages should have areas where rats may retreat from light.

Glaucoma occurs in rats as a result of uveitis, the most commonly incriminated cause being SDAV. Microphthalmos alone or accompanied by cataract or retinal dysplasia occurs as a sporadic congenital defect, possibly genetic, and must be discriminated from phthisis bulbi due to severe uveitis.

Enucleation of the eye in rats, mice, and hamsters could result in serious hemorrhage from the orbital venous plexus; careful intraoperative hemostasis is recommended.

MOUSE

The clinically relevant ocular anatomic features of the mouse are similar to those of the rat. Eyelid separation occurs at 13 to 14 days postnatally.

The important ocular problems of mice include epiphora, conjunctivitis and keratoconjunctivitis, and retinal degeneration.

Epiphora is caused by environmental contamination with ammonia, dental problems, dacryoadenitis, and infections. *Pasteurella pneumotropica* causes dacryoadenitis. Agents incriminated in murine conjunctivitis include *Pseudomonas aerugi-*

nosa, *P. pneumotropica*, *Salmonella* spp., *Streptobacillus moniliformis*, *Corynebacterium kutscheri*, Lancefield group C streptococci, *Mycoplasma pulmonis*, mousepox or ectromelia virus, Sendai virus, and lymphocytic choriomeningitis virus. As with rats, bacterial culture and sensitivity testing and systemic antibiotic therapy may be indicated in selected instances.

As in rats, cataracts in mice occur rarely as genetic defects and occasionally as a result of uveitis, retinal degeneration, and prolonged eyelid separation. Posterior lens capsule rupture in neonatal mice is inherited as a simple recessive trait in some strains.

Retinal degeneration occurs in certain strains of mice as a genetic defect. Phototoxic retinal degeneration may occur, especially in albino mice exposed to excessive light intensity or duration.

Numerous heritable ocular defects are propagated in laboratory strains of mice, which may occasionally be noted in mice kept as pets: eyelid malformations, microphthalmos, cataract, and retinal dysplasia. Autosomal recessive optic nerve hypoplasia has been reported in mice of both the waltzing and nonwaltzing Basle strains.

GUINEA PIG

Clinically relevant anatomic features of the guinea pig include (1) a rudimentary nictitating membrane, merely a fold of conjunctiva inside the medial canthus; (2) a large and extensive lacrimal gland, which occupies the lateral and anterior ventral aspects of the orbit; (3) an extensive zygomatic salivary gland, which occupies the posterior, medial, and superior aspects of the orbit; and (4) a paurangiotic retina, in which a few capillary loops extend into the retina from near the optic disk; the fundus appears avascular, however. Guinea pigs have eyelids that are open from birth.

Important ocular problems of guinea pigs include conjunctivitis; "pea eye," an inferior conjunctival mass; cataracts; and panophthalmitis.

The best-documented infectious agent causing conjunctivitis in guinea pigs is *Chlamydia psittaci*. A generally self-limiting disease, this so-called inclusion conjunctivitis is characterized by usually mild chemosis, follicular formation, and serous ocular discharge. Cyclic outbreaks of severe conjunctivitis have been seen in enzootically infected colonies. Lesions usually resolve in 3 to 4 weeks, and treatment is usually considered unnecessary. Recovered animals may be resistant to reinfection. This organism may be transmitted from genital tracts of infected animals to their offspring and cause neonatal conjunctivitis. Diagnostic confirmation may be made by identification of typical intracytoplasmic chlamydial inclusions in epithelial cells obtained by conjunctival scraping and stained with Jimenez,

Macchiavello's, or other conventional cytologic stains. The zoonotic potential of this infection is uncertain. Topical broad-spectrum antibiotic therapy of 7 to 10 days' duration may be indicated for severely affected individuals.

Bacterial conjunctivitis has been reported in association with numerous bacteria, including streptococci, *Micrococcus*, *Staphylococcus aureus*, *Pasteurella multocida*, *Bordetella bronchiseptica*, pneumococci, and *Proteus*. Typical exfoliative conjunctival cytologic findings are numerous neutrophils, with or without intracellular bacteria. Topical broad-spectrum antibiotic therapy of 7 to 10 days' duration is indicated in such instances.

Adult guinea pigs occasionally develop a nodule that protrudes from the inferior conjunctival sac unilaterally or bilaterally, described as pea eye by guinea pig fanciers. Examination of biopsy specimens has revealed that such swellings are protrusions of portions of the lacrimal or zygomatic glands. These nodules may cause minor ectropion and exposure conjunctivitis. No treatment is usually necessary. Their surgical removal for cosmetic purposes should probably be discouraged. Excision might rarely be indicated to correct significant lagophthalmos resulting in exposure keratitis.

Cortical cataracts of suspected genetic origin have been seen commonly in numerous strains of Abyssinian and English short-hair guinea pigs. Cataract occurrence in other breeds is uncertain. Dietary cataracts associated with L-tryptophan deficiency have been reported; the clinical significance of this deficiency for pet guinea pigs is uncertain.

Panophthalmitis may develop from bacterial septicemia. *Streptococcus zooepidemicus* often causes cervical and generalized subcutaneous abscesses in guinea pigs; abscess rupture or surgical manipulation may produce bacteremia with involvement of the eyes and other organs. Appropriate systemic antibiotic therapy is indicated, but prognosis for vision is guarded (Anderson, 1987; Wagner and Manning, 1976; Jacobson et al., 1983).

HAMSTER

Spontaneously occurring ocular disorders in hamsters have been rarely reported. Eyelid separation occurs at about 15 days postnatally in Syrian or golden hamsters (*Mesocricetus auratus*) and between days 10 and 14 in Chinese hamsters (*Cricetus griseus*). Keratoconjunctivitis may result from environmental trauma or filthy bedding. Facial abscesses of bacterial origin may involve the eyelids or orbit, possibly associated with dental caries and tooth root infection. Affected hamsters have periorbital or hemifacial swelling; proptosis of the globe and secondary exposure keratitis are common sequelae. Despite systemic broad-spectrum antibiotic treatment, such abscesses frequently result in death. Unfortunately, antibiotic therapy is hazardous for hamsters, as many drugs induce fatal enterocolitis. Hereditary diabetes mellitus and cataract occur in certain laboratory strains of Chinese hamsters.

OTHER RODENTS

Gerbils (*Meriones unguiculatus*) occasionally have apparent harderian gland enlargement or prolapse. Surgical excision is not recommended.

Facial dermatitis of uncertain cause affects gerbils commonly; erythema, crusting, and alopecia develop around the external nares, forepaws, and facial and periocular areas. The lesions are exacerbated by scratching and may result from reduced self-grooming. Laboratory ambient temperature influences grooming behavior; optimal temperatures for grooming in gerbils require further study. Cage bedding has also been implicated in the pathogenesis of dermatitis; sand may be superior to other materials in reducing its occurrence.

Eyelid separation in neonatal gerbils occurs at 16 to 22 days postnatally. The gerbil fundus resembles that of a pigmented rat.

Chinchillas (*Chinchilla laniger*) have a rudimentary nictitating membrane, a vertical slit pupil, and an anangiotic retina. Cataracts and asteroid hyalosis have been reported in aged animals.

Degus (*Octodon degus*) have been reported to have neonatal-onset cataracts possibly associated with diabetes mellitus. The degu retina is anangiotic.

FERRET

Clinically relevant anatomic features of the ferret include (1) a well-developed nictitating membrane; (2) a horizontally elliptic, slitlike pupil; (3) a holangiotic retina with vascular pattern similar to the dog's; (4) a well-developed tapetum; and (5) a relatively small myelinated optic disk. Eyelids separate at about 34 days after birth.

The important ocular disorders of the ferret include conjunctivitis, cataract, and lens luxation.

Infectious causes of conjunctivitis in ferrets include canine distemper virus, bacterial infections, and human influenza virus. Canine distemper is a serious, usually fatal disease in ferrets. Mucopurulent oculonasal discharge develops 7 to 10 days after exposure; severe blepharitis, corneal ulceration, and keratoconjunctivitis sicca may develop. Several days following onset of conjunctivitis, an erythematous, pruritic skin rash consistently develops on the chin, groin, and footpads. The clinical signs strongly suggest the diagnosis. Confirmation can be made

with serum antibody titers or with immunofluorescent antibody testing of conjunctival or blood smears. Mortality in infected ferrets is nearly 100 per cent; supportive care is often unsuccessful. The disease may be prevented by vaccination with modified live canine distemper vaccine of chick embryo origin at 6 to 10 weeks of age, at 10 to 14 weeks, and yearly thereafter. Ferrets are susceptible to infection with several strains of human influenza virus. Mild pneumonia and nasal and ocular discharge may develop and, in contradistinction to canine distemper infection, animals usually recover within 5 days. Treatment is not usually recommended.

Bacterial conjunctivitis is characterized by mucopurulent ocular discharge and the presence of intracellular bacteria in neutrophils noted on examination of conjunctival scrapings. Topical broad-spectrum antibiotic therapy is indicated for initial infections. Bacterial culture and sensitivity testing followed by specific antibiotic therapy is recommended for recurrent infections.

Cataracts that progress to blindness are commonly noted in ferrets; unilateral or bilateral luxation of noncataractous lenses is also occasionally noted. Both conditions are suspected to have genetic origins. Lens removal from ferrets has been unsuccessful owing to the technical difficulties inherent in manipulating their small eyes.

Corneal dermoids have been reported in ferrets. Removal by superficial keratectomy performed with the aid of magnification is indicated, followed by topical broad-spectrum antibiotic therapy that is continued until the resulting corneal ulcer has healed.

References and Supplemental Reading

Anderson, L. C.: Guinea pig husbandry and medicine. Vet. Clin. North Am. 17:1045, 1987.
Baker, H. J., Lindsey, J. R., and Weisbroth, S. H. (ed.): *The Laboratory Rat. Vol. I. Biology and Diseases.* New York: Academic Press, Inc., 1979.
Bellhorn, R. W.: Ophthalmologic disorders of exotic and laboratory animals. Vet. Clin. North Am. 3:345, 1973.
Bellhorn, R. W.: Laboratory animal ophthalmology. In Gelatt, K. N. (ed.): *Textbook of Veterinary Ophthalmology.* Philadelphia: Lea & Febiger, 1981, pp. 649–671.
Davidson, M. G.: Ophthalmology of exotic pets. Comp. Cont. Ed. Pract. Vet. 7:724, 1985.
Foster, H. L., Small, J. D., and Fox, J. G. (eds.): *The Mouse in Biomedical Research. Vol. II. Diseases.* New York: Academic Press, Inc., 1982.
Fox, J. G., Cohen, B. J., and Loew, F. M. (eds.): *Laboratory Animal Medicine.* Orlando: Academic Press, Inc., 1984.
Jacobson, E., Kollias, G., and Peters, L. J.: Dosages for antibiotics and parasiticides used in exotic animals. Compend. Cont. Ed. 5:315, 1983.
Rubin, L. F.: *Atlas of Veterinary Ophthalmoscopy.* Philadelphia: Lea & Febiger, 1974.
Wagner, J. E., and Manning, P. J. (eds.): *The Biology of the Guinea Pig.* New York: Academic Press, Inc., 1976.
Wagner, J. E., and Farrar, P. L.: Husbandry and medicine of small rodents. Vet. Clin. North Am. 17:1061, 1987.
Weisbroth, S. H., Flatt, R. E., and Kraus, A. L.: *The Biology of the Laboratory Rabbit.* New York: Academic Press, Inc., 1974.

THE OPHTHALMOLOGY REFERRAL PATIENT

PENNIE L. COOLEY, D.V.M.,
and PAUL F. DICE, II, V.M.D.

Seattle, Washington

The increase in veterinary medical knowledge and sophistication of diagnostic and surgical equipment has made it exceedingly difficult for the general practitioner to keep current in all areas of medicine and surgery. Thus specialization in limited disciplines has evolved as an extension of services offered in general practice. The public is assured that veterinarians with diplomate status in the American College of Veterinary Ophthalmologists (ACVO) have met the minimum acknowledged standards of expertise in veterinary ophthalmology. Within the United States and Canada there are individuals who have a keen interest and varied expertise in ophthalmology who are not ACVO diplomates. These individuals perform a needed service, particularly in areas where an ACVO diplomate is not located. However, it is prudent for these veterinarians to advise clients of their interest status and lack of *ophthalmology* board certification.

REFERRAL PROCESS

To expedite the referral process, the referring veterinarian should either contact the ophthalmologist by telephone or send a letter with the client so that all the pertinent history is present at the time of the referral appointment. Information regarding the owner's name, patient's name, laboratory diagnostic results, suspected diagnosis, ocular medications, ocular surgeries performed, current systemic medications, and pertinent systemic conditions should be included. Owners should be instructed to bring the currently prescribed medications to the examination. The ophthalmologist either telephones or sends a written report to the referring veterinarian, explaining the diagnosis or differential diagnosis, further diagnostic procedures required (if applicable), surgical or medical therapy, and prognosis. The ophthalmologist treats only conditions that pertain to the eyes and works closely with the referring veterinarian, especially when systemic involvement is noted. Communication between both primary care and referral veterinarians and their client is of paramount importance. The patient returns to the referring practitioner for all other veterinary care. One should not assume that an owner is unwilling to take the time or spend the money to see a specialist. People who are openly referred to a specialist in a positive manner, before their pets are beyond assistance, are much more willing to return to their referring practitioner for general veterinary care. Self-referred clients are accepted by most ophthalmologists, and all too often the ophthalmologist is asked to refer clients to another general practitioner when there is not an open and willing referral.

PATIENTS TO REFER

Which patients a veterinarian refers depends largely on the diagnostic or surgical equipment required and expertise of the general practitioner with the patient's condition. A patient should be referred if the practitioner is uncertain of the appropriate diagnosis or if the condition is not responding appropriately to prescribed therapy. Occasionally, confirmation of a diagnosis is desired. Animals with conditions that require specialized diagnostic equipment not found in the general practice should be referred, as well as those that require specialized surgical equipment and technique.

Several textbooks have been written regarding the multitude of ophthalmic diseases; thus, listing all of the specific conditions for consideration of referral is beyond the scope of this article. However, most patients presented to the veterinary ophthalmologist benefit from one or more of the following: specialized diagnostic equipment, current medical knowledge, and specialized surgical instruments and techniques.

Specialized Diagnostic Equipment

Biomicroscopy (using a slit lamp) provides minimal to high magnification, with illumination ranging from diffuse illumination to a slit beam of various intensities. Proper use of this instrument can allow detailed examination and exact localization of lesions within the anterior segment (as far posterior as the anterior vitreous face) and the adnexa. It is extremely useful in detection of ocular foreign bodies, ectopic cilia (often involved with nonhealing corneal ulcers), and detection of pathologic processes invisible to the unaided eye, to name but a few of its functions. Indirect ophthalmoscopy allows panoramic viewing of the fundus to further elucidate retinal, choroidal, optic nerve, and vitreal pathologic changes. Fundus photography aids in following progression of posterior segment disease. Tonometry (intraocular pressure measurement) and gonioscopy (detailing of the iridocorneal angle with a specialized lens) are essential to provide optimal care for many glaucoma patients. Depending on the institution or practice, other diagnostic modalities available may include electroretinography for detection of retinal degenerations, orbital radiography with various contrast studies, and ocular ultrasonography.

Current Medical Knowledge

It is the responsibility of the ophthalmologist to be knowledgeable of current information through attendance at veterinary ophthalmology conventions, perusal of ophthalmic articles in journals, and maintenance of proficiency of skills through continuing ophthalmology referrals.

Specialized Instruments and Surgical Technique

Microsurgical instruments and supplies, high-magnification optics, and advanced training are essential for performance of intraocular surgery, such as extracapsular and intracapsular lens extractions. Conjunctival pedicle grafts (for descemetoceles and perforated corneas), corneal laceration repairs, corneoscleral transpositions, placement of intraocular prostheses, and keratectomies should be performed by experienced ophthalmic surgeons on client-owned patients. Many ophthalmologists are well versed in cryosurgical procedures for glaucoma, neoplasms, and distichiasis (as well as electroepilation for the latter). A variety of types of orbital surgery can be performed. Reconstructive eyelid surgery is commonplace in the ophthalmology practice.

The liaison between ophthalmologist and general practitioner for animal eye care can be a rewarding experience if professional rapport is maintained. The ophthalmologist's aim must be to work with the general practitioner, owner, and patient to effect the best patient eye care possible.

References and Supplemental Reading

Blanchard, G. L.: The role of the primary veterinarian in the management of the referral patient. Vet. Clin. North Am. 10:249, 1980.

Ettinger, S. J., Vierheller, R. C., Lippincott, C. L., et al.: Section on referrals in veterinary medicine. J. Am. Anim. Hosp. Assoc. 12:218, 1976.

Jackson, W. F.: Editorial—Some thoughts on education and small animal specialty practice. J. Am. Anim. Hosp. Assoc. 12:436, 1976.

Rubin G. J., and Reedy L. M.: The referral practice. Comp. Cont. Ed. Pract. Vet. 5:532, 1983.

NEURO-OPHTHALMOLOGY

MARY B. GLAZE, D.V.M.

Baton Rouge, Louisiana

Neuro-ophthalmology examines the inter-relationships of the ophthalmic and central nervous systems. To the ophthalmologist, it is the foundation for explaining the array of ophthalmologic disorders that accompany neurologic disease. To the neurologist, it is a tool for pinpointing abnormalities within the nervous system. For both, neuro-ophthalmology encompasses pupillary light reflexes, vision, ocular position, and ocular movements.

Anisocoria and blindness are among the more common neuro-ophthalmologic disorders in companion animals. Simple recognition of these clinical signs is far removed from a neuro-ophthalmologic diagnosis, however. The inciting lesion must first be localized and its etiology determined. In general, the nature of neuro-ophthalmologic lesions limits treatment options and therapeutic response.

ANATOMY

Localization of the inciting lesion requires a thorough understanding of neuroanatomy. Detailed anatomic descriptions have appeared in several veterinary texts (Scagliotti, 1980; Kay, 1981; Neer and Carter, 1987). This article attempts to highlight basic, clinically relevant features (Fig. 1).

PUPILLOMOTOR PATHWAY. The afferent arm of

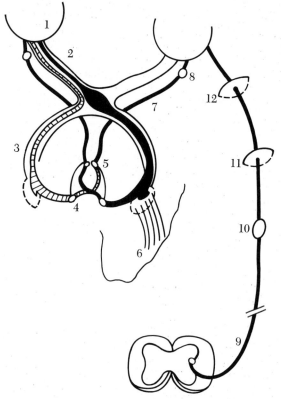

Figure 1. Diagram of the central and peripheral nervous system pathways that affect pupil size. The following structures are identified by number: 1, retina; 2, optic nerve; 3, optic tract; 4, pretectal nucleus; 5, parasympathetic nucleus of cranial nerve III; 6, occipital cortex; 7, oculomotor nerve; 8, ciliary ganglion; 9, cervical sympathetic trunk; 10, cranial cervical ganglion; 11, middle ear; 12, cavernous sinus.

the pupillary light reflex is initiated when light stimulates the retina. Impulses travel through optic nerve fibers to the optic chiasm, where 75 per cent of the fibers in the dog and 65 per cent of the fibers in the cat decussate to the contralateral side. The impulse continues along the optic tract to the midbrain's pretectal nucleus. Here the majority of fibers cross again to the original side through the posterior commissure, terminating in the parasympathetic nucleus of the third cranial nerve (i.e., the Edinger-Westphal nucleus).

The efferent portion of the pupillary light reflex is composed of uncrossed parasympathetic fibers originating in the parasympathetic nucleus of cranial nerve III. These fibers leave the midbrain with the motor efferent fibers of the oculomotor nerve but separate before synapsing at the retrobulbar ciliary ganglion. From there, short ciliary nerves (five to eight mixed nerves in the dog, two parasympathetic nerves in the cat) penetrate the globe to innervate the pupillary sphincter.

VISUAL PATHWAY. The visual pathway is identical to the afferent arm of the pupillary light reflex until the visual fibers diverge from the optic tract to enter the thalamus' lateral geniculate body. Axons course

caudally as the optic radiation of the internal capsule and terminate in the occipital lobe cortex. Clinical signs associated with lesions of the visual and pupillomotor pathways are summarized in Table 1.

EFFERENT SYMPATHETIC PATHWAY. The dilator muscle of the iris is innervated by the sympathetic nervous system, a long three-neuron chain originating in the hypothalamus. The tract descends the brainstem and cervical spinal cord to synapse at T1–T3, then passes through the anterior thorax and along the neck within the vagosympathetic trunk. After synapsing at the cranial cervical ganglion caudomedial to the tympanic bulla, the fibers traverse the middle ear and the cavernous sinus to join the ophthalmic division of the trigeminal nerve. Sympathetic fibers enter the globe as the long ciliary nerve, innervating the ciliary body and iris dilator, and also arborize within smooth muscle fibers in the superior eyelid and periorbital fascia.

OCULAR POSITION/MOVEMENT. The extrinsic eye muscles, innervated by the oculomotor, trochlear, and abducens nerves, control the position and movements of the eye. Axons of these nerves originate in the midbrain, where their nuclei receive input from the vestibular system through the medial longitudinal fasciculus. This relationship explains the effect of head position on eye movements. These and other cranial nerves pertinent to the eye are cited in Table 2.

NEURO-OPHTHALMOLOGIC DISORDERS

Anisocoria

When an animal has asymmetric pupils, it is first necessary to determine which of the two eyes is abnormal. The examiner must have an appreciation for the average pupil diameter in the normal animal evaluated under similar circumstances. A thorough ophthalmologic examination should be performed

Table 1. *Ocular Signs Associated with Lesions of the Visual and Pupillomotor Pathways*

Clinical Sign	Site of Lesion
Visual and pupillary deficits	Retina
	Optic nerve
	Optic chiasm
	Optic tract
Visual deficits only	Lateral geniculate body
	Optic radiation
	Occipital cortex
Pupillary deficits only	Pretectal nucleus (midbrain)
	Parasympathetic nucleus of oculomotor nerve
	Oculomotor nerve (cranial nerve III)
	Ciliary ganglion
	Ciliary nerve
	Iris sphincter

Table 2. *Cranial Nerves of Ophthalmic Significance*

Cranial Nerve	Function	Signs of Dysfunction
Optic (II)	Vision	Visual deficits
Oculomotor (III)	Parasympathetic fibers to iris sphincter	Fixed, dilated pupil
	Motor to superior, medial, and inferior rectus and inferior oblique muscles	Strabismus (ventrolateral)
	Motor to levator palpebrae	Ptosis
Trochlear (IV)	Motor to superior oblique muscle	Inapparent
Trigeminal (V)	Sensory to cornea	Insensitive cornea
	Sensory to lids	Decreased palpebral reflex
Abducens (VI)	Motor to lateral rectus, retractor bulbi muscles	Medial strabismus
		Impaired globe retraction
Facial (VII)	Motor to orbicularis oculi	Lagophthalmos
	Parasympathetic fibers to lacrimal gland	Inadequate tears
Vestibulo-cochlear (VIII)	Equilibrium	Nystagmus, positional strabismus

to rule out iris disorders due to anterior uveitis, glaucoma, or iris atrophy.

Neurologic causes of anisocoria may be characterized using the pupillary light reflex. When stimulated, the normal pupil constricts both directly and consensually (i.e., when the light is directed into the opposite eye). An immobile or minimally reactive pupil is clearly abnormal, although a strong light source should be used before declaring the eye unresponsive. A modification of the pupillary light response is the swinging flashlight test. The light is alternated from eye to eye at 2- to 4-sec intervals, providing a relatively constant direct or consensual stimulus. The normal animal will demonstrate minimal pupillary excursions. The pupil that dilates when the light source is switched from consensual to direct stimulation is said to exhibit a abnormal (positive) swinging flashlight test result. The initial goal is to determine whether the problem lies within the eye, within the orbit, or within the cranium. Features useful in differentiating anisocorias are summarized below and in Table 3.

AFFERENT LESIONS

1. With an afferent lesion, the anisocoria is accentuated in bright light but disappears in darkness when both pupils dilate maximally.

2. The difference in pupil size in unilateral afferent lesions is usually no more than 2 to 3 mm. Animals with bilateral, complete afferent lesions are blind, with widely dilated, fixed pupils in room light.

3. Retinal and optic nerve lesions are characterized by vision loss and an abnormal swinging flashlight test result.

4. A normal swinging flashlight test result accompanies lesions of the optic tract owing to preservation of uncrossed afferent fibers. A contralateral visual deficit results but may be clinically inapparent.

EFFERENT LESIONS

1. The degree of pupillary asymmetry is much greater in efferent than in afferent lesions. The anisocoria intensifies in light.

2. Only the pupil ipsilateral to the efferent defect demonstrates diminished response to light. Vision is unaffected.

3. Pharmacologic testing may help differentiate pre- and postganglionic parasympathetic lesions. The pupil ipsilateral to a central or preganglionic lesion will constrict much more quickly than that of the normal eye following application of 1 drop of an indirect parasympathomimetic (e.g., 0.5 per cent physostigmine). Supersensitivity (rapid constriction compared with control eye) to 2 per cent pilocarpine in the affected eye will confirm a ganglionic or postganglionic lesion. Failure to respond to pilocarpine suggests pharmacologic blockade by atropine-like drugs.

4. A syndrome of generalized dysautonomia (Key-Gaskell syndrome) with ocular manifestations has been described in cats. Affected animals may initially demonstrate anisocoria but then develop dilated, fixed pupils with no loss of vision. Other ocular signs include third eyelid protrusion and decreased tear production. Multisystemic signs include constipation, megaesophagus, bradycardia, and urinary incontinence (Bromberg and Cabaniss, 1988). Cats may also develop a pronounced, alternating anisocoria or pupillary hemidilation, believed to be associated with feline leukemia virus (FeLV) infection (Scagliotti, 1980).

EFFERENT SYMPATHETIC LESIONS

1. With efferent sympathetic lesions, the degree of pupillary asymmetry increases in the dark.

2. Sympathetic denervation is characterized by Horner's syndrome, an array of clinical signs including miosis, ptosis, narrowing of the palpebral fissure, enophthalmos, and protrusion of the third eyelid. Although the affected pupil is small, it reacts normally to light.

3. Normal mydriasis following application of 1 per cent hydroxyamphetamine (Paredrine, SmithKline & Beckman) suggests a central or preganglionic sympathetic lesion. Rapid pupillary dilation (compared with the fellow eye) following application of 10 per cent phenylephrine confirms a postganglionic lesion.

CAUSES

Conditions that may affect the retina and optic nerve include hereditary retinal atrophy; acquired

Table 3. *Differentiating Features of Pupillary and Visual Pathway Lesions*

Lesion Site	Left Eye		Right Eye		Vision Loss
	Direct	*Consensual*	*Direct*	*Consensual*	
Right retina	+	−	−	+	Complete OD
Right optic nerve	+	−	−	+	Complete OD
Optic chiasm (complete)	−	−	−	−	Complete OU
Optic chiasm (partial)	+	+	+	+	Partial OU
Right optic tract	+	+	+	+	Partial OS
Caudal commissure	+	+	+	+	No loss
Right CN III parasympathetic nucleus	+	+	−	−	No loss
Right CN III	+	+	−	−	No loss
Right lateral geniculate body	+	+	+	+	Partial OS
Right optic radiation	+	+	+	+	Partial OS
Right occipital cortex	+	+	+	+	Partial OS

CN, cranial nerve; OD, right eye; OS, left eye; OU, both eyes.

retinal and optic nerve atrophy, as a result of glaucoma or feline taurine deficiency; inflammation caused by infectious agents (mycotic diseases, toxoplasmosis, distemper, brucellosis, ehrlichiosis, protothecosis, and feline infectious peritonitis), reticulosis, trauma, or neoplasia (orbital or metastatic, such as lymphosarcoma); metabolic retinopathies; and idiopathic disease.

Disorders of the remaining afferent pupillomotor and visual pathways have similar infectious, traumatic, and neoplastic causes. The optic tract appears to be a preferential site for the demyelinating effects of canine distemper virus. Inherited storage diseases may affect the retina, lateral geniculate body, and occipital cortex.

The most common causes of damage to the parasympathetic efferent pathway are traumatic proptosis and orbital inflammation. Central nervous system disorders include early tentorial herniation, midbrain hemorrhage, and intracranial neoplasia.

In addition to pharmacologic testing, associated neurologic signs are helpful in localizing the lesion producing Horner's syndrome. Hemiplegia suggests involvement of the cervical spinal cord. Paralysis of a forelimb characterizes involvement of C8 to T2 nerve roots. Horner's syndrome without other neurologic abnormalities may occur with lesions of the vagosympathetic trunk in the neck. Middle ear disease causes concomitant vestibular deficits.

TREATMENT

Treatment is not feasible in hereditary or acquired atrophy. Prognosis for vision in infectious disorders is poor if there is extensive ocular or nervous system involvement. More focal lesions may respond to appropriate antibacterial or antimycotic therapy. *Hypertensive retinopathy*, characterized by bilateral retinal detachments, has been reported in dogs and cats. Return of vision is possible in response to systemic antihypertensive

agents (propranolol, 2.5 mg two or three times daily PO), with or without concomitant diuretic use.

Idiopathic effusive *retinal detachment* and *optic neuritis* are treated with systemic corticosteroids in high doses and for extended periods of time. Optic neuritis due to reticulosis may be treated similarly. Prednisolone is given orally at 1 to 2 mg/kg daily, tapering to 0.5 to 1 mg/kg after 10 to 14 days. Treatment may continue for as long as 6 weeks. Furosemide may be included in the management of effusive detachments, administered at a dose of 2 to 4 mg/kg orally once or twice daily. Therapy is largely empiric, and the prognosis is poor.

The benefit of treatment in storage diseases is obviously limited. In central lesions affecting the parasympathetic efferent pathway, no specific ocular therapy is available, although pupillary changes may be helpful prognostically. Proptosed eyes should be repositioned in the orbit, with systemic corticosteroid therapy instituted as for optic neuritis. *Orbital abscesses* are treated empirically with oral broadspectrum antibiotics for 10 days. Therapy in cats with *dysautonomia* is largely supportive and more often directed at the inadequate tear production than at the pupillary abnormalities.

Sympathetically denervated eyes have been treated symptomatically with topical 10 per cent phenylephrine. This is rarely indicated unless vision is affected by the degree of third eyelid protrusion. Therapy is more appropriately directed at the cause of the Horner's syndrome.

Loss of Vision

Companion animal owners seldom recognize unilateral vision loss because most animals compensate remarkably well using their normal eye and other senses. Total blindness may be suspected if inactivity, cautious gait, or unwillingness to explore a strange environment is noted. Vision loss can be relatively sudden, as with optic neuritis, or may simply reflect the culmination of multiple, chronic ocular or neurologic lesions.

Vision may be tested by observing the animal's ability to maneuver an obstacle course, react to a menacing gesture, or follow a falling cotton ball. Electroretinography and visual evoked responses may also be used to evaluate the retina and the integrity of the visual pathway.

Visual deficits may be attributable to lesions of the globe or the visual pathway. The most common are retinal and optic nerve abnormalities. The cause and therapy of these have been discussed in relation to concomitant deficits in the pupillary light reflex.

Sudden blindness due to photoreceptor degeneration has been reported in dogs. This "silent retina" syndrome is characterized initially by dilated, poorly responsive pupils and an ophthalmoscopically normal fundus. No therapy is of value (see p. 644).

Cardiac arrest, such as that following anesthetic overdose, produces cerebral ischemia and blindness which is noted on recovery, as a result of occipital lobe necrosis. Immediate therapy with 20 per cent mannitol (1.0 gm/kg IV) and dexamethasone (1 to 2 mg/kg IV) is used to reduce cerebral edema. The animal should be maintained on oral corticosteroids for 2 to 3 weeks. Cortical blindness from hypoxia may resolve in 2 to 4 weeks but is more often permanent.

Strabismus

Abnormal eye position results when the extraocular muscles are either injured or denervated (see Table 2). Orbital inflammation, trauma, and neoplasia are the more likely causes of akinesis of extraocular muscles in companion animals. Convergent strabismus related to aberrant development of the visual pathway is inherited in the Siamese cat.

The nuclei of the extraocular muscles receive input from the vestibular system through the medial longitudinal fasciculus. The position of the eyes will therefore change in response to movements of the head. In vestibular disease, positional strabismus develops, characterized by excessive ventral deviation of the ipsilateral eye as the animal's nose is tilted upward.

Nystagmus

This involuntary rhythmic movement of the eyes probably has greater neurologic than ophthalmologic significance. Spontaneous nystagmus is usually associated with an imbalance within the vestibular system. Peripheral vestibular disease is indicated by a horizontal or rotatory nystagmus whose direction and character are unchanged with varying head positions. Oscillations that change in relation to head movement or are directed vertically are more suggestive of central vestibular or brainstem lesions. Nystagmus with equal side-to-side oscillations accompanies cerebellar disease or may be seen in animals with congenital visual deficits. It may also have a genetic basis in the Siamese, similar to the neuroanatomic abnormalities responsible for strabismus.

References and Supplemental Reading

Bromberg, N. M., and Cabaniss, L. D.: Feline dysautonomia: A case report. J. Am. Anim. Hosp. Assoc. 24:106, 1988.
Kay, W. J.: Neuro-ophthalmology. In Gelatt, K. N. (ed.): Textbook of Veterinary Ophthalmology. Philadelphia: Lea & Febiger, 1981, p. 672.
Neer, T. M., and Carter, J. D.: Anisocoria in dogs and cats: Ocular and neurologic causes. Comp. Cont. Ed. Pract. Vet. 9:817, 1987.
Scagliotti, R.: Neuro-ophthalmology. In Kirk, R. W. (ed.): Current Veterinary Therapy VII. Philadelphia: W. B. Saunders, 1980, p. 510.

ADNEXAL TUMORS OF DOGS AND CATS

DENNIS V. HACKER, D.V.M.

Berkeley, California

The discussion of adnexal tumors should start with the premise that these tumors are seldom blinding, and, in dogs, neoplasms rarely cause fatalities. In dogs, metastases from adnexal neoplasms are not often encountered. This statement is not true in cats, as spread of adnexal neoplasms will occur. In both dogs and cats, distant tumors seldom metastasize to the adnexal tissue as compared with intraocular structures. This difference in metastatic rate is thought to be due to the adnexa's being less vascular than intraocular structures such as the choroid and ciliary body. The true incidence of adnexal, intraocular, and orbital neoplasms is unknown, for veterinarians infrequently submit adnexal neoplasms for histopathologic diagnoses (in an attempt to save client's money). In this discussion, both neoplastic and non-neoplastic conditions will be categorized into those of the eyelids, nictitating membrane (third eyelid), and conjunctiva.

EYELID LESIONS

A discussion of eyelid tumors would be incomplete without the discussion of chalazion. Chalazia are non-neoplastic, granulomatous lesions located within the eyelid stroma itself and are infrequently located along the eyelid margin. Single or multiple lesions may be located within the lids of the same eye. These lesions are smooth on both the skin and the conjunctival surface of the lid. Commonly, these are slowly growing, nonpainful lesions that do not ulcerate until they become quite large. These lesions are occasionally associated with sebaceous adenomata. Surgical treatment includes applying a chalazion forceps to encompass as much of the lesion as possible to minimize intraoperative bleeding. Next, one should incise the *bulbar* surface of the chalazion and débride the lesion to remove the necrotic debris. Postoperatively, an antibiotic-corticosteroid ointment should be applied to the eye three times daily for 1 week. To ensure that chalazion was indeed the correct diagnosis, tissue should be submitted for histopathologic diagnosis.

Eyelid neoplasms are probably the most commonly encountered ocular neoplasms in domestic animals. In two retrospective studies of canine eyelid neoplasms, 74 and 92 per cent of submitted tumors were benign (Krehbiel and Langham, 1975; Roberts et al., 1986). These values also are representative of the ratio of benign to malignant tumors in the author's experience. The histopathologic diagnoses of canine eyelid neoplasms are listed in Table 1. Previous reports on eyelid neoplasms have discussed the possibility of multiple cell types in canine tumors. These have been designated adnexomas. Although canine eyelid tumors may be proliferative, invasive, or ulcerative, there are no reports of metastasis from eyelid tumors that were malignant.

Eyelid neoplasms of cats, though rare, are more likely to be malignant than canine eyelid neoplasms. As yet, no retrospective study has been published concerning eyelid neoplasms of cats. Feline eyelid neoplasms are listed in Table 2.

In young dogs, histiocytoma should be considered whenever a round, white-to-pink elevated lesion exists on the eyelids. A fine-needle aspirate or excisional biopsy should be submitted for histopathologic confirmation of the tentative clinical diagnosis. Observation of these lesions without immediate surgical intervention is warranted, as they frequently involute without treatment.

Table 1. Canine Eyelid Tumors

Sebaceous adenoma
Squamous papilloma
Sebaceous adenocarcinoma
Benign melanoma
Malignant melanoma
Papilloma
Histiocytoma
Mastocytoma
Basal cell carcinoma
Squamous cell carcinoma
Fibroma
Fibropapilloma
Lipoma
Adnexal carcinoma
Hemangiopericytoma
Malignant lymphoma
Neurofibroma
Neurofibrosarcoma
Atypical epithelioma
Adnexoma
Undetermined tumors

Table 2. Feline Eyelid Neoplasms

Squamous cell carcinoma
Basal cell carcinoma
Fibroma
Fibrosarcoma
Neurofibroma
Neurofibrosarcoma
Adenoma
Adenosarcoma
Papilloma
Xanthomatosis
Hemangioma
Hemangiosarcoma
Mast cell tumors

SURGERY

For most eyelid neoplasms, surgical excision of the lesion and blepharoplastic repair of the iatrogenic defect remain the accepted method of primary treatment. The clinician is referred to standard ophthalmic surgery texts for instruction concerning surgical technique. Clients are sometimes morbidly fearful of having their pet anesthetized in spite of reassurances concerning the safety of modern anesthetic agents. Other treatment modalities are sometimes necessary when this aversion to anesthesia and surgery is paramount in the client's mind. Additionally, patients with eyelid tumors are often older and may have systemic or cardiac abnormalities, which make them anesthetic risks. Tranquilization and local anesthesia is adequate for many minor plastic procedures.

CRYOSURGERY

As most canine eyelid tumors are either benign or, even when histologically malignant, act in a relatively benign manner, cryosurgery is an acceptable alternative to surgical excision. Cryosurgery may also be efficacious in small feline eyelid tumors and in preneoplastic growths associated with squamous cell carcinoma. The patients may be anesthetized or heavily sedated with fentanyl-droperidol (Innovar-Vet, Pitman-Moore), oxymorphone (DuPont Pharmaceuticals), acepromazine (PromAce, Fort Dodge), or xylazine (Rompun, Haver). After injecting the tissue surrounding the lesion with lidocaine, the lesion may be debulked. Hemostasis by chemical or cautery means will assure that cryosurgery will be effective. The tumor is frozen using a nitrous oxide cryoprobe (Frigitronics) or a nonspray attachment on a liquid nitrogen cryogenic appliance (Brymill Corp). Although some clinicians recommend the use of a spray cryogenic appliance, spraying the area will cause excessive tissue destruction and damage. Using the spray technique, ectropion or entropion may occur to an extent that could require additional corrective surgery. Two to three freeze ($-80°C$ for 2 min)-thaw cycles are used on the area. Typical postoperative sequelae are hemorrhage from the incision site, swelling, serous to mucopurulent drainage, depigmentation and alopecia of the adjacent area, and, finally, necrosis and sloughing of the neoplastic tissue. A major complication of this technique is the extensive sloughing of tissue, which could result in a larger defect than the original lesion. Alopecia and depigmentation will occur and, depending on the extent of freezing, may be permanent. The area of the freezing procedure will be sensitive and painful. The pain and discomfort will worsen for 2 to 3 days following surgery.

IMMUNOTHERAPY

A third form of therapy that may be used on small to mid-sized lesions is immunotherapy. This is best suited for epithelial and mesenchymal derived tumor types (e.g., eyelid or conjunctival papilloma and squamous cell carcinoma). Fibrous histiocytomas have been reported to be unresponsive to this treatment regimen. Mycobacterial cell wall fractions such as Regressin (Ragland Research, Inc.) or Ribigen (Ribi-Immunochem Research, Inc.) will cause intense inflammation when injected intralesionally and into the perilesional tissue. Nonsteroidal anti-inflammatory medication should be given to ameliorate this result. Topically applied antibiotics should be prescribed to prevent secondary infection. A second set of injections may be needed to cause complete resolution of large lesions.

RADIATION THERAPY

Large eyelid tumors may be treated by debulking the neoplasm and by implantation of radioactive needles, seeds, or pellets; the use of strontium-90 applicators; cobalt or other gamma-irradiation devices; or x-irradiation. These techniques often require the referral of the patient to a university or large metropolitan referral center where clinicians trained in radiation therapy are located and where the patient may be isolated as required. Without proper training in the use of radiation techniques, the patient *and* the clinician are at great risk from radiation damage.

Unlike most canine tumors, feline eyelid squamous cell carcinomas require aggressive treatment to prevent spread to deeper ocular structures and subsequent fatal results. Cryosurgery or strontium-90 probes may be used while the lesions are small. After the lesions have encompassed a large portion of the eyelid, enucleation and biopsy of the tissue removed and possible radiation therapy postoperatively may be necessary to save the patient's life.

Recent articles have reported the lack of effect of systemic pharmacologic treatment for ocular and adnexal lesions. Azelaic acid was shown to have no effect on human adnexal and ocular malignant melanoma (Willshaw and Rubenstein, 1983). Additionally, there was no effect of 13-*cis*-retinoic acid on squamous cell carcinoma in cats (Evans et al., 1985). Although, the discipline of oncogenic pharmacology is developing rapidly, controlled studies are needed prior to using medication in lieu of surgery. Small domestic patients do well after treatment with standard surgical, cryosurgical, and radiotherapeutic measures; attempts to circumvent surgery may cause an increased risk to life.

CONJUNCTIVAL AND NICTITATING MEMBRANE LESIONS

Non-neoplastic Conditions

Non-neoplastic conditions that may mimic neoplastic disorders include fibrous histiocytoma, dermoids, and plaques. Fibrous histiocytoma, also known as granulomatous nodular episcleritis, proliferative keratoconjunctivitis, and nodular fasciitis, is commonly seen in the young collie. Young dogs of other breeds may also develop these raised pink, white, yellow, or red-gray lesions of the bulbar or third eyelid conjunctival surface. They will respond to frequent applications of topically applied potent corticosteroids, such as prednisolone acetate 1 per cent. Medical management may initially cause regression of the lesion, followed by recurrence after medication is discontinued. Intralesional corticosteroid injections, oral azothioprine (Imuran, Burroughs Wellcome), and surgical debulking of the lesion may be required to achieve resolution. The use of azothioprine as a single therapy has not resulted in permanent resolution of the lesions, and long-term oral treatment is required to prevent recurrence. These lesions do not respond well to immunotherapy (see above).

Frequently, dermoids (choristomas) are found on the conjunctiva or limbus of young dogs. These lesions are not neoplastic but are normal tissue at an abnormal site. If these lesions contain hair, they may cause keratitis and secondary uveitis. Careful sharp or blunt excision and removal combined with postoperative antibiotics and cycloplegics should yield excellent results.

Dense yellow, gray, or white residual plaques (granulomas) may remain following the subconjunctival injection of any repository corticosteroid. These masses may appear inflamed and may be confused with episcleritis, scleritis, granulomatous sclerouveitis, and focal conjunctival tumors. The plaques occasionally must be surgically excised to resolve the associated inflammation.

Neoplasia

Unlike lesions of the eyelids, conjunctival and third eyelid neoplastic growths are most commonly epithelial abnormalities. They may be malignant or benign in diagnosis and activity. Excisional biopsy of conjunctival and third eyelid lesions is easily accomplished. If the tissue is erythematous, blanching of the blood vessels with topically applied epinephrine or phenylephrine (Neo-Synephrine, Winthrop) will help assure that the topically applied anesthetic is not systemically absorbed. One should apply one drop of proparacaine (Ophthetic, Allergan) once every 2 to 3 min for three applications. Next, a cotton-tipped applicator is moistened with anesthetic and applied and held to the third eyelid. Deep anesthesia of the site is accomplished after several minutes. A small portion of the lesion is grasped with a Bishop-Harmon or other small forceps, and a small scissors is used to excise tissue for histologic diagnosis. Small, discrete lesions may be removed *in toto* using this technique. All lesions removed from the conjunctiva and third eyelid should be submitted for histologic confirmation of diagnosis.

Canine conjunctival neoplasms include angiokeratoma, hemangiosarcoma, lymphoma, fibrohistiocytoma, hemangioma, adenoma, papilloma, squamous cell carcinoma, and melanoma. Cyst development of the lacrimal gland has been reported to occur in the dog. Feline lesions may include the eyelid by extension, and malignant melanoma of the conjunctiva has been reported.

Lesions of the third eyelid may become large before being noticed because the third eyelid is not readily visible in the normal patient. Benign, non-neoplastic lesions such as plasmoma (plasmacytic-lymphocytic infiltrate) and hemangioma are occasionally found along the leading edge of the third eyelid. Plasmomas may resolve by the frequent topical use of potent corticosteroid agents, such as prednisolone acetate 1 per cent. Occasionally, an intralesional injection of a repository corticosteroid such as 10 mg of triamcinolone acetonide (Kenalog-40, E. R. Squibb), radiation therapy using a strontium-90 probe, or cryotherapy is necessary for complete resolution of these lesions.

Occasionally clinicians will mistake a prolapsed gland of the third eyelid, which may occur in older patients, for neoplastic growths. Clinically, these lesions appear exactly as in young dogs (smooth, red, nonulcerated, and nonpainful) and should be considered when a red lesion of the third eyelid occurs. If a question arises concerning the diagnosis of a lesion, an excisional biopsy is necessary. Adenocarcinoma and adenoma are often the diagnosis of third eyelid masses. In the event of neoplastic growth, the third eyelid should be excised and submitted for histopathologic examination.

Epibulbar melahomas are often seen in dogs and cats. These are nonelevated and noninvasive. They should be measured and monitored for several months to ensure that they are enlarging prior to their surgical removal. These lesions are slow growing and are relatively noninvasive. Limbal melanomas of dogs and cats should be removed while they are totally contained within the anterior stroma of the cornea. After they have deepened to include the entire corneal depth, their removal will necessitate a frozen corneal, collagen, or corneoscleral graft to repair the surgical defect. These lesions should be examined histologically to ensure the accuracy of the diagnosis. This extensive procedure should only be attempted by surgeons with the expertise and equipment to perform intraocular surgery. The differential diagnosis of epibulbar melanoma includes ciliary body melanoma that has penetrated through the sclera or cornea. Gonioscopy should be performed to differentiate these conditions.

Epibulbar lesions, such as extraocular fibroma, fibrosarcoma, and round cell sarcoma, appear to respond well to the immunotherapy described above. When injecting such lesions, care should be taken not to penetrate the globe and inject the preparations intraocularly. Inflammation is expected and should not be inhibited by the use of corticosteroids.

References and Supplemental Reading

Barron, C. N.: The comparative pathology of neoplasms of the eyelids and conjunctivae with special reference to those of epithelial origin. Acta Derm. Venereol. (Stockh) 41:1, 1962.

Bistner, S. I., Aguirre, G. D., and Batik, G.: *Atlas of Veterinary Ophthalmic Surgery.* Philadelphia, W. B. Saunders Co., 1977.

Evans, A. G., Madewell, B. R., Stannard, A. A.: A trial of 13-cis-retinoic acid for treatment of squamous cell carcinoma and preneoplastic lesions of the head in cats. Am. J. Res. 46:2553, 1985.

Gwin, R. M., Gelatt, K. N., and Williams, L. W.: Ophthalmic neoplasms in the dog. J. Am. Anim. Hosp. Assoc. 18:853, 1982.

Krehbiel, J. D., and Langham, R. F.: Eyelid neoplasms of dogs. Am. J. Vet. Res. 36:115, 1975.

Latimer, C. A., Wyman, M., Szymanski, C., et al.: Azathioprine in the management of fibrous histiocytoma in two dogs. J. Am. Anim. Hosp. Assoc. 19:155, 1983.

Martin, C. L.: Canine epibulbar melanomas and their management. J. Am. Anim. Hosp. Assoc. 17:83, 1981.

Roberts, S. M., Severin, G. A., and Lavach, J. D.: Prevalence and treatment of palpebral neoplasms in the dog: 200 cases (1975–1983). J.A.V.M.A. 189:1355, 1986.

Williams, L. W., Gelatt, K. N., and Gwin, R. M.: Ophthalmic neoplasms in the cat. J. Am. Anim. Hosp. Assoc. 17:999, 1981.

Willshaw, H. E., and Rubinstein, K.: Azelaic acid in the treatment of ocular and adnexal malignant melanoma. Br. J. Ophthalmol. 67:54, 1983.

Section
7

DISEASES
OF
CAGED
BIRDS
AND
EXOTIC
PETS

MURRAY E. FOWLER, D.V.M.
Consulting Editor

Zoonoses of Concern to Volunteers and Staff of Wild Animal
    Rehabilitation Centers...697
Basic Ornamental Fish Medicine...703
What Practitioners Should Know about Whale Strandings.................721
Preventive Medicine in Nondomestic Carnivores........................727
Llama Basics...734
Individual Care and Treatment of Rabbits, Mice, Rats, Guinea Pigs,
    Hamsters, and Gerbils...738
Medical and Surgical Care of the Pet Ferret...........................765
Update on Avian Anesthesia...776
Microbiologic Techniques for the Avian Practitioner 780
Advances in Avian and Reptilian Imaging...............................786
Repair of Injuries to the Chelonian Plastron and Carapace.............789
Vitamin A Sources, Hypovitaminosis A, and Iatrogenic
    Hypervitaminosis A in Captive Chelonians..........................791
Sexual Dimorphism and Identification in Reptiles......................796

ZOONOSES OF CONCERN TO VOLUNTEERS AND STAFF OF WILD ANIMAL REHABILITATION CENTERS

MURRAY E. FOWLER, D.V.M.

Davis, California

Many diseases are common to domestic animals, wild animals, and humans. There is no sharp line demarcating diseases associated only with wild species, but wild animals may be involved in the dissemination of most of the more than 200 diseases considered to be zoonoses.

This article is not meant to be a definitive treatise on all zoonoses; it focuses on diseases that may be a hazard to the staff, volunteers, and veterinarians serving rehabilitation centers or to the citizen who collects animals from the wild. Some rehabilitation centers may cater to only a limited group of animals such as raptors or small mammals, others may accept all types of wild animals. There are hundreds of such facilities in North America, with local and national organizations to foster better training and care of their charges.

Tables 1 through 3 list a few zoonoses and probable wild animal carriers or reservoir hosts.

AMPHIBIANS

Other than the large species of frogs, toads, and salamanders that bite, amphibians are not hazardous. Although toads have a warty skin, they are in no way responsible for the transmission of human warts.

REPTILES

SNAKES. Snakes of all shapes, sizes, and origins are kept by amateur herpetologists, and injured or diseased snakes are collected from the wild. Nonpoisonous snakes may inflict bites that are septic and produce wound infections.

TURTLES. Raising turtles is a popular hobby. Most specimens sold in the pet trade are red-eared sliders. Pet turtles are a significant hazard, particularly to children, because they may be carriers of *Salmonella*. Salmonellosis is a common infectious enteritis of children and adults caused by one of the 1300 serotypes of the genus *Salmonella*. Turtles are not the only source; others include rodents, birds, carnivores, and other reptiles.

It is estimated that over 15 million turtles are sold annually in pet shops throughout the United States. Of the over 2 million cases of salmonellosis

Table 1. *Potential Wild Host Distribution of Selected Zoonoses*

	Invertebrates	Reptiles	Birds	Mammals				
				Rodents	*Primates*	*Carnivores*	*Ungulates*	*Other*
Viral Diseases								
Arbovirus encephalitis	X	X	X	X			X	X
Cat-scratch disease (virus suspected)						X		
Lymphocytic choriomeningitis				X				
Newcastle disease			X					
Rabies				X	X	X	X	X
Vesicular stomatitis	X							
Yellow fever	X			X	X			X
Rickettsial Diseases								
Q fever			X	X				
Rocky Mountain spotted fever	X			X				
Spirochetal Diseases								
Leptospirosis				X	X	X	X	X
Rat-bite fever				X		X		

Table 2. Potential Wild Host Distribution of Selected Zoonoses

						Mammals				
	Invertebrates	Fish	Amphibians	Reptiles	Birds	Rodents	Primates	Carnivores	Ungulates	Other
Bacterial Diseases										
Anthrax					X	X		X	X	X
Brucellosis						X		X	X	X
Erysipelas		X			X	X				
Listeriosis					X	X		X		
Melioidosis						X				
Plague					X	X		X		X
Pseudotuberculosis					X	X	X	X	X	
Psittacosis						X				
Salmonellosis	X	X	X	X	X	X	X	X	X	X
Tetanus				X					X	
Tuberculosis		X			X		X	X	X	X
Tularemia					X	X		X	X	X

reported annually, approximately 280,000 (14 per cent) are associated with turtles.

Many states now have strict regulations requiring that turtles sold in pet shops be free from *Salmonella* infections. Even though great effort is expended to accomplish this, there is still the possibility of animals becoming infected after the test. Factors contributing to the continuation of infection in turtles are crowded conditions with extensive fecal contamination and transovarian passage of the *Salmonella* organism. In addition, the organism can survive and replicate in the intestine of the turtle without causing symptoms.

Prevention. Personnel should be counseled to handle turtles very carefully. Bowls and aquaria should never be cleaned in a sink in which dishes are washed or food is prepared. Hands should be washed thoroughly following any manipulation of these animals.

BIRDS

Psittacosis

Psittacosis (ornithosis) is a natural disease of birds that may be transmissible to humans. Although the disease was recognized as a clinical syndrome as early as 1874, it became a serious disease of humans only during a pandemic occurring worldwide in 1929 and 1930. The pandemic started in Argentina and was associated with the keeping of parrots as pets. The disease became so rampant that regulatory officials declared a ban on the possession of psittacine birds.

As a result, many psittacine birds in holding facilities in South America were immediately exported to other countries, including the United States. From these areas, the disease spread worldwide. Subsequently, numerous cases of atypical

Table 3. Potential Wild Host Distribution of Selected Zoonoses

			Mammals				
	Invertebrates	Birds	Rodents	Primates	Carnivores	Ungulates	Other
Fungal Diseases							
Actinomycosis			X		X	X	X
Aspergillosis		X	X	X	X		
Cryptococcosis		X		X	X	X	
Histoplasmosis		X	X		X		X
Nocardiosis			X				X
Ringworm			X	X	X	X	X
Streptothricosis						X	
Protozoan Diseases							
Amebiasis				X			
Balantidiasis				X			
Leishmaniasis			X		X		
Plasmodium infection (malaria)				X			
Sarcocystosis			X				X
Toxoplasmosis		X	X		X		X
Trypanosomiasis	X					X	X
Ascariasis					X		

pneumonia in humans have been associated with infection from birds and numerous other species. The etiologic agent is *Chlamydia psittaci*, an agent whose identity has been shifted back and forth from virus to bacterium but is now considered a bacterium.

Although the disease was originally associated primarily with psittacine birds, it is now known that the disease is common in other species as well, including raptors. In 1942, Meyer and associates demonstrated that the pigeon is important in the transmission of this disease. In the United States, in fact, the pigeon has been incriminated in more cases of human psittacosis than any other species of bird.

Psittacosis in birds varies from the asymptomatic carrier state to the peracute disease. The seriousness of the disease in birds is determined by the virulence of the organism, species resistance, and environmental factors that lower resistance. Birds may acquire the infection in the nest and carry the organism throughout life. Clinical disease may develop if the bird is placed in a stressful environment such as a cold cage or a new home in which there is a good deal of handling.

TRANSMISSION

The disease is usually acquired from an infected bird. However, bird droppings (particularly dried material that becomes caught up in dust and then is inhaled) are also an important source of infection. In addition, urine, feathers, carcasses, and droplets from nasal secretions may contain the organism.

The incubation period varies from 7 to 15 days after the initial contact, in rare cases extending up to 30 days. In humans, the disease may be characterized as an atypical pneumonia. The lungs are consistently involved in all but extremely mild cases. Headaches and afternoon fevers and chills are also common. Radiographic examination indicates that consolidation begins early in the course of the disease. No specific signs or lesions are pathognomonic of psittacosis in humans. Laboratory examination and culture for the organism rarely yield significant information. The most satisfactory diagnostic technique is the complement fixation test. An acute serum sample and a subsequent convalescent serum sample should be obtained approximately 14 to 21 days after the first sample. A rise in titer of fourfold or more provides evidence of an infection, but a diagnosis cannot be made on a single serum sample. Clinical findings plus the epidemiologic factors involved in the case are important aspects of diagnosis of psittacosis.

The following example illustrates the problem confronting the physician and the veterinarian when faced with possible psittacosis infection. The father of four young children was hospitalized with atypical pneumonia. Treated with broad-spectrum antibiotics, he made a slow recovery, ultimately returning home and to work. The physician suspected psittacosis, and acute and convalescent sera submitted for titer evaluation indicated a rise sufficient to establish a positive diagnosis.

A budgerigar was kept in the home, but it had been a pet for at least 2 years. No new birds had been brought into the house, and the budgerigar had never been taken out. The physician suggested that the bird be checked for psittacosis. Thus, a veterinarian was faced with the problem of making a specific diagnosis without sacrificing the bird. Since the disease is often latent or subclinical in birds, diagnosis depends upon serologic evidence or isolation of the organism. However, serologic methods are not infallible and require such large quantities of blood that it is virtually impossible to perform them on a tiny bird such as a budgerigar while it is alive. It must be killed and isolations taken from the spleen and the liver.

The problem was solved by giving it a course of 45 daily treatments with chlortetracycline, which eliminates the carrier state in psittacine birds. The source of infection was not ascertained, but, from the viewpoint of the family, this was a satisfactory solution to the problem.

RABBITS

Rabbits may transmit infectious diseases such as plague and tularemia and are capable of traumatic injury as well. They have sharp incisor teeth, and if restrained or handled improperly, wild species will bite. A jackrabbit can inflict severe scratches by raking with the hind feet.

Tularemia

Tularemia, an acute infectious disease of humans and numerous species of wild and domestic animals, is caused by a gram-negative bacterium, *Francisella tularensis (Pasteurella tularensis)*. The disease was first reported in the United States in 1910 and subsequently has been reported in all states.

Tularemia has been diagnosed in many species. The disease is also found in wild birds including grouse, gulls, hawks, owls, and quail. In humans, important sources of infection are the wild cottontail rabbit and hare (jackrabbit).

The disease is transmitted by the bite of blood-sucking insects, particularly ticks and fleas. Other arthropods can act as mechanical vectors for the organism. Bites from infected rabbits might also transmit the disease.

There may be several forms of the disease. The

typhoidal, or *septicemic,* form may be confused with similar diseases such as typhoid fever, influenza, brucellosis, malaria, and pulmonary tuberculosis. The septicemic form is most serious, as it may rapidly prove fatal unless treated promptly.

The organism can be cultured from blood, sputum, or material aspirated from abscesses. A direct smear may give sufficient indication of the infection to warrant beginning therapy before positive identification is made.

The *ulceroglandular* form is characterized by a papule and ulcer formation at the original site of penetration of the organism via a cut or scratch. Enlargement of regional lymph nodes also occurs. This form must be differentiated from other lymphadenitis, plague, infectious mononucleosis, parotitis, lymphoma, and leukemia. An aspiration from the node should provide direct evidence of the presence of the gram-negative organism. The oculoglandular form is conjunctivitis and associated lymphadenitis caused by splashing secretions or excretions of infected animals into the conjunctival sac or by wiping the face with a contaminated hand. Less common forms are the *glandular* (with swollen lymph nodes but no superficial lesions) and the *pulmonary,* or pneumonic, form.

An intradermal test yields positive reactions after the third or fourth day of illness. A serum agglutination test can be carried out; however, the antibodies are not likely to be evident until the tenth day after the onset of illness. This test should be rerun in order to demonstrate a rise in titer on an acute and a convalescent serum sample. In the meantime, antibiotic therapy must be instituted, particularly in the septicemic form, or the patient will die before diagnosis is completed.

RODENTS

Leptospirosis

Leptospirosis is an infectious zoonotic disease caused by the spirochete *Leptospira.* The disease is a general bacterial septicemia with a particular propensity for affecting the liver, kidneys, or both. Leptospirosis is found worldwide. Numerous species of wild animals are hosts. Rodents play a prominent part in the epidemiology of outbreaks in humans, although infections are caused by association with other species as well. The disease may exist in a rodent population in which no individuals show signs of illness. The organism may be shed in the urine of asymptomatic animals for a year or more. When the urine contaminates food or water, humans may contract the disease.

Leptospirosis organisms are extremely susceptible to desiccation; thus, infection is more likely to occur in humans in an aquatic or moist environment. The portal of entry for the organism may be the skin, especially any abraded area softened by continued immersion in water. The organism may also penetrate intact mucous membranes of the eyes, nose, and throat. Bites of wild animals have also been reported as causing leptospirosis.

The syndromes produced by this organism are so varied that in a short discussion one cannot present any significant data to assist in a diagnosis on the basis of clinical findings. Diagnosis must be established by a complete examination in conjunction with symptomatic treatment and identification of the organism in excretions. Clinical signs vary according to the species of the organism, the infective dose and the organ systems involved. Signs of hepatic insufficiency and kidney malfunction are common. The disease may be rapidly fatal without prompt and intensive treatment.

Rocky Mountain Spotted Fever

This zoonosis is caused by *Rickettsia rickettsii.* Although the disease was first described from cases in the Rocky Mountain region, it is now recognized as a disease entity in all states in which suitable tick vectors exist. It is particularly common in the central Atlantic states. The disease has a seasonal incidence, occurring with the availability of the tick vector. Most cases occur during late spring and early summer.

The disease is thought to be a primary infection of wild rodents and is spread from rodents to humans via several species of ticks. The most commonly involved vector in the western United States is the wood tick. In the east, it is most often distributed by the Eastern dog tick. However, transmission is not limited to these species.

LIFE CYCLE. The larva of the tick feeds upon a rodent and thus becomes infected. The infection in the tick is carried through the nymphal and adult stages and may be transmitted to other hosts at any stage. The adult tick survives through the winter and is infective the following year.

The incubation period for the disease is 2 to 12 days. Clinical signs include rapidly rising fever, chills, prostration, and a characteristic rash that appears between the second and fifth days after onset. The eruption is macular and rose-red, becoming fainter during the morning remission of fever early in the disease. Later, the macules become more distinct, with the appearance of petechiae. The course of the disease is usually 2 to 3 weeks. The mortality rate is as high as 20 per cent in untreated patients.

Plague

Plague is an acute infectious disease caused by a gram-negative bacterium, *Yersinia pestis (Pasteu-*

rella pestis). This disease is well-known to the medical profession through vast historical epidemics. These epidemics have now waned, and the disease is being maintained in wild rodent populations as sylvatic, or rural, plague. Wild rodents become infected but usually do not manifest clinical signs under normal conditions. Periods of stress in a population may initiate the clinical syndrome. If the population becomes overcrowded, infected animals may move to other areas where more susceptible house rodents are present, causing an epizootic in them.

Fleas are vectors of the disease. Humans acquire the disease after exposure to fleas cohabitating with rodents infected with the plague bacillus.

Although plague is carried primarily by rodents, other species of wild and domestic animals are susceptible to it. Cases have been recorded in cats, goats, deer, antelopes, kangaroos, and bats. The disease may be spread to humans from any host. In the rodent, the disease is characterized by hemorrhagic septicemia. Subcutaneous hemorrhages and hemorrhagic buboes (infected lymph nodes) are seen. Plague organisms are easily isolated from all tissues of the body.

In humans, the disease may take one of two forms: the bubonic, characterized by bacteremia and infected lymph nodes, or the pneumonic, characterized by acute lobar pneumonia, which is rapidly fatal if untreated. The approximate mortality rate for untreated cases is 70 to 80 per cent in the bubonic form and 100 per cent in the pneumonic form. It is important to realize that the pneumonic form of plague is highly communicable, and a patient suspected of having plague should be isolated. Plague is a serious infection, and early diagnosis is paramount because of the need to prevent production of toxins liberated by the organism as it multiplies in the body. Culture of blood or accessible lesions will establish a rapid diagnosis. Direct smears of such tissues should reveal the presence of large numbers of gram-negative bacilli. Therapy should be instituted upon this information even before specific identification of the organism has been made.

CARNIVORES (WOLVES, CATS, SKUNKS, HYENAS, RACCOONS)

Visceral Larva Migrans

Visceral larva migrans has been recognized as a disease entity since 1952. The larvae of a variety of intestinal nematodes from carnivores and rodents are capable of causing it. Visceral larva migrans is caused by nematodes of the following species: (1) *Toxocara canis*, found in dogs, cats, and numerous wild carnivores such as wolves, foxes, jackals, raccoons; (2) *Toxocara cati*, found primarily in cats, including the mountain lion, lynx, and bobcat; (3) *Toxascaris leonina*, found in wild carnivores; (4) *Baylisascaris transfuga*, found in bears; (5) *Ascaris columnaris*, found in skunks; and (6) *Ascaris devosi*, found in ferrets and mink.

In both primary and accidental hosts, the larvae of all these species migrate through various tissues of the body, producing clinical signs. Children are most commonly affected because they are prone to eating dirt. Children are of special risk in rehabilitation centers. When the child ingests embryonated eggs, second-stage larvae are liberated and migrate from the intestine to the liver, lungs, brain, and eyes. In these sites, the parasites cause a granulomatous eosinophilic reaction that may produce a variety of rather nonspecific clinical symptoms.

The disease presents difficulties in diagnosis. Since the larvae do not mature in this host, a diagnosis of parasitism cannot be made on the basis of fecal egg counts. The only precise method of diagnosis is via biopsy of the granulomatous lesions produced by the encysting larvae. The disease is usually not fatal. In the child, one of the more serious forms of visceral larva migrans is produced when larvae encyst in ocular structures. The lesion produced is that of an eosinophilic granuloma that may be confused with retinoblastoma.

Echinococcosis

Echinococcosis (hydatid disease) occurs worldwide. It is caused by tapeworms of the genus *Echinococcus*. *E. granulosus* is the most important species. The normal host for the adult parasite is the dog or closely related carnivores. The intermediate host for this tapeworm is a herbivorous or omnivorous animal (prey).

In a typical cycle for this disease, the adult tapeworm is found in the small intestine of the dog. Ova are passed in the feces, which contaminate the feed of sheep or other herbivores. The ova hatch in the intestine of the sheep. Larvae penetrate the wall of the intestine and are carried by the circulation to the liver, where they lodge in capillaries. Occasionally, the migrating larvae enter the blood stream and are distributed to other tissues, including the kidneys, brain, and lungs. The cycle is completed when the viscera of the infected sheep are eaten by another dog; thus, the larvae are ingested and mature into adult tapeworms.

In addition to the cycle existing with domestic dogs and sheep, there are wildlife cycles as well. The wolf and the caribou maintain a cycle. Eskimo populations are affected when dogs are fed caribou offal containing cysts. The tapeworms then develop into adults in the sled dogs, and ova are passed in the feces. Contaminated food and water are sources of infection for the Eskimo family. The coyote population in some areas of California maintains a parasite load of *E. granulosus*. There is a potential for zoonosis when coyote puppies are captured and kept as pets.

Neither the adult tapeworm in the dog nor the encysted larva in the liver of the sheep produce marked clinical signs in these hosts. This disease becomes serious when humans become accidental hosts, replacing sheep or other herbivores in the cycle. Fecal contamination in the area in which children play may result in hydatid disease.

Children are particularly susceptible to the development of cysts, and there is reason to believe that adults may have some resistance to the infection. Of cysts of the brain that are removed surgically, 64 per cent are in children younger than 15 years of age.

Rabies

Rabies is a disease dreaded by the medical profession and the population at large for centuries because of its almost universally fatal outcome. The disease is well-documented in the literature. Here, we will explore the wild animal implications of this disease.

The epidemiology of rabies in humans has changed somewhat in recent years. Extensive vaccination programs have greatly reduced the incidence of rabies in dogs. Statistics presented by the Communicable Disease Center in Atlanta, Georgia, indicate that wild animals predominate in reported cases and now provide the greatest exposure hazard to humans.

All mammals are susceptible to rabies, but certain species are more apt to spread the disease because their predatory or carnivorous habits make biting and fighting more probable. In the United States, skunks, raccoons, and foxes most often cause problems. Other species that have been implicated or in which diagnosis of rabies has occurred include the bobcat, badger, coyote, ocelot, monkey, opossum, weasel, mountain lion, and bat. Rodents are rarely involved in rabies exposures.

When a wild animal is observed, particularly one that appears friendly or docile, a human is likely to attempt to pet it or pick it up. It is axiomatic that any wild animal willing to allow a human being to pet it or pick it up is either an escaped pet or a diseased animal. In the case of species such as the skunk or any of the bat species, there is a strong likelihood that rabies is the disease involved.

Ringworm

Ringworm is a dermatomycosis in many species of domestic and wild animals and in humans. Some fungi are host specific; others are freely transmitted from one species of animal to another mechanically. The more common organisms involved in zoonoses are *Microsporum canis* and *Trichophyton mentagrophytes*.

Ringworm may be acquired easily by a human from close association with a wild animal in a rehabilitation center.

The diagnosis of this disease can be determined by a combination of microscopic examination of skin scrapings, culturing of the organism, and noting the characteristics of the lesion. Infections of *M. canis* fluoresce under a Wood's light.

Toxoplasmosis

Toxoplasmosis is caused by a protozoan parasite, *Toxoplasma gondii*. The organism was first described from an African rodent, *Ctenodactylus gundi*, in 1908. Since then, the organism has been isolated from a variety of diseased animals as well as diseased humans. Serologic methods have been used in numerous surveys. The incidence of disease has varied from none in Eskimos to 68 per cent in residents of Tahiti. The disease may be subclinical or latent in an animal and become clinical during a period of stress.

The disease syndrome in both adults and infants has been well-described in the literature. However, information has been brought to light regarding the epidemiology of this disease. Wild cats brought into rehabilitation centers are potential sources of infection in humans who come in contact with oocysts excreted in the feces of these animals. Serologic surveys of wild feline species have demonstrated that these animals develop antibody titers to toxoplasmosis.

Toxoplasma is capable of transplacental migration and, thus, is a hazard to pregnant women working in rehabilitation centers.

Trypanosomiasis

Trypanosomiasis, caused by protozoan parasites (*Trypanosoma*) of the blood, results in anemia and debility. This is a serious disease of humans and domestic and wild animals, particularly in South America and Africa. In South America, the disease is known as Chagas's disease, caused by *Trypanosoma cruzi*.

The disease maintains a life cycle in over 100 species of wild mammals, with the armadillo and the opossum important in maintaining the cycle. This parasite requires a blood-sucking insect such as the kissing bug as a vector. The wildlife cycle is broken when an animal such as the opossum comes into areas of human habitation. The vector then may transmit the parasite from the blood stream of the opossum to dogs and cats found in or around the home area. These same vectors may bite a child, causing infection. Foci of resident trypanosomiasis exist in wildlife in Texas and California. There is potential for zoonoses from these wildlife reservoirs.

Reference and Supplemental Reading

Fowler, M. E.: Diseases of children acquired from nondomestic animals. Curr. Probl. Pediatr. 4:1, 1974.

BASIC ORNAMENTAL FISH MEDICINE

SCOTT B. CITINO, D.V.M.
Miami, Florida

Ornamental fish keeping may be the most popular animal-oriented hobby in the United States. Approximately 300 million dollars is spent on pet fish in the United States each year. The growing number of ornamental fish hobbyists have few "experts" to turn to when problems arise with their aquariums. As most ornamental fish hobbyists have other pets in their households that require veterinary care, it is logical that they turn to their veterinarians for advice on fish health problems. However, the veterinary profession has historically failed to respond to the needs of its ornamental fish–keeping clientele.

Veterinarians, with excellent training in medicine and animal management, are in a unique position to help ornamental fish hobbyists with fish disease and management problems. Whether it be a sick dog, horse, or fish, there is little difference in the basic diagnostic approach taken by the veterinarian.

DIAGNOSTIC APPROACH TO FISH DISEASE

Fish diseases should be approached in a logical manner, beginning with accurate history taking and physical examination and proceeding to antemortem diagnostic techniques and postmortem examination as needed. The situation will often dictate how extensive the clinical approach must be. A good history taken over the phone may be all that is needed to solve a beginning aquarist's problems. However, a subclinical disease affecting the reproduction of an experienced aquarist's breeding stock may require an extensive clinical evaluation with outside support from a diagnostic laboratory. It is the intent of this chapter to supply the clinician with the basic supplemental information needed to begin diagnosing and treating fish diseases.

History Taking and Physical Examination

History taking and physical examination should proceed in a stepwise fashion to ensure that pertinent information is thoroughly and accurately gathered. A well-designed history and examination form is a helpful tool in this respect (Fig. 1). When collecting information about a disease problem, the entire aquarium should be scrutinized as well as the fish within it. Particular attention should be given to environmental factors surrounding the disease problem. A short discussion of a few of the more important topics to address during history taking and physical examination will follow.

THE AQUARIUM

The size, shape, composition, and location of the aquarium should be determined. The volume of an aquarium in gallons can be calculated using the formula: length (inches) × width (inches) × height (inches) ÷ 231. Knowing the volume of an aquarium allows determination of proper stocking rates, heater and filter capacities, and medication dosages. The shape of an aquarium dictates its surface area, which in turn influences the number of fish the aquarium can maintain (Leibovitz, 1980). A low, wide aquarium can support more fish than a high, narrow aquarium of the same volume owing to the superior gas exchange capabilities of the former. Because of their inert qualities, all glass aquariums are recommended over metal-framed and plastic aquariums. Aquariums should not be placed in areas where temperature extremes or drafts occur. Long periods of direct sunlight may overheat aquariums. Areas where smoke and aerosol sprays abound should be avoided, as these potential toxic agents

Client: **Date:**
Address:
Client's primary complaint: _____

Experience rating of aquarist: _____
Aquarium size: _____ gallons: _____ sq. ft. surface area: _____
Aquarium location and comments: _____
Aquarium construction: _____

History and Methods of Aquarium Set-Up
Date of aquarium set-up: _____
Gravel: size: _____, depth: _____, source: _____
Aquarium decorations: _____
Filtration used and comments: _____

Heater: functional? _____, wattage: _____,
water temperature: _____ Type of illumination: _____,
Photoperiod: _____

Water Quality
Clarity: _____, Color: _____, Odor: _____,
Algal growth: _____
Source of water: _____,
Dechlorination or other water Rx: _____
Extent of water movement: _____, Aeration quality: _____
Amount and type of organic debris: _____
Present water chemistry:
    pH: ____, O_2: ____, hardness: ____
    NH_3 ____, NO_2^-: ____, NO_3^-: ____
Water quality history: _____
Comments: _____

Aquarium Maintenance
Water changes: how often? _____, % changed: _____
Gravel stirred and siphoned regularly? _____
Filter: cleaned how often? _____, media changed? _____,
    type of media? _____
Diet fed: _____
How much and how often fed? _____ Live foods? _____

The Fish
Impression of stocking rate: _____
General impression of aquarium population: _____

Is aggression evident? _____
Have disease problems occurred before? ____, Details: _____
_____
Last addition of new fish: _____, Source of fish: _____
Are new additions quarantined? _____, Details: _____

Morbidity and mortality patterns: _____

Behavioral signs of disease: _____
_____
External signs of disease: _____
_____
Previous treatment and effect: _____
Further comments: _____

Figure 1. Example of a history and examination form for use in clinical evaluation of ornamental fish.

may be drawn into an aquarium by its air pump. Aquariums should not be cleaned with soaps, detergents, or disinfectants prior to being set up, because many of these agents may be toxic. A 5 per cent hypochlorite solution can be used to clean aquariums if the aquariums are thoroughly rinsed and allowed to dry before being set up.

The source and composition of gravel and decorative material in the aquarium should be determined. About 1 to 1.5 lb/gal of rinsed gravel provides a sufficient natural filtration bed for most aquariums. Gravel should be about 2.0 to 3.0 mm in diameter to prevent compaction and to provide adequate total surface area for biologic filtration.

An adequately-sized (5 watts per gallon), thermostatically controlled heater should be installed in the aquarium to keep water temperature within the desired temperature range of 72 to 80°F (22–27°C) for most tropical fish species. Temperature fluctuations of 5° or more can be very stressful to fish and should be avoided. Temperatures below 65°F (18°C) can severely alter metabolic rates and compromise the immune systems of warmwater species.

Closed aquarium systems should utilize biologic filtration to convert the toxic nitrogenous wastes NH_3 and NO_2^- to the less harmful NO_3^- (Spotte, 1970). The most economical and efficient method of biologic filtration in small aquariums is the undergravel filter. Undergravel filters utilize the aquarium gravel bed both as a mechanical filter to remove particulate matter and as a permanent substrate for colonization by the chemoautotrophic bacteria responsible for oxidation of nitrogenous wastes. Undergravel filters should have large-diameter lift tubes (1 inch or greater) with one lift tube for each 10 to 20 gal of water being filtered. Large flat rocks on the aquarium floor reduce the effective surface area of the filter bed. Sponge filters and trickle filters can also be used for biologic filtration in small aquariums. Various box, canister, and power filters can be used for additional mechanical filtration.

Aquariums should be illuminated by a light source with a natural spectrum to enhance both fish and plant health. Fluorescent lights are preferable to incandescent lights because of less heat production. Light should enter from the top of the aquarium to mimic natural conditions and to prevent disorientation and stress. Lights should be left on for 8 to 12 hr a day, and the light-dark cycle should follow a natural cyclic photoperiod.

WATER QUALITY AND AQUARIUM MAINTENANCE

Water is the most important and yet the most neglected aspect of a fish's environment. A high percentage of disease outbreaks in aquariums can be traced back to water quality problems, which can stress fish and lead to physiologic imbalance (Wedemeyer et al., 1976). Consequently, investigations of fish disease should include a thorough evaluation of water quality parameters.

When examining an aquarium, a subjective evaluation of water clarity, overall aquarium cleanliness, degree of algal growth, water movement, and water odor should be made initially. Water chemistry analysis should follow, with determination of pH, hardness, and dissolved oxygen and ammonia, nitrite, and nitrate concentrations. The veterinarian should encourage experienced aquarists to purchase a high-quality water chemistry test kit and to monitor and record water chemistry parameters on a routine basis.

Dissolved oxygen concentrations should always be maintained above 5.0 ppm, with concentrations that fall in the range of 6.0 to 10.0 ppm considered desirable. Increasing surface water movement and use of aeration devices will raise dissolved oxygen concentrations. Increases in temperature, altitude, and total dissolved solids all will decrease the concentration of dissolved oxygen.

Most freshwater fish can live comfortably within a pH range of 6.0 to 8.0. Extremes in pH interfere with osmoregulation and respiration in fish (Gratzek, 1980). Fish adapt well to gradual pH changes but can be seriously stressed by drastic changes. The pH of established aquariums will gradually drop if adequate buffering capacity is not present, owing to the release of hydrogen ions by the nitrification process. This gradual decrease in pH can be prevented by the addition of buffering agents such as Dolomite (Barth's) to the filter bed or by frequent partial water changes. Low pH values (below 6.0) adversely affect nitrification and will lead to increased total ammonia concentrations, which can quickly become toxic (Collins et al., 1975).

Water hardness is a measure of the concentration of the mineral carbonates calcium carbonate and magnesium carbonate in water and, consequently, reflects the buffering capacity of water. Hardness should generally be maintained between 50 to 150 ppm for most freshwater fish. Most fish tolerate slow changes in water hardness but are severely stressed by rapid changes.

Establishment of nitrification in closed aquarium systems is essential for fish health (Leibovitz, 1980). In established aquariums, the nitrification process, or nitrogen cycle, prevents the accumulation of toxic nitrogenous wastes (Fig. 2). Ammonia is the primary nitrogenous excretory product of most fish and is also added to aquarium water by the normal decomposition of proteins and amino acids. Ammonia is present in the aquatic environment in two forms, NH_3 and NH_4^+. The un-ionized form NH_3 is very toxic, whereas the ionized form NH_4^+ is relatively nontoxic. The proportion of NH_3 to NH_4^+ in aquariums is dependent primarily on water pH. The higher the pH, the greater the proportion of toxic NH_3 in the aquarium. Chronic low-level exposure to NH_3 is stressful to fish and can lead to secondary disease and chronic gill pathology (Smith and Piper, 1975). High concentrations of NH_3 (>0.3 ppm) interfere with respiration, creating a physiologic oxygen depletion in fish. NH_3 levels should never be allowed to rise above 0.2 ppm, and in established aquariums, NH_3 levels should remain below 0.02 ppm. High ammonia concentrations in an aquarium

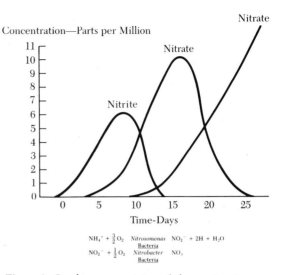

Figure 2. Graphic representation of changes in nitrogenous waste concentrations during the establishment of nitrification in a newly set-up aquarium.[3, 11] Fish deaths in the "new tank syndrome" correspond to peak ammonia and nitrite concentrations.

may be the result of overfeeding, overstocking, or insufficient nitrifying activity.

In the normal nitrification process, ammonia is oxidized to nitrites (NO_2^-) by the action of *Nitrosomonas* spp. bacteria. Nitrites at concentrations of 1.0 ppm or greater are very toxic to fish, causing methemoglobinemia and resultant physiologic oxygen depletion. Nitrites should never be allowed to exceed 0.1 ppm in aquariums. High nitrite levels usually signify a breakdown in an aquarium's nitrification capabilities.

Nitrites should be quickly oxidized to nitrates (NO_3^-) by the action of *Nitrobacter* spp. bacteria in established aquariums. Nitrates are relatively nontoxic to fish and are utilized as a nitrogen source by aquatic plants and algae. Nitrate concentrations should not be allowed to exceed 100 ppm in aquariums. A golden tinge to aquarium water often indicates high nitrate concentrations.

It is very important to determine during history taking how long an aquarium has been set up and has been housing fish. Newly set-up aquariums, which lack sufficient colonization by nitrifying bacteria, can quickly develop toxic concentrations of NH_3 and NO_2^- when fish are added too quickly. This so-called "new tank syndrome" is often the leading cause of fish mortality for the beginning aquarist (Leibovitz, 1980). Peak mortality rates generally occur 2 to 4 weeks after fish are added to an aquarium and are associated with peaks in NH_3 and NO_2^- concentrations during the establishment of nitrifying bacteria in the aquarium (Fig. 2). Certain chemotherapeutic agents such as erythromycin and methylene blue can destroy the nitrifying bacteria in an established aquarium and produce a similar catastrophic syndrome. New tank syndrome can be prevented by encouraging aquarists to add fish slowly to new aquariums while monitoring concentrations of NH_3 and NO_2^- until nitrification is established. Partial (20 per cent) water changes should be made on at least a weekly basis to dilute accumulations of NH_3 and NO_2^- during the establishment period.

Routine aquarium maintenance is essential for maintaining a healthy aquatic environment for fish. Filter systems should be cleaned routinely and filter media changed as required. Air pumps should be functioning properly, and aeration devices should be cleaned or replaced regularly to maintain correct water flow through undergravel filtration beds and good water movement in the aquarium as a whole. Aquarium gravel should be stirred on a weekly to biweekly basis to suspend detritus for siphoning and to prevent compaction or clogging of gravel filter beds. Detritus should be siphoned from the aquarium floor on a weekly basis. Partial water changes are the most important part of a routine aquarium maintenance program (Gratzek, 1980). About 10 to 20 per cent of aquarium water should be removed and replaced with fresh water on a weekly to biweekly basis to reduce concentrations of organic and nitrogenous wastes. Replacement water should be the same temperature as aquarium water and should be dechlorinated by aging or addition of a commercial preparation of sodium thiosulfate. Municipal water containing high levels of chloramines should be avoided.

STRESS

Stress may be the most important factor in the initiation of fish disease. Most outbreaks of fish disease can be associated with some form of environmental stress (Wedemeyer et al., 1976). Common stressors include poor water quality, temperature changes, abrupt fluctuations in water chemistry, oxygen depletion, overcrowding, handling, malnutrition, low-level toxins, and aggression. Acute, severe stress can result in shock and death. Prolonged low-level stress functions through the pituitary–inter-renal axis to increase plasma corticosteroids (Wedemeyer et al., 1976). Elevated plasma corticosteroids can have profound systemic effects on fish, including impairment of the inflammatory response, immunosuppression, decreased external mucous production, increased protein catabolism, and impaired wound healing. These stress effects predispose fish to secondary bacterial and fungal disease and often promote the clinical expression of subclinical disease problems. Removal of stressors alone often eliminates the clinical disease problem.

NUTRITION

Aquarists should center their fish diet around a good quality commercial staple diet. This food should contain at least 30 to 36 per cent protein and about 10 per cent fat with omega-3 fatty acids (linolenic series) incorporated. Fiber should be kept to a bare minimum in fish diets. Fish may require up to ten essential amino acids and 15 essential vitamins in their diets (Lovell, 1979). Fish can absorb much of their dietary calcium needs from the water, if the water contains at least 16 to 20 ppm calcium. Fish require about 0.5 to 0.8 per cent phosphorus in their diets, since phosphorus is not absorbed well from the water. Commercial diets should always be kept in airtight containers in a cool, dry place and should never be used past the expiration date. The commercial staple diet should be supplemented with other foods such as commercial freeze-dried and frozen foods, live food, and beef heart and liver. Supplementation ensures that fish are receiving all essential nutrients. Aquarists should not use self-collected live foods, such as daphne and tubifex worms, since many of these can act as intermediate hosts for fish parasites. Safe commercial sources for many live fishfoods are available. Aquarists should be aware that live-feeder fish can easily introduce disease-producing agents into an aquarium. Aquarists who feed their fish solely homemade diet preparations should be encouraged to have a diet analysis done.

Fish should be fed once or twice a day all they can eat in 5 to 10 min. Excess food should be removed from the tank to prevent fouling.

Nutritional diseases in ornamental fish are poorly understood but are generally of slow onset, with most fish in an aquarium involved and with young, fast-growing fish most severely affected. Signs of nutritional disease include unthriftiness, failure to grow, weight loss, pale color, ascites, anemia, growth deformities, and cataracts.

THE FISH

After acquiring all necessary background information, the veterinarian needs to ask questions about and examine the fish themselves. The entire aquarium population should first be addressed. The mixture of fish should be evaluated. Mixing aggressive and nonaggressive species may result in stress and disease in the less aggressive fish. Fish that are very territorial may become stressed if not given adequate aquarium space to establish territories. Certain species require special environmental features that, if not provided, may stress the fish. If small fish are disappearing, a large tankmate may be the culprit. The keeping of snails and other mollusks in aquariums with fish should be avoided.

Snails can act as intermediate hosts and allow completion of lifecycles for a number of digenetic trematodes that infect fish.

Overcrowding can result in stress, aggression, and oxygen depletion and can overwhelm the nitrification capabilities of an aquarium. Stocking rates for aquariums are dependent on many variables: fish size, species of fish, aquarium surface area, dissolved oxygen concentration, and water temperature. Approximately 2 to 5 inches of fish length per square foot of aquarium surface area can be used as a rule of thumb for fish stocking in closed aquariums. Morbidity and mortality patterns are sometimes helpful for disease diagnosis in aquariums (Citino, 1988). The veterinarian should determine the distribution of clinical signs and death over time. Was the onset of disease acute or gradual? Did the mortality rate peak and then decline or had the mortality rate been constant over an extended period of time? Did clinical signs or mortality begin after the addition of new fish to the aquarium? Oxygen depletion and intoxication usually present with acute onset of mortality, whereas bacterial and viral diseases usually start with a low mortality rate that rises to a peak and then declines. Parasitic diseases frequently show a continual, constant mortality rate over an extended period of time. Nutritional and environmental problems usually start with a low mortality rate that builds to a peak and remains constant until the problem is corrected. The age distribution of diseased fish is also sometimes helpful in disease diagnosis. The majority of diseases affect young fish most severely; however, some disease processes that produce hypoxia (oxygen depletion, gill parasitism) kill older and larger fish first. Sometimes, the distribution of a disease process among species can be helpful in developing a differential diagnosis. Some pathogens have definite host preferences (e.g., *Plistophora* to tetras, *Hexamita* to cichlids).

Changes in behavioral patterns and abnormal behaviors are frequently indications of disease in fish and can be helpful diagnostic clues in disease diagnosis (Francis-Floyd, 1988). The veterinarian should first examine the behavior of the entire fish population to determine behavioral patterns of disease and the incidence of disease and, then, should concentrate on individual fish with abnormal behavior. Examples of behavioral signs of disease are given in Table 1.

Many diseases are reflected externally in fish (Citino, 1988). Fish should be examined closely for abnormalities in their external characteristics. Changes in external features and external lesions can be helpful clues in developing a differential diagnosis. Examples of external signs of disease in fish are given in Table 2.

It is also very important for the veterinarian to determine, through history taking, whether the fish were treated with anything previously. Past treatments could alter the appearance of a disease process, alter water quality, produce toxic effects, and induce resistance in pathogens.

The information gathered during history taking and physical examination can be used to develop a differential diagnosis and to determine what further diagnostic procedures are needed to arrive at a definitive diagnosis.

Antemortem Diagnostics

Virtually all diagnostic techniques used in veterinary medicine can be adapted for use on fish with some inventiveness on the part of the clinician. These techniques are particularly helpful when sacrifice for postmortem examination is not possible. The following procedures should be carried out rapidly, and fish should be handled gently and kept in the water if possible.

Most of the following diagnostic tests require that the fish be anesthetized to prevent injury. Emersion in solutions of tricaine methanesulfonate (MS-222) (TMS, Crescent Research Chemicals, Phoenix, AZ) at 50 to 100 ppm or metomidate (Marinil, Wildlife Laboratories, Inc., Ft. Collins, CO) at 3 to 10 ppm will provide safe, rapid anesthesia for these short procedures. Recovery occurs rapidly in fresh, aerated water.

One of the simplest and most valuable diagnostic procedures is the cytologic examination of scrapings and biopsies taken from the external surface and gills of fish (Noga, 1988). After being anesthetized, a fish is carefully brought to the surface in a net, and the edge of a beveled glass coverslip is used to very gently scrape the surface of the fish in the direction of its scales. Mucus and possibly a few scales should be visible on the coverslip when the procedure is finished. Care should be taken not to abrade the fish. A wet-mount preparation is then prepared by placing a drop of aquarium water on the coverslip, which is then mounted on a glass slide for viewing. Wet-mount impression smears of large lesions can be made by placing a coverslip flatly on the lesion. At the same time, a small fin biopsy can be taken using delicate iris scissors, and a wet-mount squash preparation can be made between a coverslip and a slide. Gill biopsies can be taken by lifting the operculum and excising a small portion of the free border of a gill row. A wet-mount squash preparation of the gill biopsy can then be prepared, or the biopsy can be placed in 10 per cent buffered formalin for histologic examination. The wet-mounts should be examined immediately, as protozoan parasites die quickly and are much easier to identify while alive. Slides should be viewed microscopically under both low (100 ×) and high (200 to 400 ×) power. Lowering illumi-

Table 1. Behavioral Signs of Fish Disease

Behavioral Signs	Description	Possible Causes
Anorexia	Loss of normal feeding behavior	Stress; environmental causes; infectious disease; nutritional disease
Bottom sitting	Resting on bottom by a normally active species	Parasitic disease; bacterial disease; O_2 depletion; poor water quality
Circling	Unidirectional swimming in tight circles	Unilateral blindness; unilateral fin damage; skeletal muscle disease; neurologic disease
Color change	Darkening, blanching, or paleness	Blindness; stress; endocrine disorder; sporozoan disease; infectious disease
Coughing	Forceable opercular movements to flush the gills	Accumulation of debris on gills; parasitic gill infestation; bacterial or fungal gill disease
Curling	Bending of the body laterally with the tail close to the head	Skeletal muscle disease; neurologic disease; sporozoan infestation
Drifting	Moribund condition, with aimless, un-propelled motion	Environmental disease; infectious disease; toxicosis
Favoring one side	Fish always presents one side to the observer	Unilateral blindness; unilateral olfactory or lateral line damage
Fin clamping	Holding fins close to the body	Stress; environmental disease; infectious disease
Flashing	Darting, turning motion as fish scratch against objects	Ectoparasitism
Head standing	Fish assume a vertical position with head down	Gas bubble disease; gas-forming enteritis; swimbladder disease; subcutaneous emphysema; neurologic disease
Hiding	Fish conceals itself from other fish and observers	Stress; harassment; environmental disease; infectious disease
Hurdling	Drifting downward then suddenly spurting forward	Neurologic disease; toxicity
Inverted swimming	Swimming upside down, with inability to right itself	Gas bubble disease; gas-forming enteritis; subcutaneous emphysema; neurologic disease; toxicity
Lethargy	Decrease or lack of normal activity	Hypothermia; environmental disease; infectious disease; toxicity
Piping, surfacing	Gulping air at surface of water	O_2 depletion; NO_2^- toxicity; NH_3 toxicity; anemia; gill parasitism; bacterial gill disease
Shimmies	Fish stays in one place and sways back and forth	Temperature fluctuations; nutritional disease; infectious disease
Tail walking	Swimming at an oblique angle with head directed toward the surface	Swimbladder disease; skeletal muscle disease; neurological disease; sporozoan infestation
Whirling	Frenzied, tail-chasing	Neurological disease; sporozoan infestation

From Francis-Floyd, R.: Behavioral diagnosis. Vet. Clin. North Am. [Small Anim. Pract.] March 1988, p. 305.

nation and partially closing the microscope's iris give some contrast to protozoan parasites. Scanning for movement under low power helps in locating external parasites. Vital stains may be helpful in locating and identifying protozoans, while negative contrast stains are helpful in observing flagella and cilia on protozoan parasites. Lactophenol blue improves visualization of fungal structures.

While fish are anesthetized, other sampling techniques should be performed as needed. If ascites is present, a coelomic aspirate should be collected for cytology and bacterial culture and sensitivity. The aspirate can be collected by inserting a small gauge needle into the coelomic cavity just cranial and lateral to the anus. Excision or punch biopsies of external mass lesions should be taken for histologic examination. A fecal sample can be obtained by gently milking feces from the anus or by swabbing the anus. Feces can be examined in a direct wet-mount preparation for the presence of protozoans or helminth ova.

Bacterial and fungal cultures can be valuable diagnostic tools in fish medicine. Cultures are particularly helpful when abscesses or deep wounds are present. Cultures taken from the external surface of fish are often difficult to interpret because many potential pathogenic bacteria of fish are opportunistic and can normally be found in the slime layer of healthy fish. Comparison of isolates from paired cultures taken from both external lesions and aquarium water can sometimes help differentiate pathogens from environmental contaminants (Stoskopf and Citino, 1987). Samples for culture should be sent to a laboratory familiar with aquatic microbiology.

Blood sampling of live fish, even relatively small

Table 2. *External Signs of Disease in Fish*

	Possible Causes
Skin and Fin Changes	
Generalized dark color	Systemic disease; nutritional deficiency or starvation; toxicosis
Generalized reddening	Septicemia or viremia; shock
Reddened anus	Septicemia or viremia; enteritis
Dermal ulcers	Bacterial disease; mycobacteriosis; monogenetic trematodes; parasitic copepods *(Lernaea, Argulus)*
Cutaneous air bubbles	Hyperaeration
Black spots or cysts	Encysted digenetic trematode metacercaria
Large, white, raised cysts	Encysted digenetic trematode metacercaria
Large, compound, whitish cysts	Lymphocystis disease
Dermal hemorrhages	Bacterial or viral disease; trauma; monogenetic trematodes; parasitic copepods
Small, white, round spots	*Ichthyophthirius multifiliis*
Gray to bluish-white film on skin and fins	External protozoan parasites; monogenetic trematodes
Golden, speckled appearance to skin and fins	*Amyloodinium*
Frayed fins, necrosis of fins	Bacterial disease *(Flexibacter columnaris)*
Grayish-white patches on back of fish	Bacterial disease *(Flexibacter columnaris)*
Cottony appearance to localized areas of body or fins	Fungal disease *(Achlya, Saprolegnia); Epistylis*
Raised, roughened appearance of scales	Septicemia or viremia; mycobacteriosis; systemic protozoal disease
Gills	
Reddened, clubbed gills	Water quality problems; protozoan parasites; bacterial gill disease; nutritional deficiency; fungal gill disease *(Branchiomyces)*; monogenetic trematodes; toxicosis
White spots or cysts	*Ichthyophthirius multifiliis*; parasitic copepods; sporozoan parasites; encysted digenetic trematode metacercaria
Other	
Body deformities	Nutritional disease; hereditary disease; teratogenesis; mycobacteriosis; sporozoan parasites; encysted digenetic trematode metacercaria
Exophthalmus	Septicemia or viremia; mycobacteriosis; sporozoan parasites
Flared operculum	Protozoan gill disease; bacterial gill disease; fungal gill disease; oxygen depletion; poor water quality; goiter
Body wasting	Nutritional disease; chronic bacterial disease; internal protozoan parasites *(Hexamita)*; sporozoan parasites; enteric parasites; mycobacteriosis; chronic toxicosis

Reprinted with permission from Citino, S. B.: Providing veterinary care to the commercial fish farmer. Vet. Clin. North Am. [Small Anim. Pract.] March 1988, p. 449.

fish, can be done routinely with a little practice. The preferred venipuncture site is the caudal vein lying ventral to the caudal vertebrae of the tail. The vein can be approached by inserting a needle on the ventral midline of the tail down to the vertebrae or laterally a few scales below the lateral line and directed just ventral to the vertebrae. EDTA (ethylenediaminetetraacetic acid) or heparin can be used as an anticoagulant for piscine blood. Hematocrit and total solid values are easily obtained and are valuable in diagnosing anemia, hypoproteinemia, and overhydration. Stained blood smears can be used to identify hemoparasitism, to make estimates of white blood cell (WBC) counts, and to study erythrocyte and leukocyte morphology (Campbell, 1988). Quantitative hematology can be pursued using adaptations of avian techniques. Serum chemistries can be performed using standard chemistry techniques. Hematology and chemistry data from diseased fish can be compared with those from healthy specimens of the same species. If bacterial septicemia is suspected, blood cultures are often helpful in identifying the offending organism.

Radiology and ultrasound imaging are techniques that are not routinely used in fish medicine but that can be extremely useful in certain circumstances. Radiology can be performed by using ultra-detail screens or nonscreen film and standard small mammalian techniques based on thickness. Radiology is helpful in diagnosing foreign bodies and skeletal deformities or lesions, differentiating causes of equilibrium and flotation disorders, and studying the gastrointestinal tract with positive contrast agents. Real-time ultrasonography is useful for evaluating abdominal distention, for needle guidance in biopsy procedures, and for evaluation of the heart. Ultrasonography can be performed with fish still in the water if the transducer is protected in a watertight plastic bag.

Postmortem Examination

Postmortem examination is often the quickest and most valuable method of diagnosing fish diseases. Only when sacrifice of moribund fish is acceptable can postmortem examination be used to full advantage. It is suggested that clinicians become familiar with normal fish anatomy (Harder, 1975) and physiology (Hoar and Randall, 1969–71) before performing postmortem examinations on fish.

The basic equipment for postmortem examination in fish includes a scalpel handle, no. 10 and no. 15 blades, medium and delicate tissue scissors, medium and delicate tissue forceps, dissecting needles, a magnifying lens, a dissecting microscope, a good light microscope with oil immersion lens, glass slides and coverslips, syringes and needles, culturettes with transport media, sterile containers, 10 per cent buffered formalin in containers, new methylene blue stain, Gram stain, Wright-Giemsa stain, and an acid-fast stain.

If at all possible, dead fish should not be used for postmortem examination, since autolysis occurs very rapidly, and many external parasites quickly leave fish after death. Fish that are close to death are the ideal specimens for postmortem examination. When examining a large group of fish with mild disease or suspected subclinical disease, a good random sampling of fish (about 5 per cent) should be sacrificed for postmortem examination.

First, fish should be examined closely while still alive to note such signs as irregularities of motion, abnormal behavior, respiratory distress, abnormal color patterns, and external lesions. The fish should then be anesthetized. At this time, while fish are still alive, blood samples can be collected for hematology, chemistries, serology, blood parasite screening, and blood cultures, if indicated. Larger fish can be bled from the caudal vessels of the tail. Medium and small fish are most easily bled by cardiac puncture. Very small fish can be bled by cutting off the tail and collecting drops of blood with capillary tubes. The fish are then euthanized by pithing with a dissecting needle or by anesthetic overdose.

Since many fish diseases are manifested externally, a thorough external examination of the fish should be performed. Look for such signs as areas of abnormal coloration or texture, abnormal mucous production, hemorrhage, growths, nodules, and parasites associated with the integument and fins. A magnifying lens or dissecting microscope is often helpful in making this examination. Both normal- and abnormal-appearing areas of the integument should be scraped with a scalpel blade, and small sections of normal- and abnormal-appearing fins should be excised. Wet-mount and stained preparations of the scrapings and fins should be made and examined under a microscope for monogenetic trematodes, protozoa, bacteria, and fungi. Wet-mounts should be made with the water in which the fish were being kept, so delicate protozoan parasites can be kept alive. If lesions appear to be bacterial or fungal in origin, samples should be taken for culture and sensitivity. If indicated, samples of integument can also be fixed in buffered formalin for histopathology. If present, monogenetic trematodes and parasitic copepods can be preserved and saved for identification.

To examine the gills, the operculum must be removed with a pair of scissors. The gills can then be examined for gross abnormalities, using a magnifying lens or a dissecting microscope. An entire gill arch should be trimmed free and placed on a slide. The gill lamellae can be trimmed from the cartilaginous arch. A small portion of the lamellae can gently be separated with a needle and a wet-mount preparation made for microscopic examination. A gill arch should be placed in buffered formalin for histopathology, and samples should be taken for cultures if indicated.

If the fish appears ascitic, the abdominal area should be prepared or seared, and a coelomic aspirate taken for cytology and culture.

The coelomic cavity of the fish is then exposed by removing the lateral body wall. If indicated, samples of organs should be taken for culture immediately to prevent contamination. The organs of the coelomic cavity should be examined in a logical and methodic manner.

Gonads may vary in size greatly, depending on the breeding condition of the fish. Testes are generally white and smooth in appearance, with impression wet-mounts revealing motile spermatozoa. Ovaries usually appear yellowish in coloration, with eggs visible to the unaided eye. Primary diseases of the gonads are rare in fish, but secondary involvement in systemic disease processes does occur commonly. Impression smears of the gonads may be taken and stained for microscopic examination and samples placed in buffered formalin for histopathology. The gonads may need to be removed to visualize other organ systems.

Next, the entire gastrointestinal block should be examined *in situ* and then removed by severing the intestine distally at the anus and the esophagus above the stomach. While removing the gastrointestinal block, the coelomic cavity should be carefully examined for the presence of larval and adult helminths. Each portion of the gastrointestinal block should then be examined individually.

The stomach and intestinal tract should be stripped free of their mesentery and stretched out. Any visible abnormalities should be noted. The entire intestine and stomach should be opened lengthwise. Helminth parasites should be identified, and the character of the ingesta noted. The mucosa should be examined closely for lesions. Wet-mounts and stained preparations of ingesta and mucosal scrapings should be taken at several different locations to examine for helminth ova and protozoan parasites. Sections of the gastrointestinal tract can be fixed in buffered formalin for histopathology, and mucosal swabs can be taken for culture.

The liver is generally yellow-brown to dark red and is lobed. The liver and gallbladder should be examined closely for gross lesions. Bile can be aspirated and examined microscopically for protozoan parasites. Impression wet-mounts and stained preparations should be made of the liver and examined microscopically. Sections should be fixed in buffered formalin, and appropriate cultures should be taken.

The spleen is usually bright red, species dependent in shape, and located next to the fundic portion of the stomach. It should be examined closely for gross lesions, and impression smears should be made for gram, acid-fast, and Wright-Giemsa staining. Sections can be fixed in buffered formalin for histopathology, and appropriate cultures should be taken.

The heart is composed of four chambers (sinus venosus, atrium, ventricle, and bulbus arteriosus) and is located just anterior to the liver. The heart should be examined closely for gross lesions and defects. If cysts or nodules are present, smears should be made for microscopic examination. Samples should be fixed in buffered formalin for histopathology. The swim bladders are whitish, dilated sacs located retroperitoneally in the dorsal body cavity. They are generally connected to the distal esophagus or the inner ear by a pneumatic duct and are used by fish as an equilibrium-ballast device. If a fish clinically is unable to maintain its position or equilibrium in the water, these structures should be examined carefully. Helminths may sometimes be seen within these sacs.

The kidneys are dark red and are found retroperitoneally on either side of the vertebral column. The kidney is divided into two unique portions: the anterior, or head, kidney and the posterior, or trunk, kidney. The head kidney is found dorsal to and caudal to the gill arches and is a major lymphoid and hematopoietic organ in fish. The posterior kidney is found dorsal to the swim bladder and is the site of renal excretion and adrenal hormone secretion (inter-renal tissue). Both portions of the kidney should be examined for gross lesions, and appropriate smears should be taken for microscopic examination. Sections of both the head and the posterior kidney should be taken for histopathology. Since the kidney is a major site of blood filtering, it is the organ of choice for culture when bacteremia is suspected in a fish. To get an uncontaminated sample of kidney for culture, a dorsal approach can be made. The skin just caudal to the dorsal fin is prepared or seared, and an incision down to and through the vertebral column is made. The back of the fish is then split open at the incision site to expose the kidney, just under the vertebral column. A sterile loop or applicator can then be easily pushed into the kidney for a sample.

Skeletal muscle should be examined for sporozoan

parasites by making squash preparations of muscle fibers. Larval helminths encysted in skeletal muscle may be dissected free and identified under a dissecting microscope. If indicated, muscle tissue may be fixed in buffered formalin for histopathology.

The brain can be exposed by using a sharp scalpel to cut away a portion of the head. The brain should be fixed in buffered formalin and studied histologically. Other tissues should be taken for further study if indicated.

The necropsy of small fish should be performed under a dissecting microscope for adequate visualization. Very small fish and fry may be studied histologically by fixing the entire fish in buffered formalin and taking cross-sections at various levels to allow study of all major organ systems.

COMMON ETIOLOGIES OF DISEASES IN FRESHWATER ORNAMENTAL FISH

Parasitic Diseases

Ichthyophthirius Multifiliis

Also known as ich, or white spot disease, infestation with Ichthyophthirius multifiliis is one of the most common parasitisms seen in freshwater aquariums. I. multifiliis is a ciliated protozoan parasite that is usually spherical and 50 μ to 1.0 mm in diameter, with short cilia covering the entire cell surface (Fig. 3A). These short cilia give the organism its characteristic rolling motion in both the free-swimming and the encysted trophozoite forms. A large, horseshoe-shaped macronucleus is characteristic of the organism.

The complex life cycle of I. multifiliis makes treatment difficult. The mature trophozoite is encysted in the epidermis or gill epithelium of fish and appears as a white spot. After complete development, the trophozoite excysts and swims freely for a 2- to 6-hr period, after which it attaches to a suitable substrate and secretes a protective membrane around itself. Within the cyst, the organism undergoes multiple fissions, producing up to 2000 young forms called tomites (30 to 45 μ). The free-swimming, ciliated, oblong tomites are released and must find a new fish host within 24 hr or die. When a fish is found, the tomite penetrates the epithelium of the fish. After entry, the tomites develop into trophozoites and feed on cell and tissue fluids of their host until they mature and excyst. The length of the life cycle is extremely temperature-dependent, requiring 10 to 14 days for completion at the optimum temperature of 70 to 75°F (21.1 to 23.9°C).

The most common sign of infestation is the presence of small white spots on the fins, body, and gills of fish. Sometimes, only the gills are infested, making detection more difficult. Fish usually appear

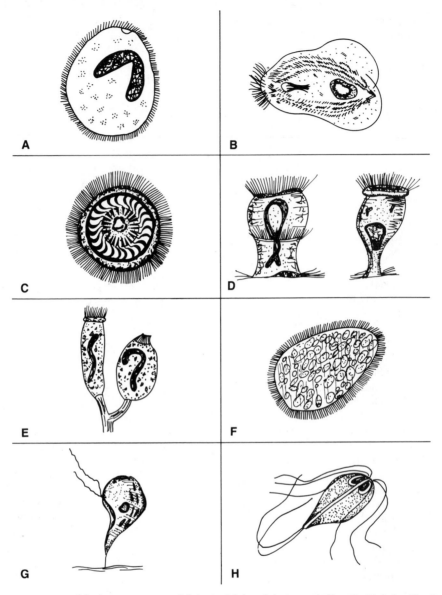

Figure 3. Common parasites of freshwater ornamental fish. A, *Ichthyophthirius multifiliis*; B, *Chilodonella*; C, *Trichodina*; D, *Scyphidia* (left), *Glossatella* (right); E, *Epistylis*; F, *Tetrahymena pyriformis*; G, *Ichthyobodo*; H, *Hexamita*.

sluggish in heavy infestations, with sudden episodes of flashing and rubbing seen early in the disease. Increased opercular movements and piping are often seen when gills are heavily infested. Sudden death may be the only clinical sign in acute outbreaks. The parasite can easily be identified on skin scrapings and gill biopsies from infested fish.

Once introduced into an aquarium, an endless cycle of infestation and re-infestation can occur until all fish are dead or fish develop an aquired immunity that stabilizes at a low-level latent infestation. The outcome of an outbreak is dependent on water quality and the level of other environmental stressors. Treatment is often difficult because the life cycle is so variable in length, and the encysted forms of the parasite are resistant to chemical treat-

ments. Treatment is based on accelerating the life cycle and preventing re-infestation of fish by free-swimming tomites. All chemical treatments should be accompanied by a concurrent elevation of aquarium temperature to 82 to 85°F (27.8 to 29.4°C), which speeds up the life cycle, kills heat-sensitive tomites, and enhances the fish's immune response to the parasite. Chemical treatments include acriflavine, malachite green, formalin, and malachite green–formalin combinations. Transferring fish to a clean aquarium every day for a week will break the life cycle. A diatomaceous earth filter can filter tomites out of the water and reduce infestations. Ultraviolet water sterilizers also reduce the number of tomites. Starting all over again with a clean aquarium often is the only way to completely elim-

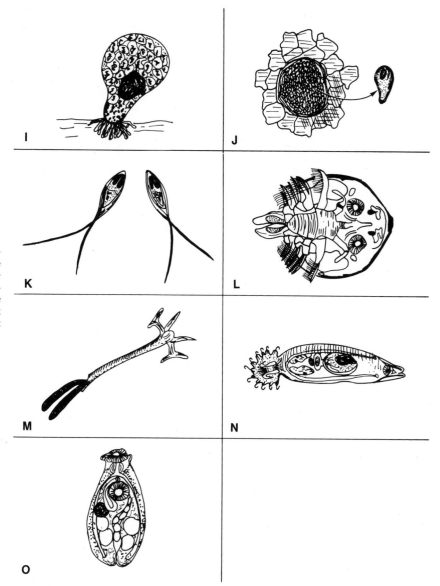

Figure 3 *Continued I, Amyloodinium; J*, pansporoblast and spore of *Plistophora hyphessobryconis; K*, spores of *Henneguya; L, Argulus; M, Lernaea; N*, monogenetic trematode, *Gyrodactylus; O*, adult digenetic trematode (drawings not to scale).

inate the parasite. To prevent parasite introductions, aquarists should be encouraged not to buy fish that appear parasitized and to quarantine new fish for at least 4 weeks.

Chilodonella

Infestations with *Chilodonella* are sometimes given the name slime disease by aquarists. *Chilodonella* is an oval to heart-shaped, ciliated protozoan parasite that is 50 to 70 μ in length, with a coarsely granular cytoplasm and oval macronucleus (Fig. 3*B*). An indentation is present at the posterior aspect of the cell. Characteristically, there are 5 to 15 parallel rows of cilia running the length of the organism, with those at the anterior end longer and forming a tuft. Another important characteristic is an extend-

able, striped oral basket that lies behind the cytostome of the parasite. The parasites are flattened dorsoventrally and, characteristically, move in a back and forth motion on tissue or in a spiraling motion when off tissue. Reproduction takes place by longitudinal fission.

The acute form of the disease, with gills primarily affected, presents as sudden death with no prior signs. Respiratory distress, clamped fins, sluggishness, paleness, and flared opercula are commonly seen in infested fish. A local or generalized increase in mucus production seen as a patchy or generalized blue-gray discoloration of fish is a common clinical sign. Shreds of cellular debris and mucus may be seen hanging from the fish. Diagnosis is made by seeing the characteristic parasite in skin scrapings and wet-mount preparations of gill and fin from infested fish. Chemical treatments include formalin, malachite green, potassium permanganate, and malachite green–formalin combinations.

Trichodinids (Trichodina, Trichodonella, Tripartiella)

Trichodinids are circular, flattened organisms that appear bell-shaped from a lateral view. Cilia line the circumference of the parasite, and a prominent denticular ring is characteristic. The size varies greatly, being anywhere from 15 to 120 μ in diameter (Fig. 3C). The parasites are very active, scurrying over the surface of the fish while in constant rotation. Reproduction is by simple fission.

Trichodinids can be found anywhere on the external surface of fish and occasionally can be found in the digestive and urinary tracts of fish. The motion and denticular ring of the parasite irritate the skin and gill epithelium, creating inflammation and increased mucus production. Trichodinids are capable of destroying all layers of the skin down to the subcutis. Clinical signs include grayish patches of excess mucus on the body surface, lethargy, respiratory distress, and small petechial hemorrhages on the gills and skin. Secondary bacterial and fungal infections are common. Diagnosis is made by looking for the characteristic parasite in skin scrapings and wet-mount preparations of gill and fin biopsies.

Trichodinid infestations are commonly associated with poor water quality and water with high organic content. Good sanitation and management of water quality will often prevent clinical outbreaks of this parasite. Chemical treatments include formalin, malachite green, acetic acid, and potassium permanganate.

Scyphidia and Glossatella

Scyphidia and Glossatella are vase-shaped, ciliated protozoa, approximately 50 × 20 μ in size. Scyphidia has two rows of cilia, one around the mouthparts and one at the midpoint of the parasite (Fig. 3D,left). Glossatella has one row of cilia around the mouthparts (Fig. 3D,right). They attach to the skin, gills, and fins of fish with an attachment organ (scopula). Reproduction is by simple longitudinal fission.

These parasites are mostly a problem in young fish kept in water with a high organic content. Since they are epiphytes, they can live away from fish, attaching themselves to substrates in the aquarium and ingesting organic matter from the water. Heavy infestations can cause respiratory distress and skin irritation, with excess mucus production. Diagnosis is made by finding the parasites in skin scrapings and wet-mount preparations of fin and gill biopsy specimens.

Improved sanitation and water quality is usually enough to eliminate the parasite in aquariums. Chemical treatments include formalin and potassium permanganate.

Epistylis

Epistylis is a stalked, ciliated protozoan with a characteristic ribbonlike macronucleus (Fig. 3E). A row of cilia is present at the apical end for drawing in food. Reproduction is by longitudinal fission.

Epistylis is an opportunistic parasite that is a problem only in aquariums with high organic content. The organisms appear as patches of white, fuzzy growths on fish and are very similar to Saprolegnia fungal growths. Hemorrhages may be associated with these patches, and heavily infested fish often flash. Fish eggs can also become infested with this parasite. Improved sanitation and water quality are important control measures for this parasite. Affected areas on fish can be swabbed with povidone iodine. Chemical treatments include formalin and malachite green.

Tetrahymena pyriformis

This free-living protozoan is pear-shaped and about 20 μ in length and has longitudinal rows of cilia (Fig. 3F). Organisms contain many cytoplasmic vacuoles that often hide the nucleus and move very rapidly with abrupt changes in direction. Reproduction is by simple longitudinal fission.

Tetrahymena pyriformis can frequently be found living in decaying organic material in aquariums. It is an opportunistic parasite of fish and usually invades wounds and bacteria-induced lesions secondarily. Tetrahymena pyriformis most frequently infest guppies and other ornamental livebearers. Infested fish are usually lethargic and lay on the bottom of the aquarium. White patches or bands intermixed with hemorrhagic areas of skin necrosis may be seen on fish. Fish may have a characteristic white rim around their eyes. The parasite occasionally invades systemically and can be found in the brain, kidneys, and other organs. Diagnosis is made by finding large numbers of the organism in skin scrapings. Chemical treatments should be accompanied by increased sanitation, improved water quality, and reduction in environmental stress. Chemical treatments include formalin, malachite green, copper sulfate, and formalin–malachite green combinations.

Ichthyobodo necatrix

Ichthyobodo necatrix is a very small, flagellated, protozoan parasite, only 7 to 14 μ in length (Fig. 3G). It is pyriform to oval, with four flagella (two long, two short). The parasite contains a central round nucleus, and its cytoplasm is highly vacuolated. It fixes itself to the epithelium of fish by its posterior end. When unattached, it moves with a characteristic, flickering, S-shaped motion. Reproduction is by simple longitudinal fission, which occurs while it is attached to a fish.

Ichthyobodo necatrix attaches itself to the skin and gills of fish. Fish tend to be lethargic and lay on the bottom of the aquarium, or pipe for air at the surface. Flashing is a common sign due to skin irritation, as is fin clamping. A bluish-gray film may be seen on the body and gills owing to increased mucus production, with reddening and hemorrhage seen on more severely infested fish. Anorexia and weight loss are seen in chronic infestations.

Ichthyobodo necatrix is sensitive to heat, so raising the water temperature to 85°F (29.4°C) will greatly reduce parasite numbers. Chemical treatments include acriflavine, formalin, malachite green, and acetic acid.

Hexamita

Hexamita is an elongated, pear-shaped, protozoan parasite that is $10 \times 5\ \mu$ in size and possesses four pairs of flagella (Fig. 3*H*). It characteristically has two nuclei and an axostyle and is highly motile, moving with a jerky motion. Reproduction is by simple longitudinal fission.

This parasitic flagellate is an important cause of mortality in certain species of ornamental fish: angelfish, discus, other cichlid species, gouramis, Siamese fighting fish, and goldfish. The disease is characterized by anorexia, weight loss, and unthriftiness. Siamese fighting fish and gouramis commonly show ascites. In cichlids, *Hexamita* is associated with the production of concave, ulcerated lesions on the head, known as "hole in the head disease," but no direct causal relationship has been found. *Hexamita* is also responsible for poor reproduction, reduced egg hatchability, and stunting and poor survival of fry in cichlid species. Antemortem diagnosis can be made by finding the highly motile flagellate in fecal samples. Postmortem examination can show catarrhal enteritis; enlarged, friable liver with black pigment present; enlarged discolored spleen; and perforated stomach with peritonitis and ascites. Organisms can be found in scrapings of gastrointestinal mucosa, liver, spleen, ascitic fluid, and heart blood.

Cichlid and anabantid breeders should be advised to quarantine new breeding stock and treat for *Hexamita* infection. Breeding stock should be periodically screened for this parasite and treated if necessary. Treatments include metronidazole, dimetridazole, and ipronidazole.

Sporozoans

Coccidiosis caused by *Eimeria* is uncommon in aquarium fish but may be seen in fish coming from pond culture. Young fish are most commonly affected, and clinical signs include emaciation, poor growth, and a yellow, fluidy diarrhea. Diagnosis is made by seeing typical *Eimeria*-type oocysts in expressed feces or intestinal mucosal scrapings. Treatments include sulfonamides, sulfa-trimethoprim or sulfa-ormetroprim combinations, and nitrofurazone.

Sporidian diseases are common in both fresh- and saltwater fish. The life cycle of sporidian parasites is complex and is not well understood. The infective and most easily recognized form of sporidian parasites is the spore. Upon the death of a host or rupture of a cyst, spores are set free into the environment. After ingestion by a new host, the spore attaches to the host's intestinal epithelium by use of a polar filament. The sporoplasm then emerges as an amoebula, which penetrates the intestinal epithelium and travels to its site of infection via the blood stream. The amoebula then enters a host cell or intercellular space and becomes a trophozoite. The parasite begins and continues division (schizogony) and fusion (sporogony), forming a mass of spores that are infective when released. The masses formed by the reproduction of these parasites are disfiguring and can result in enough tissue displacement to cause organ dysfunction. The two most common sporidian parasites infecting ornamental fish are *Plistophora* and *Henneguya*.

Plistophora is a microsporidian parasite that primarily infects the skeletal muscle cells of tetras and other species of fish. The parasite multiplies within skeletal muscle and kidney cells, forming round pansporoblasts that are 28 to 30 μ in diameter and contain many spores (Fig. 3*J*). Spores measure $6 \times 3\ \mu$, are oval, and contain one polar capsule. The first sign of infection is the development of small pale spots on fish. As the disease progresses, the entire body becomes pale. Scoliosis (curling) also occurs as a result of muscle degeneration, which leads to swimming abnormalities (tail walking). Fish segregate themselves and become emaciated late in the disease. *Plistophora* are very pathogenic because pansporoblasts rupture continually, autoinfecting the same host. Spores are shed in the urine of infected fish, allowing rapid transmission in a closed environment. Diagnosis is made by seeing the characteristic pansporoblasts in squash preparations or histologic sections of muscle and kidney. There are no effective treatments for this disease. Clinically infected fish should be isolated or destroyed to prevent transmission. Dead fish should be removed immediately to prevent spore release and cannibalism, and aquarium floors should be siphoned frequently to reduce spore concentrations. Since as many as 25 per cent of clinically normal fish in an infected group may be subclinical carriers, it may be beneficial to destroy all fish in an infected group and to start over again with a sterilized tank.

Care must be taken not to carry infective spores from one tank to another on nets and other utensils.

Henneguya is a myxosporidian parasite that infects the intercellular spaces of skin, gills, cartilage, and heart of fish and forms large, white, encapsulated masses. The masses contain many oval spores, measuring 5 to 10 μ in diameter (Fig. 3K). The spores contain two polar capsules, and the spore capsules are drawn out into long tail-like appendages (spermatozoalike). The large masses formed by the parasite are disfiguring and may cause respiratory distress if gills are heavily infected. Diagnosis is made by making Giemsa-stained smears of the masses and looking for the characteristic spores. There is no treatment for this disease. Control methods are similar to those for *Plistophora*.

Amyloodinium (Oodinium)

Amyloodinium is a parasitic dinoflagellate of both freshwater and marine fish. The trophont form is ovoid to pear-shaped and typically varies in size greatly on the same host (Fig. 3I). Its length varies from 15 to 150 μ and its width can be from 15 to 70 μ. The cell wall is chitinous and may be unpigmented to yellowish. The narrow end of the parasite has a funnel-shaped cytostome with which the organism attaches itself to the host and from which emanate plasmatic pseudopodia or rhizoids, which penetrate the epithelium of the host. An elongated red stigma is often visible near the cytostome. The cytoplasm has a foamy appearance, with numerous starch granules present and a single oval nucleus. Two species infest freshwater fish: *A. limneticum* and *A. pillularis*.

Species of *Amyloodinium* have complex life cycles. After the adult trophont form matures, it detaches from the host and sinks to the aquarium floor. There it forms a cellulose cyst wall, and cell division begins. Division occurs until 256 daughter cells are present within the original cell wall (palmella stage). The daughter cells grow flagella and break out of the cyst to become free-swimming dinospores. These dinospores again settle to the aquarium floor and develop further into infective dinospores, which again become free-swimming. The infective dinospores must find a fish host within 24 hr or they die. Once attached to the host, the flagella disappear and the trophont form develops. In a closed aquarium system, dinospores can exist in such tremendous concentrations that newly acquired fish are killed in as little as 12 hr after introduction.

Introduction of this parasite into an aquarium usually occurs through the addition of asymptomatic carrier fish. Outbreaks generally occur during periods of peak stress. If water quality is managed properly and other stress is limited, infestations are usually self-limiting, and fish gain temporary immunity to the parasite. Clinical signs include anorexia, lethargy, seclusion, flashing, fading and dull appearance, piping, congregation near the surface, and uncoordinated, darting movements. Fish often take on a yellowish dusty appearance, making them look velvety (velvet disease). The organism prefers to attach to gill epithelium but also attaches to the skin, eyes, oral cavity, and intestinal epithelium. The rhizoids of the parasite are histiolytic, which allows them to liquify host tissue and absorb it. Mortality occurs when damage to gill epithelium prevents normal respiration and osmoregulation. Diagnosis is made by seeing the trophont form of the parasite in skin scrapings and wet-mount preparations of gill and fin biopsies.

Treatment should be accompanied by improved sanitation and water quality and elimination of stress. The only effective treatment is copper. Copper is very toxic to fish and should be used with great care in freshwater aquariums. Copper should be used only when a copper test kit is available for monitoring water concentrations.

Parasitic Copepods

Parasitic copepods are crustaceans that primarily infest the external surfaces of both freshwater and marine fish (Kabata, 1970). The most commonly seen parasitic copepods in freshwater fish are *Argulus* and *Lernaea*. Both of these parasites are most frequently seen in pond-raised fish.

Argulus, or the fish louse, is a large parasite (9 to 22 mm in length) that can easily be seen as it scurries over the surface of fish. It has a flattened saucerlike shape, pointed legs, and two large sucking disks that look like eyes (Fig. 3L). A proboscis is inserted through the epidermis of fish into underlying tissues, where a cytolytic toxin is released to liquify tissues for feeding. The ulcerations that result are susceptible to secondary invasion by bacteria. *Argulus* has been implicated in the transmission of several fish diseases. Heavy infestations can kill even very large fish. If only a few parasites are present, they can be removed with forceps, but heavy infestations may require dips in potassium permanganate and treatment with organophosphates to kill juvenile forms of the parasite.

Lernaea, or the anchor worm, is 9 to 22 mm in length and has a large, branched cephalic region that enables the parasite to embed into the integument of fish (Fig. 3M). Only the straight body of the parasite and its attached egg sacs are visible protruding from fish. The ulcerations inflicted by the attachment of the parasite can easily become secondarily invaded by bacterial or fungal pathogens. Young or small fish can be killed by attachment of only a few of these parasites. These parasites can be manually removed from fish and the resulting ulcerations swabbed with povidone-iodine. Free-living juvenile forms can be killed by treating the aquarium with an organophosphate.

Monogenetic Trematodes

Monogenetic trematodes are common parasites on ornamental fish. They are 0.1 to 0.8 mm in length, possess an anterior sucker, and have a posterior holdfast armed with centrally placed hooks and surrounding hooklets. These hooks and hooklets damage the integument of fish. The two main families of monogenetic trematodes that infest ornamental fish are the Gyrodactylidae and the Dactylogyridae. The gyrodactylids (Fig. 3N) have two points on their anterior end and no eyespots; are viviparous, with juvenile trematodes visible within the adults; and most commonly parasitize the skin and fins of fish. The dactylogyrids have four points on their anterior end and four anterior eyespots, are oviparous, and most commonly parasitize the gills of fish. Monogenetic trematodes have direct life cycles requiring no intermediate host, which allow them to quickly multiply to dangerous levels in aquariums.

Clinical signs include increased activity, erratic swimming, flashing, and respiratory distress. Fish may become faded, with increased mucus production and petechial hemorrhages and ulcerations on the skin and gills. Diagnosis is made by seeing the trematodes in skin scrapings or on wet-mount preparations of fin and gill biopsy specimens. Chemical treatments include formalin, potassium permanganate, acetic acid, organophosphates, and praziquantel.

Digenetic Trematodes

Many different species of digenetic trematodes (Fig. 3, part O) may infest fish. Fish may act as definitive hosts for some species of digenetic trematodes, with the parasite located most commonly in the intestinal tract, or as an intermediate host for other species with metacercaria encysted in tissue. Metacercaria can be found encysted in almost any tissue and appear as black, white, or yellow cysts (grubs). Heavy infestations can cause disfigurement or can lead to organ dysfunction from tissue displacement. Metacercaria can be dissected out of cysts for identification. Gastrointestinal tract infestation with adult trematodes can be diagnosed by finding characteristic operculated ova in fecal samples.

All digenetic trematodes have indirect life cycles requiring one or more intermediate hosts, so most infestations are self-limiting in aquariums. Snails and other mollusks should not be kept with fish in aquariums because they can act as intermediate hosts for some digenetic trematodes. Encysted metacercaria are resistant to most chemical treatments but can be surgically extracted. Oral praziquantel may be an effective treatment for some adult digenetic trematodes.

Cestodes

Many species of cestodes are seen occasionally in wild-caught and pond-raised ornamental fish. Fish may act as definitive hosts, with the adult tapeworm in their intestinal tract, or as intermediate hosts, with pleurocercoids in their coelomic cavities. Heavy infestations may cause emaciation and debility, but most infestations are self-limiting in aquariums. Clients should be discouraged from feeding self-collected *Cyclops*, *Daphnia*, or tubifex worms, as these can act as intermediate hosts for cestodes. Adult cestodiasis can be diagnosed by finding cestode ova or segments in fecal samples. Treatments include niclosamide and praziquantel.

Nematodes

Many species of nematodes can be found infesting ornamental fish. Fish may act as definitive hosts (with adult nematodes in the gastrointestinal tract, coelomic cavity, or eye) or as intermediate hosts (with larval nematodes encysted in muscle or other tissues). Heavy infestations may cause emaciation and debility. Fish may show abdominal enlargement, and nematodes may be seen protruding from the anus. Encysted larvae may be visible in skeletal muscle. Adult nematodes in the gastrointestinal tract can be diagnosed by finding ova in fecal samples. Discourage aquarists from feeding self-collected *Cyclops*, *Daphne*, tubifex worms, and aquatic insect larvae, as these may act as intermediate hosts for nematodes. Treatments for adult nematodiasis include mebendazole, cambendazole, fenbendazole, and levamisole.

Bacterial Diseases

The diagnosis of bacterial disease in ornamental fish should always be made by exclusion. When investigating a fish disease, clinicians should first rule out managerial problems, poor water quality, nutritional disease, and parasitic disease. Most bacterial infections in fish are either stress related or secondary to some other insult (e.g., parasites, injury) that increases the susceptibility of the fish to bacterial invasion and multiplication (Bullock et al., 1970). Many bacteria can be potential pathogens in freshwater ornamental fish, with the majority being gram-negative bacteria (Bullock et al., 1970; Shotts et al., 1976). Potential pathogenic bacteria are always present on the surface of fish and in the aquatic environment. Under normal conditions, a fish's natural resistance mechanisms and immune system prevent infection and disease. Bacterial diseases of ornamental fish are difficult to categorize because the resulting lesions and clinical signs are often nonspecific. Three of the more commonly recognized bacterial disease syndromes will be discussed further.

Columnaris Disease

The main causitive agent of columnaris disease is the myxobacterium *Flexibacter columnaris*, a long, filamentous, gram-negative bacterium that moves by a creeping or flexing action. Other myxobacteria may also be involved in this syndrome. The lesions produced by *F. columnaris* are usually invaded secondarily by other opportunistic bacteria and fungi. Columnaris disease is almost always associated with stress and poor water quality.

Blanched, necrotic patches lined by a rim of hyperemia may be seen on the body of infected fish, especially around the base of the dorsal fin (saddleback disease). Fins and tail may show whitish, erosive lesions and splitting of fin rays, with hemorrhage at their base and cottony growths of opportunistic fungi (fin and tail rot). The mouths of fish may be eroded, hemorrhagic, and cottony in appearance (mouth fungus). Fish may totally lose their fins and tail as the infection progresses toward the body. Infected gills are congested and show white, discolored areas and eroded gill filaments. Diagnosis is made by seeing the characteristic, haystacklike aggregates of filamentous, gram-negative bacteria on wet-mounts, stained wet-mounts (new methylene blue), and stained smears (Gram stain) of skin scrapings, fin lesions, and gill lesions. *Flexibacter columnaris* can be isolated from lesions on Ordal's columnaris media. Treatment should consist of improved sanitation and water quality, reduction of stress, and antibiotic therapy.

Aeromonas-Pseudomonas Complex

Aeromonas hydrophila, Pseudomonas, and all gram-negative, motile bacteria are the most commonly involved organisms in this bacterial disease complex. Many other bacteria may concurrently or secondarily invade fish that have this disease. *Aeromonas* and *Pseudomonas* are often a part of the normal skin and gastrointestinal flora of fish and become disease-producing agents only when fish are stressed or injured.

The clinical signs and lesions of this disease complex are extremely variable and nonspecific. Fish may have irregular or round grayish-red ulcers, eroded fins, petechial hemorrhage of body and fins, exophthalmia, and ascites (dropsy) with abdominal distention and scale protrusion. Cases of septicemia commonly have severe peritonitis with bloody ascitic fluid and enlarged, friable abdominal organs.

Presumptive diagnosis is made by finding gram-negative rod-shaped bacteria in Gram stains of skin lesions and in impression smears of liver, spleen, and kidney.

Definitive diagnosis is made by isolating the causative organisms from aseptically taken kidney cultures (Shotts and Bullock, 1975). Treatment consists of improved sanitation, reduction of stress, and oral or parenteral antibiotic therapy.

Mycobacteriosis

A number of different mycobacteria can infect fish, including *Mycobacterium fortuitum, M. salmoniphilum, M. platypoecilus, M. piscium*, and *M. arrabanti*. All are aerobic, gram-positive, acid-fast bacteria. Mycobacteria are primarily transmitted by the fecal-oral route or by cannibalism of dead infected fish.

Piscine mycobacteriosis is generally a chronic, debilitating, systemic granulomatous disease. Clinical signs and lesions that may be seen with piscine mycobacteriosis are anorexia, emaciation, muscle wasting, skeletal deformities (scoliosis, lordosis), exophthalmia (popeye), ascites with protruding scales, ulcerations, general paleness, anemia, frayed fins, and swimming and equilibrium abnormalities. Postmortem examination of infected fish show multifocal, grayish-white granulomas throughout the abdominal viscera. Definitive diagnosis is made by seeing acid-fast bacilli in tissue smears and within histologic sections of granulomas. The piscine mycobacteria can be isolated on special medias and identified. Other granulomatous diseases that can be confused with mycobacteriosis are infections with *Nocardia asteroides, Flavobacterium*, and the fungus *Ichthyophonus hoferi*. Piscine mycobacteria are potential human pathogens, most commonly causing granulomatous skin lesions. Infected fish have a zoonotic potential and should be destroyed and carefully disposed of to prevent further disease transmission. Prophylactic treatment of fish that may have been exposed to the disease can be considered (Gratzek, 1980).

Mycotic Diseases

Saprolegniasis

Saprolegniasis is caused by members of the ubiquitous aquatic fungi family Saprolegniaceae (*Saprolegnia and Achlya*), which possess aseptate hyphal elements of variable thickness; long, cylindric, terminal septate zoosporangia with motile zoospores; and characteristic oogonia and antheridia (Neish and Hughes, 1980). Infection is almost always secondary to stress, bacterial infections, parasitic infestations, or injury (Pesut and Goldschmidt, 1983). Fish are predisposed to the disease by high organic content in water and low water temperature. The appearance of white, cottony, mycelial masses on the fins and body of fish is characteristic of saprolegniasis. Fish eggs are also commonly infected by these fungi. Treatment of saprolegniasis should be directed at the cause of the primary lesion. Fungal lesions can be swabbed with povidone-iodine. Chemical treatments include formalin, malachite green, and potassium permanganate.

Viral Diseases

The only well described and understood viral disease of ornamental fish is lymphocystis disease (Pesut and Goldschmidt, 1983). A rhabdovirus infection of Rio Grande perch (Malsberger and Loutenslayer, 1979) and an unidentified viral infection of Ramirez's dwarf cichlid (*Apistogramma ramirezi* (Leibovitz, 1980) have also been reported.

Lymphocystis Disease

Lymphocystis disease is caused by a DNA-containing iridovirus that infects dermal fibroblasts and induces them to undergo extreme hypertrophy (up to 50,000 times normal size). Focal or diffuse clusters of white, pearl-like, hypertrophied cells are seen on the fins and skin of infected fish. These lesions may become large and pedunculated. In aquariums, where the virus can become concentrated, fish may die of generalized, diffuse skin involvement. There appears to be some species predisposition to infection, and, occasionally, fish will spontaneously recover and slough the hypertrophied cell masses. Diagnosis is made by gross appearance and by seeing the pathognomonic, hypertrophied cells with thickened, hyaline cell walls; enlarged, irregular nuclei; and basophilic intracytoplasmic inclusion bodies on wet-mounts and stained preparations of lesional biopsy specimens. There is no treatment for lymphocystis disease. Since transmission is from fish to fish in water, infected fish should be destroyed or isolated from healthy fish. Ultraviolet water irradiation units will kill the virus in water and, thus, limit transmission in closed aquariums.

TREATMENT OF DISEASE IN FRESHWATER ORNAMENTAL FISH

Treatment of fish disease can be a challenging task, but one that need not be intimidating to the experienced veterinary clinician. A basic knowledge of pharmacology and fish physiology and the ability to extrapolate information are the basic tools needed to begin treating fish diseases. Treatments can be delivered to fish in a number of ways, depending on the disease being treated and the effect needed. Medications can be applied topically in several ways or administered orally or parenterally.

Medications such as a 10 per cent povidone-iodine solution and antibiotic ointments can be swabbed directly on infected wounds and, even with short contact time, produce surprisingly good results. Direct application of medications to scaleless or small-scaled species should be done with great care, as their skin burns very easily.

The most commonly used form of topical treatment by aquarists is long-term tank treatment, which consists of placing relatively low concentrations of medications directly in the fish's resident aquarium. This type of treatment has several disadvantages and should be avoided if at all possible. Disadvantages include delivery of inadequate contact concentration of medication; rapid degradation of therapeutic agents; binding of medications by substrates and organic debris; development of resistant organisms; toxicity to fish, plants, and invertebrates; and destruction of nitrifying bacteria by some medications.

Bath and dip treatments can be very effective alternatives to tank treatment. Bath and dip treatments require that fish be removed from their resident aquarium and placed in a separate container with a known volume of water. Here fish can be exposed to known concentrations of therapeutic agents for varying lengths of time, conditions can be better controlled, and the resident aquarium is spared insult. Dips are generally considered treatments of short duration (less than 15 min), whereas baths are treatments of long duration (more than 15 min). Baths and dips are excellent methods of treatment for external disease problems in fish. Using baths and dips to achieve systemic levels of therapeutic agents is questionable in all but a few instances. Only a few drugs (nifurpirinol and kanamycin) have been shown to reach therapeutic levels in fish through absorption from water.

Systemic levels of therapeutic agents in fish are best reached by oral and parenteral administration. Getting oral medication into fish can sometimes tax the resourcefulness of even the best clinician. Several flake foods for ornamental fish are commercially available with antibiotics incorporated. Flake foods can be sprayed with medications, allowed to dry, and then fed. Soaking food in medications and then feeding will work reasonably well only with fat-soluble drugs that are not leached out readily by water. Therapeutic agents and food can be mixed in liquified gelatin, allowed to solidify together, and then be fed in cubed form. Large fish can be given pills quite easily or fed medications disguised in large food items.

Therapeutic agents can be injected both intramuscularly or intracoelomically in fish. Intramus-

*Table 3. Therapeutic Agents Used in Ornamental Fish**

Drug	Dose	Dose Interval	Comments
Acetic acid (glacial)	0.5–1.0 ml/L	30–60 sec dip	
Acriflavine	5–10 ppm	Prolonged bath	Resistance has developed, kills plants
	500 ppm	30-min bath daily	
Amikacin	5.0 mg/kg	Every 48 hr IM	
Ampicillin	10–20 mg/kg	Every 24 hr PO or IM	
Carbenicillin	200 mg/kg	Every 24 hr PO or IM	
Chloramphenicol	40 mg/kg	Every 24 hr IM or IP	Destroys nitrifying bacteria
Sodium succinate	50–100 mg/kg	Every 24 hr PO	
Chlortetracycline	10–20 mg/kg	Every 24 hr PO	Resistance has developed to tetracyclines
Copper sulfate	0.25–1.0 ppm	24 to 48 hr bath	Use lower conc. in soft water; immunosuppressive
	100 ppm	1 to 5 min dip	
Dexamethasone	1–2 mg/kg	IM or IP	Shock therapy
Dimetridazole	1.5 mg/gm food	Every 24 hr PO for 5 days	
Fenbendazole	20 mg/kg	Weekly, PO, 2 treatments	
Formalin (37%)	1.0–2.0 ml/10 gal	Prolonged bath dip until fish become stressed	Oxygenate bath well
	1.0–2.0 ml/gal		
Gentamicin	3.0 mg/kg	Every 48 hr IM	
Kanamycin	20 mg/kg	Every 48 hr IM	Is absorbed from water
	50–100 ppm	24 hr bath, repeat every 48–72 hr	
Levamisole	100 mg/25 gm food	Weekly, PO, 3 treatments	
Malachite green (zinc-free)	0.1 ppm	Prolonged bath	Toxic to some fish species and fry, carcinogenic
	2.0 ppm	30 min bath	
Mebendazole	20 mg/kg	Weekly, PO, 3 treatments	
Metronidazole	10–50 mg/gm food	Every 24 hr PO for 5 days	
	5–10 ppm	Prolonged bath	
Niclosamide	200 mg/kg	PO, repeat in 2 weeks	
Nifurpirinol	2–4 mg/kg	Every 24 hr PO	Is absorbed from water, save for resistant bacteria
	0.2 ppm as bath for 24 hr, followed by 0.1 ppm as bath for 3–6 days		
Nitrofurazone	50–75 mg/kg	Every 24 hr PO	
	1–3 ppm	24 hr bath, repeat every 3 days	
Organophosphates (trichlorfon)	0.25 ppm	Prolonged bath	Handle with care, toxic to humans
Oxytetracycline	10 mg/kg	Every 24 hr IM	Increase dosage in hard water
	50–75 mg/kg	Every 24 hr oral	
	50–100 ppm	24 hr bath, repeat every 48 hr	
Potassium permanganate	1.0 gm/L	30–60 sec dip	Very caustic
Povidone-iodine	10% solution	Swab on wounds and rinse	Will burn scaleless and smooth-scaled fish
Praziquantel	100 mg/25 gm food	Every 24 hr PO, 7 days	
	10 mg/L	3 hr bath	
Sulfadimethoxine	200 mg/kg	Every 24 hr PO	
Sulfa-trimethoprim	50 mg/kg	Every 24 hr PO, IM, or IP	

*Data from Gratzek (1980); Herwig (1979); Stoskopf and Citino (1987); and the author's own experience.

cular injections should be given in the heavy back musculature under the dorsal fin. Intracoelomic injections can be given if fast systemic levels of a drug are needed. Intracoelomic injections should be given just anterodorsal to the vent, using a small-gauge needle directed anterodorsally. For small or flighty fish, anesthesia may be required for safe intracoelomic injections.

The pharmacodynamics of most therapeutic agents used on ornamental fish have not been scientifically studied, so most accepted dosages and dosage intervals are very empiric in nature. Most research on therapeutic agents focuses on economically important food fish (Setser, 1985). Many of the reported drug dosages for ornamental fish are extrapolated from dosages developed for catfish and

salmonids. Several reviews on therapeutic agents used in fish are available (Herwig, 1979; Kuhns, 1981). A short list of therapeutic agents and dosages used in ornamental fish can be found in Table 3.

References and Supplemental Reading

Bullock, G. L., Conroy, D. A., and Snieszko, S. F.: Bacterial diseases of fishes. *In* Snieszko, S. F., and Axelrod, H. R. (eds.): *Diseases of Fishes, Book 2A.* Neptune City, NJ: TFH Publications, 1970.

Campbell, T. W.: Fish cytology and hematology. Vet. Clin. North Am. [Small Anim. Pract.] March 1988, p. 349.

Citino, S. B.: Providing veterinary care to the commercial fish farmer. Vet. Clin. North Am. [Small Anim. Pract.] March 1988, p. 449.

Collins, M. T., Gratzek, J. B., Shotts, E. B., et al.: Nitrification in an aquatic recirculating system. J. Fish. Res. Board Can. 32:2025, 1975.

Francis-Floyd, R.: Behavioral diagnosis. Vet. Clin. North Am. [Small Anim. Pract.] March 1988, p. 305.

Gratzek, J. B.: An overview of the diseases of ornamental fishes. Proceedings of the Fourth Annual Kal Kan Symposium for the Treatment of Small Animal Diseases, October 1980, pp. 25–39.

Harder, W.: *Anatomy of Fishes*, Parts I and II. Stuttgart, E. Schwerzerbast'sche, 1975.

Herwig, N.: *Handbook of Drugs and Chemicals Used in the Treatment of Fish Diseases*. Springfield, IL: Charles C. Thomas, 1979.

Hoar, W. S., and Randall, D. J.: *Fish Physiology*, Vols. I–VI. New York: Academic Press, 1969–71.

Kabata, Z.: Crustaceans as enemies of fishes. *In* Snieszko, S. F., and Axelrod, H. R. (eds.): *Diseases of Fishes, Book 1*. Neptune City, NJ: TFH Publications, 1970.

Kuhns, J.: FISHDRUG/TXT: A computer-generated bibliographic index of the drugs and chemicals used in treating fish diseases. Aquariculture 2:4–18; 29–43; 45–58, 1981.

Leibovitz, L.: The aquatic environment in health and disease. J.A.V.M.A. 176:824, 1980.

Leibovitz, L.: Establishing and maintaining a healthy aquatic environment. J.A.V.M.A. 176:1234, 1980.

Leibovitz, L., Riis, R. C.: A viral disease of aquarium fish. J.A.V.M.A. 177:414, 1980.

Lovell, R. T.: Formulating diets for aquaculture species. Feedstuffs 51:29, 1979.

Malsberger, R. G., and Loutenslayer, G.: Fish viruses: Rhabdovirus isolated from a species of the family Cichlidae. Fish Health News 9:1, 1979.

Neish, G. A., and Hughes, G. G.: Fungal diseases of fishes. *In* Snieszko, S. F., and Axelrod, H. R. (eds.): *Diseases of Fishes, Book 6*. Neptune City, NJ: TFH Publications, 1980.

Noga, E. J.: Biopsy and rapid postmortem techniques for diagnosing diseases of fish. Vet. Clin. North Am. [Small Anim. Pract.] March 1988, p. 401.

Pesut, A. P., and Goldschmidt, M.: Selected integumentary diseases of tropical freshwater fish. Comp. Cont. Ed. 5:343, 1983.

Setser, M. D.: Pharmacokinetics of gentamicin in channel catfish (*Ictalurus punctatus*). Am. J. Vet. Res. 46:2558, 1985.

Shotts, E. B., and Bullock, G. L.: Bacterial diseases of fishes: Diagnostic procedures for gram-negative pathogens. J. Fish. Res. Board Can. 32:1243, 1975.

Shotts, E. B., Kleckner, A. L., Gratzek, J. B., et al.: Bacterial flora of aquarium fishes and their shipping waters imported from Southeast Asia. J. Fish. Res. Board Can. 33:732, 1976.

Smith, C. E., and Piper, R. G.: Lesions associated with chronic exposure to ammonia. *In* Ribelin, W. E., and Migaki, G. (eds.): *The Pathology of Fishes*. Madison, Univ. of Wisconsin Press, 1975.

Spotte, S. H.: *Fish and Invertebrate Culture: Water Management in Closed Systems*. New York: Wiley-Interscience, 1970.

Stoskopf, M. K., and Citino, S. B.: *Workshop on Marine Tropical Fish*. Honolulu Aquarium, Hawaii, September, 1987.

Wedemeyer, G. A., Meyer, F. P., and Smith, L.: Environmental stress and fish diseases. *In* Snieszko, S. F., and Axelrod, H. R., (eds.): *Diseases of Fishes, Book 5*. Neptune City, NJ: TFH Publications, 1976.

WHAT PRACTITIONERS SHOULD KNOW ABOUT WHALE STRANDINGS

JAY C. SWEENEY, V.M.D.

San Diego, California

Whale strandings have been recorded since the beginning of written documentation. What causes these otherwise intelligent creatures to drive themselves upon the shore remains obscure. At no time has there been more public interest in both solving the mystery of whale strandings and finding a means of preserving these magnificent animals from extinction. In North America and in many countries around the world, there are now stranding networks set up to respond to whale and other cetacean strandings. Through these networks, experts in the fields of cetacean biology and medicine have been able to share their experiences to formulate a unified plan for managing these crises. The resultant expanded capacity to deal with whale strandings has produced definitive action that has led to numerous successes in recent years. The following text represents a summary of the available written information in this area and includes some personal observations.

ORIENTATION

Through work in various oceanariums and a few centers dedicated to marine biologic research, the level of expertise in the field of marine mammal medicine has become quite sophisticated. Information has also come from the opportunistic study of cetacean strandings (Geraci et al., 1986; Dierauf, 1988; Howard, 1983). The veterinarian should become acquainted with the referenced texts before providing professional services in a whale stranding, as there are many anatomic and physiologic differences between whales and land animals. In cases of single stranded cetaceans, the practitioner frequently is involved in the diagnosis and treatment of disease. However, mass strandings usually involve animals of the same species, and disease is not thought to play a primary role. The efforts of the professional, in this case, are directed more toward the prevention of deterioration of organ functions. In either case, public sentiment demands that stranded animals be tended to, and often the local veterinarian is the first and only professional on the scene. Therefore, the veterinarian is expected to take charge and render decisions in the face of an extreme outpouring of public sentiment.

SINGLE STRANDINGS

By far, the most common strandings of cetaceans are those involving single animals. With rare exceptions, such animals are suffering from severe and life-threatening disease, and if they are alive at the time of discovery, they are in need of acute medical attention. There are many reports in the literature pertaining to the diseases found in single strandings, as well as recommendations for therapy, both at the time of stranding and in the rehabilitation phase once those animals are brought into captivity (Bain et al., 1981; Cowan et al., 1986; Stroud and Roffe, 1979; Spotte et al., 1978; Sweeney and Geraci, 1979). A further discussion on single strandings appears on page 723.

MASS STRANDINGS

Although mass strandings have been observed for centuries, the causal relationships still are debated, and there is no consensus as to the factors that lead to this phenomenon. However, what does appear clear is that certain species of dolphins and whales are probable candidates for mass strandings. These tend to be species that have strong social grouping bonds and that generally remain in groups, or pods, of many individuals. Frequently, an entire pod strands itself upon a single beach (Fig. 1). There are a number of good publications dealing with the biology of whale strandings (Martin et al., 1987; Sergent, 1982; Geraci and St. Aubin, 1979; Geraci, 1978).

By the time help arrives on the scene, the animals frequently are lying dry upon the beach as the tide withdraws and are thus exposed to the desiccating effects of the sun and wind. Dolphins and whales are covered with a thick layer of insulating blubber, and they depend upon their highly efficient thermoregulatory system, located in their appendages, to dissipate heat within the saline ocean environment (Ridgway, 1972). Without water for heat dissipation, the animals quickly generate metabolic heat, which cannot be efficiently released into the environment. Hyperthermia quickly becomes life-threatening. In addition, many animals may have suffered various forms of trauma from being battered by waves and rocks; many may have suffered from their own panic-stricken thrashing. This only hastens their demise. One of the most important

and difficult decisions made by the professionals on the scene is to determine which animals will be given the immediate care necessary for release or rescue and which are beyond salvage.

Those on the scene must critically evaluate the entire stranding episode and make the following determinations:

1. Healthy, strong animals must be immediately released and returned to deep water (Sandlofer and Craig, 1985).

2. Animals that are deemed healthy enough for survival once returned to the sea will receive treatment on the site and must be kept wet and protected from further trauma.

3. Animals that appear not to be healthy enough for expedient release back to the ocean will be transported to suitable captive facilities, where they will be given medical care and thorough rehabilitation therapy.

4. Suitable and humane euthanasia will be administered to those animals for which there is no hope of recovery.

Within the United States, the appropriate authorities (National Marine Fisheries Service) must be notified before any rescue attempts are undertaken in a cetacean stranding. Federal law mandates that no marine mammal be harassed or handled without federal authorization. This directly pertains to the handling of stranded cetaceans. Proper authorization can be obtained by notifying local officials (these differ from region to region). Usually, the phone number of the local marine mammal stranding network can be obtained by calling the local police, humane society, or wild life regulatory body. Once contacted, the local stranding networks can implement a communication scheme that notifies the proper regulatory and scientific persons, who are authorized to conduct medical treatment and specimen collection and who are experienced in dealing with public relations.

THE PUBLIC RESPONSE IN STRANDINGS

When dolphins or whales strand, the public is often the first to witness and to have access to the developing phenomena. Although there is intense interest in what is happening, rarely do those first on the scene have any intelligent knowledge about what course of action to take. Thus, when professional help arrives, frequently the first things that must be dealt with are the human chaos and the often well-intended but frequently damaging intervention already rendered to the struggling animals. There are numerous pamphlets and publications that are intended to educate the public about the basic actions of benefit to stranded whales. Ideally, those first on the scene should call authorities and then do nothing more than maintain the animals

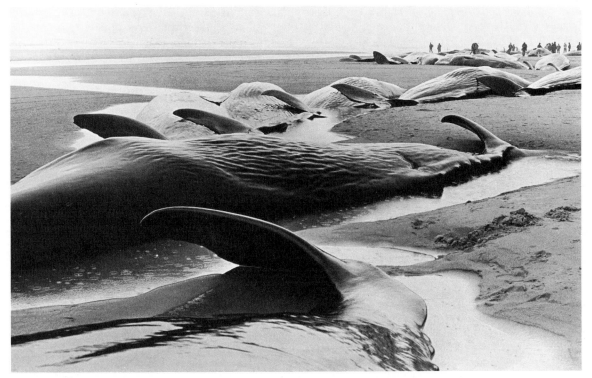

Figure 1. Sperm whales *(Physeter catodon)* stranded along the Oregon coast. (Photograph courtesy of James R. Larison, Oregon State University, © Oregon Sea Grant.)

upright, keep their skins moist, and avoid personal injury from the struggling animals. It is essential that two basic functions be sustained.

1. *Respiration.* A cetacean breathes through the blowhole located at the top of its head; therefore, it should be maintained in an upright position with the blowhole uncovered.

2. *Cooling.* A cetacean's appendages must be kept wet with a continuous supply of cold water from buckets, wet towels, or hoses (being careful to avoid the blowhole). Crowds of people around the animals and undue handling can provide additional stress in a situation where vital functions are already deteriorating rapidly. Police or other authorities may be needed to maintain order.

THE PROFESSIONAL'S RESPONSE TO THE STRANDINGS

The handling of strandings often deals as much with public relations as it does with the provision of medical expertise. Nevertheless, the animals are acutely in need of medical attention, and it is the job of the local veterinarian to provide this expertise until those experienced in strandings arrive on the scene.

Historical

Until the decade of the 1980's, the almost universal response by the public to either single or mass strandings was to return the animals to the sea with whatever resources were available. In most cases, the animals returned directly to the stranding site or were found stranded on another beach later. A recent intensive study details the appropriate response to strandings (Geraci and St. Aubin, 1979). We now know that many well-intended efforts are frequently counterproductive, since many stranded animals have already suffered biochemical alterations that, without appropriate therapy, are ultimately fatal. Experience dictates that animals be evaluated more objectively and that decisions be made based upon astute clinical evaluation. Basic physical examination parameters should be gathered first. Evaluation of respiratory rate and several reflex tests are easy to perform. Respirations should be strong and regular. In dolphins, the rate is normally less than four respirations per minute. In whales, the respiratory rate may be considerably slower. Reflexes can be evaluated by visualizing the open eye and noting a palpebral reflex upon touching the eyelid. Jaw rigidity can be evaluated by attempting to open the mouth. With this maneuver, a flaccid jaw response is an indication of advanced shock. Body temperature is critical and can be evaluated by passing a flexible thermister probe into the rectum. The probe should penetrate at least 20 cm into the colon. With a large individual, this is difficult if the animal is lying on its belly. In the usual case, the animal lies in lateral recumbency, and the anal opening is readily accessible. The normal body temperature of most cetaceans is around 97.7°F (36.5°C). Temperatures in stranded animals frequently rise well above 100.4°F (38°C) and have been noted as high as 107.6°F (42°C) (Barzdo, 1983). Rising temperature rapidly causes organ deterioration and electrolyte imbalance that, if allowed to be sustained, becomes irreversible and fatal. It should be emphasized that extreme care should be taken to avoid being injured by the struggling animals. Blood samples may be obtained from vascular grooves that lie within all the appendages (Fig. 2). The vessels lie under the dermis and can be accessed through relatively superficial venipuncture techniques. In dolphins, a 1-inch 20-gauge needle is adequate. In larger cetaceans, a 1½-inch needle is normally acceptable. In large whales, a needle of 2 inches or longer may be necessary. Rapid laboratory analysis is often not available in stranding situations. A simple blood sedimentation rate is helpful in evaluating the acute condition of individual animals. For retrospective studies, serum analyses are extremely useful in determining the physiologic status. In animals brought into captivity for follow-up care and re-acclimation, it is imperative that hematologic tests be performed immediately, so appropriate care can be rapidly provided during the immediate 24- to 48-h critical period.

Therapeutic Recommendations

The reality of dealing with strandings is that therapeutic options are often minimal, given the

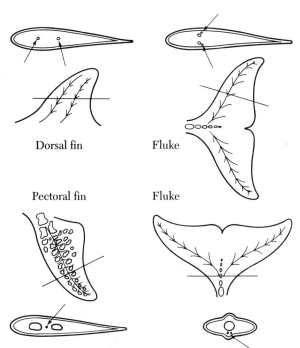

Dorsal fin   Fluke

Pectoral fin   Fluke

Figure 2. Locations for venipuncture in cetaceans.

field conditions. For determining relative dosage schedules, Table 1 is a convenient reference for length versus weight comparison in a variety of cetaceans. Therapy can be viewed in three separate situations: immediate release, captivity, and euthanasia.

IMMEDIATE RELEASE

Following an evaluation of the vital functions, immediate action should be taken to provide cooling to reduce hyperthermia. It should be assumed that these animals are under severe stress and that adrenal exhaustion is probable. For adrenal problems, short-acting corticosteroids are indicated. Refer to Table 2 for dosage recommendations for dexamethasone and prednisone. They may be given intramuscularly (IM); however, delivery via the intravenous route is preferable. Assume that dehydration is also present and administer fluids when the animal has been refloated in the water. The preferable route is via intraperitoneal (IP) injection. A variety of fluid types may be administered, including dextrose and water, saline, or half-strength saline and lactated Ringer's solution. Refer to Table 2 for recommendations on dosage. Administer IP fluids via an intracatheter needle (Abbocath, Abbott) containing a flexible catheter. In small cetaceans, this needle should be at least 5 inches in length; in larger cetaceans, longer needles are required. If this route of administration is not possible, the aforementioned fluids may be administered orally (PO) through a gastric tube, at the same dose as indicated in Table 2 for IP fluids. Tap water is also suitable. Oral administration is considered less desirable than intraperitoneal because of the debilitated condition of the animal and the possibility that the motility of its gastrointestinal tract may be impaired. In addition, fluids given this way may be vomited. In situations where immediate release is imminent, there is no indication for the administration of antibiotics. In mass strandings, it is unlikely that active infections are involved unless such infections result from the stranding process. In single

Table 1. *Weight Approximations According to Length in Cetaceans*

Total Length	Weight
1 m (3 ft 3 in)	40 kg (90 lb)
2 m (6 ft 6 in)	90 kg (200 lb)
2.5 m (8 ft)	205 kg (450 lb)
3.5 m (12 ft)	580 kg (1300 lb)
4.5 m (15 ft)	1360 kg (3000 lb)
9 m (30 ft)	10,000 kg (22,000 lb)

Modified from Ling, J. K.: Marine Mammal Strandings in Australia: Towards a National Plan. Proc. Workshop Special Committee on Marine Mammals of the Australian Mammal Society. Adelaide, Australia: South Australia Museum, 1981.

Table 2. Medication Dosages for Cetaceans

Medication	Animal Weight (kg)	Dose	Route	Repeated	Days
Corticosteroids					
Prednisone		0.5 mg/kg	IM	24 hr	3
Dexamethasone		0.15 mg/kg	IM	24 hr	2
Antibiotics					
Amoxicillin	<500	15 mg/kg	PO	24 hr	10
	>500	10 mg/kg	PO	24 hr	10
Cephalexin	<500	20 mg/kg	PO	12 hr	10
	>500	15 mg/kg	PO	12 hr	10
Gentamicin	<500	3–5 mg/kg	IM	12 hr	*
	>500	2–4 mg/kg	IM	12 hr	*
Tranquilization					
Diazepam	<500	0.2 mg/kg	IM	12 hr	†
	>500	0.15 mg/kg	IM	12 hr	†
Meperidine	<500	0.4 mg/kg	IM	6 hr	†
	>500	0.3 mg/kg	IM	6 hr	†
Fluids					
Water, saline lactated Ringer's		20 ml/kg	PO/IP	8 hr	†

*Use caution, may be nephrotoxic.
†As needed.

strandings, immediate release should not be considered an active option, since nearly all such strandings are the result of severe disease.

CAPTIVITY

Before deciding to retain an animal for captive treatment and rehabilitation, the on-site professional should consider various important factors. These include the overall condition of the animal, the availability of a suitable holding facility, and the overall size, age, and species of the animal. Very large animals are difficult to transport and may suffer unduly from the transport process itself. Very young animals are often unable to adapt to captive situations. Additionally, certain species do not fare well in captivity (e.g., *Stenella*), so care should be taken in the selection of prospective candidates. Once the decision has been made to retain an animal for captive treatment and acclimation, the same acute care therapy should be administered as previously described for animals destined for immediate release. Since prophylaxis therapy may now be considered, it becomes feasible to begin an antibiotic regimen for the prevention of secondary infections. Refer to Table 2 for a list of broad-spectrum antibiotics that have been administered by both oral and parenteral routes.

In transportation, measures must be taken to provide support for the body of these animals via stretchers, foam cushions, or both. Means must be provided for protection from agitation and self-trauma if struggling occurs. Provide continual moistening of the skin through either water sprays or skin-moisturizing ointments. When possible, provide for cooling by using ice or ice water placed over the appendages. Animals that exhibit extreme stress, struggling, or both may be sedated. Diazepam (Valium, Roche) may be administered intramuscularly for minor relaxation. Diazepam and meperidine (Demerol, Winthrop) may be given in combination for more significant sedative effects. Refer to Table 2 for dosages. With these agents avoid the intravenous route.

EUTHANASIA

Although we do not fully understand the relationships causing whale strandings, one fact remains clear: nearly all animals involved in either single or mass strandings eventually die. Selected animals within a stranding situation can be saved, but the fact remains that, even today, most stranded animals die. Even though death is the eventual outcome, there may be a considerable amount of time during which the animal appears to suffer. If a clinical evaluation indicates that an animal's condition is terminal, the veterinarian has the option to provide euthanasia. There are several options available for euthanizing dolphins and whales (Barzdo, 1983; Ling, 1981). Because of the extremely large size of stranded animals, traditional methods of euthanasia may not be applicable. Options available in field situations include:

BARBITURATES. The intravenous injection of barbiturates at 10 mg/kg is effective in inducing deep anesthesia and apnea in cetaceans. Since these animals undergo apnea for long periods in the course of deep diving, induced apnea following injections of barbiturates produces death via hypoxia without discomfort. With large cetaceans that may weigh in excess of 10,000 kg, this form of euthanasia is not practical.

SUFFOCATION. Induced suffocation by obstructing

the blowhole produces hypoxia and death without the struggling that occurs in other mammalian species. This may be the result of a tolerance to apnea, as previously discussed. Materials that physically obstruct the blowhole or that provide reservoirs for expired gases, such as large bags, produce the same effect.

EXSANGUINATION. Animals may be euthanized by strategically placed surgical wounds. Several areas for such wounds have been suggested (Sandlofer and Craig, 1985), but only wounds that penetrate the thorax to lacerate the heart and major vessels are an effective and humane method. To produce such a wound, a knife must be directed from the left or right axilla dorsally and medially between the ribs, toward the heart. For large whales, lances of 30 cm may be necessary. If the wound is directed properly, reasonably fast unconsciousness results. This method is not popular, since the public response is highly negative.

GUNSHOT. Death by gunshot may be the most practical form of euthanasia available in the field. There are several reports that provide advice for this technique (Barzdo, 1983; Ling, 1981). These include firing a low-velocity charge through the blowhole, directing the projectile downwards and posteriorly to penetrate the frontal bone of the skull. An alternative site is a position between the eye and the ear, with the projectile directed dorsally, medially, and centrally to pierce the lateral brain case. Rifles or handguns may be used. The following caliber sizes are recommended: (1) shotgun, 12 gauge, slug (2.703); (2) pistol, .32, .38, and .45 caliber; (3) rifle, .303, .308, and .375 caliber (Barzdo, 1983; Ling, 1981).

Pathobiologic Considerations

Much information on the biology and pathology of marine mammals has come from the study of strandings. The major functions of the stranding network response team are the provision of pathologic resources, including personnel to perform autopsies, and the distribution of specimens to scientists and biologists for study. In the event that no resource people are available, and dead animals are already beginning to undergo decomposition, it may be necessary for the local practitioner to provide autopsy services. In such situations, it is highly desirable to collect the following specimens from as many animals as logistically possible: blood (serum and whole blood); tissues fixed in 10 per cent formaldehyde; tissues (frozen in aluminum foil wrapped in plastic bags); bacterial cultures (cultures are usable only within 6 hr following death) of obvious pathology and of lung, liver, and kidney; and parasites fixed in alcohol-formalin-acetic acid (AFA) or 10 per cent formaldehyde. Specimens

should be retained for the preservation of skeletal remains, as the species may be desirable for anatomic study. Because of the effects of heat generated within the body tissues, the larger the species involved in the stranding, the more rapidly degeneration of tissues occurs following death. When many animals are involved, it is necessary for the veterinarian to organize dissection teams, to supervise the resection of specimens, to ensure that procedures follow proper protocol, and to ensure the safety of personnel.

Management of Survivors of Strandings

Animals that are brought into captivity require immediate and intensive medical attention. Following evaluation of both physical and biochemical parameters, treatment for specific conditions should be instituted. Stranded animals are usually dehydrated, so fluid therapy is necessary throughout the first several days. Refer to Table 2 for fluid dosages. Fluid administration may be via the intraperitoneal route; however, when possible, it should be given orally via a tube placed into the stomach. Care must be taken to avoid administering fluids too rapidly, as this induces vomiting. Prior to each fluid dosage, the presence of fluids previously administered should be evaluated by providing general suction on the tube. Fluid administration may be repeated every 8 hr. Food may be given either as an emulsified fish gruel or as whole fish, depending on the animal's ability to digest fish products. Evaluate the passage of food, to prevent the administration of additional food to an animal that is unable to digest it. Prophylactic antibiotics should be administered because we can assume that the animal's immune system is suppressed. Refer to Table 2 for antibiotic dosages and treatment schedules. Although steroids have been administered in some situations, they may further suppress the immune system and are not recommended. In the first few hours following release of the animal into a captive enclosure, it may be necessary to provide physical support, to prevent drowning. Support can be provided by a variety of slings and stretchers or by diligent handling by dedicated personnel. Generally, disequilibrium resolves rapidly, and when normal swimming is possible the animal should be allowed to acclimate on its own. Later, it will begin to accept food and acknowledge the presence of human handlers. Further medical evaluations should be performed every 48 hr until the animal stabilizes and its physical and biochemical parameters return to the normal range.

SUCCESS AND RELEASE OF SURVIVORS

The treatment of conditions resulting in or from strandings can take weeks or months. Before release of an animal back into the wild can be considered, it must be healthy, and all physical and biochemical parameters must be normal. Then, the process of reconditioning for return to the wild can begin. Normally, this process is conducted by specialized persons. It is necessary for the local clinician to work with the specialized persons to ensure a smooth transition to the wild. An animal released promptly from the stranding site or later, following captive rehabilitation, can be marked in such a way that its progress can be monitored. Simple marking procedures such as freeze-branding, cattle-tags on the dorsal fin, and spaghetti tags adhered to the skin or blubber will allow the animal to be distinguished from its wild counterparts, with whom it would be expected to re-establish social bonds. For more detailed investigative tracking, radiotelemetry transmitters can be attached to the dorsal fin to allow monitoring of movements. Such procedures should be handled by specialists with special interests in these procedures. It may be the responsibility of the local veterinarian to provide professional supervision during the attaching of marking devices, so the animal's health is ensured. If no experienced cetacean veterinary specialists are available, the local veterinarian may be asked to attend the transport of the animal back to the release site and to be responsible for the animal's condition during this release procedure. The release would be accomplished by personnel experienced in such endeavors, and thus it remains a responsibility of the local veterinarian only to monitor the patient's health.

It is hoped that through the use of current techniques, more strandings will evolve into successful release of individuals back into their natural habitat.

References and Supplemental Reading

Bain, D., Gage, L., Brick, M., et al.: On Concurrent Rehabilitation of Three Stranded Dolphins. 4th BI Conference on the Biology of Marine Mammals. December 14–18, 1981, p. 5.

Barzdo, J.: *Report of Stranded Whale Workshop: A Practical and Humanitarian Approach.* Hertfordshire, England: Whitehall College, 1983.

Cowan, D. F., Walker, W. A., and Brownell, R. L.: Pathology of small cetaceans stranded along southern California beaches. *In* Bryden, M. M., and Harrison, R. (eds.): *Research on Dolphins.* Oxford, England: Clarendon Press, 1986.

Dierauf, L. A.: *Handbook of Health, Disease and Rehabilitation in Marine Mammals.* Boca Raton, FL: CRC Press, Inc., 1988 (in press).

Geraci, J. R.: The enigma of marine mammal strandings. Oceanus 21:38, 1978.

Geraci, J. R., and St. Aubin, D. J.: *Biology of Marine Mammals: Insights through Strandings.* Washington, D. C.: U.S. Marine Mammal Commission, PB 293890, MMC-77/13, 1979.

Geraci, J. R., Cornell, L., Sweeney, J. C., et al.: Marine mammals (Cetacea, Pinnipedia, and Sirenia). *In* Fowler, M. E. (ed.): *Zoo and Wild Animal Medicine,* Vol. II. Philadelphia: W. B. Saunders Co., 1986.

Howard, E. B.: *Pathobiology of Marine Mammal Diseases,* Vols. I and II. Boca Raton, FL: CRC Press, Inc., 1983.

Ling, J. K.: Marine Mammal Strandings in Australia: Towards a National Plan. Proceedings of the Workshop Special Committee on Marine Mammals of the Australian Mammal Society. Adelaide, Australia: South Australia Museum, 1981.

Martin, A. R., Reynolds, P., and Richardson, M. G.: Aspects of the biology of pilot whales (*Globicephala melaena*) in recent mass strandings on the British coast. J. Zool. (Lond.) 211:11, 1987.

Ridgway, S. H.: Homeostasis in the aquatic environment. *In* Ridgway, S. H. (ed.): *Mammals of the Sea: Biology and Medicine.* Springfield, IL: Charles C Thomas, 1972.

Sandlofer, M. I., and Craig, A. M.: *Whale Rescue Report.* New York: North Wind Undersea Institute, 1985.

Sergent, D. E.: Mass strandings of toothed whales (Odontoceti) as a population phenomenon. Sci. Rep. Whal. Res. Inst. 34, 1982.

Spotte, S., Dunn, J. L., Kezer, L. E., et al.: Notes on the care of a beach-stranded harbor porpoise (*Phocoena phocoena*). Cetology no. 32:1, 1978.

Stroud, R. K., and Roffe, T. J.: Causes of death in marine mammals stranded along the Oregon coast. J. Wild. Dis. 15:91, 1979.

Sweeney, J. C., and Geraci, J. R.: Medical care of strandlings. *In* Geraci, J. R., and St. Aubin, D. J. (eds.): *Biology of Marine Mammals: Insights Through Strandings.* Washington, D.C.: U.S. Marine Mammal Commission, PB 293890, MMC-77/13, 1979.

PREVENTIVE MEDICINE IN NONDOMESTIC CARNIVORES

LYNDSAY G. PHILLIPS, Jr., D.V.M.

Washington, D.C.

Nondomestic carnivores, as considered in this article, include species held in zoologic collections, wild species, and those commonly maintained as pets (e.g., ferrets). This discussion of preventive medical procedures is applicable to all nondomestic carnivores. The author believes that nondomestic carnivores, as a rule, should not be held as household pets, as they do not, especially as adults, make the type of pet expected by the private owner. Too often they are presented to veterinarians with such conditions as nutritional deficiencies or as animals no longer able to be maintained because they have become too aggressive or dangerous for the owner. When they have reached this state, it is impossible to return them to the wild, and it is difficult to find a facility, such as a zoo, willing to accept them.

The author does not recommend declawing or removing the teeth in exotic carnivores, as this further decreases their chances of relocation to the wild or a zoo. Moreover, the author does not consider these practices to be part of preventive medicine; therefore, declawing and tooth removal will not be discussed.

This article provides a preventive medical program for all nondomestic carnivores intended to be housed in a healthful captive situation. Veterinarians experienced in dealing with nondomestic carnivores realize that preventive medicine is the mainstay of management of nondomestic species for several reasons. First, these mammals have the unique nature, as do most exotic species, of masking or hiding illness or distress, a behavioral attribute retained from their free-living state. Abnormal behavior attracts predators and encourages attack from other animals in the wild. By the time signs of illness are exhibited, the underlying disease condition may be advanced to a critical state. Second, it is extremely difficult to perform more than a cursory examination without the use of anesthesia. Diagnosis is limited without proper examination, and proper treatment is dependent on thorough diagnostic examination and sample collection. Thus, it is a more responsible approach to provide nondomestic carnivores with conditions designed to prevent exposure to infectious, parasitic, toxic, or traumatic agents rather than to treat pre-existing and often advanced disease.

Preventive medicine is concerned with a broad scope of factors including infectious disease, nutrition, parasitism, and physical management. All these factors must be effectively coordinated and continually monitored, improved, and updated to provide an effective program of preventive care.

INFECTIOUS DISEASE

Nondomestic carnivores are as susceptible to bacterial and fungal agents as domestic carnivores; however, susceptibility to infection increases when they are under chronic stress, are maintained with inadequate nutrition, develop heavy parasite loads, or are held in unsanitary or inadequate facilities. These conditions result in the carnivore's being exposed to potential pathogens in abnormally high concentrations or attempting to combat infections with a compromised immune system. In these instances, even common opportunistic organisms can infect the animal, resulting in localized or general disease. When species that are naturally adapted to exist in an extreme environment (desert, aquatic,

high elevation) are brought to a new environment, they are exposed to new micro-organisms. Their immune systems are naive to these organisms, and a simple infection can easily become overwhelming, systemic, and possibly fatal. Providing a proper environment, with regard to temperature, humidity, air quality, and environmental sanitation, aids in the prevention of disease by reducing exposure to potential pathogens until the animal has a chance to develop immunity to the new microflora.

The threat of infectious disease in animal collections is prevented by proper animal management and high-quality veterinary care. Early detection of disease signs is essential and is dependent on careful daily observation of individual animals by animal caretakers. At the first indication of an abnormality the veterinarian should be notified and an approach to diagnosis and treatment formulated. If it is felt that an infectious process is present, immediate examination of affected individuals is conducted to identify the disease agent, or at least its effects, and treatment is begun. Blood samples are obtained for hematology, serum chemistries, and culture if indicated. Tissue or fluid samples (e.g., swabs, aspirates, biopsies, urine) are taken for laboratory examination, bacterial and fungal cultures, and sensitivity testing. When a single animal has a localized infection, the decision to separate it from its group for treatment is dependent on the severity of the infection and the required treatment protocol. In carnivores living in family or social groups, separation of an individual from the group may result in rejection of that member when attempts are made to reintroduce the animal after 1 to 2 days. The stress of being held alone may actually be as detrimental as the condition being treated. Removal only for examination with return to the group for subsequent treatment is often the best approach. The benefit of this method of treatment is obviously weighed against the severity of the disease, its potential transmissibility to other group members, and the anticipated ability to administer medications. If a transmissible disease outbreak is detected, affected and exposed animals are isolated to prevent the spread of the infectious agent to other carnivores until treatment is completed.

Few bacterial diseases are prevented by vaccination in carnivores; tetanus and leptospirosis are the only two vaccinations regularly indicated. True protection from subsequent infection after use of these vaccines has not been established in nondomestic carnivore species, but clinical experience supports the use of these vaccines.

Susceptibility to individual viral disease is variable among the carnivore families and has not been established for all species in all families. However, the most probable viral diseases to be encountered are the viral diseases most commonly affecting domestic cats and dogs. Table 1 lists the families of

*Table 1. Suggested Immunization for Nondomestic Carnivores**

	Feline Panleukopenia	Canine Distemper	Canine Infectious Hepatitis	Feline Rhinotracheitis	Feline Calicivirus	Canine Parvovirus	Rabies
Canidae	−	+	+	−	−	+	+
Felidae	+	±	−	+	+	−	+
Procyonidae	+	+	±	−	−	−	+
Mustelidae	+	+	±	−	−	−	+
Viverridae	+	+	±	−	−	−	+
Ursidae	−	−	+	−	−	−	+
Hyaenidae	±	+	−	−	−	−	+
Ailurodae	±	+	−	−	−	−	+
Ailuropodidae	±	+	−	−	−	−	+

*Annual boosters recommended.
+Recommend immunization.
−Immunization not normally recommended.
±Susceptibility controversial.

carnivores and the commonly accepted immunizations suggested for nondomestic carnivores. These are only recommendations, as the efficacy of the vaccines has not been established in nondomestic carnivores in most cases. Also, modified-live vaccines have induced disease in some species. Because of inadequate testing to determine which vaccines are safe in each species, the use of killed vaccines should be the rule when protecting nondomestic carnivores. No killed vaccine is available for canine distemper. In most nondomestic canids, it appears that the avian-origin modified-live virus (MLV) vaccine (Fromme D, Solvay Veterinary Inc.) is safe and confers adequate protection. However, these findings cannot necessarily be carried over to other nondomestic families, as some species, such as the red panda (*Ailurus fulgens*), exhibit vaccine-induced disease with MLV canine distemper vaccine. Cooperative studies on the red panda between Cornell University and the National Zoological Park (NZP), Washington, DC, show promise for a killed canine distemper vaccine.

If a carnivore has not been shown to be susceptible to a particular viral disease, use of a vaccine containing the antigen for that disease is not recommended. In other words, use of a polyvalent vaccine containing unneeded antigen should be avoided. Choose monovalent vaccines or vaccines containing only the needed antigens for immunization of each particular species.

Use of the feline leukemia vaccine in felids is of questionable value because of the low incidence of this disease in nondomestic species.

In areas where rabies is endemic in a wild mammal population, protection of carnivores in outside enclosures affording potential contact with wildlife is indicated. Unpublished data from the NZP indicate that a killed rabies virus vaccine (Imrab, Pittman-Moore) produces high serum titers in carnivores. However, protection can only be assumed, as challenge studies in nondomestic carnivore species have not been done. It is advisable that humans

handling nondomestic carnivores be protected through the rabies pre-exposure immunization series.

All animals exposed to a suspected or confirmed rabies-positive animal should be isolated and considered potentially infected. Disposition of the exposed animal is based on the extent of human exposure and their vaccination status, the vaccination status of the exposed animal, its value (i.e., an endangered species), and the ability to quarantine it for an observation period.

The age at which to begin vaccination and the frequency of vaccination is empiric because of inadequate information for all families of carnivores. In addition, the duration of maternal passive immunity is unknown in the majority of nondomestic carnivores and obviously is dependent on the immune status of the dam. Generally, carnivores are first vaccinated at the time of weaning and receive a series of three immunizations separated by 2 to 3 weeks. Different species wean offspring at different ages, thus the difficulty in recommending immunization at particular ages. In the event of a viral disease outbreak in an animal collection, all potentially susceptible animals should be immediately vaccinated, regardless of age and last time of immunization. In such a situation, it is advisable to administer booster vaccinations to all animals 10 to 14 days later.

The importance of postmortem examination of all deaths either in an animal collection or in singly held specimens cannot be over emphasized. Not only does it provide a cause of death, but also it provides a monitor of results of treatment regimens. In addition, the postmortem examination may reveal a pathologic condition previously undiagnosed or unanticipated and thus serve as a monitor of the general health of the remaining collection. Every attempt should be made to perform a thorough necropsy in all deaths in an animal collection, including gross examinations as well as histopathologic examination to detect pathologic conditions not grossly visible. Records of all necropsy findings are maintained, as retrospective analyses can detect disease or pathologic trends not easily recognized with sporadic deaths over a long time period.

NUTRITION

Try to provide a balanced diet approximating the composition of a natural diet. There are a number of commercial products, in frozen, canned, and extruded pellet form, that provide convenience in feeding. These diets are formulated using the nutritional requirement data from domestic cats and dogs; therefore, they do not necessarily meet all the requirements for the individual families of carnivores. The research data on most carnivores is insufficient to indicate their individual nutritional requirements. Most institutions use the commercial meat products as the basis of the diet and supplement them with vitamins and minerals, live or whole carcass products (rats, mice, fowl, fish, rabbit), or vegetables or fruit for carnivores with a more omnivorous diet.

Too often, the diets of captive carnivores are formulated for cost convenience and not with the intent to approximate the natural food items of the various species. This is an area of nutrition that is in need of additional research efforts, as improper nutrition can contribute to poor general health, specific organ dysfunction or disease (e.g., hepatic, renal), poor reproductive performance, improper growth, or an impaired immune system.

Food products must be offered fresh and on a regular basis, with removal of uneaten foods to avoid consumption of spoiled materials. Every effort should be made to feed the food in an easily disinfectable container and to avoid feeding on the cage or exhibit floor, as this exposes food to bacterial, parasitic, or toxic contamination. Proper handling of food products prior to feeding is extremely important and includes (1) proper thawing of frozen products to prevent bacterial overgrowth on meat products (e.g., *Salmonella*), (2) protection from contamination by pest or other animal species, and (3) adequate storage of food materials to prevent nutrient degradation. The veterinarian should be involved in the food procurement and preparation process to serve as a check that high-quality food items are purchased and that foods received are in good condition and are maintained properly prior to utilization. In addition, the veterinarian should be involved in the formulation of diets to assist in designing a balanced ration. Periodic reviews are made of diets to confirm that the proper diet is being fed and that it is adequate for the intended species.

Records are an important part of nutrition of captive species. For each individual animal, records of daily consumption, animal weight, and stool character and output are essential. With carnivores held in pairs or groups, observations are maintained to ensure that each animal is receiving the intended diet. Dominance or aggressive behavior of some group members may result in overeating by some members and underconsumption by less dominant members. Merely offering a balanced diet does not ensure that each member will receive its intended share.

The general tendency is to overfeed carnivores. Inactivity or reduced activity in captive situations results in overconsumption of calories and excessive weight gain. Feeding regimens or diet formulations should be designed to account for the reduced caloric need in captivity. Carnivores do well with one or two fast days per week. On these fast days, bones, such as oxtails or knuckle bones, can be offered with the purpose of promoting chewing to help reduce tartar accumulation on tooth surfaces and to stimulate gingival exercise, which prevents periodontal disease.

When designing a diet for an unusual species of carnivore, consultation with zoos or individuals experienced in maintaining that species is indicated. Any time an animal is transferred to a different facility, part of the history accompanying that animal should be the diet it has been receiving and the apparent adequacy of that diet.

PEST CONTROL

Rodents and insect pests are inevitable wherever animals and their food sources are kept. They serve as potential sources of infection (e.g., leptospirosis, salmonellosis) and parasitic diseases (e.g., toxoplasmosis) for carnivores through urine and fecal contamination of cages and food and by virtue of the pests becoming food items themselves. Simple sanitation of animal quarters, proper storage of food materials, and building design that reduces harborage areas help prevent large infestations with these pests. However, a comprehensive pest control program must also incorporate trapping and the regular use of rodenticides and insecticides to keep pest populations low. These materials must be used according to label directions to be effective. More important, the carnivore must be prevented from contacting or ingesting these agents to prevent primary toxicity. The use of agents with no danger of secondary toxicity and preventing carnivores from ingesting target pests exposed to poisons are also beneficial. The veterinarian should be familiar with all pesticides used as regards the active ingredient, its mode of action, the primary treatment for exposure, and the potential for secondary toxicity. It is preferred that the veterinarian be in control of the pest control program, to monitor when and where pesticides are used. A valuable asset to a pest control program is the veterinarian who is certified as a pest control applicator or who at least consults with professional pest control personnel.

Other forms of pests include wild mammals (e.g., raccoons, skunks) that inhabit the same area and can potentially come into contact with the nondomestic carnivores. These wild species may have a capability of transmitting infectious diseases or parasites similar to that of rodents or insects plus the additional capacity to transmit more threatening mammalian diseases such as rabies.

PARASITISM

Regular examination of stool samples is conducted for the detection of internal parasites in all captive carnivores. This examination includes a direct smear, fecal flotation, and concentration methods, as all parasite ova are not detectable on a simple flotation technique. Protozoal infections are best detected on the direct saline smear; both trophozoites and cystic stages should be sought. Certain parasitic forms do not float; therefore, concentration methods such as centrifugation, sedimentation, or formalin-ether are necessary to identify the ova. To detect parasite species that are intermittent shedders, such as cestodes, it is necessary to examine consecutive daily stool samples for 3 to 5 days. Examination of all animals in a collection is routinely conducted two to four times a year to monitor for parasitic infections. More frequent examination is necessary in the case of known problems in a collection.

Special diagnostic laboratory techniques are necessary to identify certain parasitic forms. For example, cryptosporidial infection is best identified by a concentration technique followed by acid-fast staining of the material to more easily distinguish the organism from similar parasites.

Occasionally, ova, cysts, or larvae are found in fecal examinations that are nonparasitic to carnivores. One source of these parasitic forms is infected prey, such as rodents or fowl. (These include intended food animals and ingestion of pest species.) In these cases, the carnivore merely transports the parasite in its gastrointestinal tract and does not become infected. Proper identification of organisms found in a fecal examination is important in differentiating these types of ova; treatment would be unwarranted.

Treatment of identified parasitic infections is relatively simple in most carnivores. The oral administration of anthelmintics such as mebendazole (5 to 10 mg/kg), pyrantel pamoate (6.6–22 mg/kg), fenbendazole (5–10 mg/kg), and ivermectin (0.2 mg/kg) has been successful against nematode parasites. Oral praziquantel (4.5–7.7 mg/kg; lower range for felids)

and niclosamide (140 mg/kg) are effective against most cestodes. Coccidial infections respond to parenterally or orally administered sulfadimethoxine. In most cases, response to anthelmintic treatment is best if the medication is administered once daily for 3 to 5 days rather than in one single dose. In all cases, follow-up fecal examination is performed 7 to 10 days after the last treatment day to assess the success of the treatment. Efficacy is also improved if follow-up treatment is conducted, in order to act against the tissue migrating larval, egg, or developing larval stages not affected in the initial treatment. The timing of follow-up treatment depends on the life cycle of the particular parasite involved.

In cases in which there are repeated positive fecal examinations after oral anthelmintic therapy, parenterally administered levamisole hydrochloride (17 mg/kg), ivermectin (0.2 mg/kg), or disophenol (10 mg/kg) may be effective in clearing the parasitic infection. Ascarid infection, once introduced into a collection, is extremely difficult if not impossible to eradicate, particularly in felids and ursids. Regular monitoring of stool samples and periodic treatment is the best method of keeping infection levels low.

Preventive heartworm therapy may be indicated in areas where heartworm is endemic. Daily, oral diethylcarbamazine therapy during the active mosquito season is effective; monthly administration of oral ivermectin at 0.2 mg/kg has been shown to be effective against heartworm disease. In addition, diethylcarbamazine is effective in the treatment and prevention of intestinal nematode infections. Longterm effectiveness of this therapy in nondomestic carnivores is being assessed.

Animals should be watched closely for indications of external parasitism. Any time that a specimen is handled, examination of the external body surface and ears is performed to detect such ectoparasites as ticks, fleas, mites, or lice. Carbaryl, in a 3 to 5 per cent topical powder, has proved safe and effective in a wide variety of species; parenteral ivermectin has been effective in many cases for those ectoparasites feeding on body fluids.

Sanitation is an integral part of any parasite prevention program. Daily removal of fecal material and washing and disinfection of the animal's cage are necessary in eliminating exposure to infective parasitic stages. Bedding should be changed daily, and hide boxes or dens should be disinfected daily as well. An effective pest control program (covered previously in this article) is essential in removing potential sources of parasites.

Food items may act as sources of parasites in the carnivore. Muscle meat in the diet can harbor encysted parasite stages, such as *Trichinella*. Food materials can be contaminated by rodent or insect pests either at the manfacturing plant or at the site of daily diet preparation. When using whole-carcass food items, such as rats, mice, poultry, or rabbits, one must remember that they may serve as intermediate or transport hosts for parasites potentially infective to carnivores. It is a good policy, if live food animals are utilized, to perform fecal examinations periodically on these animals to detect potential problems from food sources.

TOXICITIES

Preventive programs also include monitoring for the introduction of toxic agents into animal enclosures. It has been mentioned previously that a properly designed and administered pest control program avoids primary or secondary exposure of nontarget animals to pesticides. Effective sanitation requires the use of cleaning and disinfecting agents. These agents must be used according to the label instructions, first, to be effective and, second, to avoid toxicoses. Thorough rinsing with clear water and good drainage will carry cleansing agents away from enclosures and prevent exposure to accumulations of chemicals that might build up to irritating or toxic levels. Some chemicals should be avoided around certain species because of species-specific susceptibilities (such as the susceptibility of felid species to phenolic compounds).

When live plants are used in exhibit situations, only nontoxic plants should be selected. Periodic inspection of enclosures should be made to ensure that no toxic plants have inadvertently been added. Also, the perimeter of an enclosure is periodically inspected to ascertain that no indigenous toxic plants are within reach of a cage inhabitant. A daily inspection of each cage is conducted to look for toxic or damaging materials that may have been accidentally or maliciously thrown or dropped into an animal's enclosure.

Cages should be properly located so that drainage from areas outside the cages does not pass through them. This avoids accidents in which toxic agents are used or spilled away from an enclosure, and improper drainage carries the agents into the cage without anyone being aware of it.

Another potential source of toxins is mechanical equipment around enclosures that may leak or drop fluids or materials that may be toxic if ingested or contacted.

MANAGEMENT

This area involves the veterinarian and the people responsible for the direct care of the carnivore. A team approach is utilized to provide the animal with a living environment conducive to normal activity and behavior and complemented by consistent monitoring and record keeping.

Attention is given to the design and construction of the permanent animal enclosure to prevent escape or injury, to prevent toxicity or injury from construction materials or products, and to provide shelter from environmental extremes of heat, cold, or excessive moisture or dampness. Materials used in construction should have surfaces that are easily cleaned and disinfected and are not themselves treated with toxic materials (e.g., wood preservatives). In addition, animal enclosures should have effective drainage to remove urine or water from the enclosure floor. In situations of multiple cages or displays, design should be employed to avoid contact between animals in adjacent cages to prevent fighting, disease transmission, or urinary and fecal contamination from adjacent enclosures. Proper design or employment of moats, walls, fences, or electric fencing discourages inhabitant escape as well as entry of indigenous wildlife into the enclosure. Mechanical equipment such as heat sources, air conditioning, waterers (especially the automatic type), doors and locks, and air ventilation is to be checked daily for proper function, especially during periods of extreme temperatures.

When housing more than one carnivore in an enclosure, knowledge of the natural biology of the species is essential in anticipating the compatibility of the inhabitants and the carrying capacity of the cage to avoid overcrowding (resulting in trauma, disease outbreaks, poor food intake) or detrimental dominance effects. Careful observations for compatibility are made whenever a new animal is added to a group situation or when an animal that was removed for veterinary treatment is returned. Social organization may be disrupted, resulting in unanticipated fighting or rejection of individuals.

Daily observations by the staff handling the animals are made with regard to each individual's general health and activity, its place in the social structure, wounds, body condition with respect to weight and pelage, and food consumption. Feces and urine by the group or the individual are observed, and abnormalities are noted. All these data are kept as a written daily record in the event a history is needed by the veterinarian.

PHYSICAL EXAMINATION

Newly arrived carnivores are examined prior to entry to their permanent quarters. In the case of a single animal entering a facility with no other animals, this consists of a physical examination, then release to its permanent enclosure, and close monitoring during adjustment to the new surroundings. In most instances, the arrival is to join a collection of other mammals; this animal or group of animals undergoes a predetermined quarantine period, frequently 30 days, in a site isolated from resident mammals. This has two purposes: (1) the protection of resident carnivores from infectious agents or parasites introduced by the new arrival and (2) providing a period of stabilization for the new arrival during which it can be introduced to new feeds and surroundings and can be closely observed for physical abnormalities or illness. During the quarantine stay, the animal is examined for parasites, both external and internal. Fecal examinations are conducted until three samples are negative for parasites during the quarantine period. If an animal is found to be parasitized, it is held in quarantine and treated until free of infection. In groups held in quarantine, individuals should be held separate long enough to collect fecal samples for individual parasite screening.

Each animal is weighed the day of arrival into quarantine. This provides a weight on which future treatment dosages can be based. In addition, this weighing yields an initial parameter to assess nutritional status of an animal feeding inadequately after arrival and can serve as an indicator of underlying disease if weight is lost for no apparent reason.

At approximately 2 weeks after arrival, or midway through the quarantine period, each individual receives a thorough physical examination. This procedure, in order to be complete, is performed under anesthesia, usually chemical immobilization in carnivores. The examination should include (1) complete hematology; (2) serum chemistry profile; (3) urinalysis; (4) survey radiographs of limbs, abdomen, thorax, and head; and (5) physical examination of eyes, ears, mouth (especially dental structures), auscultation, and palpation. Extra blood should be obtained for serum banking; this allows retrospective testing for pathologic conditions that may arise at a later date. Special tests that may be conducted include titers of toxoplasmosis, feline leukemia, and feline infectious peritonitis. Each carnivore is tested for the presence of dirofilariasis, either by visualizing microfilaria or an ELISA test to detect adult heartworm antigen.

This examination is preliminary. If any abnormalities are detected, the condition is treated and reassessed until the veterinarian is certain that a healthy animal can be released from quarantine.

The subject of immobilization in nondomestic species produces hesitation in some veterinarians. As stated previously, diagnosis is dependent on the ability to conduct a good physical examination. Nondomestic carnivores, as a rule, require immobilization for this to be performed, and this procedure should be done effectively, safely, and confidently by the veterinarian. A good anesthetic procedure for diagnostic data collection or at the initial signs of disease problems is infinitely better than multiple, poorly targeted or nontargeted short procedures that may be incomplete, inconclusive, stressful to the patient, or too late. The ability to perform competent anesthesia is gained through experience with multiple events. Hesitation to anesthetize a patient allows disease conditions to progress or its physical condition to deteriorate to a state in which the patient is an even poorer anesthetic risk.

Ketamine hydrochloride used alone or in combination with tranquilizing agents such as xylazine, acepromazine, or diazepam is the chemical immobilizing agent of choice for nearly all nondomestic carnivores. Doses can be found in both Fowler's and Wallach's texts on wild animals for the individual families. Tiletamine-zolazepam combination is another extremely safe immobilizing agent. Its margin of safety and effectiveness and the ability to concentrate it to achieve low-volume dosage make it an excellent agent in large carnivores.

When animals are moved or shipped from one facility to another, health certificates and the animals' complete medical histories should accompany the shipment. Thus, each newly arrived animal should be accompanied by its medical history. This history alerts the veterinarian to existing or previous medical problems, so they may be assessed in the quarantine physical examination. If uncertainty exists as to the vaccination status of an animal, it should be vaccinated before release from quarantine. Vaccination is conducted after the animal has settled into quarantine, usually at the time of the physical examination. If the animal is stressed from the shipment or the new surroundings, the competency of its immune status is questionable; vaccination at this time has the potential of being less than efficacious. Therefore, this procedure is conducted in the latter half of the quarantine period. Booster vaccination may need to be conducted after the animal is released from quarantine into its permanent enclosure.

Medical record keeping begins immediately after the animal is put into quarantine and is maintained until the animal leaves the facility or dies. These records include, but are not limited to, periodic weights, anesthetics administered and results of the procedure, diagnostic tests performed and results, vaccinations and medications administered, observations of abnormal health or behavior with presumptive diagnoses and resolutions or failures to resolve, reproductive history, and location within the collection. These should be complete and current and written in a style that can be understood by anyone. Often, medical records received with a newly arrived animal are indecipherable because they are incompletely written or are filled with abbreviations that cannot be interpreted.

No preventive medical program eliminates all the harmful situations from an animal collection, but such a program can significantly reduces them. Strict adherence to a designed preventive program results in healthy animals with fewer situations requiring veterinary attention.

References and Supplemental Reading

Appel, M.: *Virus Infections of Carnivores.* Amsterdam: Elsevier Science Publishers B.V., 1987.

Bush, M., Povey, R., and Koonse, H.: Antibody response to an inactivated vaccine for rhinotracheitis, calicivirus disease, and panleukopenia in nondomestic felids. J.A.V.M.A. 179:1203, 1981.

Bush, M., Montali, R., Brownstein, D., et al.: Vaccine-induced canine distemper in a lesser panda. J.A.V.M.A. 169:959, 1976.

Bush, M., Montali, R., Reid, F., et al.: Antibody response in zoo mammals to a killed virus rabies vaccine. Proc. Am. Assoc. Zoo Vet. 1985, p. 30.

Fowler, M. E.: *Zoo and Wild Animal Medicine,* 2nd ed. Philadelphia: W. B. Saunders, 1986.

Janssen, D., Bartz, C., Bush, M., et al.: Parvovirus enteritis in vaccinated juvenile bush dogs. J.A.V.M.A. 181:1225, 1982.

Mann, P. C., Bush, M., Appel, M., et al.: Canine parvovirus infection in South American canids. J.A.V.M.A. 187:779, 1980.

Montali, R., Bartz, C., Teare, J., et al.: Clinical trials of canine distemper vaccines in exotic carnivores. J.A.V.M.A. 183:1163, 1983.

Wallach, J. D., and Boever, W.: *Diseases of Exotic Animals.* Philadelphia: W. B. Saunders, 1983.

LLAMA BASICS

MURRAY E. FOWLER, D.V.M.
Davis, California

Companion animal practitioners are being asked to provide medical service to a new species, the llama. Some believe that the llama is a livestock species, but llamas are being maintained in suburban environments. Furthermore, numerous phone calls from small animal practitioners to the author indicate that basic information about llamas is an appropriate topic for this volume.

The general purpose of this article is to supply the veterinarian with some of the unique anatomic and physiologic aspects of the llama that have a bearing on physical examination, diagnostic procedures, surgery, and medication. This will be followed by a discussion of infectious and parasitic diseases and a few desirable preventive medicine practices.

RESTRAINT AND HANDLING

Llamas are basically gentle, easily handled animals. All llamas are capable of spitting (regurgitating stomach contents), but most do so only when severely agitated. Protection from spitting may be achieved by placing a towel or other cloth over the muzzle of a llama. Adult males have sharp, curved canine teeth that are used in fighting other males, but only the spoiled, hand-reared male will exhibit aggression toward humans. A llama can be eared as a horse is to restrain a more obstreperous animal.

EXAMINATION

Veterinarians should be cautious in weight estimations until they have gained some experience. Llama wool tends to make the animal appear much larger than it is. One cannot differentiate sex on the basis of weight, as there are little males and big females. Adult llamas weigh between 115 and 240 kg (250 to 530 lb). Normal newborn baby llamas weigh 8.2 to 18.1 kg (18 to 40 lb). Babies weighing from 3.6 to 8.0 kg (8 to 18 lb) are probably premature and may need special care.

The rectal temperature of adult llamas varies from 37.2 to 38.7°C (99 to 101.8°F). Infant body temperatures average around 39°C (102.2°F). The heart rate of a quiet, resting llama is 60 to 90 beats/min, and the respiration rate is 10 to 30 respirations/min.

The stool of the llama is pelleted and varies in character from a large cylindric mass (10 × 30 mm) to pellets of 7 to 12 mm, according to the size of the animal. Feces of a healthy llama may be voided in a compressed mass, which usually breaks apart easily into individual pellets. South American camelids use a communal dung pile for defecation and urination. Urine color varies from clear and colorless to yellowish.

VENIPUNCTURE

The jugular vein is situated deep in the neck, in juxtaposition to the carotid artery. Obtaining a blood sample or giving intravenous medication may be difficult. In all locations on the neck, extreme caution must be exercised to prevent accidental cannulation of the carotid artery. Blood can be collected either high on the neck near the jaw, or low, opposite the ventral projection of the sixth cervical vertebra. The site near the jaw is advantageous because of the separation of the jugular and carotid vessels, but the skin in this area is thick, making it virtually impossible to visualize the distended jugular. The skin is thinner lower on the neck. However, the wool precludes good visualization, and the risk of carotid penetration is greater.

Placement of an indwelling catheter for continuous medication is a challenge. Attempting to cut the skin with a large needle tip does not suffice in the adult male; the skin should be incised with a scalpel.

GASTRIC INTUBATION

Gastric intubation is frequently necessary. A piece of rubber hose may be used to serve as a Frick speculum to protect the tube as it is being inserted. A small piece of polyvinyl chloride (PVC) pipe wrapped with adhesive tape may be used as well. A standard Frick speculum is too large for the mouth of all but the largest llamas.

The speculum should be inserted over the base of the tongue. When inserting the tube, the head should be kept in a flexed position to avoid lining up with the larynx. Be aware that the llama is prone to regurgitation when a gastric tube is placed. The nasal cavity is so narrow that nasogastric intubation is not generally practiced.

SEDATION AND ANESTHESIA

The author's choice for sedation is xylazine hydrochloride, 0.25 mg/kg intravenously (IV). If the IV route is not practical, 0.40 mg/kg may be given intramuscularly (IM). This dose usually causes the llama to become recumbent. Xylazine results in significant salivation, so atropine sulfate, 0.04 mg/kg IM, should be given as soon as is practical following immobilization. Special diagnostic procedures, such as peritoneal fluid aspiration or dental examination, may be carried out using only this level of sedation.

If potentially painful procedures are to be done, the aforementioned procedure should be followed in 10 min with ketamine hydrochloride, 3 to 5 mg/kg IV. Apnea may occur if this dose is administered too rapidly.

The xylazine-ketamine combination is required for endotracheal intubation and minor surgeries such as castration. More prolonged surgeries require repeated IV doses of ketamine and xylazine or, preferably, endotracheal intubation and inhalation anesthesia with halothane or isoflurane. If endotracheal intubation is attempted without profound sedation, the llama may regurgitate and aspirate ingesta. Endotracheal intubation is not easy in the llama because of the narrow space between the mandibles and the fact that the llama is unable to open the mouth widely. Furthermore, the soft palate is elongated and must be elevated above the epiglottis with the blade of the laryngoscope.

It is usually not possible to observe the larynx when the endotracheal tube is in the passageway. Therefore, a stiff polyethylene catheter should be inserted into the trachea first, and the tube threaded over that. The head should be straightened as much as possible to facilitate exposure to the larynx.

Local anesthesia works well in llamas, but a standing laparotomy should not be attempted in a llama, because of its propensity to lie down if it is in an unpleasant situation. Epidural anesthesia may be accomplished using 1 to 2 ml of 2 per cent lidocaine hydrochloride at the sacrococcygeal junction. The epidural space is approximately 1.5 cm deep.

Surgical procedures in llamas are similar to those performed in livestock species.

DIGESTIVE SYSTEM

There are three compartments in the stomach, which are not analogous to the rumen, reticulum, omasum, and abomasum. They are appropriately called compartments 1, 2, and 3 (C-1, C-2, and C-3). Compartment 1 is divided into dorsal and ventral sacs, with each sac containing an area of glandular saccules, and is a fermentation vat. Compartment 2 is small and also is covered with glandular saccules, whereas compartment 3 is tubular and secretes digestive enzymes and hydrochloric acid. Compartment 1 occupies the entire left side of the abdominal cavity.

The small intestine lies in the right dorsal quadrant of the abdomen. There is an ileocolic orifice. The cecum is small, about 20 to 30 cm long, and pointed toward the pelvic cavity. The colon begins as a large colon and then enters a spiral, with the colon gradually diminishing to one third the diameter of the large colon. This narrowing is a common location for impaction and obstruction of the intestine.

Increased stomach motility is unusual in the llama (3 to 4 waves/min). Instead of a heavy wave rolling caudally in the left paralumbar fossa, as in cattle and sheep, the wave progresses from caudad forward. The movement is much more subtle and usually requires use of a stethoscope to hear sounds.

Digestive disorders common to the llama include stomach atony, gastric and intestinal ulcers, perforated ulcers, impactions, and, more rarely, torsions and intussusceptions. Llamas rarely bloat, and traumatic gastritis is uncommon. Llamas are not likely to engorge themselves with grain, causing gastric hyperacidity, but it has occurred.

UROGENITAL SYSTEM

Urinary catheterization of the female llama is quite easy. The external urethral opening may be palpated in a groove on the ventral vulva at the level of the hymen. While palpating the groove, the catheter should be passed dorsal to the finger. A diverticulum ventral to the urethral opening is easily entered, and passage to the urethra may appear to be blocked if this fact is not recognized. Urine samples can only be obtained from adult males by making a free catch or by cystocentesis.

The llama reproductive system and reproductive physiology are unique and beyond the scope of this article. Llamas are induced ovulators, which sets them apart from other livestock species.

MUSCULOSKELETAL SYSTEM

The foot of the llama is also unique. Instead of a firm hoof, the bearing surface of the foot has a pliable sole overlying a fibroelastic pad and an elastic encapsulated digital cushion. A small true nail is situated at the forward tip of each digit, and phalanx 2(P-2) and P-3 lie horizontally above the cushion. Hoof and nail problems are similar to those seen in other domestic ungulates.

ABDOMINOCENTESIS

A peritoneal fluid aspirate is obtained best from the midline, just caudal to the umbilicus. The sample may be obtained with the llama either standing or recumbent. The site must be clipped and prepared and local anesthesia injected. A stab incision may be made with a no. 12 scalpel blade for insertion of a 6-cm teat cannula with a quick jab. If the incision is made at the midline, penetration of the retroperitoneal fat layer does not occur.

INFECTIOUS DISEASES

The major bacterial diseases of llamas and alpacas include enterotoxemia (*Clostridium perfringens*, types A, C, and D), necrobacillosis (*Fusobacterium necrophorum*), malignant edema (*Clostridium septicum*), and abscesses (*Streptococcus zooepidemicus* and *Corynebacterium pyogenes*). Some bacterial diseases of lesser importance include listeriosis, actinomycosis, tetanus, mastitis, Johne's disease, tuberculosis, anthrax, coccidioidomycosis, cryptococcosis, and infectious keratoconjunctivitis (*Moraxella lacunata*). Viral diseases reported include rabies, contagious ecthyma, and equine herpes I. Experimental disease has been produced with foot and mouth disease (FMD) and vesicular stomatitis viruses. Naturally occurring FMD has been reported in Peru.

Llamas have not been shown to be susceptible to many of the diseases of cattle. There have been no reports of rinderpest, bovine virus diarrhea, infectious bovine rhinotracheitis, influenza, or *Pasteurella multocida* infections.

PARASITIC DISEASES

Llamas share many gastrointestinal parasites with cattle and sheep. Constant attention to these diseases is necessary, using the same principles and medication as for livestock. *Cephenemyia*, the nasopharyngeal bot of deer, may be a parasite of llamas, causing nasopharyngeal obstruction and dyspnea. *Parelephostrongylus tenuis*, the meningeal worm of white-tailed deer, causes paralysis in llamas.

PREVENTIVE MEDICINE

Llamas should be routinely vaccinated with tetanus toxoid and the toxoids for *Clostridium perfringens*, types C and D. Other *Clostridium* toxoids are given by some veterinarians. Enterotoxemia is a threat to the health of baby llamas. Vaccination of the dam 2 months before parturition, repeated 3 weeks later with type C and D toxoids, will protect the baby through the first 3 weeks of life. The vaccination of newborn llamas with toxoid is not very effective. The baby is most at risk during the first 3 weeks, but at this age it is not immunologically responsive. Annual boosters are required to maintain protection in adults. If leptospirosis is an endemic problem in the livestock of the area, appropriate serovar bacterins may be given to llamas. Killed rabies vaccines are administered in areas where rabies is endemic.

HEMATOLOGY AND CLINICAL PATHOLOGY

Hematologic and serum biochemistry parameters of llamas are compared with other species in Table 1. It is inappropriate to discuss all the variables in this text, since most hematologic responses of lamoids are similar to those of other livestock and equine species. The unique variations will be discussed.

The normal mean corpuscular volume (MCV) of llamas is less than that found in livestock species, because in the llama, higher numbers of erythrocytes are found in the approximate same or even lower packed cell volume (PCV). The mean corpuscular hemoglobin concentration (MCHC) is higher in llamas (44.5) than in livestock (30 to 35). The MCHC measures the ratio of the weight of hemoglobin (Hb) to the total volume of the erythrocytes. Since normal Hb levels in llamas are higher than those in livestock species and the PCV is slightly

Table 1. *Comparative Hemogram of Llamas, Camels, Cows, and Horses*

	Llamas	Camels	Cows	Horses
Erythrocytes (10^6 cells/μl)	9.9–17.7	7.22–11.76	5–10	6.8–12.9
Hemoglobin (gm/dl)	10.8–18.0	7.8–15.9	8–15	11–19
Packed cell volume (%)	25–44.5	25–34	24–46	32–53
MCV (fl)	21.4–29.0	35–60	40–60	37–58
MHCH (gm/dl)	38.3–47.0	36.5–50.9	30–36	31–38.6
MCH (pg)	9.4–12.0	17–22	11–17	12.3–19.7
Leukocytes (10^3 cells/μl)	7.2–22.0	11.5–16.5	4–12	5.4–14.3
Neutrophils (10^3 cells/μl)	2.9–15.0	51%	0.6–4.0	2.3–8.6
Lymphocytes (10^3 cells/μl)	0–7.4	40%	2.5–7.5	1.5–7.7
Monocytes (10^3 cells/μl)	0–1.1	4%	0.025–0.84	0–1.0
Eosinophils (10^3 cells/μl)	0–4.7	4%	0–2.4	0–1.0
Basophils (10^3 cells/μl)	0–0.3	4%	0–0.2	0.029

(Data from Kaneko, J. Clinical Biochemistry of Domestic Animals. New York, Academic Press, 1980.)

lower, a higher MCHC index results. A low MCHC in llamas is indicative of a hypochromic anemia.

The mean corpuscular hemoglobin (MCH) expresses the weight of Hb in an average erythrocyte. Normal Hb levels in llamas are slightly lower than those in other livestock species, because the erythrocytes are smaller. An excessively low value would indicate anemia. A normal leukocyte count is higher in lamoids (7000 to 22,000) than those in livestock or horses.

Table 2. *Congenital and Hereditary Conditions in Llamas*

Angular limb deformities	Medial patellar luxation
Arthrogryposis	Megaesophagus
Atresia ani and coli	Nasal agenesis
Atrial septal defect	Nonpigmented iris
Carpal ankylosis	Ovarian agenesis
Cataract	Ovarian hypogenesis
Cerebellar hypoplasia	Patent urachus
Cervical agenesis	Persistent frenulum of the
Choanal atresia	penis
Cleft palate	Polydactyly
Crooked toenails	Pyloric stenosis
Cryptorchidism	Renal agenesis
Curvature of the penis	Retention of deciduous teeth
Cyclopia	Scoliosis
Double cervix	Segmental agenesis of tubular
Ectropion	female tract
Entropion	Short ears
Eyelid hypogenesis	Supernumerary teats
Hernias	Syndactyly
Hydrocephalus	Tail agenesis
Hypoplasia of the penis	Teat agenesis
Imperforate hymen	Tendon contracture
Mandibular shortening and	Transposition of the great ves-
lengthening	sels
Maxillary shortening and	Twinning
lengthening	Ventricular septal defect

NONINFECTIOUS DISEASES

Llamas are known to be affected with white muscle diseases. Protection against these diseases in areas where the diet is deficient in vitamin E and selenium requires periodic injections of this vitamin and mineral or, preferably, feed supplementation.

A variety of congenital and hereditary defects are observed in llamas (Table 2).

CONCLUSIONS

Llamas are unique, anatomically and physiologically, so material is presented to aid the practitioner in performing a clinical examination, dealing with routine matters, and responding to emergencies.

Reference and Supplemental Reading

Fowler, M. E.: Medicine and Surgery of South American Camelids. Ames, Iowa State Univ. Press, 1989.

INDIVIDUAL CARE AND TREATMENT OF RABBITS, MICE, RATS, GUINEA PIGS, HAMSTERS, AND GERBILS

STEPHEN M. SCHUCHMAN, D.V.M.

Castro Valley, California

Diagnosis and treatment of diseases of laboratory animals are not unlike those of other, more familiar, species. The differences and similarities are neither more nor less than those between horses and cows or dogs and cats. Once this mental bridge is spanned from familiar species to laboratory species, cross-application of principles of diagnosis, treatment, and prevention of disease becomes possible.

PHYSICAL EXAMINATION

The physical examination is divided into two parts: (1) general information (Table 1) and (2) systematic examination of the animal.

General Information

The questions listed are designed to obtain basic information from the client as to the animal's care, general condition, and micro- and macroenvironment.

CHECK LIST

1. Species.
2. Sex.
3. Age.
4. Weight in grams, pounds, or ounces.
5. What kind of diet is fed and by whom?
6. How is water dispensed and by whom?
7. Room and cage temperatures.
8. Humidity.
9. Type of cage.
10. Frequency of cage cleaning.
11. Number and kind of animals owned.
12. What age group is affected?
13. What is the major complaint? How long has it been going on?
14. What does the client think is the problem?
15. Has the animal had a litter or has it been bred?
16. Has the animal been on medication in the past?
17. Is any person sick at home?

Systematic Examination of the Animal

Under each system, specific items are listed. These are guides to help identify clinical signs. It should be remembered that a high percentage of clinical illnesses seen in laboratory species are either primary or secondary to nutritionally deficient diets or poor animal husbandry practices.

EXAMINATION

The integument and hair coat should be checked for

1. General condition.
2. Signs of scratching or fighting.
3. Alopecia; distribution.
4. Pustules.
5. Fluorescence of hair shafts that are not considered normal (Wood's light examination).
6. Cutaneous swelling (neoplastic and nonneoplastic or infectious).
7. Skin scraping, cellophane tape test for mites, black paper test for mites, visible inspection for lice.

Check the digits and tail for

1. Necrosis of digits.
2. Ulcerated or abscessed footpads.
3. Circumscribed lesions or sores around base of tail.
4. Sores randomly spaced anywhere on the tail.
5. Gray-blue coloration of the tail of mice (cyanosis).
6. Fecal soiling of ventral surface of the tail near the base.
7. Congenital absence of the tail or loss of the tail, limbs, or digits.
8. Presence of ingrown toenails.

738

Table 1. Useful Information

	Hamster	Rabbit	Mouse	Rat	Gerbil	Guinea Pig
Weight at birth	2 gm	100 gm	1.5 gm	5.5 gm	3 gm	100 gm
Puberty	(F) 28–31 days (M) 45 days (best to breed 70 days)	4–9 months	35 days	50–60 days	(F) 3–5 months (M) 10–12 weeks	(F) 20–30 days (M) 70 days
Duration of estrous cycle*	4 days	Ovulation not spontaneous; stimulated by copulation, doe ovulates 10 to 13 hr after	4 days	4 days	4 days	16 days
Gestation (days)	16	28–36	19–21	21–23	24	62–72
Separation of adults during parturition and weaning	Yes	Yes	No	No	No (mates for life)	No
Number per liter	4–10	7	10	8–10	1–12	1–4
Eyes open	15 days	10 days	11–14 days	14–17 days	16–20 days	Prior to birth
Wean at	25 days	42–56 days	21 days	21 days	21 days	14–21 days or 160 gm
Postpartum estrus	Within 24 hr	14 days	Within 24–48 hr	Within 24–48 hr	Within 24–72 hr	Within 24 hr
Breeding life	11–18 months	1–3 years (maximum 6 years)	12–18 months	14 months	15–20 months	3–4 years
Adult weight	(F) 120 gm (M) 108 gm	(F) 4 kg (M) 4.3 kg	(F) 30 gm (M) 39 gm	(F) 300 gm (M) 500 gm	(F) 75 gm (M) 85 gm	(F) 850 gm (M) 1000 gm
Life span (years)	2–3	5–7	3–3½	3	4	4–5
Body temperature	97–101°F (36.1–38.3°C)	101–103.2°F (38.3–39.5°C)	96.4–100°F (35.8–37.7°C)	99.5–100.6°F (37.5–38.1°C)	100.8°F (38.2°C)	100.4–102.5°F (38–39.2°C)
Daily adult water consumption	8–12 ml/day	80 ml/kg body weight	3–3.5 ml/day	20–30 ml/day	4 ml/day	10 ml/100 gm body weight
Daily adult food consumption (varies with age and condition)	7–12 gm/day	100–150 gm/day	2.5–4 gm/day	20–40 gm/day	10–15 gm/day	30–35 gm/day
Diet	Commercial rat, mouse, or hamster chow supplemented with kale†, cabbage†, apples, milk	Commercial rabbit pellets, greens in moderation	Commercial mouse chow	Commercial rat or mouse chow	Commercial mouse or rat chow (lowest fat possible); sunflower seeds	Commercial guinea pig chow, good-quality hay, kale, cabbage, fruits (cannot rely on vitamin C levels of commercial ration)
Room temperature	65–75°F (18.3–24°C)	62–68°F (17–20°C)	70–80°F (21–27°C)	76–78°F (24.5–25.5°C)	65–80°F (18.3–26.6°C)	65–75°F (18.3–24°C)
Humidity (%)	50	50	50	50	Less than 50	50

*All species listed except rabbits are seasonally polyestrous.
†Better source of vitamin C than lettuce.

Examine the ears for
1. Condition of ear canal.
2. Scratching around the ears.
3. Sores on ears.
4. Drooping ears in rabbits (in which this is not a breed characteristic).
5. Cyanotic appearance of pinnae.
6. Congenital absence of ears or evidence of traumatic loss of part or all of the pinnae.

Observe locomotion:
1. Reluctance to move.
2. General weakness of all four limbs.
3. Paraparesis or paraplegia.
4. Palpate appendicular skeleton.
5. Lameness.
6. Favoring of a particular side when lying down (fractures or soreness on opposite side).
7. Radiographic abnormalities.

Check musculature:
1. Relative amount and condition of muscle mass.
2. Pain on palpation.

Check the central nervous system for
1. Cranial nerve deficit.
2. Spinal reflexes.
3. Postural reflexes.
4. Gross CNS disturbance (head tilt, paraplegia, circling, convulsions, flaccid or spastic paralysis).
5. Ophthalmoscopic examination (in species in which this is practical).

Evaluate the respiratory system:
1. Labored breathing.
2. Open-mouth breathing.
3. Sneezing, epistaxis.
4. Evidence of nasal discharge, staining of nares, staining of medial surface of forelegs.
5. Cyanotic coloration of pinnae and tail.

6. Auscultation of thorax.
7. Radiographic examination of thorax.

Evaluate the circulatory system:
1. Auscultation of chest.
2. Palpate pulse.
3. Radiographic examination of thorax.
4. Electrocardiogram.
5. CBC and necessary blood chemistries.
6. Color of mucous membranes.

Examine gastrointestinal system:
1. Check incisors and molars.
2. Check cheek pouches for impaction or other abnormalities.
3. Examine tongue and oral mucosa.
4. Palpate abdomen.
5. Examine anus and surrounding area for signs of diarrhea or other abnormalities.
6. Check consistency and number of fecal pellets.
7. Fecal flotation, sedimentation examination, protozoan examination, and fecal culture.
8. Radiographic examination of abdomen.

Check lymphatic system for
1. Lymphadenopathy.
2. Abscessation of nodes.
3. Neoplasms.

Examine mammary glands for
1. Neoplasm.
2. Mastitis.
3. Enlargement of glands in milk production.

Check urogenital system:
1. Determine sex.
2. Penis—sores, ulcerations.
3. Vaginal discharge.
4. Palpate for fetus.
5. Urinalysis.
6. Palpate urinary bladder for calculi.

Table 2. *Determination of the Sex of Mature and Immature Laboratory Rodents and Lagomorphs*

Male	Female
Mature Hamsters, Mice, Rats, Guinea Pigs, and Gerbils	
1. Anogenital distance longer in the male.	1. Anogenital distance shorter in the female.
2. Manipulate "genital papilla" (prepuce) to protrude penis.	2. Look for three external openings in the inguinal area:
3. Palpate for testicles either in a scrotal sac (if present) or subcutaneous in inguinal region.	(a) anus (most caudal opening),
4. Males have only two external openings in the inguinal area:	(b) vaginal orifice (middle opening)—look carefully—and
(a) anus,	(c) urethral orifice at tip of urethral papilla (most anterior opening).
(b) urethral orifice at tip of penis.	In these animals the urethral papilla is located outside the vagina (unlike dogs and cats).
In very fat males there may be a depression between the penis and anus. This depression can be obliterated by manipulating the skin in that area.	In very fat females or young females, the vaginal orifice may be either hidden by folds of skin (the former) or sealed (latter). Gentle manipulation of the skin in this area will divulge the orifice.
Mature Rabbits	
1. Protrude penis by manipulating skin of prepuce.	1. There is a common orifice for both the vagina and urethra (like dogs and cats).
2. Palpate for testicles.	2. No structure like a "penis" can be protruded from the urogenital orifice.
3. Anogenital distance is longer.	3. Anogenital distance is shorter.

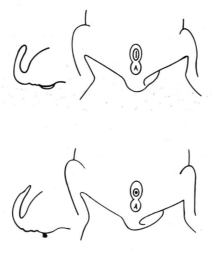

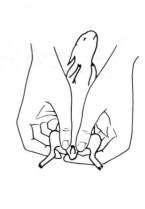

Figure 1. Sexing young rabbits. The penis of the male is a rounded protrusion 1.2 mm dorsal to the anus; a pair of reddish-brown specks occur near the vent. The vulva of the female has a slit-like opening and is less than 1.2 mm from the anus; no specks are apparent. (From Sanford: Reproduction and Breeding of Rabbits. Fur & Feather, Yorkshire, England, 1958.)

SEXING MATURE AND IMMATURE LABORATORY ANIMALS. A standard rule used to determine the sex of any mature laboratory species is that the anogenital distance is longer in the male than in the female. This is easiest to determine when both sexes are present, as is the usual case when a litter is born. To determine the sex of a mature laboratory animal, consult Table 2. To determine the sex of an immature rabbit, see Figure 1. Figure 2 illustrates sex determination in gerbils, rats, guinea pigs, and hamsters.

MANUAL RESTRAINT OF RODENTS AND LAGOMORPHS

Two basic methods are described that allow for secure and safe manual restraint of rodents. The restraining procedure for rabbits differs and is described separately. Familiarity with each species minimizes the necessity of excessive restraint.

Long-tailed rodents may be removed from their cages by gently lifting them near the base of the tail and placing them either in the hand or on a nonslip surface such as a wire cage top. Short-tailed species, if too aggressive to be picked up by the palm or cupped hands, can be removed by grasping the loose skin over the neck with long-nosed forceps.

Most routine examinations are done without any restraint other than gently holding the animal in the hand. If a procedure requires more than this, the following methods are used.

Small jumpy rodents (hamsters, mice, gerbils) should be examined at ground level to prevent injuries resulting from falls from the examining table. It is important to ensure that all exits from the examining room are closed.

Towel Method

This method is used for an aggressive animal or for one that might bite as a result of a required

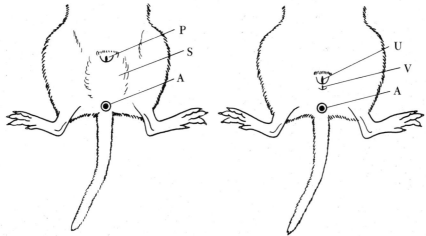

Figure 2. External genitalia of the male (A) and female (B) gerbil. Urogenital anatomy of mice, rats, guinea pigs, and hamsters is similar to that of gerbils. P, tip of prepuce; S, scrotal sac; A, anus; U, urethral orifice; and V, vaginal orifice. (From Harkness, J. E., and Wagner, J. E.: *The Biology and Medicine of Rabbits and Rodents.* Philadelphia, Lea & Febiger, 1977.)

procedure. An opened towel of desired thickness (depending on the size of the animal's teeth) is placed in the hand used to hold the patient. The rodent is allowed to walk on a wired surface while the tail (if present) is held taut. The animal is then gently grasped behind the head, using the toweled hand. Once a secure hold is established, the body can be supported in the palm of the same hand or with the free hand. Routine injections, laboratory collection of specimens, minor surgical procedures, or close examination of the oral cavity can be accomplished using this procedure.

No-towel Method

Small rodents or less aggressive large ones may be securely restrained by placing the animal on a nonslip surface and, while holding the tail or caudal end of the animal, slowly and gently grasping enough loose skin over the neck region so that the animal's head and neck are restricted in movement. The rest of the body is held in the palm or supported with the other hand.

Lifting, Carrying, and Manually Restraining Rabbits

Care should be taken when removing rabbits from their cages. The animal's quick, jerky motions can result in fracture or injury of its back. The animal is removed by grasping the loose skin over the dorsum of the neck and lifting gently while the hind legs are supported with the other hand. The animal can be carried in this manner if held close to the chest.

When ordinary means of restraint are undesirable, the following method can be used. The rabbit is placed on a nonslip surface of a table and positioned on either its back or sternum. Both fore and hind limbs are tied individually and gently but firmly stretched in their respective directions. The bindings are secured at the ends of the table. An assistant (standing in front of the animal) places each hand on the respective side of the animal's head and applies gentle but firm traction in an anterior direction. Traction is continued until the desired procedure is completed. It is thought that this procedure places the animal in a cataleptic state. Once traction is released and the animal is untied, it immediately becomes active.

BLOOD AND SERUM COLLECTION TECHNIQUES

When first using either of the following techniques, the clinician is asked to recall his or her first experience in collecting blood from a cat and how difficult it was until the technique was perfected. This experience will apply to the collection of blood from laboratory species (Tables 3 and 4). A study was done on our Hospital Colony using the technique from Table 3; the results are reported in Table 5.

Needle-hub venipuncture and orbital bleeding are two methods of blood collection that are safe, supply adequate amounts of blood, and are cosmetically acceptable. Both procedures are carried out with manual restraint only. Sedation or anesthesia is unnecessary and often contraindicated. Routine research blood collection techniques such as cardiac puncture and cutting digits or tails have a high risk factor or are otherwise unsuitable for use on a client's animal.

Total blood volume for rodents and lagomorphs averages 5 to 7 ml/100 gm of body weight. This figure is helpful in determining amounts of blood that can safely be collected.

Needle-hub Venipuncture Technique

The needle-hub venipuncture method can be used on laboratory species that have veins large enough to be cannulated with a 25-gauge needle. It can be used on rabbits, guinea pigs, mature rats, and hamsters. Each species is restrained in an appropriate manner by an assistant. A rubber band tourniquet is placed above the elbow or stifle. Rabbits and guinea pigs can be bled from the cephalic vein, while rats and hamsters are sampled from a large vein on the lateral surface of the thigh. Clipping the hair and extending the limb facilitate visualization of the vein. A 25-gauge, ⅝-inch hypodermic needle (without syringe) is inserted into the occluded vessel. Blood will flow into the hub of the needle. Collection is made (*in situ*) directly from the hub of the needle with a microhematocrit tube* or a capillary microcontainer† for serum or whole blood. If skin contamination will not affect the sample, lancing of the occluded vessel without cannulation can be done. The blood sample is then collected directly from the surface of the skin.

Orbital Bleeding Technique

The orbital bleeding technique (Riley, 1960) is used when venipuncture or lancing a vein is not practical. This is the method of choice for mice but can also be used on rats, hamsters, and gerbils. An

---

*Micro-hematocrit tubes (length, 75 mm; OD, 1.47 mm; ID, 0.56 mm; a larger size can be used accordingly), Clay Adams, a division of Becton-Dickinson and Co.

†Microtainer capillary whole blood collector, capillary blood serum separator, Becton-Dickinson, Rutherford, NJ.

Table 3. *Techniques for Performing Routine Blood Chemistries on Small Laboratory Animals*

Test	Method	Amount of Sample (λ)* Regular Plasma	or	Serum	Instrument Used	Wave Length	Comments‖
Glucose†	Ortho-toluidine (Communicable Dis. Center, U.S. DHEW, PHS, 1965)	20	or	20	Coleman 6/20	630	Plasma or serum must be removed from cells within 40 min
Glucose‡	Ortho-toluidine	25	or	25	Coleman Jr. II	595	Use Dow reagent, which uses 100 μl; can use 25 μl by cutting all solutions by 75%
BUN†	Diacetylmunoxime (Crocker, 1967)	10	or	10	Coleman 6/20	520	Use Pfizer BUN-tel, which uses 20 lambda; can use 10 lambda by cutting all solutions by 50%
BUN§	Eskalab	2	or	2	Eskalab		
Calcium or phosphorus	Harleco	—		250 100	Eskalab		Standard Harleco procedure requires twice the serum; solutions used are cut by 50%
Calcium§	Harleco calcium	—		500			Titration with EDTA
Calcium‡	O-cresophthalein complexone	—		25	Perkin-Elmer Coleman 55	565	Use Dow reagent, which uses 50 μl; can use 25 μl by cutting all solutions by 50%
SGPT†	Sigma Frankel	100	or	100	Coleman 6/20	505	Sigma Frankel uses 200 lambda; use 100 lambda by cutting all solutions by 50%
SGPT§	Eskalab	50	or	50	Eskalab		
SGPT‡	Henry et al. (1960)** (modified)	50	or	50	Chemetrics Analyzer Computer	340	
SGPT§	Eskalab	50	or	50	Eskalab		
SGOT§	Henry (1960)** Amador and Wacker (1962)** (modified)	50	or	50	Chemetrics Analyzer Computer	340	
Alkaline phosphatase§	Eskalab	—		25	Eskalab		
Alkaline phosphatase‡	Berger and Rudolph (1965)** (kinetic PNP)	—		25	Perkin-Elmer Coleman 55	405	Use of 1 ml of substrate
Sodium and potassium	Coleman flame photometer	50	or	50	Coleman flame photometer		Add 50 lambda plasma or serum to 5 ml of working diluent
Potassium and sodium	IL flame photometer	—		50	IL flame photometer		
Bilirubin, total and direct	Evelyn Malloy (diazo technique)	100 (Add 100 more for direct)	or	100	Coleman 6/20	550	Add 100 lambda to volume of 1 ml water; this is 10% of regular method and must use microcuvettes
Bilirubin, total and direct‡	Jendrassik bilirubin; Nosslin (modified)	50 (Add 50 more or direct)	or	50	Coleman Jr. II	600	

Table continued on following page

Table 3. Techniques for Performing Routine Blood Chemistries on Small Laboratory Animals Continued

Test	Method	Amount of Sample (λ)*			Instrument Used	Wave Length	Comments‖
		Regular Plasma	*or*	*Serum*			
Amylase‡	DyAmyl-L (dyed amylo-pectin)	—		50	Perkin-Elmer Coleman 55	540	For sample, dilute 50 μl with 0.95 ml saline
Amylase†	Caraway	—		50	Coleman 6/20	660	Use dilution of 50 lambda to 0.2 ml saline; use 1–5 dilution in technique
Cholesterol†	Lieberman direct	200		—	Coleman 6/20	640	
Cholesterol‡	Lieberman direct (modified)	—		25	Coleman Jr. II	625	Use 1.5 ml color reagent with microcuvettes
Cholinesterase‡	S-butyrylthiocholine hydrolysis	—		10	Perkin-Elmer Coleman 55	405	
Chloride‡	Schales and Schales	—		50			Titration with mercuric nitrate (0.01 N)
CO_2‡	Van Slyke (modified)	50 (Heparinized only)	or	50			Titration with NaOH (0.50 N) diluted 1:10 for use
Triglycerides‡	Pinter et al. (1967)** Garland and Randle (1962)**	—		200	Gilford 3400 E	340	(Worthington Biochemical Corp.)
Uric acid‡	Urica-Quant	250	or	250	Perkin-Elmer Coleman 55	405	Use BMC, which uses 500 μl; can use 250 μl by cutting reagents by 50%
LDH‡	Amador et al. (1963)** Wacker et al. (1956)** (modified)	—		25	Chemetrics Analyzer Computer	340	
Phosphorus‡	Hycel			100	Coleman Jr. II	650	Use Hycel, which uses 200 μl; can use 100 μl by cutting reagents by 50%

*10 lambda = 0.01 ml.
†Techniques of H. Weitzman, Director of Hayward Medical Laboratory, Hayward, CA.
‡Techniques of J. Alberti and L. Krusee, Veterinary Disease Laboratory, Campbell, CA.
§Technique of A. Ramans, Valley Veterinary Hospital, Ygnacio Valley Road, Walnut Creek, CA.
‖10 microliters (μl) = 0.01 ml.
**For reference details, contact author of article, Stephen Schuchman.

assistant is not required. The animal is placed on a nonslip surface to facilitate handling.

The thumb and the forefinger stabilize the head and neck and tighten the loose skin in this area. The index finger is free to lightly bulge the eye outward. With the clinician's free hand, a microhematocrit tube is placed just lateral to the medial canthus and gently but firmly slid posteriorly and medially under the globe to the venous plexus that lines the back of the orbit. A controlled thrust is required when collecting samples from rats or hamsters. In the mouse, the vessels of the plexus rupture easily when the tube contacts them. Slight withdrawal of the tube allows blood to fill the capillary tube.

When collection is completed, direct pressure over the lid expedites hemostasis. Weekly sampling has been done on the same animals without clinically affecting their health. A 40-gm mouse has a total blood volume of 2 ml. If the animal is healthy, 0.1 to 0.2 ml can be safely collected. The capacity of a microhematocrit tube is 0.02 ml.

Complete Blood Count and Plasma and Serum Collection

White blood cell pipettes (Unopette, Becton-Dickinson, Rutherford, NJ) can be filled and blood smears made directly from the pooling blood.

Specimens for routine serologic studies are obtained by using plain hematocrit tubes. When

Table 4. *Hospital Colony Study* Using Techniques† from Table 3*

Test	Species	No. of Tests Run	Mean	Units	S.D.
BUN	Mouse	3	21.0	mg/dl	2.64
	Rat	6	15.3	mg/dl	1.21
	Hamster	6	15.6	mg/dl	1.14
	Guinea pig	6	22.3	mg/dl	2.94
	Rabbit	4	15.0	mg/dl	2.58
SGPT	Mouse	2	26.0	IU/L	1.41
	Rat	4	16.7	IU/L	2.21
	Hamster	7	59.1	IU/L	26.20
	Guinea pig	6	23.0	IU/L	2.09
	Rabbit	3	39.3	IU/L	10.00
Alkaline phosphatase	Mouse	3	76.0	IU/L	2.51
	Rat	7	125.0	IU/L	20.10
	Hamster	8	54.6	IU/L	9.39
	Guinea pig	6	23.1	IU/L	4.95
	Rabbit	4	60.7	IU/L	8.53
Sodium	Mouse	2	152.0	mEq/L	2.82
	Rat	6	138.0	mEq/L	2.17
	Hamster	8	141.0	mEq/L	3.44
	Guinea pig	6	133.0	mEq/L	0.81
	Rabbit	3	144.6	mEq/L	6.11
Potassium	Mouse	2	7.00	mEq/L	0.14
	Rat	6	5.06	mEq/L	0.51
	Hamster	8	4.72	mEq/L	0.76
	Guinea pig	6	4.76	mEq/L	0.27
	Rabbit	3	4.70	mEq/L	0.45
Total protein	Mouse	3	5.90	gm/dl	0.23
	Rat	6	5.88	gm/dl	0.36
	Hamster	7	5.67	gm/dl	0.31
	Guinea pig	6	5.01	gm/dl	0.20
	Rabbit	3	6.10	gm/dl	0.51
Total bilirubin	Mouse	QNS	—	—	—
	Rat	6	0.42	mg/dl	0.14
	Hamster	6	0.77	mg/dl	0.28
	Guinea pig	6	0.57	mg/dl	0.08
	Rabbit	3	0.40	mg/dl	0.10
Cholesterol	Mouse	2	119.50	mg/dl	4.94
	Rat	3	40.00	—	3.46
	Hamster	3	88.00	mg/dl	14.70
	Guinea pig	2	60.00	mg/dl	6.36
	Rabbit	QNS	—	—	—
Creatinine	Mouse	QNS	—	—	—
	Rat	3	0.43	mg/dl	0.15
	Hamster	3	0.20	mg/dl	0.10
	Guinea pig	3	0.57	mg/dl	0.05
	Rabbit	QNS	—	—	—
Lipase	Mouse	2	0.025	Sigma-Tietz units	0.01
	Rat	6	0.072	Sigma-Tietz units	0.01
	Hamster	7	0.130	Sigma-Tietz units	0.02
	Guinea pig	6	0.060	Sigma-Tietz units	0.02
	Rabbit	3	0.190	Sigma-Tietz units	0.03

*Boulevard Pet Hospital, Castro Valley, CA.
†Techniques of J. Alberti and L. Krusee, Veterinary Disease Laboratory, Campbell, CA.
SD, Standard deviation; QNS, quantity not sufficient.

Table 5. Blood Values and Some Values of Chemical Constituents of Serum*

	Rats	Mice	Hamsters	Guinea Pigs	Rabbits	Mongolian Gerbils
SGPT (Sigma-Frankel units)	25–42	32–41	22–36	10–25	14–27	—
Alkaline phosphatase (Bodansky units)	4.1–8.6	2.4–4.0	2–3.5	1.5–8.1	2.1–3.2	—
BUN (mg/dl)	10–20	8–30	10–40	8–20	5–30	18–24
Sodium (mEq/L)	144	114–154	106–185	120–155	100–145	144–158
Potassium (mEq/L)	5.9	3.0–9.6	2.3–9.8	6.5–8.2	3.0–7.0	3.8–5.2
Bilirubin total (mg/dl)	0.42	0.18–0.54	0.3–0.4	0.24–0.30	0.15–0.20	—
Blood glucose (mg/dl)	50–115	108–192	32.6–118.4	60–125	50–140	69–119
RBC (10^6 cells/mm^3)	7.2–9.6	9.3–10.5	4–9.3	4.5–7	3.2–7.5	8.3–9.3
Hemoglobin (gm/dl)	14.8	12–14.9	9.7–16.8	11–15	10–15	10–16
Hematocrit (%)	40–50	35–50	40–52	35–50	35–45	35–45
WBC (10^3 cells/mm^3)	8–14	8–14	7–15	5–12	8–10	9–14
Segmented	30	26	16–28	42	30–50	10–20
Nonsegmented	0	0	8	0	0	0
Lymphocyte	65–77	55–80	64–78	45–81	30–50	70–89
Eosinophil	1	3	1	5	1	1
Monocyte	4	5	2	8	9	0
Basophil	0	0	0	2	0	0

*These are values found in healthy-appearing animals and can be used as guides but should not be interpreted as physiologic norms for the species listed.

plasma is needed, heparinized tubes are substituted. After the tube is filled and spun, the clot or red cell layer can be broken off and discarded, leaving a column of plasma or serum for diagnostic testing.

VIRUS DIAGNOSTIC TESTING*

Table 6 indicates viral infections that can be serologically identified and the species of laboratory animals usually tested. Testing programs such as these are used mainly for commercial colonies but have been modified for clinical application.

URINE COLLECTION

Collection techniques vary, depending upon species. Mice and rats will urinate if picked up quickly. Urine may then be collected from the table surface (if clean) with a microhematocrit tube. Animals that will not urinate spontaneously can be placed in modified metabolic cages. These can be made by placing a plastic bag or sheet of plastic on the floor of a cage that has been elevated slightly at one end. Usually within 1 hour, an adequate sample is obtained. It should be remembered that gerbils produce only two to three drops of concentrated urine a day (appreciably less than other laboratory species). Rabbits' urine may be collected either by manual expression of the bladder or by centesis. Catheterization is practical only in the male. A

*Laboratory Animal Virus Testing Service, Microbiological Associates, Inc., 4733 Bethesda Ave., Bethesda, MD 20014.

no. 3½ French urinary catheter is used, although the urethra will accommodate a larger size. Extreme caution should be used when attempting this procedure, since the urethra in this species is easily traumatized and ruptured.

URINALYSIS

Bili-Labstix (Ames, Elkhart, IN) are used to check urine for pH, protein, glucose, ketones, bilirubin, and blood. The small volume of urine obtainable in some species necessitates multiple collections to complete an analysis. Specific gravity is measured with a refractometer (Protometer B5991 or Total Solids Meter, Scientific Products, McGaw Park, IL). Centrifuged urine sediment samples can be obtained by filling a microhematocrit tube and centrifuging.

Lithuria and basic urine may be found in hamsters, guinea pigs, and rabbits. Amorphous calcium carbonate and triple phosphate crystals are the predominant types found. Rat and mouse urine is acid-reacting and comparatively free of crystals. Proteinuria is a consistent finding in these two species. Rabbit urine may have a rust color and still be normal.

ECTOPARASITE MONITORING

Mite, lice, and fungal infestations are common dermatologic problems encountered. Examination of the animal may be expedited by the use of a hand lens or binocular loupe. Scrapings, Wood's light examination, and fungal culture are the tests

Table 6. *Serologically Identifiable Viral Infections and Laboratory Animals Used**

Viral Infection	Hamster	Guinea Pig	Rat	Mouse
Reovirus, type 3	X	X	X	X
Pneumonia virus of mice (PVM)	X	X	X	X
K virus (newborn mouse pneumonitis)				X
Theiler's encephalomyelitis (GD-VIII)	X	X	X	X
Polyoma				X
Sendai virus	X	X	X	X
Minute virus of mice (MVM)			X	X
Mouse adenovirus (MAdV)			X	X
Mouse hepatitis (MHV)			X	X
Lymphocytic choriomeningitis (LCM)	X	X	X	X
Ectromelia				X
Toolan H-1		X	X	
Simian myxovirus (SV5)	X	X	X	X
Kilham rat virus			X	
Rat coronavirus			X	

*Laboratory Animal Virus Testing Service, Microbiological Associates, Inc., 4733 Bethesda Ave., Bethesda, Md. 20014.

of choice. When mite infestation is suspected but cannot be demonstrated by skin scraping, it may be helpful to place an anesthetized or chemically immobilized animal on black paper. If the test is conducted long enough and infestation is moderate to heavy, the mites will migrate from the skin to the hair shafts, where they can be seen. They may also be visible on the black paper.

FECAL ANALYSIS FOR HELMINTHS, PROTOZOA, AND BACTERIA

Analysis of feces is an important part of a laboratory animal's health program, whether the animal is used for research or as a pet. The examination should consist of (1) fecal sedimentation examination, (2) fecal flotation examination, (3) protozoan smear examination, and (4) bacterial culture of feces on selective media. The analysis should specifically check for (1) ova of *Hymenolepis nana*, (2) ova of *Syphacia, Aspicularis*, and other nematodes, (3) overgrowth of protozoa, and (4) *Salmonella* and *Pseudomonas*.

Coprophagy, feces-contaminated food or bedding, and contamination of feed during processing all contribute to heavy infestation if the life cycle of the pathogenic organism is direct. Semiyearly examinations are advised if the animal population remains closed. If new animals enter the household, testing should be more frequent.

CLINICAL SIGNS AND DISEASES MOST COMMONLY SEEN*

The following information is tabulated (Tables 7 to 11) for each species:
1. The systems most commonly affected by diseases.

*Based on the author's experience.

2. Clinical signs most commonly seen when that system is affected.
3. Description of disease.
4. Brief approach to treatment.
5. Differential diagnosis in some cases.

The systems and diseases are listed in order of decreasing frequency.*

DIAGNOSTIC RADIOGRAPHY FOR SMALL RODENTS

Diagnostic radiographs can be obtained by using the technique chart (Table 12). Individual calibration of the machine to be used is necessary for best results. Rabbits and large rats require the same technique as that for cats. Kodak Blue Brand or Sakura medical x-ray film is used in high-speed cassettes. Kodak no-screen film is also used, especially when patient movement is not a problem and greater detail is needed.

To facilitate positioning of a small mammal, four strips of adhesive tape, ½ × 12 inches long, are wrapped around the individual extremities. Thus, adequate positioning can be obtained even when the handler is wearing lead gloves. Placing small rodents in a stockinette tube or radiolucent plastic cylinder is also helpful in taking radiographs of nonanesthetized patients.

PARENTERAL ROUTES OF MEDICATION

Intramuscular and subcutaneous injections are the preferred routes of parenteral administration of medications. Accurate dosing is accomplished by using a tuberculin or a microliter syringe (Microliter syringe [0.001 to 0.1 ml], The Hamilton Co., Reno, NV) equipped with a 25- to 27-gauge needle. Mi-

Text continued on page 760

Table 7. Diseases of Rabbits

Clinical Signs	Age Group	Morbidity	Mortality	Tests	Etiologic Agent	Treatment	Comment
Respiratory System							

Unilateral or bilateral purulent nasal discharge; stained hairs around nostrils; sometimes staining of medial aspect of paws; nasal discharge may be present only on exercise; conjunctivitis; some cases may show marked dyspnea	Usually mature	H(±)	±	Culture; radiographs of thorax	*Pasteurella multocida*	A. Antibiotics
						  1. Penicillin
						  2. Furazolidone
						  3. Tetracyclines
						  4. Sulfonamides
						  5. Sulfaquinoxaline
						B. Nebulization, vaporization
							Common name: "snuffles"; primarily a respiratory disease, but same organism can cause septicemia, abscess, urogenital disease in males and females

							Other less common diseases that can cause respiratory signs:
					Pasteurella pseudotuberculosis		Pseudotuberculosis
					Vaccinia virus		Rabbitpox: Usually rash, pock-type lesions on skin and ears
					Myxoma virus		Myxomatosis: very high morbidity and mortality; may see edema of head, resulting in drooping of ears; also, in chronic cases, fibrotic nodules on nose and ears
							Nonspecific conjunctivitis (conjunctivitis only sign)

Integument and Ears

Clinical signs	Age			Diagnosis	Etiology	Treatment	Comments
Crusty accumulation in ear canals; shaking head; scratching at ears	Any	±	L	Otoscopic and microscopic examinations	Psoroptes cuniculi; Chorioptes cuniculi	Rotenone in oil; clean cage	Common name: ear canker
Crusty skin; pruritus; alopecia (patchy or generalized); usually head and ears affected but can be any place on body	Any	±	L	UV light; KOH preparations; fungal culture	Microsporum; Trichophyton	Griseofulvin	Communicable disease; Other pruritic disease: Sarcoptes
Alopecia on chest area; animal biting out hair	Mature female	0	0	Rule out other dermatologic diseases	Hair pulling for nesting behavior	Nothing	
Large subcutaneous abscess anywhere on body, usually underside of neck	Any (but more in males)	L	L	Culture	Pasteurella multocida (unless proved otherwise)	Open drain; appropriate antibiotics (penicillin)	Usually associated with fighting or from a chronically irritated area; Staphylococcus second most common cause

Digestive System

Clinical signs	Age			Diagnosis	Etiology	Treatment	Comments
Slobbering; difficulty in eating; may get teeth caught on wire cage	Usually mature	L	L	Examination of oral cavity	Probable congenital malocclusion	Routine cutting of overgrown or ingrown incisors or molars	Continuous-growing incisors must be continually worn down; if not, this condition may result. Lack of gnawing on hard objects is not a major cause; malocclusion is
Small warts on tongue and oral mucosa	Any over a month old	±	L	Biopsy	Rabbit oral papillomatosis	Remove wart or vaccinate	
Bloat; profuse mucoid diarrhea; anorexia; borborygmus; huddling	Any	+	± (young)	Fecal analysis to check for other problems	Unknown; may be 1. Due to deficiency of amylase 2. Nutritional 3. Bacterial 4. Viral 5. Irritant 6. Toxin 7. Stress	Increase roughage in diet; prevent secondary septicemia and dehydration; increase fiber in diet to 15-25%; dimetridazole powder 0.025 to 0.1% in drinking water during 3-8 weeks of age	Commonly referred to as mucoid enteritis or mucoid enteropathy; Other less common diarrhea-causing diseases: 1. Salmonellosis 2. Coccidiosis

Mammary Glands

Clinical signs	Age			Diagnosis	Etiology	Treatment	Comments
Anorexia; polydipsia; mastitis	Mature female	L	±	Culture	Streptococcus; Staphylococcus; Pasteurella	Antibiotics; drain; hot pack	Usually associated with nursing

Table continued on following page

Table 7. Diseases of *Rabbits* Continued

Clinical Signs	Age Group	Morbidity	Mortality	Tests	Etiologic Agent	Treatment	Comment
Urogenital System							
Lithuresis; pH urine 8–9; urine dries and leaves large amount of white crystals; sometimes urine may be brown or red-brown	Any; usually mature when noticed	0	0	Urinalysis	Normal rabbit urine	None	When urine dries, it has chemical consistency similar to that of boiler scale; use mild acid solution such as vinegar to clean area
Ulceration; scab-covered lesion about genitals, either sex; can have ulcers in other areas; vesicles may be on skin surrounding genitals	Mature			Look for organism in exudate using dark field microscopy	*Treponema cuniculi*	Penicillin	Not communicable disease
Miscellaneous							
Hepatomegaly; irregular surface to liver; abdominal enlargement; poor general condition; diarrhea (±); in young, mild hemorrhagic diarrhea (a healthy rabbit usually seen; hepatic lesions may be seen only as an incidental finding)	Any	±	±	Microscopic examination of feces; both types have oocysts that appear in stool	*Eimeria*; both intestinal and hepatic types occur in rabbit	Wire floors; sulfaquinoxaline; sulfamethazine; sulfaquinoxaline 0.1% solution in drinking water for 2 weeks	Other less common diseases affecting the liver 1. *Pasteurella tularensis* causes small yellow-gray necrotic foci on liver; spleen is covered with miliary necrotic foci 2. Tyzzer's disease; necrotic foci on liver, along with enteritis
Subcutaneous swellings	Any	L	L	Biopsy	Poxvirus		Shope's fibroma seen only in wild cottontails

Table 8. Diseases of Guinea Pigs

Clinical Signs	Age Group	Morbid-ity	Mortal-ity	Tests	Etiologic Agent	Treatment	Comment
Lymph System; Respiratory System							
Active, healthy-looking animal with enlarged lymph nodes; nodes may discharge pus	Usually mature	±	±	Culture	Beta-hemolytic streptococci, Lancefield type C	Antibiotics; drainage; quarantine	Called "lumps"; other diseases (less common) with same signs: pseudotuberculosis, streptobacillosis
Acute death	Any	±	H	Culture; necropsy	Beta-hemolytic streptococci		Generalized septicemia; other diseases causing acute death: salmonellosis, pseudotuberculosis
Chronic duration: anorexia, ruffled haircoat, huddling, dyspnea, nasal discharge, crusty dried mucus on medial aspect of forelegs, purulent conjunctivitis, lymphadenitis	Usually mature	±	H	Culture	Beta-hemolytic streptococci, Lancefield type C	Antibiotics; supportive care. Oxytetracycline, at a rate of 0.1 mg/ml of drinking H_2O for 7 days, can be used to control epidemic but does not eliminate condition*	*Other diseases with similar signs:*
					Bordetella bronchiseptica		*Bordetella:* usually just confined to respiratory tract
					Salmonella typhimurium or *Salmonella enteritidis*		*Salmonella:* respiratory signs usually lacking; may not have diarrhea
					Pasteurella pseudotuberculosis		Pseudotuberculosis: palpate for enlarged mesenteric lymph nodes; chronic emaciation may be only sign
							Pneumococcal pneumonia
							Virus pneumonia
							Pseudomonas
							Klebsiella
							Corynebacterium

Table continued on following page

Table 8. Diseases of Guinea Pigs Continued

Clinical Signs	Age Group	Morbidity	Mortality	Etiologic Agent	Tests	Treatment	Comment
Integument and Hair							
Alopecia (can be generalized or patchy) may be symmetric in distribution; nonpruritic	Any age	±	L	Unknown; in weanlings or females, may be due to stress; in males, a similar-looking disorder is due to grooming between two animals	Rule out other dermatologic diseases	Feed hay, cabbage, or kale or do nothing	Usually seen only in colony or heavy stress situations
Pruritus, scablike lesions, owner usually sees small, white elongated insects	Any age	±	L	Lice (*Gliricola*; *Gyropus*)	Examine hair and skin closely	Carbamate powders, dischlorvos strips	Good husbandry necessary for control
Scaly, patchy skin lesions; broken hair shafts, can be generalized; pruritic	Any	±	L	*Tricophyton*; *Microsporum*	UV light; KOH preparation culture	Griseofulvin (use cautiously, since derived from *Pencillium* cultures)	Communicable disease
Sores on hocks or plantar surface of foot; abscesses	Mature	±	L	*Corynebacterium pyogenes*	Culture	Put on softer surface; treat symptomatically (daily medicated dressings)	Problem encountered when animal is usually raised on wire
Diseases of Pregnant Females							
Sow in late pregnancy: lethargy; anorexia; huddling; may die within 24 hr	Mature	±	+	Pregnancy toxemia		Steroids; supportive care; calcium gluconate Cesarean section	Friable yellow liver on necropsy; normal fetus; may be prevented by feeding good-quality diet last part of gestation

Digestive Tract

Clinical Signs	Age			Diagnosis	Etiology	Treatment	Comments
Difficulty in chewing or moving mouth; slobbering when eating; overgrowth of molars	Mature	±	L	Physical examination; radiography	Probable congenital malocclusion; poor-quality hay diet; chronic fluorosis	Correct diet; file or cut molars to proper size	Disease of salivary glands may mimic clinical signs; chemical restraints may be needed to examine molars
Blood-tinged diarrhea; acute death sometimes in young; usually asymptomatic	Young	±	±(L)	Fecal analysis	*Eimeria caviae* or protozoan overgrowth (*Trichomonas*)	Coccidostats	Coccidiosis usually not a problem; other internal parasites not usually a problem but should check for them; nematode of cecum (*Paraspidodera*) is reported to be most common

Miscellaneous

Clinical Signs	Age			Diagnosis	Etiology	Treatment	Comments
Poor weight gain; rough coat; greater incidence of disease; increased huddling; hesitancy to move about; enlarged joints (±); subconjunctival hemorrhage (±)	Any	±	±	Serum ascorbic acid levels of feed and analysis	Ascorbic acid deficiency	Ascorbic acid in water and feed; kale, cabbage, citrus fruits, orange juice instead of water; ascorbic acid supplement 1–3 mg/100 gm/day or 100 mg tablet dissolved in 500 ml of drinking H_2O, change daily	Occurs even on fortified commercial diet 1. Poor quality control of commercial ration 2. Shelf life of guinea pig feed is short; Other diseases causing soreness of limbs or inability to move 1. Fractures 2. Muscular dystrophy (vitamin E deficiency) 3. Myositis (viral?) 4. Guinea pig paralysis (viral?)
Cachexia; generalized loss of condition	Usually mature males	±	±	Possibly radiography and/or electrolyte studies	Thought to be improper Ca:P ratio or its relationship to Mg	Put on balanced diet	Diffuse calcification of internal viscera
Straining to urinate; small amount of urine; blood-tinged urine, arching back, standing higher on hind feet	Mature males mostly	±	±	Palpate bladder for urinary calculi, x-ray abdomen	Unknown	Cystotomy	May cause intermittent or complete obstruction. It is an operable condition

*Harkness, J. E., and Wagner, J. E.; *The Biology and Medicine of Rabbits and Rodents*. Philadelphia. Lea & Febiger, 1977.

Table 9. Diseases of Hamsters

Clinical Signs	Age Group	Morbidity	Mortality	Tests	Etiologic Agent	Treatment	Comment
Gastrointestinal Tract							
Diarrhea-stained anus; lethargy; anorexia; prolapsed rectum; can die within 48 hr to 1 week after symptoms start	Any	±	H	Culture feces; fecal analysis; direct smear	Proliferative ileitis; wet tail; exact etiology unknown; overgrowth of *E. coli* and protozoan organisms (trichomonads); improper caging; overcrowding; lack of fresh water	Supportive care 1. Fluids sq. 2. Antibiotics (gentamicin) 3. Sulfonamides 4. Improve husbandry 5. Fresh food 6. Whole milk or buttermilk 7. Surgery for intussusception	Very common; guarded prognosis; normal bacteria, flora and fauna are gram-negative bacilli resembling *Bacteroides, Lactobacillus* (gram-positive type), *Streptococcus, Bacillus, Escherichia, Staphylococcus*, spirochetes, large coccus forms, *Giardia* and trichomonads; prolapsed rectum is usually accompanied by an intussusception of the colon
Mild diarrhea; animal relatively healthy in appearance	Mature	L	L	Microscopic examination of stool	Overgrowth of *Trichomonas, Giardia, Chilomastix*	High-protein diet fed for 7 days; 45% ground beef liver, 42% lean ground beef, 11% lard, 2% calcium carbonate or carbarsone per os; 15.6 mg/100 gm body weight per day for 21 days	
Constipation; diarrhea may be associated with it	Young	±	±	Palpate abdomen; x-ray abdomen	Inadequate amount of water to drink	Ensure adequate water intake; milk of magnesia	
Usually no clinical signs other than mild enteritis	Any	±	L	Fecal analysis	*Hymenolepis nana; Syphacia obvelata,* and others	Proper anthelmintic; piperazine, niclosamide (Yomesan)	*H. nana;* communicable disease

Integument

Clinical signs	Age			Diagnosis	Agent/Etiology	Treatment	Comments
Alopecia about the face, but can be generalized	Usually more	±	±	Skin scrapings	Demodex; *Notoedres*	Pyrethrum insecticides; crotamiton (Eurax)	Common; although looks like a poor prognosis, they respond; pruritus is not a major finding

Miscellaneous

Clinical signs	Age			Diagnosis	Agent/Etiology	Treatment	Comments
Paresis; inactivity; inability to lift head; crawls	Mature	±,	±	Physical examination, radiographs	Nutritional deficiency	Vitamin D	Commonly called cage paralysis; other musculoskeletal diseases: 1. Nutritional muscular dystrophy (vitamin E deficiency) 2. Polymyopathy and myocardial necrosis (congenital and genetically controlled gradual onset)
Ocular discharge; chattering; ruffled haircoat; huddling; nasal discharge ±	Young more susceptible	±	L	Possible viral etiology and/or *Pneumococcus, Streptococcus*		Antibiotics: chloramphenicol; tetracyclines	
Change in behavior; lethargy; inactivity; sleeping long periods; slow heart rate; respiratory rate slow; all animals in group may not be in this condition; low body temperature	Usually not in very old animals		±	Physical examination	Hibernation: large fluctuation in ambient temperatures; precold exposure in history	Raise environmental temperature	Animal will go into hibernation for a few days, then out; may be repeated; heart rate can be as slow as 4–15 beats/minute

Table 10. Diseases of Mice and Rats

Clinical Signs	Age Group	Morbidity	Mortality	Tests	Etiologic Agent	Treatment	Comment	Species
Integument and Appendages								
Scratching around head and ears; abrasions; scabs; bald spots	Haired animals	±	L	Skin scraping; blue paper test	*Myobia; Myocoptes; Radfordia; Notoedres*	Dichlorovos strips; ectocide; pyrethrum powder	Common in mice	Mice, rats
Sores around ears and on pinnae; scabs and wounds randomly positioned on caudal two thirds of tail	Mature males	L	L	Observation	Fighting	Separate males		Mice
Circumscribed necrotic lesion usually at base of tail	Any	±	L		Humidity too low	Adjust humidity to 50–55 per cent	Ringtail syndrome	Mice
Congenital absence of tail	At birth	0	0	Genetic studies	Hereditary			Mice
Blush or pale color of pinnae or tail	Any	±	H	Any that are necessary	Cyanosis, usually associated with severe respiratory illness or septicemia	Antibiotics; fluids; general supportive care	Poor prognostic sign	Mice
Bald spots; scaliness; pruritus (±)	Haired	+	L	Wood's light examination; KOH slide culture	*Trichophyton; microsporum*	Griseofulvin; tolnaftate cream 1 per cent	There may be some normal fluorescence of hair shafts	Mice, rats
Sloughing and/or necrosis of digits and tail; papules or pustules (±)	Any	H	H	Serology	Poxvirus (ectromelia)	Vaccination; supportive care if requested; euthanasia advised	Often a latent infection; vaccination of healthy stock	Mice

756

Respiratory System

Clinical signs	Age			Diagnosis	Etiology	Treatment/Control	Comments	Species
Sneezing; chattering; labored breathing; nasal discharge; pawing at nose; epistaxis; cachexia; unkempt coat; arching of back; generalized depression; vestibular disease; conjunctivitis	Usually mature	±	±	Culture if possible; serology	Not a specific disease entity but due to one or more of the following: enzootic bronchiectasis (rats) (probable virus); infectious catarrh (*Mycoplasma pulmonis*); disease syndrome referred to as chronic murine pneumonia	Antibiotics; long-term if necessary 1. Tylosin 2. Sulfonamides 3. Tetracycline, 2–5 mg to each ml H_2O 4. Sulfamerazine 0.02% solution	Other less common diseases with similar signs: *Pasteurella pneumotropica*; *Bordetella bronchiseptica*; pneumonia virus of mice; adenovirus; K virus; *Diplococcus pneumoniae* (common in rats); streptococcal infections	Mice, rats

Gastrointestinal Disease

Clinical signs	Age			Diagnosis	Etiology	Treatment/Control	Comments	Species
Prolapsed rectum	3 weeks and older	±	L	Fecal analysis; cellophane tape test not reliable	*Aspicularis tetraptera*; *Syphacia obvelata* or other heavy parasite infestation	Appropriate anthelmintic therapy: 1. Piperazine compounds 2. Niclosomide (Yomesan)	Pinworms and *Hymenolepis nana* are common (M)	Mice, rats
Mustard-color soiling around tail and caudal part of body; watery stools; acute death; fecal impaction	Suckling age	H	H	Fecal cultures if necessary to rule out other diseases	Epizootic diarrhea of infant mice (EDIM); epizootic diarrhea of suckling rats	Filter caps over top of cage prevent transmission; antibiotic therapy sometimes helpful	Filter caps and sanitation are effective in stopping outbreaks	Mice, rats
Mild diarrhea; usually healthy-looking animal	Any age	±	L		*Giardia* or other protozoan overgrowth	Feed apples, cabbage, ground beef; furazolidone, antibiotics		
Acute death; focal necrosis of liver (white spots); may have enteritis; diarrhea may be present	Any age	±	H	Difficult to culture; histopathology with special staining technique may demonstrate organisms	Tyzzer's disease; *Bacillus piliformes*	Antibiotics	Can be latent; other diseases with similar signs: salmonellosis, *Pseudomonas*, septicemia following stress	Mice, rats

Table continued on following page

Table 10. Diseases of Mice and Rats Continued

Clinical Signs	Age Group	Morbid- ity	Mortal- ity	Tests	Etiologic Agent	Treatment	Comment	Species
					Central Nervous System			
Head tilt; circling	Mature	L	L	Radiography; neurologic examination	*Mycoplasma* or bacterial infection of vestibular apparatus associated with upper respiratory infection	Antibiotics; steroids		Mice, rats
					Mammary Glands			
Neoplasm	Mature female	L	L	Biopsy	Mammary tumor, fibroadenoma, adenocarcinoma (M); fibrosarcoma (R)	Surgical excision	Usually recur after removal; located anywhere on body	Mice, rats
					Lymph Nodes			
Lymphadenopathy	Mature	L	±	Culture or biopsy	*Pasteurella pseudotuberculosis*	Antibiotic if bacterial		Mice, rats
					Miscellaneous			
Enlargement of salivary glands causing swelling of neck region	Mature	±	L	Biopsy	Sialodacryoadenitis; viral etiology	Steroids; antibiotics	Usually latent	Rats
Marked depression; hunched-up posture; roughened coat; conjunctivitis; anorexia; lethargy; death; stunting in surviving animals	Any; young more commonly affected	±	±	Fecal culture	*Salmonella; Pseudomonas*	Antibiotics; hyperchlorination of water (10 ppm); euthanasia advised (if communicable disease)	These are nonspecific signs of septicemia; any latent disease can cause infection if animal is stressed; examples are mouse hepatitis virus, reovirus, heavy parasitism	Mice

Table 11. *Diseases of Gerbils*

Clinical Signs	Age Group	Morbidity	Morbidity	Tests	Etiologic Agent	Treatment	Comment
Miscellaneous							
Bare spots on base of tail	Mature	±	L		Fighting due to overcrowding	Correct overcrowding	
Inflammation and ulceration around the nose and jaw	Mature			Rule out other dermatologic problems	Thought to be from mechanical abrasion	Remove source of mechanical abrasion	
Protrusion of nictitating membrane, conjunctiva, and eye itself	Older animals	?	?		Unknown		Evaluate for glaucoma or retrobulbar pressure
Scanty or patchy growth of hair	Young not weaned	?	?		Unknown	None; hair will grow in as animal gets older	
Seizures when handled: body stiffens; legs stiffen and tremble	More common in young animals				Thought to be a form of catalepsy	Phenytoin (Dilantin) has been used but may be unnecessary	Seen in some strains of mice also Seizures occur with less frequency as the animal gets older
Sneezing; chattering; labored breathing	Any	±	±	Physical; culture; radiography	Virus? Bacterial? Mycoplasm?	Penicillin tetracyclines	Usually follows stress
Diarrhea, mild	Any	±	±				No one enteric disease is prevalent but should consider enteritis due to 1. *Salmonella* 2. Unwashed vegetables 3. Parasitism, although very few natural parasites; gerbils are very susceptible to most experimental infestation 4. Protozoan overgrowth (*Entamoeba* may be a normal finding)

Data from Schwentker, V., Tumblebrook Farm, West Brookfield, MA: Personal communication.

*Table 12. Radiographic Technique for Small Mammals**

Thickness (cm)	FED (inches)	KVP	MA	Seconds	MAS
			Bone†		
0.5	36	40	100 (fine focal spot)	1/30	3.3
1		42			
2		44			
3		46			
4		48			
5		50			
6		52			
7		54			
			Soft Tissue		
1	36	38	100 (fine focal spot)	1/30	3.3
2		40			
3		42			
4		44			
5		46			
6		48			
7		50			
8		52			
9		54			
			Thoracic		
2	36	34	200	1/60	3.3
3		36			
4		38			
5		40			
6		42			
7		44			
8		46			

*Radiographic technique of R. P. Barrett, Castro Valley, CA.
†If animal is immature, it might be better to use 50 MA.
MA, milliampere; MAS, milliampere second.

croliter syringes are used when doses are 0.1 ml or less.

Intravenous injections can be given when necessary. A 25- to 27-gauge needle is chosen according to vein size. The vein of choice for an intravenous injection in each species is listed in Table 13.

INTRAGASTRIC INTUBATION AND ARTIFICIAL ALIMENTATION

Oral alimentation by eye dropper or intragastric intubation of a liquid replacement diet can help support an anorectic patient's nutritional needs. Liquid diets (Esbalic, Borden; Initol, Hill; Neo-Mull-Soy, Borden; Pet Kalorie, Haver-Lockhart), made into a slurry, fortified with baby foods (fruits, vegetables, cereals, meats) have been used satisfactorily. Usually, a volume of 2 to 3 ml/100 gm of body weight is infused at one time. Karo syrup, honey, or vegetable oil can be added if caloric requirements necessitate it. The daily caloric requirement for a healthy mature rodent is roughly 15 to 35 kcal/100 gm of body weight. The higher caloric requirement pertains to mice and hamsters, while the lower requirement is for rats, guinea pigs, and rabbits. Growth, lactation, or a febrile condition can double the daily caloric requirement. Table 14 gives several purée recipes. The purées can be given by eye dropper, gastric intubation, or free choice. Anorectic guinea pigs that would not take solid food have been fed these diets as their only source of nutrition for up to 2 months. Purées should be fed at room temperature. Refrigeration life is short, less than 2 days.

Intragastric intubation can be accomplished with either a flexible rubber tube (nos. 3 to 12 French rubber stomach tube, Davol) or a rigid metal cannula (Oral Administration Needle, Aloe Scientific, St. Louis, MO; Biomedical Needles, Animal Feeding Stainless Steel, Popper & Sons, Inc., New York) with a ball-tipped end. Sharp incisors can easily cut a flexible tube unless the jaws are manually held open. Passage of the tube through the interdental space (between incisors and molars) may help avoid this problem. If this is not possible, a tongue depressor or a small flat stick with a hole drilled in its center can be used as a mouth gag. The gag is placed on edge just behind the incisors. A tube can then be passed through the hole in the mouth gag. Specula are not needed when using metal cannulas. These are designed specifically for use in laboratory species. With a little practice, they can be passed quickly and atraumatically. With either method of gastric intubation, two points of resistance are usually encountered. The first is just before the tube reaches the esophagus, and the second is just before the tube reaches the cardia. Gentle manipulation of the tube (not pressure) will help it pass atraumatically.

DRUG DOSES

The dosages in Table 15 are ones that the author has used in his practice. They have a fair degree of safety and efficacy. Serum level studies of the chemotherapeutics have not been carried out by the author and will not be discussed here.

Table 13. Veins of Choice for Various Species

Species	Vein of Choice
Rabbit	Marginal ear vein or cephalic vein
Guinea pig	Cephalic vein
Rat	Vein on the caudolateral aspect of the thigh or the vein on the dorsal surface of the tail*
Hamster	Vein on the caudolateral aspect of the thigh
Mouse	Tail vein* (very difficult without practice)

*Wrap or immerse the tail in warm water prior to venipuncture.

Table 14. *Purée Recipes**

	Pellet	Apple	Endive	Baby Food	Esbilac†	Nutri-Cal
Main ingredient	½ cup rabbit or guinea pig pellets	1 cut-up apple (carrots or fresh corn may be substituted)	2 cups chopped endive (other greens may be substituted)	Feed from jar: Strained creamed spinach Strained pears Strained applesauce	1 tsp Esbilac powder	⅓ tsp Nutri-Cal
Amount of water	¾ cup	⅛ cup	¼ cup	None	1 tsp	⅓ tsp
Comments	Soaking pellets before blending gives best results	← ——————— Mix in blender to desired consistency ———————— →				May be fed separately or mixed with Esbilac

General Comments

A blender is suggested for preparing purées.

Amounts of liquids in the above recipes can be adjusted to change mixtures to desired consistency.

It is preferable to prepare puréed foods daily.

Use plastic medicine droppers to feed purées. If opening at tip of dropper is not large enough, it can be made bigger by cutting a little off the tip with a strong pair of scissors.

It is always advisable to present a variety of foods. A sick pet may turn away from the first entrée offered but take another with no hesitation.

Add ascorbic acid—200 mg per 500 ml of purée—for guinea pigs.

*Purée recipes from Manuel Rood, Berkeley, CA.
†Borden, Inc., Norfolk, VA.
‡EVSCO Pharmaceutical Corp., Buena, NJ.

SURGERY AND ANESTHESIA

Surgical and anesthetic procedures are routine, with just a few exceptions. Induction is accomplished by masking with halothane. Injectable anesthesia is also effective in many cases (Table 16). The author does not use nitrous oxide on rodents. Intubation is not done routinely. If it is needed, intubation is done only in the rabbit, since this is the species for which it is most practical (see *Current Veterinary Therapy VII*, p. 709, for endotracheal intubation). Planes of anesthesia can be maintained by observing respiration rate and color of the albinotic iris in those species in which it is present.

Routine surgical procedures include excision of neoplasms, débridement of abscesses, ovariohysterectomy, castration, exploratory laparotomy, and cystotomy for the removal of urinary calculi in guinea pigs.

Suturing techniques are routine except for the small size of the material needed. Preplacement of sutures during surgery of visceral organs is a helpful technique. For example, closure of the urinary bladder is easier if 4-0 catgut sutures are preplaced before the initial incision into the bladder is made. Closure of incisions is routine. Catgut is used internally and subcutaneously, and stainless steel is used in the skin. Rabbits present the main problem of chewing at incision sites. An Elizabethan collar will usually control this. Hamsters, guinea pigs, rats, and mice seem to tolerate cutaneous sutures.

Postsurgical care of laboratory animals presents particular problems. Temperature regulation and body heat conservation are paramount problems in very small rodents. Small body size and its relationship to exposed surface area make them more vulnerable to heat loss or gain. Exogenous heat sources, such as hot water bags or a well-covered heating pad on a low setting, are indicated. Take care not to overheat the animal. Full recovery from anesthesia should be accomplished before the animal is returned to its cage.

CASTRATION IN THE RABBIT*

This surgical procedure is similar to that described for the dog. Fasting prior to surgery is not necessary, since vomiting has not been encountered. The patient is placed in dorsal recumbency. The area anterior to the scrotum is carefully clipped, aseptically prepared, and draped. Use care, as rabbit skin tears easily. The incision is made on the midline just anterior to the scrotum. The subcutaneous tissue is separated, and the tunic with the testicle is located by pushing the testicle anteriorly into the incision site. The tunic is held with a forceps and then incised to expose the testis. The testicle is grasped with a forceps and pulled from the scrotum and tunic. The testicle is very friable and must be gently separated from the tunic. The tunic is replaced into the scrotum, and the ligation procedure is completed. There is little bleeding encountered in this procedure. The skin is closed with no. 34 stainless steel wire to prevent the rabbit from removing the sutures. Prophylactic antibiotics

---

*Technique of D. Montag, D.V.M.

*Table 15. Drug Dosage**

Drug	Manufacturer's Concentration	Dosage by Weight (mg/body weight)	Route	Dosage by Volume (ml/body weight)†	Comment
Fluothane	U.S.P.	Give to effect	Inhaled	Give to effect	Found to be very safe and well tolerated. I do not use nitrous oxide when anesthetizing rodents or rabbits. Halothane is my drug of choice for immobilization or anesthetization.
Innovar-Vet (Pitman-Moore)	Comes in a standard concentration containing a mixture of fentanyl, 0.4 mg/ml, and droperidol, 20.0 mg/ml	—	Intramuscular	0.02–0.05 ml/100 gm	Up to 0.15 ml/100 gm may be necessary in hamsters; 0.02–0.05 ml dose works best in rats, guinea pigs, and mice; 0.02 ml for rabbits.
Nalorphine HCL (Naline, MSD Agvet)	5 mg/ml	0.5 mg/100 gm	Subcutaneous; intramuscular; intravenous	0.1 ml/100 gm	Intravenous route for quickest response; 5 mg is the largest dose usually given.
Ketamine HCL	100 mg/ml	4.4 mg/100 gm	Intramuscular	0.05 ml/100 gm	Produces a mild form of sedation; good for minor surgical procedures and oral examination; short duration; less than 20 min.
Ketamine HCL	100 mg/ml	11 mg/kg	Intravenous	0.11 ml/kg	Used in rabbits; good for endotracheal intubation and minor surgical procedures; very short duration (less than 10 min.)
Surital (5 gm) stock bottle	2% solution	—	Intravenous	1.0 ml/2.27 kg (1.0 ml/5lb)	Used in rabbits for endotracheal intubation; use anesthetic to effect.
Atropine sulfate	1/150 gr/ml or 0.4 mg/ml	0.004–0.01 mg/100 gm	Subcutaneous; intramuscular; intravenous	0.01–0.025 ml/100 gm	More than 30% of domestic rabbits have serum atropenesterase in their bodies. This enzyme hydrolizes atropine.
Dexamethasone	1 mg/ml	0.06 mg/100 gm	Subcutaneous; intramuscular; intravenous; intraperitoneal	0.06 ml/100 gm	
Prednisone	10 mg/ml	0.05–0.22 mg/100 gm	Subcutaneous; intramuscular	0.005–0.022 ml/100 gm	
Niclosamide (Yomesan, Farbenfabriken Bayer)	500 mg tablets (active ingredients)	3–9 mg/100 gm	Oral	Feed medicated ration or a single dose per os	Mix thoroughly one pulverized tablet/1 lb of finely ground feed; small amounts of water are added to ground mixture to facilitate reshaping into a kibble type ration; air dry or feed as mash. We have used it on large numbers of mice (male, female, some pregnant) without problems; have not had opportunity to use on large numbers of other species. Medicated feed is fed for 3 days, off for 3 days, on for 3 days; repeat in 2 weeks if necessary. Procedure described can also be used in hamsters, although its efficacy has not been documented; I have no personal experience using it in guinea pigs, rabbits, or gerbils.

Table 15. *Drug Dosage** Continued

Drug	Manufacturer's Concentration	Dosage by Weight (mg/body weight)	Route	Dosage by Volume (ml/body weight)†	Comment
Piperazine citrate or adipate	500-mg tablets or in bulk	50–100 mg/100 gm	Oral	½–1 tablet/50 ml water	Put in drinking water; use the following regimen for pinworms (in mice and rats): 7 days on medication; 7 days off medication; 7 days on medication. Clean cages thoroughly just before putting animal on medication and when taking it off medication; do all animals in same room at same time. Pinworm eggs may be airborne; filter caps may help. Five percent sucrose solution may increase palatability of medicated water.
Sucrose			Oral	25 gm/487 ml of water	Used to increase palatability of medicated water.
Griseofulvin	50 mg/tablet	2 mg/100 gm	Oral	Consult chart for amount of feed consumed	Mix one (50 mg) tablet/lb of feed; follow mixing instructions for Yomesan; use cautiously in guinea pig, since griseofulvin is derived from *Penicillium griseofulvin*.
Shell Pest Strips (DDVP)		—	—	—	Place a strip 1 × 2 × 2 inches on top of average-sized mouse cage; keep it away from animal so it will not chew on it; use for 3 days; take off for 3 days. Serum cholinesterase levels will fall with long-term use but will go back to normal when strips are removed; production may be lowered. Can be used safely on mature, healthy (not systemically ill) animals.
Methyl carbamate type flea powder			—	¹⁄₁₆ tsp/100 gm if nursing; ¹⁄₆₄ tsp/adult	Put desired amount of powder into a paper bag (lunch-bag size); place animal in bag and shake; this method distributes medication evenly over animal; *only for mature animals* for lice, fleas, and superficial mites.
Crotamiton (Eurax, Westwood)	10% lotion	—	Topical	—	Apply one to two times a day.
Chloramphenicol palmitate	125 mg/4 ml	2–5 mg/100 gm	Oral	0.07–0.16 ml/100 gm	Give two to three times a day. Add 4 ml of chloramphenicol to 3 oz water.
Chloramphenicol succinate	100 mg/ml	5 mg/100 gm	Intramuscular	0.05 ml/100 mg	Give one to two times a day (dose can be doubled if needed).
Tylosin	50 mg/ml	0.2–0.4 mg/100 gm	Intramuscular	0.004–0.008 ml/100 gm	Give one to two times a day (dose can be doubled if needed).
Gentamicin sulfate (Gentocin, Schering)	50 mg/ml	0.44–0.88 mg/100 gm	Intramuscular	0.008–0.016 ml/100 gm	Give one to two times a day; has been used with good results in hamsters with wet tail.
Tetracycline (Panmycin, Upjohn)	100 mg/ml	1.5–2 mg/100 gm	Oral	0.015–0.02 ml/100 gm	Give two to three times a day or add 0.1 ml tetracycline to 3 oz water.
Sulfamerazine		5–8 mg/100 gm	Oral	30–80 mg added to sufficient quantity of water to make 100 ml of solution	Put in drinking water or administer proper dosage for weight per os.

Table continued on following page

Table 15. Drug Dosage Continued

Drug	Manufacturer's Concentration	Dosage by Weight (mg/body weight)	Route	Dosage by Volume (ml/body weight)†	Comment
Sulfaquinoxaline	Concentrate stock solution: 20 gm/ 100 ml or 20%	—	Oral	0.25–1.0 gm/ 1000 ml of water (0.025– 0.1% solution) or 0.256 gm/ 500 gm of feed (0.05% ration)	Medicate for 30 days; improve sanitation and animal husbandry methods. Add 5 ml of stock solution to 1000 ml of drinking water, giving a 0.1% solution in drinking water.
Sulfadimethoxine (Albon, Roche)	5% oral suspension	2.0–5.0 mg/ 100 gm	Oral	0.016–0.04 ml/ 100 gm	Give once a day per os or 1 ml of oral suspension to 3 oz drinking water.
	Also available in 12.5% solution	2–5 mg/100 ml	Oral	0.016–0.04 ml/ 100 gm	0.5 ml stock solution to 3 oz water.
Procaine penicillin G	300,000 units/ml	2000 units/100 gm	Intramuscular	0.0066 ml/100 gm	Has been used in all laboratory species; anaphylaxis can occur in guinea pigs; use other antibiotics if possible.
Furazolidone (Furoxone, Norden)	100 mg/ml	0.5 mg/100 gm	Oral	0.005 ml/100 gm	0.55 mg/100 ml of water, which equals 0.055% sol. or 5 mg/100 gm of feed for long-term therapy (30 days), used mainly in rabbits.
Nitrofurazone (Furacin, Norden)	0.2% solution (0.2 gm/100 ml)	8 mg/kg	Oral	4 ml/kg added to daily water	100 mg/1000 ml of water or 0.01% solution for long-term therapy in rabbits, or add 50 ml of Furacin to 1000 ml of water (2 tblsp per qt H₂O).
Vitamin A, U.S.P.	100,000 units/ml	50–500 units/100 gm	Intramuscular	0.0005–0.005 ml/ 100 gm	
Vitamin D, U.S.P.	100,000 units/ml (1 ml of stock solution can be diluted with 10 ml of saline)	20–40 units/100 gm	Intramuscular	0.002–0.004 ml of diluted stock solution/ 100 gm	
Vitamin C, U.S.P.	100 mg/ml	2–20 mg/100 gm	Intramuscular	0.02–0.2 ml/100 gm	100 mg tablet to 500 ml of water.
B complex (Vitaxin) { B₁ / B₂ / B₁₂	100 mg/ml / 2.0 mg/ml / 100 μg/ml	—	Intramuscular	0.002–0.02 ml/ 100 gm	

*Long-term antibiotic therapy (more than 5 days at therapeutic levels) may result in fatalities owing to destruction of symbiotic bacteria in the gastrointestinal tract. This is especially true in guinea pigs and hamsters. Unless otherwise stated, chemotherapeutic agents may be used on any species.

†Except where otherwise noted.

Table 16. Ketamine and Ketamine-combination Anesthetic Dosages (mg/kg/ IM)

1. Recommended dosages of ketamine:

RABBIT	GUINEA PIG	RAT	HAMSTER	MOUSE
25–55	25–55	22–24	—	22–44

2. Addition of acetylpromazine to ketamine (ketamine dosage is maintained at full strength as shown on line 1):

RABBIT	GUINEA PIG	RAT	HAMSTER	MOUSE
0.75	0.75	0.75	—	0.75

3. Xylazine dosage used in conjunction with steps 1 and 2:

RABBIT	GUINEA PIG	RAT	HAMSTER	MOUSE
2–5	2–5	2–5	2–5	2–5

(Xylazine is best administered 10 to 15 min prior to giving ketamine-acetylpromazine):

Example

Combination surgical anesthetic for a 4-kg rabbit:
    220 mg ketamine
      3 mg acetylpromazine
     20 mg xylazine

The anesthetic described in this example is usally sutiable for a surgical procedure that has the potential toelicit deep pain. Duration of anesthesia is 20 min and blood pressure is severely reduced. However, the prospect for recovery is good.

From Sedgwick, C.: Anesthesia for rabbits and rodents. *In* Kirk, R. W. (ed.): *Current Veterinary Therapy VII.* Philadelphia: W. B. Saunders Co., 1980, p. 708.

are usually not necessary. Sutures are removed in 10 days. Postoperative complications are uncommon.

COMMUNICABLE DISEASES

Dermatomycosis, salmonellosis, and hymenolepiasis are relatively common in laboratory animals. If diagnosed, the disease's public health significance should be explained to the client. Consultation with a physician familiar with communicable diseases can be helpful.

Leptospirosis, tularemia, sylvatic plague, lymphocytic choriomeningitis, and rabies can occur as natural diseases in laboratory species. Although extremely uncommon, their existence and significance should not be forgotten.

Vaccination against rabies and leptospirosis is not performed routinely unless the incidence of the disease in a specific area warrants it or an owner specifically requests it. Killed vaccines are used if they must be given.

References and Supplemental Reading

Crocker, C. L.: Rapid determination of urea nitrogen in serum or plasma without deproteinization. Am. J. Med. Techn. 33:361, 1967.

Farris, E. J., and Griffith, J. Q.: *The Rat in Laboratory Investigation.* Rpt. 1963. Philadelphia: J. B. Lippincott Co., 1967.

Green, E. L., et al.: *Biology of the Laboratory Mouse,* 2nd ed. New York: McGraw-Hill Book Co., 1966.

Hafez, E. S. E.: *Reproduction and Breeding Techniques for Laboratory Animals.* Philadelphia: Lea and Febiger, 1970.

Harkness, J. E., and Wagner, J. E.: *The Biology and Medicine of Rabbits and Rodents.* Philadelphia: Lea and Febiger, 1977.

Hoffman, R. A., Robinson, P. F., and Magalhaes, H.: *The Golden Hamster, Its Biology and Use in Medical Research.* Ames, IA: The Iowa State University Press, 1968.

Laboratory Animals. J. Lab. Anim. Sci. Assoc., Laboratory Animals Ltd., 7 Warwick Court, London, WCIR 5DP.

Laboratory Animal Science. Joliet, IL: American Association for Laboratory Animal Science.

Markowitz, J., Archibald, J., and Downie, H. G.: *Experimental Surgery,* 4th ed. Baltimore: Williams & Wilkins Co., 1959.

Melby, E. C., Jr., and Altman, N. H.: *Handbook of Laboratory Animal Science,* Vols. I and II. Cleveland, OH: CRC Press Inc., 1974.

Riley, V.: Adaptation of orbital bleeding technique to rapid serial blood studes. Proc. Soc. Exp. Biol. Med., 104:751, 1960.

Schwentker, V.: *The Gerbil: An Annotated Bibliography.* Presented by Tumblebrook Farm, West Brookfield, MA.

Wagner, J. E., and Manning, P. J.: *The Biology of the Guinea Pig.* New York: Academic Press, 1976.

Weisbroth, S. H., Flatt, R. E., and Kraus, A. L.: *The Biology of the Laboratory Rabbit.* New York: Academic Press, 1974.

Wescott, R. B.: *An Outline of Diseases of Laboratory Animals.* Columbia, MO: University of Missouri Press, 1969.

MEDICAL AND SURGICAL CARE OF THE PET FERRET

R. WAYNE RANDOLPH, V.M.D.

Flemington, New Jersey

The domestic ferret (*Mustela putorius furo*) is a fun-loving, gregarious member of the family Mustelidae that has become increasingly popular as a household pet. Because of its delightfully good-natured and inquisitive personality, this creature adapts well to human companionship, especially when raised from early age in close contact with humans. The ferret interacts well with other domestic pets (e.g., dogs, cats, and birds), and it is well suited for people seeking something a bit unusual in a pet.

Domestication of the ferret dates back to the

fourth century B.C., when ferrets were used to exterminate rats and snakes in Europe and Asia. In the mid 1870's, they were introduced into this country. Worldwide, the ferret exists only in captivity and is not a wild animal like its fellow mustelids (e.g., mink, weasels, skunks). The domestic ferret is not to be confused with America's native black-footed ferret (*Mustela nigripes*), which faces extinction. It has been estimated that 50,000 to 75,000 ferrets are sold yearly in the United States, the majority being sold as pets.

In addition to being household pets, ferrets play a major role in medical research. They serve to advance knowledge in such fields as vision research, neuroscience, virology, and toxicology. Ferrets play a minor role in the fur industry; their fur is incorporated into coats called "fitch."

In some states (e.g., California, New Hampshire, and Georgia) the keeping of ferrets is prohibited, whereas in other states there are laws regulating the possession of these animals. It is prudent to review state statutes before obtaining such a pet. The American Veterinary Medical Association has issued a cautionary statement indicating that ferrets may not make suitable pets in homes with small children.

This article describes some aspects of the medicine, surgery, husbandry, and reproductive physiology of this animal. Knowledge of these factors is helpful in keeping the ferret both well and a good pet.

SPECIES CHARACTERISTICS

Female ferrets are called jills, and they weigh 1 to 2½ lb (650 to 1100 gm). Male ferrets (called hobs) are typically twice the size of females and weigh 2½ to 4½ lb (1200 to 2000 gm). Baby ferrets are known as kits. Average body length (without the tail) measures 12 to 16 inches (30 to 40 cm).

Two color varieties are recognized. The fitch ferret is buff with a black mask, tail, and limbs; the albino ferret is white with pink eyes. Physiologic, anatomic, and reproductive data are presented in Table 1.

Hematology values (Table 2) are similar to those in cats. Serum chemistry values (Table 3) approach those in dogs and cats. Both hematology and clinical chemistry values may vary slightly with the color variety (i.e., fitch or albino). Blood can be collected by the following methods: caudal tail venipuncture, jugular venipuncture, retro-orbital puncture, and toenail clipping. Sedation is generally required except for toenail clipping. Depending on the quantity of blood required, jugular venipuncture is probably most reliable.

Mild to moderate proteinuria is often found in normal ferret urine (Table 4). Small amounts of blood may be found in the urine of estrous females. Careful cystocentesis and manual expression of the bladder both are acceptable means of collecting urine. Urine collection in ferrets can be difficult because these animals void small amounts frequently; finding a full bladder is uncommon.

With increasing diagnosis of cardiac disease in this species, it is useful to recognize the normal electrocardiogram (ECG). To obtain a ferret ECG, sedation is usually necessary. For the average-size adult ferret, administer 0.5 mg diazepam intramuscularly into one thigh; wait 5 minutes, then inject 20 mg of ketamine into the opposite thigh. The patient can be positioned in either right lateral or sternal recumbency. Table 5 provides some normal ECG data.

Table 1. *Species Information*

Parameter	Range or Value
Physiologic Data	
Life span	5–9 years (average 5–7)
Commercial breeding life	2–5 years
Body temperature	101–104°F (38–40°C)
Respiratory rate	32–36 breaths/min
Heart rate	220–250 beats/min (average 240)
Water consumption	75–100 ml/day
Chromosome number	2n = 40
Anatomic Data	
Dental formula	2 (I3/3, C1/1, P3/4, M1/2)
Vertebral formula	C-7, T-14, L-6, S-3, Cd-14 to Cd-18
Reproductive Data	
Gestation	39–46 days (average 42)
Litter size	2–17 kits (average 8)
False pregnancy	40–42 days
Placentation	Zonal
Implantation time	12–13 days
Weaning	5–6 weeks
Ovulation	30–40 hr postcoitus

Table 2. *Hematologic Values for Normal Ferrets**

Parameter	Mean	Range
Hematocrit (%)	52.3	42–61
Hemoglobin (g/dl)	17.0	15–18
Erythrocytes (10^6 cells/mm³)	9.17	6.8–12.2
Leukocytes (10^3 cells/mm³)	10.1	4.0–19
Leukocytes		
Lymphocytes (%)	34.5	12–54
Neutrophils (%)	58.3	11–84
Monocytes (%)	4.4	0–9.0
Eosinophils (%)	2.5	0–7.0
Basophils (%)	0.1	0–2.0
Reticulocytes (%)	4.6	1–14
Platelets (10^3 cells/mm³)	499	297–910
Total protein (gm/dl)	6.0	5.1–7.4

*Values are for both genders.
Reprinted with permission from Ryland, L. M., et al.: Comp. Cont. Ed. Pract. Vet. 5:25, 1983, which was adapted from Thornton et al.: Lab. Anim. 13:119, 1979.

Table 3. Serum Chemistry Values for
Normal Ferrets*

Parameter	Unit	Mean	Range
Glucose	mg/dl	136	94–207
BUN	mg/dl	22	10–45
Albumin	mg/dl	3.2	2.3–3.8
Alkaline phosphatase	IU/L	23	9–84
Aspartate aminotransferase (SAST; SGOT)	IU/L	65	28–120
Total bilirubin	mg/dl	<1.0	
Cholesterol	mg/dl	165	64–296
Creatinine	mg/dl	0.6	0.4–0.9
Sodium	mMol/L	148	137–162
Potassium	mMol/L	5.9	4.5–7.7
Chloride	mMol/L	116	106–125
Calcium	mg/dl	9.2	8.0–11.8
Phosphorus	mg/dl	5.9	4.0–9.1

*Values are for both genders.
Reprinted with permission from Ryland, L. M., et al.: Comp. Cont. Ed. Pract. Vet. 5:25, 1983, which was adapted from Thornton et al.: Lab. Anim. 13:119, 1979.

HISTORY, PHYSICAL EXAMINATION, AND RESTRAINT

Prior to bringing a ferret into the examination room, make certain the room is "ferret-proofed." Because a ferret can negotiate a hole barely 2 inches in diameter, locate and obstruct any potential avenues of escape. Be certain to examine under and around wall-mounted medical cabinets.

A complete medical history is appropriate prior to examination. Be aware that owners may not be knowledgeable about proper care, diet, or the difference between normal and abnormal conditions. Husbandry review and consultation is an important part, maybe the most important, of the office visit. If a veterinarian sees a sufficient number of ferrets, consider writing a handout on proper ferret care; be sure to include a short layman bibliography. Such a handout will save the veterinarian much time and ensure better care.

Perform a complete and thorough physical examination as one would on a cat. Evaluate all body systems as well and as extensively as possible. The biggest obstacle to thorough physical examination is the nearly perpetual motion of these patients; they are always moving. In most cases, the veteri-

Table 4. Urinalysis Results in Normal Ferrets, Based on 24-Hr Urine Samples

Parameter	Male	Female
Volume (ml/24 hr)	26	28
Sodium (mMol/24 hr)	1.9	1.5
Potassium (mMol/24 hr)	2.9	2.1
Chloride (mMol/24 hr)	2.4	1.9
pH	6.5–7.5	6.5–7.5
Protein (mg/dl)	7–33	0–32

Reprinted with permisson from Moody, K. D., et al.: Laboratory management of the ferret for biomedical research. Lab. Anim. Sci. 35:272, 1985.

Table 5. Electrocardiographic Data for
Normal Ferrets*

Parameter	Mean	Range
Rate	224 ± 51	150–340
Rhythm		
Normal sinus rhythm		
Sinus arrhythmia		
Measurements		
P wave		
Width	0.03 ± 0.009	0.015–0.04 sec
Height	0.106 ± 0.03	0.05–0.20 mv
P-R interval		
Width	0.05 ± 0.01	0.04–0.08 sec
QRS complex		
Q wave	Usually none	
R wave		
Width	0.049 ± 0.008	0.04–0.06 sec
Height	1.59 ± 0.63	0.6–3.15 mv
S wave		
Height	0.166 ± 0.101	0.1–0.25 mv
ST segment		
Width	0.030 ± 0.016	0.01–0.06 sec
QT interval		
Width	0.13 ± 0.027	0.10–0.18 sec
T wave		
Width	0.06 ± 0.01	0.03–0.1 sec
Height	0.24 ± 0.12	0.10–0.45 mv
Mean Electrical Axis (frontal plane)		+65°– +100°

*Ferrets in right lateral recumbency; sedation with ketamine and xylazine
Unpublished data from Drs. N. Joel Edwards and R. Wayne Randolph.

narian or the owner can restrain the patient by using his or her bare hands. Figure 1 depicts one suitable method. Sometimes, a small bath towel aids in this restraint. Light leather gloves are usually reserved for ferrets less than 6 months of age, which are more likely to bite. With most uncastrated males, such gloves are required. Chemical restraint is usually reserved for procedures (e.g., radiology, cystocentesis).

VACCINATIONS

Appropriate vaccination is imperative.

Canine Distemper

Ferrets are highly susceptible to canine distemper; virtually 100 per cent of patients that test positive die. Protection against this disease is afforded by vaccination with a modified live virus of chicken-embryo origin. Anecdotal evidence from veterinarians who treat ferrets suggests the use of the Fromm canine distemper vaccine (Fromm D, Solvay Veterinary, Inc.). It is a high egg passage vaccine, and it has caused no known vaccine breaks. Vaccines developed from ferret cell cultures are to be rigidly avoided, as incomplete attenuation can lead to clinical disease with canine distemper. A

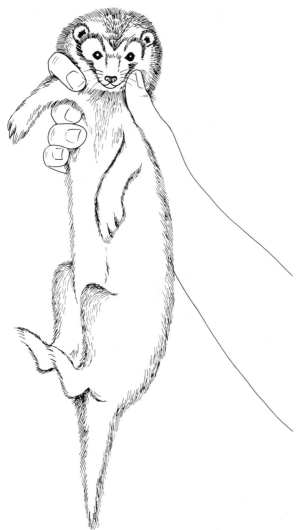

Figure 1. Proper restraint of a ferret. Use thumb and index finger to encircle the head, anterior to the forelegs; place the other three fingers just posterior to the forelegs and around the thorax. Rear legs can be supported with the other hand. Patient can be held against the body of the holder or against the table. (Modified from Kirk, R.W.: *Current Veterinary Therapy IX.* Philadelphia, W. B. Saunders, 1986.)

killed virus vaccine of high antigenicity, developed by new techniques, might be preferred over the modified live virus product, but it is not currently available.

First vaccination is administered at 6 to 10 weeks of age or at first presentation, which, in clinical practice, tends to be about 10 to 14 weeks of age (Table 6). A second dose is administered 3 to 4 weeks later; yearly boosters are given thereafter. The author empirically elects to use 4/10 cc of the 1 cc reconstituted vaccine solution; this is administered subcutaneously under the loose skin of the dorsal neck, using a 1-ml syringe with 26-gauge, ½-inch needle.

Table 6. *Schedule for Vaccination and Examination of Ferrets*

Age	Procedure
6 to 10 weeks (or first presentation)	First CDV*; fecal examination; physical examination; husbandry consultation
10 to 14 weeks (3 to 4 weeks after first presentation)	Second CDV; physical examination; husbandry review
4½ to 6 months	Spaying or castration; descenting
15 to 16 months (1 year after second CDV)	CDV (annual); fecal examination; physical examination; husbandry review

*Canine distemper vaccine; modified live virus of chicken-embryo cell culture origin; administered subcutaneously.

Rabies

The ferret is susceptible to rabies, and although rare, rabies has been reported to occur in this species. The use of rabies vaccine in ferrets remains controversial because labeling does not support its use in ferrets. This places the veterinarian in a dilemma because, in a rabies enzootic area, a decision must be made. *It is the opinion of the author that rabies vaccine should never be used in ferrets* (with the possible, single exception of a rabies epizootic inside an established zoologic park).

If a veterinarian determines that dire circumstances demand the use of rabies vaccine, only a killed product should be selected, preferably one of murine origin. *Under no circumstance should a live virus product be used.*

Other Vaccinations

For many years controversy boiled over the ferret's susceptibility to feline panleukopenia virus. Recent work has demonstrated definitively that the ferret is not susceptible to feline panleukopenia virus, canine parvovirus, raccoon parvovirus, or mink enteritis virus (Parrish et al., 1987).

It is not justified to use vaccines purported to give protection against such microbes as measles virus, canine adenovirus, canine parvovirus, canine parainfluenza virus, leptospira, feline rhinotracheitis virus, and feline calicivirus. The additional antigen burden is not warranted.

REPRODUCTIVE PHYSIOLOGY

Male

Male ferrets vary in their sexual activity according to the photoperiod; therefore, they are not sexually active year-round. Sexual maturity is reached in the spring following their birth (at about 8 to 12 months of age). Their breeding season, which begins in December and extends through July, precedes that of the female. This difference in breeding seasons is thought to be a functional adaptation allowing for proper sperm maturation.

In the nonbreeding season, testes are small, soft, and located in the subcutaneous layer of the caudoventral abdomen. As the breeding season approaches, the testes enlarge, become turgid, and descend into the scrotum. Scrotal hair is nearly lost at maximal testicular enlargement.

Body weight fluctuates widely (30 to 40 per cent) in both genders according to the photoperiod and breeding season. Subcutaneous fat accumulates in the fall and is lost in the spring. Also, in both genders the thick fur coat goes through seasonal cycles, with molting occurring in early spring.

Female

Jills are seasonally polyestrous, and they are induced ovulators. Like males, they reach sexual maturity in the spring following their birth (at about 8 to 12 months of age). Also like males, their breeding season is light dependent; it begins in March and continues through August.

Estrus is marked by profound vulvar tumescence and copious mucoserous vaginal discharge. This discharge may proceed to wet the perineum, posterior hind legs, and inguinal area in some cases; superficial perivulvar dermatitis may occur subsequent to the discharge. There is a generalized increase in body odor, and bilaterally symmetric alopecia occurs on the ventral abdomen and tail. Other than receptivity to copulation, no behavioral changes are noted.

Mating is prolonged and violent. The male batters, bites, and drags the female around by the nape of the neck. Coitus lasts 1 to 3 hr.

After coitus, ovulation occurs within 30 to 40 hr. If fertilization occurs, pregnancy continues for 42 days. In contrast to the case with other mustelids, there is no delayed implantation. Jills prefer solitude during the last 2 weeks of pregnancy. Eight kits comprise an average litter. Jills can produce a maximum of two litters per breeding season. After ovulation, the vulva decreases to normal size in 2 to 3 weeks.

If she is not bred, a jill will remain in continuous, protracted estrus until the end of the breeding season. Only spontaneous ovulation or the end of the breeding season halts this protracted estrus in nonbred females. If fertilization fails to occur after coitus, a pseudopregnancy lasting about 42 days takes place. Spontaneous ovulation also leads to pseudopregnancy.

ESTROUS BONE MARROW HYPOPLASIA

Pathogenesis

Estrous pancytopenia due to estrogen-induced bone marrow hypoplasia is a common and often fatal disease of nonspayed female ferrets in protracted estrus. This condition is known by a number of similar-sounding names. The extended estrus brings about chronically elevated estrogen levels. These high estrogen levels exert profound depressive effects on hematopoietic tissues, causing bone marrow hypoplasia. It is the bone marrow hypoplasia that is responsible for the clinical signs; these signs become evident with the depletion of erythrocytes, leukocytes, and platelets. *The ferret is one of the animals most affected by the toxic effects of estrogens. Most severely affected animals die. For this reason, all female ferrets not intended for breeding should be spayed.*

Clinical Signs

Clinical signs are multiple and vary according to the time of presentation. These signs include pale mucous membranes, cutaneous petechiae and ecchymoses, melenic stools, and moderate to severe bilaterally symmetric alopecia of the ventral abdomen and tail. Typically, the mucoserous vaginal discharge has moistened the perineum, inguinal area, and posterior ventral abdomen. Superficial perivulvar dermatitis is often present.

These animals are lethargic and anorexic; moderate to severe weight loss is common. Hypothermia is variable. Respiration is often depressed and labored. As a result of anemia, a systolic murmur and weak, rapid pulse are often noted. Systemic infection occurs occasionally. Posterior paralysis and paresis are sometimes observed. Hematologic findings include initial thrombocytosis and leukocytosis followed by thrombocytopenia, leukopenia, and anemia.

Prognosis

The prognosis for this condition remains extremely grave. It varies with the time of presentation and the rigor of therapy. Nonetheless, in patients showing clinical signs, the mortality rate can approach 100 per cent. When death occurs, it is typically from hemorrhagic anemia secondary to thrombocytopenia.

Despite a grave prognosis, some jills can be saved with timely and appropriate therapy. The earlier in the disease process a jill is presented, the better the prognosis. *No jill should be allowed to remain in estrus beyond 4 weeks.*

Treatment

There are three objectives in treating this condition: (1) to shut off the production of estrogens as quickly as possible, (2) to maintain and support the patient as the bone marrow recovers, and (3) to perform ovariohysterectomy as soon as the packed cell volume is normal or nearly normal.

Estrogen shutdown is accomplished by inducing ovulation. Rupture of the ovarian follicles can be brought about in a number of ways: (1) administration of human chorionic gonadotropin (HCG), (2) administration of gonadotropin-releasing hormone (GnRH), (3) mating, or (4) ovariohysterectomy. Mating is inappropriate at this time because it is overly stressful in this species. In the opinion of the author, ovariohysterectomy is inappropriate as well, because these patients are too fragile for anesthetic and surgical trauma. Administration of either HCG or GnRH is appropriate. Inject intramuscularly either 100 IU of HCG (Chorionic Gonadotropin, Lyphomed, Inc.) or 20 μg of GnRH (Cystorelin, CEVA Laboratories, Inc.). The injection may be repeated after 12 days; look for decreased vulvar swelling and turgidity as signs that ovulation has occurred. Of the two products, the author prefers HCG.

The second objective in treatment is maintenance and support of the patient during estrogen shutdown and subsequent bone marrow recovery. Remember that bone marrow does not recover immediately at the time of reduction of estrogen levels; such recovery proceeds slowly over weeks to months. Some marrow does not recover at all.

Useful supportive therapy includes good nursing and intensive care, fluids, appropriate pharmacologic agents, whole blood transfusions, and rigorous medical therapeutics. An incubator is ideal to combat hypothermia, but heating pads can be used as well. Medications reported to be helpful include anabolic steroids, corticosteroids, minerals and vitamins, antimicrobial agents, and lithium. Forced and assisted feedings with high-calorie nutritional products such as Ensure Plus (Ross Laboratories) or Nutri-Cal (Evsco Pharmaceuticals) are often necessary.

Multiple electrolyte solutions are used to combat dehydration. Intravenous fluid administration is possible but difficult. Instead, the author prefers subcutaneous fluid administration. The intraperitoneal route can be employed as well. It is probable that whole blood transfusions will also be required. Use only ferret blood. Usually, 2 to 5 ml of donor blood can be safely taken by jugular venipuncture with a 3- to 5-ml heparinized syringe from most larger ferrets under sedation. The preferable donor is a large male, as males are typically twice the size of females. This blood is transfused slowly into the patient's jugular vein, using a 25-gauge butterfly catheter. Transfusion into the peritoneum can also be done. Multiple transfusions (2 to 15) are often required. The time between transfusions is variable.

The third and final objective in treatment is ovariohysterectomy. This is performed only when the patient's packed cell volume is normal or nearly normal.

PARASITES

Dirofilaria

Dirofilariasis has been reported to occur both naturally and experimentally in the ferret. Microfilaremia is uncommon, as is the case in other abnormal hosts infected with *Dirofilaria immitis*. Ferrets infected with *D. immitis* may present in respiratory distress secondary to congestive heart failure.

Clinical signs prior to presentation include a progression from anorexia to depression to dyspnea. A short time interval elapses between hospital admission and death. Necropsy typically reveals severe cardiomegaly, ascites, reddish lungs (congestion), and pleural fluid. It appears that small worm burdens, as few as one, can lead to right-sided congestive heart failure.

Antemortem diagnosis is difficult because antigen detection kits are not helpful in ferrets, microfilaremia is uncommon, and patients die shortly after hospital admission. Presumptive diagnosis is based on clinical signs, thoracic radiographs, and a history of outdoor housing in an enzootic area.

The scope of this problem in ferrets is not fully appreciated. In enzootic areas, it seems reasonable to house ferrets indoors, to consider the use of a prophylactic medication, or both. The standard canine dose of diethylcarbamazine at 6.6 mg/kg or ivermectin (Heartgard, Merck), 6 μg/kg might be employed.

Ear Mites

Infestation with ear mites (*Otodectes cyanotis*) is a particularly common malady of ferrets, especially in kits obtained from a commercial source. Diagnosis is straightforward. Brown, waxy debris is observed in the opening of the external ear canal. The presence of mites is confirmed with an otoscope or by microscopic examination of waxy debris. Head shaking and ear scratching are *uncommon* signs of ear mite infestation in the ferret.

Commercial feline preparations for ear mites can be employed safely. Mitox Liquid (Norden) and Tresaderm (Merck) are two effective products. However, treatment must be diligent. Treatment failure is common and typically occurs for the following reasons: (1) the patient squirms and resists treatment, (2) the small diameter of the ear canal precludes easy application of the preparation along the canal's length, and (3) the ferret's body is not treated. Good client instruction helps to circumvent these problems. The whole body of the ferret should be treated with an appropriate flea product.

Fleas

Fleas (*Ctenocephalides*) can present a problem, especially when ferrets are housed with dogs and cats. The owner should check regularly for these parasites as one would on a dog or a cat. Moderate scratching is normal in the ferret and does not by itself constitute a diagnosis of flea infestation. When fleas are present on a ferret, the hair coat quickly becomes sparse. Those flea products safe for use on cats may be used on ferrets.

The wearing of a prescription, feline flea collar can be an effective prophylactic measure. One standard cat collar will yield three ferret collars. A cat flea collar is cut into thirds, one of these pieces is held around the ferret's neck, and the ends are sewn together with needle and thread. Most but not all ferrets will leave the collars on.

Other Parasites

Ferrets are susceptible to gastrointestinal parasites. Ascarids, coccidia, tapeworms, and *Giardia* have been reported. It is of note that gastrointestinal parasitism appears to be extremely rare with the exception of coccidia. The explanation of this rarity is not known.

Other parasites reported to occur in ferrets include *Toxoplasma*, *Sarcoptes scabei*, lungworms, and flukes. Tick infestation occurs as well but is not a common problem in pet ferrets that are housed indoors.

ANESTHESIA

Ferrets withstand anesthesia well. Many anesthetic protocols have been described for this species. Table 7 describes a regimen that has proved to be efficacious and safe. Using a 1-ml syringe with a 26-gauge, ½-inch needle, inject acepromazine subcutaneously in the dorsal neck region or intramuscularly in the posterior aspect of one thigh. Five to 30 min later, administer ketamine intramuscularly in the opposite thigh.

Ferrets can be intubated with small-bore, noncuffed endotracheal tubes, but the procedure is difficult. Instead, isoflurane or halothane is delivered to effect by small face mask in a semiopen delivery system, using low-flow technique. A small,

Table 7. Ferret Anesthetic Regimen

Drug	Dosage	Route of Administration
Acepromazine	0.1–0.25 mg/kg	Subcutaneous, intramuscular
Ketamine*	20–35 mg/kg*	Intramuscular*
Halothane or isoflurane	Low flow, low concentration, to effect	Face mask
Nitrous oxide†	Low flow, 50:50 with oxygen†	Face mask†

*Administered 5 to 30 min after the acepromazine.
†Optional.

soft towel is positioned between the rim of the face mask and the patient's neck; the towel prevents anesthetic gases from escaping into the surgery suite.

An alternative anesthetic regimen commonly employed in ferrets, especially in research laboratories, utilizes ketamine and xylazine mixed together in the same syringe and administered intramuscularly. The advantages of this system are that it is easy and there is no need for an anesthetic delivery system. Despite widespread use of this protocol, the author does not recommend its use because of concern about the cardiac arrhythmias, myocardial effects, and blood pressure changes that can occur with xylazine.

SURGERY

Indications

Two prophylactic procedures, neutering and descenting, are commonly practiced in ferrets.

All hobs not intended for breeding should be castrated. Castration is indicated to (1) diminish inappropriate urination, (2) decrease aggression toward humans and other ferrets, and (3) reduce body odor. Because body odor in intact male ferrets represents a greater problem than it does in intact females, castration is virtually mandatory.

It is strongly recommended to spay all jills not intended for breeding. Ovariohysterectomy is indicated to (1) prevent estrous bone marrow hypoplasia, (2) prevent pregnancy, (3) reduce body odor, and (4) prevent pseudopregnancy. *It is not recommended to spay a jill that is clinically ill with bone marrow hypoplasia. However, it is both appropriate and reasonable to spay a jill that is in prolonged estrus and has a packed cell volume that is normal or nearly normal.*

Both genders are descented to help alleviate body odor.

Procedures

Ferrets are hearty surgical patients. The anesthetic regimen previously described (Table 7) is employed. To curb loss of body heat, a heating pad is always placed under the patient. Leg restraints are easily fashioned from ½-inch surgical adhesive tape.

Because ferrets reach sexual maturity in the spring after their birth, they become sexually active (reach puberty) at different ages. Neutering is safely performed at 5 months of age, but it may be performed earlier or later.

The surgical instruments normally present in the veterinarian's standard surgical pack are suitable for these procedures. Additional instruments found to be helpful include a smaller needle holder, an Adson tissue forceps, and some high-quality 4½-inch Halsted mosquito hemostats.

The jill is placed in dorsal recumbency for surgery, and, after a ventral midline incision, standard feline procedure is followed. The suspensory, broad, and round ligaments are less well developed than in the queen; this facilitates exteriorization of the uterine horns. The ovaries are encased in much fat, which requires dissection before ligating the vessels.

Castration is performed according to standard, closed canine procedure. The testes will be large and descended into the scrotal sac when surgery is performed during the male breeding season (December through July). The testes will be small and located cranial to the scrotum when surgery is performed during the nonbreeding season (August through November).

Descenting, or surgical removal of the paired musk sacs lateral to the anus, is always performed *after* the neutering operation in order to preserve sterility of the instruments. Figure 2 illustrates patient positioning. A number of procedures have been described, but the author prefers the standard closed technique followed in canine and feline anal sacculectomy. The author does not recommend filling the sacs with contrast material, as cannulation of the ducts is difficult.

In both the neutering and descenting procedures, small sutures (sizes 3-0 and 4-0) of appropriate materials are selected. Excellent hemostasis and gentle tissue handling are important.

Complications

The potential surgical complications associated with these procedures parallel those described for dogs and cats. Complications are uncommon. More problems will occur if good husbandry practices are neglected, or if inattention is paid to managing the medical peculiarities of ferrets. Examples of such problems include infection with clinical canine distemper due to inappropriate vaccination, anesthetic death due to inappropriate protocol, patient escape, infection with human influenza virus from infected hospital workers, and subsequent death from estrogen-induced bone marrow suppression when the packed cell volume was not measured before surgery.

BODY ODOR

If keeping a pet ferret can be said to have one drawback, it is the animal's body odor. Three sources contribute to this odor: (1) the paired anal sacs adjacent to the anus, (2) the gonads (via hormonally sensitive sebaceous glands in the skin), and (3) sebaceous and apocrine glands in the perianal skin. Odor from the first two sources is eliminated surgically. Bathing helps to reduce odor emanating from the skin. Ferrets are bathed easily and as needed (up to one to two times per week). Select a mild baby shampoo or a hypoallergenic shampoo (Allergroom, Allerderm, Inc.).

Secretion from the paired anal sacs is probably the most foul smelling of the three sources contributing to this body odor. This offensive fluid secretion is repulsive. All mustelids and most carnivores have paired anal sacs. In a wild environment, anal sac secretions are used for scent marking, for anointing territory, and for defense. A pet ferret is most likely to express its anal sacs when frightened. The owner must understand that anal sacculectomy alone will not eliminate the animal's odor. It is necessary as well to neuter them and give them regular baths.

FERRET ATTACKS ON HUMAN INFANTS

A tragic situation exists in which apparently healthy, normal, and docile ferrets have bitten and attacked human infants, seemingly without provocation (Paisley and Lauer, 1988). The infants are usually less than 6 months old, and the attacks typically occur when the infant is in bed or sleeping. Adult supervision is absent. Injuries typically involve the face, and bites are usually numerous. Moderate to severe injury and mutilation can occur.

Why this situation occurs is not understood. Rabies has not been diagnosed in any of the cases. It is common for ferrets to lie down near napping and sleeping adult humans with no ill effect. Although very few occurrences have been reported, there is obvious cause for concern. More information needs to be forthcoming. *Therefore, it is strongly recommended that no ferret be left without adult supervision in the vicinity of awake or sleeping human infants!*

Editor's Note: The editor feels that ferrets are dangerous and inappropriate pets in households with young children.

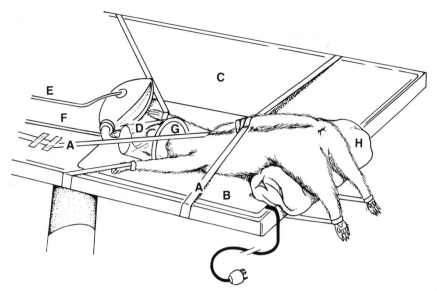

Figure 2. Patient positioning for anal sacculectomy. *A*, One-half-inch surgical adhesive tape stirrups to secure feet and tail; *B*, heating pad under whole body; *C*, surgery table tilted approximately 30°; *D*, transparent plastic anesthetic face mask with rubber gasket; *E*, anesthetic gas scavenging system; *F*, anesthetic gas delivery hose; *G*, folded paper towel or soft cloth placed between patient's ventral neck and the face mask aperture. (Reprinted with permission from Bojrab, M.J.: *Current Techniques in Small Animal Surgery*, 3rd ed. Philadelphia, Lea & Febiger, in print.)

HOUSING

Appropriate and adequate housing is necessary to promote good health and to avoid husbandry problems. Ferrets can be housed in a variety of ways, according to the needs and preferences of the owner and the number of animals involved. Outdoor housing is acceptable if properly planned and constructed to consider weather conditions and parasitism (e.g., dirofilariasis, fleas, and ticks). Most pet owners prefer to house their pet(s) indoors; this is probably preferable, especially when only a few, nonbreeding animals are kept.

Within the home, a cage is required. How much time the pet is held in the cage remains a personal decision on the part of the owner; however, most ferrets are caged at least during the night. Cages ought to be constructed of impermeable material to avoid the absorption and retention of odors. Ideal materials include plastic, fiberglass, and metal mesh. A sliding bottom tray for cleaning is helpful. Some owners choose a commercial cage designed for dogs, cats, rabbits, or mink. A small bed for sleeping is kept within the cage; it can be a small box, towel, or blanket. Ferrets love to completely wrap themselves in a towel or small blanket when sleeping. Without a bed a ferret will tend to sleep in its litter. The cage and its contents (bed, bowls, towel) ought to be easy to maintain and should be kept clean at all times.

Ferrets are easily trained to use a litter box, and one box should be maintained in the cage and at least one other within the home. Any small plastic container will do; square metal cakepans work well

also. The bottom of the litter box must be weighted to avoid spillage, and the box should always be placed in a corner. Litter material can be the white, clay cat litter or torn and shredded newspaper. Avoid the colored, scented cat litter designed to absorb odor. Litter boxes must be changed frequently and kept clean. A soiled litter box results in odor, and the ferret may choose to defecate and urinate elsewhere.

In order to maintain a ferret's safety, the owner's home must be "ferret-proofed." These small mustelids can easily crawl through an aperture 2 inches in diameter, so attention should be given to the bottom of appliances (stove, refrigerator, washer), spaces around plumbing and pipes, and openings in the walls. Without this attention, ferrets will be lost. They are the escape artists *par excellence*. It is probably prudent to supervise them when they are out of the cage.

DIET

The ferret's minimum nutritional requirements for growth, maintenance, pregnancy, and lactation have not yet been determined. Based on gastrointestinal anatomy and physiology, it is likely that these requirements parallel those of the mink and the cat. Ferrets have a poor ability to digest fiber. A desirable ferret diet is one high in both protein and fat, and low in fiber.

Commercial breeding colonies fare well on commercial mink diets. As mink diets are not readily available, experience has shown that pet ferrets do well on a diet of high-quality, dry commercial cat food. Some canned cat food may be added occasionally to increase protein intake, but this supplementation is probably not necessary except in the case of pregnant or lactating jills. They require this supplementation daily. Low protein intake has been associated with poor reproductive performance. Uncooked food is to be avoided.

Commercial ferret diets in dry form are newly available (e.g., Purina Mini Friends Ferret Chow, Purina Mills), and it is recommended that they be used in preference to commercial feline diets. These diets may not yet be available everywhere.

Ferrets eat to meet caloric requirements. They eat frequent, small meals throughout the day; therefore, they are offered free access to food. Obesity in later life associated with free choice feeding does not appear to be a problem in these animals. The owner should be aware that ferrets tend to relocate and cache their food, which can present a particular problem with canned food and table scraps.

Water must always be available. If a water bowl is used, it should have a weighted bottom to prevent spillage, as ferrets are active, messy eaters. The hanging water bottle of the rabbit or hamster type, which is less messy, is preferred. The food bowl also should have a weighted bottom or be attached to the side of the cage.

Avoid bones of all types to prevent gastrointestinal blockage. A dry, brittle hair coat with dry, scaly skin, occurring especially during the cold months, may necessitate the addition of small amounts of saturated and unsaturated fatty acids to the diet. Commercial preparations (e.g., Nutriderm, Norden) are useful for this purpose. This same hair coat condition occurring year-round suggests the need for increased protein intake. Try adding canned cat food to the diet or changing to commercial ferret chow.

CARE

When selecting a ferret, obtain a young kit (aged 5 to 6 weeks), preferably from a breeder who selects for good temperament. Ferrets get along well with dogs, cats, birds, and other animals, provided they have become accustomed to the other animals. Households with ferrets tend to keep more than one; two is probably ideal.

Claws may be trimmed by using either a human or animal nail trimmer. Declawing is neither appropriate nor needed; the claws are not retractable. A thin, lightweight pet collar (cut-down cat collar) with an identification tag or identification barrel and a bell is useful. The attached bell aids in locating the ferret. Most ferrets tolerate these collars. Some owners prefer a harness instead of a collar. Many ferrets can be trained to walk on a leash.

Ferrets have poorly developed sweat glands; therefore, they regulate heat loss by panting. When the environmental temperature exceeds 90°F (32°C), they are prone to heat exhaustion. Keep this problem in mind. Like other animals, they must not be left inside a closed automobile during warm weather.

Mature ferrets typically present on annual physical examination with brownish black, waxy debris bilaterally in the ears. Otoscopic examination reveals no ear mites. The problem appears unrelated to the ear mite problem of young kits, and it continues chronically. If not treated, the ears tend to accumulate this waxy debris and become inflamed. In affected ferrets, consider monthly cleaning with a cotton swab and one drop of mineral oil or Panolog ointment (Solvay Veterinary, Inc.).

OTHER MEDICAL CONDITIONS

Proliferative Colitis

Proliferative colitis occurs as a poorly understood disorder of ferrets. It is a disease of chronic wasting. Clinical signs include mucohemorrhagic diarrhea, weight loss, anorexia, and possible rectal prolapse. *Campylobacter jejuni* and *Campylobacter*-like bacteria are cultured from many cases. There is no successful treatment. Antimicrobial therapy is unsuccessful despite sensitivity data. Affected animals die or require euthanasia.

Campylobacter jejuni and *Campylobacter*-like bacteria can be cultured from both clinically ill animals and apparently healthy ones. Findings that this organism can be cultured from some clinically normal ferrets imply that ferrets may act as a potential reservoir of infection for human campylobacteriosis.

Aleutian Disease of Ferrets

Aleutian disease was first described in mink, caused by a parvovirus. The disease in mink is often fatal.

Aleutian disease of ferrets is also caused by a parvovirus. It is not entirely clear whether the ferret parvovirus is identical to the mink virus, or whether it is serologically distinct.

In most ferret cases infection is subclinical. Occasionally, clinical disease occurs and takes the form of a chronic, progressive wasting illness. Black, tarry feces and hypergamma-globulinemia may occur; the serum gamma-globulin fraction can exceed 20 per cent of total serum proteins. There is no treatment and no vaccine. Diagnosis is by serum counterimmunoelectrophoresis or necropsy. Clinically affected animals die or require euthanasia.

Feline Leukemia Virus

Some ferrets test positive for the feline leukemia virus when tested by the enzyme-linked immunosorbent assay (ELISA). These positive-testing ferrets include both clinically normal animals and animals ill with lymphosarcoma, severe anemia, splenomegaly, and other conditions. The nature of this relationship is not fully understood. It has been postulated that a cross-reacting retrovirus accounts for the positive tests (Gorham, 1988). Ferrets are not known to be susceptible to feline leukemia virus or related feline viruses.

Urolithiasis

Urolithiasis and lower urinary tract infection occur in both male and female ferrets. Magnesium ammonium phosphate hexahydrate (struvite) is the mineral typically encountered and may be found in the kidney, urinary bladder, or urethra. Urethral obstruction can occur in the hob. Treatment and management is the same as for the cat.

Heart Disease

A moderately wide spectrum of cardiac diseases occurs in the ferret. Congestive heart failure is known to occur. Ferrets can present with dilated (congestive) or hypertrophic cardiomyopathy. Dirofilariasis and subsequent congestive heart failure is probably the most commonly reported cardiac condition.

Management of ferret heart disease varies according to the diagnosis, and it parallels the protocols used in companion animal practice for similar conditions.

Splenomegaly

Splenomegaly occasionally occurs in ferrets. It has been demonstrated both in normal ferrets on physical examination and in clinically ill animals suffering from a variety of maladies. Such maladies include Aleutian disease, proliferative colitis, severe anemia, and splenic lymphosarcoma.

Do not empirically perform a splenectomy on finding splenomegaly. Instead, do a medical workup to establish a diagnosis. If the workup does not yield a diagnosis, consider laparotomy and splenic biopsy. Much work needs to be done to determine the causes of splenomegaly in ferrets.

Influenza

Ferrets are susceptible to a number of strains of human influenza virus. The disease is nonfatal, and the treatment is symptomatic. Initial clinical signs of infection include pyrexia, listlessness, and anorexia. These signs mimic those of canine distemper. Recovery typically occurs within 5 to 7 days. It might be wise not to handle pet ferrets when human family members suffer with the flu.

Other Problems

Ferrets are susceptible to a moderately long list of other medical problems that have been described in the literature. A number of fine reviews are listed under References and Supplemental Reading. With the increasing popularity of this pet and its continued use as a valuable laboratory research animal, more information and disease processes will be reported in the future.

References and Supplemental Reading

Bernard, S. L., Gorham, J. R., and Ryland, L. M.: Biology and diseases of ferrets. In Fox, J. G., Cohen, B. J., and Loew, F. M. (eds.): Laboratory Animal Medicine. New York: Academic Press, 1984, pp. 385–397.

Besch-Williford, C. L.: Biology and medicine of the ferret. Vet. Clin. North Am. 17:1155, 1987.

Burke, T. J.: Common diseases and medical management of ferrets. In Jacobson, E. R., and Kollias, G. V. (eds.): Contemporary Issues in Small Animal Practice: Exotic Animals. New York: Churchill Livingstone, 1988, pp. 247–260.

Fox, J. G.: Biology and Diseases of the Ferret. Philadelphia: Lea & Febiger, 1988.

Gorham, J. R.: Personal communication, 1988.

Moody, K. D., Bowman, T. A., and Lang, C. M.: Laboratory management of the ferret for biomedical research. Lab. Anim. Sci. 35:272, 1985.

Paisley, J. W., and Lauer, B. A.: Severe facial injuries to infants due to unprovoked attacks by pet ferrets. J.A.M.A. 259:2005, 1988.

Parrish, C. R., Leathers, C. W., Pearson, R., et al.: Comparisons of feline panleukopenia virus, canine parvovirus, raccoon parvovirus, and mink enteritis virus and their pathogenicity for mink and ferrets. Am. J. Vet. Res. 48:1429, 1987.

Randolph, R. W.: Ovariohysterectomy and orchiectomy in the pet ferret. In Bojrab, M. J. (ed.): Current Techniques in Small Animal Surgery. 3rd ed. Philadelphia: Lea & Febiger (in press).

Randolph, R. W.: Anal sacculectomy in the pet ferret. In Bojrab, M. J. (ed.): Current Techniques in Small Animal Surgery. 3rd ed. Philadelphia: Lea & Febiger (in press).

Ryland, L. M., and Gorham, J. R.: The ferret and its diseases. J.A.V.M.A. 173:1154, 1978.

Ryland, L. M., Bernard, S. L., and Gorham, J. R.: A clinical guide to the pet ferret. Comp. Cont. Ed. Pract. Vet. 5:25, 1983.

Sherrill, A., and Gorham, J.: Bone marrow hypoplasia associated with estrus in ferrets. Lab. Anim. Sci. 35:280, 1985.

Thornton, P. C., Wright, P. A., Sacra, P. J., et al.: The ferret, Mustela putorius furo, as a new species in toxicology. Lab. Anim. 13:119, 1979.

Williams, C. S. F.: Practical Guide to Laboratory Animals. St. Louis: C. V. Mosby, 1976, pp. 65–71.

Winsted, W.: Ferrets. Neptune City, NJ: T.F.H. Publications, 1981.

UPDATE ON AVIAN ANESTHESIA

KEVEN FLAMMER, D.V.M.

Raleigh, North Carolina

Birds have become common veterinary patients, and the need for safe and effective anesthetic regimens has gained increasing importance. The purpose of this article is to review the anesthetic techniques that have proved reliable in clinical practice. Information on the many other anesthetic agents that have been tried in birds is available in the references.

PREANESTHETIC CONSIDERATIONS

Birds are riskier candidates for anesthesia than domestic mammals. They frequently hide signs of disease and should be carefully examined before anesthesia is attempted. Special attention should be paid to their hydration, nutritional status, and how well they tolerate the stress of handling. Depending on the patient and the procedure, a complete blood count and panel of biochemical tests (e.g., aspartate aminotransferase, uric acid, total protein, and glucose) provide valuable information about the patient and also provide baseline values with which to compare postoperative tests. Whenever possible, depressed, traumatized, and dehydrated patients should be stabilized with appropriate therapy prior to anesthesia or surgery.

The crop should be empty prior to inducing anesthesia, as crop fluid may be passively regurgitated and aspirated during induction. This can be accomplished by briefly fasting the bird for 2 to 4 hr or by removing the fluid with a syringe and tube. Birds have a higher metabolic rate than mammals; if they are fasted overnight, glycogen stores in the liver will be depleted.

Care should be taken to support the patient during anesthesia. Anesthesia and handling times should be minimized by meticulous coordination and planning by the anesthetist and surgeon. Anesthetized birds lose a tremendous amount of body heat, so the operating room should be maintained at 75 to 80°F (23.9 to 26.7°C), and the patient should be placed on a water-circulating heating pad and surrounded by hot water bottles.

Little research has been conducted on the actions of preanesthetic medications in birds. In mammals, atropine sulfate (0.02 to 0.04 mg/kg IM) decreases oral and respiratory secretions, decreases gastrointestinal motility, and increases heart rate, but its effects in birds are poorly documented. Some clinicians advocate its use in birds if respiratory secretions are considered a potential problem. Diazepam (0.5 to 1.5 mg/kg IV or IM) has been used to calm fractious birds prior to induction (Taylor, 1987).

SELECTION OF THE ANESTHETIC PROTOCOL

Selection of a particular agent depends on the methods available, the effects on the species to be anesthetized, and the purpose of the anesthetic procedure. Local anesthetics are rarely used in birds, mostly because of the risk of toxicity in small patients (Altman, 1980). In addition, most procedures require restraint as well as analgesia, so general anesthesia is preferred. Both parenteral and inhalational agents are available for general anesthesia in birds.

Injectable anesthetics are relatively easy to administer and inexpensive; however, it is more difficult to control the level of anesthesia and oxygen status of the patient. Since injected drugs must be metabolized, recovery times are usually prolonged, and the bird may be depressed for many hours following the procedure. This may be a significant factor in ill birds, especially those with organ abnormalities that may prolong drug metabolism. Individual and species variability in response to injected drugs adds an additional challenge, and more extensive preoperative and postoperative monitoring may be required than with inhalation anesthesia. Injectable anesthetics are most often used for short procedures in relatively healthy birds when dosing by this method is convenient, or for surgery around the head, where intubation may be difficult and may preclude delivery of inhalational anesthetics. In these circumstances, or when inhalation anesthetics are not available, the combination of ketamine and xylazine can be used.

In ill birds, control of anesthesia is more critical, and inhalation anesthetics are usually preferred. Induction and recovery are usually smooth, with little species and individual variation. The plane of anesthesia achieved with the newer agents halothane and isoflurane can be adjusted precisely. Since little or no metabolism is required for excretion, recovery is usually faster and more complete than with injectable anesthetics. Of the three inhalation agents available to veterinary practitioners (methoxyflurane, halothane, and isoflurane), isoflurane is the agent generally preferred for avian anesthesia.

INJECTABLE ANESTHETICS

The injectable anesthetic regimen of choice for most birds is a combination of ketamine (Ketaset, Bristol) and xylazine (Rompun, Haver-Lockhart). Ketamine is a dissociative anesthetic that produces a cataleptoid state with little respiratory or cardiovascular depression. Use of ketamine alone results in poor muscle relaxation, potentially inadequate analgesia, and stormy inductions and recoveries. Combining ketamine with xylazine results in better muscle relaxation, better analgesia, and smoother recovery.

Recommended doses for ketamine are 10 to 30 mg/kg IM and 2.5 to 5 mg/kg IV and for xylazine are 1 to 4 mg/kg IM and 0.25 to 0.5 mg/kg IV (Harrison, 1986). Suggested volumes for use in common pet bird species are provided in Table 1. If the intravenous route is used, approximately one half of the recommended dose should be given, with more drug administered to effect. These doses provide anesthesia for approximately 10 to 45 min. If longer anesthesia is required, additional ketamine alone may be administered at a dose of one fourth to one third of the initial dose, or the patient may be switched to gas anesthesia.

An occasional problem encountered when using ketamine-xylazine intramuscularly is the individual and species variability in the dosage required to produce adequate anesthesia. Some birds given recommended doses remain partially awake and resist handling when stimulated. This results in time-consuming periods of waiting for the bird to become anesthetized. A number of procedures help ameliorate this problem. First, the bird should be

Table 1. *Maximum Intramuscular Doses of Ketamine (100 mg/ml) for Use with Xylazine (20 mg/ml)**

Species	Intramuscular	Intravenous
Budgerigars	0.01	0.005
Cockatiels	0.02	0.01
Conures	0.05	0.025
Lorikeets, rosellas	0.07	0.035
Amazons, miniature macaws	0.05–0.10	0.025–0.05
African greys	0.08–0.10	0.04–0.05
Cockatoos	0.12–0.15	0.06–0.07
Macaws	0.15–0.20	0.075–0.10

*Amount given in volume (ml) of ketamine to be mixed with an equal *volume* of xylazine before administering.

Reprinted with permission from Harrison, G. J.: Anesthesiology. *In* Harrison, G. J., and Harrison, L. H. (eds.): *Clinical Avian Medicine and Surgery.* Philadelphia: W. B. Saunders Co., 1986, p. 555.

placed in a quiet area in a warm, dark cardboard box immediately following injection and should not be disturbed for at least 3 to 5 min. Any disturbance may increase induction time. If halothane (Fluothane, Ayerst) or isoflurane (Aerrane, Anaquest) is available, supplying a few minutes of gas anesthesia via a mask often induces the partially awake bird. The gas can frequently be removed and the procedure continued without inhalation anesthesia. A low dose of valium (0.5 mg/kg IV) may also accomplish induction. As a final option, additional ketamine may be administered (at a rate of one fourth to one third of the original ketamine dose); however, this may prolong the recovery period.

Prolonged recovery periods are another potential problem, particularly if high doses of ketamine are required. Ketamine is excreted by the kidneys, so administering intravenous fluids (e.g., lactated Ringer's solution) will help diurese the patient and aid in the elimination of the drug. Stroking and turning the patient every 15 min may also speed recovery.

Various clinicians have reported difficulty when using ketamine-xylazine combinations in waterfowl, and some owls and accipiters (broad-winged hawks) (Redig, 1982). Special care should be used when anesthetizing these species.

INHALATION ANESTHETIC AGENTS

Delivery of Inhalation Anesthetics

Inhalation agents should be delivered with oxygen via a nonrebreathing circuit, such as a Bain's or an Ayre's T system. Induction can be accomplished by face mask or by placing the bird in an anesthetic chamber. Some avian clinicians advocate inducing birds quickly with high concentrations of anesthetic. The author has found it much safer to take a minute or two longer and induce birds with lower levels. Some of the unexplained deaths associated with halothane induction may have been due to the higher levels used.

For short procedures (less than 20 min) in healthy birds, it may be expedient simply to mask the bird. For longer procedures or when anesthetizing ill birds, it is safer to intubate the patient. Birds have complete tracheal rings, so uncuffed tubes (e.g., Cole or Magill) should be used. Inflation of cuffed tubes may cause pressure necrosis and tracheal damage. A selection of even-sized tubes ranging from nos. 4 to 22 French is adequate for most pet bird patients. Larger sizes are required for eagles and large zoologic species. The tubes should be shortened to reduce dead space.

To intubate following induction, the assistant restrains the head while the intubator opens the beak and pulls the tongue rostrally. This exposes the glottis, which is located directly behind the tongue. If the tongue is difficult to grasp, gentle digital pressure in the intramandibular space will push the tongue and glottis rostrally. The tube is gently seated in the glottis and secured by taping it to the lower beak.

Great care should be taken when birds are intubated. Slight movement of the tube within the trachea can irritate or lacerate the tracheal mucosa. This may cause bleeding or increase mucus production, which can easily plug the small-diameter tubes used in birds. The anesthetist must also be careful to monitor filling of the reservoir bag in the anesthesia circuit. The bag should be kept slightly filled. Small patients have a small tidal volume. Thus, if the bag is completely deflated, it is possible that fresh gases are bypassing the patient; if the bag is overfilled, the patient may not be able to overcome the resistance to breathing and may suffocate.

During long procedures, spontaneously breathing birds can become apneic and acidotic. Intermittent positive-pressure ventilation (IPPV) can be accomplished by bagging the patient 10 to 30 times per minute with the reservoir bag or by placing the bird on a mechanical ventilator. Pressures of 12 to 24 cm H_2O can be tolerated (Sedgwick, 1980).

METHOXYFLURANE

RECOMMENDATIONS. Induce the bird at 3 to 4 per cent, maintain at 1 to 2 per cent. Induction is variable and may take 5 to 15 min. Depending on the length of the procedure, birds usually recover to standing position in 10 to 30 min, but postrecovery depression may last several hours.

Methoxyflurane (Metofane, Pitman-Moore) is a halogenated ether that is much more soluble than halothane or isoflurane, so induction and recovery times as well as the time needed to see a response to a change in vaporizer setting are prolonged. A greater percentage of the drug must be metabolized, so postrecovery depression is prolonged and the potential for organ toxicity greater. Dose-related nephrotoxicity and hepatotoxicity have been reported in other species, and this toxicity may be potentiated if the liver and the kidneys are compromised at the time of anesthesia. Methoxyflurane is a better analgesic than halothane; however, halothane and isoflurane are generally preferred because they offer more precise control of anesthesia.

Methoxyflurane should be delivered with oxygen through a vaporizer. At one time, it was popular to administer methoxyflurane via the open drop method (e.g., place the bird's head in an 8-oz urine cup containing three cotton balls saturated with methoxyflurane). This practice is not recommended because control of anesthesia is difficult, hypoxia is

likely if the procedure is prolonged, and personnel may be exposed to gas waste.

HALOTHANE

RECOMMENDATIONS. Induce the bird at 1 to 2.5 per cent, maintain at 0.5 to 1.5 per cent. Induction usually occurs within 1 to 5 min, and recovery to standing position in 3 to 8 min, depending on the length of procedure. Postrecovery depression may last several hours.

Halothane is a halogenated hydrocarbon with much lower solubility than methoxyflurane. Induction and recovery are faster, and the plane of anesthesia can be rapidly altered. Because of this, birds receiving halothane anesthesia must be carefully monitored throughout the anesthetic procedure. Halothane sensitizes the myocardium to catecholamines, increasing the risk of arrhythmias and cardiac arrest. Birds anesthetized for more than 2 hr have a reduced rate of recovery, so caution should be exercised when using halothane for prolonged procedures in small birds.

The major advantages of halothane over methoxyflurane are faster induction and recovery times and the ability to rapidly alter the plane of anesthesia.

ISOFLURANE

RECOMMENDATIONS. Induce the bird at 2.5 to 3 per cent, maintain at 2 per cent. Induction usually occurs in 1 to 5 min, recovery in 2 to 8 min. There is little postrecovery depression.

Isoflurane is a halogenated ether that is highly insoluble, so excretion is almost entirely through the respiratory tract. Induction and recovery times are similar to halothane. However, isoflurane offers better analgesia, and there is little postrecovery depression. Birds quickly return to normal behaviors and frequently eat shortly after surgery. This is a major advantage, particularly in small birds because their high metabolic rate renders them prone to glycogen depletion and hypoglycemia following anesthesia. Other advantages include more precise control of anesthetic levels and less sensitization of the myocardium to catecholamines than with halothane. In addition, fewer problems have been noted with prolonged anesthesia. Several birds anesthetized for more than 3 hr recovered quickly and completely following isoflurane anesthesia.

Respiratory arrest is occasionally encountered with isoflurane anesthesia. Isoflurane is a respiratory depressant, and apnea may accompany high levels or rapid induction. Since respiration is required for excretion, apnea delays excretion of the drug. If apnea occurs, the chest should be thumped to stimulate respiration. If this fails, the bird should be intubated and manually resuscitated. It is fortunate that with isoflurane anesthesia the interval between respiratory and cardiac arrest is usually prolonged. Therefore, there usually is time to resuscitate the patient. Studies in spontaneously breathing cranes have indicated that respiratory acidosis occurs during isoflurane anesthesia and contributes to respiratory depression (Ludders et al., 1987). Respiratory acidosis can be reduced if breathing is assisted, either by a ventilator or by manually bagging the patient 10 to 30 times per minute.

Isoflurane is highly recommended and is used by the author for most anesthetic procedures in birds. Its wide margin of safety, rapid induction, and rapid and more complete recovery make it the ideal avian anesthetic. It is useful in routine situations when other anesthetics would be considered impractical. When performing radiography or collecting laboratory samples from fractious birds, the author frequently finds that it is less stressful to the bird to quickly mask it and deliver isoflurane than to use forceful handling. The disadvantages of isoflurane are high cost (regarding both the anesthetic and the vaporizer needed to deliver it) and the occasional episode of apnea.

MONITORING ANESTHESIA

Anesthetized birds are more challenging to monitor than are most mammals. In the author's experience, the heart and respiratory rates and character, response to positional changes, response to plucking feathers, and the withdrawal reflex provide the best constellation of signs to monitor the patient. There is much individual and species variation in what these signs indicate, so monitoring anesthetized birds is sometimes more of an art than a science. However, with a little practice, both veterinarians and veterinary technicians can readily learn to adequately monitor birds.

In the ideal situation, the bird would be at the lightest plane of anesthesia that permits the procedure to be accomplished. At a surgical plane of anesthesia, the patient should have slow, even, deep respirations and a relatively slow, even heart rate, the corneal reflex should be present, but the patient should not respond to changes in position or plucking of feathers. A slight withdrawal reflex may be present. The patient may be too deeply anesthetized if the heart rate is markedly slow or irregular, or if breathing is slow and shallow. Absence of a corneal reflex also indicates that the patient is too deeply anesthetized.

The small size of avian patients also complicates monitoring. By the time the patient is prepared for surgery, it may disappear under the drapes and the surgeon's hands. Monitoring can be aided by the use of esophageal stethoscopes, ECG oscilloscopes, cloacal temperature probes, and clear plastic drapes that allow greater visualization of the patient. Care must be taken that the weight of the drapes and the placement of the surgeon's hands and instruments do not compromise respiration. Birds lack a diaphragm and move air through the respiratory system by elevation and depression of the sternum. Effort is required for both inspiration and expiration, and pressure on the sternum may compromise respiration.

Most birds benefit from fluid administration during extended anesthesia, and fluid replacement is critical when blood loss occurs. It is difficult to maintain intravenous catheters in small birds, as their veins are thin-walled and it is easy to collapse the catheter or puncture the vessel if the position of the vessel changes. It is possible to deliver bolus fluids with repeated intravenous administration into the wing and the jugular veins. If blood loss is minimal, 10 ml/kg of lactated Ringer's with 5 per cent glucose is administered at the end of the procedure. Additional fluid and iron dextran (5 mg/kg IM) may be administered if blood loss occurs.

RECOVERY

Birds should be allowed to recover in a quiet, dark, warm, unobstructed environment. Birds that have received halothane or isoflurane anesthesia are given oxygen until they are standing and resist handling. Following methoxyflurane or injectable anesthesia, the oral cavity is wiped dry with a cotton ball to make sure secretions do not block the trachea, and the bird is loosely wrapped in a towel to restrict movement during recovery. The bird is then placed in an individual, cardboard box containing a towel for the bird to perch on. The recovery area is warmed to 70 to 75°F (21.1 to 23.9°C), and an electric heating pad set on low is placed under half of the box, allowing the bird to select a temperature gradient. This maintains the inside of the box at approximately 80 to 90°F (26.7 to 32.2°C). The patient is checked frequently to make sure that oral secretions do not accumulate. Birds must be fully recovered before being placed in a cage with other birds, as some species will attack weak and depressed individuals.

References and Supplemental Reading

Altman, R. B.: Avian anesthesia. Comp. Cont. Ed. 2:38, 1980.
Fedde, M. R.: Drugs used for avian anesthesia: A review. Poul. Sci. 57:1376, 1978.
Harrison, G. J.: Anesthesiology. In Harrison, G. J., and Harrison, L. H. (eds.): Clinical Avian Medicine and Surgery. Philadelphia: W. B. Saunders Co., 1986, pp. 549–558.

Ludders, J. W., Rode, J. A., and Mitchell, G. S.: Isoflurane ED50 and cardiopulmonary dose response during spontaneous and controlled breathing in sandhill cranes (*Grus canadensis*). ACVA:20, 1987.

Redig, P. T.: An overview of avian anesthesia. Proceedings of the Annual Meeting of the Association of Avian Veterinarians, Atlanta, GA, 1982, pp. 127–139.

Sedgwick, C. J.: Anesthesia of caged birds. *In* Kirk, R. W. (ed.): *Current Veterinary Therapy VII.* Philadelphia: W. B. Saunders Co., 1980, pp. 653–656.

Taylor, M. T.: Avian anesthesia—a clinical update. Proceedings of the First International Conference in Zoological and Avian Medicine, Hawaii, September 1987, pp. 519–524.

MICROBIOLOGIC TECHNIQUES FOR THE AVIAN PRACTITIONER

KIM LORRAINE JOYNER, D.V.M.

Loxahatchee, Florida

IMPORTANCE OF AVIAN MICROBIOLOGY

Microbiologic techniques have become an integral part of the avian practitioner's clinical program. Of the many reasons for emphasizing microbiology when dealing with avian patients, the primary one is the numerous microbial imbalances and infections seen in exotic birds. The leading causes of these imbalances are inadequate nutrition, suboptimal sanitation, and high stress situations. Basically, nutrition, sanitation, and the general environment are within the domain of managerial practices and husbandry. High stress situations occur because many exotic birds were hatched in the wild and have not adapted to captivity. In addition, the occurrence of other diseases, of which there are many, results in secondary bacterial and fungal imbalances.

The quarantine procedure in the United States also produces microbial problems. Birds that are imported into this country must undergo at least a 30-day stay in an approved quarantine station to ensure that no exotic Newcastle virus is present. In addition, these birds are given food treated with chlortetracycline to reduce the incidence of chlamydiosis. The chlortetracycline also affects the normal microfloral homeostasis, can produce resistant strains of bacteria, and causes immunosuppression. To make the situation worse, many of these birds are given antibiotics in their country of origin long before they enter the United States. This sets up a wonderful environment for pathogenic bacteria to invade the intestinal tract. In addition, these birds are highly stressed. Many of them have had improper nutrition in their countries of origin and will not eat once they arrive at a station. Moreover, when birds are housed with other birds originating from different home localities, they are exposed to micro-organisms that they have not had a chance to develop an immunity to. With all these factors and the often present overcrowding, the resulting microbial problems seen in exotic birds are not surprising.

SAMPLE COLLECTION

Gastrointestinal Samples

The most common site cultured is the cloaca. Swabs inserted into the cloaca can first be moistened with sterile saline to decrease damage to the cloacal mucosa. Inadequate penetration into the proctodeum results in a decrease in the variety and concentration of microbial species cultured. Fecal cultures should be collected almost immediately after the bird defecates, as the bacterial population will shift upon exposure to the external environment.

In the ideal situation, cloacal cultures would be taken of every bird presented, whether it was healthy or not. Such a practice gives the practitioner a baseline for making clinical decisions on future problems in a given bird or aviary. The taking of these cultures may also alert one that a possible microbial imbalance exists for the flock as a whole. In addition, cloacal cultures can be taken when a bird is suffering from any disease, as secondary microbial imbalances are more the rule than the exception. Of course, any bird suspected of having an intestinal disease should have a cloacal culture. If the bird cannot be handled easily, a fresh fecal culture will suffice. Crop cultures should be taken in birds showing crop stasis or impaction.

Respiratory Samples

The choana can be cultured by holding the beak open with various restraining devices or a third person holding strips of gauze to force the beak open. By directing the swab dorsally into the choanal slit and then rostrally, the swab can reach the distal nasal cavity. A sinus aspirate is performed by infusing sterile saline into the suborbital sinus with a needle and syringe and then recovering as much of the infused fluid as possible. One particular approach is performed by directing a needle perpendicular to the skin, in an area just ventral and rostral to the orbit.

Transglottal tracheal cultures and tracheal wash cultures can also be taken. Tracheal cultures are taken while the bird's beak is held open and a swab is placed into the upper trachea. Tracheal washes are performed by placing a sterile catheter within a sterile catheter introduced into the trachea, infusing approximately 1 ml of sterile saline (for a large macaw), and recovering the infusion by suction with a syringe. The infused fluid can be difficult to recover, but mucus usually can be obtained. These cultures are more easily taken when the bird is under gas anesthesia, preferably isoflurane.

Eye discharges are often seen in avian respiratory disease, so the conjunctival sac should be cultured by using a swab first dipped into sterile saline.

Choanal cultures are often taken when a bird is showing either upper or lower respiratory signs. Nasal discharges are heavily contaminated with environmental organisms and should be avoided. In addition, the choanal area can also be contaminated with environmental organisms, such as those seen in food. The causative agent in a sinusitis can be isolated with a choanal culture, but a sinus aspirate may be more revealing and easier to interpret. Tracheal cultures or tracheal washes can be done for suspected lower respiratory infections, but they should be carefully interpreted as well.

Environmental Cultures

Important information can be gathered from culturing a bird's environment, especially in an avicultural situation. Water or fluids can be evaluated by filtering the sample and growing the bacteria trapped on the gridded filter. The filter paper is then placed on a culture plate and incubated. This method allows for quantitative measurement, which is necessary when dealing with food or water samples. Other culture sites include incubators, hatchers, feeding utensils, and food preparation sites. Surfaces are cultured using a swab dipped in sterile saline. Exact quantitative measurements of bacterial levels in food and nesting material are beyond the scope of the veterinary laboratory, but a rough estimate can be obtained by incubating a given weight or volume of material in thioglycollate broth for approximately 4 hr and then streaking the broth onto an agar plate with a calibrated loop. Each

practitioner must use his or her own judgment when deciding the significance of environmental isolates, as no standards exist.

Environmental cultures are most often taken in an aviary or for an aviculture facility. This culturing can be especially helpful when dealing with pediatric cases. If baby birds are experiencing microbial infections, it is appropriate to culture the food, water, bedding, and so forth. If artificial incubators are used, they should also be cultured. Parent-raised birds experiencing problems should have their nesting material checked and their parents surveyed as possible sources. Water is a potential source for many organisms and, when aerosolized or exposed to the air, can carry potential infections to young birds. Hence, all water sources and containers are suspect if there are problems in a nursery, such as humidifiers, air-conditioning units, and distilled water dispensers.

Miscellaneous Samples

Cultures can be obtained of internal organs during surgery or endoscopic laparotomy. The most common sites are lesions associated with the liver, airsacs, and peritoneum. Blood cultures can be taken from larger birds, using 1 ml of blood as the minimal sample volume and inoculating blood culture tubes (Kollias et al., 1987). If organs or lesions are to cultured during necropsy, it is better to perform a sterile necropsy until all cultures are taken. This is in preference to searing the surface of organs, as many avian tissues are so small that searing may kill any possible pathogens. Carcasses that are older than a day may have contamination of intestinal microflora throughout most internal tissues. However, heart blood can be cultured from a heart puncture aspirate and does not easily become contaminated.

Eyes should be cultured when any discharge or conjunctivitis is present. Ears may also occasionally have a discharge, especially as seen in baby macaws with small external acoustic meati. This discharge may be indicative of an infection and should be cultured.

IN-HOUSE VERSUS PROFESSIONAL LABORATORY

Many avian veterinarians run their own cultures in-house because of the numbers of cultures they collect. Individual cultures can be less expensive, and the results can be obtained sooner. The disadvantage of an in-house laboratory is the initial set-up cost and the usual lack of experience of the laboratory personnel processing the samples, which is often the veterinarian or a technician. It takes years of training and experience to become proficient in microbiology. Many mistakes can happen, and possible pathogens can be overlooked when personnel are untrained. Organisms that take special techniques include *Haemophilus*, *Mycoplasma*, *Campylobacter*, anaerobes, and fastidious gram-negative organisms. Experience is also necessary to identify species of fungi, as fungi are identified by visual clues. The point is that when samples are run in-house, the veterinarian must be aware of the increased possibility of error and weigh this against the savings in time and money.

PROCESSING THE SAMPLE

A thorough discussion of avian laboratory microbiologic techniques can be found elsewhere (Drewes and Flammer, 1986) and is beyond the scope of this article. However, basic considerations will be discussed.

Care must be given to ensure proper results once the swab has been collected. The sample should be set up immediately if at all possible. The saline applied to the swab will keep the micro-organisms alive for a short time. If the swab must be transported to an outside laboratory, it should be kept refrigerated in a transport medium and kept cool even during transport. Refrigeration and speed in processing will increase the likelihood of survival of certain species of micro-organisms.

The swab is placed first on a blood agar plate, then on a MacConkey agar plate, next on a Sabouraud-dextrose plate, and finally into thiogylcollate broth. The blood agar plates will grow most aerobic organisms and are used mostly to evaluate the gram-positive growth and more selective gram-negative bacteria. MacConkey's agar inhibits the growth of most gram-positive bacteria and has a color indicator for bacteria that can ferment lactose. These two plates should be incubated for up to 48 hr at 37°F (2.8°C). A 48-hr check on the plates is necessary, as many species of bacteria seen in birds do not appear on culture plates until after 24 hr. Plates should be examined at 24 hr, so colony isolation and sensitivities can be initiated. The Sabouraud-dextrose plate can contain inhibitors such as chloramphenicol and cycloheximide. This inhibitor will decrease bacterial growth somewhat but will also inhibit the growth of *Cryptococcus neoformans* and certain species of fungi, especially those that are not usually considered pathogenic, such as various *Aspergillus*. These species of fungi can be recovered from bird samples, however, and may be important in evaluating a bird or aviary for microbial imbalances and environmental contamination. Sabouraud-dextrose plates are kept at room temperature for at least 7 days. Many species of fungi and yeast will not grow until 3 to 6 days, so these plates

should be checked daily. The thiogycollate broth is incubated for 24 hr and then checked for any bacterial growth. The broth can be gram-stained to rule out the presence of fastidious and microaerophilic organisms, as they may survive in the broth and not on conventional aerobic media. The broth can then be placed on the appropriate agar or sent to an outside laboratory if a possible pathogen is present. The broth can also be plated onto MacConkey agar to check for gram-negative bacteria that may have been present in the original sample in low numbers.

Gram-positive Bacteria Identification

Most species of gram-positive bacteria can be roughly identified as to genus from the appearance of the colony on the blood agar plate. Genus identification is usually all that is needed, unless a gram-positive bacteria is suspected of being a pathogen. Indeed, most professional laboratories have difficulty in distinguishing avian bacteria beyond the level of genus. If there is any doubt as to a colony's genus, it should be gram-stained, especially colonies that are gray or opaque. Gram-staining is important, as some gram-negative bacteria mimic the colony morphology of gram-positive bacteria and are not sustained by MacConkey's agar. The catalase test will differentiate the species that are catalase-positive from those that are catalase-negative (i.e., *Staphylococcus* from *Streptococcus*, and *Corynebacterium* and *Bacillus* from *Lactobacillus*. Alpha-hemolysis that is present should be noted and can help identify groups of *Streptococcus* and *Lactobacillus*. *Staphylococcus* colonies can exhibit different amounts of beta-hemolysis. Not all *Staphylococcus aureus* colonies are beta-hemolytic, and not all beta-hemolytic staphylococci are *Staphylococcus aureus*. Regardless, all beta-hemolytic staphylococci should have a coagulase test run. This is usually the depth of identification that is performed, but if further, more specific identification is necessary, then a good microbiologic text should be consulted (Buchanan and Gibbons, 1974).

Gram-negative Bacteria Identification

The identification of gram-negative bacteria is more involved than the identification of gram-positive bacteria. The variability of colony types within a given species can be tremendous. Therefore, colony morphology cannot be relied on, although it can be very helpful. Enterobacteriaceae grow on MacConkey's agar and usually have a typical colony morphology. Further identification of this family of bacteria can be made by noting the colony color, with pink colonies indicating lactose fermentation.

Even this is not always reliable, as some *Escherichia coli* types appear tan on MacConkey's agar, whereas they are usually pink. Differentiation among species within this family can be done quite well with the use of the API-20E strip. Colony types that do not appear to belong to Enterobacericeae (i.e., they do not have the typical pinkish or tan hue to their colonies on MacConkey's agar) can also be processed by the API-20E strip, but the results can be inconclusive. These nonlactose fermenters can often only be described as such and cannot be identified, even by the larger veterinary professional laboratories. Gram-negative bacteria that do not grow on MacConkey's agar usually cannot be easily identified by the API-20E strip. If further identification is necessary, an oxidase test should be performed and the organisms cultivated on a Triple-Sugar-Iron (TSI) agar slant, urea agar, and SIM agar. This will place an organism into one of 6 "TSI" groups, which may be all that can be done (Jang et al, 1986). If identification of these organisms is clinically important, they should be sent to a larger laboratory.

Fungi and Yeast Identification

Fungi are usually identified by colony characteristics and microscopic examination. Fungi can also have varying colony and microscopic morphology, so experience is necessary to identify this group adequately. Fungi and yeast can grow on the blood agar plate and may be confused with *Streptomyces* and other "fungoid" species of bacteria. A Gram stain or wet mount can easily differentiate these two groups of organisms. Yeasts are identified as are fungi by colony morphology, but various chemical tests are necessary to identify them to the level of genus and species. A germ tube test is used to identify *Candida albicans*, a common avian isolate.

REPORTING

This is a critical step for proper avian microbiologic techniques. Adequate reporting requires that all colony morphology types be listed. These types can be listed as they are identified (e.g., nonlactose fermenters, group 6 TSI, *Corynebacterium*, *E. coli*). Quantity should also be reported, as evaluated by the standard microbiology rating of 1 to 4+. In addition, percentages of total blood agar bacterial growth for each colony type should be calculated and reported. The need for this type of reporting will become evident when interpretation is discussed. Fungi and yeasts are simply reported as genus or genus and species and are given a 1 to 4+ rating. An example of a report is shown in Table 1.

Table 1. *Cloacal Culture Results from a Clinically Healthy Psittacine*

	Amount	Percentage
Lactobacillus	3+	20
Streptococcus	4+	60
E. coli	3+	20
Fungi and yeasts	0	0

DIRECT MICROSCOPIC EXAMINATION

Direct Gram stains can be very important when an immediate presumptive diagnosis is necessary. Sometimes only a Gram stain is used to make a diagnosis and to evaluate therapy. Gram stains do not always agree with culture results in the identification of gram-negative bacteria or yeast in a sample. Part of the reason for this is that the Gram stain can reveal anaerobes, other organisms that will not grow on conventional media, and dead organisms. The question arises as to which is better diagnostically. An adequate compromise would be to perform both whenever possible, so that the most complete medical data base can be compiled.

NORMAL INTESTINAL MICROFLORA

To be able to interpret culture results from birds, one must be aware of the concept of normal microflora. Normal microflora refers to the micro-organisms found normally in healthy birds. However, at hatching, birds are born basically sterile. As chicks grow, they come into contact with various species of bacteria in their environment. These microorganisms enter the oral and nasal cavities via food, water, nesting material, other nestmates, parents, aerosolized water, feeding utensils, human hands, and many other objects in the chick's environment. The bacteria become established in the intestinal and upper respiratory tracts. Once established, the bacteria become permanently associated with the cells lining these tracts. The bacterial species and concentrations become important for keeping pathogenic bacteria from multiplying and for digestion. Once this initial population of bacteria becomes established, it usually does not change, even with artificial attempts such as the use of antibiotics. However, this normal microfloral population is not completely static and can change. Organisms cultured one day may not be present the next day, especially in younger birds. The relative percentages will also change. For example, one day a bird may grow 2+, 80 per cent *E. coli* from the cloaca, and the next day it may grow only 1+, 5 per cent *E. coli*. These populations change because of such factors as types of food fed, levels of bacteria in the food, the use of antibiotics, diseases, and stress situations. Many times these changes are only transitory and slight, and new species of organisms in a given bird will not be cultured in overwhelming numbers. If the exposure to certain species of bacteria is high, the bacteria may eventually become established in the bird. This may represent either a benign or potentially harmful situation. An example of a benign situation would be relocating one bird to another aviary. Birds in different aviaries have different microflora (Joyner, 1988). The newly introduced bird will be exposed to new bacteria and may eventually have the bacteria as part of its normal microflora. An example of a harmful situation is the use of antibiotics in quarantine stations. Resistant bacteria, both opportunistic and pathogenic, can become established in a bird. The bacteria then becomes a source for potential primary infections and secondary imbalances for as long as the bird carries the bacteria. In young birds that have a bacteriologically naive intestinal lining, the potential for microfloral imbalances is greater, especially since they are only protected by maternal antibodies. The antibody response of a chick develops in 7 to 14 days, and maternal protection wanes from 20 to 27 days.

There is great diversity of literature discussing normal microflora in the intestinal tract of exotic birds (Joyner, 1988). This is due largely to varying methods of sample collection and lack of true controlled studies. Research in poultry concerning normal microflora is extensive and well accepted as valid. The intestinal microflora of chickens includes predominantly *Lactobacillus*, *Streptococcus*, *E. coli*, and *Clostridium welchii*, in descending order of concentration (Timms, 1968). The microflora of psittacines are similar, being predominantly gram-positive bacteria of the genera *Streptococcus*, *Staphylococcus*, *Lactobacillus*, *Corynebacterium*, and *Bacillus*. Gram-negative bacteria can also be found in healthy individuals in varying concentrations. The most common are members of Enterobacteriaceae such as *E. coli*, *Enterobacter*, *Klebsiella*, and *Citrobacter*. *Pasteurella* and *Moraxella* are also fairly common in healthy individuals. *Pseudomonas* and other non–lactose-fermenting gram-negative bacteria are found much less often but are present in healthy birds. Anaerobes have not been studied extensively in exotic birds, but in chickens several *Clostridium* species are considered to be normal flora. Many species of fungi and yeasts can be cultured from the cloaca, but they usually are present in low numbers.

The normal microflora in baby birds is similar to those in adults. At hatching, cloacal cultures reveal a no-growth pattern. In the subsequent days, *Streptococcus*, *Staphylococcus*, *Lactobacillus*, and then *Corynebacterium* will appear. Gram-negative bacteria may also be recovered in various amounts but often are only present later in the bird's growth, or if present earlier, may disappear as the bird grows.

Chicken chicks have similar developing microflora, with *Streptococcus*, *Staphylococcus*, *Lactobacillus*, and *E. coli* constituting the predominant facultative anaerobic microflora (Salanitro et al., 1978). This changing pattern reflects the developing intestinal microflora in chicks that is heavily influenced by environmental micro-organisms. As in adults, fungi and yeasts can be recovered from the cloaca and choana in low numbers in healthy chicks.

Miscellaneous Normal Microflora

Choanal microflora can vary widely, since oral and environmental contaminants are recovered as well as the flora of the upper respiratory system. The same bacteria found from cloacal cultures can be found in those of the choana. However, the day-to-day variability of species recovered is greater, as are the concentrations and percentages. Conjunctival flora of healthy psittacines consists largely of gram-positive bacteria, but often no bacteria are recovered (Zenoble et al., 1983). Gram-negative bacteria are isolated much less often. Isolates from ears are similar to eye cultures in that they grow nothing about 50 per cent of the time. Ear cultures also have the usual oral or cloacal microflora, which is predominantly gram-positive bacteria with lesser amounts of gram-negative bacteria.

Environmental sources can grow a great number of bacteria and fungi. Seeds typically fed to psittacines may contain *Bacillus*, *Enterobacter*, *Klebsiella*, *Pseudomonas*, *E. coli*, and *Acinetobacter* (Halverson and Roudybush, 1986). Fruits and vegetables are also abundant sources of bacteria and become heavily contaminated within hours with various gram-negative bacteria such as *Enterobacter*, *Pseudomonas*, and *E. coli* (Flammer, 1983). Hand feeding formulas can contain many types of bacteria, but usually only the gram-positive bacteria are in high numbers. Gram-negative bacteria increase their numbers exponentially once the food is prepared, especially if it is warmed. Food with a normal 1+, 1 to 5 per cent growth of an enteric gram-negative bacteria will grow 4+, 50 to 80 per cent gram-negative growth if allowed to stay warmed for a half hour. Water can also contain species of *Pseudomonas*, *Alcaligenes*, and other group 5 TSI organisms.

INTERPRETATION

It is obvious that normal birds and environments can contain bacteria and fungi that in some instances are considered pathogenic for birds. Whether thriving neonates or producing adults, birds can present with relatively high percentages of gram-negative bacteria and fungi and still be clinically asymptomatic and have normal blood test results. Without a doubt, it can be difficult to determine from a given culture what treatment is necessary. The practitioner must take into account several factors in deciding if the microflora cultured is pathogenically significant. The key factor is whether the bird is sick. If a baby bird is failing to thrive or has repeated crop stasis, a heavy growth of E. coli may be more suspicious than E. coli found in a healthy baby. Adults can mask their physical signs well but blood tests, behavior, a history of poor breeding performance, and a physical examination will pick up most abnormalities. If any of these tests are abnormal, heavy growths of fungi and gram-negative bacteria may become more significant. Heavy growths of potentially pathogenic organisms may occur secondary to other problems that the bird is having. However, these microbial imbalances can be the eventual cause of death in a debilitated bird, and they should be addressed. Ears and eyes that have discharges and grow predominantly gram-negative bacteria are indicative of a treatable condition, but discharges can occur without the practitioner recovering bacteria or fungi.

Aids in Interpretation

The key factor in interpreting microbiology results is whether the bird is clinically ill or whether an aviary has clinical or subclinical signs, such as poor breeding success. One must also consider the species of birds. Different species of birds have different microflora. Cockatoos are known to have larger percentages of gram-negative bacteria than most other psittacines, even when kept in the same environment. Baby cockatoos also exhibit this microfloral shift from other psittacines, even when receiving the same hand-fed diet and being housed in the same environment. Sometimes these differences are due to the varied diets and environments. Birds of prey, and any bird on a partial or complete carnivorous diet, generally grow more gram-negative bacteria than those on nonmeat diets. Waterfowl grow different bacteria than land birds because of the bacteria found in their aquatic environment.

The genus of bacteria is also important to consider. Not all gram-positive bacteria are nonpathogenic. Hemolytic Staphylococcus aureus, Listeria, and Erysipelothrix are examples, although hemolytic Staphylococcus can be found in healthy birds. Conversely, not all gram-negative bacteria are harmful. E. coli, Enterobacter, and some other bacteria in the family Enterobacericeae are often found in healthy birds. The presence of Klebsiella, especially resistant strains, is generally undesirable but can be difficult to eradicate in healthy birds. Pseudomonas is rarely found in significant numbers in healthy birds. Salmonella and Proteus are almost always associated with clinical disease. Many different species of fungi and yeasts are recovered from healthy birds and are generally considered to be opportunistic. In clinically ill birds, fungus and yeast growth can be more significant. Certain species, such as Cryptococcus neoformans and Aspergillus fumigatus, are generally more significant, even when they occur in small numbers.

The number of bacteria is also important. E. coli often grows luxuriously in healthy and clinically ill birds. This growth may be considered more significant if few other normal bacteria are found. E. coli can account for 100 per cent of the growth in healthy individuals but may be causing intestinal disturbances that cannot be detected. The cause of microbial population shifts are many and often benign, but in clinically ill birds, any microbial imbalance should be seriously considered.

Therapy

The first step in organizing a therapeutic plan is to ascertain that treatment is necessary, such as when a bird or aviary is showing clinical signs. Signs of microbial imbalances in baby birds are retained food in the crop, slow weight gain, regurgitation, constipation, and lack of feeding response. Signs of adult microbial imbalances are less distinct and often overlap with signs from the primary disease or problem. Some common signs are poor feathering, cachexia, poor breeding record, weak babies, dead-in-shell eggs, and abnormal feces.

Malnutrition is common in exotic birds and is probably the primary cause of sickness in captive birds. Poor nutrition also results in microbial imbalances; therefore, it is important to correct the diet in any bird or aviary that is experiencing problems. Parenteral vitamins should be supplemented in birds that are clinically ill.

Management techniques play a role in microbial differences between aviaries, hence it is important to correct any problems. Contaminated or spoiled food is often a cause of microbial imbalances, although all food contains micro-organisms. Food and water management should be evaluated and any necessary changes made to decrease their bacterial counts. Sources of environmental contaminants also include other birds in the aviary, rodent droppings, nest material, and humans.

Improving the diet and the environment is important for all birds that are exhibiting microbial imbalances, but more aggressive therapy is needed for those birds and aviaries more severely affected. If antibiotics are used, bacterial sensitivities should be evaluated and the appropriate drug selected. Post-treatment cultures should also be done, because the antibiotics are often not effective in eliminating the undesirable micro-organisms. Sometimes more resistant and potentially more pathogenic bacteria replace the organism at which the therapy was directed. The indiscriminant use of antibiotics not only can worsen an individual's condition but also can be detrimental to a flock. Resistant *Klebsiella* strains can be found in psittacine nurseries where prophylactic antibiotics are often used. These situations can be dangerous for young chicks or for birds experiencing other problems. If antibiotics are to be used for a long period of time, or in chicks, it is a good idea to also administer an antifungal agent such as nystatin or ketoconazole.

In recent years, *Lactobacillus* products have been used to deal with microbial imbalances. Few studies have been performed to evaluate their use in psittacines, although several studies in poultry show some benefit. In one study, psittacine chicks given *Lactobacillus* did not show obvious alterations in their normal cloacal microflora as compared to those not given *Lactobacillus* supplement but may have shown better weight gain and a lower incidence of clinical illness (Joyner, 1988).

CONCLUSION

The use of microbiologic techniques in avian medicine plays an important role in the diagnosis of disease and in developing therapeutic plans. Interpreting results requires knowledge of a host of factors, most of which are not well defined. The most important factor is whether an individual is clinically ill or whether an aviary is experiencing problems. Each case must be treated individually and with contemplation, as no standards exist for processing, interpretation, and therapy.

References and Supplemental Reading

Buchanan, R. E., and Gibbons, N. E.: *Bergey's Manual of Determinative Bacteriology*, 8th ed. Baltimore: Williams and Wilkins Co., 1974.

Drewes, L. A., and Flammer, K.: Clinical microbiology. *In* Harrison, G. J., and Harrison, L. R. (eds.): *Clinical Avian Medicine and Surgery*. Philadelphia: W. B. Saunders Co., 1986.

Flammer, K.: Environment sources of gram-negative bacteria in an exotic bird farm. Proceedings of Jean Delacour/International Foundation for the Conservation of Birds, 1983.

Halverson, J., and Roudybush, R.: The bacterial flora of psittacine seed diets. Proceedings of the Annual Meeting of the Association of Avian Veterinarians, 1986.

Jang, S. S., Biberstein, E. L., and Hirsh, D. C.: *A Diagnostic Manual of Veterinary Clinical Bacteriology and Mycology*. Davis, CA: University of California, Davis Press, 1986.

Joyner, K. L.: Clinical avian microbiology. Proceedings of the Western States Veterinary Conference, 1988.

Joyner, K. L., Swanson, J.: The use of a lactobacillus product in a psittacine hand-feeding diet: Its effect on normal aerobic microflora, early weight gain, and health. Proceedings of the Annual Meeting of the Association of Avian Veterinarians, 1988.

Kollias, G. V., Heard, D. J., Martin, H. M., et al.: Principles, techniques and clinical use of blood cultures in birds. Proceedings of the Annual Meeting of the Association of Avian Veterinarians, 1987.

Salanitro, J. P., Blake, I. G., Muirehead, P. A., et al.: Bacteria isolated from the duodenum, ileum, and cecum of young chicks. Appl. Environ. Microbiol. 35:782, 1978.

Timms, L.: Observations on the bacterial flora of the alimentary tract in three age groups of normal chickens. Br. Vet. J. 124:470, 1968.

Zenoble, R. D., Griffith, R. W., and Clubb, S. L.: Survey of bacteriologic flora of conjunctiva and cornea in healthy psittacine birds. Am. J. Vet. Res. 44:10, 1983.

ADVANCES IN AVIAN AND REPTILIAN IMAGING

SAM SILVERMAN, D.V.M.
San Francisco, California

There is a common misconception that radiographic examination of birds and reptiles is of limited value because of technical imaging problems and the paucity of information regarding radiographic interpretation for these species. Numerous recent advances in radiographic and ultrasonographic imaging systems have significantly enhanced the quality and quantity of obtainable diagnostic information on these species (Silverman, 1987). The following discussion will summarize advances in radiographic equipment, radiographic interpretation, and alternative imaging techniques applicable to reptile and avian patients.

CHEMICAL RESTRAINT

Patient restraint and immobilization have previously been unresolved problems in reptile and avian practice. The small body size of the patient, lack of patient cooperation, potential hazards of chemical restraint, and inherent danger of the exposure of humans to x-rays during manual patient restraint have discouraged many clinicians from requesting radiographic examination of reptiles and birds. Although there is no ideal anesthetic, the introduction of agents such as ketamine, diazepam, xylazine, and isoflurane have made chemical restraint more practical and safer. Isoflurane is emerging as the inhalation anesthesia of choice in birds. Its speed of induction and recovery make it a logical choice for radiographic procedures.

MECHANICAL RESTRAINT

Mechanical restraint devices have almost completely replaced chemical restraint for reptile and avian radiographic procedures in the author's practice. One important advantage of using a restraint device is that multiple radiographic exposures can be made without repositioning the patient. This is especially helpful if the radiographic exposure factors require adjustment for improved image quality. Smaller birds (i.e., less than 50 gm body weight) can be immobilized with masking tape or paper bandage tape on a sheet of processed unexposed x-ray film. Larger birds are restrained with a rigid acrylic device. The patient's neck is immobilized with a guillotinelike device, the wings are taped to the acrylic sheet, and the legs are secured with small cords, gauze, or tape. Several commercial sources are available for these devices. The same device is used for reptiles. Tape is used to immobilize the reptile's body and tail. An alternative device to use for snakes is thin-walled acrylic tubing. The snake is allowed to enter the tube, the head end of the tube is temporarily sealed with tape and the tube is placed on the x-ray cassette. Lateral projections can be made utilizing a horizontally directed x-ray beam. The author has also designed an acrylic squeeze box for small patients. The front of the box consists of an acrylic sheet that slides into grooves on the sides of the box. The distance between the front and rear of the box is adjusted so that the patient is pressed against the rear of the box. The x-ray cassette is placed against the outside rear surface of the box. This device is used to produce horizontal beam radiographs, usually of standing patients. It does not require anesthesia and is used on birds, reptiles, and small mammals.

FILM-SCREEN COMBINATIONS

The most important factor in improved radiographic image quality for the veterinary practitioner is the introduction of high speed–high resolution film screen systems (i.e., the rare earth systems). These systems offer exceptional detail, utilizing short exposure times (i.e., 1/60 sec or less). If the

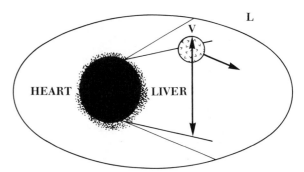

Figure 1. Hepatomegaly, ventrodorsal view. Hepatomegaly produces widening of the hepatic silhouette, caudal displacement of the ventriculus (V), and caudal movement of the central abdominal organs.

x-ray generator is capable of producing 200 ma and has an exposure time capability of 1/60 sec or shorter, it is strongly recommended that a rare earth system be used for general radiography and reptile and bird radiography. The author currently uses the Dupont Quanta Detail intensifying screens with Dupont Cronex 7 or Cronex 10 x-ray film.

AVIAN RADIOGRAPHY

Avian species are well suited for radiographic examination. The abdominal organs are relatively fixed in position, with minimal interspecies variation. Patterns of abdominal organ displacement are predictable and often well documented radiographically. Figures 1 through 4 demonstrate some of these patterns.

Gastrointestinal contrast studies are helpful in diagnosing digestive tract disease and the presence of mass effects or diseases that displace, compress, or obstruct the digestive tract. The use of mechanical restraint devices has further decreased the patient stress associated with these procedures. Double contrast gastrointestinal studies using high-density barium sulfate and room air have largely replaced the positive-contrast procedure in the author's practice. The double contrast technique usu-

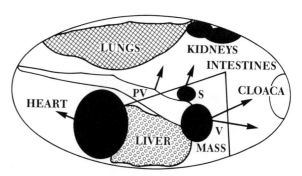

Figure 2. Hepatomegaly, lateral view. Hepatomegaly usually produces dorsal and caudal enlargement of the hepatic silhouette. This displaces the spleen (S) and the proventriculus (PV) dorsally, and the ventriculus (V) caudally.

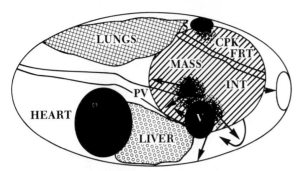

Figure 3. Dorsal abdominal mass, lateral view. The serosal surface visualization of the dorsal abdominal organs (i.e., cranial pole of the kidneys [CPK], female reproductive tract [FRT], and testes) decreases as the mass enlarges and contacts these structures. Midabdominal structures (i.e., spleen [S], ventriculus [V], and proventriculus [PV]) may be displaced away from the mass.

ally produces enhanced mucosal detail and a more accurate representation of digestive tract distensibility and proventricular wall thickness. It is less stressful to the patient, since the intestinal transit time of the air and barium sulfate is more rapid than with barium alone. The technique is based on estimating the normal crop volume of the patient. If the species does not have a crop, the proventricular volume is used. One half of this volume of 85 to 100 per cent barium sulfate is administered via a crop tube; this is followed by infusion of air via the crop tube. The volume of air administered is usually equal to twice the estimated normal crop or proventricular volume.

Conventional radiography is not without limitations in the evaluation of avian patients. The two major areas of deficiency are the respiratory tract and the skull. The avian lungs are relatively nonexpansile, are less well aerated than mammalian lungs, and are tightly adhered to the thoracic wall. High-speed computed tomography (CT) has been very effective in documenting pulmonary consolidative disease. It is unfortunate that not all scanners are capable of making thin sections with a sufficiently short exposure time. Patient motion may significantly degrade image quality, since scan times can

be several seconds. Anesthesia is strongly recommended for patients undergoing computed tomography. Skull trauma and other skull abnormalities are often difficult to diagnose with standard radiography. Computed tomography produces cross-sectional images that more clearly indicate these conditions.

ULTRASONOGRAPHY

Preliminary clinical studies have demonstrated that diagnostic ultrasonography has definite applications in avian medicine. With high-resolution transducers (i.e., 7.5 mHz or greater), it is possible to image the heart, liver, spleen, and central abdomen. Abdominal fluid enhances ultrasonographic visualization of the internal structures. Solid mass lesions can be differentiated from cystic structures. Cardiomyopathy, cystic ovaries, granulomatous liver disease, abdominal tumors, and reproductive disorders have been diagnosed ultrasonographically. It may not be necessary to remove feathers for imaging, especially when abdominal fluid is present. The ultrasound transducer is placed on the lateral thoracic and abdominal wall, alternative locations are the caudal abdominal wall and the thoracic inlet. If abdominal fluid is present, the patient can be placed in the supine or prone position to maximize visualization of the viscera. It has not been possible to visualize the gonads or kidneys ultrasonographically; however, this may be possible with improved equipment and technique.

REPTILIAN IMAGING

The reptile patient represents a unique radiographic challenge. The skin scales degrade image quality, the lack of a diaphragm and the paucity of intra-abdominal fat obscure differentiation of serosal surfaces, and the pulmonary anatomy precludes extrapolation of the conventional mammalian radiographic patterns to this group of animals. Gastrointestinal contrast studies have been helpful in diagnosing intestinal obstructive disease and the presence of large abdominal masses. The contrast medium is administered via an esophageal tube. In these patients, the double contrast procedure is performed using a technique similar to that described in birds. Distal intestinal tract obstructive disease can also be visualized with retrograde studies. There is the potential for contrast medium to be retrograded into the urinary tract and possibly produce ureteral concretions or renal damage.

Radiographs of turtles and tortoises for diagnosis of pulmonary disease should be made with a horizontally directed x-ray beam and the patient in the prone position. In the prone position, the viscera

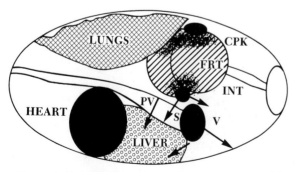

Figure 4. Central abdominal mass, lateral view. Central abdominal masses produce variable patterns of organ displacement. The spleen (S), proventriculus (PV), and ventriculus (V) usually move ventrally. Serosal surface visualization decreases.

gravitate ventrally away from the lungs. Lateral and cranial-caudal projections are made with the patient in the prone position. Radiographs for evaluation of the internal organs other than the lungs are made with a vertically directed x-ray beam and the patient in the prone position.

Computed tomography has been very helpful for imaging reptiles. The slow respiratory rate results in superior visualization of the viscera, including the lungs, as compared to most avian patients. The reptilian lung is less uniform than mammalian or avian lungs. Therefore, it is more difficult to document focal consolidative disease, but high-detail computed tomograms appear to be the most accurate method for pulmonary diagnosis.

Diagnostic ultrasound is an effective method of diagnosing urinary bladder disease in turtles and tortoises. It may also aid in the diagnosis of central abdominal abnormalities. The transducer is placed just cranial to the rear leg.

MAGNETIC RESONANCE IMAGING

Magnetic resonance imaging (MRI) exposes the patient to a high-intensity magnetic field and causes molecular reorientation of the patient's tissues. When the magnetic field is interrupted, the molecules reorient themselves, and radio frequency waves are produced. An image is constructed from the computerized analysis of these radio frequency waves. This modality is capable of demonstrating physiologic events as well as anatomic detail. It is unfortunate that imaging time is very long (e.g., several minutes). The author has done preliminary studies on avian and reptilian patients but has discovered little pathologic correlation. The applications of this technique in smaller patients is questionable.

In conclusion, reptile and avian patients present special challenges to the radiographer and the veterinarian. High-detail imaging systems are essential, and the potential of newer diagnostic modalities should be explored.

Reference

Silverman, S.: New frontiers in imaging avian and zoologic patients. Proceedings of the First International Conference on Zoological and Avian Medicine, Oahu, Hawaii, 1987, pp. 351–353.

REPAIR OF INJURIES TO THE CHELONIAN PLASTRON AND CARAPACE

GARY HARWELL, D.V.M.
Houston, Texas

Injuries and fractures of the chelonian carapace and plastron that require repair are not uncommon presentations to the small animal practitioner. Most injuries are the result of automobile-related encounters, especially in the spring months, as turtles, tortoises, and terrapins are emerging from hibernation. Vandalism of private collections, an animal being dropped, and gardening injuries such as being spaded are other causes of injury. Various repair techniques utilizing external splintage and scute restoration have been reported. However, some cases will undoubtedly depend on undescribed techniques and the clinician's ingenuity for optimum treatment.

ANATOMIC CONSIDERATIONS

The carapace (dorsal shell) and plastron (ventral shell) are composed of bony skeletal segments fused at sutures and united laterally by the bridge. In most species, the skeletal segments are overlaid by keratinized scales, or scutes, that are fused to the bone and to each other. The scute suture lines overlap the skeletal sutures, giving the shell added strength. Some species have a hinged plastron, allowing partial to complete encasement of the legs and tail when the hinge is closed. No diaphragm is present, and exposure of the coelomic cavity does not cause respiratory compromise.

CLINICAL MANAGEMENT

Minor Injuries

Minor injuries and simple fractures can be managed without anesthesia; however, care must be taken in handling some chelonians to avoid sudden bites. Since even minor injuries are usually grossly contaminated with soil or other debris, chloramphenicol succinate (Chloromycetin, Parke-Davis) is administered intramuscularly once daily for one week at a dose of 50 mg/kg.

Abraded and avulsed scutes and minor simple fractures are gently lavaged with normal saline solution, débrided with wet gauze pads, and then lavaged with dilute povidone-iodine solution. This process is repeated until all gross debris is removed. Aquatic turtles often have filamentous, symbiotic algae growing on the carapace and bridge. It is necessary to remove this algae adjacent to injury sites. Repeated scraping with a scalpel blade, drying with ether or alcohol, and abrasion with a rotary burr or disk may be necessary to dislodge the algae. After the affected scute surfaces are thoroughly cleaned and dried, a thin 1- to 3-mm layer of endodontic-grade calcium hydroxide paste (Dycal [L. D. Caulk Co., Milford, DE]) is applied over exposed skeletal bone only. Fracture crevices that result from poor bone apposition or chip avulsion are filled also. Calcium hydroxide is compatible with bone and serves to insulate and protect the bone from application of a resin-based, external splint. Stable, well-apposed scute fractures require only external splintage.

Fiberglass resins, dental acrylics, and epoxy resins have been used as external splints. Rapid polymerizing, resinous epoxy (Devcon 5 minute epoxy [Devcon Corp., Danvers, MA]) is the most economical and readily available product. The epoxy is applied thinly over the defect with a tongue depressor or applicator stick, overlapping the noninjured scute surface 1 to 3 cm. One application is usually sufficient for minor injuries. Epoxy must not cover exposed bone directly. Several hours to days after epoxy application, small fracture lines, which are of no clinical significance, may be noted in the calcium hydroxide bed.

Aquatic chelonians should be maintained out of water but in a humid environment for at least 24 hr to allow complete resin polymerization. All epoxy resins produce exothermic heat during setting, and air circulation by a fan or blower may be necessary to dissipate heat in smaller, thin-shelled specimens. Complete healing of minor injuries and fractures may require 6 months or longer. It is advisable to remove splints after 3 to 6 months in very young specimens, as expansion of the shell may be inhibited by the splint. A rotary burr or disk may be necessary to remove such splints.

Major Injuries

Exposure of the coelomic cavity by crushing fractures or avulsed fractures requires immediate antibiotic therapy as described previously, and careful débridement to prevent entry of debris into the thorax or abdomen.

Manipulation of depressed fragments and fracture edges is expedited by use of one or two double-ended dental caries explorers. Devitalized or devascularized chip fragments should be removed. After cleaning and débridement, exposed skeletal bone surfaces are lightly coated with calcium hydroxide. The prepared area and adjacent scute surfaces are then coated with epoxy. Nylon screen mesh such as screen door mesh or paint strainer screen is precut slightly larger in shape than the defect area and gently embedded in the wet epoxy. This process is repeated to create one to five layers, depending on the degree of stabilization desired. Additional layers may be added over a 24- to 48-hr period. Small air bubbles may appear in the epoxy during polymerization. These can be smoothed from the epoxy bed by gentle manipulation with a tongue depressor or applicator stick.

Large defects created from avulsed segments that cannot be replaced or that are missing can be restored by creating a prosthetic resinous scute. Exposed bone is prepared as described, and epoxy is applied to the adjacent scutes around the defect. A precut portion of screen mesh is used to cover the opening and is tacked to the wet epoxy. Then, a very thin layer of epoxy is applied to the central portion. It is imperative that epoxy does not leach through the screen and drip into the coelomic cavity.

Avulsions of periappendicular skin from its attachment at the bridge, plastron, or carapace present serious complications to repair if exposure of the coelomic cavity is apparent. Avulsed skin is difficult to attach to bone, and the slow rate of reptilian healing hinders closure of the defects. Euthanasia should be considered in patients with large defects.

DISCUSSION

Many chelonians will be released soon after repair, so in many cases, follow-up examinations are not possible. Aquatic turtles present a problem in that even the best repairs may leak at some future time, subjecting the turtle to a slow death by infection or drowning.

Assuming a successful repair is accomplished and the specimen is maintained, it is essential that proper housing, temperature, and nutrition be provided to ensure completion of the healing process.

References and Supplemental Reading

Frye, F. L.: *Biomedical and Surgical Aspects of Captive Reptile Husbandry.* Edwardsville, KS: Veterinary Medicine Pub. Co., 1981, pp. 255–258.

Frye, F. L.: Clinical evaluation of a rapid polymerizing epoxy resin for repair of shell defects in tortoises. Vet. Med. Small Anim. Clin. 68:51, 1973.

Lyvere, D. B.: Repair of the shell of a Galapagos tortoise. Mod. Vet. Pract. 47:76, 1966.

Marcus, L. C.: *Veterinary Biology and Medicine of Captive Amphibians and Reptiles.* Philadelphia: Lea & Febiger, 1981, pp. 77–78.

VITAMIN A SOURCES, HYPOVITAMINOSIS A, AND IATROGENIC HYPERVITAMINOSIS A IN CAPTIVE CHELONIANS

FREDRIC L. FRYE, B.S., D.V.M.

Davis, California

GENERAL NUTRITIONAL CONSIDERATIONS

Chelonians (turtles, tortoises, and terrapins) may be carnivorous, herbivorous, or omnivorous in their dietary preferences, depending on their species (Table 1). Marine and many semiaquatic turtle species become less carnivorous as they approach adulthood. Many sea turtles are virtually herbivorous as sexually mature adults, although as juveniles, they subsist mainly upon fish, mollusks, coelenterates (particularly, pelagic jellyfish), and marine vegetation, even silica-laden corals. Most of these animals obtain vitamin A as a preformed moiety from the tissues of their animal prey and naturally occurring carotenoids from green vegetation in the form of algae and higher plant species.

Aquatic and semiaquatic fresh and brackish water–inhabiting turtles and terrapins usually eat earthworms and other invertebrates, small whole live fish, carrion, algae, and green leafy vegetation such as pond weeds, for example, *Elodea* (*Anacharis*), *Ludwigia*, watercress, and duckweed. In captivity, many turtles and terrapins thrive on a diet that includes natural animal protein, cultured algae, pond weeds, dandelion leaves and flowers, romaine lettuce, and Swiss chard. Many semiaquatic species such as the slider and pond turtles tend to become far more herbivorous as they approach adulthood; their dietary requirements for high-density nutrients diminish as they mature. Consequently, they are able to meet these requirements more easily by eating plant materials. Adults of these species also prey on animals if they have the opportunity. Tortoises usually thrive on a diet of fresh flower blossoms (particularly those with bright-red, orange, yellow, or green petals); succulents (cactus such as the flat "beaver-tail" variety [*Opuntia*]); alfalfa leaves and flowers or dried alfalfa in the form of commercial pelleted guinea pig or rabbit chows; clover; rose petals; nasturtium and dandelion flowers and leaves; fresh corn (maize) and mixed fruits; squashes; and melons. Fresh figs are an excellent source of highly concentrated carbohydrates given prior to hibernation. A *small* amount of commercial dog or cat food usually is welcome but must not be fed to excess because its high vitamin A and D content can induce severe mineralization of soft tissues. Many tortoises avidly hunt for and eat the common brown house snail (*Helix aspersa*), eating the shell as well as the softer body parts. An occasional hard-boiled egg is a welcome treat and provides beneficial macro- and micronutrients.

HYPOVITAMINOSIS A

In reptiles, vitamin A deficiency is most frequently observed in captive semiaquatic turtles, particularly juveniles. The yolk remaining at the time of hatching usually furnishes the vitamin A required by the rapidly growing youngster for approximately 6 months even if it is fed a vitamin A–

Table 1. *Food Preferences for Selected Turtles, Terrapins, and Tortoises*

Chelonian Species	M	F	I/W/S/DF	FL	FR	V
Aldabra tortoise *Geochelone (Testudo) gigantea* *(Aldabrachelys elephantina*)*	O		O	X	X	X
Alligator snapping turtle *Macrochelys temminckii*	X	X	X			
Blanding's turtle *Emydoidea blandingii*	X	X	X	O		Pond weeds and algae
	(juveniles tend to be more carnivorous than adults)					
Box turtle *Terrapene*	X	O	X	X	X	X
Chicken turtle *Deirochelys reticularia*	X	X	X	O		Pond weeds and algae
	(juveniles tend to be more carnivorous than adults)					
Desert tortoise *Gophers agassizii*	O		O	X	X	X
		(small amts DF)				
Diamondback terrapin *Malaclemys terrapin*	O	X	X			Pond weeds and algae
Galapagos tortoise *Geochelone elephantopus*	O		X	X	X	X
Gopher tortoise *Gopherus polyphemus*	O		O	X	X	X
Greek tortoise *Testudo graeca*	O		O	X	X	X
Green turtle, marine *Chelonia mydas*						
JUVENILES: Mollusks		X	X			Algae, kelp
ADULTS:	O	O				Algae, kelp
Hawksbill turtle *Eretmochelys imbricata*						
JUVENILES: Mollusks		X				Algae, kelp
ADULTS:	O	O				X
Herman's tortoise *Testudo hermani*	O		X	X	X	X
Hinged-back tortoise *Kinixys*	O		X	X	X	X
Leatherback turtle *Dermochelys coriacea*						
JUVENILES: Jellyfish		X				Algae, kelp
ADULTS: Jellyfish		O				Algae, kelp
Leopard tortoise *Geochelone pardalis*	O		O	X	X	X
Map turtle *Graptemys*	X	X	X			Pond weeds and algae
	(juveniles tend to be more carnivorous than adults)					
Mata mata turtle *Chelys fimbriata*	O	X	O			
Mud turtle *Kinosternon*	X	X	X			Pond weeds and algae
Muhlenberg's turtle *Clemmys muhlenbergii*	X	X	X			Pond weeds and algae
	(juveniles tend to be more carnivorous than adults)					
Musk turtle *Sternotherus*	X	X	X			Pond weeds and algae
Painted turtle *Chrysemys picta*	X	X	X			Pond weeds and algae
	(juveniles tend to be more carnivorous than adults)					
Pond turtle *Clemmys*	X	X	X			Pond weeds and algae
	(juveniles tend to be more carnivorous than adults)					
Radiated tortoise *Geochelone radiata*	O		O	X	X	X

Table 1. *Food Preferences for Selected Turtles, Terrapins, and Tortoises* Continued

Chelonian Species	M	F	I/W/S/DF	FL	FR	V
Red-eared slider turtle *Trachemys scripta elegans*	X	X	X			Pond weeds and algae
	(juveniles tend to be more carnivorous than adults)					
Red-footed tortoise *Geochelone carbonaria*	O		X	X	X	X
Side-necked turtle *Chelodina*, etc.	X	X	X			Pond weeds and algae
Snapping turtle, Com. *Chelydra serpentina*	X	X	X			
Soft-shelled *Trionyx*, etc.	X	X	X			
Star tortoise *Geochelone (Testudo) elegans*	O		X	X	X	X
Yellow-footed tortoise *Geochelone denticulata*	O		X	X	X	X
Wood turtle *Clemmys insculpta*	X	O	X		O	O

*The taxonomic nomenclature regarding this animal is under reconsideration for revision (see Pritchard, 1986).

†The binomial nomenclature for this turtle was formally *Pseudemys* or *Chrysemys scripta elegans*. It has now been assigned to the genus *Trachemys*.

LEGEND: X, usual food items eaten; O, occasionally eaten; M, miscellaneous meats; F, fish; I/W/S/DF, insects, worms, slugs, snails, *small* amounts of dog food; FL, flowers, misc.; V, other vegetables; FR, fruits.

deficient diet. Once the yolk-derived vitamin A has been expended from the hepatic stores, the clinical signs of hypovitaminosis A can be expressed with alarming speed and severity.

The mucin-secreting glandular structures of the ophthalmic adnexae, pharynx, upper airway, and choanal passages rapidly exhibit squamous metaplastic alterations: Mucin production is diminished, and swelling and overgrowth of keratin is manifested (hyperkeratosis). The eyelids, conjunctivae, and ocular structures and the genitourinary tract also are involved early in the course of the disease. These mucous epithelial tissues are also more prone to invasion by pathogenic microorganisms.

High-protein diets deplete neonatal stores of yolk-derived vitamin A more rapidly than low-protein rations. Affected turtles usually have swollen eyes and, often, respiratory signs. The severity of the signs correlates with the degree of hypovitaminosis A and the length of time that the animal has been on a vitamin A–deficient diet. When the deficiency is of long duration, the widespread effects of squamous metaplasia and hyperkeratosis become more evident and difficult to treat successfully.

Treatment consists of parenteral or oral vitamin A (see the description of iatrogenic hypervitaminosis A following this discussion of hypovitaminosis A). Aquasol A (U.S. Pharmaceutical) is water miscible, and a dosage of 50 to 10,000 IU, depending on the size of the patient and the severity of the lesions,

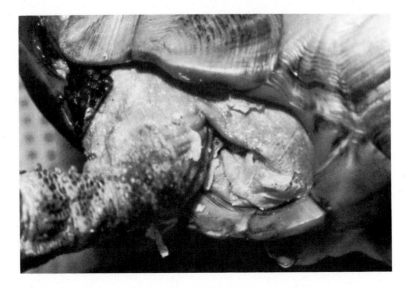

Figure 1. Appearance of tortoise's skin ten days following the intramuscular injection of approximately 75,000 IU of oil-soluble vitamin A. Note the dry and flaky appearance of the skin. (Copyright © 1987, Dr. F. L. Frye.)

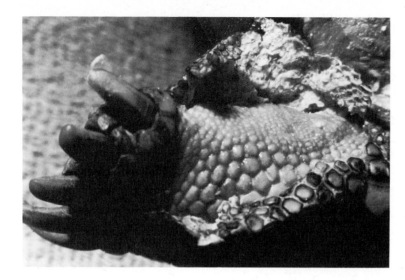

Figure 2. Same tortoise as in Figure 1 at postinjection day 14. During the intervening 4 days, the epidermis has begun to slough away from the subjacent dermis and musculature. (Copyright © 1987, Dr. F. L. Frye.)

Figure 3. Photomicrograph of tissue removed at necropsy of tortoise in Figures 1 and 2. Note the necrotizing dermatitis and denuded exterior surface (H & E stain; × 67, original magnification). (Copyright © 1987, Dr. F. L. Frye.)

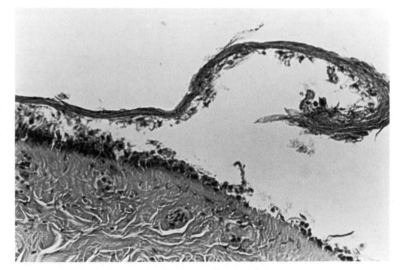

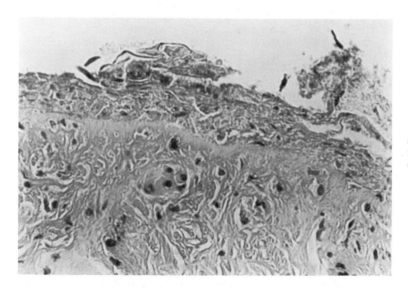

Figure 4. Photomicrograph of another area of denuded limb. Note the exposure of the skeletal muscle (H & E stain; × 67). (Copyright © 1987, Dr. F. L. Frye.)

is indicated. This very wide dosage range was arrived at empirically, but if the amount is scaled to approximately 5 IU per 10 gm of body weight, the therapeutic effect should be sufficient to reverse early lesions resulting from hypovitaminosis A. Oral administration of a product such as ABDEC Drops (Parke-Davis) may be performed on a regular basis or for correction of the captive diet responsible for the deficiency. Obviously, the diet must be corrected to include an adequate level of vitamin A or its precursor carotenoids. Here is an example in which a case can be made for the feeding of commercial dog or cat food (particularly the semimoist cat foods such as Tender Vittles, Ralston Purina). Another excellent diet that contains adequate levels of preformed vitamins and minerals is Trout Chow (Ralston Purina). Both of these products are palatable to the small turtles and are readily eaten. The diet for these small aquatic turtles may be further supplemented by feeding earthworms or small live or freshly killed whole fish.

HYPERVITAMINOSIS A

It is a common practice in clinical reptile medicine to employ injectable vitamin A, either as a sole bioactive agent or as a multiple, lipid-soluble vitamin preparation containing vitamins A, D, and E (as alpha-tocopherol or as mixed tocopherols). Often, the actual need for the patient to receive these exogenous vitamins is not adequately evaluated, and their administration has become routine for some practitioners. Sometimes, the clinical sign that is taken for a justification for using these drugs is a nasal discharge. Too often the patient is a herbivorous terrestrial tortoise whose normal vegetarian diet contains abundant natural carotenoids. It has been known for many years that the hepatic half-life for retinol(s) is long. Similarly, adipose tissue and hepatic stores of carotene are dynamic, but extended. Occasionally, these vitamins are injected with the expectation of improving a flagging appetite.

The clinical signs of hypervitaminosis A in terrestrial chelonians are subacute xeroderma followed in a few days by a florid necrotizing dermatitis (Fig. 1). These lesions typically appear on the limbs and cervical skin, but they may occur on any skin-covered surface. Usually, by the 14th day after injection, the epidermis has formed large, fluid-filled bullae and has begun to lift away from the dermis, leaving in its place variable-sized expanses of denuded moist tissue (Fig. 2). These alarming clinical signs appear to be identical to those reported and illustrated in the lay literature by Rosskopf and colleagues as being induced by the antibiotics carbenicillin and gentamicin sulfate. It is not clear whether all the cases that Rosskopf and colleagues

described also had received vitamin A injections as part of their treatment.

Histologically, hypervitaminosis A is characterized early in the process by a marked flattening of the stratum corneum and stratum germinativum. Eventually, the dermis and muscular structures are exposed (Figs. 3 and 4). Most of the tortoises affected with this disorder survive, and their damaged skin regenerates. Others resemble patients suffering from third-degree thermal burns and die as a result of the effects of having such large areas of their skin destroyed. In summary, the physical signs of hypervitaminosis A share many of the features of erythema multiforme (Stevens-Johnson syndrome) in higher vertebrates. This disorder has been associated with adverse reactions to any of several drugs.

Clinical prudence suggests that (injectable) exogenous vitamin biologicals *not* be used in reptiles *unless* the dietary history and clinical signs displayed by a particular animal clearly signal that a deficiency state exists. This appears to be particularly germane in the case of herbivorous tortoises.

If clinical judgment suggests the use of supplemental vitamin A, *oral* dosage with natural sources of carotene, preformed vitamin A, or both would seem to be the safest means for administration. Freshly grated carrots, yellow squash, green leafy vegetables, or all three are readily available and are easily given orally.

References and Supplemental Reading

Belkin, D. A.: Reduction of metabolic rate in response to starvation in the turtle, *Sternotherus minor*. Copeia 1965 3:367, 1965.

Czajka, A. F.: Gelatin-bonded food for turtles. Bull. Chicago Herp. Soc. 16:40, 1981.

Dantzler, W. H., and Schmidt-Nielsen, B.: Excretion in freshwater turtle (*Pseudemys scripta*) and desert tortoise (*Gopherus agassizi*). Am. J. Physiol. 210:198, 1966.

Dawson, W. R.: Reptiles as research models in comparative physiology. J.A.V.M.A. 159:1653, 1971.

Demovsky, R., and Greenberg, R.: Growth effect and tissue distribution of vitamin A following intravenous injection of vitamin A–rich chyle. Proc. Soc. Exp. Biol. Med. 118:158, 1964.

Derikson, W. K.: Lipid storage and utilization in reptiles. Am. Zool. 16:711, 1976.

Dessauer, H. C.: Blood chemistry of reptiles: physiology and evolutionary aspects. *In* Gans, C., and Parsons, T. S., (eds.): *Biology of the Reptilia*, Vol. 3, Morphology C. New York, Academic Press, 1970, pp. 25–26.

Dunson, W. A.: Some aspects of electrolyte and water balance in three estuarine reptiles, the Diamondback terrapin, American and "salt water" crocodiles. Comp. Biochem. Physiol. 32:161, 1970.

Dunson, W. A., and Weymouth, R. D.: Active uptake of sodium by softshell turtles (*Trionyx spinifer*). Science 149:67, 1965.

Fowler, M. E.: Metabolic bone disease. *In* Fowler, M. E. (ed.): *Zoo and Wild Animal Medicine*, Philadelphia: W. B. Saunders Co., 1978, pp. 55–76.

Fowler, M. E.: Comparison of respiratory infection and hypovitaminosis A in desert tortoises. *In* Montali, R. J., and Migaki, G. (eds.): *Pathology of Zoo Animals*. Washington, D.C.: Smithsonian Institution Press, 1980, pp. 93–97.

Fox, A. M., and Musacchia, X. J.: Notes on the pH of the Digestive Tract of *Chrysemys picta*. Copeia 1959 1959, pp. 337–339.

Frye, F. L.: The Role of Nutrition in the Successful Management of Captive Reptiles. Proceedings of the California Veterinary Medicine Association 86th Meeting and Scientific Seminar, 1974, pp. 5–20.

Frye, F. L.: *Biomedical and Surgical Aspects of Captive Reptile Husbandry.* Edwardsville, KS: Veterinary Medicine Pub. Co., 1981, pp. 23–60.

Frye, F. L.: Feeding and nutritional diseases. *In* Fowler, M. E. (ed.): *Zoo and Wild Animal Medicine,* 2nd ed. Philadelphia: W. B. Saunders Co., 1986, pp. 139–151.

Frye, F. L.: Care and feeding of some invertebrates kept as pets or study animals. Proceedings of the California Veterinary Medicine Association 99th Annual Meeting and Scientific Seminar, 1987, pp. 217–269.

Frye, F. L.: *Biomedical and Surgical Aspects of Captive Reptile Husbandry,* 2nd ed. Melbourne, FL: R.E. Krieger, 1989, (in press).

Frye, F. L., and Carney, J. D.: Parathyroid adenoma in a tortoise. Vet. Med. Small Anim. Clin. 70:582, 1975.

Frye, F. L., and Dutra, F. R.: Hypothyroidism in turtles and tortoises. Vet. Med. Small Anim. Clin. 69:990, 1974.

Frye, F. L., and Dutra, F. R.: Articular pseudogout in a turtle (*Chrysemys p. elegans*). Vet. Med. Small Anim. Clin. 71:655, 1976.

Frye, F. L., Dutra, F. R., Carney, J. D., et al.: Spontaneous diabetes in a turtle. Vet. Med. Small Anim. Clin. 71:935, 1976.

Goode, M.: *Echis colorata* (Palestine saw-scaled viper): Water economy. Herpetol. Rev. 14:120; 1983.

Haggag, G., Raheem, A., and Khalil, F.: Hibernation in reptiles. I. Changes in blood electrolytes. Comp. Biochem. Physiol. 16:457, 1965.

Haggag, G., Raheem, A., and Khalil, F.: Hibernation in reptiles. II. Changes in blood glucose, hemoglobin, red blood cell count, protein and nonprotein nitrogen. Comp. Biochem. Physiol. 17:335, 1966.

Holmes, W. N., and McBean, R. I.: Some aspects of electrolyte excretion in the Green turtle, *Chelonia mydas mydas.* J. Exp. Biol. 41:81, 1964.

Ippen, R.: Considerations on the comparative pathology of bone diseases in reptiles. Zentralbl. Allg. Pathol. 108:424, 1965.

Jackson, D. C.: Buoyancy control in the freshwater turtle, *Pseudemys scripta elegans.* Science 166:1649, 1969.

Jackson, C. G., Jr., Trotter, J. A., Trotter, T. H., et al.: An accelerated growth and early maturity in *Gopherus agassizi* (Reptilia, Testudines). Herpetologica 32:139, 1976.

Jackson, O. F., and Cooper, J. E.: Nutritional diseases. *In* Cooper, J. E., and Jackson, O. F. (eds.): *Diseases of the Reptilia,* Vol. 2 London: Academic Press, 1981, pp. 409–428.

Jarrett, A.: The Action of vitamin A on adult epidermis and dermis. *In* Jarrett, A. (ed.): *The Physiology and Pathophysiology of the Skin,* Vol. 6. London: Academic Press, 1980, pp. 2059–2091.

Jenkins, N. K., and Simkiss, K.: The calcium and phosphate metabolism of reproducing reptiles with particular reference to the adder (*Vipera berus*). Comp. Biochem. Physiol. 26:865, 1968.

Jensen, H. B., and With, T. K.: Vitamin A and carotenoids in the liver of mammals, birds, reptiles and Man, with particular regard to the intensity of the ultraviolet absorption and the Carr-Proce reaction of vitamin A. Biochem. J. 33:1771, 1939.

Kramer, D. C.: Geophagy in *Terrapene ornata ornata agassizi.* J. Herpetol. 7:138, 1973.

Medica, P. A., Bury, R. B., and Luckenbach, R. A.: Drinking and construction of water catchments by the desert tortoise, *Gopherus agassizi,* in the desert. Herpetologica 36:301, 1980.

Mettler, F., Palmer, D., Rübel, A., et al.: Gehäuft Auftretende Fälle von Parakeratrosen mit Epithelablösung der Landschildkröten. Verhandlungsber. XXIV Internat. Symp. Erkrankungen der Zootiere. Veszprem, 1982, pp. 245–248.

Palmer, D. G., Rübel, A., Mettler, F., et al.: Experimentell erzeugte Hautveränderungen bei Landschildkröten durch hohe parenterale Gaben von Vitamin A. Zbl. Vet. Med. A. 31:625, 1984.

Peaker, M.: Active acquisition of stomach stones in the American alligator, *Alligator mississippiensis* Daudin. Br. J. Herpetol. 4:103, 1969.

Peaker, M.: Some aspects of the thermal requirements of reptiles in captivity. Int. Zoo Yearb. 9:3, 1969.

Pfeiffer, C.: Foods for tortoises, I–X. Turtle Hobbyist 1,2; 5163 E. Bedford Drive, San Diego, CA 92116.

Porter, K. R.: *Herpetology.* Philadelphia: W. B. Saunders Co., 1972.

Pritchard, P. C. H.: A Reinterpretation of *Testudo gigantea* Schweigger, 1812. J. Herpetol. 20:522, 1986.

Reichenbach-Klinke, H. H., and Elkan, E.: *The Principal Diseases of Lower Vertebrates.* New York: Academic Press, 1965.

Rhodin, A. G. J.: Pathological lithophagy in *Testudo horsfieldi.* J. Herpetol. 8:385, 1974.

Schmidt-Nielsen, K.: *Desert Animals.* New York: Oxford University Press, 1964, pp. 225–251.

Schmidt-Nielsen, K., and Frange, R.: Salt glands in marine reptiles. Nature (Lond) 182:783, 1958.

Schmidt-Nielsen, K., Borut, A., Lee, P., et al.: Nasal salt excretion and the possible function of the cloaca in water conservation. Science 142:1300, 1963.

Seidel, M. E., and Smith, H. M.: *Chrysemys, Pseudemys, Trachemys* (Testudines:Emydidae): Did Agassiz have it right? Herpetologica 42:242, 1987.

Skorepa, A. C.: The deliberate consumption of stones by the ornate box turtle, *Terrapene ornata* Agassiz. J. Ohio Herp. Soc. 5:108, 1966.

Smith, H. A., *et al:* *Veterinary Pathology,* 4th Ed. Philadelphia: Lea & Febiger, 1972, pp. 1057–1071.

Sokol, O. M.: Lithophagy and geophagy in reptiles. J. Herpetol. 5:69, 1971.

Studer, A., and Frey, J. R.: Über Hautveränderungen der Ratte nach Grossen Oralen Dosen von Vitamin A. Schweiz. Med. Wochenschr. 79:382, 1949.

Van Vleet, J. F.: Comparative pathology of selenium and vitamin E deficiency and excess. Comp. Pathol. Bull. 17:1, 1985.

Wallach, J. D.: Environmental and nutritional diseases of captive reptiles. J.A.V.M.A. 159:1632, 1971.

SEXUAL DIMORPHISM AND IDENTIFICATION IN REPTILES

FREDRIC L. FRYE, B.S., D.V.M.

Davis, California

TURTLES AND TORTOISES

With a few exceptions, *grossly* observable differences between the sexes are minimal in reptiles. Generally, most terrestrial chelonian females have a plastron (lower shell) that, when viewed from the side, appears to be almost flat. In adult conspecific males, the plastron tends to be somewhat concave, or "dished" (Figs. 1 and 2). This feature allows for anatomic accommodation during copulation, when the male mounts the female from the rear in a male superior position; the concavity of the male's plastron fits neatly with the matching portion of the convex curvature of the female's carapace (Fig. 3). The flatter shape of the female's plastron also allows for the storage and early development of intracoe-

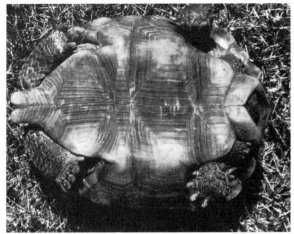

Figure 1. Plastron of a mature female desert tortoise. Note the flatness of the surface. (Copyright © 1988, Dr. F. L. Frye.)

lomic eggs prior to their oviposition. Similarly, the anal notch in the caudalmost portion of the female's plastron is larger in diameter than that of a mature conspecific male and has evolved to permit the passage of shelled ova. The cloacal vent of the female turtle is situated closer to the body than that of a conspecific male of the same size. Again, this vent location is related to the passage of shelled eggs, which often are quite large. In tortoises, the female's tail usually is quite stubby, whereas the male's is typically broad-based and much longer. This is because the penis of most male chelonians is relatively large and occupies much of the cranial portion of the male's tail. These differences can be rather subtle and may confuse those who are inexperienced in sexing these creatures. In summary, *all* external features should be carefully examined and evaluated.

Some male tortoises, especially those of the genus *Gopherus*, possess well-developed, paired sexual tubercles, or mental glands, located on each side of the ventrolateral aspects of the mandibles. These structures are modified glandular organs, histologically similar to sebaceous glands found in higher

vertebrates. These lobular-alveolar glands deliver their secretory product(s) in a holocrine fashion through short ducts to the epidermal surface. The waxy substance they secrete is believed to contain one or more pheromonelike agents that the tortoises of both sexes can detect by olfaction. Sexually active males have been observed rubbing these secretions onto objects in their territory and upon conspecific females during their courtship ritual and copulation. During and after the mating season, these mental glands become enlarged and, upon gentle digital expression, exude their secretions, which are of the consistency of soft paraffin. To the human nose, the material is odorless.

Although mental glands may be present in some females of those species known to possess them, they usually are quite rudimentary and may merely be represented as inactive remnants.

In some adult male tortoises, particularly those of the genus *Gopherus*, the twin gular plates, or projection(s) on the cranial plastron, are well developed and scooplike. With these projections, sexually aggressive males ram rivals and even prospective mates during their courtship displays. The caudal carapace of the males tends to be tucked under, whereas the female's is flared and more apronlike in shape.

In some species (e.g., *Terrapene* species box turtles), the males possess more brightly colored eyes. In many of these turtles, the iris of adult males is red; it is yellow-orange in mature females.

All male turtles and tortoises possess a single spade-shaped penis that is extended through the cloacal vent when erect. This organ is often heavily pigmented and may be erected as a defense strategy when the animal is handled: occasionally this protrusion is accompanied by forceful urination or expression of secretions from the scent glands, which augments the defensive value of this behavior. A ventral raphe, or median groove, conducts the semen to the end of the organ during intromission.

Some chelonians possess a sexually dimorphic

Figure 2. Plastron of a mature male red-footed tortoise. Note the marked convexity that is characteristically extreme in this species with its high-domed and narrow carapace. (Copyright © 1988, Dr. F. L. Frye.)

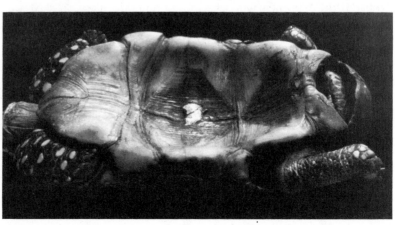

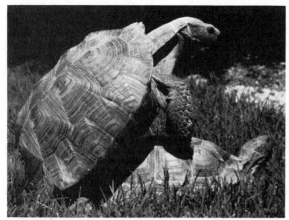

Figure 3. Mating desert tortoises. Without the plastral convexity in the male, mating would be difficult, if not impossible. (Copyright © 1988, Dr. F. L. Frye.)

transverse plastral kinesis that allows the female's plastron to partially flex or hinge and thus accommodate the passage of their often large and relatively unyielding eggs (Moll, 1985; Waagen, 1984). In some turtles, particularly the Emydid genus *Trachemys* (formerly classified as *Pseudemys* and *Chrysemys*), there is another sexually dimorphic characteristic: the adult males possess greatly elongated front claws that they wave in front of their prospective mates during courtship in order to "titillate" them. Even juvenile turtles occasionally display this behavior with each other—years before their claws have grown long enough to exhibit a sexually dimorphic difference.

LIZARDS AND SNAKES

Lizards and snakes will be discussed together because they share many of the same anatomic and behavioral characteristics.

Male lizards and snakes possess paired intromittent organs called *hemipenes*. The morphology of these organs is highly individualistic and differs between species within a given genus. These morphologic differences are employed as diagnostic characteristics by which some species are differentiated. Most hemipenes are equipped with keratinized spines, flounces, or similar adornments that, when the hemipenis is erect, tend to be directed in a retrograde direction; it is thought that these projections help hold the organ in place during intromission (which, in some snake species, may be a rather prolonged affair, often lasting more than 24 hrs; *cum staminae serpentis!*)

One hemipenis is employed at a time. The hemipenes are located distal to the cloacal vent, and each is connected by a ductus deferens to its ipsilateral testis. The testes are paired and located intracoelomically, adjacent to, or slightly posterior to, the kidneys. A scent gland and retractor penis

muscle are attached to the caudal pole of each hemipenis. Often, the paired adrenal glands are attached to the testes by a mesenterylike mesorchium; because of their yellow or orange color, they are a useful landmark during fiberoptic endoscopy of the coelomic cavity. In other species, the adrenals are attached to the kidneys; these anatomic differences are family- and genus-specific.

Sexual identification is more difficult in many lizards and snakes than in some other reptiles. In some snakes, the gradually tapering tail of the male is in marked contrast to the severely constricted postcloacal tail of the female; this is because of the absence of hemipenes in the females' tails. In some lizards, the males are more brightly colored—especially during mating season—than their conspecific females. In others, dorsal spines and cephalic armature in the form of enlarged scales or plates are more highly developed in males than in females. In the lizard species that possess femoral pores (holocrine dermal adnexal glands located on the ventral portions of the rear limbs), the pores are usually more highly developed in males. Sexually dimorphic color or pattern differences are not characteristic of snakes. In some lizards, chelonians, and crocodilians, size may be an indicator: the males tend to be larger and more robust. However, in many snake species, the females may grow larger than the males; this is well illustrated in the South American boa constrictors, anacondas, some pit vipers, and some colubrids.

In some species, such as the spectacular African Jackson's chameleon, an obvious sexual dimorphism is displayed: the males possess three highly developed, gradually tapering, keratin-covered bony horns borne in a *Triceratops* fashion on their rostrums (Fig. 4). These projections are employed during jousting and mock combat in competition with male cohorts for sexual supremacy and territorial imperatives. In captivity, such behavior be-

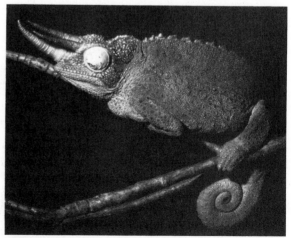

Figure 4. Head of an adult male Jackson's chameleon. Note the three prominent rostral horns that characterize the male sex in this species. (Copyright © 1988, Dr. F. L. Frye.)

tween one or more dominant lizards and lizards of lower status often leads to a failure to feed, drink and, in general, adapt to captivity by the lower-ranking animals in an enclosure. Males of some other chameleon species possess paired projections, whereas others lack rostral horns altogether and do not appear much different from their conspecific females.

Identification of the sex of some snakes and lizards may be difficult because of subtle differences and often requires the use of specialized sexing probes (FurMont Probes). These thin, elongated, yet blunt-tipped instruments are inserted *gently* (with appropriate lubrication) into the cloacal vent and directed caudally. In most female lizards, these probes will not penetrate more than a very short distance; in most males, these probes will enter the sulcus in which each of the invaginated hemipenises lies and can be inserted for a distance far longer than in females of the same species and size.

These probes must be clean and inserted very gently because they may perforate delicate tissue structures, resulting in severe wound infection. One hazard of probing lizards and snakes to determine sex is the rather high incidence of cloacal prolapse that may be induced by this procedure, particularly if metallic probes are used and if they are not inserted with delicacy. Many experienced herpetologists claim that their techniques have not created such prolapses; others have quite candidly admitted that some of their specimens have, indeed, been lost as a result of prolapse, necrotic cloacitis, or both after being probed.

Other methods for the elucidation of sex have been described. In snakes and lizards large enough to permit the maneuver, a cotton-tipped applicator stick, moistened with tap water or lubricating jelly,* may be inserted into the sulcus surrounding the inverted hemipenis (Fig. 5). In lizards and snakes that are too small to permit the insertion of a cotton-tipped applicator stick, one can use a disposable polypropylene urethral catheter (Soverign) or a plastic intravenous catheter (e.g., Abbocath, CEVA, or Jelco Labs, Raritan, NJ) with the stylet removed. These catheters are smooth-edged and are very useful as hemipenial probes. They are inserted in the same fashion as other probes. An alternative method is to gently express or evert one or both hemipenes from their inverted positions by gentle digital pressure applied to their caudal site in the tail. This method was described by Gregory (1983) and is effective in some of the larger lizards and snakes. Another very useful and safe method for determining the sex of squamates was described by

Nickerson (1970). In this technique, sterile isotonic physiologic solutions may be injected transcutaneously into the hemipenis. Such fluid injection causes immediate engorgement and eversion of one or both hemipenes (Fig. 6). The organ returns to the relaxed, flaccid state as the fluid is resorbed and spontaneously reinvaginates into its sulcus. Unless a large volume of fluid is injected, the erect organ can be replaced into its sulcus. The author has found this method particularly useful in lizards such as Gila monsters, Mexican beaded lizards, Tegus, some large skinks, and some monitors that have been reported to be particularly difficult to identify the sex by hemipenial sulcus probing. This method does not require any special equipment and is easily reproducible.

In some of the larger lizards, the twin hemipenes can be palpated as the base of the tail is rolled between the thumb and fingers of the examiner, but this technique is highly subjective and depends upon the experience of the person employing it. In some species, the circumference or diameter of the tail base has been used as a reliable indicator of sex: the tail-base diameter of a male of a given length is statistically greater than that of a conspecific female of the same length.

Direct visualization of the gonads is possible with the use of fiberoptic endoscopy, similar to that employed in birds. It can be an effective and relatively safe method if done aseptically and with care. This method also may be employed in immature chelonians. The technique requires general anesthesia, can be time consuming, and sometimes does not resolve the sex of a particular animal. In some instances, the major untoward reaction induced by this technique has been overinsufflation with the inert gas employed during the procedure to allow visualization of the coelomic viscera. Generally, some residual gas remains after withdrawing the cannula. This gas is usually absorbed within 24 hr, but if the intracoelomic pressure is sufficiently great, respiration may be impaired from iatrogenic lung compression.

In boas, anacondas, and pythons, sexual identification is much easier. Males of most genera of the family Boidae possess paracloacal *spurs*, which are actually vestigial remnants of the pelvic girdle and rear limbs (Fig. 7). These structures are located on either side of the cloacal vent. They are seen easily even in very young males of species that possess them and may be readily demonstrated on radiographs of the tail. Some female boid snakes also will be found to possess spurs, but usually these structures are much reduced in size. During courtship, the spurs are employed to produce tactile stimuli and are often quite mobile, moving in wide arcs. When not being employed in such activities, they are folded back against the body and lie within shallow grooves at right angles to the cloacal vent.

---

*Some lubricating jelly products have been found to be spermicidal and should not be employed if an immediate breeding is anticipated. Fresh raw hen's egg white (albumen) can be used in such instances.

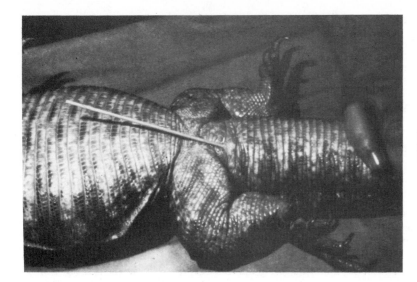

Figure 5. Use of a lubricated cotton-tipped applicator as a hemipenial sulcus probe in a lizard. (Copyright © 1988, Dr. F. L. Frye.)

Figure 6. Hemipenial eversion in a rattlesnake, induced by bilateral injection of a sterile physiologic solution. Note the fully distended hemipenis covered with caudally directed keratinized spines. (Copyright © 1972, Dr. Nathan W. Cohen. Reproduced with permission.)

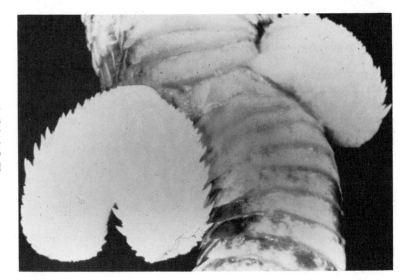

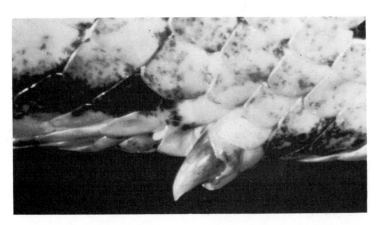

Figure 7. Paracloacal "spurs" of an adult anaconda. (Copyright © 1972, Dr. N. W. Cohen. Reproduced with permission.)

Investigators at the College of Veterinary Medicine, University of Tennessee, Knoxville, found that the sex of some male lizards of the family Varanidae (monitors) may be determined radiographically. These lizards appear to undergo soft-tissue mineralization of the hemipenes; the mineralized tissues can be readily demonstrated on radiographs. This mineralization has been confirmed by Shea and Reddacliff (1986). The biologic value of mineralization of what is normally soft erectile tissue in most other taxa is unclear and appears, at first glance, to be astonishingly paradoxic. A more parsimonious explanation may be that the stiffened cranial armature of the hemipenes may be more readily held in apposition with the caudal portion(s) of the tubular reproductive tract of conspecific females.

The author's experiences at the University of California have shown that this genus, as well as most other taxa of large lizards, can be sexed easily by the methods previously noted, particularly probing with lubricated cotton-tipped wooden applicator sticks or smooth-edged polypropylene urinary catheters (both of which are the author's preference for probing hemipenial sulci).

Histologically, the sexes of some snakes and lizards may be differentiated by the presence of *sexual segment granulation* observed in the distal convoluted tubules of the kidneys of some male lizards and snakes. Actually, the sexual segment refers to the portions of these tubules that undergo a marked columnar hypertrophy during periods of sexual recrudescence in some animals, or postmating quiescence in others. These modified renal tubules undergo a cyclic alteration that most often is seasonal. This modification consists of a change from cuboidal tubular epithelium to plump, often very tall columnar cells (Fig. 8). These cells become packed with small, round, highly eosinophilic granules that are secreted directly into the lumens of the altered tubules. The function of these granules

has been the object of much study; they are currently believed to contain pheromonelike substances. They also may contribute to the semen volume, but this is, as yet, unproved. Certainly, the product(s) of the sexual segment appear to augment and partially mediate sexually responsive behavior. Similar, if not identical, distal tubular hypertrophy and cytoplasmic granulation have been observed in histologic sections of the kidneys of some adult male *Gopherus* tortoises (Frye, 1981).

Radioimmunoassay of circulating testicular or ovarian hormones may be employed as an accurate means of determining the sex of some reptiles. This technique is relatively expensive and is limited by the availability of laboratories that can perform the assay.

Karyotype analysis has been accomplished in some reptiles, but proven heterogametic sex chromosomes have been found in only a few species. As more data accumulate, this modality may provide greater utility.

CROCODILIANS

These animals represent the most difficult common reptilian species to sex accurately—particularly as juveniles. As they grow, the task becomes much easier; in animals over 1 m long, a gloved finger can be inserted into the cloacal vent and directed cranially. In the male, a small pointed projection or papilla can be palpated; this organ, when erect, serves as a penis and tends to point caudally (Fig. 9); it is lacking in the female. Obviously, this method of sex identification is limited to reasonably large animals and carries with it some risk to the finger-bearer!

Some laboratories serving zoologic collections and commercial alligator and crocodile farms have employed radioimmunoassay of sex hormones to deter-

Figure 8. Photomicrograph of a renal section from an *Ameiva* lizard kidney. Note the massive hypertrophy of portions of the distal convoluted tubules containing densely stained intracytoplasmic granules (H & E stain; × 67, original magnification). (Copyright © 1988, Dr. F. L. Frye.)

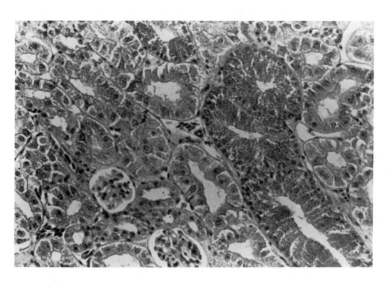

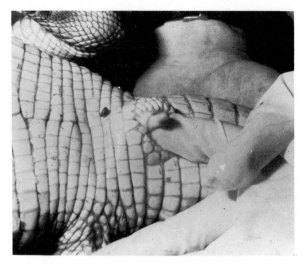

Figure 9. Caiman penis. (Copyright © 1986, Dr. F. L. Frye.)

mine the sex of these animals. Considering that these potentially dangerous creatures must be restrained in order to obtain blood specimens, it would seem more practical to employ the digital exploration of the cloaca for the presence of an erectile penis. The technique is rapid and accurate and does not require expensive equipment and reagents. Those few animals with equivocal or questionable findings can be confirmed by fiberoptic endoscopy or radioimmunoassay.

Fiberoptic endoscopy may be employed to directly visualize the gonads within the coelomic cavity. As mentioned previously, respiratory embarrassment from lung compression can be avoided by limiting the volume of inert gas used to insufflate the coelomic cavity to the minimum required to delineate the coelomic viscera.

Crocodilians possess mental glands that, histologically, are similar to those seen in some chelonians. However, in the crocodilians, these glands are surrounded by muscle fibers that facilitate expression of the fatty acid–rich holocrine secretions. These products are thought to contain pheromone(s) and are employed as territorial markers and sexual cues during courtship. These glandular structures are more highly developed in males.

One crocodilian, the gavial (gharial) is characterized by an external feature that can be used to distinguish mature males from females: the rostral, or nasal, hump is markedly larger and more bulbous in the male than in a female of the same size. The function of this structure is to produce stentorious auditory signals to receptive females.

THE TUATARA

The primitive tuatara, *Sphenodon punctatum*, is under strict protection by the government of New Zealand and is displayed in only a few carefully selected zoologic collections. Today, the largest captive breeding program in North America is at the St. Louis Zoological Park. Although with its short dorsal spines it superficially resembles an iguana, the tuatara is not a lizard, but the sole member of the order Rhyncocephalia and is characterized by several structural, physiologic, and hematologic differences that are shared by no other extant reptile. Based upon several morphologic similarities, these animals may be most closely related to primitive chelonians.

The male tuatara does not possess a true erectile penis but, rather, a small papillalike projection that serves to transfer semen to the female during copulation. Under manual restraint, this papilla can be visualized with the aid of a hand-held otoscope gently inserted into the male's cloacal vent. Alternatively, if no papilla is found and it is imperative to determine the sex of a particular specimen, a sterile fiberoptic endoscope can be inserted into the coelomic cavity through a small flank incision. Of course, this procedure must be performed by practiced hands, under aseptic surgical conditions, and using surgical anesthesia.

References and Supplemental Reading

Blair, K. D.: Sex determination in snakes. Bull. Chicago Herp. Soc. 22:150, 1987.

Brazatis, P. J.: The determination of sex in living crocodilians. Br. J. Herpetol. 4:54, 1968.

Bull, J. J.: Evolution in karyotypes: I. Sex determination. II. Chromosomes of side-necked turtles. Dissr. Abstr. Int. B. 38:1509, 1977.

Bull, J. J., and Vogt, R. C.: Temperature-dependent sex determination in turtles. Science 206:1186, 1979.

Burtner, H. J., Floyd, A. D., and Langley, J. B.: Histochemistry of the "sexual segment" granules of the male rattlesnake kidney. J. Morphol. 116:189, 1965.

Carpenter, C. C., Murphy, J. B., Mitchell, L. A., et al.: Combat bouts with spur on the Madagascar boa (*Sanzinia madagascarensis*). Herpetologica 34:207, 1978.

Charnier, M.: Action de la Temperature sur la Sex-Ratio chez l'Embryion d' *Agama agama* (Agamidae, Lacertilien). C.R. Soc. Biol. 160:620, 1966.

Chiszar, D., and Taylor, S. V.: Live snakes: Chemical cue detection and behavior. Carolina Tips 39:53, 1976.

Christiansen, J. L., and Ladman, A. J.: The reproductive morphology of *Cnemidophorus neomexicanus* X.C. *inornatus* hybrid males. J. Morphol. 125:367, 1968.

Conner, J., and Crews, D.: Sperm transfer and storage in the lizard, *Anolis carolinensis*. J. Morphol. 163:331, 1980.

Cooper, W. E., Cooper, W. E., Jr., Vitt, J. L., et al.: Responses of the skinks, *Eumeces fasciatus* and *E. laticeps*, to airborne conspecific odors: Further appraisal. J. Herpetal. 19:481, 1985.

Crews, D.: Psychobiology of reptilian reproduction. Science 189:1059, 1975.

Crews, D.: Hemipenile preference: Stimulus control of male mounting behavior in the lizard *Anolis carolinensis*. Science 199:195, 1978.

Cueller, O.: Oviductal anatomy and sperm storage structures in lizards. J. Morphol. 119:7, 1966a.

Devine, M. C.: Copulatory plugs in snakes: Enforced chastity. Science 187:844, 1975.

Devine, M. C.: Species discrimination in mate selection by free-living male garter snakes and experimental evidence for the role of pheromones. Abstr. Herpetol. Rec. 8:79, 1976.

Douglass, F. J.: Patterns of mate-seeking and burrow use in a Southern Florida population of *Gopherus polyphemus*. Abstr. Herpetol. Rec. 7:80, 1976.

Edgren, R. A.: Copulatory adjustment in snakes and its evolutionary implications. Copeia 1953, pp. 162–164.

Fitch, H. S.: Criteria for determining sex and breeding maturity in snakes. Herpetologica 16:49, 1960.

Fitch, H. S., and Henderson, R. W.: Reproduction, age, and sex differences, and conservation of *Iguana iguana*. Milwaukee Public Museum Contr. Biol. Geol. 13:1, 1977.

Ford, N. B.: Pheromone trailing behavior in three species of garter snake (*Thamnophis*). Am. Zool. (Abstract.) 16:245, 1976.

Ford, N. B.: Evidence of species specificity of pheromone trails in two sympatric garter snakes, *Thamnophis*. Herpetol. Rev. 9:10, 1978.

Frye, F. L.: *Husbandry, Medicine and Surgery in Captive Reptiles.* Bonner Springs, KS: Veterinary Medicine Pub. Co., 1973.

Frye, F. L.: Clinical obstetric and gynecologic disorders in reptiles. Proc. Am. Anim. Hosp. Assoc. 1974, pp. 497–499.

Frye, F. L.: *Biomedical and Surgical Aspects of Captive Reptile Husbandry.* Edwardsville, KS: Veterinary Medicine Pub. Co., 1981, pp. 276–310.

Fukada, H.: A method of detecting copulated female snakes. Herpetologica 15:181, 1959.

Gans, C.: Courtship, mating behavior and male combat in tuatara, *Sphenodon punctatus*. Herpetol. Rev. 18:194, 1984.

Garstka, W. R., and Crews, D.: Female sex pheromone in the skin and circulation of a garter snake. Science 214:681, 1981.

Garstka, W. R., and Crews, D.: Female control of male reproductive function in a Mexican snake. Science 217:1159, 1982.

Gehlbach, F. R., Watkins, J. F., and Kroll, J. C.: Pheromone trailing following studies of typhlopid, leptotyphlopid, and colubrid Snakes. Behavior 40:282, 1971.

Goellner, R. R.: Tuataras (*Sphenodon punctatus*) at St. Louis Zoo. Acta Zool. Pathol. Atverpiensia 78:319, 1984.

Goodenough, U.: *Genetics.* New York: CBS College Publishing Co., 1984, pp. 132–183.

Gorman, G. C.: The chromosomes of *Laticauda* and a review of karyotypic evolution in the Elapidae. J. Herpetol. 15:225, 1981.

Graham, G. L.: The karyotype of the Texas coral snake, *Micrurus fulvius tenere*. Herpetologica 33:345, 1977.

Gregory, P. T.: Identification of sex of small snakes in the field. Herpetol. Rev. 14:42, 1983.

Gutierrez, J. M., and Bolanos, R.: The karyotype of the Yellow-bellied Sea snake, *Pelamis platurus*. J. Herpetol. 14:161, 1980.

Hall, B. J.: Notes on the husbandry, behaviour and breeding of captive Tegu lizards. Int. Zoo Yearb. 18:91, 1978.

Judd, H. L., Bacon, J. P., Rüedi, D., et al.: Determination of sex in the Komodo monitor (*Varanus komodoensis*). Int. Zoo Yearb. 17:208, 1972.

Laszlo, J.: Probing as a practical method of sex recognition in snakes. Int. Zoo Yearb. 15:178, 1975.

Lilywhite, H. B.: Trailing movements and sexual behavior in Coluber constrictor. J. Herpetol. 19:206, 1985.

McBee, K., Sites, J. W., Jr., Engstrom, C., et al.: Karyotypes of four species of neotropical gekkos. J. Herpetol. 18:83, 1984.

McBee, K., Sites, J. W., Jr., Engstrom, C., et al.: First gecko reported with X and Y sex chromosomes. J. Herpetol. 21:60, 1986.

McCoy, C. J., et al.: Temperature-controlled sex determination in the sea turtle, *Lepidochelys olivacea*. J. Herpetol. 17:404, 1983.

Mengden, G. A., and Stock, A. D.: Chromosomal evolution in serpents: A comparison of G and C chromosome-banding patterns of some Colubrid and Boid Genera. Chromosoma 79:53, 1980.

Moll, E. O.: Comment: Sexually dimorphic plastral kinesis—the forgotten papers. Herpetol. Rev. 16:16, 1985.

Moon, R. G.: Heteromorphism in a kinosternid turtle. Mamm. Chromosomes Newsl. 15:10, 1974.

Muth, A.: Sex determination in desert iguanas: Does incubation temperature make a difference? Copeia 4:869, 1981.

Nickerson, M. A.: New uses for an old method used in ophidian sex determination. Br. J. Herpetol. 4:138, 1970.

Oldham, J. C., Smith, H. M., Miller, S. A., et al.: *A Laboratory Perspectus of Snake Anatomy.* Champaign, IL: Stipes Pub. Co., 1970.

Owens, D. W.: A technique for determining sex of immature *Chelonia mydas* using a radioimmunoassay. Herpetologica 34:270, 1978.

Porter, R.: *Herpetology.* Philadelphia: W. B. Saunders Co., 1972.

Reese, A. M.: The structure and development of the integumental glands of the crocodilia. J. Morphol. 35:581, 1921.

Rose, F. L.: Electrophoresis of chin gland extracts of *Gopherus* (tortoises). Comp. Biochem. Physiol. 29:847, 1969.

Rose, F. L.: Tortoise chin gland fatty acid composition. Behavioral significance. Comp. Biochem. Physiol. 32:577, 1970.

Ruedi, D., Girard, J., Heldstab, R., et al.: Testosterone for sex determination in reptiles. Proceedings of the XIX International Symposium on the Diseases of Zoo Animals. Poznan, Poland, May 18–22, 1977, pp. 141–145.

Saint-Girons, H.: Sperm survival and transport in the female genital tract of reptiles. *In* Hafez, E. S. E., and Thibault, C. G. (eds.): *The Biology of Spermatozoa.* Basel: S. Karger, 1975, pp. 105–113.

Schaefer, W. H.: Diagnosis of sex in snakes. Copeia 1934, p. 181.

Schildiger, B. J.: Endoscopic sex determination in reptiles. Proceedings of the first International Conference of Zoological and Avian Medicine, Oahu, 1987, pp. 369–375.

Shea, G. M., and Reddacliff, G. L.: Ossifications in the hemipenes of varanids. J. Herpetol. 20:566, 1986.

Sigmund, W. R.: Female preference for *Anolis carolinensis* males as a function of dewlap color and background coloration. J. Herpetol. 17:137, 1983.

Todd, S.: Egglaying by an *unmated* python (*Python molurus bivittatus*). Herpetile 3:33, 1978.

Trotter, J.: Sexing North American land tortoises (genus *Gopherus*). Turtle Hobbyist 1:2, 1976.

Tsui, H. W.: Gonadotropin control of androgen production in reptilian and avian testes. Diss. Abstr. Int. B 37:4361, 1976.

Valenstein, P., and Crews, D.: Mating-induced termination of behavioral estrus in the female lizard, *Anolis carolinensis*. Horm. Behav. 9:363, 1977.

Waagen, G. N.: Sexually dimorphic plastral kinesis in *Heosemys spinosa*. Herpetol. Rev. 15:33, 1984.

Wagner, E.: Breeding the Burmese python, *Python molurus bivittatus*, at the Seattle Zoo. Int. Zoo Yearb. 16:83, 1976.

Wagner, E.: Breeding the Gila monster, *Heloderma suspectum* in captivity. Int. Zoo Yearb. 16:74, 1976.

Weeks, H. C.: A review of placentation among reptiles with particular regard to the function and evolution of the placenta. Proc. Zool. Soc. London 1935, 1935, pp. 625–645.

Whitmore, C.: Sexing of hatchling sea turtles: Gross appearance versus histology. J. Herpetol. 19:430, 1985.

Whittaker, R.: Captive breeding of crocodilia in India. Acta Zool. Pathol. Antverpiensia. 78:309, 1984.

Wilhoft, D. C., Hotaling, E., Flanks, P., et al.: Effects of temperature on sex determination in embryos of the snapping turtle, *Chelydra serpentina*. J. Herpetol. 17:38, 1983.

Winokur, R. M., and Legler, J. M.: Rostral pores in turtles. J. Morphol. 143:107, 1974.

Winokur, R. M., and Legler, J. M.: Chelonian mental glands. J. Morphol. 147:275, 1975.

Wood, F., Plate, C., Critchley, K., et al.: Semen collection by electroejaculation of the green turtle, *Chelonia mydas*. Br. J. Herpetol. 6:200, 1982.

Section
8

NEUROLOGIC AND NEUROMUSCULAR DISORDERS

JOE N. KORNEGAY, D.V.M.
Consulting Editor

Hearing Loss in Small Animals: Occurrence and Diagnosis 805
Hypokalemic Polymyopathy of Cats 812
Canine Masticatory Muscle Disorders....................................... 816
Hereditary Myopathy of Labrador Retrievers.............................. 820
Sensory Neuropathy.. 822
Progressive Axonopathy of Boxer Dogs..................................... 828
Degenerative Myelopathy 830
Hypomyelination in Dogs... 834
Congenital Cerebellar Diseases of Dogs and Cats 838
Hydrocephalus 842
Craniocerebral Trauma... 847
Granulomatous Meningoencephalomyelitis................................... 854
Wobbler Syndrome in the Doberman Pinscher................................ 858

HEARING LOSS IN SMALL ANIMALS: OCCURRENCE AND DIAGNOSIS

MICHAEL H. SIMS, Ph.D.
Knoxville, Tennessee

Hearing is the sum total of the physiologic events that normally occur after sound waves enter the external ear canal. The best criterion for a clinical confirmation of hearing in small animals is a behavioral response (no matter how simple) to sound. This requirement is not only very practical, but ensures that we do not confuse the word *sensation* or *perception* with only an isolated portion of the physiology that supports it. It also emphasizes that cortical analysis, the so-called psychologic response, is the ultimate objective. Proper function of the individual components of the auditory system, as with the other special senses, is practically meaningless if sound is not consciously perceived by the animal. This chapter considers the different types of deafness, breed-specific hearing impairments, and the current techniques used to evaluate auditory dysfunction in small animals, specifically dogs and cats.

STRUCTURE AND FUNCTION OF THE EAR

The sensation of hearing involves three distinct series of events: (1) **conduction**, the propagation of sound energy by air and mechanical vibration through the external, middle, and inner ear cavities; (2) **transduction**, the conversion of sound energy in the environment into neural activity within receptor cells and neurons; and (3) **transmission**, the movement of action potentials through well-defined pathways in the peripheral and central nervous systems to areas that ultimately inform the animal about the quality and intensity of sound. Hearing and equilibrium, unlike other special senses, use mechanical transduction to initiate neural activity.

The pinna and external ear canal funnel and conduct pressure waves in air to the tympanic membrane (eardrum). The membrane and the attached ossicular chain vibrate in concert with the sound. The bony ossicles (malleus, incus, and stapes) contained within the air-filled middle ear cavity, together with the eardrum, promote an efficient transfer of sound energy in air to the fluid of the inner ear.

The cochlea is the coiled part of the membranous labyrinth that is enbedded within the temporal bone. The fluid-filled cochlea contains the organ of Corti, which is located on the basilar membrane and traverses the entire length of the structure. Acoustic pressure waves in the cochlea cause the basilar membrane to vibrate, leading to electrical changes across the membranes of the receptor cells. These changes, which are initiated by mechanical shearing of the cilia on the surface of the hair cells, then generate action potentials in the terminal endings of the nerve fibers composing the cochlear division of the eighth cranial nerve. From the cochlea, impulses are tonotopically transmitted to the ipsilateral and contralateral auditory cortex. The auditory pathway includes the cochlear nucleus, dorsal nucleus of the trapezoid body, lateral lemniscus, caudal colliculus, and medial geniculate body.

Much of the spectral analysis of sound is provided by the mechanics of the inner ear during the transduction phase. The hair cells in the base of the cochlea are important for high-frequency sounds, whereas low-frequency sounds preferentially affect the apex. Surprisingly, there have been few studies concerned with determining audible sound frequencies in dogs and cats. Studies using behavioral audiograms recently reported a range of 48 Hz to 85 kHz for cats and 67 Hz to 45 kHz for dogs, however. The frequency range for healthy young humans is commonly regarded as 20 Hz to 20 kHz.

DEAFNESS: CLASSIFICATION AND OCCURRENCE

Two general types of deafness, **conductive** and **sensorineural**, are recognized in dogs and cats. Conductive deafness occurs when the conduction of sound energy is compromised in the external or middle ear cavities. Deafness of this kind results when the external ear canal is occluded, the tympanic membrane is ruptured or becomes stiff, the ossicular chain is broken or becomes stiff, or there is fluid in the middle ear. Conductive deafness is usually not total, and there can be marked differences between ears. The most common cause of

805

conductive deafness is chronic otitis externa or media. In these cases, restoration of hearing may be accomplished medically or surgically.

Sensorineural deafness occurs when the physics or hydrodynamics of the inner ear are altered or when there is an abnormality in the receptor cells of the cochlea or any part of the auditory pathway from the acoustic nerve to the auditory cortex. Sensorineural deafness can be much more profound than conductive deafness. Neural deafness can occur naturally or can be induced accidentally by a variety of ototoxic drugs. Progressive cochlear damage has been reported following the use of dihydrostreptomycin, streptomycin, salicylates, neomycin, polymyxin, kanamycin, and some loop diuretics. Use of the antiseptic combination chlorhexidine/cetrimide in the external ear canal has been shown to cause cochlear and vestibular dysfunction in dogs and cats with ruptured tympanic membranes. Sensorineural deafness can also occur in conjunction with severe chronic otitis media/interna or canine distemper.

Hereditary deafness is most often of the sensorineural type and has been reported in the dalmatian, border collie, Shropshire terrier, Australian heeler, English setter, Australian shepherd, Boston terrier, collie, rottweiler, and Walker American foxhound. A predisposition for deafness in dogs is found in those breeds that have the merle gene for coat color. Dogs with auditory dysfunction that are heterozygous for dominant spotting may also have ocular defects. Congenital deafness in cats with white coat color and blue irises is common. Other causes of congenital deafness include cochlear or cochleosaccular degeneration caused by maternal exposure to ototoxic drugs or viruses. Deafness may be associated with vestibular disease, but there are no reports of electrodiagnostic evaluation in these cases.

CLINICAL EVALUATION OF AUDITORY FUNCTION

The clinical examination begins with a perceived problem in the animal's localization or discrimination of sound. Abnormal auditory function will often strain the relationship between an animal and its owner, especially with working dogs. Owners may unwittingly resort to discipline for what they consider to be inattentiveness or disobedience. Deafness is difficult to evaluate in dogs and cats, especially when there is incomplete bilateral or complete unilateral hearing loss. Therefore, a complete clinical examination should be based on both behavioral and electrophysiologic assessments.

In addition to determining the possibility of treatment, auditory evaluations will hopefully engender a pet owner's understanding of the handicap. A new consideration for the dog with nontreatable deafness

is the hearing aid. The aids are fitted into the external ear canal in compressible foam sleeves. Pet owners who are considering this type of prosthesis should be referred to a specialist or veterinary college for a complete evaluation. A dog must have some residual hearing ability to qualify for an aid. Most dogs with profound sensorineural loss would not benefit from such a device. Successful use requires an owner with an unusual commitment and a dog with a compliant temperament.

Behavioral Evaluation

One can evaluate hearing by observing an animal's behavior in response to sounds that are a part of its natural environment or sounds that are produced under artificial conditions in the clinic. Under ideal circumstances, a crude sort of audiogram could be constructed from an animal's reaction to sound of varying intensities and frequencies. Although scientists can put a great deal of confidence in psychophysical audiograms from laboratory animals, the behavioral response of pets to sound is often equivocal, and opinions from different examiners vary widely. Pets in a clinical setting are usually so apprehensive that their attentiveness to the examiner is minimal. Even animals with normal hearing will begin to ignore sounds produced by the clinician after the second or third occurrence. Some animals do, however, exhibit reflexive movement due to sound stimulation, and this can add an important dimension to a behavioral study. One such reflex, **Pryor's reflex**, consists of involuntary twitching or flicking of the ears in response to sound. One must carefully interpret reflex or volitional movement, since some movement can be initiated by an animal's keen vibratory sense.

Electrodiagnostic Evaluation

Hearing in animals can be evaluated using electrodiagnostic procedures that selectively assess the integrity of peripheral and central nervous system structures. These procedures include impedance audiometry, auditory evoked responses, and audiometric electroencephalography. Electrophysiologic recordings provide us with extended measures of auditory ability, even beyond that obtained from the trained laboratory animal. These noninvasive procedures are used not so much to establish the integrity of conscious sensibility but to affirm and explain suspected or known loss of function. A complete battery of tests allows a differentiation and characterization of conductive and sensorineural deafness. Because electrodiagnostic testing does not require conscious cooperation, it is particularly useful in testing the very young animal (1 to 2 weeks of age), in which behavioral responses are difficult to assess.

IMPEDANCE AUDIOMETRY: TYMPANOMETRY

The purpose of impedance audiometry is to assess audition based on an objective description of (1) the integrity and compliance of the eardrum, (2) the mobility of the ossicular chain, (3) the function of middle ear muscles and their attachments, and (4) the size of the external ear canal. Impedance is a measure of the rejection of energy per unit of time, and acoustic impedance is the resistance to the transmission of sound. Impedance audiometry involves the use of an impedance meter in determining the nature and degree of hearing loss. When sound waves strike the tympanic membrane in a normal ear, most of the energy is transmitted to the cochlea through movement of the ossicles in the middle ear. A small part is reflected back into the ear canal, and a small part is lost as friction. The degree to which sound is reflected is dependent on the stiffness of the tympanic membrane and associated structures. A tympanic membrane that is characterized by a high impedance accepts less energy than one that has a low impedance. The air in the external ear canal is a low impedance medium, whereas the fluid of the inner ear has a high impedance. Impedance differences between air and fluid are accommodated by the tympanic membrane and ossicular chain through a process termed impedance matching, thus allowing energy to flow more easily and efficiently from one medium to the other. Impedance is measured in cubic centimeters of air. A small volume of air is stiffer than a large volume. Therefore, the stiffness (impedance) of any medium in question can be expressed as an equivalent volume of air. Another clinically useful term that describes the stiffness of auditory structures is *compliance*. Compliance is the inverse of impedance and therefore is a convenient measure of mobility. It is also measured in cubic centimeters of air.

An electroacoustic meter determines how well the middle ear is performing its impedance-matching duties by measuring the mobility of the tympanic membrane and ossicular chain. Commercially available meters are equipped with an ear probe that contains an acoustic generator, a microphone, and a positive-negative air pump. The generator produces a continuous tone at a certain pressure in the external ear canal, and the microphone measures the resultant sound pressure level (SPL). Because a compliant eardrum and ossicular chain absorb sound, the SPL in the ear canal is inversely proportional to the complaince. A tympanogram (Fig. 1) is a graph of middle ear compliance change as air pressure is varied in the external canal from $+200$ mm H_2O to -200 mm H_2O. The pressure is measured by a transducer in series with the positive-negative air pump of the electroacoustic meter. Maximal compliance of the tympanic membrane and ossicular chain occurs when the pressure in the middle ear is offset by an external canal pressure that is equal and opposite. This normally occurs at zero or atmospheric pressure.

The maximal compliance that the meter measures is the sum of the compliance of the external ear canal and middle ear structures. Compliance contributed by the external ear canal is essentially equivalent to its actual volume. This volume is determined by a procedure termed the **physical volume test**. A positive pressure of 200 mm H_2O is applied in the external ear canal, and compliance is measured. Application of this high pressure alleviates the compliance normally contributed by the tympanic membrane and ossicular chain. As a result, the compliance measured is entirely due to the air space in the external ear canal. The compliance contributed by the tympanic membrane and ossicular chain is determined by subtracting the equivalent volume of the external ear canal from the maximal compliance.

Abnormal middle ear pressures will cause a shift in the point of maximal compliance, and changes in the stiffness of the system will alter the height of the peak. Otosclerosis and ossicular chain uncoupling are two conditions in which one might expect to encounter differences in tympanic membrane mobility. The stiff system (otosclerosis) would demonstrate low compliance, and the loose system (uncoupling) would demonstrate high compliance.

IMPEDANCE AUDIOMETRY: THE ACOUSTIC REFLEX

When a loud noise is introduced into a normal ear in human beings and animals, the muscles in the middle ear contract reflexively. This activity produces a transitory change in the impedance characteristics of the tympanic membrane and middle ear cavity (Fig. 2) and is called the **stapedial reflex**, or more properly the **intra-aural** or **acoustic reflex**. The afferent pathway of this reflex consists of the receptor cells in the cochlea and fibers of the acoustic nerve (VIII). The efferent portion consists of motor fibers in the trigeminal (V) and facial (VII) cranial nerves, which innervate the tensor tympani and stapedius muscles, respectively. The contraction of these muscles attenuates sound transmitted through the middle ear to a degree that is dependent on the frequency and intensity of the stimulus. An auditory stimulus, having an intensity well above reflex threshold and presented to one ear, will elicit contractions of intra-aural muscles in both ears. The reflex from the stimulated ear is called **ipsilateral**, and the reflex recorded from the nonstimulated ear is called **contralateral**. The time course of these

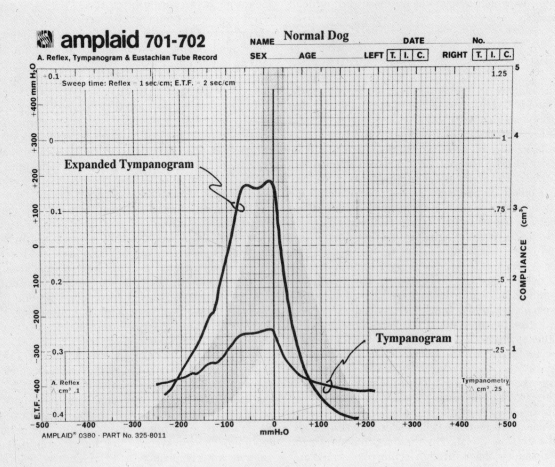

Figure 1. Tympanograms recorded from a clinically normal dog. The expanded tympanogram is produced by converting the compliance at +200 mm H_2O to 0 and displaying the graph on an expanded (inner) scale. (From Sims, M. H.: Electrodiagnostic evaluation of auditory function. Clin. North Am. [Small Anim. Pract.] 18:913–944, 1988; with permission.)

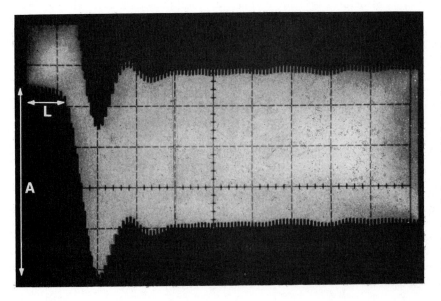

Figure 2. A recording of compliance during an ipsilateral acoustic reflex. The stimulus was a 2 kHz pure tone at an intensity of 90 dB sound pressure level. When middle ear muscles contract reflexively, compliance measured at the tympanic membrane decreases abruptly after a latent period and remains decreased until the end of the stimulus tone (not shown). Vertical arrow, stimulus onset; L, latency; A, amplitude. Vertical division = 0.5 cm^3 of air; horizontal division = 50 msec. (From Sims, M. H., and Horohov, J. E.: Effects of xylazine and ketamine on the acoustic reflex and brainstem auditory-evoked response in the cat. Am. J. Vet. Res. 47:102–109, 1986; with permission.)

reflex arcs can be determined by measuring changes in acoustic impedance (or its inverse, compliance) with the aid of an electroacoustic impedance meter and X-Y plotter or oscilloscope. The reflex can be characterized by latency, the time that lapses between stimulus application and compliance change, and amplitude, a reflection of force of contraction in middle ear muscles. Middle ear lesions profoundly alter the results of this procedure.

THE AUDITORY EVOKED RESPONSE: EARLY LATENCY COMPONENTS

Until recently, clinical methods for evaluating sensory systems in small animals were limited. Now, however, the neural components of special sensory systems can be evaluated with the use of evoked responses. Evoked responses are recordings of digitally averaged potentials arising from peripheral or central structures as a result of judiciously applied sensory stimuli. The brain responds to repetitive sensory stimuli with consistent and time-locked changes in electrical activity, which can be recorded from scalp electrodes.

Auditory evoked responses (AER) are averaged recordings of neural activity as a result of externally applied acoustic stimuli. Because AER provide highly objective information without requiring patient cooperation, investigators use them to detect neurologic, otologic, or audiologic dysfunction in animals. The AER consists of numerous waves (i.e., negative and positive peaks), each of which represents composite neuronal activity in one or more subcortical and cortical brain structures. The specific type of recording depends on the length of time that is averaged after the stimulus. Components of the AER in humans beings have been referred to as early (0 to 10 msec), middle (10 to 50 msec), late (50 to 250 msec), or long (>250 msec). Generally, the waves of successive types of AER represent the activity of neural generators at progressively more rostral levels in the neuroaxis. For the early latency components, generators are thought to be located mostly within the brain stem. Therefore, a series of waves in the 0- to 10-msec range is referred to as the brain stem AER, or BAER.

The BAER is a far-field reflection of electrical events within the brain stem as impulses ascend through the auditory pathway. This response in small animals consists of up to seven waves in the nanovolts to microvolts. The positive peaks of the BAER begin about 1.0 to 1.5 msec after stimulus application and are spaced about 1 msec apart (Fig. 3). These peaks are usually labeled with Roman numerals and characterized by latency and amplitude measurements. Latency is the time from stimulus onset to the positive peak of the wave, and

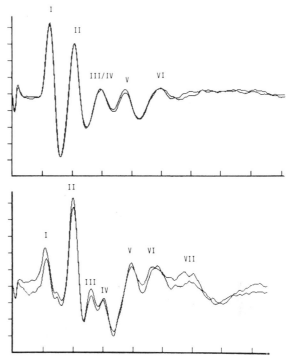

Figure 3. BAER recorded from a clinically normal dog (top) and cat (bottom). Each trace is a 10-sec average of brainstem activity after 1000 sound stimuli (clicks) presented at an intensity of 90 dB hearing level and a rate of 11.7/sec. Vertical division = 0.61 µV; horizontal division = 1 msec.

amplitude is measured from the positive peak to the following negative trough. The clinical use of these values has been well established.

The BAER can be obtained from unconscious as well as conscious animals and is generally thought to be somewhat independent of the level of arousal. Since the BAER depends on mechanical transducing mechanisms in the outer and middle ear cavities and neural mechanisms in the inner ear, peripheral nerve, and brain stem, it is particularly helpful in characterizing deafness. The BAER can also be elicited by bone conduction (Fig. 4), which does not require the participation of the external and middle ear cavities. Air–bone differences in the BAER can help distinguish between conductive and sensorineural deafness.

Studies in animals have attempted to describe, from an anatomic perspective, the neural generators of the BAER waves. However, because the pathway for sound is complex and perhaps variable among animal species, it has not been possible to associate a given wave with a single nucleus or tract. Even so, a somewhat tenable scheme has been derived from pathologic or clinical data, lesion studies, and a comparison of surface and depth recordings. There is general agreement that wave I of the BAER is generated by acoustic nerve activity. Wave II appears to be generated by the ipsilateral cochlear nucleus and the unmyelinated central terminals of the cochlear nerve. Evidence of the generator of

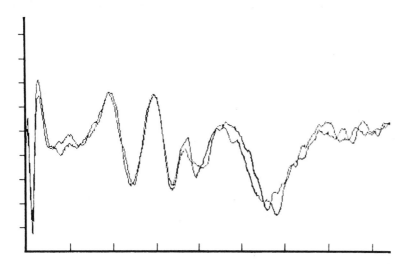

Figure 4. BAER recorded from a clinically normal dog as a result of bone stimulation. A bone vibrator was placed on the mastoid process of the temporal bone. Vertical division = 0.152 μV; horizontal division = 1 msec. (From Sims, M. H.: Electrodiagnostic evaluation of auditory function. Vet. Clin. North Am. [Small Anim. Pract.] 18:913–944, 1988; with permission.)

wave III points to the dorsal nucleus of the trapezoid body of the ipsilateral or contralateral brain stem or both. Although research supports this nuclear complex as the source of wave III, attempts to differentiate discrete nuclei of the complex have not been successful. Studies have indicated the ipsilateral or contralateral caudal colliculus is the generator of wave V, with the central nucleus as the primary source. Generators of waves IV, VI, and VII have not been clearly defined. Some investigators believe that a scheme such as the one presented above is an oversimplification of a very complex waveform.

AUDITORY EVOKED RESPONSE: COCHLEAR MICROPHONICS

The cochlea is the site of transduction for converting pressure waves in fluid to action potentials. The specific cells that accomplish this are the hair cells of the organ of Corti. The electrical responses (Fig. 5) that occur in the different parts of the cochlea (except the acoustic nerve) are referred to as the **cochlear microphonic** (CM). The CM is thought to arise from the cuticular surface of the hair cells and, within limits, is graded in accordance with audio stimulation. Although the CM is a distortion of the supplied signal, it resembles the electrical waveform enough that care must be taken not to confuse it with stimulus artifact. The CM, occurring just prior to wave I of the BAER, is best seen when the stimulus is a continuous pure tone and presented in either the rarefaction or condensation mode. The CM can be distinguished from wave I by reversing the polarity of the stimulus. When this is done, the polarity of wave I will not change but the polarity of the CM will reverse.

The CM affords a convenient monitor of the mechanical events of the cochlea by virtue of its dependence on the displacement patterns of the cochlear partition. The usefulness of the CM in audiometry is limited because it has no threshold *per se*. The potentials that comprise the CM resist the effects of anesthesia and may even be present after death. These potentials are not present in animals whose cochleae are lacking the organ of Corti and hair cells. Failure to record the CM in a young animal supports a diagnosis of hereditary deafness due to cochlear agenesis or degeneration.

AUDITORY EVOKED RESPONSE: MIDDLE LATENCY COMPONENTS

The middle latency response (MLR) in humans and animals consists of a series of vertex-positive waves occurring 10 to 50 msec after stimulus application, with wave amplitudes ranging from 0.5 to 3 μV (Fig. 6). Component waves have been designated as No, Po, Na, Pa, Nb, Pb, and occasionally Nc. Although some have indicated that the MLR is highly contaminated with reflexive muscle activity, the neural origin of these waves has been well established. Among the suggested generators of the potentials are the medial geniculate body, polysensory nuclei of the thalamus, and areas of the auditory cortex.

Although the MLR has appeal in clinical medicine because it is a noninvasive technique reported to be little affected by light sedation or sleep, very little clinical MLR research has been accomplished in animals. To date, the availability of normative data or the application of auditory evoked potentials to the diagnosis of audiologic or neurologic disorders in veterinary medicine has been focused primarily on the BAER.

ELECTROENCEPHALOGRAPHIC AUDIOMETRY

The characteristics of the electroencephalogram (EEG) pattern are dependent on the overall level

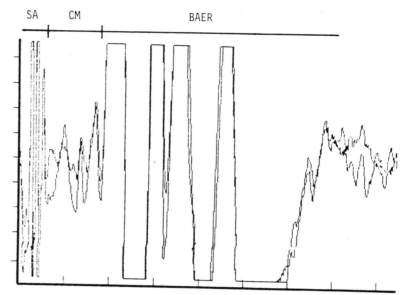

Figure 5. Cochlear microphonic (CM) activity as a result of 8 kHz pure tone stimulation. The stimulus artifact is shown by SA. Since the amplitude of the CM is much smaller than the waves of the BAER, increasing the display sensitivity caused the first four waves of the BAER to go off scale. Vertical division = 0.076 μV; horizontal division = 1 msec. (From Sims, M. H.: Electrodiagnostic evaluation of auditory function. Vet. Clin. North Am. [Small Anim. Pract.] 18:913–944, 1988; with permission.)

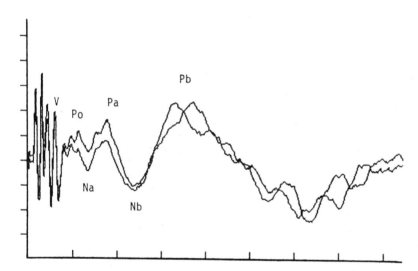

Figure 6. An MLR in a cat that resulted from monotically applied clicks at an intensity of 90 dB hearing level and a rate of 4.7/sec. Wave peaks Po to Pb are vertex-positive activities and peaks Na and Nb are vertex-negative potentials. Each trace is an average of 2000 individual responses. V, wave V of the BAER. Vertical division = 0.762 μV; horizontal division = 6 msec. (From Sims, M. H.: Electrodiagnostic evaluation of auditory function. Vet. Clin. North Am. [Small Anim. Pract.] 18:913–944, 1988; with permission.)

of consciousness. For example, when an animal is relaxed, the EEG is distinguished by low-frequency, high-voltage activity. During mental arousal, the amplitude decreases while the frequency increases. A nonstartling sound delivered to an animal in a relaxed state will cause the EEG to shift from a low-frequency, high-voltage pattern to a high-frequency, low-voltage pattern. The arousal reaction has been taken as an indication of the perception of the sound. Changes in respiratory pattern have also been used in a similar fashion.

References and Supplemental Reading

Bergsma, D. R., and Brown, K. S.: White fur, blue eyes, and deafness in the domestic cat. J. Hered. 62:171, 1971.

de Groot, E. C. B. M., and Velden, N. A. V. D.: Two types of hereditary sensorineural deafness in dogs. Vet. Pathol. 17:650, 1980.

Hayes, H. M., Wilson, G. P., Fenner, W. R., et al.: Canine congenital deafness: Epidemiologic study of 272 cases. J. Am. Anim. Hosp. Assoc. 17:401, 1981.

Mair, I. W. S.: Hereditary deafness in the dalmatian dog. Arch. Otorhinolaryngol [Suppl.] 314:1, 1973.

Marshall, A. E.: Use of brain stem auditory-evoked response to evaluate deafness in a group of dalmatian dogs. J.A.V.M.A. 188:718, 1986.

Penrod, J. P., and Coulter, D. B.: The diagnostic uses of impedance audiometry in the dog. J. Am. Anim. Hosp. Assoc. 16:941, 1980.

Rose, W. R.: Audiology. 3. Interpretation of audiograms (air-conducting testing). Vet. Med. Small Anim. Clin. 72:624, 1977.

Sims, M. H., and Moore, R. E.: Auditory evoked response in the clinically normal dog: Early latency components. Am. J. Vet. Res. 45:2019, 1984.

Sims, M. H., and Moore, R. E.: Auditory evoked response in the clinically normal dog: Middle latency components. Am. J. Vet. Res. 45:2028, 1984.

Sims, M. H., and Shull-Selcer, E.: Electrodiagnostic evaluation of deafness in two English setter littermates. J.A.V.M.A. 187:398, 1985.

HYPOKALEMIC POLYMYOPATHY OF CATS

STEVEN W. DOW, D.V.M., M.S.
and RICHARD A. LeCOUTEUR, B.V.Sc., Ph.D.

Fort Collins, Colorado

During the past several years, an idiopathic polymyopathy has been observed in a number of cats. Recent studies have linked this disorder to potassium depletion and development of severe hypokalemia. Although other primary muscle and neuromuscular junction diseases may induce similar signs, hypokalemic polymyopathy is currently thought to be one of the most common causes of generalized muscle weakness of cats.

In humans, severe hypokalemia induces muscle dysfunction ranging in severity from weakness to complete paralysis. Extremely low serum potassium concentrations may eventually result in rhabdomyolysis. Experimental potassium depletion causes muscle weakness in both dogs and cats. An idiopathic polymyopathy syndrome of cats was described in 1984 by Schunk, who noted that over two thirds of affected cats were hypokalemic. Periodic muscle weakness, apparently related to low serum potassium concentrations, has also been observed in Burmese cats in Australia and the United Kingdom. Extreme hypernatremia induced muscle dysfunction clinically indistinguishable from hypokalemia-induced polymyopathy in one cat. Normal muscle function in cats is apparently sensitive to alterations in concentrations of extracellular electrolytes, especially sodium and potassium.

CLINICAL SIGNS

In most cats examined to date, the onset of signs has been acute. However, a subclinical myopathy may exist for weeks to months without obvious clinical signs. Severely affected cats typically develop sudden signs of generalized muscle weakness. This is most often characterized by an obvious ventroflexion of the neck, apparently due to weakness of dorsal cervical muscles (Fig. 1). All affected cats have been afebrile. Other characteristic signs include reluctance to walk, sudden fatigue, a stiff and stilted gait, and apparent muscle pain when handled or palpated. Muscle weakness in cats with critically low serum potassium concentrations may progress to respiratory paralysis. This occurred in several hypokalemic cats treated with subcutaneous

or intravenous fluids, resulting in further lowering of serum potassium concentration.

BIOCHEMICAL FINDINGS

In severely affected cats, serum potassium concentration has been less than 3.5 mEq/L, and often less than 3.0 mEq/L. Hypokalemia of this magnitude damages the muscle cell membrane, as indicated by increases in serum creatine kinase (CK) activity. CK activity in affected cats is usually in the range of 500 to 10,000 IU/L. The highest CK activity observed was in a young Burmese cat (21,000 IU/L). This and the fact that others have observed a syndrome of muscle weakness associated with hypokalemia in Burmese cats suggest that this breed may be more sensitive to the effects of hypokalemia or may be afflicted with a variant of the syndrome.

Renal dysfunction has been present in all older cats with hypokalemic polymyopathy, as well as in several young cats. Increased serum creatinine concentrations, in the range of 2.5 to 5.0 mg/dl, are typical. Interpretation of urine specific gravity is difficult because hypokalemia interferes with urine-concentrating mechanisms. Mild to moderate metabolic acidosis or serum bicarbonate concentrations in the low normal range are also common. Because of the effect of pH on intracellular and extracellular redistribution of potassium, determination of acid-base status is important in interpreting serum po-

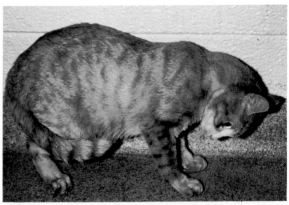

Figure 1. Characteristic cervical ventroflexion and stiff, awkward posture in a cat with hypokalemic polymyopathy.

tassium concentrations. Alkalosis tends to lower serum potassium concentration, whereas acidosis has the opposite effect. Hypophosphatemia, present in several affected cats, may, by depleting cytosolic adenosine triphosphate (ATP) stores, also have deleterious effects on muscle function and may potentiate muscle injury induced by hypokalemia.

NEUROMUSCULAR EVALUATION

There have been few morphologic abnormalities observed on light microscopic examination of muscle biopsy specimens. Mild myofiber necrosis and macrophage infiltration were present in biopsies from several cats. The relative absence of inflammation distinguishes this muscle disorder from inflammatory myopathies of cats.

Diffuse, widespread electromyographic abnormalities were present in most skeletal muscle groups tested in affected cats. Frequent positive sharp waves, fibrillation potentials, and occasional bizarre high-frequency discharges were observed. Results of motor nerve conduction testing have been normal in cats tested to date. Thus, it is very unlikely that peripheral nerve dysfunction is an important component of this disorder.

The exact mechanism by which hypokalemia induces muscle dysfunction in cats is not currently known. It is likely that hypokalemia exerts its primary effects on the muscle cell membrane. In rats and dogs, potassium deficiency alters the resting muscle cell transmembrane electrical potential difference. During potassium depletion, extracellular potassium concentration drops more rapidly than the intracellular concentration, initially inducing muscle cell membrane hyperpolarization. As potassium depletion worsens, however, further hyperpolarization is postulated to cause the sarcolemma to rapidly become more permeable to sodium, triggering muscle cell membrane hypopolarization. In dogs, severe muscle weakness ensues at this point, progressing eventually to rhabdomyolysis and paralysis. If potassium depletion has similar effects on muscle cells of cats, rapid sarcolemmal hypopolarization probably explains the sudden appearance of muscle weakness in severely hypokalemic cats.

In addition to direct effects on the muscle cell membrane, hypokalemia also has adverse effects on muscle blood flow. Following potassium depletion in dogs, the normal increase in muscle blood flow in response to exercise is greatly attenuated, leading in some instances to ischemic necrosis of muscle. Ischemic injury might also be expected to occur in muscles of severely potassium-depleted cats. Activity should be restricted as much as possible in affected cats to avoid further muscle damage.

CRITERIA FOR DIAGNOSIS

Diagnosis of hypokalemic polymyopathy in cats, as the disease is currently described, should be based on fulfilling all of the following criteria: (1) presence of typical clinical signs, (2) serum potassium concentration less than 3.5 mEq/L, (3) high CK activity, (4) electromyographic abnormalities in multiple muscle groups, (5) lack of histopathologic evidence of myositis, and (6) a favorable response to treatment with potassium. Analysis of a venous blood gas specimen to rule out metabolic alkalosis is recommended to aid in interpretation of serum potassium concentration.

Diseases that should be included in the differential diagnosis for cats with signs of generalized muscle weakness include other primary myopathies such as polymyositis, neuromuscular junction diseases (myasthenia gravis, organophosphate toxicosis, spider bite), polyneuropathies (long-standing diabetes mellitus, prolonged treatment with vincristine, polyradiculoneuritis), electrolyte-induced muscle dysfunction (particularly abnormalities of sodium and phosphorus concentration), ethylene glycol toxicosis, severe anemia, and sepsis. Most can be ruled out by neurologic examination, complete blood count, and serum biochemical analysis.

Although thiamine deficiency does induce cervical ventroflexion in cats, this is thought to be an active process and not a result of muscle weakness. Thiamine deficiency encephalopathy in cats also may induce excessive muscle tone, torticollis, and seizures, signs very different from those that develop in cats with generalized muscle weakness induced by potassium depletion. We suspect that a number of cats with hypokalemic polymyopathy have in the past been misdiagnosed as thiamine deficient.

From our experience with these cats, it has become apparent that hypokalemic polymyopathy represents only the most dramatic manifestation of chronic potassium depletion. In fact, potassium depletion and hypokalemia may be much more prevalent in cats than is generally recognized. In cats with less severe hypokalemia, clinical signs of potassium depletion may be subtle. Other less specific signs observed in hypokalemic cats include weight loss, lethargy, inappetence, poor hair coat, and chronic vomiting and constipation. Given the crucial importance of potassium to normal cell function, it is not surprising that potassium depletion has widespread adverse effects, in addition to its effects on muscle function.

CAUSES OF POTASSIUM DEPLETION IN CATS

Total body potassium content represents a balance between intake and loss via the kidneys and gastrointestinal tract. Approximately 95 per cent of body potassium is contained in the intracellular compartment, with extracellular fluid containing the balance. Under carefully controlled conditions, serum potassium concentration is a fairly accurate reflection of total body stores. However, distribution of potassium between the intracellular and extracellular compartments is influenced by a number of factors, of which metabolic alkalosis and increased serum insulin concentration are the most important. Both of these factors decrease serum potassium concentration by causing acute redistribution of potassium into the intracellular compartment. Thus, hypokalemia may represent either total body potassium depletion or transient intracellular redistribution of potassium, despite normal total body potassium content.

Studies of cats with hypokalemic myopathy have excluded the most important causes of intracellular redistribution of potassium. Hypokalemia in these cats is therefore assumed to reflect depletion of total body potassium stores. For depletion to develop, there must be either decreased intake of potassium, increased potassium losses, or both.

None of the cats studied to date had a history of gastrointestinal disease, thereby ruling out gastrointestinal potassium losses. When dietary intake of potassium was assessed, it was noted that all hypokalemic cats had been fed the same commercial cat food diet (Hill's Feline Science Diet Maintenance, as formulated before December, 1986) exclusively for periods of at least 6 months prior to development of signs. Analysis of several specimens of this food indicated that the mean potassium content was 0.34 per cent on a dry matter basis. Based on National Research Council recommendations of 0.3 to 0.4 per cent dietary potassium as the minimum necessary for maintenance in healthy adult cats, this diet was considered to be only marginally replete in potassium. Though several severely hypokalemic cats have also been fed other diets, the majority treated prior to the summer of 1987 had been fed one of two commercial cat foods (Hill's Feline Science Diet Maintenance or Hill's c/d dry cat food, as formulated before December, 1986). These two diets have since been modified so that they now contain 0.7 per cent potassium.

Urinary potassium losses have been excessive in all cats that we have studied with hypokalemic polymyopathy and concurrent renal dysfunction. In general, increased urinary potassium losses seem to occur concurrent with renal dysfunction in cats. The mechanism by which renal dysfunction in cats leads to renal potassium wasting has yet to be elucidated.

From these results, it appears that concurrent decreased dietary potassium intake and increased urinary potassium loss over a period of months may lead to severe depletion of total body potassium stores in cats. Once serum potassium concentrations decrease to a critical level, signs of hypokalemia-induced polymyopathy ensue. Other subtle effects of potassium depletion may be present for weeks to months before the more obvious signs of muscle dysfunction develop.

TREATMENT

Potassium may be administered either parenterally, as potassium chloride diluted in a balanced electrolyte solution such as lactated Ringer's, or orally, as potassium-containing elixirs or potassium salts (KCl, $KHCO_3$).

Oral treatment is recommended for all except the most severely affected cats, for the following reasons. In our early experiences with severely hypokalemic cats, administration of fluids, even those containing high concentrations of potassium (40 to 80 mEq/L) initially tended to lower serum potassium concentrations. In two cats, dramatic lowering of potassium concentrations precipitated complete paralysis, necessitating intubation and ventilatory support for 2 days before serum potassium was restored to concentrations sufficient for normal muscle function. From conversations with other veterinarians, it seems that this occurs relatively commonly. Administration of fluids is thought to decrease serum potassium concentration both by diluting extracellular potassium concentrations (this effect is potentiated by poor vascular tone characteristic of severe hypokalemia) and by accelerating renal distal tubular potassium excretion.

Parenteral administration of potassium may be required, however, for treatment of cats with profound hypokalemia and muscle weakness, particularly those in which respiratory paralysis seems imminent. In these situations, high concentrations of potassium must rapidly be administered intravenously. The recommended rate of potassium infusion in humans is 0.5 to 1.0 mEq/kg/hr. We have successfully administered KCl in lactated Ringer's solution at rates of 0.4 mEq/kg/hr in severely hypokalemic cats. However, infusions of highly concentrated potassium solutions may induce lethal cardiac arrhythmias and cause phlebitis. Therefore, these high concentration potassium solutions should be administered via a constant-rate infusion pump, with continuous electrocardiographic monitoring. Serum potassium concentrations should be determined every 3 to 6 hr and potassium infusion slowed once serum potassium concentrations reach 3.5 mEq/L. Infusion of dopamine, 0.5 µg/kg/min, can induce a transient elevation in serum potassium concentration that may be lifesaving and avoids some of the risks inherent to infusion of concentrated potassium solutions. Concurrent oral potassium supplementation must be started immediately, however, as dopamine causes only a transient redistribution of potassium from the intracellular to the extracellular fluid compartment.

Potassium can be conveniently administered orally as either potassium-containing elixirs or as KCl, which is readily available as a sodium chloride substitute. Cats apparently object to the taste of potassium chloride, as very few will continue to eat KCl-supplemented foods. Furthermore, potassium chloride is acidifying and may potentially worsen pre-existing metabolic acidosis in many of these cats. For these reasons, hypokalemic cats are usually treated initially with potassium gluconate elixir (Kaon, Adria Laboratories). The gluconate salt of potassium is not acidifying, the elixir preparation is easy to dose, and it seems to be more palatable to cats than KCl. For long-term dietary potassium supplementation, a palatable potassium gluconate powder (Tumil-K, Daniels Pharmaceuticals, Inc.) is now available.

The dose of potassium administered orally to hypokalemic cats has been determined empirically, since the total body potassium deficit cannot be calculated directly. Cats with severe hypokalemia (serum potassium <3.0 mEq/L) are given 5 to 8 mEq of potassium per day in two divided doses. Oral potassium treatment rarely has led to hyperkalemia; instead, persistent hypokalemia has been the most common problem. Serum potassium concentration is determined daily in cats with severe hypokalemia until the concentration has increased into or near the normal range (usually by 1 to 3 days after initiating therapy). At that point, serum potassium concentrations are usually monitored weekly and the dose of potassium increased or decreased to maintain serum concentrations in the normal range. A maintenance dose of 2 to 4 mEq of potassium per day has been sufficient to maintain normal serum concentration in most affected cats. However, there appears to be a great deal of individual variation in daily potassium requirements, with cats with renal dysfunction having the highest demands. In some cats, particularly young cats without evidence of renal dysfunction, feeding a diet with adequate potassium (>0.6 per cent) is often sufficient to maintain normal serum potassium concentration without the need for additional dietary potassium supplementation.

RESPONSE TO TREATMENT

A response to potassium treatment, though rarely dramatic, usually occurs within 24 hr and is manifested as an increase in muscle strength, improved appetite, and improvement in overall demeanor. Most cats are considerably improved within 2 to 3 days of instituting aggressive dietary potassium supplementation. Complete resolution of muscle weakness may take several weeks, especially in more severely affected cats. Creatine kinase activity may not return to normal for several weeks.

The prognosis for full recovery from hypokalemia-induced polymyopathy is excellent, provided an accurate diagnosis is made early and appropriate treatment instituted. Initial administration of fluids, even when supplemented with potassium, appears to be the most common reason for treatment failure. Hypokalemia and polymyopathy may recur in affected cats, especially when the diet is not continuously supplemented with potassium. Periodic monitoring of serum potassium is indicated.

References and Supplemental Reading

Bilbrey, G. L., Herbin, L., Carter, N. W., et al.: Skeletal muscle resting membrane potential in potassium deficiency. J. Clin. Invest. 52:3011, 1973.

Blaxter, A. C., Lievesley, P., Gruffydd-Jones, T., et al.: Periodic muscle weakness in Burmese kittens. Vet. Rec. 118:619, 1986.

Brown, R. S.: Potassium homeostasis and clinical implications. Am. J. Med. 77(5A):3, 1984.

Dow, S. W., Fettman, M. J., LeCouteur, R. A., et al.: Hypodipsic hypernatremia and associated myopathy in a hydrocephalic cat with transient hypopituitarism. J.A.V.M.A. 191:127, 1987.

Dow, S. W., LeCouteur, R. A., Fettman, M. J., et al.: Potassium depletion in cats: Hypokalemic myopathy. J.A.V.M.A. 191:1563, 1987.

Dow, S. W., Fettman, M. J., LeCouteur, R. A., et al.: Potassium depletion in cats: Renal and dietary influences. J.A.V.M.A. 191:1569, 1987.

Hills, D. L., Morris, J. G., Rogers, Q. R.: Potassium requirement of kittens as affected by dietary protein. J. Nutr. 112:216, 1982.

Knochel, J. P., Schlein, E. M.: On the mechanism of rhabdomyolysis in potassium depletion. J. Clin. Invest. 51:1750, 1972.

Narins, R. G., Jones, E. R., Strom, M. C., et al.: Diagnostic strategies in disorders of fluid, electrolyte and acid-base homeostasis. Am. J. Med. 72:496, 1982.

Schunk, K. L.: Feline polymyopathy. In Proceedings of the 2nd Annual Forum, American College of Veterinary Internal Medicine, Washington, D.C., 1984, pp. 197–200.

CANINE MASTICATORY MUSCLE DISORDERS

G. DIANE SHELTON, D.V.M., PH.D.
San Diego, California

and GEORGE H. CARDINET, III, D.V.M., PH.D.
Davis, California

Disorders of the muscles of mastication occur relatively commonly in clinical practice and can be of myopathic or neuropathic origin. Usual presenting signs include some combination of masticatory muscle atrophy or swelling and abnormal jaw function, manifested generally by difficulty in either opening the jaw (trismus) or closing the jaw. Although the masticatory muscles can be involved in generalized neuromuscular disease, there is preferential involvement of these muscles in selected disorders.

Recent studies on the masticatory muscles have provided insight as to why they are preferentially affected by some inflammatory disorders. There are histochemical and biochemical differences between canine masticatory and limb muscles (Orvis and Cardinet, 1981; Shelton et al., 1985a). Employing the histochemical staining method for myofibrillar adenosine triphosphatase (ATPase), which differentiates type 1 fibers (presumed slow-twitch fibers) from type 2 fibers (presumed fast-twitch fibers), it was found that type 1 and type 2 fibers of the muscles of mastication differ from those composing limb muscles. Limb muscles of dogs principally contain types 1 and 2A fibers, as well as a small number of 2C fibers, whereas masticatory muscles are predominantly composed of fibers designated as type 2M. The type 1 fibers of masticatory muscles also differ from those in limb muscles; however, they usually constitute only 10 to 20 per cent of the fiber population.

Using electrophoretic methods, the masticatory muscles were shown to contain an isoform of myosin that differs from that of limb muscles. Further, the masticatory muscles are derived embryologically from the mesoderm of the paired first branchial arches and are innervated by a cranial nerve, whereas limb muscles are innervated by spinal nerves. Given these differences, it seems plausible that humoral or cellular immune responses might be selectively mounted against proteins unique to masticatory muscles.

In an attempt to define the diversity of pathologic lesions and clinical and immunologic features of masticatory muscle disorders (MMD), a retrospective study of 29 dogs with MMD was conducted (Shelton et al., 1987). Since there has been some confusion as to whether masticatory muscle myositis (MMM) is a distinct disorder or a variant of polymyositis, four dogs with polymyositis were included as controls.

HISTOPATHOLOGIC FINDINGS

The 29 dogs with clinical signs of MMD had varied histopathologic changes on temporalis muscle biopsies. These changes were broadly grouped in four categories: (1) no pathologic changes (2 dogs, 6.9 per cent); (2) nonspecific, noninflammatory changes including fiber-type atrophy, vacuolar changes, and central nuclei (4 dogs, 13.8 per cent); (3) presumed neurogenic atrophy, as evidenced by scattered and grouped angular atrophy involving both types 1 and 2 fibers, and pyknotic nuclear clumps (7 dogs, 24.1 per cent); and (4) inflammatory muscle disease (16 dogs, 55.2 per cent). As evidenced by the foregoing, it is important to emphasize that MMD in dogs does not represent a single clinical or pathologic entity.

In acute cases of MMM, the biopsy specimen may contain myofiber necrosis, phagocytosis, and cellular infiltration with a multifocal, perivascular distribution. Autoantibodies can be demonstrated against type 2M fibers. As a result of the cellular infiltration and, presumptively, the autoantibodies, there is selective destruction of type 2M fibers, resulting in end-stage disease with only a few type 1 fibers and connective tissue remaining. Although eosinophils were frequently present among the infiltrating cell populations, large numbers were found in only two cases. Hence, the designation of eosinophilic myositis would have been appropriate in only 12 per cent of dogs with inflammatory MMD. In chronic cases of MMM, significant muscle atrophy may be evident with only modest inflammation. There is a relative increase in connective tissue, with a loss of muscle fibers. Given the focal nature of the lesion, areas of inflammation may be missed in a biopsy section.

816

CLINICAL FINDINGS

Various large breeds of dogs were affected with MMD, without an obvious age or sex predisposition. Although clinical characterization of these different disorders is imperfect, the dogs with MMM usually had either acute muscle swelling with or without trismus, or subacute to chronic muscle atrophy with or without trismus. In contrast, the dogs with neuropathic disorders most often had subacute to chronic muscle atrophy without altered jaw mobility; however, one dog with neurogenic atrophy had trismus and another had difficulty closing the jaws. All four dogs with polymyositis had normal jaw mobility, but two had masticatory muscle atrophy.

Twenty-six of the 29 dogs were evaluated by electromyography (EMG). Abnormalities, restricted to the muscles of mastication and consisting of fibrillation potentials, positive sharp waves, or bizarre high-frequency discharges, were observed in 21 dogs. Changes presumably were not identified in some dogs with advanced disease because of the nearly total loss of muscle fibers and the inability to place the recording electrodes in the proximity of the remaining damaged fibers.

IMMUNOCYTOCHEMICAL FINDINGS

Immunocytochemical staining with staphylococcal protein A–horseradish peroxidase conjugates was used for detection of immune complexes within biopsy samples and for the detection of circulating antibodies (Pflugfelder et al., 1981; Shelton et al., 1985b) (Fig. 1). Immune complex staining of type 2M fibers was identified in 87 per cent of the dogs with MMM but could not be detected in dogs without inflammatory changes or dogs with polymyositis. Antibodies directed against type 2M fibers were identified in sera from 81 per cent of the dogs with MMM, whereas sera from healthy dogs and dogs with polymyositis did not contain antibodies.

DIAGNOSTIC APPROACH

Dogs presenting with abnormalities of jaw function or atrophy or swelling of the muscles of mastication should be evaluated as shown in Figure 2. Although a large percentage of dogs with selective atrophy of the masticatory muscles have myositis, the diagnosis is not always obvious on physical examination.

Masticatory muscle myositis has been presumed to be immune mediated because of the histopathologic changes seen in affected dogs and the responsiveness of clinical signs to glucocorticoids. This hypothesis has been strengthened by the demonstration of autoantibodies against type 2M fibers in dogs with MMM. That these autoantibodies have not been found in dogs with polymyositis suggests that the pathogenesis of MMM and polymyositis may differ. The absence of antibodies in polymyositis also indicates that those seen in MMM do not result from myofiber damage alone. MMM has recently been described in a dog with systemic lupus erythematosus (Cardinet, 1988), demonstrating that MMM can occur with other immune-mediated disorders and that diagnostic tests for the presence of other autoantibodies (i.e., antinuclear antibodies) should be performed.

Serum creatine kinase (CK) may be modestly elevated in dogs with MMM; however, concentrations are significantly lower than in dogs with polymyositis. This difference probably reflects the volume of affected muscle mass in the two disorders. Although EMG may not add much information to the definition of MMM, it has been valuable in discriminating this disorder from polymyositis. In MMM, spontaneous electrical activity occurs only in the muscles of mastication, while limb muscles are electrically silent. This contrasts with polymyositis, in which there is generalized spontaneous activity affecting most muscles of the body, including those of mastication.

The presumptive diagnosis of MMM is obtained by evaluation of the histopathologic changes in a muscle biopsy sample and the demonstration of autoantibodies against type 2M fibers. This evaluation is important in defining whether the changes are neuropathic or myopathic, in anticipating recurrent episodes, and in forming a prognosis. MMM has a high incidence of recurrence, whereas neuropathies do not tend to be episodic. Immunocytochemical assay for immune complexes in type 2M fibers must be performed on muscle prepared by frozen section. Circulating antibodies against type 2M fibers can be detected by incubating an aliquot of the patient's serum with frozen sections of normal canine temporalis muscle. Serum should be collected prior to glucocorticoid therapy, as false-negative results may otherwise occur. Although current studies have provided a basis for these assays and indicated that they should aid in distinguishing the forms of MMD, larger numbers of dogs need to be tested to further establish their diagnostic value.

TREATMENT

Initiation of appropriate treatment is dependent on the histopathologic and immunocytochemical diagnosis. During the acute stage of MMM, masticatory muscle swelling and trismus usually resolve rapidly subsequent to immunosuppressive doses of glucocorticoids (prednisone, 1 to 1.5 mg/kg PO

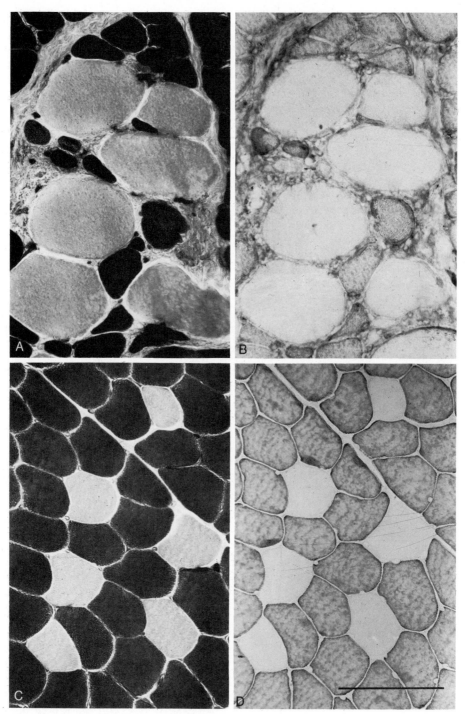

Figure 1. Paired, adjacent sections of temporalis muscle from a patient with masticatory muscle myositis (A and B) and a healthy dog (C and D) illustrate the selective localization of immunoglobulins in the patient's type 2M muscle fibers (B) and circulating antibodies against type 2M fibers in the patient's serum (D). Sections A and C were incubated and stained for myofibrillar ATPase at pH 9.8, in which type 1 fibers are lightly stained and type 2 fibers are darkly stained. Sections B and D were incubated and stained for peroxidase activity following incubation of the sections with staphylococcal protein A–peroxidase conjugates (SPA-HRPO). The type 1 fibers were unstained and normal in size or hypertrophied, whereas most type 2M fibers were positively stained and atrophic. Section D was incubated with SPA-HRPO following incubation with patient's serum. The type 1 fibers were unstained, whereas the type 2M fibers were positively stained. All fibers from the healthy dog were unstained when directly incubated with SPA-HRPO or following incubation with sera from control dogs. Bar = 100 μm. (Reprinted with permission from G. D. Shelton et al., Fiber type specific autoantibodies in a dog with eosinophilic myositis. Muscle Nerve 8:786, 1985.)

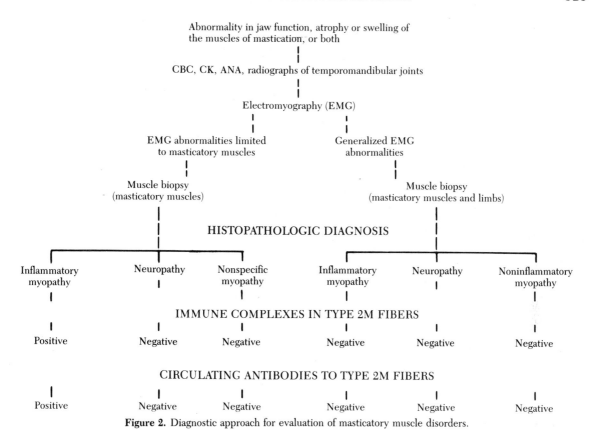

Figure 2. Diagnostic approach for evaluation of masticatory muscle disorders.

b.i.d.). Response to therapy can be determined by ability to open the jaw and serial determinations of serum CK levels. If the response is favorable, the dosage should be decreased after 3 to 4 weeks (0.5 mg/kg PO b.i.d.) and then gradually decreased to the lowest alternate-day effective dosage. Relapses are common. In chronic MMM, some have attributed trismus to an increase in connective tissue. Glucocorticoid therapy, however, may still improve jaw mobility in these dogs, suggesting that other mechanisms may contribute to the restricted movement. Serum autoantibodies can be demonstrated against type 2M fibers, further justifying the use of glucocorticoids.

Since autoantibodies against type 2M fibers can be demonstrated in both acute and chronic cases of MMM, these conditions may represent different stages of the same disorder. The course the disorder takes may relate to the animal's genetic ability to mount an inflammatory response and the inherent reactivity of the immune system. Certain breeds of dogs (i.e., Doberman pinschers and Samoyeds) tend to be severely affected and have a massive cellular infiltrate in their muscle biopsy specimens. This cellular reaction can quickly lead to myofiber destruction and end-stage myositis. If the immune response is of a lesser magnitude, the disease may take a more protracted course.

In some of the masticatory muscle disorders, unexplained changes typical of denervation may be evident. If the animal has a dropped jaw, nutrition should be maintained by feeding a gruel that the animal can lap with its tongue. Some dogs will spontaneously recover in 1 to 2 weeks. Glucocorticoids may be of benefit in some cases, although the underlying mechanisms are not fully defined. Further diagnostic procedures may reveal systemic disorders affecting the trigeminal nerves in these dogs. Therapy should be aimed at the primary disorder, if possible.

References and Supplemental Reading

Cardinet, G. H., III: Unpublished observations, 1988.

Orvis, J. S., and Cardinet, G. H., III: Canine muscle fiber types and susceptibility of masticatory muscles to myositis. Muscle Nerve 4:354, 1981.

Pflugfelder, C. M., Cardinet, G. H., III, Lutz, H., et al.: Acquired myasthenia gravis: Immunocytochemical localization of immune complexes at neuromuscular junctions. Muscle Nerve 4:289, 1981.

Shelton, G. D., Bandman, E., and Cardinet, G. H., III: Electrophoretic comparison of myosins from masticatory muscles and selected limb muscles in the dog. Am. J. Vet. Res. 46:193, 1985a.

Shelton, G. D., Cardinet, G. H. III, and Bandman, E.: Canine masticatory muscle disorders: A clinicopathological and immunochemical study of 29 cases. Muscle Nerve 10:753, 1987.

Shelton, G. D., Cardinet, G. H. III, Bandman, E., et al.: Fiber type specific autoantibodies in a dog with eosinophilic myositis. Muscle Nerve 8:783, 1985b.

HEREDITARY MYOPATHY OF LABRADOR RETRIEVERS

ROSEMARY E. McKERRELL, M.R.C.V.S.,
and KYLE G. BRAUND, F.R.C.V.S.
Cambridge, England

In 1976, Kramer and others described a condition of Labrador retriever dogs characterized by a marked deficiency of skeletal muscle mass, abnormal head posture, and a stiff hopping gait. The condition was subsequently shown to be inherited, and there were further reports in both the United States and the United Kingdom.

NOMENCLATURE

Hereditary myopathy of Labrador retrievers (HMLR) was first described as a muscle disorder characterized by a deficiency of type II muscle fibers. It has also been referred to as muscular dystrophy, myotonia, generalized muscle weakness, polyneuropathy, and hereditary myopathy.

CLINICAL SIGNS

This disease is seen only in Labrador retriever dogs. It affects both males and females and has been seen in animals of both black and yellow coat color. The age at onset and the severity of clinical signs may be variable. Some pups have clinical signs at 6 to 8 weeks of age. In others, a later onset at 6 to 7 months has been observed. Cases of both early (8 weeks) and late (6 months) onset have been observed within the same litter.

In typical cases, clinical signs become obvious at 3 to 4 months of age and include muscle weakness, abnormalities of gait and posture, and decreased exercise tolerance. Severely affected pups may have a low head posture, with ventroflexion of the neck. The back is arched, and the gait is characterized by short, stilted strides in which the hind legs are often advanced simultaneously ("bunny hopping"). The abnormality becomes more accentuated as the animal tires, and, if encouraged to continue, the pup may collapse forward with the head and neck to one side. There is no loss of consciousness or cyanosis. Exercise tolerance may be reduced to 20 yards in severely affected animals. However, mildly affected dogs may be presented because they seem to be "slow" pups that are less playful than their littermates and less willing to exercise. These dogs may

not collapse unless forcibly exercised at speed for several minutes. Rest results in some improvement, but the clinical signs rapidly recur on resumption of exercise. There is no improvement in response to administration of anticholinesterase drugs, such as edrophonium chloride.

Joint posture is often abnormal, with affected dogs having carpal overextension, carpal valgus, splaying of the digits, and a "cow-hocked" stance. As the condition progresses, generalized atrophy of skeletal muscles develops. The proximal muscles of the limbs and the muscles of the head are particularly affected, but in milder cases, the atrophy may not be dramatic.

In most cases, the clinical signs stabilize between 6 months and 1 year of age, although signs may be exacerbated by excitement or stress and particularly by exposure to cold weather. After exposure to cold, an affected dog may be unable to stand or to lift its head. Moving the animal to a warm kennel usually results in improvement within a few hours.

A less common sequel, which has been observed in three adult dogs, is the development of megaesophagus. One affected 18-month-old dog appeared to be improving in other respects. The other two dogs were affected bitches in the eighth week of pregnancy. Other sporadic complications that have been observed include the presence of a luxating patella and clinical and radiographic evidence of degenerative joint disease in the hip of one affected dog that was allowed to become obese.

NEUROLOGIC EXAMINATION

Affected dogs are bright and alert, although often poorly muscled when compared with their normal littermates. Temporal muscle atrophy is often a feature, but cranial nerve functions are otherwise normal. Muscle tone may be normal or reduced. There is no muscle pain on palpation nor dimpling on percussion. Severely affected pups are obviously weak and may have difficulty wheelbarrowing or hopping, although in less severely affected pups, postural testing may indicate no abnormalities. Proprioceptive function is normal, and no sensory deficits have been observed in affected dogs. Tendon reflexes are generally reduced or absent, even in mildly affected dogs with little muscle atrophy. There is no impairment of bladder function and no other sign of autonomic nervous system dysfunction.

DIAGNOSIS

A diagnosis of HMLR may be suspected from the signalment data, clinical signs, and results of the neurologic examination. Further procedures used in establishing the diagnosis include serology, electrodiagnosis, and muscle biopsy. Serum creatine kinase may be within normal limits or moderately elevated. Levels may increase following exacerbation of signs after exposure to cold weather but do not reach the levels reported in other degenerative muscle diseases, such as the inherited muscular dystrophy described in golden retrievers. Other routine hematologic and blood biochemical parameters are within normal limits.

Motor nerve conduction velocities are within the normal range in affected dogs, and there is no decremental response to repetitive nerve stimulation. On electromyographic examination, there frequently is spontaneous activity, particularly in the proximal limb muscles, musculature of the head, and the thoracolumbar paraspinal muscles. The most commonly recorded abnormalities are fibrillation potentials, positive sharp waves, and bizarre high-frequency discharges. Electromyographic changes may be less pronounced in mildly affected dogs and may be difficult to detect in very young dogs. Results of electrocardiographic examination of affected adults and pups have indicated no cardiac involvement.

Despite the abnormal joint posture seen in many affected dogs, there have been no abnormalities on radiography of hocks, carpi, and the vertebral column. In some cases, however, changes consistent with hip dysplasia have been present.

A wide range of morphologic features may be observed in muscle biopsies from affected dogs. The changes reported include small and large group atrophy, small angular fibers of both fiber types, and occasional fiber type grouping. All of these changes are generally considered characteristic of neurogenic disease. In other biopsies, there may be large numbers of internal nuclei, disturbances in myofiber architecture, necrosis, regeneration, and replacement of muscle fibers with fat and fibrous tissue. These changes are more commonly associated with destructive myopathies or dystrophies. Alterations in fiber type percentages are a common finding. In most muscles there is a reduction in the proportion of type 2 fibers, but in others, such as the cranial tibial, an increase in the percentage of type 2 fibers may occur. These changes

in fiber type proportions appear to become more accentuated as the disease progresses.

Preliminary biochemical data indicate significantly elevated concentrations of sodium, calcium, zinc, copper, and chloride and reduced levels of potassium and magnesium in muscles from affected adult Labrador retrievers. In addition, a significant decrease in muscle-specific proteins has been identified in the biceps femoris muscle of affected dogs.

Despite the presence of some apparently "neurogenic" features, examination of the various parts of the lower motor neuron has so far failed to identify morphologic abnormalities. The underlying pathophysiologic mechanisms involved in this disease are, therefore, still unclear.

DIFFERENTIAL DIAGNOSIS

Conditions that may present with similar signs to HMLR include skeletal problems producing abnormal gait, such as hip dysplasia, and diseases that cause exercise intolerance. The clinical signs of HMLR may particularly resemble myasthenia gravis, but other conditions resulting in lethargy or poor exercise tolerance, such as cardiopulmonary dysfunction, should also be ruled out. Differential diagnosis should include other primary muscle diseases such as polymyositis, *Toxoplasma* myopathy, myotonia, glycogen storage diseases, and hyperadrenocorticism. In severely affected dogs with marked muscle atrophy, lower motor neuron disorders, including polyradiculoneuritis and distal denervating disease, should be considered.

PROGNOSIS

In most cases, the clinical signs stabilize between 6 months and 1 year of age. There may be some improvement in ability to exercise, particularly in those dogs with the mildest signs. The atrophy of skeletal muscles persists, however, and although affected dogs may be acceptable house pets, they are not suitable for work. Owners of affected dogs should be warned that stress, including exposure to low temperatures, can result in a dramatic worsening of clinical signs, even in clinically stable adults.

The life span of affected dogs does not appear to be directly affected by the condition, although the prognosis for dogs with megaesophagus should be more guarded because of the risk of developing inhalation pneumonia.

TREATMENT

There is no definitive treatment for this condition, although various forms of medication have been used. Diazepam given orally at a dose of 10 mg twice daily was reported to have some ameliorating effect. Diphenylhydantoin had little effect, and edrophonium chloride was found to produce a worsening of clinical signs. Anabolic steroids have apparently been beneficial in some cases; however, the evidence for this is anecdotal, with no confirmatory controlled studies.

To reduce the likelihood of exacerbations, affected dogs should not be exposed to cold weather.

CONTROL

Kramer and others showed that the condition in the United States is inherited as an autosomal recessive trait. In the United Kingdom, the condition is confined to working strains of Labrador retrievers, with no cases encountered in dogs from show strains. This distinction is much less clear in the United States. Examination of pedigrees indicates that inheritance in the United Kingdom is also autosomal recessive. Because there is no way of detecting heterozygous carriers, breeders should be advised against breeding from parents or siblings of affected puppies.

References and Supplemental Reading

Hoskins, J. D., and Root, C. R.: Myopathy in a Labrador retriever. Vet. Med. Small Anim. Clin. 78:1387, 1983.
Kornegay, J. N.: Golden retriever myopathy. Proceedings of the American College of Veterinary Internal Medicine, Washington, D.C., 1984, pp. 193–196.
Kramer, J. W., Hegreberg, G. A., Bryan, G. M., et al.: A muscle disorder of Labrador retrievers characterized by deficiency of type II muscle fibers. J.A.V.M.A. 169:817, 1976.
Kramer, J. W., Hegreberg, G. A., and Hamilton, M. J.: Inheritance of a neuromuscular disorder of Labrador retriever dogs. J.A.V.M.A. 179:380, 1981.
McKerrell, R. E., Anderson, J. R., Herrtage, M. E., et al.: Generalized muscle weakness in the Labrador retriever. Vet. Rec. 115:276, 1984.
McKerrell, R. E., and Braund, K. G.: Hereditary myopathy in Labrador retrievers: A morphologic study. Vet. Pathol. 23:411, 1986.
McKerrell, R. E., and Braund, K. G.: Hereditary myopathy in Labrador retrievers: Clinical variations. J. Small Anim. Pract. 28:479, 1987.
Moore, M. P., Reed, S. M., Hegreberg, G. A., et al.: Electromyographic evaluation of adult Labrador retrievers with type II muscle fiber deficiency. Am. J. Vet. Res. 48:1332, 1987.
Simpson, S. T., Braund, K. G., and Sorjonen, D. C.: Muscular dystrophy of Labrador retrievers. Proceedings of the American College of Veterinary Internal Medicine, Salt Lake City, 1982, p. 78.

SENSORY NEUROPATHY

IAN D. DUNCAN, B.V.M.S.,
and P. A. CUDDON, B.V.Sc.
Madison, Wisconsin

The increase in knowledge of neuropathies in companion animals has made it possible to classify these diseases according to their clinical signs. Most neuropathies affect both motor and sensory function, although there are some, such as distal denervating disease (Griffiths and Duncan, 1979) and coonhound paralysis (Cummings et al., 1982), that predominantly affect motor function. Despite the fact that sensory testing in animals can often be capricious, certain neuropathies in which only sensory function is disturbed also have been recognized. This chapter will review these disorders.

SENSORY TESTING AND ITS NEUROANATOMIC BASIS

The clinical and electrophysiologic testing of sensory function in small animals is crude compared with the sophistication of sensory testing in humans (Dyck et al., 1984). Sensory modalities include proprioception (position sense), pain (nociception), touch (tactile), and temperature (hot and cold); all of these can be evaluated and quantitated in humans. In small animals, only proprioception and nociception can be evaluated accurately. Although tactile sensation can be tested in some patients, the results are sometimes spurious. Despite these limitations, proprioception and nociception are important sensory modalities, and testing of their intactness provides much information on the functional capability of a wide range of myelinated and unmyelinated fibers involved in relaying sensory information to higher centers.

All sensory modalities are relayed to the central nervous system (CNS) via a sensory receptor and its axon to a neuron in a sensory ganglion; then, from this neuron, an axon projects to the spinal cord or brain stem (Fig. 1). The sensory receptors involved in proprioception and nociception are different in both location and structure. Proprioceptors are found in muscles, joints, and tendons and in

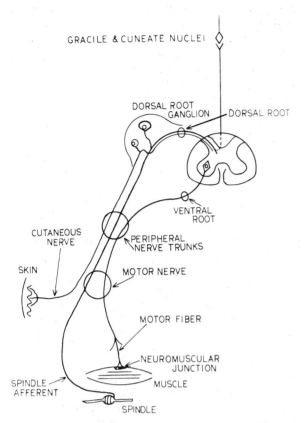

GRACILE & CUNEATE NUCLEI

DORSAL ROOT GANGLION — DORSAL ROOT

VENTRAL ROOT

CUTANEOUS NERVE

PERIPHERAL NERVE TRUNKS

SKIN

MOTOR NERVE

MOTOR FIBER

NEUROMUSCULAR JUNCTION

SPINDLE AFFERENT

MUSCLE

SPINDLE

Figure 1. Diagram of the PNS. Sensory neuropathies and neuronopathies can affect the sensory neuron and its axon at the level of the dorsal nerve root, dorsal root ganglion, mixed nerve, or cutaneous nerve.

the inner ear (special proprioception). In muscles, the receptor is the muscle spindle; in joints, there are free nerve endings (mainly nociceptors) and encapsulated receptors such as Ruffini's endings and pacinian corpuscles. Sensory fibers from muscle spindles consist of large myelinated (Aα) afferent fibers (10 to 21 μm in cats) from the annulospiral ending and smaller group (Aβ) fibers (5 to 14 μm) from secondary sensory endings. Nociceptors, which are found in skin, viscera, and so on, are pain receptors that signal tissue damage or stimuli intense enough to threaten tissue damage. They are associated with both small myelinated (Aδ) and unmyelinated (C) axons (Dyck et al., 1984). The receptors in the skin and underlying structures are most readily tested clinically and have been called "free" or "naked" endings, although ultrastructural observations show that they are actually covered by Schwann cells. Tactile sensation is perceived in the skin by a variety of low-threshold mechanoreceptors that transmit impulses to the spinal cord via medium to large myelinated fibers.

Sensory neuropathies and sensory neuronopathies affect nerve fibers or sensory neurons within the territory just described. Although sensory loss and ataxia can also be seen with lesions of the spinal cord or brain, in most instances it is possible to distinguish these on a clinical basis from lesions in the peripheral nervous system (PNS).

CLINICAL TESTING OF SENSATION

Proprioception

Conscious proprioception is evaluated using three tests: paw-position sense, reflex stepping, and the sway response. The first test is well known and involves knuckling the paw onto the dorsum and observing the expected immediate replacement. Reflex stepping involves placing a card under the paw and slowly drawing the limb away from the body. A normal dog will replace the limb quickly; loss of proprioception will lead to the limb being left abducted. The sway response is performed by placing the hind limbs together and moving the hips to one side. An animal with a proprioceptive deficit will not move the limbs appropriately to maintain balance and may fall. The latter two tests are not as frequently performed but are useful, especially when paw-position sense is equivocal.

Nociception (Pain)

The most accurate method of evaluating pain perception is to use a fine pair of hemostats and apply them to a small "tent" of raised skin. It is well known, but should be emphasized, that evidence of pain perception is judged by a cranial response and *not* the withdrawal of the limb. The initial stimulus should be as mild as possible to attempt to judge superficial pain perception. If superficial pain perception is present, deep pain sensation is too, and further testing is unnecessary. If there is no response, deeper structures, including the digits, should be squeezed to evaluate deep pain perception. When there is sensory loss, the point at which sensation is lost or diminished (sensory level) should be established, if possible. In animals with generalized loss or diminution of pain, the ear pinna and face should be evaluated. Complete and partial loss of pain sensation are referred to as analgesia and hypalgesia, respectively.

Diagnostic Tests

Examination of sensory nerve conduction can be carried out in both forelimb and hindlimb nerves (Duncan and Griffiths, 1986). These same nerves can often be biopsied, but this should be performed only if the nerve is examined using contemporary techniques (e.g., single fiber teasing, plastic embedding, and light and electron microscopy) (Dyck et al., 1984). Evaluation of H-reflexes using electromyographic equipment provides additional information on conduction through the dorsal nerve roots.

INHERITED SENSORY NEUROPATHIES

Sensory Neuropathy in English Pointers

Sensory neuropathy is inherited as an autosomal recessive trait in English pointers in the United States and shorthaired pointers in Europe (Cummings et al., 1981).

CLINICAL FINDINGS

The condition is first noticed at 3 to 5 months of age, when affected dogs begin to lick and bite at the paws of all four limbs. However, a diminution in pain perception can be noted on more thorough clinical evaluation prior to that. The paws become swollen, reddened, and ulcerated. With time, painless fractures and autoamputation can occur. On neurologic examination, there is analgesia in the digital areas of the hind paws, with hypalgesia in the forepaws. The loss of pain sensation may extend proximally up the limbs and involve the trunk. There is no ataxia, and proprioception, stretch reflexes, and muscle tone are normal. Affected dogs are not paretic. Motor nerve conduction velocity is normal, and there is no spontaneous activity on electromyographic evaluation.

PATHOLOGICAL FINDINGS

One 5-month-old pup was studied in detail at necropsy, and the lesion was located on the spinal ganglia (Cummings et al., 1981). These were reduced in size and contained a 22 to 50 per cent reduction in neurons, with a disproportionately large population of small sensory neurons. There was some degeneration of myelinated and unmyelinated fibers in ganglia, nerve roots, and peripheral nerves. In addition, there were occasional degenerating sensory neurons in the ganglia, but this was not thought to be sufficient to account for the reduction in cell bodies. In the spinal cord, there was a reduced density of fibers in the dorsolateral fasciculus. Other ascending sensory tracts were normal. Cummings and colleagues concluded that the primary problem in this disease involves a developmental deficit in nociceptive neurons. Somewhat paradoxically, however, there was an absolute increase in the smaller neurons, and the authors speculated that this might be due to retarded differentiation or growth of sensory neurons. In a later study, Cummings and associates examined the

spinal cords of affected 5- and 20-month-old pointers for the presence of substance P, the neuropeptide thought to mediate nociception at the first synapse of the axon of sensory neurons in the CNS (Cummings et al., 1984). They showed a reduction in this peptide in the spinal cord in both dogs. In older dogs there was a loss of substance P in the spinal nucleus of the trigeminal nerve. This latter finding, in addition to evidence of ongoing degeneration in the spinal cord, suggested that sensory systems, unaffected earlier in life, were involved.

PROGNOSIS

There is no treatment for this neuropathy, and despite bandaging the feet or muzzling the dog to prevent self-mutilation, infection of mutilated areas and osteomyelitis develop.

Sensory Neuropathy in Long-Haired Dachshunds

This neuropathy has been described in related dachshunds in the United Kingdom only (Duncan and Griffiths, 1982). Three affected dogs were seen, and four littermates or dogs from previous litters with identical clinical signs were reported to us. It seems likely that this neuropathy is inherited as an autosomal recessive trait, although this has not been unequivocally proven.

CLINICAL FINDINGS

The first abnormalities may be noted as early as 8 to 12 weeks of age, when owners report vague signs of posterior ataxia. Ataxia and self-mutilation of the penis are the presenting clinical signs. Affected dogs may also show intermittent dribbling of urine and have unexplained bouts of gastric disturbance, with emesis. On neurologic evaluation, a somewhat subtle hind-limb ataxia can be seen, with the dog occasionally crossing the hind legs and swaying when turning. This ataxia might be missed by some owners because of the short legs and long coat of this breed. There is neither paresis nor muscle atrophy. Proprioception is delayed or absent in all four limbs, and placing reflexes cannot be elicited. Muscle tone and patellar reflexes may be slightly reduced. Pain perception is deficient or absent over the entire body. Cranial nerve function is normal, with the exception of diminution or loss of facial sensation. The bladder is normal on palpation, and normal urination can occur, although dribbling is frequent. Results of electromyographic examination and motor nerve conduction studies are normal. There may be abnormalities on sensory nerve stimulation.

PATHOLOGICAL FINDINGS

Unlike pointers with sensory neuropathy, long-haired dachshunds show no abnormalities in the spinal ganglia. Although sensory neurons have not been quantitated, there is no evidence of cell loss or degeneration. Results of biopsies of a sensory nerve in the hindlimbs, however, indicated a profound loss of myelinated fibers on light microscopy. A 1-month-old dog was necropsied, and a notable loss of myelinated fibers in other cutaneous nerves was confirmed, whereas mixed nerves appeared comparatively normal. On electron microscopy of sensory nerves there were numerous degenerated myelinated fibers. In addition, unmyelinated fibers were abnormal, with numerous degenerating axons and axons containing abnormal organelles. Similar electron microscopic changes were identified in the thoracic portion of the vagus, suggesting autonomic involvement. As the dorsal nerve roots were normal, the predominantly distal degeneration suggested that this sensory neuropathy is a distal axonopathy. The pathologic evidence of involvement of large and small myelinated and unmyelinated fibers aids in explaining the diffuse sensory disturbances seen in these dogs. By comparison, in the pointers only small myelinated and unmyelinated fibers are affected.

PROGNOSIS

Most of these dogs live normally, although they may need to be muzzled if self-mutilation occurs. Gastric disturbances, including vomiting, which may result from autonomic nerve involvement, can lead to early death, however.

An almost identical syndrome has recently been described in a young border collie puppy (Wheeler, 1987). This dog was severely ataxic and had generalized loss of proprioception and loss of superficial pain sensation over the entire body, except on the lips and nostrils. Sensory nerve action potentials could not be elicited. Changes similar to those seen in the dachshund were seen in a cutaneous radial nerve biopsy.

Progressive Axonopathy in Boxers

Progressive axonopathy in boxers was first described in 1980 in the United Kingdom (Griffiths et al., 1980). Since then, it has been investigated in depth and has been proved to be inherited as an autosomal recessive trait. The clinical features include hindleg ataxia, proprioceptive deficits, hypotonia, patellar areflexia, and head bobbing. Although detailed electrophysiologic and pathologic studies have shown that motor fibers are affected in this disease, the predominant clinical signs are due to lesions in the peripheral sensory system. Full details of this disease are described elsewhere (Griffiths et al., 1980) (see p. 828).

ACQUIRED SENSORY NEUROPATHY

In 1983, two separate groups reported sensory disturbances in a series of dogs that on necropsy had ganglioradiculitis involving sensory ganglia of the spinal cord and head (Cummings et al., 1983; Wouda et al., 1983). A similar case has since been reported (Steiss et al., 1987); another case report documents more localized sensory loss in the face (Carmichael and Griffiths, 1981). The clinical features and the similarities and differences of all of these dogs are listed in Table 1.

A number of different breeds are represented, although it may be significant that three were Siberian huskies. There were seven females and three males. The disease occurred at 9 years of age in one dog, but most were young to middle-aged (1 to 6 years). Despite the fact that the disease onset varied from acute to chronic in nature, in all cases of generalized sensory neuronopathy there was significant progression of signs despite medical therapy. The initial signs in these affected dogs included hindleg ataxia (all dogs), difficulty in eating, regurgitation, or dysphagia (four of nine), and mutilation/hyperesthesia (three of nine). On neurologic examination there was no noticeable hindlimb paresis in any of the dogs. In five dogs, the hindlimbs had hypermetria. The patellar reflexes were diminished or absent in seven of nine dogs tested; this loss was asymmetric in some cases. In three of the cases of Cummings and colleagues, atrophy of the masticatory muscles was noted. Postural reactions were decreased in six of the dogs. Pain perception was decreased or lost over the head in six dogs. Megaesophagus was noted in two of the dogs in the Cummings's series. In the single report of localized trigeminal nerve sensory loss, the outstanding features were difficulty in eating and a bilateral decrease in pain and tactile sensation in the whole trigeminal nerve field. There was no limb involvement.

Certain ancillary examinations were of limited use. With the exception of one dog that had electromyographic evidence of scattered denervation, there was no spontaneous activity. Nerve conduction velocities in mixed nerves were slowed in some dogs. Sensory nerve velocity was delayed in the only dog tested. Results of cerebrospinal fluid evaluation were also unremarkable, except in one case in which a mild elevation in total protein and white blood cells was reported.

All of the dogs discussed in these reports were necropsied, and many similar findings were noted.

Table 1. *Clinical Neurologic Signs Observed in the Published Cases of Acquired Sensory Neuronopathy*

Breed	Onset	Ataxia	Postural Reactions	Patellar Reflexes	Muscle Tone	Muscle Bulk	Nociception Limb/Body	Nociception Face	Other Signs
1. Brittany spaniel SF, 9 yr	Subacute, progressive	++	—	0	↑↑	↓↓ (M, S)	—	↓↓	Megaesophagus, hypermetria (hind)
2. Siberian husky SF, 4 yr	Acute, progressive	+++	↓↓ (RF and hind)	0 (RH)	↑↑ (Hind)	↓↓ (LM)	—	↓ (L)	Head tilt, voice loss, hypermetria (hind)
3. Welsh corgi SF, 4½ yr	Chronic, progressive	+	↓↓ (LF, LH)	↓↓ (LH) 0 (RH)	—	↓ (M)	—	↓↓	Megaesophagus
4. Siberian husky CM, 5 yr	Chronic, progressive	+ to ++	—	0	—	N	↑↑	↓↓	—
5. Doberman pinscher F, 1½ yr	Acute, progressive	+	↓↓ to 0 (hind)	↓↓ (LH) 0 (RH)	—	N	↓↓ (Hind)	0	Anisocoria, difficulty eating, dysmetria (RH)
6. Siberian husky F, 2 yr	Acute, progressive	++	—	—	—	N	N	↑	Facial paresthesia
7. Whippet M, 5 yr	Acute, progressive	++	↓↓ (all)	N	—	N	N	0	Urinary/fecal incontinence, difficulty eating
8. Scottish terrier F, 6 yr	Chronic, progressive	++	↓↓ (hind)	0 (RH)	—	N	N	—	Dysmetria (RH)
9. Golden retriever CM, 2 yr	Chronic, progressive	+++	↓ to ↓↓ (all)	0	N	N	↑ (R)	N	Hearing loss, hypermetria
10. Rough-coated collie F, 2 yr	Acute, static	N	N	N	N	N	N	↓ (R) 0 (L)	Hypersalivation, difficulty eating

SF = spayed female, CM = castrated male; RF, LF = forelimbs, RH, LH = hindlimbs, M = masticatory muscles, S = scapular muscles, L = left side, R = right side; — = not recorded, N = normal. Increasing numbers of +, ↓, and ↑ indicates increasing severity. Cases 1–4, Cummings et al., 1983; 5–8, Wouda et al., 1983; 9, Steiss et al., 1987; 10, Carmichael and Griffiths, 1981.

The predominant lesion was seen in the sensory ganglia and nerve roots. There was widespread loss of myelinated fibers in the dorsal nerve roots but, in comparison, little or no abnormality of ventral roots. Within the dorsal root ganglia there was loss of neurons, some neuronophagia, and perivenular and perineuronal cuffing by lymphocytes and macrophages. Central nervous system changes were also seen, with degeneration and loss of fibers in the spinal tract of the trigeminal nerve and the dorsal columns of the spinal cord. All of the authors concluded that the primary lesion was a sensory neuronopathy, with resultant degeneration of peripheral sensory nerve fibers. The cause of these lesions remained unsolved, however, although the possibility of toxic, viral, immune-mediated, or genetic factors was discussed.

The case seen by Carmichael and Griffiths was somewhat different from those described above. This dog had loss of tactile and pain sensation over the entire trigeminal area but had no involvement of the mandibular nerve (motor component), with normal jaw strength and no atrophy. On necropsy, a marked loss of nerve fibers was seen in the trigeminal nerve and its spinal tract, but the motor fibers of the mandibular nerve were intact. This fiber loss was thought to be secondary to degeneration of neurons in the gasserian ganglion, which was not associated with inflammation (compare with the reports above).

In summary, the dogs with this sensory ganglioradiculitis lesion usually had a chronic-progressive problem, between 1 and 6 years of age, with ataxia as the most common presenting clinical sign. Other presenting signs included dysphagia with regurgitation and mutilation with hyperesthesia. On neurologic examination there was hindleg ataxia, sometimes with hypermetria, and there were conscious proprioception deficits. Decreased or absent patellar reflexes were common, and pain perception was frequently diminished over the head. There were no pathognomonic diagnostic ancillary tests, but sensory nerve electrophysiologic testing and biopsy may be the most useful tests to apply in future cases. In most dogs, however, it appears the disease will be progressive. There is no known treatment. Accordingly, the final diagnosis will be made at necropsy.

Note: The authors have now seen a young, female Siberian husky with progressive ataxia, hypermetria, and proprioceptive loss. At necropsy, the sensory (dorsal) nerve roots showed widespread loss of myelinated fibers, but the motor nerve roots were normal (Sawchuck, Cuddon, and Durus, in preparation).

References and Supplemental Reading

Carmichael, S., and Griffiths, I. R.: Case of isolated sensory trigeminal neuropathy in a dog. Vet. Rec. 109:280, 1981.

Cummings, J. F., de Lahunta, A., Holmes, D. F., et al.: Coonhound paralysis. Further clinical studies and electron microscopic observations. Acta Neuropathol. (Berl.) 56:167, 1982.

Cummings, J. F., de Lahunta, A., and Mitchell, W. J., Jr.: Ganglioradiculitis in the dog: A clinical, light- and electron-microscopic study. Acta Neuropathol. (Berl.) 60:29, 1983.

Cummings, J. F., de Lahunta, A., Simpson, S. T., et al.: Reduced substance P-like immunoreactivity in hereditary sensory neuropathy of pointer dogs. Acta Neuropathol. (Berl.) 63:33, 1984.

Cummings, J. F., de Lahunta, A., and Winn, S. S.: Acral mutilation and nociceptive loss in English pointer dogs. A canine sensory neuropathy. Acta Neuropathol. (Berl.) 53:119, 1981.

Duncan, I. D., and Griffiths, I. R.: A sensory neuropathy in long-haired dachshund dogs. J. Small Anim. Pract. 23:381, 1982.

Duncan, I. D., and Griffiths, I. R.: Small animal neuromuscular disorders. In Kornegay, J. N. (ed.): Neurologic Disorders—Contemporary Issues in Small Animal Practice, Vol. 5. New York: Churchill Livingstone, 1986, pp. 169–195.

Dyck, P. J., Thomas, P. K., Lambert, E. H., et al. (eds.): Peripheral Neuropathy, Vol. 1. Philadelphia: W. B. Saunders Co., 1984.

Griffiths, I. R., and Duncan, I. D.: Distal denervating disease. A degenerative neuropathy of the distal motor axons in dogs. J. Small Anim. Pract. 20:579, 1979.

Griffiths, I. R., Duncan, I. D., and Barker, J.: A progressive axonopathy of boxer dogs affecting the central and peripheral nervous system. J. Small Anim. Pract. 21:29, 1980.

Sawchuck, Cuddon, and Durus: In preparation, 1988.

Steiss, J. E., Pook, H. A., Clark, E. G., et al.: Sensory neuropathy in a dog. J.A.V.M.A. 190:205, 1987.

Wheeler, S. J.: Sensory neuropathy in a border collie puppy. J. Small Anim. Pract. 28:281, 1987.

Wouda, W., Vandevelde, M., Oettli, P., et al.: Sensory neuronopathy in dogs: A study of four cases. J. Comp. Pathol. 93:437, 1983.

PROGRESSIVE AXONOPATHY OF BOXER DOGS

IAN R. GRIFFITHS, B.V.M.S.
Glasgow, Scotland

Progressive axonopathy (PA) is a specific neurologic disease affecting the central (CNS) and peripheral nervous systems (PNS) of boxer dogs. The first clinical cases were recognized in 1977–1978, and a report of five animals was published in 1980 (Griffiths et al., 1980). Two of these animals were siblings, and this, together with the breed specificity and similarity of clinical and pathologic features, suggested an inherited basis. Further cases were soon reported, and detailed analysis of numerous pedigrees and subsequent test matings established an autosomal recessive mode of inheritance.

Following its recognition as a breed-specific disorder, the Boxer Breed Council introduced an eradication scheme that has substantially reduced the number of clinical cases. A total of approximately 30 to 40 dogs have been affected, but in the past 2 years, the author has been aware of only two new cases. The phenotypic expression of the disease is, therefore, extremely low, although there are likely to be considerably more carrier animals in the population. The disease has very recently been recognized in Norway (Presthus, 1988).

CLINICAL FEATURES

As an autosomal recessively inherited condition, PA affects both males and females equally often. The age of onset is somewhat variable, but in the vast majority of instances, signs are evident to the owner by 6 months of age and often by 3 months. The earliest abnormality is a mild bilaterally symmetric ataxia of the hindlimbs manifested as a clumsiness of gait. The ataxia gradually worsens over succeeding months, although the rate of progression varies between dogs. Hindlimb ataxia remains the major abnormality throughout the disease course. There are often periods during which the signs remain relatively static, although the overall course is progressive.

Specific abnormalities are identified on neurologic examination. Conscious proprioceptive deficits become evident as the disease develops, although in the earlier stages, proprioceptive functions such as paw-position sense are often intact. Later there is a variable loss of proprioception, with eventual absence of conscious proprioception. Muscle tone

is decreased in both front and hindlimbs. The patellar reflexes are absent. In normal young pups, it is often difficult to obtain this reflex, so its apparent absence should be considered with caution. It is still uncertain whether the patellar reflex is absent in all pups less than 2 to 3 months of age that have PA, as insufficient animals of this age have been examined. In one instance, the absence of a patellar reflex in a 4-week-old dog suggested PA, which was later confirmed. However, a second case was not diagnosed initially, as patellar reflexes appeared to be present at 6 weeks. The pedal reflexes, muscle bulk, and all other findings on clinical examination are normal. Much later in the disease, after 15 months of age, minimal forelimb weakness may be seen. Later still, mild head bobbing and fine ocular tremor can occur. Despite severe ataxia, a degree of weakness, hypotonia, and patellar areflexia, muscle atrophy does not occur.

ELECTROPHYSIOLOGY

The author has had the opportunity to follow the electrophysiologic parameters in two affected pups and their normal littermates from 1 month of age until adulthood and has also observed many sporadic cases. Motor nerve conduction velocities (NCV) and evoked compound muscle action potentials (ECMAP) were examined in sciatic/tibial and ulnar nerves, with very similar findings. There is normally an age-related maturation process, with the NCV increasing to adult values at 7 to 8 months of age. Both parameters developed normally until 3 to 4 months of age in pups with PA. The rate of increase in motor NCV then decreased, so that by 9 to 10 months, the value was at or just below the lower end of the normal range. Normal adult motor NCV is 55 to 70 m/sec, whereas dogs with PA usually have values of 40 to 55 m/sec.

The ECMAP in affected dogs decreased from the age of 3 to 4 months to less than 50 per cent of normal, whereas the duration of the potentials was often increased. As an indication of delayed conduction in ventral nerve roots, F-wave latencies were increased in affected dogs. Sensory nerve potentials, examined in the lateral cutaneous radial nerve, were also reduced in amplitude at virtually all ages. In many older dogs, no conduction could be elicited. Abnormal spontaneous activity, such as fibrillation potentials and positive sharp waves, occurred infrequently in older dogs in only distal limb muscles such as the interosseous (Griffiths, 1985).

PATHOLOGY

Abnormalities occur in both the CNS and PNS. The original term *axonopathy* was used in this disease because of the large axonal swellings (spheroids) that occur predominantly in selected areas of the CNS and PNS. Certain brainstem nuclei, including the dorsal nucleus of the trapezoid body, the cuneate, the accessory cuneate, the gracile, and the lateral lemniscus and its nucleus, contain large numbers of spheroids. Other brain stem areas contain lesser numbers, and none are identified in the cerebral hemispheres and diencephalon. The spinal cord also contains swellings, particularly in the lateral and ventral funiculi. The dorsal columns are largely, though not exclusively, spared. Occasional spheroids are also seen in the gray matter. There is no obvious tract or segmental predilection in the spinal cord. Very little axonal breakdown occurs in the brain, but affected areas of cord contain axonal breakdown products and myeloclasts.

The contents of the CNS swellings are somewhat variable. The majority contain excessive and disorganized neurofilaments, although these are absent in other swellings. Vesiculotubular profiles, vesicles, and mitochondria are other common constituents. Increased amounts of actin have been demonstrated with immunocytochemistry in many spheroids. Although the ventral horn cells appear morphologically normal by light microscopy, many contain phosphorylated neurofilaments, which are not normally found in the perikarya of these cells.

In the PNS, axonal swellings occur predominantly in the nerve roots and contain disorganized filaments and some membranous components. They are found principally at the proximal paranodes (i.e., nearer the cell bodies) and later involve more of the internode. The overlying myelin sheath is often attenuated or absent. As the disease progresses, myelin sheath changes become very prevalent in the roots, with demyelination, remyelination, and remodeling of the sheath. In the distal nerves, myelin sheath changes are far less frequent, but axonal degeneration and regeneration become progressively more obvious.

Morphometric and quantitative studies of various nerves revealed the following features: (1) The lumbar nerve roots contained a proportion of swollen axons at all ages. (2) In the more distal nerves, the larger-diameter myelinated axons did not develop to their expected maximum diameter (developmental hypoplasia). (3) Unmyelinated axons developed to their normal sizes. (4) Myelin sheath changes occurred primarily proximally, rather than distally. (5) Xenografts of affected dog nerve into nude mice failed to demonstrate any of the myelin sheath changes.

PATHOGENESIS

It is not known how the genetic abnormality causes the neural defects, but a hypothesis of the development of the lesions is possible. Postulated defects in axoplasmic transport, particularly in nerve roots, lead to the filamentous and membranous accumulations and axonal swellings. Neurofilaments are a major factor determining axonal size, and if they are not transported distally, owing to a transport defect, the larger axons in the distal nerve will not develop fully. In smaller myelinated and unmyelinated axons, neurofilaments are less important in controlling caliber, and such fibers develop normally. The temporal and spatial changes in the myelin sheath and their failure to be reproduced in the xenografts suggest they are secondary to the axonal changes. The decreased caliber of large axons and minor myelin sheath changes in limb nerves are probably the basis for the reduced NCV and ECMAP recorded electrophysiologically.

CONFIRMATION OF DIAGNOSIS

The diagnosis can be made with reasonable certainty in live animals on the basis of (1) breed, (2) age of onset, (3) clinical signs, particularly the loss of patellar reflexes in the absence of muscle atrophy, (4) slow progression of signs, (5) electrophysiologic findings, particularly the markedly reduced or absent sensory potentials and the absence of abnormal spontaneous activity, and (6) pedigree analysis.

Complete confirmation depends on the demonstration of lesions in the CNS and PNS, especially the CNS spheroids.

PROGNOSIS AND ADVICE

There is no possibility of recovery. The course of this disease is chronic with periods of stasis. Animals can function as acceptable pets for many months or years but will eventually require euthanasia because of gross gait disability. The disease is inherited as an autosomal recessive trait; therefore, both parents are carriers and siblings are possible carriers.

An advisory pamphlet detailing known carriers and advice regarding breeding is available from The Secretary, Boxer Breed Council, Farthing Ridge, 89A High Street South, Stewkley, Leighton Buzzard, Bedfordshire, U.K.

References and Supplemental Reading

Griffiths, I. R., Duncan, I. D., and Barker, J.: A progressive axonopathy of boxer dogs affecting the central and peripheral nervous systems. J. Small Anim. Pract. 21:29, 1980.

Griffiths, I. R.: Progressive axonopathy: An inherited neuropathy of boxer dogs. I. Further studies of the clinical and electrophysiological features. J. Small Anim. Pract. 26:381, 1985.

Presthus, J.: Personal communication, 1988.

DEGENERATIVE MYELOPATHY

R. M. CLEMMONS, D.V.M., Ph.D.

Gainesville, Florida

Degenerative myelopathy (DM) was first described as a specific degenerative neurologic disease in 1973 (Averill, 1973). It has also been termed chronic degenerative radiculomyelopathy (Griffiths and Duncan, 1975), German shepherd dog myelopathy (Braund and Vandevelde, 1978), and progressive myelopathy (Waxman et al., 1980a,b). Prior to 1973, the disease was considered to be related to the presence of intervertebral disk protrusion, spondylosis deformans, or osseous dural metaplasia. Although these conditions are frequently seen concurrently in dogs with DM, they do not appear to be responsible for the massive thoracolumbar demyelination and axonal loss seen in this disease. The reported age of onset is 5 to 14 years, which corresponds to the third to sixth decades of human life. There does not appear to be any sex predominance. Although a few cases have been reported in other large breeds of dogs (Averill, 1973; Griffiths and Duncan, 1975), DM appears with relative frequency largely in German shepherds, suggesting a genetic basis. This report presents findings of several studies,* many of which have not been previously published. It is hoped that they will provide perspective on the diagnosis, cause, and tentative therapy of this devastating neurologic disorder.

CLINICAL SIGNS

Clinically, DM is characterized initially by loss of proprioceptive function, which eventually leads to severe posterior ataxia. The ataxia is initially characterized by knuckling of the toes, wearing of the nails of the inner digits of the rear paws, and stumbling. Later, signs of hypermetria develop as the lateral funicular (spinocerebellar) pathways are affected. As the disease progresses, other signs of upper motor neuronal dysfunction also become more evident. The tendon reflexes become hyperactive to the point of clonus; crossed extensor reflexes become apparent, and Babinski's signs are evident. Once these signs are consistently present and easily elicited, the prognosis worsens. Pain sensation is largely spared in uncomplicated DM. The upper motor neuronal signs will continue to worsen until total physiologic transection of the spinal cord appears. At this time, afflicted dogs will develop urinary and fecal incontinence. The disease is usually progressive, although fluctuations in clinical signs are frequently seen. Rarely, classical signs of DM completely disappear but recur later. The course of the disease is reported to be 6 months to 1 year from the first appearance of clinical signs (Averill, 1973; Braund and Vandevelde, 1978; Waxman et al., 1980a). However, patients maintained beyond the loss of rear leg function eventually develop foreleg dysfunction, finally succumbing to brain stem involvement.

In a limited number of cases, signs of lower motor neuronal dysfunction may be seen. Accordingly, although these patients account for less than 10 per cent of the overall number of dogs with DM, the presence of lower motor neuronal signs cannot be used as an exclusionary test for DM. These patients have the same general abnormalities, with the addition of localized motor unit disease characterized by decreased tendon reflexes and early loss of voluntary movements. One limb is often more severely affected. Some of these dogs have abnormal signs on electromyographic studies, including spontaneous positive sharp waves and fibrillation potentials, apparently indicating ventral nerve root involvement. However, most dogs with this form of DM, originally termed chronic degenerative radiculomyelopathy (Griffiths and Duncan, 1975), have no spontaneous muscle activity and appear to have lesions predominantly in the dorsal nerve roots. It appears that this is not a separate disease but is,

---

*Clemmons, R. M., Gorman, N. T., Calderwood-May, M., and Mayhew, I. G., College of Veterinary Medicine, University of Florida, Gainesville, FL; and McDonald, T. D., University of Nebraska Medical Center, Omaha, NE.

instead, another manifestation of DM. The prognosis for this form of DM is worse, since the nerve root damage does not appear to be reversible.

DIAGNOSIS

A diagnosis of DM should be suspected in any large dog, particularly a German shepherd, with progressive spinal ataxia and weakness. This is supported by the neurologic findings of diffuse thoracolumbar spinal cord dysfunction. Early in the course of the disease, neurologic findings include hyperactive tendon reflexes in the pelvic limbs, diminished conscious proprioception, and spinal ataxia with hypermetria. Pain sensation and urinary and fecal continence are usually normal. Local hyperpathia is, for the most part, absent. Results of clinical pathologic examination are generally within normal limits, with the exception of an elevation of protein in cerebrospinal fluid (CSF) from the lumbar cistern.

It was initially determined by radial immunodiffusion techniques that dogs with DM had elevations of CSF protein secondary to increases in CSF immunoglobulin (Ig) G. However, more specific techniques using isoelectric immunofocusing failed to confirm the elevation of CSF IgG. In addition, there were no oligoclonal bands of IgG in the CSF of DM patients. However, the blood-brain barrier was found to be intact, suggesting that the elevations of CSF protein were from *de novo* synthesis. Thus, the source of the elevated proteins is still unclear.

Findings on electromyographic examination are normal, except in patients with the atypical lower motor neuronal form, supporting the localization of the disease process to the white matter pathways of the spinal cord. On the other hand, spinal cord evoked potentials recorded at the cisterna magna after stimulation of the sciatic nerve indicate a diminished amplitude and prolonged or separated N_1 wave. Moreover, these changes appear to worsen as the signs of DM progress, suggesting that abnormal spinal cord conduction may be associated with the neurologic abnormalities seen in DM.

Routine radiographic examination and myelography rule out the presence of spinal cord compression or segmental disease. However, minor disk protrusions, spondylosis deformans, and osseous dural metaplasia are commonly seen. Many DM patients also have radiographic evidence of hip dysplasia. Magnetic resonance images have recently demonstrated the presence of lesions throughout the thoracolumbar spinal cord. This may be the first visual antemortem evidence of the lesions of DM. In addition, magnetic resonance images may provide an important tool to monitor changes in DM lesions during treatment trials.

Depressed cell-mediated immune responses to conconavalin A, phytohemagglutinin P (Waxman et al., 1980a,b), and pokeweed mitogens have been found to be a reliable laboratory test, in the presence of typical clinical signs, for the diagnosis of DM. Although cell-mediated immune studies are time-consuming and expensive, they do correlate with the presence and, more important, with the severity of the disorder. It is unfortunate that ruling out the diagnosis of DM is often necessary, even when other disease states are present: Dogs with hip dysplasia or intervertebral disk protrusion may also have DM. The immune studies provide a more definitive diagnosis of DM, thus allowing for a better perspective when surgical procedures for concomitant diseases are planned. In this way, operations that potentially might cause further irreversible neurologic deterioration may be avoided. All older patients, particularly of those breeds with a predilection for DM, should be appropriately tested to make certain that DM is not present. In those cases in which the cell-mediated immune reponses were deemed normal, treatment of other diseases has usually been beneficial.

PATHOLOGIC FINDINGS

There usually are no lesions on gross pathologic examination of dogs with DM. The most striking feature is the reduction of rear limb and caudal axial musculature. Microscopic examination of the kidneys and gastrointestinal tract identifies plasma cell infiltrates. Microscopic neural tissue lesions have been described (Averill, 1973; Griffiths and Duncan, 1975; Braund and Vandevelde, 1978). The spinal cord shows widespread demyelination, with the greatest concentration of lesions in the thoracolumbar region. In severely affected areas there is also a reduced number of axons, an increased number of astrocytes, and an increased density of small vascular elements. In the thoracic spinal cord, nearly all of the funiculi are vacuolated. There are swollen axons and eosinophilic globules, representing degenerating and regenerating axons, in these areas. Macrophages and astrocytes are occasionally present within and around the borders of the vacuoles. Similar lesions are occasionally seen scattered throughout the white matter of the brains from some dogs with DM. Myelin-specific stains indicate a reduction in white matter content of myelin in the damaged areas. In DM patients who exhibit the atypical lower motor neuronal form of DM, changes similar to those in the spinal cord are seen in the spinal nerve roots.

ETIOLOGY OF DEGENERATIVE MYELOPATHY

Although the etiology of DM still remains a mystery, studies performed over the past 14 years have increased our understanding of its nature. It does not appear to be associated with a dying-back neuropathy (Braund and Vandevelde, 1978), suggesting that DM is not related to exposure to exogenous toxic substances. On the other hand, certain enteric abnormalities could lead to deficiencies of vital nutrients. One report suggested that there are decreases in serum vitamin B_{12} concentrations in 50 per cent of German shepherds with DM (Williams et al., 1984), but others failed to find reductions in urinary levels of vitamin B_{12} metabolites (Averill, 1973; Griffiths and Duncan, 1975). Serum tocopherol levels are reduced in German shepherds with DM (Williams et al., 1985). However, providing oral vitamin B complex and alpha-tocopherol acetate supplements at levels sufficient to correct the diminished serum levels does not eliminate signs of DM.

An alternative hypothesis is that DM is an immune-related neurodegenerative disease similar to other such disorders in humans, including multiple sclerosis (MS) and amyotrophic lateral sclerosis (ALS). In dogs, DM does not correlate with either disease entirely; however, from a clinical point of view, DM and MS have many similarities. The immunologic abnormalities seen in DM parallel those in MS (Lisak, 1980). In addition, one form of MS that occurs during the fourth to fifth decades is characterized as a chronic, progressive myelopathy. In both conditions, depression of cell-mediated immune responses occurs secondary to a progressive increase in circulating suppressor cells.

Dogs with DM also have 3 to 10 times more circulating immune complexes than normal dogs. Although these complexes are not specific to DM, one circulating 85,000-molecular-weight antigen has recently been recognized in dogs with DM but not in those with other neurologic disorders. Although this finding is preliminary, this may be the first indication of a serum marker for the diagnosis of DM. In addition, the use of antibodies against this antigen may provide new insights into the cause of DM. We have found that dogs that have DM together with depressed immune responses also have elevated immune complexes. The circulating immune complexes may possibly activate suppressor cells, probably macrophages, which in turn alter regulation of T-lymphocyte function. We are led to believe that circulating suppressor cells are generated by the animal in an attempt to control DM by diminishing an already activated immune system. Unfortunately, these circulating suppressor cells do not appear to be capable of reducing the inflammatory response in the central nervous system, where it would provide the most benefit.

TREATMENT

Although there is no current therapy that will resolve the lesions of DM, there is hope for control in a limited number of cases. This report will provide a strategy for the treatment of DM. However, it may first be appropriate to discuss those therapies that do not seem to have any benefit.

In the past, most practitioners have used glucocorticoids to treat DM. Although glucocorticoids are not contraindicated in DM, certain side effects occur after long-term use. For example, steroid myopathy will compound the weakness and ultimately be detrimental. Glucocorticoids should be reserved for treatment of acute exacerbations of DM, rather than for long-term treatment. When give alone, they will not alter the overall outcome of DM. If glucocorticoids are to be used, prednisone should be given at an initial level of 1 mg/kg/day in three divided doses for 3 days. This should be reduced to 0.33 mg/kg every 12 hr for 2 days. A maintenance dosage of 0.5 mg/kg every other day is continued.

Other immunosuppressive agents, including cyclophosphamide and azathioprine, have not had any long-term benefits. Immunostimulants such as levamisole, however, appear to worsen the disease and increase its rate of progression. Intravenous dimethyl sulfoxide (DMSO) has no effect on DM, at least when given in weekly injections over a 1-month period. Intramuscular injections of cobra venom have not been beneficial. Although nonsteroidal anti-inflammatory drugs appear to slow the progression of the condition, the excessive levels required invariably lead to gastrointestinal irritation. Use of vitamin E at high doses (2000 IU/day) has similar nonsteroidal anti-inflammatory actions without causing undesirable side effects. High-potency B complex vitamins may also be given twice daily.

Exercise appears to be helpful in delaying the progression of the disease. We recommend that DM patients be placed on an increasing, alternate-day exercise program including walking and swimming. If analgesia is needed after exercise, acetaminophen (5 mg/kg) is recommended.

The only treatment for DM that appears to alter the course of the disease is aminocaproic acid (EACA) (Amicar, Lederle), 500 mg every 8 hr. The beneficial effect of EACA appears to occur secondary to its antiprotease activity, suggesting that blocking the final common pathway of tissue inflammation (i.e., reducing the activation of tissue enzymes) aids in preventing tissue damage. Although nonsteroidal anti-inflammatory drugs reduce cell-to-cell interactions, thus minimizing cell-mediated inflammation, and steroid drugs stabilize lysosomal enzymes, thus preventing their release into the tissues, neither stops the progression of DM. This suggests that the activation of extracellular enzymes is the most important pathogenetic factor in DM. It appears that EACA works at this level.

Other drugs similar in action to EACA have been

useful in the treatment of human MS; however, one of these, colchicine at 0.01 to 0.02 mg/kg (or 0.3 to 0.6 mg) every 12 hr, has not shown any promise in DM. EACA has an advantage in that it can be given orally. However, the fact that it may cost the owner between $80 to $100 per month for treatment is a major limitation. Side effects are limited to gastrointestinal irritation in about one per cent of the animals treated, most of which had pre-existing irritative colitis.

Monitoring immune responses indicates that EACA does not cure DM but presumably controls the degenerative process. Because of the variability of the natural clinical course of DM, it is difficult to conduct treatment trials in a double-blinded manner. However, based on the author's clinical impressions, EACA appears to slow the progression of DM by 50 per cent in all cases. Furthermore, approximately 15 to 20 per cent of treated dogs have no further deterioration, and some even improve. Several dogs with DM have survived in excess of 4 years, which is well beyond what is typically expected in untreated affected dogs.

Interferon therapy also may ultimately be beneficial in dogs with DM, but appropriate treatment protocols must be established. Unfortunately, unlike MS, DM is a disease of years rather than decades. Because of this more rapid progression, intrathecal interferon must be given by constant infusion in patients with DM. Chronic intrathecal infusions of gamma interferon at 1,000,000 U/day in a limited number of dogs resulted in temporary cessation of progression during the infusion. However, once the infusions were stopped, the signs of DM continued to progress. There was a similar temporary improvement in spinal cord evoked potentials during this trial. These patients had fairly advanced signs of DM. Use of interferon earlier in the disease course may therefore be more beneficial.

In summary, the author currently recommends vitamin supplementation, judicious use of glucocorticoids, and trials with EACA for the treatment of DM. If EACA is to be effective, improvement will usually be seen within 8 weeks of initiation of therapy. Because of the expense of EACA, its use in dogs with posterior paralysis seems unwarranted. Accurate and early diagnosis of DM is essential, since the chances of success are markedly improved if therapy is begun early in the course of the disease.

CONCLUSION

The emphasis in this report is on providing enlightenment about a devastating neurodegenerative disease and offering hope to clients. There is reason to believe that medication discussed here can arrest the progression of DM. Although research continues to answer questions about the nature and cause of DM, treating these patients and their owners with compassion and hope may help lessen their emotional discomfort. In older patients of breeds at risk for developing DM, particularly German shepherds and Old English sheepdogs, evaluation of immune complexes or the cell-mediated immune response may improve the accuracy of diagnosis. In those patients in which no other cause of posterior ataxia can be identified, treatment trials with EACA may be indicated. However, results of treatment should be critically evaluated, using objective techniques such as spinal evoked potentials and magnetic resonance imaging, if possible. Therapy with medications that have no efficacy in DM should be avoided. New treatments must be carefully considered and tested. As research to advance our understanding of DM continues, we hope to be able to add this to the list of treatable diseases.

References and Supplemental Reading

Averill, D. R.: Degenerative myelopathy in the aging German shepherd dog: Clinical and pathologic findings. J.A.V.M.A. 162:1045, 1973.

Braund, K. G., and Vandevelde, M.: German shepherd dog myelopathy—a morphologic and morphometric study. Am. J. Vet. Res. 39:1309, 1978.

Griffiths, I. R., and Duncan, I. D.: Chronic degenerative radiculomyelopathy in the dog. J. Small Anim. Pract. 16:461, 1975.

Lisak, R. P.: Multiple sclerosis: Evidence for immunopathogenesis. Neurology 30:99, 1980.

Waxman, F. J., Clemmons, R. M., Johnson, G., et al.: Progressive myelopathy in older German shepherd dogs. I. Depressed response to thymus-dependent mitogens. J. Immunol. 124:1209, 1980a.

Waxman, F. J., Clemmons, R. M., and Hinrichs, D. J.: Progressive myelopathy in older German shepherd dogs. II. Presence of circulating suppressor cells. J. Immunol. 124:1216, 1980b.

Williams, D. A., Batt, R. M., and Sharp, N. J. H.: Degenerative myelopathy in German shepherd dogs: An association with mucosal biochemical changes and bacterial overgrowth in the small intestine. Clin. Sci. 66:25P, 1984.

Williams, D. A., Prymak, C., and Baughan, J.: Tocopherol (vitamin E) status in canine degenerative myelopathy. Proceedings of the 3rd Annual Medical Forum, American College of Veterinary Internal Medicine, 1985, p.154.

HYPOMYELINATION IN DOGS

KATHARINE F. JACKSON, B.V.M.S.,
and IAN D. DUNCAN, B.V.M.S.

Madison, Wisconsin

Hypomyelination of the central nervous system (CNS), associated with an early onset of generalized tremor, has now been described in a number of breeds of dogs. The potential causes of these disorders are inheritance, *in utero* viral infection, and intoxication. Inherited hypomyelination syndromes have been intensively studied in laboratory mice and rats, as these "myelin mutants" provide insights into the biology and pathology of myelin formation and maintenance. This article will review the current state of knowledge of hypomyelination in dogs, but normal myelination and the ways in which it can be interrupted will be discussed first.

MYELINATION AND MYELINATION DISORDERS

The formation and maintenance of myelin in the CNS or peripheral nervous system (PNS) is a complex process requiring highly organized and specific interactions between the axon and the myelin-forming cell. In the CNS, this cell is the oligodendrocyte. Before myelination can proceed, a population of functional oligodendrocytes must be produced by division and differentiation of precursor cells. The oligodendrocytes must then migrate and extend processes around axons to form the spiral lamellar arrangement of plasma membrane that becomes compacted to form mature CNS myelin. The axons have to be of an appropriate size and maturity to accept this ensheathment, and there is evidence that axons may signal oligodendrocyte division, differentiation, and myelination. Any abnormalities of the axonal or oligodendroglial populations, or the interactions between them, may result in defects of myelin formation, with resultant nervous system dysfunction.

Disorders of myelination may be termed demyelination, hypomyelination, or dysmyelination (Duncan, 1987). Demyelination refers to a situation in which previously formed myelin sheaths are lost, with sparing of axons. This is not generally a feature of congenital disease. Hypomyelination and dysmyelination are developmental disorders, resulting from an insult prior to or during myelination. In hypomyelination, axons are usually thinly myelinated, with predominantly normal myelin. They are occasionally nonmyelinated. Dysmyelination is characterized by predominantly nonmyelinated axons and occasional thinly myelinated axons, usually with abnormal myelin.

MYELINATION OF THE CANINE CNS

Most studies of CNS myelination have been carried out in rodents, particularly rats. Of the two detailed studies in dogs, one demonstrated that the corticospinal tract and fasciculus gracilis take the longest to myelinate, as in many other species, but this is complete by 6 weeks. It was also noted that myelination of the deeper areas of the lateral and ventral columns was delayed, compared with the periphery (Fox et al., 1967). A more recent study revealed that oligodendrocyte differentiation and myelination are at a peak at about 10 to 15 days postnatally in the lateral corticospinal tract of the cervical spinal cord of beagles (Lord and Duncan, 1987).

SYNDROMES OF CANINE HYPO- OR DYSMYELINATION

Hypomyelination in Springer Spaniels (The Shaking Pup)

Hypomyelination in springer spaniels was first described by Griffiths and colleagues in 1981 and has been studied in some detail (Duncan, 1987). A breeding colony for the production of shaking puppies has been successfully maintained and has demonstrated the X-linked recessive mode of inheritance of the disorder.

All affected male dogs develop a gross tremor of the head, body, limbs, and extraocular muscles at 10 to 12 days of age, and they are never able to ambulate. The tremor intensifies with excitement, diminishes with rest, and is absent during sleep. Neurologic testing is difficult, but pain sensation, withdrawal reflexes, and pupillary light reflexes are intact, and the dogs appear to have some vision. Unless intensively hand reared, affected puppies will die by 2 to 3 months of age, as they are unable

Studies on the shaking pup have been supported by grants from the NIH (NS 23124) and the NMSS (RG1791).

to feed themselves. A single shaking puppy has been maintained for 23 months and is still surviving, with very little apparent recovery of function (personal observations).

The white matter of the brain and spinal cord of shaking pups is gray and gelatinous on postmortem examination, compared with the white nerve roots and peripheral nerves. On light microscopy, a severe deficiency of myelin throughout the CNS is seen (Fig. 1). In the younger mutants, many axons are nonmyelinated and the remainder are hypomyelinated. There is somewhat more myelin in older puppies, but the defect is still severe. The PNS appears normal in all cases.

Results of electron microscopy confirm the nonmyelination and hypomyelination of CNS axons and reveal myelin sheaths that are often poorly compacted and immature. Many oligodendrocytes in the shaking pup have a striking abnormality, in which the rough endoplasmic reticulum (RER) and perinuclear envelope are distended with a floccular material. Abnormal associations of astrocytes and oligodendrocytes also are seen frequently. Quantitative studies have demonstrated reduced oligodendrocyte counts in the cervical spinal cords of 1- and 2-month-old shaking puppies, with normal astrocyte numbers and a reduction in myelin volume and thickness, compared with age-matched controls. Axonal diameters appear normal, and there is no

correlation between axonal diameter and myelin sheath thickness in the mutant.

Quantitation of myelin proteins in the CNS of shaking pups has demonstrated protein deficiencies consistent with the hypomyelination seen. However, the myelin-specific protein, proteolipid protein (PLP), and the related protein DM-20 show disproportionally low levels of expression (Yanagisawa et al., 1987).

One interesting feature of the shaking pup strain is that some female offspring of carrier dogs also develop a tremor, although this resolves with age. This is due to the existence of patches of nonmyelinated and hypomyelinated axons in the CNS of these puppies, produced by cells in which the abnormal gene on the maternal X chromosome is expressed.

Dysmyelination in Chow Chows

This condition has been described in two papers (Vandevelde et al., 1978, 1981). A total of six animals, both male and female, from four different litters were examined. It appears that the condition may be hereditary, but there is currently no direct evidence for this.

A hypermetric rocking-horse motion of the entire body was seen when the affected puppies attempted

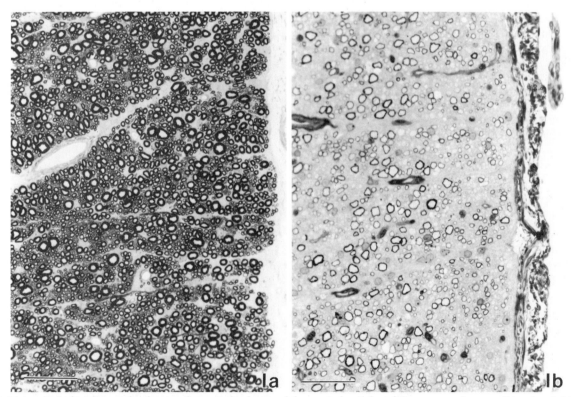

Figure 1. Light micrographs showing the ventral columns of the cervical spinal cord from a normal puppy *(A)* and a shaking puppy *(B)*. Note the paucity of myelin in the shaking pup (1 μ Epon-embedded section, toluidine blue stain. Bar = μ).

to ambulate. A tremor was present but was confined to bobbing of the head, with less severe limb involvement. There were no other significant neurologic problems. The clinical course plateaued at 6 to 8 months and then improved to the extent that the dogs were clinically normal at 12 months of age, although one 15-month-old dog did have some residual intention tremor.

On histologic examination, there was a deficiency of myelin in the CNS. This was particularly severe in the subcortical white matter, the cerebellum, the brainstem, and the periphery of the lateral and ventral columns of the spinal cord. On electron microscopy, areas of hypomyelination and nonmyelination were seen. There was no apparent decrease in the oligodendrocyte population, but some cells with features of oligodendrocytes contained astrocytelike bundles of fibrils.

On light microscopic examination of the CNS of 15-month-old and 3-year-old affected chow chows, it was apparent that myelination had continued with age in these dogs. Ultrastructural examination revealed very few naked axons, but many myelin sheaths were thin and uncompacted, and bizarre myelin formations were seen.

Hypomyelination in Samoyeds

Hypomyelination was studied in a 5-week-old male Samoyed puppy (Cummings et al., 1986). This dog was one of several affected from six litters, all of which had a common ancestor. The breeder reported a high level of perinatal mortality in these litters and recalled that many of the dead or trembling puppies were males, which suggests a possible genetic origin.

The puppy investigated in detail developed whole-body tremor at 3 weeks of age and was unable to stand or eat. The tremor worsened when the puppy was excited and diminished with rest. Postural reactions were absent or delayed and dysmetric, and patellar and flexor reflexes and pain sensation were intact. Photomotor reflexes were normal, but the menace response was absent, and there was rapid spontaneous vertical or horizontal nystagmus.

On postmortem examination there was no distinction between white and gray matter at any level of the CNS, and no myelin was seen on light microscopic examination of paraffin-embedded CNS material. Staining with antibodies specific for myelin proteins and astrocytes identified scattered myelinated fibers in all funiculi of the spinal cord and astrogliosis.

Electron microscopic examination of the CNS indicated the presence of some myelin, but it was thin and poorly compacted. Quantitation of glial cell types demonstrated a clear decrease in the oligodendrocyte population compared with controls, a normal number of astrocytes, and an increased microglial cell count. Most of the oligodendrocytes in the affected puppy were immature in appearance, and in some cells, the RER and perinuclear envelope were distended by a flocculent material.

Hypomyelination in Weimaraners

Hypomyelination was described in Weimaraners from two separate litters and was reported in another two litters (Kornegay et al.,1987). A total of eight dogs were said to be affected, including only one female. Two male Weimaraners from two different litters were examined in detail, at 4 and 6 weeks of age.

Affected dogs developed varying severities of generalized body tremor and dysmetria at 1 to 3 weeks of age, with no other apparent neurologic abnormalities. This tremor resolved with time, and dogs that were maintained were normal by 1 year of age.

In the 4- and 6-week-old puppies there was little evidence of a CNS lesion on gross pathologic examination. On light microscopy, most areas of the CNS appeared hypomyelinated, and this was most marked at the periphery of the ventral and lateral columns of the spinal cord. The PNS was normal. Results of electron microscopy confirmed that many axons in the CNS were nonmyelinated or thinly myelinated, and this was most marked in the spinal cord. There was also immaturity of myelin in the affected puppies. Counts of glial cell types indicated a preponderance of astrocytes and a deficiency of oligodendrocytes, compared with controls. The RER of a few oligodendrocytes was distended with an electron-dense material.

"Trembler," a Hypomyelinating Condition in the Bernese Mountain Dog

A condition affecting a total of 10 Bernese Mountain Dog puppies out of nine litters, both male and female, was recently described (Palmer et al., 1987). The dogs have been termed tremblers, and the authors proposed an autosomal recessive mode of inheritance.

At about 2 weeks of age, affected puppies developed a tremor of the head and limbs that worsened on excitement and diminished with rest. There were no other notable neurologic abnormalities. The tremor persisted with age but diminished in severity and was somewhat variable in older dogs. One 3½-year-old dog only trembled when excited or when sitting.

On light and electron microscopy of the spinal cord of a 9-week-old trembler, the myelin sheaths in the white matter were too thin for their associated axons, although they were ultrastructurally normal. There was also an increased glial cell count and an astrogliosis. The PNS appeared normal.

Hypomyelination in Lurcher Puppies

A tremor syndrome was described in two male crossbred lurcher puppies from the same litter (Mayhew et al., 1984). At 2 weeks of age, the puppies developed a tremor that was most marked in the hindlimbs and that worsened on excitement and resolved when the puppies slept. There were no other significant neurologic findings. One puppy recovered by 16 weeks of age, and the second one remained the same until euthanasia at 8 weeks.

Examination of plastic-embedded material revealed hypomyelination of the CNS, particularly in the peripheral areas of the lateral columns of the cord. The glial cells and most myelin sheaths appeared normal, and the PNS was not involved.

Single Case Reports

A severe tremor syndrome in a single Dalmatian puppy, associated with marked CNS hypomyelination (Greene et al., 1977), and a CNS demyelination disorder in a male spaniel (van den Akker, 1958) have been reviewed elsewhere (Duncan, 1987).

DISCUSSION

In many of the conditions described there is a strong suggestion of an inherited disorder. However, this has only been convincingly demonstrated in the shaking pup. The maintenance of a breeding colony for this mutation has provided data for a detailed family tree that demonstrates the X-linked recessive inheritance of this condition. That some females are mildly affected is not incompatible with this mode of inheritance, as described above. In the chow chow, Samoyed, Weimaraner, and Bernese Mountain Dog, a genetic basis for the disorders has been proposed but not confirmed. Unfortunately, the necessary breeding studies in dogs are time-consuming and expensive, and the particular genetic strains may be lost before enough data are collected. The clinical improvement noted in all but the Samoyeds and springer spaniels suggests that the lesions were reversible and therefore perhaps more likely to be acquired.

There is good correlation between the severity of the clinical signs in these dogs and the CNS lesions. For example, very little myelin was present in the CNS of the Samoyed, and this puppy was so severely disabled that it was unable to ambulate or eat. In contrast, trembler Bernese Mountain Dogs showed a milder tremor that improved with age, and axons in the spinal cord were myelinated, though thinly.

In the shaking pup, there is good evidence for an oligodendrocyte defect, probably with specific involvement of the PLP gene. This compares closely with the defect in the murine X-linked myelin mutant, the jimpy mouse (Duncan, 1987). Abnormal differentiation and maturation of glial cells have been suggested to underlie the defect in the chow chows, Samoyeds, and Weimaraners. There is no evidence of a primary axonal defect in any of the conditions described. An astrocytic reaction was often reported, but this could well be a secondary phenomenon.

The congenital tremor seen in these hypomyelinating disorders should be differentiated from tremor associated with various acquired conditions. These tend to occur in older dogs and are usually accompanied by other systemic or neurologic signs. Small white-coated breeds of dogs occasionally show head and body tremor, but this idiopathic condition occurs in adults, whereas the congenital disorders occur as soon as the puppies attempt ambulation. If a congenital hypomyelinating disorder is suspected, the breeding history and potential prenatal exposure to viruses or chemical or physical myelinotoxic agents should be investigated. Confirmation of the diagnosis is only possible on necropsy. Light microscopic examination of toluidine blue–stained plastic-embedded sections, as opposed to paraffin-embedded material, allows a more accurate assessment of the state of myelination of the CNS.

Treatment of the tremor is likely to prove frustrating. If a genetic disorder is suspected, breeders should be informed and eradication attempted. Many of the animals described above recovered and became essentially normal pets; therefore, if possible, affected puppies should be maintained for 3 to 4 months and observed for any clinical improvement.

Note: Molecular genetic analysis of the shaking pup has shown a severe reduction in the PLP mRNA and a point mutation in the PLP gene (Nadon et al., 1988).

References and Supplemental Reading

Cummings, J. F., Summers, B. A., de Lahunta, A., et al.: Tremors in Samoyed pups with oligodendrocyte deficiencies and hypomyelination. Acta Neuropathol. (Berl.) 71:267, 1986.

Duncan, I. D.: Abnormalities of myelination of the central nervous system associated with congenital tremor. J. Vet. Intern. Med. 1:10, 1987.

Fox, M. W., Inman, O. R., and Himwich, W. A.: The postnatal development of the spinal cord of the dog. J. Comp. Neurol. 130:233, 1967.

Greene, C. E., Vandevelde, M., and Hoff, E. J.: Congenital cerebrospinal hypomyelinogenesis in a pup. J.A.V.M.A. 171:534, 1977.

Griffiths, I. R., Duncan, I. D., McCulloch, M., et al.: Shaking pups: A disorder of central myelination in the spaniel dog. Part 1. Clinical, genetic and light-microscopical observations. J. Neurol. Sci. 50:423, 1981.

Kornegay, J. N., Goodwin, M. A., and Spyridakis, L. K.: Hypomyelination in Weimaraner dogs. Acta Neuropathol. (Berl.) 72:394, 1987.

Lord, K. E., and Duncan, I. D.: Early postnatal development of glial cells in the canine cervical spinal cord. J. Comp. Neurol. 265:34, 1987.

Mayhew, I. G., Blakemore, W. F., Palmer, A. C., et al.: Tremor syndrome and hypomyelination in lurcher pups. J. Small Anim. Pract. 25:551, 1984.

Nadon, N., Duncan, I. D., and Hudson, L.: Molecular analysis of the shaking pup mutation. Soc. Neurosci. 14:829, 1988.

Palmer, A. C., Blakemore, W. F., Wallace, M. E., et al.: Recognition of "trembler," a hypomyelinating condition in the Bernese mountain dog. Vet. Rec. 120:609, 1987.

van den Akker, S.: A case of leucodystrophia in a dog. Folia Psychiatr. Neurol. Neurochirurg. Neerland. 61:536, 1958.

Vandevelde, M., Braund, K. G., Luttgen, P. J., et al.: Dysmyelination in chow chows: Further studies in older dogs. Acta Neuropathol. (Berl.) 55:81, 1981.

Vandevelde, M., Braund, K. G., Walker, T. L., and Kornegay, J. N.: Dysmyelination of the central nervous system in the chow chow dog. Acta Neuropathol. (Berl.) 42:211, 1978.

Yanagisawa, K., Moller, J. R., Duncan, I. D., and Quarles, R. H.: Disproportional expression of proteolipid protein and DM-20 in the X-linked, dysmyelinating shaking pup mutant. J. Neurochem. 49:1912, 1987.

CONGENITAL CEREBELLAR DISEASES OF DOGS AND CATS

JOE N. KORNEGAY, D.V.M.

Raleigh, North Carolina

There have been numerous reports of cerebellar dysfunction in neonatal dogs and cats. Many of these disorders have a proven or presumed heritable basis, while others have ultimately been shown to be due to *in utero* insults. In this chapter, an overview of cerebellar functional anatomy is given, followed by a discussion of specific cerebellar diseases of neonatal dogs and cats.

FUNCTIONAL ANATOMY

The cerebellum develops embryologically from the metencephalon. It consists of a midline band termed the vermis and two larger, laterally positioned hemispheres. Two principal fissures divide the cerebellum into three lobes. Rostral and caudal lobes are demarcated by the primary fissure. The flocculonodular and caudal lobes are separated by the caudolateral fissure. There is a central medulla composed of mostly white matter and an outer cortex of gray matter. Three pairs of nuclei (deep cerebellar nuclei—dentate, interpositus, and fastigial) are located in the medulla on either side of the median plane. The cortex is composed of folds referred to as folia. Each cerebellar folium contains a central band of white matter that is bordered bilaterally by granule (inner), Purkinje (middle), and molecular (outer) neuronal cell layers. The granule cell layer is composed primarily of small granule neurons and fewer Golgi neurons. Stellate and basket neurons are present in the molecular layer. The Purkinje cell layer contains this single cell type.

Rostral, middle, and caudal cerebellar peduncles connect the cerebellum to the midbrain, pons, and medulla oblongata, respectively. The middle and caudal peduncles contain primarily afferent fibers, while the rostral peduncle contains largely efferents. There are two afferent fibers that terminate in the cerebellum. The climbing fibers originate from the olivary nuclei and terminate in a one-to-one relationship on Purkinje cells. Mossy fibers transmit all other sensory information to the cerebellum. They terminate diffusely on granule and Golgi neurons. Both of these fiber types are facilitory. With the exception of granule neurons, all cells within the cerebellar cortex are inhibitory. Efferents of the granule and Golgi neurons synapse on Purkinje cells and, to a lesser extent, on stellate and basket cells. Processes from these latter two cell types, in turn, terminate on Purkinje cells.

Purkinje cell axons are the only efferents that project from the cerebellar cortex. These inhibitory fibers synapse primarily in the deep cerebellar and lateral vestibular nuclei. Efferents from the deep cerebellar nuclei are facilitory to neurons on which they terminate in the brain stem and spinal cord. Fibers from the flocculonodular lobe project principally to the vestibular nuclei. The cerebellum integrates function, rather than either initiating or terminating it.

CONGENITAL FELINE CEREBELLAR DISEASES

Etiology and Pathogenesis

Since the latter part of the nineteenth century, there have been numerous reports of kittens with cerebellar hypoplasia (Carpenter and Harter, 1956).

The lesions in most of these kittens were initially presumed to be inherited, but investigators in the 1960's showed that cerebellar hypoplasia could be induced experimentally by inoculating pregnant cats with the panleukopenia virus (Kilham et al., 1967). Virus was also identified in brains from kittens with spontaneously occurring disease. *In utero* infection is now generally accepted as the principal cause of cerebellar hypoplasia in kittens. Although there may be heritable conditions as well, documented syndromes have not been described, to the author's knowledge.

The panleukopenia virus has a cytopathic effect on rapidly dividing cells. Involvement of the external germinal cell layer of the cerebellum late in gestation or during the immediate postnatal period prevents proper differentiation of the granule cell layer. There is a resultant marked paucity of granule cells in affected cats, and the molecular cell layer often is thin (Csiza et al., 1972). This latter effect may occur as a result of the relative absence of granule cell axons in the molecular cell layer of kittens with cerebellar hypoplasia. Purkinje cells also are affected, despite the fact that they differentiate prior to formation of the external germinal cell layer. The effect on Purkinje cells may be caused by an additional direct cytopathic effect of the panleukopenia virus.

Concomitant cerebellar hypoplasia and hydrocephalus (Kilham and Margolis, 1966; Csiza et al., 1971a) or hydranencephaly (Greene et al., 1982) have been reported in some affected kittens. Two additional cats with cerebellar hypoplasia and hydranencephaly due to *in utero* panleukopenia virus infection have recently been evaluated at the North Carolina State University College of Veterinary Medicine (NCSU-CVM) (Sharp et al., 1987). Hydrocephalus seen in affected kittens may occur as a result of temporary obstruction of cerebrospinal fluid outflow by necrotic debris arising from the inflammatory process (Csiza et al., 1971a). In support of this hypothesis, there are areas of necrosis in the thalamus and cerebrum in some kittens. Hydranencephaly could have a similar basis or might occur because of an additional *in utero* effect of the virus on vessels or other portions of the developing nervous system. In this context, whether hydrocephalus or hydranencephaly occurs could be dependent on the stage of gestation at the time of infection.

Clinical Findings

There is no apparent breed or sex predilection for cerebellar hypoplasia due to *in utero* panleukopenia virus infection. All kittens of some litters are affected, whereas only one kitten may be affected in others. Characteristic signs of cerebellar dysfunc-

tion, such as dysmetria and intention tremor, occur when the affected kitten begins to walk. These kittens have marked truncal ataxia, with a tendency to fall to either side, backward, or forward. They often have a broad-based stance and may sit on their rumps with their thoracic limbs extended. This has been referred to as tripod sitting posture (Carpenter and Harter, 1956). A hallmark of cerebellar hypoplasia due to *in utero* panleukopenia infection is the nonprogressive nature of the clinical signs. In fact, there may be slight apparent improvement, presumably as a result of accommodation through other senses such as vision and conscious proprioception. That most affected kittens have nonprogressive signs of only cerebellar involvement may aid in distinguishing this condition from lysosomal storage diseases and other encephalitides, both of which more typically cause progressive multifocal central nervous system lesions. However, kittens with hydrocephalus or hydranencephaly may have additional signs of forebrain disease.

Diagnosis

Clinical signs of pure, nonprogressive cerebellar involvement in a young kitten are very suggestive of cerebellar hypoplasia. *In utero* panleukopenia virus infection is the most likely cause. Establishing a definitive antemortem diagnosis may be difficult, as serum antibodies present in affected kittens may be maternally derived, rather than the result of active infection (Csiza et al., 1972). Results of antibody studies on cerebrospinal fluid (CSF) have not been reported, to the author's knowledge. Magnetic resonance imaging studies performed by the author on some affected kittens through collaboration with investigators at Duke University have been helpful in identifying hypoplastic or otherwise malformed cerebellums in affected kittens (Kornegay et al., 1987).

Most affected kittens have gross cerebellar hypoplasia on necropsy examination (Fig. 1). The hemispheres and dorsal portion of the vermis are

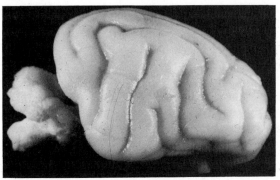

Figure 1. Marked cerebellar hypoplasia in a kitten in which *in utero* panleukopenia virus infection was suspected.

most severely involved. Cerebellar folia are usually more narrow than normal. There is a paucity of granule and Purkinje cells histologically. Some affected kittens do not have grossly evident cerebellar hypoplasia, and others do not have microscopic lesions (Csiza et al., 1972). Cysts usually are not present within the involved cerebellum but were present in two kittens evaluated at the NCSU-CVM (Kornegay et al., 1987). Isolation of the panleukopenia virus from the cerebellum or other organs provides the most definitive diagnosis. However, in one study in which secondary feline kidney cell cultures were used, this was rarely possible in kittens older than 4 weeks (Csiza et al., 1972). In another study that used direct monolayer cultures, virus was isolated in cats up to 3 years of age (Csiza et al., 1971b).

Treatment

Although there is no effective treatment for cerebellar hypoplasia, some affected kittens are functional pets. As discussed above, clinical signs may improve slightly as the kitten accommodates.

CONGENITAL CANINE CEREBELLAR DISEASES

Etiology and Pathogenesis

Congenital, noninfectious syndromes leading to cerebellar dysfunction have been described in numerous breeds of dogs (Carpenter and Harter, 1956; de Lahunta, 1983). In some of these syndromes, the cerebellum is apparently malformed at birth, with no further clinical or pathologic deterioration; in others there is progressive loss of function due to continued degeneration of differentiated cells within the cerebellum. Grossly evident forms of uniform cerebellar hypoplasia, in which clinical signs are present soon after birth and do not progress, have been reported in chow chows (Knecht et al., 1979), Irish setters (de Lahunta, 1983), and wirehaired fox terriers (de Lahunta, 1983). These dogs generally also had a reduced number of Purkinje and granule cells or marked distortion of the normal microscopic architecture of the cerebellum. A heritable basis was suspected, but not proven, in these breeds. Concomitant lissencephaly was seen in Irish setters and wirehaired fox terriers. Numerous other individual cases of grossly evident, nonprogressive cerebellar dysplasia have been described (Carpenter and Harter, 1956). Some of these dogs principally had involvement of the caudal vermis (Kornegay, 1986) (Fig. 2). There generally were not dramatic microscopic lesions in remaining differentiated portions of the cerebellum. Dogs with

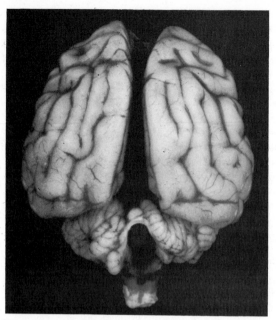

Figure 2. Cerebellar vermian hypoplasia of unknown cause in a puppy. The caudal vermis is especially affected.

cerebellar vermian hypoplasia also may have hydrocephalus. An underlying cause of this syndrome has not been defined, but the lesions are somewhat analogous to those of Dandy-Walker syndrome in humans.

Syndromes of progressive, congenital cerebellar degeneration may become clinically apparent soon after birth. In one such syndrome in Samoyeds (de Lahunta, 1983), affected dogs had signs of cerebellar dysfunction at the time of initial ambulation, and these signs then continued to progress. However, progressive degenerative cerebellar conditions more commonly do not become clinically apparent until affected dogs are several months of age or even older. These late-onset conditions are generally referred to as abiotrophies, a term that literally means loss of vital nutritional substances. Abiotrophies affecting the nervous system are collectively characterized by degeneration of differentiated neurons. Cerebellar abiotrophies have been best characterized in Kerry blue terriers (Montgomery and Storts, 1983) and Gordon setters (de Lahunta, 1980). Several other breeds appear to have analogous diseases (de Lahunta, 1983). There usually are no grossly apparent lesions, but marked neuronal depopulation is present microscopically. Purkinje cells are most severely affected. Other neurons in the cerebellum and certain other areas of the brain may also be involved. Underlying pathogenetic mechanisms are largely unknown. A simple autosomal recessive mode of inheritance has been suggested for most of the abiotrophies.

Several other breed-specific syndromes in which there are degenerative changes in the cerebellum alone or together with other portions of the central nervous system have been described in Airedale terriers (Cordy and Snelbaker, 1952), Finnish harriers (Tontitila and Lindberg, 1971), Bernese Mountain Dogs (Good, 1962), bull mastiffs (Carmichael et al., 1983), rough-coated collies (Hartley et al., 1978), Irish setters (Palmer et al., 1973), and miniature poodles (Cummings and de Lahunta, 1988).

There are no proven infectious causes of cerebellar hypoplasia in dogs. Canine herpesvirus infection may occur *in utero*, and there can be selective cerebellar involvement (Percy et al., 1971). Parvovirus infection was reported to cause diffuse encephalitis in an 8-week-old dog (Johnson and Castro, 1984). Concomitant vasculitis led to multifocal cerebral infarction in this dog. There was not preferential cerebellar involvement.

Clinical Findings

Clinical signs of cerebellar dysfunction usually predominate in affected dogs. Truncal ataxia, hypermetria, and intention tremor are most commonly seen. Involvement of other portions of the brain, as with concomitant hydrocephalus or lissencephaly, may lead to additional neurologic deficits. Signs of vestibular dysfunction are particularly common in dogs with vermian hypoplasia, apparently as a result of flocculonodular lobe involvement (Kornegay, 1986). The progression of deficits due to cerebellar hypoplasia is determined by the underlying disease process. Dogs with gross cerebellar malformation at birth usually have ataxia at the time of initial ambulation, and there is generally no further clinical deterioration. In contrast, dogs with cerebellar abiotrophies usually have a later onset of progressive neurologic dysfunction.

Diagnosis

An antemortem diagnosis of either cerebellar malformation or abiotrophy is suggested by the typical clinical course, particularly if the affected dog is a breed in which a syndrome has been characterized. There are no specific tests for either of these disease groups, although magnetic resonance imaging should be helpful in dogs with gross cerebellar malformation. Characteristic lesions are seen at necropsy. Encephalitides and lysosomal storage diseases should be included in the differential diagnosis, especially when there are deficits suggesting multifocal neurologic involvement. Serum and CSF titers are determined if canine herpesvirus infection is suspected.

Treatment

There is no specific treatment for affected dogs. Anticonvulsants may be indicated if seizures occur as a result of concomitant hydrocephalus or lissencephaly. Dogs with nonprogressive forms of cerebellar hypoplasia may be functional pets. Progressive deterioration in other dogs will lead to death or necessitate euthanasia.

References and Supplemental Reading

Carmichael, S., Griffiths, I. R., and Harvey, M. J. A.: Familial cerebellar ataxia with hydrocephalus in bull mastiffs. Vet. Rec. 112:354, 1983.

Carpenter, M. B., and Harter, D. H.: A study of congenital feline cerebellar malformations. J. Comp. Neurol. 105:51, 1956.

Cordy, D. R., and Snelbaker, H. A.: Cerebellar hypoplasia and degeneration in a family of Airedale dogs. J. Neuropathol. Exp. Neurol. 11:324, 1952.

Csiza, C. K., Scott, F. W., de Lahunta, A., et al.: Feline viruses. XIV. Transplacental infections in spontaneous panleukopenia of cats. Cornell Vet. 61:423, 1971a.

Csiza, C. K., Scott, F. W., de Lahunta, A., et al.: Immune carrier state of feline panleukopenia virus-infected cats. Am. J. Vet. Res. 32:419, 1971b.

Csiza, C. K., de Lahunta, A., Scott, F. W., et al.: Spontaneous feline ataxia. Cornell Vet. 62:301, 1972.

Cummings, J. F., and de Lahunta, A.: A study of cerebellar and cerebral cortical degeneration in miniature poodle pups with emphasis on the ultrastructure of Purkinje cell changes. Acta Neuropathol. (Berl.) 75:261, 1988.

de Lahunta, A., Fenner, W. R., Indrieri, R. J., et al.: Hereditary cerebellar cortical abiotrophy in the Gordon setter. J.A.V.M.A. 177:538, 1980.

de Lahunta, A.: *Veterinary Neuroanatomy and Clinical Neurology*, 2nd ed. Philadelphia: W. B. Saunders Co., 1983, pp. 262–278.

Good, R.: Untersuchungen uber eine Kleinhirn rindenatrophie beim Hund. Dissertation, University of Bern, Switzerland, 1962.

Greene, C. E., Gorgacz, E. J., and Martin, C. L.: Hydranencephaly associated with feline panleukopenia. J.A.V.M.A. 180:767, 1982.

Hartley, W. J., Barker, J. S. F., Wanner, R. A., et al.: Inherited cerebellar degeneration in the rough coated collie. Aust. Vet. Pract. 8:79, 1978.

Johnson, B. J., and Castro, A. E.: Isolation of canine parvovirus from a dog brain with severe necrotizing vasculitis and encephalomalacia. J.A.V.M.A. 184:1398, 1984.

Kilham, L., and Margolis, G.: Viral etiology of spontaneous ataxia of cats. Am. J. Pathol. 48:991, 1966.

Kilham, L., Margolis, G., and Colby, E. D.: Congenital infections of cats and ferrets by feline panleukopenia virus manifested by cerebellar hypoplasia. Lab. Invest. 17:465, 1967.

Knecht, C. D., Lamar, C. H., Schaible, R., et al.: Cerebellar hypoplasia in chow chows. J. Am. Anim. Hosp. Assoc. 15:51, 1979.

Kornegay, J. N.: Cerebellar vermian hypoplasia in dogs. Vet. Pathol. 23:374, 1986.

Kornegay, J. N.: Unpublished observations, 1987.

Montgomery, D. L., and Storts, R. W.: Hereditary striatonigral and cerebello-olivary degeneration of the Kerry blue terrier. Vet. Pathol. 20:143, 1983.

Palmer, A. C., Payne, J. E., and Wallace, M. E.: Hereditary quadriplegia and amblyopia in the Irish setter. J. Small Anim. Pract. 14:343, 1973.

Percy, D. H., Carmichael, L. E., Albert, D. M., et al.: Lesions in puppies surviving infection with canine herpesvirus. Vet. Pathol. 8:37, 1971.

Sharp, N. J. H.: Unpublished observations, 1987.

Tontitila, P., and Lindberg, L. A.: ETT fall av cerebellar ataxi hos finsk stovare. Svoman Elainlääkarilehti 77:135, 1971.

HYDROCEPHALUS

STEPHEN T. SIMPSON, D.V.M.

Auburn, Alabama

Hydrocephalus is the abnormal accumulation of cerebrospinal fluid (CSF) within the ventricular system. Clinical features include enlargement of the head, prominence of the forehead, divergent strabismus (sunrise sign in humans) atrophy of the brain, seizures, and mentation or behavioral abnormalities. Hydrocephalus is either acquired or congenital. Acquired forms are usually caused by obvious brain insults such as infection, trauma, or tumor and can occur at any age. Congenital hydrocephalus is a condition in which the animal is born with typical clinical signs. Toy breed dogs are often affected with the congenital forms. Recent research suggests that hydrocephalus in toy breeds may be perinatally acquired.

TERMINOLOGY

Hydrocephalus is often referred to by the patency of the affected ventricular system. Communicating hydrocephalus is present when the dilated ventricular system is patent through the normal resorption sites in the subarachnoid space (Fig. 1). Obstructive, or noncommunicating hydrocephalus, occurs when some portion of the ventricular system is occluded by a pathologic condition. Sites within the ventricular system that are particularly vulnerable to occlusion include the interventricular foramina, which connect the lateral ventricles with the third ventricle; the mesencephalic aqueduct connecting the third ventricle with the fourth ventricle; and the lateral apertures, through which CSF flows to the subarachnoid space.

Several other terms have been used to describe hydrocephalus. Terms relating to the presence or the absence of elevated intracranial pressures (hypertensive, normotensive) should be avoided unless ventricular pressure is measured. The terms internal and external have been used to denote excessive fluid within or outside the ventricular system, respectively. Most lesions associated with excessive accumulation of CSF outside the ventricular system would be more appropriately referred to as brain atrophy or cysts. In cases in which marked, diffuse brain atrophy occurs, the ventricular system is usually dilated, and the sulcate pattern may be exaggerated. This form of hydrocephalus may be referred to as hydrocephalus *ex-vacuo*.

PATHOGENESIS

Hydrocephalus may be subclassified into acquired or congenital forms, based on the nature of the causative disease. The onset of the acquired form may not always be clear. Adult-onset hydrocephalus is usually seen in older dogs and occurs subsequent to other factors such as tumor, trauma, or infection (Fig. 2). True congenital forms of hydrocephalus are evident at birth. Affected animals frequently die at a very early age, often with accompanying neurologic problems such as seizures. Causes of congenital forms of hydrocephalus include *in utero* infec-

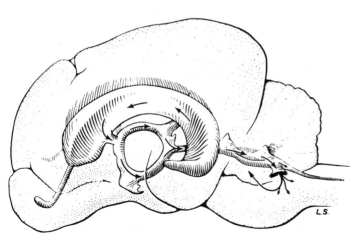

Figure 1. The normal flow of CSF from a rostral to a caudal direction begins in the lateral ventricles and continues through the interventricular foramina to the third ventricle. From there, CSF passes through the mesencephalic aqueduct to the fourth ventricle and through the lateral apertures into the subarachnoid space. It is eventually reabsorbed across arachnoid villi into the cerebral venous sinuses and veins. (Reprinted with permission from de Lahunta, A.: *Veterinary Neuroanatomy and Clinical Neurology*, 2nd ed. Philadelphia, W. B. Saunders Co., 1983.)

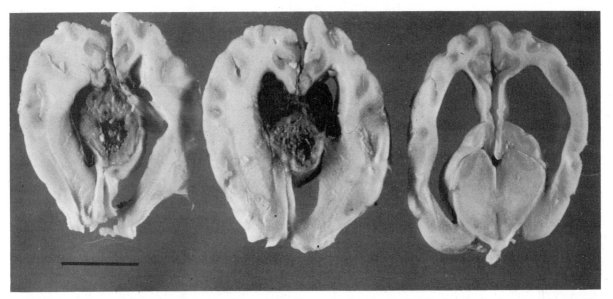

Figure 2. Sections of brain from a mature boxer dog with an ependymoma in the third ventricle that created a rapidly decompensating obstructive hydrocephalus. The dog's clinical signs consisted of marked depression and confusion, ataxia, aimless walking (pacing), and head pressing. Postural reactions were poor to absent, and spinal reflexes were slightly exaggerated. The only cranial nerve deficit was an absent menace response (bar = 2 cm).

tions with a variety of viruses, *Toxoplasma*, and possibly *Mycoplasma*. Exposure to a number of potentially teratogenic drugs or chemicals at particular stages of gestation also may cause hydrocephalus in puppies and kittens.

Toy breed dogs have an increased incidence of hydrocephalus. Breeds at high risk include Chihuahua, toy poodle, Pomeranian, and Yorkshire, Manchester, and Maltese terriers. Puppies of these breeds are very small at birth, often have only 60 to 61 days of gestation, and have a higher amount of stress at birth (dystocia). Hereditary contributions to the formation of hydrocephalus in these and other breeds cannot be discounted, but they have not been clearly defined. Maldevelopment of the mesencephalic aqueduct has been reported to be a cause of congenital hydrocephalus. In the author's experience, this occurs mostly in brachycephalic breeds, such as bulldogs. Maldevelopment of absorptive sites of CSF is another potential cause of hydrocephalus in toy breed dogs. Vitamin A deficiency may cause congenital hydrocephalus. While hydrocephalus in toy breeds appears to have a familial component, other factors that may contribute to its development (e.g., size of dam, gestational age, maturity at term, and size at birth) also have a hereditary basis. Therefore, it is misleading to unequivocally say that hydrocephalus is inherited.

Perinatally acquired hydrocephalus may resemble true congenital forms of hydrocephalus. Potential causes of perinatally acquired hydrocephalus include brain damage at birth, infection, and trauma. There is a 40 per cent incidence of intraventricular hemorrhage and brain necrosis in preterm or undersized babies. Hydrocephalus, as well as varying degrees of mental retardation and other neurologic deficits, is a common sequela to intraventricular hemorrhage. Newborn beagle puppies have been used as models for neonatal intraventricular hemorrhage.

Data based on electroencephalographic and computed tomography (CT) (discussed later) indicate that hydrocephalus in the Maltese appears to be caused by a neonatal event that produces progressive dilation of the ventricles for about 2 years and results in varying degrees of mental incapacitation. Intraventricular hemorrhage conceivably could be involved. Despite the progressive ventricular enlargement, clinical signs improve over the first 2 years of life, with many of these dogs becoming satisfactory pets as long as little is demanded of them. The author has observed that, later in life, with the occurrence of concomitant central nervous system (CNS) or metabolic diseases, these compensated hydrocephalic dogs may suddenly again have neurologic dysfunction. The acuteness of these clinical signs is confusing, in that a chronic underlying disease is often not suspected. The clinician must exclude other factors, such as tumor, encephalitis, toxin, or trauma.

In all experimental models of hydrocephalus, regardless of cause, the ependymal lining of the ventricular system is affected in dilated regions. It becomes flattened and denuded, with shortened and matted cilia. The ependymal cell lining has been shown to have poor regenerative capabilities. Astrocytic subependymal gliosis occurs, and the ependymal layer becomes permeable to CSF. It is possible that this breakdown of ependymal integrity is the fundamental cause of the progressive dilation of the ventricular system; this etiology would also support the fact that most hydrocephalic animals have normal intracranial pressure.

CLINICAL FINDINGS

Clinical signs of acquired hydrocephalus may be complicated by signs of the causative disease. Signs of the hydrocephalic component include decorticate activity such as pacing, aimless walking, purposeless activity, restlessness, and head pressing. Marked behavioral changes, seizures, or both may be evident. Gait may be normal or severely affected if brainstem or cerebellar structures are compromised. Acute elevations of intracranial pressure may produce severe obtundation or very erratic and frantic behavior. Signs of blindness may be evident. Chronically affected animals may exhibit more subtle signs, such as changes in water drinking, house training, or responsiveness and endocrine dysfunctions.

Many cases of hydrocephalus in toy breeds are recognized by 2 to 3 months of age because of clinical signs of unthriftiness, abnormal cranial structure, persistent fontanelles, seizures, abnormal ambulation, or other obvious neurologic abnormalities. They are often smaller than their littermates and may have multiple congenital defects. Many cases are not diagnosed until years later, when a neurologic syndrome develops that requires veterinary attention. A complete neurologic evaluation, including electroencephalography, plain skull radiographs, and CT will confirm evidence of hydrocephalus.

A detailed study of a series of hydrocephalic Maltese dogs revealed a varied clinical presentation. Less than 20 per cent of them had seizures; when seen, the seizures usually occurred during the first year of life. Seizures did not persist in adults. Owners most commonly complained about behavioral problems in these dogs. Most dogs demonstrated erratic behavior, usually associated with environmental changes (other dogs or people visiting the household) or with factors related to reproduction (estrus, whelping, mothering, or breeding). Seventy-five per cent of the Maltese dogs could not be house trained or were extraordinarily difficult to house train despite the use of appropriate methods.

DIAGNOSIS

Hydrocephalus is difficult to diagnose. Signalment and history are important considerations. Toy and brachycephalic breeds are at higher risk than other breeds. Dogs that are small at birth or are born prior to 61 days of gestation also appear to be at greater risk. Litter size, whelping sequence, and

stresses such as dystocia or neonatal injury are other factors that may contribute to the occurrence of hydrocephalus. The preceding information is usually not known by the owner but may be acquired from the breeder. The veterinarian should determine gestational age, weight at birth, size and number of animals in the litter, type of delivery, and whether any complications were noted. Physical abnormalities may or may not be evident. Skull abnormalities, including persistence of fontanelles after 3 weeks of life and domed calvaria, have been associated with hydrocephalus. The presence of strabismus, and other neurologic abnormalities previously discussed, should heighten the index of suspicion of hydrocephalus.

The electroencephalograph (EEG) is the best and most economical way of confirming hydrocephalus in dogs less than 18 months of age. It is not as specific in older or mildly affected dogs. Electroencephalographs of affected Maltese dogs younger than 1 year of age had synchronous, high-voltage, slow wave activity typical of hydrocephalus (Fig. 3A). In older Maltese dogs, the EEG gradually changed to a nonspecific, low-voltage, slow-wave pattern (Fig. 3B).

Open sutures and fontanelles that were not evident on physical examination and an homogeneous (ground-glass) appearance of the cranium may be seen on plain radiographs of the skull. The loss of detail of the sulcate impressions on the skull causes the ground-glass appearance. Contrast ventriculography has been used to confirm hydrocephalus; however, CT has become the best method of confirmation. Repeated computed tomograms in Maltese dogs indicated gradual enlargement of the ventricular system until it became stable at approximately 2 years of age (Fig. 4A and B). Ultrasonography through the central fontanelle has been used to diagnose and monitor hydrocephalus and other intracranial events in human neonates and would also be of use in dogs with persistent fontanelles. Determination of intracranial pressure elevations by CSF tap may lead the clinician to consider temporary or permanent shunting techniques, discussed under treatment. However, in the author's experience, by the time most congenital or neonatal hydrocephalus is detected, the intracranial pressure is normal.

TREATMENT

Therapy for hydrocephalus is usually dictated by clinical signs, the age of the animal at time of evaluation, and concomitant problems. The prognosis for acquired forms of hydrocephalus is dependent on an accurate diagnosis and successful treatment of the initiating cause. Palliative treatment with glucocorticoids, osmotic diuretics, and

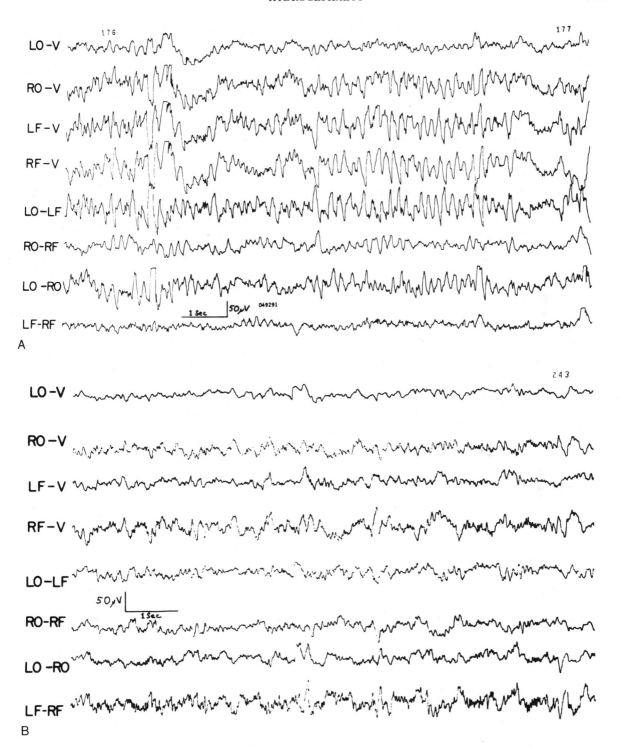

Figure 3. Electroencephalograms from a male Maltese with confirmed hydrocephalus at 4 months *(A)* and 25 months *(B)* of age. The EEG in *A* contains synchronous, high-voltage waves that are typical of many cases of hydrocephalus. The depressed amplitude in the left occipital to vertex lead is an artifact. The EEG in *B* is considered abnormal but does not contain the synchronous, high-voltage waves that are more typical of hydrocephalus. *Key (A and B):* LO, left occipital; RO, right occipital; LF, left frontal; RF, right frontal; V, vertex.

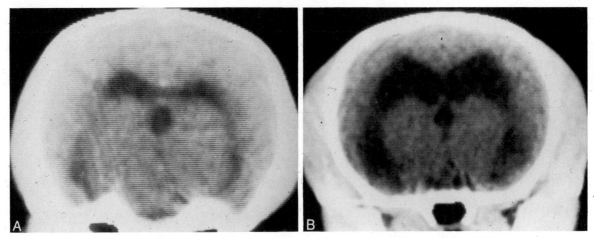

Figure 4. Computed tomography (CT) scans of the dog in Figure 3 at 4 months (A) and 25 months (B) of age. The hydrocephalus is more evident on the scan at 25 months, despite being less evident at this age by EEG examination (Fig. 3B).

general supportive measures may lead to temporary resolution of some signs. However, a diagnosis of the underlying disease should be sought. In the event of an underlying disease that completely resolves, there may be minimal residual effects of hydrocephalus. However, compensation may not occur for several weeks. When the underlying disease process cannot be resolved, dysfunction arising from hydrocephalus and other complications of the underlying disease will usually cause death or necessitate euthanasia.

Treatment of true congenital hydrocephalus, accompanied by severe cranial distortions, is usually ineffective because of the massive amount of brain damage present at birth. Use of glucocorticoids reduces CSF production, so it may be effective in dogs without significant cranial defects. The empirical use of dexamethasone, 0.25 mg/kg PO t.i.d. or q.i.d., has been effective in toy breed dogs with hydrocephalus. The dose should be slowly reduced over 2 to 4 weeks. Prednisone, 0.25 to 0.5 mg/kg PO b.i.d., also has been used. This dosage should be continued if clinical improvement occurs and should be reduced at weekly intervals to eventually 0.1 mg/kg every other day. The final dosage should be maintained for at least a month. If clinical improvement does not occur within a week, alternative treatments should be sought. Complete withdrawal of medication is the goal, but some animals will require repeated treatments or continuous alternate-day treatment.

Acetazolamide, a carbonic anhydrase inhibitor, is a diuretic that has been shown to reduce CSF pressure by reducing CSF production. It would be of use in patients with elevated intracranial pressure and should be used at a dosage of 10 mg/kg every 6 to 8 hr. Since it causes severe renal potassium loss, care must be taken not to intoxicate the patient.

The prognosis for lasting resolution of clinical signs is poor. Exacerbations and the need for repeated treatments should be expected in dogs younger than 2 years of age. Clinical stabilization may not occur until after this age. In the aged, otherwise stable hydrocephalic, the effects of other diseases often exacerbate clinical signs. These conditions must also be managed in hydrocephalic dogs.

Hydrocephalics that have seizures may require anticonvulsants. Phenobarbital, 2 to 5 mg/kg PO b.i.d., is often adequate, with the dosage being adjusted to maintain a blood level between 15 and 40 μg/ml to achieve seizure control.

Hydrocephalic dogs are frail, and minor medical conditions can be life-threatening. Additionally, these dogs have a very poor tolerance to many drugs commonly used to treat nonspecific illnesses, such as diarrhea, vomiting, and coughing. The author has observed severe decompensation of clinical signs as a result of dehydration from vomiting or diarrhea. Moreover, rapid clinical decompensation can occur from drugs used to empirically treat these nonspecific illnesses. Clinical signs include seizures, coma, hysteria, and gait disturbances.

Surgical treatment has been advocated for hydrocephalus. If clinical signs do not improve within 2 to 3 weeks, or if deterioration occurs while glucocorticoid therapy is attempted, removal of CSF through a ventricular tap has been advocated. The author believes that this would benefit only those few dogs with severely increased intracranial pressure.

Shunting of CSF to the right atrium or peritoneal cavity using systems designed for use in humans has also been advocated. Whether this procedure has greater utility than medical management has not been proved. In cases in which the procedure has been performed, the dogs' lateral ventricles have not returned to normal size, but clinical function has improved. The clinical response of these animals is similar to that of compensated hydrocephalics.

References and Supplemental Reading

Barber, D. L., Oliver, J. E., Jr., and Mayhew, I. G.: Neuroradiography. *In* Oliver, J. E., Jr., Hoerlein, B. F., and Mayhew, I. F. (eds.): *Veterinary Neurology.* Philadelphia: W. B. Saunders Co., 1983, pp. 91–106.
Braund, K. G.: Diseases of the nervous system. *In* Oliver, J. E., Jr.,
Hoerlein, B. F., and Mayhew, I. F. (eds.): *Veterinary Neurology.* Philadelphia: W. B. Saunders Co., 1983, pp. 194–196.
de Lahunta, A.: *Veterinary Neuroanatomy and Clinical Neurology,* 2nd ed. Philadelphia: W. B. Saunders Co., 1983, pp. 30–52.
Oliver, J. E., Jr., and Hoerlein, B. F.: Cranial surgery. *In* Oliver, J. E., Jr., Hoerlein, B. F., and Mayhew, I. F. (eds.): *Veterinary Neurology.* Philadelphia: W. B. Saunders Co., 1983, pp. 486–488.
Pasternak, J. F., Groothuis, D. R., Fischer, J. M., et al.: Regional cerebral blood flow in the beagle puppy model of neonatal intraventricular hemorrhage: Studies during systemic hypertension. Neurology 33:559, 1983.
Thorburn, R. J., Lipscomb, A. P., Reynolds, E. O. R., et al.: Accuracy of imaging of the brains of newborn infants by linear-array real-time ultrasound. Early Hum. Dev. 6:31, 1982.

CRANIOCEREBRAL TRAUMA

ANDY SHORES, D.V.M., Ph.D.
East Lansing, Michigan

The most frequent cause of craniocerebral trauma in small animals is motor vehicle trauma. Other causes include falls from heights, injuries from animal fights, blunt trauma, and gunshot wounds. Small animals with head injuries are evaluated relatively frequently by most small animal practitioners. The incidence of head injury among all traumatic injuries in a study of one urban area was 20 per cent in dogs and 35 per cent in cats. Craniocerebral trauma in small animals requires emergency management consisting of a rapid and thorough assessment of the patient, initiation of therapy for any life-threatening conditions, localization of neurologic injuries, and continuation of therapy and patient monitoring.

PATHOGENESIS

Brain Injury

The most important consideration in craniocerebral injuries is the nature and extent of brain injury. Brain injuries can consist of concussion (a transient loss of consciousness, without structural damage), contusions and lacerations, intracranial hemorrhage, and cerebral edema.

Concussion probably occurs in most patients that sustain head injury of any severity. A loss of consciousness occurs for a few seconds or minutes and may be followed by a period of confusion or disorientation. In humans, this period is frequently accompanied by temporary amnesia. At the moment of impact, a small, transient rise in intracranial pressure and marked electrical discharge in the brain occur. These events may be partially responsible for the loss of consciousness. Recovery from a simple concussion is usually complete unless complicated by more severe intracranial injuries. Unconsciousness for more than a few minutes indicates more severe brain involvement. Contusions and lacerations of the cerebrum are accompanied by edema, petechial or ecchymotic hemorrhage, and parenchymal damage. Cerebral edema is the manifestation of vascular stasis and congestion, with pericellular and perivascular fluid accumulation. The edema is initially focal but may become generalized as a result of the escape of fluids (proteins, blood) into the parenchyma.

Intracranial hemorrhage can be subarachnoid, intraparenchymal, epidural, or subdural. Subarachnoid and intraparenchymal hemorrhage occur most commonly. Neither is an indication for surgical intervention unless accompanied by depressed or compound skull fractures. However, intraparenchymal hemorrhage may lead to seizures. Epidural hemorrhage (bleeding between the calvaria and dura) occurs with any skull fracture secondary to meningeal artery laceration. Subdural hemorrhage (between the arachnoid and dura) is of venous origin and, therefore, develops slowly. Clinical signs are usually more severe unilaterally and worsen steadily over a period of hours to days. Surgical intervention is usually indicated to evacuate the hematoma and control hemorrhage. Epidural and subdural hematomas that significantly increase intracranial pressure are rare in small animals.

Skull Fractures

Skull fractures can be linear, elevated, or depressed, and some are compound (open). Simple linear fractures or elevated fractures of the cranial vault do not require fracture management and are generally associated with less severe brain injury than fractures of the base of the skull (basilar fractures); however, severe and even fatal intracranial injuries can occur in craniocerebral trauma without skull fracture. Basilar fractures often extend into the ear, orbit, nasal cavity, or sinuses, opening portals for bacterial contamination of the central nervous system (CNS). Basilar fractures may also contuse or lacerate one or more cranial nerves. Bleeding from the external ear canal is a frequent manifestation of basilar fractures. Hemorrhage from the nose or nasopharynx or into the orbit can also occur.

Depressed and compound skull fractures require fracture management. Any compound skull fracture should be treated as soon as the patient's general condition permits. Surgery for skull fractures that are depressed more than the thickness of the calvaria and are not compound can be delayed for 24 to 48 hr in the absence of neurologic deterioration.

MANAGEMENT

Initial Evaluation

Owners are instructed to transport the injured animal on a plywood stretcher or similar system to avoid complicating any spinal injuries. The airway, breathing, and cardiac function (ABCs) should be evaluated first. A patent airway is maintained in the unconscious animal by gently extending the head and neck and pulling the tongue forward. A rapid but thorough physical examination is essential but may be pre-empted to allow treatment of any life-threatening conditions. Shock frequently accompanies craniocerebral trauma caused by motor vehicle accidents but occurs less frequently with other causes. Intravenous fluids are initially necessary. Subsequent recordings of vital signs and evaluation of all organ systems are necessary.

During the initial evaluation, a neurologic history is taken (Table 1). Brainstem hemorrhage, the most frequently encountered lesion in severe craniocerebral trauma, usually produces unconsciousness immediately after the accident. Unlike simple concussions, in which loss of consciousness is transient, brainstem hemorrhage often results in persistent coma. Signs develop more slowly with cerebral injuries that are accompanied by severe edema.

These injuries may eventually lead to foramen magnum or transtentorial brain herniation, with resultant brainstem compression. Transtentorial herniation can be associated with unilateral or bilateral signs.

Neurologic Examination

The initial neurologic assessment should include evaluation of the level of consciousness, motor activity, brainstem reflexes, and respiratory pattern. Respiratory patterns associated with brain injury are listed in Table 2. A coma scale modified from the Glasgow Coma Scale used for humans (Fig. 1) is helpful in grading the initial neurologic status of the patient and then in serially monitoring improvement or deterioration. The coma scale also assists in determining prognosis. Each category (level of consciousness, motor activity, brainstem reflexes) receives a score of 1 to 6, according to the descriptions for each grade. A total score of 3 to 8, without signs of improvement, indicates a grave prognosis; 9 to 14, a poor to guarded prognosis; and 15 to 18, a good prognosis. Further evaluation of the nervous system is necessary to exclude additional injuries. Concomitant conditions, such as limb or spinal fractures and dyspnea, may preclude performing some portions of the neurologic examination. However, cranial nerve and spinal reflex evaluations can be performed on most animals.

LEVEL OF CONSCIOUSNESS. Decreasing levels of consciousness indicate abnormal function of the cerebral cortex or interference with transmission of sensory stimuli by the brainstem ascending reticular activating system (ARAS) to the cerebral cortex. Consciousness and wakefulness are initiated by sensory stimuli that act through the ARAS on the cerebral cortex and are maintained by a positive feedback system. Descriptions of the levels of consciousness are listed in Table 3.

MOTOR ACTIVITY. Animals that are not comatose, but have an altered state of consciousness, usually maintain some voluntary motor activity. Some degree of hemiparesis or tetraparesis may be exhibited. Voluntary motor activity is absent in the comatose animal. Reflexes may be exaggerated in all four limbs, but severely affected comatose animals lose muscle tone and reflex activity.

Table 2. *Respiratory Patterns Associated with Craniocerebral Trauma*

Lesion	Associated Respiratory Pattern
Diencephalon	Cheyne-Stokes respiration
Mesencephalon	Hyperventilation
Medulla	Irregular or ataxic respirations*

*Usually associated with slowing of the pulse rate and a poor prognosis.

Coma Scale

Motor Activity

Normal gait, normal spinal reflexes	6
Hemiparesis, tetraparesis or decerebrate activity	5
Recumbent, intermittent extensor rigidity	4
Recumbent, constant extensor rigidity	3
Recumbent, constant extensor rigidity with opisthotonus	2
Recumbent, hypotonia of muscles, depressed or absent spinal reflexes	1

Brain Stem Reflexes

Normal pupillary light reflexes and oculocephalic reflexes	6
Slow pupillary light reflexes and normal to reduced oculocephalic reflexes	5
Bilateral unresponsive miosis with normal to reduced oculocephalic reflexes	4
Pinpoint pupils with reduced to absent oculocephalic reflexes	3
Unilateral, unresponsive mydriasis with reduced to absent oculocephalic reflexes	2
Bilateral, unresponsive mydriasis with reduced to absent oculocephalic reflexes	1

Level of Consciousness

Occasional periods of alertness and responsive to environment	6
Depression or delirium, capable of responding to environment but response may be inappropriate	5
Semicomatose, responsive to visual stimuli	4
Semicomatose, responsive to auditory stimuli	3
Semicomatose, responsive only to repeated noxious stimuli	2
Comatose, unresponsive to repeated noxious stimuli	1

Figure 1. Small Animal Coma Scale (SACS). Neurologic function is assessed for each of the three categories and a grade of 1 to 6 is assigned according to the descriptions for each grade. The total score is the sum of the three category scores. This scale is designed to assist the clinician in evaluating the neurologic status of the craniocerebral trauma patient. As a guideline and according to clinical impressions, a consistent total score of 3 to 8 represents a grave prognosis, 9 to 14 a poor to guarded prognosis, and 15 to 18 a good prognosis. (Modified from the Glasgow Coma Scale used in humans.)

Decerebrate rigidity (Fig. 2) is frequently seen in animals that are recumbent secondary to craniocerebral trauma. This extensor rigidity in all limbs may be intermittent (being exacerbated by stimulation) or constant and possibly accompanied by opisthotonus. Development of decerebrate rigidity signifies unfavorable progression (refer to the coma scale).

BRAINSTEM REFLEXES. Various neuro-ophthalmologic changes are seen, depending on the level of brainstem or diencephalic injury. Ocular trauma should first be excluded as a cause of abnormal pupil size. Diencephalic lesions, particularly those in the hypothalamus, may cause miosis because of involvement of the origin of the sympathetic pathway. Lesions involving the midbrain can lead to either widely dilated or midposition unresponsive pupils. Pupils are widely dilated when there is involvement of the oculomotor nerves or nuclei. Concomitant involvement of both the sympathetic

pathway descending the brainstem (tectotegmentospinal tract) and the oculomotor nerve(s) or parasympathetic nuclei leads to midposition pupils. Oculomotor lesions may also cause ventrolateral strabismus. Unilateral signs are usually seen with oculomotor nerve lesions, as with midbrain compression that occurs because of transtentorial herniation, whereas nuclear involvement is generally associated with bilateral signs. Focal pontine hemorrhage commonly produces pinpoint pupils as a result of selective involvement of the descending tectotegmentospinal tracts. Oculocephalic reflexes (physiologic nystagmus, "doll's-eye reflex") also may

Table 3. Levels of Consciousness

Normal: Bright, alert, and responsive to environment and all external stimuli

Depression: Lethargic, despondent, but capable of responding to environment in a normal manner

Delirium: Disoriented, irritable, or fearful; capable of responding to environment, but response may be inappropriate

Semicomatose (stupor): Semiconscious; responsive only to noxious stimuli; dementia; unconscious vocalization

Coma: Unconscious and unresponsive to repeated noxious stimuli

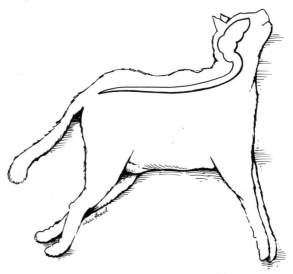

Figure 2. An illustration of a cat exhibiting decerebrate rigidity posture and opisthotonos.

Outline of Emergency Management and Therapy for Cranio-Cerebral Trauma

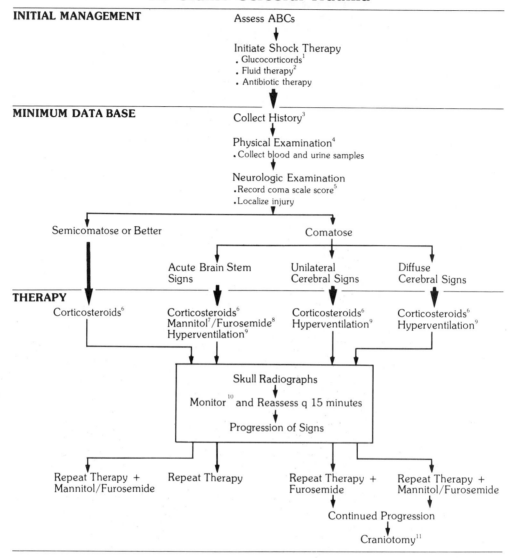

INITIAL MANAGEMENT

Assess ABCs

Initiate Shock Therapy
- Glucocorticords[1]
- Fluid therapy[2]
- Antibiotic therapy

MINIMUM DATA BASE

Collect History[3]

Physical Examination[4]
- Collect blood and urine samples

Neurologic Examination
- Record coma scale score[5]
- Localize injury

Semicomatose or Better

Comatose

Acute Brain Stem Signs   Unilateral Cerebral Signs   Diffuse Cerebral Signs

THERAPY

Corticosteroids[6]

Corticosteroids[6]
Mannitol[7]/Furosemide[8]
Hyperventilation[9]

Corticosteroids[6]
Hyperventilation[9]

Corticosteroids[6]
Hyperventilation[9]

Skull Radiographs

Monitor[10] and Reassess q 15 minutes

Progression of Signs

Repeat Therapy + Mannitol/Furosemide

Repeat Therapy

Repeat Therapy + Furosemide

Repeat Therapy + Mannitol/Furosemide

Continued Progression

Craniotomy[11]

1 Sodium Prednisolone Succinate or Phosphate, 5-10 mg/kg IV
2 Lactated Ringer's Solution 20 ml/kg (dog)/10 ml/kg (cat) for hypovolemic shock;
   over 1 hour period; Repeat if necessary, then reduce to 44 ml/kg/day
3 See Table 1
4 Vital signs, evaluate all systems, emergency therapy as needed
5 See Figure 1
6 Dexamethasone, 2 mg/kg IV
7 20% Mannitol, 2 g/kg IV
8 Furosemide: Dog - 2-4 mg/kg IV not to exceed 50 mg total
             Cat - 2-3 mg/kg IV not to exceed 10 mg total
9 Via tracheal or tracheostomy intubation
10 See Table 3
11 See Figure 4

Figure 3. This outline is a flow-chart–style guide to the management of craniocerebral trauma. (Adapted from Shores, A., and Simpson, S.T.: Coma and stupor. *In* Ford, R.B. (ed.): *Clinical Signs and Diagnosis in Small Animal Practice.* New York, Churchill Livingstone, 1987.)

be impaired with brainstem lesions as a result of either involvement of cranial nerve nuclei that innervate the extraocular eye muscles or the interconnecting medial longitudinal fasciculus.

Ancillary Diagnostic Methods

The minimum data base for animals with motor vehicle trauma should include thoracic radiographs, an electrocardiogram, and blood and urine analyses. Skull radiography is an important ancillary procedure in craniocerebral trauma, as many skull fractures cannot be palpated. Computed tomography (CT) and magnetic resonance imaging (MRI) are the optimal ancillary diagnostic procedures but are available only in some veterinary institutions or by special arrangement with human radiology facilities. Cerebrospinal fluid (CSF) collection is *contraindicated* in acute craniocerebral trauma. The sudden loss of even small amounts of CSF from the cerebellomedullary cistern can precipitate brain herniation in these animals.

Therapy

The importance of a thorough examination and initiation of therapy for life-threatening injuries, shock, or airway obstruction has been emphasized. Figure 3 outlines the emergency management of craniocerebral trauma. If the patient is in hypovolemic shock, 10 mg/kg of sodium prednisolone succinate or phosphate and lactated Ringer's solution (LRS) is given through an intravenous catheter. Fluid therapy should be sufficient to control shock; however, because the blood-brain barrier is disrupted with craniocerebral trauma, overhydration is avoided. Excessive fluid therapy contributes to cerebral edema. An initial amount of 40 ml/kg LRS in dogs and 20 ml/kg LRS in cats is given over a 1-hour period, and then the patient is re-evaluated. If the patient continues to exhibit signs of hypovolemic shock, this dosage is repeated. If the patient does not exhibit signs, the fluid administration rate is reduced to 44 ml/kg/day (two thirds of the daily maintenance level).

Oxygen is administered by mask or nasal catheter or in an oxygen cage. Tracheal or tracheostomy intubation should be considerations in the comatose patient. Hypoxia will contribute to cerebral edema.

Glucocorticoids, diuretics (mannitol, furosemide), dimethyl sulfoxide (DMSO), and hyperventilation all have been advocated for reduction and control of cerebral edema. There are studies that support and others that discount the efficacy of each of these medications, including some studies in humans that suggest an increased mortality rate associated with the use of glucocorticoids in the treatment of head trauma. The author routinely uses glucocorticoids and, when indicated, mannitol (Fig. 3). Furosemide has been shown to decrease CSF production and is frequently used in humans with craniocerebral trauma. Both mannitol and furosemide are contraindicated in the presence of shock and hypovolemia because of their diuretic effects. A study of cerebral edema in cats demonstrated that combined furosemide and albumin therapy was as effective as mannitol or furosemide alone in reducing cerebral edema.

Because of the oncotic stabilizing effect of albumin, the hematocrit did not increase with the combined therapy, suggesting that it would be safe and efficacious in the presence of shock and hypovolemia. The use of DMSO has been shown to reduce cerebral edema experimentally. However, based on clinical impressions, it does not seem to be any more effective than other approved parenteral drugs. Broad-spectrum antibiotic therapy is indicated for patients with shock, open wounds, open skull fractures, or a need for intracranial surgery.

If the patient's condition does not improve within 30 min of the administration of water-soluble glucocorticoids, dexamethasone, 2 mg/kg given by slow IV administration, is recommended. Continued unfavorable progression warrants additional therapy. In the comatose or semicomatose animal, hyperventilation should be considered. Hyperventilation with oxygen is accomplished by tracheal or tracheostomy intubation. Arterial carbon dioxide partial pressure (P_{CO_2}) is directly related to cerebral blood flow. Therefore, hypercapnia increases cerebral blood flow and intracranial pressure. In humans, intracranial pressure monitoring is frequently used to evaluate the effectiveness of therapy. When arterial blood gas analysis is available, the P_{CO_2} should be maintained in the range of 25 to 30 mm Hg.

The use of mannitol is controversial when the differentiation between intracranial hemorrhage and edema has not been made. Mannitol is efficacious if the vascular system is intact but may seep into an area of hemorrhage, drawing more fluids into the extravascular space. Reducing brain edema in the presence of epidural or subdural hemorrhage also

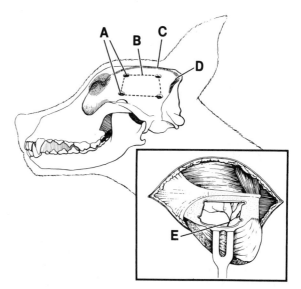

Figure 4. Anatomic guidelines for bur holes and a lateral rostrotentorial craniotomy in the treatment of craniocerebral trauma. *A*, Rostral pair of bur holes; *B*, lines for connecting bur holes to perform the craniotomy; *C*, dorsal sagittal venous sinus; *D*, transverse venous sinus; *E*, middle meningeal artery.

Monitoring Form: Cranio-Cerebral Trauma

Case No.: _____ Date: _____/_____/_____

Name: _____ Clinician: _____

Species: _____ Brief History: _____

Breed: _____ _____

Sex: _____ _____

Neurologic Localization:

Ancillary Diagnostics/Results:

Previous Therapy (Drug/Dose/Time):

Time / Temp	HR[1] / RR[2]	MM[3] / CRT[4]	U/O[5]	COMA SCALE				Therapy/Notes
				Motor Activity[6]	Brain Stem Reflexes[6]	Level of Consciousness[6]	Total Score[7]	

1   Heart rate/min
2   Respiratory rate/min
3   Mucous membrane color
4   Capillary refill time (sec)
5   Urinary output (ml/min)
6   Graded 1 to 6 (see Coma Scale)
7   Total coma scale score

Figure 5. An example of a form used to record monitoring information for craniocerebral trauma patients.

can create more space for hemorrhage, resulting in an exacerbation of signs. In the author's opinion, mannitol, 2 gm/kg IV, should be administered when clinical signs indicate further deterioration after glucocorticoid administration, particularly if the clinical signs indicate brainstem, rather than cerebral, injuries, and there is no evidence of hemorrhage.

Increasingly unfavorable signs indicate progressive cerebral edema, with impending brain herniation. At this point, a craniotomy is considered, except in cases of acute brainstem hemorrhage. A balanced anesthetic protocol should be used to limit the anesthetic effects on cerebral autoregulatory mechanisms. Induction with a narcotic-barbiturate combination and maintenance with these agents or isoflurane and a nondepolarizing muscle relaxant has been recommended. Halothane anesthesia is strictly contraindicated, since it can precipitate brain herniation. Surgical management of craniocerebral trauma is indicated for evacuation of subdural hematomas, hemostasis of lacerated meningeal arteries, relief of uncontrolled cerebral edema, decompression of skull fractures, and removal of bone fragments from the brain parenchyma. Surgery to elevate depressed skull fractures can be delayed for 24 to 48 hr in patients with a stable neurologic status. Anatomic guidelines for creating bur holes and performing a lateral rostrotentorial craniotomy are illustrated in Figure 4.

After the surgical approach to the lateral aspect of the cranial vault, a gas-powered, high-speed surgical drill or a gas-sterilized hobby drill is used to make the bur holes. This allows the initial evacuation of an epidural hematoma. The bur holes are then connected to perform the craniotomy. Lacerated meningeal vessels are ligated with 4-0 synthetic absorbable suture. Severely contused, hemorrhagic cortical tissue is removed by gentle suction. Bone fragments and foreign material are removed. Lacerated meningeal tissue is closed, if feasible, or patched with temporalis muscle fascia. The skull flap is replaced and secured with 22-gauge wire sutures, unless excessive cerebral edema precludes its replacement. Textbooks listed in the supplemental reading list give detailed descriptions of intracranial surgical procedures.

Patient Monitoring and Continued Therapy

The semicomatose or comatose patient is monitored continuously and re-evaluated every 15 to 60 min, depending on initial patient status. Monitoring includes consistent, time-regulated evaluations that usually include heart rate, respiration, temperature, mucous membrane color, and neurologic function. The coma scale is useful in monitoring improvement or deterioration of neurologic status. Urinary output is monitored if the patient is presented in shock or if diuretic therapy is used. Figure 5 is an example of a form used to monitor craniocerebral trauma patients.

The comatose patient is positioned so that the head is elevated to assist venous return from the head. Pressure on the jugular veins may result in increased cerebral perfusion pressure, increased cerebral blood flow, and subsequent increased intracranial pressure. Continued therapy for the semicomatose or comatose patient includes frequent turning to prevent hypostatic lung congestion, adequate cage padding to prevent decubitus ulcers, maintenance of fluid and electrolyte balance, maintenance of urinary and bowel functions, and proper nutrition. Antibiotic therapy is usually continued as long as the patient is debilitated. Glucocorticoids are continued for 1 to 2 days at low levels (dexamethasone, 0.2 to 0.4 mg/kg IV daily). The caloric requirements for the craniocerebral trauma victim are elevated, so nutritional supplementation is an essential component of prolonged therapy. Pharyngostomy or nasogastric tubes require minimal maintenance and are indicated in patients incapable of eating. Surgical wounds should be bandaged to prevent additional trauma and contamination.

Anticonvulsant therapy is instituted if the patient has seizures. Diazepam (5 to 10 mg IV) is usually effective in stopping the seizure and should be followed by phenobarbital (2 mg/kg IM or PO b.i.d.). Oral anticonvulsants should be continued for 6 months and then slowly withdrawn. If additional seizures occur, life-long therapy is usually required. The author routinely prescribes prophylactic anticonvulsant therapy (phenobarbital, 2 mg/kg PO b.i.d.) for at least 6 weeks in severely affected patients that do not have seizures, and then slowly withdraws the medication. Anticonvulsant therapy is reinstituted if seizures recur.

Coma persisting for longer than 48 hr despite medical or surgical therapy warrants a poor prognosis. Continued nursing care for 2 to 4 weeks may be rewarding in rare instances. Establishing a prognosis early in the therapy of severe craniocerebral trauma is the subject of numerous research projects. Correlation of intracranial pressure monitoring, serum catecholamine levels, or multimodality evoked potential testing with neurologic status is one of the promising prognostic tools of the future.

References and Supplemental Reading

Albright, A. L., Latchaw, R. E., and Robinson, A. G.: Intracranial and systemic effects of osmotic and oncotic therapy in experimental edema. J. Neurosurg. 60:481, 1984.
Davis, R. A., and Cunningham, P. S.: Prognostic factors in severe head injury. Surg. Gynecol. Obstet. 159:597, 1984.
de Lahunta, A.: Veterinary Neuroanatomy and Clinical Neurology. Philadelphia: W. B. Saunders Co., 1983, p. 356.
Kolata, R. J., Krant, N. H., and Johnston, O. E.: Patterns of trauma in urban dogs and cats: A study of 1000 cases. J.A.V.M.A. 164:499, 1974.
Oliver, J. E.: Intracranial injury. In Kirk, R. W. (ed.): Current Veterinary Therapy VII. Philadelphia: W. B. Saunders Co., 1980, p. 815.
Oliver, J. E., and Hoerlein, B. F.: Cranial surgery. In Oliver, J. E., Hoerlein, B. F., and Mayhew, I. G. (eds.): Veterinary Neurology. Philadelphia: W. B. Saunders Co., 1987, p. 470.
Shores, A.: Neuroanesthesia: A review of the effects of anesthetic agents on cerebral blood flow and intracranial pressure in the dog. Vet. Surg. 14:254, 1985.
Shores, A., and Simpson, S. T.: Coma and stupor. In Ford, R. B. (ed.): Clinical Signs and Diagnosis in Small Animal Practice. New York: Churchill Livingstone, 1987, p. 269.
Vick, N. A.: Cranio-cérebral trauma. In Vick, N. A. (ed.): Grinker's Neurology, 7th ed. Springfield, IL: Charles C. Thomas Pub., 1976, p. 648.
Woolf, P. O., Hamill, R. W., Louyse, A. L., et al.: The predictive value of catecholamines in assessing outcome in traumatic brain injury. J. Neurosurg. 66:875, 1987.
Young, B., Ott, L., Twyman, D., et al.: The effect of nutritional support on outcome from severe head injury. J. Neurosurg. 67:668, 1987.

GRANULOMATOUS MENINGOENCEPHALOMYELITIS

KYLE G. BRAUND, B.V.Sc.

Auburn, Alabama

Granulomatous meningoencephalomyelitis (GME) is a sporadic, idiopathic, inflammatory disease of the central nervous system (CNS) of dogs and, rarely, cats. This disease appears to have a worldwide distribution, with recent reports coming from the United States, Australia, New Zealand, Switzerland, and the United Kingdom.

NOMENCLATURE

Lesions of GME may be disseminated or focal. The *disseminated* form has been described previously as inflammatory reticulosis, granulomatous reticulosis, and histiocytic encephalitis. The *focal* form of GME has been described previously as neoplastic reticulosis.

PATHOLOGY

Macroscopic lesions are not observed in organ systems outside the CNS. In brain or spinal cord, soft, gray, oval lesions with irregular or well-defined margins may be discerned on gross sectioning. Sometimes, the cut surface of the CNS has a granular, mottled appearance, with fingerlike projections. Meninges may appear thickened and cloudy, and occasionally, optic nerves are grossly enlarged. Internal hydrocephalus may be present in some dogs.

Microscopic lesions are restricted to the CNS. The lesions are characterized by dense aggregations of mesenchymal cells arranged in a whorling perivascular pattern (Fig. 1). The perivascular cuffs are composed of histiocytes (i.e., macrophages) and varying numbers of lymphocytes, monocytes, and plasma cells set in nets of reticulin fibers (Fig. 2). In some areas, the perivascular cells are predominantly lymphocytic, whereas in other regions, histiocytic cells are most numerous. Many, if not all, the histiocytes are derived from circulating blood monocytes rather than from CNS histiocytic cells such as microglial, adventitial, and leptomeningeal cells. Neutrophils and multinucleate giant cells are sometimes present in small numbers. Aggregates of histiocytic cells (granulomatous nodules), apparently unrelated to blood vessels, may also be seen at the center of the most severe lesions. Many granulomas appear to develop eccentrically from a previously formed lymphocytic cuff. Granulomatous lesions may compress and invade adjacent CNS parenchyma, resulting in necrosis, glial cell reaction, and edema.

DISTRIBUTION

In the *disseminated* form of GME, lesions are usually widely distributed throughout the CNS, but primarily in white matter of the cerebrum, caudal brainstem, cerebellum, and cervical spinal cord. Comparable lesions may be found in gray matter and in leptomeningeal and choroid plexus vasculature. Coalescence of granulomatous lesions from a large number of adjacent blood vessels may produce a true space-occupying mass, which represents the *focal* form of GME (Fig. 3). The cells of this mass may have neoplastic features, such as a variable mitotic index and varying degrees of pleomorphism. Focal lesions are usually single and most commonly occur in the brainstem, especially in the pontomedullary region, and cerebral white matter. Animals with focal GME often have accompanying disseminated lesions. In some dogs, an *ocular* form occurs, with granulomatous cuffs initially involving the optic nerves, optic disk, or retina. In these dogs, either or both disseminated and focal lesions in the CNS may develop subsequently.

ETIOLOGY AND PATHOGENESIS

The cause of GME is unknown. The results of bacteriologic and mycologic cultures of blood and cerebrospinal fluid (CSF) have been negative, as have special-agent tissue stains including Gram, Giemsa, Ziehl-Neelsen, periodic acid–Schiff, methenamine silver, and Young's fungal stain. That the lesion resembles experimental allergic encephalomyelitis supports a possible immunologic basis for the disease. Immunohistologic studies have indicated that many lymphocytic and lymphoblastic cells are immunoglobulin-bearing. There are also morphologic similarities between GME and viral encephalomyelitis. It is possible that GME repre-

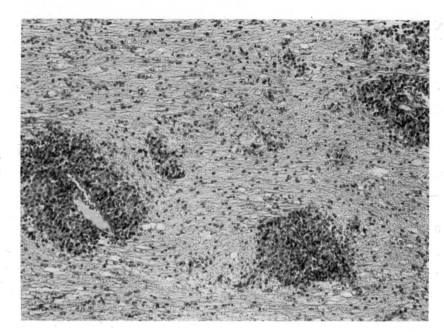

Figure 1. Multifocal perivascular cuffs in the cerebrum of a dog with disseminated GME (H & E stain; × 33).

sents an altered host reponse to an infectious agent. Distemper and rabieslike inclusion bodies and *Toxoplasma*-like organisms have been described in CNS lesions of some dogs with GME. It is of interest that the onset of signs of GME in two dogs was believed to be related to administration of the anthelmintic drug levamisole, a known immunostimulant. This observation, together with the reported occurrence of CNS lesions in normal dogs after levamisole administration, suggests that levamisole may have activated an immune response against latent or incomplete antigens present in nervous tissue. However, most dogs with GME have been vaccinated aginst canine distemper and rabies. No correlation has been noted between onset of signs and the time of previous vaccination against distemper or rabies. In other animal species, viruses are known to produce similar granulomatous reactions within the CNS (e.g., equine infectious anemia, visna in sheep, and feline infectious peritonitis).

The question of neoplastic transformation remains enigmatic. It has been suggested that the initial inflammatory process may become transformed to a neoplastic one. The role of a cell-associated virus in this transformation process remains to be proved.

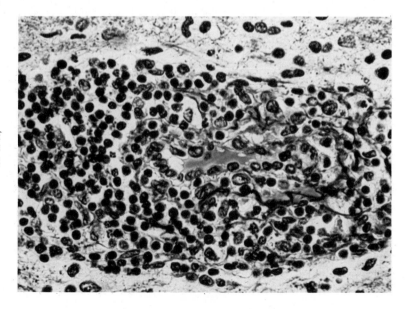

Figure 2. Perivascular cuff composed of histiocytes and lymphocytes set in fine nets of reticulin fibers (Wilder's reticulin stain; × 132).

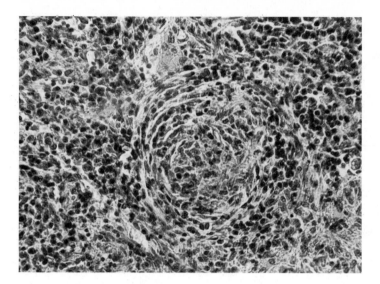

Figure 3. Coalescence of granulomatous lesions in the cerebrum of a dog with focal GME. H & E stain; × 66).

INCIDENCE

The incidence of GME relative to other CNS disorders may be more common than the literature would suggest. At Auburn University College of Veterinary Medicine, GME represents approximately 1.2 per cent (20 of 1688) of neurology postmortem cases. At the University of Pennsylvania, an incidence of 0.57 per cent (24 of 4200) of all postmortem cases has been reported. Disseminated and focal GME are more common than the ocular form. A compilation of 138 cases of GME from recent literature indicates that approximately 60 per cent are disseminated, 35 per cent are focal, and about 5 per cent are ocular.

BREED. Approximately 80 per cent of cases of GME occur in small (toy) breed dogs, of which 30 per cent are poodles.

AGE. The majority of confirmed cases occur in young to middle-aged dogs, with a mean age just under 5 years (ranging from 8 months to 10 years).

SEX. GME occurs in both sexes; however, there appears to be a higher incidence in females.

CLINICAL COURSE

The onset of *disseminated* GME is usually acute, with a progressive course over a 1- to 8-week period. In approximately 25 per cent of dogs, there is rapid deterioration of clinical signs, leading to death within 1 week. In more than 50 per cent of all cases of GME, the clinical course is from 3 to 8 weeks. The *ocular* form also tends to have a sudden onset and may remain static or be progressive, especially if disseminated lesions coexist. The *focal* form of GME has a more insidious onset and slowly progresses over a longer period. In 10 to 20 per cent of patients, death occurs within 3 to 12 months. The rate of progression of focal lesions in the caudal

brainstem and cervical spinal cord may be slower than that of focal lesions within the cerebrum.

CLINICAL SIGNS

Clinical signs are variable and reflect lesion localization. The *ocular* form of GME is characterized by acute onset of visual impairment and dilated pupils that are unresponsive to light stimulation, as a result of unilateral or bilateral optic neuritis. A hyperemic and edematous disk may be seen on ophthalmic examination. Vessels may be dilated and focal hemorrhage may be present.

Focal GME usually produces signs suggestive of a single, space-occupying lesion. These signs vary according to the location of the lesion, as described in the following examples:

1. *Cerebral Syndrome.* Behavioral or mental status change, circling, pacing, head pressing, and central visual impairment with normal pupillary reflexes.

2. *Midbrain Syndrome.* Mental depression or coma, rigid extension of all limbs, ventrolateral strabismus, mydriatic pupil(s) unresponsive to light with normal vision, and drooping of the upper eyelid(s).

3. *Pontomedullary Syndrome.* Hemiparesis ranging to tetraplegia and multiple cranial nerve deficits such as depressed palpebral reflex, medial strabismus, and jaw, facial, pharyngeal-laryngeal, or tongue paralysis.

4. *Vestibular Syndrome.* Head tilt, circling/falling/rolling, and nystagmus.

5. *Cerebellar Syndrome.* Spastic, goose-stepping gait, intention tremor, wide-based stance.

In animals with *disseminated* GME, clinical signs usually reflect several, that is, multifocal, syndromes (e.g., cerebral, brainstem, and spinal cord syndromes) as a result of the scattered distribution of lesions. Common clinical signs may include incoordination; ataxia and falling; cervical hyperesthesia; head tilt; nystagmus; facial or trigeminal nerve paralysis or both; circling; visual deficits; seizures; and depression. Occasionally, fever will accompany the clinical neurologic signs.

DIAGNOSIS

A tentative diagnosis of GME may be suggested by signalment data, the clinical course of the disease, and clinical signs. Hematology, serum chemistry, and radiographic studies are usually normal, and electroencephalographic recordings are frequently nonspecific. Computed tomography, magnetic resonance imaging, or both may detect a mass lesion in dogs with the focal form of GME. The most useful diagnostic aid is CSF analysis. In most dogs, CSF is abnormal, with mild to pronounced pleocytosis ranging from 50 to 900 white blood cells/mm^3. Cells are predominantly mononuclear, including lymphocytes (60 to 90 per cent), monocytes (10 to 20 per cent), and variable numbers of large anaplastic mononuclear cells with abundant lacy cytoplasm. While neutrophils typically comprise from 1 to 20 per cent of the cell type differential, they may be the predominate cell type on rare occasions. A marked decrease in CSF cellularity after glucocorticoid administration has been reported by some workers, but not by others. Protein in CSF is usually mildly or moderately elevated, ranging from 40 to 400 mg/dl. Occasionally, protein is elevated without pleocytosis. The high CSF protein apparently results from both blood-brain barrier disturbance and local IgG production. Cerebrospinal fluid pressure may be normal or increased. Lumbar-derived CSF reportedly contains fewer cells and less protein than CSF derived from cisternal puncture. CSF protein and cellularity is not necessarily influenced by the degree of meningeal involvement or the extent of necrosis within the granulomatous lesions.

DIFFERENTIAL DIAGNOSIS

Granulomatous meningoencephalomyelitis cannot be distinguished from other common neurologic diseases on the basis of clinical signs alone. *Disseminated* GME should be differentiated from other inflammatory CNS diseases. Bacterial meningoencephalomyelitis is often characterized by cervical hyperesthesia, cervical rigidity, and fever. Results of CSF analysis are abnormal, with very high protein levels (ranging from 100 to 1000+ mg/dl) and extreme polymorphonuclear pleocytosis (ranging from 100 to over 1000 cells/mm^3). Cases of *Toxoplasmosis* and fungal (cryptococcosis, blastomycosis,

and histoplasmosis) encephalomyelitis usually produce a mixed mononuclear and polymorphonuclear pleocytosis that ranges from 40 to 100 cells/mm^3. Organisms are often identified in CSF. Furthermore, systemic signs of toxoplasmosis or mycosis may be present, and serum titers may be elevated. Distemper viral encephalomyelitis and Rocky Mountain spotted fever usually result in a mild mononuclear pleocytosis, ranging from 8 to 40 cells/mm^3. Either or both positive serum and CSF titers and fluorescent antibody testing on conjunctival smears (e.g., canine distemper virus) help confirm these diseases. In addition, distemper most commonly occurs in dogs younger than 1 year of age. Cervical intervertebral disk disease and cervical trauma also need to be considered in animals with cervical hyperesthesia. Radiography should confirm the diagnosis in such cases.

Ocular GME needs to be differentiated from other causes of optic neuritis, including canine distemper, systemic mycosis, toxoplasmosis, and acute toxicity such as lead poisoning. Historical evidence of exposure to toxins and CSF analysis may aid in the differential diagnosis; however, in many cases, the final diagnosis is only established at necropsy.

Differential diagnostic considerations of *focal* GME include other primary and metastatic CNS tumors and severe focal, granulomatous lesions, sometimes seen with toxoplasmosis and mycotic infections. Again, CSF analysis and serum titers may help confirm a diagnosis. Results of CSF evaluation are variable in dogs with primary and secondary CNS tumors. Some dogs have increased protein without an associated pleocytosis, whereas others with more biologically aggressive tumors may have a marked pleocytosis. Definitive diagnosis may be established only after postmortem examination.

PROGNOSIS AND TREATMENT

The prognosis for permanent recovery is poor. The shortest survival periods, ranging from several days to weeks, are seen with the *disseminated* and *ocular* forms. Longer survival periods of from 3 to 6 months, or longer, are more suggestive of a *focal* lesion. Long-term therapy is generally unsatisfactory, although temporary remission of signs is often achieved with glucocorticoid administration, such as oral prednisone, 1 to 2 mg/kg/day initially for several days, then reducing the dosage to 2.5 to 5 mg on alternate days. Most dogs require continued therapy to prevent recurrences of signs. Improvement may last for several months in some dogs, although most eventually die of the disease. Cessation of glucocorticoid therapy is invariably associated with rapid and dramatic clinical deterioration. The ocular form of GME may be treated initially with retrobulbar glucocorticoid (betamethasone, 2.5 mg) in conjunction with oral prednisone therapy.

References and Supplemental Reading

Alley, M. R., Jones, B. R., and Johnstone, A. C.: Granulomatous meningoencephalomyelitis of dogs in New Zealand. N.Z. Vet. J. 31:117, 1983.

Bailey, C. S., and Higgins, R. J.: Characteristics of cerebrospinal fluid associated with canine granulomatous meningoencephalomyelitis: A retrospective study. J.A.V.M.A. 188:418, 1986.

Braund, K. G., Vandevelde, M., Walker, T. W., et al.: Granulomatous meningoencephalomyelitis in six dogs. J.A.V.M.A. 172:1195, 1978.

Cordy, D. R.: Canine granulomatous meningoencephalomyelitis. Vet. Pathol. 16:325, 1979.

Fankhauser, R., Fatzer, R., Luginbuhl, H., et al.: Reticulosis of the central nervous system (CNS) in dogs. Adv. Vet. Sci. Comp. Med. 16:35, 1972.

Russo, M. E.: Primary reticulosis of the central nervous system in dogs. J.A.V.M.A. 174:492, 1979.

Sarfaty, D., Carrillo, J. M., and Greenlee, P. G.: Differential diagnosis of granulomatous meningoencephalomyelitis, distemper, and suppurative meningoencephalitis in the dog. J.A.V.M.A. 188:387, 1986.

Sutton, R. H., and Atwell, R. B.: Nervous disorders in dogs associated with levamisole therapy. J. Small Anim. Pract. 23:391, 1982.

Vandevelde, M., Fatzer, R., and Fankhauser, R.: Immunohistologic studies in primary reticulosis of the canine brain. Vet. Pathol. 18:577, 1981.

WOBBLER SYNDROME IN THE DOBERMAN PINSCHER

H. B. SEIM, III, D.V.M.

Fort Collins, Colorado

Caudal cervical spondylopathy (wobbler syndrome) has been reported as a relatively common disease in breeds of large dogs. About 80 per cent of the cases are seen in Doberman pinschers and Great Danes. The exact etiology is unknown. Multiple factors, including improper nutrition, trauma, and heredity, are probably involved. Wobbler syndrome has recently been subdivided into five relatively distinct syndromes based on the location of the compression lesion with respect to the vertebral canal: (1) chronic degenerative disk disease, (2) "hourglass" compression, (3) ligamentum flavum disease, (4) congential bony malformation, and (5) vertebral tipping. There is resultant dorsal (ligamentum flavum), lateral (facets and joint capsule), and/or ventral (dorsal longitudinal ligament and dorsal annulus fibrosus) compression on the spinal cord. The ligamentous enlargement is felt to occur subsequent to either chronic degenerative disk disease or cervical vertebral instability resulting in ligamentous hypertrophy. The syndrome of chronic degenerative disk disease is most commonly seen in adult Doberman pinschers and will be the major emphasis of this article.

DIAGNOSIS

History

Affected Doberman pinschers usually have slowly progressive incoordination over a period of months to years. All four limbs are affected, but signs are generally more pronounced in the rear legs. Recent acute deterioration, precipitated by minor trauma, may be the owner's principal complaint. However, upon thorough questioning, owners usually will describe previous insidious paraparesis or tetraparesis. Hyperpathia is occasionally seen, with or without concurrent paraparesis or tetraparesis.

Neurologic Examination

Results of the neurologic examination vary with the site of the lesion. There is usually ambulatory tetraparesis, with retention or exaggeration of spinal reflexes in all four limbs. The front legs generally are advanced in a short, choppy manner at gait and are often held in extension when the dog is in lateral recumbency. This phenomenon is thought to reflect caudal cervical location of the lesion. Flexor muscles of the thoracic limbs are selectively paralyzed, while extensors are released from upper motor neuron inhibition.

The neck is often carried in flexion. Because of the dynamic nature of the lesion (see following discussion), this position results in the least amount of cord compression. Extension of the neck often causes hyperpathia or, more important, accentuates cord compression with consequent worsening of motor deficits. Moderate to severe atrophy of the infraspinatus and supraspinatus muscles is often seen.

Radiology

Plain radiographs of the neck are not diagnostic for the affected interspace or exact location within the vertebral canal of the compressive mass. On myelography, one may see (1) ventral midline spinal cord compression due most commonly to hypertrophied dorsal longitudinal ligament and dorsal annulus fibrosus, (2) dorsal compression due to ligamentum flavum enlargement, or (3) circumferential (hourglass) compression due to the previous two problems plus lateral impingement upon the cord by facet osteophytes and joint capsule enlargement. The compression is often dynamic. Strong linear traction on the head usually alleviates the compression if it is ligamentous in origin. Similarly, ventral flexion partially alleviates the compression, whereas dorsal extension makes it worse. Without this information, one cannot realistically plan the proper decompressive procedure (Fig. 1).

CLINICAL MANAGEMENT

Treatment options are generally divided into medical and surgical. Conservative medical man-

agement consists of strict confinement, a neck brace to help immobilize the caudal cervical spine, and anti-inflammatory medications. This treatment regimen should be continued for 3 to 4 weeks. If the patient responds favorably during the treatment period, gradual return to normal activity should be encouraged. Care should be taken not to allow excessive movement of the head and neck. If there is minimal, or no, response to conservative medical management, or if the patient's condition deteriorates in the face of therapy, surgery should be considered.

Several techniques for surgical treatment of this syndrome have been previously described. These include ventral interbody screw stabilization without decompression, dorsal decompressive laminectomy with facet fusion or dorsal spinal plating, ventral decompression and fusion, and ventral spinal plating. In many instances, treatment was not based on a myelographic study; therefore, critical evaluation of the preoperative status, surgical therapy, and postoperative progress in these cases is difficult. The author believes that preoperative evaluation of each patient by myelography is essential to determining the site of the lesion, the number of involved interspaces, the true significance of plain

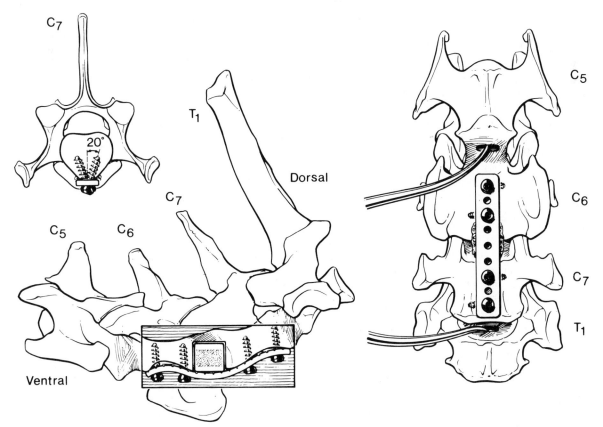

Figure 1. Ventral decompression with bone graft and Lubra plate stabilization. The screws are angled at 20° to the midline to prevent penetration of the vertebral canal. The vertebral spreaders are inserted into the fenestrated disk spaces so that traction can be applied to stretch the affected disk space 2 to 4 mm.

film "abnormalities," and the dynamics of the lesion. These features are important in planning appropriate surgical decompression and stabilization.

In choosing an appropriate surgical technique, the author has focused on the use of cervical traction to relieve spinal cord compression caused by hypertrophied dorsal annulus fibrosus. Two surgical techniques will be described that allow ventral decompression by linear traction and subsequent stabilization with cortical cancellous bone grafts and either a Lubra plate (Lubra, Ft. Collins, Co) or Steinmann's pins and Methylmethacrylate (Howmedic, Rutherford, NJ). These techniques were devised to achieve cervical spinal interbody fusion, with the affected interspace in traction and the spinal cord decompressed. They are intended for solitary lesions in which there is dynamic ventral spinal cord compression. When multiple lesions are present, the most significant site should be operated on, or an alternative surgical procedure should be considered.

The dog is premedicated with dexamethasone phosphate, 1 mg/kg body weight IV. Broad-spectrum antibiotics are given immediately preoperatively, and for 7 days postoperatively. Patients with any degree of tetraparesis are placed on a ventilator or have intermittent positive-pressure respiration during anesthesia.

SURGICAL PROCEDURES

In each procedure discussed, symmetric positioning of the patient in dorsal recumbency is critical. Care is taken to prevent hyperextension of the neck when placing the anesthetized dog on the surgery table. The head is secured to the table with a rope tied around the muzzle, caudad to the upper canine teeth. The front legs are directed caudally, with sufficient tension to create linear traction on the head and neck, and are then securely taped to the table. Tape is used to stabilize lateral motion of the head and body. The ventral neck and heads of the humeri must be draped into the sterile field. A routine ventral cervical approach is performed to expose the longus colli muscles. Lateral subperiosteal elevation of the longus colli muscles from the ventral aspect of the vertebral bodies adjacent to the affected interspace(s) allows adequate visualization for screw or pin placement.

A defect is created over the affected interspace with a pneumatic drill. The shape of the defect varies, depending on the procedure utilized. The cervical vertebral interspaces have a slightly caudal to cranial slant. In order to center the defect over the intervertebral space at the level of the vertebral canal, the slot is begun slightly craniad to the interspace. The depth of the defect can be gauged by visualizing three distinct layers of bone as one

drills: (1) the hard outer cortical layer of the vertebral body, (2) the softer, more vascular marrow layer, and (3) the inner cortical layer of the vertebral body. The middle layer is more easily drilled than the outer cortical layers and should be reached at each end of the defect. Once the inner cortical layer is visualized, the appropriate depth has been reached. Entering the vertebral canal is not necessary if the lesion is dynamic.

Ventral Decompression with Bone Graft and Lubra Plate Stabilization

The size and the shape of the vertebral defect are critical in this technique. The defect must perfectly accommodate a solid bone graft, when the cervical spine is placed in linear traction. Applying traction to the spine requires two assistants; one to grasp the dog's head just behind the ears, and the other to grasp the front legs. When gentle traction is placed on the head and front legs, the interspace can be expected to increase 2 to 4 mm. This variability depends upon the size of the dog and the degree of degenerative disk disease present. Alternatively, vertebral spreaders can be used to spread the interspace. This requires fenestration of the disk spaces craniad and caudad to the affected interspace. It is important to remove the ventral annulus fibrosus to the level of the nucleus pulposus. This is easily accomplished with a no. 11 Bard-Parker scalpel blade or pneumatic drill. Vertebral spreaders are inserted into the fenestrated disk spaces and gentle traction is applied to allow a 2- to 4-mm increase in the affected interspace. The graft is gently tapped into the defect, and the vertebral spreaders are removed to lock the graft in place. Excess graft that protrudes from the ventral surface of the vertebral bodies is drilled away. Several types of bone grafts have been successfully used in this procedure; Keil bone plugs (12.5 mm in diameter) or full cortical tibial allografts from the middle one third of a 25- to 30-lb donor harvested and preserved as described by Henry and Wadsworth are both appropriate.

Once the graft is in place, a single straight Lubra plate is placed on the ventral aspect of the vertebral bodies craniad and caudad to the graft (Fig. 1). Two holes are drilled with a 2.0-mm drill bit in each vertebral body at a 20 to 25° angle to the midline. The depth of the hole and the length of the screw vary with the size of the vertebral body. This measurement can generally be made on a lateral radiograph by estimating the distance from the ventral vertebral body to the ventral aspect of the vertebral canal. The screw holes are not tapped prior to placement. Fully threaded cortical screws that are 3.5 mm in diameter and of appropriate length are placed to hold the plate securely to the

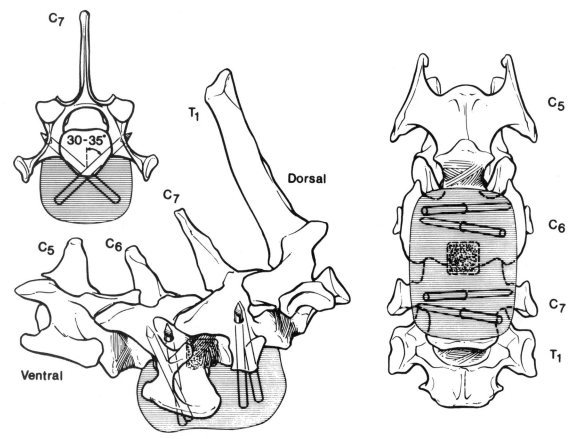

Figure 2. Ventral decompression with bone graft, Steinmann's pins and methylmethacrylate stabilization. The pins are placed at a 30 to 35° angle to the midline to allow penetration of two cortices without entering the vertebral canal. Methylmethacrylate is placed over all four protruding pins to accomplish stabilization.

vertebral bodies. The plate should assume the undulating shape of the interspace and cover the bone graft. Autogenous cancellous bone is harvested from the humeral head. This graft is packed into any remaining gaps in the defect created and should cover the Lubra plate at the level of the affected interspace. The longus colli muscles are apposed with interrupted mattress sutures. A snug closure over the autogenous cancellous bone graft helps hold it in place. The remaining closure of soft tissues is performed in routine fashion.

Use of an interbody screw for stabilization instead of the Lubra plate should be avoided, as use of the screw results in excessive stress on the vertebral body, with resultant fracture instability, and spinal compression.

Ventral Decompression with Bone Graft, Steinmann's Pins, and Methylmethacrylate Stabilization

The size and the shape of the defect are not as critical with this technique. Generally, the defect should extend no further than one half to three fourths of the width of the interspace, and no more

than one fourth the length of the vertebral body cranially or caudally. Two 7/32-inch Steinmann's pins are placed in the vertebral bodies craniad and caudad to the defect, at diverging angles, approximately 25 to 30° to the midline. The pins are placed to engage two cortices and are cut 2.5 to 3 cm from the vertebral body surface (Fig. 2). The interspaces craniad and caudal to the defect are prepared for insertion of the vertebral spreaders, as previously described. The interspace is distracted 2 to 4 mm and held in place by the vertebral spreaders. Autogenous cancellous bone is harvested from the humeral head and is packed into the defect. Medical-grade methylmethacrylate powder is gently mixed with the catalyst. When the cement begins to assume a puttylike consistency (i.e., when handled, it does not adhere to the surgeon's gloves), it is carefully molded around the protruding pins. Care is taken to cover each pin with the methylmethacrylate. As the cement begins to harden, the heat of polymerization is dissipated by lavaging the site with sterile physiologic saline solution. The time from mixing to complete polymerization is approximately 5 min. It is imperative that the vertebral spreaders remain in place until the cement has completely hardened. The mass of cement is often so large that it cannot be completely covered by the longus colli muscles. The muscle edges are approximated at the cranial and caudal aspects of the cement. The remainder of the closure is routine.

POSTOPERATIVE CARE

The patient recovers in a neck brace until there is radiographic evidence of fusion. Some dogs have difficulty in rising with the neck brace in place; others react violently to its presence and attempt to remove it. If the brace is not tolerated, it should be removed. Whether or not the patient will tolerate the neck brace can usually be determined in the first 24 to 48 hr. Ambulatory patients are discharged 24 to 48 hr postoperatively. Nonambulatory patients are treated with frequent hydrotherapy, physiotherapy, elevated padded cage racks, frequent turning, and bladder expression three to four times a day. The use of a supporting cart is helpful in nursing patients to an ambulatory status. Some advantages of a cart include unhindered eating, drinking, micturition, and defecation. Animals with motor function also can be encouraged to ambulate, and the erect position facilitates physiotherapy. Skin sutures are removed in 14 days. Patients should have radiographs taken at 1, 3, 6, and 12 months postoperatively to assess the degree of fusion.

PROGNOSIS

An accurate prognosis is difficult to make, even in patients that present with similar neurologic deficits. This difficulty arises from the inability to predict the compensatory capacity of the spinal cord in each patient at the time of evaluation and immediately postoperatively. However, based on the results of neurologic examination at the time of presentation and the number of lesions present myelographically, certain general prognostic criteria can be given. Patients that have one lesion and are ambulatory upon presentation generally have a favorable prognosis. Patients that have one lesion but are nonambulatory at the time of presentation have a guarded prognosis. Patients that have two lesions and are ambulatory at the time of presentation have a favorable to guarded prognosis; however, if they are nonambulatory, the prognosis is guarded to unfavorable.

There are many variables that must be taken into consideration in the patient that presents with wobbler syndrome. It is for this reason that the preoperative findings and operative techniques utilized can be used only as guidelines for discussing the potential outcome with clients.

References and Supplemental Reading

Henry, W. B., and Wadsworth, P. L.: Diaphyseal allografts in the repair of long bone fractures. J. Am. Anim. Hosp. Assoc. 17:525, 1981.

Seim, H. B., III, and Withrow, S. J.: Pathophysiology and diagnosis of caudal cervical spondylo-myelopathy with emphasis on the Doberman pinscher. J. Am. Anim. Hosp. Assoc. 18:241, 1982.

Seim, H. B., III, and Withrow, S. J.: Ventral decompression for treatment of herniated cervical intervertebral disk in the dog. In Bojrab, M. J. (ed.): Current Techniques in Small Animal Surgery, 2nd ed. Lea & Febiger, 1983, pp. 544–548.

Swaim, S. F.: Ventral decompression of the cervical spinal cord in the dog. J.A.V.M.A. 164:491, 1979.

Withrow, S. J., and Seim, H. B., III: Caudal cervical spondylopathy and myelopathy in large breed dogs. In Bojrab, M. J. (ed.): Current Techniques in Small Animal Surgery, 2nd ed. Lea & Febiger, 1983, pp. 541–544.

Section
9

GASTROINTESTINAL DISORDERS

DAVID C. TWEDT, D.V.M.

Consulting Editor

Endoscopy..864
Feline Hepatic Lipidosis...869
Serum Bile Acid Concentrations for Hepatobiliary Function
   Testing in Cats...873
Drug-Induced Hepatic Disease of Dogs and Cats 878
Cholelithiasis and Cholangitis..884
Copper Metabolism Defect in West Highland White Terriers.............889
Management of Hepatic Copper Toxicosis in Dogs.......................891
Feline Pancreatitis 893
Effects of Glucocorticoids on the Gastrointestinal System.................897
Esophageal Strictures 904
Reflux Esophagitis...906
Medical Therapy for Gastrointestinal Ulcers 911
Antral Pyloric Hypertrophy Syndrome 918
Canine Lymphocytic-Plasmacytic Enteritis.................................922
Exocrine Pancreatic Insufficiency...927
Chronic Intestinal Bacterial Overgrowth 933
Plasmacytic-Lymphocytic Colitis in Dogs 939
Campylobacter Enteritis 944
Extraction and Oral Nasal Fistula 948
Oral Diagnosis...951
Endodontics 954

ENDOSCOPY

TODD R. TAMS, D.V.M.
West Los Angeles, California

The word *endoscopy* is derived from Greek by combining the prefix *endo-*, "within," and the verb *skopein*, "to view, to observe intently, to monitor." The result is a most appropriate term for the procedure of peering into the recesses of the living body for diagnostic and therapeutic purposes. Endoscopy is one of the best and most fundamental methods of examining the gastrointestinal tract. The opportunity to examine directly and obtain tissue samples from the esophagus, stomach, and small and large intestine has revolutionized the clinical approach to diagnosis and has facilitated more accurate treatment of disorders of the digestive system. When used judiciously, endoscopy offers a valuable alternative to exploratory surgery for procurement of biopsies and retrieval of foreign bodies.

Endoscopy is now a well-established procedure in veterinary medicine. Endoscopic equipment is no longer considered a luxury that only large referral centers or veterinarians practicing in affluent areas can justify purchasing. An endoscope is one of the most versatile and diagnostically valuable pieces of equipment that a veterinary practice can have in its armamentarium. The purpose of this chapter is to familiarize veterinarians with the principles of flexible fiberoptic instrumentation and to review indications for use of endoscopy in patients with gastrointestinal disorders (for a discussion on endoscopic examination of the respiratory tract, see p. 219).

INSTRUMENTATION

The flexible fiberoptic endoscope works on the principle of the image-carrying fiber bundle, which transmits an image through the instrument from the structure being examined to the observer. The fiber bundle contains thousands of individual, ultra-thin (8 to 12 μm in diameter) glass fibers, each of which has the ability to transmit efficiently light entering the distal end of the fiber with minimal loss of brightness or change in color. The condition of total internal reflection is what enables glass fibers to transmit light. A ray of light is reflected each time it hits along the boundary surfaces of the fiber until it emerges at the other end. For this to occur, a long cylindrical glass fiber must be surrounded by a medium with a lower refractive index. This is accomplished by placing a thin layer of glass

of lower index than the fiber core glass around each glass fiber. The cladding glass prevents leakage of light from the fiber, a loss in transmission, and the transfer of light from the fiber to other objects with which it comes in contact. Light that does not enter the face of the fiber at or greater than a set angle (called the critical angle) will not undergo internal reflection and will be lost. Light may be reflected tens of thousands of times in traveling 1 m.

Flexible endoscopes contain two separate fiber bundles, an image guide (viewing) bundle and a light guide (light transmission) bundle. Image guide bundles are much more expensive to produce because the thousands of fibers in the bundle need to be spatially arranged precisely. For the image at one end of the bundle to duplicate the image at the other end, the ends of each individual fiber must occupy the same relative position in both ends of the bundle. A bundle's resolving power, the amount of image detail that the bundle can convey, depends on the diameter of the fiber core, the thickness of the fiber cladding, and the alignment and orderliness of the packing of the fibers within the bundle. Fiber alignment greatly affects the quality of the image. Imperfect alignment results in distorted images and dark areas in the image.

Individual fibers in the bundle that have been broken or damaged produce black or gray dots in the image. An isolated glass fiber is surprisingly strong and resistant to damage. However, when thousands of fibers are arranged into a bundle that is then packed into the body of an endoscope with other mechanical parts, the fibers are more susceptible to damage. Meticulous technical care in design and determining positioning arrangements of fibers and demanding durability tests are required to ensure maximum safety and resistance to damage of the fiber bundle. Better-quality endoscopes are more expensive, but they offer higher-quality optics and maneuverability.

A lens system at the tip of the fiberscope forms an image of the object in view; the light representing this image is transmitted through the image guide. A duplicate image is formed on the proximal end of the bundle near the eyepiece. Because the entire image guide bundle is no more than 0.5 to 3.0 mm in diameter, depending on the size of the endoscope, the image that arrives at the proximal bundle is too small to view with the unaided eye. The fiberscope eyepiece serves as an ocular lens that creates an enlarged image of the tiny image presented to the proximal bundle. The direct internal transmission of light through the fiber bundle provides an accurate reproduction of the object in view regardless of the straight, curved, or coiled configuration of the endoscope during an examination.

Light guide bundles are designed to maximize light-carrying ability rather than to produce an image. They are much less expensive to produce because light fibers can be randomly packed in the light guide bundle. Light guide fibers are much thicker (30μm) than image guide fibers (8 to 12 μm) and are much more efficient at carrying light. Image fibers must be small to maximize resolution. Light for illumination is supplied from an external light source. A variety of endoscopic light sources are available, ranging from low-power halogen light sources to sophisticated high-intensity xenon units. The halogen units are quite adequate for use in animals and supply light that provides excellent visualization and sufficient capabilities for photography.

Flexible endoscopes also have channels for water flushing, air insufflation, and suction. These capabilities greatly improve the endoscopist's ability to perform a thorough examination. Air is supplied by a pump within the light source and is emitted from a nozzle in the distal tip. Air is used to distend the walls of the organ being examined so that they do not obstruct examination by collapsing around the tip of the endoscope. Water is forced through a pressurized water container and serves to flush mucus and other debris away from the tip of the endoscope. Fluid and air can be suctioned through the working channel of the endoscope into a suction unit attached to a port on a section of the light source connector.

Most flexible endoscopes have two-stage flexibility, with the most distal portion (approximately 6 cm) being more flexible than the proximal portion. Depending on the endoscope, the distal tip can be deflected using knobs on the control housing in either two or four directions. Tip deflection enhances maneuverability as the endoscope is advanced through the various curves and angles of the body system being examined. Four-direction deflection capability allows for endoscope tip excursion through a variety of planes. The endoscopist then has the opportunity to perform a more thorough examination and to obtain samples from any mucosal area within reach. Four-direction capability is preferred over two-direction for gastrointestinal endoscopy.

A working channel housed in the endoscope is used to pass biopsy forceps, cytology brushes, foreign body graspers, and other ancillary instruments. The same channel is used for suction. Depending on the size of the endoscope, the working channel diameter generally varies from 2.0 to 2.8 mm.

Instruments are advanced through the working channel port, which is located near the control section.

In addition to the endoscope and light source, a suction pump, biopsy forceps, foreign body grasper, and brushes for obtaining cytology samples should be available. The ancillary instrument used most often for gastrointestinal endoscopic examinations is the biopsy forceps. The most common reason for performing gastrointestinal endoscopy is to both examine *and* obtain biopsies from the areas being examined, regardless of gross appearance. Examination without biopsy may result in inaccurate diagnosis.

SELECTION OF AN ENDOSCOPE

The author's recommendation to veterinarians interested in purchasing their first endoscope is to purchase a single high-quality endoscope that may be used for a variety of procedures (e.g., esophagogastroduodenoscopy, colonoscopy, bronchoscopy, reproductive endoscopy) in small cats and dogs as well as in large dogs. A pediatric endoscope with four-way tip deflection capability meets these criteria. The insertion tube diameter should range from 6.0 to 7.9 mm (preferred range) to 9.0 mm. The major limitation of a large insertion tube (9.0 mm or greater) is that there is more difficulty in passing it through the pyloric canal to the duodenum in cats and small dogs. The larger 9.0- to 9.5-mm endoscopes can be used quite effectively in many animal patients, but there are inherent difficulties in performing a complete examination in very small patients. This becomes an important consideration for any urban practice in which many feline and small canine patients are seen. A standard working length of 100 cm or more is adequate for performing a thorough examination in dogs and cats.

INDICATIONS FOR GASTROINTESTINAL ENDOSCOPY

During its early development, fiberoptic endoscopy was used primarily as an adjunct to other diagnostic methods, especially barium contrast x-rays. However, in recent years many veterinary gastroenterologists have come to regard endoscopy as one of the most sensitive methods of evaluating gastrointestinal tract symptoms. This has resulted in a substantial increase in the use of endoscopy in many specialty hospitals, corresponding with a decrease in the number of barium series that are performed. This trend is expected to continue as more veterinarians become familiar with the distinct diagnostic advantages of endoscopy.

Table 1. *Possible Indications for Gastrointestinal Endoscopy*

Initial	Follow-up
Regurgitation	Repeat esophageal stricture bougie-
Dysphagia	nage
Retching	Follow-up biopsies in patients with
Unexplained salivation	moderate to severe gastritis, in-
Unexplained nausea	flammatory bowel disease, colitis
Vomiting	(i.e., assess progression of disease,
Hematemesis	efficacy of therapy)
Diarrhea	Serial assessment during ulcer heal-
Melena	ing
Dyschezia	Serial assessment of mucosal healing
Constipation	and examination for possible stric-
Possible foreign body	ture formation following esophageal
	mucosal damage from a foreign
	body

Most of the commonly encountered disorders of the gastrointestinal tract involve either the mucosa of the organ in question or disrupted mucosal anatomy. Endoscopy offers the clear advantage of complete mucosal examination of the esophagus, stomach, descending duodenum (in cats and small dogs, the ascending duodenum as well), and colon. Endoscopic biopsies provide rapid assessment and evaluation of many disorders. In addition, endoscopy plays an important therapeutic role in foreign body removal, guided bougienage or balloon dilation of esophageal strictures, and placement of gastric feeding tubes. Well-established indications for endoscopy are listed in Table 1. Disorders that can be reliably diagnosed via endoscopy are listed in Table 2.

Diagnosis of Esophageal Abnormalities

Esophagoscopy should be considered for any patient with signs of esophageal disease. The decision whether or not to actually perform an endoscopic examination of the esophagus is based on clinical impression and a review of any indicated laboratory tests and radiographic studies. Common signs of esophageal disease include regurgitation, dysphagia, excessive salivation, and change in appetite, which may be either increased or decreased.

In the esophagus, as elsewhere in the gastrointestinal tract, endoscopy is most effective in diagnosis of disorders that affect the mucosa. Hence, it can be expected that diagnosis of inflammatory, neoplastic, and obstructive lesions (e.g., stricture, foreign body) will be relatively precise. While survey or contrast radiography is useful for identifying an obstructive lesion, esophagoscopy provides a means of obtaining a definitive diagnosis and in some cases offers important therapeutic options. Esophageal foreign bodies (including fishhooks, bones, and other objects) can often be successfully removed using graspers that are passed through or alongside the endoscope. Any erosive damage to the esophagus can be assessed after a foreign body has been removed. Bougienage or balloon dilation procedures to dilate esophageal strictures are most safely performed under endoscopic visualization. Esophageal tumors can be diagnosed by guided biopsy. In human medicine, endoscopic laser therapy has been successfully used for ablation of neoplastic tissue. This is a palliative measure under-

Table 2. *Gastrointestinal Disorders Amenable to Diagnosis by Endoscopy*

Site of Disorder	Type of Disorder			
	Inflammatory	*Infectious/Parasitic*	*Anatomic*	*Neoplastic*
Esophagus	Esophagitis Chemical injuries (acid, al- kali)		Strictures Foreign bodies Hiatal hernia Diverticula Megaesophagus (endos- copy rarely necessary for diagnosis)	Squamous cell carci- noma Adenocarcinoma Metastases Others
Stomach	Gastritis (e.g., lympho- cytic-plasmacytic, eosin- ophilic, histiocytic) Chemical injuries Ulcer-benign and malig- nant	Physaloptera	Foreign bodies Hypertrophic gastropa- thies Pyloric mucosal hyper- trophy Polyps	Lymphosarcoma Adenocarcinoma Others
Duodenum	Inflammatory bowel dis- ease Lymphangiectasia Duodenal ulcer	Giardiasis Histoplasmosis		Lymphosarcoma Adenocarcinoma Others
Colon	Colitis	Trichuriasis Cestodiasis Protozoal infections (ex- amine mucosal brushings) Histoplasmosis	Polyps Strictures Cecal inversion	Lymphosarcoma Adenocarcinoma Others

taken in esophageal cancer patients primarily to relieve luminal obstruction and hemorrhage.

The diagnosis of reflux esophagitis cannot be made consistently based solely on gross examination, because in some cases changes are limited to microscopic inflammation. Certain endoscopic "clues" may be observed by an experienced endoscopist; however, that will suggest the likelihood of reflux esophagitis (e.g., distal esophageal erythema, gastroesophageal sphincter dilation, pooling of fluid in the distal esophagus). Monitoring distal esophageal pH with a probe and obtaining a suction biopsy of the distal esophageal mucosa provide a more sensitive means of diagnosis of reflux esophagitis than visualization alone.

In most patients with megaesophagus, endoscopic examination is not necessary for diagnosis and is rarely of benefit in determining a cause of the disorder. Megaesophagus is a specific syndrome characterized by generalized esophageal dilation and hypoperistalsis, and it is differentiated from other causes of esophageal dilation such as esophageal foreign body, vascular ring anomaly or other stricture disorders, and neoplasia. Esophageal motility disorders in which there is not easily detected radiographic evidence of marked esophageal dilation are best recognized by esophageal fluoroscopy and manometry studies. If this equipment is not available, esophagoscopy may be beneficial; in some cases, pooling of fluid or mild esophageal dilation can be identified.

Diagnosis of Gastric Abnormalities

Indications for gastroscopy include signs referable to gastric diseases, including nausea, salivation, vomiting, hematemesis, and melena. Gastroscopy mainly defines abnormalities of the gastric mucosa, but it may also reveal distortion of the stomach's normal anatomic relationships. Using proper technique, the entire mucosal surface of the stomach and the antral-pyloric canal can be examined. The most common disorders diagnosed include chronic gastritis, gastric foreign bodies, and gastric motility disorders. Ulcers, neoplasia, and pyloric hypertrophy are less commonly found. Special therapeutic considerations include foreign body removal and endoscopy-guided percutaneous tube gastrostomy placement. Gastrostomy tube placement is a quick and simple procedure and provides an excellent means of temporarily feeding an anorectic or debilitated patient.

In evaluating a patient with signs suggestive of a gastric disorder, gastric mucosal biopsies should be obtained even if gross lesions are not present. It is common for a patient with chronic gastritis to have lesions only identifiable on microscopic examination. Different classifications of gastritis (e.g., lym-

phocytic-plasmacytic, eosinophilic, histiocytic) and degree of involvement (e.g., mild, moderate, severe) can be determined from mucosal biopsy samples; these findings are extremely important in determining specific therapeutic regimens. If gross lesions are identified (e.g., localized hyperemic areas, superficial erosions, raised follicular-like changes, nodules, or masses), forcep biopsies should be obtained from these areas as well as from several normal areas. Four to six biopsy samples are obtained from different areas of the gastric body if the stomach is grossly normal. Biopsies are best obtained from the surface of a gastric fold. The size of the tissue samples obtained may be inadequate if the stomach is too distended with air, because the folds become too flattened. When the endoscope is first advanced to the stomach during the course of an examination, air is insufflated to distend the gastric walls so that thorough mucosal evaluation is enhanced. Suctioning most of the air out just prior to taking biopsies greatly increases the gastric fold surface area from which samples can be obtained. It is more difficult to obtain a tissue sample of adequate size from the gastric antrum than it is from other parts of the body, unless there is hypertrophy or discrete raised or cratered lesions.

Clues that a gastric motility disorder may be present include pooling of bile or gastric fluid, or finding undigested food in the stomach of an animal that has fasted 8 to 10 hours or more. The stomach normally empties within 6 to 8 hours after a meal. There is often mucosal hyperemia due to superficial irritation from bile, but despite this gross abnormality gastric biopsies in idiopathic gastric motility disorders are usually normal.

Because biopsies obtained from some masses with standard biopsy forceps are relatively small, sufficient tissue for confident diagnosis is sometimes not obtained. The same site of a mass should be biopsied several times, each time extending the biopsy forceps more deeply into the tissue. If only the surface of a neoplastic mass is biopsied, a mistaken diagnosis of granulomatous or fibrous disease may be made. Samples from ulcerative lesions are best taken by grasping the wall or the junction of the wall and the gastric mucosa. Gastric polyps are reliably diagnosed on endoscopic biopsy in dogs and cats.

A major shortcoming of gastroscopy is that neoplastic diseases involving the serosa or deep layers of the gastric wall cannot be identified or definitively diagnosed on mucosal biopsy. If endoscopic findings do not correlate with clinical signs or if there is a poor response to therapy, exploratory surgery should be recommended.

Diagnosis of Duodenal Abnormalities

Using a flexible pediatric endoscope (9.0 mm diameter or less), the duodenum can be directly examined in most cats and dogs. An endoscope with a diameter of 7.9 mm can consistently be advanced to the duodenum in cats and dogs as small as 4 lb. The distal duodenum or proximal jejunum can often be reached in cats and small dogs. Certain portions of the duodenum, including the area immediately beyond the pylorus and the medial wall of the descending segment, are sometimes difficult to view other than tangentially. In small patients (especially cats), care must be taken to not be too forceful in advancing the endoscope through areas where there is increased resistance.

Clinical signs of small intestinal disease include vomiting, diarrhea, melena, and weight loss. By far the greatest value of duodenoscopy is its capability of definitively diagnosing inflammatory small bowel disorders via biopsy. Frequently the only major sign in inflammatory bowel disease patients is vomiting. If only gastric biopsies are obtained from these animals, the diagnosis may be missed. In inflammatory disease, the small bowel mucosa may appear normal, or it may have varying degrees of irregularity, fissures, or folliclelike changes.

Endoscopy offers an alternative approach to obtaining small bowel biopsies in cases of protein-losing enteropathy when there is concern that full-thickness surgical biopsy sites may heal slowly. Multiple biopsies can be safely obtained. Duodenal fluid can be aspirated into tubing passed through the endoscope to obtain specimens for detection of *Giardia*. Diagnostic yield for giardiasis is much higher with this method than when testing is limited to stool examinations.

Neoplasms that involve the small bowel mucosa can be reliably diagnosed on biopsy. It is occasionally difficult for a pathologist to differentiate lymphocytic enteritis from lymphosarcoma; in this situation, full-thickness surgical biopsies may be necessary to clarify the diagnosis.

Diagnosis of Large Intestinal Disorders

Flexible colonoscopy provides a means of thoroughly examining the entire colon to the level of the ileocolic junction. In some dogs, the endoscope can be guided into the ileum. Indications for colonoscopy include signs of inflammatory disease (e.g., hematochezia, dyschezia, increased frequency of defecation), chronic diarrhea, constipation, fecal incontinence, and evaluation of a rectal or colonic mass. The most commonly diagnosed disorders include a variety of mucosal inflammatory disorders (lymphocytic-plasmacytic colitis is the most common) and rectal polyps. Colonic strictures, histoplasmosis, parasitic typhlitis, inverted cecum, and neoplasia are seen less commonly but can be reliably diagnosed by colonoscopy. Colonoscopy is much more accurate than contrast radiography in obtaining a definitive diagnosis of large intestinal disorders.

A majority of patients with idiopathic colitis have grossly normal mucosa. Confirmation of the diagnosis requires that the colon be properly prepared so that high-quality biopsy samples can be obtained from various levels of the colon. If the ileocolic area can be reached, an attempt should be made to obtain biopsies from the ileum as well. Even if the endoscope cannot be advanced to the ileum, the biopsy forceps can often be guided into the ileum; blind biopsies can then be procured. In patients with chronic diarrhea that is not clearly limited to large bowel signs, it is best to obtain biopsies from both the small and the large intestine.

References and Supplemental Reading

Happé, R. P., and van der Gaag, I. V.: Endoscopic examination of esophagus, stomach, and duodenum in the dog. J. Am. Hosp. Assoc. 19:2, 1983.

Kawahara, I., and Ichikawa, H.: Fiberoptic instrument technology. *In* Sivak, M. V. (ed.): *Gastroenterologic Endoscopy*. Philadelphia: W. B. Saunders Co., 1987, pp. 20–41.

Leib, M. S.: Colonoscopy. *In* Tams, T. R. (ed.): *Small Animal Endoscopy*. St. Louis: C. V. Mosby Co. (in press).

Mathews, K. A., and Binnington, A. G.: Percutaneous incisionless placement of a gastrostomy tube utilizing a gastroscope: Preliminary observations. J. Am. Hosp. Assoc. 22:5, 1986.

Tams, T. R.: Gastrointestinal endoscopy—instrumentation, handling technique, maintenance. *In* Tams, T. R. (ed.): *Small Animal Endoscopy*. St. Louis: C. V. Mosby Co. (in press).

FELINE HEPATIC LIPIDOSIS

LARRY M. CORNELIUS, D.V.M., PH.D.,
and GILBERT JACOBS, D.V.M.

Athens, Georgia

Hepatic lipidosis (fatty liver) is a fairly common hepatobiliary disorder of cats that is seen also in several other species including humans, dogs, horses, and cows. Fatty liver in humans is generally defined as an acquired disorder of metabolism resulting in accumulation of triglycerides within hepatocytes in quantities sufficient to be visible by light microscopy (Vierling, 1982). It is generally believed that most of the accumulated fat in the hepatocytes is triglyceride (neutral fat), but analyses for fatty acids and cholesterol have not been reported.

Many processes may lead to fat accumulation in the liver. It should be stressed that triglyceride accumulation in the liver *per se* is not usually thought to be harmful to hepatocytes, will not cause inflammation, fibrosis, or cirrhosis, and is a potentially reversible lesion. Why some people and animals with hepatic lipidosis develop severe liver failure is unknown. Excessive fatty acid accumulation in hepatocytes might cause cellular damage, but this has not been proved.

Fatty liver occurs both with and without evidence of intrinsic liver disease. In normal animals there is constant cycling of fatty acids between the liver and adipose tissue, and normally there is a delicate balance between the two. For several reasons, distortion of this balance may occur, leading to hepatic lipidosis. First, hepatic uptake of fatty acids from the blood is a function of their concentration. As the blood concentration of fatty acids increases, the liver takes up more fatty acids. Second, the liver has only two ways to dispose of fatty acids—oxidation within mitochondria or peroxisomes or re-esterification to triglycerides. There are limits to the rate of fatty acid oxidation in the liver, but there are probably no limits to the amounts that can be esterified to triglyceride. Thus, the liver accumulates triglycerides easily but has a relatively limited capacity to secrete triglyceride in the form of very low density lipoproteins (VLDL). In short, the normal liver can remove fatty acids from the blood and re-esterify them at a rate that exceeds its capacity for synthesis and secretion of VLDL (Zakim, 1982).

Hepatic lipidosis can occur because of derangement in hepatic triglyceride synthesis, fatty acid oxidation, triglyceride transport from the liver as VLDL, changes in nutritional or hormonal status, or toxic influences on hepatocellular function that can adversely influence the balance of triglyceride deposition and dispersal from the liver (Center, 1986).

In obese people, mild fatty liver is common, and this is thought to be the result of the inability of the liver to secrete all of the fatty acids delivered to it. This finding is a physiologic consequence of the obese state and *per se* signifies nothing about the functional status of the liver. Information regarding the liver of normal obese cats is unavailable but is probably similar. Hepatic lipidosis can be produced, also, by feeding large amounts of carbohydrate or infusing excessive glucose in parenteral hyperalimentation regimens. Hepatic triglyceride accumulation, in these instances, results from stimulation of hepatic synthesis of fatty acids caused by excessive ingestion or administration of carbohydrates. The increased fatty acid synthesis exceeds the capacity of the liver to secrete VLDL.

Transport of long-chain fatty acids into the hepatic mitochondrion for oxidation is dependent on coupling to carnitine, a quaternary amine synthesized mainly in the liver, and certain enzymes of the carnitine transport mechanism. In humans, deficiencies of carnitine or its associated enzymes cause long-chain fatty acids to accumulate in the hepatocyte cytosol, resulting in hepatic lipidosis and, in certain cases, severe hepatic failure (Chapoy et al., 1980). Acute episodes of hepatic failure occur intermittently despite constantly low carnitine levels and are associated with fasting or semistarvation. It has been hypothesized that mobilization and hepatic uptake of free fatty acids in the face of a limited capacity for oxidation somehow has an initiating role, perhaps as a result of toxic effects of certain fatty acids on the liver and other tissues (McGarry and Foster, 1980).

Fatty liver is common in patients with certain endocrine disorders such as diabetes mellitus. Diabetes leads to enhanced lipolysis as a result of relative or absolute insulin deficiency, a reaction that is normally suppressed by insulin. The excessive blood fatty acids are taken up by hepatocytes, and some are stored as triglycerides. Fatty liver associated with diabetes mellitus is apparently of little functional consequence in humans and dogs but may be associated with hepatic failure in cats, although the exact relationship of liver failure to the fat accumulation is unclear.

Starvation, hypercortisolemia (stress or glucocor-

869

ticoid administration), and catecholamines (stress) may also cause hepatic fat accumulation by similar mechanisms. They stimulate lipolysis in adipocytes and cause mobilization of fatty acids, resulting in increased hepatic uptake, synthesis, and storage of triglyceride. Although fatty liver in patients starved for relatively brief periods can be explained by increased delivery of fatty acids to the liver, the situation is more complex in chronic starvation or in protein-calorie malnutrition (ingestion of carbohydrate with little or no protein). In the latter condition, there is evidence that the liver is not adequately secreting VLDL, probably as a result of protein deficiency resulting in decreased hepatic apoprotein levels. Since apoproteins are necessary for the formation of hepatic VLDL, protein deficiency can cause fat to accumulate in the liver. Thus, fatty liver in severely malnourished patients may reflect not only increased fatty acid mobilization and uptake by the liver, but also diet-induced decreases in hepatic triglyceride secretion in the form of VLDL.

Synthesis and secretion of VLDL are complicated processes, and the failure of either can lead to hepatic lipidosis. The role of dietary protein deficiency in impairing VLDL synthesis has already been discussed. Agents that interfere with protein synthesis, such as ethionine, or with assembly of VLDL, such as orotic acid, cause fatty liver in the absence of destruction of hepatocytes. Other toxins, such as carbon tetrachloride, cause a defect in synthesis of VLDL and lead to fatty liver. In these instances, hepatic lipid accumulation is a reflection of toxic injury to the liver (Zakim, 1982).

IDIOPATHIC HEPATIC LIPIDOSIS IN THE CAT

This following discussion will be limited to those cats with fatty liver for which a definitive cause cannot be established (idiopathic hepatic lipidosis, or IHL).

Clinical Description

IHL occurs almost exclusively in very obese or formerly obese cats. In some cases, obesity may at first be somewhat inapparent, but the distribution of fat appears to be such that there is a large amount of intra-abdominal adipose tissue. Muscle wasting may be somewhat obscured by the obesity but is often severe. There is sometimes a history suggestive of one or more stressful episodes recently preceding the onset of illness. The syndrome is characterized by depression, usually complete anorexia, dehydration, developing icterus, and a progressive and relentless course. Many cats develop signs of severe hepatic failure including central nervous system (CNS) signs (stupor, coma, headpressing) indicative of hepatoencephalopathy (HE) and clotting/bleeding disorders (melena, hematomas after venipuncture). Laboratory findings on a screening initial data base commonly include a mild nonregenerative anemia, moderately to markedly increased serum alkaline phosphatase (alk phos, 5 to 15 times normal), mildly to moderately increased serum alanine aminotransferase (S-alt, 2 to 5 times normal), and sometimes decreased blood urea nitrogen (BUN) and serum albumin values. Other laboratory abnormalities may include increased serum bilirubin, bile acid, and ammonium levels and prolonged clotting times. Glucose intolerance has been documented in a few cases.

Diagnosis

A definitive diagnosis can only be established by liver biopsy. It is important to realize that IHL increases the risk of anesthesia in affected cats. Also, clotting function should be assessed prior to biopsy and abnormalities treated appropriately. Percutaneous hepatic biopsy can usually be accomplished with a Tru-Cut needle, using ketamine, 22 to 33 mg/kg IM, for sedation, by personnel experienced with the technique. However, the liver is only slightly enlarged in IHL, and it is not easy to biopsy by the blind, percutaneous method. If ultrasound instrumentation is available, ultrasonically guided percutaneous hepatic biopsy is safer and more effective.

It may be preferable to perform an exploratory celiotomy and obtain a wedge biopsy of the liver. Using this procedure also allows for the placement of a pharyngostomy or gastrostomy tube during the same period of anesthesia (see p. 33). After premedication with an anticholinergic drug such as atropine or glycopyrrolate (Robinul, A. H. Robins), it is preferred to use inhalant induction with isoflurane (Forane, Anaquest) utilizing an induction chamber. The cat is then intubated, and anesthesia is maintained with a mixture of isoflurane, oxygen, and nitrous oxide. Every effort should be made to expedite surgery and avoid prolonged anesthesia time. Characteristic findings are large amounts of intraabdominal fat and a liver with a diffuse mustard color and a finely reticulated pattern. Confirmation of IHL must be done by histopathologic examination. Since routine processing removes lipid, the pathologist should be asked to prepare one section of liver to check for lipid (in addition to routine H & E staining). This is done by freezing a portion of the formalin-fixed biopsy specimen, sectioning, and staining with a fat stain such as oil red O. The diagnosis is confirmed by finding diffuse accumulation of lipid in hepatocytes without other significant hepatic lesions.

Pathophysiologic Mechanisms

The pathophysiologic mechanisms of IHL in cats are unknown at present. Since obesity, anorexia, and stress are nearly always present, speculation has involved various possibilities associated with these disorders, as well as the unique nutritional requirements of cats as best as they are currently understood.

As previously discussed, excessive caloric intake will cause fat to accumulate in the liver, and it is likely that obese cats have a mild fatty liver. Stress hormones (cortisol, epinephrine, glucagon, growth hormone) cause lipolysis in adipose tissue, resulting in delivery of excessive fatty acids to the liver, where they are taken up and converted into triglycerides. Once the cat becomes anorectic, a different set of metabolic events begins. These changes are dictated by two separate but related needs:

1. The CNS's unique requirement for glucose must be met, first by conversion of hepatic glycogen to glucose (glycogenolysis), and after 24 to 48 hr by catabolism of muscle protein and conversion to glucose (gluconeogenesis). Cats are known to catabolize body proteins more rapidly than other species during fasting, apparently because hepatic transaminases and urea cycle enzymes continue to be active (Morris and Rogers, 1983).

2. All the tissues of the body require a source of energy, which must come from stored calories. Fatty acids become the main fuel in the fasted state in order to minimize the amount of amino acid, and hence tissue protein that must be converted to glucose. As fasting becomes prolonged, the CNS lessens its dependence on glucose for energy and can utilize ketones instead.

Two observations on cats with IHL may be relevant to understanding pathophysiologic mechanisms: (1) Body fat stores appear to be relatively unused considering the prolonged anorexia, and (2) Ketonuria is seldom observed (ketones are derived from hepatic oxidation of fat). Both of these findings would appear to indicate that fat is not being appropriately utilized as an energy source. If this is so, it is not surprising that severe muscle wasting is observed in cats with IHL. In most species during fasting, gluconeogenesis from muscle protein can supply glucose for the CNS for several weeks since other tissues acquire their energy source from fat breakdown. Failure to properly utilize fat for energy would obviously make the fasting animal more dependent on muscle protein breakdown.

As previously discussed, fasting cats have an additional demand for muscle protein catabolism because of the continued activity of hepatic transaminases and enzymes of the urea cycle. Another potential complicating factor for fasting cats is their absolute requirement for a source of arginine. Cats cannot synthesize arginine as can most other species and during fasting must obtain it from muscle protein catabolism. Depletion of muscle protein may cause relative or absolute arginine deficiency. Arginine is an important component of the urea cycle for conversion of ammonia to urea, and a deficiency has been reported to cause decreased ornithine production, increased carbamoyl phosphate and orotic acid synthesis, and hyperammonemia (Morris and Rogers, 1983). As previously discussed, orotic acid has been reported to be hepatotoxic, resulting in fatty liver (Alpers and Isselbacher, 1975). Protein depletion might also result in decreased lipoprotein apoprotein synthesis, with subsequent decrease in hepatic fat mobilization and transport (Burrows et al., 1981).

If cats with IHL do not properly oxidize fat for energy (speculative at this point), what are potential causes and why does only the occasional obese, anorexic, stressed cat develop the syndrome? The answers to these questions are unknown at present. In humans, carnitine deficiency syndromes are recognized causes of decreased fat oxidation (Chapoy et al., 1980). Carnitine is a quaternary amine synthesized mainly in the liver from lysine using methionine as a methyl donor. Carnitine is essential for the transport of long-chain fatty acids into the mitochondrion. Failure of the transport mechanism due to carnitine deficiency or abnormalities in the carnitine acyl transferase enzymes means that long-chain fatty acids cannot be used to produce energy in cells. Two forms are reported—skeletal muscle, in which fat accumulates diffusely in skeletal muscle, and systemic, resulting in lipid deposition in liver, heart, and nervous tissue. Acute hepatic failure, characterized by hypoglycemia, hyperammonemia, HE, and severe hepatic lipidosis, is associated with systemic carnitine deficiency. Episodes frequently are precipitated by a bout of fasting. Carnitine deficiency is documented by measuring plasma and tissue carnitine levels. Human patients often respond to oral carnitine supplementation. Similar studies in cats have not been reported.

Treatment

Until the cause(s) and pathophysiologic mechanisms of IHL are better understood, treatment will continue to be mainly supportive. The most important consideration is to maintain adequate fluid and caloric intake until the cat starts drinking and eating enough voluntarily. This often requires a long period of time (1 to 12 weeks). Daily fluid requirements are 50 to 60 ml/kg. Total caloric intake should be 80 to 100 Kcal/kg/day, and the diet should be nutritionally balanced. Administration of insufficient calories, especially as carbohydrate, and infusion of glucose may worsen IHL (Center, 1986). Recommendations for the food to be used vary. If hyperammonemia or signs of HE are present, prescription diet Feline k/d (Hill's Pet Products) is recommended because its restricted protein content is of high biologic value. Otherwise, prescription diet Feline c/d (Hill's Pet Products) is advised because of its moderate fat and protein levels, which appear to be well assimilated. Only the enteral route should be considered, and several methods have been used.

Appetite stimulants can be tried and may be successful in a few cats in which IHL is diagnosed very early. Several benzodiazepine compounds have been shown to stimulate appetite in animals including cats. Diazepam (Valium, Roche), 0.05 to 0.15 mg/kg IV or 1.0 mg PO s.i.d. or b.i.d., and oxazepam (Serax, Wyeth), 0.2 to 0.5 mg/kg PO s.i.d. or b.i.d., often induce eating in anorectic cats. However, cats given these drugs usually eat only small amounts, and marked sedation and ataxia may be seen as side effects (Rogers and Cornelius, 1985).

Force-feeding by mouth is usually unacceptable because of the additional stress to the cat. Nasogastric intubation can be accomplished with local anesthesia and a size 5 or 6 French feeding tube (Peditube, Biosearch Medical Products) (Crowe, 1986). Only fluids and liquid nutritional supplements can be administered through this relatively small-diameter tube. Commercial products such as Vivonex (Norwich Eaton) can be used for short periods of time but may cause diarrhea. Diluting such products in half with water may lessen this tendency. Vivonex is a high-protein supplement and should not be used if the cat shows signs of HE. This technique may be most useful when only a few days of caloric supplementation are needed, such as when trying to stabilize the patient prior to anesthesia and liver biopsy.

Placement of a pharyngostomy or gastrostomy tube allows the enteral administration of well-balanced commercial cat food gruels (Feline K/D or C/D), which are prepared by using an electric blender and mixing with enough water to make a slurry thin enough to be administered through the tube (Rogers and Cornelius, 1985). The gruel should first be administered at the rate of about 5 ml/kg six to eight times per day. If vomiting occurs, the amount administered per feeding should be reduced by about half and gradually increased over a period of a few days. The objective is to reduce the daily tube-feeding frequency to three times per day. If vomiting is a problem with this regimen, administration of metoclopramide (Reglan, A. H. Robins), 0.4 mg/kg t.i.d. SC, 30 min. prior to feeding often helps. Unfortunately, many cats tolerate pharyngostomy tubes poorly, and persistent gagging and regurgitation are common.

Better success has been achieved in our hospital by the surgical placement of a gastrostomy tube. Cats usually tolerate the gastrostomy tube exceptionally well, and complications have been minimal. A Foley catheter (of a size from no. 16 to no. 24, depending on the size of the cat) is inserted into the stomach by gastrostomy during general anesthesia, and celiotomy (a liver biopsy can be done immediately prior to tube placement) and a gastropexy are performed. The balloon on the Foley catheter is inflated for additional anchoring during the first few postoperative days. After a few days, the balloon usually ruptures, but by this time adhesions have formed at the site of the gastropexy, and this is sufficient to prevent leakage of stomach contents into the peritoneal cavity. The site of entry of the tube through the skin into the stomach should be covered with a 4×4 in gauze sponge to which an antibiotic ointment has been applied. A light wrap is then used to cover the incision site, and it is made wide enough to prevent exposure of the tube entry even if some slippage of the bandage occurs. The end of the tube is tightly stoppered and left exposed so that gruel can be administered. After each administration of gruel, the tube should be flushed with water. If the cat bothers the tube, an Elizabethan collar should be applied to prevent tube removal. The bandage should be changed and the wound cleaned every 3 to 5 days. The owner should be instructed to offer a highly palatable food to tempt the cat to eat frequently. Sometimes it is necessary to withhold tube-feeding temporarily in order to see if the patient is interested in eating. The gastrostomy tube must be left in place until the cat is eating and drinking adequate amounts on its own (usually 1 to 12 weeks).

Balanced electrolyte solutions such as lactated Ringer's are recommended if parenteral fluids are required to help maintain hydration. As previously mentioned, administration of parenteral glucose solutions without adequate oral caloric intake may worsen hepatic lipid accumulation.

B complex and fat-soluble vitamins can be mixed into the oral feeding preparations. Coagulation abnormalities are sometimes present and can be the result of either malabsorption of vitamin K, as a result of prolonged cholestasis, or decreased hepatic synthesis of various clotting factors. Administration of vitamin K_1 (Aquamephyton, Merck, Sharp & Dohme), 2 to 5 mg/kg/day SC divided t.i.d. for 5 to 7 days, is indicated if abnormalities of coagulation are documented.

The use of lipotrophic compounds containing choline and methionine is not justified. In dogs with hepatic insufficiency, it has been shown that methionine may precipitate HE.

Stress on the patient should be minimized. The cat should be sent home as soon as it is feasible for the owner to provide the daily care required. The dedication and amount of time and patience required of both the owner and veterinarian must be understood from the outset.

Other treatment measures have been tried but are *unproved* at this time. Carnitine (USA International), 250 to 500 mg s.i.d., may be supplemented in the gruel during the time the cat is being tube-fed. No adverse effects have been observed, and this drug is discontinued when the patient starts to eat adequately on its own. Some clinicians have advocated low doses of insulin to help prevent lipolysis and improve hepatic secretion of VLDL. Because of the sensitivity of cats to insulin and the potential for hypoglycemia, the use of insulin is not advised unless the cat is diabetic. Glucocorticoids should probably be avoided since they will worsen muscle catabolism and wasting and stimulate lipolysis, causing increased delivery of fatty acids to the liver.

Prognosis

Better success is now being achieved in cats with IHL, but the prognosis should still be considered guarded at best. Early diagnosis and aggressive management are essential if the disorder is to be reversed. Otherwise, most severely affected cats die of hepatic failure. Especially important is early, meticulous, consistent caloric and fluid replacement until the cat will eat and drink adequate amounts on its own. With early diagnosis, a dedicated owner, and appropriate management, many of these patients will completely recover. Recurrence of IHL in a cat appears to be uncommon, but the owner should be warned that obesity is a risk factor. Weight control achieved by not overfeeding is strongly advised.

References and Supplemental Reading

Alpers, D. H., and Isselbacher, K. J.: Fatty liver: biochemical and clinical aspects. *In* Schiff, L. (ed.): *Diseases of the Liver*, 4th ed. Philadelphia: J. B. Lippincott Co., 1975, p. 818.

Burrows, C. F., Chiapella, A. M., and Jezyk, P.: Idiopathic feline hepatic lipidosis: The syndrome and speculations on its pathogenesis. Fla. Vet. Winter: 18–20, 1981.

Center, S. A.: Hepatic lipidosis in the cat. Proc. of Fourth Annual ACVIM Forum, 1986, pp. 13–71 through 13–79.

Chapoy, P. R., Angelini, C., Brown, W. J., et al.: Systemic carnitine deficiency—a treatable inherited lipid storage disease presenting as Reye's syndrome. N. Engl. J. Med. 303:1389, 1980.

Crowe, D. T.: Clinical use of an indwelling nasogastric tube for enteral nutrition and fluid therapy in the dog and cat. J. Am. Anim. Hosp. Assoc. 22:675, 1986.

McGarry, J. D., and Foster, D. W.: Systemic carnitine deficiency (editorial). N. Engl. J. Med. 303:1413, 1980.

Morris, J. G., and Rogers, Q. R.: Nutritional implications of some metabolic anomalies in the cat. Proc. Am. Anim. Hosp. Assoc. 50:325, 1983.

Rogers, K. S., and Cornelius, L. M.: Feline icterus. Comp. Cont. Ed. Pract. Vet. 7:391, 1985.

Vierling, J. M.: Hepatobiliary complications of ulcerative colitis and Crohn's disease. *In* Zakim, D. and Boyer, T. C. (eds.): *Hepatology: A Textbook of Liver Disease*. Philadelphia: W. B. Saunders Co., 1982, pp. 797–824.

Zakim, D.: Metabolism of glucose and fatty acids by the liver. *In* Zakim, D., Boyer, T. C. (eds.): *Hepatology: A Textbook of Liver Disease*. Philadelphia: W. B. Saunders Co., 1982, pp. 76–109.

SERUM BILE ACID CONCENTRATIONS FOR HEPATOBILIARY FUNCTION TESTING IN CATS

S. A. CENTER, D.V.M.

Ithaca, New York

Liver disease is a common diagnosis in feline patients. Clinical signs are often vague and have an insidious onset. Signs commonly include lethargy, weight loss, intermittent vomiting or diarrhea, inappetence, unkempt appearance due to decreased grooming, pyrexia, behavior changes, ptyalism, hepatomegaly, and jaundice. A presumptive diagnosis of liver disease is made on the basis of screening observations derived from history, physical examination, and routine laboratory tests. The definitive diagnosis is confirmed by hepatobiliary function testing and biopsy.

ROUTINE LABORATORY TESTING

Hematologic abnormalities may include alterations in erythrocyte morphology (poikilocytosis), anemia (regenerative or nonregenerative), and changes in the leukogram indicating inflammation, sepsis (leukocytosis ± left shift), or endotoxemia (leukopenia). Mild thrombocytopenia develops in certain instances.

The most commonly used screening tests include the serum activities of liver enzymes: alkaline phosphatase (ALP), gamma-glutamyltransferase (GGT), alanine aminotransferase (ALT, formerly SGPT), aspartate aminotransferase (AST, formerly SGOT), and measurement of total bilirubin. Increased serum activity of the transaminases is common. These enzymes have high sensitivity but only moderate specificity for the detection of clinically important hepatobiliary disorders. Increased serum activity of ALP is highly specific for feline liver disease, but it is relatively insensitive. The serum activity of GGT is more sensitive but less specific than ALP. Simultaneous evaluation of ALP and GGT improves the diagnostic efficacy of each enzyme in the cat.

Hyperbilirubinemia is common in cats showing clinical signs of liver disease. The detection of bilirubinuria may precede the recognition of hyperbilirubinemia or jaundice. The consistent detection of bilirubin in feline urine is undeniably abnormal at any urine specific gravity. Although bilirubin is a useful test of liver function, anicteric liver disease is common enough in cats to warrant the availability of more sensitive testing methods.

LIVER FUNCTION TESTS

Tests designed to evaluate the functional integrity of the hepatobiliary system are indicated when screening tests provide a high index of suspicion for liver disease. These tests are especially appropriate in the anicteric patient. Once nonhemolytic jaundice is recognized, liver function testing is usually superfluous. The detection of functional hepatobiliary impairment requires the measurement of substances synthesized, regulated, metabolized, or excreted by this system. Exogenous or endogenous substances may be used as function tests. The cholephilic organic anion dyes, sulfobromophthalein (BSP) and indocyanine green (ICG), have been used extensively in dogs. ICG seems to be a better test in cats than is BSP, although the use of either substance in cats is limited by the rapid rate of plasma dye clearance in cats at the conventional canine doses. Since bilirubin competes with the hepatic uptake, metabolism, and excretion of the organic anion dyes, these dyes are invalid for testing liver function in the presence of hyperbilirubinemia.

Several endogenous substances that fulfill the criteria for function testing include glucose, albumin, cholesterol, fibrinogen, bilirubin, ammonia, and bile acids. Unfortunately, the first five of these

substances undergo other important metabolic interactions that invalidate strict interpretation of their serum concentrations as indicators of hepatocellular function. The serum activity of liver enzymes cannot be considered to be function tests since liver enzymes may increase as a result of transient reversible or irreversible alterations in the permeability of hepatocellular membranes, cell death, or enzyme induction.

The estimation of ammonia tolerance is considered a sensitive method for assessment of hepatic function. Unfortunately, baseline ammonia concentrations are unreliable indicators of ammonia tolerance. Patients showing signs consistent with hepatic encephalopathy may have normal baseline blood ammonia values, since there are many other toxins responsible for hepatoencephalopathic signs. Inability to regulate blood ammonia is best assessed by a provocative test of ammonia tolerance completed by the oral or rectal administration of ammonium chloride (100 mg/kg). This test challenges the integrity of the portal circulation and hepatocellular function. There are, however, several major drawbacks in the use of the ammonia tolerance test (ATT). Ammonium chloride is unpalatable and therefore must be given by orogastric tube, in a gelatin capsule, or by rectal administration as a retention enema. The oral administration of ammonium chloride may induce vomiting, which will invalidate the provocative nature of the test. Rectal administration is cumbersome and requires a cleansing enema before instillation of the ammonium chloride. Diarrhea precludes this avenue of ammonium chloride delivery. In addition, administration of exogenous ammonia runs the risk of inducing encephalopathic signs, although this is rare. The analysis of blood ammonia requires strict attention to the expediency of sample collection, management, and analysis. A control sample *must* be evaluated with each set of clinical samples as quality control against sample mismanagement and as a guarantee of optimal assay performance. Ammonia is labile in blood, and consequently blood samples must be expediently transported to the laboratory on ice for plasma separation, preferably completed in a refrigerated centrifuge. Plasma should be assayed immediately (within hours), as plasma frozen for 24 to 72 hr gives variable results. The assay of blood ammonia cannot at present be completed on blood handled in a routine manner or mailed to a laboratory. Because of the inconveniences encountered with the use of the ATT, further investigations into more practical and convenient methods of assessing hepatobiliary function have been completed. The search for other methods that have equivalent sensitivity to the ATT has led to the adaptation of serum bile acid concentrations as a test of liver function.

SERUM BILE ACIDS

The use of serum bile acids as a test of liver function has become increasingly popular in humans and in companion animals because they are endogenous substances that may be routinely and conveniently measured. They have been shown to be equal in sensitivity to the ATT in patients with portosystemic vascular anomalies, to be more dependable than testing with BSP or ICG, and to be more convenient for use in clinical practice. They may be used in hyperbilirubinemic patients when liver function testing seems necessary to differentiate the cause of jaundice as they do not compete with bilirubin for transport or metabolism as do the organic anion dyes (BSP and ICG). It is important to realize that the serum bile acid test is not meant to be used alone but, rather, in an adjunctive capacity with the other routine screening tests. Many clinicians are currently using the bile acid test to detect portosystemic vascular anomalies and severe occult liver disease, in decision analysis in assessing the need for hepatic biopsy, and to follow the progress of patients under treatment for liver disease.

BILE ACID METABOLISM

Understanding the normal physiologic role and metabolism of bile acids improves the clincian's ability to interpret bile acid concentrations as a measure of hepatic function.

The primary bile acids (cholic acid and chenodeoxycholic acid) are synthesized in the liver from cholesterol. A small portion of the primary bile acids are converted to the secondary bile acids (cholic acid → deoxycholic acid, chenodeoxycholic acid → lithocholic acid) by the endogenous intestinal flora. Bile acids are conjugated to an amino acid (taurine in cats) in the liver. The bile acid conjugation with amino acid is physiologically important in that it increases their water solubility and miscibility. Clinically, the amino acid conjugation is important in that it affects the validity of bile acid analysis completed by radioimmunoassay. The measurement of glycoconjugates by radioimmunoassay in dogs and cats cannot be recommended, as these species do not primarily conjugate their bile acids to glycine. An enzymatic procedure in common use measures total serum bile acid concentrations. In this assay, the amino acid conjugation is irrelevant.

Following synthesis and amino acid conjugation, bile acids are secreted into the biliary network and transported to the gallbladder, where they are stored and concentrated. At mealtimes, neurohumoral and hormonal mediators stimulate bile flow and contraction of the gallbladder. The bile acids are expelled into the intestinal lumen, where they facilitate fat digestion and absorption. Reabsorption occurs throughout the small bowel, but most occurs

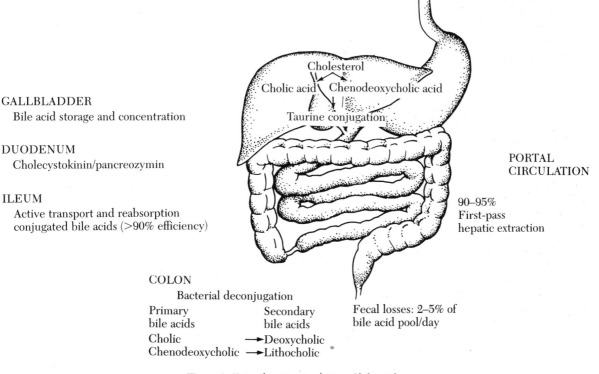

GALLBLADDER
Bile acid storage and concentration

DUODENUM
Cholecystokinin/pancreozymin

ILEUM
Active transport and reabsorption
conjugated bile acids (>90% efficiency)

Cholesterol
Cholic acid   Chenodeoxycholic acid
Taurine conjugation

PORTAL CIRCULATION

90–95%
First-pass
hepatic extraction

COLON
Bacterial deconjugation

Primary bile acids	Secondary bile acids
Cholic	→ Deoxycholic
Chenodeoxycholic	→ Lithocholic

Fecal losses: 2–5% of bile acid pool/day

Figure 1. Enterohepatic circulation of bile acids.

by an efficient active process in the ileum resulting in loss of only 2 to 5 per cent of the bile acid pool in the feces each day. After intestinal absorption, bile acids enter the portal circulation and are directly transported to the liver, where they are extracted on first pass in a system that is 90 to 95 per cent efficient. During and immediately after meals, the bile acid pool recycles between two and five times. This highly efficient enterohepatic circulation allows a small bile acid pool to satisfy normal physiologic functions (Fig. 1).

The extremely efficient enterohepatic circulation of bile acids results in only a very small amount of bile acids "spilling over" into the systemic circulation. In health, fasting bile acid concentrations are usually below postprandial values. Although bile acids are exclusively synthesized in the liver, hepatic failure does not seem to limit their serum concentration. There is a tremendous reserve capacity for bile acid synthesis that is rarely if ever maximally utilized. Liver disease or interruptions in the portal circulation result in increased serum bile acid concentrations.

In health, serum bile acid values increase 2 hours following a meal. The postprandial values represent the ability of the hepatobiliary system to cope with the provocative bile acid challenge following meal-induced gallbladder contraction and efficient intestinal absorption. The postprandial values may be more discriminant in the detection of hepatobiliary dysfunction than are the fasting values. It is recommended that a 12-hr fasting and a 2-hr postprandial concentration be measured to maximize the diagnostic utility of bile acids, since it appears that the relative change or pattern observed after eating may have some predictive capabilities.

Although controversial, it has been shown that certain bile acids accumulate in association with particular types of hepatobiliary injury (e.g., cholestasis) and may be used to predict the type of disease processes prior to hepatic biopsy. Nevertheless, the quantification of specific bile acid moieties in humans and animals with liver disease has not shown them to be more informative than measurement of the total serum bile acid concentration in the detection of hepatobiliary dysfunction. Furthermore, discrimination of specific bile acid moieties requires methodologies too laborious and expensive for routine clinical application.

Technique for Performing the Bile Acid Test

To maximize the diagnostic information from total serum bile acid measurement, a 12-hr fasting and a 2-hr postprandial serum sample should be obtained. The diet used to stimulate gastric emptying and subsequent gallbladder contraction should be similar in protein and fat content to p/d (dogs) and c/d

(cats) (Hill's Pet Products). These diets contain formulations for which the 2-hr postprandial interval seems to work optimally. Diets with lower fat and protein content do not seem to consistently challenge the bile acid enterohepatic circulation at the 2-hr postprandial interval. If a patient is inappetent, a small amount of food may be force-fed (1 to 2 tsp/cat). If a patient has encephalopathic tendencies, a low-protein meal mixed with a few milliliters of corn oil has proved sufficient. Avoid excess oil in the food, because extreme lipemia complicates the chemical analysis of bile acids. If a patient is vomiting, measurement of a random fasting value is recommended. In these cases, the shortcomings of a single fasting bile acid concentration must be considered when test results are interpreted.

Since bile acids are stable in serum at room temperature for several days, samples may be delivered or mailed to the laboratory without the haste required with measurement of blood ammonia. Serum samples may be frozen at $-20°C$ until they are routinely mailed for analysis. Hemolysis complicates the enzymatic method of total serum bile acid analysis, and serum should therefore be separated from whole blood prior to shipping.

Determinants of the Serum Bile Acid Concentration

Use of serum bile acids as an endogenous test of liver function necessitates consideration of the variables influencing their serum concentration. Delayed gastric emptying may delay gallbladder contraction and hence the presentation of bile acids to the intestines. Delayed intestinal transit may also interfere with presentation of bile acids to the ileum, where maximal absorption occurs. These variables may influence the serum concentrations attained after a 12-hr fast and during the 2-hr postprandial interval. In addition to these variables, ileal diseases associated with fat malabsorption may interfere with bile acid absorption, leading to reduced serum bile acid concentrations. Intestinal diseases involving the ileum and causing steatorrhea, however, are rare in dogs and seem even more uncommon in cats.

It is important to remember that the bile acid test relies on the integrity of the enterohepatic circulation as well as on hepatobiliary function. With the exception of intestinal (ileal) malabsorption, any aberration in the enterohepatic circulation of bile acids causes an increase in their serum concentration—that is, portosystemic vascular anomalies, intrahepatic arterioportal fistulae, acquired portosystemic shunts, and acquired hepatic dysfunction including (but not limited to) such conditions as diffuse lipidosis, cholangiohepatitis, severe fibrosis, and cirrhosis. No matter how severe liver dysfunction seems, bile acid concentrations will *always* be increased. Synthetic failure is never reflected in a subnormal serum bile acid concentration.

Bile Acid Concentrations: Normal vs. Abnormal

In cats, normal fasting serum concentrations are ≤ 5 μmol/L, whereas normal 2-hr postprandial bile acid concentrations are ≤ 10 μmol/L, using the enzymatic procedure for measuring 3-alpha hydroxylated bile acids. As with all laboratory tests, there is a "gray zone" that is prudent to respect when interpreting test results. On the basis of laboratory evaluation of more than 75 cats with histologically confirmed liver disease, values between 10 and 20 μmol/L warrant a conservative approach of watchful waiting, whereas values greater than 20 μmol/L have dependably been associated with substantial morphologic evidence of hepatic disease or disruptions in the portosystemic circulation.

Application of Bile Acid Concentrations in Feline Liver Disease

Bile acid concentrations exceeding 20 μmol/L indicate the need for liver biopsy in our clinical patients. In patients with increased liver enzymes, the bile acid test helps decide whether aggressive diagnostic efforts are appropriate early in the course of the disease. If bile acid values are normal, we

recommend supportive therapy; watch and wait and *recheck the values in 2 weeks*. If the bile acid values exceed 20 μmol/L in the cat, a liver biopsy should be considered. In patients with normal bile acid concentrations but persistently increased liver enzymes (> 2 to 4 weeks), hyperthyroidism is ruled out on the basis of serum T_4 concentration, and a careful re-examination of history, physical, and laboratory data is completed to identify secondary disorders such as systemic infection or gastrointestial disease that could influence the hepatic enzyme activity. If secondary disorders are not identified, a liver biopsy is recommended. In cats with portosystemic shunts or cirrhosis, the serum bile acid test is as sensitive, as reliable, more convenient, and probably safer for the patient than the ammonia tolerance test.

Bile acid concentrations in cats with various forms of liver disease are shown in Figure 2. There is a wide variation and overlap of values between different diseases. There is no indication that varying magnitudes of difference correlate with different degrees of hepatobiliary dysfunction.

Patients with portosystemic shunts or cirrhosis may have fasting bile acid concentrations that are either markedly increased or within the normal range. The basic functional disturbances in these conditions are similar in that there is reduced functional hepatic mass and shunting of blood around normal sinusoidal pathways. With a prolonged fast, the chance for continued circulation of systemic blood (hepatic arterial supply) to the liver

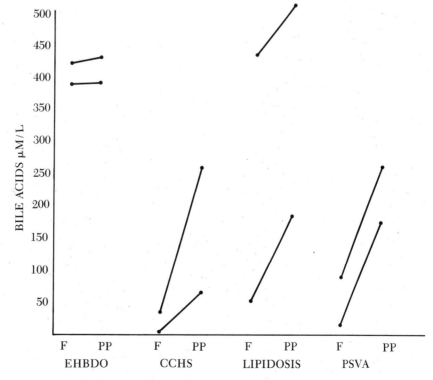

Figure 2. Serum bile acid concentrations in cats (n = 2 for each disease) with extrahepatic bile duct obstruction (EHBDO), cholangitis cholangiohepatitis syndrome (CCHS), hepatic lipidosis, and portosystemic vascular anomaly (PSVA) (F, 12-hr fasting; PP, 2-hr postprandial). (New York State College of Veterinary Medicine, Cornell University, 1987.)

provides a route by which functioning hepatocytes have the opportunity to extract bile acids. This continued extraction during a prolonged fast explains the normal values observed in some patients with severely reduced hepatic function or altered hepatoportal circulation. However, following a meal, the time-limited interval restricts the opportunity for continued bile acid extraction from the systemic circulation. In this circumstance, the serum bile acid concentration increases dramatically. Patients with severe cholestasis have markedly increased fasting bile acid concentrations that may remain unchanged or increase only slightly following a meal. This pattern is typical of extrahepatic bile duct obstruction and certain other disorders associated with severe cholestasis (hepatic lipidosis in cats). Other feline hepatobiliary disorders associated with cholestasis have associated circulatory or hepatocellular dysfunction that also may influence the bile acid concentrations, and hence different patterns of relative change may be observed between the fasting and postprandial intervals.

In conclusion, the relative changes in bile acid concentrations between the fasting and 2-hr postprandial samples may allow prediction of shunting lesions (cirrhosis, portosystemic vascular anomalies) or severe cholestasis. Further diagnostic extrapola-

tions from the serum bile acid concentrations are not recommended. A definitive diagnosis cannot be made on the basis of this test. It must be accepted that hepatic function tests are best used adjunctively with other routine tests for the detection of liver disease. Their major clinical utility should be to support a definitive diagnosis of hepatobiliary disease, to indicate the need for hepatic biopsy, and to monitor a patient's response to treatment.

References and Supplemental Reading

Barnes, S., Gallo, G. A., Trash, D. B., et al.: Diagnostic value of serum bile acid estimations in liver disease. J. Clin. Pathol. 28:506, 1975.

Center, S. A.: Feline liver disorders and their management. Comp. Cont. Ed. Pract. Vet. 8:889, 1987.

Center, S. A., Baldwin, B. H., deLahunta, A., et al.: Evaluation of serum bile acid concentrations for the diagnosis of portosystemic venous anomalies in the dog and cat. J.A.V.M.A. 186:1090, 1985.

Center, S. A., Baldwin, B. H., Erb, H., et al.: Bile acid concentrations in the diagnosis of hepatobiliary disease in the cat. J.A.V.M.A. 189:891, 1986.

Center, S. A., Bunch, S. E., Baldwin, B. H., et al.: Comparison of sulfobromophthalein and indocyanine green clearances in the cat. Am. J. Vet. Res. 44:727, 1983.

Festi, D., Morselli Labate, A. M., Roda, A., et al.: Diagnostic effectiveness of serum bile acids in liver diseases as evaluated by multivariate statistical methods. Hepatology 3:707, 1983.

Kaplowitz, N., Kok, E., and Javitt, N. B.: Postprandial serum bile acid for the detection of hepatobiliary disease. J.A.M.A. 225:292, 1973.

Meyer, D. J.: Liver function tests in dogs with portosystemic shunts: Measurement of serum bile acid concentration. J.A.V.M.A. 188:168, 1986.

DRUG-INDUCED HEPATIC DISEASE OF DOGS AND CATS

SUSAN E. BUNCH, D.V.M.
Raleigh, North Carolina

It has been said that adverse drug reactions represent one of the penalties that the medical profession pays for progress. It is the intent of this chapter to review, and put into perspective, adverse drug reactions in dogs and cats for which the target organ is the liver. Only medicinal agents, defined as any chemical compound used in the diagnosis or treatment of disease in humans or animals, will be considered.

GENERAL CONCEPTS OF DRUG-ASSOCIATED ADVERSE HEPATIC REACTIONS

The liver is susceptible to toxic injury directly and indirectly as a result of its critical role in metabolism of foreign substances. Intense exposure to high concentrations of ingested compounds via generous portal circulation, as well as essential participation in biotransformation of many orally and parenterally administered agents, accounts for the vulnerability of the liver to adverse drug reactions. Generation of potentially toxic metabolites from otherwise harmless parent compounds is the mechanism believed to be the basis of hepatic injury caused by many therapeutic agents in human medicine. Factors known to contribute to formation of toxic metabolites include genetic predisposition, age, sex, concurrent administration of glutathione-depleting or microsomal enzyme-altering chemicals, and nutritional imbalances.

Drugs are an important cause of both acute and

chronic hepatic disease in human medicine and can produce histologic lesions that mimic any primary hepatobiliary disease. A classification scheme for hepatotoxic substances based on mechanism of action and typical histologic lesion was first devised by Zimmerman in 1968 and remains useful for most acute adverse hepatic reactions today (Table 1). **Intrinsic** hepatotoxins according to this scheme predictably cause dose-dependent hepatic injury in both humans and in experimental animals. Adverse reactions usually are observed soon after administration. *Direct intrinsic* hepatotoxins, which damage hepatocytes structurally, generally are not in clinical use today. *Indirect intrinsic* hepatotoxic agents, however, cause hepatic injury by alteration of specific metabolic pathways, the ultimate result of which may be hepatocellular dysfunction (e.g., cholestasis) or cell death. Some drugs that are classified in the intrinsic category but that do not behave as purely direct or indirect hepatotoxins are categorized as *mixed*. **Idiosyncratic reactions** are the result of unique susceptibility, so dosage and duration of treatment are not important contributing elements. Instead, immunologic interactions may be responsible, manifested by classic signs of allergy such as fever, skin rash, lymphadenopathy, eosinophilia, and autoantibody production. In nonhypersensitive individuals, genetically influenced metabolic aberrations in drug-metabolizing enzyme systems may account for more rapid generation of injurious toxic intermediates. There is no adequate scheme to categorize chronic drug-induced adverse hepatic reactions, so they are classified primarily by histologic lesion.

COMPARATIVE ASPECTS OF HUMAN AND ANIMAL HEPATOTOXICTY

Several studies of human patients have determined the overall frequency of drug-induced adverse hepatic reactions to be relatively low. Such investigations have not been carried out in veterinary medicine, but it is reasonable to suggest on the basis of published literature and clinical experience that clinically significant adverse hepatic reactions to drugs in small animals are unusual. As a cause of fulminant hepatic failure in human patients, however, therapeutic agents assume a much more important role, with up to 25 per cent of these cases attributable to drug therapy.

All drugs documented as having adverse effects on the human liver as of 1983 were recently compiled. The list totaled more than 120 drugs, half of which are also currently used in veterinary medicine. More than ten of these, as well as certain drugs used only in animals (e.g., mibolerone), are believed to be hepatotoxic in dogs and, occasionally, in cats (Table 2). When an adverse hepatic reaction is suspected to be associated with a drug not known to cause hepatic damage in animals, the attending clinician customarily reviews the human literature to learn whether such a response has been observed in human patients and whether a valid association might be made. Conversely, the presumption under which most toxicologic studies of drugs for human use are conducted is that drug-induced hepatic injury in experimental animals is predictive of what will occur in human patients. An investigation was conducted to determine, retrospectively, whether results of laboratory animal toxicity studies could be reliably extrapolated to humans. It is interesting to note that of eight therapeutic agents for which there was information about responses of both humans and laboratory dogs or cats, only three of these eight drugs caused significant histologic or clinicopathologic evidence of hepatic injury, and five drugs caused minimal to no histologic changes in the liver and mild to no abnormalities in clinical chemistry test results. The findings from this study support the conclusion that assigning hepatotoxicity by extrapolating data between species may be misleading, and that species' reactions should be considered separately.

Most adverse hepatic reactions described in client-owned dogs and cats have been idiosyncratic or indirect intrinsic reactions associated with demonstrable parenchymal injury. When hepatic tissue has been obtained for histologic examination, the lesion is most often one of necrosis, regardless of the agent suspected. Indirect intrinsic hepatotoxins that cause rapidly reversible "benign" or "bland" cholestasis in human patients, without histologic or ultrastructural evidence of injury, have been stud-

Table 1. Mechanisms of Hepatic Injury Due to Drugs in Humans

Category	Mechanism	Lesion	Example
Intrinsic toxicity			
Direct	Direct cellular injury	Necrosis, steatosis, or both	CCl_4
Indirect (cytotoxic)	Interference with metabolic pathways leading to cell damage	Steatosis or necrosis	Ethanol MTX*
Indirect (cholestatic)	Interference with bile excretion	Bilirubin casts	MT*
Host idiosyncracy			
Increased sensitivity	Drug allergy	Necrosis or cholestasis	Phenytoin
Metabolic aberration	Enzyme defect?	Necrosis or cholestasis	Isoniazid

*MTX, methotrexate; MT, methyltestosterone.

Table 2. *Contemporary Drugs Known or Suspected to be Hepatotoxic in Dogs and Cats*

Mebendazole (dogs)
Diethylcarbamazine (*Dirofilaria immitis* microfilariae positive-dogs)
Thiacetarsemide (dogs)
Diethylcarbamazine-oxibendazole (dogs)
Halothane (dogs)
Methoxyflurane (dogs)
Trimethoprim-sulfadiazine (dogs)
Griseofulvin (cats)
Acetaminophen (dogs, cats)
Glucocorticoids (dogs)
Mibolerone (dogs)
Megesterol acetate (cats)
Primidone, phenytoin (dogs)

---

ied in animals experimentally but have not been incriminated in spontaneous cases of hepatotoxicity.

CLINICALLY SIGNIFICANT DRUG-INDUCED HEPATOTOXICITY IN DOGS AND CATS

Acute Hepatic Injury

Anthelmintics

First approved for use as a broad-spectrum anthelmintic for dogs in 1977, **mebendazole** (Telmintic, Pitman-Moore) was considered safe and effective according to results of toxicologic studies. Several clinical reports have been published since then, describing serious adverse hepatic reactions. In one report, the hepatic status of six of nine dogs changed after mebendazole was given at recommended dosages. Four of six dogs developed jaundice, vomiting, and biochemical evidence of hepatobiliary disease within 2 weeks after administration. Coagulopathy was detected in two of four dogs during routine testing before hepatic biopsy. Two dogs died, and two dogs recovered with supportive care. Identical histologic lesions consisting of severe centrilobular necrosis were observed in hepatic tissue specimens from three of four dogs. Laboratory testing of five asymptomatic dogs from the same kennel identified slowly reversible abnormal hepatic enzyme activities in two dogs. Another case report about one dog that died was published 1 year later, with similar clinical signs, laboratory test results, and histologic findings as the earlier report. During the first 3 years after mebendazole was released for use in the United States, the Food and Drug Administration's Center for Veterinary Medicine (CVM) received 57 complaints regarding 544 treated dogs, 228 of which had adverse reactions including poor response to treatment and hepatotoxicity. There were 23 deaths among the adverse reactions believed to be directly related to drug use. Repeat toxicologic studies conducted in poodles, Irish setters, and mixed-breed dogs failed to confirm predictable toxicity despite high long-term dosages and conditions known to alter hepatocellular function and integrity (e.g., use of carbon tetrachloride or barbiturates, glutathione depletion, and hypoxia). It is interesting to note that all five of the most severely affected published clinical cases were females, two of which were siblings. Failure to reproduce the clinical syndrome experimentally under recommended conditions and in the presence of hepatic compromise suggests that the infrequent adverse hepatic reaction to mebendazole is idiosyncratic, perhaps the result of metabolic aberration.

Diethylcarbamazine (DEC) generally is used with impunity in dogs for heartworm prophylaxis. There is no evidence to indicate that DEC is directly injurious to the liver. When given to dogs with patent *Dirofilaria immitis* infections, however, an adverse drug reaction characterized by potentially fatal hypovolemic shock may be observed. Recent investigations have clarified the pathogenesis of this reaction, which results from DEC-stimulated release of substances from microfilariae that induce hepatic vein constriction. Signs of depression, hyporesponsiveness, inappropriate defecation, and vomiting are seen within the first 30 to 60 min after DEC is given. Cardiac depression, manifested by bradycardia and poor pulse quality, immediately precedes obvious signs of shock. In dogs that survive, most signs regress within 3 hr of onset. Published morbidity and mortality rates are variable and may be attributable to biochemical characteristics of the microfilariae.

Vomiting, depression, hyperbilirubinuria, and jaundice associated with high hepatic enzyme activities in dogs given **thiacetarsemide** (Caparsolate, Ceva Labs) for adult heartworm treatment have been reported in the scientific literature as well as to the CVM. In human patients who react adversely to treatment for filariasis, it is not clear whether the mechanism is one of direct hepatocellular injury, which seems likely in animals, or of hypersensitivity. Single high doses of organic arsenic certainly can cause hepatic necrosis. There is no reason to believe that abnormal pretreatment hepatic enzyme activities predict adverse drug reactions or contraindicate use of thiacetarsamide, assuming a primary hepatobiliary disease has been ruled out. Therapy should be stopped if persistent emesis or jaundice develops or if bilirubinuria becomes excessive after the first or second dose (see p. 265).

Prevention of heartworm and hookworm infection in dogs is the indication for use of a combination product containing DEC and **oxibendazole** (Filaribits Plus, Norden). Within 1 year after its release, periportal hepatitis associated with use of this drug in seven dogs had been documented. Clinical signs of depression, anorexia, vomiting, diarrhea, polydipsia, polyuria, and weight loss were observed 2 to 4 weeks after drug administration. Improvement in clinical signs and serum biochemical abnormalities was seen soon after the drug was discontinued. In an additional six dogs, ongoing hepatic injury was suspected on the basis of persistent biochemical abnormalities. More severe hepatic damage may be related to continued administration of the drug past the time of onset of clinical signs, prompted by the importance of heartworm prevention having been underscored to clients by veterinarians. The Food and Drug Administration changed the product label as a result of some 300 reports to the CVM of adverse drug reactions of all kinds during the 1½ years following marketing. As with the related benzimidazole mebendazole, the adverse hepatic reaction is believed to be idiosyncratic.

Inhalation Anesthetics

Despite the frequent use of halogenated inhalation anesthetics in contemporary veterinary medicine, there have been only isolated reports of hepatic disease linked with their use in animals. **Methoxyflurane** (Metofane, Pitman-Moore) has been reported to have contributed in some way, either directly or indirectly, to the deaths of two dogs after repeated exposure. A similar sequence of events was purported to have caused the death of a dog after **halothane** (Fluothane, Ayerst) use. In all cases, illness developed within 1 week after the most recent exposure, and the major histologic lesion in the liver was centrilobular necrosis with a mixed inflammatory infiltrate. Considering other factors involved at the time in each case (e.g., multiple drug use, undetected concurrent illness, prolonged time of anesthesia), it is difficult to state with confidence that the inhalation anesthetic caused hepatic failure. Changes in hepatic blood flow, microsomal enzyme induction, generation of reactive halothane metabolites that bind covalently to cellular macromolecules, and hypoxia are some of the factors now well known to contribute to the development of "halothane hepatopathy" in human patients. Each of these is a possible contributing factor in many veterinary patients receiving halothane. Halothane is considered no more hepatotoxic than other halogenated inhalation anesthetics, and patients with pre-existing hepatic disease are at no greater risk of having an adverse hepatic reaction. It would be prudent to select another inhalation anesthetic for a patient with a history of unexplained jaundice following previous exposure to halothane or to methoxyflurane.

Antimicrobials

Oral forms of **tetracycline** rarely cause hepatic dysfunction in human patients, although mild degrees of fatty infiltration can be seen in liver biopsy specimens. Derivatives of tetracycline, especially when given in large doses intravenously, are known to cause overt hepatic disease with a characteristic form of microvesicular fatty change in the liver of humans and laboratory dogs. Development of the lesion depends on maintenance of high blood levels, which are not achieved by oral administration, the route most commonly used in animals. The likelihood of iatrogenic hepatic disease caused by tetracycline in dogs and cats seems remote, unless clearance is delayed by renal or bile secretory failure. Documented reports of adverse hepatic reactions to tetracycline in treated dogs and cats are not available. Until the effects of orally administered tetracycline on the canine and feline liver are known, however, tetracycline use should be avoided in dogs or cats with diseases of which hepatic steatosis is a component, such as diabetes mellitus, hypothyroidism in dogs, and idiopathic fatty liver syndrome in cats.

Two separate anecdotal reports of jaundice in two dogs following 3 weeks of treatment with **trimethoprim-sulfadizaine** (TMS; Tribrissen, Coopers) have appeared in the veterinary literature. In one case, a drug-drug interaction may have been responsible for the adverse hepatic reaction, since two other medications were being given concurrently with TMS. Both dogs recovered rapidly after drug withdrawal. Another adverse drug reaction that has been ascribed to the sulfadiazine element of TMS affects Doberman pinschers in particular, causing immune-mediated vasculitis of the eyes, skin, muscles, kidneys, and joints. The liver apparently is spared in such cases. The clinical and histologic features of human patients with TMS-induced hepatic injury suggest that true hypersensitivity is responsible in most cases. Equivalent information is not available to allow precise characterization of TMS as a hepatotoxin in dogs and cats.

Commonly used for treatment of dermatophytosis in dogs and cats, **griseofulvin** (Fulvicin, Schering) has been reported to have caused undesirable side effects in seven cats given standard dosages for recommended periods of time. In two of seven cats, the liver was a target organ. Subsequent attempts to determine whether the hematologic (e.g., leukopenia) or hepatic biochemical test abnormalities described earlier would develop in clinically healthy cats failed to recreate the clinical syndrome. Existing information suggests that the most important unfavorable effect of griseofulvin in cats is teratogenicity rather than hepatotoxicity.

Analgesics

Acetaminophen is an effective nonnarcotic analgesic that is found in the medicine cabinet of many homes. Owners' sincere desire to relieve their pet's discomfort, coupled with lack of knowledge that overdose causes methemoglobinemia and hepatic necrosis and that there are marked species differences in susceptibility to toxicity, accounts for most cases of iatrogenic acetominophen toxicity in dogs and cats. At therapeutic doses, a majority of administered acetaminophen is excreted in the urine as glucuronide conjugates. Small quantities of reactive electrophilic metabolites are converted to a harmless substance by conjugation with glutathione in the liver. Toxicity results when glutathione stores are consumed to 30 per cent of normal, allowing reactive metabolites to bind covalently to vital cellular macromolecules. Dogs and cats can tolerate doses up to 100 mg/kg and 60 mg/kg, respectively, given once with minimal clinical and hematologic consequences and with no change in blood levels of glutathione. Significant illness occurs in dogs at a dose of 200 mg/kg and in cats at a dose of 120 mg/kg. Though microscopic lesions (centrilobular necrosis and congestion, hydropic degeneration, bile stasis) in the canine liver are more severe than in the feline liver, clinical toxicity is certainly more severe in cats. When they receive more than a certain dosage, cats are unable to increase excretion of acetaminophen by forming glucuronide conjugates because of a relative deficiency of hepatic glucuronyl transferase activity, leading to a relative overproduction of reactive metabolites that rapidly deplete available liver and erythrocyte glutathione. Despite the central role of the liver in the cause and effects of acetaminophen toxicity, the most devastating and potentially lethal effect in both dogs and cats that first prompts owners to seek veterinary care is cyanosis from severe methemaglobinemia. Hepatotoxic effects become apparent 24 to 36 hr later.

Chronic Hepatic Injury

Steroids

Results of experimental and retrospective clinical studies of dogs have shown that administration of various **glucocorticoids** or excess endogenous cortisol predictably induces a specific hepatic disorder in dogs as young as 11 weeks. Most dogs respond to excess glucocorticoids with high alkaline phosphatase (AP; 5- to 64-fold) and alanine transaminase (ALT; 3- to 10-fold) activities that may persist for as long as 42 days after drug withdrawal. The high AP activity is not stimulated by cholestasis, but by factors not yet understood. Modest delays in excretion of sulfobromophthalein (BSP) and retention of conjugated bile acids (usually < 50 μmol/L) have been observed in clinical cases of hypercortisolism and in some, but not all, experimentally created cases. The pattern of largely reversible histologic changes of centrilobular vacuolization and glycogen accumulation and rare hepatocyte necrosis seems unique to this exclusively canine syndrome. It is extremely unusual for steroid hepatopathy to progress to the point of hepatic failure.

Rare reports of jaundice and hepatotoxicity in cats given **megesterol acetate** (Ovaban, Schering) and in dogs given **mibolerone** (Cheque, Upjohn) for a prolonged time have been received by the CVM. Complications of megesterol treatment in cats are most often related to endocrine dysfunction rather than to hepatic disease. Mibolerone appears to be relatively safe in bitches, although hepatotoxicity and thyrotoxicity have been noted in cats after chronic administration. Current recommendations for use of mibolerone in bitches include evaluation of hepatic function at 6-month intervals.

Anticonvulsants

A wealth of information has become available in recent years about the hepatic effects of short- and long-term administration of anticonvulsant drugs in dogs. Results of early experimental studies in which phenytoin, primidone, or phenobarbital were given at low to recommended dosages for less than 90 days agree that increases in serum AP and ALT activities observed in a majority of dogs were not associated with morphologic evidence of serious hepatic injury. A more recent study, using recommended and excessive dosages of commonly used anticonvulsant drugs, was designed to resemble the clinical setting, in which dogs with seizure disorders usually require long-term drug therapy and often need increasing dosages of antiseizure medications because seizures are progressively more difficult to control. Dogs given conventional dosages of primidone or phenytoin remained clinically healthy throughout the 6-month treatment period. Fatal toxic hepatopathy did develop in three of eight dogs given primidone and phenytoin in combination at higher dosages and for longer periods of time than in the previous studies. In the same study, dogs given phenytoin or primidone alone did not have as severe ultrastructural changes in the liver as did dogs given both drugs at the same time. It is interesting to note that two clinical reports have described jaundice and hepatic failure in four dogs in a manner nearly identical to the three dogs of the experimental investigation. To determine the overall frequency of compromised hepatic function in anticonvulsant-treated dogs with seizure disorders, the hepatic status of 48 dogs that had received primidone, phenytoin, or a combination of anticonvulsant drugs for 6 months or longer was evaluated. The proportion of dogs believed to have serious hepatic consequences from extended anticonvulsant drug therapy estimated from this retrospective analysis was 6 to 15 per cent. In this series of dogs, abnormalities of liver-specific enzyme activities and BSP excretion were noted most often in dogs given primidone or a combination of anticonvulsant drugs. Another infrequent manifestation of chronic anticonvulsant drug therapy is cirrhosis, which has been seen in dogs given primidone for several years. From the findings in these studies, it is clear that hepatic disease associated with long-term use of anticonvulsant drugs does occur in dogs, with a relatively low overall frequency.

DIAGNOSIS

The basis for diagnosis of adverse hepatic reactions often is circumstantial evidence. Since the clinical signs, laboratory test results, and histologic findings of drug-induced hepatic disease in dogs and cats are unique only to the type and degree of hepatic injury, a detailed, accurate history becomes the fundamental principle of diagnosis. All therapeutic agents given, including those approved for human use that the owner has administered for symptomatic relief, as well as those to which the animal has been exposed in the veterinary hospital, should be identified. The dosage, duration of treatment, and onset and progression of clinical signs all are important in determining whether a valid association might be made between drug use and development of illness. A reasonable temporal sequence of events following the administration of a drug and a known pattern of response to the drug are firm support for a link. Because most drug-induced hepatic diseases are potentially reversible, as compared with other primary canine and feline hepatopathies, the temptation to overinterpret the drug history must, however, be resisted. Improvement in hepatic status following withdrawal of the offending agent, provided the extent of hepatic injury has not been massive, contributes further support that the cause of ongoing, active hepatic injury has been removed. If recovery is slow, hepatic biopsy assumes greater importance in gaining prognostic information and in ruling out other hepatic diseases if possible.

Specific methods to identify animals that are susceptible to toxicity are not available at this time. The most conclusive evidence of drug toxicity is return of hepatic disease on rechallenging the patient. This practice becomes rational only when the drug is one for which there is no substitute or the initial adverse hepatic reaction had been mild. For most of the drugs that are known or suspected to be hepatotoxic in dogs and cats, there are alternative choices that offer similar therapeutic benefit, so that reinstitution of the causative agent is indicated only to document and characterize the reaction.

TREATMENT

Immediate suspension of drug administration is the treatment of choice for most drug-induced hepatopathies of dogs and cats. Lack of documentation of immune-mediated hypersensitivity reactions to drugs in animals precludes logical use of corticosteroids, when time and supportive care would be as beneficial. In dogs with anticonvulsant drug-induced hepatic disease in which antiseizure medication must be sustained, gradual conversion over 7 to 10 days to single-drug therapy with phenobarbital while monitoring serum phenobarbital levels (therapeutic range: 15 to 45 μg/ml) is indicated.

There is only one drug for which there is a specific antidote in the event of overdose, especially in cats: acetaminophen. Replacement of depleted glutathione prevents binding of reactive metabolites to essential macromolecules, if started early enough. If poisoning has occurred within 2 hours, vomiting should be induced, activated charcoal should be given (2 gm/kg body weight), and a sodium sulfate cathartic administered (0.5 gm/kg body weight as a 20 per cent slurry PO). If cyanosis is already present, oxygen should be given and stress minimized. Oral or intravenous administration of glutathione precursors such as N-acetylcysteine (NAC; Mucomyst, Bristol) should be initiated as soon as possible: NAC, 140 mg/kg PO or IV as a 20 per cent solution for the first dose, regardless of time since poisoning, repeated in 6 hr and every 6 hr thereafter at a dosage of 70 mg/kg for a *total* of seven treatments. Ascorbic acid should be given at the same time intervals as NAC (30 mg/kg PO).

USE OF DRUGS IN ANIMALS WITH HEPATIC DISEASE

In animals with hepatic disease, drug kinetics and ultimate effect may be modified by altered extraction, by impaired metabolizing enzyme activity or biliary excretion from hepatocellular injury, by changes in hepatic blood flow, by hypoalbuminemia, or by interaction among these factors. Because most clinically significant canine and feline hepatic diseases are characterized by a mixture of hepatocellular, biliary, and vascular lesions, it is unrealistic to expect to achieve therapeutic benefit with a simple adjustment in drug dosage or frequency. A simple, reliable method to evaluate hepatic drug-metabolizing capability that could be used clinically to determine appropriate drug dosage is not available. It is certainly simplistic to assume that any drug should not be used in animals with pre-existing hepatic disease if it has the liver as the major means of biotransformation or if it has been implicated as hepatotoxic. It generally is not necessary to adjust drug dosages when therapy is started in animals with hepatic disease, except for those with significant congenital or acquired portosystemic shunting of blood. Concurrent variable degrees of hepatocellular dysfunction theoretically could complicate drug disposition further, resulting in therapeutic failure or drug toxicity. The most important drugs for which dosages should be reduced by up to 50 per cent are anesthetic drugs such as diazepam, meperidine, thiamylal, and thiopental. Methionine-containing products, which are converted to mercaptans by intestinal flora, should not be given to animals with serious hepatic dysfunction to avoid precipitating hepatic encephalopathy. Until a predictable marker of drug disposition has been developed, monitoring blood levels of drugs and clinical response must suffice.

CONSIDERATIONS FOR THE FUTURE

What needs to be accomplished first to determine the true significance of adverse hepatic reactions caused by drugs in veterinary medicine is uniform, accurate, detailed reporting of suspected cases to a central agency that would critically review the data. Chronic adverse hepatic reactions can be especially difficult to confirm, since other drugs often have been given simultaneously, and the histologic lesions may resemble those of other chronic hepatopathies. The CVM Drug Surveillance Program (telephone number: 301-443-4095 **collect** from 7:00 AM to 4:00 PM, or 301-443-1209 to leave a recorded message after hours) receives and evaluates such reports. If the CVM were aware of all well-charac-

terized, suspect, adverse hepatic reactions, the frequency of drug-induced hepatotoxic reactions could be determined in the general population and this information combined with adequate characterization of the reaction (e.g., silent, with reversible abnormal hepatic enzyme activity, or fulminant, with severe hepatic injury) so that use of therapeutic agents could be as educated as possible.

References and Supplemental Reading

Benson, G. J., Brock, K. A.: Hepatic necrosis and halothane. J.A.V.M.A. 185:368, 1984.

Bunch, S. E., Baldwin, B. H., Hornbuckle, W. E., et al.: Compromised hepatic function in dogs treated with anticonvulsant drugs. J.A.V.M.A. 184:444, 1984.

Cullison, R. F.: Acetaminophen toxicosis in small animals: Clinical signs, mode of action, and treatment. Comp. Cont. Ed. 6:315, 1984.

Hardy, R. M., O'Brien, T., Adams, L. G., et al.: Periportal hepatitis associated with the use of a heartworm-hookworm preventive (diethylcarbamazine oxibendazole) in thirteen dogs. J. Am. Anim. Hosp. Assoc. (in press).

Hayes, A. W., Fedorowski, T., Balazs, T., et al.: Correlation of human hepatotoxicants with hepatic damage in animals. Fund. Appl. Toxicol. 2:55, 1982.

Kaplowitz, N.: Drug-induced hepatotoxicity. Ann. Intern. Med. 104:826, 1986.

Muller, G. H., Kirk, R. W., Scott, D. W.: *Small Animal Dermatology*, 4th ed. Philadelphia: W. B. Saunders Co., (in press).

Papich, M. G., Davis, L. E.: Drugs and the liver. Vet. Clin. North Am. 15:77, 1985.

Polzin, D. J., Stowe, C. M., O'Leary, T. P., et al.: Acute hepatic necrosis associated with the administration of mebendazole to dogs. J.A.V.M.A. 179:1013, 1981.

Rogers, W. A., Ruebner, B. H.: A retrospective study of probable glucocorticoid-induced hepatopathy in dogs. J.A.V.M.A. 170:603, 1977.

Sutton, R. H., Atwell, R. B., Boreham, P. F. L.: Liver changes, following diethylcarbamazine administration, in microfilaremic dogs infected with *Dirofilaria immitis*. Vet. Pathol. 22:177, 1985.

Zimmerman, H. J.: Drug-induced liver disease. Drugs 16:25, 1978.

CHOLELITHIASIS AND CHOLANGITIS

SUSAN E. JOHNSON, D.V.M.

Columbus, Ohio

Cholelithiasis occurs infrequently in dogs and cats (Hirsh and Doige, 1983; Schall et al., 1973; Wales et al., 1982). In many cases, clinical signs are absent and cholelithiasis is an incidental finding. Less frequently, choleliths lead to cholestatic liver disease when they are associated with cholecystitis or cholangitis, obstruction of the cystic or common bile duct, or perforation of the gallbladder or bile ducts (Harris et al., 1984; Hirsch and Doige, 1983; Lipowitz and Poffenbarger, 1984; Mullowney and Ten-

nant, 1982; Wolf, 1984). Choleliths may be present in the gallbladder (cholelithiasis), common bile duct (choledocholithiasis), or rarely in the hepatic and lobar ducts.

Choleliths in dogs and cats are usually greenish-brown to black and may be single or multiple. They consist of predominantly insoluble bile pigments, although other components including calcium, bile salts, protein, magnesium, phosphorus, iron, carbonate, and cholesterol have also been reported

(Mullowney and Tennant, 1982; Wales et al., 1982). Quantitative analysis is necessary to characterize the predominant chemical component. Cholesterol choleliths, the most common type of stone in humans, are less likely to form in dogs because the cholesterol content of dog bile is lower than in humans, and dogs have a better capability to maintain biliary cholesterol in solution (Nakayma, 1969). Little is known about the cholesterol content of cat bile, but choleliths predominantly consisting of cholesterol have been reported (Jorgensen et al., 1987; O'Brien and Mitchum, 1970).

ETIOLOGY

The cause of spontaneous cholelithiasis in dogs and cats is unknown. Factors that theoretically could predispose to cholelith formation include bile stasis, altered composition of the bile, and biliary infections. Sludged bile and pigment choleliths form in the gallbladder of dogs with experimentally induced cystic duct ligation (Bernhoft et al., 1983). Choleliths can also be produced experimentally in dogs by feeding a diet that is low in protein and fat, high in carbohydrates, and supplemented with cholesterol (Englert et al., 1977). This diet is deficient in the amino acid taurine, which may contribute to cholelithiasis by causing precipitation of bile acids. Recent evidence suggests that gallbladder epithelial injury and hypersecretion of mucus that binds bilirubin may be important factors in cholelith formation (Lee and Nicholls, 1986). Bacteria such as *Escherichia coli* that contain beta-glucuronidase have been incriminated in the pathogenesis of calcium bilirubinate stones in humans. Beta-glucuronidase deconjugates bilirubin to a less-soluble form that precipitates with calcium.

Inspissated or "sludged bile" does not represent true cholelithiasis, but it may be an evolutionary stage in cholelith formation (Bernhoft et al., 1983). Bile sludge consists predominantly of mucin complexed with solids such as bilirubin, cholesterol, or calcium salts (Bernhoft et al., 1983). Bile sludge appears grossly as viscous, greenish-black bile that may contain sandlike gritty material. The consistency of the bile appears to be altered secondary to chronic cholestasis or bacterial infection. Sludged bile may occur in the gallbladder, common bile duct, and intrahepatic ducts and in severe cases can lead to mechanical biliary obstruction. This is most commonly seen as a complication of cholangiohepatitis complex of cats.

Cholecystitis and cholangitis may be found in association with cholelithiasis. Clinical signs of biliary tract disease are more likely when this occurs. Cholangiohepatitis complex, consisting of cholangitis, cholangiohepatitis, and biliary cirrhosis, is common in cats but rare in dogs (Cornelius, 1985;

Hirsch and Doige, 1983; Prasse et al., 1982; Zawie and Garvey, 1984). This disorder is occasionally associated with concurrent cholelithiasis; sludging of the bile is a more frequent finding (Hirsch and Doige, 1983; Zawie and Garvey, 1984). The etiology of cholangiohepatitis complex is unknown, but most likely there are multiple causes. Lesions of cholangiohepatitis complex are seen clinically in association with biliary bacterial infections, chronic pancreatitis, cholelithiasis, liver fluke infection, and anatomic abnormalities of the biliary tract.

When concurrent cholelithiasis and inflammation of the extrahepatic biliary tract are identified, it is difficult to determine whether choleliths formed as a consequence of bile stasis, inflammation, and bacterial infection or whether cholelithiasis initiated the inflammation, which led to secondary biliary stasis and bacterial infection (Fig. 1). Regardless of the inciting cause, treatment is directed at removal of choleliths, relief of obstruction, and control of bacterial infection. Chronic biliary tract inflammation and cholelithiasis that result in partial to complete obstruction can result in end-stage hepatic disease with histologic characteristics of biliary cirrhosis.

CLINICAL MANIFESTATIONS

Dogs and cats with cholelithiasis are often asymptomatic. Clinical signs are most likely when cholelithiasis is complicated by bacterial infection of the bile ducts and gallbladder, extrahepatic bile duct obstruction, rupture of the extrahepatic biliary tract, or secondary hepatic involvement (cholangiohepatitis or biliary cirrhosis). Icterus, vomiting, anorexia, weight loss, and dehydration are the most consistent clinical findings when dogs and cats with choleli-

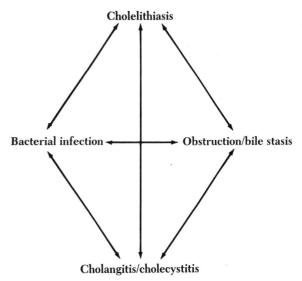

Figure 1. Relationship of cholelithiasis to cholangitis and cholecystitis.

thiasis are symptomatic. With overt jaundice, the urine usually appears dark yellow to orange as a result of marked bilirubinuria. These signs may be acute or chronic. An acute onset is most likely with sudden obstruction of the cystic or common bile duct by the cholelith, or rupture of the gallbladder. Intermittent icterus and vomiting over a period of months to years may occur with long-standing cholelithiasis.

Other potential physical examination findings include fever, abdominal pain, abdominal fluid accumulation, hepatomegaly, acholic feces, and excessive bleeding. Fever is usually indicative of primary or secondary bacterial biliary infection or of septic or bile peritonitis. Abdominal pain may be caused by peritonitis or distention of an obstructed gallbladder. With complete common bile duct obstruction, the feces may be clay colored because of a lack of bile pigments entering the intestine. Hepatomegaly may occur secondary to marked bile engorgement associated with acute extrahepatic bile duct obstruction. Rarely, a distended, obstructed gallbladder may be palpated. Excessive bleeding may be noted with chronic common bile duct obstruction (more than 2 weeks) because of a deficiency of bile acids in the gut leading to malabsorption of vitamin K.

DIAGNOSIS

Although uncommon, cholelithiasis should be considered in the differential diagnosis of any cat or dog with cholestatic hepatobiliary disease. Biochemical evaluation of symptomatic patients is not specific for the underlying biliary tract disorder but suggests cholestatic liver disease. Biochemistries are characterized by moderate to marked increases in serum alkaline phosphatase activity, gamma-glutamyl transferase activity, cholesterol, serum bile acids, and total and conjugated serum bilirubin. Serum alanine aminotransferase activity is also usually elevated, indicating secondary hepatocyte damage associated with severe cholestasis. Cats with marked cholestasis may have only mild increases in serum alkaline phosphatase activity as compared with dogs because of the lower enzyme content of their liver and the shorter half-life of serum alkaline phosphatase in this species. Hypercholesterolemia is a common finding with acute cholestasis because of increased hepatic cholesterol synthesis and decreased hepatic conversion to bile acids. Sulfobromophthalein retention is usually prolonged but does not provide any additional diagnostic information about liver function in the presence of overt jaundice.

Potential hematologic findings include a neutrophilia and left shift, which usually indicates bacterial cholangitis or cholecystitis or complications such as rupture of the gallbladder with septic or bile peritonitis. A mild nonregenerative anemia is also common. Hemostatic abnormalities are most likely to occur with chronic extrahepatic bile duct obstruction. With vitamin K deficiency, the one-stage prothrombin time (OSPT) is usually prolonged. The activated partial thromboplastin time (APTT) and activated clotting time (ACT) may also be abnormal.

The urinalysis usually indicates marked bilirubinuria. The absence of urine urobilinogen in a hyperbilirubinemic animal suggests complete extrahepatic bile duct obstruction. This is caused by failure of bile pigments to enter the intestinal tract where bacteria convert the bilirubin to urobilinogen. However, the concentration of urine urobilinogen is affected by numerous nonhepatic factors (e.g., urine pH, intestinal bacterial population, urine concentration) and is considered an unreliable test in clinical patients.

Abdominal fluid accumulation may occur with complications of cholelithiasis such as biliary tract rupture or septic peritonitis. Abdominocentesis should be performed. With bile peritonitis, the fluid has a characteristic dark-brown to black appearance. Chemical tests for bilirubin are positive, and concentrations are higher in abdominal fluid than in serum. Cytologic examination of the fluid reveals a mixture of inflammatory cells that include bile-laden macrophages. If sepsis complicates bile peritonitis, bacteria may also be seen. Aerobic and anaerobic bacterial cultures of blood and abdominal fluid should be obtained in such cases. Hypoglycemia may occur as a complication of septic peritonitis.

Choleliths may appear as radiopaque densities in the area of the gallbladder or bile ducts on a routine abdominal radiograph. Pigment stones, however, are usually radiolucent unless they contain calcium (e.g., calcium bilirubinate). Hepatomegaly may be seen with biliary obstruction and hepatic bile engorgement or cholangiohepatitis. A distended gallbladder is infrequently identified on survey radiographs. When emphysematous cholecystitis complicates cholelithiasis, the gallbladder is outlined by gas accumulation in the lumen and wall. Abdominal detail may be lost if peritonitis is caused by rupture or infection of the gallbladder or bile ducts.

Real-time ultrasonography provides a unique diagnostic modality for evaluating disorders of the biliary tract (Nyland and Hager, 1985; Nyland and Park, 1983). Hepatic ultrasonography is especially useful as a noninvasive procedure to help differentiate intrahepatic and extrahepatic biliary obstruction. It also can provide information about the underlying cause of obstruction (e.g., cholelithiasis, intraluminal or extraluminal mass lesions, pancreatitis) and whether primary hepatic disease is present. With extrahepatic bile duct obstruction, the gallbladder is usually enlarged and the cystic and common bile duct, which are not normally seen, are distended and tortuous. Similar changes may be detected in the intrahepatic bile ducts. Thickening of the gallbladder with cholecystitis may also be seen. Both radiolucent and radiopaque choleliths can be detected ultrasonographically and appear as hyperechoic densities within the gallbladder and bile ducts (Nyland and Park, 1983). Choleliths are differentiated from mural masses by the presence of acoustic shadowing and movement of the density with changes in position of the animal. Inspissated or sludged bile also appears in the gallbladder as an echogenic substance, but sludge does not cause acoustic shadowing. Sludged bile may indicate biliary stasis, but the significance of this finding should not be overinterpreted, since sludging of the bile can be seen on ultrasonography in sick, anorexic animals without clinical biliary tract disease.

If long-standing biliary obstruction and cholangiohepatitis lead to biliary cirrhosis, biochemical evidence of hepatocyte dysfunction may be detected, such as hypoalbuminemia, decreased blood urea nitrogen concentration, hyperammonemia, and a coagulopathy that is not responsive to parenteral vitamin K_1 therapy. Microhepatica is a typical finding in dogs with biliary cirrhosis. However, in cats with cirrhosis, the liver is usually normal to increased in size.

Exploratory laparotomy is usually required for definitive diagnosis and treatment of cholelithiasis and accompanying cholangitis. When choleliths are identified radiographically or ultrasonographically, the history, clinical signs, and laboratory tests should be critically evaluated to determine whether choleliths are *clinically significant*. Since the majority of choleliths do *not* cause clinical signs, surgical removal may not always be warranted.

Biopsies of the liver, gallbladder, and affected bile ducts should be obtained at surgery. Histopathologic changes may be absent with uncomplicated cholelithiasis. However, mild cholangitis and cholecystitis are common. Suppurative cholangitis or cholecystitis is most likely when bacterial infection, whether primary or secondary, plays a role in the inflammation. Necrosis and mucosal ulcerations are common with acute cholecystitis. As the inflammation becomes more chronic, the bile ducts and gallbladder wall may become thickened and histologically there is increased fibrous connective tissue. Infiltrates of lymphocytes, plasma cells, and neutrophils in and around the bile ducts are present with chronic cholangitis. The gallbladder mucosa also shows mononuclear infiltrates in the submucosa and lamina propria. Cystic hyperplasia of the gallbladder mucosa is sometimes described in dogs with cholelithiasis but may also be found in asymptomatic animals. If cholangitis secondarily involves the hepatocytes (cholangiohepatitis), findings include portal inflammation with infiltration of neutrophils, lymphocytes, or a mixed pattern; proliferation and distention of intrahepatic bile ducts; periportal hepatocyte degeneration and necrosis; and portal fibrosis. With long-standing inflammation, fibrosis may connect adjacent portal areas, resulting in biliary cirrhosis.

TREATMENT

Supportive therapy to correct fluid, electrolyte, and acid-base imbalances is indicated prior to surgery. A balanced electrolyte solution such as lactated Ringer's solution should be infused intravenously to supply maintenance requirements (40 to 60 ml/kg/day) and correct dehydration. Since hypokalemia is a common finding secondary to anorexia and vomiting, the fluids should be supplemented with potassium chloride (20 mEq/L), with adjustments in potassium supplementation based on daily serum potassium concentrations. Blood gas analysis should be performed when possible to characterize and quantitate acid-base imbalances. Metabolic acidosis is most common and unless very severe (pH < 7.1) can be controlled with the lactate provided in lactated Ringer's solution. When septic peritonitis is a complication, hypoglycemia is prevented or controlled by adding 50 per cent dextrose to the fluids to make a 2.5 to 5 per cent concentration (50 to 100 ml of 50 per cent dextrose/L bottle).

If a coagulopathy is detected, vitamin K_1 (AquaMEPHYTON, Merck Sharp & Dohme), 5 to 15 mg IM repeated every 12 hr, should be given for 24 to 48 hr prior to surgery. If vitamin K deficiency is the cause of the coagulopathy, hemostatic parameters should improve after 12 to 24 hr of therapy. If anemia (PCV < 20 per cent) is present, a blood transfusion should be given prior to surgery.

Systemic antibiotics are routinely used when evidence of inflammatory biliary tract disease and cholelithiasis is identified. Ideally, the choice of antibiotic should be based on culture and sensitivity testing of bile and hepatic tissue obtained at surgery. In patients with peritonitis or septicemia, infected peritoneal fluid or blood cultures may provide similar information. Antibiotic therapy may be initiated on a presumptive basis if life-threatening peritonitis or sepsis is detected, surgical exploration is delayed, or results of bacterial culture and sensitivity testing are pending. Antibiotics used for treatment of biliary infections should be effective against both gram-negative aerobic and anaerobic bacteria. The most common bacteria isolated from biliary infections are aerobic, gram-negative organisms such as E. coli, *Klebsiella*, *Enterobacter*, *Proteus*, and *Pseudomonas*. It is presumed that these enteric organisms ascend the biliary tract, resulting in infection. Anaerobic bacteria such as *Bacteroides* and *Clostridia* are common infecting organisms in human biliary tract infections (Dooley et al., 1984); however, little is known about the role of anaerobes in cats and dogs with biliary tract inflammation. Gas-producing organisms such as *Clostridium* and *E. coli* have been incriminated as causes of emphysematous cholecystitis in dogs.

The ideal antibiotic for treatment of biliary infections should also be excreted in an active form in therapeutic concentrations in the bile (Dooley et al., 1984). Antibiotics routinely used include ampicillin, 20 mg/kg every 6 to 8 hr PO, or 10 mg/kg every 6 to 8 hr IV, IM, or SC; amoxicillin, 22 mg/kg every 12 hr PO; cephalexin (Keflex, Dista), 20 mg/kg every 8 hr PO; or cephadroxil (Cefa-Tabs, Bristol), 22 mg/kg every 12 hr PO. Choramphenicol and tetracycline are alternative choices that are effectively excreted in the bile. However, these antibiotics should not be used if primary hepatocellular dysfunction is detected, since chloramphenicol is highly dependent on hepatic metabolism for excretion and tetracycline is potentially hepatotoxic. In addition, resistance of enteric bacteria to tetracyclines probably limits their usefulness (Dooley et al., 1984). With complete biliary obstruction, antibiotics do not enter the bile in therapeutic concentrations.

When cholelithiasis is complicated by cholecystitis, peritonitis, or septicemia, gentamicin, 2 mg/kg every 8 hr IM or SC for 5 days, is given in combination with parenteral ampicillin, 10 mg/kg every 6 to 8 hr IV, IM, or SC, or a cephalosporin such as cephalothin (Keflin, Lilly), 20 to 35 mg/kg every 8 hr IV, for broad-spectrum coverage until results of culture and sensitivity are available. The dose of gentamicin should be reduced in the presence of azotemia, and renal function should be monitored on an alternate-day basis during therapy since nephrotoxicity is an important complication. When an anaerobic organism is confirmed by culture or emphysematous cholecystitis is detected, antibiotics most likely to be effective include penicillin G, 20,000 U/kg every 4 to 6 hr IV, metronidazole (Flagyl, Searle & Co.), 10 to 15 mg/kg every 8 hr PO, or clindamycin, 5 to 10 mg/kg PO every 12 hr. Antibiotic therapy should be continued for at least 10 to 14 days.

Techniques for biliary tract surgery are described elsewhere (Blass, 1983; Breznock, 1983). Surgery should be performed as soon as the patient is medically stable. Diagnostic and therapeutic procedures performed during exploratory laparotomy include evaluation of the patency of the gallbladder and bile ducts, removal of choleliths for chemical analysis and bacterial culture, identification and repair of secondary biliary rupture, and collection of samples of affected tissue (liver, gallbladder) and bile for aerobic and anaerobic cultures and biopsy.

A cholecystotomy is indicated to remove choleliths or inspissated bile from the gallbladder and to allow tube exploration of the extrahepatic biliary tract for obstructing lesions (Breznock, 1983). Samples of bile are first obtained for culture, and then choleliths and inspissated or normal bile are removed and the gallbladder is lavaged. When extensive cholecystitis or rupture of the gallbladder is present, a cholecystectomy is recommended (Breznock, 1983). Choleliths in the common bile duct can be removed via duodenotomy or, if the common bile duct is dilated, a choledochotomy (Breznock, 1983). Biliary bypass procedures such as cholecystoduodenostomy or cholecystojejunostomy may be indicated in some cases of obstruction (Breznock, 1983). If bile peritonitis is present, aerobic and anaerobic bacterial cultures should be obtained and the abdomen should be lavaged with large volumes of saline.

Antibiotics and intravenous fluid therapy are continued postoperatively. The hemogram and biochemistries are evaluated on an alternate-day basis until parameters such as neutrophilia, hyperbilirubinemia, and increases in liver enzymes resolve. With relief of biliary obstruction, a progressive decrease in serum bilirubin concentration to normal occurs over the following 3 to 5 days. The patient should be monitored daily for fever, vomiting, and abdominal pain, which may indicate postoperative complications such as septic peritonitis, wound dehiscence with bile peritonitis, or pancreatitis. If vomiting occurs, serum lipase or amylase activity should be evaluated to rule out pancreatitis. Abdominocentesis or peritoneal lavage may be useful if peritonitis occurs. Any fluid obtained should be evaluated cytologically and cultured. Gram staining is useful as a preliminary guide to identifying the type of organism and thus selecting an appropriate antibiotic while culture results are pending. Ultrasonography may be useful to detect complications such as pancreatitis and recurrent biliary obstruction.

The bile acid dehydrocholic acid (Decholin, Miles Pharmaceuticals), 10 to 15 mg/kg PO every 8 hr, has been recommended empirically to prevent bile sludging because of its hydrocholeretic properties. It is primarily used when inspissated bile is present. Potential side effects with long-term therapy or higher doses include pruritus due to bile salt deposition in the skin and diarrhea (Greene, 1984). Cholesterol choleliths in humans can be dissolved by giving bile acids such as chenodeoxycholic acid, which improve cholesterol solubility by lowering biliary cholesterol secretion. However, these drugs are unlikely to be useful in dogs and cats since most choleliths consist of predominantly bile pigments rather than cholesterol.

Little is known about the likelihood of recurrence of cholelithiasis in dogs and cats. If the underlying mechanism of cholelith formation is not reversed, recurrence is possible. Since bacterial infection may be a cause of cholelithiasis, antibiotic therapy may be effective in preventing recurrences. After cholelith removal and treatment of infection, the patient should be re-evaluated periodically (e.g., complete blood count, serum biochemistries) to determine if inflammatory cholestatic liver disease persists. A liver biopsy should be performed to document persistent cholangitis or cholangiohepatitis. This situation is especially likely in cats, since cholangiohepatitis complex is a common disorder that could either be a cause or effect of cholelithiasis. Biopsy findings of suppurative cholangitis would suggest recurrences of bacterial infection and warrant antibiotic therapy. Ascending biliary infections may also be a complication of biliary tract surgery such as cholecystoduodenostomy. On the other hand, immune mechanisms are suspected to play a role in the pathogenesis of lymphocytic cholangitis of cats (Prasse et al., 1982). Lymphocytic cholangitis in cats may be controlled with prednisolone, 1 to 2 mg/kg every day PO.

When long-standing cholelithiasis, cholangiohepatitis, and partial to complete biliary obstruction result in biliary cirrhosis, the long-term prognosis is poor, even with removal of choleliths and control of infection. Symptomatic treatment for liver failure is indicated depending on the clinical manifestations of complications.

References and Supplemental Reading

Bernhoft, R. A., Pellegrini, C. A., Broderick, W. C., et al.: Pigment sludge and stone formation in the acutely ligated dog gallbladder. Gastroenterology 85:1166, 1983.

Blass, C. E.: Surgery of the extrahepatic biliary tract. Comp. Cont. Ed. 5:801, 1983.

Breznock, E. M.: Surgery of hepatic parenchymal and biliary tissues. In Bojrab, M. J., (ed.): Current Techniques in Small Animal Surgery. Philadelphia: Lea & Febiger Co., 1983, pp. 212–225.

Cornelius, L. M.: Cholangiohepatitis in cats. Mod. Vet. Pract. 66:626, 1985.

Dooley, J. S., Hamilton-Miller, J. M. T., Brumfitt, W., et al.: Antibiotics in the treatment of biliary infections. Gut 25:988, 1984.

Englert, E., Harmon, C. G., Freston, J. W., et al.: Studies on the pathogenesis of diet-induced dog gallstones. Am. J. Dig. Dis. 22:305, 1977.

Greene, C. E.: Gastrointestinal, intra-abdominal, and hepatobiliary infections. In Greene, C. E. (ed.): Clinical Microbiology and Infectious Diseases of the Dog and Cat. Philadelphia: W. B. Saunders Co., 1984, pp. 247–268.

Harris, S. J., Simpson, J. W., Thoday, K. L.: Obstructive cholelithiasis and gallbladder rupture in a dog. J. Small Anim. Pract. 25:661, 1984.

Hirsch, V. M., Doige, C. E.: Suppurative cholangitis in cats. J.A.V.M.A. 182:1223, 1983.

Jorgensen, L. S., Pentlarge, V. W., Flanders, J. A., et al.: Recurrent cholelithiasis in a cat. Comp. Cont. Ed. 9:265, 1987.

Lee, S. P., Nicholls, J. F.: Nature and composition of biliary sludge. Gastroenterology 90:677, 1986.

Lipowitz, A. J., Poffenbarger, E.: Gallbladder perforation in a dog. J.A.V.M.A. 184:838, 1984.

Mullowney, P. C., Tennant, B. C.: Choledocholithiasis in the dog: A review and a report of a case with rupture of the common bile duct. J. Small Anim. Pract. 23:631, 1982.

Nakayma, F.: Composition of gallstone and bile: Species difference. J. Lab. Clin. Med. 73:623, 1969.

Nyland, T. G., Hager, D. A.: Sonography of the liver, gallbladder, and spleen. Vet. Clin. North Am. 15:1123, 1985.

Nyland, T. G., Park, R. D.: Hepatic ultrasonography in the dog. Vet. Radiol. 24:74, 1983.

O'Brien, T. R., Mitchum, G. D.: Cholelithiasis in a cat. J.A.V.M.A. 156:1015, 1970.

Prasse, K. W., Mahaffery, E. A., DeNovo, R., et al.: Chronic lymphocytic cholangitis in three cats. Vet. Pathol. 19:99, 1982.

Schall, W. D., Chapman, W. L., Finco, D. R., et al.: Cholelithiasis in dogs. J.A.V.M.A. 163:469, 1973.

Wales, E. E., Englert, E., Peric-Golia, L., et al.: The spontaneous amorphous black pigment gallstone of the domestic dog. J. Comp. Pathol. 92:381, 1982.

Wolf, A. M.: Obstructive jaundice in a cat resulting from choledocholithiasis. J.A.V.M.A. 185:85, 1984.

Zawie, D. A., Garvey, M. S.: Feline hepatic disease. Vet. Clin. North Am. 14:1201, 1984.

COPPER METABOLISM DEFECT IN WEST HIGHLAND WHITE TERRIERS

LARRY P. THORNBURG, D.V.M.

Columbia, Missouri

The copper metabolism defect in West Highland white terriers (WHWTs) is associated with excess copper accumulation in the liver. The disease is independent of diet. The defect is familial, but the mode of inheritance is not established. Normal dogs (of all breeds) have a liver copper concentration less than 400 parts per million on a dry weight basis (ppm dw). A WHWT is declared to have increased hepatic copper when the concentration in the liver exceeds 400 ppm dw. WHWTs can tolerate a moderate excess of hepatic copper without any adverse effects. No damage occurs in the liver until the copper concentration exceeds approximately 2000 ppm dw.

WHWTs rarely accumulate excess copper throughout their lifetime. By 6 months of age, a WHWT has reached its upper limit of excess copper. Some WHWTs that have excess hepatic copper at 6 months will return to the normal range when a second liver biopsy specimen is analyzed after 1 year of age.

A multifocal hepatitis with associated mild to moderate elevation of liver enzymes (alanine aminotransferase and alkaline phosphatase) is the earliest abnormality. The early hepatitis does not alter the sulfobromophthalein excretion, bile acid concentration, or ammonia tolerance. The liver enzyme abnormalities that occur are in no way characteristic nor diagnostic of the copper metabolism defect, but merely reflect liver damage. The hepatitis may persist for months without evidence of clinical illness. Neither fibrosis nor cirrhosis results from the persistent hepatitis.

It appears that dogs become clinically ill only when the copper-loaded liver suffers widespread necrosis. The mechanism that initiates the necrosis is unknown. Stressful events such as whelping or showing have been incriminated as causes. The hepatic necrosis results in a dramatic rise in liver enzymes, in particular the alanine aminotransferase. The sulfobromophthalein excretion is prolonged, bile acid concentrations elevated, and there may be an abnormal ammonia tolerance. The clinical signs that are associated with the widespread necrosis are not specific and include some degree of inappetance, vomiting, diarrhea, lethargy, and in approximately half of the dogs, icterus. Neither blood clotting abnormalities nor hemolytic anemia has yet been observed to be associated with the widespread necrosis.

The liver enzymes return to the normal range during the few weeks following necrosis, although some abnormalities in the function tests usually persist. Fibrosis or, in some dogs, cirrhosis forms as the areas of necrosis undergo repair. As the repair progresses and cirrhosis develops, function tests may worsen, albumin level decreases, and liver enzymes may again show elevations. Dogs with cirrhosis may develop icterus, ascites, or both.

The copper metabolism defect in WHWTs can be diagnosed only by atomic absorption analysis of copper in liver tissue. Copper, even when in excess, is uniformly distributed throughout all lobes of the noncirrhotic liver. A biopsy specimen from any part of the liver will result in an accurate diagnosis.

The treatment of choice is the copper chelator penicillamine. This is a safe, effective drug. Not all WHWTs with abnormal hepatic copper concentration need treatment. The minimal hepatotoxic concentration is approximately 2000 ppm dw. WHWTs that have something less than the minimal hepatotoxic concentration at the time of biopsy may not need treatment with penicillamine, since copper accumulation rarely is continuous throughout life. Results from three dogs indicate that penicillamine, when given at a dose of 22 mg/kg/day at least 20 minutes before a meal, removes copper from the liver at the rate of approximately 1000 ppm/year. When the drug is given with the meal the efficacy decreases by about one-half. Once treatment is discontinued, the copper slowly reaccumulates in the liver at the rate of approximately 400 ppm/year. Following the initial decoppering, a periodic regimen of treatment should be pursued.

Some WHWTs cannot tolerate penicillamine on an empty stomach. They have violent episodes of vomiting. These dogs must be given the drug with a meal. Two male WHWTs developed an autoimmune-like vesicular disease of the mucocutaneous junctions while receiving penicillamine. In both dogs, complete remission was achieved by drug withdrawal. In one dog, the mucocutaneous lesions reappeared when challenged with penicillamine.

References and Supplemental Reading

Thornburg, L. P., Shaw, D., Dolan M., et al: Hereditary copper toxicosis in West Highland white terriers. Vet. Pathol. 23:148, 1986.

Thornburg, L. P.: A study of canine hepatobiliary disease, Part 4: Copper and liver disease. Companion Anim. Pract. 2:3, 1988.

MANAGEMENT OF HEPATIC COPPER TOXICOSIS IN DOGS

DAVID C. TWEDT, D.V.M.,
and ELIZABETH L. WHITNEY, D.V.M.

Fort Collins, Colorado

Hepatic copper toxicity was first identified in Bedlington terriers in 1975. It has subsequently been shown that affected dogs have an inherited autosomal recessive defect, causing expression of an abnormal hepatic metallothionein (copper-binding protein). The defect results in reduced biliary excretion of copper secondary to hepatic metallothionein sequestration of the metal in hepatic lysosomes. Clinically there is a progressive accumulation of hepatic copper ranging from 1000 to 12,000 parts per million (ppm) per dry weight of liver (normal hepatic copper is less than 400 ppm). The extent of damage that occurs in the liver parallels the increasing hepatic copper concentrations. The morphologic changes extend from focal to chronic hepatitis, which may lead to cirrhosis. In some cases, acute hepatic necrosis may develop, releasing excess copper into the plasma and causing a hemolytic anemia.

During the past decade an increasing number of breeds other than the Bedlington terrier have been identified as having hepatic disease and a concurrent increase in the hepatic copper content. Whether the excess in hepatic copper is the cause of the liver disease or a result of it is unknown. It is probable that many of these defects, though unlikely to be identical to that of the Bedlington terrier, are genetically transmitted and result in progressive hepatic copper accumulation. Copper may also concentrate in the liver secondary to certain primary liver diseases, especially those that involve biliary tract disorders. Liver disease with concurrent copper accumulation is reported in the Bedlington terrier, Doberman pinscher, West Highland white terrier, cocker spaniel, and Labrador retriever, as well as other purebred and mixed-breed dogs.

COPPER METABOLISM

Copper is an important essential trace element that must be supplied daily through the diet, but like all heavy metals it is also potentially toxic. In response to this duality, homeostatic mechanisms have evolved to control both the absorption and excretion of copper. It is these mechanisms that operate to offset excesses or deficiencies of copper in disease states.

Copper is found universally in the diet. Approximately half of the daily copper intake is not absorbed but rather is excreted in the feces. Absorbed copper is transported into the intestinal epithelial cells through a speculated active transport process. Upon entering the plasma, copper is bound to albumin for transport to the liver. The copper is rapidly dispersed in the liver and becomes temporarily bound to hepatic cytosol proteins. The major proteins binding to copper include ceruloplasmin and metallothioneins. Ceruloplasmin is the exclusive transport ligand involved in carrying copper from the liver via the blood to the tissues where it is used for various body functions. The metallothioneins are proteins, found not only in the liver, that function in copper storage and thus in tissue detoxification. Such liver-bound copper becomes packaged in hepatic lysosomes and is eventually excreted into the bile, thus maintaining a constant balance of the metal within the body. Copper excreted through bile is not available for resorption in the intestine because of its binding to bile and amino acids.

TREATMENT

The therapy for copper hepatotoxicity can be divided into two basic categories. The first category comprises dogs that are known to be affected with an inherited defect resulting in progressive accumulation of hepatic copper (i.e., Bedlington terriers), but as yet without evidence of serious hepatic injury. In this situation, dietary copper restriction or therapy to limit copper absorption may be very important in preventing abnormal hepatic copper sequestration. However, such management alone is as yet unproven, and the use of intermittent or long-term copper chelator therapy is at this time indicated. It is advisable for these animals to have periodic monitoring of their hepatic copper concentrations in order to direct the course and duration of therapy. The second category includes dogs with abnormal hepatic copper and evidence of significant hepatocellular damage with or without outward signs of liver disease. These dogs require aggressive copper chelator therapy. Additional supportive therapy is often required in the management of these cases. Dietary copper restriction or drugs to reduce copper absorption appear to be of little immediate benefit in the management of these dogs.

DIETARY RESTRICTION. The restriction of dietary copper probably does little to lower hepatic copper concentrations in diseased dogs. This is because their livers already contain large amounts of copper and copper-restricted diets alone have a very minimal effect in causing a net depletion of copper. It is difficult to limit dietary copper because commercial dog foods contain supplemental copper that meets or more frequently exceeds the minimal dietary requirements established by the National Research Council. These standards require that there be at least 0.8 mg of copper per 1000 Kcal of metabolizable energy, a level considered by some to be far in excess of what is needed for the normal dog. Most commercial foods contain concentrations in excess of 7 mg/kg diet on a dry weight basis. Unfortunately, many manufacturers do not list the copper content in their diets, making dietary selections difficult. There are no proven nutritionally balanced commercial diets that are substantially low in copper content to recommend for use in affected dogs.

Homemade diets that do not contain excess copper can be prepared. These diets should exclude liver, shellfish, organ meats, and cereals that all are high in copper content. Available references for home diets give formulations that fit these requirements. Mineral supplementations or dog treats containing copper are to be avoided. Providing distilled water that is free of copper may also be instituted but is probably not necessary. Diets low in copper will not reduce existing hepatic copper but will be of benefit in slowing further hepatic copper accumulation. Low-copper diets have most potential when managing young dogs known to be affected with an inherited hepatic copper metabolism defect (i.e., Bedlington terriers and West Highland white terriers).

REDUCING COPPER ABSORPTION. There are several therapies prescribed for humans to reduce copper absorption, but these are of unproven benefit in animals. Ascorbic acid given with meals may reduce intestinal copper absorption. Ascorbic acid is also said to augment copper excretion through urine, but this is not well documented. A dose of 500 to 1000 mg/day is suggested.

Zinc therapy appears to show the most promise in dogs. Zinc given as either the acetate or sulfate salt has been proved effective in preventing copper reaccumulation in the livers of humans with Wilson's disease. These patients had previously been depleted of hepatic copper with chelators and, when given oral zinc, maintained previous hepatic copper

concentrations. Oral zinc therapy has also been shown to reduce tissue copper levels in normal laboratory animals. Dietary zinc works by causing an induction of the intestinal copper-binding protein metallothionein. Dietary copper binds to the metallothionein with a high affinity that prevents its transfer from the intestine into the blood. When the intestinal cell dies and is sloughed, the metallothionein-bound copper is excreted through the stool. A dose of 5 to 10 mg/kg body weight of zinc is given twice a day. This therapy is unproven and may not be as effective in dogs, since hepatic copper concentrations in affected dogs usually far exceed concentrations found in humans or laboratory animals. Care must be taken when prescribing zinc, since an excess will inhibit iron absorption and toxic levels may result in a hemolytic anemia. Although zinc therapy may indirectly prevent copper accumulation in the liver, it probably has little if any effect in "decoppering" dogs that already have excess copper in their livers. Projections made from laboratory animals treated with zinc suggest that it may take longer than an entire lifetime to lower hepatic copper levels significantly. Hopefully the question of zinc therapy for affected dogs will be answered in the near future. A final concern is indiscriminate zinc therapy given to young Bedlington or West Highland white terriers. Both breeds are known to have individuals affected with a defect that results in progressive copper accumulation. To detect affected animals, hepatic copper concentrations must be obtained at approximately 1 year of age. Dietary zinc supplementation given prior to biopsy may mask proper identification of these dogs.

COPPER CHELATORS. Treatment with copper chelators has a proven beneficial effect in dogs with abnormal hepatic copper concentrations. Chelators bind with copper either in the blood or the tissues and promote its removal through the kidneys. Penicillamine (Cuprimine, 250-mg capsules [Merck Sharp & Dohme], or Depen, 250-mg tablets [Wallace]) is the copper chelator most often recommended for use in dogs. Therapy with this drug is usually slow and takes months to years to cause a substantial reduction in hepatic copper. There are limited reports on the effectiveness of penicillamine as a copper chelator in dogs. The authors have treated a limited number of Bedlington terriers that had substantial abnormal hepatic copper concentrations. On the average, they lost 900 ppm of copper per dry weight of liver per year when given the recommended dosage of penicillamine. Penicillamine therapy is not beneficial for the rapid treatment of the acutely ill patient or one suffering from a hemolytic crisis with elevated serum copper concentrations. A recommended dose for penicillamine is 10 to 15 mg/kg given twice a day. The drug should be given on an empty stomach, since a considerable amount will not be absorbed when given with meals. A host of *side effects* of this drug are reported in humans. In dogs, a very common side effect is vomiting. This problem may be alleviated in some cases by reducing the dose and giving it more frequently. Some dogs experience both reversible renal disease and cutaneous skin eruptions with this drug. In human patients, penicillamine therapy may cause a pyridoxine deficiency, but this has not been identified in dogs. To avoid this complication, the diet should contain the B vitamin pyridoxine or it should be supplemented. Periodic liver biopsies are suggested to monitor hepatic copper levels and response to therapy.

Tetramine cupretic agents appear to be promising alternative copper chelators in dogs. Trientine (Cuprid, 250 mg capsules [Merck Sharp & Dohme]) is a 2,2,2-tetramine that is the alternative drug for humans intolerant to penicillamine. In treating a number of normal control dogs and dogs with abnormal hepatic copper, we have yet to experience any objectionable side effects. The copper chelating ability of trientine at a recommended dose of 10 to 15 mg/kg given twice a day appears to be comparable to that of penicillamine. A urinary loss of approximately 0.5 mg of copper per day should be expected at this dose. Dog studies have shown this drug to be an effective copper chelator without a significant influence on zinc or iron concentrations. Experimental studies suggest that trientine is an active chelator of copper in the blood and may be of benefit when treating dogs with an acute hemolytic crises due to elevated serum copper concentrations.

The authors have used another tetramine chelator, 2,3,2-tetramine, both in normal control dogs and in affected Bedlington terriers. This compound is four to nine times more potent than trientine and resulted in mean reduction of 3282 ppm of hepatic copper after approximately 200 days of therapy in five affected Bedlington terriers given a dose of 15 mg/kg body weight. At this dose there was an approximate daily loss of 2 mg of copper in the urine. This drug was also effective in one Bedlington terrier with acute hepatic necrosis and hemolytic anemia. This compound is not commercially available as a drug, but it can be obtained from chemical supply companies as *N,N'*-bis(2-aminoethyl)-1,3-propanediamine and then prepared as a salt to be given orally.

SYMPTOMATIC THERAPY. Supportive therapy should be given in all cases as deemed necessary. The reader should refer to chapters on acute and chronic liver disease in *Current Veterinary Therapy IX.*

References and Supplemental Reading

Allen, K. G. D., Hunsaker, H. A., and Twedt, D. C.: Tetramine cupruretic agents: A comparison in dogs. Am. J. Vet. Res. 48:28, 1987.
Cook, C. S., Hardy, R. M., Heyman, L., et al.: Understanding copper toxicosis. Gazette 104:66, 1987.
Hardy, R. M.: Copper-associated hepatitis in Bedlington terriers. *In* Kirk, R. W. (ed.): *Current Veterinary Therapy VIII.* Philadelphia: W. B. Saunders Co., 1983, pp. 834–836.
Twedt, D. C., Hunsaker, H. A., and Allen, K. G. D.: The use of 2,3,2-tetramine as a hepatic copper chelating agent for the treatment of copper hepatotoxicosis in Bedlington terriers. J.A.V.M.A. 192:52, 1988.

FELINE PANCREATITIS

DENNIS W. MACY, D.V.M.

Fort Collins, Colorado

Pancreatitis in domestic animals occurs most frequently in dogs, followed by cats, cows, pigs, and horses. In cats, the incidence of pancreatitis ranges from 1.5 to 35 cases per 1000 animals. Despite this relatively frequent occurrence, pancreatitis is seldom diagnosed clinically in cats.

PATHOLOGY

Evidence of previous pancreatic inflammation is a fairly common lesion of older cats. Pancreatitis is categorized into acute, chronic-active, and chronic forms.

Acute pancreatitis is characterized by infiltration of neutrophils, moderate to severe pancreatic necrosis, edema or hemorrhage or both, and absence of fibrosis. **Chronic-active pancreatitis** is characterized by the presence of neutrophil infiltration, necrosis, and evidence of chronicity: fibrosis, nodular hyperplasia, and mononuclear infiltration. **Chronic pancreatitis** is characterized by mononuclear infiltration and extensive fibrosis.

In a large series of necropsied cats with histopathologically confirmed pancreatitis, 33 per cent of cases were acute, 25 per cent chronic-active, and 41 per cent chronic. In addition to pancreatic lesions, cats with pancreatitis consistently have lesions in the liver and kidney. Histopathologic evidence of cholangiohepatitis has been seen in 64 per cent of cats with pancreatitis. The concurrent pathologic involvement of both the biliary tree and the pancreatic duct should be expected, because in cats the common bile duct and the main pancreatic duct cojoin before entering at the major duodenal papilla. Several clinical studies have found evidence of significant renal pathology associated with pancreatitis in cats. In the same series, renal pathology was found in 68 per cent of the cats examined. Because there was no consistent single histopathologic feature of the renal lesions, it is difficult to hypothesize a cause-and-effect relationship. Other diseases that occur concurrently in cats with pancreatitis include feline infectious peritonitis, diabetes mellitus, panniculitis, and pancreatic insufficiency. Although feline infectious peritonitis (FIP) was observed in 7 per cent of affected cats, FIP was not considered the cause of pancreatitis since many of the pancreatic lesions were chronic. Diabetes mellitus occurred in 8 per cent of cats with evidence of pancreatitis and was associated with chronic pancreatic destruction and atrophy of islet cells. Panniculitis has also been associated with pancreatitis, and one case of pancreatic insufficiency associated with pancreatitis has been described.

ETIOLOGY

As in dogs and humans, many etiologies have been advanced to explain development of pancreatitis in cats: traumatic injury, FIP, toxoplasmosis, systemic leukodystrophies, and a variety of parasitic infections, including pancreatic fluke, *Eurytrema procyonis*, and aberrant migration of liver flukes, *Amphimerus pseudofelineus* and *Opisthorchis felineus*. The common-channel theory of reflux of bile into the pancreas is supported by the presence of significant cholangiohepatitis in 64 per cent of cats with pancreatitis. The presence of azotemia and renal pathology in many cats with pancreatitis also suggests a possible causal relationship. However, the etiology of most cases of feline pancreatitis is classified as idiopathic.

CLINICAL DISEASE

Pancreatitis has been reported to affect cats ranging in age from 5 weeks to 18 years. Males may be affected more often than females. Although pancreatitis has been found most commonly in domestic long- or short-hair breeds, Siamese cats were reported to represent 39 per cent of affected cats in one large series. Most cats with pancreatitis are of average weight, unlike dogs, in which obesity is reported to be a predisposing factor. The history and clinical signs of cats with naturally occurring or spontaneous pancreatitis are similar to those reported for dogs and include the following, in decreasing order of frequency: anorexia (70 per cent), vomiting (41 per cent), weight loss (23 per cent), icterus (23 per cent), diarrhea (12 per cent), fever (7 per cent), and polydipsia/polyuria (5 per cent).

Shock, dyspnea, and pleural and peritoneal effusions have been reported, but less frequently. In experimentally induced acute pancreatitis in cats, vomiting, depression, abdominal pain, tachycardia, and fever are the predominant features. There is a low frequency of abdominal pain reported in spontaneous cases of pancreatitis as compared with experimental pancreatitis, which can be explained by the subclinical or chronic nature of spontaneous pancreatitis in most cats. Polydipsia and polyuria in cats with pancreatitis occurred only in cats with diabetes mellitus.

LABORATORY FINDINGS IN CATS WITH PANCREATITIS

Pancreatitis is seldom diagnosed antemortem, and the reported laboratory abnormalities associated with the disease are limited to small clinical series or individual case reports and one model of experimentally induced pancreatitis in cats. Hematologic abnormalities are usually nonspecific. Mild normocytic normochromic anemia may be observed in cats with any category of pancreatitis and should be considered a nonspecific change. White blood cell counts are more variable and do not necessarily correlate with the acuteness of the disease process. Cats with experimentally induced acute pancreatitis demonstrated wide variation in their white blood cell counts, but mean values were not considered significantly different from normal values over the 7-day period of the study. In dogs, elevated lipase and amylase concentrations have been used to confirm pancreatitis. Little is known about amylase tissue origins and normal clearance mechanisms in cats. Although elevated serum amylase levels have been reported in spontaneous pancreatitis, experimentally induced pancreatitis in cats has been associated with decreased serum amylase concentrations. Low serum amylase concentrations have been observed in people with concurrent pancreatitis and pancreatic exocrine insufficiency (PEI). However, PEI is rare in cats and rarely a consequence of pancreatitis. Based on the discordant nature of the reported serum amylase levels associated with pancreatitis and uncertainty of its metabolism, serum amylase levels probably have limited utility in the diagnosis of pancreatitis in cats. Elevated serum lipase levels may be more useful in confirming pancreatitis in cats. Despite the fact that little is known about the tissue origin of lipase in cats, it is likely to be similar to that in dogs and humans and specific for pancreatic lesions. In experimentally induced acute pancreatitis in cats, serum lipase increases sixfold initially and remains markedly elevated for 12 to 24 hr following lesion induction, then decreases to three times normal levels for 2 to 3 days and remains two times normal levels for a period of a week. Reports of elevated serum lipase concentrations in cats with spontaneous pancreatitis are rare, and many cats with chronic pancreatitis or chronic-active pancreatitis have normal serum lipase concentrations. Comparison of serum and peritoneal lipase levels has been reported as a means of confirming a diagnosis of pancreatitis in cats. Based on experimental data and clinical reports, elevated serum lipase concentrations appear to be the most sensitive means of confirming a diagnosis of acute pancreatitis. However, because normal lipase concentrations may be observed in chronic pancreatitis, the presence of normal serum lipase concentrations should not rule out a diagnosis of pancreatitis.

The most frequently reported laboratory abnormality in cats with pancreatitis is elevated blood urea nitrogen levels. Although azotemia may be due to dehydration secondary to vomiting or diarrhea, significant renal pathology has been found in two-thirds of the cats with pancreatitis. More importantly, azotemia may potentially alter interpretation of serum amylase and lipase concentrations. In dogs, both serum amylase and lipase concentrations may be elevated in azotemic animals. Similar studies in cats have not been conducted. In general, azotemia should be corrected before determining lipase concentration to avoid spurious results.

In both experimentally induced and spontaneous pancreatitis in cats, significant increases in blood glucose levels have also been observed. Hyperglycemia may be transient or permanent and must be differentiated from elevated glucose concentrations due to excitement during sample collection. Simultaneous urine glucose determination is suggested in order to aid interpretation of hyperglycemia. Serum protein levels may be abnormal as a result of compartmental shifts with pancreatitis. Hypoalbuminemia and hypoproteinemia have been noted in experimentally induced pancreatitis in cats, presumably secondary to leakage of albumin from the surface of inflamed pancreas. Hypoalbuminemia may in turn induce hypocalcemia in some cats with acute pancreatitis but has not been associated with hypocalcemic tetany. Elevations in serum cholesterol have been observed in cats with experimentally induced pancreatitis during the first week, but cholesterol elevation in naturally occurring disease has not been reported. Because of the lack of specificity of cholesterol for pancreatic lesions, it is doubtful that changes in serum cholesterol will ever be very valuable in the diagnosis of pancreatitis.

Hypokalemia has frequently been reported in cats with spontaneous pancreatitis; the etiology of hypokalemia is unknown but may be associated with renal dysfunction, vomiting, or other mechanisms. Although hypokalemia has little diagnostic specificity for pancreatitis, its recognition is important for managing the patient.

Diarrhea was observed in 12 per cent of the cats with pancreatitis in one series and was reported in several other clinical reports. Although diarrhea has been previously attributed to exocrine pancreatic insufficiency (EPI) caused by destruction of the exocrine pancreas, one study found diarrhea equally frequent in cats with acute and chronic pancreatitis. This suggests that a cause other than EPI is responsible for diarrhea in cats with pancreatitis. Although the PABA absorption test (a test of pancreatic exocrine function) has resulted in variable results in normal cats (see p. 929), when it was used to evaluate exocrine function 1 week to 1 month after induction of experimental pancreatitis, little to no change was found. Icterus is a common clinical finding in cats with pancreatitis, present in 23 per cent of cats with pancreatitis in one report. Icterus was found most often in cats with chronic-active pancreatitis but has also been seen in cats with both the acute and chronic forms of pancreatitis. The presence of icterus is not surprising, given the prevalence of concurrent cholangiohepatitis. Radiographic evaluation of the abdomen may on rare occasions be helpful in making a diagnosis of pancreatitis. The pancreas is not visualized in normal cats, although occasionally a soft tissue mass in the area of the pancreas or a gas-filled anterior duodenal segment may be seen in cats with acute pancreatitis.

TREATMENT

Limiting Food Intake

Cats that develop pancreatitis often become anorectic during acute stages of the disease. Food should not be made available for 2 to 4 days when managing cats with pancreatitis. In order to allow time for resolution of inflammatory lesions, guidelines for return to a normal feeding regimen in dogs with pancreatitis are usually tied to cessation of vomiting and return to normal white blood cell or serum lipase levels. Since vomiting occurs in less than 50 per cent of cats with pancreatitis, serum lipase elevation is inconsistent and the presence of leukocytosis is variable, an arbitrary 2- to 4-day period of nothing *per os* (NPO) appears to be a more practical approach. The NPO period should be followed by tapering of parenteral fluid administration, reintroduction of water, and feeding of small amounts of food. Cats that remain persistently anorectic following this NPO period should have a white cell count, another serum chemistry profile, and serum lipase levels re-evaluated. If the results of these tests are normal, appetite stimulants may be used in the patient.

Antibiotics

Antibiotic therapy in the management of pancreatitis is an unsettled issue. In some species, such as dogs, the benefit of antibiotic therapy has been documented. However, antibiotic therapy in people with pancreatitis has been shown to be of limited or no value. There are no studies of the effectiveness of antibiotic therapy in the management of cats with pancreatitis. Since many cats are azotemic on presentation, nephrotoxic aminoglycosides such as gentamicin should *not* be used. Amoxicillin plus clavulanate is suggested, being effective against anaerobes and enteric organisms, which are frequently incriminated as causing abscesses following pancreatitis.

Glucocorticoids

A short course of glucocorticoid therapy is often indicated in cats with pancreatitis. In addition to membrane-stabilizing properties and beneficial effects on blood flow, their anti-inflammatory properties may be especially beneficial in cats with concurrent cholangiohepatitis. Five milligrams of prednisolone given once daily for 5 consecutive days is recommended. Although long-term steroid therapy has been shown to be detrimental in some species with pancreatitis, short-term steroid therapy has not been shown to have an adverse side effect and may be quite beneficial.

Fluid Therapy

Cats with pancreatitis may be dehydrated as a result of prolonged anorexia, vomiting, or diarrhea. Correction of dehydration followed by maintenance fluid therapy will help increase pancreatic blood flow and ameliorate potential ischemic changes. Lactated Ringer's solution should be used for the correction of dehydration and maintenance fluid therapy. Many cats with pancreatitis are hypokalemic, and addition of potassium chloride (20 mEq/L fluids) is recommended provided the patient has normal renal function. Cats have a high vitamin B requirement, and B vitamin complex should be added to lactated Ringer's during the maintenance fluid therapy.

PROGNOSIS

Cats with pancreatitis generally have a good prognosis provided they do not have serious secondary diseases such as FIP, cholangiohepatitis, or renal failure. Cats tend to respond quickly to therapy but may be subject to repeated clinical or subclinical attacks of pancreatitis. Most cats that develop pancreatitis survive, even with repeated episodes. It is uncertain whether most cats with pancreatitis are subclinical or whether transient anorexia allows resolution of lesions, or both. Fortunately, the general therapy for cats with vague clinical signs associated with pancreatitis is similar to specific therapies for the disease.

References and Supplemental Reading

Anderson, N. V., Strafuss, A. C.: Pancreatitis in dogs and cats. J.A.V.M.A. 159:885, 1971.

Duffell, S. J.: Some aspects of pancreatic disease in the cat. J. Small Anim. Pract. 16:365, 1975.

Fox, J. N., Mosley, J. G., Vogler, G. A., et al.: Pancreatic function in domestic cats with pancreatic fluke infection. J.A.V.M.A. 178:54, 1981.

Garvey, M. S., Zawie, D. A.: Feline pancreatic disease. Vet. Clin. North Am. [Small Anim. Pract.] 14:1235, 1984.

Holzworth, J., Coffin, D.: Pancreatic insufficiency and diabetes mellitus in a cat. Cornell Vet. 43:502, 1985.

Hoskins, J. D., Turk, J. R., Turk, M. A.: Feline pancreatic insufficiency. Vet . Med. Small Anim. Clin. 77:1745, 1982.

Jubb, K. V. F., Kennedy, P. C.: Pathology of Domestic Animals, 2nd ed. Vol. 2. New Academic Press, 1985, pp. 314–326.

Kelly, D. F., Baggott, D. G., Gaskell, C. J.: Jaundice in the cat associated with inflammation of the biliary tract and pancreas. J. Small Anim. Pract. 16:163, 1975.

Kitchell, B. E., Strombeck, D. R., and Cullen, V.: Clinical and pathologic changes in experimentally induced acute pancreatitis in cats. Am. J. Vet. Res. 47:1170, 1986.

Macy, D. W.: Feline pancreatitis: Some clinical and pathologic features of 96 histologically confirmed cases. J. Small Anim. Pract. (submitted).

Owens, J. M., Drazner, P. H., Gilbertson, S. R.: Pancreatic disease in the cat. J.A.V.M.A. 11:83, 1975.

Rothenbacher, H., Lindquist, W. D.: Liver cirrhosis and pancreatitis in a cat infected with Amphimerus pseudofelineus. J.A.V.M.A. 143:1099, 1963.

Ryan, C. P., Howard, E. B.: Systemic lipodystrophy associated with pancreatitis in a cat. Feline Pract. 11:31, 1981.

Schaer, M.: A clinicopathologic survey of acute pancreatitis in 30 dogs and 5 cats. J. Am. Anim. Hosp. Assoc. 15:682, 1979.

Smart, M. E., Downey, R. S., Smith, J. R., et al.: Toxoplasmosis in a cat associated with cholangitis and progressive pancreatitis. Can. Vet. J. 14:313, 1973.

Smith, F. W. K.: Feline pancreatitis: A review. Compan. Anim. Pract. 1:4, 1987.

Suter, P. F., Olsen, S. E.: Traumatic hemorrhagic pancreatitis in the cat: A report with emphasis on radiographic diagnosis. J. Am. Vet. Radiol. Soc. 10:4, 1969.

Wagner, A., Macy, D. W.: Nephelometric determination of serum amylase and lipase in spontaneous azotemia in the dog. Am. J. Vet. Res. 43:697, 1982.

Wilken, R. J., Hurvitz, A. L.: Profiling in veterinary clinical pathology. Dog and Cat. New York: New York Instruments Corp., 1978.

Zontine, W. J.: Acute pancreatitis in dogs and cats. Small Anim. Clin. 2:136, 1962.

EFFECTS OF GLUCOCORTICOIDS ON THE GASTROINTESTINAL SYSTEM

RAY DILLON, D.V.M.
Auburn, Alabama

The clinical effects of corticosteroids are divided into those of metabolism and fluid balance, negative feedback on the hypothalamus and pituitary, and anti-inflammatory and immunosuppressive reactions (see *Current Veterinary Therapy IX*, p. 954). An understanding of the biochemical mechanisms of inflammation has provided the rationale for altered clinical indications and dosage. The differences in mechanism of action and pharmacokinetics of synthetic corticosteroids are germane to the use of corticosteroids in the clinical treatment of disorders of the gastrointestinal tract.

INFLUENCES ON CORTICOSTEROID THERAPY

Anti-Inflammatory and Immunosuppressive Effects

The empiric use of glucocorticoids is based on the palliative effects of inhibition of both the early and late manifestations of inflammation—for example, the initial redness, pain, and edema and also the proliferative effects of chronic inflammation. The ability to decrease the inflammatory reaction regardless of the insult (e.g., pathogens, chemical or physical insult, appropriate or hypersensitive immune responses) is attributed to (1) stabilization of microvascular permeability and fluid exudation, (2) decreased accumulation of leukocytes at the site, (3) inhibition of mononuclear phagocytes in tissue, (4) decreased protease secretion from macrophages, and (5) decreased activity of fibroblasts, with reduced production of collagen and glycosaminoglycans in chronic disease and healing. In the face of cell-mediated immune reaction, decreased production of lymphokines is required for mobilizing and activating macrophages.

Based on IgG and IgM concentrations, the humoral response of dogs administered even high doses of glucocorticoids is generally normal. Inhibition of antigen-antibody complexes does not seem to occur in dog sera after glucocorticoid administration. There is no direct inhibition of complement action in canine serum or tissue after administration of prednisolone or dexamethasone, but a functional decrease in serum complement does occur after therapeutic doses of dexamethasone. This continues for 6 days after therapy. The species-specific activity of decreased C3 is a direct effect of hepatic protein synthesis in dogs, and the decreased complement cocentrations (not inhibition of action) correlate with clinical response to inflammatory diseases.

The effects of glucocorticoids on lymphocytes vary in different species. Laboratory testing indicates that lymphocyte blastogenesis (transformation) is generally not altered in dogs receiving chronic prednisolone. In steroid-susceptible animals (rabbits, rats, mice), lympholysis with a decrease in both T- and B-cells occurs after corticosteroid treatment. In steroid-resistant species (humans, monkeys, guinea pigs, dogs, cats), there is little or no lympholysis of normal lymphocytes. The transient lymphocytopenia that occurs following a single dose of glucocorticoids in steroid-resistant species is believed to be due to redistribution of cells, affecting T-cells more than B-cells. Confusion about the effects of steroids on lymphocytes was based on *in vivo* studies in mice and the use of extremely high concentrations of steroids *in vitro*. Using therapeutic concentrations, corticosteroids do result in a decreased proliferative response of human lymphocytes to mitogens and antigens *in vitro*. It is generally believed that a steroid-induced decrease in production of T-cell growth factor, interleukin-2 (the hormone produced by a clone of lymphocytes when an antigen is recognized), causes glucocorticoids to suppress the initiation and generation of a "new" immune response more efficiently than an immune response that is already established.

Biologic Activity Related to Plasma Binding

Glucocorticoids are reversibly bound to corticosteroid-binding globulin (CBG), which has a high affinity and a low capacity for cortisol. Concentrations exceeding CBG binding capability (one site per mole of CBG) are bound to plasma albumin, which has a low affinity but a high binding capacity

897

(1 to 20 sites per mole of albumin). Only the unbound portion of cortisol or synthetic corticosteroids that exceeds the binding capacity of both CBG and albumin is biologically active. In normal human plasma cortisol, about 80 per cent is bound to CBG, 10 per cent is bound to albumin, and 10 per cent is unbound and biologically active. The CBG and albumin normally serve as buffers and reservoirs and can be affected by other hormones (progesterone, estrogen, oral contraceptives, thyroxine, and androgens). The total concentration of cortisol may vary, but the unbound portion usually remains the same in species in which CBG is influenced by physiologic changes.

This finely tuned system is designed for nanograms per deciliter, and following therapeutic doses, is challenged with milligrams of medication. Since the relation of dose and effect is not linear, a moderate increase in prednisolone results in a marked increase in active product (if albumin-binding sites are saturated or altered by other drugs or if hypoalbuminemia is present). Thus, in hypoalbuminemic states, a dose of prednisolone will have a much more significant biologic effect than the same dose in a dog with normal albumin levels. Similarly, drugs with significant albumin binding have the ability to dislocate bound (inactive) corticosteroid and make it available to the target cells. Dosages of corticosteroids should always be altered in relation to the serum albumin.

Because plasma binding dictates the amount of available active steroid for diffusion into target cells, the peak plasma concentration of corticosteroid is important and may be more important than the total dose. At the same dose, parenteral administration has a higher biologic effect on certain target cells than oral administration. This effect occurs because the concentration exceeding the binding capacity is higher even though the total "bioavailability" and the area under the plasma curve are the same. The biologic effect of increased dosage of corticosteroids is not based on a simple linear relationship.

Further complications to seeking a simple clinical protocol for finding the correct immunosuppressive versus anti-inflammatory dose of corticosteroids include the marked differences in the plasma-binding capabilities of different synthetic products. Albumin affinity is inversely related to the number of polar groups in the steroid. Although prednisolone has a relatively high affinity for albumin, dexamethasone has a low affinity for albumin. Dexamethasone has a corresponding low hepatic clearance compared with prednisolone, and the clearance of dexamethasone is capacity limited and binding sensitive. Thus, dexamethasone is altered by hepatic insufficiency to a greater degree than prednisolone.

Metabolism of Corticosteroids

The sum of all the metabolites of prednisolone or prednisone in the feces and urine accounts for only 50 per cent of the administered drug; the other half presumably is metabolized by target organs. Each corticosteroid has a different metabolism and affinity for target cell receptors (Tables 1, 2, and 3). However, steroids are small lipophilic molecules that enter the target cells by simple diffusion. This is dictated by the concentration of unbound steroid. Hydrocortisone has a plasma half-life of 90 min, but its main biologic effects occur only after 2 to 8 hr. Thus, utilization and inactivation of unbound products are dictated by metabolism in the liver and other target organs. Metabolism is slowed if there is a double bond C1-C2 (methylprednisolone, prednisolone, dexamethasone, betamethasone) and if there is a fluorine atom at C9 (dexamethasone, betamethasone). Although prednisone is inactive until converted to prednisolone by the liver, the ratio of prednisolone to prednisone is constant even after first-time passage through the liver. This is true whether prednisolone or prednisone is administered and regardless of the route of administration. The ratio of prednisolone to prednisone varies but usually is about 20:1. The maximum prednisone concentration in dogs is the limiting factor. In dogs, clearance of prednisolone does not increase with increased dose. Elderly humans have decreased renal and nonrenal clearance and have longer biologic effects from corticosteroids. The ratio and conversion of most glucocorticoids are not altered by severe hepatic disease but are influenced by microsomal enzyme induction (e.g., phenobarbital, phenytoin, and phenylbutazone).

Activity of Glucocorticoids

Most steroid effects involve interaction with intracellular receptors (with the possible exception of the hypothalamic-pituitary axis and adipose tissue). In most tissues, glucocorticoids diffuse into the cells and bind to specific receptors in the nucleus. All tissues have receptors with a high affinity for glucocorticoids, but the receptor number and the protein induced by messenger RNA (mRNA) vary with the target cell. The reversible reaction results in exposure of nuclear binding sites, which results in binding to both DNA and chromatin protein. The receptor determines the specificity for a particular DNA sequence and hence regulates the formation of specific mRNAs that direct the synthesis of specific proteins. Thus, the plasma half-life may have no relationship to the biologic effects. The receptor binding in the nucleus is reversible, as is the binding of steroid to receptor. Glucocorticoids in-

Table 1. Comparison of Corticosteroid Agents

Drug	Affinity for Glucocorticoid Receptors	Potency, Anti-Inflammatory	Potency, Sodium Retaining	Duration of Action After Dose†
Hydrocortisone*	1.0	1.0	1.0	S
Cortisone	0.01	0.8	0.8	S
Corticosterone	0.85	0.3	15.0	S
Prednisolone	2.2	4.0	0.8	I
Prednisone	0.05	4.0	0.8	I
Methylprednisolone	11.9	5.0	Minimal	I
Triamcinolone	1.9	5.0	None	I
Dexamethasone	7.1	30.0	Minimal	L
Betamethasone	5.4	30.0	Minimal	L
Desoxycortisone	0.19	Minimal	50.0	—
Fludrocortisone	3.5	15.0	150.0	S
Aldosterone	0.38	None	500.0	—

*Hydrocortisone is standard of 1.
†Duration of action: S = 8 to 12 hr, I = 12 to 36 hr, L = 36 to 72 hr.

duce the formation of polypeptides that have anti-inflammatory effects. Macrocortin, a small polypeptide of macrophage origin, and lipomodulin, one of leukocyte origin, have an inhibitory effect on phospholipase A_2 and therefore act as a "brake" on inflammatory cells. Recent studies have emphasized the importance of the steroid-induced proteins' ability to modulate the inflammatory response.

Lipocortin is a term used collectively for anti-inflammatory protein mediators of glucocorticoid action. The gene for lipocortin has been cloned. In some humans with severe inflammatory disease, autoimmune disease, or both, plasma antibodies to lipomodulin decrease the activity of lipomodulin, blocking the natural suppression of inflammation by cortisol or synthetic glucocorticoids and allowing intense inflammatory responses to occur (e.g., rheumatoid arthritis and systemic lupus). The action of stabilization of liposomal membranes and decreased blood vessel permeability may be independent of phospholipase A_2. It varies with the species of animal.

Corticosteroid Receptors

Glucocorticoid receptors in target cells are subject to up regulation and down regulation. After exposure to corticosteroid, the receptor binding capacity declines significantly, but it returns to normal within 12 hr of hormone removal. The responsiveness of target cells is also influenced by the concentration of receptors. Chronic exposure to corticosteroids may cause increased side effects because of the decrease in target cell receptors. Thus, the side effects of Cushing's syndrome would be more common in tonic cortisol secretion or repository glucocorticoids, as compared with intermittent or alternate-day massive doses. It is not known if sustained down regulation of receptors is required

Table 2. Types of Corticosteroid Preparations

Parenteral preparations
1. Aqueous solutions of soluble steroid esters
   a. Sodium succinate and sodium phosphate (rapid absorption with hours of action)
      Dexamethasone, betamethasone, hydrocortisone, methylprednisolone, prednisolone, prednisone
2. Solutions of free steroid alcohols (insoluble solution in polyethylene glycol)
   a. Dexamethasone (Azium, Schering) flumethasone (Flucort, Diamond) (slower than esters, CNS problems with high dose IV)
3. Suspensions of insoluble steroid esters (short-acting drugs in complex with dissolution of particles being the rate-limiting step)
   a. Acetates, diacetates, acetonides, pivalates (local release of drug in tissue site [e.g., joint])
   b. Methylprednisolone acetate suspension (Depo-Medrol, Upjohn)
   c. Isoflupredone acetate suspension (Predef 2X, Upjohn)
   d. Triamcinolone acetonide suspension (Vetalog, Squibb)
   e. Triamcinolone diacetate suspension (Aristocort, Lederle)

Table 3. Initiation and Maintenance of Glucocorticoid Therapy

1. Decrease the end-product effects of inflammation, 1 to 2 mg/kg/day of short-acting divided b.i.d. or t.i.d. for 5 to 10 days
   Prednisolone, prednisone, methylprednisolone PO
2. If clinical response occurs, consolidate the total daily dose to s.i.d. for 1 week.
3. Reduce the s.i.d. dose to 0.5 to 1.0 mg/kg/day or less for 5 to 7 days
4. Convert to alternate-day therapy
5. Reduce dose by half each week until minimally effective dose can be determined. Discontinue steroid therapy if possible.

for effective suppression of immune cell function by corticosteroids. The buffering effects of albumin binding, which are observed with prednisolone, are less in dexamethasone and other glucocorticoids with low-affinity binding. The influence of target cell receptors is believed to be minimal in pituitary feedback and adipose tissue, where the activity of unbound corticosteroids is initially related to plasma or cytosol receptors and only later directly related to nuclear receptors.

LIVER

The liver is the main site of conversion of inactive prednisone to the biologically active prednisolone and the conversion of prednisolone to prednisone. The ratio of prednisolone to prednisone is relatively stable, each maintaining a bound and unbound fraction, and is usually noted by first passage through the liver regardless of which product is given. Except in very severe hepatic dysfunction, hepatic conversion is unaffected by disease. Further, in cirrhosis, a slight impairment of the conversion of prednisone into prednisolone (but not of the conversion of prednisolone into prednisone) is noted. However, although hepatic disease does not alter the dose of corticosteroids when low levels of serum albumin are present in cirrhosis patients, there is an increased amount of unbound corticosteroid. In addition, *in vitro* experiments have implied that increased bilirubin concentration would increase the unbound concentrations by displacing steroids from the albumin-binding sites, thereby increasing the biologic activity. Increased biologic activity can be assumed in icteric animals, especially those with unconjugated bilirubin and hypoalbuminemic serum. Except in severe hepatic failure, the metabolism of corticosteroids seems to be unaffected.

Induction of microsomal liver enzymes causes clinical failure of corticosteroid maintenance therapy in humans. Administration of rifampicin, barbiturates, and phenytoin requires the dose of prednisolone to be doubled to suppress plasma levels of cortisol. Changes in the ratio of prednisolone to prednisone, the amount of unbound drug, and the percentage of steroid metabolized have all been altered by drugs inducing hepatic enzymes. The addition of one of these drugs may result in the failure of a corticosteroid to suppress a disease because of altered hepatic metabolism. However, not all inhibitors of the P-450 system influence the metabolism of prednisolone. Cimetidine is an important example of a drug without effect on prednisolone metabolism.

Indications in Hepatic Disease

The continued lack of clear diagnostic and etiologic information about inflammatory hepatic disease in dogs prevents accurate recommendations of therapy for most clinical cases of "chronic hepatitis" (see *Current Veterinary Therapy IX*, p. 939). The apparent beneficial effects of decreasing bilirubin, decreasing patient discomfort, and stimulating appetite have not been associated with increased survival, decreased hospital time, or increased intervals between relapses. The corticosteroid therapy may cause a temporary remission and even predispose to complications. Hepatic abscess formation is uncommon in dogs but usually is the result of steroid therapy when bacterial endocarditis is misdiagnosed as an immune-mediated disease. Based on clinical evaluation in humans with virus-induced (hepatitis A or hepatitis B) chronic hepatitis, corticosteroid therapy has not been associated with any improvement in long-term prognosis and may be contraindicated in acute viral hepatic failure.

The role of corticosteroids in chronic hepatitis is unclear. Recommended initial dosages of prednisolone for dogs (1 to 2 mg/kg daily) are gradually decreased until maintenance levels of 0.4 mg/kg/day are reached. Given the hepatic side effects of corticosteroids and the relapsing and unpredictable nature of most chronic hepatic disorders in dogs, chronic corticosteroid administration may not control the inflammation or immune destruction of hepatic tissue. Corticosteroids' ability to induce independent hepatic disease further confuses sequential biochemical testing and hepatic biopsies.

Steroid-induced Hepatopathy

There are such differences in metabolism of corticosteroids and their availability to diffuse into target and hepatic cells that even a single dose may induce hepatic disease. Although glucocorticoids can induce a separate isoenzyme of alkaline phosphatase (AP) of hepatic origin, the initial and major increase in serum AP (SAP) is a result of hepatic insult, not a benign steroid-induced enzyme. The steroid-induced enzyme of AP in dogs has been associated with bile canaliculi and has been identified in hyperadrenocorticism, after corticosteroid administration, in hepatic lipidosis, diabetes mellitus, and neoplasia without any hepatic metastasis, and as a minor fraction in normal dogs.

The morphologic lesion of steroid-induced hepatopathy is variable but includes hepatic vacuolation and necrosis. Sometimes there is a more diffuse and subtle vacuolation. Prednisolone, prednisone, dexamethasone, and repository corticosteroids may cause the lesions. They may occur in the absence of abnormal hepatic enzymes (ALT and SAP) and may be present for weeks after elevated enzyme activity has returned to normal. Repository corticosteroids and alternate-day prednisolone frequently cause mild lesions without elevations in

SAP. In experimental studies, there was no difference in the hepatopathy when the same dose of prednisolone or prednisone was administered; however, the hepatopathy was more severe when the same dose of prednisolone was administered IM compared with PO. The peak concentration after IM dosage is higher than that following PO dosage. Following injection, the unbound portion is higher, and biologic effects and subsequent side effects are more conspicuous. Hepatopathy is more likely to occur in hypoalbuminemic dogs for the same reasons. The hepatopathy is generally considered to be reversible, although histologic lesions persist for weeks after therapy has been discontinued.

The common use of corticosteroids and the routine screening of dogs with biochemical profiles emphasize the need for a careful history of medications when evaluating increased values for SAP and alanine aminotransferase (ALT). A dog with steroid-induced hepatopathy commonly may have an elevated SAP and abnormal ALT and sulfobromophthalein (BSP) excretion, but this is rarely accompanied by an abnormal resting ammonia level. Careful monitoring of suspected hepatopathies with biochemical evaluation 1 month after discontinuing the steroids will avoid unnecessary hepatic biopsy. If corticosteroid therapy has been part of the medical history (even within the previous 6 weeks), the pathologist should be alerted if surgical biopsy is required for some other condition. Hepatic enzyme induction by barbiturates or inhibition by cyclophosphamide, erythromycin, or other drugs, and the combined use of corticosteroids with other hepatotoxic drugs (e.g., primidone, mebendazole, thiacetarsamide) is of clinical concern in many complicated cases.

GLUCOCORTICOIDS IN THE BOWEL

The effects of glucocorticoids on the bowel are probably time, dose, and product specific. At normal serum concentrations, hydrocortisone would seem to have a dose-dependent protective effect on human enterocytes. Thus, glucocorticoids at physiologic levels may maintain the digestive, absorptive, and cellular function of human jejunum and may explain the diarrhea in the glucocorticoid-deficient state of Addison's disease. The duodenum has the highest concentration of glucocorticoid receptors in the bowel. In addition, the effects of glucocorticoids on the net Na^+ and water absorption and K^+ secretion by the colonic epithelium are of uncertain clinical significance.

An initial enhanced absorptive capacity of the small bowel after corticosteroids may be mediated by an increase in carrier transport and activation of brush-border enzymes. Studies indicate that there is an enhanced synthesis of enterocyte membrane proteins, with the implication of a direct action on mature enterocytes to increase absorptive and digestive capacities. However, the ability of chronic steroid administration to decrease crypt cell turnover results in hypoplasia and decrease in enterocyte numbers and an implied decrease in villous regeneration after damage. The clinical significance of these observations might help explain the rapid response of some bowel diseases to corticosteroids and the possible liabilities of chronic corticosteroid administration.

Inflammatory Bowel Disease

The inability to establish a specific infectious etiology or specific environmental etiology (related to such factors as foods or toxins) has led to the initial conclusion that inflammatory bowel disease (IBD) is an immunologic disorder. In humans, autoantibodies reactive with mucin-associated antigens or with colonic epithelial cell antigens have been identified in ulcerative colitis. Circulating and intestinal lymphocytes from humans with IBD were cytotoxic for colonic epithelial cells and are antibody dependent. The hypothesis that IBD is caused by autoantibodies that arm natural killerlike cells that are cytolytic is consistent with a steroid-responsive disease. IBD may be the result of a poorly regulated immune response to one or more mucosal or bacterial antigens, leading to the influx of inflammatory cells that are the actual cause of tissue injury.

The responsiveness of IBD to corticosteroids is probably related to the chronicity and severity of the chronic inflammatory disease. The reversibility of ulcerative colitis, for example, is dependent not on the degree of inflammation but on the degree of fibrosis before therapy is started. This dependence emphasizes the need for early diagnosis and therapy.

Most steroids probably are absorbed from the small intestine by simple passive diffusion. In studies of humans with IBD, the absorption of prednisolone was extremely variable. Some patients with severe malabsorption had incomplete absorption. The site and the severity of the bowel disease will influence the diffusion, so the clinician must calculate the dose according to the clinical signs instead of using a standard dose of 1 to 2 mg/kg b.i.d. A standard dosage is further complicated by the hypoalbuminemia that frequently is associated with a protein-losing enteropathy. The unbound and biologically active portion would be significantly higher in the patient with low serum albumin levels. Side effects and delayed healing after surgery would likewise be a consequence of the same dose in a hypoalbuminemic dog.

Prednisolone would have a higher local biologic effect than would prednisone in the bowel, but the systemic effects would be identical. Patients with IBD of the lower bowel may benefit from the use of enteric-coated prednisolone, so the release in the terminal ileum and colon would have a more pronounced local effect. If local effects are desired, the use of enteric-coated corticosteroids would apply only to biologically active metabolites and not to prodrugs (prednisone, hydrocortisone).

In addition to IBD, an excessive immunologic response has been associated with gluten-sensitive enteropathy, food allergy, and an ill-defined eosinophilic-plasmacytic enteritis. Identification and removal of the offending stimuli are difficult in the average clinical practice. However, elimination of potential pathogens such as parasites (e.g., *Giardia, Campylobacter, Histoplasma*) is important before a malabsorption syndrome is treated with corticosteroids. Exacerbation of a fungal or parasitic disorder may occur after corticosteroids are given. The clinical responses of IBD and eosinophilic-plasmacytic enteritis to corticosteroids are often quite remarkable. Initial high doses (prednisolone, 1 to 2 mg/kg b.i.d. for 5 days) should be tapered to low doses (0.5 mg/kg s.i.d. for 7 to 14 days). The initiation of prednisolone therapy is delayed for 1 week after full-thickness bowel biopsy. Because of the variables of absorption and plasma binding, the dose is frequently adjusted, depending on clinical response. In severe diffuse infiltrative small bowel disease, parenteral prednisolone is used for the first 3 days. Increasing the dose to extremely high concentrations does not enhance the duration or intensity of immunosuppression and increases the likelihood of side effects. In dogs, there appears to be no advantage in maintaining therapy after an initial response. The malabsorption will often abate without any clinical recurrence in dogs between the ages of 1 to 3 years. The clinical signs of ulcerative colitis may often return despite therapy; and when clinical signs return, the effects of sulfasalazine (Azulfidine, Pharmacia) for maintenance are augmented by corticosteroids. The clinical experience in cats with IBD indicates that chronic corticosteroids are frequently necessary to control clinical signs. The clinical side effects are minimal.

Dogs with severe hypoproteinemia and malabsorptive small bowel diarrhea from IBD can respond with weight gain and normal plasma protein levels within weeks of corticosteroid therapy. The rapid return of normal absorptive test results emphasizes that corticosteroids may block the end effect of the inflammatory response in the bowel rather than inhibit antibody formation or dissociation of antigen-antibody complexes or alter the initiating cause. The growing evidence that IBD is often the result of increased concentration of leukotriene B4 from activated neutrophils, but without evidence of increased arachidonic acid metabolism, explains why this defective metabolism may be normalized by

steroids, sulfasalazine, and 5-aminosalicylic acid, all of which inhibit steps in arachidonic acid metabolism. Steroids induce the synthesis of phospholipase inhibitors (lipocortin), and sulfasalazine and 5-aminosalicylic acid inhibit the activity of lipoxygenase, a more specific enzyme for leukotrienes. The direct effect of the glucocorticoid on enterocyte function may provide another key.

Gastrointestinal Complications of Corticosteroids

High doses of dexamethasone have been associated with gastric bleeding and ulcers. However, the evidence that corticosteroids alone predispose to gastric or colonic ulcers is unclear.

Although glucocorticoids rarely are the sole cause of gastrointestinal ulceration or bleeding, experimental studies indicate that decreased gastrointestinal mucus production and altered mucus barrier are the result of high doses. Stimulation of the G-cells to produce gastrin, combined with impaired blood flow to the mucosal layers of the stomach, will promote acid back-diffusion, with the potential for gastric erosion and ulcer formation. The potential for ulcer formation is promoted by decreased epithelial repair, which predisposes the dog to the ulcerogenic effects of other drugs, especially nonsteroidal anti-inflammatory agents. Careful consideration should be given to combining of ulcerogenic drugs, especially with high doses of corticosteroids. Most dogs receiving high doses of corticosteroids develop occult blood in the stool, usually without clinical or endoscopic signs.

Gastrointestinal hemorrhage, gastric and colonic ulcers and perforation, and pancreatitis are complications of high doses of dexamethasone, used in many neurosurgical patients. Gastric erosions are a frequent occurrence even after only 2 days of dexamethasone therapy. However, colonic perforation characterized by depression, anorexia, and vomiting and resulting in death 4 to 8 weeks after surgery is a serious sequela. The perforation usually occurs in the proximal descending colon on the antimesenteric border. The neurologic disorder probably results in altered bowel motility, causing physical trauma to mucosa, alteration in bacterial flora, and abnormal microcirculation, which causes ischemia. The experimental combination of dexamethasone and severe hypotension and hemilaminectomy did not increase the incidence of gastric or colonic erosions or bleeding as compared with dexamethasone alone. This emphasizes the neurologic dysfunction that contributes to the clinical complication of corticosteroid therapy. The continued use of corticosteroids in the presence of a perforated bowel is usually fatal because of the decreased ability of white blood cells to destroy bacteria at the site of perforation, the blunted systemic inflammatory response to the stimuli, and the delayed healing and repair. There may also be a delay in diagnosis because of the blunting of the febrile response from blocking interleukin-2. The high doses of dexamethasone exacerbate the problem because of the poor plasma binding and the long biologic effects even after the drug is discontinued. Dexamethasone requires four to five half-lives before 95 per cent of the drug is removed, and its biologic effect continues well beyond the disappearance of the drug.

Recommendations to prevent gastrointestinal complications of corticosteroid administration in dogs (especially patients with neurologic impairment) include the following: (1) Use prednisolone or prednisone; (2) use short-term therapy; (3) do not use ulcerogenic drugs such as aspirin concomitantly; (4) correct fecal retention before surgery and avoid enemas immediately after surgery; (5) avoid repeated manual expression of the urinary bladder by using indwelling catheterization. The use of an H_2 antagonist is common but of unknown clinical benefit. The route of administration (PO versus IM) does not appear to be a significant factor in the development of gastric or colonic complications.

ROLE OF CORTICOSTEROIDS IN PANCREATITIS

Corticosteroid therapy has been incriminated as a predisposing cause of acute pancreatitis in humans and dogs. However, experimental evidence in dogs and humans has indicated that increased serum lipase activity can be the consequence of high doses of corticosteroids in the absence of histologic evidence of pancreatitis. Increased enzyme activity could be the result of increased pancreatic synthesis, increased cellular permeability to pancreatic enzymes, and extrapancreatic release of lipase from liver or adipose tissue. Although anecdotal reports of the occurrence of pancreatitis after steroid therapy abound, a critical review of human cases and experimental studies has not established a pattern. The pancreatic acinar lesions after glucocorticoids in rabbits and mice are species specific and have not been observed in guinea pigs, rats, or dogs. The production of viscous proteinaceous secretions that obstruct the pancreatic duct and induce pancreatitis after corticosteroid use has not been confirmed in dogs. Studies of exocrine pancreatic secretion and evaluation of trypsin, bicarbonate, and morphologic changes after corticosteroid administration in intact dogs and in the isolated canine pancreas are often conflicting.

Experimental studies have indicated that glucocorticoids can stimulate formation of zymogen granules, resulting in overfilling of the cells with secretory products even though secretions were unchanged. Further studies have indicated that glucocorticoids can increase the cholecystokinin (CCK) receptors on cells without changing their affinity for CCK, resulting in increased sensitivity to CCK and increased amylase secretion with minimal CCK stimulation.

Although consequences of lipid and carbohydrate metabolism associated with corticosteroids could presumably predispose to pancreatitis, serum cholesterol and triglyceride levels were unchanged after chronic administration of dexamethasone or prednisolone in experimental dogs. Triglyceride electrophoresis was not altered after long-term prednisolone treatment in dogs.

The lack of convincing clinical or experimental studies in dogs, the absence of a consistent tissue-injury pattern in steroid-treated dogs, the elevation of serum lipase in the absence of disease, and the absence of secretory abnormalities lead one to question whether steroid-induced pancreatitis is a common singular clinical entity. Although the author and others can cite apparent cases of steroid-induced pancreatitis, the experimental evidence does not support such a contention, and a rare relapse of pancreatitis after steroid challenge has been mentioned. Given the common administration of corticosteroids for allergic and dermatologic conditions and the rarely documented pancreatitis after therapy, the incrimination of glucocorticoids as a single cause of pancreatitis in dogs would seem to be overemphasized.

Further, the potential beneficial role of corticosteroids in necrotizing pancreatitis to decrease the production of lymphokines and proteases, decrease edema, and improve microcirculation in the pancreas should be considered an adjunct to fluid therapy. Because experimental studies of intact and isolated canine pancreas with ductal infusion of oleic acid have failed to provide evidence for the use of steroids in this chemical model of pancreatitis, the use of corticosteroids in mild pancreatitis is not recommended. In human pancreatitis, the potential benefits of corticosteroids have received new emphasis. The use of corticosteroids (prednisolone, 3 to 5 mg/kg) in conjunction with fluid therapy for shock in the treatment of necrotizing pancreatitis *is* indicated when the consequences of release of pancreatic proteases and lymphokines are the major concern.

References and Supplemental Reading

Batt, R. M., Scott, J.: Response of the small intestinal mucosa to oral glucocorticoids. Scand. J. Gastroenterol. [Suppl] 74:75, 1982.

Bencosme, S. A., Lazonarus, S. S.: Pancreas of cortisone-treated rabbits. Arch. Pathol. 62:285, 1956.

Bergrem, H., Groitum, P., Rugstad, H. E.: Pharmacokinetics and protein binding of prednisolone after oral and intravenous administration. Eur. J. Clin. Pharmacol. 24:415, 1983.

Bergrem, H., Opedal, I.: Bioavailability of prednisolone in patients with intestinal malabsorption: The importance of measuring serum protein-binding. Scand. J. Gastroenterol. 18:545, 1983.

Davis, M., Williams, R., Chakroborty, J., et al.: Prednisone or prednisolone for the treatment of chronic active hepatitis? A comparison of plasma availability. Br. J. Clin. Pharmacol. 5:501, 1978.

Dillon, A. R., Sorjonen, D. C., Spano, J. S., et al.: Effects of dexamethasone and surgical hypotension on hepatic morphologic features and enzymes of dogs. Am. J. Vet. Res. 44:1996, 1983.

Dillon, A. R., Spano, J. S., Powers, R. D.: Prednisolone induced hematologic, biochemical and histologic changes in the dog. J. Am. Anim. Hosp. Assoc. 16:831, 1980.

Eckersall, P. D., and Nash, A. S.: Isoenzymes of canine plasma alkaline phosphatase: An investigation using isoelectric focusing and related to diagnosis. Res. Vet. Sci. 34:310, 1983.

Frey, B. M., Frey, F. J.: Phenytoin modulates the pharmacokinetics of prednisolone and the pharmacodynamics of prednisolone as assessed by the inhibition of the mixed lymphocyte reaction in humans. Eur. J. Clin. Invest. 14:1, 1984.

Frey, F. J., Frey, B. M., Benet, L. Z.: Inequality of clearance values obtained by IV bolus and by steady state infusion: Prednisolone studies in dogs. Pharmacology 24:246, 1982.

Frey, F. J., Frey, B. M., Greither, A., et al.: Prednisolone clearance at steady state in dogs. J. Pharmacol. Exp. Ther. 215:287, 1980.

Frey, F. J., Ruegsegger, M. K., Frey, B. M.: The dose-dependent systemic availability of prednisone, one reason for the reduced biological effect of alternate-day prednisone. Br. J. Clin. Pharmacol. 21:183, 1986.

Korkor, A. B., Kuchiboltla, L., Arrieh, M., et al.: The effects of chronic prednisone administration on intestinal receptors for 1,25-dihydroxyvitamin D_3 in the dog. Endocrinology 117:2267, 1985.

Madsbad, S., Bjerregaard, B., Henriksen, J. H., et al.: Impaired conversion of prednisone to prednisolone in patients with liver cirrhosis. Gut 21:52, 1980.

Milne, E. M., and Doxey, D. L.: Alkaline phosphatase and its isoenzymes in the tissues and sera of normal dogs. Vet. Res. Commun. 10:229, 1986.

Milsap, R. L., George, D. E., Szefler, S. J., et al.: Effect of inflammatory bowel disease on absorption and disposition of prednisolone. Dig. Dis. Sci. 28:161, 1983.

Moore, M. R., and Robinette, J. D.: Cecal perforation and adrenocortical adenoma in a dog. J.A.V.M.A. 191:87, 1987.

Moore, R. W., Withrow, S. J.: Gastrointestinal hemorrhage and pancreatitis associated with intervertebral disk disease in the dog. J.A.V.M.A. 180:1443, 1982.

Muller-Peddinghaus, R., Niepold, D., Hillebrand, W., et al.: Glucocorticosteroid effects on dog and rat serum complement. Immunopharmacology 7:567, 1985.

Nielsen, O. H., Ahnfelt-Ronne, I., Elmgreen, J., et al.: Abnormal metabolism of arachidonic acid in chronic inflammatory bowel disease: Enhanced release of leucotriene B_4 from activated neutrophils. Gut 28:181, 1987.

Olivesi, A.: Nonabsorption of enteric-coated prednisolone. Normal absorption of nonenteric-coated prednisolone in a patient with Crohn's disease and massive intestinal resection. Therapie 40:5, 1985.

Parent, J.: Effects of dexamethasone on pancreatic tissue and serum amylase and lipase activities in dogs. J.A.V.M.A. 108:743, 1982.

Pickup, M. E., Farah, F., Lowe, J. R., et al.: Prednisolone absorption in coeliac disease. Eur. J. Drug Metab. Pharmacokinet. 2:87, 1979.

Renner, E., Horber, F. F., Jost, G., et al.: Effect of liver function on the metabolism of prednisone and prednisolone in humans. Gastroenterology 90:819, 1986.

Rose, J. Q., Yurchak, A. M., Meikle, A. W., et al.: Effect of smoking on prednisone, prednisolone and dexamethasone pharmacokinetics. J. Pharmacokinet. Biopharm. 9:1, 1981.

Rose, J. Q., Yurchak, A. M., Jusko, W. J.: Dose-dependent pharmacokinetics of prednisone and prednisolone in man. J. Pharmacokinet. Biopharm. 9:389, 1981.

Schalm, S. W., Summerskill, W. H. J., Co, V. L. W.: Prednisone for chronic active liver disease: Pharmacokinetics, including conversion to prednisolone. Gastroenterology 72:910, 1978.

Scott, J., Peters, T. J.: Protection of epithelial function in human jejunum, cultured with hydrocortisone. Am. J. Physiol. 83:532, 1983.

Sorjonen, D. C., Dillon, A. R., Powers, R. D., et al.: Effects of dexamethasone and surgical hypotension on stomach of dogs: A clinical, endoscopic and pathologic evaluation. Am. J. Vet. Res. 44:127, 1983.

Tanner, A. R., Halliday, J. W., Powell, L. W.: Serum prednisolone levels in Crohn's disease and coeliac disease following oral prednisolone administration. Digestion 21:310, 1985.

Thomas, P., Richards, D., Richards, A., et al.: Absorption of delayed-release prednisolone in ulcerative colitis and Crohn's disease. J. Pharm. Pharmacol. 37:757, 1985.

Tsang, S. Y., Garovoy, M. R., Benet, L. Z.: Immunosuppressive activity of prednisone and prednisolone and their metabolic interconversion in the mixed lymphocyte reaction. Therapie 40:5, 1985.

Tsang, S. Y., Garovoy, M. R., Benet, L. Z.: Immunosuppressive activity of prednisone and prednisolone and their metabolic interconversion in the mixed lymphocyte reaction. Int. J. Immunopharmacol. 7:731, 1985.

Uribe, M., Schalm, S. W., Summerskill, W. H. J., et al.: Oral prednisone for chronic active liver disease: Dose responses and bioavailability studies. Gut 19:1131, 1978.

Wellman, M. L., Hoffman, W. E., Dorner, J. L., et al.: Immunoassay for the steroid-induced isoenzyme of alkaline phosphatase in the dog. Am. J. Vet. Res. 43:1200, 1981.

ESOPHAGEAL STRICTURES

DENNIS A. ZAWIE, D.V.M.

Farmingville, New York

Acquired intraluminal esophageal stricture in small animals is a sequela to severe, acute esophagitis (Strombeck, 1979). Strictures generally involve the entire circumference of the esophageal wall, often reducing the lumen to only a few millimeters in diameter.

Cicatrix formation can be found at any location in the esophagus. Most strictures are found at the thoracic inlet because of pooling of gastric fluid in this region, especially if reflux occurs during an anesthetic procedure (Hardie et al., 1987; Zawie, 1985). In the majority of cases, a solitary, fibrous band is noted, but multiple ringlike strictures can occasionally be seen. Success of therapy is often dependent on the length of the stricture. Generally, the longer the stricture, the more difficult it is to manage and the more guarded the prognosis becomes.

PATHOGENESIS OF ESOPHAGEAL STRICTURES

Esophagitis can result from the ingestion of a strong acid or alkali, thermal burns, trauma secondary to foreign bodies, or reflux of gastric fluid into the esophagus.

Esophagitis associated with gastric reflux primarily occurs during procedures requiring general anesthesia and is the most common cause of esophagitis in small animals (Pearson et al., 1978). Drugs such as diazepam, atropine, and certain narcotic analgesics interfere with proper function of the lower esophageal sphincter (Strombeck, 1979). As a result, destructive components within gastric juice are refluxed into the esophagus and promote the inflammatory process. Hydrochloric acid reduces esophageal pH to 2.0 and causes protein denaturation of esophageal mucosa (Pope, 1983). Pepsinogen is activated to pepsin at a low pH. The proteolytic properties of this enzyme cause further tissue destruction (Pope, 1983). Bile acids and pancreatic enzymes also enhance the erosion of esophageal epithelium (Pope, 1983). Furthermore, anesthetic agents suppress normal esophageal motility, thereby increasing contact time between esophageal mucosa and destructive elements in gastric juice (Pope, 1983). When this occurs, esophagitis becomes severe and the likelihood of stricture formation increases. Poor patient preparation (food-filled stomach) and tilting the surgery table also predispose an animal to reflux esophagitis (Zawie, 1985).

When the inflammatory process extends beyond the mucosal layer, through the lamina propria and into the muscle layers, scar tissue formation occurs. Once the deeper layers of the esophagus are affected by the inflammatory process, fibroblastic activity begins almost immediately (Strombeck, 1979). It can take up to a week or more for collagen fibers to form and for a mature stricture to develop. Therefore, clinical signs may not be apparent until some time after the initial insult (Strombeck, 1979).

CLINICAL SIGNS

Regurgitation of solid food is the predominant clinical sign associated with esophageal strictures. Affected animals can only handle gruels or liquids. In spite of having a ravenous appetite, these animals lose weight because of decreased caloric intake associated with chronic regurgitation. Signs of pain or discomfort are uncommon.

DIAGNOSIS

Although endoscopic examination can be helpful in evaluating esophageal strictures, it must be emphasized that the diameter of the esophageal lumen is less than the diameter of the average endoscope (7.5 to 9.0 mm) in many cases of stricture. Thus, in these instances, the endoscope cannot be advanced through the stricture and the extent of scar tissue

formation cannot be assessed. A routine esophagogram using liquid barium remains one of the best methods of evaluating the number, length, and location of esophageal strictures.*

TREATMENT

The treatment for esophageal strictures includes surgery or bougienage. Surgical resection of esophageal strictures is difficult and requires considerable expertise. Furthermore, a number of complications including restricture at the surgical anastomosis can arise (Strombeck, 1979). Surgery for this condition is reported to have less than a 50 per cent success rate (Harvey, 1985).

Dilatation of the esophagus can be accomplished by using graduated steel-stemmed or mercury-filled dilators (bougies) (Hardie et al., 1987). This technique, called bougienage, must be performed under general anesthesia. Proper equipment is essential to assure successful dilatation.

Initially, small-diameter dilators are passed through the esophageal lumen. As the fibrous ring stretches, progressively larger dilators are passed until the stricture is completely broken down. Considerable damage can be done to the esophageal wall, and care must be taken not to undermine the esophageal mucosa or perforate the esophagus entirely. Bougienage must often be repeated if restricture occurs. This procedure is best left to those veterinary clinicians who have developed this particular skill. If multiple strictures are present, another technique using a guide wire and stainless steel "olives" is recommended.

A new method of managing esophageal strictures using balloon catheters has recently been described (Hardie et al., 1987; Burke et al., 1987). A specially treated polyethylene catheter (Rigiflex Dilator, Microvasive) is advanced to the stricture site under fluoroscopic or endoscopic control. General anesthesia is required. Once the center of the balloon is properly positioned at the stricture site, it is inflated with dilute contrast medium. Luminal pressure is monitored with a manometer. When adequate distention occurs, the stricture visibly dilates. Postdilatation evaluation with an endoscope is necessary to assess damage to the esophageal mucosa and assure adequate distention of the esophagus. Balloon catheter dilatation is superior to bougienage, because radial stretch forces rather than longitudinal shearing forces are generated at the stricture site (Dawson et al., 1984). Other advantages of balloon dilatation are a decreased risk of perforation,

---

***Editor's Note**: In some instances, Barium paste or Barium meal is required to demonstrate an esophageal stricture, as liquid barium may easily pass undetected through all but the most narrow strictures.

a longer period free of clinical signs, and a decreased number of procedures required to dilate the stricture (Dawson et al., 1984).

After bougienage or balloon dilatation is completed, intensive therapy for esophagitis is instituted. First, cimetidine (Tagamet, SmithKline) is initiated at 10 mg/kg every 8 hours to decrease acid secretion. Cimetidine is usually given by intramuscular injection in the hospital and changed to oral administration upon release. Second, an anti-inflammatory dosage of prednisone, 0.5 mg/kg daily, is given to decrease fibroblastic activity and prevent further stricture formation. Metoclopramide (Reglan, A. H. Robins) can also be used to help prevent further gastroesophageal reflux. The drug can be given orally or by subcutaneous injection at a dosage of 0.2 to 0.5 mg/kg three times daily. Therapy is generally continued for approximately 2 weeks.

Gastrostomy tubes may be necessary to provide nutritional support in debilitated animals or if food intake is restricted for any length of time because multiple dilatation procedures are indicated.

References and Supplemental Reading

Burke, R. L., Zawie, D. A., and Garvey, M. S.: Balloon catheter dilation of intramural esophageal strictures in the dog and cat: A description of the procedure and a report of six cases. Semin. Vet. Med. Surg. (Small Anim.) 2:241, 1987.

Dawson, S. L., Mueller, P. R., Ferruci, J. T., et al.: Severe esophageal strictures: Indications for balloon catheter dilitation. Radiology 153:631, 1984.

Hardie, E. M., Greene, R. T., Ford, R. B., et al.: Balloon dilatation for treatment of esophageal stricture: A case report. J. Am. Anim. Hosp. Assoc. 23:547, 1987.

Harvey, C. E.: Esophagus. In Slatter, D. H. (ed.): *Textbook of Small Animal Surgery*. Philadelphia: W. B. Saunders Co., 1985, pp. 661–662.

Pearson, H., Darke, P. G. G., Gibbs, C., et al.: Reflux oesophagitis and stricture formation after anesthesia: A review of seven cases in dogs and cats. J. Small Anim. Pract. 19:507, 1978.

Pope, C. E.: Gastroesophageal reflux. In Sleisenger, M. H., and Fordtram, J. S. (eds.): *Gastrointestinal Disease*. Philadelphia: W. B. Saunders Co., 1983, pp. 449–475.

Strombeck, D. R.: *Small Animal Gastroenterology*. Davis, CA: Stonegate Publishing, 1979, pp. 50–67.

Zawie, D. A.: Medical diseases of the esophagus. AAHA 1985 Scientific Proceedings. 52:267, 1985.

REFLUX ESOPHAGITIS

TODD R. TAMS, D.V.M.
West Los Angeles, California

The term *reflux* refers to movement of gastric or duodenal contents into the esophagus without associated eructation or vomiting. Reflux esophagitis is a disorder in which esophageal inflammation of variable degree occurs as a result of mucosal contact with gastric or duodenal fluid or ingesta. In many cases, the inflammation may not be visible grossly. A variety of factors can contribute to its development in individual patients. The incidence of reflux esophagitis in dogs and cats is unknown, but it is thought to occur more commonly than is currently recognized. It can be particularly difficult to diagnose without special instrumentation (e.g., pH probe monitoring, endoscopy), because in many animal cases clinical signs are quite subtle. History and recognition of suggestive clinical signs constitute the basis for performing diagnostic procedures or instituting empiric therapy. Because significant discomfort can result from reflux episodes, it is important that reflux esophagitis be diagnosed and treated without delay.

Normal lower esophageal sphincter (LES) function is essential in the prevention of gastroesophageal reflux and esophagitis. The LES is located at the gastroesophageal junction and is a zone of high resting pressure that acts to prevent reflux of gastric contents into the esophagus. In response to esophageal peristaltic contractions, the LES undergoes a phase of initial relaxation that is followed by postdeglutition contraction. Initial relaxation begins when an esophageal peristaltic contraction is in the proximal esophagus. Postdeglutition contractions prevent reflux of a food bolus following its passage into the stomach.

Reflux of small amounts of fluid is considered a normal physiologic phenomenon in both animals and people. Functional defense mechanisms prevent esophageal mucosal damage when these minor reflux episodes occur. These defenses include acid clearance by means of one or two esophageal peristaltic sequences that empty all or most of the acid from the esophagus and neutralization of any postperistaltic residual acid by bicarbonate-rich saliva. It has been shown in human patients that some individuals can experience significant reflux episodes without developing demonstrable esophageal mucosal changes. Although clinical signs of reflux may be experienced (heartburn, indigestion, dyspepsia), significant sequelae such as esophagitis, esophageal stricture, and chest pain often never develop.

Although the relationships and factors responsible for individual variations in response to reflux are unknown, a number of factors are likely involved in determining how significant a problem reflux episodes will be in an individual. These include volume and frequency of reflux, character of the refluxed material, competency of esophageal clearing mechanisms, and gastric emptying patterns. It has been estimated that up to 7 per cent of the general human population has symptoms of heartburn daily, and a much larger percentage monthly. Many humans never seek medical attention for what they consider a minor problem or normal physiologic event. The frequency of mild reflux in animals is unknown, since signs of mild reflux are extremely difficult to detect.

MECHANISMS OF GASTROESOPHAGEAL REFLUX

Manometric measurements of the LES have shown that a decrease in resting pressures is the major factor in the pathogenesis of gastroesophageal reflux. Reflux primarily occurs by three different mechanisms: transient complete relaxation of the LES, a transient increase in intra-abdominal pressure, or spontaneous free reflux associated with a low resting pressure of the LES. Human studies have shown that in normal individuals reflux episodes are almost always caused by transient sphincter relaxation. The predominant reflux mechanism in reflux esophagitis patients varies, although transient LES relaxation seems to predominate. This transient relaxation mechanism may explain why some patients with reflux esophagitis have resting LES pressure values that overlap those of normal controls.

Transient changes in intra-abdominal pressure may intermittently overcome a hypotensive LES; however, complete sphincter relaxation alone does not guarantee that significant reflux will occur. Factors that may influence reflux in this situation include body position, intragastric volume, intragastric pressure, and relaxation of the diaphragmatic hiatus. Significant reflux can occur in animals that undergo general anesthesia, especially when ingesta or fluid is retained in the stomach. Anesthetic agents promote relaxation of the LES, and any procedure that involves positioning the patient with the rear quarters elevated can promote gravitational flow of gastric contents to the esophagus. Mild to severe esophagitis may result, and in some cases esophageal stricture formation occurs. Clinical situations in which a reflux episode may be enhanced must be recognized and preventive measures used to decrease the chances of occurrence of serious sequelae.

MECHANISMS OF ESOPHAGEAL MUCOSAL DAMAGE

Although both acid and pepsin have been implicated in the past as the major injurious agents in reflux disease, it now appears that the importance of acid has been overemphasized and that of pepsin minimized. Recent animal studies have shown that pepsin, rather than acid, is a major causative agent of erosive esophagitis caused by reflux of acid gastric contents.

Of the potentially injurious agents in *acid* gastric contents (acid, bile salts, pepsin, trypsin, others), pepsin produces a mucosal injury consistent with both the macroscopic and microscopic appearance of reflux esophagitis in symptomatic human patients. Hydrochloric acid at physiologic pH values does not appear to break the esophageal squamous mucosal barrier to hydrogen ion back-diffusion or cause esophagitis. Pepsin, however, can cause mucosal permeability changes resulting in severe hydrogen ion back-diffusion. Rabbit esophageal perfusion studies demonstrated that pepsin causes significantly more esophageal injury than does bile, trypsin, or acid alone. The extent of injury increased in a dose-dependent manner as pepsin concentration was increased. Pepsin injury was characterized by mucosal erosion and ulceration with submucosal hemorrhage. Acid, bile, and trypsin damage was generally limited to submucosal edema without mucosal disruption.

Excessive *alkaline* gastroesophageal reflux produces inflammatory changes comparable to excessive acid gastroesophageal reflux. The alkaline nature of refluxed material alone does not appear to produce mucosal damage. Rather, in the presence of alkaline reflux, the pancreatic enzyme trypsin has been shown to be the factor that causes the most significant damage. Pepsin causes minimal esophageal changes in the presence of an alkaline environment. Trypsin is present in the gastric contents of human patients with decreased pyloric tone and duodenogastric reflux. The pH of the refluxate appears to control which agent will be the most active in causing esophageal damage. Pepsin's optimal pH range for proteolytic activity is 2 to 4.5, and it is the most injurious agent when the refluxate is acid. Trypsin's optimal pH range for proteolytic activity is 5 to 8.

The bile salt taurodeoxycholate was found to protect the esophageal mucosa from the injurious effects of acid and pepsin, but the effect of trypsin in the alkaline medium was potentiated. Bile salts decrease pepsin's proteolytic activity, and the protective bile salt effect is dose related. The combination of bile, trypsin, and an alkaline refluxate could potentially cause the most severe degree of esophageal injury. Bile salts may play an important role in modulating the injurious effect of acid and pepsin in certain clinical settings. The concentration of injurious agents in the refluxed gastric fluid and the duration of their contact with the esophageal mucosa are the major factors determining the likelihood and severity of mucosal injury.

FACTORS THAT PROMOTE GASTROESOPHAGEAL REFLUX

Pharmacologic agents that have been associated with decreased LES pressure and reflux include atropine, morphine, meperidine, diazepam, and pentobarbital. Phenothiazine-derivative tranquilizers can also decrease LES pressure. Pregnancy in humans is associated with an increased frequency of heartburn, a sensation of chest pain that is due to esophageal pain from mucosal contact with refluxate. This was originally thought to be due to reflux enhanced by increased gastric pressure from an enlarging uterus. However, it is now recognized that elevated progesterone levels decrease LES pressure, increasing the likelihood of reflux. Reflux esophagitis in humans can also be stimulated by high-fat or spicy foods, chocolate, alcohol, and nicotine.

The most common causes of reflux esophagitis in dogs and cats are general anesthesia, persistent vomiting due to any cause (e.g., pancreatitis, gastric or intestinal foreign body), and hiatal hernia disorders. Delayed gastric emptying and duodenogastric reflux are less commonly associated with reflux esophagitis episodes. During anesthesia, there is suppression of normal esophageal motility as well as decreased LES pressure. As a result, acid and other refluxed agents cannot be cleared as quickly as in an awake animal with normal esophageal defenses. In addition to the use of anesthetic agents, elevation of the animal's abdomen relative to the thorax if the surgery table is tilted and improper preparation (e.g., incompletely evacuated stomach) also can play a major role in enhancing reflux. Moderate to severe esophagitis can result in esophageal stricture formation (see the previous article, entitled Esophageal Strictures).

Most hiatal hernia patients have some degree of reflux esophagitis. Decreased LES pressure leads to esophageal reflux in most patients with sliding hiatal hernias. Hiatal hernia patients are often presented for evaluation because of clinical signs that suggest a significant degree of esophagitis (e.g., salivation, inappetance, decreased activity, regurgitation). Treatment involves both management of esophagitis and medical management or surgical correction of the hiatal hernia.

Gastric emptying and gastric motility may be reduced in some patients with gastroesophageal reflux. Delayed emptying of liquids or solids would be expected to increase esophageal reflux. However, only a fraction of human patients with reflux esophagitis have delayed gastric emptying. Detailed studies have not been performed in animals, but clinical signs and endoscopic evidence of esophagitis in patients with gastric motility disorders have not been commonly observed by the author. The most important clinical situation regarding patients with gastric motility disorders probably involves general anesthesia. Every effort must be made to ensure that there is sufficient time for the stomach to empty before anesthetic induction, since the combination of anesthesia and an incompletely evacuated stomach increases the likelihood of a reflux episode and subsequent development of esophagitis.

Duodenogastric reflux may be damaging for two reasons. It increases the gastric volume available for gastroesophageal reflux and it adds bile and other potentially damaging duodenal fluid components to the gastric contents. Animals that have a chronic intermittent pattern of vomiting bile fluid may have duodenogastric reflux and should be watched carefully for signs of esophagitis.

DIAGNOSIS

The clinical signs of reflux esophagitis vary depending on the degree of inflammation present. The clinician must maintain a high index of suspicion, because in many cases only subtle clinical signs may be evident. With mild esophagitis, there may be increased swallowing motions, salivation, and inappetance. In more severe cases, there may be regurgitation, dysphagia, total anorexia, and signs such as reluctance to move, standing with the head extended, reluctance to lie down, and trembling, suggesting esophageal pain. Heartburn pain in humans can be quite intense, and it is suspected that a similar situation exists in animals. Esophageal hemorrhage may occur in severe cases.

The immediate past medical history must be reviewed carefully and may provide important clues regarding both diagnosis and etiology. Signs such as increased attempts at swallowing, salivation, regurgitation, and inappetance that occur within 1 to 4 days of an anesthetic procedure strongly suggest reflux esophagitis. Coughing may indicate aspiration pneumonia. Animals with persistent vomiting should be observed carefully for signs of esophagitis. Severe esophagitis must be identified and treated early, since one of the potential sequelae is stricture formation.

Chronic reflux esophagitis occurs most commonly in animals with hiatal hernia disorders. Clinical signs include hypersalivation, regurgitation, and vomiting, often noted shortly after eating. There may also be coughing, dyspnea, and exercise intolerance. Hiatal hernias are most commonly identified in immature animals.

Radiographic contrast studies are often normal in cases of mild to moderate esophagitis. Survey films may show increased esophageal density in moderate to severe esophagitis. Segmental narrowing and irregularity of luminal contour may occasionally be identified on contrast studies. Persistence of contrast in the thoracic esophagus or esophageal dilation suggests the possibility of gastroesophageal reflux. In hiatal hernia, the gastric cardia, fundus, and LES will be cranial to the esophageal hiatus. A definitive diagnosis may not always be possible in sliding hiatal hernia, and fluoroscopy may be needed to confirm the diagnosis.

A definitive diagnosis of esophagitis is most often made by endoscopic visualization of the esophageal mucosa. Variable degrees of mucosal erythema or isolated patches of eroded mucosa may be seen. Mucosal friability may be evidenced by bleeding caused by gentle manipulation with the endoscope tip or biopsy forceps. Pooling of fluid in the esophagus or a markedly dilated gastroesophageal junction or both are not diagnostic, but these findings should alert the endoscopist to the possibility of a reflux disorder.

Numerous human studies have reported that 50 to 60 per cent of patients with symptoms suggesting gastroesophageal reflux have an endoscopically normal esophagus. Symptom severity often does not predict the degree of endoscopic abnormality. When esophagitis is suspected in the absence of visible diagnostic changes in the mucosal surface, an esophageal mucosal biopsy should be obtained from an area 2 to 5 cm proximal to the gastroesophageal junction. With proper technique, adequate mucosal biopsies can be obtained with the standard flexible forceps. Alternatively, biopsies can be obtained with a suction biopsy instrument. Histologic changes appear before significant symptoms and endoscopically observable changes and persist after the endoscopic indicators have disappeared in response to therapy. An endoscopically demonstrable hiatal hernia is nearly always associated with reflux esophagitis.

TREATMENT

Because there are a variety of pathophysiologic mechanisms that contribute to reflux esophagitis, an individualized treatment program for each patient is often necessary. Treatment may include dietary modification, antacids, histamine H_2 receptor antagonists, gastric promotility agents, antiinflammatory drugs, and mucosal protectant therapy. Single or combination drug therapy may be

required. Most canine and feline patients are managed with H_2 receptor blockers, bland low-fat diets, and motility modification.

Mild reflux esophagitis is often asymptomatic and generally resolves without therapy. If clinical signs suggestive of reflux esophagitis occur within several days of an anesthetic procedure, treatment should be instituted whether endoscopy is available for definitive diagnosis or not. Treatment in this situation usually includes antacids and the H_2 receptor antagonist cimetidine (Tagamet). In addition to acid-neutralizing effects, antacids have also been shown to increase LES pressure and decrease reflux episodes. Antacids irreversibly inactivate pepsin if the gastric pH can be elevated over 6. Antacids need to be given frequently (every 2 to 4 hr), however, because infrequent administration may result in a rebound hypersecretion of acid. This limits their practicality for use in animal patients.

Histamine H_2 receptor antagonists such as cimetidine, ranitidine (Zantac, Glaxo), and famotidine (Pepcid, Merck) are used to decrease gastric acid production, thereby decreasing acid volume available for reflux. There is no adverse effect on resting or stimulated LES pressure levels. Large multicenter human clinical trials have shown that H_2 receptor blocker therapy results in consistent improvement in symptoms of reflux esophagitis. Cimetidine, 5 mg/kg t.i.d., or ranitidine, 2 mg/kg b.i.d. is generally used for 2 to 3 weeks in dogs and cats with acute reflux esophagitis. Long-term therapy should be used in hiatal hernia patients with chronic reflux esophagitis if corrective surgery either is not performed or is unsuccessful.

Prokinetic drug therapy in the form of metoclopramide (Reglan) provides several beneficial effects. Metoclopramide increases LES pressure, thereby decreasing reflux, and stimulates more rapid gastric emptying by increasing gastric contractions. It also enhances relaxation of the pylorus for more effective aboral movement of gastric contents and increases distal esophageal contractions. Two human studies have shown that metoclopramide was as effective as cimetidine or ranitidine in decreasing reflux symptoms. One disadvantage of metoclopramide is that it may cause bothersome side effects such as restlessness, hyperactivity, and occasionally aggressive behavior. In the author's experience, these side effects are not common in dogs and cats, but clients should always be forewarned of the possibility that side effects may occur. If side effects do occur, they usually will be noted within 1 hour of the first or second dose and usually subside within 3 to 4 hours. Unfortunately, lowering the dose does not usually alleviate side effects. The dose of metoclopramide is 0.2 to 0.4 mg/kg (maximum starting dose 10 mg) two to three times daily 30 to 45 min before feeding and at bedtime. Cimetidine and metoclopramide are often used concurrently. Side effects of metoclopramide will occasionally be increased when it is used with cimetidine.

One of the newest forms of reflux esophagitis therapy involves use of sucralfate (Carafate, Marion) to provide an esophageal mucosal cytoprotective effect. Sucralfate is an aluminum salt that has been shown to bind selectively to areas of injured gastrointestinal tract mucosa and to form a local protective layer that binds pepsin and bile and prevents them from causing further mucosal damage. Sucralfate has previously been used primarily to treat erosive gastritis and gastric and duodenal ulcers. In addition, a *gastric cytoprotective effect* of sucralfate has been demonstrated in animals against ethanol, bile, histamine, aspirin, and indomethacin. Until recently, little was known about any effect that sucralfate might have in prevention of esophageal mucosal injury.

Sucralfate cytoprotection against pepsin-induced esophageal lesions has been demonstrated using a liquid preparation in short-term experiments in rabbits. A recent study in cats demonstrated a protective effect of liquid sucralfate against intermittent, repeated esophageal exposure to acid over a period of days. It appears that sucralfate acts not only by a mucosa-adhering effect on damaged tissue but also by enhancing normal mucosal defenses. The exact mechanism is unknown. Based on this recent information, it seems reasonable to recommend that use of sucralfate in a liquid form be considered for patients with evidence of esophagitis. Its greatest value may be in treatment of acute reactions in the esophagus and in prevention of further damage. Sucralfate should also be considered for use as a preventive medication in situations in which a significant reflux episode could potentially be expected to occur (e.g., emergency surgery in a patient with an incompletely evacuated stomach). The recommended dose is 1 gm/30 kg q.i.d. Treatment should be timed to prevent inactivation of other oral medications.

A short course (2 to 3 weeks) of corticosteroid therapy (e.g., prednisone, 0.5 mg/kg b.i.d.) may be indicated in severe reflux esophagitis to minimize fibrosis and possible stricture formation.

Patients with evidence of reflux esophagitis following anesthesia should be treated aggressively, since there is potential for esophageal stricture formation (see p. 904). Patients with reflux esophagitis secondary to persistent vomiting are treated with injectable cimetidine or ranitidine and an antiemetic agent to control vomiting. In general, oral medications should not be used in vomiting patients; however, if there is significant esophagitis, use of liquid sucralfate should be considered. Animals with hiatal hernia disorders will require long-term medical therapy if surgery is not performed. A combination of cimetidine or ranitidine, metoclopramide, and a low-fat diet is usually used. Fats empty from the stomach more slowly than do carbohydrates and protein. Low-fat diets are also used in patients with gastric motility disorders. Metoclopramide and dietary management are usually sufficient to control signs in animals with both reflux esophagitis and decreased gastric motility. Therapy in acute cases of reflux esophagitis is generally continued for 2 to 3 weeks beyond signs of clinical improvement. Patients with severe esophagitis should be followed endoscopically and histologically to ensure complete resolution of inflammatory changes.

References and Supplemental Reading

Behar, J.: The role of the lower esophageal sphincter in reflux prevention. J. Clin. Gastroenterol. (Suppl. 1) 8:2, 1986.

Ellison, G. W., Lewis, D. D., Philips, L., et al.: Esophageal hiatal hernia in small animals: Literature review and a modified surgical technique. J. Am. Anim. Hosp. Assoc. 23:391, 1987.

Johnson, L. F., and Harmon, J. W.: Experimental esophagitis in a rabbit model. J. Clin. Gastroenterol. (Suppl. 1)8:26, 1986.

Katz, P. O., Geisinger, K. R., Hassan, M., et al.: Acid-induced esophagitis in cats is prevented by sucralfate but not synthetic prostaglandin. Dig. Dis. Sci. 33:217, 1988.

Lieberman, D. A., and Keeffe, E. B.: Treatment of severe reflux esophagitis with cimetidine and metoclopramide. Ann. Intern. Med. 104:21, 1986.

Magne, M. L.: Esophageal motility disorders in the dog. Proc. 4th Annu. A.C.V.I.M. Meet. 4:12, 1986.

Schweitzer, E. J., Bass, B. L., Johnson, L. F., et al.: Sucralfate prevents experimental peptic esophagitis in rabbits. Gastroenterology 88:611, 1985.

Zawie, D. A.: Medical diseases of the esophagus. Comp. Cont. Ed. Pract. Vet. 9:1146, 1987.

MEDICAL THERAPY FOR GASTROINTESTINAL ULCERS

MARK G. PAPICH, D.V.M.

Saskatoon, Saskatchewan

Among the most popular prescription and non-prescription drugs for people in North America are those used to treat gastric and duodenal ulceration. Although antacids, histamine H_2-receptor antagonists, and mucosal protectants are intended specifically for gastrointestinal (GI) ulcerative disease or other hypersecretory conditions, they have been administered to small animals for a broader group of disorders that include gastritis, esophagitis, vomiting, GI bleeding, and ulcer prophylaxis associated with certain surgical procedures. Until the past few years, attention has focused on drugs that neutralize stomach acid or decrease its secretion (e.g., antacids and cimetidine). Ulcer therapy is today shifting attention to drugs that are cytoprotective rather than antisecretory (Thomson and Mahachai, 1987).

GUT MUCOSAL PROTECTIVE BARRIER

The stomach and intestines are protected from physiochemical insults such as acid, bile salts, digestive enzymes, and mechanical shear force by mucus and bicarbonate secretion, epithelial cell turnover and repair, a rich mucosal blood supply, and prostaglandin secretion.

Mucus–Bicarbonate Barrier

The mucus secreted by the epithelial cells is composed of an adherent layer of gel glycoprotein that protects the epithelium. Continuity of the gel is important for its protective effect against acid and pepsin. The mucus gel layer has been referred to as the mucus–bicarbonate barrier (Garner et al., 1987), because epithelial alkali secretion has an important protective influence on the mucosa (Fromm, 1987; Richardson, 1985). Bicarbonate is incorporated into the mucosal gel layer to neutralize the effects of acid on the mucosa. A pH gradient is formed that maintains a near physiologic pH at the mucosal surface; near the lumen, the pH approaches that of stomach acid (pH 1 to 3).

Epithelial Cell Turnover

GI mucosal cells have a very high rate of turnover in comparison with most cells in the body. This rapid turnover provides a protective effect, particularly against shear forces in the GI tract, and allows for rapid healing following chemical (e.g., acid and pepsin) or mechanical injury. Cells in the crypts of the mucosa migrate to the luminal surface and provide continual replacement of cells that have sloughed.

Mucosal Blood Flow

Nutrients and oxygen are provided for the gastric and intestinal mucosa via a rich vascular supply. The GI mucosa has a high metabolic rate and a large requirement for oxygen and precursors to maintain the protective mucus–bicarbonate layer and support the rapid turnover rate of epithelial cells. Mucosal blood flow appears to correlate with rates of bicarbonate secretion. Influences that may temporarily impair or disrupt mucosal blood flow (e.g., shock or microvascular thrombosis) can lead to loss of mucosal integrity, erosion, and ulceration. Microscopic studies show that a component of mucosal injury induced by nonsteroidal anti-inflammatory drugs (NSAIDs) is a focal ischemia caused by blood flow stasis in injured areas (Fromm, 1987).

Role of Prostaglandins in Mucosal Protection

Stimulation or perturbation of the GI mucosa stimulates a release of arachidonic acid, which is converted by the enzyme cyclo-oxygenase to various prostanoids: prostaglandins (PGs), prostacyclin (PGI_2), and thromboxane (TXA_2). The prostanoids that have a protective role in the GI tract are PGs of the E type, particularly PGE_2, although PGI_2 and $PGF_{2\alpha}$ also may play a role (Richardson, 1985; Cohen, 1987).

In experimental studies, PGs were shown to inhibit gastric acid secretion, increase mucosal bicarbonate secretion, and maintain mucosal blood flow via their vasodilating properties (Rask-Madsen, 1987; Sontag, 1986; Garner et al., 1987). PGs are involved in both the secretion and the composition of healthy, protective mucus. Additionally, PGs may be the intercellular messenger for the stimulus of mucosal cell turnover and migration. Some have

911

suggested that human ulcer patients have reduced gastric and duodenal PG concentrations. Whether this is through a reduced level of synthesis or an increase in mucosal PG degradation is not known.

Evidence for the above propositions stems from studies performed in experimental animals or patients that have received PG-inhibiting drugs (NSAIDs). It is well known that NSAID administration is a cause of GI ulceration. Aspirin (parenteral) administered to dogs resulted in a reduction in the content of mucus of the gastric mucosa; aspirin, indomethacin, and ibuprofen administration resulted in a decrease in gastric and duodenal bicarbonate secretion (Garner et al., 1987; Fromm, 1987). In addition, NSAIDs appear to inhibit mucosal cell turnover and repair, and mucus loses its ability to maintain a pH gradient after exposure to NSAIDs. Further evidence for the role of prostaglandins in the GI tract comes from experimental and clinical studies that have demonstrated that new synthetic analogues of PGE administered orally can inhibit gastric acid secretion, maintain the integrity of protective mucus, increase mucosal alkali secretion, and protect against NSAID-induced injury (Sontag, 1986; Garner et al., 1987).

APPROACH TO ULCER THERAPY

The incidence, pathogenesis, and clinical signs of GI ulceration and gastritis have been thoroughly reviewed in previous editions (Twedt and Magne, 1986; Twedt, 1983). Veterinarians have employed antiulcer medications for a variety of GI diseases, many of which may not involve mucosal ulceration *per se*. Despite a lack of well-controlled clinical trials, there is a general impression among veterinarians that antiulcer therapy is effective for the following diseases: chronic superficial gastritis, chronic hypertrophic gastritis, bilious vomiting, reflux esophagitis, uremic gastritis, gastritis associated with neurologic disease, and gastric and duodenal ulcers.

A successful response to ulcer treatment can be anticipated if aggressive therapy is begun early, but the long-term prognosis will vary depending on the initial cause.

Importance of Acid Suppression

It is generally recognized that acid suppression is important for treating GI ulcers in human patients. The "no acid, no ulcer" recommendation still persists in current textbooks. The exact degree and duration of acid suppression needed for ulcer healing, however, have not been clearly defined. Results from clinical studies of humans have suggested that complete acid suppression is not necessary for

ulcer healing to occur; suppression in the range of 55 to 60 per cent during a 24-hr period appears to be effective. Higher doses of either cimetidine or ranitidine that suppress acid secretion to a greater degree have failed to show an increased therapeutic benefit. A recent study demonstrated that there is a clear relationship between acid suppression and the rate of ulcer healing, but that a reduction in nocturnal acidity was the most important factor. The suppression of gastric acidity for nonspecific, nonulcerative gastritis in small animals can clearly be questioned. There is no current evidence that dogs and cats with gastritis, gastric erosions, or GI ulcers have excess acid secretion and will benefit from drugs that decrease stomach acid, but there is a clinical impression that acid suppression in these patients is beneficial, and on that basis, acid-suppressing drugs are administered.

ANTACID DRUGS

The common antacids are bases of aluminum, magnesium, or calcium: magnesium hydroxide [$Mg(OH)_2$, milk of magnesia]; aluminum hydroxide [$Al(OH)_3$]; and calcium carbonate ($CaCO_3$). These drugs effectively neutralize hydrochloric acid without systemic absorption and cause a minimum of adverse side effects. Antacids also are of benefit in that they bind to bile acids and decrease pepsin activity in the stomach.

Sodium bicarbonate ($NaHCO_3$, baking soda) has been a common home remedy for many years, but its use should be discouraged because the alkali can be absorbed and, with repeated administration, lead to systemic alkalosis.

Magnesium hydroxide has a laxative effect as it increases bowel motility, and $Al(OH)_3$ has a constipating effect related to a decrease in motility of intestinal smooth muscle. These effects will counteract one another, and most formulations are mixtures of $Mg(OH)_2$ and $Al(OH)_3$; some also contain $CaCO_3$. The active ingredients in common antacids are shown in Table 1.

An additional advantage of combining $Mg(OH)_2$ and $Al(OH)_3$ is to optimize the extent and rate of acid neutralization. Magnesium salts and $CaCO_3$ have a short but rapid neutralizing effect, and $Al(OH)_3$ has a slow rate of acid neutralization that persists longer. All antacid products are not equally active. The measure of an antacid's activity is the acid neutralizing capacity (ANC), which can vary as much as threefold among various brands. For the products listed in Table 1, most manufacturers recommend a standard dose of 5 to 10 ml, regardless of the patient's size or the product's ANC. Dosages of 5 to 10 ml four to six times a day are the recommended regimen for dogs and cats. Antacid tablets will not be as effective in dogs and cats as

Table 1. *Composition of Common Antacids*

Trade Name	Active Ingredients	ANC*
Amphogel 500 liquid	$Al(OH)_3$, $Mg(OH)_2$	32
Amphogel tablet	$Al(OH)_3$	22
Amphogel liquid	$Al(OH)_3$	10
Amphogel Plus tablet	$Al(OH)_3$, $Mg(OH)_2$, simethicone	18
Camalox liquid	$Al(OH)_3$, $Mg(OH)_2$, $CaCO_3$	18
Camalox tablet	$Al(OH)_3$, $Mg(OH)_2$, $CaCO_3$	18
DiGel liquid	$Al(OH)_3$, $Mg(OH)_2$	12
DiGel tablet	$Al(OH)_3$, $Mg(OH)_2$, $MgCO_3$, dimethicone	10
Gelusil liquid	$Al(OH)_3$, $Mg(OH)_2$	12
Gelusil II liquid	$Al(OH)_3$, $Mg(OH)_2$	24–32
Gelusil tablet	$Al(OH)_3$, $Mg(OH)_2$	11
Maalox liquid	$Al(OH)_3$, $Mg(OH)_2$	13.5
Maalox Plus liquid	$Al(OH)_3$, $Mg(OH)_2$, simethicone	13.6
Maalox TC liquid	$Al(OH)_3$, $Mg(OH)_2$	27
Maalox tablets	$Al(OH)_3$, $Mg(OH)_2$	23
Maalox Plus tablets	$Al(OH)_3$, $Mg(OH)_2$, simethicone	12
Mylanta liquid	$Al(OH)_3$, $Mg(OH)_2$, simethicone	13
Mylanta II liquid	$Al(OH)_3$, $Mg(OH)_2$, simethicone	25–32
Mylanta tablets	$Al(OH)_3$, $Mg(OH)_2$, simethicone	7.5–11.5
Mylanta II tablets	$Al(OH)_3$, $Mg(OH)_2$, simethicone	19–23
Phillip's milk of magnesia	$Mg(OH)_2$	14
Riopan liquid	Magaldrate	11&15
Riopan tablets	Magaldrate	12–13.5
Rolaids tablets	Aluminum sodium carbonate	8
Titralac liquid	$CaCO_3$	20
Titralac tablets	$CaCO_3$	8.5
Tums tablets	$CaCO_3$	10

*ANC, Acid neutralizing capacity in mEq/5 mL or mEq/tablet.

liquid formulations because they do not have as high an ANC as most liquids; tablets probably should be crushed (chewed) to ensure complete dissolution and maximal buffering effect.

It is recognized that many people take less than the recommended dosage, and even on a schedule of every 4 hr, antacids do not provide continuous buffering. Nevertheless, clinical trials have documented a benefit from antacid administration with this schedule. This observation has raised questions about the possibility that the healing effect from antacids is related to other factors in addition to the ANC of the antacid. Results of recent studies have suggested that the aluminum component of antacid formulations has a cytoprotective role on the GI mucosa related to local synthesis of PGs, particularly PGE_2 (Szelenyi et al., 1986; Berstad, 1987). It is reasonable to suggest, therefore, that the acid-neutralizing ability of antacids is not the only mechanism by which antacids promote ulcer healing.

Acid Rebound

Acid rebound is a sustained hypersecretion of gastric acid following the administration of an antacid. The question has been asked whether acid rebound reduces the efficacy of an antacid that is not administered frequently enough to provide continuous buffering. Recent studies have shown that acid rebound is the result of parietal cell stimulation by divalent cations. This effect is seen primarily with calcium-containing antacid products; magnesium cations are capable of stimulating acid secretion as well, but to a lesser degree. The effect appears to be mediated by the local action of the cation on the parietal cell and is independent of intraluminal pH.

Although acid rebound is a real phenomenon, there are no data to suggest that it adversely affects ulcer healing or pain relief (Holtermuller, 1982). Acid rebound will be mitigated during much of the dosing interval by the buffering capacity of the product. Also, as mentioned earlier, antacids appear to have ulcer healing effects that are not correlated with the amount of acid neutralized during a dosing interval.

Adverse Effects and Drug Interactions

Some adverse effects were mentioned earlier—diarrhea with magnesium-containing compounds and constipation with aluminum-containing products. Other adverse effects are uncommon, but veterinarians should be aware of possible drug interactions that can decrease the systemic availability of another drug administered orally with an antacid (e.g., in humans, it is known that antacids will decrease the oral absorption of digoxin, tetracyclines, phenothiazines, glucocorticoids, and cimetidine).

HISTAMINE H$_2$-RECEPTOR ANTAGONISTS

Histamine H$_2$-receptor antagonists effectively block the secretion of stomach acid via their blockade of the gastric parietal cell histamine H$_2$ receptor. Three stimulatory receptors have been associated with the parietal cell—the histamine H$_2$ receptor, a muscarinic cholinergic receptor, and a gastrin receptor (Fig. 1). An interrelationship between all three receptors appears to be involved in gastric acid secretion. The histamine receptor activates membrane adenylate cyclase, and increased intercellular levels of cyclic AMP stimulate acid secretion. The cholinergic receptor and gastrin receptor, on the other hand, appear to mediate their effects on acid secretion via increasing cytosolic concentrations of free calcium, although the exact mechanism by which they do this is probably different (Wollin, 1987). The histamine H$_2$ receptor is the dominant receptor for stimulation of acid secretion. Evidence for this has come from studies that show histamine H$_2$-receptor blocking drugs to be potent inhibitors of cholinergic- and gastrin (or pentagastrin)-stimulated acid secretion, whereas antimuscarinic or gastrin-blocking drugs only partially suppress histamine-stimulated secretion.

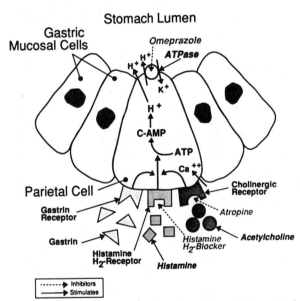

Figure 1. Gastric mucosal cells and parietal cell. The parietal cell secretes hydrogen ions (H$^+$) via the H$^+$/K$^+$ ATPase (proton pump). The parietal cell is stimulated by an interaction of three receptors: gastrin receptor, histamine H$_2$-receptor, and cholinergic receptor. Stimulation leads to increased intracellular calcium (Ca^{++}) and cyclic-AMP (c-AMP), which subsequently stimulate H$^+$ secretion. Acid secretion can be suppressed by blocking the histamine H$_2$-receptor with drugs such as cimetidine, by blocking the cholinergic receptor with drugs such as atropine, or by inhibiting the ATPase with drugs such as omeprazole.

Cimetidine and Ranitidine

The histamine H$_2$-receptor antagonists that have been used in veterinary medicine are cimetidine (Tagamet, SmithKline) and ranitidine (Zantac, Glaxo). In numerous clinical trials comparing cimetidine and ranitidine for treating gastric or duodenal ulcers in humans, there was no advantage of one drug over another.

The comparative pharmacokinetics for cimetidine and ranitidine in dogs are listed in Table 2. The pharmacokinetics are comparable to what has been described in humans, except that both drugs have a higher degree of systemic availability following oral absorption in dogs. If dosages are calculated on the assumption that a 50 per cent reduction in acid secretion is needed for ulcer healing, a cimetidine dose of 5 mg/kg (IV or PO) in dogs will suppress acid secretion for 3 to 5 hr (the EC$_{50}$* is 0.5 to 1.0 µg/ml). Ranitidine has no therapeutic advantage over cimetidine, but the longer half-life combined with a greater potency in dogs may allow for a decreased frequency of administration and improved compliance. Ranitidine dosed at a rate of 2 mg/kg (PO or IV) every 8 hr in dogs will provide continuous acid suppression.

Effects of Histamine H$_2$-Receptor Antagonists Not Related to Acid Suppression

Histamine H$_2$-receptor antagonists also appear to have beneficial effects that are independent of acid secretion. Although exact mechanisms are not known and results of studies have been disputed, cimetidine may increase the luminal bicarbonate secretion in dogs, increase mucus production, and increase mucosal blood flow. Some or all of these effects may be related to stimulation of local PG synthesis.

Adverse Drug Effects

Several adverse effects have been attributed to histamine H$_2$-receptor antagonists. In view of the widespread use of these drugs in human medicine, adverse effects fortunately are quite uncommon. The incidence of such reactions is unknown in veterinary medicine, but the following are descriptions of adverse effects reported in humans (Zimmerman and Schenker, 1985; Somogyi and Gugler, 1982).

ENDOCRINE EFFECTS. Gynecomastia and an antiandrogenic action have been the most common endocrine effect. A decrease in sperm count has

---

*EC$_{50}$ is the effective plasma concentration required for a 50 per cent reduction in acid secretion.

Table 2. Comparative Pharmacokinetics of Cimetidine and Ranitidine

Species	Drug	T½* (hr)	Vd† (L/kg)	Cl‡ (L/kg/hr)	F§ %	Recommended Dosage
Humans‖	Cimetidine	1.9	0.9	0.32	74	800 mg every 24 hr to 300 mg every 6 hr¶
Dogs**	Cimetidine	1.3	1.2	0.6	95	5 mg/kg every 4–6 hr
Humans‖	Ranitidine	2.5	1.5	0.52	53	150–300 mg every 12–24 hr¶
Dogs**	Ranitidine	2.2	2.6	0.8	81	2 mg/kg every 8 hr

*T½: elimination half-life
†Vd: Apparent specific volume of distribution
‡Cl: Total systemic clearance
§F: Systemic availability following an oral dose.
‖Value represents the mean from several studies.
¶The dose represents total dose per person.
**Data from Papich, M. G., Davis, C. A., and Davis, L. E.: Pharmacokinetics of cimetidine and ranitidine in dogs (in preparation).

also been noted in some males. It appears that ranitidine is less antiandrogenic than cimetidine. Cimetidine administration has caused decreased circulating levels of parathyroid hormone, but the clinical significance is not known. There is no evidence to support the administration of cimetidine for treating hyperparathyroidism.

CENTRAL NERVOUS SYSTEM TOXICITY. In some patients, cimetidine has caused mental confusion, lethargy, vomiting, and seizures. The mechanism for these reactions is unknown, but they are more common in elderly patients and patients with renal disease. Therefore, it may be related to impaired drug elimination and subsequent high blood levels. It is recommended that dosages be decreased in patients with renal disease.

GASTROINTESTINAL EFFECTS. It is not known what effect long-term suppression of acid secretion may have on normal digestive function. Chronic acid suppression may affect the natural defense mechanisms that prevent bacterial colonization in the stomach. In human patients who are maintained on acid-suppressing drugs for prolonged periods, there are higher levels of gram-negative bacteria in gastric aspirates and a higher rate of bacterial overgrowth. Additionally, bacterial overgrowth in the stomach can potentially lead to formation of carcinogenic substances, because bacteria can convert dietary nitrites to carcinogenic nitrosamines. Although hypoacidity and bacterial overgrowth may theoretically be a possibility, there is no clinical evidence to support a serious concern.

There is no evidence that rebound hypersecretion of acid occurs after suddenly stopping cimetidine or ranitidine.

Drug Interactions

Extensive reviews are available describing drug–drug interactions between H₂-receptor antagonists and other drugs administered (Somogyi and Gugler, 1982; Zimmerman and Schenker, 1985). These interactions have been described in humans (Table 3), but similar clinical data are not available for dogs and cats. The adverse effects can be described as effects on GI absorption caused by raising the stomach pH and effects on metabolizing or excretory systems. Cimetidine is recognized as an inhibitor of hepatic metabolizing P450 enzymes, and certain drugs metabolized via this mechanism may be cleared more slowly. Ranitidine does not affect the P450 enzymes as does cimetidine, and ranitidine may be preferred in a patient who is receiving multiple drugs.

Newer H₂-Receptor Antagonists: Famotidine and Nizatidine

Famotidine (Pepcid, Merck) and nizatidine (Axid, Lilly) recently have become available in tablets, suspension, and injectable solution formulations for use in human medicine. Famotidine has had only limited use in veterinary medicine, but the drug has a theoretic advantage of increased potency (32 times more potent than cimetidine), and in humans the effect of a single dose persists for 12 hr. Despite the increased potency, there are no studies to indicate that famotidine has better efficacy than ranitidine or cimetidine in humans. Nizatidine has a potency similar to that of ranitidine but has not been used in veterinary medicine. There are no recommended dosages for dogs and cats; famotidine dosages are now extrapolated from human dosages of 20 to 40 mg per person twice daily.

SUCRALFATE

Sucralfate (Carafate, Marion; Sulcrate, Nordic) is a complex molecule consisting of a combination of sucrose octasulfate and aluminum hydroxide. Systemic absorption of sucralfate is minimal, and the beneficial effects of sucralfate are attributed to local effects on the GI tract. Because the drug is not

Table 3. *Possible Drug Interactions with Cimetidine (in Humans)*

Drug	Effect on Plasma Drug Concentration	Mechanism of Drug Interaction
Ketoconazole	Decreased	Requires acidity in stomach for maximal oral absorption.
Warfarin	Decreased elimination	Decreased hepatic metabolism caused by enzyme inhibition.
Diazepam	Decreased elimination	Decreased hepatic metabolism caused by enzyme inhibition.
Carbamazepine	Decreased elimination	Decreased hepatic metabolism caused by enzyme inhibition.
Phenytoin	Decreased elimination	Decreased hepatic metabolism caused by enzyme inhibition.
Theophylline	Decreased elimination	Decreased hepatic metabolism caused by enzyme inhibition.
Digitoxin	Decreased elimination	Decreased hepatic metabolism caused by enzyme inhibition.
Propranolol	Increased peak concentrations	Decreased metabolism caused by decreased hepatic blood flow.
Lidocaine	Increased peak concentrations	Decreased metabolism caused by decreased hepatic blood flow.
Morphine	Increased peak concentrations	Decreased metabolism caused by decreased hepatic blood flow.
Tetracycline	Increased	Better oral absorption when stomach acid is low (acid-labile drug).
Erythromycin	Increased	Better oral absorption when stomach acid is low (acid-labile drug).
Penicillin G	Increased	Better oral absorption when stomach acid is low (acid-labile drug).
Procainamide	Increased	Competitive inhibition of renal tubular secretion.

absorbed systemically, it is extremely well tolerated, and early experience with its use in veterinary medicine looks promising.

Sucralfate's efficacy for treating GI ulcers is attributed to several effects. In the acid milieu of the stomach, sucralfate dissociates to aluminum hydroxide ions and sucrose octasulfate. Sucrose octasulfate polymerizes to a viscous sticky substance that adheres to the gastric mucosa, protects against H^+ back-diffusion, and promotes ulcer healing. Because of electrostatic charges, sucralfate preferentially adheres to ulcerated tissue. The affinity of sucralfate for injured, ulcerated mucosa is five times greater than that for normal tissue (Hardin et al., 1987).

In addition to sucralfate's mucosal protective effect, it is also beneficial because it inactivates pepsin and absorbs bile acids, and the aluminum hydroxide released has an acid-neutralizing effect. Moreover, several studies have indicated that sucralfate has a significant cytoprotective role—an effect that is probably caused by a stimulation of PGs (PGE$_2$, PGI$_2$) (Rask-Madsen, 1987; Thomson and Mahachai, 1987).

There are no clinical reports of sucralfate's efficacy in dogs and cats. In humans, numerous studies have reported that sucralfate is as effective as histamine H$_2$-receptor antagonists or antacids for ulcer healing. Sucralfate may be particularly useful for treating and preventing NSAID-induced ulcers. In horses, sucralfate protected against phenylbutazone-induced GI toxicity; and in rats, the protection from sucralfate was so complete that NSAIDs were no more toxic to the stomach than saline if sucralfate was administered before the NSAID (Hardin et al., 1987).

Dosing Recommendations

Dosages administered to people are not precise. Sucralfate is available as a 1-gm tablet and usually is administered as a 1-gm dose three to four times daily. We have administered sucralfate to large dogs at a dosage of 1 gm per dog every 8 hr, and 0.5 gm to smaller dogs. Cats should receive one-half to one-quarter of a tablet every 8 to 12 hr. There are very few side effects associated with sucralfate administration, the most common of which is constipation resulting from the aluminum hydroxide component.

Sucralfate may have the ability to adsorb other drugs that are administered orally (e.g., tetracyclines, phenytoin, cimetidine, digoxin), but there are no clinically important drug interactions reported. Because sucralfate requires an acid environment for dissolution, it is recommended that administration of histamine H$_2$-receptor antagonists and sucralfate be separated by 30 min.

ANTICHOLINERGIC DRUGS

Antimuscarinic, anticholinergic drugs will decrease acid secretion by blocking the cholinergic receptor on the parietal cell (Fig. 1). At dosages that do not produce significant side effects, however, the antimuscarinic drugs are only moderately effective.

Antimuscarinic drugs include the tertiary ammonium compounds atropine and scopolamine and the quaternary ammonium compounds glycopyrrolate (Robinul-V, Robins), methscopolamine bromide (Pamine, Upjohn), propantheline bromide (Pro-Banthine, Searle), isopropamide (Darbazine, Norden), and pirenzepine. For systemic use, quaternary ammonium compounds are preferred because they do not have effects on the central nervous system owing to poor penetration of the blood–brain barrier. Pirenzepine is more selective than other anticholinergic drugs, and it inhibits acid secretion at lower dosages than are required to affect other tissues. Side effects still occur, however. Clinical use of pirenzepine has not been reported in veterinary medicine.

The antimuscarinic drugs have a profound effect on many functions of the GI tract. Although they may decrease acid secretion, they also can decrease stomach emptying, decrease mucosal secretion of bicarbonate, and decrease the secretion of protective mucus. Bowel motility is also decreased, and chronic treatment can lead to bowel atony. Antimuscarinic drugs do not have a significant effect on pancreatic exocrine secretion and probably are not useful for the management of pancreatitis in small animals.

Other side effects of antimuscarinic drugs include photophobia, urine retention, and xerostomia. Although antimuscarinic drugs may have a place in the treatment of rare cases, for most patients the doses required for acid suppression can produce significant side effects to a degree that makes routine use undesirable for ulcer treatment. The side effects listed above also should be considered if these drugs are used as antiemetics.

PROTON PUMP INHIBITORS: OMEPRAZOLE

Following stimulation of parietal cell membrane receptors, acid (H^+) is secreted into the lumen by the H^+/K^+ ATPase (gastric proton pump) (Fig. 1). The ATPase is located in the membrane of the parietal cell, and it actively exchanges K^+ for H^+ at the luminal interface (Sachs, 1986). The experimental drug omeprazole, a substituted benzimidazole, is capable of blocking the H^+/K^+ ATPase and is one of a new class of drugs called the proton pump inhibitors. Omeprazole is a potent (ten times more than cimetidine) drug in dogs and has a long duration of action. Although the plasma half-life is approximately 1 hr in dogs, it has a duration of effect lasting 24 hr or more, which is attributed to selective accumulation of omeprazole in the acidic parietal cell.

Omeprazole is not available clinically, and concerns regarding its long-term effects have raised questions about its safety. Chronic suppression of acid secretion has caused hypergastrinemia in experimental animals, and the trophic effects of gastrin on the gastric mucosa have been associated with mucosal cell hyperplasia, rugal hypertrophy, and development of carcinoids.

CYTOPROTECTIVE DRUGS

Synthetic Prostaglandins

As mentioned earlier, PGs have an important protective effect on the GI mucosa. They inhibit

gastric acid secretion and at lower doses are associated with improved mucosal blood flow, mucus–bicarbonate secretion, strengthening of the mucosal barrier, and mucosal cell turnover and repair. It is likely that no single mechanism fully explains cytoprotection and that a number of factors act together.

The orally administered PGs enprostil and arbaprostil are synthetic derivatives of PGE_2. Misoprostol is a derivative of PGE_1. Most clinical use of synthetic PGs has focused on misoprostol (Cytotec, Searle). At the time of this writing, misoprostol is licensed for use in humans in Canada but is not available in the United States. Misoprostol, as expected, has a cytoprotective effect as well as an antisecretory effect. In several studies, however, it was shown that at dosages that were cytoprotective, misoprostol was not as effective as other antiulcer drugs; at higher dosages that suppress acid secretion, equal efficacy can be expected. The ulcer-healing effects of synthetic PGs apparently are more closely correlated with their acid-suppressing action than with their cytoprotective effects (Rask-Madsen, 1987; Sontag, 1986; Fromm, 1987).

Oral synthetic PGs are not without side effects. The side effects reflect the action of PGs on the GI tract. Abnormal bowel movements, diarrhea, and abdominal pain were reported in human studies. These drugs are absolutely *contraindicated in pregnancy* because they can cause termination of pregnancy.

Licorice Products

A group of drugs that have interesting and promising properties are extracts from natural licorice or synthetic licorice compounds. Carbenoxolone is a synthetic compound that has been used in Europe for ulcer treatment, but it is not yet available in North America. These drugs appear to have significant cytoprotective properties: increasing secretion and viscosity of GI mucus, stabilizing GI cellular membranes, and stimulating epithelial cell renewal and repair. Their action is mediated in part by an increased local concentration of PGs.

The only significant side effect of carbenoxolone is a mineralocorticoid effect resulting in fluid retention and, in some patients, potassium loss. Efforts are underway to produce other synthetic licorice compounds that lack aldosterone-like activity.

SUMMARY

Several antiulcer drugs have been used in small animal patients to treat GI ulcers as well as nonspecific gastritis and for ulcer prophylaxis. Acute GI ulceration occurs in small animals, but fortunately the incidence is rare. The cause can often be associated with NSAID administration.

Magnesium and aluminum antacid compounds, although popular in human medicine, are used infrequently in veterinary medicine because they can be difficult to administer to our patients and frequent administration may be a reason for less than optimum compliance. Acute ulceration and prophylaxis against ulceration can best be managed with the administration of either sucralfate, histamine H_2-receptor antagonists, or both. Although other drugs are becoming available, there is no information to suggest that they have superior efficacy over H_2-receptor antagonists or sucralfate. No clinical reports are available, but most veterinarians have been satisfied with the efficacy of sucralfate or H_2-receptor blockers. For acute ulceration, both drugs may have a synergistic effect, although this has not been proved. If both drugs are administered together, administer sucralfate 30 min before cimetidine or ranitidine, as an acid environment is needed for sucralfate's action.

There are no conclusive studies that show cimetidine to be superior to ranitidine, or vice versa. Ranitidine, however, may be preferred in a patient that is receiving multiple drugs or when compliance may be a problem.

References and Supplemental Reading

Berstad, A.: Enhancement of mucosal defence by antacids. Scand. J. Gastroenterol. (Suppl. 128) 22:44, 1987.

Cohen, M. M.: Role of endogenous prostaglandins in gastric secretion and mucosal defense. Clin. Invest. Med. 10:226, 1987.
Fromm, D.: How do non-steroidal anti-inflammatory drugs affect gastric mucosal defenses? Clin. Invest. Med. 10:251, 1987.
Garner, A., Allen, A., and Rowe, P. H.: Gastroduodenal mucosal defence mechanisms and the action of non-steroidal anti-inflammatory agents. Scand. J. Gastroenterol. (Suppl. 127) 22:29, 1987.
Hardin, C. K., Sexton, C. R., and Peoples, J. B.: Efficiency of sucralfate in preventing peptic ulceration induced by nonsteroidal anti-inflammatory drugs. Am. Surg. 53:373, 1987.
Holtermuller, K. H.: Acid rebound: Fact or fiction. Hepatogastroenterology 29:135, 1982.
Rask-Madsen, J.: The role of eicosanoids in the gastrointestinal tract. Scand. J. Gastroenterol. (Suppl. 127) 22:7, 1987.
Richardson, C. T.: Pathogenic factors in peptic ulcer disease. Am. J. Med. (Suppl. 2C) 79:1, 1985.
Sachs, G.: The parietal cell as a therapeutic target. Scand. J. Gastroenterol. 21:1, 1986.
Somogyi, A., and Gugler, R.: Drug interactions with cimetidine. Clin. Pharmacokinet. 7:23, 1982.
Sontag, S. J.: Prostaglandins in peptic ulcer disease: An overview of current status and future directions. Drugs 32:445, 1986.
Szelenyi, I., Engler, H., and Beck, H.: Aluminum hydroxide inhibits acetylsalicylic acid-induced gastric erosions in cats with Heidenhain pouch. Agents Actions 18:372, 1986.
Thomson, A. B. R., and Mahachai, V.: Pharmacological management of patients with peptic ulcer disease: Prospects for the late 1980's. Clin. Invest. Med. 10:152, 1987.
Twedt, D. C., Magne, M. L.: Chronic gastritis. In Kirk, R. W. (ed): Current Veterinary Therapy IX. Philadelphia: W. B. Saunders Co., 1986, pp. 852–855.
Twedt, D. C.: Gastric ulcers. In Kirk, R. W. (ed): Current Veterinary Therapy VIII. Philadelphia: W. B. Saunders Co., 1983, pp. 765–770.
Wollin, A.: Regulation of gastric acid secretion at the cellular level. Clin. Invest. Med. 10:209, 1987.
Zimmerman, T. W., and Schenker, S.: A comparative evaluation of cimetidine and ranitidine. Ration. Drug Ther. 19:1, 1985.

ANTRAL PYLORIC HYPERTROPHY SYNDROME

ROBERT C. DeNOVO, D.V.M.

Knoxville, Tennessee

Partial pyloric obstruction results in delayed gastric emptying and chronic vomiting. Intrinsic lesions of the pylorus that cause obstruction include mural thickening such as muscular hypertrophy, neoplasia, eosinophilic granuloma, or infiltrative mycoses. Gastric and duodenal ulcers and antral mucosal hyperplasia can also cause obstruction of the pylorus. These disorders are similar grossly, and definitive diagnosis requires biopsy. Foreign bodies commonly cause pyloric obstruction and can be removed by endoscopy or gastrotomy. Lesions external to the pylorus such as pancreatic abscesses or neoplasia will infrequently compress the pylorus, causing delayed gastric emptying. Of the multiple causes of obstructive pyloric disease, antral pyloric hypertrophy syndrome is being identified as an important etiology.

Antral pyloric hypertrophy is an obstructive narrowing of the pyloric canal caused by hypertrophy of the pyloric circular smooth muscle or hyperplasia of the pyloric mucosa or both. Two clinical syndromes of antral pyloric hypertrophy occur. Congenital pyloric muscular hypertrophy, also known as congenital pyloric stenosis, occurs most frequently in brachycephalic dogs such as the boxer and Boston terrier. In this instance, the luminal diameter of the pylorus is decreased as a result of concentric hypertrophy of the circular smooth muscle. Several reports have recently characterized a syndrome of acquired pyloric obstruction in predominantly middle-aged, small breeds of dogs with chronic gastric retention. Lesions described consist of varying degrees of benign muscular hypertrophy or mucosal hyperplasia involving the pyloric antrum. The contribution of the muscular and mucosal components varies in the individual dog. This syndrome has been called acquired pyloric stenosis, multiple polyps of the gastric mucosa, hypertrophic gastritis, and chronic hypertrophic pyloric gastropathy. These conditions are probably variations of the same disease process and will be collectively referred to here as antral pyloric hypertrophy syndrome.

ETIOPATHOGENESIS

The cause and pathogenesis of antral pyloric hypertrophy are unknown. As in dogs, both congenital and acquired antral pyloric hypertrophy occur in humans. Clinical observations in humans indicate that genetic predisposition, environmental factors, and chronic inflammation are important factors in the development of this condition. Familial aggregations of congenital pyloric stenosis occur frequently in humans, with males being affected approximately four times more often than females. Being born to professional parents appears to predispose to this condition. Acquired antral pyloric hypertrophy in adults can occur secondary to gastritis, pyloric ulcers, or gastric neoplasia. Chronic stress from psychic influences, inflammatory diseases, and ulcers is believed to stimulate sympathetic tone to the stomach, which in turn causes decreased gastric motility and retention of gastric contents. When the pyloric antrum becomes distended, G cells in the antral mucosa are stimulated to produce gastrin. Gastrin, in addition to stimulating the production of hydrocholoric acid, has potent trophic effects on both gastric mucosa and smooth muscle. Over a prolonged period, the trophic effects of gastrin are believed to result in pyloric mucosal and muscular hypertrophy. Antral pyloric hypertrophy occasionally occurs in adults without predisposing disease. In this instance, the condition is believed to be the same congenital disorder seen in children, but as a milder form and later in clinical appearance.

Experimental data indicate that gastrointestinal hormones, neural dysfunction, or an interplay of both is involved in the development and maintenance of antral pyloric hypertrophy. Dodge (1976) showed that injection of pentagastrin into pregnant bitches produced pyloric stenosis in approximately 28 per cent of their pups. Histopathology of the pylorus in affected pups showed hypertrophy of circular smooth muscle that closely resembled that found both in children and in pups with congenital pyloric stenosis. Additionally, ganglion cells in the myenteric plexus of affected experimental pups were decreased in number and showed changes in size and configuration similar to ganglion cell changes seen in children with pyloric stenosis. Other studies have shown that selective destruction of the pyloric myenteric plexus also causes antral distention, muscular hypertrophy, and pyloric stenosis (Okamoto et al., 1967).

The experimental studies indicate that neuroendocrine mechanisms are important in the pathogenesis of antral pyloric hypertrophy. However, the relationship between spontaneously occurring antral pyloric hypertrophy in dogs and the experimental findings or the human disease process is unclear. It is possible that a congenital or acquired neural defect of pyloric function could cause chronic gastric retention and subsequent distention. Dogs with mild defects might initially be asymptomatic. However, distention of the stomach increases gastrin production. The trophic effects of hypergastrinemia could, over a prolonged period, induce pyloric hypertrophy and contribute to outflow obstruction. Additionally, persistent hyperacidity from high gastrin concentrations stimulates release of secretin and cholecystokinin. These enteric hormones are also trophic to the pylorus and stimulate pyloric contraction, which likely contributes to muscular hypertrophy. Measurements of serum gastrin concentrations in affected dogs might provide more insight into the pathogenesis of this disorder.

CLINICAL PRESENTATION

Antral pyloric hypertrophy occurs most commonly in small, purebred middle-aged dogs. Matthiesen (1986) reported that of 45 affected dogs, 88.8 per cent weighed less than 10 kg. Of those, the Lhasa apso, Shih Tzu, and miniature poodle were most commonly affected. This syndrome occurs infrequently in large breeds such as German shepherds and Doberman pinschers. The mean age at presentation is 8.8 years, with a range of 3 to 15 years. Approximately twice as many male dogs as female dogs are affected.

The most frequent owner complaint is chronic, intermittent vomiting occurring within a few hours of eating. The history of signs prior to presentation can vary from several days to 6 months; however, intermittent vomiting for a year or longer is not unusual. The frequency of vomiting tends to increase with time. Abrupt projectile vomiting typical of gastric outflow obstruction does not commonly occur with antral pyloric hypertrophy. The character of the vomitus varies from undigested to partially digested food mixed with gastric fluid and mucus. The vomitus rarely contains bile. Most dogs are normal between vomiting episodes; however, some will have progressive anorexia and weight loss. Afflicted dogs occasionally have postprandial eructation, abdominal distention, and signs of discomfort that are relieved by vomiting. Antiemetics and promotility drugs such as metoclopramide do not relieve the signs.

Most dogs with antral pyloric hypertrophy have no consistent physical or laboratory abnormalities. Moderate weight loss, abdominal distention, and dehydration may be seen on physical examination. Abdominal palpation may identify an enlarged stomach and elicit some discomfort. Although protracted vomiting can cause large losses of water, sodium, chloride, hydrogen, and potassium ions, electrolyte depletion and acid-base imbalance are uncommon with antral pyloric hypertrophy. Mild acidosis may occur from dehydration. Vomiting is usually not severe enough to cause hypochloremic alkalosis, which is more characteristic of complete pyloric obstruction. Because concurrent illness due to renal disease, liver disease, or hypoadrenocorticism can complicate the clinical presentation, complete hematologic, biochemical, and urinary tests are necessary for accurate diagnosis.

DIAGNOSIS

A tentative diagnosis of antral pyloric hypertrophy is based on signalment, history, physical examination findings, and the exclusion of metabolic diseases that could cause chronic vomiting. Radiology is most useful in the diagnosis of antral pyloric hypertrophy. Depending on the severity and duration of antral pyloric hypertrophy, survey radiographs will show a normal to markedly enlarged stomach. In chronic partial obstruction of the pylorus, survey radiographs show a distended, fluid-filled stomach. This is in contrast to the gaseous distention that typically occurs with gastric volvulus. Contrast radiography using barium sulfate should be used to outline the lumen of the stomach and to evaluate gastric emptying. A standard dosage using 15 ml/kg for dogs less than 14 kg and 10 ml/kg for dogs greater than 14 kg administered via stomach tube is recommended. The time interval between the administration of barium and the presence of barium in the duodenum (the gastric emptying time) is about 15 min in most normal dogs. Gastric emptying of liquid barium sulfate is usually complete in 1 to 4 hr (Barber, 1986). An initial delay in gastric emptying of barium may be of no clinical significance, since anxiety, fear, or the pain of gastric intubation and physical restraint can significantly delay gastric emptying. However, retention of most of the contrast within the stomach after 4

hr or the presence of any barium within the stomach for longer than 12 to 24 hr is abnormal and indicates gastric retention. Radiographic findings must be interpreted in light of medications given within the last 24 to 36 hr. Drugs having anticholinergic effects, such as atropine, propantheline (Pro-Banthine, Searle), isopropamide (Darbazine, Norden) and methscopolomine (Pamine, Upjohn) can cause gastric atony with prolonged retention of gastric contents.

Fluoroscopy helps to visualize sequential changes in the shape of the stomach and pylorus. Contractility of the stomach and pylorus is usually normal with antral pyloric hypertrophy; however, barium has little forward movement through the pylorus. In general, restrictive mural diseases of the pylorus such as muscular hypertrophy, inflammation, or neoplasia produce annular narrowing of the pylorus. In such instances, barium may fill only the entrance to the pyloric lumen, resulting in what has been called a beak sign, describing the beaklike appearance of barium projecting into the pyloric antrum. A narrow stream of barium may be observed to fill the entire length of the narrowed pyloric lumen. Polyplike filling defects of the pyloric lumen caused by marked mucosal hyperplasia occur in some instances of antral pyloric hypertrophy. Other causes of filling defects that could occlude the pyloric lumen include foreign bodies, eosinophilic granuloma, and neoplasia.

Endoscopic examination of the stomach can be helpful in diagnosing antral pyloric hypertrophy and eliminating other causes of pyloric disease. In antral pyloric hypertrophy, the mucosa is typically a normal color and is nonulcerated. Grossly enlarged folds of redundant mucosa may be observed occluding the pylorus, and insufflation with air fails to distend the pyloric canal.

Definitive diagnosis is based on operative findings and histopathology of full-thickness pyloric biopsies. When palpated, the pyloric region will feel firm and enlarged. A longitudinal incision made on the ventral border of the pylorus and extending into the lumen will help to determine the extent of the lesion. Grossly, lesions vary from focal or multifocal mucosal polyps to a diffuse pattern of rugal thickening that involves the circumference of the antrum. The thickness of the pyloric wall will vary from normal to markedly thickened, depending on the extent of muscular hypertrophy. The lesions of antral pyloric hypertrophy can easily be mistaken for neoplasia on the basis of gross appearance; however, the presence of ulceration is more typical of malignancy.

Microscopic examination of excised tissue reveals variable degrees of mucosal hyperplasia or hypertrophy of the circular smooth muscle of the pylorus. Histologically, these lesions have been classified into one of three categories depending on the extent of mucosal and muscular involvement (Matthiesen, 1986; Sikes et al., 1986). The most commonly described type of lesion is characterized by diffuse mucosal hyperplasia with cystic dilatation of gastric glands and foveolar hyperplasia. Smooth muscle hypertrophy is absent to mild, and there are varying degrees of chronic inflammatory cell infiltration, with lymphocytes, plasma cells, and neutrophils in the lamina propria. Small foci of mucosal ulceration may occasionally be seen. A second type of lesion is characterized by both mucosal hyperplasia and marked thickening of the circular muscular layer, with irregular bundles of hypertrophied fibers. The third and least frequently described lesion is characterized primarily by smooth muscle hypertrophy of the pylorus, with minimal mucosal involvement.

TREATMENT

Successful treatment of antral pyloric hypertrophy requires surgery to improve gastric outflow. Many surgical techniques have been described for the correction of pyloric obstruction (Grandage, 1988). Of these surgical options, the Heineke-Mikulicz (H-M) pyloroplasty (Matthiesen, 1986), the Y-U antral flap pyloroplasty (Bright, 1988), and pylorectomy with gastroduodenostomy (Billroth I) (Walter et al., 1985b) result in the most favorable outcome. An incision should be made longitudinally into the ventral surface of the pylorus. The incision should extend from the antrum to the duodenum and should completely penetrate the mucosa. The pyloric area can then be examined visually and palpated to determine the extent of abnormal tissue. The decision on which surgical procedure to use is made after inspection of the pylorus and depends on the amount of tissue to be excised, the tissue pliability, and the diameter of the pyloric canal. If mucosal involvement is minimal, the H-M pyloroplasty usually provides adequate enlargement of the pyloric outflow. If focal mucosal folds or polyps are obstructing the pylorus, the most effective treatment is excision of the redundant mucosa followed by H-M pyloroplasty. An alternative technique that has been clinically effective in the treatment of pyloric antral hypertrophy is the Y-U pyloroplasty (Bright, 1988). This technique provides better exposure to the distal stomach and proximal duodenum and has recently been shown to improve gastric emptying while preventing duodenogastric reflux (Stanton et al., 1987). In dogs with severe changes, especially those with extensive mucosal involvement or generalized thickening of the pyloric wall with loss of antral pliability, complete pylorectomy and gastroduodenostomy are usually required to adequately relieve the gastric outlet obstruction. Although this latter procedure is technically more demanding and is more likely to result in biliary tract damage, suture line leakage, and iatrogenic pancreatitis, favorable results have been achieved in dogs when previous H-M pyloroplasty has failed (Sikes et al., 1986).

PROGNOSIS

With appropriate surgical management, most dogs with antral pyloric hypertrophy will have complete resolution of their clinical signs. About 80 per cent of afflicted dogs reportedly have had excellent clinical response on long-term follow-up. In general, the best results were achieved by either a Y-U antral flap pyloroplasty or by complete resection of the pylorus followed by a gastroduodenostomy. When clinical signs persist following H-M pyloroplasty, complete pyloric and antral resection is recommended.

References and Supplemental Reading

Barber, D. M., and Mahaffey, M. B.: The Stomach. *In* Thrall, D. E. (ed.): *Textbook of Veterinary Diagnostic Radiology.* Philadelphia: W. B. Saunders Co., 1986, pp. 473–492.

Bright, R. M.: Personal communication, 1988.

Bright, R. M., Richardson, D. C., and Stanton, M. E.: Y-U antral flap pyloroplasty in the dog. Comp. Cont. Ed. Pract. Vet. (in press).

Dodge, J. A., and Karim, A. A.: Induction of pyloric hypertrophy by pentagastrin. Gut 17:280, 1976.

Grandage, J.: The Stomach. *In* Slatter, D. H. (ed.): *Textbook of Small Animal Surgery.* Philadelphia: W. B. Saunders Co., 1985, pp. 703–712.

Happé, R. P., Van Der Gaag, I., and Wolvekamp, W. Th.: Multiple polyps of the gastric mucosa in two dogs. J. Small Anim. Pract. 18:179, 1977.

Happé, R. P., Van Der Gaag, I., Wolvekamp, W. Th.: Pyloric stenosis caused by hypertrophic gastritis in three dogs. J. Small Anim. Pract. 22:7, 1981.

Kelly, K. A.: Motility of the stomach and gastroduodenal junction. *In* Johnson, R. L. (ed.): *Physiology of the Gastrointestinal Tract.* New York: Raven Press, 1981, pp. 393–410.

Matthiesen, D. T., and Walter, M. C.: Surgical treatment of chronic hypertrophic pyloric gastropathy in 45 dogs. J. Am. Anim. Hosp. Assoc. 22:241, 1986.

Mroz, C. T., and Kelly, K. A.: The role of extrinsic antral nerves in the regulation of gastric emptying. Surgery 45:369, 1977.

Okamoto, E., Iwasaki, I., Kakutani, T., et al.: Selective destruction of the myenteric plexus: Its relation to Hirschsprung's disease, achalasia of the esophagus and hypertrophic pyloric stenosis. J. Pediatr. Surg. 2:444, 1967.

Sikes, R. I., Birchard, S., Patnaik, A., et al.: Chronic hypertrophic pyloric gastropathy: A review of 16 cases. J. Am. Anim. Hosp. Assoc. 22:99, 1986.

Stanton, M. E., Bright, R. M., Toal, R., et al.: Effects of the Y-U pyloroplasty on gastric emptying and duodenogastric reflux in the dog. Vet. Surg. 16:392, 1987.

Walker, P. J., Beauchamp, R. D., and Townsend, C. M.: Regulation of growth of gut and pancreas. *In* Thompson, J. C. (ed.): *Gastrointestinal Endocrinology.* New York: McGraw-Hill Book Co., 1987, pp. 136–140.

Walter, M. C., Goldschmidt, M. H., Stone, E. A., et al.: Chronic hypertrophic gastropathy as a cause of pyloric obstruction in the dog. J.A.V.M.A. 186:157, 1985a.

Walter, M. C., Matthiesen, D. T., and Stone, E. A.: Pylorectomy and gastroduodenostomy in the dog: Technique and clinical results in 28 cases. J.A.V.M.A. 187:909, 1985b.

CANINE LYMPHOCYTIC-PLASMACYTIC ENTERITIS

MICHAEL L. MAGNE, D.V.M.

Santa Rosa, California

Inflammatory bowel diseases are characterized by inflammatory cellular infiltrate within the lamina propria of the gastrointestinal tract. This infiltrate may consist of lymphocytes, plasma cells, eosinophils, macrophages, neutrophils, or combinations of these cells. Lymphocytic-plasmacytic enteritis (LPE), often referred to as idiopathic inflammatory bowel disease, is the most common chronic inflammatory intestinal disease seen in dogs.

PATHOGENESIS

In order to understand the possible pathogenesis of LPE, we must first appreciate normal function of the gut immune system, since it is hyperactivity or dysfunction of this system that is believed to play a central role in inflammatory bowel disease.

Gut-associated lymphoid tissue (GALT) constitutes approximately 25 per cent of the intestinal mucosa and functions to protect against invasion by potential pathogens as well as to modify potentially pathogenic responses to ingested antigens. The major components of GALT include duodenal lymphoid follicle aggregates (Peyer's patches), lymphocytes and plasma cells present in the intestinal lamina propria, and intraepithelial lymphocytes predominantly of T-cell origin. Lymphocytes in mesenteric lymph nodes and the hepatic reticuloendothelial system also function as integral parts of the intestinal immune system.

Dogs and cats have approximately 20 Peyer's patches, each containing a prominent B-cell–dependent area and a smaller T-cell–dependent area. The epithelium overlying these lymphoid aggregates consists of specialized lymphoepithelial cells referred to as membranous (M) cells, which function in the uptake of antigens from the intestinal lumen and their subsequent presentation to underlying lymphocytes. M cells may also serve as a portal of entry for certain viruses and as attachment sites for enteropathogenic bacteria. Antigens are processed by the M cells and then presented to lymphocytes and macrophages in the lymphoid aggregates or passed to mesenteric lymph nodes. Antigen-specific B cells, especially IgA-producer precursors, are stimulated and respond by clonal expansion. These stimulated lymphocytes pass into the systemic circulation via the mesenteric lymph nodes and tho-racic duct. Following a 4- to 6-day migration, in which they mature into IgA-secreting plasma cells, these cells "home" to subepithelial connective tissues of the intestinal mucosa, bronchial epithelium, mammary glands, and salivary glands. Antigenic stimulation of intestinal lymphoid aggregates also results in IgG-specific suppressor cells, which become systemically distributed and function to suppress systemic responses to ingested antigens. Intestinal IgA also inhibits systemic responses to ingested antigens by minimizing antigen uptake from the gut, as well as enhancing hepatic antigen clearance.

IgA is produced by plasma cells in the lamina propria of the gut and other secretory mucosae and is also secreted in large amounts in the bile. This immunoglobulin serves two roles in mucosal protection: **antigen neutralization** and **inhibition of microbe and parasite attachment**. Other immunocompetent cells serve complementary or synergistic roles. Although important in mucosal defense, IgA does not appear to be essential for survival.

Selective IgA deficiency is relatively common in humans, occurring in 1 of 500 persons, most of whom are asymptomatic. Intestinal biopsy samples of affected individuals reveal increased numbers of IgM-secreting plasma cells, suggesting that IgM may be capable of substituting for IgA. However, IgA-deficient patients are more prone to develop food allergy, presumably secondary to increased antigen access to the systemic circulation. Additionally, IgA deficiency has been associated in human patients with Crohn's disease, gluten enteropathies, and various autoimmune disorders. The relationship between IgA production, food allergy, and inflammatory intestinal diseases in small animals has not been adequately studied.

The precise role of cell-mediated immunity in gut immune reactions and defense has been poorly elucidated. It is known that oral antigen administration stimulates T cells, which mediate helper, suppressor, or cytotoxic functions. Large numbers of killer (K) and natural killer (NK) cells, which mediate cell-mediated cytotoxicity, are found in the intestinal tract and, in some species, account for up to 50 per cent of intraepithelial lymphocytes. These cells can destroy enterocytes infected with certain viruses but may also serve as replication sites for other viral agents. Intestinal macrophages are bactericidal for IgA-coated organisms, and IgE can initiate antibody-dependent cytotoxicity by eosinophils and macrophages located within the intestinal lamina propria. The precise role this antibody-mediated cytotoxicity plays in normal immune defense as well as disease states remains to be clarified.

The most commonly incriminated causative factors in LPE are **dietary** and **microbial** antigens. Implicated dietary factors include specific meat proteins, additives, preservatives, or food colorings. Gluten has been shown to produce an inflammatory enteropathy in hypersensitive persons, and it has also been shown that certain Irish setter dogs manifest a wheat-sensitive enteropathy. Dietary intolerances have long been known to occur in dogs and cats, and these may, in fact, represent hypersensitivity responses to specific antigenic substances within the particular offending diet. Infectious organisms may play a role in the development of LPE by various means. It is known that *Giardia* can produce inflammatory changes in the gut wall. Other organisms that may produce similar changes include *Salmonella* and *Campylobacter*. Slow-growing strains of *Mycobacteria* have been implicated in the pathophysiology of Crohn's disease in humans, a disease with similarities to inflammatory bowel disease in small animals. Whether these, or other, infectious organisms are etiologic factors in canine LPE is unknown.

Emphasis has recently been focused on the possibility that LPE represents an immune-mediated disorder in which tissue injury results from lymphocyte and antibody-mediated cytotoxicity. Excessive antigen exposure or prolonged mucosal-antigen contact can lead to the formation of immune complexes with either IgG or IgM in the lamina propria and submucosa. These immune complexes initiate a local inflammatory reaction resulting from complement activation and the attraction of phagocytic cells into the area. The release of proteolytic and lysosomal enzymes from these phagocytic cells results in local tissue destruction and inflammatory disease. It has been shown that certain T-cell–dependent immune responses can result in intestinal mucosal damage characterized by villus atrophy and crypt hyperplasia. Additionally, humans with inflammatory bowel disease may demonstrate serum antibodies to colonic epithelial cell antigens, certain milk proteins, RNA proteins, and viral antigens. Tissue damage in LPE patients may be an unfortunate sequela of an immune response to an environmental (dietary, microbial?) antigen, or the immunologic damage may be truly autoimmune and directed against self-components that cross-react with the environmental antigen. An immune-mediated basis for LPE is supported by the inability to document a primary etiology, the chronic and recurrent nature of the disorder, and the consistent clinical response seen with the use of corticosteroids and other immunosuppressive drugs.

HISTORY AND CLINICAL SIGNS

The animal with LPE typically presents with a history of chronic vomiting, diarrhea, or weight loss. Symptoms are often intermittent initially, with periods of weeks or months separating bouts. Affected individuals are usually anorectic during exacerbations, but some animals exhibit a ravenous appetite. Diarrhea is often watery, but the stools may also be soft or semiformed. Frank blood or mucus may be present in the stool in individuals with colonic involvement. Hematochezia may also be seen in patients with ileal inflammation, but without colitis. Melena occurs in a small percentage of cases and is indicative of either severe intestinal or gastric involvement. Vomiting is a common clinical sign and most often occurs with no relationship to feeding. There is no consistent correlation between vomiting and the presence of gastric inflammatory disease, since approximately two-thirds of the dogs that are vomiting have histologically normal gastric mucosa. Vomiting in these patients results either from visceral stimulation due to intestinal inflammation or from gastric motility dysfunction leading to delayed gastric emptying. Hematemesis may be present with either gastric or duodenal involvement. As time passes, clinical bouts usually occur at closer intervals, and many individuals become persistently symptomatic. Paradoxically, some animals with chronic severe disease may present with acute symptoms.

Other clinical signs that are less commonly reported include borborygmus, abdominal pain and cramping, pica, polyuria, or polydipsia.

Physical examination may reveal a cachectic, depressed patient; on the other hand, the animal may appear perfectly healthy with no obvious signs. Thickened intestinal loops may be palpated, and some dogs exhibit pain on abdominal palpation. Mesenteric lymphadenopathy is not uncommon and results from reactive nodal hyperplasia. Common nonspecific findings include elevated body temperature and poor coat.

There appears to be no specific age predilection for the onset of LPE in dogs, although most affected individuals are over 2 years of age. I have, however, diagnosed LPE in animals as young as 8 months. There also is no apparent breed predilection, with the possible exception of the immunoproliferative enteropathy reported in the basenji breed.

DIAGNOSIS

Clinical pathology findings are nonspecific. Leukocytosis, usually mature neutrophilic, is relatively common; a significant left shift may occasionally be seen. Peripheral eosinophilia is common in individuals with a mixed inflammatory infiltrate of lymphocytes, plasma cells, and eosinophils. Normocytic, normochromic anemia, attributable to chronic inflammatory disease, is also common. I have also observed microcytic, hypochromic, iron-deficiency anemia in three dogs, all with histologically severe disease. Vitamin K–responsive hypoprothrombinemia and coagulopathy have been reported in cats with LPE, but I have not observed this in affected dogs. Protein-losing enteropathy may be manifested by panhypoproteinemia due to malabsorption and protein loss through the inflamed gut wall. Conversely, some individuals may exhibit hypoalbuminemia but normal to elevated globulin levels, which presumably result from chronic systemic antigenic stimulation. The presence of protein-losing enteropathy and panhypoproteinemia correlates with a more chronic or severe clinical course. Mild to moderate increases in serum liver enzymes may be noted and are associated with a periportal mononuclear infiltrate, attributed to inflammatory efflux from the gut.

Other tests that may be helpful in the diagnosis of LPE include serum cobalamin (B_{12}) and folate assays and the D-xylose absorption test. Although D-xylose absorption is a good indicator of intestinal absorptive capability, there are several limitations to its usefulness. Delayed gastric emptying and intestinal bacterial overgrowth can affect results, and it has also been shown that individuals with chronic enteropathies may have normal absorption of D-xylose. When further biochemical tests of intestinal function are indicated, I recommend a panel that measures serum trypsin-like immunoreactivity (TLI), cobalamin, and folate levels. Assay of serum TLI assesses pancreatic function, while measurement of serum cobalamin and folate levels tests for intestinal absorption as well as intestinal bacterial overgrowth. It must be emphasized that all of these tests may be unaffected by LPE, and the presence of normal results does not rule out inflammatory bowel disease.

Radiography is usually not helpful in establishing a definitive diagnosis; rather, the value lies in ruling out other causes of chronic vomiting, diarrhea, or weight loss. Survey abdominal radiographs in dogs with LPE usually appear normal, although some patients may show intestinal dilatation, often within the proximal duodenum. Contrast studies may show mucosal irregularities, bowel wall thickening, or delayed gastric emptying, but frequently no abnormalities are seen. False-positive findings may also be seen in individuals with normal gastrointestinal function. Abnormal radiographic findings unfortunately do not yield a specific diagnosis in these cases, but merely confirm the necessity of mucosal examination and biopsy. Clinical studies of humans with signs of upper gastrointestinal disease indicate that gastrointestinal contrast studies should be reserved for those patients in whom endoscopic examination and biopsy fail to yield a diagnosis.

The **differential diagnosis** for LPE is lengthy and includes other infiltrative bowel diseases (eosinophilic enteritis, lymphosarcoma, histoplasmosis), lymphangiectasia, giardiasis, *Campylobacter* infection, salmonellosis, gastrointestinal motility disturbances, pancreatic exocrine insufficiency, and intestinal bacterial overgrowth.

Definitive diagnosis of LPE is established by intestinal mucosal biopsy, procured either endoscopically or via exploratory laparotomy. Although a presumptive diagnosis may be based on history, physical examination, and laboratory studies, intestinal biopsy is strongly recommended in order to determine the type and severity of the disease, thus allowing accurate prognostication and therapy. As with any disease, the earlier a diagnosis is made, the better the prognosis for satisfactory control or cure.

Endoscopy is the recommended method of obtaining intestinal biopsies in suspected LPE patients, because of its minimally invasive nature and lower cost. A significant advantage of endoscopic biopsy over full-thickness biopsies obtained by laparotomy is the ability to obtain diagnostic samples in hypoproteinemic patients without fear of poor tissue healing or dehiscence. Multiple tissue biopsies can be taken, allowing an accurate assessment of disease extent. With experience and good endoscopic equipment, it is possible to routinely obtain biopsy samples from the stomach, duodenum, proximal jejunum (small dogs), colon, and ileum. Possible disadvantages are the inability to visualize and biopsy the jejunum in larger dogs and the procurement of biopsy samples that extend no deeper than the muscularis mucosa. Since most cases of LPE involve the entire small intestine and the inflammatory changes always involve the mucosa, duodenal biopsies obtained by endoscopy are usually representative. In some cases, newer suction biopsy instruments that are advanced under endoscopic or fluoroscopic guidance may yield a larger tissue sample for evaluation.

In affected individuals, the endoscopic appearance of the intestinal mucosa may range from completely normal to severely inflamed and ulcerated. The mucosa is often thickened and friable in advanced cases. Biopsies are always taken, regardless of the gross appearance of the mucosa. Because of the small tissue sample obtained, multiple biopsies, usually four to eight, are recommended. As previously mentioned, many dogs with chronic vomiting due to LPE do not have gastric disease; thus, it is essential that the small intestine be examined and biopsied.

If endoscopic equipment is unavailable, exploratory laparotomy to obtain biopsy samples is indicated. It is not uncommon for the entire gastrointestinal tract to appear grossly normal, even in severe cases, and biopsies should be taken regardless of the gross appearance. Full-thickness biopsies are taken from the duodenum, jejunum, and ileum. Complications of full-thickness biopsy include dehiscence and stricture formation. Biopsy of mesenteric lymph nodes is also recommended.

HISTOLOGIC FINDINGS

The normal intestinal lamina propria may contain occasional inflammatory cells, usually consisting of small lymphocytes or plasma cells. Other cells, such as eosinophils, neutrophils, or macrophages, are not observed in normal intestinal mucosa. As already mentioned, LPE is characterized by the presence of an infiltrate within the lamina propria consisting predominantly of lymphocytes and plasma cells, often with smaller percentages of eosinophils, neutrophils, or macrophages. Histopathologic changes are commonly reported as mild, moderate, moderate to severe, or severe, and the relative percentages of inflammatory cells should be noted. An experienced pathologist is very helpful.

Histologic changes noted as mild are often indicative of other clinical disorders such as bacterial overgrowth, giardiasis, or diarrhea due to other causes. Therefore, when intestinal mucosal biopsies reveal mild inflammatory changes, diagnostic effort should be redirected to these areas. Moderate to severe histologic changes characterized by a heavy inflammatory cell infiltrate, villus blunting or atrophy, and fibrosis within the lamina propria are significant changes indicative of "primary" LPE. The histologic severity provides valuable information as to specific therapy and long-term prognosis for control. Some patients initially diagnosed as having LPE subsequently have been found to have lymphosarcoma.

THERAPY

Treatment of patients with LPE must be individualized to the particular case and depends on the type, severity, and extent of inflammatory disease present. Treatment failure most often results from either inadequately aggressive therapy or failure to accurately stage the extent of the disease process. Therapeutic agents include corticosteroids, metronidazole, immunosuppressive agents, and dietary management.

Corticosteroids are indicated for their anti-inflammatory and immunosuppressive actions. Additionally, it has been shown that corticosteroids enhance the absorption of fluid and electrolytes by the small intestinal mucosa. Another beneficial effect is their nonspecific appetite-stimulating activity in certain individuals. Immunosuppression and catabolic ef-

fects are possible complications of long-term or high-dose use. Mild to moderate cases will usually respond to prednisone given at a dosage of 0.5 to 1.0 mg/kg twice daily for 2 weeks. Administration frequency is then reduced to once daily for 2 to 4 weeks. Alternate-day therapy is continued, with dosages reduced in 50 per cent increments at 4-week intervals. In milder cases, treatment can sometimes be discontinued after 3 to 6 months. In more severe cases, high doses (e.g., 1.0 to 1.5 mg/kg b.i.d.) should be given for the first 2 to 4 weeks, and dosages are subsequently reduced in 50 per cent increments at 4-week intervals. Dogs with severe disease will require long-term corticosteroid therapy, either months, years, or lifelong. To minimize corticosteroid side effects, dosages are adjusted to the minimum amount necessary to control clinical signs.

Metronidazole is a unique pharmacologic agent that, in addition to antiprotozoal and anaerobic antibacterial activities, exerts profound immunosuppressive activity, specifically against cell-mediated immune responses. I have found this drug useful in conjunction with corticosteroids and, in some cases, as a single agent. Indications for metronidazole use include refractoriness or relapse while on corticosteroids, moderate to severe histologic changes, or excessive side effects due to high steroid dosages. The recommended dosage is 10 mg/kg, initially given three times daily. After 2 to 4 weeks, administration can be reduced to twice daily. Side effects are very rare, although I have observed anorexia in occasional animals, more commonly in cats than in dogs.

The use of more potent immunosuppressive drugs such as **azathioprine** or **cyclophosphamide** is indicated in very severe cases (e.g., protein-losing enteropathy) or if corticosteroids are poorly tolerated or inadequate to achieve remission. I prefer azathioprine for use in dogs because it has fewer side effects than cyclophosphamide. The recommended dose is 2.0 to 2.5 mg/kg given once a day. In these cases, prednisone is given at 2.0 to 2.5 mg/kg per day for 2 weeks; then, assuming there is clinical improvement, prednisone dosages may be decreased in 50 per cent increments at 4-week intervals, using alternate-day therapy. When clinical remission is achieved, the azathioprine dose may be reduced by 50 per cent, which is easily accomplished by administering on an alternate-day basis. Azathioprine is generally continued for 3 to 6 months. Side effects of azathioprine are uncommon in dogs, but anorexia, hepatic damage, and bone marrow suppression have been reported. Because of this, a complete blood count should be performed every 2 weeks for the first 2 months of use and then once a month thereafter. Evidence of anemia, leukopenia, or jaundice is an indication for discontinuation.

Dietary management is an essential component in the rational treatment of LPE. Although the use of controlled diets does appear to be beneficial in the long-term management of these cases, dietary manipulation alone is usually inadequate to control signs in the symptomatic individual. In fact, many clinically affected animals will already have been treated with controlled diets, and owners will report either temporary or insignificant resolution of clinical signs. In symptomatic patients, particularly those with moderate to severe disease, pharmacologic intervention is almost always necessary to bring about remission. The beneficial role of high-quality, controlled diets is in maintaining clinical remission. Recommended commercial diets include Hill's Prescription Diet i/d, ANF, Nutromax, Eukanuba, Science Diet Canine Growth, and Gaines Cycle 3 or Cycle 4. Low-fat diets such as Prescription Diets r/d and i/d or Cycle 3 are recommended if malabsorption is significant. Homemade diets based on boiled rice or potatoes, poultry, cottage cheese, and eggs can also be used. Feeding small amounts several times daily is recommended to maximize dietary assimilation. It is recommended that dietary management be continued for the remainder of the animal's life.

Supplementation of medium-chain triglycerides (MCT Oil, Mead Johnson; Portagen, Mead Johnson) to the diet may benefit some individuals with severe malabsorption in which long-chain triglycerides are poorly absorbed. Medium-chain triglycerides are transported by the portal venous system following direct absorption by enterocytes; thus, their absorption is not affected by lymphatic obstruction as occurs in lymphangiectasia and many cases of LPE. MCT Oil is supplemented at a dosage of 1 to 2 ml/kg body weight daily, with 1 ml supplying approximately 8 Kcal. Portagen is a powdered elemental diet supplement; 1½ cups is added to water to make 1 quart of a mixture supplying 30 Kcal/fluid ounce (1 Kcal/ml). However, this mixture is hypertonic and may induce vomiting or exacerbate diarrhea.

Vitamin depletion, especially of fat-soluble vitamins, can result in individuals with malabsorption or prolonged anorexia or diarrhea. Vitamin supplementation with a commercial preparation is recommended in dogs with LPE until resolution of clinical symptoms. Folate deficiency may occur in animals with chronic, severe disease and requires specific supplementation. When low serum folate levels are documented, folic acid is supplemented at a dose of 2.5 to 5.0 mg/day.

LPE is a disorder that is most often controlled by therapy, but rarely cured. A decision to alter or discontinue treatment should be based on a thorough review of the patient's clinical response and, ideally, repeated examination and biopsy of the intestinal mucosa. If corticosteroids alone, given at low doses two to three times weekly, have kept the animal asymptomatic over a period of 3 months, it is rational to attempt discontinuation of therapy. Relapse is treated by daily medication for 2 weeks, followed by gradual reduction to maintenance levels. It is interesting to note that some individuals, irrespective of histologic severity, will show a dramatic clinical response, yet rebiopsy of the intestine shows little histologic improvement. Other cases may show complete histologic resolution.

References and Supplemental Reading

August, J. R.: Dietary hypersensitivity in dogs: Cutaneous manifestations, diagnosis, and management. Comp. Cont. Ed. Pract. Vet. 7:469, 1985.

Batt, R. M.: Chronic small intestinal disease in the dog. Proceedings of the 8th Kal Kan Symposium, 1984, pp. 93–103.

Batt, R. M.: Wheat-sensitive enteropathy in Irish setters. In Kirk, R. W. (ed.): Current Veterinary Therapy IX. Philadelphia: W. B. Saunders Co., 1986, pp. 893–896.

Batt, R. M., Bush, B. M., and Peters, T. J.: Subcellular biochemical studies of a naturally occurring enteropathy in the dog resembling chronic tropical sprue in human beings. Am. J. Vet. Res. 44:1492, 1983.

Breitschwerdt, E. B.: Immunoproliferative enteropathy of basenjis. Proc. 5th Annu. ACVIM Meet. 5:683, 1987.

Buffington, C. A.: Therapeutic use of vitamins in small animals. In Kirk, R. W. (ed.): Current Veterinary Therapy IX. Philadelphia: W. B. Saunders Co., 1986, pp. 40–47.

Burrows, C. F.: The treatment of diarrhea. In Kirk, R. W. (ed.): Current Veterinary Therapy VIII. Philadelphia: W. B. Saunders Co., 1983, pp. 784–790.

DeNovo, R. C.: Therapeutics of gastrointestinal disease. In Kirk, R. W. (ed.): Current Veterinary Therapy IX. Philadelphia: W. B. Saunders Co., 1986, pp. 862–872.

Donaldson, R. M.: Crohn's disease. In Sleisenger, M. H., and Fordtran, J. S. (eds.): Gastrointestinal Disease: Pathophysiology, Diagnosis, Management. Philadelphia: W. B. Saunders Co., 1983, pp. 1088–1121.

Gitnick, G.: Evidence for infectious agents in IBD. In Gitnick, G. (ed.): Current Gastroenterology. Vol. 7. Chicago: Year Book Medical Publishers, 1987, pp. 305–313.

Greenberger, N.: Allergic disorders of the intestine and eosinophilic gastroenteritis. In Sleisenger, M. H., and Fordtran, J. S. (eds.): Gastrointestinal Disease: Pathophysiology, Diagnosis, Management. Philadelphia: W. B. Saunders Co., 1983, pp. 1069–1082.

Kagnoff, M. F.: Immunology and disease of the gastrointestinal tract. In Sleisenger, M. H., and Fordtran, J. S. (eds.): Gastrointestinal Disease: Pathophysiology, Diagnosis, Management. Philadelphia: W. B. Saunders Co., 1983, pp. 20–44.

O'Brien, T. R.: Small intestine. In O'Brien, T. R. (ed.): Radiographic Diagnosis of Abdominal Disorders in the Dog and Cat. Philadelphia: W. B. Saunders Co., 1978, pp. 270–351.

Pollock, R. V. H., and Zimmer, J. F.: Intestinal immunity. Proceedings of the 8th Kal Kan Symposium, 1984, pp. 81–86.

Sherding, R. G.: Intestinal lymphangiectasia. In Kirk, R. W. (ed.): Current Veterinary Therapy IX. Philadelphia: W. B. Saunders Co., 1986, pp. 885–888.

Strombeck, D. R.: Dietary allergies, eosinophilic gastroenteritis, and gluten-induced enteropathy. In Strombeck, D. R. (ed.): Small Animal Gastroenterology. Davis, CA: Stonegate Publishing, 1979, pp. 230–239.

Tams, T. R.: Chronic canine lymphocytic plasmacytic enteritis. Comp. Cont. Ed. Pract. Vet. 9:1184, 1987.

Tams, T. R., and Twedt, D. C.: Canine protein-losing gastroenteropathy syndrome. Comp. Cont. Ed. Pract. Vet. 3:105, 1981.

Trier, J. S.: Celiac sprue. In Sleisenger, M. H., and Fordtran, J. S. (eds.): Gastrointestinal Disease: Pathophysiology, Diagnosis, Management. Philadelphia: W. B. Saunders Co., 1983, pp. 1050–1069.

Williams, D. A.: New tests of pancreatic and small intestinal function. Comp. Cont. Ed. Pract. Vet. 9:1167, 1987.

Zimmer, J. F.: Nutritional management of gastrointestinal diseases. In Kirk, R. W. (ed.): Current Veterinary Therapy IX. Philadelphia: W. B. Saunders Co., 1986, pp. 909–916.

EXOCRINE PANCREATIC INSUFFICIENCY

DAVID A. WILLIAMS, Vet. M.B., Ph.D.
Gainesville, Florida

ETIOLOGY

The most common cause of exocrine pancreatic insufficiency in dogs is pancreatic acinar atrophy. This disease most commonly affects dogs 1 to 5 years of age and is characterized by atrophy of the acinar cells with minimal inflammation. Cells of the endocrine pancreas become disorganized but are otherwise unaffected. Nutritional imbalance, pancreatic duct obstruction, toxicosis, ischemia, viral infection, immune-mediated disease, and a primary congenital abnormality in the pancreas itself all have been suggested as potential causes, but the etiology remains unknown. A genetic predisposition to development of pancreatic acinar atrophy has been reported in German shepherd dogs, but many other breeds are also affected.

End-stage chronic pancreatitis is a much less common cause of exocrine pancreatic insufficiency in dogs, although it is probably the most common cause in cats. In chronic pancreatitis, both endocrine and exocrine pancreatic cells are progressively destroyed; thus, exocrine pancreatic insufficiency is often accompanied by diabetes mellitus. Chronic pancreatitis is probably the underlying cause of most cases of exocrine pancreatic insufficiency in older dogs and may be particularly prevalent in miniature schnauzers and Yorkshire terriers.

Exocrine pancreatic insufficiency may develop as a result of obstruction to the flow of juice secondary to adenocarcinoma, although this is uncommon. In cats, exocrine pancreatic insufficiency can occur as a complication of proximal duodenal resection and cholecystoduodenostomy. In this species, dual pancreatic ducts are absent and therefore damage to the major duodenal papilla blocks pancreatic secretion.

Extremely rare causes of exocrine pancreatic insufficiency in children include congenital deficiencies of individual pancreatic digestive enzymes or of intestinal enteropeptidase. These have not yet been reported in dogs or cats.

PATHOPHYSIOLOGY

Nutrient malabsorption in canine exocrine pancreatic insufficiency does not arise simply as a consequence of failure of intraluminal digestion. Studies of both naturally occurring and experimental exocrine pancreatic insufficiency in several species have revealed abnormal activities of mucosal enzymes and impaired function as indicated by abnormal transport of sugars, amino acids, and fatty acids. Morphologic changes in the jejunal mucosa are seen in some cases, but functional abnormalities often occur in animals with no histologic evidence of mucosal damage. The cause of this mucosal pathology is unknown, but the absence of the trophic influence of pancreatic secretions, concurrent overgrowth of bacteria in the small intestine, and endocrine and nutritional factors all may be contributory.

Bacterial overgrowth in the duodenum of dogs with exocrine pancreatic insufficiency is common. Potential factors that may predispose to overgrowth include absence of the antibacterial factors present in pancreatic juice and changes in intestinal motility or immunity secondary to malnutrition.

The effect of bacterial overgrowth on mucosal enzymes and morphology depends on the type of bacteria present. When the overgrowth includes obligate anaerobes, activities of many jejunal mucosal enzymes are often markedly decreased, and partial villus atrophy sometimes occurs (Fig. 1). The reductions in mucosal enzyme activities probably arise because obligate anaerobic bacteria produce proteases that release and destroy exposed brush-border enzymes. When obligate anaerobes are not present, mucosal enzyme activities are generally normal or increased. Similar changes are seen in dogs with exocrine pancreatic insufficiency but without bacterial overgrowth. These changes have been attributed to reduced degradation of exposed brush-border enzymes by intraluminal pancreatic proteases. Even when mucosal abnormalities are minimal, bacterial overgrowth may be of pathophysiologic significance, since microbial deconjugation of bile salts and hydroxylation of fatty acids may exacerbate fat malabsorption and diarrhea.

CLINICAL SIGNS

Animals with exocrine pancreatic insufficiency most commonly present with polyphagia and weight

927

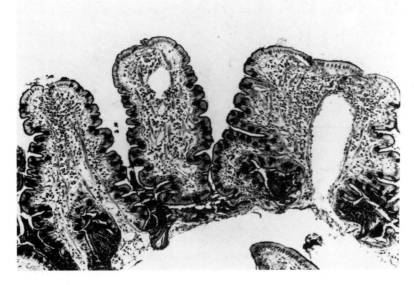

Figure 1. Partial villous atrophy in a jejunal biopsy specimen from a dog with exocrine pancreatic insufficiency due to pancreatic acinar atrophy. Villi are short and stumpy, with a broadened plateau at the extrusion zone, and there is evidence of folding or fusion of villi. (Reprinted with permission from Williams, D. A., Batt, R. M., and McLean, L.: Bacterial overgrowth in the duodenum of dogs with exocrine pancreatic insufficiency. J.A.V.M.A. 191:201, 1987.)

loss. Although often dramatic, weight loss may be minimal in some cases, and not all animals are obviously polyphagic. Pica and coprophagia are often reported, as are excessive borborygmus and apparent abdominal discomfort. In many cases, large amounts of semiformed feces are passed, but intermittent severe watery diarrhea may also occur. Feces are sometimes reported to be normal. The feces may become more normal in appearance when a low-fat or highly digestible diet is fed. All these signs are nonspecific and may occur with malabsorption due to any cause.

DIAGNOSIS

Routine laboratory test results are generally not helpful in establishing the diagnosis of exocrine pancreatic insufficiency. Serum alanine aminotransferase activity is often mildly to moderately increased, while total lipid, cholesterol, and polyunsaturated fatty acid concentrations are usually reduced. Dogs with exocrine pancreatic insufficiency show a remarkable ability to maintain normal serum protein concentrations even when severely malnourished. Mild lymphopenia and eosinophilia occasionally occur, but complete blood count results are usually within normal limits, and major abnormalities should be pursued as evidence of additional or alternative underlying disorders.

Several laboratory tests for the diagnosis of exocrine pancreatic insufficiency have been described, but in many cases their reliability has not been demonstrated and is highly questionable. Dogs with exocrine pancreatic insufficiency can be readily identified by radioimmunoassay of serum trypsinlike immunoreactivity in a single fasting serum sample. The bentiromide (N-benzoyl-L-tyrosyl-p-aminobenzoic acid [BT-PABA]) test and assay of fecal proteo-

lytic activity using an azoprotein-based method will also identify most affected dogs, but these latter tests give false-positive results in a small proportion of cases.

Serum Trypsinlike Immunoreactivity

Serum trypsinlike immunoreactivity (TLI) refers to the concentration of proteins recognized by antibodies raised against the pancreatic digestive enzyme trypsin. In healthy animals, serum TLI results from the presence of trypsinogen, the inactive zymogen form of the enzyme, which leaks out of the pancreas in trace amounts. Serum TLI can be detected in all normal dogs provided that a species-specific assay is used (Diagnostic Products Corp., Los Angeles, CA). In 100 normal dogs, serum TLI concentrations ranged from 5.2 to 34.0 μg/L (Williams and Batt, 1988).

TLI is a pancreas-specific marker, since trypsinogen is synthesized and stored only in pancreatic acinar cells. In contrast, canine amylase and lipase activities are not exclusively pancreatic in their origin. Quantitation of a putative pancreas-specific isoenzyme of amylase using either electrophoresis or selective inhibition has not yet proved reliable in the identification of dogs with exocrine pancreatic insufficiency.

Pancreatic acinar atrophy is associated with almost total absence of pancreatic acinar cells. It is therefore not surprising that serum TLI concentrations are dramatically reduced (<2.5 μg/L) in affected dogs (Fig. 2). In contrast, serum TLI concentrations in dogs with small intestinal disease are not significantly different from those in healthy controls (Fig. 2). Intestinal disease does not affect serum TLI, because pancreatic enzymes enter the blood

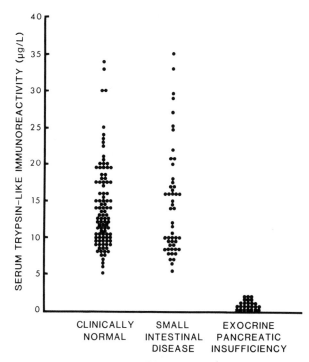

Figure 2. Serum trypsin–like immunoreactivity in 100 clinically normal dogs, 50 dogs with small intestinal disease, and 25 dogs with exocrine pancreatic insufficiency. (Reprinted with permission from Williams, D. A., and Batt, R. M.: Sensitivity and specificity of radioimmunoassay of serum trypsin–like immunoreactivity for the diagnosis of canine exocrine pancreatic insufficiency. J.A.V.M.A. 192:195, 1988.)

Bentiromide Absorption Test

The synthetic substrate bentiromide contains a bond that is cleaved by the pancreatic enzyme chymotrypsin, releasing *p*-aminobenzoic acid (PABA). Chymotrypsin activity in the small intestine may be indirectly assayed *in vivo* by oral administration of this substrate. Free PABA is absorbed from the gut lumen and subsequently excreted in the urine. Absorption is assessed by measuring sequential PABA concentrations in either plasma or urinary excretion. The relatively high cost of the substrate, the requirement for either multiple blood sampling or collection of urine in a metabolism cage, and the laboratory expertise required for the PABA assay have largely restricted the use of this test to specialty centers.

Although often considered the most reliable test for the diagnosis of exocrine pancreatic insufficiency, this test is not highly specific. A proportion of dogs with small intestinal disease have subnormal PABA absorption; thus, results from dogs with exocrine pancreatic insufficiency overlap somewhat with those from dogs with small intestinal disease (Fig. 3). Nonetheless, extremely low PABA absorp-

directly from the pancreas and are not absorbed intact from the intestinal lumen.

A very small proportion of samples submitted for assay of TLI have borderline subnormal concentrations in the range of 3.0 to 5.0 μg/L. These dogs have not been available for further investigation using alternative tests, but on retesting, results have usually been either clearly normal or diagnostically subnormal. A few dogs with exocrine pancreatic insufficiency exhibit a transient rise in serum TLI following a meal. Failure to take serum after withholding food for at least 3 hr may explain initial equivocal results in dogs that clearly have exocrine pancreatic insufficiency on retesting. The return to normal in some dogs may reflect regeneration of acinar cell function following an episode of pancreatic disease.

Very rarely, serum TLI is consistently subnormal but above the 2.5 μg/L value considered diagnostic for exocrine pancreatic insufficiency. On follow-up of the few such patients seen so far, none has shown signs of persistent weight loss or diarrhea. Such animals may have chronic subclinical pancreatic disease, as was confirmed in one case in which severe chronic pancreatitis was found as an incidental finding at necropsy.

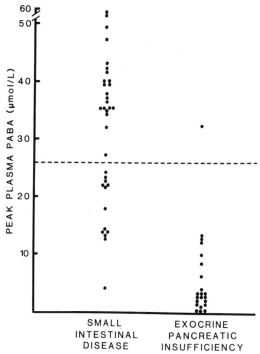

Figure 3. Peak plasma PABA concentration after combined bentiromide-xylose absorption testing of 35 dogs with small intestinal disease and 22 dogs wtih exocrine pancreatic insufficiency. The dashed line indicates the lower limit of the range of peak plasma PABA concentrations in clinically normal dogs. (Reprinted with permission from Williams, D. A., and Batt, R. M.: Sensitivity and specificity of radioimmunoassay of serum trypsin–like immunoreactivity for the diagnosis of canine exocrine pancreatic insufficiency. J.A.V.M.A. 192:195, 1988.)

tion usually indicates exocrine pancreatic insufficiency.

Bentiromide test results in normal cats have been reported, but their diagnostic value in distinguishing cats with exocrine pancreatic insufficiency from those with small intestinal disease is not known.

Fecal Proteolytic Activity

Fecal proteolytic activity (often inaccurately referred to as fecal "trypsin") has been used as an index of pancreatic enzyme activity for many years. Unfortunately, the x-ray film gelatin digestion test as widely used is an unreliable assay of fecal proteolytic activity and gives many false-negative and false-positive results. Fecal proteolytic activity assayed using substrates such as azocasein is more reliable, and results are consistently low in most dogs with exocrine pancreatic insufficiency (Fig. 4). At least three fecal specimens should be assayed, because normal dogs (and cats) also occasionally pass feces with low protease activity. Dogs with exocrine pancreatic insufficiency rarely exhibit normal fecal proteolytic activity as assessed by this type of assay. This type of test is probably the most reliable

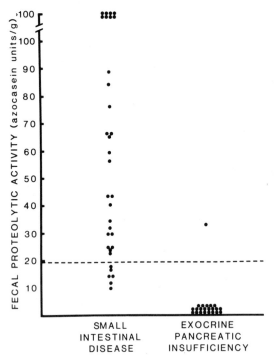

Figure 4. Fecal proteolytic activity, assayed using an azocasein substrate, in 34 dogs with small intestinal disease and 22 dogs with exocrine pancreatic insufficiency. Results represent the mean value of determinations in samples collected on at least 3 days, or the activity of a pooled 3-day collection. The dashed line indicates the lower limit of the range of values in control dogs. (Reproduced with permission from Williams, D. A., and Batt, R. M.: Sensitivity and specificity of radioimmunoassay of serum trypsin–like immunoreactivity for the diagnosis of canine exocrine pancreatic insufficiency. J.A.V.M.A. 192:195, 1988.)

approach to diagnosis in cats and can be applied to other species.

Other Tests

Microscopic examination of feces for evidence of undigested food (fat droplets, starch grains, muscle fibers) has long been used as a test for exocrine pancreatic insufficiency. This approach is subjective and imprecise, and interpretation is complicated by the variation in fecal characteristics that occurs with different diets and with changes in intestinal transit time.

Although exocrine pancreatic insufficiency is usually associated with severe steatorrhea, this is not always apparent on examination of Sudan III stained samples. Quantitative assessment of fecal fat output is a more sensitive indicator of steatorrhea, but neither qualitative nor quantitative tests reliably differentiate exocrine pancreatic insufficiency from other causes of fat malabsorption.

Oral and intravenous glucose tolerance is often abnormal in dogs with exocrine pancreatic insufficiency. However, glucose intolerance does not occur in all cases, nor is it unique to dogs with exocrine pancreatic insufficiency.

Starch tolerance test results are usually abnormal in dogs with exocrine pancreatic insufficiency, but abnormal results are also found in some patients with small intestinal disease.

Plasma turbidity (lipemia) after oral administration of fat is often diminished or absent in dogs with fat malabsorption. Exocrine pancreatic insufficiency can theoretically be distinguished from other causes of fat malabsorption by repeating the test after addition of pancreatic extract to the fat meal. However, some dogs with exocrine pancreatic insufficiency develop visually detectable lipemia after a fatty meal without addition of pancreatic extract, and other factors such as variation in gastric emptying times make this test difficult to evaluate reliably.

Summary

Assay of serum TLI, the bentiromide test, and quantitative assay of fecal proteolytic activity all are sensitive tests for exocrine pancreatic insufficiency in dogs. Serum TLI is a more specific test, however, since the other tests give a higher proportion of abnormal results in dogs with small intestinal disease. Microscopic examination of feces for undigested food, assessment of fecal proteolytic activity by x-ray plate gelatin digestion, starch tolerance, plasma turbidity, and glucose tolerance all are unreliable and have limited value. Quantitative assay of fecal proteolytic activity is probably the test of choice for use in cats and other species, but there is little available clinical information.

TREATMENT

Most dogs with exocrine pancreatic insufficiency can be managed successfully by simply supplementing each meal with pancreatic enzyme extracts. In a small proportion of cases, weight gain is suboptimal even though other signs such as diarrhea and polyphagia abate. The explanation for this is not known, but chronic bacterial overgrowth may lead to irreversible mucosal damage in some cases. Additional measures that may be required for optimal response in such individuals include antibiotic therapy to treat associated bacterial overgrowth in the small intestine, dietary modification, vitamin supplementation, inhibition of gastric acid output, and glucocorticoid therapy.

Enzyme Replacement

Enzyme replacement using an initial dose of 2 tsp of powdered non–enteric-coated pancreatic extract (Gastrizyme, Schering; Pancrezyme, Daniels; Viokase-V, A. H. Robins) with each meal per 20 kg of body weight is generally effective. Animals that do not show an optimum response to this dose do not benefit by increasing the amount of extract. Other dietary modifications (see following) may benefit such animals. Tablets, capsules, and enteric-coated preparations are either ineffective or no more effective than powdered extracts and are not recommended. The extract should be mixed with a maintenance dog food immediately prior to feeding. Two meals a day are usually sufficient to promote weight gain of 0.5 to 1.0 kg/week; diarrhea generally resolves within 2 to 3 days, and coprophagia and polyphagia also often disappear within a few days.

As soon as clinical improvement is apparent, owners can determine a minimum effective dose of enzyme supplement that prevents return of clinical signs. This varies slightly between different enzyme preparations, and also from dog to dog. Most affected animals need at least 1 tsp of extract with each meal. One meal per day is enough for some dogs, whereas some do better when fed twice daily.

Chopped healthy ox or pig pancreas, 3 to 4 oz per meal, is sometimes an economical alternative to feeding of relatively expensive dried extracts. Pancreas can be stored frozen at −20°C for at least 3 months, and enzyme activity will be adequately maintained.

Addition of bile salts or antacids and preincubation of enzymes with the food prior to feeding do not increase the effectiveness of enzyme supplements. Inhibition of gastric acid secretion by cimet-

idine probably reduces intragastric destruction of lipase, but it is expensive and rarely improves the clinical response.

Dietary Modification

Fat absorption does not return to normal despite appropriate enzyme therapy. Dogs compensate by eating slightly more than usual, so approximately 20 per cent more than calculated maintenance requirements should initially be fed. This amount of food may need to be adjusted later to maintain ideal body weight.

Most dogs with exocrine pancreatic insufficiency do well when fed regular maintenance diets. Experimental studies indicate that dietary fiber impairs pancreatic enzyme activity, and high-fiber diets should therefore probably be avoided. Highly digestible diets (Hill's Prescription Diet i/d) may be beneficial, particularly in those individuals in which weight gain is poor. These patients may also benefit from supplementation with readily digested medium-chain triglyceride oil (MCT Oil, Mead Johnson) to further facilitate fat absorption.

Vitamin Supplementation

Serum concentrations of cobalamin (vitamin B_{12}) and of fat-soluble vitamins are often severely subnormal in dogs with exocrine pancreatic insufficiency and do not necessarily increase in response to treatment with enzymes, even though the clinical response may otherwise be excellent. Clinical deficiency states are rarely recognized, but vitamin K–responsive coagulopathies have been documented in both dogs and cats with exocrine pancreatic insufficiency. Although appropriate doses are not established, it is reasonable to give oral supplements containing fat-soluble vitamins as well as parenteral cobalamin. Parenteral vitamin K_1, 5 to 20 mg every 12 hr, should be given when there is clinical or laboratory evidence of a coagulopathy. Tocopherol (Vitamin E), 250 to 500 mg/day with food, and cobalamin, 250 µg IM or SC per week for 1 month, will normalize serum concentrations of these vitamins.

Antibiotic Therapy

In most cases, bacterial overgrowth is a subclinical complication of exocrine pancreatic insufficiency, and antibiotic therapy need not be routinely given to affected dogs. Bacterial overgrowth can contribute to malabsorption and diarrhea, however, and some animals that do not respond fully to routine enzyme supplementation may benefit from antibiotic therapy.

Oral oxytetracycline, 10 to 20 mg/kg every 12 hr for 14 days, is a reasonable initial antibiotic of choice. Metronidazole, 10 to 20 mg/kg q 12 hr for 7 to 14 days, may be more effective if obligate anaerobes are present.

Glucocorticoid Therapy

In the few dogs that respond poorly to the aforementioned treatments, oral prednisolone (or prednisone) at an initial dosage of 2 to 4 mg/kg for 7 to 14 days may be beneficial. In one such case, lymphocytic-plasmacytic enteritis was documented. Long-term glucocorticoid administration is generally unnecessary.

CONCLUSION

The underlying cause of development of exocrine pancreatic insufficiency is generally irreversible, and lifelong treatment is necessary. If owners are willing to accept the cost of enzyme replacement, the prognosis is generally good. A few dogs fail to regain normal body weight in spite of all therapeutic measures. Even in these cases there usually is complete remission of diarrhea and polyphagia and affected animals are acceptable pets. Clinical observations in cats are poorly documented, but as in dogs, a generally favorable response is expected.

References and Supplemental Reading

Batt, R. M., and Mann, L. C.: Specificity of the BT-PABA test for the diagnosis of exocrine pancreatic insufficiency in the dog. Vet. Rec. 108:303, 1981.

Hawkins, E. C., Meric, S. M., Washabau, R. J., et al.: Digestion of bentiromide and absorption of xylose in healthy cats and absorption of xylose in cats with infiltrative intestinal disease. Am. J. Vet. Res. 47:567, 1986.

Hill, F. W. G.: Malabsorption syndrome in the dog: A study of thirty-eight cases. J. Small Anim. Pract. 13:575, 1972.

Pidgeon, G.: Exocrine pancreatic disease in the dog and cat. Part 2: Exocrine pancreatic insufficiency. Canine Pract. 14:31, 1987.

Rogers, W. A., Stradley, R. P., Sherding, R. G., et al.: Simultaneous evaluation of pancreatic exocrine function and intestinal absorptive function in dogs with chronic diarrhea. J.A.V.M.A. 177:1128, 1980.

Sherding, R. G., Stradley, R. P., Rogers, W. A., et al.: Bentiromide:xylose test in healthy cats. Am. J. Vet. Res. 43:2272, 1982.

Strombeck, D. R., and Harrold, D.: Evaluation of 60-minute blood p-aminobenzoic acid concentration in pancreatic function testing of dogs. J.A.V.M.A. 180:419, 1982.

Watson, A. D. J., Church, D. B., Middleton, D. J., et al.: Weight loss in cats which eat well. J. Small Anim. Pract. 22:473, 1981.

Westermarck, E., and Sandholm, M.: Fecal hydrolase activity as determined by radial enzyme diffusion: A new method for detecting pancreatic dysfunction in the dog. Res. Vet. Sci. 28:341, 1980.

Williams, D. A., and Batt, R. M.: Sensitivity and specificity of radioimmunoassay of serum trypsin-like immunoreactivity for the diagnosis of canine exocrine pancreatic insufficiency. J.A.V.M.A., 192:195, 1988.

Williams, D. A., Batt, R. M., and McLean, L.: Bacterial overgrowth in the duodenum of dogs with exocrine pancreatic insufficiency. J.A.V.M.A. 191:201, 1987.

Zimmer, J. F., and Todd, S. E.: Further evaluation of bentiromide in the diagnosis of canine exocrine pancreatic insufficiency. Cornell Vet. 75:426, 1985.

CHRONIC INTESTINAL BACTERIAL OVERGROWTH

M. D. WILLARD, D.V.M.

East Lansing, Michigan

Intestinal bacterial overgrowth (IBO), also referred to as contaminated bowel, is a syndrome that typically develops secondary to various gastrointestinal diseases, although some patients have no obvious predisposing cause. This syndrome may be clinically inapparent or may cause varying degrees of weight loss, vomiting, and diarrhea. IBO is usually defined as greater than 10^5 bacteria per milliliter of 12-hr fasting distal duodenal or proximal jejunal fluid in a patient that has not been on antibiotics for at least 4 to 8 days.

CAUSES

The significance of IBO was established when it was identified as the cause of the vomiting, diarrhea, and weight loss in the stagnant loop or blind loop syndrome of human beings and animals. Due to inability to properly propel ingesta along the intestinal tract, blind or stagnant loops allow bacterial proliferation and colonization. This retained ingesta provides a continuing source of nutrition for both ingested bacteria as well as the normally low numbers of bacteria in the duodenum or jejunum (e.g., $< 10^4$ bacterial per milliliter), allowing them to proliferate dramatically. Blind loops may be caused by intestinal neoplasia (Fig. 1), diverticuli, surgery such as the Billroth II procedure, adhesions secondary to abdominal trauma or surgery or neoplasia. Stagnant loops are segments of intestine with impaired motility. Such areas of hypomotility may be due to intestinal fibrosis/scarring, extramural adhesions, or partial obstruction from an intestinal stricture (Fig. 2) or foreign object or neoplasia. Rarely, pseudoobstruction due to sclerosis of the intestinal tunica muscularis may occur. This has been reported in dogs and could be associated with IBO.

Gastritis with achlorhydria may also predispose patients to IBO. Gastric acid typically kills the majority of bacteria that are swallowed. If adequate gastric acid is not present, these bacteria may gain access to the small intestines in sufficient numbers to establish and perpetuate IBO. However, not all people with achlorhydria have IBO, and some patients with achlorhydria have intestinal motility deficits that may also predispose to IBO. Achlorhydria has not yet been convincingly documented in dogs, but gastric hyposecretion has been confirmed by use of pentagastrin-stimulation tests. This decreased gastric acid production may be sufficient to predispose to IBO. It is interesting to note that approximately one-third of the dogs reported to have gastric acid hyposecretion also had enteritis or diarrhea or both. There is also at least one report of IBO in a dog with chronic gastritis in which gastric acid secretion was not evaluated. Finally, long-term use of potent H_2 antagonists (e.g., cimetidine or ranitidine) has resulted in IBO in humans and can probably do the same in dogs and cats.

Exocrine pancreatic insufficiency (EPI) is also associated with IBO. Approximately 70 per cent of dogs with EPI have IBO that may be severe enough to prevent otherwise appropriate enzyme replacement therapy from effectively controlling diarrhea and weight loss. It is interesting that this association has not been recognized in human beings. The reasons for the high prevalence of IBO in canine EPI are uncertain, but the lack of bacteriostasis due to the absence of exocrine pancreatic secretions and

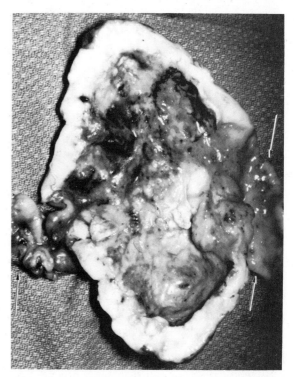

Figure 1. A resected section of small intestine with lymphosarcoma that has been opened longitudinally. The intestinal lumen is dilated, allowing stasis of contents, and the mucosa is grossly necrotic, probably because of the bacteria that have proliferated. Normal intestine is seen at either end of the dilated section (arrows).

933

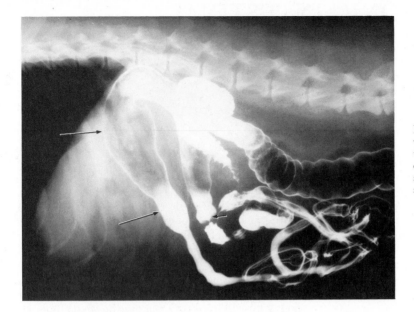

Figure 2. A lateral barium contrast-enhanced radiograph of the abdomen of a dog with repeated bouts of explosive diarrhea that was partially controlled with tetracycline therapy. A partial obstruction of the small intestine (short arrow) is causing a stagnant loop (long arrows).

immunodeficiency secondary to deficient nitrogen balance are possibilities.

There is probably always an underlying, predisposing cause of IBO. However, this cause can apparently be occult, as in patients with IBO despite normal gross gastrointestinal anatomy and motility. In humans, IBO has been associated with diverse disease states such as severe malnutrition (e.g., kwashiorkor), intestinal lymphosarcoma, old age, and diarrhea due to other causes, even that which is experimentally induced by intestinal fluid administration. Microscopic lesions of the intestinal mucosa may be present in patients with IBO, but it is unclear whether the lesions were caused by the IBO or whether the IBO was caused by the lesions. Defects of local immunity (e.g., IgA or IgM) seem a logical cause of IBO; however, selective IgA and IgM deficiencies are relatively common in humans yet these individuals apparently do not have an increased incidence of IBO. However, agammaglobulinemia in humans seems to be associated with IBO. Finally, defects in intestinal mucin have recently been hypothesized as a predisposing cause of IBO. Mucin is believed to be important in protecting the intestinal mucosa by carrying away bacteria that have IgA or IgM attached, preventing adherence and colonization.

Many but not all reported cases of IBO in companion animals have been in German shepherds. German shepherds subjectively seem to have a disproportionately high incidence of chronic gastrointestinal disease, have been suggested as having relatively less serum IgA than some other breeds, and seem to have lymphocytic-plasmacytic enteritis and eosinophilic gastroenteritis more often than expected. Rarely, certain families of German shepherds seem to have a greater incidence of gastrointestinal disease than other families. (Statistics have

not yet been generated to prove or disprove these clinical impressions.) Even if these impressions are correct, it will still be uncertain whether IBO is in fact the cause of some of these diseases, or whether these diseases allow IBO to occur. It may be noteworthy that IBO has not yet been reported in cats, although it seems reasonable that it eventually will be documented.

PATHOPHYSIOLOGY

Enteric microorganisms and anaerobes (especially *Escherichia coli* and *Clostridium species*, respectively) are commonly involved in canine IBO. However, many different bacteria alone or in various combinations may be present in any given patient with IBO. It is therefore intuitively obvious that IBO may have diverse clinical signs in different patients because of the characteristics of the various bacterial populations. Some patients with culture-confirmed IBO are asymptomatic. However, when clinical signs do accompany IBO, there are some pathophysiologic mechanisms that seem to be relatively consistent. Deconjugated bile salts and hydroxylated fatty acids are probably important mechanisms in most IBO patients that have diarrhea. These substances are produced by bacterial metabolism in the small intestine. Both are detergents and act as intestinal secretagogues. In addition, deconjugated bile acids are absorbed in the jejunum instead of only being absorbed in the ileum. This inappropriately early absorption prevents them from aiding fat digestion and absorption, thereby resulting in steatorrhea. Finally, both deconjugated bile acids and hydroxylated fatty acids may directly injure intestinal epithelium. Certain bacteria, particularly *Clostridium species*, also produce enzymes that damage the mucosa and degrade intestinal brush-border enzymes. Loss of these brush-border enzymes results in malabsorption of disaccharides, with their subsequent metabolism by the bacteria in the small intestine. Volatile fatty acids and alcohols produced by metabolism of these unabsorbed carbohydrates also injure the intestinal brush border. Villus blunting, damaged enterocyte microvilli, and mucosal mononuclear cell infiltrates may be secondary to the enzymes, deconjugated bile acids, hydroxylated fatty acids, volatile fatty acids, or alcohols produced by the bacteria. In severe cases, there may be permanent intestinal mucosal damage due to these substances. Finally, altered intestinal motility may also occur. Regardless of whether these motility changes are primary or secondary to the IBO, they perpetuate or worsen the diarrhea by disrupting the normal migrating motor complexes (the so-called intestinal housekeeper). This disruption can potentially cause further stagnation and retention of intestinal contents, perpetuating the bacterial overgrowth.

Fat malabsorption often occurs because of the ease of disrupting the complex digestion that lipids require. This causes loss of the most calorie-dense nutrients and allows further hydroxylation of fatty acids in the colon, resulting in colonic hypersecretion and diarrhea. Vitamin B_{12} malabsorption usually occurs, ostensibly because many bacteria bind to or metabolize cobalamin. Red blood cell changes because of the resulting vitamin B_{12} deficiency have been reported in humans but not dogs. Finally, patients with IBO may be hypoproteinemic. Many bacteria can ferment proteins. In addition, there may be increased fecal and urinary nitrogen excretion, decreased hepatic protein synthesis, or increased intestinal loss of endogenous proteins. As a patient's nitrogen deficiency progresses, it becomes less able to repair the intestinal mucosa. Fortunately, many dogs with IBO have normal or nearly normal serum albumin concentrations.

DIAGNOSIS

Clinically, IBO should be considered in dogs (and presumably cats) with chronic small intestinal diarrhea. Steatorrhea does not always occur, and some patients have diarrhea without weight loss. In the same manner, severe weight loss without diarrhea (due to occult malabsorption) has been reported in humans and probably occurs in dogs. Rarely, several related dogs may be affected, suggesting a familial predisposition. Mild to severe gastrointestinal disease with intermittent to constant diarrhea with or without vomiting may occur. Treatment with various drug combinations may or may not help. In particular, failure to respond to orally administered aminoglycoside antibiotics such as neomycin or kan-

amycin does not rule out IBO, as these drugs have no activity against anaerobic bacteria.

In a dog with chronic small intestinal diarrhea, EPI should be ruled out, preferably by the serum trypsin-like immunoreactivity assay or bentiramide (PABA) absorption tests. If EPI is present, appropriate pancreatic enzyme replacement will usually resolve the diarrhea and weight loss. However, a dog with EPI may have concurrent IBO. If a dog with definitively diagnosed EPI does not respond to appropriate pancreatic enzyme replacement and dietary management with antacids, IBO should be considered and appropriate antibiotics should be used.

If EPI has been ruled out in a patient with chronic small intestinal diarrhea and IBO is possible, several tests may be considered (Table 1). The nitrosonaphtol test for urinary tyrosine metabolites has been used but appears unreliable in dogs. Fasting serum vitamin B_{12} and folate concentrations seem to be reasonably good screening tests. There currently are five main recognized syndromes that cause persistently and significantly decreased serum vitamin B_{12} concentrations: IBO, EPI (with or without bacterial overgrowth), small intestinal villus atrophy, severe ileal disease or resection, and pernicious anemia. Pernicious anemia has never been convincingly documented in dogs, and severe disease limited to the ileum (or ileal resection) is rare. EPI may be definitively diagnosed by other tests. Once these three entities have been ruled out, IBO and villus atrophy are the most likely diagnoses. However, some dogs with decreased serum vitamin B_{12} concentrations have shown relatively normal results on duodenal mucosal biopsies, have had normal numbers of duodenal bacteria, and have apparently responded to dietary change or therapy for giardiasis. Although these latter patients may have had occult IBO that was not diagnosed by the culture techniques used, they may also have had decreased serum vitamin B_{12} concentrations secondary to other, undetected intestinal disease. Therefore, decreased serum vitamin B_{12} concentrations cannot be used to definitively diagnose IBO. In addition, some patients with normal serum B_{12} concentrations have had increased duodenal bacterial counts. Therefore, it is uncertain how sensitive the measurement of serum B_{12} concentration is for detecting IBO. To make matters more confusing, there is marked variation in the reference values determined by different laboratories even though they all may be using radioimmunoassays. Therefore, one must not extrapolate normal values from one laboratory to another. Finally, many bacteria can synthesize folate, resulting in increased serum folate concentrations in patients with IBO. Increased serum folate concentrations appear to be less consistent in canine IBO than are decreased serum vitamin B_{12} concentrations.

Table 1. *Comparison of Tests Currently Used to Diagnose IBO in Patients with Chronic Small Intestinal Diarrhea*

	Specificity of a Positive Reaction	Sensitivity of a Negative Reaction	Availability
Nitrosonaphtal test on urine	Doubtful	Doubtful	Readily available
Serum B_{12}/folate concentrations	Good if also eliminate villus atrophy and EPI	Occasional false negatives known to occur. Unsure of frequency	Readily available
Quantitated duodenal cultures	Excellent	Unsure, but false negatives known to occur	Difficult to perform correctly
D-Xylose absorption (pre- and postantibiotics)	Good	Poor, many dogs with IBO known to have normal values	Readily available
Expired H_2 after disaccharide ingestion	Good	Unsure	At institutions
Expires $^{14}CO_2$ after ^{14}C-xylose ingestion	Good	Unsure	At institutions
Duodenal cytology/histopathology	Unsure	Very poor	Readily available
Trial with appropriate antibiotics	Probably good	Unsure	Readily available

The most definitive test for canine IBO at this time is the quantitated aerobic and anaerobic culture of distal duodenal or proximal jejunal fluid. The fluid may be collected at exploratory laparotomy or by endoscopy. If intestinal fluid is collected at laparotomy, a syringe with a 20- or 22-gauge needle is inserted into an isolated distal duodenal or proximal jejunal loop and the contents are aspirated. One should avoid aspirating air and must quickly eliminate any air in the syringe in order to prevent strict anaerobic bacteria from dying. If an endoscope is used, a sterile tube is passed through the biopsy channel of a properly cleaned and disinfected (or preferably gas-sterilized) endoscope so that distal duodenal or proximal jejunal secretions can be aspirated. If the endoscope is equipped with a water source to wash off the viewing port, the water container should be sterilized before use and sterile water should be used. The endoscopist must also take care to avoid contamination of the biopsy channel and must not insufflate excessive air into the duodenum lest the strict and fastidious anaerobes (e.g., *Bacteroides*) die. Once duodenal fluid is obtained, it must be carefully and immediately cultured. It is best if the first milliliter of aspirated fluid can be discarded, as it is most likely to have contaminants. Anaerobes may be the predominant bacteria present; therefore, one should use prereduced media. The bacterial counts must be quantitated. Less than 100,000/ml (and often less than 20,000) alpha-hemolytic *Streptococcus* organisms, enterics, or *Staphylococcus* organisms are expected in normal dogs. Bacteria in excess of 100,000/ml or a few clostridia will occasionally be found in an otherwise normal dog's duodenum.

Some dogs have very little duodenal fluid, especially if atropine is used as a preanesthetic. In such cases, one may be unable to discard the initial portion of the collected fluid. As an alternative to duodenal fluid, duodenal mucosa could be cultured and the results expressed as the number of bacteria per gram of mucosa. At this time, it is uncertain whether culturing duodenal fluid or duodenal mucosa would be the best test, but most studies have used fluid. One must be aware that IBO may occur sporadically in focal areas of the intestines. This is why normal numbers of bacteria cultured from up to three different sites in the intestine may be required to rule out IBO.

Another test for IBO is comparison of intestinal D-xylose absorption before and after antibiotic therapy. D-Xylose is a five-carbon sugar that many (but not all) bacteria metabolize. Deficient D-xylose absorption may be due to intestinal disease (e.g., infiltrative or neoplastic) or IBO. If a previously deficient D-xylose absorption curve returns to reference values after antibiotic therapy, one can presumptively diagnose IBO. However, the D-xylose absorption test is cumbersome. Furthermore, many dogs with IBO will have normal D-xylose absorption curves before antibiotic therapy. Whether or not this is due to the fermentation characteristics of the bacteria causing IBO is unknown. Therefore, normal D-xylose absorption does not eliminate IBO (or other malabsorptive disorders for that matter).

Measurement of expired hydrogen gas concentrations in dogs after ingestion of carbohydrates (especially disaccharides) has recently been described. If the concentration of expired hydrogen gas increases in the first 2 to 4 hr after eating, small intestinal bacterial overgrowth may be presumptively diagnosed, whereas increased expired hydrogen gas after that time suggests small intestinal carbohydrate malabsorption with subsequent colonic bacterial metabolism. Chromatographs dedicated to detecting expired hydrogen gas are available. Expired gas may be collected from dogs by using a face mask and a 60-ml syringe with a three-way stopcock. Some bacteria do not produce large amounts of hydrogen gas, however, so false-negative tests are possible.

Similar tests are used in humans including one

in which ^{14}C-D-xylose is ingested and concentrations of expired $^{14}CO_2$ are measured as a marker for IBO. This test has yet to be evaluated in dogs. Despite the fact that some bacteria do not metabolize xylose, many do. Detection of radioactive gases requires additional equipment and is only available in institutes with a license to use isotopes. Nonetheless, breath tests measuring hydrogen or $^{14}CO_2$ are probably better because they evaluate the entire small intestine instead of a relatively small area as occurs with cultures.

Evaluation of serum concentrations of specific unconjugated bile acids seems useful in humans. When bile acids are deconjugated, they are more readily absorbed in the small intestine. Increased serum concentrations of certain unconjugated bile acids have been correlated with IBO. The assay is tedious, however, and dogs have different patterns of bile acids compared with human beings. It may nonetheless become a worthwhile test in dogs.

Histopathology and duodenal cytology are unreliable for diagnosing IBO. There may be no detectable histologic changes, or those present may be nonspecific (e.g., flattening of enterocytes, villus blunting, or mononuclear cell infiltrates). Bacteria are rarely reported either histologically or cytologically in dogs with IBO. This is because the bacteria causing canine IBO apparently do not have K-88, K-99, or 987P receptors as do the adherent enterotoxigenic *E. coli* of piglets and calves.

Trial antibiotic therapy is sometimes used as a diagnostic aid in patients with chronic small intestinal diarrhea. It is reasonable to use antibiotics for 7 to 10 days in a patient with chronic small bowel diarrhea before starting an in-depth diagnostic workup, just as it is appropriate to suggest a dietary trial and to treat for parasites (especially *Giardia*). The trial is quick, simple, and cheap; however, it has unknown reliability. Some patients with diarrhea will have spontaneous resolution that coincides with antibiotic therapy, whereas some patients with IBO will not have clinical resolution because of an underlying intestinal disease that allowed IBO to occur. If clinical response occurs, the patient should be treated for at least 2 to 3 weeks to ensure that the antibiotics are effective and that the response was not a fortuitous transient phenomenon.

TREATMENT

When IBO is diagnosed in a patient with diarrhea, vomiting, or weight loss, the next question is whether underlying intestinal disease is also present. If it is, it should be treated whenever possible. In patients with readily treatable intestinal disease (e.g., eosinophilic enteritis), the IBO may or may not be treated initially. Correction or control of underlying diseases (e.g., EPI or intestinal lym-

phangiectasia) may alleviate the clinical signs and perhaps the IBO. However, in severely ill patients or those without a treatable or identifiable underlying disease, antibacterial therapy is indicated. Since anaerobes are often an important component in IBO, it is desirable to use drugs that kill both aerobic and anaerobic organisms. Amoxicillin, tetracycline, and tylosin (Tylan-Plus, Elanco) are three reasonable choices. Amoxicillin should be given twice daily at 20 mg/kg/treatment, and tetracycline should be administered twice daily 1 hr before eating, at a dose of 20 mg/kg/treatment. Tylan-Plus is administered three times per day mixed in with the meals. The dose of Tylan-Plus is empiric but 30- to 50-kg dogs are given 1 heaping teaspoon per meal, 15- to 30-kg dogs ¾ tsp per meal, 10- to 15-kg dogs ½ tsp per meal, and dogs less than 10 kg receive ¼ to ½ tsp per meal. Metronidazole is effective against anaerobes and can be used if they are suspected; however, this drug has no effect on aerobes.

Effective therapy will usually cause resolution or improvement in clinical signs within 7 to 14 days and sometimes within 5 days. It is noteworthy that some dogs with IBO experience resolution of signs when treated with antibiotics to which the bacteria are resistant, according to standard disk-diffusion methods. This clinical response might occur because high concentrations of the antibiotic in the duodenum overcome bacterial resistance. Alternatively, if a mixed flora is necessary to cause clinical signs, then an antibiotic that inhibits only one or two of the bacteria might be sufficient. If there is no apparent response to appropriate antibiotics, the clinician should reconfirm that parasites (especially *Giardia*) and EPI have in fact been ruled out. Then, small intestinal biopsy must be considered to determine if there is underlying intestinal disease that is responsible for the continuation of signs. Chronic IBO can produce irreversible intestinal mucosal changes or can occur secondary to other intestinal diseases (e.g., intestinal lymphosarcoma, lymphocytic-plasmacytic enteritis, intestinal lymphangiectasia, and others).

In summary, dogs with chronic small intestinal disease not due to parasites and unresponsive to dietary therapy should be screened for IBO (Fig. 3). Measurement of serum vitamin B_{12} concentrations and measuring expired hydrogen gas after ingestion of disaccharides currently seem to be the best screening tests available. Quantitated cultures of fasting, distal duodenal, or proximal jejunal contents are the most definitive tests and should be performed if possible. However, most clinicians will not be able to perform these cultures. Patients with IBO due to blind or stagnant loops should be treated surgically. Patients diagnosed as having IBO plus EPI should be treated with antibiotics only if it appears that the IBO is inhibiting appropriate en-

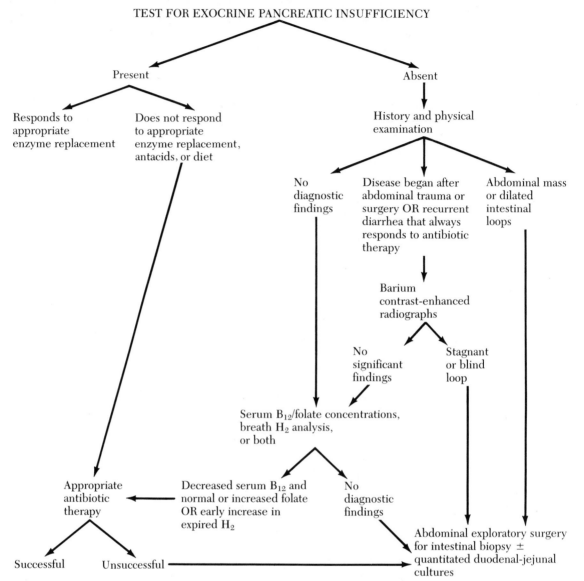

Figure 3. Diagnostic approach for intestinal bacterial overgrowth in patients with chronic small intestinal diarrhea or unexplained weight loss.

zyme replacement therapy. If IBO is diagnosed in a patient without a clearly identifiable underlying cause, appropriate antibiotic therapy should be recommended.

References and Supplemental Reading

Batt, R. M., and Morgan, J. O.: Role of serum folate and vitamin B_{12} concentrations in the differentiation of small intestinal abnormalities in the dog. Res. Vet. Sci. 32:17, 1982.

Batt, R. M., Needham, J. R., and Carter, M. W.: Bacterial overgrowth associated with a naturally occurring enteropathy in the german shepherd dog. Res. Vet. Sci. 35:42, 1983.

Bjorneklett, D., Hoverstad, T., and Hovig, T.: Bacterial overgrowth. Scand. J. Gastroenterol. [Suppl.] 109:123, 1985.

Happé, R. P.: Investigations into disorders of canine gastroduodenal function. Ph.D. Thesis, University of Utrecht, 1982.

King, C. E., and Toskes, P. P.: Comparison of the 1-gram [^{14}C] xylose,

10-gram lactulose-H_2, and 80-gram glucose-H_2 breath tests in patients with small intestine bacterial overgrowth. Gastroenterology 91:1447, 1986.

Mathias, J. R., and Clench, M. H.: Review: Pathophysiology of diarrhea caused by bacterial overgrowth of the small intestine. Am. J. Med. Sci. 289:243, 1985.

Rumessen, J. J., Gudmand-Hoyer, E., Bachmann, E., et al.: Diagnosis of bacterial overgrowth of the small intestine. Comparison of the ^{14}C-D-xylose breath test and jejunal cultures in 60 patients. Scand. J. Gastroenterol. 20:1267, 1985.

Setchell, K. D. R., Harrison, D. L., Gilbert, J. M., et al.: Serum unconjugated bile acids: Qualitative and quantitated profiles in ileal resection and bacterial overgrowth. Clin. Chim. Acta. 152:297, 1985.

Stockbrugger, R. W.: Bacterial overgrowth as a consequence of reduced gastric acidity. Scand. J. Gastroenterol. [Suppl.] 111:7, 1985.

Washabau, R. J., Buffington, C. A., and Strombeck, D. R.: Evaluation and management of carbohydrate malassimilation. *In* Kirk, R. W. (ed.): *Current Veterinary Therapy IX.* Philadelphia: W. B. Saunders Co., 1986, pp. 889–892.

Williams, D. A., Batt, R. M., and McLean, L.: Bacterial overgrowth in the duodenum of dogs with exocrine pancreatic insufficiency. J.A.V.M.A. Assoc. 191:201, 1987.

PLASMACYTIC-LYMPHOCYTIC COLITIS IN DOGS

MICHAEL S. LEIB, D.V.M.,
WILLIAM H. HAY, D.V.M.,
and LOIS ROTH, D.V.M.
Blacksburg, VA

Plasmacytic-lymphocytic colitis (PLC) is a common cause of large bowel diarrhea in dogs. It is poorly understood, imprecisely defined, and the subject of controversy. The etiology is not understood, but the characteristic histologic lesion of a plasmacytic, lymphocytic infiltrate of the mucosa suggests an underlying immunologic mechanism. Clinical response to dietary manipulation suggests that hypersensitivity to food antigens plays an important role in the pathogenesis of this disease, although parasitic hypersensitivity and bacterial hypersensitivity are also possible causes.

The pathogenesis is subject to speculation. It is thought that the mucosal inflammatory cell infiltrate leads to alterations in colonic motility, decreased absorption of water and electrolytes, and production of excessive secretions. Inflammation of the rectum stimulates the defecation reflex, causing frequent defecation of small volumes of stool. Colonic inflammation leads to excess mucus production. Hematochezia is caused by hemorrhage from friable colonic mucosa or, in rare instances, from erosion or ulceration. (See p. 922 for further discussion of inflammatory bowel disease.)

This chapter summarizes the authors' experience with PLC in dogs, accounting for approximately 15 per cent of referral cases of large bowel diarrhea in our practice. As most of this chapter is based on subjective clinical impressions, further study is needed to elucidate the etiology and pathogenesis and evaluate the treatment of PLC.

HISTORY AND CLINICAL SIGNS

Most cases of PLC occur in young dogs (less than 3 years of age), although the authors have occasionally seen older dogs (8 years or older) with this syndrome. No breed or sex predilection has been recognized. The following clinical signs, in decreasing order of frequency, have been observed: hematochezia, tenesmus, increased frequency of defecation, small volume of stool per defecation, and excess mucus production. Weight loss, vomiting, anorexia, and lethargy occur infrequently. In many cases, diarrhea is intermittent, occurring between periods of normal stool. Predisposing events triggering bouts of diarrhea have not been identified.

Physical examination is usually normal. Careful abdominal palpation should be performed to rule out the possibility of an abdominal mass. A digital rectal examination may suggest that other causes of large bowel diarrhea are present if sublumbar lymphadenopathy, rough and corrugated rectal mucosa, or a rectal mass is detected.

DIFFERENTIAL DIAGNOSIS AND DIAGNOSTIC PLAN

There are many causes of chronic diarrhea in dogs. The veterinary clinician must follow a complete and logical diagnostic plan in order to discover the cause of the diarrhea. It is especially important for the clinician to localize the diarrhea to the large bowel or small bowel (Table 1). Small bowel diarrhea is characterized by a mild increase in frequency of defecation, a large amount of stool per defecation, and occasional steatorrhea. It is often accompanied by weight loss.

Signs of small and large bowel diarrhea may occur simultaneously; however, signs of either large or small bowel diarrhea most often predominate. Mixed signs occur, because some diseases can affect both the small and large intestines. In addition, many small intestinal disorders result in malassimilation of nutrients, leading to the delivery of irritating substances (e.g., hydroxy fatty acids) to the colon, causing a secondary colitis.

Table 2 lists many of the causes of chronic large

Table 1. *Localization of Chronic Diarrhea*

Sign	Small Bowel	Large Bowel
Frequency of defecation	Mild to moderate increase	Moderate to severe increase
Quantity per defecation	Normal to increased	Scant to decreased
Weight loss	Common	Rare
Excess mucus production	Absent	Present
Blood	Melena	Hematochezia
Tenesmus	Absent	Present

939

Table 2. *Causes of Chronic Large Bowel Diarrhea*

Inflammatory
  Plasmacytic-lymphocytic
  Histiocytic ulcerative
  Eosinophilic
  Granulomatous
  Suppurative

Parasitic
  Trichuris vulpis
  Giardia
  Ancylostoma species
  Uncinaria stenocephala
  Entamoeba histolytica
  Balantidium coli

Neoplastic
  Benign polyp (adenomatous or hyperplastic)
  Leiomyoma
  Adenocarcinoma
  Lymphosarcoma
  Leiomyosarcoma
  Plasmacytoma
  Mast cell tumor

Noninflammatory
  Noninflammatory colonic disease (irritable bowel syndrome)
  Cecal inversion
  Ileocolic intussusception
  Small bowel malassimilatory disorder (secondary colitis)

Infectious
  Histoplasma capsulatum
  Salmonella species
  Yersinia enterocolitica
  Prototheca species
  Heterobilharzia americana
  Clostridium difficile

bowel diarrhea in dogs. Chronic diarrhea can also accompany metabolic disorders such as uremia, relapsing acute pancreatitis, hypoadrenocorticism, and hypothyroidism. Primary metabolic disorders often produce clinical signs such as polyuria-polydipsia, severe vomiting, hypovolemic shock, and nonpruritic alopecia, which are suggestive of noncolonic disorders.

In the authors' experience, the most common causes of chronic large bowel diarrhea are (in decreasing frequency) *Trichuris vulpis* infestation, noninflammatory colonic disease (irritable bowel disease), PLC, neoplasia, giardiasis, and histiocytic-ulcerative colitis. Noninflammatory colonic disease (irritable bowel syndrome) represents a large percentage (approximately 40 per cent) of referral cases seen by the authors. The etiology and pathophysiology are unknown in dogs. In humans, abnormal myoelectrical activity leads to colonic dysfunction. Affected persons often develop diarrhea during stressful periods. Although stress can be implicated in dogs with irritable bowel syndrome, other affected dogs appear to be relatively stress free. Until colonic motility studies are clinically available, this disorder can only be suspected after ruling out other causes of diarrhea.

Neoplastic lesions of the colon and rectum fre-

quently cause large bowel diarrhea in older dogs. The most common benign lesions are adenomatous or hyperplastic polyps. Polyps may be single or multiple. Endoscopically, they may appear as sessile or polypoid masses. Ulceration producing hematochezia can occur. In humans, adenomatous polyps have the potential for malignant transformation.

The most common malignant tumors of the large bowel are adenocarcinoma and lymphosarcoma. Adenocarcinomas may form infiltrative annular lesions and are seen more often in male dogs (1.5 to 2:1 ratio). They occur more frequently in the rectum than in the colon. Lymphosarcoma may also occur as a singular mass, although it usually is seen as a diffusely infiltrative lesion in the colonic wall.

Histiocytic ulcerative colitis occurs most frequently in boxers. This syndrome can be distinguished from PLC by mucosal ulceration, visible endoscopically, and the histologic lesion characterized by the mucosal infiltration by macrophages containing PAS-positive granules.

All dogs with chronic large bowel diarrhea should have a complete blood count, biochemical profile, and urinalysis performed. Primary metabolic disorders causing diarrhea should be easily identified. Dogs with PLC often have normal laboratory values, although chronic blood loss may result in mild anemia and hypoproteinemia. Severe anemia and hypoproteinemia suggest that ulcerative colitis or an ulcerated tumor may be present. Eosinophilia may indicate parasitic infection, such as *T. vulpis* or less commonly *Giardia*, or *Ancylostoma*, or eosinophilic colitis.

Because *T. vulpis* is the most common cause of chronic large bowel diarrhea, multiple fecal samples should be examined as the presence of ova may be intermittent. Although *Giardia* is primarily a small bowel pathogen, it occasionally may produce signs of large bowel diarrhea. Fecal examination techniques such as zinc sulfate flotation or formol-ether concentration can be used to identify cysts. To perform a zinc sulfate flotation test, 0.5 to 1.0 gm of feces and five drops of Lugol's iodine are thoroughly mixed in a tube with 33 per cent zinc sulfate solution. The tube is covered with a cover slip and centrifuged in a free-swinging head centrifuge for 5 minutes at 1,500 rpm. The *Giardia* cysts will migrate toward the coverslip, which can then be examined microscopically. In addition, examination of fresh fecal smears with saline may identify *Giardia* trophozoites.

Rectal cytology has frequently been recommended as part of the diagnostic plan for large bowel diarrhea. This procedure is inexpensive and simple to perform. Cytologic impressions can be made by rubbing the rectal wall with a gloved finger and gently rolling the finger across a microscope slide, which can be routinely stained with a Romanovsky's stain. Colonic epithelial cells and a mixed bacterial population are normally seen. Abnormal findings include erythrocytes, neutrophils, eosinophils, macrophages, or plasma cells. Malignant cells, parasite ova, or histoplasma organisms may be seen. The authors are currently evaluating the usefulness of this technique in the diagnosis of chronic large bowel diarrhea. Preliminary data suggest that this technique is of limited value, as a specific cytologic pattern for PLC has not been observed.

Before pursuing a further diagnostic workup, an anthelmintic such as fenbendazole should be administered to eliminate occult *T. vulpis*. Additionally, the patient should be restricted to a high-quality diet (eliminate table scraps and foreign material) for 2 to 3 weeks. The authors often recommend ID (Hill's Prescription Diet) or Eukanuba (Iams) for the diet trial.

COLONOSCOPY

If the diarrhea continues despite therapeutic deworming and maintenance on an acceptable diet, colonoscopy and mucosal biopsy should be performed. Food should be withheld for 24 hr prior to colonoscopy. A cathartic such as Golytely (Braintree Laboratories) should be given to cleanse the large intestine and allow optimal endoscopic visualization. Although the dosage and dosing interval of this product have not been established for dogs, the authors have found that 30 ml/kg body weight given via orogastric tube two times 2 hr apart the afternoon before colonoscopy and repeated once the morning of colonoscopy gives acceptable results.

Because the lesions of PLC are usually present in the descending colon, either rigid or flexible colonoscopy is useful in obtaining a diagnostic tissue sample. Flexible colonoscopy offers the advantage of being able to evaluate the entire colon and cecum. Using flexible colonoscopy, it is possible to visualize tumors or inflammatory lesions in the transverse and ascending colon and whipworms or cecal inversion in the cecocolic region. However, general anesthesia is often needed. Rigid colonoscopy requires relatively inexpensive equipment and can usually be performed with narcotic sedation. Using rigid colonoscopy, it is possible to evaluate only the distal colon.

For flexible colonoscopy, the dog should be placed in left lateral recumbency; for rigid colonoscopy, the animal may stand or may be examined in sternal or left lateral recumbency. The endoscope should be advanced slowly into the colon as air is insufflated to distend mucosal folds. The endoscope should be advanced only if the lumen is clearly visible, reducing the possibility of colonic perforation. After advancing the endoscope as far into the colon as possible, a thorough visual examination of the entire luminal circumference can be performed as the endoscope is slowly withdrawn.

Normal colonic mucosa is smooth and pale pink. Submucosal blood vessels can be visualized. Dogs with PLC usually have increased mucosal granularity. It is often difficult to visualize the submucosal blood vessels because of infiltration of inflammatory cells or edema. Hyperemia is common. This endoscopic lesion must be carefully assessed, as a warm-water enema can cause hyperemia. The mucosa may spontaneously bleed or bleed excessively (friability) after contact with the endoscope. In most cases of PLC, the entire colon is not uniformly affected. Some areas can appear normal. Erosion and ulceration occur rarely in dogs with PLC. Multiple tissue samples of all abnormal regions should be taken. In addition, biopsies of normal-appearing regions of colon should be taken, as they can assist the pathologist in interpreting specimens.

The major histologic feature of this disease is a moderate to severe infiltrate of plasma cells and lymphocytes into the lamina propria (Fig. 1). There occasionally is an increase in globular leukocytes. In most cases, the inflammatory infiltrate seems to be confined to the mucosa, with minimal infiltration into the submucosa. Erosions seen in the most

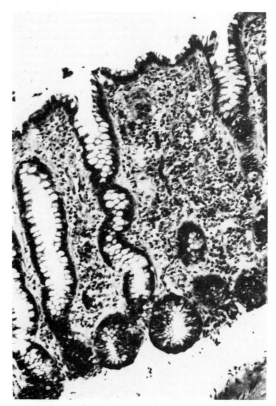

Figure 1. Colonic mucosa from a 3-year-old female Irish setter with plasmacytic-lymphocytic colitis. There is an increased population (grades 3–5) of plasma cells and lymphocytes in the lamina propria. The muscularis mucosa has been artifactually detached.

severe cases are characterized by the adherence of cellular debris to the surfaces devoid of epithelium, along with a superficial neutrophilic infiltrate into the lamina propria. Specimens that include only mucosa and muscularis mucosa are often too small for further assessment.

In evaluating biopsy specimens, normal morphology must be considered. Any individual sample may include discrete lymphoid aggregates in the submucosa, along with a small but diffusely distributed population of plasma cells and lymphocytes, which are normally present in the lamina propria (Fig. 2). One must realize that "normal" constitutes a range of cellularity and that a distinct division between normal and abnormal cannot easily be made. It requires an experienced pathologist to differentiate these normal cell populations from inflammatory cell infiltrates. Overzealous evaluation of the cellularity of a colonic biopsy specimen can lead to an erroneous diagnosis of PLC and result in failure to determine the dog's true problem. Severe infiltration of inflammatory cells must occasionally be differentiated from colonic lymphosarcoma, in which the cellular infiltrate is usually homogeneous and has a greater propensity to distort mucosal glands and infiltrate the submucosa.

THERAPEUTIC PLAN

The treatment of canine colitis has historically been directed at the administration of medications

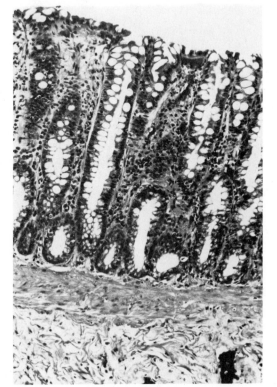

Figure 2. Normal colonic mucosa from a 7-year-old male beagle. A normal complement (grades 2–5) of plasma cells and lymphocytes is present in the lamina propria.

to reduce inflammation, alter bacterial flora, and normalize colonic motility. The authors' recent clinical experience suggests that dietary modification is useful in the treatment of colitis.

As controlled clinical therapeutic trials have not been conducted in dogs with PLC, therapeutic recommendations are based on subjective clinical impressions. To rationally manage dogs with PLC, the therapeutic trial should be followed by thorough clinical evaluation and follow-up colonoscopy with mucosal biopsy. Complete cure is rarely achieved. More often, the clinician's goal should be to reduce the severity and frequency of diarrhea, improving the dog's quality of life.

Dogs with PLC are initially placed on a hypoallergenic diet for 3 to 4 weeks. A mutton-based diet may be provided by d/d[R] (Hill's Prescription Diet) or as a homemade ration. Consumption of all other foods must be eliminated. If significant clinical improvement occurs, the dog should be challenged with its original diet. The return of diarrhea suggests that a diagnosis of PLC secondary to dietary hypersensitivity be made. Approximately 30 per cent of cases of PLC seen by the authors respond favorably to a hypoallergenic diet.

Ingredients (e.g., ground beef, powdered milk, soybean meal, wheat flour) can be individually added to the hypoallergenic diet to help identify the offending allergen. Each additional ingredient should be fed for 7 to 10 days. If the offending allergen can be identified, a commercial diet lacking the incriminated ingredient can often be found. However, many clients are so delighted by the clinical improvement produced with the hypoallergenic test diet that they are unwilling to challenge their dog or test individual ingredients.

Dogs that exhibit a partial response to the hypoallergenic diet may benefit from fiber supplementation. The authors recommend that 1 to 3 tbsp of a fiber supplement such as Metamucil (Searle) be added to the hypoallergenic diet. Fiber absorbs fluid and binds fecal material in the colon. It also increases colonic segmentation, thereby increasing fecal transit time. This allows additional absorption of water from the colon and ultimately reduces defecation frequency. In humans, high-fiber diets may decrease the risk of colorectal cancer, possibly by binding dietary resins and bile salts in the large intestine.

Dogs that fail to respond favorably to dietary manipulation may be returned to their original diet and treated with sulfasalazine. Sulfasalazine has for many years been the treatment of choice for canine colitis. It is composed of sulfapyridine and 5-aminosalicylic acid joined by an azo bond, which is broken by bacteria in the aboral ileum and oral colon. Sulfapyridine is absorbed and excreted by the kidneys, whereas 5-aminosalicylic acid possesses topical anti-inflammatory action. Proposed mechanisms of action for 5-aminosalicyclic acid include inhibition of prostaglandin synthesis, alteration of prostaglandin metabolism, alteration of polymorphonuclear and macrophage function, enhancement of colonic absorption of sodium and water, and reduction of colonic secretion.

Because sulfasalazine frequently causes side effects (Table 3), therapy must be monitored carefully. Side effects have been attributed to the sulfa component. Shirmer tear tests are recommended prior to administration of sulfasalazine and should be reevaluated after 1, 3, and 6 months of therapy. Early recognition of decreased tear production and cessation of therapy often result in resumption of tear production. Although bone marrow suppression is uncommon in dogs, a complete blood count can be performed at the same intervals.

The reported dosage for sulfasalazine in dogs is 15 to 50 mg/kg every 8 hr (not to exceed 3 to 5 gm/day). We have found that 50 mg/kg every 8 hr (up to 3 gm/day) is often necessary to achieve significant clinical improvement. The dosage should be reduced after 4 weeks if acceptable stool consistency is maintained. If the animal's feces remain normal or near normal for several months, the dog may be completely weaned off medication. However, most dogs with PLC will need long-term treatment, with approximately 50 per cent of the initial dose given every 8 to 12 hr.

Several newer drugs have been evaluated in humans with ulcerative colitis and have been found to be effective and not to produce the side effects associated with sulfasalazine. A sulfasalazine analogue, olsalazine, will be marketed under the name Dipentum (Pharmacia Co.). This drug consists of two salicylate radicals joined by the same azo bond as in sulfasalazine. This drug will result in the release of two salicylate compounds in the colon. A pH-sensitive polymer-coated 5-aminosalicyclic acid, Asacol (Tillotts Laboratories), was recently found to be effective in treating humans with mild to moderate ulcerative colitis. The protective coating allows the drug to be delivered to the colon, rather than being inactivated or absorbed in the stomach and small intestine. Clinical trials are necessary to evaluate the potential value of these drugs in dogs with PLC.

Dogs that fail to respond to treatment with a hypoallergenic diet, additional dietary fiber, and sulfasalazine may benefit from therapeutic trials with a combination of the following treatments: further dietary modification, glucocorticoids, immunosuppressants, tylosin, and metronidazole. Diets such as ID (Hill's), Eukanuba (Iams), Science Diet (Hill's), and ONE (Purina) should be tried to obtain clinical improvement in refractory cases.

Corticosteroids have been used in the treatment of canine and human colitis, especially during acute flare-ups, and in patients refractory to sulfasalazine. Corticosteroids may decrease the dosage of sulfasalazine necessary for control of clinical signs, thus reducing the possibility of toxic side effects. Prednisolone, 1 to 2 mg/kg every 24 hr, may reduce or eliminate diarrhea. The dose should be gradually tapered to the lowest alternate-day dose required to control clinical signs.

Since corticosteroids have frequent side effects (e.g., polyuria, polydypsia, polyphagia, hepatopathy), they may not be suitable for long-term patient management. Azathioprine, a thiopurine antimetabolite, has successfully been used for maintenance therapy of canine colitis in corticosteroid-intolerant dogs. The dosage may be gradually reduced from 2 mg/kg every 24 hr to 0.5 mg/kg every 48 hr. Neutropenia and thrombocytopenia can occur, and a complete blood count should be monitored frequently.

Tylosin is a macrolide antibiotic that has been reported to be effective in treating some dogs with colitis. It has an unknown mechanism of action but probably alters colonic bacterial flora. In the authors' experience, it has limited clinical efficacy. The suggested dosage varies greatly, depending on the form available, although 20 to 40 mg/kg every 12 hr is frequently suggested. The long-term effects of this antibiotic on colonic bacterial flora and colonic function are unknown.

Metronidazole is an antibiotic that has antiprotozoal activity against *Giardia* and is effective against anaerobic bacteria. Studies in humans have shown that metronidazole decreases the cell-mediated immune response in granulomatous colitis. A dosage of 10 to 30 mg/kg every 8 to 24 hr for 2 to 4 weeks has been suggested to help control refractory cases of canine colitis. Side effects are infrequent but may include neurologic signs such as seizures, neutropenia, nausea, vomiting, and diarrhea.

Retention enemas with corticosteroids or 5-aminosalicyclic acid (Row-Asa enemas, Reid Rowell Inc.) are useful in humans with distal ulcerative colitis. These enemas are administered prior to bedtime, and clinical improvement is often evident the next day. Their mechanism of action is thought to be via topical anti-inflammatory effects, but systemic absorption of corticosteroids does occur. This treatment has rarely been used by the authors in dogs with PLC, but potential benefits exist and clinical trials should be instituted. (An additional description of therapy for colitis can be found in *Current Veterinary Therapy IX*, pp. 896–903. An expanded discussion of the pathogenesis of inflammatory

Table 3. *Side Effects of Sulfasalazine*

Keratoconjunctivitis sicca	Oligospermia
Vomiting	Allergic dermatitis
Exacerbation of colitis	Anemia
Cholestasis	Leukopenia
Fever	

bowel disease can be found in this volume on page 922.)

References and Supplemental Reading

August, J. R.: Dietary hypersensitivity in dogs: Cutaneous manifestations, diagnosis, and management. Comp. Cont. Ed. Pract. Vet. 7:469, 1985.

Burrows, C. F., Kronfeld, D. S., Banta, C. A., et al.: Effects of fiber on digestibility and transit time in dogs. J. Nutr. 112:1726, 1982.

Burrows, C. F., and Merritt, A. M.: Influence of α-Cellulose on myoelectric activity of proximal canine colon. Am. J. Physiol. 245:G301, 1983.

Canfield, P. J., Bennett, A. M., and Watson, D. J.: Large intestinal biopsies from normal dogs. Res. Vet. Sci. 28:6, 1980.

Ewing, G. O., and Gomez, J. A.: Canine ulcerative colitis. J. Am. Anim. Hosp. Assoc. 9:395, 1973.

Holt, P. E., and Lucke, V. M.: Rectal neoplasia in the dog: A clinicopathological review of 31 cases. Vet. Rec. 116:400, 1985.

Krook, A., Danielsson, P., Kjellander, J., et al.: The effect of metronidazole and sulfasalazine on the fecal flora in patients with Crohn's disease. Scand. J. Gastroenterol. 16:182, 1981.

Morgan, R. V., and Bachrach, A.: Keratoconjunctivitis sicca associated with sulfonamide therapy in dogs. J.A.V.M.A. 180:432, 1982.

Ridgway, M. D.: Management of chronic colitis in the dog. J.A.V.M.A. 185:804, 1984.

Sandberg-Gertzén, H., Jäamerot, G., and Kraaz, W.: Azodisal sodium in the treatment of ulcerative colitis. Gastroenterology 90:1024, 1986.

Schroeder, K. W., Tremaine, W. J., and Ilstrup, D. M.: Coated oral 5-aminosalicyclic acid therapy for mildly to moderately active ulcerative colitis. N. Engl. J. Med. 317:1625, 1987.

Schwartz, A. G., Targan, S. R., Saxon, A., et al.: Sulfasalazine-induced exacerbation of ulcerative colitis. N. Engl. J. Med. 306:409, 1982.

Sherding, R. G.: Canine large bowel diarrhea. Comp. Cont. Ed. Pract. Vet. 2:279, 1980.

Sutherland, L. R., Martin, F., Greer, S., et al.: 5-Amino-salicylic acid enema in the treatment of distal ulcerative colitis, proctosigmoiditis and proctitis. Gastroenterology 92:1894, 1987.

Van Kruiningen, H. J.: Granulomatous colitis of boxer dogs: Comparative aspects. Gastroenterology 53:114, 1967.

Van Kruiningen, H. J.: Clinical efficacy of tylosin in canine inflammatory bowel disease. J. Am. Anim. Hosp. Assoc. 12:498, 1976.

CAMPYLOBACTER ENTERITIS

DEBORAH J. DAVENPORT, D.V.M.

Blacksburg, Virginia

Veterinarians have recognized *Campylobacter* species as pathogens of importance since the early 1900's—primarily as the etiologic agents of "vibrionic infertility" in ruminants. However, it was not until the 1970's that the importance of *Campylobacter* as an enteropathogen was widely accepted by veterinarians and physicians (Skirrow, 1981). In humans, *Campylobacter jejuni* is currently recognized as one of the leading bacterial causes of gastroenteritis, and *Campylobacter pylori* appears to be an important marker for and perhaps a cause of inflammatory gastroduodenal disease (Blaser, 1987). *C. jejuni* also appears to be an important enteropathogen in companion animals, as demonstrated by recent reports of spontaneous and experimentally induced *Campylobacter* enteritis in dogs, cats, and ferrets (Fox et al., 1983b; Fox et al., 1987; Macartney et al., 1981; Prescott and Munroe, 1982).

ETIOLOGIC AGENT

The earlier obscurity of *Campylobacter* enteric infections was probably attributable to the fastidious nature of *Campylobacter* and the lack of sophisticated culture techniques necessary for isolation of the organism from feces. In addition, confusing changes in taxonomy also contributed to a lack of recognition of *Campylobacter* species as enteropathogens. The organisms of the genus *Campylobacter* were previously classified as *Vibrio*. A new genus, *Campylobacter*, was created in 1963 on the basis of biochemical, serologic, and DNA characteristics. Subsequent taxonomic changes resulted in renaming of the organism *Campylobacter fetus* subspecies *jujuni* as *C. jejuni*, and the identification of the organism *C. pylori*.

Campylobacter organisms are small (1.5 to 3.5μ × 0.2 to 0.4μ), curved, gram-negative rods that have a single polar flagellum at one or both extremities. This flagellum is responsible for the peculiar corkscrewlike motility exhibited by *Campylobacter* species. Approximately 50 *C. jejuni* serotypes have been identified; however, only three serotypes are commonly isolated from humans and domestic animals (Shane and Montrose, 1985). All serotypes are characterized by thermophilia, susceptibility to desiccation, and microaerophilic culture requirements. The organism must be kept moist and sheltered from atmospheric oxygen in order to survive outside the body. Survival times of 3 to 5 weeks in feces, milk, water, bile and urine have been reported at cooler temperatures (4°C) (Shane and Montrose, 1985).

EPIDEMIOLOGY

C. jejuni is a ubiquitous organism that can be isolated from nearly all mammalian and avian species. The organism has been associated with diarrhea in dogs, cats, ferrets, calves, lambs, foals, monkeys, and humans. Prevalence rates of 1.6 to 75 per cent in dogs and 0 to 45 per cent in cats have been reported (Fox et al., 1983b; Prescott and Munroe, 1982; Holt, 1981). The large variability in prevalence rates can probably be ascribed to differences in geography, population tested (age, state of health, source), and culture techniques. These high prevalence rates have generated controversy over the importance of C. jejuni in animals. Several studies have shown no difference in the frequency of fecal C. jejuni isolates from normal and diarrheic animals. More recent studies do find significantly higher prevalence rates in diarrheic animals (Fox et al., 1983b; Holt, 1981; Prescott and Munroe, 1982).

The highest numbers of positive fecal isolates are identified in young animals from pounds or shelters. High prevalence rates are also noted in rural animals exposed to livestock and in stray animals trapped near meat- or poultry-processing plants. The lowest prevalence rate is expected in adult household pets.

These findings parallel prevalence studies in humans in less developed countries where there are high numbers of positive fecal isolates in both healthy and diarrheic children. In more developed countries, numbers of positive fecal isolates are significantly higher in diarrheic patients.

PATHOGENESIS

The fecal-oral route of transmission of C. jejuni is probably most important in pets, based on the high prevalence of Campylobacter infections in animals, raised in crowded, unsanitary quarters. Consumption of contaminated food (particularly poultry products) and water is also an important route of disease transmission in humans and animals. Farm animals may be exposed directly to manure or to water contaminated by livestock or avian excreta. House flies (Musca domestica) have recently been implicated as mechanical vectors in transmission of C. jejuni to uninfected animals (Shane and Montrose, 1985).

Companion animals appear to be more resistant to C. jejuni enteritis than do humans, in whom a 200 to 500 organism oral inoculum is sufficient to cause clinical disease. In order to produce Campylobacter-associated enteritis experimentally in gnotobiotic puppies, conventional puppies, kittens, and adult dogs, at least 10^{10} organisms must be administered orally (Macartney et al., 1981; Prescott and Munroe, 1982).

Once ingested, Campylobacter organisms proliferate in the small bowel and, by poorly understood mechanisms, cause disease in 1 to 7 days. Despite some evidence of direct tissue invasion (bacteremia, mucosal erosions, intestinal inflammatory infiltrates), C. jejuni is believed to attach to and colonize the intestinal mucosa without invasion of the enterocyte. Cytolytic, heat-labile enterotoxins that have been isolated from C. jejuni experimentally cause intestinal edema (Shane and Montrose, 1985). In addition, the gram-negative Campylobacter contains lipopolysaccharides that may cause diarrhea by secretory mechanisms.

High fecal Campylobacter isolation rates have been identified in young animals; in animals with concurrent salmonellosis, parvoviral enteritis, and gastrointestinal parasites; and in stressed or debilitated animals. The association of C. jejuni infections with immunoincompetence and other disease states suggests that the organism is an opportunistic pathogen that may act synergistically with other enteric pathogens.

CLINICAL SIGNS

Clinical signs of campylobacteriosis are nonspecific and typical of any acute gastroenteritis. Most severe clinical signs are seen in young, debilitated, or immunocompromised animals. The acute onset of diarrhea is the most prominent and consistent clinical manifestation of experimental and naturally occurring C. jejuni infections. Diarrhea may predominately affect the small or large bowel or may be indeterminate. Stools are soft to watery and often contain blood and mucus. Tenesmus is a frequent finding. Rarely, severe bloody diarrhea typical of hemorrhagic gastroenteritis is encountered.

Vomiting is less consistently reported in C. jejuni infections than is diarrhea, but may be severe. Other clinical manifestations may include pyrexia, depression, lethargy, dehydration, and inappetence. Some animals may exhibit abdominal discomfort and gas- or fluid-distended bowel loops. Rarely, animals may develop Campylobacter septicemia and exhibit signs consistent with septicemia or endotoxemia.

Chronically affected Campylobacter cases may have intermittent chronic diarrhea, weight loss, and mild lymphadenopathy. These signs parallel those reported in the protracted form of Campylobacter enteritis in humans.

Clinical signs typically appear 1 to 7 days after exposure, with most animals exhibiting clinical signs for 3 to 10 days if untreated. The disease appears to be self-limiting in most cases, but in a small number of patients, bacteremia or chronic, recurrent infections may develop.

LABORATORY FINDINGS

Clinicopathologic changes in spontaneous and experimentally induced Campylobacter enteritis have not been well studied but appear to be nonspecific. Laboratory evidence of dehydration, manifested by elevations in packed cell volume (PCV), total protein (TP), serum and urine osmolality, serum sodium, creatinine, blood urea nitrogen (BUN), and urine specific gravity, is often present. Mild to moderate leukocytosis with a left shift is not uncommon. Leukopenia may be identified with concomitant parvoviral or *Salmonella* infections but only rarely in uncomplicated campylobacteriosis. Hypokalemia is an expected finding secondary to inappetence and gastrointestinal potassium losses. Hypoglycemia may complicate *Campylobacter* enteritis in young puppies and kittens.

DIAGNOSIS

Diagnosis of *C. jejuni* enteritis is based on history, clinical signs, cytologic techniques, and culture of the organism. Important historic factors to consider include the date of acquisition and source of the affected pet, the degree of sanitation exercised in its environment, exposure to other diarrheic animals, and whether any human members of the household are affected.

Cytologic examination can be performed on fresh saline smears or on thin, air-dried, stained preparations. Saline smears can be prepared by mixing equal volumes of fresh diarrheic feces with saline on a slide. Once the coverslip is in place, the slide can be examined using light, phase, or dark-field illumination. *Campylobacter* organisms can be identified by their small size, spiral or corkscrew shape, tapered ends, and rapid darting motility. Thin air-dried preparations can be stained with Wright's or Gram stain and examined under light microscopy. Again, the organism can be identified by its small size and typical seagull wing appearance. Both red and white blood cells are also common findings in fecal smears from patients with *Campylobacter* enteritis. Inexperienced observers must be careful not to confuse larger, motile spirochetes commonly found in feces with *C. jejuni*. In the hands of experienced observers, cytologic examination is a relatively insensitive but specific tool for the presumptive diagnosis of *C. jejuni* infections. Thus, a positive cytologic identification of *Campylobacter* organisms justifies the expense and difficulty of specific *Campylobacter* culture.

Culture of *Campylobacter* species is difficult and requires a laboratory experienced in isolation and identification of *Campylobacter*. Appropriate samples for culture include thickly coated rectal swabs, fresh feces, and blood. Tissue samples tend to contain only small numbers of organisms and generally are not suitable for culture.

Rectal swabs should be transported in Cary-Blair or Stuart medium and refrigerated at 4°C until submitted. Feces should also be refrigerated if delivery to the laboratory is delayed.

Campylobacter species are best propagated using commercial isolation and enrichment media designed specifically for *Campylobacter* (*Campylobacter* Agar, BBL Microbiological Systems; *Campylobacter* CVA Agar, Gibco Laboratories). Selective *Campylobacter* media contain a number of antibiotics that reduce the overgrowth of other enteric bacteria. Culture of *Campylobacter* species requires thermophilic (42 to 43°C) and microaerophilic conditions (3 per cent O_2, 10 per cent CO_2, 85 per cent N at 1 atmosphere).

Growth of *C. jejuni* is expected in 2 to 5 days. Cultures should be examined every 48 hr for flat, pink mucoid colonies.

Serologic testing of acute and convalescent sera has been used in humans for the diagnosis of campylobacteriosis. Dogs, cats, and ferrets have been experimentally shown to seroconvert following *Campylobacter* enteritis (Fox et al., 1987; Prescott and Munroe, 1982; Macartney et al., 1981). These agglutination and immunofluorescent techniques have not been widely studied in companion animals.

HISTOPATHOLOGY

Gross pathologic findings are generally nonspecific and typical of acute enteritis. Thickening and congestion of bowel loops, fluid bowel contents, and mesenteric and colonic lymphadenopathy may be seen.

Histologic findings in experimental and spontaneous *Campylobacter* enteritis are similar and include reduction in epithelial height, blunted villi, focal exfoliation of the brush border and goblet cells, mononuclear cell infiltration of the lamina propria, mucosal edema, mild lacteal dilation, hyperplasia of epithelial glands, reactive hyperplasia of lymph nodes, and Peyer's patches. Lesions are usually limited to the jejunum, ileum, and colon except in cases of gastric *C. pylori* infection in humans and ferrets (Blaser, 1987; Fox et al., 1987). Warthin-Starry stain can be used to identify the *Campylobacter* organisms on the epithelial surface in crypts and rarely within enterocytes.

THERAPY

Therapy of *Campylobacter* enteritis in companion animals must include both supportive and specific measures. Maintenance of fluid, electrolyte, and acid-base balance is vital. An isotonic, balanced electrolyte solution such as lactated Ringer's is usually the fluid of choice. Glucose and potassium should be supplemented as necessary, based on serial serum determinations. Physiologic saline may be indicated in animals with severe vomiting and resultant hyponatremia and hypochloremia. The volume of fluid administered should be sufficient to replace volume deficits, meet maintenance requirements, and replace ongoing losses.

If vomiting becomes excessive, antiemetics can be used judiciously to limit fluid and electrolyte losses. Prochlorperazine, 0.5 mg/kg SC or IM every 6 to 8 hr, or metoclopramide, 0.2 to 0.4 mg/kg SC every 8 hr, would be suitable.

Specific antibiotic therapy is indicated in the treatment of C. jejuni. In humans, early antibiotic treatment has been shown to reduce the signs and severity of Campylobacter-associated diarrhea (Salazar-Lindo et al., 1986). Similar findings have been reported in dogs and cats (Holt, 1981).

Additionally, suitable antibiotic therapy will eliminate fecal shedding of C. jejuni (Holt, 1981; Salazar-Lindo et al., 1986). The duration of fecal shedding in dogs and cats has not been well studied but has been demonstrated to be as long as 40 days. Because of the risk of exposure of susceptible animals and the potential for zoonotic infections, antibiotic therapy can be justified solely on the basis of elimination of fecal shedding. Antibiotic therapy has not been demonstrated to result in a chronic carrier state or resistant strains, as it does in Salmonella enteritis.

Selection of antibiotics is most suitably based on culture and sensitivity. Admittedly, the fastidious nature of the organisms can make sensitivity testing difficult to perform and interpret. While awaiting culture and sensitivity results, erythromycin appears to be the drug of choice for treating C. jejuni. Erythromycin should be administered at a dose of 10 to 15 mg/kg PO every 8 hr for 5 days. If vomiting occurs following the administration of erythromycin, the use of enteric-coated products may be helpful. Other antibiotics with expected efficacy against C. jejuni include tylosin, tetracycline, aminoglycosides, chloramphenicol, furazolidine, and clindamycin. Parenteral use of these agents is recommended in animals whose gastrointestinal signs preclude the use of oral antibiotics.

Antibiotics with variable efficacy against C. jejuni include metronidazole, ampicillin, and sulfonamides. Antibiotics with no expected efficacy include penicillin, trimethoprim, vancomycin, and cephalosporins. Several of these antibiotics are incorporated in the selective Campylobacter culture media in order to limit the overgrowth of C. jejuni isolates by enteric commensals.

Resolution of clinical signs is expected within 48 to 72 hr after initiation of antibiotic therapy. Failure to respond suggests the wrong diagnosis, poor choice of antibiotics, or late initiation of therapy. Fecal culture and sensitivity testing should be repeated 1 week and 1 month after therapy to ensure clearance of the organism.

In chronic, recurrent cases of C. jejuni enteritis, longer antibiotic courses appear to be more effective. Three to 6 weeks of erythromycin therapy may be required.

PREVENTION

Because the most important modes of transmission are the ingestion of contaminated food and water and the fecal-oral route, routine hygienic measures should be sufficient to prevent spread. Isolation of Campylobacter-affected animals is recommended because of potential zoonotic infections.

Campylobacter is susceptible to most commonly used disinfectants, including bleach, phenolic compounds, 70 per cent ethyl alcohol, iodophors, and quaternary ammoniums.

ZOONOTIC POTENTIAL

Transmission of Campylobacter species from dogs to humans has been recognized in the United States and Europe (Holt, 1981; Prescott and Munroe, 1982; Fox et al., 1983b; Shane and Montrose, 1985). Cats have less frequently been associated with transmission of Campylobacter enteritis. Despite these reports, less than 5 per cent of Campylobacter-associated diarrhea in humans is believed to be attributable to exposure to pets (Skirrow, 1981). The overwhelming majority of human cases are associated with consumption of contaminated foodstuffs.

References and Supplemental Reading

Blaser, M. J.: Gastric Campylobacter-like organisms, gastritis and peptic-ulcer disease. Gastroenterology 93:371, 1987.

Fox, J. G., Ackerman, J. I., and Taylor, N.: Campylobacter jejuni infection in the ferret: An animal model of human campylobacteriosis. Am. J. Vet. Res. 48:85, 1987.

Fox, J. G., Moore, R., and Ackerman, J. I.: Canine and feline campylobacteriosis: Epizootiology and clinical and public health features. J. Am. Vet. Med. Assoc. 183:1420, 1983a.

Fox, J. G., Moore, R., and Ackerman, J. I.: Campylobacter jejuni-associated diarrhea in dogs. J.A.V.M.A. 183:1430, 1983b.

Holt, P. E.: The role of dogs and cats in the epidemiology of human Campylobacter enterocolitis. J. Small Anim. Pract. 22:681, 1981.

Macartney, L., McCandlesh, A. P., Al-Mashat, R. R., et al.: Natural and experimental enteric infections with Campylobacter fetus ssp jejuni in dogs. In Newell, D. G. (ed.): Campylobacter: Epidemiology, Pathogenesis and Biochemistry. Hingham, MA: MTP Press, Inc., 1981.

Prescott, J. F., and Munroe, D. L.: Campylobacter jejuni enteritis in man and domestic animals. J.A.V.M.A. 181:1524, 1982.

Salazar-Lindo, E., Sack, R. B., Chea-Woo, E., et al.: Early treatment with erythromycin of Campylobacter jejuni-associated dysentery in children. J. Pediatr. 109:355, 1986.

Shane, S. M., and Montrose, M. S.: The occurrence and significance of Campylobacter jejuni in man and animals. Vet. Res. Commun. 9:167, 1985.

Skirrow, M. B.: Campylobacter enteritis in dogs and cats: A "new" zoonosis. Vet. Res. Commun. 5:13, 1981.

EXTRACTION AND ORAL-NASAL FISTULA

PETER P. EMILY, D.D.S.

Fort Collins, Colorado

Animals with oral signs such as excessive drooling, mouth shyness, changes in eating habits, facial swelling, loose teeth, and traumatic injuries certainly need dental attention.

Extraction (exodontia), when absolutely necessary, is made much easier if proper technique and high-speed dental equipment are employed.

Tooth sectioning, root tip elevation, and atomization constitute an easily employed dental procedure, not only to facilitate and speed up exodontia but to reduce postoperative trauma, pain, and complication such as oral-nasal fistula formation associated with poor surgical technique and equipment.

Oral-nasal fistula formation is a common complication of exodontia or periodontal disease. Proper closure of the fistula has been poorly understood. If the closing flaps are placed under tension in an attempt simply to pull the two sides of the defect together, the result is unsatisfactory. A tension-free double-flap procedure has consistently produced fistula closure.

INDICATIONS FOR EXODONTIA

Extraction is most often warranted in severe cases of periodontal disease and bone loss, in slab fractures such as those seen in the upper fourth premolars, for supernumerary teeth, for coronal fractures, for retained root tips, and when client preference prevails.

Many alternatives to tooth extraction are available. Root canal therapy, restorations, orthodontics, and periodontal surgery may be employed to save teeth that would otherwise be removed.

Teeth that are involved with periodontal disease are easier to extract than those that have normal bony support. The bone and connective fibers of periodontally involved teeth are either lost or diseased, resulting in a poorly supported tooth.

PROCEDURE FOR EXTRACTION OF SINGLE-ROOTED TEETH

Single-rooted teeth are the easiest to extract. These include the upper and lower incisors and the upper and lower first premolars. An exception to this rule are the canines, which have extremely long roots proportional to the crown.

The extraction of single-rooted teeth is begun with the use of a no. 15 blade directed at a 45° angle to the long axis of the tooth, severing the epithelial attachment. A small dental elevator is then placed between the tooth and the crestal alveolar bone and rotated approximately 90° caudally and rostrally. Step away for a few minutes after elevation to allow for periodontal ligament hemorrhage to take place. The hydraulic pressure created from bleeding around the tooth will aid in root removal. With the use of dental forceps, the tooth is rotated on its long axis and lifted out of the alveolus. Care must be taken not to bend the coronal portion laterally. This can result in tooth fracture and root retention.

The socket is cleared of debris or fibrous granulation tissue that may be present. A bone file or bone rongeur may be necessary for bony fragment removal. The alveolar bone should be filed or smoothed (alveolectomy). Sharp bony ridges or protrusions result in osseous ischemia or osseous necrosis.

Normal extraction does not call for the use of sutures unless the gingiva was torn during the extraction or a flap procedure was used. A Gelfoam pack and tetracycline powder are packed into the tooth socket to reduce postoperative bleeding and promote bacteriostasis. It has been shown that tetracycline is effective in reducing postoperative osteitis and promoting osteogenesis. Tetracycline powder is also conducive to osseous growth. Hand pressure applied to the area with a gauze sponge for a few minutes will reduce the hemorrhage and compress the alveolar plates expanded during extraction.

PROCEDURE FOR EXTRACTION OF MULTI-ROOTED TEETH

Tooth extraction of multi-rooted teeth is best accomplished with the use of a high-speed dental handpiece with 700 or 701 tapered cross-cut fissure burs. Cutting diamond disks in a slow-speed hand piece are less desirable. They are much broader in diameter and difficult to control. An uncontrolled cutting disk can severely lacerate a practitioner's hand or the animal's lip, cheek, palate, or gingiva.

The upper fourth premolar will be used as a teaching example. The epithelial attachment of the upper fourth premolar is severed in the manner described for single-rooted teeth. Since the upper fourth premolar has three roots, it is sectioned to create the equivalent of three single-rooted teeth. All tooth sectioning is carried down to the root furcation. First the palatal root is separated with a diagonal cut from medial caudal to lateral rostral through the furcation. The palatal root and the lateral rostral root are approximately parallel to each other; a diagonal cut can be directed to the furcation separating the two roots. It is very difficult to elevate the palatal root mechanically without root fracture. A fractured segment of the palatal root can be removed with the use of the high-speed bur (330L) directed from the top of the palatal root and down along its long axis. The high-speed bur will atomize the remaining root segment to the apex. Atomization is easily accomplished under water spray and proper light. The caudal and rostral roots are next separated with a 701 fissure bur and high-speed hand piece. The crown is divided along the buccal groove through to the furcation. Next, a 701 tapered fissure bur is employed to remove approximately 1 to 2 mm of the labial alveolar bony crest circumferentially around the remaining two roots. A slightly deeper cut is made on the caudal and rostral aspect of the tooth at the junction of the root and the bony alveolar crest. A 701 fissure bur is used to cut a 1-mm-deep groove at the caudal and rostral base of each respective root. This groove serves as a purchase point for the dental elevator. Using a straight elevator placed between the previously sectioned crown, lightly wedge the two sections apart to ensure that they are completely separated. Next, the lateral side of a straight elevator is placed into the caudal root purchase point or groove. The caudal root is elevated rostrally, using the first molar as a fulcrum point. The straight elevator in like manner is placed in the purchase point of the rostral root and elevated caudally. The labial or lateral bony plate has not been sacrificed. There remain three separated sockets. The use of Gelfoam or a Gelfoam pad impregnated with tetracycline powder works well for providing both hemostasis and osseous repair. A plug of Gelfoam and tetracycline is placed in each of the root sockets, filling them to the subgingival margin.

CANINE TOOTH EXTRACTIONS

Canine teeth, because of their length and possible postoperative oral-nasal complications, can pose difficult problems. Make a triangular incision from the distal (caudal) gingival sulcus to the mesial (rostral)

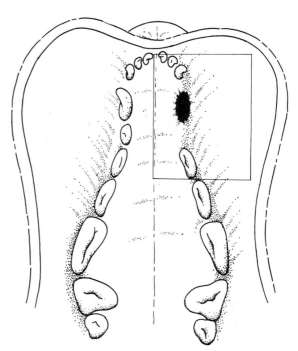

Figure 1. Defect and flap outline.

gingival sulcus to the apex on the mesial aspect of the canine. This full-thickness gingival mucoperiosteal flap is reflected caudally with the use of a small periosteal elevator, exposing the entire lateral canine eminence of buccal bone.

Use a 701 bur in a high-speed dental hand piece to incise the labial plate of bone to midroot depth

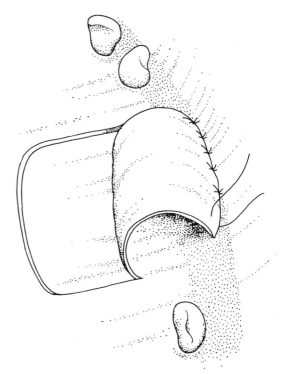

Figure 2. Placement and suture of palatal flap.

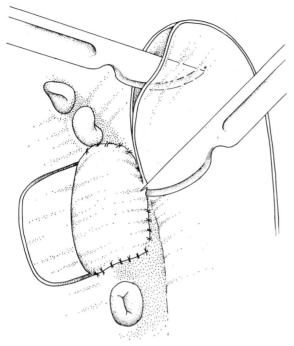

Figure 3. Scarification of lateral epithelium and harvesting of mucosal covering flap.

around the entire border of the root. The incision of bone is best performed under water irrigation. The upper canine is elevated at the midbody points and in total laterally. Take care not to elevate from the coronal palatal aspect, which would result in tipping the apex into the turbinates and possibly oral-nasal fistula formation.

The irregular bony alveolar edges are removed,

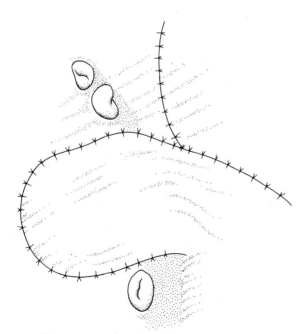

Figure 4. Completed flap placement and suture.

and the socket is examined for granulation tissue and debris. The socket is packed with tetracycline and Gelfoam and sutured along the rostral and gingival border.

ORAL-NASAL FISTULA

Total healing by first intention is the goal when turbinate exposure is encountered during exodontia, but invariably there are occasional failures. A secondary fistula at the original site is usually the result of primary closure failure.

The fistulous tract becomes epithelialized, with resultant avascular scarring around the defect. Common causes of fistula are (1) inadequate approximation of the opposing raw surfaces, (2) failure to evert one or both edges of the wound, (3) necrosis of the end of a flap used in closure, (4) flap tension (all flaps must be absolutely tension free at the time of closure), (5) infection, (6) careless suturing, and (7) traumatic disruption of the wound.

The most effective closure of oral-nasal fistula is in two layers without tension or infection, using proper suturing techniques, and ensuring an adequate blood supply and protection during healing.

Oral-nasal fistula allows fluid and food to escape into the turbinates to perpetuate nasal discharge and chronic infection.

Closure of a fistula can be very difficult for the same reasons that caused its primary occurrence. This is compounded by the inadequacy of local tissue and subsequent postoperative care.

Preoperative cultures should be taken, especially if the presence of *Staphylococcus*, *Bacteroides*, or hemolytic *Streptococcus* is suspected. If this microbacterial state exists, surgical remission is greatly impaired. Long-term antibiotic therapy should be employed to render the fistula site as free of bacteria as possible prior to surgical closure.

Surgical Procedure

Fistula closure is a modification of a two-layer closure method outlined by Wassmund, a maxillofacial surgeon. A description of an upper left canine fistula procedure will be used to outline and detail a double-flap closure. Figure 1 shows the defect and flap outline.

A full-thickness mucoperiosteal flap is raised from the palatal aspect of the defect. The incision line begins slightly rostral and medial to the defect, progressing medial to a midpoint approximating the width of the defect. The incision turns caudally, paralleling the defect to the caudal extent of the defect, then continues laterally to the edge of the defect. This full-thickness mucoperiosteal palatal flap is elevated to the edge of the defect, turned upside down so that the oral epithelium is turned to the turbinates, and released of tension. The lateral aspect of the defect is freshened by shaving the margin to the rostral and caudal midline of the defect, leaving the medial half of the defect untouched. This provides a raw surface on the lateral side to oppose the palatal flap. This palatal flap is sutured to the fresh lateral surface of the defect, raw surface to raw surface (Fig. 2). A partial-thickness mucosal flap approximately 1 mm thick by 1.5 cm wide (this is an arbitrary width contingent on the width of the defect to be covered) and approximately 3 cm long (again, an arbitrary length contingent on the length of defect to be covered) is raised lateral to the defect and in the buccal mucosa, beginning at the caudal edge of the defect and continuing to the predetermined length needed to cover the defect in a tension-free manner. The incision line is carried laterally and then caudally to the caudal edge of the defect. *If the mucosal flap is to cover epithelialized or keratinized tissue lateral to the defect and medial to the mucosal flap, this short zone of tissue must be scarified to provide a raw surface under the repositioned mucosal flap* (Fig. 3).

The fingerlike flap is raised and brought medially over the palatal flap and donor site, covering them *in toto*, and sutured completely in place (Fig. 4).

The two sides of the mucosal donor site are sutured together. All sutures are absorbable suture material of choice.

This procedure has produced a double or pancake flap where the surface oral epithelium of the palatal and labial gingival flap is now inside the nasal turbinates and the lateral mucosal epithelium of the covering flap remains outside, producing a consistently effective fistula closure.

ORAL DIAGNOSIS

PETER P. EMILY, D.D.S.

Fort Collins, Colorado

Dentistry in veterinary medicine utilizes all the disciplines practiced in human dentistry, such as orthodontics, periodontics, endodontics, oral surgery, restorative techniques, intraoral radiology, and crown and bridge work.

A complete oral examination includes evaluation of both hard and soft tissues for pathology, anatomy, and genetic considerations.

The hard tissue consists of the teeth and osseous structures. The soft tissue includes the lips, cheeks, tongue, palate, gingiva, and oral mucosa.

This article deals with hard tissue evaluation as related to anatomy, genetics, and pathology.

DEVELOPMENTAL EVALUATION

Hard tissue evaluation, in terms of growth and bite relationships, is undertaken in the branch of dentistry called orthodontics. Orthodontics, by definition, is the proper positioning and relationship of the teeth: the correction or placement of malaligned teeth into their proper relationship in the dental arches through mechanical and occasionally surgical means.

Orthodontics cannot begin without first understanding proper tooth alignment, genetic relation-

ship, and developmental defects and their etiologies. These factors become immediately evident on initial clinical examination and evaluation of the mouth.

Brachygnathic (overshot), prognathic (undershot), and wry bites are genetic defects. At this time, the only method to distinguish genetic from developmental bite relationships is based on A. H. Angle's classification developed before the turn of the century, prior to radiographic and cephalometric evaluation of skeletal growth patterns as related to the teeth and their arrangement in the mouth.

Until we can properly evaluate the total arrangement of the skeletal and dental patterns by establishing normal cephalometric standards for all the breed types (mongrels excluded), we will use only A. H. Angle's classification for bite relationships based on dentition only. Bite types will be divided into class I, class II, and class III relationships. Class I occlusion is normal (Fig. 1), class II is brachygnathic or overshot (Fig. 2), and class III is prognathic or undershot (Fig. 3). These classifications are based on molar-premolar relationships. In a normal or class I premolar-molar relationship, the lower posterior (cheek) teeth are rostral (anterior) to their counterparts, the cusp tips pointing to the center of the opposing interproximal space. Thus,

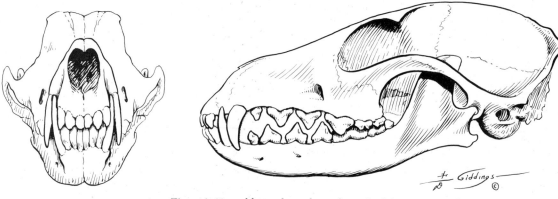

Figure 1. Normal bite relationship—class I (angle).

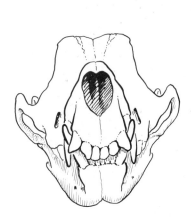

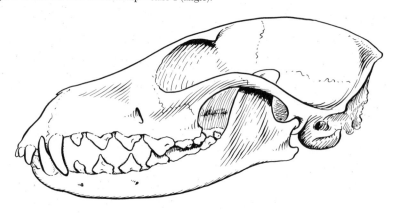

Figure 2. Brachygnathia—class II (angle).

the lower first premolar is rostral to the upper first premolar, the lower second premolar is rostral to the upper second premolar, and so forth. In a class II brachygnathic (overshot) bite, the upper first premolar opposes the lower premolar, and so forth. The degree of upper premolar rostral displacement is contingent on the degree of involvement.

In a class III mandibular prognathism (undershot), the opposite premolar relationship is seen, in that the upper premolars are caudal to their normal position (e.g., the upper first premolar opposing

the lower second premolar). Again, these bite relationships in Angle's classifications are based solely on tooth position, with no reference to skeletal relationship.

There is no equivalent human classification for wry bite, because this malocclusion does not occur in humans. A wry bite produces tooth relationships and a unilateral prognathism that affect not only the teeth but also the whole head. The affected dentition on the wry side can be prognathic, open, or any degree of both. There is a deviation of the

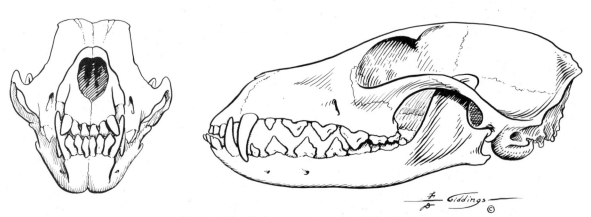

Figure 3. Mandibular prognathia—class III (angle).

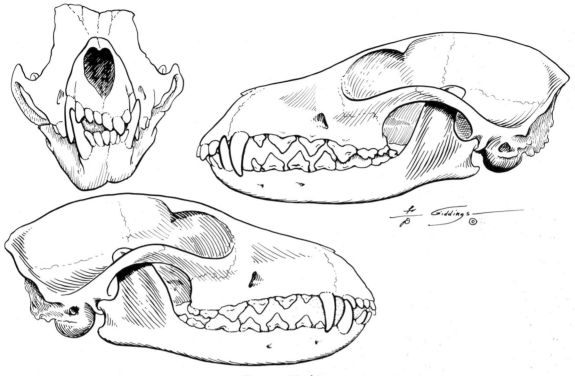

Figure 4. Wry bite.

midline that can be traced from midskull through the dentition. In advanced cases, the head also appears asymmetric. One side of the head becomes larger than the other side, giving the head a lopsided appearance. Wry bites are the most difficult to diagnose because of the degree of deformity. A wry bite can be an additional complication of other bite relationships, such as seen in brachycephalic (undershot) head types (Fig. 2).

All dogs have the same number of teeth, whether the head is brachycephalic or dolichocephalic. Teeth are easiest to count by considering them in block sections. All incisors, premolars, and molars can be categorized into groups. Missing teeth then become obvious by group asymmetry. By the same asymmetry, supernumerary, or extra, teeth become apparent. Supernumerary teeth are removed only when there is crowding, creating either a malocclusion or a periodontal problem. The reason that longheaded (dolichocephalic) breeds often have room enough for several supernumerary teeth or have missing teeth is not clearly understood. Of the six modes of genetic inheritance, the autosomal recessive mode is the most probable.

Many forms of malocclusion are developmental rather than genetic. Most developmental defects are the result of primary teeth retained beyond their normal time of exfoliation. Removal of the primary canines and incisors prior to or at their normal exfoliation time would eliminate the largest cause of anterior cross-bites—upper canines in rostral version and lower canines in medial version, traumatizing the palate. This occurs when the upper permanent canine enters the mouth rostral to the primary canine. The lower permanent canine enters the arch medial to the primary canine. The combination of retained primary upper and lower canines can cause the lower permanent canine to be deflected medially by the retained lower primary canine and the upper permanent canine to be deflected rostrally by the retained primary upper canine. The lower canine is locked medially, traumatizing the palate whenever the mouth is closed. This can eventually lead to oral-nasal fistula formation.

INTERCEPTIVE ORTHODONTICS

Interceptive procedures such as serial extraction of the primary incisors are often effective in preventing deflection of the permanent teeth into a malocclusion. The permanent incisors erupt into the mouth caudal to the primary incisors. One or more incisors can be deflected by retained primary teeth. Removal of the primary incisors before their normal time of exfoliation will allow the permanent incisors to advance rostrally without primary tooth retardation, thereby eliminating the chance of caudally displaced permanent teeth (anterior crossbite). Selective extraction of the entire upper or lower primary incisors is a method of promoting additional advancement of the permanent dentition. The incisors that need to be advanced in the arch are removed in serial or selective extractions (e.g., extraction of the upper primary incisors in a mandibular prognathic puppy). It is important to note that serial extraction will not be effective if malocclusion is of genetic origin. Ethically, orthodontics to correct malocclusions should be used only to correct bites resulting from nongenetic (developmental) origins. True genetic malocclusion should rarely be corrected unless there is a complication such as periodontal disease resulting from the malocclusion. Animals with genetic malocclusion should not be corrected unless they are neutered.

ENDODONTIC EVALUATION

Hard tissue pathology is usually endodontic. It may be seen as broken cusp tips or crowns and can occur on all teeth, but especially the canines and carnasials. These teeth have exposed pulp chambers. Discolored teeth (purple, red, gray), intraoral or extraoral swellings, and sinus tracts due to tooth abscessation are the result of tooth pathology.

Endodontic lesions are the second most common oral problem. Endodontic involvement is largely the result of trauma. The lack of treatment not only perpetuates pain and generalized complications for the pet but also removes a large source of practice revenue for veterinarians.

ENDODONTICS

THOMAS W. MULLIGAN, D.V.M.
San Diego, California

Endodontic therapy, treatment of the soft tissue of the tooth, is commonly misunderstood in veterinary medicine. The term *hidden lesion* is certainly appropriate for most periapical abscesses in our dogs and cats. The fact they are not readily visible does not make them any less real.

Pulpal necrosis, infection, and exposure to the oral flora are considered indications for endodontic therapy. Unfortunately, pets usually do not exhibit noticeable clinical signs of pain when these insults first occur. This has led to the general misconception that an animal patient's teeth are somehow "different" from our own—that is, that they are not painful and will not develop periapical abscesses.

There are three primary ways endodontic therapy is accomplished: coronal approach, surgery, and pulpotomy. The most conservative is the coronal approach.

The desired end result of root canal therapy is to perfect a seal in the apical third of the root canal.

This will prevent the nidus, the infected dentin, from chronically seeding into the periapical tissue of the periodontium.

PATHOGENESIS AND DIAGNOSIS

The endodontic system can be exposed to the environment in a variety of ways. Coronal fractures and rapid attrition are probably the leading causes of exposure in dogs. Cervical line erosions in cats and, to a lesser degree, caries in dogs also commonly lead to root chamber exposure.

When the pulp is no longer surrounded by the tooth's protective dentin, it becomes infected by the mouth's abundant flora. This infection occurs, as with all soft tissue, within 4 to 6 hr. The usual soft tissue pathophysiology follows, and the tissue swells. The problem is compounded in the root chamber because the pulp is surrounded by the hard tissue of the tooth, which does not allow room for expansion. As a result, a tremendous internal pressure is placed on the tissue, and bacteria exert their destructive influence.

Does it hurt? Anatomic and histopathologic studies clearly demonstrate the trigeminal nerve innervation of the teeth. There can be no doubt that our charges get toothaches, exactly as humans do. If you have ever probed a recently insulted tooth, you got an instant reaction from the patient.

Reluctance to chew, excessive salivation, mouth shyness, and lack of biting power in working and security dogs all are common histories noted by the keen observer.

After a period of a week or two, the pulp can no longer withstand the pressure and infection. Necrosis is completed, and the pain subsides. This is when the second, and most destructive, stage of pathology begins: the so-called hidden infection formation of a periapical abscess.

The second scenario can be pulpal necrosis without demonstrable external exposure. The etiology is usually unknown. The common causes are infection by the hematogenous route or tooth trauma without visible fracture or erosion.

The clinical sign of this problem is discoloration of the crown. As necrosis progresses, the integrity of the vessel walls is lost and blood soaks into the porous dentin. The result is either a bluish or red tooth. A gray tooth usually indicates strangulation of tissue.

Fistulation is another indication for root canal therapy. We are all familiar with the fistula that can form just ventral to the eye. These fistulas are due to a periapical abscess from either the upper fourth premolar or, occasionally, the first or second molar.

Other commonly seen fistulas are from the labial vestibule (usually an upper canine source). The lower canine will fistulate directly ventral to the apex through the skin under the chin.

A fistula will occasionally be present from the gingival area, with no apparent damage to the dentition. A good rule is: If the fistula is coronal to the mucogingival line, the problem is periodontal; if the opening is on or apical to the mucogingival line, it is endodontic.

If a surgical flap is performed and the fistula has bone on all sides, it is endodontic. Beware of combination lesions!

Because of the internal hidden nature of endodontic lesions, radiology is in many ways a useful adjunct to endodontic therapy:

1. For confirmation of pathology.
2. To pinpoint the location of the source of involvement.
3. To determine the diameter of the root chamber and canal.
4. To evaluate the extent of the periapical and apical destruction.

5. To search for anatomic deviations of the endodontic system.

6. For postoperative evaluation.

Relatively recent periapical involvements may not always have had time to exhibit radiographic apical lucencies. As a result, negative radiographic findings should not be completely relied on to rule out periapical abscess formation.

Intraoral, bisecting technique radiographs are strongly recommended whenever possible.

Regardless of the cause of the lesion, once pulpal exposure or necrosis occurs, endodontic therapy is indicated. The necrotic tissue becomes infected either immediately, as in the case of exposure, or eventually by hematogenous means in the case of primary necrosis.

The infection of the pulp leads to contamination of the surrounding porous dentin. Once the dentin harbors microorganisms, it is impossible to sterilize the interior of the tooth. Thus, the contaminated tooth acts as a chronic nidus. The infection inevitably infiltrates through the apices of the tooth, and a periapical abscess will form. This abscess will continue to be active and worsen as long as the tooth remains intact.

How soon the abscess forms, as well as how destructive it becomes, will depend on a number of factors. The virulence of the microorganisms will obviously help determine the severity of the infection.

Another factor is the size of the apical opening. Deciduous teeth of our patients have large apical openings. As a result, severe periapical abscesses form quite rapidly in young animals—sometimes in 2 or 3 weeks. Since adult animals tend to have small openings or delta foramina (multiple small openings) at their apical ends, the abscess formation is usually slower—but just as inevitable.

The thickness of bone surrounding the infected root tip determines when the abscess becomes obvious in the form of a fistula. Most animal teeth are set deeply in bone, and the gases produced from suppuration will take the line of least resistance. As a result, the gas vents through the coronal access hole and slows fistula formation. This factor becomes apparent if a root canal procedure fails to produce the desired seal at the apices of the tooth. When the access hole is sealed, a fistula always forms in a very short time.

The periapical abscesses created by infected carnassial teeth readily develop draining fistulas. This is because the mesial root tip is very close to the maxillary sinus, with only a thin sheet of bone separating them. It is easy for the periapical abscess to dissect quickly into the sinus and cause a severe and obvious fistula to form from the subsequent sinusitis. The fourth upper premolar is no more susceptible to abscessations than any other tooth. It only demonstrates a fistula more readily than the others.

As the abscess remains hidden over a period of time, three primary lesions develop. The periodontal tissues surrounding the root tip are destroyed in an increasingly larger zone. The root tip itself starts to dissolve. Most of the tooth root and the surrounding tissue eventually dissolve, and along with probable fistulation, the tooth is lost.

The other serious sequela is that the abscess tends to leach toxins and bacteria systemically throughout the body. A correlation has been demonstrated between endodontic lesions and pyelonephritis, endocarditis, bacterial hepatitis, and septic arthritis, as well as general poor health.

Since sterilization of the infected dentin cannot be accomplished, only one or two courses of treatment are available to the veterinary dentist. The offending tooth must either be extracted or a seal must be perfected in the distal third of the root canal to entrap the contamination inside the tooth. If the infection can no longer leak out the apices, the periapical abscess will heal itself. The tooth will then be serviceable, even though dead, for the life of the host.

ROOT CANAL THERAPY BY THE CORONAL APPROACH

Access

The entry location depends on the particular tooth. The object is to allow an unobstructed entry to the apex of each root canal.

In general, as much remaining crown tissue should be spared as possible to retain maximum strength. Common openings in multiple-root teeth are discouraged for this reason. Whenever possible, entry sights are thus aligned directly over the root canal itself.

CANINE TEETH. The crown is occasionally fractured close enough to the gingiva to allow entry directly into the apex. Thus the access hole is already available for entry.

Because of the curvature of most canals, the creation of your own access is recommended. If excess lateral stress is put on an endodontic file (especially Hedstrom), the file commonly breaks in the tooth while filing.

The usual entry site in canine teeth is on the mesial surface, just coronal to the gingiva. This location usually allows unobstructed access to the distal end of the canal.

INCISORS. If the crown is fractured, it is usually possible to enter directly into the exposed canal. In cases in which entry creation is necessary, the usual site is directly through the labial surface just coronal to the gingiva. For cosmetic purposes, the central incisors can also be penetrated from the lingual surface.

UPPER FOURTH PREMOLARS. These teeth have usually sustained a slab fracture of the buccal surface. As they are already weakened, a common access hole is not recommended.

The endodontic system of this tooth, as in all teeth with multiple roots, interconnects from each canal into the central root chamber. As a result, all canals of any involved tooth must be addressed.

In general, entry should be made with three small holes, one over each individual root. It can be difficult for the inexperienced clinician to locate the canals of this tooth. The entry into an already extracted tooth is recommended for practice, and this tooth should be kept as a model.

The palatine root can be handled in two ways. It can be entered and treated as any other root. An alternative method is to amputate it from the main body of the tooth and extract. The two remaining roots still supply adequate support. It is important to emphasize that there is a tendency to attempt mesial root entry too lingual.

MOLARS AND PREMOLARS. These teeth have a low incidence of disorders requiring endodontics. If the need arises, entry is made as described previously. In general, the entries are through the occlusal cusps of the crown.

The bur should be either round or a no. 330 pear. The usual round size varies from no. ½ to no. 2, whichever is most appropriate.

The bur should be turning at full speed before contacting the enamel. Enter the tooth at a 90° angle from the surface of the enamel. If initial entry is attempted at an angle, crazing of the enamel will often occur. You will feel the bur drop into the root chamber as it is advanced through the dentin.

Once entry is accomplished, the angle of the access hole can be sculptured to accommodate the angle and appropriate diameter to allow straight unobstructed entry to the tooth's apices.

If desired, a root canal explorer or small-diameter endodontic file can be used to confirm entry into the root chamber.

Endodontic Files

Files vary in length, diameter, and flute configurations. The common lengths used in humans are 20, 25, and 30 mm. These files are long enough for all teeth in the pet population, except the canine teeth of large dogs. Larger dogs and some exotic breeds have root canals longer than 30 mm. For these teeth, the 55-mm files are required to allow complete penetration to the distal apex.

The diameter sizes commonly used range in increments of 0.15 mm at the tip of the file through 0.80 mm. Various sizes are usually color coded for easy identification. Sizes 90 through 140 are available but rarely needed. A set of 15 through 80 diameters in both 30 mm and 55 mm are recommended as a part of your instrumentation.

Flutes at the ends of the files are available in various configurations. The ones most commonly used in veterinary dentistry are either K or Hedstrom. The K files are currently available only in lengths used in human endodontics. The Hedstrom files are available in 55-mm length as well as in the shorter sizes for humans. The Hedstrom files are machined instead of twisted and are more brittle than the K files. The author prefers K files when available.

Debriding the Canal

The soft tissue must be completely removed from the root chamber. If necrosis of the nerve is relatively recent, it often can be removed intact. This can be accomplished by introducing a barbed broach into the canal and, after entangling the pulp tissue, pulling the tissue from the tooth. This often can be accomplished with an endodontic file of appropriate size.

Once the bulk of the soft tissue has been removed, the canal must be filed to remove all remaining soft tissue and necrotic dentin.

The filing is accomplished by introducing into the canal a small-diameter file that will go all the way to the distal tip. Unlike human teeth, our patients' teeth will usually have an apical foramen that will allow us to introduce the file as far as possible with no concern of penetration of the periapical tissues through the apices.

Progressively larger-diameter files are employed until only clean dental shavings are being returned. A chelating product known as CSPE Premier will assist your filing efforts. This product lubricates the files and also softens the dentin, helping to ensure a more efficient filing.

TWISTING VS. IN AND OUT. When filing with K files, the endodontist should enter the file full distance, make a one-quarter turn, and pull out. By overrotating the file, you run the risk of embedding the file tip too firmly and fracturing the file in the canal.

Hedstrom files should never be rotated. They are designed for in-and-out filing only.

It is essential that dentinal filings do not become impacted in the root tip. To ensure cleanliness, the root canal must be flushed frequently with bleach (sodium hypochlorite). This solution can be used from full strength to a 50:50 dilution. The more dilute form will cause less chemical irritation to mucous membranes. This fluid will dissolve dentinal filings. As a final rinse, it is recommended to use three solutions. Flush well with bleach followed by

hydrogen peroxide. A final flush of copious amounts of saline should accomplish satisfactory cleansing.

WHEN TO CHANGE FILES. Endodontic files, like all mechanical things, have to be changed periodically. It is prudent to change files on a routine basis. The flutes at the tip of the file often tend to stretch—a sure sign of metal fatigue.

FILING THE PROXIMAL END. Debriding the chamber coronal to the entry hole in a canine tooth is unnecessary. The same is true of the interconnecting canals of teeth with multiple roots. Our objective is to seal the distal third of the canal. Filing these proximal areas is not only time-consuming but pointless, and it weakens the crown.

Determine Apical Diameter

Apical diameter must be determined when the apical seal is eventually perfected. Begin by introducing a small file that obviously will go to the maximum depth of the canal. Measure this distance. Now introduce larger-diameter files until you determine the largest-diameter file that will still extend completely to the distal apex. This is the lumen size of the tooth's apex. Record this size for future use.

Drying the Canal

The canal must be completely dry before introducing any sealing materials. This is accomplished with absorbent paper points. These points are supplied in lengths for both human and veterinary use, and both should be kept on hand. Fine, medium, and coarse diameters in human lengths and medium and coarse diameters in veterinary lengths are recommended. Fine diameters in veterinary lengths are not available.

The points are inserted to the bottom of the canal to absorb the moisture. New points are introduced until the point comes out completely dry. The diameter of the apex frequently is too small to allow full introduction of the veterinary medium-size paper point. This leaves the most critical area of the procedure damp. A wisp of cotton on a barbed broach will solve the dilemma. The tooth is now ready to be sealed.

Sealing the Root Canal

A large variety of materials and methods for endodontic sealing are available to the veterinary dentist. Because of the relatively enormous size of our patients' root canals, some of the commonly employed methods in human dentistry are not applicable.

The combination of zinc oxide and eugenol (ZOE) is considered the reagent of choice by the author. This material has many attractive properties:

1. It is bacteriostatic.
2. Mixing ratios are not critical.
3. It permits a long working time.
4. It is highly compatible with the periapical tissues.
5. It is economical.

As you become more experienced with endodontic therapy, you may wish to employ some other modalities. The use of ZOE is highly recommended initially.

Appropriate amounts of the two reagents are spatulated together on a glass mixing slab. The desired consistency is reached when a strand approximately ½ inch is left when the spatula is pulled free. Since the point of the whole root canal procedure is to seal the distal third of the canal, it is essential that no air, debris, or water be retained in the distal end. To ensure a complete fill, the use of one of the two following methods is advised.

The most efficient method is to use a spiral paste filler. These coils are available in the usual lengths used in human and veterinary practice.

The spiral filler is driven by a low-speed hand piece. If using an air turbine, a 1:10 reduction gear is recommended to ensure very slow rotation. The spiral must turn in a clockwise direction when viewed from the rear. Choose a spiral that is smaller in diameter than the lumen of the apex.

The spiral is dipped into the filling paste and introduced the full length of the canal. This is done without rotation. Once the spiral is completely inserted, start the rotation and "pump" the spiral back and forth to ensure that all the air bubbles are removed. Draw the filler out while still rotating. Keep repeating this process until the canal is completely full.

An alternate method is to use an endodontic file as a spiral filler. The technique is the same, except that the files are rotated manually counterclockwise.

Use of Gutta-Percha

Gutta-percha is a material made from a plant of that name. This material has been found to be ideal for endodontic use. It is compressible, allowing it to be adapted to the walls of the prepared root canal during condensation, and it is dimensionally stable, undergoing little or no dimensional change during intraoral temperature variations. Equally important, it is easily removed from the canal should retreatment of the tooth become necessary. It can be softened by immersion in chloroform or by subject-

ing it to heat. These properties are sometimes used in human dentistry (i.e., the chlorpercha technique) but are not commonly recommended techniques for veterinary use at this time.

It has been shown that filling with a spiral filler is extremely efficient. Even so, using gutta-percha in conjunction with filling paste will raise the success rate even higher. The gutta-percha will effectively seal the apices and push the ZOE outward into all the small surrounding deficits and lateral canals of the dentinal walls by hydrostatic pressure. It acts as a cork in the apices.

Gutta-percha is available in the same diameters as endodontic files. Unfortunately, varying diameters in the veterinary lengths are not available. Using the human-length gutta-percha, choose the diameter that corresponds to the apical lumen size. Enter the paste-coated gutta-percha into the lumen of the prefilled tooth and push completely into the distal tip, perfecting the seal. In the case of canine teeth, this can be accomplished by pushing with a ramrod such as an old file shaft or an endodontic plugger.

Once the initial gutta-percha is in place, continue to introduce more into the chamber until the tooth cannot accept any more. Use endodontic spreaders to help ensure maximum packing. Excess gutta-percha left protruding from the entrance is removed with heat. Heat a beaver tail with a cigarette lighter and wipe off the unneeded ends.

Sealing the Access Opening

Sealing of the access opening is usually accomplished with composite or silver amalgam. With the advent of modern materials, amalgam is not as widely used. Composite is normally set chemically but can also be obtained in the light-setting form. Neither composite nor amalgam adheres to either dentin or enamel. The first step is to undercut the opening so the composite will mechanically interlock. This is most easily accomplished with a no. 330 pear bur or an inverted cone (usually 33½ or 35 size). These burs will automatically accomplish the undercut by introducing the bur into the hole and simply rotating around the entry hole with the bur's shaft.

It is recommended to undercut and seal the exposed proximal access hole in canine teeth, even though debriding is not usually done in this portion of the canal.

Clean any residual ZOE and gutta-percha from the access area. If ZOE mixes with composite, the composite will not harden completely.

Mix the composite as the manufacturer recommends and introduce it into the prepared opening. A composite carrier is very handy for this purpose.

Pack relatively tightly with a packing instrument and finish the area off flush with the tooth's surface. Excess can be easily removed with a surgical sponge moistened with alcohol.

It is recommended to smooth the finished surface once the composite is set in the same manner as any restoration. This will give a professional appearance and eliminate an area predisposed to plaque accumulation.

If amalgam is used, the same principles apply. Mix the amalgam in an amalgamator and introduce it to the access site with an amalgam carrier. Pack tightly with a ball burnisher condenser. Dentinal varnish is not necessary in this application. It is necessary only to seal the dentin with varnish in vital tooth restorations. Varnish is used *only* under amalgam, never under composite.

Proper technique and attention to detail when performing endodontic procedures cannot be overemphasized. Shortcuts and lack of attention to detail will greatly lower your success rate.

Section
10

ENDOCRINE
AND
METABOLIC
DISORDERS

MARK E. PETERSON, D.V.M.
Consulting Editor

Common Endocrine Diagnostic Tests: Normal Values and
Interpretation 961
Guidelines for Collection, Storage, and Transport of Samples for
Hormone Assay 968
Diabetes Insipidus 973
Canine Growth Hormone–Responsive Dermatosis 978
Feline Acromegaly (Growth Hormone Excess)........................... 981
Canine Primary Hyperparathyroidism..................................... 985
Hypercalcemia of Malignancy... 988
Treatment of Canine Hypothyroidism 993
Canine Myxedema Stupor and Coma....................................... 998
Feline Hypothyroidism 1000
Treatment of Feline Hyperthyroidism......................................1002
Dietary Therapy for Canine Diabetes Mellitus 1008
Insulin-resistant Diabetes Mellitus 1011
Medical Treatment of Neuroendocrine Tumors of the
Gastroenteropancreatic System with Somatostatin 1020
Therapy for Spontaneous Canine Hyperadrenocorticism 1024
Radiation Therapy for Canine ACTH-Secreting Pituitary Tumors........1031
Mitotane (O,P'-DDD) Treatment of Cortisol-Secreting Adrenocortical
Neoplasia..1034
Feline Hyperadrenocorticism...1038
Feline Hypoadrenocorticism..1042
Hyperlipidemia..1046

COMMON ENDOCRINE DIAGNOSTIC TESTS: NORMAL VALUES AND INTERPRETATION

R. J. KEMPPAINEN, D.V.M.,
and C. A. ZERBE, D.V.M.
Auburn, Alabama

The following list of endocrine testing procedures represents protocols in relatively common use in small animal veterinary medicine. Emphasis has been placed on procedures involving the direct measurement of hormones in serum or plasma. The list is not meant to be exhaustive, nor does the absence of a particular test mean that the authors object to its use. Instead, this guide is designed to act as a brief reference to methods for and interpretation of the more frequently used endocrine tests. Some sources of substances employed in endocrine tests are listed in Table 1. Except where indicated, the procedures and normal values represent those recommended by the Endocrine Diagnostic Laboratory, Auburn University College of Veterinary Medicine. Users of endocrine tests must interpret their results based on reference values and protocols provided by the diagnostic laboratory analyzing their samples. In turn, these reference laboratories should be able to assure users of the validity of each analytic method used to estimate hormone concentrations in samples from a particular species.

SAMPLE HANDLING

Endocrine reference laboratories vary in their sample collection, storage, and submission recommendations. Because of the potential for loss of certain hormones after blood collection, we generally prefer collecting blood samples into EDTA- or heparin-containing tubes and centrifuging the blood as soon as possible after collection. The plasma is stored frozen or at 4°C and shipped to the laboratory in insulated containers with frozen gel packs. Exceptions to these recommendations include the submission of samples for thyroxine (T_4) or tri-iodothyronine (T_3) measurement, which do not require cold conditions for shipment, and the submission of samples for insulin measurement, for which serum is utilized in our assay. Some samples (e.g., plasma endogenous adrenocorticotropic hormone [ACTH]) require even more stringent collection and shipment handling, including in some cases shipment

of frozen samples on Dry Ice using overnight mail delivery service.

TESTS OF THE HYPOTHALAMIC-PITUITARY-ADRENOCORTICAL (HPA) AXIS

Basal or Resting Plasma or Serum Cortisol

USE. This test is not generally recommended for any purpose; however, it is still requested by some clinicians.

PRINCIPLE. Cortisol is the major glucocorticoid secreted by the adrenal cortex in dogs and cats.

METHOD. A serum or plasma sample collected from an animal in a resting condition is tested using radioimmunoassay (RIA).

NORMAL VALUES. In dogs, normal cortisol values are 0.5 to 4.0 µg/dl (1 µg/dl = 10 ng/ml). In cats, the range is 0.3 to 5.0 µg/dl.

INTERPRETATION. A single basal plasma or serum cortisol determination is of limited diagnostic usefulness, since levels overlap in samples taken from animals with HPA disease and those with no disease of this axis.

Stress associated with sample collection or normal episodic secretion of cortisol in certain individuals may yield higher than normal values in samples taken from animals with normal HPA function.

Recent administration of glucocorticoids such as hydrocortisone, prednisolone, or prednisone may yield elevated values as a result of cross-reactivity in many cortisol RIAs.

ACTH Stimulation Test

USES. The ACTH stimulation test is used to screen for hyperadrenocorticism; to distinguish hyperadrenocorticism from iatrogenic Cushing's disease (i.e., secondary adrenocortical insufficiency with clinical signs of hyperadrenocorticism); to diagnose Addison's disease; and to monitor the response to mitotane (Lysodren) (o,p'-DDD) therapy.

PRINCIPLE. Administration of a maximal stimula-

Table 1. *Possible Sources for Substances Used in Endocrine Testing*

Substance	Source	Trade Name
Natural ACTH	Armour Pharmaceutical Suite 200 920 Harvest Drive Blue Bell, PA 19422	H. P. Acthar Gel
Synthetic ACTH	Organon Pharmaceuticals 375 Mt. Pleasant Ave. West Orange, NJ 07052	Cortrosyn
Thyroid-stimulating hormone (TSH)	Coopers Animal Health 520 West 21st St. P. O. Box 419167 Kansas City, MO 64141–0167	Dermathycin
Gonadotropin-releasing hormone (Gn-RH)	Ceva Laboratories 10551 Barkley St. Overland Park, KS 66212	Cystorelin
Dexamethasone	Schering Corporation Animal Health Division Kenilworth, NJ 07033	Azium solution
Xylazine	Haver Mobay Corporation Animal Health Division Shawnee, KS 66201	Rompun
Clonidine	Boehringer Ingelheim Pharmaceuticals 90 East Ridge P. O. Box 368 Ridgefield, CT 06877	Catapres
Metyrapone	Ciba Pharmaceutical Co. 556 Morris Ave. Summit, NJ 07901	Metopirone

tory dose of exogenous ACTH tests adrenocortical secretory capacity. ACTH is needed by the adrenal zona fasciculata and zona reticularis to synthesize and release cortisol and to maintain adrenocortical responsiveness.

METHOD. In dogs, collect a pre-ACTH blood sample for plasma or serum cortisol determination. Inject 2.2 IU/kg ACTH gel IM, and collect a post-ACTH sample 2 hr later. Alternatively, inject 0.25 mg per dog of synthetic ACTH intravenously and collect a post-ACTH sample 1 hr later. In cats, collect a pre-ACTH blood sample for plasma or serum cortisol determination. Inject 2.2 IU/kg ACTH gel IM and collect two post-ACTH samples, one at 1 hr and another at 2 hr post-ACTH. Alternatively, inject 0.125 mg per cat of synthetic ACTH intramuscularly and collect two post-ACTH samples, one at 30 min and another at 60 min post-ACTH. Two post-ACTH samples are recommended, since some cats will show peak cortisol concentrations with the first post-ACTH sample but the value may be much lower in the second sample.

NORMAL VALUES. In dogs, normal pre-ACTH cortisol values are 0.5 to 4.0 µg/dl (plasma or serum cortisol); post-ACTH normal values are 8 to 20 µg/dl. In cats, pre-ACTH normal values are 0.3 to 5.0 µg/dl; post-ACTH normal values are 5 to 15 µg/dl (peak cortisol concentration in either of the two post-ACTH samples).

INTERPRETATION. A normal response to ACTH suggests functional integrity of the HPA axis. However, approximately 15 to 20 per cent of dogs with hyperadrenocorticism show a normal response to ACTH. When this occurs in a dog suspected of having the disease, a low-dose dexamethasone suppression test (DST) is recommended.

A reduced response is seen in Addison's disease. Usually, both pre- and post-ACTH cortisol values are less than 0.5 µg/dl. Slightly greater values may occur, but the post-ACTH concentrations will be reduced compared with normal.

Reduced responses to ACTH are also seen in association with adrenocortical suppression resulting from glucocorticoid treatment (which may or may not be causing clinical signs of Cushing's disease) or during or after mitotane therapy.

Exaggerated responses to ACTH (i.e., post-ACTH cortisol of greater than 20 µg/dl) are seen in approximately 85 per cent of dogs with pituitary-dependent hyperadrenocorticism (PDH), whereas about 50 per cent of dogs with functional adrenocortical tumors (ATs) show excessive responses to ACTH. Exaggerated responses to ACTH have been documented in dogs with chronic illness not directly involving the HPA axis (Chastain et al., 1986).

The ACTH stimulation test is the recommended initial screening procedure for use in a dog with clinical signs of hyperadrenocorticism and known or possible treatment in the recent past with glucocorticoids.

Low-Dose DST (Dexamethasone Suppression Test)

USE. The low-dose DST is used as a screening test for hyperadrenocorticism.

PRINCIPLE. This test is designed to distinguish animals with hyperadrenocorticism from those not affected with this disorder. A low dose of the potent glucocorticoid dexamethasone is administered to act as a negative feedback signal suppressing ACTH and consequently cortisol.

METHOD. In dogs and cats, a pre-dexamethasone blood sample is collected for plasma or serum cortisol determination. Inject 0.01 or 0.015 mg/kg dexamethasone IV, and collect two post-dexamethasone samples, one at 4 hr and another at 8 hr post-dexamethasone. It is often advantageous to dilute the dexamethasone (1:10 dilution with sterile saline) before use to allow for accurate dosing.

NORMAL VALUES. In dogs, normal pre-dexamethasone cortisol values are 0.5 to 4.0 µg/dl; normal post-dexamethasone values are less than 1.5 µg/dl (at both 4 and 8 hr). In cats, normal pre-dexamethasone cortisol values are 0.3 to 5.0 µg/dl; normal post-dexamethasone values are less than 1.5 µg/dl (at both 4 and 8 hr).

INTERPRETATION. Approximately 90 per cent of dogs with hyperadrenocorticism fail to show normal suppression of cortisol in the low-dose DST.

Some laboratories (Peterson, 1986) recommend using a lower cortisol concentration (1 μg/dl) for the cutoff for normal at 8 hr post-dexamethasone. This value may be more accurate when the 0.015 mg/kg dose of dexamethasone is used.

Chronic non-HPA axis illness or recent or concurrent therapy with certain drugs (e.g., glucocorticoids, anticonvulsants) may be associated with a reduced suppressive effect of dexamethasone.

Suppression of cortisol concentrations to a value less than 1 μg/dl at 4 hr, with a rebound to a value greater than 1.5 μg/dl at 8 hr, would be consistent with PDH.

High-Dose DST

USE. The high-dose DST is used to differentiate PDH from AT as causes of hyperadrenocorticism.

PRINCIPLE. A high dose of dexamethasone is expected to suppress cortisol concentrations in animals with PDH, but not in those with AT.

METHOD. In dogs and cats, collect a pre-dexamethasone blood sample for plasma or serum cortisol determination. Inject 0.1 or 1.0 mg/kg dexamethasone IV, and collect two post-dexamethasone samples, one at 4 hr and another at 8 hr post-dexamethasone. We recommend using the 1.0 mg/kg dose of dexamethasone in dogs if cortisol concentrations were not suppressed in response to a previous dose of dexamethasone. The 1.0 mg/kg dose of dexamethasone should be used with caution in a dog with diabetes mellitus and, in our opinion, in dogs with basal cortisol concentrations in excess of approximately 12 μg/dl.

EXPECTED VALUES. This test is designed for use only in animals with confirmed hyperadrenocorticism (previously diagnosed based on the results of the low-dose DST, ACTH stimulation, or combined DST–ACTH stimulation test). A cortisol concentration that is less than one-half (50 per cent) of the pre-dexamethasone value at either 4 or 8 hr post-dexamethasone is consistent with PDH.

INTERPRETATION. In our experience, up to 20 per cent of dogs with PDH do not show suppression of cortisol to high doses of dexamethasone. Therefore, failure to suppress adequately to high doses of dexamethasone cannot be taken to confirm AT. Instead, further diagnostic procedures are required (such as endogenous ACTH measurement, metyrapone suppression test, imaging evaluation).

Some researchers (Peterson, 1986) who recommend the use of 1.0 mg/kg dexamethasone for the high-dose DST state that cortisol concentrations should be suppressed below 1.5 μg/dl in one of the post-dexamethasone samples to support a diagnosis of PDH.

In cats, the 1.0 mg/kg dose of dexamethasone would likely be of greater diagnostic value in the differential diagnosis of hyperadrenocorticism.

Combined DST–ACTH Stimulation Test

USE. The combined DST–ACTH stimulation test principally serves as a screening test for hyperadrenocorticism. The addition of dexamethasone suppression permits (1) identification of a percentage of animals with hyperadrenocorticism that respond normally to ACTH but fail to show normal cortisol suppression in response to dexamethasone and (2) immediate diagnosis of PDH in some animals.

PRINCIPLE. This test examines both negative feedback and adrenocortical secretory capacity in a relatively short time period.

METHOD. In dogs and cats, collect a pre-dexamethasone blood sample for plasma or serum cortisol determination. Inject 0.1 mg/kg dexamethasone IV and collect a post-dexamethasone sample 4 hr later. Immediately after collection of the post-dexamethasone sample, administer ACTH (see ACTH stimulation test protocol). Collect a post-ACTH sample (two post-ACTH samples in cats).

NORMAL VALUES. In dogs, normal pre-dexamethasone cortisol values are 0.5 to 4.0 μg/dl (plasma or serum cortisol); normal post-dexamethasone values are less than 1.0 μg/dl; and normal post-ACTH values are 8 to 20 μg/dl. In cats, normal pre-dexamethasone cortisol values are 0.3 to 5.0 μg/dl; normal post-dexamethasone values are less than 1.5 μg/dl; and normal post-ACTH values are 5 to 15 μg/dl.

INTERPRETATION. In a dog, lack of suppression in response to dexamethasone (post-dexamethasone cortisol value greater than 1.0 μg/dl), an exaggerated response to ACTH (post-ACTH cortisol value greater than 20 μg/dl), or both would be consistent with hyperadrenocorticism.

A post-dexamethasone cortisol value that is less than 50 per cent of the pre-dexamethasone value, together with an exaggerated response to ACTH, is consistent with PDH. In the authors' experience, this response pattern occurs in approximately 40 per cent of dogs with hyperadrenocorticism.

Inadequate suppression of cortisol to dexamethasone, together with an exaggerated response to ACTH, is consistent with hyperadrenocorticism. However, further tests (e.g., 1.0 mg/kg high-dose DST, endogenous ACTH measurement, metyrapone suppression) are required to differentiate PDH from AT. Similarly, further evaluation is required in a dog that exhibits a lack of suppression in response to dexamethasone but has a normal response to ACTH. The lack of cortisol suppression by dexamethasone is highly suggestive of hyper-adrenocorticism, provided that the dog has not received glucocorticoids in the recent past.

Normal results on this combined test do not absolutely rule out a diagnosis of hyperadrenocorticism. The authors recommend the low-dose DST as the next procedure if equivocal results are obtained with the combined test or if normal results are observed in a dog strongly suspected of having hyperadrenocorticism. Conversely, abnormal test results are possible in animals with chronic non–HPA-axis disease or in animals treated with certain drugs.

Plasma Endogenous ACTH Measurement

USES. Plasma endogenous ACTH measurement is used to differentiate PDH from AT as a cause of hyperadrenocorticism and to distinguish primary from secondary hypoadrenocorticism.

PRINCIPLE. Plasma ACTH concentrations are higher in animals with PDH than in those with AT, and higher in animals with primary as compared with secondary hypoadrenocorticism.

METHOD. ACTH is measured using RIA of a plasma sample. Blood should be collected from animals in a nondisturbed state into tubes with EDTA or heparin and ideally should be centrifuged at 4°C immediately after collection. Plasma should be rapidly harvested and stored frozen in plastic tubes for shipment. The samples should remain frozen until the time of assay at the laboratory. Therefore, this usually requires Dry Ice packing (several pounds) and the use of an overnight mail service.

NORMAL VALUES. In dogs, normal plasma endogenous ACTH levels are 10 to 70 pg/ml. In cats, normal values range from less than 5 to 85 pg/ml.

INTERPRETATION. Plasma ACTH concentrations are generally less than 20 pg/ml in animals with AT and in animals with secondary hypoadrenocorticism. Plasma ACTH concentrations are generally greater than 40 pg/ml in animals with PDH and usually much higher (often greater than 500 pg/ml) in animals with primary hypoadrenocorticism.

Plasma ACTH determination is of little diagnostic value for the initial diagnosis of hyperadrenocorticism. It is best used as a differentiating test once hyperadrenocorticism has been diagnosed.

Proper collection, storage, and shipment of samples are critical in obtaining accurate information with this test. Use of a reference laboratory with a validated assay for dog or cat samples is also mandatory. Users should contact the reference laboratory before collecting the sample for endogenous ACTH measurement to obtain recommendations on collection and handling.

Determination of plasma ACTH concentrations provides a more accurate means of separating PDH from AT as the cause of hyperadrenocorticism compared with the high-dose DST. Plasma ACTH measurement provides the differential diagnosis from a single determination in more than 90 per cent of the cases studied. Therefore, it is one of the most useful differentiating tests and is recommended as the initial test for this purpose. Cost and availability remain problems.

Metyrapone Suppression Test

USE. The metyrapone suppression test is used to differentiate PDH from AT as the cause of hyperadrenocorticism in dogs.

PRINCIPLE. Metyrapone inhibits the 11β-hydroxylase enzyme, thereby decreasing cortisol synthesis. After metyrapone treatment, dogs with PDH have accumulation of the precortisol metabolite 11-deoxycortisol (11-DOC), with a decrease in plasma cortisol concentrations. Dogs with AT show little or no change in 11-DOC concentrations and a decrease in cortisol values.

METHOD. Cortisol and 11-DOC are measured by RIA of EDTA plasma. Collect a pre-metyrapone sample for cortisol and 11-DOC determination. Administer metyrapone at 25 mg/kg PO every 6 hr for four consecutive treatments (the authors recommend a schedule of noon, 6 PM, midnight, and 6 AM or 1 PM, 7 PM, 1 AM, and 7 AM). Collect a post-metyrapone sample 6 hrs after the last dose of metyrapone.

EXPECTED VALUES (Michigan State University, Endocrine Diagnostic Laboratory, 517-353-0621). This test should only be used in dogs known to have hyperadrenocorticism. Ideally, post-metyrapone cortisol concentrations should be less than 50 per cent of the pre-metyrapone cortisol values. After metyrapone, 11-DOC concentrations equal to or greater than 2 μg/dl (range 2 to 12.5 μg/dl) are consistent with PDH. In contrast, 11-DOC concentrations are less than or equal to 1.2 μg/dl (range 0.1 to 1.2 μg/dl) in dogs with AT.

INTERPRETATION. If after metyrapone administration there is inadequate cortisol suppression but an increase in 11-DOC (> 2 μg/dl), a diagnosis of PDH can be made. If, however, 11-DOC concentrations are less than 2 μg/dl without appropriate cortisol suppression, the results cannot be accurately interpreted and the test should be repeated.

In dogs with extremely high pre-metyrapone cortisol concentrations (> 13 μg/dl), results of the metyrapone suppression test may be invalid. However, in our experience, all dogs with 11-DOC concentrations less than or equal to 1.2 μg/dl following metyrapone have had an AT. Only one dog with a confirmed AT had test results consistent with PDH.

If post-metyrapone 11-DOC values are between 1.2 and 2.0 μg/dl, if there is inadequate post-metyrapone cortisol suppression with an 11-DOC value of less than 2.0 μg/dl, or if the pre-metyrapone cortisol value is greater than 13 μg/dl, it is then recommended either to repeat the test or to use another method (e.g., ACTH assay or the high-dose DST) to distinguish PDH from AT.

The potential for acute adrenal insufficiency exists after metyrapone administration. However, of the more than 60 dogs tested by the authors, only 4 have experienced weakness or depression following metyrapone treatment. If these signs occur and are severe, the authors recommend discontinuing the metyrapone. Immediately collect a post-metyrapone blood sample for cortisol and 11-DOC and then administer a suitable glucocorticoid IV or IM.

Like the endogenous plasma ACTH assay, this test has the advantage of positively identifying dogs with AT. Furthermore, hospitalization of the dog for testing is not required.

TESTS OF THYROID FUNCTION

Basal or Resting Plasma or Serum Thyroxine (T_4) or Tri-iodothyronine (T_3)

USE. The basal or resting plasma or serum T_4 or T_3 test is used for initial screening for hypo- or hyperthyroidism.

PRINCIPLE. T_4 is the main secretory product of the thyroid. T_3 is also secreted by the thyroid and is additionally formed by conversion from T_4 in peripheral tissues.

METHOD. A plasma or serum sample is tested with RIA or another method.

NORMAL VALUES. In dogs, normal T_4 values are 1.0 to 4.0 μg/dl and normal T_3 values are 45 to 150 ng/dl. In cats, normal T_4 values are 0.8 to 4.0 μg/dl and normal T_3 values are 30 to 150 ng/dl.

INTERPRETATION. Measurement of T_4 provides a better assessment of thyroid function than T_3, since it is the major thyroid secretory product and its levels are less likely to be modified by nonthyroid factors.

Hypothyroidism is improbable in a dog that has a basal T_4 value of 1.5 μg/dl or greater.

Certain nonthyroidal illnesses (e.g., chronic renal failure, hyperadrenocorticism) or treatment with certain drugs (e.g., dilantin, primidone, glucocorticoids) may be associated with reduced T_4 and T_3 concentrations (but a normal thyroid). Thyroid hormone replacement therapy is not recommended in these cases.

Thyroid function in animals with borderline low T_4 concentrations, in patients affected with chronic illness, or in those animals receiving drugs that may alter T_4 values should be evaluated using another method, usually the TSH stimulation test.

T_4 and T_3 concentrations are usually elevated above the normal range in cats with hyperthyroidism. However, in some cats with this disease, T_4 and T_3 concentrations fluctuate into and out of the normal range over a period of days (Peterson et al., 1987). Therefore, if T_4 values are in the normal range and if hyperthyroidism is suspected, repeat determinations of T_4 and T_3 should be performed over a period of several days. Alternatively, the T_3 suppression test described by Peterson and Ferguson (1989) could be used.

Therapeutic monitoring for adequacy of thyroxine replacement therapy can be performed by determining the T_4 concentration in a sample collected 4 to 8 hr after a dose of the drug. T_4 concentrations should be near peak levels at this time ("ideal" post-pill T_4 concentration of 2.5 to 4.5 μg/dl).

TSH Stimulation Test

USE. The major use of the TSH stimulation test is to diagnose primary hypothyroidism in dogs.

PRINCIPLE. Although basal levels of T_4 may overlap between euthyroid and hypothyroid dogs and basal T_4 levels may be suppressed by illness or drugs, dogs with primary hypothyroidism fail to show an increase in T_4 concentrations in response to exogenous TSH, since they have reduced or no functional thyroid tissue. In contrast, the normal thyroid responds to exogenous TSH by increasing the secretory rate of T_4.

METHOD. In dogs, collect a pre-TSH blood sample for plasma or serum T_4 determination. Inject 0.25 IU/kg TSH IV or IM. (A study has shown that reconstituted TSH solutions can be effectively stored at 4°C for up to 3 weeks [Bruyette et al., 1987].) A total dose of 5 IU is recommended for dogs weighing over 20 kg. Collect a post-TSH sample at 6 to 8 hr if the TSH was given IV, or at 8 to 12 hr if the TSH was given IM.

In cats, collect a pre-TSH blood sample for plasma or serum T_4 determination. Inject a total dose of 2.5 IU TSH intramuscularly and collect a post-TSH sample at 8 to 12 hr.

NORMAL VALUES. In dogs, normal pre-TSH T_4 values are 1.0 to 4.0 μg/dl; post-TSH T_4, greater than 3.5 μg/dl. In cats, normal pre-TSH T_4 values are 0.8 to 4.0 μg/dl; post-TSH T_4, greater than 3.0 μg/dl.

INTERPRETATION. A normal response to TSH virtually rules out a diagnosis of primary hypothyroidism.

A low pre-TSH value with very little response to TSH (T_4 increase of less than 0.5 μg/dl) would be typical of primary hypothyroidism.

Borderline responses (i.e., low to low-normal pre-TSH value; some increase of T_4 in response to TSH but absolute value less than 3.5 μg/dl in a dog) may occur in association with nonthyroidal illness, treatment with certain drugs, secondary hypothyroidism, or possibly in the early stages of primary hypothyroidism. Evaluation of these results should be made with consideration of historical and clinical observations. The response to TSH should be diminished in a subsequent test if the animal is developing primary hypothyroidism.

Thyroid hormone replacement therapy is not indicated in those animals with reduced basal T_4, post-TSH T_4, or basal T_3 resulting secondarily from nonthyroidal illness (euthyroid sick syndrome) or from therapy with certain drugs (Ferguson, 1986).

TEST OF PANCREATIC ENDOCRINE FUNCTION

Measurement of Fasting Serum Insulin

USE. The measurement of fasting serum insulin assists in the diagnosis of an insulin-secreting pancreatic tumor.

PRINCIPLE. Insulin concentrations are inappropriately elevated relative to the prevailing blood glucose level in animals with insulin-secreting pancreatic tumors. Insulin concentrations are best evaluated under fasting conditions and in conjunction with blood glucose concentrations determined at the same time.

METHOD. Serum insulin is generally measured in a sample collected from an animal in a fasting condition. Our RIA method requires serum, since anticoagulants interfere in the assay. To evaluate for the presence of an insulin-secreting pancreatic tumor, a recommended procedure is to draw a blood sample in the morning and begin fasting the dog (Feldman and Nelson, 1987). Measure glucose in this sample (using a reagent strip) and in subsequent samples collected at hourly intervals. When the glucose concentration declines below 60 mg/dl, additional serum is collected for insulin and glucose (using a more refined analytic method) measurement. In most dogs, hypoglycemia will occur with 8 hr of fasting, but an occasional dog may require more than 24 hr before developing low blood glucose concentrations.

NORMAL VALUES. In dogs, fasting serum insulin ranges from 5 to 25 μU/ml and fasting serum glucose from 70 to 100 mg/dl. For cats, we have no established values in our laboratory. Our insulin RIA is invalid for cat samples.

INTERPRETATION. In a dog with normal pancreatic endocrine function, fasting serum insulin values would be expected to be in the low-normal to nondetectable range when serum glucose is less than 60 mg/dl.

A serum insulin concentration greater than the normal range (i.e., >25 μU/ml) measured in a sample with a serum glucose of less than 60 mg/dl is consistent with the presence of an insulin-secreting pancreatic tumor. An insulin concentration in the mid to upper range of normal measured under these conditions is suggestive but not diagnostic of an insulin-secreting pancreatic tumor, and the test should be repeated.

The amended insulin-to-glucose ratio is probably not a useful manipulation of insulin and glucose values for diagnosis of insulin-secreting tumors (Feldman et al., 1986).

TESTS OF GONADAL FUNCTION

Measurement of Serum or Plasma Progesterone Concentrations

USE. The major use of serum or plasma progesterone determinations is to detect ovulation.

PRINCIPLE. Progesterone is principally secreted by the corpora lutea in the bitch and queen.

METHOD. RIA of serum or plasma is the standard technique.

NORMAL VALUES. In female dogs, progesterone concentrations vary with the stage of the estrous cycle. Progesterone is low (<1 ng/ml) during anestrus and early proestrus. Progesterone begins to rise in late proestrus and continues to increase during estrus, reaching 3 to 8 ng/ml near the time of ovulation. Highest concentrations of progesterone occur about 2 to 4 weeks after ovulation and are in the range of 15 to 70 ng/ml. In later diestrus, progesterone concentrations gradually decline, reaching values near 1 ng/ml about 8 to 15 weeks after ovulation. In female cats, since the queen is an induced ovulator, progesterone concentrations remain low (<1 ng/ml) during estrus and increase after ovulation (naturally or artificially induced). Progesterone concentrations are detectably increased (above 1 ng/ml) 3 days after a successful mating stimulus and reach peak concentrations (15 to 80 ng/ml) in 2 to 3 weeks. In cases of pseudopregnancy, progesterone declines to basal concentrations (approximately 1 ng/ml or less) 5 to 6 weeks after ovulation. With pregnancy, progesterone concentrations are maintained at relatively high concentrations until approximately 3 weeks before parturition, when they begin to decline gradually (Banks, 1986). Progesterone concentrations are low at the time of parturition. Progesterone concentrations are less than 0.2 ng/ml in male dogs and cats.

INTERPRETATION. The main value of progesterone measurement is to determine whether a bitch or queen ovulated. A progesterone concentration greater than 10 ng/ml 2 to 3 weeks after estrus indicates that ovulation has likely occurred.

Determination of progesterone concentrations for the diagnosis of pregnancy is of little value, since individual profiles of progesterone overlap between pregnant bitches and bitches who have ovulated but not conceived.

Serial measurements of progesterone could potentially be used to detect deficient luteal function during an estrous cycle or pregnancy.

Other Gonadal Hormones: Testosterone and Estrogen

Testosterone circulates at a concentration of approximately 0.3 to 6.0 ng/ml in plasma of male dogs and cats. It is secreted in an episodic fashion. Testosterone concentrations are generally less than 0.1 ng/ml in female dogs except during estrus, when levels may reach 1 ng/ml. Evaluation of concentrations of this hormone for purposes of assessing fertility have generally been unrewarding. Measurement of testosterone in our experience is of limited clinical usefulness. Determination of plasma testosterone could potentially be of use in the detection of lesions in the hypothalamic-pituitary-testicular axis, or possibly to diagnose cryptorchidism.

Estrogen concentrations have been determined in the dog and cat, and fluctuations in levels of this hormone (usually estradiol 17_β is measured) have been documented during the estrous cycle. However, because absolute levels of this hormone vary between stages of the cycle, isolated determinations of estrogen appear to be of limited usefulness in documenting a particular stage of the estrous cycle in an individual dog (Concannon, 1986). Possible diagnostic uses of estrogen measurement include detection of Sertoli cell tumors in a male dog or the presence of functional ovarian tissue in a presumably spayed female.

EVALUATION OF GROWTH HORMONE

Basal Growth Hormone Concentrations, Xylazine and Clonidine Stimulation Tests

USES. Basal growth hormone concentrations and xylazine and clonidine stimulation tests are used to evaluate for the presence of acromegaly, to aid in the diagnosis of pituitary dwarfism, and to screen for adult-onset growth hormone deficiency (alopecia and hyperpigmentation).

PRINCIPLE. Growth hormone, a protein hormone secreted by the pituitary, has diverse metabolic activities in the body. In dogs, disorders involving growth hormone include acromegaly, pituitary dwarfism, and adult-onset growth deficiency (growth hormone-responsive dermatosis, or hyposomatotropism).

METHOD. In dogs, growth hormone is measured in serum samples collected before and at intervals after the injection of xylazine or clonidine. A basal blood sample is collected for serum growth hormone measurement, and xylazine, 0.3 mg/kg (Lothrop, 1987) or clonidine, 10 μg/kg (Eigenmann and Eigenmann, 1981), is given IV. Samples are collected at 15, 30, 45, and 60 min for serum growth hormone determination. Serum should be frozen and samples shipped on Dry Ice using an overnight mail service.

NORMAL VALUES (University of Tennessee Endocrine Diagnostic Laboratory, 615-546-6092). In dogs, pre-xylazine or pre-clonidine growth hormone values are 1 to 7 ng/ml, and peak-value post-xylazine or post-clonidine (usually at 15 to 30 min) values are 5 to 27 ng/ml.

INTERPRETATION. Growth hormone concentrations are generally reduced in pituitary dwarfism and adult-onset growth hormone deficiency and raised in acromegaly. However, basal levels overlap between normal dogs and those with growth hormone deficiency. Therefore, provocative testing (such as with clonidine or xylazine) provides a better method to evaluate the status of this hormone when a deficiency is suspected.

In dogs with pituitary dwarfism or adult-onset growth hormone deficiency, little or no response of plasma growth hormone concentrations to xylazine or clonidine is observed.

Basal growth hormone concentrations, and to some degree the secretory response of growth hormone to xylazine and clonidine, may be reduced in dogs with hypothyroidism or hyperadrenocorticism.

Basal growth hormone concentrations are generally elevated in acromegaly (in dogs, usually associated with endogenous or exogenous progesterone exposure). In some animals, however, it is necessary to demonstrate nonsuppressibility of growth hormone concentrations after glucose administration (1 gm/kg glucose) (Eigenmann, 1986).

OTHER HORMONES

Hormones such as luteinizing hormone, follicle-stimulating hormone, prolactin, parathyroid hormone, epinephrine, norepinephrine, glucagon, gastrin, and aldosterone have been measured in serum, plasma, or urine samples from dogs and cats. Certain endocrinology reference laboratories offer these assays for veterinarians, and users should contact these laboratories for advice on usefulness of the test, sample collection methods, and shipment requirements.

References and Supplemental Reading

Banks, D. R.: Physiology and endocrinology of the feline estrous cycle. *In* Morrow, D. A. (ed.): *Current Therapy in Theriogenology II.* Philadelphia: W. B. Saunders Co., 1986, pp. 795–800.

Bruyette, D. S., Nelson, R. W., and Bottoms, G. D.: Effect of thyrotropin storage on thyroid-stimulating hormone response testing in normal dogs. J. Vet. Intern. Med. 1:91, 1987.

Chastain, C. B., Franklin, R. T., Ganjam, V. K., et al.: Evaluation of the hypothalamic-pituitary-adrenal axis in clinically stressed dogs. J. Am. Anim. Hosp. Assoc. 22:435, 1986.

Concannon, P. W.: Clinical and endocrine correlates of canine ovarian cycles and pregnancy. *In* Kirk, R. W. (ed.): *Current Veterinary Therapy IX.* Philadelphia, W. B. Saunders Co., 1986, pp. 1214–1224.

Eigenmann, J. E.: Disorders associated with growth hormone oversecretion: Diabetes mellitus and acromegaly. *In* Kirk, R. W. (ed.): *Current Veterinary Therapy IX.* Philadelphia, W. B. Saunders Co., 1986, pp. 1006–1014.

Eigenmann, J. E., and Eigenmann, R. Y.: Radioimmunoassay of canine growth hormone. Acta Endocrinol. 98:514, 1981.

Feldman, E. C., and Nelson, R. W.: Hypoglycemia. *In* Feldman, E. C., and Nelson, R. W. (eds.): *Canine and Feline Endocrinology and Reproduction.* Philadelphia: W. B. Saunders Co., 1987, pp. 304–327.

Feldman, E. C., Schall, W. S., Kruth, S. A., et al.: Amended insulin:glucose ratio. (Letter.) J.A.V.M.A. 188:1227, 1986.

Ferguson, D. C.: Thyroid hormone replacement therapy. *In* Kirk, R. W. (ed.): *Current Veterinary Therapy IX.* Philadelphia, W. B. Saunders Co., 1986, pp. 1018–1025.

Leifer, C. E., Peterson, M. E., and Matus, R. E.: Insulin-secreting tumor: Diagnosis and medical and surgical management in 55 dogs. J.A.V.M.A. 188:60–64, 1986.

Lothrop, C.: Personal communication, 1987.

Peterson, M. E.: Canine hyperadrenocorticism. *In* Kirk, R. W. (ed.): *Current Veterinary Therapy IX.* Philadelphia, W. B. Saunders Co., 1986, pp. 963–972.

Peterson, M. E., and Ferguson, D. C.: The thyroid. *In* Ettinger, S. J. (ed.): *Textbook of Veterinary Internal Medicine.* Philadelphia, W. B. Saunders Co., 1989.

Peterson, M. E., Graves, T. K., and Cavanagh, I.: Serum thyroid hormone concentrations fluctuate in cats with hyperthyroidism. J. Vet. Intern. Med. 1:142, 1987.

GUIDELINES FOR COLLECTION, STORAGE, AND TRANSPORT OF SAMPLES FOR HORMONE ASSAY

THOMAS J. REIMERS, Ph.D.

Ithaca, New York

Estimation of hormone concentrations in blood samples by immunoassay techniques has become very useful in diagnosis of endocrine diseases and monitoring of therapy (e.g., post-pill testing for hypothyroidism) in small animal medicine. Several private, state, and university diagnostic laboratories now provide radioimmunoassay services for quantifying hormones in biologic samples collected from animals. Because very few radioimmunoassay reagents and kits were developed by manufacturers for use on serum or plasma samples from small animals, considerable effort, time, and expense have been contributed by these diagnostic endocrinology laboratories to establish reliability of radioimmunoassays. However, these laboratories, which use excellent assay procedures and provide reliable test results, are confronted daily with poor-quality samples. An accurate, specific, and precise immunoassay cannot give a diagnostically reliable test result if the sample being analyzed was collected, stored, or transported to the laboratory in a manner that destroys the hormone.

A considerable amount of information has been gathered in the human medical literature regarding proper procedures for collection and handling of samples for radioimmunoassay. However, data from studies of humans cannot always be extrapolated to other animal species. Some hormones are quite stable in blood samples from one species but deteriorate rapidly in samples from another.

This article describes some of the information that is known about correct and incorrect procedures for collecting, storing, and transporting samples for hormone analysis. It also recommends practical guidelines for sample collection and handling based on day-to-day experience obtained at the Diagnostic Laboratory at Cornell University and on research conducted at Cornell and elsewhere. Most of the guidelines apply to thyroxine (T_4), 3,5,3'-triiodothyronine (T_3), cortisol, and insulin because these are the most commonly assayed hormones in small animal medicine. Likewise, most of the information serving as a basis for the guidelines was obtained from studies of dogs.

COLLECTION OF BLOOD SAMPLES FOR ENDOCRINOLOGY TESTING

Effects of Anticoagulants, Hemolysis, and Lipemia

Several reports have been published on differences in concentrations of hormones between plasma and serum samples obtained from humans and animals (Kubasik and Sine, 1978, 1979; Bauman, 1980; Vahdat et al., 1981; Olson et al., 1981; Reimers et al., 1982b, 1983). Generally, the differences have been small or nonexistent for T_3, T_4, cortisol, insulin, and progesterone. However, many diagnostic endocrinology laboratories prefer receiving serum rather than plasma samples because they often use automated pipetting equipment that may become obstructed by fibrin clots. Regardless of the anticoagulant used, plasma samples frequently form clots after freezing and thawing.

Evacuated serum separator tubes, which have a self-contained serum separator and clot activator, are often used for collection of blood samples. The material inside the tube is inert and causes no significant effect on concentrations of T_3, T_4, cortisol, insulin, luteinizing hormone (LH), progesterone, or prolactin in serum (Reimers et al., 1982b, 1983).

Large amounts of heparin have been reported to adversely affect determination of concentrations of adrenocorticotropin (ACTH) in plasma. Apparently, heparin (at least in large amounts) traps ACTH molecules, promoting formation of high-molecular-weight aggregates that interfere with the direct radioimmunoassay of ACTH (Dupouy et al., 1980). ACTH also deteriorates rapidly in samples without anticoagulant. Therefore, to prevent significant errors in ACTH determinations, sodium or potassium ethylenediaminetetraacetic acid (EDTA) should be used as an anticoagulant and blood cells should be removed from plasma as soon as possible after collection.

Cellular elements of anticoagulated or untreated blood from cows rapidly metabolize progesterone (Holdsworth, 1980; Owens et al., 1980; Vahdat et al., 1981, 1984; Oltner and Edqvist, 1982; Reimers et al., 1983). However, no significant effect of storage on progesterone concentrations could be demonstrated in heparinized whole blood from dogs (Oltner and Edqvist, 1982).

Significant effects of hemolysis on hormone concentrations were observed in EDTA-treated blood samples collected from dogs (Reimers et al., 1982b). Neither T_4 nor cortisol concentrations were affected by hemolysis in this study. However, storage of hemolyzed blood samples for 18 hr (i.e., overnight) before centrifugation caused a dramatic decrease in concentrations of insulin (Fig. 1). This effect was seen after storage at 4°C (36 per cent decrease) as well as at room temperature (68 per cent decrease). Reductions in insulin concentrations in samples from individual dogs ranged from 42 per cent to 93 per cent when stored 18 hr at room temperature.

The effect of hemolysis on insulin is apparently enzymatic and not due to nonspecific interference by hemoglobin or other cellular products in the insulin radioimmunoassay that was used. For accurate determination of insulin concentrations, avoid

hemolysis in samples from dogs. If the plasma or serum is hemolyzed to the extent of being brick red but still translucent, discard the sample and collect another. Although not examined in great detail, lipemia does not affect concentrations of T_3, T_4, or cortisol in serum or plasma. However, if possible, avoid submitting heavily lipemic samples for analysis.

Effects of Fasting, Reproductive State, Stress, Pulsatile Secretion, Circadian Rhythms, and Drugs

Besides anticoagulants, lipemia, and hemolysis, other more subtle factors should be considered when collecting blood samples from animals for hormonal analyses. Many studies of humans and rats have shown the importance of nutritional state on evaluation of endocrine functions. In euthyroid humans, fasting caused a significant, rapid decrease in serum concentrations of T_3 without affecting T_4 concentrations (Vagenakis et al., 1975). However, basal concentrations of T_3, T_4, and cortisol in the serum of dogs were not affected by fasting for 36 hr (Reimers et al., 1986). Furthermore, fasting did not affect thyroidal and adrenocortical reserves of these hormones because results of ACTH-response and thyrotropin (TSH)-response tests were not different among fed dogs and those fasted 12, 18, 24, or 36 hr. Therefore, whether or not dogs are fasted overnight before being subjected to thyroid or adrenal functions tests will not affect reliability of the test results.

Reproductive state of animals may be an important factor to consider when examining endocrine functions of the thyroid gland and adrenal cortex. Uptake of radioiodine by the thyroid gland and its release from the gland were greater in pregnant and diestrous bitches than in anestrous bitches (Monty et al., 1979). Concentrations of T_4 were similar in serum from euthyroid diestrous (metestrous) and pregnant bitches but were greater than those in anestrous, proestrous, lactating, and male dogs before and after intravenous injection of TSH (Reimers et al., 1984). Concentrations of T_3 were greater in serum from diestrous bitches before and after TSH injection than in serum from dogs in other reproductive states. Kemppainen and Sartin (1984) reported a higher mean concentration of T_4 in anestrous females than in males from which samples were collected every 20 min for 25 hr.

Basal concentrations of cortisol did not differ among dogs of different reproductive states (Reimers et al., 1984). However, concentrations after intramuscular injection of ACTH were different (anestrus = diestrus > lactation = pregnancy = male > proestrus). In contrast, Kemppainen and Sartin (1984) observed higher 24-hr mean concen-

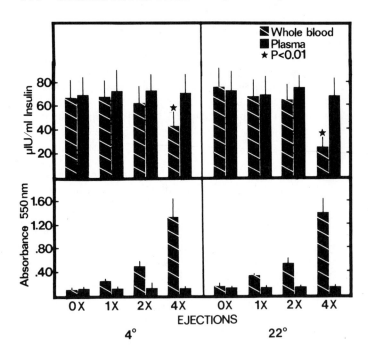

Figure 1. Mean concentrations ± SEM (n = 6 dogs) of insulin in plasma from hemolyzed blood. Whole blood or plasma was ejected through a syringe and needle once (1X), twice (2X), or four times (4X) to produce varying degrees of hemolysis (0X, no ejection). Subsamples were stored for 18 hours at 4°C or room temperature (22°C) before centrifugation and hormone assays. Relative hemolysis of all subsamples was quantified by determining absorbance at 550 nm in a spectrophotometer.

trations of cortisol in plasma samples from anestrous females than from males. The mean concentration of plasma ACTH was also higher in females. Insulin concentrations in the serum of dogs are quite variable and may be affected by reproductive state also (Reimers et al., 1982a).

Many hormones, especially cortisol and ACTH, are secreted in an episodic or circadian fashion (Kemppainen and Sartin, 1984; Peterson, 1986) and are significantly affected by stress (De Silva et al., 1986). In dogs, episodic secretion of ACTH, cortisol, and T_4 was evident, with an average of 9.0 ACTH peaks, 10.1 cortisol peaks, and 3.3 T_4 peaks in a 24-hr period (Kemppainen and Sartin, 1984). Because of this rapidly changing secretory pattern, quantification of these hormones in a single baseline sample is of little, if any, diagnostic value. Basal concentrations of ACTH and cortisol in dogs with hyperadrenocorticism are frequently within the normal range (Peterson, 1984), and normal dogs may exhibit elevated concentrations of these hormones simply because of the effect of stress on the hypothalamic-pituitary-adrenocortical axis.

In humans, the circadian rhythm of ACTH and cortisol secretion is an important consideration for timing of diagnostic tests (Cryer, 1979). Pigs, horses, humans, sheep, cattle, and monkeys generally have the highest serum or plasma concentrations of cortisol in the early morning and lowest concentrations in the evening (Weitzman et al., 1971; Bottoms et al., 1972; McNatty et al., 1972; Challis et al., 1980; Thun et al., 1981; Johnson and Malinowski, 1986). In contrast, circadian rhythms of cortisol in dogs and cats could not be detected (Johnston and Mather, 1978, 1979; Kemppainen

and Sartin, 1984; Reimers et al., 1986). In a clinical situation, the adrenocortical response to stressful effects of handling, an unfamiliar environment, and blood collection would probably override any circadian secretory pattern if it existed. Circadian rhythmicity of plasma or serum T_4 concentrations in dogs also was not evident (Kemppainen and Sartin, 1984; Reimers et al., 1986). Therefore, it is probably not necessary to begin testing thyroid or adrenocortical function in the morning or always at a consistent time of day.

A variety of drugs and hormones affect concentrations of T_3, T_4, and cortisol in blood samples regardless of the medical condition of the glands (Cryer, 1979; Cavalieri and Pitt-Rivers, 1981; Wenzel, 1981; McDonald, 1982; Ferguson, 1984). Drugs and hormones that may affect plasma or serum concentrations of T_3 or T_4 are shown in Table 1. These drugs may affect TSH secretion, synthesis of T_4 by the thyroid gland, synthesis of plasma binding proteins by the liver, binding of T_3 and T_4 to binding proteins, or peripheral deiodination of T_4 to biologically active T_3. Testing of thyroid or adrenal function while the patient is being treated with medications may give misleading results, and medications should be avoided if possible.

STORAGE OF SERUM AND PLASMA SAMPLES

Once blood is properly collected and serum or plasma is separated from cellular elements of blood, most hormones routinely analyzed for diagnostic purposes are very stable. Storage of canine serum

ble 1. *Drugs and Hormones Used in Veterinary edicine That May Affect Serum Concentrations of T_3 and T_4*

Drug	Increase T_3	Increase T_4	Decrease T_3	Decrease T_4
lrogens			X	X
bamazepine			X	X
zepam			X	X
henylhydantoin			X	X
rogens	X	X		
luorouracil	X	X		
cocorticoids			X	X
othane	X	X		
parin			X	X
ide			X	X
ilin		X		
oprusside			X	X
nobarbital			X	X
nothiazine				X
nylbutazone			X	X
nidone			X	X
pranolol			X	X
staglandins		X		
iocontrast agents		X		
cylates			X	X
onylureas			X	X
azides	X			

From Ferguson, D. C.: Vet. Clin. North Am. 14:783, 1984; nzel, K. W.: Metabolism 30:717, 1981.)

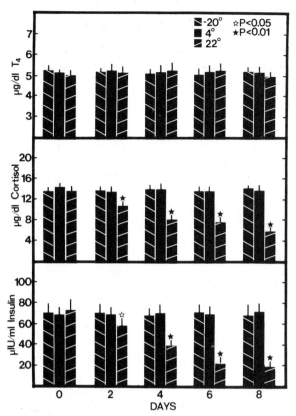

Figure 2. Mean concentrations ± SEM (n = 6 dogs) of T_4, cortisol, and insulin in canine serum stored at −20°C, 4°C, and room temperature (22°C) for 0, 2, 4, 6, and 8 days.

nples up to 8 days at 4°C did not affect concentions of T_4, cortisol, and insulin (Fig. 2); storage bovine samples for 8 days also did not affect these ee hormones or T_3, LH, prolactin, and progesone. Concentrations of T_3, T_4, LH, and prolactin l not change even when samples of serum were red at room temperature for 8 days. However, tisol concentrations in canine serum stored at)m temperature decreased 21 per cent by 2 days, per cent by 4 days, 44 per cent by 6 days, and per cent by 8 days (Fig. 2). Storing samples at)m temperature caused a 20 per cent reduction serum insulin by 2 days, a 46 per cent reduction 4 days, a 70 per cent reduction by 6 days, and a per cent reduction by 8 days. Because of this tability, serum and plasma samples must not be)red at room temperature for any significant igth of time (i.e., >12 hr). For most hormones at have been examined, it appears that storage of um samples in the refrigerator is as good as rage in the freezer, at least for 8 days (Fig. 2).)wever, it is recommended that storage time at ⊃ be minimal before freezing or submitting the nple to a diagnostic endocrinology laboratory.

Most hormones are very stable in frozen (−20°C sufficient) serum or plasma, and concentrations not change appreciably in tightly closed conners. It is standard practice for the Endocrinology .boratory at Cornell University to freeze many iall aliquots of pooled serum for monitoring reatability of a particular assay over a long period of time. Some of these aliquots are stored for nearly a year without any noticeable decrease (or increase) in hormone concentrations. Freezing and thawing (at room temperature) of serum samples up to eight times has no detrimental effects on concentrations of T_4, cortisol, or insulin (Reimers et al., 1982b).

TRANSPORTING SAMPLES FOR ENDOCRINE TESTING

Samples for endocrine testing should be submitted to the testing laboratory by the fastest possible means in order to avoid deterioration. The U.S. Postal Service has several different options for submitting samples quickly. Courier services such as UPS, Purolator, Airborne, Federal Express, Emery, and Flying Tigers also provide next-day and second-day delivery services in the United States, including Hawaii and Puerto Rico, and Canada.

Samples should be securely packaged to prevent breakage of containers or leakage of samples. Sample tubes made of polypropylene with tightly fitting caps are very resistant to breakage and serve well for submitting serum or plasma samples. Polystyrene and glass containers should be avoided. Postal service workers may refuse to handle any package that shows signs of internal breakage.

Samples that will arrive at the testing laboratory within 2 to 3 days usually do not need to be shipped with dry ice. However, it is recommended that serum or plasma samples be sent with ice packs. It is preferable to ship samples early in the week so they do not sit in a post office, airport, warehouse, or other facility over the weekend.

SUMMARY

1. Follow the laboratory's instructions regarding use of anticoagulants, storage conditions, transporting procedures, and so on. To save time and money, contact the laboratory before submitting samples of questionable quality (e.g., hemolyzed serum).

2. For T_3, T_4, cortisol, insulin, progesterone, testosterone, and estradiol, collect blood samples without anticoagulant. Store samples in the refrigerator for 6 to 8 hr to allow clotting. Centrifuge and recover serum for analysis.

3. For ACTH, collect the sample in an evacuated glass tube containing EDTA and transfer the whole blood immediately into a plastic container or collect the sample with a plastic syringe and transfer to a plastic tube containing EDTA. Centrifuge the sample immediately, collect the plasma, and freeze in a plastic container. Submit the frozen sample to the laboratory.

4. Hemolysis causes rapid deterioration of insulin in canine blood samples. For accurate test results, avoid hemolysis. Discard a hemolyzed plasma or serum sample and collect another.

5. Because reproductive state can have significant effects on concentrations of thyroid hormones, cortisol, and insulin in blood samples from dogs, the reproductive state of the patient should be noted when testing for thyroid, adrenocortical, or pancreatic function.

6. Store serum or plasma samples at 4°C or lower until submitted to the laboratory for analysis. Freeze samples when storage is expected to be longer than 3 days. Do not store samples at room temperature.

7. When possible, avoid administering medications, especially analgesics, anesthetics, and hormones, to the patient before testing thyroid or adrenocortical function.

8. Ship serum or plasma samples (never whole blood) with ice packs. Special circumstances (e.g., ACTH analysis) may require submission of samples packed in dry ice.

9. Be aware of nonspecific effects of drugs, reproductive state, fasting, secretory patterns, and other factors on hormone concentrations.

10. Avoid shipping samples on Fridays. Rather, ship samples early in the week to avoid layovers in post offices, airports, and so on.

References and Supplemental Reading

Bauman, J. E.: Comparison of radioimmunoassay results in serum and plasma. Clin. Chem. 26:676, 1980.

Bottoms, G. D., Roesel, O. F., Rausch, F. D., et al.: Circadian variation in plasma cortisol and corticosterone in pigs and mares. Am. J. Vet. Res. 33:785, 1972.

Cavalieri, R. R., and Pitt-Rivers, R.: The effects of drugs on the distribution and metabolism of thyroid hormones. Pharmacol. Rev. 33:55, 1981.

Challis, R. G., Socol, M., Murata, Y., et al.: Diurnal variations in maternal and fetal steroids in pregnant rhesus monkeys. Endocrinology 106:1283, 1980.

Cryer, P. E.: Diagnostic Endocrinology, 2nd ed. New York: Oxford University Press, 1979, pp. 55–94.

De Silva, M., Kiehm, D. J., Kaltenbach, C. C., et al.: Comparison of serum cortisol and prolactin in sheep blood sampled by two methods. Domest. Anim. Endocrinol. 3:11, 1986.

Dupouy, J. P., Chatelain, A., and Godaut, M.: Influences of heparin on ACTH distribution and immunoreactivity in plasma of the rat. In vivo and in vitro studies. J. Physiol. (Paris) 76:631, 1980.

Ferguson, D. C.: Thyroid function tests in the dog. Vet. Clin. North Am. 14:783, 1984.

Holdsworth, R. J.: Measurement of progesterone in bovine plasma and preserved whole blood samples by a direct radioimmunoassay. Br. Vet. J. 136:135, 1980.

Johnson, A. L., and Malinowski, K.: Daily rhythm of cortisol, and evidence for a photo-inducible phase for prolactin secretion in nonpregnant mares housed under non-interrupted and skeleton photoperiods. J. Anim. Sci. 63:169, 1986.

Johnston, S. D., and Mather, E. C.: Canine plasma cortisol (hydrocortisone) measured by radioimmunoassay: Clinical absence of diurnal variation and results of ACTH stimulation and dexamethasone suppression tests. Am. J. Vet. Res. 39:1766, 1978.

Johnston, S. D., and Mather, E. C.: Feline plasma cortisol (hydrocortisone) measured by radioimmunoassay. Am. J. Vet. Res. 40:190, 1979.

Kemppainen, R. J., and Sartin, J. L.: Evidence for episodic but not circadian activity in plasma concentrations of adrenocorticotrophin, cortisol and thyroxine in dogs. J. Endocrinol. 103:219, 1984.

Kubasik, N. P., and Sine, H. E.: Results for serum and plasma compared in 15 selected radioassays. Clin. Chem. 24:137, 1978.

Kubasik, N. P., and Sine, H. E.: A further comparison of radioassay results for serum and plasma. Clin. Chem. 25:135, 1979.

McDonald, L. E.: Hormones affecting metabolism. In Booth, N. H., and McDonald, L. E. (eds.): Veterinary Pharmacology and Therapeutics. Ames, Iowa: Iowa State University Press, 1982, pp. 553–592.

McNatty, K. P., Cashmore, M., and Young, A.: Diurnal variation in plasma cortisol levels in sheep. J. Endocrinol. 54:361, 1972.

Monty, D. E. Jr., Wilson, O., and Stone, J. M.: Thyroid studies in pregnant and newborn beagles, using ^{125}I. Am. J. Vet. Res. 40:1249, 1979.

Olson, P. N., Bowen, R. A., Husted, P. W., et al.: Effects of storage on concentrations of hydrocortisone (cortisol) in canine serum and plasma. Am. J. Vet. Res. 42:1618, 1981.

Oltner, R., and Edqvist, L. -E.: Changes in plasma progesterone levels during storage of heparinized whole blood from cow, horse, dog and pig. Acta Vet. Scand. 23:1, 1982.

Owens, R. E., Atkins, D. T., Rahe, C. H., et al.: Time-dependent loss of radioimmunoassayable levels of progesterone following ambient temperature incubation of heparinized bovine blood. Theriogenology 13:305, 1980.

Peterson, M. E.: Canine hyperadrenocorticism. In Kirk, R. W. (ed.): Current Veterinary Therapy IX. Philadelphia: W. B. Saunders Co., 1986, pp. 963–972.

Reimers, T. J., Cowan, R. G., McCann, J. P., et al.: Validation of a rapid solid-phase radioimmunoassay for canine, bovine, and equine insulin. Am. J. Vet. Res. 43:1274, 1982a.

Reimers, T. J., McCann, J. P., and Cowan, R. G.: Effects of storage times and temperatures on T_3, T_4, LH, prolactin, insulin, cortisol and progesterone concentrations in blood samples from cows. J. Anim. Sci. 57:683, 1983.

Reimers, T. J., McCann, J. P., Cowan, R. G., et al.: Effects of storage, hemolysis, and freezing and thawing on concentrations of thyroxine, cortisol, and insulin in blood samples. Proc. Soc. Exp. Biol. Med. 170:509, 1982b.

Reimers, T. J., McGarrity, M. S., and Strickland, D.: Effect of fasting on thyroxine, 3,5,3'-triiodothyronine, and cortisol concentrations in serum of dogs. Am. J. Vet. Res. 47:2485, 1986.

Reimers, T. J., Mummery, L. K., McCann, J. P., et al.: Effects of reproductive state on concentrations of thyroxine, 3,5,3'-triiodothyronine and cortisol in serum of dogs. Biol. Reprod. 31:148, 1984.

Thun, R., Eggenberger, E., Zerobin, K., et al.: Twenty-four-hour secretory pattern of cortisol in the bull: Evidence of episodic secretion and circadian rhythm. Endocrinology 109:2208, 1981.

Vagenakis, A. G., Burger, A., Portnay, G. I., et al.: Diversion of peripheral thyroxine metabolism from activating to inactivating pathways during complete fasting. J. Clin. Endocrinol. Metab. 41:191, 1975.

Vahdat, F., Hurtgen, J. P., Whitmore, H. L., et al.: Decline in assayable

progesterone in bovine plasma: Effect of time, temperature, anticoagulant, and presence of blood cells. Am. J. Vet. Res. 42:521, 1981.

Vahdat, F., Sequin, B. E., Whitmore, H. L., et al.: Role of blood cells in degradation of progesterone in bovine blood. Am. J. Vet. Res. 45:240, 1984.

Weitzman, E. D., Fukushima, D., Nogeire, C., et al.: Twenty-four hour pattern of the episodic secretion of cortisol in normal subjects. J. Clin. Endocrinol. 33:14, 1971.

Wenzel, K. W.: Pharmacological interference with in vitro tests of thyroid function. Metabolism 30:717, 1981.

DIABETES INSIPIDUS

RHETT NICHOLS, D.V.M.

New York, New York

Diabetes insipidus (DI) is a disorder of water metabolism characterized by polyuria, urine of low specific gravity or osmolality (so called insipid, or tasteless urine), and polydipsia. It is caused by defective secretion or synthesis of the antidiuretic hormone arginine vasopressin (central DI) or by the inability of the renal tubule to respond to this hormone (nephrogenic DI). Deficiency of vasopressin (also commonly referred to as antidiuretic hormone [ADH]) or diminished responses to vasopressin at receptor sites on the distal renal tubule and collecting duct can be partial or complete.

PHYSIOLOGY OF VASOPRESSIN (ANTIDIURETIC HORMONE)

ADH plays a fundamental role in the regulation of osmotic homeostasis. The primary effect of ADH is to conserve body fluids by reducing the rate of urine production. This antidiuretic action is achieved by promoting the reabsorption of solute-free water in the distal and collecting tubules of the kidney. The combination of ADH release and thirst mechanism ensures the maintenance of normal water and osmotic concentration of body fluids.

ADH is formed in the supraoptic and paraventricular nuclei of the hypothalamus and stored in the posterior lobe of the pituitary. Probably the most important stimulus for ADH secretion under physiologic conditions is the influence of plasma osmolality on hypothalamic osmoreceptors. At plasma osmolalities below a certain minimum or threshold level, plasma ADH is suppressed to low or undetectable levels. Above this point, plasma ADH increases dramatically in direct proportion to increases in plasma osmolality. In humans, a change in plasma osmolality of only 1 per cent is sufficient to evoke a significant change in ADH secretion.

The secretion of ADH can also be affected by changes in blood volume or pressure, nausea, hypoglycemia, the renin-angiotensin system, and nonspecific factors such as pain, emotion, and physical exercise. In addition, a large number of drugs and hormones have been implicated in the alteration of ADH secretion or the effects of ADH at the level of the renal tubule.

ADH exerts its effect by binding to specific receptors on the renal tubular cell. ADH-sensitive adenylate cyclase is then stimulated, resulting in the generation of cAMP within the cell. These intracellular events increase the number of aqueous channels on the luminal membrane. The net effect is free water reabsorption.

ETIOLOGY OF DIABETES INSIPIDUS

Central diabetes insipidus is characterized by an absolute or relative lack of circulating ADH and is classified as primary (idiopathic) or secondary in nature. The idiopathic forms of central DI are the most common in veterinary medicine. Secondary central DI usually results from head trauma or neoplasia. Although hypothalamic and pituitary tumors have been reported as potential causes of central DI, head trauma in small animals appears to be the most common cause of transient or permanent central DI in this second category.

Nephrogenic DI refers to the condition in which the renal tubule is resistant to the actions of ADH. This end-organ unresponsiveness may be related to receptor and postreceptor defects. In human patients, the rare congenital form of nephrogenic DI is believed to be an X-linked recessive disorder. Only three cases of congenital nephrogenic DI have been reported in dogs, whereas it has not been documented in the cat. Causes of acquired (secondary) nephrogenic DI, both complete and partial, include a variety of renal and metabolic disorders. These disorders include pyelonephritis, chronic renal failure, hypercalcemia, hypokalemia, hyperadrenocorticism, hyperthyroidism, hepatic failure, and pyometra.

CLINICAL FEATURES OF DIABETES INSIPIDUS

Age, Breed, Sex

Central DI may appear at any age in any breed and can affect either sex. Primary nephrogenic DI tends to be a rare congenital defect and therefore is diagnosed in young animals.

Clinical and Historical Signs

The physical examination in most dogs or cats with DI is unremarkable despite owner complaints of polyuria, polydipsia, nocturia, and incontinence. Insatiable thirst forces these animals to drink any liquid within reach, including their own urine. Because these pets are constantly seeking water, many become restless and partially anorexic and lose weight. Those animals with acquired central DI secondary to a growing pituitary or hypothalamic neoplasm may have additional signs. These include anything from visual deficits, incoordination, aimless wandering, and seizures to vague owner complaints of "ain't doing right."

Routine Laboratory Findings

Recommended initial diagnostic studies include a complete blood count (CBC), urinalysis with a urine culture, and a serum chemistry profile. Routine CBC, serum biochemical, and electrolyte profiles are generally unremarkable in dogs and cats with DI. When abnormalities are present, they are usually secondary to dehydration from water restriction by the pet owner. Such abnormalities may include a slightly increased hematocrit or hypernatremia.

The urinalysis is a major key in establishing the presence of a polyuric state. A urine specific gravity less than 1.030 in dogs and less than 1.035 in cats suggests that a concentration defect and hence polyuria exist. Most dogs with DI have a water diuresis (≤ 1.007). Urine specific gravities in cats with DI generally are in the isosthenuric range (1.008 to 1.012). Unfortunately, previously mentioned causes of acquired nephrogenic DI as well

as psychogenic polydipsia, may also present with a water diuresis.

Differential Diagnosis

In approaching the problem of polyuria and polydipsia, the clinician should keep in mind that DI is one of the least common conditions to rule out. Therefore, a practical diagnostic approach to the animal with polyuria and polydipsia is to initially rule out more common causes. For example, in the middle-aged to older dog presented with polyuria and polydipsia, a water diuresis (urine specific gravity ≤ 1.007), and normal blood work, early Cushing's syndrome and pyelonephritis are primary considerations when developing a differential diagnosis. Once Cushing's disease and pyelonephritis have been ruled out with the appropriate diagnostic testing or therapeutic trials, then less common causes such as DI and psychogenic polydipsia should be pursued.

TESTS TO DIAGNOSE DIABETES INSIPIDUS

Random Plasma Osmolality

Dogs and cats with DI have a primary polyuria with a secondary polydipsia; these animals drink excessively because they urinate excessively. Loss of free water through the kidneys results in volume contraction and increased serum osmolality. The psychogenic drinkers, on the other hand, have a primary polydipsia with a secondary polyuria; these animals urinate excessively because they drink excessively. Psychogenic drinkers tend to have lower values for serum osmolality because of chronic water overload when compared with animals with DI. It has therefore been suggested that a single random plasma osmolality test can be used to differentiate psychogenic polydipsia from DI. Unfortunately, this generalization concerning plasma osmolality is true only in a minority of so-called classic cases; most animals with DI or psychogenic polydipsia show a considerable overlapping of values. Under no circumstances should random plasma osmolality be used to distinguish nephrogenic DI from central DI.

Modified Water Deprivation Test

The modified water deprivation test is the time-honored procedure commonly used to confirm the diagnosis of DI. This test is designed to determine whether endogenous ADH is released in response to dehydration and whether the kidneys can respond to ADH. When the test is properly performed, one can differentiate central DI from nephrogenic DI and from psychogenic polydipsia. Again, all other more common differential diagnoses for polyuria and polydipsia should be ruled out prior to this procedure. Failure to recognize polyuric syndromes such as pyometra, pyelonephritis, chronic renal insufficiency, or hyperadrenocorticism prior to water deprivation may lead to an incorrect or inconclusive diagnosis or cause significant patient morbidity.

The protocol for the modified water deprivation test has been the subject of several recent reviews. The test is performed in two stages—an abrupt water deprivation test followed by a vasopressin (ADH) response test. To start the modified water deprivation test, animals are confined to a cage with no food or water and are weighed at 1- to 2-hr intervals. When greater than 5 per cent of body weight has been lost, the urinary bladder should be completely emptied and the urine checked for specific gravity or osmolality or both. Failure to concentrate urine adequately indicates that the animal has either central or nephrogenic DI with or without renal medullary washout.

If the animal fails to concentrate urine adequately following abrupt water deprivation, a vasopressin (ADH) stimulation test can be performed to help determine the cause of the disorder (central versus nephrogenic DI). Immediately following the end point of the abrupt water deprivation test, aqueous ADH (Pitressin, Parke Davis) is administered at a dose of 0.5 U/kg of body weight IM (maximum dose, 5 units). Water deprivation should be continued and the bladder emptied 30, 60, and 120 min following the ADH injection. Specific gravity or osmolality or both are determined on these urine samples. The test is now complete, and the dog or cat is then offered small amounts of water over the next few hours.

Most dogs and cats with DI lose 5 per cent of their body weight within 3 to 10 hr. Dogs and cats with complete central DI cannot concentrate urine osmolality greater than plasma osmolality (290 to 310 mOsm/kg) even with severe dehydration; however, the increase in urine osmolality after ADH administration ranges from 50 to 800 per cent greater than preinjection level. Animals with partial central ADH deficiency can increase their urine osmolality above 300 mOsm/kg after dehydration, followed by a further 10 to 50 per cent increase in urine osmolality after ADH administration. Animals with primary nephrogenic DI cannot concentrate urine to levels greater than plasma osmolality after dehydration or increase urine osmolality after ADH administration.

At times, results obtained from the modified water deprivation test are difficult to interpret and may even lead to misdiagnosis. Factors that may alter proper interpretation include renal medullary washout, enhanced antidiuretic response to low levels of ADH in patients with central DI, and abnormally elevated osmolar set points for ADH release. Some have even suggested that the use of urine osmolality as an index of plasma ADH concentration is questionable. They argue that a number of hormones such as prostaglandins, atriopeptins, and antidiuretic substances distinct from ADH can influence urine osmolality. Probably the most common problem in interpretation leading to misdiagnosis involves the unsuspected case of canine hyperadrenocorticism. Distinction between animals with partial DI and psychogenic polydipsia and those with Cushing's syndrome can be difficult to impossible based on results of the modified water deprivation test. These patients may show either (1) complete ability to concentrate urine after dehydration (suggesting psychogenic polydipsia) or (2) incomplete ability to concentrate urine after dehydration followed by a further increase of 10 to 50 per cent in urine concentration after aqueous ADH injection (suggesting partial central DI). Misdiagnosis of hyperadrenocorticism is most easily avoided by screening for this disorder (using ACTH stimulation or low-dose dexamethasone suppression testing) prior to water deprivation. At the Animal Medical Center, because of the high incidence of Cushing's syndrome in our patient population, diagnostic testing for hyperadrenocorticism is a routine consideration in the workup of a dog presented with polyuria and polydipsia. Although the modified water deprivation test may have some shortcomings, it remains a relatively safe and valuable test in the diagnostic workup of polyuria and polydipsia in small animals.

Gradual Water Deprivation

To minimize the possible effects of renal medullary washout on test results, progressive water restriction prior to abrupt water deprivation is recommended by some authorities as a standard procedure. One method is to begin water restriction three days before abrupt water deprivation. The patient is allowed twice its normal daily water requirement (120 to 150 ml/kg), divided into six to eight small portions during the initial 24 hr. Over the next 48 hr, the animal is given gradually decreasing amounts of water until normal maintenance requirements are reached (60 ml/kg).

The ADH Trial

In those cases in which owners are reluctant to hospitalize their animals for water deprivation testing, an outpatient ADH trial can be considered. Again, all other common causes of polyuria and polydipsia should first be ruled out, limiting the differential diagnosis to central DI, nephrogenic DI, psychogenic polydipsia, and various causes of medullary washout. The pet owner should measure the animal's 24-hr water intake for 2 to 3 days before the test is initiated, allowing free choice water intake. Long-acting ADH (Pitressin Tannate in Oil, Parke-Davis) is then given SC or IM. A dramatic reduction in water intake or an increase in urine concentration greater than 50 per cent would strongly suggest a deficit in ADH synthesis or release and a diagnosis of central DI. Animals with nephrogenic DI (and some cases of severe medullary washout) will not respond to ADH. Psychogenic drinkers may exhibit a mild decline in water intake because the chronically low serum osmolality from chronic water overload tends to depress ADH production.

Plasma ADH Concentrations

Endogenous plasma ADH determinations have been extremely useful in distinguishing nephrogenic DI, central DI, and psychogenic polydipsia in human patients, especially when incorporated into the water deprivation test. Such assays are currently available at several medical schools. However, because of high cost and limited availability, this test is impractical for most veterinarians.

The Hickey-Hare Test

The Hickey-Hare test first appeared in the veterinary literature in 1977 as a method to more clearly distinguish polyuric states in which medullary washout was a suspected complication. This test assesses the pituitary and renal tubular ability to reduce urine volume in response to increasing plasma osmolality. The standard protocol involves quantitating changes in urine production after intravenous administration of hypertonic saline (2.5 per cent) to a water-loaded animal. In theory, hypertonic saline administration creates a hyperosmolar environment that stimulates ADH release as well as replenishing a "washed out" medullary interstitium. A significant reduction in urine flow rate ($\leq$ 25 per cent) is indicative of a normal pituitary-renal tubule concentrating axis. Animals with psychogenic polydipsia should have reduced urine volume in response to the administration of hypertonic saline, whereas those with central DI and nephrogenic DI should not. The Hickey-Hare test appears most useful in the unusual situation of a nondiagnostic water deprivation test. The test, however, cannot be recommended on a routine basis for workup of polyuria and polydipsia because the water deprivation test is safer, easier to perform, and provides consistent and diagnostic information in the majority of cases.

TREATMENT OF DIABETES INSIPIDUS

Once the diagnosis of DI is established, specific therapy can be instituted. Animals with central DI are initially treated with long-acting ADH preparations. If the degree of polyuria remains unacceptable to the owner, the additional use of nonhormonal therapy then can be considered. Dogs and cats with nephrogenic DI are ADH resistant and therefore are not candidates for hormone replacement. The thiazide diuretics, by paradoxically decreasing urine volume, remain the only available and acceptable therapeutic option for nephrogenic DI (other than no treatment at all).

Hormonal Replacement Therapy

VASOPRESSIN TANNATE IN OIL

The most effective treatment of ADH deficiency (complete and partial central DI) is hormone replacement. Standard therapy in veterinary medicine has long been the parental administration of vasopressin tannate in oil (Pitressin Tannate in Oil, Parke-Davis). This agent is a purified preparation of ADH in repository form. Available in 1-ml ampules containing 5 U/ml, the drug can be administered by either SC or IM injection. In general, 3 to 5 units in dogs (1 to 2 units in cats) every 24 to 72 hr will give satisfactory relief of polyuria and polydipsia in most cases of central DI. It is important to vigorously shake and warm the vials prior to administration to ensure proper suspension of the active hormone, which should be visible as a brown precipitate at the bottom of the ampule. Failure to do so constitutes a common cause of treatment failure with this agent. Adverse side effects are rarely noted. Reported side effects include skin reactions, abdominal pain, and hematuria. To avoid water overload the hormone should not be given at fixed intervals but only after polyuria recurs. However, owner noncompliance with this suggestion has rarely caused problems.

DESMOPRESSIN ACETATE (DDAVP)

A synthetic ADH analogue, desmopressin acetate (DDAVP, USV Laboratories), has been approved for use in humans and now appears to be the drug of choice in the treatment of central DI. This compound, which is derived from arginine vasopressin, has increased antidiuretic activity, decreased pressor actions and side effects, and prolonged duration of action when compared with natural ADH. Experimental studies with normal dogs and spontaneous cases of central DI in dogs and cats indicate that the drug is safe for use in small animals. Slow metabolic clearance, absorption through the nasal mucosa or conjunctival lining, stability in aqueous preparations, and lack of side effects make DDAVP an excellent drug for the treatment of central DI.

DDAVP is currently available as both intranasal and injectable preparations. The intranasal form is supplied in 2.5-ml vials containing 0.1 mg/ml of solution. A small, calibrated plastic catheter comes with each ampule so that exact amounts can be measured and deposited intranasally or in the conjunctival sac. Although administration of medication to animals via the intranasal route is possible, it is not well tolerated in most cases. Drops placed into the conjunctival sac are a more suitable alternative. The dose of DDAVP in humans is usually independent of body weight. Two to four drops administered once to twice daily appear sufficient to control signs of central DI in dogs and cats. The maximal effect of the drug occurs 2 to 8 hr after administration, and the duration of DDAVP varies from 8 to 24 hr. Some animals may require only evening administration of the medication to control nocturia. In humans, a few instances of resistance to prolonged therapy with DDAVP have been reported; this has not been reported in dogs or cats.

Injectable DDAVP (DDAVP Injection, USV Laboratories) is used in humans for chronic therapy of central DI and management of temporary polyuria following head trauma or surgery in the pituitary region. However, because of its short duration of action (12 to 24 hr), which would require repeated injections, and its high cost, injectable DDAVP is not suitable for long-term management of central DI in veterinary medicine. For similar reasons, other short-acting ADH preparations such as aqueous ADH (Pitressin, Parke-Davis) and lysine vasopressin (Diapid Nasal Spray, Sandoz Pharmaceuticals) play virtually no role in the chronic therapy of central DI.

Nonhormonal Therapy

Nonhormonal therapy includes the use of agents such as chlorpropamide (Diabinese, Pfizer) and thiazide diuretics. These drugs used alone or in combination with each other or as an adjunct to hormone therapy have been efficacious in some animals with DI. Thiazide diuretics are especially useful in the treatment of nephrogenic DI.

CHLORPROPAMIDE

Chlorpropamide is an oral sulfonylurea hypoglycemic agent that has been shown to be effective in reducing polyuria in persons with partial central DI by up to 50 per cent. Chlorpropamide appears to potentiate the renal tubular effects of ADH by increasing cAMP within the cells of the tubules and collecting ducts.

The effectiveness of chlorpropamide in the treatment of canine central DI has been variable. Some clinicians report a 20 to 50 per cent reduction in urine output, while others report no effect at all. The drug has been used successfully in a cat with central DI. In humans, optimal antidiuretic activity is seen 3 to 10 days after beginning treatment. Perhaps more consistent therapeutic results may require several consecutive days of therapy. The suggested dosage of chlorpropamide is 10 to 40 mg/kg/day. Since this drug stimulates insulin secretion regular feeding schedules should be established to avoid problems with hypoglycemia. Chlorpropamide is ineffective in the treatment of nephrogenic DI.

THIAZIDE DIURETICS

Therapeutic success with ADH-resistant polyuria (nephrogenic DI) and central DI has been achieved with the use of the thiazide diuretics hydrochlorothiazide (Hydrodiuril, Merck Sharp & Dohme) and chlorothiazide (Diuril, Merck Sharp & Dohme). In some cases, daily fluid requirements have been reduced by as much as 50 to 85 per cent. Thiazides reduce total body sodium concentration by inhibiting sodium reabsorption in the ascending loop of Henle. Resultant decreased plasma sodium and osmolality inhibit the thirst center, thereby reducing water consumption. This leads to extracellular fluid volume contraction, decreased glomerular filtration rate, increased proximal tubular sodium and water reabsorption, and decreased delivery of water to the distal tubule. The net effect is a reduction in urine volume.

The dose of these drugs must be individualized for each patient. Suggested dosages for hydrochlorothiazide and chlorothiazide are 2.5 to 5.0 mg/kg b.i.d. and 20 to 40 mg/kg b.i.d., respectively. Side effects are rare but may include occasional hypokalemia.

No Therapy

Some owners elect not to treat their pets. The untreated DI patient appears to survive well as long as water is always available. In general, these are outdoor animals with free access to water at all times. Humans with untreated or poorly treated DI may suffer from hydronephrosis secondary to chronic urinary retention. This complication has not been reported in dogs or cats.

PROGNOSIS OF DIABETES INSIPIDUS

The idiopathic or congenital central DI patient has a favorable prognosis with treatment. These animals usually become asymptomatic with appropriate therapy and have normal life spans. The untreated central DI patient, on the other hand, has a guarded prognosis. These animals are constantly at risk for life-threatening dehydration from accidental water restriction or water loss. Even minor illnesses such as nonspecific vomiting and diarrhea may lead to severe dehydration. Animals with expanding hypothalamic or pituitary tumors have a grave prognosis, especially if neurologic signs are present. Central DI secondary to head trauma has a variable prognosis; spontaneous recovery may occur.

The prognosis with acquired nephrogenic DI depends on its etiology. For example, the dog with early Cushing's disease has a better prognosis than the animal with hypercalcemia of malignancy or severe pyelonephritis. Successful therapy of primary nephrogenic DI is less than ideal. Much like the untreated central DI patient, these animals are predisposed to severe dehydration after mild illness or accidental water restriction.

References and Supplemental Reading

Biewenge, W. J., vanden Brom, W. E., and Mol, J. A.: Vasopressin in polyuric syndromes in the dog. Front. Horm. Res. 17:139, 1987.

Breitschwerdt, E. B.: Clinical abnormalities of urine concentration and dilution. Comp. Cont. Ed. Pract. Vet. 3:413, 1981.

Breitschwerdt, E. B., Verlander, J. W., and Hribernik, T. N.: Nephrogenic diabetes insipidus in three dogs. J.A.V.M.A. 179:235, 1981.

Edwards, C. R.: Vasopressin analog DDAVP in diabetes insipidus, clinical and laboratory studies. Br. Med. J. 3:375, 1973.

Feldman, E. C., and Nelson, R. W.: Polydipsia and polyuria. In Feldman, E. C., and Nelson, R. W. (eds.): Canine and Feline Endocrinology and Reproduction. Philadelphia: W. B. Saunders Co., 1987, pp. 1–28.

Greene, C. E., Wong, P. L., and Finco, D. R.: Diagnosis and treatment of diabetes insipidus in two dogs using two synthetic analogues of antidiuretic hormone. J. Am. Anim. Hosp. Assoc. 15:371, 1979.

Hardy, R. M., and Osborne, C. A.: Water deprivation test in the dog: Maximal normal values. J.A.V.M.A. 174:479, 1979.

Joles, J. A., and Gruys, E.: Nephrogenic diabetes insipidus in a dog with renal medullary lesions. J.A.V.M.A. 174:830, 1979.

Kosman, M. E.: Evaluation of a new antidiuretic agent desmopressin acetate (DDAVP). J.A.M.A. 240:1896, 1978.

Lage, A. L.: Nephrogenic diabetes insipidus in a dog. J.A.V.M.A. 163:251, 1973.

Lage, A. L.: Apparent psychogenic polydipsia. In Kirk, R. W. (ed.): Current Veterinary Therapy VI. Philadelphia: W. B. Saunders Co., 1977, pp. 1098–1102.

Lage, A. L.: Nephrogenic diabetes insipidus. In Kirk, R. W. (ed.): Current Veterinary Therapy VI. Philadelphia: W. B. Saunders Co., 1977, pp. 1102–1106.

Miller, M., Moses, A. M., and Streeten, D. H. P.: Recognition of partial defects in antidiuretic hormone secretion. Ann. Intern. Med. 73:721, 1970.

Mulnix, J. A., Rijnberk, A., and Hendricks, H. J.: Evaluation of a modified water deprivation test for diagnosis of polyuric disorders in dogs. J.A.V.M.A. 169:1327, 1976.

Randall, R. V., Clark, E. C., and Bahn, R. C.: Classification of the causes of diabetes insipidus. Mayo Clin. Proc. 34:299, 1959.

Rogers, W. A., Valdex, H., Anderson, B. C., et al.: Partial deficiency of antidiuretic hormone in a cat. J.A.V.M.A. 170:545, 1977.

Schwartz-Porsche, D.: Diabetes insipidus. In Kirk, R. W. (ed.): Current Veterinary Therapy VII. Philadelphia: W. B. Saunders Co., 1980, pp. 1005–1011.

Zerbe, R. L., and Robertson, G. L.: A comparison of plasma vasopressin measurements with a standard indirect test in the differential diagnosis of polyuria. N. Engl. J. Med. 305:1539, 1981.

CANINE GROWTH HORMONE–RESPONSIVE DERMATOSIS

CLINTON D. LOTHROP, JR., D.V.M.

Knoxville, Tennessee

Canine growth hormone-responsive dermatosis, first described by Siegel in 1977, is a rare endocrine alopecia of mature dogs. The primary clinical features of this syndrome are bilaterally symmetric alopecia and hyperpigmentation occurring mainly on the trunk, caudal thighs, collar area, pinna, and tail, while sparing the head and legs. The alopecia is characterized by a retention of the secondary hairs (undercoat) with a loss of primary hairs (guard). Siegel coined the term pseudo-Cushing's syndrome to describe this disorder, because the alopecia resembles that in Cushing's syndrome. However, dogs with uncomplicated growth hormone-responsive dermatosis have normal hemograms, serum chemistries, urinalyses, and normal results of adrenal and thyroid function tests. Skin biopsies from dogs with growth hormone-responsive dermatosis are characterized by histopathologic changes consistent with an endocrine dermatosis; orthokeratotic hyperkeratosis, epidermal melanosis, dermal and epidermal thinning, follicular keratosis and telogenization, and sebaceous gland atrophy. Decreased dermal elastin content has been suggested to be a histopathologic abnormality specific for growth hormone–responsive dermatosis but is routinely seen only in dogs that have clinical signs for at least 2 years. In addition, a decreased dermal elastin content can rarely be seen in other catabolic endocrine skin disorders, such as diabetes mellitus and hyperadrenocorticism.

Growth hormone-responsive dermatosis occurs predominantly in Pomeranian, chow chow, poodle, water spaniel, keeshond, and Samoyed breeds but can occur in any breed of dog. The age of onset of growth hormone-responsive dermatosis is most commonly between 1 and 2 years but can occur at any age. There appears to be an increased incidence in male dogs of certain breeds. The hallmark of growth hormone-responsive dermatosis is the correction of integumentary abnormalities with growth hormone replacement. Growth hormone-responsive dermatosis has been suggested to be due to growth hormone deficiency occurring in the adult dog, but the pathogenesis of this syndrome has yet to be defined. Necropsy results for two dogs with growth hormone-responsive dermatosis showed moderate atrophy of the pituitary gland in one case and no pituitary abnormalities in the second case. There is no proof of a genetic inheritance of this syndrome, but the predisposition of certain breeds suggests there may be hereditary influences.

Endocrine alopecia and dwarfism occur with growth hormone deficiency in the immature dog. Pituitary dwarfism occurs most commonly in the German shepherd and Carnelian Bear Dogs and appears to be inherited as an autosomal recessive trait. This disorder differs from adult-onset growth hormone responsive dermatosis in that partial to complete deficiencies of adrenocorticotropin, thyrotropin, and gonadotropins are found along with the somatotropin deficiency. Pituitary dwarfs often appear normal until 2 or 3 months of age, at which time failure to grow is noticed. The hair coat often remains short because of inadequate development of primary hairs. The typical truncal alopecia and hyperpigmentation develop in dwarf dogs with growth hormone deficiency. Most dwarf dogs have a colloid-filled pituitary cyst at necropsy, with secondary changes in other endocrine glands. The alopecia of dwarf dogs will respond to growth hormone supplementation, but longitudinal bone growth and increased stature do not occur owing to closure of the growth plates. If concurrent hypothyroidism is present, thyroxine replacement is necessary to obtain optimal results. Although the endocrine alopecia in dwarf dogs and dogs with adult-onset growth hormone-responsive dermatosis responds to growth hormone supplementation, the presence of multiple pituitary abnormalities in dwarf dogs and differences in pituitary histopathology in these two syndromes suggests that the pathogenesis of these syndromes may be different.

DIAGNOSIS OF GROWTH HORMONE DEFICIENCY

The diagnosis of growth hormone deficiency can be confirmed by measurement of serum or plasma growth hormone. Measurement of a basal growth hormone concentration is inadequate to correctly diagnose growth hormone deficiency, since many normal dogs have a low basal growth hormone concentration. Therefore, a growth hormone response test should be performed using the alpha-adrenergic agonist clonidine (10 µg/kg) or its structural analogue xylazine (100 to 300 µg/kg). These agents stimulate growth hormone release by inducing production of endogenous growth hormone releasing factor (GRF). Alternatively, human GRF (1 to 5 µg/kg) can be used to stimulate growth hormone production. To perform a growth hormone response test, 2 to 4 ml of blood should be collected before and 15, 30, 45, 60, and 120 min after intravenous administration of either clonidine, xylazine, or GRF. After collection, the blood should be promptly centrifuged and the plasma (EDTA) or serum frozen at $-20°C$ until assayed for growth hormone. Homologous canine growth hormone radioimmunoassays are used to determine the plasma or serum growth hormone concentration. The absence of a significant increase in the plasma or serum growth hormone concentration is consistent with the diagnosis of growth hormone deficiency.

Both clonidine and xylazine are potent hypotensive agents and should be used cautiously. Side effects, at the recommended doses, range from mild drowsiness and bradycardia to complete collapse, and last from 15 to 60 min. If necessary, atropine can be used to correct the bradycardia and the alpha-adrenergic antagonists phentolamine or yohimbine can be used to antagonize the hypotensive effects of clonidine and xylazine. Hypothyroidism and hyperadrenocorticism should be ruled out with appropriate thyroid and adrenal function tests prior to performing a growth hormone response test in a dog with suspected adult-onset growth hormone-responsive dermatosis, since these disorders can potentially induce a reversible growth hormone deficiency.

CLINICAL FINDINGS IN ADULT-ONSET GROWTH HORMONE–RESPONSIVE DERMATOSIS

A growth hormone response test (using either xylazine or GRF as a provocative stimulus) was evaluated in 95 dogs with suspected adult-onset growth hormone-responsive dermatosis. All animals were in apparent normal health, except for the typical moderate to severe truncal alopecia and hyperpigmentation. Thyroid and adrenal function

Table 1. *Reproductive Status and Growth Hormone Levels in 95 Dogs With Suspected Growth Hormone-Responsive Dermatosis*

Breed*	Reproductive Status†				Normal GH Response	Diminished GH Response
	M	MC	F	FS		
Poodle (n = 14)	5	4	1	4	2	12
Pomeranian (n = 15)	7	3	1	4	0	15
Chow Chow (N = 19)	9	4	1	5	14	5
Water spaniel (n = 4)	0	0	1	3	2	2
Keeshond (n = 4)	1	1	1	1	3	1
Samoyed (n = 4)	2	1	0	1	1	3
Mixed breed (n = 4)	1	0	1	2	1	3
Other breeds (n = 25)	14	3	7	7	9	22
Total	39	16	13	27	32	63

*n = the number of different animals evaluated.

†M, male; MC, male castrate; F, female; FS, female spayed.

test results were determined to be normal in each animal. A complete or partial lack of a growth hormone response was observed in 63 of the 95 animals (Table 1). A total of 32 breeds of dogs were represented in the 95 animals suspected to have adult-onset growth hormone-responsive dermatosis. Several breeds of dogs appeared to be predisposed to adult-onset growth hormone-responsive dermatosis, including the chow chow, poodle, Pomeranian, water spaniel, keeshond, and Samoyed.

These results suggest a decreased risk in intact female dogs and an increased incidence in male dogs of the poodle, chow chow, Pomeranian, and Samoyed breeds. The finding of normal growth hormone response test results in 32 of 95 animals with suspected adult-onset growth hormone-responsive dermatosis suggests that a true growth hormone deficiency may not be present in some dogs with this syndrome of clinical alopecia. This is particularly true in the chow chow and keeshond breeds. Although these dogs usually respond to growth hormone supplementation, other causes of the alopecia must be considered.

TREATMENT

Treatment of adult-onset growth hormone-responsive dermatosis is by subcutaneous growth hormone administration. Human, porcine, and bovine growth hormone are effective in treatment. Ovine growth hormone was not effective in treating dogs, one of which subsequently responded to bovine growth hormone. Growth hormone should be administered at a dose of 0.1 U/kg three times per week for 4 to 6 weeks.

Alternatively, dogs can be treated with 2 to 5 U (<14 kg body weight) or 5.0 units (>14 kg body weight) growth hormone administered every other day for 10 treatments. Hair growth should be seen within 4 to 6 weeks after completion of therapy with either treatment protocol.

Growth hormone is diabetogenic in all species, and dogs treated with exogenous growth hormone can potentially develop transient or permanent diabetes mellitus. A fasting blood glucose level should be determined prior to and at weekly intervals during growth hormone supplementation. Growth hormone therapy should be stopped if persistent hyperglycemia develops, or else permanent diabetes mellitus may occur. Remission of clinical signs following growth hormone therapy is variable and ranges from 6 months to more than 3 years.

Growth hormone-responsive dermatosis is an endocrine alopecia of adult dogs of undefined etiology. Although most dogs respond to growth hormone replacement, it is unlikely that a true growth hormone deficiency exists in all dogs diagnosed as having adult-onset growth hormone-responsive dermatosis. Therefore, new treatment modalities will likely be developed as the etiologies of this syndrome are defined.

References and Supplemental Reading

Eigenmann, J. E.: Diagnosis and treatment of dwarfism in a German shepherd dog. J. Am. Anim. Hosp. Assoc. 17:798, 1981.

Eigenmann, J. E.: Growth hormone and insulin-like growth factor I in the dog: Clinical and experimental investigations. Domest. Anim. Endocrinol. 2:1, 1985.

Eigenmann, J. E.: Growth hormone-deficient disorders associated with alopecia in the dog. In Kirk, R. W. (ed.): *Current Veterinary Therapy IX*. Philadelphia: W. B. Saunders Co., 1986, p. 1015.

Eigenmann, J. E., and Patterson D. F.: Growth hormone deficiency in the mature dog. J. Am. Anim. Hosp. Assoc. 20:741, 1984.

Hampshire, J., and Altszuler, N.: Clonidine or xylazine as provocative tests for growth hormone secretion in the dog. Am. J. Vet. Res. 42:1073, 1981.

Lothrop, C. D., Jr.: Growth hormone response to growth hormone releasing factor in normal and suspected growth hormone deficient dogs. Pro. Am. Coll. Vet. Intern. Med. 14–42, 1986.

Parker, W. H., and Scott, D. W.: Growth hormone-responsive alopecia in the mature dog: A discussion of 13 cases. J. Am. Anim. Hosp. Assoc. 16:824, 1980.

Scott, D. W.: Growth hormone-related dermatoses in the dog. In Kirk, R. W. (ed): Current Veterinary Therapy VIII. Philadelphia: W. B. Saunders Co., 1983, p. 852.

Scott, D. W., and Walton, D. K.: Hyposomatotropism in the mature dog: A discussion of 22 cases. J. Am. Hosp. Assoc. 22:467, 1986.

FELINE ACROMEGALY (GROWTH HORMONE EXCESS)

MARK E. PETERSON, D.V.M.

New York, New York

Chronic hypersecretion of growth hormone (GH) results in acromegaly, a disease characterized by overgrowth of connective tissue, bone, and viscera. In 1975, Gembhardt and Loppnow reported an association between diabetes mellitus and acidophilic pituitary adenomas in two cats and proposed that GH oversecretion from these pituitary adenomas was responsible for the diabetic state; however, circulating GH concentrations were not determined to confirm the diagnosis of acromegaly. More recently, acromegaly has been documented in eight cats in which the diagnosis was confirmed by the demonstration of high circulating concentrations of GH, as well as the finding of an acidophilic pituitary tumor at necropsy (Eigenmann et al., 1984; Lichtensteiger et al., 1986; Peterson et al., 1986).

ETIOLOGY

In cats, as in humans, acromegaly is most often caused by a GH-secreting tumor of the pituitary gland (Lichtensteiger et al., 1986, Peterson et al., 1986). As opposed to dogs (Eigenmann, 1986), in which progestogen treatment or the increased circulating progesterone concentrations that occur during diestrus can stimulate pituitary GH overproduction (without the development of a pituitary tumor), progestogens do not appear to stimulate GH secretion in cats. We have previously reported a preliminary study of a cat that developed diabetes associated with high circulating GH values following therapy with megestrol acetate (Peterson et al., 1981). However, in that cat, the acromegalic state failed to resolve after cessation of progestogen administration, as occurs in progestogen-induced acromegaly in dogs. In addition, we have since reported that administration of relatively high dosages of megestrol acetate to normal cats for periods of 12 months also failed to produce detectable rises in circulating GH concentrations, despite the development of a diabetogenic state (Peterson, 1987).

CLINICAL FEATURES

Acromegaly results from the excessive secretion of GH in the mature animal. As in humans, feline acromegaly appears to be associated with middle or old age (approximately 8 to 14 years). All reported cases of feline acromegaly have been mixed-breed cats (domestic short- and long-hair). Seven of the eight reported cats with acromegaly have been males, suggesting a possible sex predilection.

General Appearance

In humans, the earliest recognizable signs of acromegaly are soft tissue swelling and hypertrophy of the face and extremities. Similarly, alterations in facial features and body dimensions are observed in some cats with acromegaly. GH-induced proliferation of connective tissue results in an increase in body size, most frequently manifested as marked weight gain and enlargement of the abdomen and face (Table 1). The increases in body weight may occur despite the presence of the catabolic state of unregulated diabetes mellitus. The skin may become thickened and may develop excessive folds, particularly around the head and neck. Growth and hypertrophy of all organs in the body (e.g., heart, liver, kidneys, tongue) is also a characteristic sign of acromegaly (Table 1).

Table 1. *Frequency of Clinical Signs and Abnormal Laboratory Findings in Eight Cats with Acromegly*

	No. (%) of Cats
Clinical signs	
Polyuria/polydipsia	8 (100%)
Heart murmur	7 (88%)
Cardiomegaly	7 (88%)
Hepatomegaly	7 (88%)
Nephromegaly	5 (63%)
Renal failure	5 (63%)
Large head	5 (63%)
Weight gain	4 (50%)
Arthritis	4 (50%)
Spondylosis	4 (50%)
Large mandible (prognathia inferior)	4 (50%)
Large endocrine organs	3 (38%)
Potbelly	3 (38%)
Large tongue	2 (25%)
Circling	2 (25%)
Laboratory findings	
Hyperglycemia/glycosuria	8 (100%)
Hyperproteinemia	6 (75%)
Azotemia	5 (63%)
Hyperphosphatemia	4 (50%)
Hypercholesterolemia	3 (38%)
Increased SGPT (alanine aminotransferase)	3 (38%)
Erythrocytosis	3 (38%)
Increased serum alkaline phosphatase	1 (13%)
Ketonuria	1 (13%)

Diabetes Mellitus

The most commonly recognized clinical manifestation of acromegaly in cats is insulin-resistant diabetes mellitus (Table 1). GH, especially in carnivores (particularly cats and dogs), displays powerful diabetogenic activity and appears to provoke hyperglycemia mainly by inducing peripheral insulin resistance. Excessive GH has been shown to decrease insulin receptor numbers, increase receptor binding affinity, and induce a post-receptor insulin defect similar to that observed with cortisol-induced insulin antagonism. All cats with acromegaly thus far reported have exhibited severe, persistent hyperglycemia that was relatively refractory to insulin therapy and could be controlled only with extremely large doses of exogenous insulin (30 to 130 U/day of an intermediate- or long-acting insulin). Despite the presence of such uncontrolled diabetes mellitus, the development of ketoacidosis is rare in cats with acromegaly.

Skeletal System

In some cats with acromegaly, articular changes (associated with degenerative arthritis) may be severe and crippling (Table 1). The changes result from fibrous thickening of the joint capsule and related ligaments, as well as bony overgrowth and articular cartilage proliferation. Radiographic evidence of acromegalic arthropathy includes an increase in joint space secondary to thickening of the articular cartilage, cortical thickening, osteophyte proliferation, and tufting of the terminal phalanges. Other bony changes that may occur in acromegaly include enlargement of the mandible, leading to prognathism and an overbite of the lower incisors. There also may be increased spacing between the teeth, as commonly occurs in acromegalic dogs (Eigenmann, 1986). Finally, the bony ridges of the calvarium may be thickened, and marked spondylosis deformans of the spine may be evident in some cats.

Cardiovascular System

Another prominent manifestation of acromegaly in some cats is cardiomyopathy. Cardiovascular abnormalities that may be detected on physical examination include the presence of a systolic murmur, gallop rhythm, and, especially late in the course of the disease, signs of congestive heart failure (e.g., dyspnea, muffled heart sounds, ascites) (Table 1). Radiographic findings may include mild to severe cardiomegaly, pleural effusion, and pulmonary edema. The cause of cardiac disease in acromegaly is not clear but may be related to the general growth-promoting effect of excess GH on tissues.

Nervous System

In human patients with acromegaly, peripheral neuropathy is common and results from a combination of (1) nerve entrapment (median nerve, spinal nerves, cauda equina) due to overgrowth of the surrounding ligamentous and fibrous tissue and (2) axonal demyelination of peripheral nerves associated with a proliferation of the perineurial and subepineurial elements. Central nervous system signs can also develop as a result of the extrasellar expansion of the pituitary tumor. Peripheral neuropathies have not been documented in cats with acromegaly, possibly because of the difficulty in detecting mild paresthesias, sensory losses, and muscle weakness in the cat. Although CNS signs caused by the mass effect of the expanding tumor can develop in feline acromegaly, overt neurologic signs appear to be unusual even when a large pituitary tumor is compressing and invading the hypothalamus (Table 1).

Renal System

Polyuria and polydipsia are common signs of feline acromegaly and appear to develop primarily because of the associated diabetic state. However, acromegaly also produces several other alterations in renal function. The kidney is hypertrophied, and the glomerular filtration rate and renal plasma flow may increase. The nephromegaly is also associated with an increase in both secretory and absorptive functions. In long-standing acromegaly, however, development of azotemia and clinical signs of renal failure may develop in some cats. The mechanism of impairment of renal function in feline acromegaly is not clear.

SCREENING LABORATORY TESTS

Clinicopathologic features of feline acromegaly include severe hyperglycemia and glycosuria without ketonuria, increases in hepatic serum enzyme concentrations, hyperphosphatemia, hyperproteinemia, hypercholesterolemia, and mild erythrocytosis (Table 1). Mild elevations in the serum concentrations of alanine aminotransferase and alkaline phosphatase appear to develop secondary to the hepatic lipidosis associated with the GH-induced diabetes mellitus. Hyperphosphatemia is caused by a GH-induced increase in the renal tubular reabsorption of phosphate (Corvelain et al., 1964). The mechanism of the hyperproteinemia (which is associated with a normal pattern of distribution on serum protein electrophoresis) is unclear. Mild erythrocytosis, which also develops in some cats with acromegaly, probably represents another manifestation of the anabolic effects of GH excess.

DIAGNOSIS

Feline acromegaly should be suspected in any cat that has severe insulin-resistant diabetes mellitus (persistent hyperglycemia despite daily insulin doses > 25 U/day), especially if other characteristic signs of acromegaly (especially arthropathy or cardiomyopathy) are also present. The definitive diagnosis of acromegaly generally can be established by demonstrating markedly elevated circulating GH concentrations. In mild acromegaly, however, basal GH concentrations may be only slightly elevated or may fall into the normal range. In addition, at least in human patients, it has been shown that disease conditions other than acromegaly may increase GH secretion (e.g., chronic renal failure, cirrhosis, starvation). Therefore, confirmation of a presumed acromegaly may require evaluation of pituitary GH responsiveness to a glucose suppression test. Administration of a glucose load (1 gm/kg), either orally or intravenously, normally results in suppression of circulating GH concentrations to less than 5 ng/ml within 60 min, whereas GH concentrations remain elevated in acromegaly. If circulating GH

concentrations are clearly elevated in the presence of severe hyperglycemia, as they usually are in most cats with acromegaly, such glucose suppression tests are unnecessary. Unfortunately, serum (plasma) GH determinations are not routinely performed by most veterinary commercial laboratories (at present, a validated assay for feline GH is only available at the University of Tennessee Endocrine Diagnostic Laboratory, 615-546-6092). It may be difficult for the practicing veterinarian to obtain reliable results because of the unavailability of GH radioimmunoassays that have been validated for use in cats (GH assays designed for humans will not accurately measure feline GH).

Computerized tomography (CT), if available, is a useful means to identify a mass in the region of the pituitary and hypothalamus, a finding that supports the diagnosis of acromegaly. In addition to documenting the presence of a pituitary tumor, determining the size and location of the tumor from the CT is helpful in establishing the mode of therapy (i.e., surgery, medical therapy, radiotherapy) and in monitoring the tumor response to therapy.

TREATMENT

Acromegaly can be treated in three ways—with surgery, irradiation, or medical (pharmacologic) means. In human patients, surgical excision of GH-secreting tumors is a rapid and effective treatment for acromegaly. Use of surgery has not been evaluated in cats with GH-secreting pituitary tumors. However, surgical cure is most likely to result if the pituitary tumor is small and noninvasive. Large, invasive pituitary tumors, like in the reported cats with acromegaly, are only rarely cured by surgery. Therefore, before hypophysectomy is considered as treatment, localization and determination of tumor size are critical, since surgery would be of little to no value in cats with large, invasive pituitary tumors.

Pituitary radiation therapy provides a viable alternative to neurosurgical therapy. Radiation therapy is an effective treatment for most human patients with acromegaly, with GH concentrations falling to normal or nearly normal levels in 60 to 75 per cent of patients. However, the major disadvantage of radiation treatment is that clinical improvement is slow in onset and may extend over 2 years or more. As with surgery, radiation is less effective in destroying large, invasive pituitary tumors. In one acromegalic cat treated with radiation therapy (cobalt irradiation), a dramatic decrease in the size of the tumor with remission of neurologic signs and near normalization of the serum GH concentration occurred within 2 months of therapy. Unfortunately, in that cat, relapse of the acromegalic state developed 6 months after radiation therapy. In another cat, however, radiation therapy was totally ineffective in reducing tumor size or GH secretion. Although this form of therapy may offer the best chance for control of feline acromegaly, the availability of radiation is limited.

Medical treatment for acromegaly in humans has included estrogen therapy, dopaminergic agents (e.g., bromocriptine, levodopa), and long-acting somatostatin analogues (Lamberts et al., 1985). Long-acting somatostatin derivatives have recently attracted much attention because of their efficacy in inhibiting GH secretion in human patients with acromegaly. In two cats with acromegaly, a somatostatin analogue (SMS 201-995) was administered (10 to 20 μg b.i.d. SC) for a few weeks, but no decrease in serum GH concentrations was observed in either cat. It is possible, however, that a higher daily dose and a more frequent dosing interval would be more successful in lowering circulating GH values. In support of that, three to four daily injections of SMS 201-995 (100 to 300 μg/day) are necessary in some human patients to induce maximal inhibition of GH release. However, in a third cat with acromegaly treated with SMS 201-995, daily doses as high as 200 μg/day failed to decrease serum GH concentrations (Morrison et al., 1988).

PROGNOSIS

The severity of clinical signs and the clinical course of feline acromegaly are related to both the rise in circulating GH concentrations and the duration of GH hypersecretion. The short-term prognosis for feline acromegaly appears to be relatively good. Mild to moderate cardiac disease responds well to diuretic therapy. Severe insulin-resistant diabetes mellitus can generally be satisfactorily controlled using large doses of insulin in divided daily doses, as described above. In cats with severe insulin resistance, use of an intermediate-acting insulin (e.g., NPH) is generally preferred over a longer-acting insulin (such as PZI) because the intermediate-acting insulins have a more rapid onset of action, are more rapidly absorbed into the bloodstream, and therefore have a more potent glucose-lowering effect than do the longer-acting insulin preparations. In some cats, use of a combination of regular insulin with NPH or PZI at a 1:2 ratio (one-third of total dose given as regular and two-thirds administered as NPH or PZI) may be required to control severe hyperglycemia (see p. 1019).

Despite the possibility that acromegaly may have been diagnosed late in the natural course of the disease, survival times for cats with acromegaly have ranged from 8 to 30 months. However, all of the cats do eventually die or are euthanized because of the development of severe congestive heart failure, renal failure, or an expanding pituitary tumor. Further investigations of medical, surgical, and radiation treatment of feline acromegaly are needed, as are investigations into early diagnosis of this disorder.

References and Supplemental Reading

Corvilain, J., Abramow, M., Bergans, A.: Effect of growth hormone on tubular transport of phosphate in normal and parathyroidectomized dogs. J. Clin. Invest. 43:1608, 1964.

Eigenmann, J. E.: Disorders associated with growth hormone oversecretion: Diabetes mellitus and acromegaly. In Kirk, R. W. (ed.): Current Veterinary Therapy IX. Philadelphia: W. B. Saunders Co., 1986, pp. 1006–1014.

Eigenmann, J. E., Wortman, J. A., and Haskins, M. E.: Elevated growth hormone levels and diabetes mellitus in a cat with acromegalic features. J. Am. Anim. Hosp. Assoc. 20:747, 1984.

Gembardt, C., and Loppnow, H.: Zur pathogenese des spontanen Diabetes Mellitus der katze II. Mitteilung: Azidophile adenome des hypophysenvorderlappens und diabetes mellitus in zwei Fallen. Berl. Munch. Tieraztl. Wochenschr. 89:336, 1976.

Lamberts, S. W. J., Uitterlinden, P., Verschoor, L., et al.: Long-term treatment of acromegaly with the somatostatin analogue SMS 201-995. N. Engl. J. Med. 313:1576, 1985.

Lichtensteiger, C. A., Wortman, J. A., and Eigenmann, J. E.: Functional pituitary acidophilic adenoma in a cat with diabetes mellitus and acromegalic features. Vet. Pathol. 23:518, 1986.

Morrison, S. A., Randolph, J., Lothrop, C. D.: Hypersomatotropism and insulin-resistant diabetes in a cat. J.A.V.M.A., 1988 (in press).

Peterson, M. E.: Effects of megestrol acetate on glucose tolerance and growth hormone secretion in the cat. Res. Vet. Sci. 42:354, 1987.

Peterson, M. E., Javanovic, L., and Peterson, C. M.: Insulin resistant diabetes mellitus associated with elevated growth hormone concentrations following megestrol acetate treatment in a cat. Scientific Proceedings of the American College of Veterinary Internal Medicine, 1981, p. 63.

Peterson, M. E., Taylor, R. S., Greco, D. S., et al.: Spontaneous acromegaly in the cat. Proceedings of the Fourth Annual Veterinary Medical Forum, American College of Veterinary Internal Medicine, p. 48, 1986.

CANINE PRIMARY HYPERPARATHYROIDISM

EDWARD C. FELDMAN, D.V.M.

Davis, California

DIFFERENTIAL DIAGNOSIS AND DIAGNOSTIC PLAN

Severe hypercalcemia (serum calcium > 12 mg/dl) is usually, if not always, a serendipitous finding identified in a dog's serum biochemical profile. If hypercalcemia is an animal's only problem, as usually occurs with primary hyperparathyroidism, there may be no obvious clinical signs. Clinical signs due to hypercalcemia, when present, typically consist of mild listlessness, muscle weakness, polyuria, polydipsia, or inappetence. More worrisome clinical signs are usually related to the underlying cause of hypercalcemia.

Once hypercalcemia is identified, the abnormality should be confirmed by analyzing a second blood sample. Confirmed hypercalcemia should be investigated in a logical sequence of diagnostic steps directed at identifying the associated disease that would account for the disturbance. A suspicion of any of the differential diagnoses of hypercalcemia must be maintained until a definitive diagnosis is established. Among the disorders associated with hypercalcemia are lymphosarcoma, renal failure, apocrine gland carcinoma of the anal sac, primary hyperparathyroidism, metastasis to bone of a mammary tumor or multiple myeloma, blastomyosis, hypoadrenocorticism, hypervitaminosis D, septic osteomyelitis, and disuse osteoporosis.

The initial investigative procedure should be to repeat a thorough physical examination. Of specific interest are palpation of the peripheral lymph nodes searching for lymphadenopathy to support a diagnosis of lymphosarcoma; palpating the anal sac area and performing a rectal examination in search of an anal sac carcinoma; testing the flexibility of the mandible by compressing the canine teeth, looking for laxity suggesting chronic renal disease and renal osteodystrophy; palpating as much of the skeleton as possible, looking for bone pain caused by a metastatic cancer; and checking for mammary tumors that might have metastasized to bone. The complete blood count (CBC) should be reviewed for evidence of leukemia, and the biochemistry profile should be reviewed for a variety of abnormalities including the following: (1) hyperglobulinemia, which might reflect the presence of a multiple myeloma; (2) elevation in blood urea nitrogen (BUN), creatinine, and phosphorus suggestive of renal failure or hypervitaminosis D (urine specific gravity is usually < 1.015 in dogs regardless of the cause of hypercalcemia); (3) normal or low phosphorus, which reduces the likelihood of renal failure but is encountered in a variety of other causes for hypercalcemia; (4) elevation in liver enzymes, which may be associated with neoplasias metastasizing to the liver; and (5) elevation in serum potassium and depression in serum sodium, associated with hypoadrenocorticism.

If the diagnosis is still in doubt, radiographs of the thorax are warranted. The primary purpose of this study is to rule out the presence of a cranial mediastinal mass, which would be most suggestive of lymphosarcoma. The radiographs can also be studied for abnormalities suggestive of blastomycosis or neoplasia and for skeletal abnormalities (bone lysis). Lack of definitive findings should be followed by lymph node and bone marrow biopsies, again attempting to include or rule out a diagnosis of lymphosarcoma. The next diagnostic step is ultrasonography of the abdomen, especially the liver, searching for evidence of neoplasia. When all these studies fail to identify a cause of hypercalcemia, we recommend exploratory surgery of the thyroid/parathyroid areas in searching for a functioning parathyroid tumor (primary hyperparathyroidism).

An alternative to performing lymph node and/or bone marrow biopsies, ultrasonography, or "exploratory" neck surgery would be assessment of the serum PTH concentration (Allegro Intact PTH, Nichols Institute Diagnostics). Early results from work with this assay have been promising as an aid in identifying the cause of hypercalcemia. This assay is currently being performed by the University of California, Davis, and Michigan State University. Its availability will probably continue to improve over the next few years (see next section).

NEW DIAGNOSTIC AIDS

Several new diagnostic tools deserve mention as being potentially useful. Ionized (versus total serum) calcium is the actual substance used in the multitude of intracellular functions that calcium serves. In the past, ionized blood calcium concentrations have been cumbersome to measure and unreliable, but current instrumentation offers precise and easy evaluation of this divalent cation. Thus, measurement of ionized calcium concentrations provides a more accurate and sensitive method of establishing hypercalcemia, although it is not often needed for this purpose. Rather, in cases of primary hyperparathyroidism, measurement of ionized calcium concentrations offers a more accurate means of assessing potentially life-threatening hypocalcemia following parathyroid tumor removal.

Measurement of serum immunoreactive parathyroid hormone (PTH) concentrations may provide definitive biochemical evidence in support of primary hyperparathyroidism in human beings. Recent developments in PTH assays have resulted in commercially available radioimmunoassays specific for the intact hormone, and which have been validated for canine PTH.

Finally, measurements of 1,25-dihydroxycholecalciferol (1,25[OH]$_2$D) may be useful, albeit more difficult to obtain. Since PTH is a major stimulus for the renal biosynthesis of this important dihydroxylated vitamin D metabolite, the concentration of 1,25(OH)$_2$D may be indirect evidence supporting the diagnosis of primary hyperparathyroidism (Nesbitt and Lobaugh, 1987).

Before any of these tests are recommended for use in clinical practice, we await their application to a variety of spontaneously hypercalcemic and hypocalcemic dogs to assess their usefulness. Comparison of serum calcium concentration with a simultaneously obtained serum PTH concentration has become a reliable aid in diagnosing primary hyperparathyroidism.

PRIMARY HYPERPARATHYROIDISM

In our current series, the clinical signs most often identified in 28 dogs with primary hyperparathyroidism included polydipsia/polyuria, listlessness, muscle weakness, and inappetence. Although such clinical disturbances sound obvious, one striking feature of the dogs afflicted with this hormonal disorder was a lack of easily recognized signs. Most owners who noticed problems did not consider them to be severe. Rather, they were subtle and often not mentioned on the initial history. After the laboratory abnormalities were identified and specific questions asked, some owners did relate that their dogs "might" have one or more of the signs that were pointed out.

Hypercalcemia may be related to the presence of urinary tract infections, urolithiasis with or without infection, nephrocalcinosis, and/or renal insufficiency in humans. A canine counterpart to this syndrome was noted in 14 dogs (50 per cent) in this series. Eleven dogs had urinary tract infections (which were caused by a variety of bacteria); eight had bladder, ureteral, urethral and/or renal calcium uroliths; and four had renal insufficiency.

The only consistent abnormality on CBC and serum biochemical analyses from our 28 dogs with primary hyperparathyroidism was hypercalcemia. The serum phosphorus concentration appeared to be of limited value in the diagnosis of primary hyperparathyroidism in dogs. Seventeen dogs in this series had serum phosphorus values within the reference range. Seven dogs had low serum phosphorus concentrations, and four dogs with renal insufficiency had high levels. Eleven dogs in this series had high alkaline phosphatase activities without increases in ALT (SGPT) or radiographic evidence of excessive bone resorption. Surprisingly, electrocardiograms performed on 12 of these dogs when they were hypercalcemic were not significantly different from repeated studies obtained when their serum calcium concentrations had decreased into the reference range.

Exploratory cervical surgery on 25 dogs in this series (3 dogs did not have surgery) proved to be a diagnostic and therapeutic procedure. The aim of surgery should be to identify and remove a parathyroid tumor (adenoma). This goal can be accomplished by performing a complete medical evaluation, as previously described, prior to considering cervical exploration. The surgeon should be experienced in recognizing normal versus abnormal parathyroid anatomy (Nesbitt et al., 1985). The removal of a functioning parathyroid adenoma or carcinoma results in rapid decline in PTH concentrations if glomerular filtration rate and hepatic function are normal. The serum calcium concentration usually decreased to or below the reference range within 12 to 72 hr of surgery.

Prophylactic, postsurgical vitamin D therapy using dihydrotachysterol (Hytakerol, Winthrop-Breon) is recommended. From our experience, dogs should receive dihydrotachysterol at a rate of 0.02 mg/kg/day for 3 days beginning as soon as the dog recovers from anesthesia and then 0.01 mg/kg/day for 1 week. After this time, the dose should be reduced by 25 to 50 per cent every week until it is discontinued 8 to 12 weeks later. Calcium carbonate, given orally, is also recommended. Dosage is not critical, and 1.0 to 4.0 gm/day, divided, is easily administered. The calcium dosage is tapered down at a rate consistent with the reducing vitamin D doses.

Dogs with primary hyperparathyroidism should be monitored after surgery for signs of hypocalcemia and by measuring serum calcium concentrations daily for 5 to 7 days. Dogs that did not develop tetany had a mean serum calcium concentration before surgery of 14.1 mg/dl, versus a mean of 16.6 mg/dl in dogs that did develop tetany. The likelihood of hypocalcemic tetany after surgery increases with the severity of presurgical hypercalcemia. Dogs that develop signs of hypocalcemia will usually do so 2 to 6 days after removal of a parathyroid tumor. Postoperative hypocalcemia most likely is the result of depressed secretory activity of normal parathyroid chief cells due to their long-term suppression and atrophy secondary to chronic hypercalcemia.

Clinical signs of tetany develop with various degrees of hypocalcemia. If signs of tetany are observed and hypocalcemia confirmed, calcium gluconate diluted to a 5 per cent solution can be given subcutaneously two to three times daily once any acute signs are relieved with intravenous calcium. Total intravenous dose required is variable, and calcium should be administered slowly and to effect. The dose administered SC should be that needed IV, initially. Oral administration of calcium and vitamin D should be initiated or continued as described previously. Cessation of all hypocalcemic signs usually will occur within minutes of IV calcium replacement, but restoration of serum calcium concentrations above 8.5 to 9.0 mg/dl may take several days. Subcutaneous calcium gluconate therapy should be continued for 2 to 5 days.

After surgery and release from the hospital, the animal should have serum calcium concentration monitored twice weekly for 2 weeks and then weekly for 1 month. The rate of vitamin D administration in our dogs was tapered weekly, attempting to maintain serum calcium concentrations in the low-normal reference range. Low-normal serum calcium concentrations should stimulate return of parathyroid gland function. Once the vitamin D dose is progressively reduced over a period of weeks without development of hypocalcemia, the dog may be given a trial period without medication. If signs of hypocalcemia develop, therapy can be reinstituted. Most dogs in this series were treated for 6 to 12 weeks, and therapy was reinstated in only one dog.

A potential complication of vitamin D replacement therapy is hypercalcemia from vitamin D toxicosis. Prolonged hypercalcemia may cause nephrocalcinosis, leading to renal tubular damage and irreversible renal failure. PTH or the depressed serum phosphorus concentrations or both appear to have a renal protecting effect in dogs with hypercalcemia due to primary hyperparathyroidism. Iatrogenic hypercalcemia with an associated hyperphosphatemia caused by vitamin D toxicosis is more likely to cause renal problems than is spontaneous primary hyperparathyroidism. Dogs may develop vitamin D toxicosis at any time during the postsurgery supplementation period. When hypercalcemia is discovered in a dog without evidence of renal failure, treatment with vitamin D and calcium should be discontinued and the serum calcium, BUN, and creatinine concentrations monitored. Dogs that develop both hypercalcemia and abnormal renal function also should be treated intravenously with saline solution and furosemide. This should aid in protecting renal function and decrease serum calcium concentrations. Once serum calcium concentrations decline to the reference range, daily monitoring of serum calcium will determine whether vitamin D supplementation needs to be reinstituted.

In dogs, the most common primary parathyroid lesion responsible for excessive PTH secretion is a solitary noninvasive adenoma composed of active chief cells. Twenty-six of the 28 dogs in this series had a single adenoma in one of the cervical parathyroid glands. Parathyroid carcinomas are rare but were identified in two dogs. Spontaneous primary parathyroid hyperplasia has been reported in dogs, but it is also rare (Thompson et al., 1984).

References and Supplemental Reading

Berger, B., and Feldman, E. C.: Primary hyperparathyroidism in dogs: 21 cases (1976–1986). JAVMA 191:350, 1986.

Feldman, E. C., and Nelson, R. W.: *Canine and Feline Endocrinology and Reproduction.* Philadelphia: W. B. Saunders Co., 1987, pp. 328–356.

Krook, L.: Spontaneous hyperparathyroidism in the dog. Acta Pathol. Microbiol. Scand. 41:(Suppl. 122)27, 1957.

Nesbitt, T., Crane, S. W., and Aronsohn, M.: The parathyroid. *In* Slatter, D. H., (ed.): *Textbook of Small Animal Surgery.* Philadelphia: W. B. Saunders Co., 1985, pp. 1874–1881.

Nesbitt, T., and Lobaugh, B.: Primary hyperparathyroidism in dogs (letter). J.A.V.M.A. 191:917, 1987.

Thompson, K. G., Jones, L. P., Smylie, W. A., et al.: Primary hyperparathyroidism in German shepherd dogs: A disorder of probable genetic origin. Vet. Pathol. 21:370, 1984.

Torrance, A. G., and Nachreiner, R.: Intact parathormone assay validation, sample handling, and parathyroid function testing in dogs. Proc. Am. Coll. Vet. Intern. Med. p. 725, 1988 (abstract).

HYPERCALCEMIA OF
MALIGNANCY

ROBERT E. MATUS, D.V.M.,
New York, New York

and ELEANOR C. WEIR, B.V.M.S.
New Haven, Connecticut

Malignancy-associated hypercalcemia (MAHC) is the most common cause of hypercalcemia in veterinary small animal medicine. It is a serious clinical problem that frequently leads to renal failure, encephalopathy, coma, and death early in the course of the disease. MAHC has been reported in association with spontaneously occurring tumors in dogs, cats, and horses. The canine tumors most often associated with hypercalcemia include lymphosarcoma, which is associated with hypercalcemia in 20 per cent of cases, and apocrine cell adenocarcinoma of the anal sac, in which hypercalcemia occurs with a frequency of 80 to 90 per cent. Isolated examples of other tumors associated with hypercalcemia have been reported, including adenocarcinomas of the mammary gland and nasal cavity, squamous carcinomas of the stomach and mammary gland, thyroid carcinoma, epidermoid carcinoma, and testicular interstitial cell tumors.

GENERAL PATHOGENIC MECHANISMS IN MALIGNANCY-ASSOCIATED HYPERCALCEMIA

Regardless of the species of animal afflicted or the tumor type, two general mechanisms are believed to precipitate MAHC. The first of these is local osteolytic hypercalcemia, which is thought to result from invasion of bone or bone marrow by tumor cells that elaborate locally acting bone-resorbing factors. Tumors that cause hypercalcemia via this mechanism are often hematologic in origin. Examples include multiple myeloma and, in some cases, tumors of the lymphosarcoma-leukemia complex.

Solid tumors with bone metastases are also thought to cause local osteolytic hypercalcemia, and in human patients metastatic breast cancer is frequently associated with hypercalcemia. Although hypercalcemia associated with metastatic bone disease appears to be rare in veterinary cancer patients, it has been described in canine mammary gland adenocarcinomas with bone metastases.

The precise mechanism of bone resorption in local osteolytic hypercalcemia is unclear. Rather than simple physical destruction of bone by malignant cells themselves, it is likely that local factors produced at the metastatic site stimulate osteoclastic resorption. Proposed factors include prostaglandins and, in the case of lymphoreticular malignancies, a family of proteins known as osteoclast-activating factors (OAF). These latter factors are secreted from normal and neoplastic lymphocytes *in vitro* and appear to include interleukin-1, tumor necrosis factor, lymphotoxin, and other unidentified factors.

The second mechanism of MAHC, which has recently received wide attention in human and veterinary medicine, is known as humoral hypercalcemia of malignancy (HHM). In this syndrome, the attendant hypercalcemia results from the elaboration, by tumor tissue remote from bone, of a circulating factor which causes hypercalcemia by stimulating osteoclastic bone resorption. Leading candidates for HHM factor include parathyroid hormone(PTH)-like peptides and transforming growth factor-like peptides. A protein with biologic activities similar to PTH has recently been purified from three human HHM-associated tumors, and the gene encoding this protein has been cloned (Moseley et al., 1987; Mangin et al., 1988). Although amino acid sequence analysis of this PTH-like peptide reveals significant amino-terminal sequence homology with human PTH, the remainder of the molecule is structurally different from PTH. The amino-terminal sequence homology with PTH accounts for its PTH-like properties *in vivo*. Since this protein exhibits *in vitro* bone resorption and causes hypercalcemia when infused into animals, it is likely that it is the mediator of, or plays a major role in, the syndrome of HHM.

An alternative hypothesis is that tumor-derived growth factors are mediators of bone resorption in HHM, based on the observation that these factors stimulate bone resorption *in vitro*. Evidence for their role in HHM includes demonstration of transforming growth factor activity in some HHM-associated tumors, copurification of this activity with bone-resorbing activity in tumor tissue extracts and conditioned medium, and the ability to block tumor-induced bone resorption *in vitro* with antibodies to the epidermal growth factor receptor.

PATHOGENESIS OF HYPERCALCEMIA IN CANINE LYMPHOSARCOMA AND CANINE APOCRINE CELL ADENOCARCINOMA OF THE ANAL SAC

Lymphosarcoma is the most common hematopoietic tumor and the most common cause of hypercalcemia in dogs. Studies on the pathogenesis of hypercalcemia in canine lymphosarcoma have led to conflicting results regarding the mechanism of the hypercalcemia. In one study of 18 hypercalcemic dogs with lymphosarcoma (Meuten, 1983a), bone histomorphometry showed increased osteoclastic bone resorption in only those hypercalcemic dogs with infiltration of bone marrow by neoplastic cells, suggesting that local osteolytic hypercalcemia is the pathogenic mechanism in this disease. In a second study of 19 hypercalcemic and 17 nonhypercalcemic dogs with lymphosarcoma (Weir et al., 1988), bone histomorphometry revealed increased parameters of bone resorption in those dogs with no evidence of tumor at the biopsy site, suggesting that the hypercalcemia may be humorally mediated. In the same study, the hypercalcemic dogs demonstrated an increase in fractional phosphorus excretion and in nephrogenous cAMP excretion compared with the nonhypercalcemic group, whereas plasma 1,25-dihydroxyvitamin D (1,25[OH]$_2$D) and immunoreactive PTH levels were in the low-normal range in both groups. These *in vivo* findings suggest that in some instances the hypercalcemia associated with canine lymphosarcoma is humorally mediated by a factor that is PTH-like in its ability to stimulate nephrogenous cyclic AMP excretion and to inhibit proximal tubular phosphate reabsorption. The factor appears to differ from PTH in its inability to stimulate formation of 1,25[OH]$_2$D in the kidneys, and in its lack of cross-reactivity with PTH antiserum. Studies *in vitro* have also shown that tumor tissue extracts from hypercalcemic dogs with lymphosarcoma contain a PTH-like protein, whereas tumor tissue from nonhypercalcemic do not, further suggesting that a PTH-like protein is related mechanistically to the hypercalcemia (Weir et al., 1988).

In apocrine cell adenocarcinoma of the anal sac, the mechanism of hypercalcemia is clearly humoral, since tumor resection results in normocalcemia and local or metastatic recurrence results in recurrent hypercalcemia. In a recently reported series of dogs, urinary cAMP levels and fractional phosphorus excretion were elevated, serum PTH levels were suppressed, and bone histomorphometry revealed increased bone resorption with no compensatory increase in formation, again indicating that the responsible mediator is PTH-like in some respects but non-PTH-like in others (Meuten et al., 1983b). Recent *in vitro* studies using an apocrine cell adenocarcinoma line established in nude mice have also demonstrated that tumor tissue extracts contain a PTH-like biologic activity (Rosol et al., 1986). These unfractionated extracts also exhibit *in vitro* bone-resorbing activity and transforming growth factor-like activity.

PATHOPHYSIOLOGY

In most cases of MAHC, intense bone resorption is the major source of calcium contributing to the hypercalcemic state. Intestinal calcium absorption is frequently suppressed as a result of low circulating levels of 1,25[OH]$_2$D, which is the vitamin D metabolite responsible for calcium absorption under normal circumstances. This, combined with intense bone resorption, leads to a state of severe negative calcium balance. This is in contrast to primary hyperparathyroidism, where a high plasma concentration of 1,25[OH]$_2$D contributes to hypercalcemia by increasing intestinal calcium absorption.

One additional mechanism contributing to the hypercalcemia seen in MAHC is increased renal calcium reabsorption. This is similar to although less pronounced than that in primary hyperparathyroidism in dogs, suggesting that the HHM factor causes less distal tubular calcium reabsorption than PTH.

A final mechanism of hypercalcemia that has been reported in a small number of human patients with lymphoma is the apparent secretion by the tumor of 1,25[OH]$_2$D, which causes hypercalcemia by both intestinal calcium absorption and bone resorption. Although this mechanism has not yet been reported in dogs, it should be suspected in any case of MAHC with elevated plasma concentrations of 1,25[OH]$_2$D.

From a general standpoint, hypercalcemia supervenes in MAHC when the body's compensatory ability to increase calcium excretion is overwhelmed. Early in the course of the disease, increased excretion of calcium via the kidneys and suppressed intestinal calcium absorption maintain a state of normocalcemia. The capacity of the kidneys to excrete the excess calcium load is eventually overwhelmed, and hypercalcemia develops. This process may be accelerated by reduced renal function, which develops as a result of toxic effects of calcium on the kidneys.

APPROACH TO DIAGNOSIS AND TREATMENT

The clinical management of hypercalcemia presents an interesting challenge. This abnormality has classically been considered to be a medical emergency requiring immediate treatment. We have found this paraneoplastic syndrome to be highly variable with respect to clinical signs and severity. Although hypercalcemia is commonly associated with marked alteration in renal function, the resulting changes are often insidious and chronically progressive rather than acute. We have observed fluctuations in serum calcium concentrations that may vary from day to day in dogs with hypercalcemia. A dog with lymphoma and historic moderate hypercalcemia of 12 to 13 mg/dl as adjusted for serum albumin concentration (measured calcium − measured albumin + 3.5) may demonstrate normal calcium levels of <11.5 mg/dl on referral for treatment several days later without any therapeutic intervention.

The most common clinical signs associated with hypercalcemia are polydipsia and polyuria, which are probably caused by a partial lack of response to antidiuretic hormone at the level of the distal tubule. The exact mechanism is unknown, but experimentally hypercalcemia does cause a reduction of cAMP in cells that are normally responsive to antidiuretic hormone. Prolonged hypercalcemia with hypercalciuria may also cause a decrease in renal concentration ability secondary to decreased sodium-chloride reabsorption and the occurrence of medullary washout.

As the disorder progresses, however, clinical signs such as anorexia, lethargy, neurologic disturbances, and vomiting are noted. In these dogs, serum calcium levels often exceed 15 mg/dl and associated increases in serum creatinine and urea nitrogen may also be observed. Serum phosphorus concentrations are highly variable and are associated more with glomerular filtration rate than with hypercalcemia itself. Hypercalcemic nephropathy is considered to be both a proximal and distal tubular disorder in which actual nephron degeneration occurs secondary to calcium deposition, and to this extent it is progressively irreversible at the level of the individual nephron. Renal function, however, may be stabilized at an acceptable level following appropriate treatment, depending on the extent of overall damage to the kidney.

Acute renal failure may occur secondary to prolonged hypercalcemia. Dehydration due to anorexia and vomiting or water deprivation will exacerbate renal insufficiency. Soft tissue mineralization of renal parenchyma may occur when the calcium phosphorus product exceeds 60 mg/dl and may further enhance the severity and magnitude of renal dysfunction.

Cardiac abnormalities such as shortened QT intervals and prolonged PR intervals may also be demonstrated. However, life-threatening arrhythmias are not commonly observed in dogs with calcium concentrations of less than 15 mg/dl when azotemia is not marked. Certainly, metabolic changes associated with acute renal failure and soft tissue mineralization will make the cardiac abnormalities associated with hypercalcemia more severe.

The approach to diagnosis and treatment of hypercalcemia is dictated by the physical status of the individual animal. Emergency intervention is not usually indicated, but supportive care should be instituted based on the degree of associated metabolic abnormalities observed, while proceeding with appropriate diagnostic testing to determine the underlying cause of hypercalcemia.

DIAGNOSIS OF HYPERCALCEMIA OF MALIGNANCY

In many instances, the cause of hypercalcemia will be readily apparent to the astute clinician. Lymphoproliferative disorders are the most common cause of hypercalcemia in dogs and cats. Hypercalcemia is present in approximately 20 per cent of dogs with lymphoma and 17 per cent of dogs with multiple myeloma (Weller, et al., 1982; Matus et al., 1986). In cats, hypercalcemia is extremely rare and is usually observed only in association with an advanced clinical stage of disease in lymphoma.

In lymphoma, physical examination may reveal generalized lymphadenopathy; radiographs may demonstrate an anterior mediastinal mass, hepatic or splenic enlargement, or internal lymphadenopathy; bone marrow aspiration may show infiltration by malignant lymphocytes, even in the absence of marked lymphadenopathy. Lymph node biopsy will confirm the diagnosis in the majority of cases. However, we have observed several dogs with hypercalcemia due to lymphoma in which the only demonstrable physical abnormality was moderate renomegaly. In these dogs, renal biopsy was necessary to confirm the diagnosis of lymphoma. We would now consider the use of ultrasonography to examine visceral organs for echogenic patterns consistent with infiltrative disease to be appropriate in the diagnostic evaluation of animals with hypercalcemia of unknown origin.

In myeloma, radiographs may demonstrate lytic bony lesions of the long bones, pelvis, ribs, vertebral bodies, or cranium, and biochemical profiles usually reveal a high total protein concentration with low albumin and elevated globulin levels.

Subsequent serum electrophoresis will demonstrate a monoclonal gammopathy. If myeloma is suspected, a urine sample should be analyzed for the presence of light chains of myeloma (Bence Jones) protein by either the heat precipitation method or protein electrophoresis. Bone marrow aspiration will confirm the diagnosis in the majority of cases, showing an infiltration of malignant plasma cells.

In older female dogs and occasionally in castrated male dogs, perianal or apocrine gland adenocarcinoma of the anal sac is not an uncommon cause of hypercalcemia. Routine rectal examination will reveal a space-occupying perianal mass that may be invasive and occasionally ulcerated. Careful digital rectal palpation is necessary to evaluate the sublumbar area for the presence of lymph node enlargement. Thoracic and abdominal radiographs should be performed to evaluate for any potential lymph node enlargement, pulmonary masses, or lytic bony lesions that may indicate metastasis.

Other uncommon causes of hypercalcemia of malignancy in dogs include tonsillar carcinoma, pulmonary epidermoid carcinoma, and mammary gland adenocarcinoma. Metastatic bony lesions have rarely been associated with hypercalcemia of malignancy in dogs. We have observed hypercalcemia in association with malignant mammary gland adenocarcinoma or prostatic carcinoma with bony metastases in only a few dogs.

DIFFERENTIAL DIAGNOSIS

Other, nonneoplastic diseases that may be rarely associated with hypercalcemia in dogs include the following: primary hyperparathyroidism, hypoadrenocorticism, renal disease, and more recently the infectious disease blastomycosis. Four dogs with blastomycosis demonstrated serum calcium concentrations greater than 15 mg/dl, in association with pulmonary granulomatous lesions and lymphadenopathy (Dow et al., 1986). It is possible that the production of a lymphokine or monokine associated with immune stimulation and granulomatous inflammation somehow caused the observed hypercalcemia in these dogs.

Primary hyperparathyroidism due to parathyroid adenoma is an uncommon disease in dogs. Physical examination and subsequent radiographic and biochemical evaluation are usually unremarkable, with the exception of repeatable hypercalcemia. Plasma immunoreactive PTH levels should be obtained if possible to document a marked increase in circulating PTH. A reliable midregion radioimmunoassay for PTH in dogs is currently available through the University of Minnesota, College of Veterinary Medicine, Veterinary Diagnostic Laboratory, 1943 Carter Ave., St. Paul, MN, 55108. Surgical exploration of the neck and removal of the involved parathyroid gland is the diagnostic and therapeutic procedure of choice in dogs in which primary hyperparathyroidism is suspected. The major complication of surgery is the occurrence of hypocalcemia (Weir et al., 1986).

SUPPORTIVE MANAGEMENT OF HYPERCALCEMIA

Clinically, volume expansion is the most appropriate treatment for hypercalcemia. Administration of NaCl intravenously at maintenance levels (approximately 20 to 40 ml/kg divided t.i.d.) should be instituted following initial replacement of estimated loss due to dehydration. The use of NaCl promotes renal calcium excretion because of the relationship of sodium and calcium reabsorption. Should the animal demonstrate adequate ability to handle this increased fluid and solute load over 24 hr, the fluid administration may be increased to 5 per cent above maintenance levels and furosemide (Lasix) added to the treatment regimen at a dosage of 2 mg/kg IV b.i.d. to t.i.d. Furosemide enhances calcium excretion by the inhibition of chloride reabsorption and concurrent decrease in calcium absorption by the renal tubule. Furosemide should not be administered until adequate hydration is achieved and assessment of renal function is established. Inappropriate use of this diuretic in the absence of adequate fluid administration may potentiate dehydration and initiate a vicious cycle of decreased renal perfusion, potentiating hypercalcemia-induced nephropathy. Thiazide diuretics should never be used because they cause decreased urinary excretion of calcium and therefore may potentiate hypercalcemia.

Glucocorticoids are useful agents in the treatment of hypercalcemia but should not be used initially in the management of an animal with hypercalcemia of unknown origin. Although agents such as prednisone and dexamethasone cause decreased intestinal absorption and increased urinary excretion of calcium, their use may make the definitive diagnosis of the cause of hypercalcemia difficult. The most common cause of hypercalcemia of malignancy in dogs and cats is lymphoma. Glucocorticoids are lymphocytolytic and may alter lymph node architecture and patterns of lymphocyte infiltration in bone marrow, making the pathologic diagnosis extremely uncertain. We cannot recommend the use of a clinical trial of glucocorticoids as a diagnostic procedure in the pursuit of a cause of hypercalcemia of unknown origin.

Diphosphonates have recently been used in human and veterinary medicine to control unrelenting hypercalcemia. These compounds decrease calcium levels, primarily by blocking osteoclast-mediated bone resorption. The use of the investigational agent dichloromethylene diphosphonate (10 to 30 mg/kg

PO b.i.d. to t.i.d.) resulted in improvement of hypercalcemia in two dogs with parathyroid adenomas in which serum calcium concentrations were decreased from greater than 15 ng/dl to less than 12 mg/dl after 3 to 4 days of therapy (Couto and Chew, 1987). Another dog with hypercalcemia of malignancy associated with a nonresectable perianal gland adenocarcinoma demonstrated a decrease in serum calcium concentration from 15 mg/dl to 10 mg/dl following 10 days of diphosphonate treatment. This allowed palliative chemotherapy of the malignancy to be instituted (Couto and Chew, 1987). The diphosphonate etidronate disodium, IV infusion (Didronel, Norwich Eaton), is commercially available but to our knowledge has not been clinically evaluated in the treatment of hypercalcemia in dogs or cats. The use of diphosphonate treatment is apparently contraindicated in the face of severe azotemia (creatinine >5 mg/dl) in humans, as the drug is excreted by the kidney.

Other agents that may be of potential benefit in the supportive treatment of hypercalcemia include the prostaglandin inhibitors; aspirin, indomethacin (Indocin, Merck Sharp & Dohme), and piroxicam (Feldene, Pfizer). Studies in dogs, however, have not shown that the prostaglandins are a major factor in the occurrence of hypercalcemia of malignancy in either lymphoma or apocrine gland adenocarcinoma. Perhaps the most logical use of these analgesics would be in the treatment of hypercalcemia of malignancy associated with metastatic carcinoma to bone. This condition is rare in dogs. Potential complications of the use of these antiprostaglandin agents include severe gastrointestinal ulceration and hemorrhage and aggravation of existing renal failure.

The antineoplastic agent mithramycin (Mithracin, Miles Pharmaceuticals) has occasionally been used in the treatment of hypercalcemia of malignancy in dogs with lymphoma and perianal or apocrine gland adenocarcinoma. Although effective in lowering serum calcium concentration, the drug is highly toxic to the hematopoietic system and, in our experience, causes severe thrombocytopenia. The drug is administered once a day for 2 to 4 days at a dosage of 25 μg/kg IV, in combination with fluid therapy. The use of this drug should be restricted to dogs with otherwise refractory hypercalcemia in which other palliative treatment to reduce tumor volume may be attempted following successful short-term management of acute, severe hypercalcemia.

In human medicine, a promising approach to the supportive treatment of hypercalcemia associated with malignancy is the combined use of glucocorticoids and calcitonin. The hypocalcemic effect of the polypeptide hormone calcitonin is principally due to an inhibition of bone resorption. It is initially extremely effective in rapidly lowering serum calcium concentration, but an "escape" phenomenon is observed after several days of administration. The use of glucocorticoids in combination with calcitonin has allowed for a more sustained lowering of serum calcium concentrations in human patients and is considered by some physicians to be first-line therapy for short-term control of severe hypercalcemia. The use of calcitonin for treatment of hypercalcemia has not been evaluated in veterinary medicine.

PROGNOSIS FOLLOWING PRIMARY TREATMENT OF MALIGNANCY

In dogs with lymphoma and myeloma associated with hypercalcemia, the prognosis for response and survival following chemotherapy is considerably worse than in those dogs that have lymphoma and normal serum calcium concentrations (Weller et al., 1982; Matus et al., 1986). However, the individual response to treatment and subsequent survival may vary greatly. Other factors such as clinical stage of disease, degree of renal insufficiency, and coagulation abnormalities all affect the prognosis in dogs with lymphoma and hypercalcemia. Appropriate fluid administration and blood product support may allow for the successful induction of treatment. However, the severely compromised animal with marked azotemia, hypercalcemia, and a large clinical tumor burden is prone to acute renal failure, thrombosis, disseminated intravascular coagulation, and possible death despite supportive care.

The prognosis for dogs with perianal or apocrine gland adenocarcinoma of the anal sac must be guarded. In our experience, successful surgical removal of the tumor may be associated with prolonged normalization of serum calcium concentrations. The malignancy is prone to recur, however, and metastasis to regional lymph nodes may either be present at the time of diagnosis or may occur within a few months following surgical removal. Successful surgical resection of the involved sublumbar lymph nodes can be accomplished in approximately 50 per cent of those dogs with radiographic evidence of lymph node enlargement. In many instances the nodes are invasive, however, and only biopsy for confirmation of malignancy is possible. Distant pulmonary metastasis is an uncommon occurrence. We have used chemotherapy to treat only a few dogs with inoperable apocrine gland adenocarcinoma and have not been overly impressed with our ability to control the malignancy. It is possible that in certain cases, the use of carefully planned radiation therapy may be of benefit in the control of local disease and regional metastasis, with chemotherapy reserved for the treatment of distant metastasis.

References and Supplemental Reading

Chew, D. J., and Meuten, D. J.: Disorders of calcium and phosphorus metabolism. Vet. Clin. North Am. 12:411, 1982.

Couto and Chew: Personal communication, 1987.

Dow, S. W., Legendre, A. M., Stiff, M. S., et al.: Hypercalcemia associated with blastomycosis in dogs. J.A.V.M.A. 188:706, 1986.

Fields, A., Josse, R. G., and Bergsagel, D. E.: Metabolic Emergencies. In DeVita, V. T., Hellman, S., and Rosenberd, S. A. (eds.): Cancer, Principals and Practice of Oncology, 2nd ed. Philadelphia: J. B. Lippincott Co., 1985, pp. 1866–1872.

Insogna, K. L., and Broadus, A. E.: Hypercalcemia of malignancy. Ann. Rev. Med. 38:241, 1987.

Mangin, M., Webb, A. C., and Dreyer, B. E.: Identification of a parathyroid hormone-like peptide from a human tumor associated with humoral hypercalcemia of malignancy. Proc. Natl. Acad. Sci. (in press).

Matus, R. E., Leifer, C. E., MacEwen, E. G., et al.: Prognostic factors for multiple myeloma in the dog. J.A.V.M.A. 188:1288, 1986.

Meuten, D. J.: Hypercalcemia. Vet. Clin. North Am. 14:891, 1984.

Meuten, D. J., Kociba, G. J., Capen, J. J., et al.: Hypercalcemia in dogs with lymphosarcoma: Biochemical, ultrastructural and histomorphometric investigations. Lab. Invest. 40:553, 1983a.

Meuten, D. J., Segre, G. V., Capen, C. C., et al.: Hypercalcemia in dogs with adenocarcinoma derived from apocrine glands of the anal sac. Lab. Invest. 48:428, 1983b.

Moseley, J. M., Kubota, M., Diefenbach-Jagger, H., et al.: Parathyroid hormone-related protein purified from a human lung cancer cell line. Proc. Natl. Acad. Sci. 84:5048, 1987.

Mundy, G. R., Ibbotson, K. J., D'Souza, S. M., et al.: The hypercalcemia of cancer. N. Engl. J. Med. 310:1718, 1984.

Rosol, T. J., and Capen, C. C.: In vitro bone resorption and transforming growth factor activities in hypercalcemic canine adenocarcinoma tumor line (CAC-8) maintained in nude mice. (Abstract.) J. Bone Min. Res. 1(Suppl. 1):180, 1986.

Rosol, T. J., Capen, C. C., and Brooks, C. L.: Bone and kidney adenylate cyclase-stimulating activity produced by a hypercalcemic canine adenocarcinoma line (CAC-8) maintained in nude mice. Cancer Res. 47:690, 1987.

Rosol, T. J., Capen, C. C., Minkin, C., et al.: In vitro bone resorption activity produced by a hypercalcemic adenocarcinoma line (CAC-8) in nude mice. Calcif. Tissue Int. 39:3361, 1986.

Weir, E. C., Norrdin, R. W., Barthold, S. W., et al.: Primary hyperparathyroidism in a dog: Biochemical, bone histomorphometric, and pathologic findings. J.A.V.M.A. 189:1471, 1986.

Weir, E. C., Norrdin, R. W., Matus, R. E., et al.: Humoral hypercalcemia of malignancy in canine lymphosarcoma. Endocrinology 122:602, 1988.

Weller, R. E., Theilen, G. H., and Madewell, B. R.: Chemotherapeutic responses in dogs with lymphosarcoma and hypercalcemia. J.A.V.M.A. 181:891, 1982.

TREATMENT OF CANINE HYPOTHYROIDISM

RICHARD W. NELSON, D.V.M.

W. Lafayette, Indiana

Thyroid hormone supplementation is indicated for the treatment of confirmed hypothyroidism and for tentatively diagnosing hypothyroidism through clinical response to trial therapy. The initial therapeutic approach is similar for both situations and involves the administration of thyroid hormone preparations that are either synthetic or of animal origin (Table 1).

Preparations of animal origin include desiccated thyroid and thyroglobulin. The variable biologic activity and shelf life of these preparations may result in a poor initial response to therapy or relapse of clinical signs despite owner compliance (Devlin and Watanabe, 1966; Rosychuk, 1982). Because of these potential problems, thyroid preparations of animal origin are not routinely recommended for the treatment of hypothyroidism, especially if response to trial therapy is being used to establish a diagnosis.

The pharmaceutical and clinical problems associated with thyroid preparations of animal origin led to the development of synthetic preparations of thyroxine (T_4), 3,5,3'-triiodothyronine (T_3), or a combination of both. Synthetic preparations are sodium salts of T_4 and T_3 and have better stability and standardization of potency when compared with the products of animal origin. They are preferred for the treatment of hypothyroidism.

INITIAL THERAPY WITH SODIUM LEVOTHYROXINE

Synthetic levothyroxine (synthetic T_4) is the initial thyroid hormone supplement of choice for treating hypothyroidism. The oral administration of synthetic T_4 should result in normal serum concentrations of both T_4 and T_3, attesting to the fact that these products are able to be converted to the more metabolically active T_3 by peripheral tissues. The plasma half-life of sodium levothyroxine is between 12 and 16 hr, and peak plasma concentrations are reached from 4 to 12 hr after administration (Nesbitt et al, 1980; Rosychuk, 1982). The plasma half-life and time of peak plasma concentration vary, and this variability has led to a wide range of recommendations for dosage and frequency of administration. Remember, however, that the initial dosage and frequency of administration are merely a starting point. Because of variability in absorption and

Table 1. *Some of the Thyroid Hormone Replacement Products Currently Available for Use in Dogs*

Synthetic Products
Levothyroxine
Synthroid (Flint)
Soloxine (Daniels)
Levothroid (Rorer)
Levoid (Nutrition Control Products)
Noroxine (Vortech)
Thyro-Tab (Vet-A-Mix)
Liothyronine
Cytobin (Norden)
Cytomel (SmithKline)
Levothyroxine and Liothyronine
Euthroid (Warner/Chilcott)
Thyrolar (Armour)
Animal Products
Desiccated Thyroid
Thyroid (Lilly)
Armour Thyroid (Rorer)
Thyroid Strong (Marion)
Thyrar (Rorer)
S-P-T (Fleming)
Thyroglobulin
Proloid (Parke-Davis)

metabolism, the dosage and frequency may require alterations before a complete clinical response is observed.

A brand name rather than a generic T_4 product should be used initially, because some dogs do not seem to respond as well to generic brands. Generic T_4 should be used only after a clinical response is observed following the administration of brand name T_4 products. Our initial dosage of sodium levothyroxine is 20 μg/kg body weight (0.1 mg/4.5 kg) every 12 hr. Some dogs require sodium levothyroxine twice a day to prevent clinical signs, but others only require it once a day. By initially administering the hormone twice daily, both groups of dogs should benefit. Conversely, once-daily therapy will only benefit the group of dogs with slower metabolism and longer duration of effect of the hormone supplement. The large therapeutic index (i.e., margin of safety) will prevent the development of thyrotoxicosis in most dogs that are receiving twice-daily T_4 supplements but that really only need once-daily treatment. Once clinical signs of hypothyroidism have completely resolved after treatment with twice-daily T_4 supplements, a once-daily regimen (using a T_4 dose of 20 μg/kg/day) should then be evaluated.

The dosage of sodium levothyroxine should initially be reduced to 5 μg/kg twice daily in dogs with concurrent cardiac problems. Thyroid supplementation increases basal cellular metabolism and oxygen consumption, increases heart rate, and may reduce ventricular filling time. A sudden increase in demand for oxygen delivery to peripheral tissues, plus the chronotropic effects of T_4, may place undue stress on a poorly functioning heart, causing decom-

pensation and signs of congestive heart failure. In addition, adjustments in the dosage of digitalis may be necessary in a patient that had previously compensated congestive heart failure and that is placed on thyroid hormone supplementation (Eichelbaum, 1976). For these dogs, the lower dosage of sodium levothyroxine may be gradually increased over the ensuing 3 to 4 weeks to allow compensation for the alterations in cellular metabolism.

RESPONSE TO THERAPY

With appropriate therapy, all of the clinical and clinicopathologic alterations associated with hypothyroidism are reversible. Clinical improvement should be seen within 4 to 6 weeks of initiating therapy, and some changes may be noted within the first week, depending on the thyroid hormone-responsiveness of the tissue. Increases in mental alertness, activity, and appetite are usually the initial signs of improvement and are seen within the first week, followed by noticeable improvement in the skin within the first month. Although some hair regrowth usually occurs within the first month, complete regrowth and a significant reduction in hyperpigmentation of the skin may be delayed for several months. The hair coat may in fact worsen initially, as old hair is shed in large quantities. Obesity, if due to hypothyroidism, should also be improving within a month after initiating therapy. Reproductive abnormalities, especially hypospermia and anestrus, are usually the last alterations to normalize. Clinicopathologic alterations (e.g., nonregenerative anemia, hyperlipidemia) also frequently do not resolve for several months.

THERAPEUTIC MONITORING

Therapeutic monitoring includes evaluation of the clinical response to thyroid hormone supplements and, if necessary, the measurement of serum thyroid hormone concentrations prior to and following sodium levothyroxine administration. Thyroid supplementation should be continued for a minimum of 1 to 3 months before evaluating the effectiveness of treatment. Further monitoring of therapy is probably not needed in dogs with confirmed hypothyroidism if clinical improvement is observed in conjunction with a lack of complications. If a diagnosis of hypothyroidism is being established by evaluating response to trial therapy, the thyroid hormone supplement should be withdrawn once the clinical signs have resolved. If clinical signs begin to recur, hypothyroidism should be suspected and either thyroid hormone testing should be performed to confirm the diagnosis or thyroid supplementation should be reinitiated. If the clinical signs do not recur following withdrawal of thyroid hormone supplementation, thyroid hormone-responsive disease and not hypothyroidism should be suspected. Thyroid hormone supplementation should not be reinitiated in this situation.

The primary indications for measuring serum thyroid hormone concentrations following initiation of therapy are lack of response to therapy and the development of thyrotoxicosis. A poor response to therapy may be due to an incorrect diagnosis, inappropriate dose or frequency of administration of sodium levothyroxine, use of thyroid supplements of animal origin, poor intestinal absorption of levothyroxine, serum antithyroid hormone antibodies, and possibly peripheral conversion defects. Measuring serum thyroid hormone concentrations while the dog is receiving the thyroid hormone supplement will help identify the cause of the poor response. Before measuring serum thyroid hormone concentrations, however, inadequate owner compliance in administering the hormone or use of outdated preparations should be investigated.

Another indication for measuring serum thyroid hormone concentrations is the development of thyrotoxicosis. Fortunately, excessive administration of thyroid supplements resulting in signs of thyrotoxicosis (e.g., polyuria, polydipsia, polyphagia, weight loss, panting, nervousness, aggressive behavior) is unusual in dogs owing to the rapid catabolism and excretion of thyroid hormone by the liver and kidneys. Nevertheless, thyrotoxicosis may develop in a dog with concurrent renal or hepatic dysfunction or following excessive administration of thyroid hormone supplements. If signs suggestive of thyrotoxicosis develop in a dog receiving thyroid supplementation, the medication should be discontinued. The signs should resolve within 1 to 3 days if they are due to the thyroid medication. Once the signs have resolved, a lower dosage should be initiated and serum thyroid hormone concentrations evaluated in 2 to 4 weeks.

When monitoring therapy, serum thyroid hormone concentrations should be measured prior to and 6 to 8 hours following sodium levothyroxine administration. Ideally, this will allow the clinician to evaluate the peak and trough of the serum concentrations and thus enable assessment of dosage, frequency of administration, and adequacy of intestinal absorption. Serum T_3 concentrations can also be evaluated concurrently. Although serum thyroid hormone concentrations may be measured once the hormone has been given for at least five times the plasma half-life of the hormone (i.e., 5 to 10 days for T_4, 1 to 2 days for T_3), it is preferable to wait at least a month after beginning therapy since the increased metabolic rate may change the rate of T_4 and T_3 catabolism (Rogers et al., 1975). Possible results for pre- and postpill serum thyroid hormone concentrations and recommendations

for changes in therapy are given in Table 2. If the dose of thyroid hormone supplement and the dosing schedule are appropriate, the serum thyroid hormone concentrations (both T_3 and T_4) should be within or above the normal basal range in all blood samples evaluated. Adjustments should be made in the dosage, frequency of administration, or type of thyroid hormone supplement (i.e., sodium liothyronine) if the dog has a poor response to therapy and one or more serum thyroid hormone concentrations are below the normal basal range. Conversely, the diagnosis of hypothyroidism should be reconsidered if the dog has a poor response to therapy and all serum thyroid hormone concentrations are within or above the normal basal range.

Postpill serum thyroid hormone concentrations (especially T_4) are frequently above the normal range. In our experience, approximately 50 per cent of dogs receiving 20 μg sodium levothyroxine/kg body weight once or twice daily will have postpill serum T_4 concentrations in excess of 50 ng/ml (normal 15 to 35 ng/ml). Of these, approximately 20 per cent will have serum T_4 concentrations in excess of 75 ng/ml, with no apparent deleterious effects or signs of thyrotoxicosis. Documentation of serum thyroid hormone concentrations above the normal range, without concurrent clinical signs of thyrotoxicosis, is not an absolute indication to reduce the dosage of sodium levothyroxine. However, we recommend a reduction in dosage whenever postpill serum T_4 concentrations exceed 100 ng/ml.

Perhaps the biggest diagnostic dilemma is presented by a dog in which trial therapy is used to tentatively establish a diagnosis of hypothyroidism, the clinical response to thyroid hormone supplementation is poor, and serum T_4 concentrations are normal but serum T_3 concentrations remain low despite therapy. In our experience, the majority of these dogs are euthyroid and the clinical signs are due to another problem. Low serum T_3 concentrations are frequently found in euthyroid dogs and are most likely due to the thyroid's minimal secretion of T_3 compared with T_4, the primary intracellular location of T_3, the influence of concurrent illness on thyroid hormone physiology and metabolism (i.e., sick euthyroid syndrome), and possibly anti-T_3 antibodies that interfere with the radioimmunoassay used for measuring serum T_3 (Feldman and Nelson, 1987). Trial therapy with sodium liothyronine may be tried, but it will usually be ineffective in producing a beneficial response in a dog that has failed to respond to sodium levothyroxine and that has serum T_4 concentrations in the normal range.

THERAPY WITH SODIUM LIOTHYRONINE

Sodium liothyronine (synthetic T_3) is not the initial thyroid supplement of choice. Sodium lioth-

Table 2. *Therapeutic Recommendations Based on Results of Evaluation of Serum Thyroid Hormone Concentrations in Dogs Receiving Synthetic Thyroid Hormone Supplements*

Serum Thyroid Hormone Concentration		Daily Frequency of Administration	Clinical Signs of Thyrotoxicosis	Recommendation
Prepill	Postpill			
Normal	Normal	—	—	No change; re-evaluate diagnosis if signs still present
Normal or increased	Increased	—	Absent	No change unless $T_4 > 100$ ng/ml, then reduce dosage 25 per cent; re-evaluate diagnosis if signs still present
Normal or increased	Increased	—	Present	Reduced dosage 25 per cent; re-evaluate diagnosis if signs still present
Low	Normal or increased	Once (T_4)	—	Increased frequenxy to b.i.d.
		b.i.d.(T_3)	—	Increase frequency to t.i.d.
Low	Normal or increased	b.i.d. (T_4)	—	Increase dosage
		t.i.d. (T_3)	—	Increase dosage
Low	Low	—	—	Increase dosage; consider intestinal malabsorption, antithyroid hormone antibodies

yronine supplementation results in normal serum T_3 but low to nondetectable serum T_4 concentrations, whereas sodium levothyroxine therapy results in normal serum levels of both T_3 and T_4. It is currently believed that normalization of both serum T_4 and T_3 provides the most nearly normal intracellular concentrations of T_3 in all tissues, thus producing euthyroidism (Larsen et al., 1981). Nevertheless, liothyronine therapy is indicated when levothyroxine therapy has failed to achieve a response in a dog with confirmed hypothyroidism.

The most plausible explanation for failure to respond to a T_4 supplement is impaired absorption of levothyroxine from the intestinal tract. The majority of intestinal absorption of orally administered levothyroxine occurs in the ileum and colon (Cottle and Veress, 1965; Chung and Van Middlesworth, 1967). Absorption is influenced by the form in which the hormone is administered (e.g., gelatin capsule versus albumin carrier) and by intraluminal contents, including plasma proteins, soluble dietary factors, and intestinal flora (Brennan, 1980). All of these bind thyroid hormone and impair absorption. In humans, between 40 and 80 per cent of orally administered levothyroxine is absorbed into the circulation, the remainder being excreted in the feces. Excessive intraluminal binding of T_4 could limit the absorption of T_4 by the intestinal tract. Impaired absorption of sodium levothyroxine should be suspected when basal serum T_4 and T_3 concentrations are low and there is no increase in serum concentrations following oral levothyroxine administration. Antithyroid hormone antibodies that interfere with the radioimmunoassay technique should also be considered in this situation. Liothyronine therapy may help if impaired intestinal absorption is suspected. In contrast to thyroxine, T_3 is almost completely absorbed from the human intestine (95 per cent versus 40 to 80 per cent). This more complete absorption reflects less binding affinity of intestinal contents for T_3, especially plasma proteins secreted into the bowel lumen (Hays, 1970).

Another theoretic indication for liothyronine therapy is impaired ability to convert T_4 to T_3 by peripheral tissues, thus greatly reducing the formation of the metabolically active form of thyroid hormone. Conversion defects should be suspected when (1) basal serum T_4 is normal or increased, T_3 is nondetectable, and there is an adequate response in serum T_4 but no measurable serum T_3 following thyroid-stimulating hormone (TSH) administration or (2) when serum T_4 is normal or increased, serum T_3 is nondetectable, and there is an increase in T_4 but not T_3 in serial blood samples evaluated following sodium levothyroxine administration. Unfortunately, conversion abnormalities have not been documented in either humans or dogs and are probably rare, if they exist at all. The clinician must be careful when evaluating serum T_3 concentrations. They should not take precedence over T_4 concentrations. Triiodothyronine is primarily an intracellular hormone; serum concentrations do not necessarily reflect intracellular concentrations. In our experience, the majority of dogs with normal serum T_4 and low serum T_3 concentrations are euthyroid. If trial therapy is contemplated in these dogs, sodium levothyroxine is still the supplement of choice for reasons previously discussed. Only after a dog fails to respond to sodium levothyroxine should sodium liothyronine therapy be initiated.

The plasma half-life of sodium liothyronine is approximately 5 to 6 hr, with peak plasma concentration occurring 2 to 5 hr after administration (Nesbitt et al., 1980; Fox and Nachreiner, 1981). As with sodium levothyroxine, the plasma half-life and time of peak plasma concentration are variable from dog to dog, so the dose and frequency of administration of sodium liothyronine are subject to change. Our initial dosage of liothyronine is 4 to 6 μg/kg body weight every 8 hr. As with sodium levothyroxine, some dogs need less frequent hormone supplementation. Therefore, once clinical improvement is observed (usually within 4 to 6 weeks), the frequency of administration may be reduced to twice a day. If clinical signs recur, three daily doses should be reinstituted.

Re-evaluation of the original diagnosis or alterations in the dosage based on evaluation of serum T_4 and T_3 concentrations may be necessary in dogs that fail to respond. If sodium liothyronine is being used, blood samples should be obtained just prior to and 2 to 4 hr after administration. Evaluation of serum T_3 is mandatory with this supplement. Serum T_4 concentrations will be low to nondetectable with adequate T_3 supplements owing to the negative feedback suppression on the remaining functional thyroid tissue and an inability of T_3 to be converted to T_4. Guidelines for adjustments in T_3 therapy are similar to those for T_4 supplements (Table 2). Serum T_3 concentrations prior to and following T_3 administration should be within or above the normal range in a dog receiving an adequate dosage of a T_3 supplement.

ANTITHYROID HORMONE ANTIBODIES

Circulating antithyroid hormone antibodies have been described in humans and in dogs (Beckett et al., 1983; Young et al., 1985). The primary importance of these antibodies is their interference with radioimmunoassay techniques for measuring serum T_4 and T_3 concentrations. If antithyroid hormone antibodies are present in a dog receiving thyroid hormone supplementation, measurement of serum thyroid hormone concentrations cannot be used to monitor therapy. The clinician must rely on clinical response to assess therapy. The presence of these antibodies also raises some interesting questions concerning therapy. In our limited experience and in human beings with hypothyroidism, the presence of antithyroid hormone antibodies does not seem to interfere with the physiologic actions of thyroid hormone supplements (Pearce et al., 1981; Beckett et al., 1983). A clinical response should occur with appropriate therapy. Antithyroid hormone antibody interference with the thyroid supplement should be considered, however, if the hypothyroid dog with these antibodies fails to respond to appropriate therapy.

References and Supplemental Reading

Beckett, G. J., Todd, J. A., Hughes, G. J., et al.: Primary hypothyroidism with grossly elevated plasma total thyroxine and triiodothyronine levels. Clin. Endocrinol. 19:295, 1983.
Brennan, M. D.: Thyroid hormones. Mayo. Clin. Proc. 55:33, 1980.
Chung, S. J., and Van Middlesworth, L.: Absorption of thyroxine from the intestine of rats. Am. J. Physiol. 21:97, 1967.
Cottle, W. H., and Veress, A. T.: Absorption of biliary thyroxine from loops of small intestine. Can. J. Physiol. Pharmacol. 43:801, 1965.
Devlin, W. F., and Watanabe, H.: Thyroxine-triiodothyronine concentrations in thyroid powders. J. Pharm. Sci. 55:390, 1966.
Eichelbaum, M.: Drug metabolism in thyroid disease. Clin. Pharmacokinet. 1:339, 1976.
Feldman, E. C., and Nelson, R. W.: *Canine and Feline Endocrinology and Reproduction.* Philadelphia: W. B. Saunders Co., 1987.
Fox, L. E., and Nachreiner, R. F.: The pharmacokinetics of T_3 and T_4 in the dog. Proceedings of the 62nd Conference of Research Workers in Animal Disease, 1981, p. 13.
Hays, M. T.: Absorption of triiodothyronine in man. J. Clin. Endocrinol. Metab. 30:675, 1970.
Larsen, P. R., Silva, J. E., and Kaplan, M. M.: Relationships between circulating and intracellular thyroid hormones: Physiological and clinical implications. Endocrinol. Rev. 2:87, 1981.
Nesbitt, G. H., Izzo, J., Peterson, L., et al.: Canine hypothyroidism: A retrospective study of 108 cases. J.A.V.M.A. 177:1117, 1980.
Pearce, C. J., Byfield, P. G., Edmonds, C. J., et al.: Autoantibodies to thyroglobulin cross reacting with iodothyronines. Clin. Endocrinol. 15:1, 1981.
Rogers, W. A., Donovan, E. F., and Kociba, G. J.: Lipids and lipoproteins in normal dogs and in dogs with secondary hyperlipoproteinemia. J.A.V.M.A. 166:1092, 1975.
Rosychuk, R. A.: Thyroid hormones and antithyroid drugs. Vet. Clin. North Am. (Small Anim. Pract.) 12:111, 1982.
Young, D. W., Sartin, J. L., and Kemppainen, R. J.: Abnormal canine triiodothyronine-binding factor characterized as a possible triiodothyronine autoantibody. Am. J. Vet. Res. 46:1346, 1985.

CANINE MYXEDEMA STUPOR AND COMA

MICHAEL J. KELLY, D.V.M.

San Diego, California

Myxedema stupor and coma is a rare syndrome representing the extreme expression of severe hypothyroidism. As the name suggests, this condition involves a diminished level of consciousness in association with severe hypothyroidism. Although it is well characterized in human hypothyroid patients, there have been only a few reports of the condition in dogs. Because of the extremely high mortality associated with untreated myxedema coma, it is essential that treatment be instituted promptly and vigorously as soon as the diagnosis is made.

CLINICAL FINDINGS

The reported dogs with myxedema coma have been middle-aged dogs (average age 5 years). The Doberman pinscher breed seems to have a higher than normal representation. There does not appear to be any sex predilection.

The most common client historic complaints are mental dullness, depression, unresponsiveness, inappetence, anorexia, and a dry, coarse, sparse, hair coat. These signs result from an overall reduction of the oxidative processes and a slowing of metabolic activity. Although inappetence is a common clinical complaint, dogs may present with slightly to moderately increased body weight related to limited physical activity coupled with fluid retention. The cerebral depression is further aggravated by hypoventilation and carbon dioxide retention. As in dogs with hypothyroidism not associated with myxedema coma, the hair changes can be dramatic. The dermis is typically dry, rough, and thickened, with the hair being brittle and standing out from the body. Histologically, there is thickening of the stratum corneum and thinning of the underlying strata to one or two cell layers. Hair follicles are often lacking hair shafts and distended with laminated keratin plugs. Follicular epithelium and adnexal glands are atrophic.

Physical findings, in addition to the historic ones, include weakness; hypothermia, with an absence of shivering; nonpitting edema of the skin, face, and jowls; peritoneal effusion; bradycardia; and cyanotic mucous membranes. The dog may be so weak and depressed that the chin rests on the floor as if it were being used as a fifth appendage to support the body. In severe hypothyroidism, a dramatic reduction in oxygen consumption and in heat production develops. This is clinically reflected by a lower basal metabolic rate, an extreme sensitivity to cold, and a decreased body temperature. The failure to shiver might result from impaired hypothalamic temperature regulation or from impaired calorigenesis.

The nonpitting edema characteristic of the myxedema stupor and coma syndrome is most prominent in the face and jowls. Histochemically, the dermal connective tissue is infiltrated by a metachromatically staining, periodic acid-Schiff positive material. Chemical studies of deposits of this material reveal mixtures of protein in complex with mucopolysaccharides and hyaluronic acid. Dermal swelling is further aggravated by abnormal accumulations of water and sodium that result from the high osmotic pressure of thee mucinous deposits. Myxedema results from abnormal connective tissue metabolism. Kinetic studies demonstrate that the degradation of hyaluronic acid is decreased by myxedema to a greater degree than is its synthesis. The net result is an increase in hyaluronic acid in the tissue. These skin modifications are directly related to lack of thyroid hormones. The skin alterations disappear after 4 to 8 weeks of replacement therapy.

The peritoneal serous effusion reflects extreme instances of extracellular accumulation of myxedematous fluid. The effusions develop slowly and have a high protein content. Pleural and pericardial effusions will frequently accompany peritoneal effusions. These can be diagnosed with both radiology and ultrasonography. The cyanotic mucous membranes are secondary to bradycardia and hypoventilation resulting in anoxia and increased carbon dioxide concentration.

The bradycardia characteristic of myxedema coma can also be associated with distant and faint cardiac sounds, cardiomegaly, and mild hypotension. Hemodynamic investigations show decreased cardiac output and stroke volume coupled with prolonged circulation time. Long-standing, severe hypothyroidism may also be associated with a dilatative type of cardiomyopathy.

LABORATORY FINDINGS

The most important screening laboratory abnormalities are hypercholesterolemia, dilution hyponatremia, anemia, and increased protein content of serous effusions. In addition, resting serum T_4 concentrations are subnormal and fail to increase normally after administration of thyroid-stimulating hormone (TSH). Histologic studies reveal that the thyroid tissue mass in dogs with myxedema is reduced by more than 75 per cent. This results in severe depression of circulating thyroid hormone and an inability of the remaining thyroid tissue to respond to endogenous or exogenous TSH.

Hypercholesterolemia, hypertriglyceridemia, and elevation of total lipids result from decreased metabolism and clearance of these substances from the blood. Further increases in the serum cholesterol concentration occur because there is reduced secretion of cholesterol into the bile. Cholesterol values exceeding 1000 mg/dl may occur in canine myxedema.

The dilutional hyponatremia may be due to decreased blood volume to the distal diluting segment of the nephron, and/or inappropriate secretion of antidiuretic hormone. An abnormality of the sodium pump (the cellular mechanism that maintains the intracellular concentration of sodium and potassium ions) may also contribute to the altered blood sodium level. In the euthyroid subject, part of the body's oxygen consumption and adenosine triphosphate synthesis provide energy for the sodium pump. This active process is highly calorigenic and is controlled by the level of circulating thyroid hormones. The low basal metabolic rate associated with hypothyroidism is primarily explained by the decreased function of the sodium pump. The hyponatremia can contribute to the progressive dementia of the dog with myxedema.

The classic hematologic finding associated with canine hypothyroidism is a normocytic, normochromic, nonregenerative anemia. This phenomenon is considered to be a physiologic adaption to the diminished oxygen requirement of the peripheral tissues, possibly resulting from decreased erythropoietin secretion. Finally, the increased protein content of serous effusions results from increased capillary permeability to albumin and the large increase of the total exchangeable pool of albumin despite a reduction of plasma volume.

DIAGNOSIS

The diagnosis of myxedema stupor and coma is suspected on the basis of historic findings of progressive mental dullness, unresponsiveness, depression, and weakness. It is supported by the physical findings of hypothermia; nonpitting edema of the face and jowls; a coarse, dry, brittle hair coat; and occasional bradycardia. It is confirmed by the laboratory findings of hypercholesterolemia and dilutional hyponatremia together with low resting serum T_4 concentrations that increase little (if at all) after administration of TSH.

DIFFERENTIAL DIAGNOSIS

Myxedema stupor and coma should be added to the list of metabolic, neuromuscular, cardiovascular, and neoplastic diseases that present with weakness as a prominent sign. The metabolic causes include hypoglycemia, electrolyte abnormalities, hepatoencephalopathy, endogenous cortisol deficiencies, ketoacidic diabetes mellitus, and uremic encephalopathy. The neuromuscular etiologies include myasthenia gravis, polyradiculoneuritis, and progressive myopathies. The cardiovascular diseases to be considered are the bradyarrhythmias, the tachyarrhythmias, and third-degree heart block. The most common neoplasms to be considered are bleeding hemangiosarcoma and lymphosarcoma causing hypercalcemia.

THERAPY

Treatment of myxedema stupor and coma is divided into three areas—maintaining vital function, replacing thyroid hormone, and treating precipitating factors.

Hypoventilation can lead to surprisingly severe carbon dioxide retention, which contributes to narcosis. When possible, arterial blood gases should be measured and ventilation assisted. Hypotension usually responds rapidly to replacement of thyroid hormone. Vasopressor agents are not recommended except in severe cases. No attempt should be made to warm the dog with external heat, which can result in increased oxygen requirements and decreased peripheral tone, both of which exacerbate existing cardiovascular failure. Parenteral fluids should be given only with extreme caution so as to prevent fluid excess and circulatory failure.

It is debatable whether adrenocortical insufficiency exists concurrently with hypothyroidism in myxedema stupor and coma. Cortisol is secreted at a reduced rate, but its disposal is decreased to the same extent. Consequently, the circulating cortisol concentrations remain within normal limits, with a normal amount of hormone available for use by the peripheral tissues. In human patients, the standard adrenocorticotropic hormone (ACTH) stimulation test yields varying responses—sometimes reduced, but more often delayed. In human myxedematous patients, it is believed that even if adrenal insufficiency is not present, the rapid restoration of normal levels of plasma T_4 via intravenous administration may produce relative adrenal insufficiency. Therefore, hydrocortisone is given intravenously at therapeutic doses until the myxedema is controlled.

Levothyroxine sodium (Synthroid, Flint) for parenteral administration is commercially available. This is the single most important therapy for the disease. It replaces the defect that exists and can, if given in time, reverse all of the pathology associated with myxedema coma. A single dose of 100 to 200 μg can be administered intravenously. This can restore the peripheral pool of T_4 to normal and can make normal amounts of T_4 immediately available for metabolic use. Improvement of vital signs is usually evident within 6 hr. As soon as the dog stabilizes, oral levothyroxine sodium should be initiated.

Myxedema coma is often precipitated by infection, central nervous system depressants, and stress such as trauma or cold exposure. Sedatives, tranquilizers, narcotics, and anesthetics should be strictly avoided because of the risk of further respiratory depression.

References and Supplemental Reading

Chastain, C. B.: Canine hypothyroidism. J.A.V.M.A. 181:349, 1982.

Chastain, C. B., Graham, C. L., and Riley, M. G.: Myxedema coma in two dogs. Canine Pract. 9:20, 1982.

Kelly, M. J., and Hill, J. R.: Canine myxedema stupor and coma. Comp. Cont. Ed. Pract. Vet. 6:1049, 1984.

FELINE HYPOTHYROIDISM

MARK E. PETERSON, D.V.M.

New York, New York

Naturally occurring hypothyroidism is an extremely rare clinical disorder in cats. Although surveys of the histologic evaluation of the feline thyroid gland have revealed several pathologic abnormalities consistent with the development of hypothyroidism (thyroid atrophy, lymphocytic thyroiditis, and goiter), spontaneous acquired primary (thyroidal) hypothyroidism has yet to be convincingly documented in adult cats (Clark and Meier, 1958; Lucke, 1964). Despite the apparent nonexistence of adult-onset feline hypothyroidism, congenital or juvenile-onset hypothyroidism appears to develop with some frequency in cats. One kitten with congenital hypothyroidism associated with thyroid gland enlargement (goiter) resulting from a suspected defect in thyroid hormone biosynthesis (defective peroxidase activity resulting in an iodine organification defect) has been reported (Arnold et al., 1984). In addition, we have recently identified five other cats with congenital hypothyroidism. One of these cats also had a goiter associated with an iodine organification defect (which was documented on the basis of a thyroid scan, radioiodine uptake studies, and a perchlorate discharge test), whereas the other four cats had thyroid dysgenesis confirmed by thyroid biopsy. As in hypothyroid dogs, it is likely that congenital hypothyroidism results in early death in most affected kittens and therefore goes undiagnosed. Neither secondary (pituitary) nor tertiary (hypothalamic) hypothyroidism has been described in either the juvenile or mature cat.

The most common cause of feline hypothyroidism is iatrogenic destruction or removal of the thyroid gland (following radioiodine or surgery) for treatment of hyperthyroidism. Although antithyroid drug overdosage could also produce hypothyroidism, this appears to be uncommon. As discussed in the chapter on feline hyperthyroidism, cats treated with methimazole that develop subnormal T_4 concentrations usually maintain normal circulating T_3 concentrations and thus fail to demonstrate any clinical signs of hypothyroidism.

CLINICAL FEATURES

The clinical signs associated with iatrogenic primary hypothyroidism in adult cats usually include lethargy and nonpruritic seborrhea sicca. Matting of hair over the back (because of failure to groom) and hair loss over the lateral and medial distal halves of both pinnae may also develop. Bilateral, symmetric alopecia, with the exception of the pinnal involvement, does not appear to develop. In addition, hair removed by clipping usually will regrow. Obesity, although it may develop, is not a consistent sign (Thoday, 1986).

Cats with congenital hypothyroidism typically

have signs of disproportionate dwarfism, with an enlarged, broad head but short neck and limbs. Severe lethargy, mental dullness, constipation, hypothermia, and bradycardia have been observed in most cats. Hair is usually present all over the body but consists mainly of undercoat with primary hairs scattered throughout. Obesity is generally not present. Radiographic examination has revealed almost complete absence of ossification centers in long bones (Arnold et al., 1984).

DIAGNOSIS

Diagnosis of iatrogenic hypothyroidism can be difficult because of the vague clinical signs that these cats usually display. The tentative diagnosis in these cats should be based on the clinical signs described above, together with a history of surgical thyroidectomy or treatment with radioiodine for hyperthyroidism. Congenital or juvenile-onset hypothyroidism should be suspected in any young cat with stunted growth and other clinical signs characteristic of cretinism (mental dullness). Because of the multiple factors that can falsely lower baseline serum thyroid hormone values in cats with diseases other than hypothyroidism, the definitive diagnosis of iatrogenic or spontaneous feline hypothyroidism should be confirmed by the finding of a subnormal resting serum T_4 concentration that fails to rise adequately 6 hr after administration of bovine TSH using a dosage of 1.0 IU/kg IV (Hoenig and Ferguson, 1983). Alternatively, the TSH can be administered intramuscularly using a dosage of 2.5 units per cat, and the post-TSH T_4 sample collected at 8 to 12 hr after injection (Kemppainen et al, 1984). Using either protocol, a normal response is a post-TSH T_4 concentration that either is 2.0 to 3.0 μg/dl higher than the basal serum T_4 value or exceeds the normal range of basal T_4 concentrations (approximately 4 μg/dl in most laboratories). In kittens with documented hypothyroidism, other procedures (e.g., thyroid scanning, radioiodine uptake studies, perchlorate discharge testing, thyroid biopsy, biochemical analysis of thyroid tissue) should be considered to help better classify the underlying causes of the congenital feline hypothyroidism (Stanbury, 1986).

TREATMENT

As in dogs, the recommended treatment for feline hypothyroidism is daily administration of levothyroxine, using an initial dose of 10 to 20 μg/kg/day. This dosage should subsequently be adjusted on the basis of the cat's clinical response and postpill serum T_4 evaluation. Complete resolution of clinical signs can usually be expected in cats with adult-onset iatrogenic hypothyroidism. Thyroid hormone is crucial for normal growth and development of the central nervous system and skeleton. Consequently, the dwarfism and mental dullness that develop in kittens with hypothyroidism usually persist because of the delayed period of time from onset to diagnosis in these cats.

References and Supplemental Reading

Arnold, U., Opitz, M., and Grosser, I.: Goitrous hypothyroidism and dwarfism in a kitten. J. Am. Anim. Hosp. Assoc. 20:753, 1984.

Clark, S. T., and Meier, H.: A clinicopathological study of thyroid disease in the dog and cat. Part 1. Thyroid pathology. Zentralbl. Veterinarmed. [A]5:17, 1958.

Hoenig, M., and Ferguson, D. C.: Assessment of thyroid functional reserve in the cat by the thyrotropin-stimulation test. Am. J. Vet. Res. 44:1229, 1983.

Kemppainen, R. J., Mansfield, P. D., and Sartin, J. L.: Endocrine responses of normal cats to TSH and synthetic ACTH administration. J. Am. Anim. Hosp. Assoc. 20:737, 1984.

Lucke, V. M.: An histological study of thyroid abnormalities in the domestic cat. J. Small Anim. Prac. 5:351, 1964.

Stanbury, J. B.: Inherited metabolic disorders of the thyroid system. In Ingbar, S. H., and Braverman, L. E. (eds.): The Thyroid, 5th ed. Philadelphia: J. B. Lippincott, 1986, p. 687.

Thoday, K. L.: Differential diagnosis of symmetric alopecia in the cat. In Kirk, R. W. (ed.): Current Veterinary Therapy IX. Philadelphia: W. B. Saunders, 1986, p. 545.

TREATMENT OF FELINE HYPERTHYROIDISM

MARK E. PETERSON, D.V.M.

New York, New York

Hyperthyroidism (thyrotoxicosis) is a multisystemic disorder resulting from excessive circulating concentrations of the two thyroid hormones thyroxine (T_4) and triiodothyronine (T_3). In most cats with hyperthyroidism, functional thyroid adenomatous hyperplasia (or adenoma) involving one or both thyroid lobes is responsible for thyroid hormone oversecretion. In about 70 per cent of hyperthyroid cats, both thyroid lobes are enlarged; the remaining cats have involvement of only one lobe. Thyroid carcinoma only very rarely causes hyperthyroidism in cats, with a prevalence of approximately 1 to 2 per cent. Although first documented within the past decade, hyperthyroidism has become the most common endocrine disorder of middle-aged to old cats and is one of the most frequently diagnosed disorders in small animal practice.

In cats with hyperthyroidism, the aim of treatment is to control the excessive secretion of thyroid hormone from the adenomatous (or rarely, carcinomatous) thyroid gland. Feline hyperthyroidism can be treated in three ways—surgical thyroidectomy, radioactive iodine (^{131}I), or chronic administration of an antithyroid drug. Antithyroid drug therapy is also extremely useful as short-term treatment (3 to 6 weeks) in the preparation of the hyperthyroid cat prior to thyroidectomy. The treatment of choice for an individual cat depends on several factors, including the age of the cat, the presence of associated cardiovascular diseases or other major medical problems, the availability of a skilled surgeon or nuclear medicine department, and the owner's willingness to accept the form of treatment advised. Of the three forms of treatment available, it must be emphasized that only surgery and radioactive iodine remove and destroy the adenomatous thyroid tissue, respectively, and thereby "cure" the hyperthyroid state. Use of an antithyroid drug (e.g., methimazole) will block thyroid hormone synthesis; however, since antithyroid drugs do not destroy adenomatous thyroid tissue, relapse of hyperthyroidism invariably occurs within 24 to 72 hr after the medication is discontinued. The advantages and disadvantages of each form of treatment are summarized in Table 1 and should always be considered when selecting the most appropriate treatment.

ANTITHYROID DRUGS

Methimazole (Tapazole) and propylthiouracil (PTU) are the two thiourylene antithyroid drugs available for use in the United States. After administration, these drugs are actively concentrated by the thyroid gland, where they act to inhibit the synthesis of thyroid hormones. Antithyroid drugs do not interfere with the thyroid gland's ability to concentrate, or "trap," inorganic iodine, nor do they block the release of stored thyroid hormone into the circulation.

Advantages of long-term antithyroid drug treatment over other available treatment modalities (surgery and radioactive iodine) include absence of certain complications such as permanent hypothyroidism and postsurgical hypoparathyroidism (Table 1). In addition, unlike surgery or radioiodine therapy, use of antithyroid drugs requires no advanced skills, training, or special licensing and is a practical treatment choice for most practitioners.

Although both PTU and methimazole are effective in decreasing serum thyroid hormone concentrations into the normal or low range, PTU produces a high incidence of mild to serious adverse effects, which include anorexia, vomiting, lethargy, immune-mediated hemolytic anemia, thrombocytopenia, and the development of serum antinuclear antibodies (ANA) in both normal and hyperthyroid cats (Aucoin et al., 1985; Peterson et al., 1984). Because of the prevalence of severe hematologic complications, use of PTU for control of feline hyperthyroidism can no longer be recommended. We recently reported the results of a 3-year evaluation of the efficacy and safety of methimazole in 262 cats with hyperthyroidism (Peterson et al., 1988). Overall, our studies show that methimazole is better tolerated and safer than PTU in cats and can be considered the antithyroid drug of choice for both the preoperative and long-term medical management of feline hyperthyroidism.

Initial Treatment

Methimazole should initially be administered at a dose of 10 to 15 mg/day, depending on the severity of the hyperthyroid state. This methimazole dosage

Table 1. *Advantages and Disadvantages of Treatment Modalities for Feline Hyperthyroidism*

	Methimazole	Surgery	Radioiodine
Persistent hyperthyroidism	Low (dose-related)	Rare	Low (dose-related)
Complications			
Hypoparathyroidism	Never	Common	Never
Permanent hypothyroidism	Never	Intermediate	Rare (dose-related)
Anorexia, vomiting	Common	Rare	Never
Hematologic effects	Rare (thrombocytopenia, agranulocytosis, serum ANA)	Never	Rare (only with very high doses)
Neurologic damage	Never	Rare (vocal cord paralysis, Horner's syndrome)	Never
Hospitalization time required	None	1–3 days	1–4 weeks
Time until euthyroid	1–3 weeks	1–2 days	1–12 weeks
Relapse/recurrence	High	Intermediate	Low
Ease of treatment	Simple	Most difficult	Intermediate (not readily available)

ensures that serum T_4 concentrations will decrease to normal or low values within 2 to 3 weeks of treatment in most cats. During the first 3 months of therapy (the time period when the most serious side effects associated with methimazole therapy develop), the cats should be examined every 2 to 3 weeks in order to make necessary dose adjustments and to monitor for adverse effects. At each of these rechecks, serum T_4 concentrations and complete blood and platelet counts should be determined. If little to no decrease in serum T_4 concentration occurs during this initial treatment period, the daily methimazole dosage should be gradually increased in 5-mg increments (after poor compliance by owners or difficulty in giving the medication has been ruled out as the cause of persistent hyperthyroidism). Although a few cats appear to be "resistant" to the effects of the drug, euthyroidism can be restored in virtually all cats if a high enough dosage of methimazole (25 to 30 mg/day in a few cases) is reliably administered on a daily basis.

If methimazole is given as preoperative preparation, surgical thyroidectomy can be performed once serum T_4 concentrations decrease to normal or low values (usually within 2 to 4 weeks). Surgical risks in cats with subnormal circulating T_4 concentrations do not appear to be increased, probably because normal serum T_3 concentrations are maintained in these cats (see below). The last dose of methimazole should be administered on the morning of surgery.

Long-Term Treatment

In cats in which long-term methimazole treatment is planned, the goal of treatment is to maintain serum T_4 values within the low-normal range with the lowest possible daily dosage, since some side effects (at least serum ANA development, see below) appear to develop less frequently with lower doses of methimazole. Therefore, if serum T_4 concentrations fall to low or low-normal values during methimazole treatment in these cats, the daily drug dosage should be decreased by 2.5- to 5-mg decrements and further testing continued at 2- to 3-week intervals until the lowest daily dose is found that will effectively maintain serum T_4 concentrations within the low-normal range. Although a few cases of feline hyperthyroidism can be effectively controlled on a long-term basis with a daily dose as low as 2.5 to 5 mg, the great majority will require a dosage of 7.5 to 10 mg/day. Other cats may continue to require dosages of 15 to 20 mg/day to maintain serum T_4 concentrations within normal range.

Although subnormal serum T_4 concentrations commonly develop during both short- and long-term treatment with methimazole, serum T_3 values usually remain within the normal range, and clinical signs suggestive of hypothyroidism have not been observed. Unlike PTU, methimazole does not appear to inhibit the 5'-deiodination of T_4 to T_3. Since

Table 2. *Clinical Side-Effects and Hematologic and Immunologic Abnormalities Associated with Methimazole Treatment in 262 Cats with Hyperthyroidism*

Sign	No. (%) of Cats	Time When Signs Develop (Days)	
		Range	Median
Anorexia	29 (11.1)	1–78	18.0
Vomiting	28 (10.7)	7–60	15.0
Lethargy	23 (8.8)	1–60	21.0
Excoriations	6 (2.3)	6–40	19.0
Bleeding	6 (2.3)	15–50	22.5
Hepatopathy	4 (1.5)	15–60	41.0
Thrombocytopenia	7 (2.7)	14–90	24.0
Agranulocytosis	4 (1.5)	26–95	62.5
Leukopenia	12 (4.7)	10–41	23.0
Eosinophilia	30 (11.3)	12–490	21.0
Lymphocytosis	19 (7.2)	14–90	18.5
Antinuclear antibodies*	52 (21.8)	10–870	46.0
Positive Coombs' test*	3 (1.9)	45–60	50.0

*Antinuclear antibodies determined in 239 cats and direct antiglobulin (Coombs') tests performed in 160 cats.

Modified from data in Peterson, M. E., et al.: Methimazole treatment of 262 cats with hyperthyroidism. J. Vet. Intern. Med. 2:150–157, 1988.

T_3 appears to be the most metabolically active thyroid hormone, normal circulating T_3 concentrations explain the absence of clinical signs of hypothyroidism.

Although divided doses of methimazole, given every 8 or 12 hours, tend to be most effective in controlling the hyperthyroid state, euthyroidism can often be maintained when the necessary dose is given only once daily. Despite a serum half-life for methimazole of only 4 to 6 hr, studies in human hyperthyroid patients have shown that the drug has an intrathyroidal residence time of approximately 20 hr. Since antithyroid drugs act to inhibit thyroid hormone synthesis only after they are concentrated within the thyroid gland, serum half-life of these drugs is of lesser importance than the intrathyroidal drug concentration for adequate control of the hyperthyroid state. In addition, many cat owners, especially those using methimazole on a long-term basis, may find a treatment regimen of once-daily medication easier to maintain than having to give medication two or three times daily. However, methimazole must be given at least once daily or serum thyroid hormone concentrations will again rise into the thyrotoxic range. Consequently, elevated circulating T_4 concentrations will develop in many cats treated with methimazole on a long-term basis because of a decrease in compliance by the owners or increased difficulty in giving daily medication.

Adverse Effects Associated with Methimazole Treatment

Mild clinical side effects associated with methimazole treatment are relatively common (approximately 15 per cent of cats) and include anorexia, vomiting, and lethargy (Table 2). In most cats, these adverse signs are transient and resolve despite continued administration of the drug. Severe gastrointestinal signs persist in some cats, however, necessitating discontinuation of the drug. Self-induced excoriations of the face and neck also may develop in a few cats within the first 6 weeks of therapy (Table 2). Although these cutaneous lesions tend to be partially responsive to treatment with systemic glucocorticoids, cessation of methimazole administration is usually required for complete resolution of these excoriations. Finally, hepatic toxicity is an uncommon but serious reaction that can develop during drug treatment. Methimazole-induced hepatopathy is characterized by the development of marked increases in serum concentrations of alanine aminotransferase, alkaline phosphatase, and total bilirubin. Clinical improvement, with resolution of anorexia, vomiting, and lethargy, usually occurs within a few days after cessation of methimazole, but jaundice and abnormal serum biochemical tests indicative of liver disease may not resolve for several weeks. Rechallenge with the drug will again induce clinical signs and serum biochemical abnormalities indicative of hepatic disease within a few days. A variety of hematologic abnormalities may develop in cats during treatment with methimazole (Table 2). Those abnormalities that do not appear to be associated with any adverse effects include eosinophilia, lymphocytosis, and transient leukopenia with a normal differential count. As with PTU treatment, more serious hematologic reactions that develop in a few cats treated with methimazole include severe thrombocytopenia (platelet count <75,000 cells/mm^3) and agranulocytosis (severe leukopenia with a total granulocyte count <250 cells/mm^3). Immune-mediated hemolytic anemia, a major side effect associated with PTU treatment (Aucoin et al., 1985; Peterson et al., 1984), has not been observed with methimazole therapy. Most cats that develop severe thrombocytopenia also show concomitant overt bleeding (epistaxis, oral hemorrhage). Development of agranulocytosis during methimazole treatment predisposes to severe bacterial infections, systemic toxicity, and fever. If serious hematologic reactions develop during methimazole therapy, the drug should be stopped and supportive care given; these adverse reactions should resolve within 5 days after the methimazole is withdrawn. Since most life-threatening side effects (e.g., hepatopathy, thrombocytopenia, agranulocytosis) caused by methimazole treatment usually develop again quickly after rechallenge with the drug, alternative therapy with either surgery or radioiodine should be considered in these cases.

During methimazole therapy, serum ANA develop in a high percentage of cats after treatment with methimazole. The risk of developing ANA appears to increase with the duration of methimazole treatment, with ANA developing in approximately half of cats treated for longer than 6 months in our study (Peterson et al., 1988). The risk of developing serum ANA also appears to be greater for cats treated with higher daily methimazole doses, since most cats that develop ANA are receiving doses ≥15 mg/day, and ANA will disappear in most cats after the dosage is decreased. Despite the high prevalence of ANA development during long-term treatment with methimazole, clinical signs associated with a lupuslike syndrome (dermatitis, polyarthritis, glomerulonephritis, hemolytic anemia or fever) have not been observed in any of these cats. However, the potential for lupus development in cats with methimazole-induced ANA still exists. The daily drug dose should therefore be decreased to as low as possible (while still maintaining serum T_4 values within the low-normal range), since ANA tests will become negative in many cats when the methimazole dosage is decreased.

Although the most serious adverse effects of methimazole treatment usually develop during the first few weeks of drug administration, side effects can potentially occur at any time during treatment. After the first 3 months of methimazole therapy, one should continue to measure serum T_4 concentrations at 3- to 6-month intervals in order to monitor dosage requirements and response to treatment. Although it does not appear to be necessary to continue to monitor complete blood and platelet counts during these rechecks, the cell counts should be performed if agranulocytosis or thrombocytopenia is suspected. In addition, although methimazole-induced lupus has not been detected in cats that develop ANA during treatment, periodic monitoring of serum biochemical screening values and urinalysis, as well as serum ANA determinations, are also recommended if signs consistent with a lupuslike syndrome develop.

SURGERY

Surgical thyroidectomy is a highly effective treatment for feline hyperthyroidism. Although thyroidectomy is most often successful, it can be associated with significant morbidity and mortality. Hyperthyroidism is a systemic illness that affects all body systems; although thyroidectomy in itself is a relatively simple procedure, cardiovascular, hepatic, and gastrointestinal dysfunctions associated with hyperthyroidism greatly increase anesthetic and surgical risks. All hyperthyroid cats should therefore be prepared for surgery by administration of an antithyroid drug, propranolol, or iodide to decrease the metabolic and cardiac complications associated with hyperthyroidism.

Preoperative Preparation

Use of the antithyroid drug methimazole, as described above, is the method of choice for the preoperative preparation of a hyperthyroid cat. After methimazole treatment has maintained euthyroidism for 1 to 3 weeks, most systemic complications associated with hyperthyroidism will have improved or resolved, and the anesthetic and surgical complications will be greatly minimized. The last dose of methimazole should be administered on the morning of surgery.

In hyperthyroid cats that cannot tolerate antithyroid drug treatment, alternate preoperative preparation with propranolol or stable iodine, alone or in combination, should be used. Although propranolol, a beta-adrenergic blocker, does not lower elevated serum thyroid hormone concentrations, this drug blocks many of the cardiovascular and neuromuscular effects of excess thyroid hormone and controls the tachycardia and hyperexcitability associated with feline hyperthyroidism. In addition, treatment with a beta-adrenergic blocker helps prevent arrhythmias that commonly develop during the anesthetic period in untreated cats with hyperthyroidism (Peterson, 1987). Propranolol should be administered for 7 to 14 days before surgery at a dosage of 2.5 to 5.0 mg every 8 hours, as required to decrease resting heart rate within the normal range and control hyperexcitability. In cats with congestive heart failure secondary to chronic thyroid hormone excess, propranolol should not be initiated until cardiac failure has been stabilized with diuretics (and digitalis when indicated). In these cases, propranolol should be used with caution, since the drug depresses myocardial function.

Large doses of stable iodine block T_4 and T_3 release from the thyroid gland and lower serum thyroid hormone concentrations. In addition, iodine treatment will cause a reduction in the size and vascularity of the adenomatous thyroid gland. Iodine has major limitations as antithyroid therapy, however, since serum T_4 and T_3 concentrations may not ever completely normalize during iodine treatment, and the drug often loses its antithyroid effect within a few weeks. Therefore, iodine should not be used as sole therapy in preparation for thyroidectomy but can be given in conjunction with propranolol or an antithyroid drug. Iodine should be administered as either oral potassium iodide (saturated solution of potassium iodide [SSKI]), Lugol's solution, or intravenous sodium iodide at a dosage of 50 to 100 mg/day for 7 to 14 days prior to surgery. Common side effects of oral potassium iodide treatment include excessive salivation and decreased appetite; such adverse signs appear to result from the unpleasant taste of iodine. To prevent this adverse effect, the dose of SSKI can be placed within a small gelatin capsule and immediately administered.

Anesthesia

Anesthetic management of the hyperthyroid cat should include the judicious use of agents that have minimal cardiac arrhythmic effects. A variety of anesthetic agents and techniques can be used, and none has advantages that exclude use of all others, especially if the hyperthyroid state has been controlled with methimazole prior to surgery.

Premedication with acetylpromazine is useful because this drug reduces autonomic manifestations of hyperthyroidism and may prevent arrhythmias induced by thiobarbiturates and inhalation agents (Peterson, 1987). Use of xylazine (Rompun, Haver-Lockhart) is contraindicated because it potentiates the development of cardiac arrhythmias induced by inhalation or barbiturate anesthesia. Atropine should also be omitted because it stimulates adrenergic activity and may induce tachycardia and arrhythmias. If an anticholinergic agent is used, glycopyrrolate (Robinul-V, Robins) is the drug of choice because it has minimal effects on cardiac rate and rhythm. Because hyperthyroid cats are particularly sensitive to catecholamine-induced arrhythmias, anesthetic agents that stimulate sympathoadrenal activity, such as ketamine, should be avoided. Thiobarbiturates are acceptable induction agents because they possess antithyroid activity and do not stimulate catecholamine secretion. Many inhalation agents are acceptable for maintaining anesthesia in cats with hyperthyroidism. If available, enflurane or isoflurane is preferred over methoxyflurane and halothane because they sensitize the heart to catecholamine-induced arrhythmias to a lesser extent (Peterson, 1987).

During the anesthetic period, continuous monitoring of the anesthetic level and electrocardiogram is essential. Ventricular arrhythmias are common, especially in cats not rendered euthyroid prior to surgery. If arrhythmias develop, the anesthetic concentration should be lowered and the cat ventilated with a higher concentration of oxygen. If the arrhythmias persist, small doses (0.1 mg) of intravenous propranolol usually restore normal sinus rhythm (Peterson, 1987).

Surgical Considerations

Prior to and during surgical thyroidectomy, a number of factors must be considered to ensure a successful outcome. About 30 per cent of hyperthyroid cats have disease in only one thyroid lobe, whereas the remaining 70 per cent have bilateral thyroid lobe involvement. In cats with unilateral thyroid tumors, the contralateral lobe is in normal position and either small or normal in size when inspected at surgery. Hemithyroidectomy corrects the hyperthyroid state in these cats, and relapse resulting from the development of adenomatous changes in the remaining "normal" thyroid lobe is extremely rare and takes years to develop. In cats with bilateral thyroid adenomas (adenomatous hyperplasia), removal of both lobes with preservation of parathyroid function is necessary to control hyperthyroidism and avoid postoperative hypocalcemia. With bilateral thyroid tumors, enlargement of both lobes can easily be identified at surgery in most cats; however, about 15 per cent of cats with bilateral lobe involvement have one lobe that is only slightly enlarged and may be mistaken as normal. Preoperative thyroid imaging is helpful in defining the extent of thyroid lobe involvement in these cases (Peterson and Becker, 1984). If thyroid imaging is not feasible, we recommend removal of the obviously enlarged lobe with preservation of

the associated external parathyroid gland in all cats with suspected unilateral lobe involvement. If bilateral lobe involvement was initially present, relapse of hyperthyroidism will usually occur within 12 months of surgery. Preservation of the external parathyroid gland during hemithyroidectomy minimizes the risk of hypoparathyroidism should removal of the contralateral lobe be required.

Techniques for unilateral and bilateral thyroidectomy have been reported for cats with hyperthyroidism (Birchard et al., 1984; Black and Peterson, 1983; Flanders et al., 1987; Peterson and Randolph, 1989). Both intracapsular and extracapsular methods designed for removal of thyroid tissue while preserving parathyroid function have been used. With the intracapsular technique for thyroidectomy, however, it can be difficult to remove the entire thyroid capsule (and therefore all abnormal thyroid tissue) while concurrently preserving parathyroid function. Small remnants of thyroid tissue that remain attached to the capsule may regenerate and produce recurrent hyperthyroidism. The main advantage of the extracapsular, as compared with the intracapsular, technique is that the incidence of relapse is much less because the entire thyroid capsule is removed together with the thyroid lobe.

Postoperative Complications

There are many potential complications associated with thyroidectomy, including hypoparathyroidism, Horner's syndrome, and laryngeal paralysis (most commonly, voice change). The most serious complication is hypocalcemia, which develops after the parathyroid glands are injured, devascularized, or inadvertently removed in the course of bilateral thyroidectomy. Since only one parathyroid gland is required for maintenance of normocalcemia, hypoparathyroidism develops only in cats treated with bilateral thyroidectomy. After bilateral thyroidectomy, the serum calcium concentration should be monitored on a daily basis until it has stabilized within the normal range. In most cats with iatrogenic hypoparathyroidism, clinical signs associated with hypocalcemia will develop within 1 to 3 days of surgery. Although mild hypocalcemia (6.5 to 7.5 mg/dl) is a common finding during this immediate postoperative period, laboratory evidence of hypocalcemia alone does not require treatment. However, if accompanying signs of muscle tremors, tetany, or convulsions develop, therapy with vitamin D and calcium is indicated (Peterson, 1986). Although hypoparathyroidism may be permanent in some cats, spontaneous recovery of parathyroid function may occur weeks to months after surgery. In most cases, such transient hypocalcemia probably results from reversible parathyroid damage and ischemia incurred during surgery. Alternatively, accessory parathyroid tissue may compensate for the damaged parathyroid glands and maintain normocalcemia.

Long-Term Management

Serum thyroid hormone concentrations fall to subnormal levels for 2 to 3 months after hemithyroidectomy for unilateral thyroid lobe involvement. However, thyroxine supplementation is rarely required during this period. If bilateral thyroidectomy has been performed, thyroxine (0.1 to 0.2 mg/day) should be started 24 to 48 hr after surgery. Although thyroxine supplementation at this dosage can be safely continued indefinitely, the low serum concentrations of T_4 and T_3 that develop 24 to 48 hr after bilateral thyroidectomy may spontaneously increase to within normal range weeks to months postoperatively. Thyroxine administration can then be discontinued. Because of the potential for recurrence of hyperthyroidism, all cats treated with surgical thyroidectomy should have their serum thyroid hormone concentration monitored once or twice a year. In cases of recurrent thyrotoxicosis after bilateral thyroidectomy, treatment with either methimazole or radioiodine is favored over reoperation since the incidence of surgical complications (especially permanent hypoparathyroidism) is considerably higher in subsequent operations than in the initial procedure (Birchard et al., 1984).

RADIOACTIVE IODINE

Radioactive iodine provides a simple, effective, and safe treatment for cats with hyperthyroidism. The basic principle behind treatment of hyperthyroidism with radioiodine is that thyroid cells do not differentiate between stable and radioactive iodine; therefore, radioiodine, like stable iodine, is concentrated by the thyroid gland after administration. In cats with hyperthyroidism, radioiodine is concentrated primarily in the hyperplastic or neoplastic thyroid cells, where it irradiates and destroys the hyperfunctioning tissue. Normal thyroid tissue, however, tends to be protected from the effects of radioiodine, since the uninvolved thyroid tissue is suppressed and receives only a small dose of radiation (unless very large doses are administered).

The radioisotope most frequently used to treat hyperthyroidism is radioiodine-131 (^{131}I). Radioiodine-131 has a half-life of 8 days and emits both beta particles and gamma radiation. The beta particles, which cause 80 per cent of the tissue damage, travel a maximum of 2 mm in tissue and have an average path length of 400 μm. Therefore, beta particles are locally destructive but spare adjacent hypoplastic thyroid tissue, parathyroid glands, and other cervical structures.

The ideal goal of ^{131}I therapy is to restore euthyroidism with a single dose of radiation without producing hypothyroidism. Three major methods have been used to estimate the activity of ^{131}I required to destroy the hyperfunctioning thyroid tissue in cats with hyperthyroidism. With any of these three methods, the ^{131}I will be more effective in destroying hyperfunctioning tissue if the cat has not been treated with methimazole (or if antithyroid medication has been discontinued for at least a week).

With the first method of ^{131}I dose determination, various parameters of thyroid kinetics are determined with a small "tracer" dose of radioiodine (Turrel et al., 1984). Using an estimated desired radiation dose of 15,000 to 20,000 rads per gram of thyroid tissue, the therapeutic dose of ^{131}I is calculated from the following parameters: (1) the effective half-life of ^{131}I (which accounts for both the physical half-life and duration of radioiodine retention by the thyroid); (2) the fraction of ^{131}I deposited in the thyroid gland (the percentage of thyroid uptake); and (3) estimated thyroid gland weight. Using this method, the calculated ^{131}I dose may range from 1 to 10 mCi, which can be administered either orally or as a single subcutaneous or intravenous injection. With this ^{131}I dose method, approximately 80 per cent of hyperthyroid cats become euthyroid within 3 months (most within 2 weeks) after a single dose of radioiodine, while the remaining cats require a second ^{131}I treatment for complete resolution of the hyperthyroid state. Very few cats develop hypothyroidism from ^{131}I overdosage and require thyroid hormone supplementation with this regimen. The major disadvantage of this method of dose determination is that the procedures used may necessitate sedating the cat on one or multiple occasions.

The second method of dose determination is to select a relatively low dose of ^{131}I without determining thyroid gland kinetics. Administration of 2 to 6 mCi of ^{131}I (based on the size of the thyroid nodule and the T_4 value) will produce euthyroidism in the majority of cats with hyperthyroidism. However, use of this approach will also result in under- or overtreatment of a number of cats, resulting in persistent hyperthyroidism or hypothyroidism, respectively. The advantage of this method is that nuclear medicine equipment is not needed, the time required to determine thyroid kinetics is eliminated, and sedation of the cat is not required.

The third method of radioiodine therapy is to administer extremely large doses of radioiodine (10 to 30 mCi). These doses of ^{131}I will almost always totally destroy the adenomatous thyroid tissue as well as normal thyroid tissue. Thus, this method is effective in curing the hyperthyroidism in almost all cats but will increase the risk of hypothyroidism.

In general, we recommend use of such large doses of ^{131}I only in cats with hyperfunctioning thyroid adenocarcinoma to ensure complete destruction of the malignant tissue.

Regardless of the method of dose determination selected, there are certain radiation safety restrictions and procedures that must be followed. The cats should be confined to restricted areas of the hospital that have minimal traffic and should be housed in metabolic cages so that urine and feces can be collected safely. All personnel handling the cats, cages, food dishes, and excreta should wear long laboratory coats, disposable plastic gloves, and film badges. All material removed from the cage must be handled as radioactive waste and be disposed of accordingly. The cats are discharged from the hospital when the radiation dose rate has decreased to a safe level that has been determined by the state radiation control office (usually after a 1- to 3-week period).

Overall, use of radioiodine may be the optimum treatment for feline hyperthyroidism when nuclear medicine facilities are available. Radioactive iodine treatment involves a single, nonstressful procedure that is without associated morbidity or mortality. Untoward systemic effects have not been observed. Unlike surgery, it does not require anesthesia. A single ^{131}I treatment will restore euthyroidism in most cats with hyperthyroidism, whereas cats that remain persistently hyperthyroid can be successfully retreated with radioiodine and those that become hypothyroid can be readily supplemented with thyroxine. At present, the major disadvantage of radioiodine therapy is the unavailability of facilities that can safely handle ^{131}I and accurately determine the ideal dose to administer.

References and Supplemental Reading

Aucoin, D. P., Peterson, M. E., Hurvitz, A. I., et al.: Propylthiouracil-induced immune-mediated disease in cats. J. Pharm. Exp. Ther. 234:13, 1985.

Birchard, S. J., Peterson, M. E., and Jacobson, A.: Surgical treatment of feline hyperthyroidism: Results of 85 cases. J. Am. Anim. Hosp. Assoc. 20:705, 1984.

Black, A. P., and Peterson, M. E.: Thyroid biopsy and thyroidectomy. In Bojrab, M. J. (ed.): Current Techniques in Small Animal Surgery. Philadelphia: Lea & Febiger, 1983, pp. 388–396.

Flanders, J. A., Harvey, H. J., and Erb, H. N.: Feline thyroidectomy: A comparison of postoperative hypocalcemia associated with three different surgical techniques. Vet. Surg. 16:362, 1987.

Peterson, M. E.: Hypoparathyroidism. In Kirk, R. W. (ed.): Current Veterinary Therapy IX. Philadelphia: W. B. Saunders Co., 1986, pp. 1039–1045.

Peterson, M. E.: Considerations and complications in anesthesia with pathophysiologic changes in the endocrine system. In Short, C. E. (ed.): Veterinary Anesthesiology. Baltimore: Williams & Wilkins, 1987, pp. 251–270.

Peterson, M. E., and Becker, D. V.: Radionuclide thyroid imaging in 135 cats with hyperthyroidism. Vet. Radiol. 25:23, 1984.

Peterson, M. E., Hurvitz, A. I., Leib, M. S., et al.: Propylthiouracil-associated hemolytic anemia, thrombocytopenia, and antinuclear antibodies in cats with hyperthyroidism. J.A.V.M.A. 184:806, 1984.

Peterson, M. E., Kintzer, P. P., and Hurvitz, A. I.: Methimazole treatment of 262 cats with hyperthyroidism. J. Vet. Intern. Med. 2:150, 1988.

Peterson, M. E., and Randolph, J. F.: Endocrine diseases. In Sherding, R. G. (ed.): Diseases of the Cat: Diagnosis and Management. New York: Churchill Livingstone, 1989, pp. 1095–1161.

Turrel, J. M., Feldman, E. C., Hayes, M., et al.: Radioactive iodine therapy in cats with hyperthyroidism. J.A.V.M.A. 184:554, 1984.

DIETARY THERAPY FOR CANINE DIABETES MELLITUS

RICHARD W. NELSON, D.V.M.

W. Lafayette, Indiana

Dietary therapy, in conjunction with exogenous insulin, plays an integral role in the successful management of diabetes mellitus in humans. Unfortunately, dietary therapy has received minimal attention in the management of diabetes mellitus in dogs, despite the frequent inability of exogenous insulin to maintain good glycemic control. In our experience, the initiation of dietary therapy in conjunction with insulin injections has reduced daily insulin requirements, improved glycemic control, and seemingly decreased the frequency of diabetic complications in many of our diabetic dogs. The factors that should be considered when formulating an appropriate dietary regimen include the correction and prevention of obesity, the establishment of an appropriate feeding schedule, and the selection of diets that minimize postprandial hyperglycemia and enhance the actions of insulin.

CALORIC INTAKE AND OBESITY

Obesity decreases tissue responsiveness to insulin and creates glucose intolerance by causing down-regulation of peripheral insulin receptors, impairing insulin receptor binding affinity, and causing post-receptor defects in insulin action. A relative tissue insensitivity to exogenous insulin may also exist in the obese diabetic dog. The severity of obesity directly correlates with the severity of glucose intolerance. Fortunately, obesity-induced alterations in insulin responsiveness are reversible. As obesity resolves, up-regulation of peripheral insulin receptors occurs and insulin receptor binding affinity improves.

Obviously, the daily caloric intake of the diabetic dog should be designed to correct and prevent obesity. By correcting and preventing obesity, exogenous insulin therapy should become more effective, and daily insulin requirements may decline. Excellent in-depth discussions on canine caloric requirements and the management of obesity are available (Lewis et al., 1987). Daily caloric intake should be based on the dog's ideal body weight, age, and necessity for weight reduction. As a general rule, the daily caloric requirement for dogs less than 8 years of age is 60 to 80 Kcal/kg of ideal body weight, and for dogs 8 years and older it is 40 to 60 Kcal/kg of ideal body weight. A rough approximation of ideal body weight should be based on the size of the dog and general breed standards. This ideal body weight should then be compared with the dog's current body weight and overall appearance. If obesity is present, the calculated daily caloric requirement should be reduced an additional 40 per cent to promote weight loss.

Once the daily caloric requirement is established, the daily quantity of food can be determined by dividing the daily caloric requirement by the amount of calories per can or cup of food to be fed. Feeding a low-calorie dense diet specifically intended for weight reduction, such as Prescription Diet r/d, will reduce begging by the dog and improve the chances of success. Prescription Diet r/d provides 260 Kcal per can or 200 Kcal/8-oz measuring cup of dry food. The initial quantity of food is an estimate that frequently needs adjustment to obtain and maintain ideal body weight for that particular dog. Adjustments in caloric intake should take place after the first month and should be based on weekly determinations of the dog's body weight. Incremental changes by 10 per cent of daily caloric intake are recommended until ideal body weight is maintained. Adjustments in daily insulin requirements may also be necessary as the obese diabetic dog loses weight.

FEEDING SCHEDULE

The hypoinsulinemic diabetic dog cannot secrete endogenous insulin in response to postprandial increases in portal blood glucose and must rely on exogenous insulin to minimize postprandial hyperglycemia. The development of postprandial hyperglycemia is dependent, in part, on the amount of food consumed per meal and the effectiveness of exogenous insulin at the time nutrients are absorbed from the intestine. Feeding several small meals minimizes the amount of nutrients absorbed from the intestine at any one meal and is preferable to feeding one large meal. In addition, the time when these meals are consumed should be manipulated to coincide with the time when the exogenous insulin is active in metabolizing assimilated nutrients. For the diabetic dog receiving one insulin injection per day, our ideal feeding schedule consists of three equal-sized meals fed at 6-hr intervals, beginning at the time of the insulin injection. For the diabetic dog receiving insulin twice a day, the ideal schedule consists of four equal-sized meals fed at the following times: immediately following each insulin injection, midafternoon, and late evening. Feeding multiple meals at specified times represents the ideal situation, and although these feeding schedules should be used whenever possible, the owner's schedule must be considered and the feeding protocol altered to comply with what is feasible. Many owners who are administering insulin twice a day, for example, are satisfied with the results of feeding their pets two equal-sized meals, one meal immediately after each insulin injection.

Subsequent adjustments in the time of feeding are based on results of serial blood glucose determinations obtained every 1 to 2 hr for 14 to 24 hr following the insulin injection. If the meals are consumed while exogenous insulin is still metabolically active, there is minimal to no increase in the postprandial blood glucose concentration. In contrast, a postprandial increase in the blood glucose concentration, usually within 2 hr of consuming food, is an indication of waning insulin activity. If this occurs, the time between insulin administration and feeding should be shortened.

COMPOSITION OF THE DIET

Ideally, the diet for the diabetic dog should be designed to maximize gastrointestinal transit time, prolong the intestinal absorption of nutrients (especially monosaccharides), and minimize the postprandial increase in the blood glucose concentration. Of the three commercial forms of pet food, soft-moist, canned, and dry food, postprandial hyperglycemia is most apt to develop following consumption of soft-moist foods. This is partly because the carbohydrate in soft-moist food is primarily sucrose in the form of corn syrup, a disaccharide requiring minimal digestion prior to intestinal absorption.

In contrast, the carbohydrates in dry and canned

foods are primarily starches (e.g., corn, wheat, barley), which are complex carbohydrates requiring intraluminal digestion to monosaccharides before absorption can take place. The more complex carbohydrates in canned and dry foods increase gastrointestinal transit time, delay absorption of nutrients, and reduce postprandial fluctuations in blood glucose. The increased amounts of animal fat in canned foods and increased fiber in dry foods may also delay gastrointestinal transit time and help reduce postprandial hyperglycemia. These properties make most dry and canned foods more acceptable diets for diabetic dogs. Soft-moist foods should not be fed because of their greater propensity for inducing postprandial hyperglycemia, which makes glycemic regulation more difficult.

The ideal percentage of carbohydrate, protein, and fat in the diet has not been established for the diabetic dog. The recommended diet for humans with diabetes consists of 55 to 60 per cent complex carbohydrates, 20 per cent protein, and 20 to 25 per cent fat. These diets high in complex carbohydrates and moderately restricted in fats seem to improve glucose tolerance, enhance tissue sensitivity to insulin, and lower plasma cholesterol, triglyceride, and lipoprotein concentrations. Comparable guidelines would seem appropriate for diabetic dogs. Most commercial dry foods contain 45 to 60 per cent carbohydrate, 22 to 30 per cent protein, and 7 to 13 per cent fat, whereas commercial canned foods contain 30 to 55 per cent carbohydrate, 30 to 40 per cent protein, and 10 to 25 per cent fat. Although these diets are acceptable, most do not contain ideal quantities of carbohydrate and some may contain excessive amounts of fat, especially the canned foods.

Prescription Diets (Hill's Pet Products) offer an interesting alternative to commercial foods. Prescription Diet g/d most closely resembles the recommendations for human diabetics. Prescription Diet g/d contains 60 to 65 per cent carbohydrate, 19 per cent protein, and 11 to 15 per cent fat. Prescription Diet w/d is also similar to human recommendations, containing 55 per cent carbohydrate, 16 per cent protein, and 7 to 12 per cent fat. In addition, Prescription Diet w/d contains 13 to 16 per cent fiber, which has been shown to be beneficial in improving glucose tolerance. Although Prescription Diet r/d has been recommended for the dietary management of canine diabetes mellitus because of its increased fiber (22 to 25 per cent) and reduced fat content (7 per cent), the carbohydrate content (36 to 39 per cent) of this diet is below recommendations established for humans. The beneficial effects of the increased fiber content of r/d, however, may outweigh that lost from lowering the carbohydrate content.

DIETARY FIBER

Several studies have emerged during the past decade evaluating the influence of dietary fiber on improving glycemic control in both insulin-dependent and non–insulin-dependent diabetes mellitus in humans. Although controversial, soluble fiber (e.g., guar gum, pectin) rather than insoluble fiber (e.g., cellulose, lignins) is believed primarily responsible for this glycemic improvement. By increasing daily soluble fiber consumption from levels of 3 to 10 gm/day to greater than 35 gm/day, an improvement in glycemic control is observed, including a decrease in fasting and postprandial blood glucose concentrations, urine glucose excretion, glycosylated hemoglobin concentrations, daily insulin requirements, and adverse insulin reactions. Soluble fibers are believed to exert their effects on glycemic control by altering gastrointestinal transit time, carbohydrate absorption, and the secretion of gastrointestinal hormones and by enhancing tissue sensitivity to insulin. Carbohydrates have a synergistic influence on increased fiber intake. For increased fiber intake to be effective, daily carbohydrate intake must exceed 40 per cent of the diet and must be mixed intimately with the fiber prior to ingestion.

Increased soluble fiber intake also affects lipid metabolism in human diabetics. Total blood cholesterol concentrations and the low-density lipoprotein cholesterol fraction decrease, whereas the high-density lipoprotein cholesterol fraction increases with consumption of diets high in soluble fiber. Although somewhat controversial, increased intake of soluble fiber also seems to lower plasma triglyceride concentrations, especially in patients with hypertriglyceridemia. The beneficial effects on plasma triglyceride concentrations are more apparent on postprandial rather than fasting concentrations. High-fiber diets also reduce the total lipid and triglyceride content of the liver in experimental animals. These alterations in lipid metabolism are beneficial in diabetes mellitus, in which derangements in cholesterol metabolism and hypercholesterolemia are frequently found.

Fiber-induced alterations in lipid metabolism probably result from binding of bile salts to fiber in the intestinal lumen, enhanced bile salt excretion, and impaired cholesterol and triglyceride absorption. In addition, short-chain fatty acid metabolites of fiber and decreased portal glucose and insulin concentrations may alter hepatic synthesis and peripheral metabolism of triglycerides and cholesterol.

Despite obvious improvement in blood glucose and lipid parameters following the acute consumption of soluble fiber, the benefit obtained from chronic increased fiber intake remains controversial. Some investigators have found continued improvement in glucose and lipid parameters with chronic increased fiber intake, whereas others have been unable to document measurable improvement. In addition, the role of increased fiber intake in minimizing chronic complications of diabetes mellitus is still unanswered.

Studies involving increased fiber intake in humans with diabetes mellitus have interesting implications for the diabetic dog. The influence of increased soluble and insoluble dietary fiber intake on glycemic control in dogs with insulin-dependent diabetes mellitus is currently under investigation. Preliminary results would suggest comparable improvement in glycemic control in the diabetic dog as has been reported in humans. We have also had some success in improving glycemic control by feeding Prescription Diet r/d or w/d to a few poorly regulated diabetic dogs. Of these, Prescription Diet w/d appears preferable because the carbohydrate content of this diet is more in accord with levels found to be beneficial in human studies, the palatability is better, the frequency of defecation is less, and owner compliance with the use of this diet seems better. Both diets are restricted in calories, enhancing weight reduction. It is interesting that the fiber in these diets is primarily insoluble fiber, which is not believed to be as effective in improving glycemic control as soluble fiber. Nevertheless, until controlled studies dictate otherwise, the use of these high-fiber diets is indicated.

CONCURRENT PANCREATITIS

Problems in other organ systems frequently accompany the diagnosis of diabetes mellitus, including hyperadrenocorticism, infection, pancreatitis, congestive heart failure, and liver and renal insufficiency. Dietary therapy plays a role in many of these disorders and may force the clinician to modify the diet of the diabetic dog. This is especially evident with concurrent pancreatitis.

Chronic recurring pancreatitis is one of the most common complications of diabetes mellitus in dogs. Fortunately, many of the principles governing the dietary management of pancreatitis are similar to those for diabetes mellitus, including feeding several small meals per day rather than one large meal, restricting dietary fat consumption, feeding digestible high-quality protein, and relying on carbohydrates for calories. A highly digestible diet consisting of low-fat cottage cheese mixed 1:2 by volume with cooked white rice has proved successful in the initial dietary management of pancreatitis. Once the clinical signs of pancreatitis have resolved and the dog is stable on a cottage cheese and rice diet, a more nutritionally complete diet (e.g., the dry form

of Prescription Diets w/d or g/d) can be substituted. If recurring pancreatitis becomes a problem, we have had success feeding a 1:1 mixture of cooked white rice and dry food. For finicky eaters, we recommend mixing rice and lean meat such as chicken, turkey, or fish with dry food. Canned foods are not routinely used because of their fat content, and soft-moist foods are strictly avoided.

SUMMARY

Currently recommended guidelines for feeding diabetic dogs are as follows:

1. Daily caloric intake should maintain the dog at its ideal body weight. If the diabetic dog is obese, a weight reduction program should be initiated.

2. The daily caloric requirement should be between 40 and 80 Kcal/kg of ideal body weight, depending on the dog's age and activity. If the dog is obese, the calculated daily caloric requirement should be reduced an additional 40 per cent to promote weight loss.

3. An ideal initial daily feeding schedule consists of three meals fed at 6-hr intervals, beginning at the time of the insulin injection. Subsequent adjustments in the time of feeding should be based on results of serial blood glucose determinations.

4. Soft-moist foods should not be fed to diabetic dogs; dry and canned foods are more acceptable diets.

5. Based on recommendations for humans with diabetes, the diet should contain 55 to 60 per cent complex carbohydrates, 20 per cent protein, and less than 25 per cent fat. Prescription Diets g/d and w/d meet these requirements. Although some commercial dog foods are acceptable, most do not contain ideal quantities of carbohydrate or fiber and some contain excessive amounts of fat.

6. The influence of increased dietary fiber intake on improving glycemic control has not been completely established in diabetic dogs. Improvement in glycemic control has been documented in some diabetic dogs fed Prescription Diets w/d and r/d, which contain increased amounts of fiber.

7. Dietary therapy may need modification depending on the presence of concurrent disorders, most notably pancreatitis.

References and Supplemental Reading

Anderson, J. W., and Chen, W.: Plant fiber. Carbohydrate and lipid metabolism. Am. J. Clin. Nutr. 32:346, 1979.
Anderson, J. W., Chen, W., and Sieling, B.: Hypolipidemic effects of high carbohydrate, high fiber diets. Metabolism 29:551, 1980.
Crapo, P. A.: Carbohydrate in the diabetic diet. J. Am. Coll. Nutr. 5:31, 1986.
El-Beheri, B. B.: Rationale for changes in the dietary management of diabetes. J. Am. Diabetic Assoc. 81:258, 1982.
Feldman, E. C., and Nelson, R. W.: *Canine and Feline Endocrinology and Reproduction*. Philadelphia: W. B. Saunders Co., 1987.

Gatti, E., Catenazzo, G., Camisasca, E., et al.: Effects of guar-enriched pasta in the treatment of diabetes and hyperlipidemia. Ann. Nutr. Metab. 28:1, 1984.

Lewis, L. D., Morris, M. L., and Hand, M. S.: *Small Animal Clinical Nutrition*, 3rd ed. Topeka: Mark Morris Associates, 1987.

Mattheeuws, D., Rottiers, R., Kaneko, J. J., et al.: Diabetes mellitus in dogs: Relationship of obesity to glucose tolerance and insulin response. Am. J. Vet. Res. 45:98, 1984.

Reaven, G., Coulston, A., and Marcus, R.: Nutritional management of diabetes. Med. Clin. North Am. 63:927, 1979.

Riccardi, G., Rivellese, A., Pacioni, D., et al.: Separate influence of dietary carbohydrate and fiber on the metabolic control in diabetes. Diabetologia 26:116, 1984.

Vinik, A. I., Crapo, P. A., Brink, S. J., et al.: Nutritional recommendations and principles for individuals with diabetes mellitus: 1986. Diabetes Care 10:126, 1987.

INSULIN-RESISTANT DIABETES MELLITUS

KAREN J. WOLFSHEIMER, D.V.M.

Baton Rouge, Louisiana

Continued study of diabetes mellitus in humans and animals has shown the disease to have multiple causes. Classification according to these causes has been proposed by the National Diabetes Data Group (Table 1). Although this classification is based on human diabetes, it does have relevance to veterinary diabetes. We now recognize that diabetes mellitus may result from not only an absolute deficiency of insulin (spontaneous type I diabetes and certain groups of secondary diabetes), but also from a relative deficiency of insulin (spontaneous type II, certain groups of secondary diabetes, and impaired glucose tolerance class).

Another classification has been proposed in dogs, based on glucose and insulin response to an IV glucose tolerance test. In this classification, type I diabetics have no insulin secretion in either the fasted state or with glucose stimulation. Type II diabetic dogs are subdivided according to whether they are obese or nonobese dogs. Nonobese type II diabetics have fasted insulin concentrations that are within normal range but are unable to increase insulin secretion on glucose stimulation. Obese type II diabetics have elevated fasted insulin concentrations but are also unable to increase insulin secretion on glucose stimulation. Type III diabetic dogs are only mildly hyperglycemic (< 200 mg/dl) and are also subdivided into nonobese and obese dogs. Nonobese type III diabetics have fasted insulin concentrations within the normal range, and their glucose-stimulated insulin secretion is subnormal. Obese type III diabetics have elevated fasted insulin concentrations, as well as hypersecretion of insulin in response to glucose stimulation.

Insulin resistance exists whenever normal concentrations of insulin produce a less than normal biologic response. Insulin-resistant states include (1) those in which a maximal response to insulin is decreased no matter what dose is given (decreased responsiveness), (2) those in which a maximal response is obtained, but only by giving greater than normal amounts of insulin (decreased sensitivity), and (3) those in which there is a combination of decreased responsiveness and decreased sensitivity. Proposed mechanisms for insulin resistance include abnormal insulin molecule, increased insulin degradation, insulin antibodies, insulin receptor antibodies, high circulating levels of counterregulatory hormones, insulin receptor defects (altered numbers or affinity) and postreceptor defects.

In a clinical setting, it may be difficult to determine the nature of the insulin resistance. In humans, insulin resistance has been subdivided into mild to moderate insulin resistance and extreme insulin resistance. There are specific syndromes and metabolic conditions that are recognized to cause

Table 1. *The National Diabetes Data Group Classification**

Spontaneous diabetes mellitus
    Type I: Insulin-dependent diabetes mellitus (IDDM)
    Type II: Non–insulin-dependent diabetes mellitus (NIDDM)
        Nonobese
        Obese

Secondary diabetes mellitus
    Pancreatic disease: Pancreatitis, pancreatectomy
    Hormonal: Excessive secretion of counterregulatory hormones (glucocorticoids, glucagon, growth hormone, catecholamines, thyroid hormone) and progesterone
    Drugs: Exogenous administration of glucocorticoids, progesterone, others

Impaired glucose tolerance (IGT)

Gestational diabetes: Glucose intolerance that begins during pregnancy

(*From* National Diabetes Data Group: Classification and diagnosis of diabetes mellitus and other categories of glucose intolerance. Diabetes 25:1039, 1979.)

mild to moderate insulin resistance in humans, dogs, and cats (Table 2). Extreme insulin resistance is recognized to occur with acanthosis nigricans in humans and may be due to primary target cell resistance (type A) or autoimmune (antiinsulin receptor antibodies) (type B) mechanisms. Clinical syndromes of extreme insulin resistance have not yet been documented in dogs and cats. It remains a diagnostic challenge to the veterinary clinician to detect the cause in individual cases in which insulin resistance is suspected.

In diabetic dogs and cats, insulin resistance has been arbitrarily defined to exist when therapeutic doses of insulin exceed 2 to 2.5 units/kg of body weight per day (Feldman and Nelson, 1987). The clinician should be concerned that insulin resistance is a problem if there are persistent signs that insulin therapy is inadequate. These signs include persistent glycosuria, ketonuria, polyuria, polydipsia, polyphagia, or weight loss. If these signs are present, then an insulin response test should be performed to document and differentiate the cause of persistent hyperglycemia. The insulin response test is performed by collecting a fasted blood glucose level in the early morning prior to insulin administration. Then insulin is administered at the regular dose and time; feeding is allowed according to the animal's regular schedule, and blood glucose concentrations are determined every 2 hr for the following 12 to 24 hr (24 hr is preferred). The data obtained from this test can be plotted to aid in differentiating the cause of the hyperglycemia. Results will aid in differentiating insulin resistance from the Somogyi overswing, rapid metabolism of insulin, and the dawn phenomenon as causes for the hyperglycemia. Typical curves for these causes of hyperglycemia are described elsewhere (Wolfsheimer, 1986). If an essentially flat curve is obtained or there is minimal response to the insulin, then one should consider underdose or insulin resistance. If the given dose is greater than 2 to 2.5 units/kg, then insulin resistance should be considered.

Table 2. *Clinical Diseases Associated with Mild to Moderate Insulin Resistance*

Disease	Humans	Dogs	Cats
Insulin antibodies	Yes	Yes?	?
Type I diabetes mellitus	Yes	Yes*	?
Type II diabetes mellitus	Yes	Yes	?
Obesity	Yes	Yes	Yes?
Acromegaly	Yes	Yes	Yes
Cushing's syndrome	Yes	Yes	Yes
Pregnancy	Yes	?	?
Ketoacidosis	Yes	?	?
Uremia	Yes	Yes*	?
Liver disease	Yes	?	?
Sepsis	Yes	Yes*	?

*Demonstrated in experimentally induced diabetes mellitus.

Insulin resistance has also been shown to occur with normal blood glucose concentrations or mild to moderate hyperglycemia and hyperinsulinemia in both experimental conditions using euglycemic clamp infusions and in spontaneous diseases in dogs. Normoglycemia with hyperinsulinemia has been recognized by the author in a family of schnauzers with hyperchylomicronemia. Other investigators have recognized insulin resistance with normoglycemia and hyperinsulinemia in obese dogs (Mattheeuws et al., 1984) and in certain dogs with Cushing's syndrome (Peterson, 1984).

The mechanism for the endogenous hyperinsulinemia is uncertain in most cases. Hyperinsulinemia may occur to compensate for receptor defects (insulin insensitivity) or postreceptor defects (insulin unresponsiveness). In some cases, it may be due to hypersecretion of insulin as the primary event (due to stimulation of the beta cells by secretagogues such as glucagon or growth hormone) with secondary down-regulation of receptors at the target organ. In either event, prolonged overstimulation of beta cell secretion can lead to exhaustion, with resulting absolute insulin deficiency.

If the clinician has a suspicion that a particular normoglycemic patient may be at high risk for having insulin resistance that could lead to overt diabetes mellitus, an intravenous glucose tolerance test (IVGTT) may be performed. Blood samples for glucose and insulin determinations are collected before and at frequent intervals up to 1 to 2 hr after the administration of 500 mg/kg of dextrose (Wolfsheimer, 1986). Glucose clearance and total insulin secretion can be determined to document insulin resistance. If insulin resistance can be detected early and the underlying condition causing it can be determined and successfully managed, overt diabetes mellitus may be delayed or avoided.

The flow chart provided in Figure 1 can be used to rule out various recognized causes of insulin resistance in dogs and cats. Prior to performing an in-depth and expensive workup for insulin resistance, one should eliminate client management problems including improper storage, handling, or administration of the insulin product. A thorough history should include emphasis on drug therapy of any kind. A complete physical examination may reveal abnormal physical findings, which may help to prioritize laboratory diagnostic tests performed on the individual patient. The following discussion is a description of the proposed mechanisms and management recommendations for several of the causes of insulin resistance listed in Table 2.

TYPE I VERSUS TYPE II DIABETES MELLITUS

Dogs with experimentally induced type I (insulin-dependent) diabetes mellitus with absolute insulin

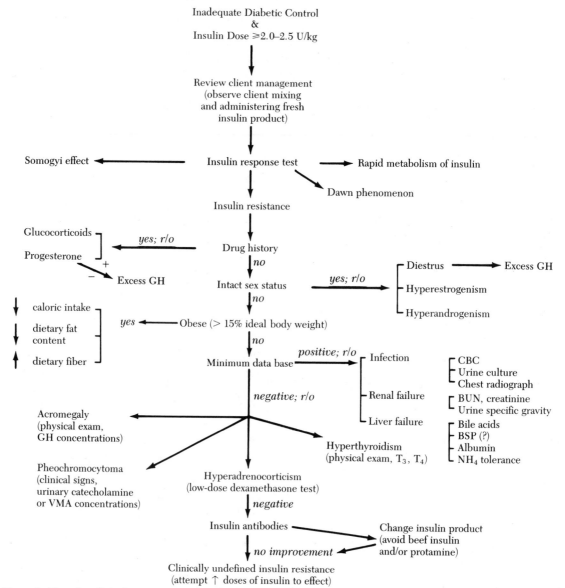

Figure 1. Flow chart for ruling out causes of insulin resistance (r/o, rule out; GH, growth hormone; BSP, Bromsulphalein; VMA, vanillylmandelic acid).

deficiency exhibit insulin resistance (Bevilacqua et al., 1985). Ketoacidosis and hypophosphatemia may contribute to the insulin resistance, which involves both the liver and peripheral tissues. With the initiation of exogenous insulin therapy, these dogs should show improvement in insulin sensitivity.

It is widely recognized that type II (non–insulin-dependent) diabetes mellitus in humans may be associated with a variable degree of insulin resistance. Fasted insulin concentrations may be normal or increased. The insulin response to hyperglycemia may be normal or increased, although the majority of patients have an impaired response. This type of diabetes may occur in dogs and may account for an increasing number of the diabetic cats diagnosed in practice (Feldman and Nelson, 1987). These cats

maintain a sustained hyperglycemia during periods of stress and often require insulin therapy. However, once the stress (usually of some other disease) is resolved, insulin therapy may no longer be necessary.

SECONDARY DIABETES MELLITUS

In addition to spontaneous diabetes mellitus, there are a variety of secondary causes of diabetes in dogs and cats (see Table 1). The previous discussion pertaining to absolute and relative insulin deficiency in spontaneous type I and type II diabetes mellitus also applies to secondary diabetes. By mechanisms previously described, progression of a specific disease syndrome causing diabetes mellitus can initially involve relative insulin deficiency and then absolute insulin deficiency.

Cushing's Syndrome or Hyperadrenocorticism

Hyperadrenocorticism, either spontaneous or iatrogenic, can result in insulin resistance and glucose intolerance. The resulting hyperglycemia may be due to increased hepatic glucose production from gluconeogenesis (hepatic insulin resistance) as well as decreased glucose utilization in peripheral tissues (peripheral insulin resistance) (Amatruda et al., 1985).

Healthy dogs given 1 to 2 mg/kg/day of prednisolone for 3 weeks had no significant changes in glucose tolerance or insulin secretion, although fasting blood glucose concentrations were mildly but significantly increased (Wolfsheimer, 1986). Cats given 2 mg/kg/day of prednisolone for 8 days developed significant decreases in glucose tolerance, and some cats developed fasting hyperglycemia (Middleton, 1985). Diabetes has been reported to occur following glucocorticoid therapy in clinical case reports and is most likely to occur in animals with subclinical diabetes prior to the onset of glucocorticoid therapy. The development of glucose intolerance may also depend on the duration and dose of glucocorticoid.

Dogs with spontaneous hyperadrenocorticism may develop significant hyperinsulinemia, glucose intolerance, or overt diabetes mellitus. In a study of 60 dogs, approximately 85 per cent of the dogs had hyperinsulinemia (Peterson, 1984). Only about 10 per cent of the dogs were overtly diabetic, but 40 per cent had fasting hyperglycemia. Although overall glucose utilization is impaired, hepatic glucose overproduction appears to play the major role in development of hyperglycemia (Peterson et al., 1986).

The mechanisms responsible for glucose intolerance seen with hyperadrenocorticism are not completely understood. Erythrocyte insulin receptor binding has been shown to be decreased (decreased number of receptors) in dogs with spontaneous hyperadrenocorticism and hyperinsulinemia (Wolfsheimer and Peterson, 1987). This could be a primary abnormality, but is more likely to reflect down-regulation of receptors secondary to hyperinsulinemia. Hyperinsulinemia may be due to direct stimulation of pancreatic beta cells by glucocorticoid or a postreceptor alteration in insulin target cells, resulting in insulin resistance. As the hyperadrenocorticism persists, insulin resistance worsens and hyperglycemia may develop. If the hyperinsulinemia persists, pancreatic beta cell exhaustion occurs, so that plasma insulin concentrations decrease and overt diabetes mellitus develops.

Correction of the hyperadrenocorticism will improve insulin resistance so that insulin requirements are decreased in those cases of overt diabetes mellitus with no pancreatic beta cell reserve. Correction of the hyperadrenocorticism during the early stages may resolve insulin resistance and glucose intolerance in dogs that still have pancreatic reserve, negating the need for insulin therapy.

Dogs and cats developing glucose intolerance after a short course (< 4 weeks) of glucocorticoid therapy should be immediately withdrawn from glucocorticoids. Animals receiving longer courses of glucocorticoid therapy should receive a rapid tapering dose (0.2 to 0.4 mg/kg every other day over 2 to 3 weeks) to minimize side effects due to adrenal suppression by glucocorticoids. Animals with blood glucose concentrations greater than 250 mg/dl should receive insulin therapy and the dose decreased as indicated during the withdrawal of glucocorticoids. Some animals that were subclinically diabetic prior to glucocorticoid therapy may require lifelong insulin therapy even when glucocorticoid therapy is withdrawn.

A diagnosis of spontaneous hyperadrenocorticism can be made from the appropriate history, physical examination, and diagnostic test findings. If a patient has overt diabetes mellitus, the low-dose dexamethasone test may be preferred over the adrenocorticotropic hormone (ACTH) stimulation test for making a diagnosis of spontaneous hyperadrenocorticism. Poorly regulated diabetic dogs may have elevated resting cortisol concentrations, making interpretation of the ACTH stimulation test difficult. Dogs with blood glucose concentrations in excess of 250 mg/dl should be started on insulin therapy as soon as a diagnosis of diabetes has been made.

Once a diagnosis of hyperadrenocorticism is made, specific therapy with o'p'-DDD (mitotane) should be instituted. Because of the rapid decrease in daily insulin requirement, the institution of a lower initial dose of o'p'-DDD has been recommended (Eigenmann and Peterson, 1984). A dose of 25 to 35 mg/kg/day is given in conjunction with 0.4 mg/kg/day of prednisone to prevent rapid reduction in circulating glucocorticoid concentrations and insulin requirements. When normal plasma cortisol concentrations are reached, o'p'-DDD can be continued at the standard dose of 50 mg/kg/week (given once weekly or split into twice weekly).

Acromegaly or Excess Growth Hormone

Acromegaly in dogs and cats is characterized by overgrowth of soft tissue or bony structures and is due to chronic elevations in growth hormone (GH) concentrations. Some agromegalic patients may also develop glucose intolerance and diabetes mellitus.

Excess GH production may be due to a pituitary adenoma or progestogen exposure.

In dogs, the most common reason for excess GH production is either the administration of progestogens or the naturally occurring exposure to endogenous progesterone during the luteal phase of the estrous cycle in intact bitches (Eigenmann and Peterson, 1984). Most normal dogs do not develop elevated GH concentrations during their luteal (progesterone) phase, but the mechanism by which progesterone triggers excess GH production is not known.

Those dogs with excess GH may exhibit mild to marked hyperglycemia, hyperinsulinemia, increased circulating insulin-like growth factors (somatomedins), and marked insulin resistance. The mechanism for GH-associated insulin resistance is not fully understood. Studies support that resistance occurs in both the liver and peripheral tissues and is predominantly due to postreceptor alterations. Studies of receptor binding in acromegalic patients have yielded conflicting results. It is also possible that progesterone may directly contribute to hyperglycemia by increasing hepatic glucose production and peripheral insulin resistance owing to its steroidal nature.

From a clinical management standpoint, the sooner the condition of excess GH production can be recognized and resolved, the better the chances are to preserve pancreatic beta cell function. The definitive treatment would be withdrawal of exogenous progestogens or spaying the intact bitch or both. In dogs treated with exogenous progestogens, GH concentrations remain elevated for a longer period of time than do GH levels in intact bitches experiencing elevations of progesterone during the luteal phase.

It is often helpful to determine the fasted plasma insulin concentration or insulin response to the IVGTT. The observance of high plasma insulin concentrations carries a better prognosis for recovery than the observance of low or absent plasma insulin concentrations.

The decision to institute insulin therapy will depend on the degree of hyperglycemia (Eigenmann and Peterson, 1984). Recommendations are to administer insulin if the blood glucose level is greater than 150 mg/dl in dogs with progestogen therapy and is in excess of 200 mg/dl in bitches in the luteal phase. Insulin therapy seems to improve both insulin resistance and the recovery of beta cell function. Initially, very large doses of insulin may be required (> 2.5 units/kg). After progestogen withdrawal or spaying, insulin therapy will gradually change. Frequent monitoring of the patient's blood glucose determinations is necessary to dictate modifications in insulin dose over the course of days to weeks. Urine glucose determinations may be helpful but often are misleading and should only be used in conjunction with blood glucose determinations.

The duration of excess GH production and the plasma insulin concentrations should theoretically be helpful in predicting whether a patient will fully recover. The owner should be aware that each dog must be considered individually in its ability to regain normal glucose tolerance.

Excess GH production in cats is most often associated with pituitary adenomas (Peterson, 1987). Clinical signs may include glucose intolerance and hyperglycemia with marked insulin resistance, weight gain, organomegaly, cardiomyopathy, arthropathy, spondylosis deformans, macroglossia, prognathia inferior, and abdominal enlargement. Although the administration of progestogens to cats can result in hyperglycemia (Mansfield et al., 1986), the role of progestogens in the development of naturally occurring GH excess is unknown but is unlikely to be significant (Peterson, 1987). Management of diabetes mellitus with insulin therapy in these patients is difficult and often requires very large doses (> 30 units/day). The use of radiation therapy, bromocriptine, or somatostatin analogues to decrease GH production needs to be evaluated in these cats in the future.

Hyperthyroidism

Hyperthyroidism can occur simultaneously with diabetes mellitus in cats and may play a role in the development of diabetes. Increased thyroid hormone results in increased gluconeogenesis and glycogenolysis, both of which may contribute to hyperglycemia. The role of thyroid hormone in insulin resistance is less certain, and experimental evidence is contradictory. Administration of exogenous T_3 to human patients resulted in an increased secretion and clearance of insulin in association with postreceptor defects in the liver and peripheral tissues (Dimitriadis et al., 1985). Studies of naturally occurring hyperthyroidism in humans have demonstrated hyperinsulinemia, decreases in receptor binding, and postreceptor defects. The increases in measured total immunoreactive insulin may be in part due to increases in proinsulin, which is not as biologically active as insulin.

The role that insulin resistance plays in hyperthyroid states needs to be evaluated in animals, especially cats. Medical or surgical control of hyperthyroidism should theoretically decrease insulin requirements or possibly eliminate the need for daily insulin.

OBESITY

Obesity is a metabolic imbalance in which ingestion of energy is in excess of that being used, resulting in an excess of body fat. Obesity is considered to be present when body weight is greater than 15 per cent of ideal body weight. It is the most common nutritional disease and is often accompanied by derangements in carbohydrate and lipid metabolism. Obese patients may have alterations in insulin secretion as well as insulin resistance.

Multiple theories are proposed to explain the insulin resistance encountered in obesity (Amatruda et al., 1985). It may be due to a decrease in insulin sensitivity or insulin responsiveness, although the predominant alteration appears to be a postreceptor defect. It is unclear what causes the hyperinsulinemia that occurs in obesity. Some studies support a primary abnormality in the central nervous system and endocrine-pancreas axis, resulting in increased beta cell secretion of insulin with a secondary hyperphagia. In other studies, the hyperinsulinemia has been shown to occur as a result of hyperphagia. In this case, increases in plasma free fatty acids from diet or increased hepatic production cause a target cell postreceptor alteration. Increased free fatty acids result in decreased glucose uptake and utilization by cells, so that hyperglycemia occurs.

In humans, the degree of insulin resistance can be directly correlated with the degree of obesity. In dogs, obesity has been shown to cause insulin resistance in normoglycemic and type II diabetic dogs (Mattheeuws et al., 1984). Decreasing body weight by decreasing caloric intake will improve insulin resistance. In addition, insulin resistance has been shown to be improved in obese humans by lowering plasma free fatty acids.

Weight reduction in the obese diabetic patient should be achieved by a closely regulated reduction in caloric intake. To avoid hypoglycemia, blood glucose should be monitored more frequently in those dogs on a weight-reduction program since insulin requirements are expected to decrease.

The role of the fiber, fat, and carbohydrate content of diets in glucose and lipid homeostasis needs to be evaluated in dogs and cats. At this time, it would seem practical to limit caloric intake in obese diabetic patients. A low-fat, high-fiber commercial diet (Prescription Diet r/d, Hill's Pet Products) has been designed for use in obese canine and feline patients. This diet is recommended for the obese diabetic patient, and its use in thin diabetic dogs has resulted in undesirable weight loss. A less fat-restricted diet (Prescription Diet w/d, Hill's Pet Products) may be used in thin or normal-weight diabetic dogs. In those diabetic patients with finicky appetites, well-balanced homemade diets with limited fat seem useful. Soft-moist diets, which contain glucose rather than starch as a source of carbohydrate, should be avoided in diabetic pets. Reduced-fat diets should be recommended for those schnauzers with hyperchylomicronemia and diabetes or mild glucose intolerance.

Exercise has been shown to improve glucose tolerance by directly improving insulin resistance, as well as aiding in weight loss by increasing daily caloric requirements. However, in diabetics with blood glucose concentrations greater than 300 mg/dl, especially if associated with ketonuria, exercise will only result in deterioration of metabolic control (Kemmer and Berger, 1986). If extra exercise is anticipated, the insulin dose should be decreased by up to 50 per cent of the usual dose, depending on the duration and intensity of the exercise. If exercise is spontaneous, then an increase in carbohydrate ingestion should be allowed before, during, and after exercise. Exercise should be performed postprandially to blunt the postprandial rise in blood glucose.

RENAL FAILURE

Mild glucose intolerance is recognized to occur in chronic renal failure in "nondiabetic" human patients (Amatruda et al., 1985). This glucose intolerance can be due to both a decrease in beta cell secretion of insulin as well as a peripheral insulin resistance. Insulin receptor binding is normal, and the resistance is due to a postreceptor defect. Insulin resistance is thought to be mediated by a dialyzable circulating small-molecular-weight peptide that works by a protein synthesis–dependent mechanism and is unique to uremic patients. The insulin resistance results in a hyperinsulinemia to maintain normal glucose concentrations. However, when elevated parathormone (PTH) concentrations occur, normal insulin secretion by the beta cells is decreased by altering calcium balance within the beta cell. Glucose intolerance, and in some cases hyperlipidemia, can then occur in some patients with renal failure. As renal function declines, the metabolic clearance rate of insulin decreases and glucose tolerance may actually improve. In diabetic patients with chronic renal failure, insulin requirements increase early in renal failure and then decline as the glomerular filtration rate (GFR) is markedly decreased. Diabetic patients with severe uremia may experience episodes of hypoglycemia.

Elevated concentrations of glucagon and GH have been observed in the blood of uremic patients, but the role they play in the insulin resistance of uremia is uncertain. Elevations in glucagon may contribute to hyperglycemia by increased gluconeogenesis.

Normalization of PTH concentrations by a low-phosphate diet and phosphate binders has been shown to improve beta cell secretion of insulin and glucose tolerance in children. Insulin resistance can be improved by hemodialysis or peritoneal dialysis. Therapeutic management of the uremic diabetic patient can be difficult, and the clinician should be aware that insulin requirements may either increase or decrease, depending on the degree of renal failure.

LIVER DISEASE

Insulin resistance is recognized to occur in both acute liver failure and chronic liver diseases, including cirrhosis. Although acute liver failure is most often associated with severe hypoglycemia, mild to moderate insulin-resistant hyperglycemia can occur (Vilstrup et al., 1986). Impaired glucose tolerance occurs in at least 50 per cent of human cirrhosis patients. The incidence of glucose intolerance in dogs and cats with liver disease is poorly documented. The hyperinsulinemia that is recognized with liver disease is due to increased secretion of insulin and possibly a decreased clearance of insulin by the liver (Cavallo-Perin et al., 1985). The trigger mechanism for the increased insulin secretion is not known, and there is disagreement about the significance of increased concentrations of stimulators of beta cell secretion such as glucagon, GH, and catecholamines. It is unknown whether the primary defect is hypersecretion of insulin with secondary down-regulation of receptors or if the primary defect is insulin insensitivity or unresponsiveness in the liver and peripheral tissues with secondary hypersecretion of insulin.

SEPSIS

Sepsis occurring in clinical patients can result in either hypoglycemia or hyperglycemia. Experimentally induced sepsis in dogs resulted in increases in plasma glucose, insulin, and glucagon (Raymond et al., 1985). Septic dogs had a blunted response to insulin infusions, as evidenced by a decreased ability of insulin to promote glucose uptake in peripheral tissues. This insulin unresponsiveness was found to be a result of postreceptor defects.

Treatment for insulin resistance during sepsis should be oriented toward adequate fluid therapy to maintain blood pressure and tissue perfusion, together with appropriate antimicrobial therapy. Insulin therapy in septic diabetic patients should be closely monitored because of the potential alterations in insulin requirements. Use of regular insulin at 4- to 8-hr intervals, low-dose IM injections hourly, or constant-rate IV infusion will allow for closer titration of insulin needs.

INSULIN ANTIBODIES

Several components of insulin products may be antigenic, including insulin, proinsulin, and protamine. Today's insulin products, especially the pur-

ified products, contain minimal contamination with proinsulin, which is more antigenic than insulin. The development of insulin resistance due to antiinsulin antibodies is relatively uncommon in humans and not well documented in dogs and cats. Since pork and canine insulin have identical amino acid sequences, pork insulin should be less antigenic than beef insulin in dogs. Although antibody formation against insulin has been shown to be higher in diabetic dogs given beef insulin than in those given pork insulin, the importance in management of diabetic dogs is not known (Feldman and Nelson, 1987). A disadvantage of pure pork insulin is a shorter duration of action compared with beef-pork insulin. A change in insulin products from a beef-pork to pure pork or from protamine to nonprotamine-containing products should only be considered after other reasons for insulin resistance have been ruled out.

PREGNANCY

The role of progesterone in the production of excess GH in dogs has been previously discussed. Although progesterone elevations during pregnancy do not routinely result in excess GH production, this could potentially occur, resulting in hyperglycemia. In addition, estrogens and progesterone can directly antagonize the effects of insulin. Production of insulinase by the placenta, which occurs in pregnant women and results in increased degradation of insulin, may also occur in pregnant dogs and cats (Feldman and Nelson, 1987). Because these potential complications could result in insulin resistance and because of the potential for familial transmission of diabetes, breeding should be discouraged and owners should be counseled to spay intact bitches and queens.

MISCELLANEOUS CONDITIONS

Other less common clinical syndromes not listed in Table 2 that can cause insulin resistance include hyperandrogenism and pheochromocytoma. Hyperandrogenism may be diagnosed on the basis of clinical signs and measurement of plasma androgen concentrations. Castration and ovariohysterectomy are specific treatments. Pheochromocytoma may be diagnosed on the basis of clinical signs due to excessive catecholamine secretion or tumor invasion and measurement of urinary catecholamines or vanillylmandelic acid. Surgery is required for definitive diagnosis and removal of the tumor.

Insulin resistance is recognized to occur in malnourished cancer patients (Bennegard et al., 1986). These patients show decreased fasting plasma insulin concentrations, receptor alterations, and postreceptor alterations. It is not known whether the insulin resistance is due to the tumor, anorexia, or a combination of both.

Defects in the absorption of subcutaneous insulin have been proposed as an explanation for insulin resistance (Schade, 1986). Specific insulin proteases within the subcutaneous tissue may be involved in rapid insulin degradation. However, this syndrome has not been well documented in human, canine, or feline diabetic patients.

In summary, there are many potential causes of insulin resistance in a clinical setting. Many of these causes can be determined by a thorough history and physical examination, if the clinician is aware of those concomitant diseases or drug therapies that can result in insulin resistance. There are several diagnostic tests that can be performed to determine whether underlying metabolic diseases or endocrinopathies are contributing to insulin resistance.

The clinician may elect to manipulate insulin therapy, diet, or life-style of the patient to aid in better diabetic control. By increasing the frequency of insulin administration from once to twice daily or by changing from an intermediate insulin product (NPH Iletin, Lily; Lente, Squibb-Novo) to a longer-acting insulin product (Protamine, Zinc, and Iletin, Lily; Ultralente, Squibb-Novo), improved diabetic control can often be gained. By coordinating the time of peak insulin activity with meals or by adding regular insulin at the time of meals, postprandial hyperglycemia can be minimized. In spite of attempts to rule out causes of insulin resistance, a specific cause may not be apparent and the amount of insulin administered may have to be maintained at high levels to control diabetes in certain patients.

References and Supplemental Reading

Amatruda, J. M., Livingston, J. N., and Lockwood, D. H.: Cellular mechanisms in selected states of insulin resistance: Human obesity, glucocorticoid excess and chronic renal failure. Diabetes Metab. Rev. 1:293, 1985.

Bennegard, K., Lundgren, F., and Lundholm, K.: Mechanisms of insulin resistance in cancer associated malnutrition. Clin. Physiol. 6:539, 1986.

Bevilacqua, S., Barrett, E. J., Smith, D., et al.: Hepatic and peripheral insulin resistance following streptozotocin-induced insulin deficiency in the dog. Metabolism 34:817, 1985.

Cavallo-Perin, P., Cassader, M., Bozzo, C., et al.: Mechanism of insulin resistance in human liver cirrhosis. J. Clin. Invest. 75:1659, 1985.

Dimitriadis, G., Baker, B., Marsh, H., et al.: Effect of thyroid hormone excess on action, secretion and metabolism of insulin in humans. Am. J. Physiol. 248:E593, 1985.

Eigenmann, J. E., and Peterson, M. E.: Diabetes mellitus associated with other endocrine disorders. Vet. Clin. North Am. [Small Anim. Pract.] 14(4):837, 1984.

Feldman, E. C., and Nelson, R. W.: Diabetes mellitus. In Feldman, E. C., and Nelson, R. W. (eds.): Canine and Feline Endocrinology and Reproduction. Philadelphia: W. B. Saunders Co., 1987, pp. 229–267.

Kemmer, F. W., and Berger, M.: Therapy and better quality of life: The dichotomous role of exercise in diabetes mellitus. Diabetes/Metabolism Reviews. 2:53, 1986.

Mansfield, P. D., Kemppainen, R. J., and Sartin, J. L.: The effects of megestrol acetate treatment on plasma glucose concentration and insulin response to glucose administration in cats. J. Am. Anim. Hosp. Assoc. 22:515, 1986.

Mattheeuws, D., Rottiers, R., Kaneko, J. J., et al.: Diabetes mellitus in dogs: Relationship of obesity to glucose tolerance and insulin response. Am. J. Vet. Res. 45:98, 1984.

Middleton, D. J., and Watson, A. D. J.: Glucose intolerance in cats given short-term therapies of predisolone and megestrol acetate. Am. J. Vet. Res. 46:2623, 1985.

Peterson, M. E.: Decreased insulin sensitivity and glucose tolerance in spontaneous canine hyperadrenocorticism. Res. Vet. Sci. 36:177, 1984.

Peterson, M. E.: Effects of megestrol acetate on glucose tolerance and growth hormone secretion in the cat. Res. Vet. Sci. 42:354, 1987.

Peterson, M. E., Winkler, B., Kintzer, P. P., et al.: Effect of spontaneous hyperadrenocorticism on endogenous production and utilization of glucose in the dog. Domest. Anim. Endocrinol. 3:117, 1986.

Raymond, R. M., Klein, D. M., Gibbons, D. A., et al.: Skeletal muscle insulin unresponsiveness during chronic hyperdynamic sepsis in the dog. J. Trauma 25:845, 1985.

Schade, D. S., and Duckworth, W. C.: In search of the subcutaneous insulin-resistance syndrome. N. Engl. J. Med. 315(3):147, 1986.

Vilstrup, H., Iversen, J., and Tygstrup, N.: Glucoregulation in acute liver failure. Eur. J. Clin. Invest. 16:193, 1986.

Wolfsheimer, K. J.: Diabetes: Mechanisms and therapy. Scientific Proceedings, 53rd Meeting, American Animal Hospital Association, New Orleans, 1986, pp. 218–223.

Wolfsheimer, K. J., Flory, W., and Williams, M. D.: Effects of prednisolone on glucose tolerance and insulin secretion in the dog. Am. J. Vet. Res. 47:1011, 1986.

Wolfsheimer, K. J., and Peterson, M. E.: Erythrocyte insulin receptor binding in dogs with Cushing's syndrome. (Abstract.) ACVIM Scientific Proceedings, San Diego, 1987, p. 882.

MEDICAL TREATMENT OF NEUROENDOCRINE TUMORS OF THE GASTROENTEROPANCREATIC SYSTEM WITH SOMATOSTATIN

CLINTON D. LOTHROP, JR., D.V.M.

Knoxville, Tennessee

The coordinated interaction of the gastroenteropancreatic system in the digestion, absorption, and assimilation of nutrients is controlled by a network of neuroendocrine cells located diffusely throughout the alimentary tract.

The ability of these neuroendocrine cells to uptake and decarboxylate biogenic amines is a characteristic of this group of cells. Hence, historically these cells are referred to as APUD cells, an acronym for Amine, Precursor, Uptake, Decarboxylation. Since the earlier cytochemical classification of the APUD cell network, more than 36 different peptide hormones produced by APUD cells have been identified by biochemical and immunologic techniques. The physiologic role for many of the newly identified peptide hormones in gastrointestinal function is unknown. Our current knowledge of the physiologic actions of many of the gastrointestinal hormones has largely been derived from the symptomatology of hormonally active neuroendocrine tumors. The clinical syndromes of hormone excess associated with the major endocrine tumors of the gastroenteropancreatic system are summarized in Table 1.

Insulinoma (β-cell tumor) is the most commonly diagnosed endocrine tumor of the gastrointestinal tract in dogs. It is rare in cats and apparently is a common endocrine tumor in ferrets. Gastrinomas are less common, but the occurrence of these tumors is well documented in dogs. There is only one report of a gastrinoma in a cat. Carcinoid tumors have been reported to occur in dogs and in one cat, but without the characteristic carcinoid syndrome seen in approximately 50 per cent of human carcinoid patients. The less common gastrointestinal endocrine tumors such as VIPoma, glucagonoma, and somatostatinoma have not been reported in dogs or cats.

Clinical symptoms of neuroendocrine tumors most commonly are secondary to excessive hormone production or interference with normal alimentary function due to development of a large neoplasm. A number of excellent reviews, retrospective studies, and case reports of veterinary gastroenteropancreatic tumors have been reported and therefore will not be repeated in this review (see References and Supplemental Reading). The purpose of this review is to discuss medical treatment of gastroenteropancreatic tumors with a long-lasting somatostatin analogue, SMS201-995 (Sandostatin*).

---

*Sandostatin is an investigational new drug produced by Sandoz Inc., East Hanover, New Jersey, and is not yet commercially available. For information regarding availability and use, contact C. D. Lothrop, Jr.

Table 1. *Major Endocrine Tumors of the Gastroenteropancreatic System*

APUDoma	Peptide/Hormone	Cell Type*	Syndrome/Symptom
Gastrinoma	Gastrin	G	Zollinger-Ellison syndrome
VIPoma	Vasoactive intestinal peptide	?	Watery diarrhea syndrome (Verner-Morrison syndrome, watery diarrhea, hypokalemia, achlorhydria)
Carcinoid	Serotonin, substance P, neurotensin	—	Flushing, diarrhea
Insulinoma	Insulin	B	Hypoglycemia
Glucagonoma	Glucagon	A	Diabetes, dermatosis
Somatostatinoma	Somatostatin	D	Diabetes, malabsorptive diarrhea, cholelithiasis
Pancreatic peptidoma	Pancreatic polypeptide	PP	Asymptomatic

*Cell type refers to the cell producing that peptide.

SOMATOSTATIN

Somatostatin is a tetradecapeptide (SS-14) that is found in most vertebrate tissues. Its highest concentrations are found in the cerebral cortex and the duodenum. Somatostatin was originally identified in hypothalamic extracts as a potent growth hormone inhibitor and later as an insulin inhibitory factor. Somatostatin is present in blood and tissues not only as SS-14 but also as somatostatin-28 (SS-28), the preprohormonal forms and a variety of smaller fragments of both SS-28 and SS-14. Peptides containing the SS-14 fragment have biologic activity. Somatostatin exerts a wide range of physiologic effects in the alimentary tract, including inhibition of secretion of all known gut peptides, gut and pancreatic exocrine secretions, nutrient absorption, blood flow, and motor activity. Glucagon, secretin, gastrin, and bombesin stimulate somatostatin production by gastroenteropancreatic delta cells. The interactions of somatostatin with other gut peptides suggest that somatostatin has a central regulatory role in coordinating nutrient digestion and absorption.

Initial investigations with SS-14 and SS-28 indicated that pharmacologic doses of somatostatin inhibited hormone secretion from normal, hyperplastic, and neoplastic endocrine cells. However, continuous intravenous infusions were necessary to obtain optimal activity owing to a half-life of only 2 to 3 min. The extremely short half-life limited the usefulness of somatostatin in chronic therapy.

The cyclic octapeptide SMS201-995 is an analogue of somatostatin with a longer duration of action and an increased potency for inhibiting secretion of growth hormone and glucagon in humans and animals. The elimination half-life of SMS201-995 following subcutaneous administration varies—40 min in rats, 75 min in dogs, and 102 min in humans. SMS201-995 is completely bioavailable following subcutaneous administration. SMS201-995 is effective in blocking hormone secretion when administered intravenously or subcutaneously because of a longer half-life, increased potency, and excellent bioavailability. SMS201-995 caused significant clinical improvement to complete resolution of all clinical signs when administered subcutaneously two to three times daily at doses of 50 to 200 μg in human patients with a variety of neuroendocrine tumors (gastrinoma, VIPoma, glucagonoma, pituitary somatotropic adenomas). After chronic SMS201-995 treatments, a decrease in tumor mass was observed (based on computed tomography) in several human patients with pituitary tumors. SMS201-995 was ineffective in slowing the growth of large, rapidly growing undifferentiated gastroenteropancreatic endocrine tumors and has been effective in only 50 per cent of human insulinoma patients. It was recently reported that only 50 per cent of human insulinomas express membrane receptors for somatostatin. Therefore, the ineffectiveness of SMS201-995 in some insulinoma patients is presumably due to the absence of somatostatin receptors on the tumor cells. This is in contrast to other gastroenteropancreatic endocrine tumors (gastrinoma, VIPoma, glucagonoma), which appear consistently to express membrane receptors for somatostatin. Nevertheless, SMS201-995 appears to be a well-tolerated and extremely effective drug for long-term treatment of some gastroenteropancreatic endocrine tumors. In addition, it appears that SMS201-995 may also be useful in the treatment of acute pancreatitis because of its ability to inhibit pancreatic exocrine function.

INSULINOMA

Functional β-cell tumors, insulinomas, are the most common gastroenteropancreatic endocrine tumor in dogs. Insulinomas occur predominantly in middle-aged or older dogs but have been reported in dogs as young as 4 years old. There is no gender predilection. Insulinomas can occur in any breed of dog, but the incidence appears higher in Irish setters, German shepherds, boxers, collies, and golden retrievers. Benign adenomas are rare in dogs but not in humans. Most insulinomas appear to be malignant β-cell carcinomas in dogs.

Clinical signs of insulin-secreting tumors are the result of decreased serum glucose concentrations. The severity and duration of clinical signs are related to the serum glucose concentration, the rate of decline in the serum glucose concentration, and the duration of hypoglycemia. In response to hypoglycemia, cortisol, glucagon, epinephrine, and growth hormone are released. Symptoms therefore result from neuroglycopenia and increased plasma catecholamines. Clinical signs include seizures, weakness, ataxia, collapse, exercise intolerance, muscle fasiculations, shaking, trembling, abnormal behavior, attitude changes, and polyphagia.

Treatment of β-cell tumors (which are almost always malignant in dogs) should initially be surgical exploration and resection of primary tumor and metastatic lesions. Metastatic sites include regional lymph nodes, liver, spleen, and portal vessels. Animals with nonresectable malignancies should not necessarily be euthanatized, because some patients respond well to medical therapy alone.

Medical therapy of dogs with β-cell tumors should begin with frequent feeding of complex carbohydrate-rich meals in small amounts several times a day. Frequent feeding of small meals may be helpful in managing clinical signs for short periods of time but is unlikely to be effective as the only treatment in chronic therapy of β-cell tumor patients.

Prednisolone, a short-acting glucocorticoid, is a

well-tolerated and often effective drug that can be used in chronic treatment of β-cell tumors. Prednisolone should be administered initially at 1 mg/kg divided twice daily and the dose decreased to the minimal effective dose. Dogs that are on high doses of prednisolone for long periods of time can be expected to develop signs of iatrogenic Cushing's syndrome. Glucocorticoids do not block insulin production or decrease tumor mass but inhibit the action of insulin in peripheral tissues, resulting in an increase in the blood glucose concentration.

Diazoxide, a benzothiadiazide compound, inhibits insulin secretion by blocking calcium mobilization and stimulates the beta-adrenergic system, resulting in increased hepatic gluconeogenesis, glycogenolysis, and decreased peripheral glucose utilization. Diazoxide should be initially administered at 10 mg/kg divided twice daily and given with meals. The dose may be increased up to 60 mg/kg as needed to alleviate clinical signs, as long as adverse reactions do not occur. Side effects of diazoxide are primarily gastrointestinal and include anorexia, vomiting, and diarrhea. Other potential side effects include diabetes mellitus, bone marrow suppression, sodium and fluid retention, and cardiac arrythmias. Thiazide diuretics, which reportedly potentiate the effects of diazoxide, can be administered concurrently (hydrochlorothiazide, 2 to 4 mg/kg) to enhance the hyperglycemic effects of diazoxide.

Streptozotocin, a naturally occurring nitrosurea compound, is selectively cytotoxic to pancreatic β-cells and therefore potentially valuable for chemotherapy of β-cell tumors. However, its usefulness in dogs is severely limited because of severe nephrotoxicity. Alloxan, a uric acid derivative, is also directly β-cell cytotoxic. Alloxan was administered once (65 mg/kg IV) to five dogs with hyperinsulinism, with reported good results. Nephrotoxicity developed in one of the five dogs treated with alloxan. Other drugs that have been suggested to be helpful in alleviating the hypoglycemia associated with β-cell tumors but that have not been evaluated in dogs include phenytoin, propranolol, and L-asparaginase.

The treatment of canine β-cell tumors with the somatostatin analogue, SMS201-995, was investigated in five dogs with surgically confirmed relapsing β-cell tumors (Table 2). All five dogs treated with SMS201-995 had been previously treated by surgical resection and prednisolone supplementation. In addition, three of five dogs were also treated with diazoxide. All five dogs had moderate to severe clinical symptoms of hypoglycemia and were refractory to previous treatments at the initiation of SMS201-995 treatment. SMS201-995 (10 to 20 μg) was administered two to three times daily in each dog. Two dogs initially showed a positive response but subsequently became refractory to SMS201-995

after 1 to 2 weeks of therapy. One dog was maintained free of clinical signs for more than 9 months before relapsing hypoglycemia occurred. This dog was nonresponsive to increased doses of SMS201-995 (40 μg t.i.d.) at that time. One dog responded positively to SMS201-995 and was free of clinical signs for 1 month, until euthanasia because of severe pneumonia. One dog treated concurrently with prednisolone and SMS201-995 responded positively to both drugs. The SMS201-995 treatment was stopped after 1 week, and the dog has subsequently been maintained clinically normal on prednisolone alone for more than 1 year. The results of these initial studies with SMS201-995 treatment, although mixed, suggest that it may be useful for treatment of some β-cell tumors in dogs. All dogs that had metastatic β-cell tumors were relatively refractory to standard treatment modalities and were clinically symptomatic. The finding that SMS201-995 caused significant improvement in even two of five cases is encouraging. It is likely that SMS201-995 may be more efficacious in dogs with less severe β-cell tumors. SMS201-995 is without significant side effects at recommended doses and should be useful in the medical treatment of β-cell tumors in the dog.

GASTRINOMA

Gastrin-secreting tumors (Zollinger-Ellison syndrome) of the gastroenteropancreatic tract are rare in humans and animals. The clinical signs associated with gastrin-secreting tumors are due to excessive secretion of gastric hydrochloric acid secondary to chronic hypergastrinemia. Gastric hyperacidity results in duodenal and gastric ulcers and causes a reflux esophagitis. The resulting clinical signs are moderate to severe vomiting, weight loss, anorexia, depression, abdominal pain, and diarrhea. Hematemesis and melena may occur in association with gastrointestinal ulcers. The diarrhea associated with gastrin-secreting tumors is due to hyperacidity, which causes inactivation of pancreatic enzymes, damage to the intestinal mucosa with associated malabsorption, and precipitation of bile salts. The diagnosis of gastrinoma can be confirmed with an elevated fasting serum gastrin level, a positive secretin stimulation test, documentation of gastric acid hypersecretion, or surgical exploration, biopsy, and tumor resection.

Prior to the development of the H_2 receptor antagonists, treatment of malignant nonresectable gastrin-secreting tumors was limited to gastric resection (partial to total gastrectomy) to decrease gastric hyperacidity. The H_2 receptor antagonists bind to histamine receptors on the gastric parietal cells and block gastrin-stimulated hydrochloric acid secretion but do no decrease serum gastrin concen-

Table 2. *Treatment of Canine β-Cell Tumors with the Somatostatin Analogue SMS201-995*

Case	Breed	Age (years)	Tumor Classification	Previous Treatment*	Response to SMS201-995†	Outcome
1	Bernese mountain dog	9	Metastatic β-cell tumor	1, 2, 3	±	Good response for 2 weeks, then nonresponsive to SMS201-995.
2	West Highland white terrier	8	Metastatic β-cell tumor	1, 2, 3	+ + +	Euthanized after 9 months because of uncontrolled seizures.
3	West Highland white terrier	13	Metastatic β-cell tumor	1, 2, 3	+ + +	Euthanized after 1 month because of pneumonia.
4	Poodle	10	Isolated β-cell tumor	1	−	Normal on prednisolone alone for > 1 year; no response to SMS201-995.
5	Cairn terrier	9	Metastatic β-cell tumor	1, 2	±	Good response for 2 weeks, then euthanized because of nonresponsiveness to SMS201-995.

*1, Surgical resection of tumor; 2, prednisolone supplementation; 3, diazoxide supplementation.

†±, Transient improvement of clinical signs; + + +, complete resolution of clinical symptoms for a significant period of time; −, no response to SMS201-995.

trations. Combination of an anticholinergic drug with an H_2 blocker is necessary to control hyperacidity in patients with conditions not controlled by H_2 blockers alone.

The clinical signs seen in the nine previously reported cases (eight dogs; one cat) and the one additional case described in this report include vomiting, diarrhea, weight loss, anorexia, depression, polydipsia, abdominal pain, hematemesis, and melena. At the time of initial examination, all animals were found to be extremely ill, and four were euthanized shortly after examination. Medical treatment with cimetidine was attempted in only one of the nine previously reported cases. Treatment with cimetidine was associated with temporary subjective clinical improvement. The four untreated animals and the one treated animal died within 4 1/2 months of initial examination and treatment.

The recommended cimetidine dose is 5 to 10 mg/kg given three to four times daily. This dose should be adjusted as necessary to control clinical signs. Ranitidine, also a histamine H_2 receptor antagonist, can be used in place of cimetidine and should be administered orally twice daily at 2.0 to 4.0 mg/kg. Omeprazole, an H^+,K^+ ATPase inhibitor that blocks parietal cell H^+ secretion, is a newer, longer-lasting, more potent inhibitor of gastric acid secretion that offers promise for improved treatment of hyperacidity associated with gastrinomas in humans and animals. In human patients with Zollinger-Ellison syndrome, omeprazole was well tolerated and was more effective than either cimetidine or ranitidine in decreasing gastric hyperacidity. In

addition, omeprazole is active when administered once daily, rather than the four to six daily treatments needed with the H_2 antagonists. The somatostatin analogue SMS201-995 has recently been shown to be highly effective in ameliorating gastrinoma-associated symptoms in human patients. Somatostatin blocks gastric acid production by blocking G-cell gastrin secretion and by directly inhibiting parietal cell H^+ secretion.

A 12-year-old mixed-breed dog with persistent anorexia, hematemesis, diarrhea, and weight loss was found to have a malignant gastrinoma based on surgical biopsy, duodenal ulcers, and an extremely elevated fasting serum gastrin concentration (>10,000 pg/ml). The animal was nonresponsive to treatment with carafate, cimetidine, and anticholinergics and continued to have persistent vomiting, anorexia, and depression. Treatment with 10 μg SMS201-995, administered subcutaneously three times daily was begun after 5 days of incomplete response to conventional medical therapy. The animal improved significantly with SMS201-995 treatment and was discharged after 1 week. The animal was managed effectively with few clinical signs for more than 10 months with SMS201-995 (10 to 20 μg t.i.d.), carafate, and cimetidine. Two attempts to stop SMS201-995 were made over the 10-month treatment period, and both times severe vomiting and radiographically evident duodenal ulcers recurred. The animal was euthanized as a result of seizures of unknown origin after 10 months of therapy. The remarkable results obtained with SMS201-995 treatment of human gastrinoma patients and the one dog in this study suggest that effective medical therapy for chronic treatment of malignant gastrinomas is now possible.

The results of treating four canine insulinomas and one gastrinoma with SMS201-995 are similar to the results obtained during experimental drug trials with larger numbers of human patients and demonstrates that SMS201-995 is an important advance in medical treatment of neuroendocrine tumors in dogs.

References and Supplemental Reading

Bauer, W., Briner, U., Doepfner, W., et al.: Life Sci. 31:1133, 1982.
Bonifils, S.: New somatostatin molecule for management of endocrine tumours. Gut 26:433, 1985.
Brazeau, P.: Somatostatin: A peptide with unexpected physiologic activities. Am. J. Med. 81(Suppl. 6B):8, 1986.
Ellison, E. C., Gower, W. R., Elkhammas, E., et al.: Characterization of the in vivo and in vitro inhibition of gastrin secretion from gastrinoma by a somatostatin analogue (SMS 201-995). Am. J. Med. 81(Suppl. 6B):56, 1986.
Feldman, E. C., and Nelson, R. W.: Canine and Feline Endocrinology and Reproduction. Philadelphia: W. B. Saunders Co., 1987, pp. 375–398.
Gyr, K., Beglinger, C., Kohler, E., et al.: Circulating Somato-statin—physiological regulator of pancreatic function? J. Clin. Invest. 79:1595, 1987.
Hawkins, K. L., Summers, B. A., Kuhajda, F. P., et al.: Immunocytochemistry of normal pancreatic islets and spontaneous islet cell tumors in dogs. Vet. Pathol. 24:170, 1987.
Leifer, C. E., Peterson, M. E., and Matus, R. E.: Insulin-secreting tumor: Diagnosis and medical and surgical management in 55 dogs. J.A.V.M.A. 188:60, 1986.
McArthur, K. E., Collen, J. J., Maton, P. N., et al.: Omeprazole: Effective, convenient therapy for Zollinger-Ellison syndrome. Gastroenterology 88:939, 1985.
McMillan, F. D., Barr, B., and Feldman, E. C.: Functional pancreatic islet cell tumor in a cat. J. Am. Anim. Hosp. Assoc. 21:741, 1985.
Mehlhaff, C. J., Peterson, M. E., Patnaik, A. K., and Carillo, J. M.: Insulin-producing islet cell neoplasms: Surgical considerations and general management in 35 dogs. J. Am. Anim. Hosp. Assoc. 21:607, 1984.
Nelson, R. W., and Foodman, M. S.: Medical management of canine hyperinsulinism. J.A.V.M.A. 187:78, 1985.
O'Dorisio, T. M.: Gut endocrinology: Clinical and therapeutic impact. Am. J. Med. 81(Suppl. 6B):1, 1986.
Park, J., Chiba, T., and Yamada, T.: Mechanisms for direct inhibition of canine gastric parietal cells by somatostatin. J. Biol. Chem. 262:14190, 1987.
Reichlin, S.: Secretion of somatostatin and its physiologic function. J. Lab Clin. Med. 109:320, 1987.
Vinik, A. I., Tsai, S., Moattari, A. R., et al.: Somatostatin analogue (SMS 201-995) in the management of gastroenteropancreatic tumors and diarrhea syndromes. Am. J. Med. 81(Suppl. 6B):23, 1986.
Wolfe, M. M., and Jensen, R. T.: Zollinger-Ellison syndrome: Current concepts in diagnosis and management. N. Engl. J. Med. 317:1200, 1987.

THERAPY FOR SPONTANEOUS CANINE HYPERADRENOCORTICISM

EDWARD C. FELDMAN, D.V.M.,
DAVID S. BRUYETTE, D.V.M.
Davis, California

and RICHARD W. NELSON, D.V.M.
Lafayette, Indiana

Several therapeutic options are available for the treatment of spontaneous hyperadrenocorticism (Cushing's syndrome) in dogs, including sophisticated surgery as well as medical treatments. The therapeutic approach chosen by the veterinarian is dependent, in part, on the underlying etiology. Approximately 80 to 85 per cent of dogs with spontaneous hyperadrenocorticism have pituitary-dependent hyperadrenocorticism (PDH). The available options for treating PDH include o,p'-DDD, ketoconazole, hypophysectomy, and bilateral adrenalectomy. Cobalt teletherapy may be recommended if a pituitary macroadenoma is present. The remaining 15 to 20 per cent of dogs with spontaneous hyperadrenocorticism have functional adrenocortical tumors (AT), of which approximately 50 per cent are benign. The most commonly recommended therapy for these dogs is surgical removal of the tumor. If surgery is not allowed by an owner or if metastatic disease is present, o,p'-DDD or ketoconazole may provide short or, in some dogs, long-term relief of clinical signs.

The differentiation between PDH and AT requires the evaluation of one or more of the following: high-dose dexamethasone suppression test (DST), basal adrenocorticotropic hormone (ACTH) concentration, abdominal radiographs, ultrasonography of the adrenal glands, corticotropin-releasing hormone (CRH) test, metyrapone test, computerized tomography (CT scan), or magnetic resonant imaging (MRI) of the pituitary gland or adrenal glands. Unfortunately, many veterinarians cannot or do not proceed diagnostically beyond confirming the diagnosis of hyperadrenocorticism. This may be because of unfamiliarity with tests that distinguish PDH from AT, owner financial constraints, lack of facilities to perform some of the tests, or tests that are completed but are inconclusive. How does the veterinarian proceed in these situations? One alternative is to refer the patient to a colleague or institution that can proceed with the required tests. The second alternative is to realize that most dogs with hyperadrenocorticism have pituitary-dependent disease with bilateral adrenal hyperplasia, which is usually responsive to therapy with o,p'-DDD. One may choose, therefore, to initiate o,p'-DDD treatment without establishing whether a dog has pituitary-dependent Cushing's or an adrenocortical tumor.

Regardless of the therapeutic option chosen, excellent rapport must be established between the veterinarian and owner for successful long-term management of these animals. The surgical and medical options should be discussed in detail, including what is expected of the owner. The goal is to return these dogs to a normal endocrine state, but this is not always possible, and all potential complications should be discussed. These dogs may have endocrine excesses or deficiencies after treatment, and the prepared owner can accept these setbacks. Time spent explaining the pathophysiology in lay terms is well worth the effort to improve client understanding and to establish a good basis for future communications.

MEDICAL THERAPY OF PITUITARY-DEPENDENT HYPERADRENOCORTICISM USING o,p'-DDD

Induction Therapy

Since development of the o,p'-DDD treatment protocol first suggested by Schechter and colleagues (1973), chemotherapy using o,p'-DDD has been the most commonly employed treatment for hyperadrenocorticism. There are two phases of therapy: an initial induction phase designed to gain control of the disorder and a lifelong maintenance phase designed to prevent recurrence of the signs of the disease.

THE CUSHING'S DOG WITH OVERT POLYDIPSIA

After in-hospital diagnostic studies have been completed, polydipsic dogs with hyperadrenocorticism are returned to their owners for monitoring of water intake. If an owner has more than one pet, the water intake of the pets at home can be determined while the suspect dog is in the hospital. In this manner, the dog with hyperadrenocorticism can be returned to its normal environment for water intake monitoring, and the owner can determine approximately how much to subtract from the total water consumed by all dogs to determine the patient's water intake. Admittedly, the presence of more than one pet in the home may eliminate water intake monitoring. Water intake is determined for several 24-hr periods to eliminate errors in measuring and to achieve a reliable average figure from which therapy can begin. Dogs with polydipsia due to hyperadrenocorticism usually drink quantities of water that exceed 100 ml/kg of body weight/24 hr.

Once polydipsia has been confirmed and the daily quantity of water consumption established, therapy may be initiated at home with the owner administering o,p'-DDD (mitotane; Lysodren [Bristol-Myers]) at a dosage of 25 mg/kg b.i.d. Glucocorticoids are not routinely administered but are dispensed so the owner has a small supply at home should they be needed in the future. The owner should receive thorough instructions on the actions of o,p'-DDD and should also have specific instructions about when the drug should be discontinued. Mitotane administration should be stopped when (1) the polydipsic dog's daily water consumption approaches 60 ml/kg; (2) the dog simply takes longer to consume a meal, and certainly if it develops partial or complete inappetance; (3) the dog vomits; (4) the dog has diarrhea; or (5) the dog is unusually listless. The occurrence of any of these signs is an indication for the owner to stop daily o,p'-DDD therapy and have the dog examined by the veterinarian. Usually the induction phase of therapy is complete when *any* reduction in appetite is noted or when daily water consumption falls to or below 60 ml/kg of body weight. The water intake in polydipsic dogs may fall to the normal range in as few as 2 days or in as long as 35 days (average is 5 to 14 days).

Because of the potency of o,p'-DDD, the veterinarian is encouraged not to rely solely on the instructions given to an owner. This drug is highly successful in eliminating the signs of hyperadrenocorticism because of its potency coupled with *close communication between the owner and the veterinarian.* Either the veterinarian or a technician should call the owner every day beginning with the second day of therapy. In this way, the owner will be impressed with the veterinarian's concern and will observe the animal closely. We advise our clients to feed their dogs two small meals each day. The dog's appetite should be observed *prior to* each o,p'-DDD administration. If food is rapidly consumed, medication can be given. If food is consumed slowly, incompletely, or not at all, the medication should not be given until the veterinarian is notified and an ACTH response test is performed.

In addition to making daily phone calls, the veterinarian should see the dog 8 to 9 days after beginning therapy. At this time, a thorough history should be taken and a physical examination and an ACTH response test should be performed. Dogs that have responded clinically to the medication (or if the owner is not certain about response) should have further therapy withheld until results of the ACTH response test can be evaluated. Dogs that have failed to respond clinically should have an ACTH response test performed but should also remain on daily therapy.

The goals of therapy with o,p'-DDD are to achieve resolution of the clinical signs and an ACTH response test result that is suggestive of *hypoadrenocorticism*. In our laboratories, successful response to o,p'-DDD is indicated by a pre-ACTH plasma cortisol concentration that is less than 5 μg/dl and a post-ACTH plasma cortisol concentration that is also less than 5 μg/dl. A dog that has a normal or exaggerated response to ACTH prior to therapy and a *normal* response to ACTH following the initial phase of therapy usually remains clinically hyperadrenal.

The maintenance phase of therapy with o,p'-DDD may be initiated once a hypoadrenal response to ACTH is obtained. If the dog with hyperadrenocorticism has a normal or exaggerated response to ACTH following the initial 8 to 9 days of o,p'-DDD therapy, daily medication should be continued. It is usually continued for 3 to 7 additional days, the shorter time period being used for dogs that have shown some reduction in post-ACTH cortisol concentrations compared with pretreatment values. ACTH response tests should be repeated every 7 to 10 days until a low post-ACTH plasma cortisol concentration is achieved. It is important to emphasize that each dog must be treated as an individual. There appears to be no reliable method of predicting the length of time required for a response or the amount of o,p'-DDD necessary to destroy enough of the adrenal cortex for a response to be seen. Most dogs, however, respond within 5 to 9 days of daily o,p'-DDD therapy. It is unusual for a dog to require more than 14 consecutive days of o,p'-DDD.

THE CUSHING'S DOG WITHOUT OVERT POLYDIPSIA

Approximately 20 per cent of dogs with PDH are not polydipsic. Like the polydipsic dogs, they can and should be treated at home by their owners. Absence of polydipsia simply eliminates one of the factors that can be monitored during the initial phases of therapy. Before beginning therapy, an ACTH response test must be obtained. Alterations in therapy will be based on history, physical examination, and the comparison of current ACTH response test results with those obtained before treatment. These dogs must be closely monitored by the owner. The most important monitoring guide in these dogs is their appetite. Reduction in appetite in any dog receiving o,p'-DDD is an indication that the induction phase is completed or that overdosage is imminent.

The therapeutic approach in these dogs is similar to that previously outlined. The dose of 50 mg/kg/day (25 mg/kg b.i.d.) is used. Instead of an initial 9-day plan, o,p'-DDD is given for 7 consecutive days, unless the owner observes signs that suggest that adequate dosage has been given before the 7 days have elapsed. Close communication, as previously described, is mandatory. An ACTH response test is performed at the end of this time and o,p'-DDD discontinued until the results of the response test are known. The o,p'-DDD treatment protocol is repeated until results of the ACTH response test are suggestive of hypoadrenocorticism (values < 5 μg/dl). At that time, the maintenance phase of therapy is initiated. Most dogs will respond during the initial 7 days of therapy. If listlessness, inappetence, vomiting, or diarrhea is observed by the owner during a treatment cycle, o,p'-DDD should be discontinued and the veterinarian contacted. The veterinarian can then perform an ACTH response test. If the dog is clinically ill and rapidly responds to glucocorticoid treatment (within hours), o,p'-DDD overdosage is likely, but an ACTH response test is needed to confirm this suspicion. Glucocorticoid therapy must be stopped for 48 hr prior to performing the ACTH response test.

THE CUSHING'S DOG WITH CONCURRENT DIABETES MELLITUS

Approximately 10 per cent of dogs with hyperadrenocorticism also have diabetes mellitus. In most situations, diabetes mellitus is first diagnosed and hyperadrenocorticism is suspected because of abnormalities found on physical examination (e.g., endocrine alopecia; potbellied appearance) or because of apparent insulin antagonism after insulin therapy is initiated. Both the diabetes and hyperadrenocorticism should be treated. However, attempts at extremely good control of the diabetes mellitus should be delayed until the hyperadrenocorticism has been controlled. A dosage of insulin adequate to prevent ketoacidosis and severe hyperglycemia (> 500 mg/dl) is advised. An NPH insulin dose of 0.5 to 1.0 U/kg body weight administered twice daily is a conservative initial dosage. The insulin dosage should be reduced into this range when initiating o,p'-DDD therapy in dogs receiving large doses of insulin.

The therapeutic approach to hyperadrenocorticism in dogs with concurrent diabetes mellitus is the same as that described for the dog with hyperadrenocorticism and no polydipsia. Hyperadrenocorticism causes insulin antagonism in many of these dogs. Therefore, as control of the hyperadrenocorticism is achieved, insulin antagonism usually resolves and insulin requirements decrease. To help minimize hypoglycemic reactions, owners are asked to obtain urine samples from their pet at least three times daily during the induction phase of o,p'-DDD therapy. Each sample is checked for glucose. Any urine sample found to be negative for glucose should be followed by a 10 to 20 per cent reduction in the subsequent insulin dose. Approximately one-third of our dogs do not require exogenous insulin following successful therapy. An additional one-third require significantly less insulin and have better control of the diabetes mellitus following o,p'-DDD therapy. The insulin requirement in the remaining dogs may be minimally reduced by control of the hyperadrenocorticism, but their serial blood glucose levels are invariably improved. Good regulation of the diabetes mellitus should be attempted once the hyperadrenocorticism is controlled.

Maintenance Therapy

Once the initial daily protocol with o,p'-DDD completes adequate destruction of the adrenal cortex, as determined by clinical signs, reduced water intake, and ACTH stimulation test results, maintenance therapy should begin. Mitotane does not affect the pituitary; therefore, the excessive ACTH secretion associated with PDH continues or becomes exaggerated (Nelson et al., 1985). Failure to continue o,p'-DDD therapy will result in regrowth of the adrenal cortices and return of clinical signs. This recurrence of the disease typically occurs within 6 to 24 months of stopping therapy.

Maintenance therapy involves choosing an o,p'-DDD protocol and altering that regimen as required by the dog. Dogs that respond to daily o,p'-DDD therapy within 10 days are classified as sensitive and begin a maintenance schedule of 25 mg/kg of o,p'-DDD every 7 days or 12.5 mg/kg twice weekly. Those that initially require more than 10 days of therapy are classified as resistant and receive 50 mg/kg every 7 days. An ACTH response test is performed 1 and 3 months after beginning the maintenance therapy and every 3 to 6 months thereafter. These test results dictate whether a dose change is warranted. If the plasma cortisol concentration after ACTH administration is normal or elevated, the o,p'-DDD dosage or the frequency of administration is increased. Some dogs remain stable for months or years on a conservative dosage, whereas others receive o,p'-DDD every 2 or 3

days. Return of clinical signs suggestive of hyperadrenocorticism should be managed by performing an ACTH stimulation test to confirm disease recurrence, followed by raising the dose of o,p'-DDD. Obvious recurrence of hyperadrenocorticism should be treated with daily o,p'-DDD therapy as initially suggested, whereas any dog with returning signs should also at least be assessed for other diseases, such as renal disease and diabetes mellitus.

Adverse Reactions to o,p'-DDD

Problems with o,p'-DDD therapy usually fall into two categories: those related to reactions to the drug and those resulting from excessive administration and the development of glucocorticoid and, if severe, mineralocorticoid deficiency.

A small percentage of dogs will demonstrate mild gastric irritation from the drug 2 to 4 days after medication has been started. If this occurs, the medication should be discontinued until the veterinarian can evaluate the dog. If the gastric upset occurs because of drug sensitivity and not because the treatment is complete (as would be suggested by little or no change in an ACTH response test result), dividing the dose further may be helpful. In some dogs, discontinuing the medication may be necessary for a few days.

Some dogs are quickly overdosed with o,p'-DDD, developing hypocortisolism and weakness, lethargy, vomiting, diarrhea, and anorexia within a few days of beginning therapy. In our experience, this is uncommon, but it is recommended that the induction phase of therapy be initiated on a Saturday so that if illness develops after 2 to 4 days, the veterinarian is available during the regular working week rather than on a weekend. If signs of hypocortisolism develop, glucocorticoid therapy is warranted. Clinical improvement is usually seen within 3 hr following the administration of prednisolone, 0.25 to 0.5 mg/kg of body weight. Although administration of glucocorticoids is not recommended during o,p'-DDD therapy, we routinely send prednisolone home with the owner to be used if o,p'-DDD overdosage occurs. If an overdosage is suspected and the dog responds to glucocorticoid therapy, it should be continued for 3 to 5 days and then tapered over a period of 1 to 2 weeks. Mitotane (o,p'-DDD) therapy should be withheld until the dog is able to remain asymptomatic without receiving glucocorticoids for 1 or 2 weeks. A decrease in the dose or frequency of o,p'-DDD administration should be made when therapy with o,p'-DDD is reinitiated. Alternatively, an ACTH response test can be performed at 4- to 8-week intervals, withholding o,p'-DDD until the post-ACTH plasma cortisol concentration approaches or exceeds 5 μg/dl.

If a dog fails to respond to glucocorticoid medication, it should be examined by the veterinarian. In addition to a complete physical examination, one should obtain at least blood urea nitrogen (BUN) and serum electrolyte determinations and perform an ACTH stimulation test. If oral therapy is not possible because of vomiting, parenteral fluids and glucocorticoids are warranted.

Glucocorticoid therapy is also indicated for any dog receiving o,p'-DDD and undergoing stress (e.g., illness, trauma, elective surgery). The adequately treated dog has sufficient adrenocortical reserve for day-to-day living, but not enough to handle major stresses. During these times, prednisolone should be administered at 2.2 mg/kg/day for 2 days and the dosage then gradually reduced over the next week.

TIME SEQUENCE FOR IMPROVEMENT IN CLINICAL SIGNS

The most obvious and rapid response to o,p'-DDD therapy is a reduction in water intake, urine output, and appetite. These signs usually improve within the initial 5- to 14-day induction phase of therapy. Activity may improve quickly as well. Other signs take longer to resolve. Muscle strength improves within a few days to as long as 2 months, as does a reduction in the potbellied appearance. It often takes 1 to 6 months before there is significant improvement in alopecia, thin skin, acne, bruising, calcinosis cutis, and panting. Dogs with coat abnormalities may go through a phase of severe seborrhea associated with worsening alopecia and pruritus, which may last 1 or 2 months before the hair coat shows significant improvement. Some dogs go through a phase of puppy hair coat before the normal adult coat returns. A few dogs have dramatic changes in coat color following successful therapy.

FAILURE TO RESPOND TO o,p'-DDD

It is uncommon for o,p'-DDD to fail to help a dog with PDH. The drug is quite potent, and its effect on destroying the zone fasciculata and zona reticularis is consistent. The following are potential reasons for an apparent treatment failure: (1) Adrenocortical tumors (adenomas or carcinomas) are less sensitive to the cytotoxic effects of o,p'-DDD. (2) Drug malabsorption may occur. (3) The drug batch may not be potent, and replacing the owner's tablets with o,p'-DDD obtained from a new bottle may solve an apparent treatment failure. (4) One often begins to worry about a treatment failure after 14 to 21 consecutive days of therapy without a response, but a small percentage of dogs require 30 to 60 consecutive days of therapy or they require 100 to 150 mg of o,p'-DDD/kg/day rather than the usual dosage of 50 mg/kg/day to obtain a response. (5) The diagnosis of hyperadrenocorticism may be incorrect. (6) The dog may have iatrogenic Cushing's syndrome secondary to excessive exogenous glucocorticoid administration (as would be confirmed with a pretreatment ACTH response test).

The various causes of an apparent treatment failure must be considered before abandoning the use of o,p'-DDD. However, if treatment failure has occurred, either ketoconazole therapy, bilateral adrenalectomy, or hypophysectomy should be considered.

MEDICAL THERAPY USING KETOCONAZOLE

Ketoconazole (Nizoral, Janssen) is an imidazole derivative that has antifungal properties. Its antifungal activity is linked to the inhibition of ergosterol synthesis and to interference with other membrane lipids. In addition to its antifungal activity, ketoconazole has been shown to interfere with gonadal and adrenal steroid synthesis both *in vitro* and *in vivo* (Pont et al., 1982; Willard et al., 1985, 1986). This information has led to the suggestion that ketoconazole administration might be of value in the treatment of hyperadrenocorticism.

We have evaluated the use of this drug in dogs with pituitary-dependent Cushing's as well as those with Cushing's secondary to an adrenocortical tumor. Most ketoconazole-treated dogs have shown a rapid reduction in serum cortisol concentrations and a reduction in adrenocortical responsiveness to ACTH. Plasma testosterone concentrations have fallen markedly, with variable changes in plasma concentrations of estrogen and progesterone. In the dogs treated for more than 2 months, there has been significant improvement in their clinical condition as evidenced by a reduction in water intake, urine production, appetite, weight, and regrowth of hair.

Ketoconazole, with its low incidence of toxicity, reversible inhibition of adrenal steroidogenesis, and negligible effects on mineralocorticoid production, promises to be an attractive (albeit expensive) alternative in the management of canine hyperadrenocorticism. Ketoconazole is useful in the following circumstances: (1) medical management of those dogs that have malignant adrenal tumors and for whom surgical intervention is not an option, but palliative therapy is desired; (2) as initial therapy prior to adrenalectomy in an attempt to control the hyperadrenocorticism for 4 to 8 weeks, thus reducing the risks of anesthesia and surgery; (3) as a treatment option for owners who refuse surgery; (4) as a test therapy for 4 to 8 weeks to provide evidence for or against a diagnosis of hyperadrenocorticism in dogs with vague test results; and (5) as primary therapy in dogs that cannot be treated with o,p'-DDD because of drug sensitivity.

The dosage of ketoconazole that the authors have used to treat hyperadrenocorticism has been 5 mg/kg b.i.d. for 7 days; then 10/mg/kg b.i.d. for 7 to 14 days; and, if necessary, 15 mg/kg b.i.d. Dogs seem to tolerate the drug better when the dosage is gradually increased to 15 mg/kg. Adverse reactions are usually a result of hypocortisolism, although 0.1 to 1 per cent of dogs may have an idiosyncratic hepatopathy with icterus as well as abnormal liver enzymes and function tests. Discontinuation of the drug and supportive care should resolve the problem. The drug should be discontinued if anorexia, depression, vomiting, or diarrhea is observed. Glucocorticoid treatment may be needed if an overdosage is suspected. An ACTH response test, without stopping the drug, should be performed after 10 to 14 days of treatment. The goals in therapy are the same as with o,p'-DDD: lack of adrenocortical response to ACTH and clinical improvement without causing illness. Rechecks are recommended every 3 to 4 months. Because this drug is an enzyme blocker, twice-daily medication has been necessary in the long-term management of these patients.

SURGICAL THERAPY: ADRENALECTOMY

Adrenalectomy may be unilateral for an adrenocortical tumor or bilateral as a mode of therapy for PDH. The surgical approach has been well described elsewhere and will not be discussed here (Johnston, 1983). It is recommended, however, that this surgery be performed by specialists operating in facilities capable of handling the potential postoperative complications that may develop.

Preoperative Evaluation

Once the diagnosis of hyperadrenocorticism due to an adrenal tumor has been confirmed, attempts should be made to localize the tumor and rule out metastasis. Methods of tumor localization include abdominal radiographs, ultrasonography, CT scans, and gamma camera imaging. Abdominal radiographs may identify a mass craniomedial to the kidney or, in approximately 50 per cent of dogs with adrenal tumors, demonstrate adrenal calcification. Adrenocortical carcinomas frequently metastasize to the liver and lungs. Ultrasonography has proved valuable for localizing the tumor and detecting hepatic metastasis. If metastasis is suspected, an ultrasound-guided biopsy of the liver can be performed to confirm this suspicion. Thoracic radiographs should

also be evaluated for metastatic disease in the lung parenchyma.

All dogs undergoing adrenal surgery to correct a state of hyperadrenocorticism can be assumed to be immunosuppressed and to have poor wound healing secondary to the chronic excesses in circulating glucocorticoids. Therefore, these dogs should be treated with ketoconazole for 4 to 8 weeks prior to surgery. Following such therapy, the dog is a better anesthetic and surgical risk. Ketoconazole is also recommended as the sole therapy for dogs with inoperable tumors and those with obvious metastasis.

Patient Management During and After Surgery

Steroids should not be administered prior to anesthesia, as they predispose the patient to overhydration and an increased risk of thromboembolic episodes. Beginning with anesthesia, parenteral isotonic fluids (e.g., lactated Ringer's) should be administered at a surgical maintenance rate. After the adrenal tumor is identified, dexamethasone is placed in the IV infusion bottle at a dose of 0.02 to 0.04 mg/kg of body weight. This dose should be given over a 6-hr period and should be repeated q.i.d. for the first day and then b.i.d. thereafter until the dog is eating and drinking normally, not receiving IV fluids, and considered stable. Once the dog is eating and drinking, the glucocorticoid supplement should be switched to prednisone or prednisolone, 1.0 mg/kg PO b.i.d. for 2 days. The dosage is then gradually reduced over the ensuing 6 to 8 weeks. If a unilateral adrenalectomy has been performed, glucocorticoid supplementation can be discontinued once the contralateral normal adrenocortical tissue becomes functional. With bilateral adrenalectomy, most dogs will remain stable on a prednisolone dosage of 0.1 mg/kg administered once or twice daily.

Mineralocorticoid supplementation was once considered mandatory with bilateral adrenalectomy. Before production of this drug was halted, desoxycorticosterone acetate was administered at a dose of 0.02 to 0.04 mg/kg of body weight, IM when the adrenal glands were excised. Good success is now achieved using dexamethasone IM as previously described, or hydrocortisone hemisuccinate (0.5 to 1.0 mg/kg IV q.i.d.). Once the dog is eating and drinking, oral mineralocorticoids (e.g., Florinef, Squibb) given twice daily may be substituted for the parenteral drugs. Oral hydrocortisone may also be administered at a dose of 0.5 to 1.0 mg/kg/day.

Approximately 50 per cent of dogs undergoing unilateral adrenalectomy develop alterations in serum electrolytes as a result of a transient mineralocorticoid deficiency that develops within 48 hr of surgery. Serum electrolytes should be monitored daily for 3 to 4 days after surgery. If hyperkalemia and hyponatremia develop, hydrocortisone hemisuccinate therapy should be initiated as previously described. Therapy can usually be discontinued within 1 week. Alternatively, this therapy can be initiated at the time of surgery in all dogs undergoing adrenalectomy. Hydrocortisone therapy should then be discontinued after 2 days of therapy, to be given again only if hyperkalemia or hyponatremia is documented.

SURGICAL THERAPY: HYPOPHYSECTOMY

Surgery to remove the pituitary gland, and thus the source of ACTH in PDH, has been successfully performed in dogs. Hypophysectomy as a treatment modality for PDH has several advantages, including removal of the pituitary tumor, preventing expansion of the tumor into the central nervous system, and eliminating the frequent re-evaluations and complications associated with medical therapy or bilateral adrenalectomy. Although the surgical procedure has been described (Lubberink, 1980), it requires specialized equipment and considerable experience. As such, hypophysectomy is not readily available.

In addition to the standard preoperative diagnostic evaluation of the patient, a CT scan with positive contrast enhancement should be obtained of the pituitary region prior to hypophysectomy to evaluate for the presence of a macroadenoma or hydrocephalus. If present, these are contraindications to performing the surgery. Brachycephalic dogs are poor candidates for this surgery because of their venous sinus anatomy.

If hypophysectomy is successful, the Cushing's dog will lose all clinical features of the disease. Using an intraoral transsphenoidal approach to remove the pituitary gland, the authors have found it difficult to remove the corticotrophs located along the base of the brain. As such, normal ACTH secretion may be re-established following hypophysectomy, and chronic glucocorticoid supplementation may not be necessary. Dexamethasone, 1.0 mg/kg IV, is recommended during hypophysectomy, however, and should be followed with decreasing dosages administered once daily during the ensuing week.

A complete hypophysectomy results in the loss of several pituitary hormones. Fortunately, diabetes insipidus is transient because ADH can be secreted by remaining tissue. In our experience, renal concentrating capabilities are re-established within 2 weeks of surgery. Postsurgical polyuria/polydipsia, however, should be controlled with vasopressin, beginning at surgery. Failure to re-establish renal concentrating capabilities with exogenous ADH may result in severe hypernatremia and life-threatening hypertonic dehydration. Vasopressin supplementation may be discontinued, as a trial, 1 to 2 weeks following hypophysectomy. Hypothyroidism from a TSH deficiency is permanent, requiring lifelong thyroid hormone supplementation following hypophysectomy. Similarly, growth hormone (GH) deficiency seems to be permanent, but the need for exogenous growth hormone supplementation is yet to be determined. Although clinical manifestations of adult-onset GH deficiency have not yet developed in any of our dogs, studies of long duration (i.e., years) will be necessary before the question of GH supplementation can be answered. The anabolic actions of GH are a result of GH-induced somatomedin C secretion by the liver. It is interesting that in one study, somatomedin C concentrations returned to normal 1 month following hypophysectomy, despite a persistent deficiency in circulating GH concentrations (Eigenmann et al., 1977).

RADIATION THERAPY: PITUITARY MACROADENOMA

Approximately 5 to 10 per cent of dogs with PDH have clinical signs caused by a growing pituitary tumor that expands dorsally into the hypothalamus. The most common signs associated with large pituitary tumors include mental dullness, inappetence, lethargy, and apparent disorientation. Some owners have also reported that their pets pace aimlessly, appear blind, are ataxic, head-press, circle, appear "trapped" in the corner of a room, develop Horner's syndrome, urinate or defecate in the home, or convulse. Less common signs include aggressive behavior, loss of thermoregulatory capability, wide fluctuations in body temperature, or coma. A small number of dogs are initially evaluated because any of the previous mentioned signs are noted by the owner. Most of the dogs with neurologic clinical signs have been previously diagnosed and treated for PDH.

The diagnosis is difficult to confirm and is initially made by ruling out other causes of neurologic disturbances. The primary differential diagnosis for the presence of a large pituitary tumor includes the drug-induced neurologic signs occasionally caused by o,p'-DDD therapy, which are transient in nature and typically last 24 to 48 hr following each dosage. The diagnosis of pituitary macroadenoma can be confirmed with a CT scan using positive-contrast enhancement.

Modes of therapy are limited. Some dramatic success has been obtained with the use of cobalt irradiation. Cobalt irradiation has successfully reduced tumor size and caused a reduction in or elimination of the neurologic clinical signs in several of our dogs and in those in a recent report (Dow et al., 1986). However, reduction of the secretory nature of the pituitary tumors is variable, and secretion may even increase despite a confirmed reduction in tumor size.

References and Supplemental Reading

Dow, S. W., LeCouteur, R. A., Rosychuk, R. A. W., et al.: Results following radiation therapy of functional pituitary neoplasms in dogs. (Abstract.) American College of Veterinary Internal Medicine Scientific Proceedings, Washington, D.C., 1986.

Eigenmann, J. E., Becker, M., Kammerman, B., et al.: Decrease of non-suppressible insulin-like activity after pancreatectomy and normalization by insulin therapy. Acta Endocrinol. (Copenh.) 85:818, 1977.

Feldman, E. C., Nelson, R. W.: *Canine and Feline Endocrinology and Reproduction.* Philadelphia: W. B. Saunders Co., 1987, pp. 137–194.

Johnston, D. E.: Adrenalectomy in the dog. *In* Bojrab, M. J. (ed.): *Current Techniques in Small Animal Surgery.* Philadelphia: Lea & Febiger, 1983, pp. 386–388.

Lubberink, A. A. M. E.: Therapy for spontaneous hyperadrenocorticism. *In* Kirk, R. W. (ed.): *Current Veterinary Therapy VII.* Philadelphia: W. B. Saunders Co., 1980, p. 979.

Nelson, R. W., Feldman, E. C., and Shinsako, J.: Effect of o,p'-DDD therapy on endogenous ACTH concentrations in dogs with hypophysis-dependent hyperadrenocorticism. Am. J. Vet. Res. 46:1534, 1985.

Pont, A., Williams, P. L., Loose, D. S., et al.: Ketoconazole blocks adrenal steroid synthesis. Ann. Intern. Med. 97:370, 1982.

Schechter, R. D., Stabenfeldt, G. H., Gribble, D. H., et al.: Treatment of Cushing's syndrome in the dog with an adrenocorticolytic agent (o,p'-DDD). J.A.V.M.A. 162:629, 1973.

Willard, M. D., Nachreiner, R., McDonald, R., et al.: Ketoconazole-induced changes in canine steroidogenesis. (Abstract.) American College of Veterinary Internal Medicine Proceedings, San Diego, 1985.

Willard, M. D., Nachreiner, R. F., McDonald, R., et al.: Hormonal and clinical pathologic changes with long-term ketoconazole therapy in the dog and cat. American College of Veterinary Internal Medicine Scientific Proceedings, Washington, D.C., 1986, pp. 13-25 and 13-27.

RADIATION THERAPY FOR CANINE ACTH-SECRETING PITUITARY TUMORS

STEVEN W. DOW, D.V.M., M.S.
and RICHARD A. LeCOUTEUR, B.V.Sc.

Fort Collins, Colorado

Pituitary-dependent hyperadrenocorticism (PDH), a relatively common endocrinopathy of dogs, is usually recognized when systemic abnormalities induced by prolonged hypercortisolemia develop. Hyperadrenocorticism results most often from oversecretion of adrenocorticotropic hormone (ACTH) by a small, functional tumor (microadenoma) of the pars distalis or pars intermedia of the pituitary gland. There is a small subset of dogs, however, with PDH caused by a large, functional adenoma (macroadenoma) or carcinoma of the pituitary gland. In these animals, neurologic abnormalities induced by space-occupying effects of a large pituitary neoplasm may precede, or develop concurrently with, obvious endocrinologic abnormalities. Large, nonfunctional pituitary tumors have also been reported in dogs.

DIAGNOSIS OF LARGE PITUITARY TUMORS

Unfortunately, from a diagnostic viewpoint, neurologic signs induced by a large pituitary neoplasm in dogs are relatively nonspecific. Mental depression, excessive somnolence, and behavioral changes may be observed. Other abnormalities include seizures or cranial nerve deficits, especially facial paralysis. The occurrence of neurologic abnormalities indicative of an intracranial space-occupying lesion in a dog with PDH suggests the presence of a large pituitary macroadenoma or carcinoma.

High-dose dexamethasone suppression testing or endogenous plasma ACTH assay can be used to confirm the existence of PDH, although neither test permits distinction between a microadenoma and a large pituitary tumor. At present, only x-ray computed tomographic (CT) evaluation of the head reliably distinguishes dogs with PDH caused by a pituitary microadenoma from dogs with a large (> 5 mm) pituitary tumor (Fig. 1). CT does not, however, allow differentiation of a macroadenoma from a pituitary carcinoma in dogs.

For CT evaluation of the head, a dog is anesthetized, intubated, and positioned in ventral recumbency on the patient-handling table. A series of nonenhanced CT images of the head may be made initially, after which contrast medium is administered. A slow intravenous bolus of diatrizoate meg-

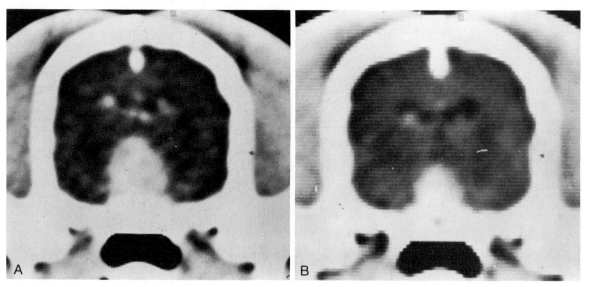

Figure 1. *A,* Postcontrast transverse CT images of the head of a dog with a large functional pituitary adenoma before radiation therapy. *B,* Four months after radiation therapy tumor size has decreased approximately 50 per cent.

lumine and diatrizoate sodium (Renograffin 76, Squibb Diagnostics) is given over 5 to 10 min, and the CT examination is repeated. The pituitary gland of a dog is located (in the transverse plane) at the level of the temporomandibular joints. A contrast-enhancing mass that measures 5 mm or more in diameter and is located in the region of the pituitary fossa in a dog with PDH is most likely either a pituitary macroadenoma or carcinoma. Each tumor type appears to occur with approximately equal frequency in dogs.

Other techniques such as optic thecography and cerebral angiography may be used to localize large pituitary tumors in dogs; however, these techniques do not provide precise information regarding extent of a neoplasm. In the future, magnetic resonance imaging may allow better characterization of pituitary tumors in dogs and may permit further differentiation of tumor types, but at present it does not provide an advantage over CT in terms of tumor localization.

TREATMENT OPTIONS

Treatment options for a dog with a large pituitary tumor are limited. Traditional therapy of PDH in dogs involves treatment with o,p'-DDD or, more recently, with the adrenal steroid synthesis-inhibitor ketoconazole. Each of these treatments effectively controls adverse systemic effects of hypercortisolemia but does not slow growth of a pituitary neoplasm. In fact, by removing the negative feedback effects of cortisol, growth of a pituitary tumor may be accelerated, at least in some dogs. This phenomenon, known in humans as Nelson's syndrome, has appeared to occur in a few dogs with

large, functioning pituitary neoplasms after initiation of adrenolytic therapy. The sudden occurrence of signs of central nervous system dysfunction or rapid worsening of pre-existing neurologic abnormalities soon after initiating adrenal suppressive treatment is often the first indication that a large, rapidly growing pituitary tumor may be present.

To be successful, therapy of dogs with a large pituitary tumor must control both the space-occupying effects of the tumor as well as the adverse endocrinologic effects of excessive tumor ACTH secretion. Two treatment options are currently available: surgery and radiation treatment.

Hypophysectomy

Surgical hypophysectomy has been advocated as a treatment for PDH in dogs. Cures have been reported following hypophysectomy in some dogs with microadenomas. The surgery is difficult, however, and associated with high morbidity and mortality, even when performed by experienced surgeons.

Hypophysectomy, though routinely performed in humans, is unlikely to be successful in dogs with a large pituitary neoplasm. The anatomy of the canine pituitary gland is such that the surgical approach is difficult and visualization of a tumor is severely limited. In addition, suprasellar extension of a pituitary tumor in dogs is common, owing to incomplete development of the diaphragma sellae and lack of resistance to dorsal tumor extension. When suprasellar tumor extension has occurred there is little chance of complete surgical extirpation of a pituitary tumor. Tumor debulking is unlikely to provide more than very transient benefit.

Radiation Therapy

Radiation therapy offers the best treatment currently available for dogs with a large pituitary tumor. Six dogs with PDH caused by a large, functional pituitary tumor and one cat with a large, nonfunctional acidophilic macroadenoma have been successfully treated with pituitary irradiation by the authors, and there are reports of successful pituitary irradiation in one dog and in one cat. Successful radiation treatment of a variety of other primary central nervous system tumors of dogs has also been reported.

There are several advantages of radiation therapy over surgical treatment. Perhaps most important, pituitary irradiation provides a means of achieving direct, noninvasive tumor control, unassociated with serious treatment-related morbidity or mortality. Radiation therapy, at least in humans, is more effective in preventing tumor recurrence than is surgery alone. In addition, pituitary irradiation may decrease excessive pituitary ACTH secretion while preserving normal pituitary gland function.

Radiation sources capable of delivering megavoltage radiation are required for pituitary irradiation. High-energy radiation is necessary to penetrate to the depth of the pituitary gland without seriously injuring overlying soft tissues. Cobalt 60 sources and linear accelerators, available at several veterinary facilities, are capable of delivering megavoltage radiation.

In the protocol used at Colorado State University Veterinary Teaching Hospital, 6-MV photon teletherapy was delivered to the pituitary gland through bilaterally opposed portals, directed temporally. A portal width of 4×4 or 5×5 cm was used, depending on the size of the dog's head and on the dimensions of the tumor. These portal widths include at least a 1-cm margin of brain tissue in the irradiated volume. Each dog received a total of 40 Gy given in 10 equal 4-Gy fractions over 22 days. More recently, protocols delivering 45 Gy to the tumor in 15 equal fractions have been used.

RESPONSE TO PITUITARY IRRADIATION

A dramatic response to radiation therapy has been observed in all dogs treated to date. In several dogs, a marked treatment response, evidenced by increased alertness and responsiveness to naturally occurring stimuli, was observed after fewer than half of the radiation treatments had been given. This improvement was attributed to a direct radiation-induced tumor effect. In all dogs, a decrease in both pituitary tumor size and peritumoral edema was observed on follow-up CT images done within 3 to 6 months of completion of radiation therapy. Resolution of neurologic abnormalities paralleled the decrease in tumor size, and all dogs were neurologically normal within 6 months of completion of pituitary irradiation. Further decreases in tumor size continued over the next 1 to 2 years. In agreement with the experience following pituitary irradiation in humans, a small residual tumor mass can be expected. Although the natural course of growth of a pituitary tumor is unknown at this time, in one dog treated with o,p'-DDD alone and followed by us by means of serial CT scans, a pituitary tumor continued to enlarge slowly and by 20 months had doubled in size.

Despite an obvious decrease in pituitary tumor size following radiation, plasma ACTH concentrations initially remained high in five of six dogs. In four dogs treated with radiation therapy only, basal ACTH concentrations in three of the dogs declined to normal at 5, 11, and 17 months, while in the fourth dog, ACTH concentration remained increased at 12 months. Basal ACTH concentration was nearly normal at 14 months in one dog treated with o,p'-DDD and irradiation, whereas basal ACTH concentration remained increased at 8 months in a second dog treated with o,p'-DDD and pituitary irradiation. In a third dog treated with a combination of o,p'-DDD and irradiation, plasma ACTH concentrations were initially normal but increased to high concentrations by 8 months after completion of radiation treatment.

The single death in this group of dogs occurred at 5 months in a dog treated with pituitary irradiation alone. Development of diabetic ketoacidosis and pulmonary thromboembolism in this dog was attributed to the adverse effects of uncontrolled hyperadrenocorticism.

ADVERSE EFFECTS OF PITUITARY IRRADIATION

Several adverse effects have been attributed to pituitary irradiation. Hearing impairment, ranging in severity from partial to complete deafness, has been observed in most dogs. Portals were such that the dog's middle and inner ears were unavoidably included in the irradiated field. Use of orthogonal portals or dorsal and ventral portals that largely spare one or both middle and inner ears is being investigated in an effort to minimize this problem. Acute onset of signs suggestive of central vestibular disease occurred in three dogs within 12 to 24 months of pituitary irradiation. Signs resolved rapidly over 1 to 2 weeks. One dog developed signs of unilateral trigeminal nerve dysfunction 3 years after pituitary irradiation. During radiation treatment, particularly in dogs with very large tumors, an initial worsening of neurologic status may occur, probably as a result of radiation-induced cerebral edema or early tumor necrosis. Dexamethasone or prednisone, administered at anti-inflammatory doses for 1 to 2 weeks, has been successful in controlling these signs. Mild, localized hair depigmentation may also occur in the irradiated field. Hypopituitarism has not been observed in any dogs treated by means of pituitary irradiation. In persons, normal pituitary corticotrophs are known to be more resistant to the effects of irradiation than are neoplastic pituitary cells. They may therefore survive the effects of radiation treatment, whereas neoplastic cortico-trophs are rapidly killed.

TREATMENT RECOMMENDATIONS

Pituitary irradiation presently offers the most effective treatment available for dogs with a large pituitary tumor. CT examination is mandatory for diagnosis of these tumors and for treatment planning and follow-up evaluation. Pituitary hypersecretion of ACTH can be expected to persist for at least 6 months after completion of pituitary irradiation. Concurrent treatment to normalize serum cortisol concentrations (either o,p'-DDD or ketoconazole) is recommended for at least the first 6 to 12 months after radiation therapy, especially for dogs initially manifesting severe, hypercortisolemia-related adverse effects. Periodic measurement of ACTH concentration at 3- to 6-month intervals is necessary to determine accurately when adrenal suppressive therapy can be discontinued. Irradiation-induced hypopituitarism is apparently uncommon in dogs, at least within the first 1 to 2 years after treatment. Until more dogs have been treated, however, serum cortisol and thyroxine concentrations should be measured at 6- to 12-month intervals to determine whether supplementation of these hormones is necessary.

References and Supplemental Reading

Dow, S. W., LeCouteur, R. A., Rosychuk, R. A., et al: Radiation therapy of functional canine pituitary tumors. (Abstract.) 7th Annual Conference, Veterinary Cancer Society, Madison, October 26–28, 1987, p. 21.

Eigenmann, J. E., Lubberink, A. A. M. E., and Koemann, J. P.: Panhypopituitarism caused by a suprasellar tumor in a dog. J. Am. Anim. Hosp. Assoc. 19:377, 1983.

Feldman, E. C., Turrel, J. M., and Nelson, R. W.: Radiation therapy of an ACTH-secreting pituitary/hypothalamic mass—a case report. (Abstract.) Proceedings of the A.C.V.I.M. 3rd Annual Medical Forum, San Diego, 1985, p. 140.

LeCouteur, R. A., Gillette, E. L., Dow, S. W., et al: Radiation response of autochthonous canine brain tumors. (Abstract.) Int. J. Rad. Oncol. Biol. Phys. 13(Suppl. 1):166, 1987.

Leibel, S. A., and Sheline, G. E.: Tolerance of the central and peripheral nervous system to therapeutic irradiation. Adv. Rad. Biol. 12:257, 1987.

Peterson, M. E.: Hyperadrenocorticism. Vet. Clin. North Am. 14:731, 1984.

Post, K. D., and Muraszko, K.: Management of pituitary tumors. Neurol. Clin. 4:801, 1986.

Sheline, G. E.: Radiation therapy of pituitary tumors. In Givens, J. R. (ed.): Hormone-secreting Pituitary Tumors. Chicago: Year Book Medical Publishers, 1982, pp. 121–143.

Turrel, J. M., Fike, J. R., LeCouteur, R. A., et al.: Radiotherapy of brain tumors in dogs. J.A.V.M.A. 184:82, 1984.

Turrel, J. M., Fike, J. R., LeCouteur, R. A., et al: Computed tomographic characteristics of primary brain tumors in 50 dogs. J.A.V.M.A. 188:851, 1986.

MITOTANE (O,P'-DDD) TREATMENT OF CORTISOL-SECRETING ADRENOCORTICAL NEOPLASIA

PETER P. KINTZER, D.V.M.
North Grafton, Massachusetts

and MARK E. PETERSON, D.V.M.
New York, New York

In dogs, adrenocortical tumors are the underlying cause of 10 to 15 per cent of cases of naturally occurring hyperadrenocorticism. Approximately half of these cortisol-secreting tumors are malignant, and many have metastasized by the time of diagnosis. Mitotane (o,p'-DDD; Lysodren, Bristol-Myers Oncology Division) is a potent adrenocorticolytic agent that causes a selective, marked, progressive destruction of the adrenal cortices in normal dogs and dogs with adrenocortical hyperplasia. Unlike ketoconazole and metyrapone, two drugs that lower circulating cortisol concentrations by inhibiting enzymes for glucocorticoid synthesis, o,p'-DDD is directly cytotoxic to adrenal cortical tissue. Although the efficacy of o,p'-DDD in the therapy of pituitary-dependent hyperadrenocorticism is well established, its use in the treatment of adrenal tumors has not been well described.

Unilateral adrenalectomy is the treatment of choice for an adrenal adenoma or carcinoma (if metastasis has not occurred), since complete cure is attainable. However, if the tumor is unresectable, if the owner refuses surgery, if the dog is an unsuitable surgical candidate, or if gross metastasis is detected prior to surgery (using radiography, ultrasonography, or computed tomography), medical adrenalectomy with o,p'-DDD should be considered. In addition, o,p'-DDD may be useful as preoperative preparation for surgical adrenalectomy, since control of hypercortisolism may decrease anesthetic risks and help minimize such complications as thromboembolism, sepsis, and poor wound healing.

DIAGNOSIS OF CORTISOL-SECRETING ADRENAL TUMOR

Once the diagnosis of hyperadrenocorticism has been confirmed with a low-dose dexamethasone suppression test or an adrenocorticotropic hormone (ACTH) stimulation test, a high-dose dexamethasone suppression test should next be performed to help determine the etiology of the cortisol excess (see p. 963). In our laboratory, serum cortisol values generally remain above 1.5 µg/dl at all sampling times in dogs with adrenal tumors; therefore, suppression of the serum cortisol concentration below 1.5 µg/dl is diagnostic of pituitary-dependent hyperadrenocorticism, rules out an adrenal tumor, and obviates the need for additional diagnostic testing.

Unfortunately, approximately 15 to 20 per cent of dogs with pituitary-dependent hyperadrenocorticism also fail to demonstrate adequate suppression during the high-dose dexamethasone suppression test (using a dexamethasone dose of 1.0 mg/kg). Because pituitary-dependent disease is so much more common than functional adrenal neoplasia (80 per cent versus 20 per cent), this means that an individual dog showing inadequate suppression of serum cortisol values after 1.0 mg/kg dexamethasone has about a 50 per cent chance of having an adrenal tumor versus nonsuppressible pituitary-dependent hyperadrenocorticism. Because of the relatively high morbidity and mortality associated with surgical exploration of the adrenal glands, other less invasive procedures to differentiate nonsuppressible pituitary-dependent hyperadrenocorticism from a cortisol-secreting adrenal tumor are recommended before exploratory celiotomy is considered.

Measurement of the endogenous plasma ACTH concentration is very useful in making this distinction, especially in these dogs that fail to demonstrate adequate serum cortisol suppression during the high-dose dexamethasone test. Plasma ACTH concentrations are normal to high in dogs with pituitary-dependent hyperadrenocorticism, but values are undetectable to low normal in dogs with adrenal tumors. The accurate determination of plasma ACTH concentration requires careful sample collection and handling and use of a reliable, validated radioimmunoassay for canine ACTH. It is recommended that blood for ACTH assay be collected using chilled syringes and EDTA-containing tubes. The samples should be spun immediately (preferably at 4°C) and the plasma stored in plastic vials and kept frozen (ideally at −70°C) until assayed. Since ACTH is unstable in unfrozen plasma, samples should be sent by air express in a styrofoam container with sufficient quantities of dry ice (see p. 972).

An adrenal mass is occasionally detectable on abdominal radiographs. Mineralization is apparent in about 25 to 50 per cent of the tumors seen on radiographs and is, in our experience, usually indicative of malignancy. Ultrasonography has recently emerged as a useful means of screening for adrenal neoplasia. It appears to be more sensitive than plain radiographs, and, furthermore, the liver can be concurrently evaluated for metastatic disease. Computed tomography can, in most instances, reliably differentiate between normal adrenal glands, bilateral adrenal enlargement (suggestive of pituitary-dependent hyperplasia), and unilateral adrenal cortical tumors and can also accurately detect hepatic metastasis. Its use, however, is hampered by limited availability, expense, and the need for anesthesia.

Overall, it is very important to distinguish pituitary-dependent from primary adrenal forms of hyperadrenocorticism before use of o,p'-DDD is considered, because different therapeutic o,p'-DDD protocols are used depending on the cause of the hyperadrenocorticism (see below).

TREATMENT OF ADRENAL TUMORS WITH MITOTANE

In treatment of dogs with proven adrenocortical neoplasia, o,p'-DDD is used as a true chemotherapeutic agent with the goal of therapy being to destroy all neoplastic tissue. Although destruction of all neoplastic adrenocortical tissue is probably not necessary in treatment of adrenal adenomas, most dogs with adrenal tumors treated with o,p'-DDD either will have known adrenal carcinoma or will not have been surgically explored (and therefore have about a 50 per cent chance of having adrenal carcinoma). The induction of overt hypoadrenocorticism (as reflected by undetectable basal and post-ACTH serum cortisol concentrations) is not discouraged, since this generally indicates that all neoplastic adrenocortical tissue has probably been destroyed. The limiting factor in the production of complete adrenal insufficiency in many dogs is the development of direct o,p'-DDD toxicity (see p. 1037).

Initial Therapy

Initially, o,p'-DDD should be administered at a dosage of 50 to 75 mg/kg PO daily in divided doses for 10 to 14 days. Glucocorticoid supplementation with prednisone or prednisolone, 0.2 mg/kg/day PO, can be given concurrently and may help reduce adverse effects. Although side effects associated with o,p'-DDD are rare during this initial period, the o,p'-DDD should be discontinued and the dog evaluated as soon as possible should severe adverse effects develop (e.g., anorexia, vomiting, weakness).

After completion of this initial loading period with o,p'-DDD, the dog should be examined and the effectiveness of treatment evaluated using an ACTH stimulation test. If glucocorticoid supplementation is being given, it must be withheld on the morning of the test, since both prednisone and prednisolone will cross-react in most cortisol assays, resulting in spuriously elevated values.

The therapeutic objective of the induction period is to decrease both basal and post-ACTH cortisol concentrations to undetectable or low values (e.g., less than 1.0 µg/dl). Should the basal and post-ACTH cortisol concentrations fall slightly but remain within or above the normal resting range, daily o,p'-DDD should be continued (50 to 75 mg/kg/day) and ACTH stimulation testing repeated at 7- to 14-day intervals until cortisol concentrations fall to below the normal resting range (less than 1.0 µg/dl). Once low to undetectable serum cortisol concentrations are documented, o,p'-DDD should be continued at a weekly maintenance dosage of 100 to 200 mg/kg.

Occasionally, initial o,p'-DDD treatment using a daily dosage of 50 to 75 mg/kg is relatively to totally ineffective in destroying neoplastic adrenocortical tissue, and the serum cortisol response to ACTH remains greatly elevated or unchanged from pretreatment test results. In these dogs, the loading dosage of o,p'-DDD should be increased to 100 mg/kg/day and ACTH stimulation testing continued at 7- to 14-day intervals. Should serum cortisol concentrations remain greatly elevated, one should increase the o,p'-DDD dosage by 50 mg/kg/day increments (every 7 to 14 days, if necessary) until ACTH stimulation testing reveals that the serum cortisol concentrations have decreased to at least some extent or until intolerance to the drug develops. If these incremental increases in drug dosage have lowered cortisol concentrations considerably but values remain within or above the normal resting range, daily o,p'-DDD is continued at the previous week's dosage and ACTH stimulation testing continued at 7- to 14-day intervals until circulating cortisol values fall below normal resting range (less than 1.0 µg/dl). If a direct drug reaction develops (not secondary to low serum cortisol concentration), daily o,p'-DDD is continued at the highest tolerated dosage until cortisol levels have fallen. Maintenance o,p'-DDD therapy is begun once serum cortisol concentrations fall to undetectable to low values.

Maintenance Therapy

Once undetectable to low-normal serum cortisol concentrations are documented by ACTH stimulation testing, o,p'-DDD should be continued at an initial maintenance dosage of 100 to 200 mg/kg/week, in divided doses, together with daily maintenance glucocorticoid supplementation given as either prednisone or prednisolone, 0.2 mg/kg/day. To ensure that serum cortisol concentrations remain suppressed to desired levels, an ACTH stimulation test should be repeated 1 to 2 months after initiation of maintenance o,p'-DDD therapy.

The original weekly maintenance o,p'-DDD dosage should be continued if basal and post-ACTH serum cortisol concentrations remain at undetectable to low values at the time of follow-up evaluations. If circulating cortisol concentrations rise into the normal resting range (1 to 4 µg/dl), however, the weekly maintenance o,p'-DDD dosage should be increased by 50 per cent. If basal or post-ACTH serum cortisol concentrations rise above normal resting range (greater than 4 µg/dl), daily o,p'-DDD induction treatment is reinstituted (usually 50 to 100 mg/kg/day) until cortisol concentrations fall to low or undetectable values; the weekly maintenance dosage is then increased by 50 per cent. Such adjustments in o,p'-DDD dosage are followed by repeat ACTH stimulation testing in 1 month to ensure an adequate response to the new maintenance dose. Subsequent dosage adjustments are based on periodic ACTH stimulation tests at 3- to 6-month intervals, as well as on the dog's tolerance of the medication itself.

Side Effects

The most common side effects noted during o,p'-DDD treatment of dogs with adrenal tumors include partial to complete anorexia, weakness, and lethargy. These adverse reactions usually appear to result from a direct toxic effect of the high doses of o,p'-DDD being administered. In most dogs, side effects do not appear to be related to low circulating cortisol concentrations for the following reasons: (1) The dogs are receiving at least maintenance daily glucocorticoid supplementation, (2) no resolution in adverse signs occurs in most dogs when the glucocorticoid dosage is increased, and (3) many dogs do not have undetectable post-ACTH cortisol concentrations when adverse effects develop. Moreover, a similar drug reaction occurs in human adrenal carcinoma patients receiving large doses of o,p'-DDD.

If severe side effects develop during treatment with o,p'-DDD, the o,p'-DDD should be stopped, the glucocorticoid supplementation continued, and the dog re-evaluated as soon as possible. An ACTH stimulation test together with serum electrolyte determinations should be performed at this time (to rule out glucocorticoid and mineralocorticoid deficiency, respectively).

If serum electrolyte concentrations are normal but serum cortisol concentrations are found to be below normal range, the daily glucocorticoid dosage is increased (to approximately 0.4 mg/kg/day) to rule out cortisol deficiency as the cause of the adverse side effects. If adverse side effects recur after the maintenance o,p'-DDD is reinstituted despite such an increase in daily glucocorticoid supplementation, however, a direct toxic drug effect is likely.

In dogs suspected of suffering from a direct toxic effect of o,p'-DDD, the maintenance o,p'-DDD is reinstituted after signs of toxicity have resolved but at a 25 to 50 per cent lower dose. As a consequence of this lower weekly maintenance dose, cortisol concentrations will usually rise to within or above the normal resting range on repeat ACTH stimulation testing. The resting and post-ACTH cortisol concentrations must, however, be kept below 4 to 5 μg/dl to prevent recurrence of signs of hyperadrenocorticism. Restitution of the higher weekly maintenance dose of o,p'-DDD can be attempted at a later date; unfortunately, recurrence of adverse signs associated with o,p'-DDD toxicity is likely.

Although rare, complete glucocorticoid and mineralocorticoid deficiency (Addison's disease), characterized by low basal and post-ACTH cortisol concentrations as well as serum electrolyte disturbances of hyperkalemia and hyponatremia, can develop in some dogs treated with high doses of o,p'-DDD. If iatrogenic Addison's disease does develop, o,p'-DDD should be stopped and supplementation with appropriate doses of glucocorticoid and fludrocortisone acetate (Florinef, Squibb) given. Further o,p'-DDD is not usually required in these dogs unless hypoadrenocorticism resolves and serum cortisol concentrations increase into or above normal resting range. As previously mentioned, the induction of an addisonian state is not undesirable. In fact, such an occurrence may enhance the dog's long-term prognosis, since all functional neoplastic adrenocortical tissue (as well as any remaining normal adrenal tissue) has probably been destroyed.

PROGNOSIS OF MITOTANE-TREATED ADRENAL NEOPLASIA

The overall long-term prognosis for dogs with an adrenocortical adenoma treated with o,p'-DDD ranges from fair to good. Attainment of undetectable to low serum cortisol concentrations is usually possible without undue toxicity. Resolution of clinical signs of hyperadrenocorticism occurs in most cases; however, maintenance o,p'-DDD therapy and daily replacement of glucocorticoid generally must be continued for the life of the dog.

Most dogs that have small adrenal carcinomas without widespread metastasis carry at least a fair prognosis. Adequate control of serum cortisol concentrations and resolution of clinical signs is often achieved, though it is sometimes less complete and shorter in duration than in cases of adenomas. On the other hand, dogs with large adrenocortical carcinomas and those with widespread metastasis have, in the vast majority of cases, a poor to grave prognosis. Although a favorable outcome is possible, most cases will only partially respond to o,p'-DDD, respond temporarily, or respond only to high doses (with the attendant unacceptable side effects). There may be short-term palliation of clinical signs of hyperadrenocorticism despite progressive tumor growth and spread. Dogs with carcinomas that show no response to large loading doses of o,p'-DDD administered daily for weeks generally have an ominous prognosis.

References and Supplemental Reading

Hoffman, D. L., and Mattox, V. R.: Treatment of adrenocortical carcinoma with o,p'-DDD. Med. Clin. North Am. 56:999, 1972.
Hogan, T. F., Citrin, D. L., Johnson, B. M., et al.: o,p'-DDD (mitotane) therapy of adrenal cortical carcinoma. Cancer 42:2177, 1978.

FELINE
HYPERADRENOCORTICISM

CAROLE A. ZERBE, D.V.M.

Auburn, Alabama

Hyperadrenocorticism (Cushing's syndrome), a disorder resulting from excessive production of cortisol by the adrenal cortex, appears to be relatively uncommon in cats. Although this syndrome was first recognized in 1975, 14 of the 16 cases that have been described in the literature have only recently been reported (1986 and 1987). Thus, as with any newly recognized syndrome, the best means of diagnosis and treatment are not yet clearly defined.

Although canine and feline hyperadrenocorticism appear similar in many respects, there are major differences in the manifestations between cats and dogs. As in dogs, reported causes of spontaneous (naturally occurring) hyperadrenocorticism in cats include pituitary-dependent hyperadrenocorticism (PDH, approximately 81 per cent incidence) and adrenal tumors (approximately 19 per cent incidence). Of the three cats with adrenal tumors, one had a carcinoma and two had an adrenal adenoma. Iatrogenic Cushing's syndrome has been described in cats but will not be included in this discussion.

CLINICAL FEATURES

Signalment

Cats with hyperadrenocorticism are middle-aged or older (average 10.4, range 7 to 15 years). Hyperadrenocorticism in cats, unlike in dogs, occurs more frequently in females (69 per cent) and has no apparent breed predilection, with the disease being reported in domestic short- and long-haired, mixed-breed, Siamese, and one Burmese.

Clinical Signs

Polyuria, polydipsia, a pendulous abdomen, and polyphagia are the most frequently observed clinical signs of feline hyperadrenocorticism (Table 1). Cutaneous abnormalities such as truncal and abdominal alopecia, unkempt hair coat, thin skin, bruising, and abscesses are also common. Additional abnormalities include muscle wasting, weight gain or loss, hepatomegaly, other infections, and depression.

Although polyuria and polydipsia are common in both canine and feline hyperadrenocorticism, the cause and time of onset of the polyuria and polydipsia differ. In dogs, the polyuria and polydipsia occur early in the syndrome and are secondary to glucocorticoid inhibition of the secretion or action of antidiuretic hormone. In cats, the polyuria and polydipsia result from a glucocorticoid-induced hyperglycemia with subsequent glucosuria and osmotic diuresis. Indeed, 81 per cent of reported cats with hyperadrenocorticism had concurrent overt diabetes mellitus (only 10 to 15 per cent of dogs with hyperadrenocorticism develop diabetes mellitus). In addition, the onset of polyuria and polydipsia in cats appears to be delayed. Therefore, it is possible that hyperglycemia, and thus polyuria and polydipsia, may not be detected in the early stages of hyperadrenocorticism.

Recurrent infections may be life threatening and include facial abscesses, bacterial and fungal cystitis, pyothorax, bronchitis, rhinitis, pancreatitis, and enteritis. One cat had demodicosis. As in other species, this apparent predisposition to infections suggests that cats with hyperadrenocorticism are immunosuppressed. The concurrent diabetes mellitus may also contribute to the development of the infections.

Table 1. *Incidence of Historic and Clinical Signs of Spontaneous Feline Hyperadrenocorticism*

Sign	No. (%) of Cats
Polyuria/polydipsia	15/16 (94%)
Pendulous abdomen	15/16 (94%)
Polyphagia	14/16 (88%)
Hair loss	11/16 (69%)
Muscle wasting	10/16 (63%)
Weight gain	9/16 (56%)
Hepatomegaly	9/16 (56%)
Thin skin	7/16 (44%)
Infections	6/16 (38%)
Depression	4/16 (25%)
Weight loss	3/16 (19%)
Easy bruising	3/16 (19%)

Compiled from data in the following references: Fox and Beatty, 1975; Meijer et al., 1978; Peterson and Steele, 1986; Zerbe et al., 1987a; Feldman and Nelson, 1987; Drazner, 1987; and from personal communication with some of those authors.

LABORATORY FINDINGS

Complete Blood Count

The most common abnormalities noted on the hemogram are lymphopenia, eosinopenia, and neutrophilia, but these findings are inconsistent (Table 2).

Serum Biochemistries

The most common biochemical abnormalities in cats with hyperadrenocorticism are hyperglycemia and hypercholesterolemia (Table 2). The hyperglycemia, common in dogs and cats with hyperadrenocorticism, results from a glucocorticoid-induced glucose intolerance and insulin resistance. However, cats develop hyperglycemia more frequently and have higher glucose concentrations (usually in the diabetic range) than do dogs. The hypercholesterolemia is probably related to the poorly controlled diabetic state rather than to the glucocorticoid excess *per se*.

Mild to moderate increases in alanine aminotransferase (ALT) and serum alkaline phosphatase (SAP) develop in 50 and 40 per cent of the cats, respectively. Increased SAP is found in most dogs with hyperadrenocorticism and results from induction of a steroid-induced isoenzyme, whereas cats appear to lack this isoenzyme. The increases in SAP and ALT in cats are probably related to the diabetes mellitus rather than to the glucocorticoid excess.

Urinalysis

Glucosuria is common (Table 2) and is the cause of the primary polyuria. Despite the high incidence of polyuria, the urine specific gravity of cats with

Table 2. *Incidence of Laboratory Abnormalities in Spontaneous Feline Hyperadrenocorticism*

Laboratory Finding	No. (%) of Cats*
Hyperglycemia	14/15 (93%)
Glucosuria	13/15 (87%)
Hypercholesterolemia	10/13 (77%)
Lymphopenia	10/14 (71%)
Eosinopenia	9/14 (64%)
Neutrophilia	9/14 (64%)
Increased alanine amino transferase	7/14 (50%)
Increased serum alkaline phosphatase	5/15 (40%)
Mature leukocytosis	3/14 (21%)
Decreased blood urea nitrogen (BUN)	3/15 (20%)

Compiled from data in the following references: Fox and Beatty, 1975; Meijer et al., 1978; Peterson and Steele, 1986; Zerbe et al., 1987a; Feldman and Nelson, 1987; and Drazner, 1987; and from personal communication with some of those authors.

*Not all cats received all tests.

hyperadrenocorticism ranged from dilute to concentrated.

Radiographs

Hepatomegaly was noted in 11 of the 16 cats on which radiographs were performed. Although calcification of the adrenal glands occurs in up to 30 per cent of normal cats and is occasionally apparent radiographically, none of these cats had radiographic evidence of adrenal calcification. One cat had evidence of pulmonary infiltrates on thoracic radiographs.

EVALUATION OF PITUITARY ADRENAL FUNCTION

Resting Cortisol Concentrations

Some cats with nonadrenal illness have increased basal cortisol values, and some hyperadrenocorticoid cats have normal basal cortisol concentrations. Therefore, as in other species, a basal cortisol determination is not useful in the diagnosis of hyperadrenocorticism.

ACTH Stimulation Tests

The adrenocorticotropic hormone (ACTH) stimulation test, a test of adrenocortical reserve, is used for diagnosing hyperadrenocorticism. This test can be accomplished by collecting blood for determination of plasma (or serum, depending on the laboratory used) cortisol concentrations before and 1 and 2 hr after IM injection of ACTH gel (2.2 U/kg). Alternatively, synthetic ACTH (cosyntropin, 0.125 mg/cat) may be administered IM and samples collected at 30 and 60 min. It is imperative that both post-ACTH cortisol samples be collected in cats, since 30 to 40 per cent of cats will peak at the time of the first post-ACTH sample (often with cortisol values much lower in the second sample) but others will peak at the time of the second post-ACTH sample.

Ten of the 12 cats with hyperadrenocorticism evaluated using the ACTH stimulation test showed an exaggerated response. Two cats (17 per cent) had normal responses to ACTH despite the presence of hyperadrenocorticism. This is similar to canine hyperadrenocorticism, in which approximately 15 to 20 per cent of dogs show a normal response to ACTH. Thus, if a cat is suspected of having the disease but results of an ACTH stimulation test are normal, a high-dose dexamethasone suppression test (0.1 mg/kg IV) is recommended (see following). Additionally, cats with nonadrenal illness (e.g., renal failure, diabetes mellitus) may have exaggerated cortisol responses to ACTH (though not usually to the same degree as cats with hyperadrenocorticism). Therefore, test results should be cautiously interpreted in these animals. As in dogs, the ACTH stimulation test is a screening test only and test results will not distinguish PDH from adrenal tumor.

Low-Dose Dexamethasone Suppression Test

The low-dose dexamethasone suppression test (0.01 to 0.015 mg/kg IV), a test of the integrity of the cortisol negative-feedback pathway, is the most accurate screening test available for use in dogs. In normal cats, an IV dose of dexamethasone ranging from 0.010 to 0.015 mg/kg will suppress serum cortisol concentrations to low or undetectable values in most cats for more than 8 hr. However, with the 0.01 mg/kg dose, 14 to 20 per cent of these normal cats showed escape from cortisol suppression by 8 hr. Of the five cats with hyperadrenocorticism that were evaluated using the low-dose dexamethasone suppression test (0.01 mg/kg IV), four (80 per cent) were resistant to cortisol suppression and thus had results consistent with hyperadrenocorticism. One cat, however, had good cortisol suppression and would have been falsely considered normal based on this test alone. Therefore, it appears that this test may not be as useful for diagnosis of hyperadrenocorticism in cats as it is in dogs.

High-Dose Dexamethasone Suppression Test

The high-dose dexamethasone suppression test (0.1 to 1.0 mg/kg IV), a differentiating test, is used in dogs to distinguish PDH from adrenal tumors. In normal cats, dexamethasone doses of 0.1 and 1.0 mg/kg given IV cause consistent and reliable suppression of cortisol values. Five cats with hyperadrenocorticism were evaluated before and 2 hr after the administration of IV dexamethasone (0.1 mg/kg) as part of the combined dexamethasone suppression–ACTH stimulation test (see following). None of these cats had adequate suppression of cortisol at 2 hr (presumably indicating hyperadrenocorticism). In addition, although all of these cats had PDH, only two cats had cortisol suppression that would have been considered consistent with PDH. In one of these cats, when the dose of dexamethasone was increased to 1.0 mg/kg and samples were collected at 0, 2, 6, and 8 hr, serum cortisol concentrations significantly decreased and were consistent with a diagnosis of PDH. As in dogs with adrenal tumor, dexamethasone doses ranging from 0.1 to 1.0 mg/kg failed to suppress cortisol concentrations in one cat with an adrenal tumor.

Thus it appears that a dexamethasone suppression test using a dose of 0.1 mg/kg may be a reliable screening test for feline hyperadrenocorticism (and may be preferred over the low-dose dexamethasone suppression test), while a dexamethasone suppression test using a dose of 1.0 mg/kg may be appropriate for distinguishing PDH from adrenal tumor in cats.

Combined Dexamethasone Suppression–ACTH Stimulation Test

The combined dexamethasone suppression–ACTH stimulation test, although controversial, is used as a screening test for hyperadrenocorticism in dogs and has the added advantage of immediate diagnosis of PDH in approximately 40 per cent of dogs tested. This test is accomplished by collecting a blood sample, injecting dexamethasone IV (0.1 mg/kg), collecting a post-dexamethasone sample at 2 hr, immediately giving ACTH, and collecting two post-ACTH samples (see ACTH Stimulation Tests, previously discussed). The dexamethasone suppression portion of the test may be extended to 4 hr.

Some normal cats and cats with nonadrenal illness may be resistant to dexamethasone suppression of cortisol or have an exaggerated response to ACTH. However, of the five cats with hyperadrenocorticism that were evaluated using this test, all had markedly exaggerated responses to ACTH and either no cortisol suppression or less than 50 per cent suppression of baseline cortisol after dexamethasone (possibly indicating PDH as it does in the dog), but not suppression into the normal range (thus still indicating hyperadrenocorticism). Therefore, this test would appear to be a good screening test for hyperadrenocorticism in cats and may have the added benefit of identifying PDH in a percentage of these cats.

Endogenous ACTH Determinations

Endogenous plasma ACTH concentrations should be high in cats with PDH and low or nondetectable in cats with adrenal tumor. All five of the cats with PDH that were evaluated using this test had high or normal values that were consistent with PDH. One cat with an adrenal adenoma had undetectable ACTH concentrations, as would be expected. Thus, this test appears to be useful in distinguishing PDH from an adrenal tumor. As in other species, this test can only be used after hyperadrenocorticism has been confirmed.

Selecting the Appropriate Test

There is a paucity of information regarding adrenal function testing in cats with hyperadrenocorticism and nonadrenal illness. Since feline hyperadrenocorticism is an uncommon disease, it will probably be some time before firm recommendations can be made as to the best endocrine tests to use when screening for and differentiating between the etiologies of hyperadrenocorticism in cats. However, at this time it would seem that the ACTH stimulation test, the combined dexamethasone suppression–ACTH stimulation test, and the high-dose dexamethasone suppression test (0.1 mg/kg IV) are the most useful screening tests. It is important to realize the limitations of these tests, and the veterinarian should carefully consider clinical signs and laboratory abnormalities as well as results of the adrenal function tests before making a diagnosis of hyperadrenocorticism. For example, if a cat has a normal response to one of the screening tests but hyperadrenocorticism is still suspected, a different screening test then should be used or the testing repeated at a later date (in 3 to 4 weeks). Likewise, caution must be used before diagnosis of hyperadrenocorticism in a cat with equivocal test results, since some normal cats and cats with nonadrenal illness may have similar results.

Once a diagnosis of hyperadrenocorticism is made, differentiating tests can be used to determine if the cat has PDH or adrenal tumor. The ACTH assay and possibly the 1.0 mg/kg dexamethasone suppression test appear to be useful for this. It could be argued, however, that it is not necessary to distinguish PDH from adrenal tumor in cats, since the current recommended treatment of feline hyperadrenocorticism is unilateral adrenalectomy for adrenal tumor and bilateral adrenalectomy for PDH.

TREATMENT

Treatment of hyperadrenocorticism includes both surgical and medical modalities and has been attempted in cats with PDH and in cats with adrenal tumors. These therapies have met with varying degrees of success.

Adrenal Tumor

Of the three cats with adrenal tumors, one cat was not treated and was diagnosed at necropsy and two cats underwent unilateral adrenalectomy. At a 6-week recheck, clinical signs of hyperadrenocorticism were resolving in one cat. The remaining cat progressively improved, lost its insulin dependence, and survived 14 months before being killed by a car.

Pituitary-Dependent Hyperadrenocorticism

Of the 13 cats with PDH, 6 were not treated, 5 underwent bilateral adrenalectomy, 1 was treated with o,p′-DDD and then cobalt irradiation, and 1 received metyrapone. The use of o,p′-DDD in cats has generally been discouraged because of the sensitivity of this species to chlorinated hydrocarbons. We have used o,p′-DDD in a limited number of normal cats, and the drug was well tolerated by most of them; however, the dosage used (25, 37, and 50 mg/kg, PO) caused adrenocortical suppression in only half of the cats. In one cat with hyperadrenocorticism, treatment with o,p′-DDD was ineffective in controlling clinical signs, and its use was not associated with any side effects or adrenocortical suppression. Cobalt irradiation of the pituitary tumor was then unsuccessfully attempted in this cat. The cat subsequently was euthanized 1 month later. Metyrapone, a drug that decreases cortisol synthesis by inhibiting 11-β-hydroxylase, the enzyme that converts 11-deoxycortisol to cortisol, was administered to one cat at a dosage of 65 mg PO t.i.d. for 6 months. Clinical improvement was noted, but the cat was lost to follow-up.

Bilateral adrenalectomy, followed by mineralocorticoid and glucorticoid replacement therapy, appears to be the most successful treatment for PDH. This surgery was performed in five cats, all of which showed clinical improvement with resolution of polyuria and polydipsia and regrowth of hair. Four of these hyperadrenocorticoid cats had concurrent diabetes mellitus. After surgery, three cats no longer required insulin therapy. One cat remained a diabetic but was controlled on approximately 1 U of PZI insulin per day. One cat was lost to follow-up, one cat is still doing well at time of this writing (4 years), and two cats died of unrelated problems after 10 and 30 months. The other cat developed acute signs of circling, wandering aimlessly, and apparent blindness 2 months after surgery. Euthanasia was performed, but necropsy was not permitted. An expanding pituitary tumor was the probable cause of the neurologic abnormalities.

It is noteworthy that all cats that were treated with adrenalectomy for either PDH or adrenal tumor survived the surgery and experienced no reported complications. In contrast, dogs that undergo this type of operation have significant morbidity and mortality. Four of five diabetic cats that were successfully treated for their hyperadrenocorticism no longer required insulin therapy, a success rate that is not paralleled in dogs.

PROGNOSIS

Untreated or unsuccessfully treated spontaneous feline hyperadrenocorticism appears to be a progressive disorder with a grave prognosis. In all reported cases that were not treated, cats died of severe infection, uncontrolled diabetes mellitus, or euthanasia. With proper treatment, cats with adrenal adenomas or PDH appear to have a good to excellent prognosis. One cat, however, did develop neurologic abnormalities presumably related to an expanding pituitary tumor. Since this is a disease of middle-aged to older cats, it is not unreasonable to expect that some will die or be euthanized because of problems unrelated to their hyperadrenocorticism (as occurred with four of these seven successfully treated cats). The one cat with an adrenal carcinoma was not treated. It is likely, however, that cats with adrenal carcinoma will have a grave prognosis, as do dogs.

References and Supplemental Reading

Drazner, F. H.: The adrenal cortex. *In* Drazner, F. H. (ed.): *Small Animal Endocrinology*. New York: Churchill Livingstone, 1987, p. 201.

Feldman, E. C., and Nelson, R. W.: Hyperadrenocorticism. *In* Feldman, E. C., and Nelson, R. W. (eds.): *Canine and Feline Endocrinology and Reproduction*. Philadelphia: W. B. Saunders Co., 1987, p. 137.

Fox, J. G., and Beatty, J. O.: A case report of complicated diabetes mellitus in a cat. J. Am. Anim. Hosp. Assoc. 11:129, 1975.

Johnston, S. D., and Mather, E. C.: Feline plasma cortisol (hydrocortisone) measured by radioimmunoassay. Am. J. Vet. Res. 40:190, 1979.

Kemppainen, R. J., Mansfield, P. D., and Sartin, J. L.: Endocrine responses of normal cats to TSH and synthetic ACTH administration. J. Am. Anim. Hosp. Assoc. 20:737, 1984.

Medleau, L., Cowan, L. A., Cornelius, L. M., et al.: Adrenal function testing in the cat: The effect of low dose intravenous dexamethasone administration. Res. Vet. Sci. 42:260, 1987.

Meijer, J. C., Lubberink, A. A. M. E., and Gruys, E.: Cushing's syndrome due to adrenocortical adenoma in a cat. Tijdschr. Diergeneeskd. 103:1048, 1978.

Peterson, M. E., Altszuler, N., and Nichols, C. E.: Decreased insulin sensitivity and glucose tolerance in spontaneous canine hyperadrenocorticism. Res. Vet. Sci. 36:177, 1984.

Peterson, M. E., and Graves, T. K.: Effects of low dosages of intravenous dexamethasone on serum cortisol concentrations in the normal cat. Res. Vet. Sci. 44:38, 1988.

Peterson, M. E., Kintzer, P. P., Foodman, M. S., et al.: Adrenal function in the cat: Comparison of the effects of cosyntropin (synthetic ACTH) and corticotropin gel stimulation. Res. Vet. Sci. 37:331, 1984.

Peterson, M. E., and Steele, P.: Pituitary-dependent hyperadrenocorticism in a cat. J.A.V.M.A. 189:680, 1986.

Scott, D. W., Manning, T. O., and Reimers, T. J.: Iatrogenic Cushing's syndrome in the cat. Feline Pract. 12:30, 1982.

Smith, M. C., and Feldman, E. C.: Endogenous ACTH and plasma cortisol response to synthetic ACTH and dexamethasone sodium phosphate in normal cats. Am. J. Vet. Res. 48:1719, 1987.

Zerbe, C. A., Nachreiner, R. F., Dunstan, R. W., et al.: Hyperadrenocorticism in a cat. J.A.V.M.A. 190:559, 1987a.

Zerbe, C. A., Refsal, K. R., Peterson, M. E., et al.: Effect of nonadrenal illness on adrenal function in the cat. Am. J. Vet. Res. 48:451, 1987b.

FELINE HYPOADRENOCORTICISM

DEBORAH S. GRECO, D.V.M.,
College Station, Texas

and MARK E. PETERSON, D.V.M.
New York, New York

Adrenocortical insufficiency, or hypoadrenocorticism, results from deficient adrenal production of glucocorticoids, mineralocorticoids, or both. Either destruction of the adrenal cortex (primary adrenocortical insufficiency; Addison's disease) or deficient pituitary adrenocorticotropic hormone (ACTH) production (secondary adrenocortical insufficiency) can impair adrenocortical function and produce hypoadrenocorticism.

In cats, the cause of the complete destruction or atrophy of all three zones of each adrenal cortex in primary hypoadrenocorticism is not known (idiopathic atrophy), but the condition may result from immune-mediated destruction of adrenal tissue (Johnessee et al., 1983). Secondary hypoadrenocorticism develops because of deficient ACTH production associated with an underlying hypothalamic-pituitary disorder, or may result from administration of drugs that suppress pituitary ACTH production. Secondary hypoadrenocorticism has not yet been reported as a naturally occurring disorder in cats but has been induced by the administration of glucocorticoids and progestogens (Chastain et al., 1983; Peterson, 1987).

PATHOPHYSIOLOGY OF ADRENOCORTICAL INSUFFICIENCY

Adrenocortical hormones exert a myriad of effects on body fluid balance, gastrointestinal function, cardiac performance, renal excretion of electrolytes, and neurologic function. Deficiency of the adrenocortical hormones may result in profound changes in blood pressure, renal function, cardiac performance, gastrointestinal function, and mental status.

Without aldosterone, renal reabsorption of sodium and chloride and renal excretion of potassium and hydrogen ions are impaired, resulting in hyponatremia, hypochloremia, hyperkalemia, and metabolic acidosis. Hyponatremia can lead to extracellular volume depletion, vascular volume contraction, circulatory collapse, reduced tissue perfusion, prerenal azotemia, and metabolic acidosis. Release of vasopressin (antidiuretic hormone) secondary to severe volume contraction causes an increase in renal water reabsorption that further exacerbates hyponatremia. Hyperkalemia causes decreased neuromuscular activity, which is manifest clinically as profound weakness and decreased myocardial contractility. Decreased myocardial contractility coupled with suppression of cardiac conduction (secondary to hyperkalemia) further contributes to circulatory collapse. Metabolic acidosis occurs as a result of hyperkalemia, reduced tissue perfusion, and prerenal azotemia, which causes retention of organic acids. The net effect of mineralocorticoid deficiency is an imbalance in serum electrolytes, leading to cardiovascular shock.

Glucocorticoid deficiency causes anorexia, vomiting, decreased vascular sensitivity to catecholamines, depressed mentation, and decreased gluconeogenesis and glycogenolysis. Cortisol deficiency may also result in an inability of the kidneys to excrete a free water load, further aggravating hyponatremia caused by aldosterone deficiency. Calcium ions are retained by the renal tubules, resulting in mild hypercalcemia.

In primary hypoadrenocorticism (Addison's disease), deficiency of both glucocorticoids and mineralocorticoids causes the clinical signs observed. Because the primary insult is to the adrenal glands, pituitary production of ACTH continues unhindered. In fact, in primary hypoadrenocorticism, reduced cortisol production results in decreased negative feedback at the pituitary, with increased release of ACTH and greatly increased circulating concentrations of ACTH.

In secondary hypoadrenocorticism, the deficient ACTH secretion results in atrophy of the zona fasciculata and zona reticularis and a subsequent decrease in glucocorticoid production. Because ACTH has little stimulatory effect on mineralocorticoid production, however, the adrenal zona glomerulosa is generally preserved in secondary adrenocortical insufficiency. The deficiency in glucocorticoid production results in clinical signs similar to those observed in primary hypoadrenocorticism, except that the derangements associated with mineralocorticoid deficiency (and subsequent electrolyte disturbances) are absent.

CLINICAL FEATURES OF PRIMARY ADRENOCORTICAL INSUFFICIENCY

The clinical signs associated with primary hypoadrenocorticism in cats are relatively nonspecific and are similar to those found in a variety of disorders (Table 1). Primary hypoadrenocorticism has been reported in eight neutered, domestic short-hair cats ranging in age from 1 to 9 years (Johnesse et al., 1983; Peterson and Greco, 1986). There appears to be no sex predilection. Like dogs with spontaneous primary adrenal insufficiency, cats affected with mild primary adrenocortical insufficiency may show intermittent, mild illness that exacerbates during periods of stress and that resolves with supportive treatment (i.e., parenteral fluid therapy, cage rest). When adrenal impairment becomes severe, clinical signs such as anorexia, lethargy, weakness, hypothermia, and depression develop. In addition, weight loss, vomiting, polydipsia, and polyuria may be observed. Again, there may be a history of response to the administration of fluids, corticosteroids, or both.

Physical examination of a cat suffering from adrenocortical insufficiency commonly reveals lethargy, depression, and hypothermia (Table 1). Less commonly, weakness, prolonged capillary refill time, dehydration, weak pulse, and bradycardia may be observed. Radiographic examination of the thorax reveals the presence of microcardia in approximately half of the reported cases.

Table 1. *Clinical Signs and Abnormal Laboratory Findings in Eight Cats with Primary Hypoadrenocorticism (Addison's Disease)*

	No. (%) of Cats
Clinical signs	
Lethargy	8 (100%)
Anorexia	8 (100%)
Weight loss	8 (100%)
Dehydration	7 (88%)
Weakness	6 (75%)
Slow capillary refill time	5 (63%)
Weak pulse	4 (50%)
Microcardia	4 (50%)
Vomiting	2 (25%)
Polyuria/polydipsia	2 (25%)
Bradycardia	1 (13%)
Laboratory findings	
Hyperkalemia	8 (100%)
Hyponatremia	8 (100%)
Hypochloremia	8 (100%)
Azotemia	8 (100%)
Hyperphosphatemia	7 (88%)
Lymphocytosis	3 (38%)
Anemia	2 (25%)
Eosinophilia	1 (13%)
Hypercalcemia	1 (13%)

ROUTINE LABORATORY FINDINGS

Diagnosis of feline hypoadrenocorticism requires laboratory evaluation to confirm and support historic and clinical findings. The lack of specific clinical signs makes laboratory evaluation critical in differentiating hypoadrenocorticism from other more common disorders.

Cats with primary hypoadrenocorticism usually exhibit a mild normocytic, normochromic nonregenerative anemia; however, the anemia may be masked by dehydration. Lymphocytosis and eosinophilia are observed in approximately one-third of the reported cases (Table 1). Normal to elevated eosinophil and lymphocyte counts in an ill cat with signs suggestive of hypoadrenocorticism are significant, because the expected response to stress would result in eosinopenia and lymphopenia.

Classic electrolyte changes such as hyponatremia, hypochloremia, and hyperkalemia are consistent features of primary feline hypoadrenocorticism. Sodium:potassium ratios of less than 27:1 are highly suggestive of hypoadrenocorticism; however, serum electrolyte levels may be normal in cats with secondary adrenocortical insufficiency or early hypoadrenocorticism, or after recent parenteral fluid therapy. Mild hypercalcemia may be present as a result of increased renal tubular calcium resorption.

The extracellular fluid volume contraction (and subsequent decreased renal perfusion) associated with feline primary adrenocortical insufficiency often results in prerenal azotemia and hyperphosphatemia. As in cases of canine primary hypoadrenocorticism, pretreatment urine specific gravities are variable but may be lower than would be expected in an animal with prerenal azotemia. The cause of this apparent loss of renal concentrating ability is poorly understood but may be secondary to renal sodium depletion with resultant medullary washout.

Hypoglycemia is not a common manifestation of hypoadrenocorticism in cats or dogs, although gluconeogenesis and glycogenolysis are impaired as a result of cortisol deficiency. Metabolic acidosis is often observed as a result of decreased hydrogen ion secretion in the distal renal tubule, increased generation of metabolic acids secondary to reduced tissue perfusion, and renal retention of organic acids.

DIAGNOSIS OF ADRENAL INSUFFICIENCY

The most accurate test for definitive diagnosis of feline hypoadrenocorticism is an ACTH stimulation test. The finding of a low basal serum cortisol concentration with a subnormal or negligible response to ACTH is indicative of adrenocortical insufficiency. When interpreting results of ACTH stimulation testing, it is important to remember that the protocol for this test in cats differs slightly from that in dogs; at least three samples must be collected to ensure detection of the peak cortisol response (see following). In addition, because cats tend to respond to ACTH with a lesser rise in peak serum cortisol concentrations than that seen in dogs, it is imperative to compare test results to reference values obtained in normal cats.

Two regimens for ACTH stimulation testing have been described (Peterson et al., 1984). One method is to collect blood for determination of serum (or plasma) cortisol concentration before and at 60 and 120 min after intramuscular administration of ACTH gel (2.2 U/kg). With this regimen, the maximal rise in cortisol concentrations occurs at 2 hr after ACTH gel administration in about 60 per cent of normal cats, whereas the remaining cats have peak values at 1 hr postinjection. Alternatively, the ACTH stimulation test may be performed by injecting synthetic ACTH (cosyntropin) and measuring serum cortisol before and at 30 and 60 min after intravenous or intramuscular administration (0.125 mg). As with the ACTH gel test, the time at which the peak cortisol response occurs is also variable with the cosyntropin test.

A subnormal serum cortisol response to ACTH administration accompanied by serum electrolyte findings of hyperkalemia and hyponatremia is consistent with primary hypoadrenocorticism. If there are no serum electrolyte changes, one of the following may be present: (1) early primary hypoadrenocorticism with at least some residual mineralocorticoid secretion; (2) secondary hypoadrenocorticism resulting from pituitary or hypothalamic disease; or, most commonly, (3) secondary hypoadrenocorticism resulting from the administration of drugs such as glucocorticoids or megestrol acetate. If steroid or progestogen usage cannot be documented, a plasma ACTH concentration should be determined. Plasma ACTH concentrations in cats with primary hypoadrenocorticism are extremely elevated, whereas plasma ACTH concentrations in cats with secondary hypoadrenocorticism are inappropriately decreased (in low to low-normal range) when compared with subnormal circulating cortisol concentrations.

TREATMENT OF ADRENAL INSUFFICIENCY

In cats with acute adrenal failure, initial therapy should be aimed at restoring the circulating blood volume, correcting severe acid-base imbalances, providing an immediate source of glucocorticoid, correcting serum electrolyte disturbances (i.e., hyperkalemia, hyponatremia), and treating hyperkalemic myocardial toxicity, if present.

The intravenous fluid of choice is 0.9 per cent

saline, which should be initially administered at rate of 40 ml/kg/hr through an indwelling intravenous catheter. The jugular vein is the preferred site of fluid administration in cats because of the large volumes of fluid that may be needed. The estimated dehydration deficit, based on skin turgor, packed cell volume, and total serum protein concentration, should be administered over a 2- to 6-hr period. As soon as fluid deficits have been restored, the rate of fluid administration should be decreased to 60 ml/kg/day, given as a continuous intravenous infusion or in boluses of fluid delivered two to three times daily. Fluid therapy may be curtailed as soon as the cat is eating and drinking on its own and when azotemia and serum electrolyte abnormalities have been corrected.

Rapid administration of a glucocorticoid is extremely important in the initial management of severe adrenocortical insufficiency in order to restore tissue perfusion and alleviate clinical signs such as depression, anorexia, vomiting, and diarrhea. Dexamethasone administered intravenously at a dosage of 0.5 to 1.0 mg/kg is adequate initial glucocorticoid replacement and will not interfere with ACTH stimulation testing. Glucocorticoid replacement should then be continued as prednisone (or prednisolone) at a dosage of 0.2 mg/kg/day either parenterally or orally (when possible).

In those cats with serum electrolyte imbalances associated with primary adrenocortical insufficiency, mineralocorticoid replacement therapy should be provided using desoxycorticosterone acetate in oil (DOCA; Percorten Acetate [Ciba]), administered intramuscularly at the initial dosage of 0.5 to 1.0 mg once daily. The mineralocorticoid effects of this drug enhance renal potassium excretion and sodium resorption. The DOCA dosage is adjusted on the basis of daily serum electrolyte determinations and is continued until oral fludrocortisone acetate (Florinef Acetate, Squibb) or injectable reposital desoxycorticosterone pivalate (DOCP; Percorten Pivalate [Ciba]) can be initiated. As opposed to dogs, in which the major clinical signs of primary hypoadrenocorticism usually resolve within a day or two of treatment, cats with adrenocortical insufficiency may have signs of weakness, lethargy, and anorexia that persist for 3 to 5 days despite proper management.

If severe and life-threatening, metabolic acidosis should be treated with sodium bicarbonate, which may be added to the intravenous fluids. The dosage of sodium bicarbonate should be based on laboratory blood gas analysis. If blood gas analysis is not available, the base deficit may be approximated by subtracting the cat's venous CO_2 from normal venous CO_2 (22 mEq/L) concentration. The total dosage of bicarbonate in milliequivalents can be calculated by using the following formula: Deficit (mEq) = 0.3 × body weight (kg) × base deficit. One-quarter of the calculated bicarbonate dosage should be administered with the intravenous fluids during the first 6 hr of therapy, after which time the cat's acid-base status should be re-evaluated. Appropriate fluid, glucocorticoid, and mineralocorticoid therapy should generally correct any remaining acid-base imbalances.

Once the animal is stabilized, maintenance therapy for the cat with primary adrenocortical insufficiency consists of lifelong mineralocorticoid and glucocorticoid supplementation. Either oral fludrocortisone acetate (0.1 mg/day) or intramuscular injections of reposital desoxycorticosterone pivalate (12.5 mg/month) can be given for chronic mineralocorticoid therapy. The dosage of mineralocorticoid supplementation is adjusted (as needed) based on serial serum electrolyte concentrations, determined every 1 to 2 weeks during the initial maintenance period. Glucocorticoid supplementation can be provided as oral prednisone or prednisolone (1.25 mg/day) or intramuscular methylprednisolone acetate (Depo-Medrol, Upjohn) (10 mg/month). Overall, the long-term prognosis for feline primary hypoadrenocorticism (Addison's disease) is excellent. With appropriate glucocorticoid and mineralocorticoid supplementation, cats suffering from adrenocortical insufficiency may have a normal life expectancy. The owner should be made aware of the clinical signs of relapse and advised that continuous glucocorticoid and mineralocorticoid therapy will be necessary for the rest of the cat's life.

References and Supplemental Reading

Chastain, C. B., Graham, C. L., and Nichols, C. E.: Adrenocortical suppression in cats given megestrol acetate. Am. J. Vet. Res. 42:2029, 1981.

Johnessee, J. S., Peterson, M. E., and Gilbertson, S. R.: Primary hypoadrenocorticism in a cat. J.A.V.M.A. 183:881, 1983.

Peterson, M. E., Kintzer, P. P., Foodman, M. S., et al.: Adrenal function in the cat: Comparison of the effects of cosyntropin (synthetic ACTH) and corticotropin gel stimulation. Res. Vet. Sci. 37:331, 1984.

Peterson, M. E., and Greco, D. S.: Primary hypoadrenocorticism in the cat. Proceedings of the Fourth Annual Veterinary Medical Forum (American College of Veterinary Internal Medicine), sec. 14, 1986, p. 42.

Peterson, M. E.: Effects of megestrol acetate on glucose tolerance and growth hormone secretion in the cat. Res. Vet. Sci. 42:354, 1987.

Zemer, R. L.: An experimental study of the adrenal cortex. I. The survival value of the adrenal cortex. Am. J. Physiol. 79:641, 1927.

HYPERLIPIDEMIA

P. JANE ARMSTRONG, D.V.M.,
and RICHARD B. FORD, D.V.M.

Raleigh, North Carolina

Over the past two decades there has been an explosive increase in knowledge about serum lipids, their transport, and their physiologic determinants. In humans there is an undisputed risk of coronary heart disease associated with increased serum cholesterol concentrations, particularly low-density lipoprotein cholesterol. Emphasis on the importance of serum triglyceride and cholesterol determination in human medicine has made these parameters commonly included components of canine and feline serum biochemical profiles. Total serum cholesterol and triglyceride concentrations can be useful indicators of metabolic abnormalities involving organs such as the thyroid, kidney, pancreas, and liver. Lipid profiling (quantitative analysis of the various lipoprotein subfractions) offers clinicians the opportunity to further scrutinize hyperlipidemic patients.

Although increases in blood lipid levels are certainly recognized in dogs and cats, there is a paucity of literature to aid the practitioner in interpreting results. In this emerging area of clinical investigation, additional studies will undoubtedly expand our knowledge about the significance of hyperlipidemic states in companion animals. At the present time, at least four facts are clear: (1) Hyperlipidemia in the fasted (> 12 hr) dog or cat is abnormal; (2) there appears to be significant morbidity, and occasional mortality, associated with hypertriglyceridemia in dogs and cats; (3) specific dietary or drug intervention can diminish or eliminate the morbidity associated with hypertriglyceridemia; and (4) there is little evidence linking hypercholesterolemia with clinical disease in dogs or cats.

TERMINOLOGY

Hyperlipidemia is a broad descriptive term that implies a concentration of any lipid in the blood of a fasted patient that exceeds the upper range of normal for that species. Hyperlipidemia includes both hypercholesterolemia and hypertriglyceridemia. Serum or plasma separated from blood that contains an excess concentration of triglyceride will appear turbid and is said to be *lipemic*. *Lactescence* is the opaque, milklike appearance of serum or plasma that contains even higher concentrations of triglyceride. The most common cause of lipemic serum in dogs and cats is postprandial hyperlipidemia. Lactescence is characteristically seen in animals with extreme elevations in triglyceride, well beyond the levels caused by a recent meal.

Hyperlipoproteinemia is the type of hyperlipidemia that results from accelerated synthesis or retarded degradation of lipoproteins. Hyperlipoproteinemia is synonymous with fasting hyperlipidemia. Disturbances of lipoprotein metabolism occur as a result of some underlying metabolic disease (i.e., *secondary*, or acquired, hyperlipoproteinemia). Some of the conditions known to cause secondary hyperlipoproteinemia in dogs and cats are discussed below. In *primary*, or familial, hyperlipoproteinemia, hyperlipidemia occurs in the absence of underlying disease and a heritable basis for the disorder can be documented. Although primary and secondary forms of hyperlipoproteinemia are poorly described in the veterinary literature, it appears that both exist in the dog and cat.

LIPOPROTEINS

Since lipids are insoluble in water, the blood lipids must be transported in association with plasma proteins. Lipoproteins, the complex macromolecules that perform this function, are spherical particles composed of an inner core of nonpolar lipids (triglyceride and cholesteryl esters) and a surface coat of phospholipids, free cholesterol, and apoproteins. Apoproteins bind to specific enzymes or transport proteins on cell membranes, thereby directing the lipoprotein to its sites of metabolism.

Four major lipoprotein classes can be identified in the blood of most species, including dogs and cats. The current designations for these classes are chylomicrons, very low-density lipoproteins (VLDLs), low-density lipoproteins (LDLs), and high-density lipoproteins (HDLs). All four classes contain both triglyceride and cholesterol, but in varying amounts. The higher the proportion of triglyceride, the less dense the lipoprotein particle. Chylomicrons, the largest and lightest of the lipoprotein classes, are synthesized within the intestinal mucosa. They are the primary transport system for dietary fat and should not be present in the serum of a fasted patient. VLDLs are also triglyceride-rich, but they are synthesized within the liver from endogenous triglyceride. LDLs are degradation products of VLDLs and are composed primarily of cholesterol. HDLs are the major cholesterol carriers in canine and feline blood and quantitatively are the major lipoprotein class in the fasting state in dogs and cats. HDLs contain an insignificant amount of triglyceride. The reader is referred to the reviews by Zerbe and DeBowes for more comprehensive discussions on lipoprotein metabolism and lipid transport.

DIAGNOSIS OF HYPERLIPIDEMIA

Hyperlipidemic patients may be recognized by the presence of fasting lipemia or by laboratory diagnosis of hypertriglyceridemia or hypercholesterolemia or both.

Visual Inspection

It should be emphasized that visible lipemia does not define hyperlipoproteinemia, since not all blood lipid increases are evident from gross examination of the sample. Only the larger lipoprotein particles, chylomicrons and VLDLs, are of sufficient size to scatter transmitted light when they are present in the serum in excessive amounts. Increased concentrations of triglyceride will cause lipemia, but hypercholesterolemia will not. Visual inspection of a turbid serum or plasma sample can provide some information about its lipid content. Lipemia is generally evident when the triglyceride concentration exceeds 200 mg/dl. An abundance of triglyceride, usually in excess of 1000 mg/dl, is required to impart lactescence to a sample. If a sample is allowed to stand under refrigeration for 8 to 12 hr, chylomicrons will float to the surface to form an opaque "cream layer" (positive chylomicron test). The persistence of chylomicrons in the blood after a 12-hr fast indicates that the patient has abnormal triglyceride metabolism. If a lipemic sample has a negative chylomicron test or if the sample remaining below the cream layer is still turbid, VLDLs are likely to be increased.

Laboratory Tests

Until procedures for separation of the various lipoprotein classes become standardized and commercial laboratories are able to provide comprehensive lipoprotein profiles for animals, diagnosis of hyperlipidemia should be based on laboratory determination of serum triglyceride and total cholesterol. In humans, lipoprotein concentrations are known to be influenced by genetic and environmental factors, including diet. Although not proven,

it is likely that similar factors are operational in dogs and cats. Reference ranges for serum triglyceride and total cholesterol are given by most laboratories. It must be assumed that these values apply only to adult dogs and cats in the fasted state; lipid values in patients less than 6 months of age have not been reported. Cats appear to have lower total cholesterol and lower fasting serum triglyceride concentrations than those in dogs. Although standardized values for these analytes have not been strictly defined in veterinary medicine, an adult dog can be considered to be hyperlipoproteinemic when the serum triglyceride concentration exceeds 150 mg/dl or the total cholesterol concentration exceeds 300 mg/dl. A cat may be considered to be hyperlipoproteinemic if the triglyceride and cholesterol concentrations exceed 100 mg/dl and 200 mg/dl, respectively.

Some reference laboratories that provide services to both physicians and veterinarians include HDL or estimated LDL cholesterol levels (mg/dl) as part of a standard biochemical profile on dogs and cats. In human medicine, these values are important in risk assessment for coronary heart disease; the clinical value of these test results in veterinary medicine has not yet been determined.

Some reference laboratories offer lipoprotein electrophoresis (LPE) as a means of further characterizing abnormalities of lipid metabolism in animals. The value of LPE has been in question in human medicine for several years and is justifiably questioned in veterinary medicine. Compared with the quantitative assays currently available, LPE appears to have limited value in the routine evaluation of lipid disorders in dogs and cats. The reviews by Ford and Zerbe will provide the reader with more information on LPE.

The distribution of the lipoprotein classes in serum can be measured by differential ultracentrifugation, which separates the classes by density characteristics. Each fraction (VLDL, LDL, and HDL) can then be analyzed as to cholesterol and triglyceride content. This technology is not routinely available to the practitioner and has only recently been applied to spontaneous lipid disorders in dogs and cats. It is anticipated that subclassification of hyperlipoproteinemic patients by lipoprotein phenotype will facilitate diagnosis and treatment.

Laboratory Considerations

Veterinarians attempting to assess a dog or cat for hyperlipidemia should submit serum, rather than plasma or whole blood. The laboratory should *not* clear lipemic serum prior to performing assays for triglyceride and cholesterol; doing so can reduce triglyceride levels significantly and, to a lesser extent, lower cholesterol levels. Serum on which LPE or differential ultracentrifugation is to be performed should not be stored for longer than 3 to 5 days and must not be frozen, as freezing damages the lipoprotein structure.

The presence of excess triglyceride, particularly chylomicrons, is an important source of either positive (falsely increased) or negative (falsely decreased) interference for analytes determined by colorimetric methods. Lipemia also causes *in vitro* hemolysis, a phenomenon induced by the effect of lipid on erythrocyte membrane fragility. Hemolysis also may interfere with certain biochemical tests. The type and extent of interference by lipemia and hemolysis vary considerably from one laboratory to another, depending on the analytic instrumentation and methodology used.

Some laboratories routinely attempt to clear lipemic serum prior to performing any assays, but others do not. When interpreting test results reported on biochemical profiles, the clinician must know whether the serum sample was lipemic and, if so, whether the sample was cleared prior to testing.

HYPERTRIGLYCERIDEMIA

The most prevalent, and perhaps the most clinically significant, form of hypertriglyceridemia recognized in companion animals is hyperchylomicronemia. Affected animals have lipemic blood that yields a positive chylomicron test. Serum triglyceride (TG) levels are invariably increased, since chylomicrons are the lipoprotein class principally responsible for triglyceride transport.

Most cases of mild to moderate hypertriglyceridemia encountered in practice can be attributed to hyperchylomicronemia subsequent to a recent (within 4 to 6 hr) meal—that is, postprandial or physiologic hyperlipidemia. Hypertriglyceridemia in the fasted (> 12 hr) dog or cat is an abnormal finding that justifies further clinical study. Not only does fasting hypertriglyceridemia indicate an underlying disorder affecting lipid metabolism, but affected animals are at risk of developing serious clinical disease, particularly acute pancreatitis. Abdominal distention and distress, abdominal pain, diarrhea, xanthoma formation, lipemia retinalis, uveitis, seizures, peripheral neuropathies, and behavioral changes have also been observed in hypertriglyceridemic patients. The correlation between clinical signs and serum lipids is based on the fact that clinical signs resolve as TG levels reach normal and recur as TG levels become excessive.

Miniature Schnauzer Hyperlipidemia

Several reports have been published suggesting that the miniature schnauzer breed is predisposed to primary, or familial, hyperlipidemia. Although it is not definitively known that hyperlipidemia is an inherited disorder of miniature schnauzers, there appears to be a higher than expected incidence of hypertriglyceridemia in the breed.

Although there is no sex predisposition, the majority of affected dogs are middle-aged and older. The incidental discovery of opaque serum in a healthy schnauzer is common. When clinical signs occur, they characteristically include abdominal distress, pain, and diarrhea *not* associated with elevated amylase or lipase or with acute pancreatitis. Lipid profiles of affected dogs reveal dramatic elevations of serum TG ranging from 500 mg/dl to over 8000 mg/dl, composed predominantly of chylomicrons. Our studies have not shown any correlation between triglyceride concentration and the severity of clinical signs. Nonetheless, dogs with triglyceride levels of 500 mg/dl or higher are considered to be at risk and, as such, are candidates for dietary intervention (see treatment, discussed later).

It should also be noted that the occurrence of primary hyperlipidemia in dogs is by no means limited to the miniature schnauzer breed. Several other purebred dogs as well as mixed breeds have been identified as having fasting hyperchylomicronemia without detectable underlying disorders.

Hyperchylomicronemia in Cats

Familial hyperchylomicronemia has been described in domestic cats in New Zealand (Jones et al., 1986). Clinical signs in 20 related cats included peripheral neuropathies, cutaneous xanthomata, and the formation of lipid granulomas in abdominal organs. Most affected kittens, however, failed to show signs other than the presence of fasting hyperlipidemia and lipemia retinalis. Kittens that showed clinical signs in addition to hyperlipidemia generally did not do so until 8 to 9 months of age. Lipoprotein fractionation revealed a marked increase in chylomicrons and a smaller increase in VLDL. The defect was attributed to deficient lipoprotein lipase activity. An autosomal recessive mode of inheritance of this trait is suspected.

Similar lipoprotein abnormalities have been recognized in two 3-week-old male Himalayan kittens and in two unrelated young adult cats in North America. Lipemia retinalis, lipemic aqueous, uveitis, and cutaneous xanthoma formation were the clinical abnormalities in the two adult cats.

Diabetes Mellitus

Hyperlipidemia secondary to diabetes mellitus in dogs and cats is usually characterized by marked hypertriglyceridemia with less severe hypercholesterolemia. In insulin-deficient states, the clearance of chylomicrons is impaired because of insufficient activation by insulin of lipoprotein lipase situated in vascular endothelial cells. Examination of lipid profiles of affected dogs reveals that there is an increase in both chylomicrons and VLDL. Lipemia retinalis and cutaneous xanthomatosis may be observed in diabetic dogs and cats with severe hypertriglyceridemia. The hyperlipidemia associated with diabetes mellitus usually improves or resolves as glycemic control is achieved.

HYPERCHOLESTEROLEMIA

Hypercholesterolemia of Unknown Etiology

In veterinary medicine, hypercholesterolemia is most commonly recognized as a secondary hyperlipidemia associated with an underlying disorder. A limited survey of dogs, however, suggests that Doberman pinschers and rottweilers may have a higher than expected incidence of hypercholesterolemia, characterized by increased LDL cholesterol. It is not known whether hypercholesterolemia in these dogs is associated with clinical illness. At this time, treatment specifically intended to lower serum cholesterol does not appear to be indicated.

Hypothyroidism

In human medicine, it is well recognized that alterations in thyroid status result in changes in serum concentrations of cholesterol and triglyceride. Hypercholesterolemia is associated with hypothyroidism, partly because of decreased catabolism of LDL. The relationship of triglyceride concentration to thyroid status is more variable, but triglyceride level is usually elevated in association with myxedema. Hypercholesterolemia is present in about two-thirds of hypothyroid dogs, leading to the suggestion that cholesterol be included in initial screening for hypothyroidism (Larsson, 1988). Canine hypothyroid patients may also have increased triglyceride concentrations, particularly if hyperlipidemia is marked. Atherosclerotic-type arterial lesions have occasionally been reported in hypothyroid dogs. Alterations in the lipoprotein profile of hypothyroid dogs have not been characterized. Therapy should be directed toward correcting the thyroid hormone deficiency. In human medicine, patients who have hypothyroidism often show a dramatic lowering of lipid levels once hormone replacement therapy is started.

Diabetes Mellitus

Patients with insulin-dependent diabetes mellitus (IDDM) are susceptible to several disorders of lipid metabolism as well as carbohydrate metabolism. Clinically, the most common finding is hypertriglyceridemia (see earlier), yet there appears to be a distinct subset of dogs with IDDM that have a normal triglyceride concentration but increased total cholesterol and LDL cholesterol. The value of distinguishing between hypertriglyceridemic and hypercholesterolemic diabetes mellitus is being studied at this time.

Nephrotic Syndrome

Hyperlipidemia may be detected in patients with proteinuria due to glomerulonephritis or amyloidosis. It is believed that diminished plasma oncotic pressure stimulates hepatic lipoprotein synthesis, although urinary loss of plasma protein factors regulating lipoprotein synthesis or catabolism may also play a role. Hypercholesterolemia occurs inconsistently in dogs with heavy proteinuria. There are a few isolated case reports of nephrotic syndrome in cats. Even though renal amyloidosis in cats primarily affects the medulla, hypercholesterolemia has been reported in Abyssinian cats with this condition. In nephrotic syndrome in human patients, LDL cholesterol is elevated most frequently, but as hypoalbuminemia progresses, VLDL triglyceride also rises. The lipid profile in dogs and cats with nephrotic syndrome has not yet been characterized. The influence of hyperlipidemia on morbidity and mortality in nephrotic syndrome is not known.

COMBINED HYPERLIPOPROTEINEMIA

Disorders associated with combined hyperlipoproteinemia (i.e., hypertriglyceridemia and hypercholesterolemia) do occur in dogs and cats but have not been studied. Canine hyperadrenocorticism has been associated with elevated VLDL triglyceride and LDL cholesterol. Recognition of this lipoprotein phenotype may ultimately prove to be a valuable parameter in the diagnosis of Cushing's syndrome in dogs. Since total triglyceride values seldom exceed 500 mg/dl, triglyceride-induced lipid disorders are unlikely to occur in affected patients.

TREATMENT

In the management of hyperlipidemia of dogs and cats, it is at least as important to know *when* to treat as it is to know *how* to treat. Primary, or familial, hyperlipidemic states do appear to exist among dogs and cats, yet the majority of lipid disorders recognized in practice are secondary to an underlying disorder, most often an endocrine disease. The lipid disorder generally resolves if the underlying disorder is properly diagnosed and treated.

Hypertriglyceridemic patients, particularly those with fasting triglyceride concentrations greater than 500 mg/dl, should be treated. Therapeutic intervention is indicated to reduce the risks associated with elevated levels of triglycerides, particularly acute pancreatitis. A realistic goal of therapy is a triglyceride concentration consistently below 200 mg/dl.

The first line of treatment is reduction of dietary fat. Commercially available prescription diets (r/d and w/d, Hill's Pet Products) have proved to be consistently effective in reducing excessive serum triglycerides as long as fat supplementation is restricted by the owner. The beneficial effects of commercially available low-fat diets are probably also due, in part, to their high-fiber content. It is recognized in human medicine that dietary fiber can interfere with fat assimilation and improve insulin receptor performance.

Feeding fat-restricted diets can result in undesirable weight loss over time, particularly if the diet fed is formulated to reduce body weight (e.g., Prescription Diet r/d, Hill's Pet Products) rather than to maintain optimal weight. Caloric supplementation may eventually be indicated and can be accomplished through trial-and-error addition of a maintenance-type diet. Specific recommendations regarding the amount of dietary fat, as a percentage of total calories, for hypertriglyceridemic patients are not available.

Fish oils are an important source of linolenic acid, an omega-3 polyunsaturated fat, and have recently been recognized for their ability to reduce serum lipids, particularly triglycerides, in human patients. In veterinary medicine, neither the short- nor long-term effects of administering fish oils, which are available in capsule form at health food stores, are known.

Clofibrate, gemfibrozil, and niacin are known to reduce triglyceride levels in human patients. None of these drugs is without some side effects. Indiscriminate use of these products in either dogs or cats cannot be recommended until such time that dosage and therapeutic efficacy can be established.

References and Supplemental Reading

DeBowes, L. J.: Lipid metabolism and hyperlipoproteinemia in dogs. Comp. Cont. Ed. Pract. Vet. 9:727, 1987.

Ford, R. B.: Clinical Application of Serum Lipid Profiles in the Dog. College Station, TX: Gaines Veterinary Symposium, 1977, pp. 12–16.

Jones, B. R., Johnstone, A. C., and Hancock, W. S.: Inherited hyperchylomicronemia in the cat. Vet. Ann. 26:330, 1986.

Larsson, M. G.: Determination of free thyroxine and cholesterol as a new screening test for canine hypothyroidism. J. Am. Anim. Hosp. Assoc. 24:209, 1988.

Mahley, R. W., and Weisgraber, K. H.: Canine lipoproteins and atherosclerosis. Circ. Res. 35:713, 1974.

Rogers, W. A.: Lipemia in the dog. Vet. Clin. North Am. 7:637, 1977.

Rogers, W. A., Donovan, E. F., and Kociba, G. J.: Idiopathic hyperlipoproteinemia in dogs. J.A.V.M.A. 166:1087, 1975.

Rogers, W. A., Donovan, E. F., and Kociba, G. J.: Lipids and lipoproteins in normal dogs and in dogs with secondary hyperlipoproteinemia. J.A.V.M.A. 166:1092, 1975.

Schaefer, E. J.: When and how to treat the dyslipidemias. Hosp. Pract. 23:69, 1988.

Zerbe, C. A.: Canine hyperlipidemias. In Kirk, R. W. (ed.): Current Veterinary Therapy IX. Philadelphia: W. B. Saunders Co., 1986, pp. 1045–1053.

Section
11

INFECTIOUS
DISEASES

CRAIG E. GREENE, D.V.M.
Consulting Editor

Panel on Feline Leukemia Virus Vaccination 1052
Alternative Testing Procedures for FeLV 1065
Management of the FeLV-Positive Patient...............................1069
Clinical Significance of Antigenic Variation in Canine Parvovirus........1076
Bacteremia in Dogs and Cats..1077
Anaerobic Infections in Dogs and Cats.................................1082
Canine Lyme Borreliosis...1086
Plague 1088
Group G Streptococcal Infections in Kittens...........................1091
Group A Streptococcal Infections in Dogs and Cats 1094
Clinical and Public Health Significance of Antimicrobial-resistant
    Enteric Bacterial Infections 1096
Cat-scratch Fever 1099
Systemic Antifungal Chemotherapy 1101
Nasal Aspergillosis...1106
Feline Cryptococcosis...1109
Feline Toxoplasmosis...1112

PANEL ON FELINE LEUKEMIA VIRUS VACCINATION

Introduction

CRAIG E. GREENE, D.V.M.

Athens, Georgia

Vaccination for feline leukemia virus (FeLV) infection is one of the more important subjects that veterinarians evaluate in practice today. The development of a vaccine (Leukocell, Norden) against retroviral infection is a major achievement. Never before has there been a vaccine available for a disease with such a protracted incubation period. Nor has it been possible to test for an infectious disease prior to vaccination. Furthermore, no vaccine is 100 per cent protective. It is possible that some FeLV-vaccinated cats may still become infected—something clients need to understand. Therefore, the use of feline leukemia vaccine involves a more conscious effort by practitioners to explain the FeLV situation to their clients before administering the vaccine. The veterinarian must also consider whether or not animals to be vaccinated should always be tested.

Because of the uncertainties that practitioners see as being associated with use of the FeLV vaccine, the editors have sought the opinions of three authorities on the subject. These experts were asked to provide answers, when possible, to some of the following questions: Should all cats be tested prior to vaccination? Should FeLV-positive cats be vaccinated? Can FeLV-vaccinated cats be placed in contact with FeLV-positive cats? Can FeLV vaccination be used as part of a testing-and-elimination program? Does FeLV vaccine prevent transient or persistent viremia following exposure to virulent virus? Does FeLV vaccine prevent latent infections? Does the vaccine generate FOCMA antibodies and protection against neoplasia? Are three vaccinations essential for initial immunity? If the initial vaccination series is stopped prior to completion and the animal is presented later, should the regimen be started over? Are there complications associated with vaccination? Are antibody titers helpful in determining the response to vaccination? Should cats be revaccinated yearly?

The answers to these and other questions are provided in the three separate articles that follow. Each article is the viewpoint of its author and is supported by his interpretation of the available scientific research on the subject. Many of their opinions correspond; however, the lack of uniform agreement is the clue that more definitive research on some aspects of feline leukemia vaccination needs to be performed.

Discussion 1

ALFRED M. LEGENDRE, D.V.M.

Knoxville, Tennessee

Since the introduction of the first vaccine against feline leukemia virus (Leukocell, Norden) in early 1985, many questions have arisen about the efficacy and safety of the vaccine. In the first 2 years of clinical use, modifications have been made in the vaccine that have largely eliminated the adverse effects of pain at the injection site, malaise, depression, and vomiting. There is no evidence that the vaccine suppresses the immune system. The main issue to be resolved is the efficacy of the vaccine in the field. The cost of vaccination must be considered in relation to the degree of protection in specific risk situations.

EFFICACY OF THE VACCINE

Before considering specific risk situations, the efficacy of the feline leukemia virus (FeLV) vaccine needs to be considered.

A major question about FeLV vaccination is the extent of protection. Does vaccination protect absolutely? Does it prevent latent infection as well as transient infection following exposure? Does it protect against viremia as well as against the development of neoplasia induced by FeLV? Studies are in progress to answer these questions.

The prototype of the Leukocell vaccine, when given weekly for 5 weeks, protected 81 per cent of cats from oronasal challenge with virulent virus (Lewis et al., 1981). In studies done at Norden Laboratories (Sharpee and Olsen, 1986), Leukocell vaccination greatly reduced the likelihood of persistent viremia and the development of neoplasia. Only 20 per cent of vaccinated cats were persistently viremic compared with 70 per cent of control subjects. Only 8 per cent of vaccinates developed neoplasia compared with 60 per cent of control subjects. The oronasal challenge system used was a severe but unrealistic one. Immunosuppressive doses of corticosteroids were used to increase the percentage of viremic cats over that achieved by oronasal inoculation of virus alone. The resistance to infection should theoretically be better in cats that are not immunosuppressed.

The extent of protection of vaccinated pet cats to street virus is still undetermined. Some field studies have been done (Henley et al., 1986), but these were not well-controlled studies. With a low incidence of persistent viremia (1 to 2 per cent) in random source cats, it would take an excessively large number of cats in a vaccination study to determine the efficacy of vaccination. Evaluation of the vaccine can be done best by the introduction of susceptible kittens into a multiple-cat household infected with FeLV. To mimic a household with multiple cats, the author housed adult asymptomatic viremic cats with vaccinated and control kittens in a large room. This natural model for evaluation of protection was used to evaluate the Leukocell vaccine available in 1987, which was licensed for three-dose subcutaneous administration. The author gave the kittens only <u>two</u> doses of the vaccine in this study because many clients often do not return kittens for the third dose of vaccine. The author found that when only two doses of the vaccine were administered, the vaccine did <u>not</u> protect kittens living with viremic cats. Another study by Pedersen and colleagues (1985) using an oronasal challenge and immunosuppression did not show protection with two doses of vaccine. Because two doses of the vaccine is more practical, Norden Laboratories is currently attempting to license a modified two-dose vaccine. The lack of protection from two doses of a three-dose vaccine is not too surprising because most of the antibody response noted in a study of antibody responses in pet cats occurred after the third dose of the vaccine. The protection afforded by three doses of the vaccine was not evaluated in the author's study.

There are no data available in client-owned ani-

mals to indicate the protective value of the FeLV vaccine when it is administered according to manufacturer's recommendations. In discussions with veterinarians, a few practitioners have identified cats that were leukemia virus–negative at the time of vaccination that subsequently developed viremia and FeLV-associated disease. The possibility of early infection or activation of latent infection cannot be excluded in these anecdotal observations.

ANTIBODY RESPONSES TO GP70

The only acceptable way to evaluate FeLV vaccine responses in client-owned cats is to evaluate serum antibody responses to vaccination, since challenge by virulent virus is obviously not acceptable. Antibodies play a major role in protecting cats against FeLV viremia. In the author's studies of client-owned cats vaccinated with Leukocell, a total of 84 cats completed the vaccine trial. Production of antibodies to the major antigens believed necessary for protection against viremia (GP70) and neoplasia (feline oncornavirus cell membrane antigen) was measured.

The major virus envelope glycoprotein GP70 is felt to be important in the attachment and infection of cells by FeLV virus. Administration of hyperimmune serum to cats experimentally infected with FeLV prevented the development of viremia (Haley et al., 1985). Neutralizing antibodies are directed against GP70, but, as has been shown using monoclonal antibodies to GP70, not all anti-GP70 antibodies are virus neutralizing (Grant et al., 1983). This makes direct correlation of anti-GP70 antibodies to protection tenuous, but antibody response to vaccination is still a valuable tool in evaluating immune response. Because of technical difficulties in measuring serum neutralizing antibody concentrations, most antibody determinations are done against purified GP70 in an ELISA system. After three doses of Leukocell vaccine, there was a significant increase in antibodies to GP70 in pet cats that were seronegative before vaccination. About 55 per cent of the cats had what the author considers adequate levels of antibodies to GP70. Therefore, slightly over half the pet cats might be protected against FeLV viremia (Stallman and Legendre, 1986). This level of seroconversion to GP70 is similar to a study by Pedersen and associates (1985).

ANTIBODY RESPONSES TO FOCMA

The protective value of feline oncornavirus cell membrane antigen (FOCMA) antibody is clearly established. Antibodies against FOCMA have been shown to prevent tumor development in kittens infected with feline sarcoma virus (Essex et al.,

1971). Cats with high FOCMA antibody concentrations did not develop lymphosarcoma induced by FeLV (Essex et al., 1975). In client-owned cats, the rise in mean antibody titers after three doses of vaccine was significant. Nearly 50 per cent of cats receiving three doses of vaccine developed what we consider protective titers (1:16 or greater) of FOCMA antibodies. FOCMA antibodies do not confer protection against viremia or FeLV-associated non-neoplastic disease but are protective against FeLV-induced malignancies.

ANTIBODY RESPONSES TO BOTH GP70 AND FOCMA

When the antibody responses in apparently naive cats (seronegative before vaccination) of all ages were evaluated, 37 per cent developed what the author considers adequate titers to both GP70 and FOCMA (Stallman and Legendre, 1986). In our studies of client-owned cats vaccinated with Leukocell, 17 per cent of the cats had pre-existing antibodies to GP70 or FOCMA. In this group with serologic evidence of exposure prior to vaccination, 50 per cent of the cats had what the author regards as adequate levels of antibodies to both GP70 and FOCMA before vaccination. However, after vaccination, 93 per cent of the cats with some pre-existing antibodies had developed adequate antibody concentrations to both antigens. In summary, the vaccine is capable of bolstering antibody concentrations in aviremic cats and in a greater percentage of those with previous exposure. If all cats (seropositive and seronegative before vaccination) are included, 46 per cent of the cats in the study had what the author considers adequate antibody concentrations to both antigens after vaccination. The protection, as inferred from the serologic data, is certainly not absolute or comparable to other feline vaccines (e.g., panleukopenia, rabies). There may well be other mechanisms of immune protection that were not identified in these studies.

ANTIBODY RESPONSES TO YEARLY REVACCINATION

Fifty-six of the original 84 cats were available for rechecking and revaccination 1 year after the third dose of vaccine (Legendre, Stallman, and Potgieter, unpublished studies). No vaccinated cat was viremic upon testing, but the low number of cats precludes making a statement that the vaccine had protected against persistent viremia. There was a decrease in GP70 and FOCMA antibody concentrations at 1 year postvaccination. Revaccination produced a higher titer than that measured after the initial vaccination series. There was a significant rise in

FOCMA antibody titers after the yearly booster; however, GP70 titers were not significantly increased by revaccination. These data suggest that the responses to the FOCMA component are more consistent than the antibody responses to GP70. After the yearly booster, approximately half the cats had what the author regards as adequate levels of antibodies to both GP70 and FOCMA. Yearly revaccination increases antibody concentrations.

FeLV TESTING BEFORE VACCINATION

In the ideal situation, testing of all cats for FeLV infection would be done prior to vaccination, even though this increases the cost of vaccinating a cat against FeLV. Testing eliminates vaccination in cats shown to be virus positive and alerts the client and veterinarian to the possible development of FeLV-related diseases. Knowing the prevaccination viral status of cats prevents the veterinarian being blamed for vaccine failure. A positive enzyme-linked immunosorbent assay (ELISA) should be confirmed with an indirect fluorescent antibody (IFA) test. The confirmatory IFA test minimizes the likelihood of a false-positive reaction. Do all cats need to be tested? Young kittens are unlikely to be infected with FeLV unless they are born of virus-infected queens. Cats in isolated environments that have been previously tested are also at low risk; however, when there is a doubt about exposure, testing should be done.

VACCINATION OF VIREMIC CATS

Cats identified as viremic pose a difficult problem for the veterinarian. Owners often insist that the veterinarian initiate some sort of treatment. The question of vaccination of FeLV-positive cats is difficult because there are no reports on the benefits or risks of vaccination of viremic cats. Controlled double-blind survival studies are necessary to establish benefits of vaccination. Published data about the survival times of asymptomatic, FeLV-positive cats may not reflect the expected survival of a pampered pet cat. In one study (Hardy, 1981), 83 per cent of FeLV-infected healthy cats died within 3 years of diagnosis. Most studies such as this have been done in multiple-cat households where exposure to a myriad of feline diseases would probably have shortened the life of the immunosuppressed, viremic cat. Cats in a sheltered environment would be expected to live longer. In the absence of data, the author believes that it is unlikely that vaccination will benefit an asymptomatic viremic cat. FeLV is immunosuppressive, thereby reducing the likelihood of a strong immune response. The viremic cat, if immunoresponsive, should be able to eliminate the viremia without vaccination.

AGE CONSIDERATIONS

Because of cost considerations, the veterinarian must consider which cat would benefit most from vaccination and encourage those clients to vaccinate their cats. Excluding kittens that are infected perinatally, most kittens become exposed to FeLV when they begin going outside. Serologic evaluation of free-roaming cats for antibodies against FeLV showed that 6 per cent of cats younger than 5 months of age had antibodies, compared with 74 per cent of cats older than 3 years of age. Most cats had been exposed to FeLV by 1 year of age (Rogerson et al., 1975). Experimentally, young cats have been shown to be more susceptible to FeLV infection after exposure than are adult cats (Hoover et al., 1976; Grant et al., 1980). These risk factors make kittens a high-priority group for vaccination before exposure to FeLV. In the author's study of humoral responses of pet cats, 75 per cent of cats between 2 and 6 months of age developed antibodies to at least one major antigen of the Leukocell vaccine, compared with 50 per cent of cats older than 5 years of age. The magnitude of antibody response was also greatest in the 2- to 6-month-old cats (Stallman and Legendre, 1986). If solid immunity could be achieved prior to FeLV exposure, either or both transient and latent virus infection could be prevented.

While young cats are in a high-priority group, cats of all age groups should be vaccinated against FeLV unless they are in a completely isolated environment. Adult cats are more resistant to infection than young cats, requiring long, intense exposure to produce infection. In spite of these experimental data, many young adult and middle-aged cats are presented to veterinarians with FeLV-related diseases. The age at initial exposure is not known in these cases. Even though a middle-aged free-roaming aviremic cat would be expected to have had exposure to FeLV infection, it cannot be assumed that the cat has immunity from previous exposure. A neighborhood previously free of viremic cats may be changed by the introduction of an asymptomatic carrier. Therefore, cats that were thought to have had exposure may be immunologically naive. The vaccination of older cats is less likely to produce a strong immune response. However, the immunity of cats with borderline antibody levels will be bolstered, and some of the seronegative cats will produce substantial antibody responses.

HIGH-INTENSITY EXPOSURE SITUATIONS

Certain exposure situations create ambiguity for the veterinarian. When can a vaccinated FeLV-negative cat be safely introduced into a household containing virus-positive cats? It is probably never safe to introduce an aviremic cat into a high-exposure situation. With less than half of pet cats having concentrations of antibodies considered to be adequate to both FOCMA and GP70 after three doses of vaccine, the safety of a cat cannot be assured. Furthermore, the protective value of vaccine-induced antibodies is still unproven. The vaccine produces excellent antibody responses in some cats, but because of the variability in response to vaccination, clients should be advised not to put FeLV-negative cats with FeLV-positive cats. In situations in which the housing together of virus-positive and virus-negative cats is unavoidable, virus-negative cats should be vaccinated according to the manufacturer's recommendations. Cats with pre-existing antibodies against FeLV should respond with increased amounts of antibodies. Some seronegative pet cats from environments containing viremic cats were able to mount an immune response after vaccination (Stallman and Legendre, 1986). There may be benefit from vaccination of aviremic cats in intense-exposure situations.

In FeLV-free catteries, it is probably wise to vaccinate cats against FeLV, in conjunction with periodic testing and elimination of viremic cats. These animals have the potential for exposure at shows and in breeding situations. To ensure maximum protection, vaccination would be advised.

The vaccination of all cats entering a humane shelter is a questionable practice from the aspect of cost-benefit analysis. It would seem to be better to test all incoming animals to reduce the likelihood of FeLV exposure at the shelter. If the period of stay at the shelter is less than 3 months, there would probably be insufficient time to mount an adequate immune response to protect against exposure at the shelter. Vaccination at shelters may not be cost effective.

EVALUATION OF ANTIBODY CONCENTRATIONS

The testing of cats for virus-neutralizing antibodies is not generally available to the practitioner. Testing for anti-GP70 antibodies is available. However, there is not a standardized assay, and the results vary considerably from laboratory to laboratory. The protective value of anti-GP70 antibodies is still not established. The testing for anti-FOCMA antibodies is more available and consistent, but this assay does not measure protection against viremia. Because most cats with FeLV infection die of non-neoplastic infections, the expenditure to identify cats resistant to neoplasia is probably not justified. The FOCMA antibody concentration may also decrease over time, resulting in a loss of protection against FeLV induced neoplasia.

INTERRUPTED VACCINATION SERIES

The vaccination schedule that produces the highest titers is not known. It is still unclear what concentration of antibodies is necessary for protection. If it were known that a specific cat had not developed an adequate antibody response to vaccination, further vaccines could be given. If a cat has not received all three doses of the vaccine, it is probably not protected. A cat that did not receive the third dose of vaccine should probably restart the series. This may not be absolutely necessary, but no data exist about antibody response to the vaccine given by another schedule.

It has become apparent that the vaccine against FeLV does not produce the consistent antibody responses that are seen with other feline vaccines. This is a new vaccine that will undoubtedly continue to be improved. A two-dose modification of the vaccine is being evaluated. The current vaccine has been shown in an experimental situation by Norden Laboratories to reduce the incidence of persistent viremia and to reduce the likelihood of development of FeLV-induced neoplasia. The modifications of the vaccine have virtually eliminated the side effects noted with the early vaccine. Three doses of the vaccine (Leukocell, Norden) may protect some cats, especially young cats vaccinated before their first exposure to FeLV. Yearly revaccination substantially increases the antibody concentrations. Ongo-

ing studies will clarify the role of vaccination in the prevention of FeLV infection.

References and Supplementary Reading

Essex, M., Jakowski, R. M., Hardy, W. D., et al.: Feline oncornavirus-associated cell membrane antigen. III. Antibody titers in cats from leukemia cluster households. J. Natl. Cancer Inst. 54:637, 1975.

Essex, M., Klein, G., Snyder, S. P., et al.: Correlation between humoral antibody and regression of tumors induced by feline sarcoma virus. Nature 233:195, 1971.

Grant, C. K., Ernisse, B. J., Jarrett, O., et al.: Feline leukemia virus envelope GP 70 of subgroups B and C defined by monoclonal antibodies with cytotoxic and neutralizing function. J. Immunol. 131:3042, 1983.

Grant, C. K., Essex, M., Gardner, M. B., et al.: Natural feline leukemia virus infection and the immune response of cats of different ages. Cancer Res. 40:823, 1980.

Haley, P. J., Hoover, E. A., Quackenbush, S. L., et al.: Influence of antibody infusion on pathogenesis of experimental feline leukemia virus infection. J. Nat. Cancer Inst. 74:821, 1985.

Hardy, W. D.: The feline leukemia virus. J. Am. Anim. Hosp. Assoc. 17:951, 1981.

Henley, J. P., Stewart, D. C., and Dickerson, T. V.: Evaluating the efficacy of feline leukemia vaccination in two high-risk colonies. Vet. Med. 81:470, 1986.

Hoover, E. A., Olsen, R. G., Hardy, W. D., et al.: Feline leukemia virus infection. Age-related variation in response of cats to experimental infection. J. Nat. Cancer Inst. 57:365, 1976.

Lewis, M. G., Mathes, L. E., and Olsen, R. G.: Protection against feline leukemia by vaccination with a subunit vaccine. Infect. Immun. 34:888, 1981.

Pedersen, N. C., Johnson, L., and Ott, R. L.: Evaluation of a commercial feline leukemia virus vaccine for immunogenicity and efficacy. Feline Pract. 15:7, 1985.

Rogerson, P., Jarrett, W., and Mackey, L.: Epidemiological studies on feline leukaemia virus infection. Int. J. Cancer 15:781, 1975.

Sharpee, R. L., and Olsen, R. G.: Feline leukemia vaccine: Evaluation of safety and efficacy against persistent viremia and tumor development. Comp. Cont. Ed. 8:267, 1986.

Stallman, C. G., and Legendre, A. M.: Field trials of Leukocell, a commercial subunit feline leukemia vaccine. Proceedings of a Symposium on Feline Leukemia Virus and Vaccine, Eastern States meeting, 1986, pp. 20–29.

Discussion 2

RICHARD L. OTT, D.V.M.

Pullman, Washington

Feline leukemia virus (FeLV) infection is a potentially devastating condition in cats not only because of the diseases that may be caused by the virus (e.g., lymphosarcomas, myeloproliferative diseases, anemias) but also because of the disease states that may occur as a result of the immunosuppressive effects of FeLV infection. Intense research efforts have been devoted toward the development of an effective vaccine. The first such vaccine to be licensed in the United States was Leukocell, marketed by Norden Laboratories, Lincoln, Nebraska. Leukocell is based on a prototype vaccine developed by investigators at the Ohio State University (Lewis et al., 1981; Olsen, 1985). The prototype vaccine

contained, as does Leukocell, soluble, nonassembled, noninfectious FeLV proteins plus preservatives and adjuvant material.

INTERRUPTED VACCINATION SERIES

The Leukocell vaccine protocol recommends vaccination of healthy cats 9 weeks of age or older. Primary vaccination consists of two doses of vaccine administered intramuscularly or subcutaneously 2 to 3 weeks apart. The manufacturers have indicated that maximum serologic response occurs following two doses of vaccine but that a third dose given 2 to 4 months after the second dose will prolong, though not necessarily enhance, the protective effect of the vaccine. Annual revaccination with a single dose of vaccine is recommended (A User's Manual for "Leukocell" Feline Leukemia Vaccine, 1985).

If a cat receives two doses of vaccine (primary vaccination) and for some reason does not receive the third dose within the recommended 4-month period, it would seem, based on the manufacturer's observations, that it would be unnecessary to start the vaccination series anew. The third dose of vaccine would be administered when the cat is next presented, and subsequently a single-dose annual revaccination would be administered 1 year following the third dose. Conversely, if a cat receives only a single dose of vaccine and is not presented for the second dose within a 2-month period, it would seem appropriate to start the series anew when the cat is next presented.

PREVACCINATION ANTIGEN TESTING

It is strongly recommended that cats be tested for FeLV infection prior to vaccination. If an untested cat is vaccinated and is subsequently found to be FeLV-positive, it would be impossible to determine whether the cat was viremic prior to vaccination or whether the vaccine failed to prevent subsequent infection. In such cases, the owner might mistakenly assume that the vaccine produced the FeLV infection.

An enzyme-linked immunosorbent assay (ELISA), conducted as a prevaccination screening test, is a rapid, specific test for FeLV infection. Cats whose ELISA results are positive on first examination should be retested in 3 to 4 weeks. If the results are still strongly positive, the cats should not be vaccinated. Such a cat may have an indirect fluorescent antibody (IFA) performed. Positive results of an IFA test indicate bone marrow infection has occurred, and the vast majority of such cats will be persistently viremic.

Many veterinarians conduct FeLV ELISAs in their offices on a weekly to biweekly schedule. With both in-office testing and testing by a commercial laboratory, there is a time delay before the results are available. If the owner is informed of the significance of the test results, the cat presented for FeLV vaccination is in apparent good health on physical examination, and the cat is not from a high-risk area, a prevaccination sample may be collected and the first dose of vaccine administered at that visit. Subsequently, if the result of the ELISA is negative, vaccination proceeds on the regular schedule. If, on the other hand, the ELISA result is positive, the second dose of vaccine is withheld and the ELISA-positive cat is retested 3 to 4 weeks after

the first sample was drawn. If the result of the second ELISA is negative, the cat was presumably transiently infected, has developed natural resistance, and further vaccination may be unnecessary. However, it may be considered desirable to complete the vaccination series. If the result of the second ELISA is strongly positive, further vaccination is unwarranted.

It must be borne in mind that a negative ELISA does not rule out the possibility that either a cat has been very recently exposed to FeLV or the cat is latently infected with FeLV.

Some authorities have questioned the value of prevaccination testing in low-risk situations (e.g., single cats in a household, cats in FeLV-tested and FeLV-negative catteries) on the basis that only 1 to 9 per cent of this population will be FeLV-positive and that prevaccination testing will not prevent vaccination of latently infected cats (Macy, 1988). Prevaccination testing of cats in the low-risk category could be considered to be non–cost-effective. However, if prevaccination testing is not performed, one must then assume that any cat that, subsequent to vaccination, shows signs of FeLV infection and is FeLV test positive was obviously infected prior to vaccination. The additional assumption here is that the vaccine is 100 per cent effective in preventing FeLV infection. Neither assumption is borne out by facts.

POSTVACCINATION ANTIBODY TESTING

Tests that measure serum antibodies to FeLV are offered by several veterinary diagnostic laboratories. Most of these tests utilize IFA or ELISA procedures. Not only is the specificity of such tests extremely questionable but also no correlation between antibody titers as determined by these tests and protection against FeLV infection is currently available (Pedersen, 1986). Only virus-neutralizing antibodies have been correlated with protection. Neutralizing antibody titers of 1:10 or greater protect a cat against infection (Hardy, 1986). It is unfortunate that virus-neutralizing antibodies against FeLV are difficult to measure and such tests are not usually available to practitioners.

Feline oncornavirus cell membrane antigen (FOCMA) antibody tests are of little or no practical value. FOCMA antibody, if present to a significant degree, protects cats from FeLV-induced tumors but does not protect against the far more frequently occurring FeLV-induced anemias and immunosuppressive disorders (Hardy, 1986). In addition, FOCMA antibody titers seem to vary significantly with time.

It is theoretically possible that testing of FeLV and FOCMA antibody titers would offer some information regarding the effect of vaccination. It is unfortunate that, given the lack of specificity of such tests and the lack of correlation between the antibody titers and protection, the test results are apt to be extremely confusing, misleading, and certainly not cost-effective.

Adverse Postvaccination Reactions

Leukocell (Norden) is a noninfectious vaccine that, by itself, will not produce FeLV infection in cats, will not activate a latent infection, will not harm an FeLV-infected cat, and will not result in a vaccinated cat's showing positive results to FeLV ELISA or IFA testing because of vaccination alone.

Adverse reactions to Leukocell vaccination may vary from mild, local reactions characterized by discomfort, pain, or lameness immediately following vaccination to systemic reactions marked by fever, depression, anorexia, vomiting, and diarrhea lasting 6 to 24 hr after vaccination. There have been reports of severe reactions including abortions in vaccinated pregnant queens and seizures; however, such reports are rare. A survey involving 1029 intramuscular vaccinations reported 31.4 per cent local or systemic reactions (Rosenthal and Dworkis, 1987). Even with this relatively high rate of adverse reactions, the researchers considered the vaccine to be safe. The subcutaneous route of vaccination may well reduce the number of local adverse reactions.

A potential significant adverse reaction to Leukocell vaccination has been reported infrequently. Several cats that had received one or two doses of the vaccine died within 1 to 2 weeks after vaccination as a result of feline infectious peritonitis (FIP), confirmed by pathologic and laboratory examination (Pedersen, 1988). Clinically healthy cats persistently infected with FeLV and FIP virus, when vaccinated with bacille Calmette-Guérin (BCG) tuberculosis vaccine, died as a result of confirmed FIP shortly after the second dose of BCG (Ott, 1980). BCG is a potent nonspecific immunostimulant. The humoral immune response to BCG in a cat with nonclinically apparent FIP infection may be sufficient to exacerbate clinical FIP. It has been suggested that the adjuvant in Leukocell may produce a similar effect. There is insufficient evidence to unequivocally state that such is the case.

VACCINE SAFETY AND EFFICACY

The ideal FeLV vaccine obviously would not cause infection or disease in vaccinated cats nor would it produce positive FeLV antigen test results in vaccinated cats that previously had negative test results. Adverse reactions to the vaccine would be minimal, so it could be used safely, although perhaps not effectively, in FeLV-infected cats whether that infection was demonstrable or latent. The ideal vaccine would produce strong immunologic responses involving both the humoral and the cell-mediated immune systems. A high proportion of vaccinated cats should be able to withstand challenge, either natural or artificial, and neither become viremic nor develop disease in response to the challenge.

Leukocell qualifies as a safe vaccine. It does not produce FeLV infections, and antigen tests do not show positive results following vaccination. Leukocell does not appear to exacerbate the course of FeLV infection if viremic cats are inadvertently vaccinated, and it does not seem to activate a latent infection. Adverse reactions to Leukocell are more frequent than similar reactions to other commonly used feline vaccines; however, it is considered a safe vaccine. Leukocell does not seem to interfere with immune responses to other commonly used feline vaccines (panleukopenia, rabies, herpes, or calicivirus) when these vaccines are used concurrently with Leukocell.

It has been shown that only a relatively small percentage of cats developed virus-neutralizing antibodies after vaccination with Leukocell and prior to challenge (Pedersen et al., 1985). A somewhat higher percentage developed FOCMA antibodies after vaccination. In contrast, both virus-neutralizing and FOCMA antibodies rise rapidly after challenge with virulent virus (Pedersen et al., 1985). Nonspecific lymphocyte blastogenesis does not change after two doses of the vaccine which could indicate a lack of cell-mediated immunity response to the vaccine (Olsen, 1986). It would appear that the humoral and cell-mediated immunity responses to Leukocell do not conclusively demonstrate the efficacy of the vaccine.

Experiments involving the vaccination and subsequent challenge of cats that had never been exposed to FeLV and had negative FeLV test results prior to vaccination yielded extremely variable findings. Reported protection by vaccination against persistent viremia, disease, or both varied from approximately 25 to 80 per cent protection (Sharpee et al., 1986; Pedersen et al., 1985). Although 80 per cent of cats were protected against persistent viremia in one study, 52 per cent of the vaccinated cats did show a transient viremia after challenge (Sharpee et al., 1986). These cats may well have developed a transient latent infection. It has not been conclusively demonstrated that Leukocell vaccination prevents latent infections.

The clinical trials of Leukocell that have been reported seem to be of questionable validity (Henley et al., 1986; Jacob, 1986). These trials often lack controls, and in some cases, vaccination was combined with a test and removal of FeLV-infected cats. A test and removal program is, by itself, effective in controlling FeLV infections in infected multiple-cat facilities. Thus, in this situation, it is difficult to demonstrate that the vaccine had any effect whatsoever. Reports that cast the vaccine in a less favorable light may be criticized on the basis that vaccinated cats may have been in contact with infected cats prior to the completion of vaccination (Jacob, 1986). The results of the report would indicate that it is not completely safe to place a vaccinated cat in an infected household.

Unconfirmed reports from veterinarians in the field are ambiguous; however, several cats, which had negative FeLV test results prior to vaccination, received three doses of vaccine and yearly revaccination, have later been presented with a persistent FeLV viremia and some have developed FeLV-related disease.

INDICATIONS FOR VACCINATION

Based on the available data on the efficacy of Leukocell, it is difficult to strongly recommend the vaccination of all cats. It does seem reasonable to suggest the vaccination of cats with negative FeLV test results that come from households (single or multiple-cat households) where such cats are allowed a degree of freedom to roam. It must be emphasized to the owner that the vaccination series should be completed before young cats are allowed to roam, that yearly revaccination is necessary, and that the vaccine is perhaps only 50 per cent effective. Owners may then make their own cost-effective evaluations.

A case can possibly be made for the vaccination of cats entering a high-risk environment such as an infected cattery or a multiple-cat household where the owners do not wish to remove the healthy, but persistently viremic, cats. In such unusual circumstances, it would be essential that incoming cats be completely isolated from resident cats until the vaccination series is completed. Although it is not recommended that a vaccinated cat be kept in intimate cat-to-cat contact with infected cats, such situations do occur and will provide a real challenge to the efficacy of the vaccine.

Multiple-cat facilities in which there is considerable movement of cats in and out and the chances for FeLV exposure are reasonably high might well wish to consider FeLV vaccination as an adjunct to testing and removal of FeLV-infected cats.

In essentially closed catteries that are free from FeLV infection and that routinely retest to maintain that status, vaccination does not seem to be economically warranted and is apt to produce a complacency regarding regular testing.

It is hoped that ongoing studies will clarify the role of Leukocell in the prevention of FeLV infections. New and possibly improved vaccines will appear. In the meantime, FeLV vaccination with Leukocell may be recommended, with reservations, in some situations.

References and Supplemental Reading

Hardy, W. D., Jr.: The oncogenic viruses of cats: The feline leukemia and sarcoma viruses. In Holzworth, J. (ed.): Diseases of the Cat, Medicine and Surgery Philadelphia: W. B. Saunders Co., 1987, pp. 246–268.

Hardy, W. D., Jr.: Feline immunology: A look into the controversy surrounding FeLV—the immune response, vaccine and testing. Vet. Forum, August 1986, p. 9.

Henley, J. P., Stewart, D. C., and Dickerson, T. V.: Evaluating the efficacy of feline leukemia vaccination in two high-risk colonies. Vet. Med. 81:470, 1986.

Hoover, E. A., Olsen, R. G., and Hardy, W. D., Jr., et al.: Feline leukemia virus infection: Age-related variation in response of cats to experimental infection. J. Nat. Cancer Inst. 57:365, 1976.

Jacob, M.: Report on FeLV vaccinations. Cats Magazine 43:EE4, 1986.

Jarrett, O.: Feline leukemia virus. In Pract. 7:125, 1985.

Lewis, M. G., Mathes, L. E., and Olsen, R. G.: Protection against feline leukemia by vaccination with a subunit vaccine. Infect. Immun. 34:888, 1981.

Macy, D. W.: Feline leukemia virus. In Barlough, J. E. (ed.): Manual of Small Animal Infectious Diseases. New York: Churchill Livingstone, 1988, pp. 79–99.

Olsen, R. G.: An innovative technic produces a feline leukemia virus vaccine. Vet. Med. 80:61, 1985.

Olsen, R. G.: New information on feline leukemia vaccination. Proceedings of the 11th World Small Animal Veterinary Association Congress, Paris, France, 1986.

Ott, R. L.: Unpublished report, 1980.

Pacitti, A. M., and Jarrett, O.: Duration of the latent state in feline leukemia virus infections. Vet. Rec. 117:472, 1985.

Pedersen, N. C.: Feline immunology: The value of serological tests for the measurement of antibodies to FeLV and FIPV. Vet. Forum, October 1986, pp. 29–30.

Pedersen, N. C.: Feline infectious peritonitis: Letter to the editor. Reprinted in Cats Magazine 45:EE21, 1988.

Pedersen, N. C., Johnson, L., and Ott, R. L.: Evaluation of a commercial feline leukemia virus vaccine for immunogenicity and efficacy. Feline Pract. 15:7, 1985.

Pedersen, N. C., Meric, S. M., Ho, E., et al.: The clinical significance of latent feline leukemia virus infection in cats. Feline Pract. 14:32, 1984.

Rojko, J. L.: Biology of the feline leukemia virus. Proceedings of the 10th Annual Kal Kan Symposium for the Treatment of Small Animal Diseases, Kal Kan Foods Inc., 1987, pp. 89–95.

Rosenthal, R. C., and Dworkis, A. S.: Adverse reactions to Leukocell. J. Am. Anim. Hosp. Assoc. 23:515, 1987.

Sharpee, R. L., Beckenhauer, W. H., Baumgartener, L. E., et al.: Feline leukemia vaccine: Evaluation of safety and efficacy against persistent viremia and tumor development. Comp. Cont. Ed. Pract. Vet. 8:267, 1986.

A User's Manual for "Leukocell" Feline Leukemia Vaccine. Norden Laboratories, Lincoln, Nebraska, 1985.

Discussion 3

RICHARD G. OLSEN, Ph.D.

Columbus, Ohio

The long search for a successful feline leukemia virus (FeLV) vaccine culminated in 1985 with the introduction of a commercial subunit vaccine (Leukocell, Norden). At the time, the vaccine, and to a lesser extent the disease, were unconventional and, therefore, poorly understood. This article addresses some of the key issues that veterinary practitioners most often inquire about regarding feline leukemia vaccination.

Infection with FeLV results in two conditions—viremia and tumors. Persistent viremia initially results in immunosuppression and a variety of non-neoplastic diseases. These "associated diseases" are the cause of death in the majority of affected cats. Those that survive eventually die of neoplastic disease. Neoplastic cells transformed by FeLV express a tumor-specific protein known as feline oncornavirus-associated cell membrane antigen (FOCMA). Thus, in order for a vaccine to be effective, it must elicit FeLV-specific antibodies to prevent viremia, and FOCMA antibodies to prevent neoplastic disease.

Investigators at the Ohio State University developed the prototype of the first successful feline leukemia vaccine (Lewis et al., 1981). It was derived from a feline lymphoid tumor persistently infected with the Kawakami-Theilen strain of FeLV. This virus-cell system expressed both FeLV and FOCMA (Wolff et al., 1979), making it a convenient source of viral and tumor-specific antigens.

It was discovered that when the virus-cell system was propagated in serum-free media, FeLV replication was not driven to completion. Instead, individual viral proteins were expressed as soluble subunits into the culture media. The solubilized FeLV proteins were noninfectious but still immunogenic. Unlike intact FeLV (either live or inactivated), the soluble viral proteins also had the important distinction of being nonimmunosuppressive. This preparation was eventually patented and became the basis for a safe and effective commercial feline leukemia vaccine.

DIAGNOSTIC TESTING PRIOR TO VACCINATION

Reliable in-clinic diagnostic tests are now available for detection of FeLV-positive cats. These include serum tests and, more recently, a saliva enzyme-linked immunosorbent assay (ELISA)

(Lewis et al., 1987). Although testing can be valuable for detecting FeLV-positive cats prior to vaccination, it is probably not necessary to test in all situations. Specifically, testing of low-risk cats is discretionary, whereas testing of high-risk cats is advisable.

A low-risk cat is one that is clinically healthy (the single most important factor in the decision to either test or vaccinate), has a normal health history, comes from a single-cat household, lives indoors, and has had minimal exposure to other cats. A high-risk cat is clinically suspect, has a chronic susceptibility to infectious disease, and lives in a multiple-cat setting or otherwise has frequent contact with other cats and, therefore, an increased chance of FeLV exposure.

To an extent, feline leukemia is age related. Neonatal and geriatric cats tend to be less immunocompetent and more susceptible to FeLV (particularly after experimental exposure). However, the age of the cat has little bearing on the decision to test. The juvenile cat is more likely to develop progressive FeLV disease once infected, but the adult cat is more likely over time to be exposed and become persistently viremic. In assessing the need to test, the risk profile just described is much more important than the cat's age.

VACCINATION OF FeLV-POSITIVE CATS

There are circumstances when vaccination of an FeLV-positive cat is an acceptable practice. An FeLV-positive cat with a low-risk profile may have been the subject of an occasional false-positive diagnostic test, or the animal may have a transient infection, which occurs in about 40 per cent of cats that have been exposed to FeLV. In such cases, it is justified to initiate the primary vaccination regimen, pending a retest 4 to 6 weeks later.

Consecutive positive test results, especially when an immunofluorescent antibody test corroborates the results of an earlier ELISA test, indicate that the cat is persistently infected. Vaccination is of no value in such cases. However, there is no evidence that infected cats are adversely affected when feline leukemia vaccination is administered.

Of greater importance than vaccination of the clinically healthy but FeLV-positive cat is vaccination of a clinically affected cat, whether it is FeLV-positive or FeLV-negative. An anemic, gaunt cat showing signs of some infectious process is a poor candidate for vaccination of any kind. The cat will not respond immunologically to the maximum extent, nor will it be protected if it is affected by the disease for which it is vaccinated. In addition, the stress of vaccination may exacerbate any existing disease. For these reasons, vaccination of the clinically affected cat may jeopardize the practitioner's standing in the eyes of the client.

MAINTAINING AN FeLV-FREE COLONY

In infected cat colonies or those of unknown status, feline leukemia vaccination is an important tool for establishing and maintaining an FeLV-free facility. Vaccination should be preceded by diagnostic screening to eliminate FeLV-positive cats (a "test-and-elimination" program). The remaining (FeLV-negative) cats should then be vaccinated and maintained in an isolated setting. A retest should be done 4 to 6 weeks later to identify cats that had previous false-negative test results or that were incubating disease. Such cats should, of course, be eliminated from the colony. The test and elimination program should continue until the entire colony tests FeLV-negative.

There have been convincing reports that a program of vaccination and testing is effective in limiting the spread of FeLV in a humane shelter or closed colony that is FeLV-infected (Henley et al., 1986). In an Ohio humane shelter, vaccination of FeLV-negative cats was coupled with elimination of FeLV-positive cats and was followed by diagnostic screening of all incoming cats. During the year after this procedure was implemented, the incidence of FeLV infection was reduced from 14.3 per cent to 1.5 per cent. Of 400 vaccinated cats at the shelter, only six tested FeLV-positive after vaccination, and it was suspected that some of those that had positive test results were exposed prior to vaccination.

In a similar example involving a closed colony of 46 cats, diagnostic testing revealed that ten were FeLV-positive. All cats were vaccinated but were allowed to continue to have unrestricted access to each other. During the ensuing year, only one FeLV-negative vaccinated cat became FeLV-positive. However, that cat was clinically suspect at the time of vaccination and received only two of the recommended three primary doses. The cat died 11 weeks after the initial dose, which suggests that it had been incubating disease at the time vaccination was initiated.

The latter case demonstrated that properly vaccinated cats will be protected if placed in contact with FeLV-positive cats. However, to knowingly allow healthy vaccinated cats to mingle with suspect or infected cats is poor management and should be avoided whenever possible. Nevertheless, the pre-

ceding reports of protection from contact exposure to FeLV were indicators of vaccine efficacy under field conditions and corroborated the much more severe challenge-of-immunity tests conducted during vaccine development (Lewis et al., 1981; Sharpee et al., 1985).

Once an FeLV-free colony is established, vaccination and testing may be performed selectively. A truly closed colony with restricted access is a low-risk environment. Vaccination can be discontinued, and diagnostic screening can be confined to paired tests for cats entering the colony after a suitable quarantine period has elapsed. A humane shelter, on the other hand, is a high-risk setting because animals are continually introduced into the colony. If the shelter is FeLV-free, only incoming cats need be tested. All FeLV-negative cats accepted by the shelter should be vaccinated. Clients adopting cats prior to completion of primary vaccination should be instructed to have the initial regimen completed by a licensed veterinarian.

PREVENTION OF FELINE LEUKEMIA VIREMIA

Protection against feline leukemia viremia was evaluated in controlled challenge-of-immunity tests conducted prior to licensing of the feline leukemia vaccine (Sharpee et al., 1985). To enhance their susceptibility to FeLV infection, 25 vaccinated cats and ten nonvaccinated control cats were artificially immunosuppressed with a corticosteroid at the time of challenge. A challenge dose consisting of $10^{5.7}$ focus-forming units of the virulent Rickard strain of FeLV was then administered oronasally on two successive days. Clearly, the conditions of this experimental challenge were far more severe than what would be expected in nature. The results are shown in Table 1. Of the vaccinated cats, 80 per cent were protected against persistent viremia, and 48 per cent against transient viremia. In contrast, 70 per cent of the control subjects developed persistent viremia.

Persistent feline leukemia viremia precedes progressive disease. Thus, the result of the challenge-of-immunity test is sometimes interpreted as indicating that the vaccine was 80 per cent effective. However, test cats were artificially immunosuppressed and were subjected to a challenge dose far exceeding what would occur under natural conditions. This was affirmed by the fact that nonvaccinated control subjects experienced a 70 per cent rate of persistent viremia, considerably higher than the 30 per cent rate estimated to occur following contact exposure. Eighty per cent protection in vaccinated cats under the experimental conditions described is tantamount to a much higher efficacy in a typical field situation.

Table 1. *Results of FeLV Challenge after Three IM Vaccine Doses*

Results	Prevalence in Vaccinated Cats		Prevalence in Control Cats	
Viremia Incidence				
Persistent	5/25	(20%)	7/10	(70%)
Transient	13/25	(52%)	2/10	(20%)
Aviremic	6/25	(24%)	1/10	(10%)
Undetermined*	1/25	(4%)		
Tumor Incidence				
Overall	2/25	(8%)	6/10	(60%)
In persistently viremic cats	2/5	(40%)	6/7	(86%)
Mortality				
FeLV-related	5/25	(20%)	7/10	(70%)
In cats with tumors	2/2	(100%)	6/6	(100%)
Overall	7/25	(28%)	9/10	(90%)
Protection				
Against persistent viremia*	20/25	(80%)	3/10	(30%)
Against tumor development	23/25	(92%)	4/10	(40%)
Against death resulting from FeLV	20/25	(80%)	3/10	(30%)

*The viremic status of one FeLV-positive vaccinated cat was undetermined because of death from nonFeLV causes at postchallenge week 11.

Following experimental challenge, the transiently infected vaccinated cats all reverted to aviremic status. Of the 20 vaccinated cats that survived challenge (Table 1), 17 were still alive 4 years later, three having died of non-FeLV causes. After approximately one fourth of their normal lifespan had elapsed, these vaccinated cats remained FeLV-negative and in good health. This study duplicated earlier results with the prototype vaccine (Lewis et al., 1981). Together, these development studies indicated that properly vaccinated cats will be reliably protected from persistent feline leukemia viremia following natural exposure, although transient infection may occur in a small percentage of cases.

PREVENTION OF FeLV LATENCY

Even occasional transient feline leukemia viremia in vaccinated cats would be of concern if latent infection occurred as a result. In latent (nonproductive) FeLV infection, virus is not produced in bone marrow or peripheral blood lymphocytes. However, the FeLV genome is still present in target cells and capable of reactivation under certain conditions, most notably the administration of corticosteroids (Rojko et al., 1979). If the vaccine would reliably protect cats from latent infection, its value as a immunizing agent would be enhanced considerably.

A recent study demonstrated that vaccinated cats are, in fact, protected from latent FeLV infection (Haffer et al., 1987). A total of 17 cats were assembled from various vaccine development studies. All had received the recommended three primary doses and were challenged as previously described (Sharpee et al., 1985). In an attempt to activate latent FeLV 24 to 35 months after challenge, methylprednisolone was administered to all cats once a week for 4 consecutive weeks at the rate of 7.5 mg/kg of body weight. The corticosteroid treatment resulted in a mean 69 per cent reduction in lymphocyte count, indicating that immunosuppression did, in fact, occur. Latency was assessed by culturing bone marrow aspirates from femoral shafts prior to immunosuppressive treatment and 1 week after the last treatment.

The results of this latency assessment are shown in Table 2. Cat ED-3 was persistently infected, as indicated by the presence of the FeLV group-specific antigen p27 in its serum. This cat also yielded virus from bone marrow, which is typical of persistently viremic cats. Cat KC-3 was a true case of latent infection. Serum diagnostic test results were negative, but bone marrow cultures revealed the presence of p27. The remaining 15 cats had negative results throughout the 21-day incubation period. Even though eight of these vaccinated cats were transiently viremic following severe challenge, none were latently infected. This result indicated that genome integration occurred in the transiently infected cats but was subsequently eliminated at a result of the host immune response.

Table 2. *Determination of Latency: Presence of FeLV in Serum and Bone Marrow of Vaccinated Cats Following Challenge and Artificial Immunosuppression*

Cat No.	FeLV Isolation before and after Methylpredisolone Treatment			
	Serum		Bone Marrow	
	Pre	Post	Pre	Post
2435*	−	−	−	−
2450	−	−	−	−
2460	−	−	−	−
2395*	−	−	−	−
2451*	−	−	−	−
2440*	−	−	−	−
2448*	−	−	−	−
2377	−	−	−	−
2482*	−	−	−	−
2417*	−	−	−	−
2432	−	−	−	−
2375*	−	−	−	−
ED-3†	+	+	+	+
BA-1	−	−	−	−
CA-4	−	−	−	−
LD-3	−	−	−	−
KC-3‡	−	−	+	+

*Had transient postchallenge viremia.
†Had persistent postchallenge viremia.
‡Had latent postchallenge infection.

PREVENTION OF FeLV-INDUCED NEOPLASIA

To a great extent, the term feline leukemia is a misnomer because only a relatively small minority of affected cats (perhaps 20 per cent) survive FeLV-associated disease and go on to develop a neoplastic disorder. (Hindsight suggests that "feline retrovirus infection" would have been a more appropriate and less sensationalistic name than the one adopted.) Nevertheless, a comprehensive feline leukemia vaccine must prevent neoplastic disease as well as persistent viremia. Antibodies to the tumor-specific antigen FOCMA are the best known correlate to protection against FeLV-induced neoplasia. In an FeLV-transformed cell, FOCMA is expressed as a viral epitope on the cell membrane. Cytotoxic antibodies destroy the tumor cell by recognizing FOCMA on the surface of transformed cells (Grant et al., 1977).

The development tests described earlier demonstrated conclusively that vaccinated cats develop a strong FOCMA antibody response and are effectively protected against tumor development (Lewis et al., 1981; Sharpee et al., 1985). As seen in Table 1, vaccinated cats showed 92 per cent protection against tumor development (versus 40 per cent protection in control subjects), despite artificial immunosuppression and administration of a massive FeLV challenge dose on 2 successive days.

RECOMMENDED VACCINATION SCHEDULE

The original vaccine development studies showed that a primary regimen consisting of three intramuscular (IM) doses was superior to two IM doses in terms of the rates of protection against persistent viremia and tumor development (Sharpee et al., 1985). These results served as the basis for the vaccine's original label recommendation for three primary IM doses. Subcutaneous (SC) administration of the vaccine has since been shown to elicit serum antibody values equivalent or superior to those following IM vaccination. As a result, the vaccine is now indicated for either IM or SC administration. Annual revaccination with a single dose is recommended. No duration-of-immunity study has been done, but the single annual dose has proved to be clinically adequate in cases in which contact exposure occurred (Henley et al., 1986).

On occasion, completion of the initial three-dose vaccination regimen may be interrupted or delayed. The effect of extending primary vaccination beyond the recommended intervals has not been studied and is not known with certainty. As with all vaccines, practitioners place themselves at risk by not following label recommendations. Thus, veterinarians are best advised in such cases to re-initiate the complete three-dose series. This recommendation is made, in part, because the vaccine is inactivated, not a modified live-virus preparation. Its inability to replicate *in vivo* means that successive doses are needed to achieve a maximum immune response.

POSTVACCINATION REACTIONS

After the feline leukemia vaccine was introduced, systemic postvaccination reactions were an occasional but continuing problem (Sharpee et al., 1985). These reactions were characterized most often by fever, anorexia, and depression occurring 6 to 12 hr after vaccination and lasting 24 to 48 hr. Such sequelae were reported, for example, in slightly more than 3 per cent of the cats in the prelicensing field trial. More serious hypersensitivity reactions occurred in 0.44 per cent of the field trial cats.

To minimize and reduce postvaccination reactions, the manufacturing process was altered in two respects. Neither alteration affected vaccine potency in terms of antigenic content or serologic response. The first change consisted of an additional purification step. The second change was removal of a nonessential preservative. In vaccine serials manufactured prior to these product alterations, the rate of reported reactions was 17.8 per 100,000 doses sold. After the manufacturing changes, reported reactions declined to 2.8 per 100,000 doses sold, a level that compares favorably with that for any commercial vaccine.

A safety issue of far greater importance than the low incidence of transitory postvaccination reactions is immunosuppression. Feline leukemia virus is immunosuppressive in either live or killed form. The envelope protein p15e, which is common to all retroviruses, is the immunosuppressive antigen. This p15e has a profound effect on feline cellular immunity, reducing lymphoblast transformation by as much as 68 per cent (Mathes et al., 1979). When purified p15e is added to feline neutrophils *in vitro*, neutrophil production is immediately curtailed. It is noteworthy that the author has found that clinically normal cats with latent FeLV infection exhibit some neutrophil dysfunction, making the vaccine's efficacy against latent infection all the more significant.

We know that the feline leukemia vaccine contains p15e (as well as all other FeLV proteins) in some form because vaccinated cats respond to it serologically (Mastro et al., 1986). However, it has been conclusively shown that the vaccine produces no immunosuppressive effect. Vaccine does not impair lymphocyte blastogenesis, either *in vivo* when given at a tenfold concentration or *in vitro*. A 50-fold concentration of vaccine did not suppress white blood cell counts of vaccinated cats below normal levels, and vaccinated cats responded serologically to concurrent administration of other feline vaccines (Sharpee et al., 1985). The latter finding is, in itself, a significant indicator of the absence of immunosuppressive effect. In the author's laboratory it has been shown that purified p15e impairs antiviral and anti-FOCMA responses and that such immunosuppression occurs rapidly following p15e administration (Mathes et al., 1979).

Absence of an immunosuppressive effect indicates that p15e is present in the vaccine as an analogue or in a precursor form that is nonpathogenic. Recent studies at the National Cancer Institute suggest how this occurs (Henderson et al., 1984). During retrovirus assembly, viral proteins undergo molecular restructuring within the host cell. One of the structural changes that occurs is cleavage by cellular enzymes of a peptide bond between p15e and a p2e molecule. This alteration is apparently necessary for p15e to become immunosuppressive. Because the feline leukemia vaccine consists of soluble viral proteins but not infective whole FeLV, it probably contains p15e with an intact p2e protein in a nonimmunosuppressive precursor assemblage.

RELEVANCE OF ANTIBODY RESPONSE TO VACCINATION

A strong and consistent serologic response to vaccination is desirable, but certainly not the sole or even the most critical indicator of protection, particularly protection that results from cellular immunity. A variety of immune cells are activated following FeLV exposure. Some are antibody-producing cells and some are not. A serologic response indicates that a primordial cell, driven by an immunogen, has been activated. Antibody is the final, not the primary, expression of the immune process.

Is a vaccinated cat that does not express virus-neutralizing antibody resistant to disease? In all probability it is, because antibody precursor cells have been sensitized and will exhibit a strong serologic response when natural exposure occurs. This is illustrated by the marked anamnestic response that occurred in many vaccinated cats following challenge (Sharpee et al., 1985). The initial serologic response in some animals was modest, but challenge was followed by much more pronounced antibody titers and protection.

Perhaps as important as conventional serum antibodies is the complement-dependent cytotoxic (CDC) antibody response to FeLV exposure. Studies have shown that feline CDC antibodies in the presence of cat complement will lyse homologous FeLV-infected tumor cells (Grant et al., 1977). This may be particularly important in the case of FeLV. Unlike herpes virus or coronavirus, for example, FeLV is a nonlytic virus. Thus, an infected cell produces virus for the normal life of the cell. Lysis interrupts cell transformation or viral replication. Virus-neutralizing antibody neutralizes cell-free FeLV but has no effect on FeLV transformation of cells or viral replication within those cells. It appears that lysis of infected cells is the role of CDC antibody.

Testing conducted by the manufacturer in a limited number of cats demonstrated that the vaccine consistently elicited marked levels of CDC antibodies after each of three vaccine doses. It is interesting that CDC antibody responses were vigorous in all cats after the initial dose, whereas anti-FeLV titers at that test interval were still modest. Thus, the vaccine's immunizing properties should not be assessed on the basis of anti-FeLV or anti-FOCMA values alone. Nor should a veterinarian feel compelled to measure postvaccination antibody response as an indicator of immunogenicity. This is a test with limited relevance, and qualified laboratories that use standardized methods are few in number.

The author thanks Mark Dana (Norden Laboratories) for assisting in the preparation of this report.

References and Supplemental Reading

Grant, C. K., DeBoer, D. J., Essex, M., et al.: Antibodies from healthy cats exposed to feline leukemia virus lyse feline lymphoma cells slowly with cat complement. J. Immunol. 119:401, 1977.

Haffer, K. N., Sharpee, R. L., and Beckenhauer, W. H.: Feline leukaemia vaccine protection against viral latency. Vaccine 5:133, 1987.

Henderson, L. E., Sowder, R., Copeland, T. D., et al.: Quantitative separation of murine leukemia virus proteins by reversed-phase high-pressure liquid chromatography reveals newly described gag and env cleavage products. J. Virol. 52:492, 1984.

Henley, J. P., Stewart, D. C., and Dickerson, T. V.: Evaluating the efficacy of feline leukemia vaccination in two high-risk colonies. Vet. Med. 81:470, 1986.

Lewis, M. G., Mathes, L. E., and Olsen, R. G.: Protection against feline leukemia by vaccination with a subunit vaccine. Infect. Immun. 34:888, 1981.

Lewis, M. G., Wright, K. A., Lafrado, L. J., et al.: Saliva as a source of feline leukemia virus antigen for diagnosis of disease. J. Clin. Microbiol. 25:1320, 1987.

Mastro, J. M., Lewis, M. G., Mathes, L. E., et al.: Feline leukemia vaccine: Efficacy, contents, and probably mechanism. Vet. Immunol. Immunopathol. 11:205, 1986.

Mathes, L. E., Olsen, R. G., Hebebrand, L. C., et al.: Immunosuppressive properties of a virion polypeptide, a 15,000-dalton protein, from feline leukemia virus. Cancer Res. 39:950, 1979.

Rojko, J. L., Hoover, E. A., Mathes, L. E., et al.: Influence of adrenal corticosteroids on the susceptibility of cats to feline leukemia virus infection. Cancer Res. 39:3789, 1979.

Sharpee, R. L., Beckenhauer, W. H., Baumgartner, L. E., et al.: Feline leukemia vaccine: Evaluation of safety and efficacy against persistent viremia and tumor development. The Compendium 8:267, 1986.

Wolff, L. H., Mathes, L. E., and Olsen, R. G.: Recovery of soluble feline oncornavirus-associated cell membrane antigen from large volumes of tissue culture fluids. J. Immunol. Methods 26:151, 1979.

ALTERNATIVE TESTING PROCEDURES FOR FeLV

ELEANOR C. HAWKINS, D.V.M.

West Lafayette, Indiana

The ability to detect the presence of feline leukemia virus (FeLV) infection in cats is important for the diagnosis of FeLV-related syndromes and is critical for the prevention of transmission of the disease. The presence of persistent viremia with FeLV is associated with a grave prognosis, and over 80 per cent of such cats die within 3 years. There is no specific treatment for FeLV infection, although many related diseases can be successfully managed as they occur. The clinical signs associated with FeLV infection are extremely variable and nonspecific, making a diagnosis of FeLV infection impossible based on clinical signs alone. It is fortunate that the development of FeLV infections can be successfully prevented. The critical step in the prevention of FeLV infections is the identification of FeLV-infected cats. The FeLV is not stable in the environment and requires close contact for transmission. Noninfected cats can be maintained free from disease by preventing their contact with infected cats.

Practical testing methods for the detection of FeLV infection through the identification of FeLV antigens have been available since the development of the indirect immunofluorescent antibody (IFA) test in 1972 by W. D. Hardy and colleagues. The later development of enzyme-linked immunosorbent assay (ELISA) techniques that use monoclonal antibodies against the p27 core antigen of the leukemia virus has resulted in a number of commercially available test kits. For clinical testing, the IFA test and the ELISA traditionally have been performed on whole blood (IFA) or serum (ELISA). Alternative methods for FeLV detection have become available. These alternative tests rely on ELISA technology but use saliva or tears as specimens for antigen detection.

RELATIONSHIP OF ANTIGEN TESTS TO STAGE OF INFECTION

The primary difference between testing methods (blood IFA, and serum, tear, and salivary ELISAs) is the stage of infection, which may be detected by the identification of FeLV antigens in the various specimens. Discrepancies in the results of the various testing methods would be seen because of this difference even if the testing methods were faultless. Therefore, it is necessary to understand the sequential pathogenesis of FeLV infection.

Several stages of infection have been characterized in the cat (Rojko et al., 1979; Jarrett, 1983). Following oral exposure, the virus infects the lymphoid tissue of the pharynx. The virus undergoes a short period of multiplication in lymphoid tissue cells and then enters the systemic circulation within blood mononuclear cells. First, lymphoid tissues throughout the body become infected. Next, the bone marrow becomes involved as the virus infects stem cells. The virus multiplies extensively in the bone marrow, and virus-laden neutrophils and platelets as well as free virus are released into the systemic circulation. Last, glandular and mucosal epithelia become infected, and the virus then may be shed in body secretions. The bone marrow infection is detectable 1 to 3 weeks following exposure. Infected neutrophils and platelets can be detected in the peripheral blood 2 to 4 weeks or longer after exposure, and infection of epithelial tissues at high concentrations occurs in 4 to 8 weeks or longer.

The majority of cats that are exposed to FeLV successfully eliminate the infection or suppress the expression of the virus. Cats that do not develop persistent viremias appear to abort the infection during the time of lymphoid and bone marrow involvement. In a few experimental cases, virus has been identified in the blood by IFA and serum ELISA for up to 8 weeks following exposure even in cats that apparently recover from infection (Jarrett, 1983; Jarrett et al., 1982). Virus also can be isolated from the oropharynx in these cats for approximately the same period of time. In the majority of cases, seroconversion occurs either without viremia or with a viremic stage of only a few days (Jarrett, 1983; Lutz et al., 1983).

Serum ELISA can detect free viral antigens in the circulation of infected cats. It appears to be sensitive enough to detect early infections prior to bone marrow involvement in some cases and, therefore, can be transiently positive in cats that subsequently eliminate infection. The most strongly positive results occur following infection of the bone marrow, where extensive multiplication of the virus occurs followed by the release of particles into the circulation both within blood elements and free in the plasma.

The IFA test detects the same viral antigens as does the ELISA but tests for their presence within circulating neutrophils and platelets. This test would not be expected to be positive prior to involvement of the bone marrow and release of infected cells into the circulation. A period of up to 3 months may be required following exposure before detection by this method is possible. However, once a cat is positive for FeLV based on IFA testing, the cat is unlikely to ever successfully eliminate the infection.

Tests utilizing saliva or tears would not be expected to be strongly positive until the virus is amplified within the marrow, is released into the circulation, and finally has infected the epithelial tissues. A period of several months following exposure may be required for detection of infection using these methods. In most cases, once a cat has a positive result for FeLV based on saliva or tear testing, it is unlikely to eliminate the infection. A transient, weak reaction may be obtained from saliva shortly after oral exposure and is probably related to local infection of the lymphoid tissues.

It is unfortunate that the various test methods are not faultless in their ability to identify FeLV antigen. The methods available for saliva and tear testing will be discussed, and comparisons will be made between results obtained by these alternative methods of testing and the traditional tests.

ALTERNATIVE TESTING METHODS

Saliva

Saliva can be collected and tested using a variety of techniques. Several test kits are available. Two of the test kits are CITE Feline Leukemia Virus Test Kit with STACPAK (Agritech Systems, Inc., Portland, ME) and Diasystems FeLV Flex II (Fermenta Animal Health [formerly Tech America Diagnostics] Kansas City, MO). These kits provide swabs or filter paper strips on which to collect saliva. The specimens are then assayed for FeLV antigen using slight modifications of the procedures for testing serum.

When using the modified serum kits, antigens in the saliva are bound to antibodies attached to the test well or test membrane and are also bound to enzyme-conjugated antibodies. A color change demonstrates that enzyme is present and, therefore, that FeLV antigens are present in the saliva. If FeLV antigens are not present in the saliva, the enzyme-conjugated antibodies have no antigens on which to bind, and they are eliminated in the wash procedures.

One kit (ClinEase-Virastat FeLV Viral Antigen Saliva Assay, Norden) provides a hard, plastic swab (ball) that actually contains monoclonal antibodies directed against FeLV antigen. The plastic ball acts like the antibody-coated test well of the traditional serum ELISA kits. The antibodies on the ball are protected by a sugar coating that is broken down by soaking prior to performing the test. Saliva is obtained by placing the ball into the oral cavity, and the reaction with FeLV antigens present in the saliva occurs directly on the ball. The ball is incubated in a test tube containing a solution of monoclonal antibodies against FeLV antigens that have been conjugated with an enzyme. A strict washing procedure must then be performed to ensure that all conjugated antibody that has not binded to FeLV antigens is removed from the ball. If FeLV antigens are present in the saliva, the antigens are bound to the antibodies on the ball and, in turn, bind the enzyme-conjugated antibodies from the solution to the ball. Finally, the ball is placed in a tube containing a substrate for the enzyme and a color indicator. The presence of enzyme and therefore the presence of antigen are demonstrated by a color change.

Tears

Until recently, there has been no commercially available test kit produced specifically for the evaluation of tears for the presence of viral antigen. The author and colleagues have developed a practical technique utilizing an FeLV test kit marketed for serum testing (Diasystems FeLV) for this purpose (Hawkins et al., 1986). Tears are collected using a single Schirmer's tear test strip. These standardized, sterilized strips of filter paper are readily available for the detection of keratoconjunctivitis sicca in humans and animals. A single strip is folded 90° at the notched end and is placed in the ventral conjunctival sac in the same position used to measure tear production. However, instead of timing the collection period, the strip is left in place until it is filled to within 2 to 5 mm of the far end with tears. A moisture line is clearly visible. If the tear strip cannot be assayed immediately following collection, the strip can be dried at room temperature following collection and will remain reactive for up to 7 days. The collection procedure is simple to perform and, in most cats, can be performed by just one person.

The dried strip is assayed in an ELISA test well coated with monoclonal antibody against FeLV antigen, with the following modifications of the routine serum procedure. The tear strip is pressed down into a test well with a wooden applicator stick. Three drops, instead of one, of the enzyme-conjugated antibody solution are added to the test well. The extra reagent is necessary to provide an adequate volume of solution so viral antigen can elute off the test strip and react with the antibodies coating the well. The well is covered with transparent tape and is placed in the refrigerator for 24 hr. The prolonged incubation period is necessary to increase the sensitivity of the test procedure. After the incubation period, the test well is emptied and is thoroughly rinsed according to the test kit directions. The substrate and color indicator solutions are added to the test well as directed. The presence of viral antigen will be demonstrated by a visible green color change. Any noticeable green color should be considered a positive result. Positive and negative control sera are provided with the test kits and should be run with each assay, using the standard incubation periods to ensure the proper functioning of the reagents.

Commercial test kits are now available for testing tears (CITE Feline Leukemia Virus Test Kit with STACPAK, and Diasystems FeLV Flex II). Tears are collected on tear test strips as previously described. However, a much shorter incubation period is recommended. Data have not been published demonstrating the sensitivity and the specificity of these kits.

TEST COMPARISONS

There appears to be good correlation between saliva or tear tests for FeLV and serum ELISA or IFA tests performed at the same time, although extensive clinical trials have not been performed. The major discrepancy is a tendency for negative saliva or tear test results in cats that are positive for FeLV by serum ELISA. Ninety-five per cent of cats with experimentally induced infections and 83 per cent of clinical cases that had positive results for FeLV by serum ELISA had positive results by the tear test previously described (Hawkins et al., 1986). Seventy-seven per cent of cats that had positive results for FeLV by serum ELISA had positive results for FeLV antigen in their saliva (Lutz and Jarrett, 1987). This disagreement in results can be explained by factors relating to the test procedures themselves and by the variability of the viral infection within individual cats. There is some degree of discrepancy between serum and IFA test results, and explanations proposed for these discrepancies also may explain some of the differences between results from alternative and traditional testing methods.

Alternative testing methods may fail to detect the presence of antigen in saliva or tears (false-negative results) because of problems with the test methods. In the case of saliva testing using the plastic ball containing antibodies, inadequate soaking of the ball prior to collection of saliva may fail to destroy the protective seal and may prevent a reaction from

occurring. If the ball is not tested immediately following collection, the reagents may dry and provide inaccurate results. No controls are provided. When testing saliva or tears using the other methods, antigen may fail to elute off the swab or test strip into solution, and elution is necessary to allow binding with the antibodies. Furthermore, all the alternative testing methods rely on a relatively smaller and less consistent volume of material than is evaluated by serum ELISA.

Alternative testing results may be inconsistent with serum test results because of the peculiarities of the body fluids being tested. The course of the viral infection may be variable in individual cats, so that saliva or tears do not contain detectable virus. Although the alternative test procedures are designed to have enhanced sensitivity as compared with that of serum tests, the concentration of virus particles in the secretions may be inconsistent. Interfering compounds, such as immunoglobulins, may be present in saliva or tears and may block the antigen-antibody test reaction. In addition, it is possible that intermittent shedding of virus into body secretions may occur in some cats in spite of persistent viremia.

Some FeLV-infected cats are persistently positive for FeLV by serum ELISA but are negative or only transiently positive for FeLV by IFA. These cats, which may account for 5 to 10 per cent of serum ELISA–positive cats (Lutz et al., 1983) may also have false-negative results on saliva or tear tests when compared with results from serum ELISA. One explanation proposed for the discordant test results is the restriction of infection to certain areas of the body of a partially effective immune response (Lutz et al., 1983). This compartmentalization of infection may prevent the release of virus particles in body secretions, whereas virus may be detectable in serum. The release of incomplete virus particles into the blood without the release of complete virions may cause a positive result by serum ELISA but negative tear or saliva test results. Similarly, cats with early infections may be tested prior to the involvement of epithelial tissues.

Positive tear or saliva test results have been rare in cats that are FeLV-negative by serum ELISA or IFA. Over 200 cats that were serum ELISA–negative for FeLV were tested by the tear method described. In no case were the tears found to be positive (Hawkins et al., 1986). Only 1 per cent of cats that had serum ELISA–negative results had positive results by saliva testing (Lutz and Jarrett, 1987). Explanations for false-positive results of saliva testing include cross-reactions with proteins from the microbial flora of the oral cavity and the detection of transient infections during the early oral stage.

A serious source of false-positive test results using any of the ELISA techniques is inadequate washing of the test system. Inadequate washing allows for the persistent presence of conjugated antibody that is not specifically bound to antigen. A color change will result even in the absence of antigen.

CLINICAL APPLICATIONS

The saliva and tear tests cannot be recommended as routine screening tests for the individual pet cat. A good screening test should be rapid, simple, inexpensive, and very sensitive, allowing for the rapid identification of high-risk patients. Then more specific testing methods can be employed. The serum ELISA test is the most sensitive test and is recommended for the routine screening of cats. The alternative testing methods often fail to identify cats with early infections and miss a portion of cats with stable disease. Even serum ELISA tests may miss incubating infections and should be re-evaluated in 12 weeks (Lutz and Pedersen, 1986).

The saliva and tear tests are rapid, simple techniques for confirming the presence of infection. A patient that has positive results by serum ELISA and is then found to have positive results by tear or saliva testing is more likely to be at a later stage of infection, more likely to be persistently viremic, and less likely to appear positive as a result of laboratory error than a patient found to have positive results by serum ELISA alone. The alternative ELISA tests are more convenient than the traditional IFA confirmation, since they can be performed within the practice setting.

It should be re-emphasized that there are transient periods of time during which cats that do *not* remain persistently viremic have positive results for FeLV by serum ELISA and IFA and during which virus isolation tests from the oropharynx have had positive results. Therefore, no single positive test should be used to condemn a cat that is already an established member of an household. Repeat testing should be performed in 12 weeks. However, extreme caution should be exercised when a potential new addition to a household has a positive result by any method or when performing test and elimination protocols within a cattery.

Another use for the alternative testing methods is the determination of the potential of a cat for shedding virus. Cats that have a positive result for

FeLV antigen in their saliva or tears certainly should be considered infectious. It still is prudent to consider cats that have serum ELISA positive results and tear or saliva negative test results as potential shedders of the virus until repeated testing is performed. Many questions remain unanswered about the infectivity of cats that test positive for serum ELISA but test negative for tear or saliva IFA and about the possibility of intermittent virus shedding.

Although not the ideal screening test under certain circumstances, tear testing offers some advantages as a screening test under certain circumstances that may outweigh its relative lack of sensitivity. Many catteries are reluctant to bring all their cats to the veterinarian for annual FeLV testing because of logistic and economic reasons. Tears can be collected in the home by nonprofessionals, and the strips are stable after drying for up to 1 week. Therefore, specimens can be collected at a cattery site and can be carried or mailed to the veterinarian or laboratory for assay. The ease and inexpensiveness of this procedure may allow some catteries to perform regular FeLV testing of their cats. It is likely that if infection exists within a cattery it will be detected by testing all cats annually with alternative methods, since catteries that have FeLV tend to have a high percentage of FeLV-positive cats. Repeated negative testing of all cats makes the likelihood of active disease within a cattery very small. If FeLV is detected by a positive tear test in any one of a cattery's cats, the necessity of a rigorous test and elimination program based on traditional testing methods should be obvious.

References and Supplemental Reading

Hawkins, E. C., Johnson, L., Pedersen, N. C., et al.: Use of tears for diagnosis of feline leukemia virus infection. J.A.V.M.A. 188:1031, 1986.
Jarrett, O.: Recent advances in the epidemiology of feline leukemia virus. Vet. Ann. 23:287, 1983.
Jarrett, O., Golder, M. C., and Stewart, M. F.: Detection of transient and persistent feline leukemia virus infections. Vet. Rec. 110:225, 1982.
Lutz, H., and Jarrett, O.: Detection of feline leukemia virus in saliva. J. Clin. Microbiol. 25:827, 1987.
Lutz, H., and Pedersen, N. C.: Immunodiagnosis of feline leukemia virus infection. *In* Kirk, R. W. (ed.): *Current Veterinary Therapy IX.* Philadelphia: W. B. Saunders Co., 1986, pp. 448–452.
Lutz, H., Pedersen, N. C., and Thielen, G. H.: Course of feline leukemia virus infection and its detection by enzyme-linked immunosorbent assay and monoclonal antibodies. Am. J. Vet. Res. 44:2054, 1983.
Rojko, J. L., Hoover, E. A., Mathes, L. E., et al.: Pathogenesis of experimental feline leukemia virus infection. J. Nat. Cancer Inst. 63:759, 1979.

MANAGEMENT OF THE FeLV-POSITIVE PATIENT

DENNIS W. MACY, D.V.M.

Fort Collins, Colorado

The feline leukemia virus (FeLV) along with its associated diseases is the number one infectious cause of morbidity and mortality in cats. The management of feline patients persistently infected with the feline leukemia virus is largely based on opinion, is often controversial, and requires clinicians to be prepared to address five issues:

1. Determination of the type of FeLV infection.
2. Providing the client with the appropriate prognosis, based on the type of infection and disease that is present.
3. Instituting appropriate medical management for the disease or diseases associated with the infection.
4. Making management recommendations to the owners to prevent the spread of the virus to noninfected cats.
5. Giving opinions on public health considerations in managing FeLV positive cats.

TYPES OF FELINE LEUKEMIA INFECTION

Following exposure to the feline leukemia virus, it is estimated that as many as 30 per cent of cats become persistently viremic. Of the remaining 70 per cent, 40 per cent develop immunity after transient infections, and 30 per cent are insufficiently exposed either to develop immunity or to become infected and, thus, remain susceptible to the virus. New evidence indicates that many exposed cats might be latent carriers of FeLV and test negative for circulating virus antigen but have sequestered virus present in their bone marrow. Latently infected cats might inappropriately be placed into immune or susceptible categories. The duration of viral latency has not been firmly established, but viral latency may last several months to possibly, years. Following glucocorticoid therapy or possibly stress, latently infected cats may become persistently viremic. Since FeLV latency cannot be routinely evaluated, uncertainty has been raised about the ability of routine ELISA tests to establish the presence of virus in all cats. The recognition of a viral latency category may explain how the isolated

apartment cat that tested negative for years may suddenly test positive.

CONFIRMATION OF FeLV INFECTIONS

There are four types of tests for evaluating cats for evidence of FeLV exposure. The first two, IFA (immunofluorescent antibody) and ELISA (enzyme-linked immunosorbent assay) detect antigen. The second two include antibody detection by various methods and bone marrow culture to detect viral antigen. Viral latency is a state in which virus is integrated into the host genome but is not replicating and cannot be detected by ELISA or IFA. The detection of virus latency requires bone marrow culturing techniques, usually in the presence of glucocorticoids or neonatal kitten macrophages, and is technically difficult and not available to the practitioner.

Both IFA tests and ELISAs for FeLV detect the presence of the viral protein p27. IFA is the first test developed for FeLV detection and identifies p27 in circulating infected white blood cells and platelets. The required sample for IFA evaluation is a thin blood film or a thin buffy coat smear, the latter being preferable in the leukopenic patient. The principal advantage of the IFA test is the good correlation with viremia and virus shedding (97 per cent). Its disadvantages include the facts that (1) the test must be performed in a commercial reference laboratory, which means that results may not be immediately available; (2) false-positive results may occur as a result of thick smears, platelet clumping, or the presence of eosinophilia; and (3) false-negative results may occur because of leukopenia or thrombocytopenia. IFA-positive cats generally remain positive for life. Only 3 per cent become negative over a period of time. Clinicians should be aware that cats undergoing transient infections may become IFA-positive for several weeks before they eliminate the virus.

ELISA is the most commonly used procedure in clinical practice for detecting FeLV. The ELISA test detects soluble p27 viral antigen in body fluids. The most frequently evaluated sample is blood, but serum, tears, and saliva may also be used. ELISA is more sensitive than IFA testing, is seldom associated with false-negative results, and may detect infections up to 5 weeks sooner than the IFA procedure. The disadvantages of ELISA include the subjectivity associated with a colorimetric procedure and the technical errors that may result in false-positive results. Weak color changes may result from technical error and the presence of antimurine antibodies. The antimurine antibodies associated with false-positive results can be eliminated by the CITE procedure (Agritech, Portland, ME), which contains an internal control that indicates the presence of antimurine antibodies, or by preincubation with murine antigen (Virachek [Synbiotic, San Diego, CA]).

The results of any of these ELISAs may not always correlate with persistent viremia. Five to 30 per cent of cats with positive ELISA results may not be viremic but, instead, may have local infections in regional lymph nodes or mammary or salivary tissue that shed enough viral p27 antigen to produce a positive colorimetric reaction when blood or serum is assayed. Positive ELISA results indicate that the cat harbors replicating virus but do not necessarily mean that the cat is viremic. Because ELISA findings may be falsely positive or may be discordant with IFA results, positive ELISA results in otherwise healthy cats (or weakly positive results) should be evaluated for IFA to confirm shedding of the virus. A negative IFA result indicates that the cat is not viremic at the time of the test, is not shedding the virus, and, thus, is not contagious. However, a cat with negative IFA results may have positive ELISA results. Cats with this pattern of test results are frequently referred to as discordant. Cats may be transiently discordant or persistently discordant. Fifty per cent of the discordant cats have negative findings on both ELISA and IFA testing, and 50 per cent remain discordant over a long period of time. Persistently discordant cats may be potential immune carriers, sequestering the virus in regional lymph nodes or other tissue. The feline immunodeficiency virus (FIV) causes many clinical manifestations similar to those of FeLV. Thus, practitioners should test for FeTLV in sick cats that exhibit FeLV-like clinical signs and have been found negative for FeLV by available methods. The rate of concurrent (FIV) and FeLV infections is unknown.

Depending on the test used, antibody testing may be of short-term prognostic value. However, antibody levels tend to decrease if not restimulated; thus, these levels do not provide a basis for long-term prognosis. Results of the indirect membrane immunofluorescent (IMI) assay for antibody to FOCMA and FeLV group C, gp 70-related antigens are of the highest prognostic value. Depending on the laboratory, titers of 1:4 to 1:32 are considered protective against tumor development. A high antibody titer in an unvaccinated cat with negative ELISA results is suggestive of virus latency or continual exposure to an FeLV-positive cat.

THERAPY FOR FeLV VIREMIA

Passive Immunotherapy

There is no effective means of clearing established FeLV infection with passive antibody therapy. Antibodies from immune cats (passive immunotherapy) are effective in eliminating infections only when they are administered prior to the establishment of infection in the bone marrow. Kittens born to FeLV-immune queens receive protection from the colostric antibodies, but maternal colostric antibodies should be expected to wane by 6 to 12 weeks of age. However, the administration of serum from FeLV-immune cats may induce complete or partial remission or prolonged remission in cats receiving chemotherapy for lymphoma, without altering virus status.

Biological Response Modifiers, Immunoabsorption, and Transplantation

The use of nonspecific immune stimulants such as levamisole has not been shown to be effective in reversing viremia. Blood constituents have been shown to have antitumor effects in a variety of species. The active constituent appears to be a tissue plasma protein called fibronectin, and its antitumor activity appears to be associated with macrophage activation. Fibronectin administered six times every 2 weeks to cats with lymphosarcoma resulted in a complete or partial remission rate of 38 per cent (Hayes et al., 1980). Extracorporeal immunoabsorption therapy removes circulating immune complexes that may act as blocking factors to normal tumoricidal or viral responses. The results of extracorporeal immunoabsorptions have been nonuniform, although complete remission and reversal of viremia have been reported in infected cats. Recently, bone marrow transplantation using a combination of whole body radiation and immune donors has resulted in reversal of viremia in four of seven cats with established experimental FeLV infections. Although a promising development, bone marrow transplantation requires specialized facilities and equipment and is not widely available.

Antiviral Drugs

Most antiviral drugs for retrovirus act by inhibiting reverse transcriptase; several antiviral drugs have been evaluated in cats with FeLV infections.

Suramin has been shown to inhibit FeLV replication in tissue culture. It is unfortunate that suramin has failed to be effective in preventing FeLV infections or in reversing established FeLV infections and has significant toxicity in the cat. Zidovudine (Retrovir, Burroughs Wellcome) (formerly AZT) has been shown to be more effective than suramin in FeLV infections but is expensive and has a time limitation (Traveres et al., 1987). If cats are administered 10 to 20 mg/kg AZT in the first 14 to 21 days after exposure to FeLV for six weeks, they are protected from bone marrow infections and persistent viremia. However, administration of AZT to cats with established FeLV infections has failed to reverse viremia but reduces the amount of p27 in infected leukocytes.

ASSOCIATED INFECTIONS

Cats persistently infected with FeLV have a fivefold increase in secondary infections such as bacterial stomatitis, abscesses, pyothorax, upper respiratory infections, feline infectious peritonitis, toxoplasmosis, haemobartonellosis, and cryptococcosis. Any cat presented with a history of chronic infection should be evaluated for FeLV and FIV. Secondary infections may be seen with or without anemia or leukopenia. The immunosuppressive effects of the feline leukemia virus are seen in virtually all parts of the immune system. *In vitro* lymphocyte blastogenesis assays may be depressed as much as 90 per cent from normal levels in infected cats, although there may be a long preclinical period before significant changes are detectable. Leukopenic cats frequently have atrophied thymuses and defects in neutrophil and macrophage functions. FeLV-infected cats have defects in humoral immunity, characterized by delayed or suboptimal transition from an IgM to an IgG antibody response. Although many of the alterations in the immune system have been attributed to the viral envelope protein p15e, the mechanisms of others are unknown. The *in vitro* immunosuppressive effects of p15e have been shown to be blocked in part by the use of nonsteroidal anti-inflammatory agents. The safety and the dose of these agents, in order to block the effects of p15e *in vivo*, have yet to be established. Although FeLV-negative cats may resolve many infections with or without therapy, FeLV-positive cats tend to fail to limit or resolve even minimal bacterial, fungal, or protozoal invasions and require early aggressive and often prolonged prophylactic treatment for these opportunistic infections in order to survive. Upper respiratory viral infections may be exacerbated as a result of FeLV infections. Rhinotracheitis frequently results in destruction of the turbinates and normal respiratory defense mechanisms, leading to

secondary bacterial rhinitis. These severe infections are characterized by the presence of marked tissue necrosis and anaerobic bacterial proliferation, which may account for their poor response to systemic antibiotic therapy. Topical 2 per cent chloramphenicol concentration in a fluocinolone acetonide–dimethyl sulfoxide solution (Synotic Syntex) applied to both nostrils twice a day, is useful in the management of chronic rhinitis in FeLV-infected cats. Orally administered metronidazole (Flagyl, Searle), which diffuses well into necrotic tissues and is effective against anaerobes, may also be useful. Clinicians should be aware that some animals develop hepatotoxicity, diarrhea, anorexia, and reversible cerebellar or vestibular toxicities associated with metronidazole therapy.

Seventy-five per cent of feline cryptococcosis cases are associated with persistent FeLV infections. *Cryptococcus* infections are characterized most frequently by nasal granuloma formation in the cat, but *cryptococcus* may also infect a wide variety of other tissues, including the lungs. Ketoconazole, 10 mg/kg divided b.i.d. daily for 2 to 3 months, is well tolerated by most cats and is effective in eliminating the infection. However, thereafter, long-term, low intermittent administration of ketoconazole may be required to prevent recurrence. CNS infections with *Cryptococcus* pose a special challenge because of the blood-brain barrier. A combination of flucytosine (150 mg/kg divided t.i.d.) with amphotericin B (0.25 mg/kg every other day), for an accumulative dose of 4 mg/kg, helps prevent development of resistant strains that frequently develop with the use of flucytosine alone, and provides adequate antifungal levels in the CSF. Alternately, high-dose ketaconazole, 40 mg/kg divided b.i.d., provides adequate antifungal CSF levels but may be associated with increased risk of hepatotoxicity (see p. 1103).

Toxoplasmosis in cats is frequently associated with persistent FeLV infections. Diagnosis of this disease is usually made by biopsy. Treatment includes sulfonamides and pyrimethamine or clindamycin (see p. 1114).

Stomatitis and gingivitis are often seen in cats with FeLV and may be associated with autoimmune plasmocytic lymphocytic infiltration or chronic calicivirus infections, with or without secondary anaerobic bacterial infections. FeLV-associated stomatitis is treated with supportive therapy, including a good anaerobic antimicrobial such as clindamycin or metronidazole, or topical application of 2 per cent chloramphenicol and Synotic preparation on infected tissues. Topical therapy frequently reduces the swelling and pain associated with this condition and allows the animal to eat. Cats with lymphocytic plasmacytic infiltration sometimes respond to a combination of oral prednisolone, 2.2 mg/kg/day, and azathioprine, 1.1 mg/kg PO every other day. Gold salt therapy was also reported to be effective in chronic gingivitis.

FEVER

Whether FeLV alone causes fever is controversial. However, it has been the author's observation that FeLV may induce fevers that are not associated with obvious secondary infections. A fever may be a positive sign following exposure to FeLV, in that the author has observed that experimentally infected cats that develop fevers following bone marrow transplantation are more likely to eliminate the virus than are cats that become persistently infected. Enhanced release of the endogenous pyrogen interleukin-1 from infected macrophages may be the mechanism for some of the observed fevers in FeLV-infected cats. Antibiotics should be administered if there is doubt as to the cause of the fever episode. The use of antipyretics in FeLV-positive cats is questionable and may actually be contraindicated.

CACHEXIA ASSOCIATED WITH FeLV INFECTION

Many cats persistently infected with FeLV develop a rough hair coat and have an unthrifty appearance. This general "poor doer" condition may last for several years and frequently progresses to a cachexic state despite normal caloric intake. Although the exact mechanism of the FeLV-associated cachexia is unknown, it may be associated with the monokines (tumor necrosis factor) cachectin, which may be released from FeLV-infected monocytes. Tumor necrosis factor is known to be a potent catabolic agent. In anorexic cats or cats with poor appetites, diazepam (Valium, Roche) 0.2 mg/kg IV frequently temporarily induces feeding, usually within seconds. Oxazepam (Serax, Wyeth) 2.5 mg orally usually induces feeding in 20 min in anorexic cats. It is unfortunate that the appetite-stimulating properties of benzadiazepine derivatives appear to wane after repeated dosage in sick cats. Nasogastric tubes or gastrostomy tubes may be necessary to provide nutritional requirements for these cats. Anabolic steroids are often helpful in more prolonged stimulation of appetite and are of more value in appetite stimulation than in correcting the anemias for which they are frequently prescribed in cats with this disease.

HEMATOLOGIC ABNORMALITIES

Anemia

Seventy-five per cent of all anemic cats carry FeLV. Ten per cent of the FeLV-associated anemias

are hemolytic and regenerative in character. The hemolytic processes thought to be associated with immunosuppression are associated with FeLV subgroup A infections. Immunosuppression associated with this subgroup is thought to facilitate haemobartonellosis and to predispose cats to anemias that yield positive Coombs's test results. Although the exact mechanism of the latter is unknown, FeLV is known to alter red blood cell membranes, and antibodies to red blood cell membranes have been described in cats that carry FeLV.

Hemolytic anemias may be transient or progressive in these cats. Transfusions should be avoided until the packed cell volume (PCV) drops to 10 per cent or below. To take advantage of any potential therapeutic effects of passive immunotherapy, blood donors should be vaccinated for FeLV (Leukocell, Norden).

Haemobartonella may be effectively treated with oxytetracycline, 20 mg/kg t.i.d., or longer-acting doxycycline, 1 mg/kg b.i.d. for 21 days. Immune-mediated hemolytic anemias should be treated with prednisone, 2.2 mg/kg per day, and in more resistant cases, with azathioprine (Imuran, Burroughs Wellcome) 0.5 to 1 mg/kg every other day. Nonregenerative anemias may occur secondary to myeloproliferative disease, medullary fibrosis, or osteosclerosis. Myeloproliferative disease is frequently associated with FeLV subgroup B. Bone marrow evaluation is usually characterized by a hypercellular response, which may be associated with megaloblastic changes. The anemia is unresponsive to hematinics, vitamin B_{12}, or folic acid. Temporary clinical improvement may be seen with blood transfusions. However, duration of clinical improvement becomes shorter with each transfusion. Erythroid aplasia (pure red blood cell aplasia) and aplastic anemia are the most frequent types of anemia associated with FeLV infections and are thought to be caused by FeLV subgroup C. Cats affected with aplastic anemia are frequently young (2 to 3 years of age). The anemia is characterized by destruction of erythroid precursors and relative unresponsiveness of the remaining bone marrow elements. The unresponsiveness of the bone marrow is associated with serum erythropoietin concentrations, which are normal or elevated. The anemia is usually characterized as normocytic to macrocytic and normochromic. Although there are anisocytotic and macrocytotic changes, there is an absence of polychromasia. Bone marrow rubricytes and rubriblasts may be megaloblastic, and myeloid to erythroid ratios are frequently abnormal. Similar to the anemias found with myeloproliferative disease, anemias associated with erythroid aplasia are unresponsive to hematinics, vitamin B_{12}, or folic acid. Theoretically, glucocorticoids and immunosuppressive agents such as cyclosporine and cyclophosphamide should be useful, but experimental evidence suggests that they are not helpful in the treatment of this form of anemia in infected cats. Supportive blood transfusions are the most valued means of managing these cats.

Neutropenia

Another hematologic abnormality associated with FeLV is neutropenia. The proliferation of some strains of FeLV in myeloid precursors is possibly cytopathic and may be the mechanism responsible for the observed neutropenias. Neutropenia may follow a stressful episode in both viremic and latently infected cats and may be transient, persistent, or cyclic. Neutropenias associated with FeLV should be considered preneoplastic; some neutropenic cats progress to myeloproliferative disease or aplastic anemia. Glucocorticoids (2 mg/kg PO) may result in normalization of peripheral neutrophil counts by causing premature release of neutrophils from the maturation pool in the bone marrow but may impair the neutrophils' normal phagocytic ability. Bacterial infections are frequently seen in neutropenic patients, and cats should be monitored closely for infection and treated properly when the disease condition develops. If prophylactic antibiotics are to be used, trimethoprim sulfa is a good choice (33 mg/kg divided dose). FeLV-associated neutropenias may also be associated with signs of diarrhea, which may mimic panleukopenia caused by parvovirus infections in cats. Cats with panleukopenia can be differentiated from cats with neutropenia associated with FeLV in that they usually have a more chronic clinical course and have a history of vaccination against panleukopenia. Because the enteritis is associated with destruction of the normal intestinal barrier, these cats are highly susceptible to gram-negative septicemia. Patients with a panleukopenialike syndrome associated with FeLV need to be treated aggressively with parenteral fluids, gentamicin, 2 mg/kg/t.i.d., and a combination of amoxicillin and clavulanic acid, 14 mg/kg/b.i.d.

Thrombocytopenia

Thrombocytopenia may also be observed in cats infected with FeLV. Megakaryocytes are persistently infected in viremic cats. Thrombocytic half-life is subsequently reduced, which may be one reason for the macrocytic platelets observed in these cats. Despite the presence of absolute thrombocytopenia, the presence of bleeding is infrequently observed clinically.

ABORTION AND INFERTILITY

Abortion and infertility have been associated with FeLV infections. Reproductive failure in cats is observed most frequently as infertility and occasionally as abortion. Between 60 and 70 per cent of queens with infertility problems carry FeLV, although other viruses such as FIV have also been incriminated. FeLV-related abortions are most frequently observed in the second trimester. The mechanism is unknown but may be associated with FeLV tropism from rapidly growing cells in the placenta or neonate. In the absence of an effective antiviral agent, a test and removal program is the best means of controlling abortion and infertility problems associated with FeLV infections in catteries.

GLOMERULONEPHRITIS

The persistent antigenemia associated with FeLV infection is thought to be responsible for the high incidence of glomerulonephritis associated with persistent FeLV infections. More than 70 per cent of cats with evidence of glomerulonephritis have persistent FeLV infections. It is fortunate that most glomerulopathies associated with FeLV are subclinical, although, occasionally, nephrotic syndrome will develop. The mechanism of the glomerulonephritis appears to be associated with IgG production against FeLV-related antigens and antigens related to FOCMA/FeLV group C.

Extracorporeal immunoabsorption, which is effective in removing antibody-antigen complexes associated with FeLV, would seem to be the ideal treatment, but it is not practical in most situations. The use of immunosuppressive therapy to block antibody production is a double-edged sword in an already immunocompromised patient. Management of the nephrotic syndrome is similar to that used in patients with glomerulopathies caused by other etiologies.

POLYARTHRITIS

FeLV immune complexes have been associated with chronic progressive polyarthritis in both young and old cats. In young cats, the disease is characterized by fibrous ankylosing arthritis, and in older cats by lymphocytic and plasmacytic synovitis. Affected cats are infected with both FeLV and feline syncytium-forming virus (FeSFV). Prednisone, 2 mg/kg per day, and azathioprine 1 mg/kg every other day, may be helpful in reducing the clinical signs associated with these conditions.

NEUROLOGIC DISEASE

A variety of neurologic signs have been associated with persistent FeLV infections, without obvious tumor infiltration or impingement. Alternating anisocoria, spastic pupil syndrome, urinary incontinence, and progressive rear leg weakness are most frequently observed. FeLV infects cells of the central nervous system and is believed to be responsible for these signs. FIV has also been associated with a variety of neurologic signs and cats may need to be tested for FIV as well as FeLV. No effective therapy has been reported for neurologic abnormalities associated with FeLV.

OSTEOCHONDROMATOSIS

Osteochondromatosis, or multiple cartilaginous exostosis, associated with FeLV occurs in adult cats. Lesions are most frequently seen in flat bones. The exact role that FeLV plays in the pathogenesis of osteochondromatosis is not known. Surgical removal will not prevent recurrence of the lesions or prevent development in other sites. This disease differs from osteochondromatosis in other animals in that it develops in adult animals after epiphyseal closures.

FADING KITTEN SYNDROME

New kittens affected with FeLV frequently develop what is termed fading kitten syndrome, which is characterized by marked lethargy, poor hair coat, cachectic body state, secondary infections, and death, usually within 20 weeks of birth. Necropsy findings are distinguished by marked thymus atrophy. Therapeutic intervention in these young kittens is usually unrewarding. Testing and removal of cats with positive results should be the principal means of management of this disease in catteries.

LYMPHADENOPATHY IN YOUNG CATS

Distinctive lymphadenopathy of young cats (distinctive peripheral lymph node hyperplasia) has been recently reported in cats younger than 2 years of age (Moore et al., 1986). Many of these affected cats are otherwise clinically normal, whereas others show nonspecific signs such as fever, lethargy, anorexia, and hepatomegaly. Lymphadenopathy does not result from neoplastic proliferation but, rather, from lymphoid hyperplasia in response to the persistent FeLV infection. In most affected cats, the lymphadenopathy resolves in 30 days without therapy. Antibiotic and glucocorticoid therapy may have utility in resolving the lymphadenopathy, although some infections *are* resistant to therapy. Cats with distinctive lymphadenopathy are at risk of developing lymphosarcoma. Distinctive lymphadenopathy of young cats is thought to be similar to the pre-AIDS lymphadenopathy observed in humans affected with human immunodeficiency virus (HIV).

LYMPHOSARCOMA

Seventy per cent of cases of lymphosarcoma in cats are associated with FeLV. Combination chemotherapy is considered to be superior to single-drug therapy in the management of lymphosarcoma. Several combinations of drug regimens using vincristine, cyclophosphamide, and prednisone have been used for the management of these diseases. Cyclophosphamide is supplied in 25- and 50-mg tablets and is administered in a dose of 2.2 mg/kg for 4 consecutive days each week. The principal toxicity is myelosuppressive, which usually peaks at 7 to 10 days. Cystitis, although common in dogs treated with this drug, is rarely seen in cats. Cyclophosphamide should be withheld when neutropenia is below 1000 cells/ml. Prednisone or prednisolone is given daily in a dose of 2 mg/kg. Cats are more resistant to the adverse effects of glucocorticoids than are dogs and tolerate higher doses for more prolonged periods. Vincristine is supplied in 1-mg vials and is given intravenously (0.75 mg/m^2) once weekly for two to three consecutive treatments and then often is reduced to once every 3 to 4 weeks thereafter. This drug is a vesicant and causes sloughing when it is deposited outside the vein. Neurotoxicities are rare in cats, and the drug is considered nonmyelosuppressive. All antineoplastic drug therapies should be continued until relapses are seen.

LYMPHOID LEUKEMIA

Lymphoid leukemia carries a poor prognosis and a 27 per cent remission rate, as opposed to solid lymphoid tumors in other locations. This may be due in part to the severe anemia and pancytopenia that frequently accompany lymphoid leukemias. Blood transfusions should be given to severely anemic cats (PCVs below 10 per cent).

PROGNOSIS

The prognosis in cats carrying FeLV varies, depending on the testing pattern, the strain of virus, and the type of disease that develops. In general, the distribution of diseases that develop following FeLV infections includes 50 per cent immunosuppressive, 25 per cent anemias, 10 per cent FeLV-associated (such as feline infectious peritonitis [FIP]), and 5 per cent lymphomas. These percentages are approximate and vary, depending on the strain(s) of the virus in a particular geographic location. Of the persistently viremic cats, as determined by IFA, 83 per cent will die within 3½ years, and only 16 per cent of the non–FeLV-positive cats will die in the same time period. Persistently discordant cats (ELISA-positive/IFA-negative) are at less risk, and 50 per cent may be expected to develop disease. However, it is estimated that only 10 per cent of the latently infected cats can be expected to develop FeLV-related disease. Only the cats that totally eliminate all forms of the virus infection following exposure may be considered to have no risk associated with FeLV exposure. Untreated cats with lymphosarcoma usually die within 1 to 2 months. Although lymphosarcoma is not a curable disease, complete remission can be obtained in 80 per cent of these cats, with a median survival time of 5 months. Anatomic sites influence expected remission rates (mediastinal, 92 per cent; alimentary, 82 per cent; multicentric, 100 per cent; leukemic, 27 per cent; and extranodal, 50 per cent). One in four cats may have lengthy remission periods of a year or longer. The prognosis in individual cases is adversely affected by the degree of debilitation and the severity of hematologic abnormalities (e.g., leukopenia, anemia, thrombocytopenia). Thirty per cent of lymphosarcomas are negative for FeLV, and histologic classification of the tumor does not appear to significantly alter the prognosis in the management of cats with lymphosarcoma.

PREVENTION OF FeLV

In the ideal situation, FeLV-positive cats would be quarantined and would not be allowed outside, where they can come in contact with other cats. As a result of contact outdoors with other cats, viremic felines may spread FeLV to contact cats, may develop life-threatening abscesses from fighting, or may contract debilitating contagious diseases, such as rhinotracheitis. In multiple-cat households, testing and removal remain the best protection against this disease. In the testing and removal management system, cats are tested every 3 months, and cats with positive results are immediately removed. When all cats in the household have had two consecutive negative tests, the household may be classified as FeLV-free. All new cats to be introduced into the household should be quarantined for a period of three months and should have negative results after two FeLV tests. The testing and removal system has been shown to reduce the infection rate from 19 per cent to less than 1 per cent when it is followed. Although the system is effective in reducing the FeLV infection rate, it is not foolproof. Neither the ELISA nor the IFA test is sensitive enough to pick up latently infected cats that may pass through the quarantine procedure

and later have recrudescence of the infection as a result of stress or glucocorticoid administration.

VACCINATION

Since 1985 there has been a USDA-approved, commercially available FeLV vaccine (Leukocell, Norden). Although the efficacy of this vaccine has been challenged by some, it remains the only available product for FeLV immunoprophylaxis at this time (see p. 1052 for viewpoints of FeLV vaccination).

Since cats younger than 1 year of age are the most susceptible to FeLV infection and there is an increased exposure with age, vaccine programs should be targeted at, but not limited to, kittens and young cats. Prevaccination testing for FeLV is ideal, and a combination of FeLV vaccination and a testing-and-removal program is the best possible means of controlling the disease. However, prevaccination testing should not be considered mandatory. Mandatory testing of single-cat households with no known previous exposure to FeLV is questionable because of (1) the cost associated with the testing, (2) the test's limited ability to identify latently infected cats, (3) the lack of documented harm in vaccinating cats with positive results, and (4) the low yield of cats with positive results (1 to 9 per cent) in the general population. However, in multiple-cat households (where the infection rate is frequently 30 per cent or higher) or in cats known to have previous exposure to FeLV, prevaccination testing is cost-effective and should be recommended. Because persistently viremic cats may be immunosuppressed, they should not receive modified live-virus rabies vaccine.

PUBLIC HEALTH CONSIDERATIONS

Controversy still exists regarding public health aspects of FeLV infections. In the natural setting, most retroviruses are considered species-specific, although there is laboratory evidence that FeLV can produce lymphosarcoma in neonatal puppies under experimental situations and that some subgroups of FeLV replicate in human tissue lines *in vitro*. It is fortunate that FeLV is readily inactivated by human complement. However, humans with low complement levels may be theoretically at risk. Young children and patients with various neoplastic or immune-mediated diseases generally have low complement levels.

Despite these theoretical concerns, in more than a decade and a half of investigation there is no conclusive evidence that FeLV has caused disease in a single human. Yet, with the contradictory serologic data, hypothetical situations, and natural history of some retroviruses infecting alternate hosts, the possibility of this virus eventually infecting a human cannot be eliminated. Given the scientific uncertainties regarding this issue, one can either strongly condone or deny an owner's wish for euthanasia of an FeLV-positive cat, based on public health considerations as we know them today. However, if euthanasia is to be considered, an IFA test should be performed to confirm that the cat is, in fact, probably persistently infected.

References and Suggested Reading

Boyce, J. T., Kociba, G. J., Jacobs, R. M., et al.: Feline leukemia virus–induced thrombocytopenia and macrothrombocytosis in cats. Vet. Pathol. 23:16, 1986.

Essex, M., Cotter, S. M., Sliski, A. H., et al.: Horizontal transmission of feline leukaemia under natural conditions in a feline leukaemia cluster household. Int. J. Cancer 19:90, 1977.

Haley, P. J., Hoover, E. A., Quackenbush, S. L., et al.: Influence of antibody infusion on pathogenesis of experimental feline leukemia virus infection. J. Nat. Cancer Inst. 74:889, 1985.

Hayes, A. A., MacEwen, E. G., Matus, R. E., et al.: Antileukemic activity of plasma cryoprecipitate therapy in the cat. Dev. Cancer Res. 4:245, 1980.

Hoover, E. A., Kociba, G. J., Hardy, W. D., Jr., et al.: Erythroid hypoplasia in cats inoculated with feline leukemia virus. J. Nat. Cancer Inst. 53:1271, 1974.

Kociba, G. J.: Hematologic consequences of feline leukemia virus infection. In Kirk, R. W. (ed.): Current Veterinary Therapy VIII. Philadelphia: W. B. Saunders Co., 1986, pp. 488–490.

Kociba, G. J., Lange, R. D., Dunn, C. D., et al.: Serum erythropoietin changes in cats with feline leukemia virus–induced erythroid aplasia. Vet. Pathol. 20:548, 1983.

Lewis, M. G., Fertel, R. H., and Olsen, R. G.: Reversal of feline retroviral suppression by indomethacin. Leuk. Res. 9:1451, 1985.

Lutz, H., Pedersen, N. C., and Theilen, G. H.: Course of feline leukemia virus infection and its detection by enzyme-linked immunosorbent assay and monoclonal antibodies. Am. J. Vet. Res. 44:2054, 1983.

Madewell, B. R., and Jarrett, O.: Recovery of feline leukemia virus from non-viremic cats. Vet. Rec. 112:339, 1983.

Moore, F. M., Emerson, W. E., and Cotter, S. M., et al.: Distinctive peripheral lymph node hyperplasia of young cats. Vet. Pathol. 23:386, 1986.

Rojko, J. L., Hoover, E. A., and Mathes, L. E., et al.: Influence of adrenal corticosteroids on the susceptibility of cats to feline leukemia virus infection. Cancer Res. 39:3789, 1979.

Rojko, J. L., Hoover, E. A., Quackenbush, S. L., et al.: Reactivation of latent feline leukaemia virus infection. Nature 298:385, 1982.

Swenson, C., Kociba, G. J., O'Keefe, D., et al.: Cyclic hematopoiesis in feline leukemia virus–infected cats. J.A.V.M.A. 191:93, 1987.

Travares, L., Rasker, C., Johnson, K., et al.: 3'-Azido-3-deoxythymidine in feline leukemia virus infected cats: A model for therapy and prophylaxis of AIDS. Cancer Res. 47:3190, 1987.

CLINICAL SIGNIFICANCE OF ANTIGENIC VARIATION IN CANINE PARVOVIRUS

LELAND E. CARMICHAEL, D.V.M.,
and COLIN R. PARRISH, Ph.D.

Ithaca, New York

Antigenic and genomic analyses of canine parvovirus (CPV) isolates from the United States, Europe, Australia, and Japan collected since 1978 reveal that viruses circulating after 1980 were, in many cases, different from the earlier isolates. The newer virus type is now the most prevalent one in the world dog population. Analysis of viruses isolated between 1978 and 1987 with monoclonal antibodies (MAbs) reveal two distinct antigenic types of CPV. Some MAbs reacted only with the "old" (1978–79) type, some were specific for the post-1980 type, and several others reacted equally well with both viruses. Both viruses are neutralized equally by sera from dogs immunized with the earlier strains, but sera from dogs with the variant CPV neutralizes the post-1980 types to a somewhat greater (approximately two- to three fold) extent.

The DNAs from wild-type, pre-1980 viruses and the antigenically variant post-1980 isolates from widely different geographic locations also differed in their restriction enzyme digestion profiles. There was remarkable homogeneity in the restriction enzyme digestion patterns ("DNA fingerprints") of the earlier viruses; however, the viral DNAs of the post-1980 viruses, though similar to the earlier isolates, have restriction site differences.

It is theorized that the CPVs now most commonly isolated (> 95 per cent of recent isolates) from dogs arose naturally around 1980 from a single variant virus. The new type has gradually replaced the original strain. The epidemiologic significance of these findings is not yet fully known, but the appearance of a variant virus that seems to have largely replaced the original virus in the global canine population suggests a remarkable selective advantage of the new CPV type over the original virus. Similar variation was observed with mink enteritis parvovirus (MEV), where three antigenically and genomically variant types were observed among stored MEV isolates obtained over a 30-year period. Cross-protection tests with the mink viruses showed that inactivated vaccines protected equally against the homologous and the variant forms of MEV.

Preliminary data suggest that the recent CPV types are more virulent; viral titers in the feces of infected dogs are generally higher than those of dogs infected with the original virus. Also, the incubation period seems to be shorter with the variant CPV—around 4 to 5 days rather than 6 to 8 days. In recent studies done in the authors' laboratory, severe hemorrhagic enteritis developed in specific pathogen free (SPF) beagles following oral infection with a 1984 isolate, signs that had not been observed in experiments with original isolates. Beagle puppies given relatively low doses of a recent (variant) isolate did not die but, after an incubation period of 4 to 5 days, exhibited signs including marked depression or collapse, diarrhea, anorexia, lymphopenia, and substantial weight loss. The sudden collapse, resembling shock, was unexpected, but further studies are required to define the comparative virulence of the viruses.

Since virtually all commercial CPV vaccines are produced from the 1978–79 isolates or from the heterologous feline panleukopenia virus (FPV), the question has often been asked whether the current vaccines protect against the more recent CPV isolates. This question has been tested by experiments in the authors' laboratories using inactivated CPV vaccine, live homologous (CPV) vaccine, and an experimental recombinant vaccine. The experimental recombinant vaccine consisted of noninfectious CPV empty virions (capsids) produced in murine cells transformed by a bovine papilloma virus DNA vector that contained the complete CPV capsid gene. Others (Dees et al., 1985) have obtained similar results with a commercial inactivated FPV vaccine. In all instances, the genomic and antigenic changes in post-1980 CPV appeared to be of no practical significance with respect to vaccination success. Existing CPV vaccines of proven efficacy protect susceptible dogs efficiently against both types of virus, and other explanations (e.g., interference by inhibiting levels of maternal antibodies) must be sought for immunization failures.

References and Supplemental Reading

Appel, M. J. G., and Carmichael, L. E.: Protection of pups with a commercial vaccine against a recent field isolate of canine parvovirus. Vet. Med. Small Anim. Clin. Oct. 1987, p. 1091.
Carmichael, L. E., and Binn, L. N.: New enteric viruses in the dog. Adv. Vet. Sci. Comp. Med. 25:1, 1981.
Dees, C., Stroh, S., and Bartkoski, M.: Post-1980 canine parvovirus: Immunodiagnosis and vaccination procedures. Abstract (#72) from Conference of Research Workers in Animal Diseases, Chicago, IL, 1985.
Parrish, C. R., O'Connell, P. H., Evermann, J. F., et al.: Natural variation of canine parvovirus. Science 230:1046, 1985.
Parrish, C. R., Gorham, J. R., Schwartz, T. M., et al.: Characterization of antigenic variation among mink enteritis virus isolates. Am. J. Vet. Res. 45:2591, 1984.
Parrish, C. R., Have, P., Foreyt, W. J., et al.: The global spread and replacement of canine parvovirus strains. J. Gen. Virol. 69:1111, 1988.

BACTEREMIA IN DOGS AND CATS

STEVEN W. DOW, D.V.M., M.S.
Fort Collins, Colorado

Although generally considered a very serious event, bacterial invasion of the bloodstream actually occurs often but is rarely of consequence in the healthy individual. Host defenses must be severely compromised for overwhelming bacteremia to develop, usually as a consequence of either an underlying disease or surgical or medical intervention. When bacteremia does develop, the severity of the animal's predisposing illness is the single most important factor influencing survival. Death from bacteremia is much less probable when the infection occurs in an individual that was previously healthy.

Despite medical advances, the incidence in humans of bacteremia, especially gram-negative bacillary bacteremia, has remained steady or has increased, in parallel with the advent of more invasive and aggressive patient monitoring and treatment. Because blood cultures are done infrequently in dogs and cats, it is difficult to estimate accurately the prevalence of bacteremia in companion animals.

In two previous reviews of blood culture results from dogs with suspected bacteremia, approximately 25 per cent had positive culture results, whereas in a recent study completed by the author, nearly 50 per cent of critically ill dogs and cats with suspected sepsis had positive blood culture results.

ETIOLOGY

Dogs

In two reviews of blood cultures from dogs, *Staphylococcus* was found to be the most common bloodstream isolate, followed by bacteria of the family Enterobacteriaceae (especially *Escherichia coli* and *Klebsiella*) and streptococci. Coagulase-positive staphylococci (usually *S. intermedius*) are frequent isolates from the blood of dogs with endocarditis and diskospondylitis. Skin wounds or infections are thought to provide the portal by which most staphylococci enter the bloodstream. Coagulase-negative staphylococcal bacteremia usually originates from infection of intravenous (IV) catheters. Beta-hemolytic streptococci, another relatively common bloodstream isolate in dogs, tend to enter via skin infections and are also associated with endocarditis and diskospondylitis. Enterococci gain access to the bloodstream via either the urinary or the gastrointestinal (GI) tract.

Aerobic, gram-positive bacilli (diphtheroids), though often found as contaminants in improperly collected blood cultures, apparently are important causes of endocarditis in dogs. Both *Corynebacterium* and *Erysipelothrix* have been associated with aortic valve endocarditis in dogs.

Bloodstream invasion by gram-negative bacilli usually represents opportunistic infection. *E. coli*, one of the most common bloodstream isolates in humans, dogs, and cats typically originates from the urinary tract as well as from intestinal, cutaneous, and respiratory sources. *Klebsiella* and *Enterobacter* are also common bloodstream pathogens. In the case of gram-negative bacillary bacteremia occurring in neutropenic patients or in those with hematologic malignancy, these bacteria probably gain access to the bloodstream via small ulcers in the gastrointestinal tract. *Pseudomonas aeruginosa*, like bacteria of the Enterobacteriaceae family, is an opportunist. Dogs with hematologic malignancy, especially those that become neutropenic after aggressive chemotherapy, seem particularly susceptible to *Pseudomonas* bacteremia. Also predisposed to *Pseudomonas* infection are dogs with extensive burn wounds or tracheostomies and those treated extensively with antibiotics.

Anaerobic bacteremia was demonstrated in 31 per cent of critically ill dogs and cats in a recent study (Dow et al., manuscript in preparation). The importance of anaerobic bacteremia may have been underestimated previously when blood culture specimens were not routinely processed for isolation of anaerobes. *Clostridium perfringens* and *Bacteroides*, the most common bloodstream isolates from dogs, usually originate from the lower intestinal tract. Nearly 16 per cent of positive blood cultures from dogs have been polymicrobial, frequently containing *E. coli* and an obligate anaerobe.

Cats

There are distinct differences between dogs and cats with respect to bacteremia. Gram-positive cocci are rarely isolated from the bloodstream of cats. Enterobacteriaceae, particularly *Salmonella*, are common isolates, as are obligate anaerobes (*Bacteroides* and *Fusobacterium*). Polymicrobial infection is frequent, occurring in up to 30 per cent of cats with positive blood culture results. In most instances, bloodstream infection in cats appears to originate from the gastrointestinal tract. Bacteremia may be a more frequent occurrence in cats than is generally appreciated, judging from the observation that 71 per cent of blood cultures drawn from critically ill cats with suspected sepsis were positive.

PATHOGENESIS

Bacteria entering the bloodstream from extravascular sites of infection generally do so via lymphatics. In healthy individuals, these bacteria are rapidly removed, primarily by fixed tissue macrophages residing in the liver and the spleen. Persistent bacteremia ensues only when bacteria enter the bloodstream more rapidly than the reticuloendothelial system can remove them or when phagocyte function is impaired. Neutrophils, although important in limiting extravascular multiplication of bacteria, are not directly involved in clearing bacteria from the bloodstream. In addition, serum from healthy individuals is itself bactericidal.

In dogs, common sources from which bacteria enter the bloodstream include urinary tract infection, skin and wound infections, abscesses, and peritoneal infection. Infected intravenous catheters have also been shown to serve as portals of entry in both humans and dogs. Peritoneal and gastrointestinal infections are common sources of bacteremia in cats. Factors known to predispose to the development of bacteremia in humans include malignancy, neutropenia, cytotoxic chemotherapy, burns, splenectomy, diabetes mellitus, catheterization, and renal or hepatic failure. In dogs and cats, prior urinary tract infection, leukemia, portosystemic shunts, and diabetes mellitus all are associated with high rates of bacteremia.

Three patterns of bacteremia occur: transient, intermittent, and continuous. Bacteria may transiently enter the bloodstream any time infected tissues or heavily contaminated mucous membrane surfaces are manipulated. Frequently, bacteria shower into the bloodstream during dental procedures or débridement of wounds or abscesses. Normally, these bacteria are cleared from the bloodstream within minutes. However, animals with pre-existing valvular heart disease may be at increased risk of developing endocarditis and persistent bacteremia.

Intermittent bacteremia, the most common clinical pattern, is usually associated with the presence of undrained abscesses. A fever spike, which typically occurs 30 to 40 min after bacteria enter the bloodstream, is of little use clinically in timing the collection of blood cultures from patients with intermittent bacteremia.

Continuous bacteremia characterizes intravascular infection, resulting from either endocarditis or catheter-associated infection. Bacterial endocarditis is an uncommon sequela to bacteremia and generally develops only when there is pre-existing cardiac valve damage, allowing bacteria to adhere to and proliferate on the valve surface.

DIAGNOSIS

Despite the fact that antimicrobial therapy is usually instituted before blood culture results are available, the effort and the expense of blood culture can, in most instances, be justified. Broad-spectrum, combination antibiotic treatment, usually including an aminoglycoside, is initially administered to patients with suspected bacteremia. Subsequent susceptibility testing of bloodstream isolates facilitates effective antimicrobial treatment and, in some cases, allows discontinuation of potentially toxic antibiotics. Initial antibiotic therapy may in some cases prove to be ineffective. In one study (Dow et al., manuscript in preparation), a change in antibiotic treatment was ultimately made in 18 per cent of animals shown by blood culture results to have been initially treated empirically with ineffective antibiotics. Bacterial isolation and susceptibility testing is crucial for effective long-term management of animals with bacterial endocarditis. Blood culture also constitutes an important part of the diagnostic workup of animals with fevers of unknown origin, particularly when immunosuppressive therapy is contemplated.

Blood cultures are indicated in dogs or cats manifesting any of the following: acute illness with fever (or hypothermia), abnormal leukogram (especially with a severe left shift or neutropenia), shock, and unexplained hypoglycemia, hypotension, icterus, depression, or thrombocytopenia. Concurrent cultures of urine and exudates from other potential sites of infection should be obtained. Blood cultures are also indicated in the diagnostic workup of dogs with intermittent or shifting leg lameness, recent or changing cardiac murmur, or other signs of bacterial endocarditis.

A minimum of two blood cultures should be done, as it is nearly impossible to accurately interpret a single culture, whether positive or negative. Blood should be collected from a peripheral vein, if possible, after the skin has been clipped and thoroughly disinfected with alternating swabs of alcohol and either iodine or an iodophore. Specimens need not be drawn from multiple veins unless phlebitis or catheter-associated infection is suspected. Blood can also be carefully collected from recently placed indwelling central venous catheters.

Guidelines for timing and number of cultures are given in Table 1. Prior administration of antibiotics has not been shown to decrease the likelihood of isolating bacteria from the bloodstream of both animals and humans. Bacteria are usually present in the bloodstream in very low numbers, often less than 10 bacteria per ml of blood. Therefore, the volume of blood cultured is critical—a minimum of 5 to 10 ml of blood per specimen should be cultured, if possible. Commercial liquid blood culture media, packaged in diaphragm-stoppered bottles, is recommended for routine blood culture. Most of these media are suitable for the isolation of both aerobic and anaerobic bacteria. Blood culture bottles should be warmed to room temperature prior to and after inoculation with blood. Table 2 is presented as an aid to interpretation of blood culture results.

THERAPY

In most instances, antibiotics are selected empirically for treatment of animals with suspected bacteremia. It is imperative to conduct a thorough search for the source of infection before starting antibiotic treatment. Cytologic examination of gram-stained smears of wound exudates and urine and careful inspection of intravenous catheters may reveal the source of infection and facilitate selection of appropriate antimicrobials prior to return of blood culture results.

The efficacy of regimens utilizing combination, broad-spectrum antibiotics for treatment of bacteremia in humans, compared to that of single-antibiotic regimens, has been debated widely, and multiple studies have failed to adequately resolve the issue. In general, the clinician should select a treatment regimen based on the characteristics of the individual infection rather than rely on empiric combinations of antibiotics. Vigorous diagnostic efforts and limited use of appropriate antibiotics gen-

Table 1. *Recommendations for Blood Culture*

Patient's Clinical Status	No. of Cultures	Interval Over Which Cultures Collected	Interval Between Each Culture	Timing of Culture
Fever of unknown origin	3	24 hr	At least 1 hr	Preferably prior to predicted fever spike
Subacute bacterial endocarditis	2–3	24 hr	At least 1 hr	Unimportant
Overwhelming acute sepsis	3	30 min–1 hr	15 min	At least two cultures prior to antibiotics
Subacute sepsis	3	24 hr	At least 1 hr	Prior to fever spike if possible
Patient currently receiving antibiotics	3–6	48–72 hr	12–24 hr	Prior to fever spike if possible

(With permission from Dow, S. W., et al.: Bacteremia: Pathogenesis, etiology, diagnosis. Compend. Cont. Ed. November 1988.)

erally prove more effective than routine combination antibiotic treatment.

The timing of initiation of antibiotic treatment constitutes one of the most important variables influencing the prognosis of bacteremic patients. A single initial loading dose of antibiotic(s) should be given, regardless of renal function; potential nephrotoxicity becomes a less important consideration in the case of life-threatening sepsis. All antibiotics are administered intravenously, as systemic absorption after subcutaneous or intramuscular injection is unreliable in animals in septic shock. Where identifiable, treatment of surgically correctable sources of infection, such as undrained abscesses, should not be delayed. The patient's condition will rarely improve greatly until the source of continued bloodstream infection has been eliminated. Intravenous catheters must be removed if they are suspected as a source of infection.

Antibiotic selection is based on a determination of the most probable source of infection and the most probable pathogen(s). If the source is unknown, particularly in neutropenic animals, broad-spectrum coverage, including an aminoglycoside, is warranted in order to adequately cover Enterobacteriaceae and *Pseudomonas*.

For treatment of bacteremic infections that are likely to be caused by gram-positive cocci (especially endocarditis, diskospondylitis, and acute osteomyelitis), antibiotics effective against coagulase-positive

Table 2. *Interpretation of Blood Culture Results*

Organism Isolated	Probable Source	Interpretation
Staphylococcus aureus, intermedius (coagulase-positive)	Skin, IV catheter, endocarditis, diskospondylitis	Significant
Staphylococcus (coagulase-negative)	Skin, IV catheter	Possible contaminant*
Streptococcus (beta-hemolytic)	Skin, endocarditis, diskospondylitis	Significant
Streptococcus (alpha-hemolytic)	Skin, mouth	Possible contaminant*
Enterococcus (enteric *Streptococcus*)	GI tract	Significant
Corynebacterium	Skin, endocarditis	Probably significant
Erysipelothrix	Skin, endocarditis	Probably significant
Bacillus	Skin	Possible contaminant*
Enterobacteriaceae†	GI, urinary, respiratory tracts	Significant
Pseudomonas	Skin, GI, urinary tracts	Significant
Bacteroides	GI tract, abscesses	Significant
Clostridium	Skin, GI tract, abscesses	Significance uncertain

*Unless isolated from multiple cultures.
†Enterobacteriaceae family includes *E. coli, Salmonella, Klebsiella, Enterobacter, Proteus*, and *Serratia*.
(With permission from Dow, S. W., et al.: Bacteremia: Pathogenesis, etiology, diagnosis. Compend. Cont. Ed. November 1988.)

Table 3. *Antibiotic Selection for Treatment of Animals with Suspected Bacteremia*

Site of Primary Infection	Most Probable Organism(s)	Antibiotic Regimen
Skin	Gram-positive cocci	PRP, cephalosporin
Urinary tract	*Escherichia coli*, gram-positive cocci	Aminoglycoside, cephalosporin
GI tract	Enterobacteriaceae, anaerobes	Penicillin (or clindamycin or metronidazole) plus aminoglycoside
Respiratory tract	Enterobacteriaceae, gram-positive cocci	Penicillin plus aminoglycoside; cephalosporin
Bone	Gram-positive cocci	PRP or cephalosporin
Heart valves	Gram-positive cocci	PRP plus aminoglycoside
Neutropenic, unknown source	Enterobacteriaceae, *Pseudomonas*	Ticarcillin (or carbenicillin) plus aminoglycoside

PRP, penicillinase-resistant penicillin (nafcillin, oxacillin)

staphylococci (usually *S. intermedius* in dogs) must be administered initially. *Staphylococcus intermedius* is much more likely to be resistant to penicillins than are beta-hemolytic streptococci. In most cases, either a parenterally administered penicillinase-resistant penicillin, such as oxacillin or nafcillin, or a first-generation cephalosporin (cefazolin, cephapirin, cephalothin) is preferred. In dogs with life-threatening endocarditis, an aminoglycoside is initially added to the treatment regimen, pending blood culture results.

Animals with bacteremia that is thought to be caused by gram-negative bacilli other than *Pseudomonas* are best treated with an aminoglycoside (or possibly a second- or third-generation cephalosporin), pending culture results. Parenterally administered trimethoprim-sulfonamide combinations are effective against most Enterobacteriaceae, with the exception of some strains of *Klebsiella*.

Pseudomonas bacteremia is an extremely ominous development and demands aggressive antibiotic treatment. Clinically, *Pseudomonas* bacteremia cannot be readily distinguished from bacteremia caused by bacteria of the Enterobacteriaceae family. This necessitates empiric treatment against *Pseudomonas* for animals at high risk of developing *Pseudomonas* sepsis (e.g., animals with hematologic malignancy, severe neutropenia, burn wounds). If *Pseudomonas* bacteremia is considered probable (e.g., prior *Pseudomonas* urinary tract infection) or positive culture results have confirmed *Pseudomonas* bacteremia, treatment regimes utilizing an aminoglycoside (gentamicin or amikacin) in combination with an expanded-spectrum penicillin (ticarcillin, carbenicillin) are recommended. Alternatively, some of the newer third-generation cephalosporins may be effective.

Anaerobic infections are often polymicrobial and generally require broad-spectrum antibiotic treatment. Anaerobic bacteremia is most probable in animals with peritonitis and other infections related to the gastrointestinal tract. Adequate coverage for most obligate anaerobes can be achieved by parenteral administration of penicillins (penicillin G, ampicillin, amoxicillin). Chloramphenicol and metronidazole can be used as alternatives to penicillins, as both are effective against obligate anaerobes, including those resistant to penicillins, and both reach effective serum concentrations when given orally. An aminoglycoside is often included in the treatment regimen for peritonitis and other mixed infections because of the likelihood of concurrent infection with coliform bacteria. Several cephalosporin antibiotics, especially cefoxitin, provide broad coverage for both obligate anaerobes and gram-negative bacilli and can be used effectively as single agents for mixed infections. Cefoxitin (Mefoxin, Merck), 11 to 22 mg/kg/day IV in three divided doses) has proved very effective as single-agent antibiotic treatment in animals with a variety of mixed infections and avoids the potential nephrotoxicity of aminoglycosides. Antibiotic treatment recommendations, based on probable source of infection, are given in Table 3.

References and Supplemental Reading

Bodey, G. P., Bolivar, R., Fainstein, V., et al.: Infections caused by *Pseudomonas aeruginosa*. Rev. Infect. Dis. 5:279, 1983.
Calvert, C. A.: Valvular bacterial endocarditis in the dog. J.A.V.M.A. 180:1080, 1982.
Calvert, C. A., Greene, C. E., and Hardie, E. M.: Cardiovascular infections in dogs: Epizootiology, clinical manifestations and prognosis. J.A.M.A. 187:612, 1985.
Dow, S. W., Curtis, C. R., Jones, R. L., et al.: Results of blood culture from dogs and cats: 100 cases (1985–1987). J.A.V.M.A. 1988 (in press).
Duma, R. J.: Gram-negative bacillary infections: Pathogenic and pathophysiologic correlations. Am. J. Med. 78:154, 1985.
Hirsch, D. C., Jang, S. S., and Biberstein, E. L.: Blood culture of the canine patient. J.A.V.M.A. 184:175, 1984.
Reller, R. B., Murray, P. R., and MacLowery, L. D.: Cumitech 1A. Blood cultures II. American Society for Microbiology, Washington, D.C., 1982.
Sisson, D., and Thomas, W. P.: Endocarditis of the aortic valve in the dog: J.A.V.M.A. 184:570, 1984.
Sullam, P. M., Drake, T. A., and Sunde, M. A.: Pathogenesis of endocarditis. Am. J. Med. 78:110, 1985.
Tilton, R. C.: The laboratory approach to the detection of bacteremia. Ann. Rev. Microbiol. 36:467, 1982.
Weinstein, M. P., Murphy, J. R., Reller, E. B., et al.: The clinical significance of positive blood cultures: A comprehensive analysis of 500 episodes of bacteremia and fungemia in adults. II. Clinical observations with special reference to factors influencing prognosis. Rev. Infect. Dis. 5:54, 1983.

ANAEROBIC INFECTIONS IN DOGS AND CATS

STEVEN W. DOW, D.V.M., M.S.

Fort Collins, Colorado

Results of recent studies indicate that anaerobic bacteria are an important cause of infections in animals. Although anaerobic bacteria have been familiar to microbiologists for over a century, recent improvements in anaerobic culture methods have made anaerobic bacteriology technically easier, with the result that isolation of obligate anaerobes from clinical specimens has increased. In addition, as awareness of the importance of anaerobic infection has increased, more specimens are now processed for isolation of anaerobes. There is a growing appreciation of the significance of anaerobic infection in both humans and animals.

BACTERIOLOGY

Most clinically important anaerobic bacteria are classified as obligate anaerobes. These bacteria do not utilize oxygen for metabolism, relying instead on fermentative metabolism. They are able to tolerate exposure to atmospheric concentrations of oxygen for several minutes. The most important bacteria in this group are *Bacteroides*, *Fusobacterium*, and *Peptostreptococcus*. *Clostridium* and *Actinomyces*, although anaerobes, are much more oxygen-tolerant than obligate anaerobes. Facultative anaerobes, such as *Escherichia coli*, can survive and grow either anaerobically or aerobically.

Very dense populations of obligate anaerobes are found in the colon, oropharynx, and female reproductive tract, and many anaerobic infections occur in or near these locations. With the exception of bite wounds and some clostridial infections, most anaerobic infections arise endogenously.

PATHOGENESIS

Intact epithelial barriers normally provide a very effective defense against anaerobic infection. However, when these barriers are disrupted, anaerobic bacteria gain access to underlying tissues and may, in the presence of favorable environmental conditions, establish infection. Healthy tissues are resistant to infection by anaerobes by virtue of both high redox potential and oxygen tension. These defenses are impaired when blood supply to tissues is decreased, when tissue necrosis has developed, or when there has been prior infection with oxygen-utilizing bacteria.

Pathogenic anaerobes are capable of elaborating a number of virulence factors, including potent toxins and enzymes. Both *Bacteroides* and *Clostridium* elaborate a number of these factors. Tissue necrosis, white blood cell lysis, and decreased opsonization of bacteria result from the effects of anaerobe-produced virulence factors.

CLINICAL FEATURES

Anaerobic infection is more likely to occur in certain body sites, especially those likely to be contaminated by endogenous flora. These sites include the oropharynx, skin, respiratory tract, abdomen, reproductive tract, musculoskeletal system, and central nervous system (CNS). Tissue contamination resulting from open wounds or surgery is responsible for initiating most clostridial infections, which may range in severity from localized abscesses to rapidly fatal clostridial myonecrosis. *Clostridium perfringens* is responsible for most cases of clostridial myonecrosis. This uncommon infection develops quickly and is characterized by marked toxin production and muscle necrosis. However, unlike many other clostridial infections, *C. perfringens* infection of muscle may not exhibit the clinical feature of gas production. Toxins produced by rapidly dividing clostridia frequently precipitate septic shock. Clostridial cellulitis and fasciitis, both more common infections than clostridial myonecrosis, are associated with marked liberation of gases into subcutaneous tissues and production of a putrid, thin, serosanguineous wound exudate.

Infected wounds in and around the oropharynx often contain anaerobic bacteria. This is not surprising, given the high concentrations of obligate anaerobes present on oropharyngeal mucous membrane surfaces. Examples include submandibular and retrobulbar abscesses and necrotizing, ulcerative gingivitis. Bite wounds are invariably contaminated with oropharyngeal bacteria, and infection very often results, especially following cat-bite wounds. The bacterial flora of bite-wound abscesses closely resembles the oropharyngeal flora, typically containing a mixture of obligate anaerobes (*Bacteroides*, *Fusobacterium*) and facultative bacteria (*Pasteurella* and *Escherichia coli*).

The pleural space provides a favorable environment for growth of anaerobes. Bacteriologic specimens collected from animals with pyothorax contain predominantly obligate anaerobes. Pyothorax usually involves bacteria of oropharyngeal origin. Bacteria are thought to gain access to the pleural space following thoracic wall penetration (foreign bodies, bite wounds) or after foreign bodies have penetrated oropharyngeal tissues and migrated caudally. Lung abscesses and chronic, consolidating aspiration pneumonia are other examples of anaerobic pleuropulmonary infections.

Anaerobic infection of the peritoneal cavity is frequent, particularly when the initial source of infection is bowel leakage. Often, these are mixed infections, containing coliform bacteria together with obligate anaerobes (especially *Bacteroides*, *Peptostreptococcus*, and *Clostridium*). *Clostridium* is also a relatively frequent isolate from liver abscesses in dogs.

Obligate anaerobes also figure prominently in chronic bone infections, particularly slowly developing osteomyelitis that occurs after open fractures and internal fracture fixation. Bone sequestration and the presence of chronic draining tracts suggest anaerobic osteomyelitis.

Other infections in dogs and cats that may be associated with anaerobic bacteria include pyometra, pyogenic CNS infection (brain abscess, subdural empyema), chronic sinusitis, and infections of malignant tumors.

DIAGNOSIS

Anaerobic infections have a number of characteristics that allow a tentative diagnosis to be reached before culture results are available (Table 1). Cytologic examination of gram-stained tissue exudates is crucial to an accurate, early diagnosis of anaerobic infection. The presence of multiple morphologic types of bacteria, together with purulent inflammation, is strong presumptive evidence of anaerobic infection. Cytologic examination of tissue exudates also facilitates empiric selection of antibiotics, allows detection of culture contamination, serves as a check on culture accuracy, and, in some instances, can eliminate the need for culture.

Proper specimen collection and transport is critical if anaerobes are to be successfully cultured. Exposure to oxygen and environmental extremes must be minimized. Exudates can be collected simply by aspiration into a syringe, which is then emptied of air and sealed. Large volumes of fluid are preferred for anaerobic culture, and tissue biopsies are also suitable. Specimens should not in most

Table 1. *Clinical Hints Suggesting Anaerobic Infection*

1. Foul-smelling exudate
2. Necrotic tissue; gangrene
3. Gas in wounds
4. Infections after bite wounds
5. Chronic osteomyelitis, especially after open fractures
6. Infections from penetrating foreign bodies
7. Infections associated with solid tumors
8. Bacteria seen on a Gram stain that fail to grow on routine culture
9. Endocarditis with negative routine blood cultures
10. Blackish discoloration of exudate; may fluoresce red under ultraviolet light if *Bacteroides melaninogenicus* is present
11. Sulfur granules in discharges (actinomycotic granules)
12. Infections nonresponsive to aminoglycosides, polymyxins, sulfonamides
13. Delayed-onset pneumonia after aspiration
14. Bacteremia with icterus
15. Closed-space infections: pyothorax, pyometra, brain abscess, lung abscess, intra-abdominal abscess
16. Infections characterized by very high fever and white blood cell counts
17. Subacute onset of inflammation in a previously contaminated area (e.g., following bowel surgery)

(Reprinted with permission from Dow, S.W., et al.: Anaerobic infections. Comp. Cont. Ed. 9:828, 1987.)

instances be collected on swabs; this method procures very small specimen volumes and often does not provide an anaerobic environment. Commercial anaerobic transport devices are necessary for transport of specimens if a delay in shipping or processing is probable. Specimens should be maintained at room temperature prior to and during transport.

TREATMENT

Surgical Management

With few exceptions, the mainstay of treatment includes surgical débridement and drainage. Thorough removal of infected, devitalized tissues and collections of purulent exudation have several important effects: (1) tissue oxygenation is improved, making the local environment less hospitable for anaerobic growth; (2) necrotic tissues, which provide very favorable conditions for proliferation of anaerobic bacteria, are eliminated; and (3) tissue blood flow is increased, accelerating delivery of white blood cells and antimicrobials. The net effect is to eradicate local infection and reduce the likelihood of local spread. In general, surgical débridement of tissues in which anaerobic infection is present should be aggressive and complete, for these infections have a tendency to recur if infected tissues are not adequately débrided.

Antimicrobial Treatment

Antibiotic treatment is generally combined with surgical treatment, particularly when surgery alone is unable to eliminate all residua of anaerobic infection or when there is the possibility of systemic infection. Higher doses of antimicrobials are usually given, and for longer periods of time, than in treatment of aerobic infections.

Initial selection of antibiotics is nearly always made empirically because anaerobic bacteria tend to grow slowly in culture, delaying culture results, and because routine antibiotic susceptibility testing cannot be done on anaerobic isolates. In addition, most anaerobic infections are polymicrobial, and it is not always clear which bacteria are pathogenic and which are merely commensal. Isolation of *Bacteroides* from culture is usually considered significant, especially in view of the apparent prevalence of resistance to penicillins and first-generation cephalosporins among *Bacteroides* isolates in both humans and animals.

Prompt antibiotic administration is essential, as delay in treatment is associated with poor response. Complication rates in small animals were shown to be higher when initial treatment did not include an antibiotic effective against anaerobes. Cytologic examination of gram-stained wound specimens, the most effective means of making an initial diagnosis of anaerobic infection, greatly facilitates rational empiric selection of antimicrobials.

Five types of antimicrobials are considered routinely effective against obligate anaerobes: penicillins, chloramphenicol, clindamycin, metronidazole, and some cephalosporins.

Penicillins remain one of the most effective drugs for treatment of anaerobic infections. Penicillin G is considered the drug of choice for most clostridial infections and for infections caused by anaerobic streptococci (Table 2). The spectrum of activity of amoxicillin against anaerobic bacteria is similar to that of penicillin G. Expanded-spectrum penicillins such as ticarcillin may be somewhat more effective than penicillin G against *Bacteroides fragilis*.

In humans, many *Bacteroides* strains, especially *B. fragilis*, are resistant to penicillins. Resistance to penicillins and first-generation cephalosporins has

also been observed in *Bacteroides* isolates from animals, although the frequency of resistance appears to be lower than that in humans. When *Bacteroides* is isolated from a severe anaerobic infection, particularly when the response to treatment with a penicillin is less than expected, alternatives to penicillins should be sought.

Chloramphenicol is active against most strains of *Bacteroides*, is well-absorbed orally, and penetrates well into most tissues. However, it appears clinically that *in vivo* efficacy of chloramphenicol may not always parallel *in vitro* activity.

Clindamycin has antibacterial characteristics similar to those of chloramphenicol and has been widely used in humans for treatment of anaerobic infection. Tissue penetrability, especially into abscesses and white blood cells, exceeds that of chloramphenicol. Clinically, clindamycin appears to be very effective in treatment of chronic pleuropulmonary infections (pyothorax, lung abscess) in dogs. Side effects generally are limited to gastrointestinal irritation.

Metronidazole is the only readily available antimicrobial with consistent bactericidal activity against *B. fragilis* and most other clinically important anaerobes, except *Actinomyces* and some streptococci. Oral absorption is excellent, as is tissue penetrability. Metronidazole has been proved very effective in humans for treatment of chronic anaerobic infections in relatively inaccessible sites, as deep bone infection and brain abscess. The oral dose of metronidazole for treatment of anaerobic infection in dogs has not been determined. Until such studies are done, it is recommended that dogs be treated with a total daily dose of 30 mg/kg, divided every 6 to 8 hr. At higher doses severe neurotoxicity, manifested as central vestibular or cerebellar disease, has been seen in dogs.

First-generation cephalosporins and most second-generation cephalosporins are relatively ineffective against *Bacteroides*. An exception is cefoxitin (Mefoxin, Merck), a second-generation cephalosporin effective against most obligate anaerobes, including *B. fragilis*. Cefoxitin is also active against most

Table 2. *Susceptibility of Pathogenic Anaerobes to Various Antimicrobials*

	Anaerobic Cocci	Bacteroides	B.[a] fragilis	Fusobacterium	Actinomyces Eubacterium	Clostridium	C. perfringens
Penicillins[b]	4+	3+	1+	3+	3+	3+	4+
Cephalosporins[c]	3+	2+−3+	1+	2+−3+	3+	2+	3+
Cefoxitin	3+	3+	3+	2+	3+	2+−3+	3+
Clindamycin	2+−3+	3+	3+	3+	3+	2+	3+
Chloramphenicol	3+	3+	3+	3+	3+	3+	3+
Metronidazole	1+−2+	3+	3+	3+	1+	3+	3+
Erythromycin	2+−3+	2+−3+	1+−2+	2+−3+	3+	2+−3+	3+
Tetracycline	1+−2+	2+−3+	1+−2+	2+−3+	2+−3+	2+	2+

1+, Poor to inconsistent activity. 2+, Moderate activity. 3+, Good activity. 4+, Drug of choice.
[a]Anaerobe most likely to be resistant to penicillins and cephalosporins.
[b]Includes penicillin G and aminopenicillins (ampicillin, amoxicillin).
[c]First-generation cephalosporins.
(Reprinted with permission from Dow, S.W., et al.: Anaerobic infections. Comp. Cont. Ed. 9:836, 1987.)

bacteria of the Enterobacteriaceae family. Therefore, very broad-spectrum coverage for both anaerobes and coliform bacteria, particularly suitable for treatment of peritonitis, can be achieved with cefoxitin alone. Cefoxitin has been used effectively in dogs for treatment of mixed infections caused by obligate anaerobes and bacteria of the Enterobacteriaceae family.

Two categories of antimicrobials, aminoglycosides and polymixins, are completely ineffective for treatment of anaerobic infections. Sulfonamides, although active *in vitro* against anaerobic bacteria, are considered relatively ineffective *in vivo* because of inactivation by substances released from lysed white blood cells and necrotic tissues.

Specific Treatment Recommendations

Aggressive, radical surgical débridement of infected tissues, combined with intravenous administration of penicillin G, is indicated for treatment of all serious clostridial infections. Surgical débridement of tissues is also recommended for treatment of soft tissue infections. Well-encapsulated soft tissue abscesses, without evidence of tissue spread, often do not warrant adjunctive antibiotic treatment. Amoxicillin plus clavulanic acid is very effective for both prophylaxis and treatment of bite-wound infections.

Effective pleural drainage is crucial for successful management of pyothorax in dogs and cats. Chest tube drainage and lavage alone is sufficient in most cases, though thoracotomy and pleural stripping may hasten resolution in dogs with long-standing pyothorax. Long-term treatment with penicillins or clindamycin is recommended. Clindamycin is recommended as initial treatment for lung abscess in dogs, followed by lobectomy if radiographic evidence of treatment response is not observed after several weeks of treatment.

In addition to broad-spectrum antibiotic treatment, peritonitis usually warrants exploratory laparotomy to locate and correct the source of infection.

A penicillin given with an aminoglycoside will usually provide adequate initial coverage for both obligate anaerobes and *E. coli*.

Pyometra, the most common anaerobic urogenital tract infection of dogs and cats, is best managed by ovariohysterectomy. Prostaglandin-induced uterine emptying, combined with chloramphenicol treatment, is recommended for treatment of pyometra in valuable breeding animals.

Successful treatment of pyogenic infection of the CNS (brain abscess, subdural empyema) in dogs and cats requires accurate lesion localization and identification. Computed tomographic examination of the head is currently the diagnostic procedure of choice. Antibiotic treatment alone (penicillin plus metronidazole, penicillin plus chloramphenicol, or metronidazole plus cefotaxime) may be sufficient for well-circumscribed lesions not associated with severe neurologic deficits. Otherwise, surgical drainage is indicated, in conjunction with antibiotic treatment. Anaerobic endocarditis is best managed by prolonged, high-dose antibiotic treatment, preferably based on antibiotic susceptibility testing of the bloodstream isolate.

References and Supplemental Reading

Abramowicz, M.: Drugs for anaerobic infections. Med. Lett. Drugs Ther. 26:87, 1984.

Anderson, C. B., Marr, H. H., and Ballinger, W. F.: Anaerobic infections in surgery: Clinical review. Surgery 79:313, 1976.

Bartlett, J. G.: Recent developments in the management of anaerobic infections. Rev. Infect. Dis. 5:235, 1983.

Bartlett, J. G.: Experimental aspects of intra-abdominal abscess. Am. J. Med. 76:91, 1984.

Cline, K. A., and Turnbull, T. L.: Clostridial myonecrosis, Ann. Emerg. Med. 14:129, 1985.

Dow, S. W., Jones, R. L., and Adney, W. F.: Anaerobic bacterial infections and response to treatment in dogs and cats: Review of 36 cases (1983–1985). J.A.V.M.A. 189:930, 1986.

Finegold, S. M., Bartlett, J. G., and Chow, A. W.: Management of anaerobic infections. Ann. Int. Med. 83:375, 1975.

Hirsch, D. C., Biberstein, E. L., and Jang, S. S.: Obligate anaerobes in clinical veterinary practice. J. Clin. Microb. 10:1188, 1979.

Hnatko, S. I.: Epidemiology of anaerobic infections. Surgery 93:125, 1983.

Lerner, P. I.: Antimicrobial considerations in anaerobic infections. Med. Clin. North Am. 58:533, 1974.

Sheperd, W. E.: Cumitech 5: Practical Anaerobic Bacteriology. Washington, D.C.: American Society for Microbiology, 1977.

CANINE LYME BORRELIOSIS

RUSSELL T. GREENE, D.V.M.

Raleigh, North Carolina

ETIOLOGY

Lyme borreliosis is one of the most commonly reported human tick-borne illnesses in the United States. Clinical cases are also being recognized in dogs. It is a complex, multi-organ disorder caused by a spirochete, *Borrelia burgdorferi*. The primary vectors in the United States are *Ixodes dammini* in the Northeast and upper Midwest, *I. pacificus* in the West, and possibly *I. scapularis* in the Southeast. The nymphal stage is thought to be the most important in the transmission of the spirochete to dogs and humans.

Persistence of the spirochete within the host is postulated to be important in the pathogenesis of the disease. Although controversial, it is proposed that lipopolysaccharides in the cell wall of *B. burgdorferi* cause the release of interleukin-1 from macrophages. This acute phase reactant is thought to then lead to inflammation and the tissue damage that is responsible for the clinical signs. Host factors also are probably important, since only a small percentage of dogs that become exposed develop clinical signs.

CLINICAL SIGNS

Canine clinical manifestations are categorized as being either acute or chronic. Fever, inappetence, lethargy, lymphadenopathy, and acute onset of lameness or pain are variably observed in acute infections. Often, these acutely affected dogs do not have swollen joints, and it is frequently difficult to localize the origin of the pain. Lameness may be intermittent and often migratory from one leg to another.

Recurrent, intermittent, nonerosive arthritis is considered the primary chronic manifestation of canine Lyme disease. This has been the primary clinical manifestation reported in dogs. The majority of affected dogs have recurrent episodes of lameness and often have two or more joints involved. The carpus is commonly affected.

The characteristic skin lesion, erythema chronicum migrans, as frequently observed in human cases, has not been documented in dogs. In endemic areas, expanding lesions, often visualized on the abdomen or other sparsely haired areas, are suspicious. The expanding nature of these lesions differentiate them from the localized reaction to a tick bite.

Neurologic and cardiac manifestations also have not yet been reported in canine infections. There are suspicions in endemic areas that signs of meningitis or encephalitis may be manifestations of canine Lyme disease. In addition, atrioventricular (A-V) block has been observed in seropositive dogs, but definite documentation of *B. burgdorferi* as the cause has not yet been successful. With time and increased awareness of these disease syndromes, these manifestations are likely to be reported in the veterinary literature.

There is evidence that renal lesions may develop secondary to *B. burgdorferi* infections in dogs. Proteinuria, glomerulonephritis, and tubular damage have been observed in seropositive dogs, but documentation of a causal relationship is difficult.

DIAGNOSIS

The results of hematologic, biochemical, and immunologic testing are often within reference ranges. Joint fluid examined in chronically lame dogs is characterized by a purulent exudate and rarely contains spirochetes. The mean cell count is approximately 46,000 cells/mm³, with the majority of these cells being polymorphonuclear leukocytes. In acute infections, the volume of synovial fluid often is not enough to obtain an adequate sample.

Cerebrospinal fluid (CSF) analysis in humans with neurologic signs often reveals a mild increase in cells and protein. The majority of the cells are mononuclear. Occasionally, spirochetes have been cultured from the CSF of affected humans. Also, documentation of increased intrathecal antibody titers may be a useful diagnostic aid, especially when compared with serum levels early in the disease.

Attempts to identify or culture *B. burgdorferi* from the blood, CSF, and joints in affected humans and dogs are rarely successful. A special medium, Barbour-Stoenner-Kelly II, is required to grow *Borrelia* spirochetes. Blood samples anticoagulated with citrate can be submitted to an appropriate laboratory for isolation. Positive identification of isolated organisms using monoclonal antibodies is required. Isolation of *B. burgdorferi* may be an incidental finding, in that it has been isolated from the sera, urine, and tissues of asymptomatic wildlife, laboratory animals, and seropositive dogs.

Histologic samples can be evaluated for the presence of pathogenic spirochetes. Special stains and monoclonal antibodies are necessary for specific identification, since nonpathogenic spirochetes and artifacts may be detected. The organism has been observed in tissues of asymptomatic animals. Thus, the presence of spirochetes would seem to be a significant finding when they are surrounded by an inflammatory process.

Antigen detection methods may be useful in the diagnosis of this disease, since there is persistence of the organism within the host. These tests are currently being evaluated.

Both indirect fluorescent assays (IFAs) and enzyme-linked immunosorbent assays (ELISAs) are used for diagnosis in humans and dogs. There are interlaboratory differences among the absolute titer results. There is also considerable overlap between the antibody titers of dogs with clinical infections versus those with subclinical infections. This has made interpretation of a single serum titer of any magnitude difficult. An IFA IgG titer greater than 1:64 has often been considered significant or indicative of past or present *Borrelia* infection, although dogs in endemic areas can be asymptomatic and have IgG titers of 1:8192. IFA titers of clinically affected dogs have ranged from 1:256 to 1:16,384. After a single intravenous experimental inoculation of *B. burgdorferi* into dogs by the author, IgM titers remained increased for approximately 2 months, whereas specific IgG titers increased rapidly and persisted for up to 8 months. In serologic tests for *Borrelia*, there is little cross-reactivity with *Leptospira*.

TREATMENT

Tetracycline, ampicillin, or, less desirably, erythromycin, all at standard doses for 10 to 14 days, are utilized for treatment of acute canine cases. Ceftriaxone has been shown to be an effective antibiotic *in vitro*, but its cost may prohibit its use. Acute infections often resolve within 24 hr of instituting antibiotic therapy. Chronic infections are sometimes more difficult to treat. In human cases in which the arthritis does not resolve after appropriate therapy, high doses of intravenous penicillin G (22,000 units IV/kg repeated every 6 hr for 10 days) is recommended. This may be beneficial in dogs too.

Aspirin or other nonsteroidal anti-inflammatory drugs may be helpful for pain relief during episodes of synovitis, but treatment is not useful during asymptomatic periods. Glucocorticoids may give rapid pain relief, but there is evidence that they may interfere with the response to antibiotics and may cause a recrudescence of spirochetemia.

PREVENTION

In dogs, many aspects of the disease are probably still unrecognized. A better understanding of the serology or improved isolation techniques will allow for increased efficiency of diagnosis of the disease. Rapid removal of the tick will help prevent the disease, since it takes approximately 24 hr of tick feeding before the organism can be transmitted in tick saliva. Commercial vaccines are not available. However, the prospects for their production appear to be promising, as hamsters were actively and passively protected by a killed preparation. Until an effective canine model is developed, efficacy of such a vaccine will be difficult to demonstrate.

References and Supplemental Reading

Burgess, E. C.: Natural exposure of Wisconsin dogs to the Lyme disease spirochete (*Borrelia burgdorferi*). Lab. Anim. Sci. 36:288, 1986.

Burgess, E. C.: Borreliosis (Lyme disease). *In* Barlough, J. (ed.): *Manual of Small Animal Infectious Diseases*. New York: Churchill Livingstone Inc., 1988.

Greene, R. T., Levine, J. F., Breitschwerdt, E. B., et al.: Clinical and serologic evaluations of induced *Borrelia burgdorferi* infection in dogs. Am. J. Vet. Res. 49:752, 1988.

Habicht, G. S., Beck, G., and Benach, J. L.: Lyme disease. Sci. Am. 257:78, 1987.

Kornblatt, A. N., Urband, P. H., and Steere, A. C.: Arthritis caused by *Borrelia burgdorferi* in dogs. J.A.V.M.A. 186:960, 1985.

Lissman, B. A., Bosler, K. E. M., Camay, H., et al.: Spirochete-associated arthritis (Lyme disease) in a dog. J.A.V.M.A. 185:219, 1984.

Magnarelli, L. A., Anderson, J. F., Kaufmann, A. F., et al.: Borreliosis in dogs from southern Connecticut. J.A.V.M.A. 186:955, 1985.

Steere, A. C., Green, J., Hutchinson, G. J., et al.: Treatment of Lyme disease. Zentralbl. Bakteriol. Mikrobiol. Hyg. [A] 263:352, 1986.

PLAGUE

DENNIS W. MACY, D.V.M.

Fort Collins, Colorado

Plague (pest, black death, pestilent fever) is caused by *Yersinia pestis*. In the past 2000 years, three pandemics of plague have occurred: (1) in 542, Justinian plague killed an estimated 100 million people, including one fourth of the European population; (2) the pandemic of 1346, which lasted for 300 years, resulted in 25 million deaths; and (3) a smaller pandemic of 1874, which continued through 1930, established natural infection foci in North America, South America, West Africa, and South Africa. In the United States, the number of cases of human plague have increased since 1965. A total of 105 cases were reported from 1970 to 1979, the largest number in a decade since 1904 to 1909. In 1983 alone, 40 cases of human plague were reported in the United States. At present, natural foci of plague in animal populations exist on all continents except Australia. In the United States, plague is endemic in foci in the semiarid regions of 15 Western states, from the High Plains west to the Pacific Ocean, including Hawaii. Although plague foci within this region exist from Mexico to the Canadian border, 90 per cent of the human cases have been reported in New Mexico, Arizona, and California. New Mexico has accounted for more than 50 per cent of the human cases of plague reported each year in the United States since 1949.

OCCURRENCE IN ANIMALS

A total of 230 species of wild rodents have been naturally infected with the plague organism (sylvatic plague), and over 1500 species of fleas have been shown to transmit *Y. pestis*. In the natural foci, wild plague is perpetuated through circulation of *Y. pestis* by fleas from one rodent to another. Rodent species vary tremendously in their degree of susceptibility to infection with the plague organism. The California ground squirrel, rock squirrels of various species, and prairie dogs are frequently infected. Prairie dogs have an extremely high mortality rate (approaching 100 per cent). Birds and other vertebrates do not play a regular role in the natural cycle of plague. Lagomorphs usually are not permanent reservoirs for infection; however, they become infected during high rodent-plague infections and serve as an important source of infection to hunters. Raptors, although resistant to infection, may distribute the organism by transporting in-

fected prey or fleas. Humans and carnivores are accidental hosts and do not play a role in the maintenance of the disease in nature. Carnivores, with the exception of the cat, are relatively resistant to infection but may be important in transmitting infected fleas from rodents to humans. In 1984, 10 per cent of human cases of plague were associated with exposure to infected cats.

ANIMAL-TO-HUMAN TRANSMISSION

The most common mode of transmission to humans is through fleas that have been feeding on plague-infected rodents. After ingestion of a blood meal from a bacteremic host, *Yersinia pestis* multiplies in the proventriculus of the flea. When the flea attempts to feed again, it regurgitates bacteria intradermally into the new host. Fleas may remain infected for over a year, which allows the disease to be transmitted long after the death of the host that infected them. Dogs and cats may serve to transport the vector (fleas) from plague-infected wildlife to humans. Fleas of other species found on dogs and cats increase the chances that the animals have come in contact with species in which plague is endemic. Dogs and cats may also bring sick, infected rodents home. Handling plague-infected animals may result in transmission of the plague organism through breaks in the skin or through mucous membrane contact. Finally, pets (particularly cats) may become bacteremic and may transmit the organism through bites or scratches, or with pneumonia through droplet formation from sneezing or coughing. Because many cats and dogs are allowed to roam in plague-enzootic areas, veterinarians and animal health technicians in these areas are at increased risk for potential exposure to the plague organism. Since 1977, plague has been confirmed in two veterinarians and one animal health technician in the United States.

Rodent-to-Dog and Rodent-to-Cat Transmission

In contrast to the disease in humans, in which the flea is the major vector for transmission, the infection in cats and dogs is acquired through oral mucous membrane contact with infected rodents or lagomorphs. Dogs and wild carnivores (coyotes, raccoons, skunks) regularly seroconvert after ingestion of a plague-infected animal but rarely develop clinical signs of disease or die. As many as 38 per cent of the dogs in one plague-enzootic region were reported to have antibodies against plague, whereas only 18 per cent of the cats in the same area had titers to the plague organism. Experimental infections in cats have shown that the mortality rate following ingestion of plague-infected mice is 50 per cent, suggesting that half the cats exposed to the plague organism in nature die.

DISEASE IN DOGS AND CATS

Dogs, like wild carnivores, are relatively resistant to the clinical disease following exposure. However, like rodents, there is heterogeneity to this resistance. Some dogs develop high fevers and lymphadenopathy following exposure to the plague organism, and an occasional fatal case of plague has been reported. Cats are more susceptible than dogs, and numerous case reports of the disease in cats have been described. Infected cats are usually hunters, and following ingestion of a plague-infected rodent, they develop an acute febrile response (103 to 106°F; 39.4 to 41.1°C) concurrent with a bacteremia. Bacteremic cats are frequently anorexic, depressed, and dehydrated and may have respiratory signs. In more chronic cases of plague, marked submandibular or cervical lymph node lymphadenopathy (bubo) develops, which forms abscesses and may ulcerate and drain. Although abscesses are most frequently observed in areas that are draining sites of inoculation such as the head and neck, they may appear elsewhere on the body in association with a septicemic dissemination of the organism. These abscesses cannot be differentiated clinically from those caused by *Pasteurella* organism. Septicemia may lead to severe suppurative pneumonic plague. The clinical course of plague varies with individual cats. Acutely septicemic animals die within 1 to 2 days, whereas others may survive for several weeks.

HUMAN PLAGUE

The human disease has been classified into three clinical forms and is similar to that described in the cat: the bubonic, septicemic, and pneumonic forms. Humans usually acquire the disease from a flea bite or through broken skin or mucous membrane contact with infected tissues or body fluids of rodents. Inhalation of organisms contained within droplets from infected individuals or animals with pneumonic plague is rare. The incubation period for plague is 2 to 6 days, and the symptoms and signs are similar in all three forms of the disease, starting with fever, chills, nausea, achiness, diarrhea, and vomiting. In *septicemic* plague, endotoxemia, shock, disseminated intravascular coagulation (DIC), and a variety of CNS signs may develop. *Bubonic* plague is the most common disease manifestation and is characterized by draining lymph node abscesses (bubos) in sites draining the flea bite, usually the extremities. Inguinal or axillary lymphadenopathy is also common. Septicemic plague may develop from any form of the disease, but it occurs especially in individuals in whom the disease is not confined to regional lymph nodes or in patients for whom treatment has been delayed. Septicemia tends to occur more frequently in the young and in the elderly. *Pneumonic* plague may result from inhalation of infected droplets secondary to hematogenous or lymphatic spread from bubonic or septicemic plague. Primary pneumonic plague in humans is now contracted most often through contact with animals with plague pneumonia. If left untreated, bubonic plague has a mortality rate of 25 to 60 per cent; the mortality rate in pneumonic and septicemic plague is close to 100 per cent. The death rate in the United States for all forms of treated plague currently is 17 per cent.

DIAGNOSIS

Early diagnosis is important for both the health of the animal and the protection of the client, veterinarian, and his or her staff. All free-roaming cats in enzootic areas should be considered at risk for exposure to plague. Radiographic findings of pneumonia in a cat in an endemic area should alert clinicians to the possibility of plague and the need to take precautionary measures to prevent droplet transmission associated with caring for animals with plague pneumonia. A marked leukocytosis is characteristic of acute septicemic plague but is not in itself diagnostic. Even when the clinician has a strong suspicion that a patient has plague, the diagnosis must be confirmed by identification of the organism in culture or in tissue by fluorescent antibody (FA), or by demonstrating a fourfold rise in antibody titer to *Y. pestis*.

Yersinia pestis is usually found in large numbers in infected tissues. Needle aspirates from enlarged lymph nodes or purulent material from abscesses should be collected prior to initiation of therapy and submitted for evaluation to a *qualified reference laboratory*. (Veterinarians are advised to contact the laboratory before sending samples.) Gram stains of aspirations from infected animals contain large numbers of gram-negative coccobacilli. The bipolar "safety pin" appearance is best demonstrated with Giemsa but is not pathognomonic for *Y. pestis*. Nonstained, air-dried smears of aspirated material or refrigerated tissue specimens are suitable for fluorescent antibody testing for *Y. pestis*. Blood, tissue, or aspirates may be submitted for culturing and organism identification. Fresh samples should be refrigerated (4 to 8°C; 39.2 to 46.4°F) but not frozen, and double-wrapped in plastic to prevent leakage during mailing or transport to the reference laboratory. If significant delays in transport are anticipated or temperature ensurance is questionable, the specimen should be inoculated into transport media (Stuart's or Cary-Blair are suitable). Blood culture bottles containing trypticase soy broth should be inoculated with blood from animals suspected of having septic plague. Because dogs and cats in endemic areas frequently have high titers to *Y. pestis* that persist for a year or longer after exposure, a single titer is of little value in differentiating active disease from previous exposure. However, a fourfold increase in paired titers taken 10 to 14 days apart is indicative of recent plague infection.

TREATMENT

Because plague can be a rapidly fatal zoonotic disease, care must be taken to protect those caring for animals infected with this disease. When plague is suspected based on clinical and epidemiologic information, specimens for diagnostic tests should be obtained and specific antimicrobial therapy started immediately. Do not wait for laboratory confirmation of the disease. Cats with plague-carrying fleas should be treated immediately with carbamates or pyrethrins. Cats with pneumonic clinical signs should be kept in strict isolation because droplet formation following their coughing or sneezing may infect those caring for them. Veterinarians and their assistants should wear surgical masks, gloves, and gowns while caring for animals with pneumonic plague. Surgical gloves should be worn while treating animals with the septicemic or bubonic form of the disease. All body fluids and tissues should be double-wrapped in plastic and incinerated as a routine disposal management procedure. The organism is subject to desiccation and survives only 2 to 3 hr in the environment unless it is contained within organic material such as pus and other body excreta or in an animal carcass. In such cases, it may be viable for several months. Routine disinfectants are effective in killing the plague organism and should be used as a precautionary measure on cages and examination tables employed in the care of infected animals. *Y. pestis* is not extremely resistant to antimicrobial therapy and is susceptible to a wide range of common antibiotics. Streptomycin is considered the most effective antibiotic against the plague organism. However, streptomycin is bactericidal. Thus, caution should be used in administering the drug in the pneumonic form of the disease because it may precipitate endotoxemic shock and

a DIC crisis. Chloramphenicol is also very effective in the treatment of plague and is especially useful in the treatment of patients with central nervous system involvement because it penetrates the blood-brain barrier. Although *Y. pestis* shows *in vitro* sensitivity to penicillin and ampicillin, it demonstrates *in vivo* resistance to these antibiotics, and penicillin or ampicillin should *not* be used. Tetracyclines, including tetracycline, chlortetracycline, and oxytetracycline, are used primarily for the bubonic form of plague and for prophylactic antibiotic therapy. Infected animals should be treated for a minimum of 10 days to 2 weeks. Other animals exposed to plague-infected animals should be treated prophylactically with tetracycline for a minimum of 7 days. Gentamicin, kanamycin, and trimethoprim-sulfamethoxazole are used less frequently for plague. All persons that have participated in the care of plague-infected animals should be advised to contact their physician immediately.

CONTROL

Plague is so involved in our ecosystem that preventing or eliminating all risk of human exposure from the wild rodent population is not usually feasible. Plague may exist in an area without human cases because of a lack of exposure to the rodent sources or their fleas. Dogs and cats have been used as sentinel animals to determine the presence of plague in various areas of the country because they are more likely to come in contact with endemic rodent species. Up to 38 per cent of dogs on a New Mexico Indian Reservation endemic for plague were found to have antibodies against the plague bacillus. The primary means of plague control is education of people living in the plague enzootic areas to the modes of transmission. Veterinarians should educate their assistants and staff members as to the modes of transmission and should have a heightened sensitivity to the possibility of plague infections existing in the sick cats that they treat. Examination of fleas on patients may quickly determine if they are of rodent origin, suggesting contact with a reservoir species for plague. Flea control in pets should be stressed in plague enzootic areas, to prevent vector transmission to pet owners. Residents in endemic areas can help by eliminating food and shelter for wild rodents or rats (e.g., preventing accumulation of brush piles and old cars in and around the house, and insisting upon proper disposal of garbage). The public should be advised to avoid rodent burrows, especially those in which flies may be over the surface. The presence of flies suggest that a dead rodent may exist in the burrow and that hungry fleas may be looking for a new host. Local health officials may institute selective rodent control measures but not before flea control has been instituted.

References and Supplemental Reading

Human plague associated with domestic cats—California, Colorado MMWR 30:265, 1981.

Kaufman, A. F., Mann, I. M., Gardiner, T. M., et al.: Public health implications of plague in domestic cats. J.A.V.M.A. 179:875, 1981.

Poland, J., and Barnes, A.: Plague. In Steele, J. H. (ed.): CRC Handbook Series in Zoonoses. Boca Raton, FL: CRC Press, 1979, pp. 515–579.

Poland, J. D., Barnes, A. M., and Herman, J. J.: Human bubonic plague from exposure to a naturally infected wild carnivore. Am. J. Epidemiol. 197:332, 1973.

Rollag, O. J., Skeels, M. R., Nims, L. J., et al.: Feline plague in New Mexico: Report of five cases. J.A.V.M.A. 179:1381, 1981.

Rosser, W. W.: Bubonic plague. J.A.V.M.A. 191:406, 1987.

Rust, J. H., Cavanaugh, R., and Marshall, J. D.: The role of domestic animals in the epidemiology of plague: I. Experimental infection of dogs and cats. J. Infect. Dis. 124:522, 1971.

Thilsted, J. P.: Plague. In Barlough, J. E. (ed.): Manual of Small Animal Infectious Diseases. New York: Churchill Livingstone, 1988.

Von Reyn, C. F., Barnes, A. M., Weber, N. S., et al.: Bubonic plague from direct exposure to a naturally infected wild coyote. Am. J. Trop. Med. Hyg. 25:626, 1976.

Weniger, B. G., Warren, A. J., Forseth, V., et al.: Human bubonic plague transmitted by domestic cat scratch. J.A.M.A. 251:927, 1984.

Werner, B. S., Curtis, W. E., Nelson, B. C., et al.: Primary plague pneumonia contracted from a domestic cat at South Lake Tahoe, California. J.A.M.A. 251:929, 1984.

GROUP G STREPTOCOCCAL INFECTIONS IN KITTENS

PATRICIA BLANCHARD, D.V.M.

Tulare, California

and DENNIS WILSON, D.V.M.

Davis, California

Beta-hemolytic streptococci are also considered part of the normal flora of the pharynx, skin, and upper respiratory and genital tracts of cats. They have been isolated from a variety of suppurative processes in cats. Beta-hemolytic streptococcal infections are generally sporadic and are associated most often with the respiratory tract, the female genital system, and the integument. In cats, outbreaks of streptococcal infections have been described only in association with tonsillitis and cervical lymphadenitis in juvenile patients. Neonatal infections in kittens with group G streptococci have not been previously described but can be an important cause of neonatal mortality, especially in breeding catteries.

PATHOGENESIS AND IMMUNITY

Neonatal infections with group G streptococci arise from initial contamination of the umbilicus, which most probably occurs at birth. The source of the bacteria is most probably the vagina of the queen. Fatal infections probably develop when the inoculated dose of bacteria exceeds the ability of the natural defenses (neutrophils and colostral antibodies) to limit and destroy the organism.

Survey studies of an endemically affected cattery indicate that 100 per cent of young, nulliparous queens carry larger numbers of group G streptococci as part of their normal flora. As the queens age and following multiple pregnancies, the number of organisms and the rate of carriage declines (68 per cent). In addition, the carriage rate and the colonization density in older, multiparous queens drop dramatically during gestation and remain low postpartum when compared with those of nulliparous queens younger than 2 years of age (Table 1). Such low carriage rates and colonization densities result in a lower incidence of exposure and a smaller dose of bacteria in kittens born to older queens, which may explain the higher incidence of infection in the first litters of young queens. Group G streptococci are also part of the normal flora of the prepuce of male cats, which can contribute to the rapid spread of the organism in a naive breeding colony.

CLINICAL SYNDROME

Most kittens infected at birth have no clinical signs but gain less weight than littermates. Death usually occurs between 7 and 11 days of age. Within

Table 1. *The Effects of Age, Gestation, and Parturition on Vaginal Colonization by Streptococcus canis in Queens*

	Age in Months		
	16	**30–40**	**40+**
Number in group	13	7	11
Mean plate scores* at			
Prebreeding	2.8*	2.4*	1.8*
Gestation (4–7 weeks)	2.2	1.1	0.14
Parturition	0.8	0.14	0.23
4 wk postpartum	1.8	0.4	0.3
8 wk postpartum	1.6	0.14	0

*Mean plate score is the average growth zone value of the entire group. The growth zone is the highest dilution streak zone in which five colonies or more of *S. canis* were present. This was determined on a bovine blood agar plate with a four-zone streak pattern.

24 hr prior to death, kittens develop a transient fever in excess of 100°F (37.8°C). Occasionally, kittens in the litter will have a visibly swollen and infected umbilicus. More than one kitten in a litter can be affected, although the whole litter is not usually affected. In kittens born to queens with minimal prior exposure to the organism, death may occur at less than 3 days of age.

Most affected kittens are from the first litter of queens younger than 2 years of age. Group G streptococci have also been isolated from the uterus of periparturient young queens with metritis or endometritis. There was a high mortality rate among the kittens of some of these queens, but no postmortem examinations of the kittens were done to determine the cause of death. Generally, queens with kittens that have streptococcal infections remain healthy.

Infected kittens develop an initial neutrophilia and regenerative left shift followed by a severe neutropenia with degenerative left shift and myeloid depletion of the bone marrow. Occasionally, toxic neutrophils with intracellular cocci are present in the peripheral blood.

A high kitten mortality rate may be seen on initial entry of the organism into a naive cattery, but the mortality rate due to streptococcal infections should decline to less than 5 per cent within 1 year in the absence of immunosuppressive environmental factors and viruses. New additions to an affected cattery may exhibit a high mortality rate among their first litters. Although the disease may be more prevalent in catteries, litters of household cats are also susceptible. Similar to litters in catteries, the litters of young household queens are most often affected.

A low rate of cervical lymphadenitis due to group G streptococci in 3- to 6-month-old kittens is also seen in affected catteries and, sporadically, in household cats. Previous research into this condition indicates that the infection begins as tonsillitis, which then spreads via lymphatics to the local lymph nodes. In some untreated patients, the lymphatic spread continues with entry of the bacteria into the circulation via the thoracic duct. Kittens with thoracic cavity involvement may present in respiratory distress due to pleuritis and embolic pneumonia but are more often found dead with minimal premonitory signs.

NECROPSY FINDINGS

The most common postmortem lesions in kittens between 7 and 11 days of age are sanguinopurulent peritonitis and suppurative omphalophlebitis that extends into the liver via the ductus venosus and spreads throughout the portal venous system, resulting in thromboembolic hepatitis. Occasionally, pulmonary thromboemboli with hemorrhagic infarcts are also present. Histologically, in addition to the aforementioned lesions, most kittens have myocardial necrosis associated with colonies of streptococci.

In 3- to 6-month-old kittens that die following untreated lymphadenitis, the jugular groove frequently contains a diffuse purulent exudate and the thoracic cavity is filled with red purulent fluid. The lungs are swollen, with multiple infarctions and purulent emboli within pulmonary vessels. Histologically, all kittens also have myocardial necrosis associated with bacterial colonies.

DIAGNOSIS

Definitive diagnosis is based on culture results. In fatal neonatal infections, most organs yield positive culture results, although the liver, lung, umbilicus, and peritoneal cavity are the most easily cultured and most likely to yield positive results. In juvenile cats with lymphadenitis, the preferred site for culture is the cervical lymph node, from which a needle aspirate is drawn. Pharyngeal swabs from this group do not always yield the organism and are frequently overgrown by normal flora.

Group G streptococci in cats are beta-hemolytic on bovine blood agar and grow well at 37°C (98.6°F) in air. They are gram-positive cocci and catalase negative. The majority of feline isolates ferment lactose but not trehalose or sorbitol.

A tentative diagnosis can be made on Gram stains of the umbilical or peritoneal exudate of neonatal kittens and from needle aspirates of the cervical lymph node in cats with lymphadenitis. Single bacteria and chains of small gram-positive cocci are present on Gram stains of clinical exudates. *Staphylococcus*, which is also a gram-positive coccus, does not cause lymphadenitis and usually does not form chains.

Other causes of omphalophlebitis in neonates are

hemolytic *Escherichia coli*, which is a gram-negative rod and may be present with *Streptococcus* and in some cases with *Staphylococcus*. The latter is much less common than *Streptococcus* or *E. coli*.

Differential diagnoses for cervical lymphadenitis in cats should include *Yersinia pestis*, which is a gram-negative coccobacillus (see p. 1089), lymphosarcoma, and metastatic tumors of the head. The latter two are uncommon in cats between 3 and 6 months of age, although that is the most common age range for cats with streptococcal lymphadenitis. Cytology and Gram stains of needle aspirates should allow adequate differentiation of an infectious problem from a neoplastic disease and distinguish between *Streptococcus* and *Yersinia*.

TREATMENT AND CONTROL

Group G streptococci of cats have been uniformly sensitive to penicillin, which is the drug of choice. Most kittens that develop neonatal streptococcal infections are found dead with minimal premonitory signs, so treatment is not effective except in prevention of infection among littermates. Amoxicillin pediatric drops given every 12 hr for 5 days have been used effectively in preventing further infections of littermates. In one large breeding colony with a significant incidence of neonatal streptococcal infections, routine antibiotic usage and navel dipping with 2 per cent tincture of iodine at birth have prevented the problem. Newborn kittens receive a single, 0.25-ml subcutaneous injection of a 1:6 dilution in sterile 0.9 per cent saline of a product containing 150,000 IU benzathine penicillin and 150,000 IU of procaine penicillin per ml. The queen receives a single, 1-ml subcutaneous injection of the same product undiluted. Over the past 3 years, no ill effects have been seen in kittens or queens with routine single-dose penicillin therapy.

Juvenile kittens with lymphadenitis receive 0.5 ml of the undiluted penicillin formulation subcutaneously at the time of detection. A second treatment is rarely required, since the benzathine is a long-acting penicillin. Kittens that do not fully respond within 24 hr receive a second treatment at 2 to 3 days.

Elimination of the vaginal and preputial carrier state has been unsuccessful, since antibiotics do not reach effective levels at these sites. The bacteria are also carried in the pharynx, probably associated with the tonsils in a lower percentage of cats. Streptococci also can be cultured from the feces.

Several cesarean-derived, closed, specific pathogen-free cat colonies have remained free of streptococci for over 7 years. Initial introduction of the bacteria in one such colony resulted in a high incidence of neonatal mortality. Privately owned catteries are very unlikely to be free of the organism.

PUBLIC HEALTH SIGNIFICANCE

In humans, group G streptococci have received increasing attention as a cause of pharyngitis, neonatal sepsis, cellulitis, arthritis, puerperal sepsis, and endocarditis. *Streptococcus canis* sp. nov. has been proposed as the official name for animal beta-hemolytic group G streptococci. This proposal is based on biochemical and DNA similarities of canine and bovine strains and their differences from human strains of group G streptococci. Feline strains are similar to the animal isolates biochemically but have not been examined for DNA homology. No evidence has been found to indicate that infections in humans have arisen from animal sources.

References and Supplemental Reading

Blanchard, P. C.: Group G streptococcal infections in kittens: Pathogenesis, immunity and maternal carrier state. Ph.D. thesis (comparative pathology), University of California, 1987.

Blanchard, P. C., and Wilson, D. W.: Spontaneous *Streptococcus canis* infections of neonatal kittens in a closed cat colony. Vet. Pathol. (submitted).

Devriese, L. A., Homme, J., Kilpper-Balz, R., et al.: *Streptococcus canis* sp. nov.: A species of group G streptococci from animals. Int. J. Syst. Bacteriol. 36:422, 1986.

Fox, E. N.: M protein of group A streptococci. Bacteriol. Rev. 38:57, 1974.

Reitmeyer, J. C., and Steele, J. H.: The occurence of beta-hemolytic streptococcus in cats. Southwest. Vet. 36:41, 1984.

Swindle, M. M., Narayan, O., Luzarraga, M., et al.: Contagious streptococcal lymphadenitis in cats. J.A.V.M.A. 177:829, 1980.

Swindle, M. M., Narayan, O., Lazarraga, M., et al.: Pathogenesis of contagious streptococcal lymphadenitis in cats. J.A.V.M.A. 179:1208, 1981.

Timoney, J. F., and Trachman, J.: Immunologically reactive proteins of *Streptococcus equi*. Infect. Immun. 48:29, 1985.

GROUP A STREPTOCOCCAL INFECTIONS IN DOGS AND CATS

CRAIG E. GREENE, D.V.M.

Athens, Georgia

Streptococci are gram-positive, nonmotile, facultative anaerobic bacteria that cause localized to widespread pyogenic infections in animals and humans. Many species of streptococci are normal microflora of the oral cavity, nasopharynx, skin, and genital and gastrointestinal tracts. Strain differences of streptococci are responsible for the varying host ranges and degrees of pathogenicity.

Lancefield's group A are the most important disease-producing beta-hemolytic streptococci in humans. Dermatitis, pharyngitis, scarlet fever, and rheumatic fever are the main clinical syndromes associated with infection. In contrast, in dogs and cats, groups G, C, and L are the primary pathogenic species, whereas groups A and M cause nonsymptomatic infections.

Humans are the principal natural reservoir hosts of group A streptococci, which cause a majority of human streptococcal infections. In cases of pharyngitis, the greatest concentration of group A streptococci occurs on the caudal aspects of the pharynx and tonsillar region. The primary means of spread of this infection is by large airborne droplets, thereby necessitating close contact between individuals. These factors explain why an increased risk of infection is associated with crowding and lack of good personal hygiene. Diseased or convalescent carriers excrete large numbers of organisms. Having contracted the organism, untreated individuals can harbor it in the presence or absence of clinical illness for 4 months or longer.

Prevalence rates for group A streptococci are higher in children younger than 10 years of age, especially those in day-care or classrooms, since the group situation provides a constant reservoir for infection. Symptomatic rather than carrier children are more likely to bring infection into the home, and when children become ill, the isolation rate in other household members can be as high as 50 per cent.

A high rate of recurrence of group A streptococcal infections in some children is most likely due to factors such as mistakes in, or lack of, patient compliance with use of prescribed antimicrobial therapy; decreased antibody production to the specific strain or other existing immunodeficiency; and the presence of a reservoir for reinfection within immediate family members or close contacts. Dogs and cats have been suggested as possible sources of reinfection under such circumstances.

Whenever streptococcal typing of oropharyngeal isolates from dogs and cats has been performed, groups G, C, L, and M have been present, in decreasing order of frequency. Group A streptococcal isolations are uncommon on random sampling of household pets. However, a higher prevalence of infected pets has been shown by some screening studies for group A streptococcal colonization of tonsils of dogs and cats from households in urban environments where strep throat had recently been present.

The most probable scenario concerning the spread of group A streptococcal infections between humans and dogs and cats in households where recurrent infections develop is as follows: Domestic pets that come into close contact with infected humans can develop pharyngeal colonization with group A streptococci. These infected animals are clinically asymptomatic. If these animals are overlooked during treatment, they may be a reservoir of reinfection of family members. It should not be assumed that these animals are the primary or a permanent source of infection, since, in three infected pets studied by the author, group A streptococci were cultured for only 2 to 3 weeks after the animals were removed from the households. Pets might be involved in the transient spread of infection in a household; however, their contribution to the persistence of group A streptococci in nature is probably minimal. Other humans in the household are more likely than the pets to be harboring the organism on a more permanent basis.

Culture and isolation of group A streptococci have been the main methods of confirming infections in humans. Detection of group A streptococci on pharyngeal culture in the presence of clinical signs is only presumptive proof of clinical streptococcal pharyngitis. As many as 15 to 20 per cent of school-aged children (whether asymptomatic or clinically affected) are pharyngeal carriers of group A streptococci. In conclusion, a negative culture result eliminates the need for treatment, whereas a positive result regarding group A streptococci does not differentiate between clinical and asymptomatic infections.

The bacitracin sensitivity test is the most com-

1094

monly used method to screen for group A versus non–group A infections. The growth of most (approximately 95 to 99 per cent) but not all human isolates of group A streptococci is inhibited by 0.01 unit bacitracin disks. The greatest source of error with the use of bacitracin sensitivity testing on human isolates has been to misclassify groups B, C, and G streptococci as group A, because up to 22 per cent of these isolates have been shown to be inhibited by bacitracin. Because most isolates of streptococci in dogs and cats are non–group A types, the frequency of false-positive reactions using this means of identification is much higher.

Antigen detection test kits are now marketed as being relatively specific for rapid detection of group A streptococcal infections in humans. However, their sensitivity varies between 60 to 95 per cent, depending on the cultural methods used to make a comparison. Although these kits are in widespread use by pediatricians, their accuracy in detecting animal infections is uncertain. Therefore, when requested, the veterinarian should swab and culture for accurate detection of infection in a household pet.

The recovery of group A streptococci from throat swab specimens of dogs and cats is affected by the extent of infection, the method used in swabbing the throat, and the inadvertent collection of indigenous microflora that inhibit the growth of group A streptococci. Sedation or light anesthesia may be required to obtain proper pharyngeal specimens. Under good illumination, cotton or dacron sterile swabs should be rubbed over the surface of exposed tonsils or in the tonsillar crypts, avoiding contact with other areas of the oral cavity. Keeping swabs at cool temperatures (approximately 50°F; 10°C) during transport ensures recovery of streptococci regardless of the humidity of the transport swab. Swabs that cannot be refrigerated should be kept dry.

In humans, the drug of choice for treatment of streptococcal pharyngitis due to group A and other forms of streptococcal illnesses is penicillin. Broader spectrum or more expensive penicillins or cephalosporins are unnecessary, owing to the unusual development of penicillin resistance, but these drugs are more readily available in oral formulations than is penicillin. Erythromycin can be used in patients that have penicillin allergies; however, the gastrointestinal side effects are problematic. Tetracyclines and sulfonamides are poor choices for treating group A streptococci because of the development of drug resistance.

The antimicrobial spectrum for group A streptococcal infections in pets is the same as for human strains. Although infected dogs and cats are carriers, it is judicious to treat them when they may be a source for recurrent infection of household members. Isolates of group A streptococci from dogs have shown the greatest sensitivity to penicillin, erythromycin, and chloramphenicol. In dogs and cats, the recommended total daily dosages for penicillin, erythromycin, and chloramphenicol are 10,000 to 100,000 IU, 3 to 20 mg/kg, and 10 to 50 mg/kg, respectively. In addition, daily dosages of cephalosporins (10 to 40 mg/kg) have also been used to treat resistant group A streptococcal infections.

References and Supplemental Reading

Biberstein, E. L., Brown, C., and Smith, T.: Serogroups and biotypes among beta-hemolytic streptococci of canine origin. J. Clin. Microbiol. 11:558, 1980.

Copperman, S. M.: Cherchez le chien—household pets as reservoirs of persistent or recurrent streptococcal sore throats in children. N.Y. State J. Med. 82:1685, 1982.

Crowder, H. R., Dorn, C. R., and Smith, R. E.: Group A *Streptococcus* in pets and group A streptococcal disease in man. Int. J. Zoonoses 5:45, 1978.

Greene, C. E.: Zoonotic aspects of group A streptococcal infection in dogs and cats. J. Am. Anim. Hosp. Assoc. 24:218, 1988.

Mayer, G., and Van Ore, S.: Recurrent pharyngitis in family of four. Postgrad. Med. 74:277, 1983.

Wuori, L. A.: What's new pussy cat? Cornell Feline Health Center Communication, November 1986.

CLINICAL AND PUBLIC HEALTH SIGNIFICANCE OF ANTIMICROBIAL-RESISTANT ENTERIC BACTERIAL INFECTIONS

DWIGHT C. HIRSH, D.V.M.

Davis, California

The clinical and public health significance of antimicrobial-resistant enteric bacteria (members of the family Enterobacteriaceae) is determined by both the agent itself and the genes encoding the resistance. Resistant enteric agents that infect and produce disease in both humans and other animals have clinical relevancy because of inherent difficulties in the treatment of such diseases.

CLINICAL AND PUBLIC HEALTH SIGNIFICANCE OF RESISTANCE GENES

Enteric bacteria become resistant to antimicrobial agents by acquiring DNA that encodes proteins that protect the micro-organism from harm by the antimicrobial. These proteins inactivate the antimicrobial, change the permeability of the bacterial cell, or result in a change or a by-pass of the target within the bacterial cell. The genes responsible for these proteins are more often than not located on autonomously replicating pieces of extrachromosomal DNA called plasmids. Plasmids carry genes that encode proteins that fulfill a variety of functions, from toxicity to substrate utilization. When plasmids carry genes that encode resistance to antimicrobials, they are called R plasmids. Although any number of resistance genes may be carried on an R plasmid, the usual number is three to four. Examples of R plasmids isolated from enteric microorganisms found in the feces of clinically normal dogs are shown in Table 1. Plasmids may also encode the information enabling them to transfer, by conjugation, to other members of the family. Thus, some R plasmids have the potential to move from one strain of enteric bacteria to another (from one species or from one genus to another) carrying resistance to multiple antimicrobials. Not only may the entire plasmid be mobile, but the genes themselves have the property of moving from segment to segment of DNA (e.g., from plasmid to plasmid

or from plasmid to chromosome and vice versa). These mobile genes, or transposable elements (transposons), account for the multiplicity of resistance genes on R plasmids, being added or deleted as the need arises.

The main environmental reservoir for these resistance genes is the intestinal tract of humans and other animals receiving antimicrobials. The genes move throughout the environment inside of enteric bacteria that are shed by these animals. Since the plasmids found in enteric bacteria isolated from humans are the same as those found in other animals, it is highly probable that human enteric organisms and other animal enteric micro-organisms participate in the same genetic pool of resistance genes.

In general, there are two types of animal reservoirs for genetic material encoding resistance to antimicrobial agents: animals receiving antimicrobials for therapeutic reasons and those receiving antimicrobials for growth-promoting (prophylactic) reasons. Approximately 200 million prescriptions for antimicrobials are written for humans in the United States annually. It is unknown how many prescriptions for these drugs are written for other animals. Most of the antimicrobials, as well as the

Table 1. *Resistance Encoded by R Plasmid Found in* Escherichia coli *in the Feces of Normal, Untreated Dogs*

Frequency (%)	Resistance Spectrum
18	Ap Cm Km Sm Su Tc
18	Km Sm Su Tc
13	Ap Cp Cm Km Sm Su Tc
10	Sm Tc
5	Ap Sm Su Tc
5	Ap Sm Tc
5	Sm Su Tc

Ap, ampicillin; Cm, chloramphenicol; Km, kanamycin; Sm, streptomycin; Su, sulfonamides; Tc, tetracycline; Cp, cephalothin.

resistant enteric micro-organisms are excreted by humans and other animals (companion and captive) receiving antimicrobials and end up in a sewage-treatment system. Antimicrobials will select for R plasmid–containing micro-organisms in such an environment.

In the hospital environment, the concentration of R plasmids is more critical because of the constant selective pressure exerted by antimicrobial agents on enteric bacteria. To survive in this environment, these bacteria must have the genes to inactivate the antimicrobials. They do this by acquiring R plasmid DNA. It is the rare exception that an enteric micro-organism in the hospital environment is relatively susceptible to antimicrobials. They almost always contain an R plasmid encoding resistance to multiple antimicrobials. In the author's hospital, a strain of *Klebsiella pneumoniae* is endemic. This micro-organism contains a conjugal R plasmid encoding resistance to ampicillin, cephalothin, chloramphenicol, gentamicin, kanamycin, streptomycin, and trimethoprim-sulfonamides.

The other major environmental source of genes encoding resistance to antimicrobials is the intestinal tract of food-producing animals receiving feed into which antimicrobials have been added for growth promotion or to prevent disease. The magnitude of this problem is realized from the following data. There are about 100 million cattle and about 40 million pigs receiving antimicrobials (the most commonly used are penicillin and tetracycline) per year in the United States. Animals receiving antimicrobials will excrete approximately 10^8 R plasmid–carrying bacteria per gram of feces. This selection takes place regardless of the amount of antimicrobial that is used (prophylactic or therapeutic amounts). If a cow and a pig excrete approximately 70 lb and 4 lb of feces a day, respectively, the numbers of R plasmid–bearing enteric micro-organisms going into the environment untreated is immense. These data do not take into account the amount of biologically active antimicrobial that finds its way into the environment.

The clinical and public health risk of this environmental pool (community, hospital, food-producing animals) of genetic information encoding resistance to antimicrobial agents comes about in the following way. R plasmid–bearing pathogenic bacteria (e.g., *Salmonella*) are obviously of clinical relevance in themselves. However, R plasmid–bearing potential pathogens or nonpathogenic enteric micro-organisms also pose a significant threat. When the potential pathogens infect a compromised site, they produce disease that is difficult to treat. The R plasmid–bearing nonpathogens act as reservoirs from which R plasmid genes can move to pathogen and potential pathogen alike.

COMMUNICABILITY OF ENTERIC BACTERIA

Contact of an animal with an infectious agent may or may not lead to infection. For infection to occur, the bacteria must contend with the innate immunity of the surface that is to be infected. For enteric micro-organisms, the surface most likely to be involved is the mucosa of the alimentary canal. The most important parts of the innate immunity of this surface are the normal flora residing throughout the tract, gastric acidity, and the peristaltic activity of the small intestine.

The normal flora is acquired shortly after birth. Once established, this flora is remarkably stable. This is so because each site or location along the tract is inhabited by micro-organisms most aptly suited to live at that location. Competitors are excluded from that particular site. Exclusion may be passive (the niche dweller simply competes more effectively for nutrients) or active, as evidenced by the excretion of substances (e.g., volatile fatty acids, bacteriocins, microcins) that are lethal for potential competitors.

Another important aspect of restricted colonization of a mucosal surface is the ability of the micro-organism to adhere to receptors on or associated with an epithelial cell lining the tract. If the receptor to which the prospective colonizer is to attach is already occupied by another micro-organism, colonization (infection) is prevented. If the micro-organism cannot adhere, it will be swept away.

Gastric acidity is an efficient barrier to the entry of ingested micro-organisms into the intestinal tract. Infectious agents that are potential colonizers of the intestinal tract either must be resistant to the low pH of this environment or must be ingested in numbers large enough to allow them to successfully compete for a site along the tract distal to the stomach.

If the ingested micro-organism is to colonize the small intestine, it must adhere tightly to receptors on the surface or associated with the surface of epithelial cells of this area.

If a normal animal becomes exposed to an infectious agent from an exogenous source, the chances are excellent that infection will not occur. However, there are a number of circumstances that will influence the outcome of this interaction, especially stress and antimicrobial agents. Stress brought about by psychologic, dietary, or physiologic influences changes the composition of the normal flora of the alimentary tract. In the oral cavity, the amount of fibronectin coating epithelial cells decreases following exposure of an animal to a stressful situation. Fibronectin contains receptors for gram-positive members of the normal flora in this and adjoining areas. When this substance is decreased, receptors for gram-negative micro-organisms are exposed. Thus, following stress, the oral cavity is recolonized with gram-negative micro-organisms, mainly enteric organisms.

As is the case in the oral cavity, stressfull events cause changes in the makeup of the normal flora of the distal small and the large intestines. The main change is a reduction in the numbers of obligate anaerobic bacteria, which comprise 99 per cent of the flora in this location. Subsequent to the fall in the numbers of these micro-organisms, an increase in the numbers of enteric organisms takes place. The reason for the drop in the number of obligate anaerobes is not known. As a result of this drop, the concentration of fatty acids decreases, resulting in the overgrowth of enteric organisms.

Certain antimicrobials affect the normal flora as well. Gram-positive cocci on buccal and gingival surfaces, obligate anaerobes in the gingival sulcus, and obligate anaerobes in the distal portions of the intestinal tract are important regulating influences of the alimentary canal. A reduction in any of these results in an increased number of enteric micro-organisms along the tract. In addition, the infective dose of enteric micro-organism is greatly reduced. For instance, it takes approximately 10^8 salmonellae to infect a normal animal, but after reduction in the normal flora (the obligate anaerobes), the number of salmonellae needed to infect is less than 10^2. In practical terms, this means that animals receiving antimicrobials, for whatever reason, are vulnerable to colonization by an enteric micro-organism provided the prospective colonizer is resistant to the antimicrobial being used. In the author's small animal clinic, animals receiving antimicrobials (especially ampicillin) were shown to be approximately 40 times more likely to become infected with salmonellae than nontreated animals.

If the reduction of colonization resistance is due to antimicrobials, the colonizing enteric micro-organism will be resistant to the drug being used. If resistant, the micro-organisms will contain R plasmids and will be resistant to other antimicrobials as well. If the reduction of colonization resistance is due to stress, the colonizing enteric organisms may or may not be resistant (contain an R plasmid). This would depend on the environment of the animal. If the environment were one in which antimicrobials were in use, the likelihood of colonization with an enteric containing an R plasmid would be great, as it would be for animals in the hospital. It is important to keep in mind that the number of R plasmid–containing enteric micro-organisms in the intestinal tract of humans and other animals *not* receiving antimicrobials is considerable (fluctuating between 0 and 10^8 organism/gm feces), although not nearly as significant as in those receiving antimicrobials (constant level of 10^8 organism/gm feces).

Colonizing micro-organisms may be pathogens, may have pathogenic potential, or may be nonpathogenic. If colonization occurs with a pathogenic micro-organism, such as *Salmonella*, that requires treatment, antimicrobial effectiveness will be compromised if the agent contains an R plasmid. It has been shown that the case fatality rate for humans with invasive R plasmid–bearing *Salmonella* was 21 times higher than that for humans with invasive disease caused by susceptible strains. It should be stressed that the disease itself usually is not influenced by the R plasmid, only the treatment. However, there are transposable elements encoding virulence determinants. If these elements were to insert onto an R plasmid, as has been demonstrated with strains of enterotoxigenic *Escherichia coli*, the disease and the treatment would be influenced.

The risk to the host following colonization with an enteric micro-organism with no pathogenic potential is minimal, even if it contains an R plasmid. What risk there is stems from the potential of the R plasmid to move to other enteric micro-organisms that have increased virulence potential.

SUMMARY

Enteric bacteria in our environment are in contact with a very mobile gene pool that encodes resistance to multiple antimicrobial agents. Some of these bacteria are able to infect and produce disease in humans and other animals. Other species have the potential to infect and produce disease only if the site becomes compromised. Finally, there are enteric organisms that do not have the ability to produce disease at all. This latter group serves only as a source of resistance genes, as do all enteric organisms regardless of their potential to produce disease.

The fact that an enteric organism possesses an R plasmid has little to do with infection or disease unless the genes for these functions are also on the R plasmid. The major consequence of the acquisition of an R plasmid is compromise of treatment. This consequence can be greatly reduced by measures aimed at shrinking the size of the environmental pool of resistance genes. Antimicrobials should be used for treatment of disease or for short periods for protection of a compromised site(s). To do otherwise is unwise and irrational because such activity places unneeded selective pressures on naturally occurring resistance genes in our environment. Since the level of resistance genes will fall following the removal of antimicrobials, cessation of all nontherapeutic drug administration (except for prophylaxis proven to be beneficial) would result in a decrease in the numbers of R plasmid–possessing enteric bacteria. Therefore, it follows that disease produced by enteric micro-organisms would be easier to treat.

References and Supplemental Reading

Cohen, M. L., and Tauxe, R. V.: Drug-resistant *Salmonella* in the United States: An epidemiologic perspective. Science 234:964, 1986.

Falkow, S.: *Infectious Multiple Drug Resistance.* London: Pion Limited, 1975.

Finkel, M. J.: Magnitude of antibiotic use. Ann. Int. Med. 89:791, 1978.

Hirsh, D. C., Ling, G. V., and Ruby, A. L.: Incidence of R-plasmids in fecal flora of healthy household dogs. Antimicrob. Agents Chemother. 17:313, 1980.

Holmberg, S. D., Wells, J. G., and Cohen, M. L.: Animal-to-man transmission of antimicrobial-resistant *Salmonella*: Investigations of U.S. outbreaks, 1971–1983. Science 225:833, 1984.

Levy, S. B.: Playing antibiotic pool: Time to tally the score. N. Engl. J. Med. 311:663, 1984.

Mercer, H. D., Pucurull, D., Gaines, W., et al.: Characteristics of antimicrobial resistance of *Escherichia coli* from animals: Relationship to veterinary and management uses of antimicrobial agents. Appl. Microbiol. 22:700, 1971.

O'Brien, T. F., Hopkins, J. D., Gilleece, E. S., et al.: Molecular epidemiology of antibiotic resistance in *Salmonella* from animals and human beings in the United States. N. Engl. J. Med. 307:1, 1982.

van der Waaij, D.: *Antibiotic Choice: The Importance of Colonization Resistance.* Letchworth, England: Research Studies Press, 1983.

CAT-SCRATCH FEVER

JOHNNY D. HOSKINS, D.V.M.

Baton Rouge, Louisiana

Cat-scratch fever, also known as cat-scratch disease, cat-scratch syndrome, or benign lymphoreticulosis, is a benign, self-limiting, "presumed" infectious disease affecting humans. Following a cat scratch or bite, this syndrome exhibits any or all of the following signs: an erythematous, crusted papule; a granuloma of the eye with or without conjunctivitis; and a mucous membrane lesion (canker sore, abrasion, or gingivitis) at the site of injury. In the majority of patients, the illness is mild, and signs may include painful regional lymphadenopathy; fever (38.3 to 41.1°C; 100.9 to 105.98°F); malaise or fatigue; headache; anorexia, emesis, and weight loss; splenomegaly; sore throat; conjunctivitis; exanthem (maculopapular, petechial, erythema nodosum); and parotid swelling (Margileth, 1987).

Skin lesions develop 3 to 10 days after a scratch or bite from a cat and usually persist for 1 to 3 weeks, with a few remaining for 8 to 10 weeks. The primary inoculation lesion always heals without scar formation. Persistence of a lymphadenopathy for several months in a generally healthy patient with gradual spontaneous resolution of enlarged lymph nodes is the natural course of cat-scratch fever. Most commonly, the enlarged lymph nodes are found in the head, neck, or axillary areas. Less frequently, brachial, breast or chest, epitrochlear, inguinal, femoral, and occipital areas are involved. The lymphadenopathy usually develops about 2 weeks after a scratch or bite and may last for 2 to 5 months before gradual resolution.

ETIOLOGY

Various feline and human infectious agents have been proposed as the cause of cat-scratch fever, including mycobacteria, *Chlamydia*, and several viruses. Because extensive efforts to demonstrate a bacterial cause were unsuccessful, a viral etiology was assumed. All attempts at viral isolations from several samples of human lymph node biopsies have been unsuccessful, as have electron microscopic examinations of these tissues. Serologic studies also failed to yield positive results. However, the long-awaited breakthrough may have come in reports by Wear and coworkers, who propose a bacterium as the cause of cat-scratch fever.

After studying a single case in 1981, in which a small, gram-negative, silver-staining bacterium was seen in lymph node tissue, Wear and coworkers (1983) began a study of lymph nodes from additional cases of cat-scratch fever. Morphologically identical bacilli were found in lymph nodes sections from 34 of 39 patients with cat-scratch fever from October 1982 to March 1983, but not in sections of the lymph nodes from 91 patients with other diseases. These identical bacteria were subsequently found in primary skin lesions of cat-scratch fever patients. Further evidence that the bacilli are the causative agents in cat-scratch fever is to be seen in the occurrence of these small, pleomorphic, gram-negative, non–acid-fast, intracellular bacilli in capillary walls and in macrophages in lymph node tissue of involved areas; their disappearance as the disease process resolved; and immunofluorescent staining of the bacilli by fluorescein-tagged convalescent serum from cat-scratch fever patients. Furthermore, humans with Parinaud's oculoglandular syndrome (POGS) have the same bacilli in their conjunctival lesions, indicating a common cause of the two diseases. Biochemical and physiologic analyses of one isolate suggested that it was a member of the genus *Rothia*. However, this finding has been disputed. It is believed that the causative agent of cat-scratch fever, when successfully cultured, will probably be a previously unknown bacterium.

THE DISEASE IN HUMANS

Cat-scratch fever occurs worldwide in all races and more often in males than in females. It tends to be seasonal, with the majority of patients being recognized in the fall and winter months; however, in warmer climates, the disease is more often observed during July and August. Most patients affected with cat-scratch fever are younger than 21 years of age. In the family, more than one member may, on occasion, be affected, usually a sibling and rarely a parent. When this happens, the individuals are affected within a 2- to 3-week period of each other. Human-to-human transmission has not been reported, and common exposure to the same cat is most probably the source of infection. Patients with cat-scratch fever do not require isolation or quarantine.

Cat-scratch fever does not stir fears of widespread epidemics, severe morbidity, or high fatality rates as do many diseases. It can have a significant impact, however. The financial burden and inconvenience of medical care and surgery may be large, and complications may occur, including oculoglandular syndrome of Parinaud, severe systemic disease, erythema nodosum, thrombocytopenic purpura, osteolytic lesions, encephalopathy or encephalitis, and other neurologic manifestations. Less often recorded, but no less significant for the patient and the family, is the fear that the signs and symptoms may represent lymphoma or other more serious diseases, until it is diagnosed only as cat-scratch fever.

The Role of the Cat

In cat-scratch fever, human patients have generally had direct contact with a cat, with documented scratches or bites in about 90 to 95 per cent of the confirmed cases. The exact role the cat plays is unknown. Cats that transmit cat-scratch fever are not ill and have no distinctive features. The length of time during which they are capable of transmitting the disease is unknown. Most suspected cats are younger than 1 year of age. The cat living in the household may not necessarily be the transmitter of the causative agent. Therefore, inquiry must be made concerning those in the homes of relatives, close friends, and neighbors.

Cats that transmit cat-scratch fever may merely be a mechanical vector, inoculating the causative agent by scratch, lick, or bite. In rare cases, the disease develops following a scratch from a thorn, crab claw, or wood splinter or is associated with insect bites. In each case, the patient usually remembers that a cat had more than likely licked the skin abrasion.

Diagnosis

Diagnosis of cat-scratch fever presents very little difficulty in a majority of patients if the physician inquires about the patient's contact with cats and especially cat scratches or bites. Diagnosis can be made, based on the criteria: (1) the patient had contact with a cat; (2) the patient has scratches, a primary inoculation papule, or both; (3) the result of a skin test (described later) is positive; (4) test results show negative aerobic and anaerobic bacterial cultures and negative serologies for infectious mononucleosis, brucellosis, cytomegalovirus disease, tularemia, toxoplasmosis, histoplasmosis, or herpes simplex; and (5) the lymph nodes have characteristic histologic lesions of cat-scratch fever. There are no diagnostic laboratory tests for cat-scratch fever. A few patients have been reported to have eosinophilia; rarely, minimal leukocytosis may occur initially with an increased number of polymorphonuclear cells.

When available, the cat-scratch fever skin test with a nonstandardized antigen prepared from human lymph node aspirates (with differing recommendations for its preparation and differing criteria for interpreting a positive reaction) is recommended. The skin test reaction becomes positive about the time the clinical signs are manifest. Occasionally, conversion may be delayed for 4 weeks; therefore, a second skin test should be considered if cat-scratch fever is still suspected. In a baffling, atypical case of cat-scratch fever, biopsy specimens of skin, lymph node, or both should be taken by an experienced surgeon, the specimen handled properly, and interpretation of results performed by a pathologist who is familiar with the special stains needed to detect the causative bacilli.

Treatment and Prevention

In the majority of patients, no active therapy is needed. Treatment consists of close observation, analgesics for pain, aspiration of the enlarged lymph node if suppuration occurs and reassurance that the skin lesion and lymphadenopathy will subside spontaneously. Aspiration relieves painful lymphadenopathy, and with one or two aspirations the patient usually becomes asymptomatic within 24 to 48 hr. Antimicrobial agents are not recommended for typical cases of cat-scratch fever, because patients consistently do not respond to them. If moderate to severe acute lymphadenitis is present, particularly with redness and increased heat of the overlying skin, an antimicrobial agent may be given for 7 to 10 days. Application of moist, warm compresses to the primary skin lesion may facilitate drainage and shorten the duration of lymphadenopathy. Patients generally recover within 2 to 5 months of its diagnosis.

There are no diagnostic laboratory tests to determine if a particular cat is in fact a carrier of the cat-scratch fever agent. Because the involved cat is invariably healthy, disposal of the suspected cat is not recommended nor is declawing recommended. It is also advisable to wash cuts, bites, and scratches promptly and not to allow the cat to lick an open wound. It would seem prudent to prevent a suspected carrier cat from coming into close contact with sick children and immunocompromised persons.

References and Supplemental Reading

Carithers, H. A.: Cat scratch disease: An overview based on a study of 1,200 patients. Am. J. Dis. Child. 139:1124, 1985.
Emmons, R. W.: Cat scratch disease: The mystery finally solved? Ann. Int. Med. 100:303, 1984.
Gerber, M. A., MacAlister, T. J., Ballow, M., et al.: The aetiological agent of cat scratch disease. Lancet 8840:1236, 1985.
Hadfield, T. L., Malaty, R. H., Van Ellan, A., et al.: Electron microscopy of the bacillus causing cat scratch disease? J. Infect. Dis. 152:643, 1985a.
Hadfield, T. L., Wear, D. J., Margileth, A. M., et al.: Letter to editor. Is Rothia dentocariosa the cause of cat scratch disease? Lancet 8840:720, 1985b.
Margileth, A. M.: Cat scratch disease: A therapeutic dilemma. Vet. Clin. North Am. 17:91, 1987.
Margileth, A. M., Wear, D. J., Hadfield, T. L., et al.: Cat-scratch disease: Bacteria in skin at the primary inoculation site. J.A.M.A. 252:928, 1984.
Wear, D. J., Margileth, A. M., Hadfield, T. L., et al.: Cat scratch disease: A bacterial infection. Science 221:1403, 1983.
Wear, D. J., Raga, H. M., Zimmerman, L. E., et al.: Cat scratch disease bacilli in the conjunctiva of patients with Parinaud's oculoglandular syndrome. Ophthalmology 92:1282, 1985.

SYSTEMIC ANTIFUNGAL CHEMOTHERAPY

JAMES O. NOXON, D.V.M.

Ames, Iowa

The ideal antifungal agent for systemic use would have a broad spectrum of activity, be fungicidal, have widespread tissue distribution, be available in oral and injectable forms, have low toxicity, and be reasonably priced. It is unfortunate that currently available drugs are less than ideal in many respects; however proper patient management requires an understanding of these drugs. Amphotericin B (AMB), the standard antifungal treatment for 30 years, has limited use because of toxicities. The imidazoles are fungistatic and reach subtherapeutic concentrations in some tissues. Other antifungal drugs have similar limitations. The continued development of new antifungal agents offers promise for the future of antifungal chemotherapy. This article will review the properties and indications of the antifungal drugs available for systemic chemotherapy.

AMPHOTERICIN B

Amphotericin B (Fungizone, Squibb) is a polyene macrolide antibiotic isolated from the actinomycete, *Streptomyces nodosus*. Amphotericin B irreversibly binds to ergosterol, the principal sterol in the cell wall of fungal organisms, altering the integrity and permeability of the cell membrane. Rapid metabolic deterioration and cell death of susceptible organisms follow. The drug binds less avidly to cholesterol, the principal sterol of mammalian cell membranes, thus reducing the effects of AMB in animal tissues.

Amphotericin B is available in vials containing 50 mg of the drug as a lypholized powder, sodium desoxycholate to effect colloidal distribution of the drug, and buffers. Sterile water is mixed with the contents of the vial to yield a solution with a concentration of 5 mg/ml. This solution is stable for 1 week when refrigerated. Dilutions of the stock solution for clinical use are made with 5 per cent dextrose, since solutions containing electrolytes, preservatives, or acids reportedly cause precipitation of the drug. When properly prepared, the drug may be given intravenously, intrathecally, intra-articularly, or subconjunctivally.

Amphotericin B is detectable in the serum of dogs, where it is strongly bound to plasma proteins, for up to 12 days following a single intravenous dose. The effects of AMB appear to be cumulative following multiple injections. The drug is widely distributed to most body tissues, although low concentrations of AMB are found in cerebrospinal fluid (CSF), bronchial secretions, and aqueous humor. The mechanisms of metabolism and excretion of AMB are unclear, although there is significant clearance by renal and biliary routes.

A wide variety of mycotic agents are susceptible to AMB, including *Blastomyces*, *Histoplasma*, *Cryptococcus*, *Candida*, *Coccidioides*, *Sporothrix*, and *Aspergillus*. The minimum inhibitory concentration of AMB may vary within each group of fungi. Some species or subtypes are susceptible to concentrations reached in clinical use, whereas others are resistant.

Two regimens for AMB therapy may be used (Table 1). The first is a rapid infusion technique with the dose of AMB diluted into approximately 30 ml of 5 per cent dextrose and administered over 5 to 10 min. A butterfly catheter works well for IV infusion. This technique is recommended in most cases of systemic mycotic infections and is expedient for animals treated on an outpatient basis. The second technique involves dilution of the drug into 250 to 500 ml of 5 per cent dextrose and infusion of this solution over a 4- to 6-hr time span. This slow infusion technique is useful for debilitated patients and animals with impaired renal function.

In each technique, the dose is given three times each week until a total accumulated dosage of 9 to 12 mg/kg is achieved. The therapeutic efficacy of AMB does not appear to be altered by the infusion of lower individual doses, as long as the total accumulated dosage is sufficient. Relapses are less probable with higher accumulated dosages.

Table 1. *Techniques for Administration of Amphotericin B*

Rapid IV Infusion Technique
1. Prepare stock solution of AMB, using 10 ml sterile water for injection.
2. Dilute 0.25 mg/kg of AMB into 30 ml 5% dextrose.
3. Place butterfly catheter, and flush with 10 ml 5% dextrose.
4. Infuse AMB solution over 5 min.
5. Flush catheter with 10 ml of 5% dextrose.
6. Remove butterfly catheter.
7. Subsequent doses of AMB will be with 0.5 mg/kg, repeated three times each week until an accumulated dosage of 9–12 mg/kg is reached.

Slow IV Infusion Technique
1. Prepare stock solution of AMB by adding 10 ml sterile water for injection to one vial (50 mg).
2. Calculate initial dose of AMB at 0.25 mg/kg, and add to 250–500 ml 5% dextrose.
3. Place an indwelling catheter in a peripheral vein, and administer total volume over 4 to 6 hr.
4. Flush the catheter with 10 ml 5% dextrose, and remove the catheter.
5. Subsequent doses of AMB at 0.5 mg/kg will be given three times each week until an accumulated dosage of 9–12 mg/kg is reached.

Amphotericin B is a relatively toxic antifungal agent. Nephrotoxicosis is the most severe and limiting of the adverse effects. Amphotericin B causes renal vasoconstriction and subsequent diminished glomerular filtration rate and may have direct toxic effects on tubular epithelial cells. The renal damage seen in dogs following AMB therapy seems to be more severe and to occur more frequently when higher individual doses are given. Most canine patients show some degree of renal dysfunction while receiving AMB.

Patients should be monitored by pretreatment determinations of serum urea nitrogen (SUN) or creatinine concentrations. Amphotericin B is discontinued when the patient's SUN exceeds 30 mg/dl and is not reinstituted until the SUN falls within normal levels. Pretreatment intravenous sodium loading with 0.9 per cent sodium chloride solution may help decrease the nephrotoxic effects of AMB and is recommended if the patient develops evidence of renal toxicosis. Fluid therapy may also expedite the drop in SUN concentration after renal damage occurs. Pre-existing renal disease does not affect clearance of AMB, but patients may be more susceptible to the nephrotoxic effects of the drug.

Reduced nephrotoxicity of AMB has been found in dogs when 12.5 gm of mannitol were simultaneously infused with AMB; however, dogs with blastomycosis receiving this combination have had lower overall cure rates compared with dogs receiving AMB alone. The addition of mannitol to AMB is best reserved for patients with underlying renal disease.

Other adverse effects of AMB therapy include fever, anorexia, vomiting, hypokalemia, and phlebitis. Also, extravasation of the drug results in severe irritation of the perivascular tissues. Phlebitis has a limiting effect on therapy, since it may interfere with subsequent infusions of the drug. Concurrent aspirin therapy or heparin flushes of the infusion catheter have been advocated to decrease the phlebitis, but there is no conclusive evidence that these measures are effective. The author feels that careful venipuncture technique and rotation of injection sites will minimize the phlebitis.

Cats seem to be more sensitive than dogs to the adverse effects of AMB. Lower individual doses (0.25 mg/kg) help decrease the severity and frequency of these reactions. The rapid infusion technique is preferred in cats.

IMIDAZOLES

The imidazoles are a rapidly expanding group of antifungal agents. Their mechanism of action appears to be primarily fungistatic, although fungicidal activity has been reported at high drug concentrations. The imidazoles interfere with ergosterol synthesis and incorporation into fungal cell membranes. They also appear to have direct effects on membrane fatty acids and interfere with enzymes required for cellular respiration and metabolism. Several imidazoles have been developed and used in veterinary medicine. Those commercially available for systemic use include miconazole and ketoconazole (KTZ). Miconazole is available as an intravenous preparation but has seen minimal use because of toxicities and limited efficacy.

Ketoconazole (Nizoral, Janssen) is the principal imidazole derivative that is used in humans and animals. It is well absorbed from the gastrointestinal tract and widely distributed in the dog following oral administration. Concentrations of KTZ in the CSF and brain are lower than those in other tissues; however, they exceed the reported minimum inhibitory concentrations for most pathogenic fungi when the drug is administered at 30 mg/kg daily. Ketoconazole is metabolized and excreted primarily by the liver.

Several pathogenic fungi are susceptible to KTZ, including, to varying degrees, *Candida*, *Histoplasma*, *Blastomyces*, *Coccidioides*, *Cryptococcus*, *Sporothrix*, and *Aspergillus*. Clinical success has been reported following KTZ therapy in canine blastomycosis, canine coccidioidomycosis, canine and feline cryptococcosis, feline histoplasmosis, canine aspergillosis, and canine sporotrichosis. Treatment failures have also been reported in these same diseases. Treatment regimens involving combinations of KTZ and other antifungal drugs have had encouraging results and will be discussed later.

The recommended daily dose of KTZ in the dog is 10 to 30 mg/kg, divided into two or three doses. Animals with central nervous system, skin, or bone involvement may require a higher dosage in order to reach therapeutic concentrations in affected tissues. The minimum treatment period is 2 months. Ketoconazole therapy is generally continued for 1 to 3 months beyond clinical recovery of the patient. In cats, a daily total of 10 to 15 mg/kg, divided into two or three doses, has been effective for various systemic mycoses.

Ketoconazole may cause anorexia, depression, transient alopecia, vomiting, and increased hepatic enzyme activity. Reduction of the dose or dividing the dosage into two or three daily doses will alleviate these adverse effects in most cases. Cats with increased hepatic enzyme activity and anorexia have responded well to alternate-day drug administration. Ketoconazole inhibits enzymes in the pathway of steroid hormone production. Hormone profiles of dogs receiving KTZ are altered significantly (e.g., lowered cortisol values); however, adverse clinical effects resulting from these changes have not been observed. Ketoconazole should not be used in pregnant animals.

Clinical response to KTZ therapy is generally not seen for at least 5 to 10 days following the onset of therapy. Use of KTZ as the sole therapeutic agent should be avoided if the patient is in critical condition, is debilitated, or has malabsorption due to gastrointestinal involvement.

Long-term KTZ therapy is necessary to control some mycotic infections in both animals and humans. In humans, indefinite therapy may be necessary to control fungal meningitis caused by *Coccidioides immitis*. In dogs, pulmonary coccidioidomycosis requires therapy of at least 6 months duration in most cases. Animals with bone involvement or disseminated disease may require KTZ therapy for 12 months or longer to avoid relapse.

Two promising imidazole derivatives under investigation are itraconazole and fluconazole. Itraconazole is well absorbed following oral administration, is insoluble in aqueous fluids and highly protein bound, and sustains plasma levels following a single dose much longer than KTZ. Like KTZ, itraconazole is found in minimal concentrations in the CSF. However, experimental studies showed itraconazole to be effective in cryptococcal meningitis in rabbits. *In vitro* activity has also been demonstrated against *Aspergillus* and *Sporothrix* organisms. Itraconazole is currently under investigation for use in mycotic infections in dogs and has shown encouraging results in blastomycosis and nasal aspergillosis (Legendre, 1987).

Fluconazole, another investigational imidazole, is given orally and reaches high concentrations in the CSF and urine. The drug has shown promise in experimental studies of several mycotic infections.

FLUCYTOSINE

Flucytosine (5-FC; Ancobon, Roche) is a fluorinated pyrimidine with a narrow range of antimycotic activity, limited primarily to yeastlike fungi such as *Cryptococcus*. The drug is well absorbed following oral administration and is distributed to most organs. Concentrations of 5-FC in the CSF approach 60 to 70 per cent of serum concentrations. Flucytosine is deaminated in the cytoplasm of susceptible fungi into 5-fluorouracil, which competitively inhibits thymidylate synthetase activity. Consequently, DNA and cellular protein synthesis are inhibited. Resistance that may develop during long-term administration of 5-FC has been attributed to deficiencies in enzyme pathways necessary for proper metabolic degradation of the drug, increased synthesis of competitive pyrimidines by the fungal cell, and other mechanisms. The majority of 5-FC is excreted unchanged in the urine.

Flucytosine is given orally at 25 to 50 mg/kg every 6 hr. The duration of treatment is based on clinical factors and response to therapy. In general, 5-FC should be administered for several weeks beyond clinical remission. Adverse effects of 5-FC include gastrointestinal disturbances, cutaneous reactions, hepatotoxicity, and bone marrow suppression. Patients receiving 5-FC should be monitored for leukopenia and thrombocytopenia, which may occur within days of the onset of treatment. The drug should be discontinued if adverse effects are seen. Flucytosine is most often used in conjunction with other antifungal agents such as AMB.

IODIDES

Both sodium and potassium iodide have been used successfully to manage cutaneous and lymphocutaneous forms of sporotrichosis. The precise mechanism of action of these salts is unknown. A 20 per cent solution of sodium iodide is given orally at 20 to 40 mg/kg every 8 to 12 hr. Cats are more susceptible to iodide toxicosis; therefore, the dosage should be reduced and the drug administered only once daily. Adverse effects include vomiting, anorexia, cardiomegaly, and cutaneous reactions. They are generally reversible when the dosage is decreased or the drug discontinued.

COMBINATION CHEMOTHERAPY

Antifungal chemotherapy may be enhanced by using combinations of drugs that demonstrate synergism or advantageous additive effects. Benefits of combination chemotherapy include increased therapeutic efficacy against some fungal organisms, less toxicity, shorter treatment times, and, in some cases, lower cost of therapy. The potential for drug antagonism should be considered before combinations are used. Experimental studies and clinical trials have demonstrated clear advantages in some mycoses when drug combinations are used instead of single-drug therapy.

Combination therapy using AMB plus 5-FC has been shown to be superior to AMB alone for cryptococcal infections, especially when the central nervous system is involved. It has not been clearly established whether the advantages observed by combining the two therapies result from synergism or from additive effects of the drugs. In this regimen, AMB is given as described previously until an accumulated dose of 4 to 6 mg/kg is achieved. Flucytosine is given, as previously described, beginning on the first day of AMB therapy. Some investigators advocate administration of AMB at 0.25 mg/kg once a month after the induction dose of 4 to 6 mg/kg is reached (Greene et al., 1984). The duration of therapy should be individualized for each patient.

The combination of AMB and KTZ allows a rapid response to therapy while avoiding the toxicosis associated with prolonged administration of AMB. The effects of these drugs are most probably additive, although in vitro synergism has been demonstrated against some organisms. Amphotericin B is given, as previously described, until an accumulated dosage of 4 to 6 mg/kg is reached. The patient is placed on KTZ at 10 mg/kg daily, beginning on the first day of AMB treatment and continuing for 2 to 3 months. Higher dosages of KTZ are recommended with bone, central nervous system, or disseminated disease.

A similar regimen produced a 61 per cent cure rate in canine blastomycosis (Legendre et al., 1984). Canine histoplasmosis and coccidioidomycosis have also been reported to respond to combination AMB/KTZ treatment (Richardson et al., 1983). Disseminated histoplasmosis and cryptococcal meningitis, diseases associated with poor prognoses, have been successfully managed at the Iowa State University Veterinary Teaching Hospital using this drug combination. Intermittent AMB therapy or prolonged KTZ therapy may be necessary in some cases.

Experimental studies have suggested an additive or synergistic effect against *Aspergillus* with combinations using AMB and 5-FC or AMB and rifampin. It is unfortunate that extremely high concentrations of the drugs are necessary to achieve these effects. There has been speculation that lower, nontoxic concentrations levels may exhibit synergism *in vivo*. However, the clinical value of such combinations in dogs or cats has not been established.

MONITORING THERAPY

The proper duration of therapy is difficult to determine in systemic fungal infections. The time required to eliminate the infection depends on the organism, the antifungal agent, the site and extent of involvement, and the clinical condition of the patient. Present recommendations are based on experimental studies and clinical trials and may vary with disease conditions. Drug toxicities and the high cost of therapy may also limit the treatment period. Patients should be routinely evaluated for drug-induced toxicosis and for evidence that the therapy is effective.

Efficacy of therapy is judged by clinical improvement of the patient, radiographic resolution of disease, declining serologic titers, and the failure to isolate the infective agent. Clinical improvement generally precedes elimination of the causative agent and may be sustained over a long time period in the absence of a cure, as in coccidioidomycosis. Generally, therapy should extend well beyond (generally months) clinical recovery of the patient. Radiographic improvement may precede or follow

Table 2. Guidelines for Systemic Antifungal Chemotherapy

Regimen	Dosage	Route	Minimum Duration of Treatment	Advantages	Disadvantages
AMB	(D) 0.5 mg/kg three times weekly	IV	6–8 weeks*	Rapid onset of action	Nephrotoxic; phlebitis
	(C) 0.25 mg/kg three times weekly	IV	4–8 weeks		
KTZ	(D) 10–30 mg/kg daily	PO	2–3 months	Oral administration; broad spectrum of activity; low toxicity	Fungistatic; slow onset of action; long-term therapy‡
	(C) 10–30 mg/kg daily to every other day	PO	2–3 months		
Na Iodide	(D) 20–40 mg/kg two to three times daily	PO	4–6 weeks		Poor tolerance in some animals; narrow spectrum (*Sporothrix*)
	(C) 20 mg/kg once daily	PO	4–6 weeks		
AMB/KTZ	(D) 0.25 mg/kg AMB three times weekly	IV	3–4 weeks†	Rapid onset of action; broad spectrum of activity	
	10–30 mg/kg KTZ once daily	PO	2–3 months		
AMB/5-FC	(D) 0.5 mg/kg AMB three times weekly	IV	4–5 weeks†	Rapid onset of action; penetrates CSF	Narrow spectrum (*Cryptococcus*); leukopenia (5-FC); thrombocytopenia (5-FC); nephrotoxicosis (AMB)
	25–50 mg/kg 5-FC four times daily	PO	6 weeks		
	(C) 0.25 mg.kg AMB three times weekly	IV	3–4 weeks		
	25–50 mg/kg 5-FC four times daily	PO	4–6 weeks		

(D), dog; (C), cat; IV, intravenous; PO, *per os*.
*Until a total accumulated dosage of 9–12 mg/kg is reached.
†Until a total accumulated dosage of 4 mg/kg is reached.
‡May be necessary for coccidioidomycosis.

elimination of the organism by several weeks. Radiographic improvement is a good prognostic indicator but should not be the sole basis for determining the duration of antifungal therapy.

Several immunologic techniques are available for the detection of fungal antigens or antibodies against certain organisms (Jackson, 1986). The latex agglutination test for cryptococcal antigen is a useful diagnostic tool because it detects fungal *antigen* in serum and CSF and does not depend on an immunologic response of the host. The test has also been used to monitor treatment in canine and feline cryptococcosis, with therapy discontinued when antigen is no longer detected in the patient's serum. Declining serial titers indicate effective therapy and justify a favorable prognosis. However, the test may not detect localized infections, and high cryptococcal antigen titers may persist following elimination of viable organisms (Scholer, 1985). Titers were also reported to decline just prior to death in some human patients with severe cryptococcosis; therefore, declining titers should be correlated with clinical signs.

Antibody titers may be measured by several immunologic techniques. These titers are dependent on the immune response of the host and may persist for months after the agent is eliminated. Antibody titers have primarily been used for diagnosis of fungal infections. The value of antibody

titers in determining the duration of antifungal therapy has not been established.

Histology and cytology, as well as fungal cultures, may be used to monitor the presence of viable organisms. Demonstration of organisms by these techniques supports continued therapy; negative findings are of dubious value. These procedures are of limited value in most cases because of the deep-seated nature of mycotic infections.

All these procedures, as well as routine clinical pathologic tests, may be used to determine the efficacy of the treatment regimen and the duration of antifungal chemotherapy. The incidence of relapse is high in patients with systemic fungal infections, even when recommended treatment regimens are followed (Table 2). Patients should have routine evaluations for at least 1 year following remission of a systemic mycotic infection, and owners should be advised of the possibility of disease recurrence.

References and Supplemental Reading

Graybill, J. R., and Craven, P. C.: Antifungal agents used in systemic mycoses: Activity and therapeutic use. Drugs 25:41, 1983.
Greene, C. E., O'Neal, K. G., and Barsanti, J. A.: Antimicrobial chemotherapy. *In* Greene, C. E. (ed.): *Clinical Microbiology and Infectious Diseases of the Dog and Cat.* Philadelphia: W. B. Saunders Co., 1984, pp. 144–188.

Hellebusch, A. A., Salama, F., and Eadie, E.: The use of mannitol to reduce the nephrotoxicity of amphotericin B. Surg. Gynecol. Obstet. 134:241, 1972.

Jackson, J. A.: Immunodiagnosis of systemic mycoses in animals: A review. J.A.V.M.A. 188:702, 1986.

Legendre, A. M.: Personal communication, 1987.

Legendre, A. M., Selcer, B. A., Edwards, D. F., et al.: Treatment of canine blastomycosis with amphotericin B and ketoconazole. J.A.V.M.A. 184:1249, 1984.

Richardson, R. C., Jaeger, L. A., and Wigle, W.: Treatment of systemic mycoses in dogs. J.A.V.M.A. 183:335, 1983.

Roudebush, P.: Mycotic pneumonias. Vet. Clin. North Am. 15:949, 1985.

Scholer, H. J.: Diagnosis of cryptococcosis and monitoring of chemotherapy. Mykosen 28:5, 1985.

Stevens, D. A.: Problems in antifungal chemotherapy. Infection 15:87, 1987.

NASAL ASPERGILLOSIS

NICHOLAS SHARP, B. VET. MED.

Raleigh, North Carolina

Canine nasal aspergillosis is one of the two major disease conditions that cause severe destruction of nasal turbinate tissue. (The other is nasal neoplasia). Nasal aspergillosis is said to occur more frequently in young dogs and is distinct from nasal neoplasias, which tend to occur in the older population. However, a number of geriatric dogs with aspergillosis have now been seen, so age alone can be a misleading criterion. Dolichocephalic and mesaticephalic breeds are affected, but the condition is very rare in brachycephalic dogs. The condition is also rare in cats.

ETIOLOGY

The etiologic agent is nearly always *Aspergillus fumigatus*; occasionally, *A. nidulans*, *A. niger*, or *A. flavus* are incriminated. *Penicillium* are known to cause an identical disease and will be considered under the general term of nasal aspergillosis. The pathogenesis is unclear. Affected animals rarely have an obvious predisposing cause for colonization with this ubiquitous organism. A few dogs have a history of previous cranial trauma or surgery that has left a bone sequestrum to act as a nidus for infection. It is unclear whether the immunosuppression frequently seen in this disorder is the cause or the result of infection. Immunosuppressed cancer patients do not seem predisposed to nasal aspergillosis, and concurrent opportunistic infections do not occur.

In addition to the aforementioned fungi, a wide variety of gram-positive and gram-negative bacteria can be cultured from the nasal discharge. These organisms comprise the nasal microflora and generally require no treatment.

CLINICAL SIGNS

The history is frequently one of chronic nasal discharge of several months' duration, which progresses from serous to mucopurulent then to sanguinopurulent, with or without epistaxis or bilateral involvement. Some dogs have a rapid progression over 2 or 3 weeks, whereas others have a very gradual worsening of signs. The presence of sanguinopurulent nasal discharge or epistaxis signifies that a destructive process has occurred within the nose. The cause will usually be fungal or neoplastic disease but may occasionally result from extension of dental disease or extranasal causes such as a coagulopathy. Important features that help distinguish aspergillosis from neoplasia are the often profuse and continuous nature of the discharge and a continued ability to breathe through the nose in most dogs with aspergillosis. Although the disease is somewhat variable, many dogs with nasal neoplasia have a discharge that is less profuse, and the ability to breathe through the nose is lost because of replacement of turbinate tissue with solid tumor. Features that are more suggestive of aspergillosis are an ulceration around the external nares; the presence of pain or discomfort on palpation of the frontal sinus, nasal chamber, or rhinarium; and a reluctance to play with, or carry, objects in the mouth.

In nasal aspergillosis, the organism destroys the delicate turbinate scrolls and replaces them with a few fungal colonies. An inflammatory discharge results. The predominant finding on radiologic examination of the nasal chambers is an increase in radiolucency, with loss of turbinate pattern. Erosion of the nasal vault is rare but can occur. Fungal invasion of the frontal sinus(es) is common, is easily overlooked, and may be the sole site of infection in some dogs. Frontal sinus aspergillosis may be associated with chemosis, and penetration into the soft tissues of the orbit may occur. When available, computed tomographic examination can be very helpful in demonstrating the disease but often adds little information to that obtained by good-quality radiographs.

If not effectively treated, aspergillosis may extend into the calvarium or orbital area or may cause severe epistaxis and anemia. However, most dogs do not seem to suffer these severe complications.

Diagnosis is based on a combination of the aforementioned findings. To further strengthen a clinical suspicion, serologic evaluation is very useful; detection of serum antibodies to *Aspergillus* with ELISA or agar gel immunodiffusion techniques can give reliable results.* No exact figures exist but the false-positive rate for either technique is approximately 15 per cent for both clinically normal dogs and those with nasal neoplasia. The radiologic features help distinguish aspergillosis from nasal neoplasia and, together with the appropriate clinical features and positive results from serologic tests, are usually sufficient data for diagnosis. However, for definitive diagnosis, it is highly desirable to see the organism on rhinoscopy and to confirm the organism by direct culture of fungal plaques. Rhinoscopy allows noninvasive biopsy and is performed with a flexible pediatric bronchoscope that is 4- or 5-mm in diameter, an arthroscope, or an otoscope. Histologic or cytologic evidence of fungal hyphae can also be used to confirm the diagnosis.

CLINICAL MANAGEMENT

Therapy for nasal aspergillosis is difficult, and until recently, a high proportion of dogs remained infected despite multiple medical and surgical treatments. Because of these frustrations, the discomfort of the dog, and the antisocial nature of the profuse nasal discharge, euthanasia was frequently requested.

Surgery

The author strongly believes that rhinotomy and turbinectomy have no value in the diagnosis or treatment of nasal aspergillosis. In some cases, surgery may reduce the overall success of systemic thiabendazole. In addition, the exudation that often occurs after rhinotomy and turbinectomy may leave the animal with a nasal discharge even if the organism is eliminated.

Systemic Therapy

Of the currently available systemic antimycotic agents, the two most useful for nasal aspergillosis

are thiabendazole (Mintezol, Merck) and ketoconazole (Nizoral, Janssen). An 8-week course of ketoconazole or thiabendazole for a 30-kg dog costs approximately $140 to $160. Neither drug is completely efficacious, probably because the majority of the imidazoles are much more effective against yeasts, such as *Candida*, than against the filamentous fungi. Both drugs appear to eliminate infection in 40 to 50 per cent of dogs. In some dogs, ketoconazole has been found effective when thiabendazole has failed. Thiabendazole is commonly used at a dose of 20 mg/kg, divided every 12 hr for 6 to 8 weeks, but may cause inappetence and nausea. This can usually be managed by drug withdrawal and then gradual reintroduction to the full dose over several days (Harvey, 1984). The drug should be given with food to enhance absorption and reduce inappetence.

Ketoconazole is administered for 6 to 8 weeks at 10 mg/kg, divided every 12 hr, with food to enhance absorption. The median lethal dose (LD_{50}) for ketoconazole is 80 mg/kg, and minimal inhibitory concentration (MIC) values initially suggested that doses of 40 mg/kg were necessary to inhibit *Aspergillus*. The results of therapy at this dose have been no better than with the lower dose, and side effects were more severe. Even at 10 mg/kg, mild hepatopathy occurs, as manifested by a transient reversible elevation in liver enzyme activities. Mild inappetence and gastrointestinal upset may also occur but less frequently than with thiabendazole. Fulminant hepatic failure has been rarely reported in humans receiving ketoconazole therapy.

Of the newer systemic antifungal drugs, fluconazole (Pfizer) and itraconazole (Janssen) appear to be the most promising in treating clinical cases. Neither are, as yet, commercially available. Fluconazole has been employed by the author at 2.5 or 5.0 mg/kg total daily dose, divided every 12 hr and given with food. Infection has been eliminated in 60 per cent of dogs, which suggests that this drug will have only minor advantages over ketoconazole in the treatment of aspergillosis. The minimum follow-up period in these cases was at least 6 months. Limited experience with itraconazole has suggested that it may be effective in up to 70 per cent of animals with aspergillosis when used at doses of 10 mg/kg (Legendre, 1988). If further studies are as promising, itraconazole may prove to be the most efficacious of the systemic antifungals, and it is certainly less toxic than ketoconazole.

Topical Therapy

A number of topical therapies have been anecdotally employed in this condition, including amphotericin B, Lugol's iodine, nystatin, miconazole, clotrimazole, and thiabendazole. Of these, topical

---

*ELISA testing is currently available through the Clinical Immunology Laboratory, Veterinary Hospital of the University of Pennsylvania, 3850 Spruce Street, Philadelphia, PA 19104.

amphotericin B and, perhaps, miconazole warrant more formal evaluation for useful therapeutic effects.

The most successful topically applied drug employed for nasal aspergillosis is enilconazole (Imaverol, Pitman-Moore). It is not absorbed after oral administration and has an acute LD_{50} in excess of 640 mg/kg. In chronic toxicity studies, dogs that were given 20 mg/kg orally for 2 years experienced little ill effect other than variable inappetence. The drug is well suited for therapy against *Aspergillus* because it is fungicidal at low concentrations, often at an MIC of less than 3 μg/ml. Enilconazole has activity in the vapor phase, which must enhance its penetration of the nasal cavity. To be successful as a topical therapy, enilconazole must be adequately distributed to the affected areas of the nasal chamber(s) or frontal sinus(es). Therefore, the tube arrangement shown in Figure 1 is suggested, having been successfully employed in 23 dogs. Bilateral tube placement is recommended even in dogs with unilateral disease. Furthermore, an additional tube into the frontal sinus is necessary in dogs with frontal sinus disease. Fluoroscopic studies with contrast media have shown inadequate delivery of the drug to the frontal sinus when a fenestrated tube that terminates in the nasal chamber is used.

For tube placement, a short incision is made over each frontal sinus. The skin and periosteum are reflected, and a hole is made into the sinus using an air drill, intramedullary pin, or rongeurs. If no fungus is found in the sinus, a single length of intravenous drip tubing is measured from the female Luer fitting, to extend from the sinus to the level of the midnasal chamber. The tubing is cut and fenestrated. A separate stab incision is made through the skin for the tubing, which is then passed into the sinus and through the connecting ostium into the nasal chamber. This ostium may need to be enlarged with a blunt instrument. The procedure is performed bilaterally. If infection exists in one or both frontal sinuses, a separate tube for each sinus is placed in identical fashion but is not passed through the ostium into the nasal chamber. The subcutaneous tissue and skin are closed in routine fashion, and the tubing is then securely anchored to the skin of the head using nonabsorbable suture material. The suture should be tied both around the tube itself and to tape butterflies attached to the tube. An extension set is connected to each of the surgically implanted tubes and anchored to the outside of a plastic Elizabethan collar. The anchorage should allow sufficient slack for movement and twisting of the collar, and each tube should be labeled as to its destination.

The first drug treatment is made the day following tube placement, when the dog is conscious and able to protect its larynx. The total daily dose per animal is 20 mg/kg divided every 12 hr. The stock solution of enilconazole (100 mg/ml) is mixed with an equal volume of water and is then divided equally for flushing down the tubes. The instilled volume should be kept deliberately low, preferably less than 10 ml, to lessen risk of inhalation. The resultant emulsion that forms with water solidifies after 5 min and so should be made fresh for each treatment.

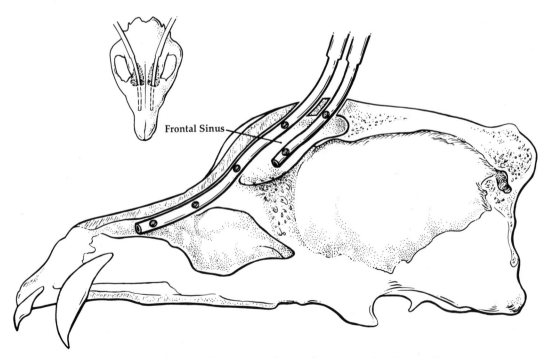

Frontal Sinus

Figure 1. Diagram showing tube placement for topical treatment of nasal aspergillosis.

Drug that remains in the tubing should be evacuated using air. The dog's nose is lowered during the flushing to decrease the volume of drug wasted by swallowing, to ensure that drug appears at both nostrils after administration, and to be sure tubes ending in the frontal sinus(es) do not block sinus drainage. Sneezing is usually profuse, and salivation may occur because of the foul taste of the preparation. Most animals learn to tolerate the procedure well, and in some cases, the treatments may be undertaken by the owner. Occasionally, animals are inappetent or have mild gastrointestinal upsets during treatment. After 7 to 10 days, the tubes are removed, and within a further 2 or 3 days if therapy has been successful, the discharge should stop almost completely. Infection was not successfully eliminated in only three dogs of 26 dogs treated by the author. In two of these three dogs, fungal invasion of the orbital soft tissues had occurred. In such cases, it would seem advisable to combine enilconazole with a systemic antifungal, as the hyphae in this location will not be adequately exposed to the topical treatment. Indications of success are a lack of nasal discharge, healing of the ulcerated nostril, and an absence of nasal pain. Because of the extensive destruction caused by the fungus, many animals will have persistent crusting of mucopurulent discharge at one or both nostrils and occasional sneezing. A bacterial rhinitis has occurred in a few dogs following the successful elimination of fungus, but each responded completely to a short course of antibiotic therapy based on sensitivity testing. Re-evaluation using rhinoscopy is best performed 4 weeks or more after the end of therapy. An absence of fungal colonies and the dog's clinical status are the best indications of elimination of infection. Antibody titers may persist for up to 5 years and are of little prognostic value, although they usually decrease over the first 12 months following successful treatment.

NASAL ASPERGILLOSIS IN CATS

Enilconazole has not been used therapeutically in feline nasal aspergillosis, and no data exist on this species's tolerance of the drug. However, cats appear to tolerate ketoconazole well at doses up to 30 mg/kg, and it would seem prudent to use this as the initial drug of choice. If enilconazole is used topically in the cat, care should be taken with drug injection, as some cats tolerate flushing of any liquid into the upper airway poorly and may suffer respiratory obstruction.

References and Supplemental Reading

Harvey, C. E.: Nasal aspergillosis and penicilliosis in dogs: Results of treatment with thiabendazole. J.A.V.M.A. 184:48, 1984.

Legendre, A.: Personal communication, University of Tennessee, 1988.

Sharp, N. J. H., and Sullivan, M.: Medical treatment of canine nasal aspergillosis using ketoconazole. J.A.V.M.A. (accepted).

Sharp, N. J. H., Harvey, C. E., and O'Brien, J.: Treatment of canine nasal aspergillosis with fluconazole. 1988 (unpublished).

Sharp, N. J. H., Sullivan, M., Harvey, C., et al.: Medical treatment of canine nasal aspergillosis using enilconazole. 1988 (unpublished).

Sharp, N. J. H., Burrell, M. H., Sullivan, M., et al.: Canine nasal aspergillosis: Serology and treatment with ketoconazole. J. Small Anim. Pract. 25:149, 1984.

Sullivan, M.: Rhinoscopy, a diagnostic aid? J. Small Anim. Pract. 28:839, 1987.

Sullivan, M., Lee, R., Jakovljevic, J., et al.: The radiological features of aspergillosis of the nasal cavity and frontal sinuses in the dog. J. Small Anim. Pract. 27:167, 1986.

FELINE CRYPTOCOCCOSIS

LINDA MEDLEAU, D.V.M.
Athens, Georgia

ETIOLOGY

Cryptococcosis is a worldwide systemic fungal infection of humans and animals. Although there are several different species of *Cryptococcus*, only one species, *C. neoformans*, causes the disease. Cryptococcosis usually presents as a subacute or chronic disease. It is the most common systemic fungal disease of cats.

Cryptococcus neoformans is a round, encapsulated, yeastlike fungus that ranges from 3.5 to 7 μ in diameter. Capsule size ranges from 1 to 30 μ in diameter. The fungus reproduces by forming one to two blastoconidia (buds) that are connected to the parent cell by a narrow isthmus. In contrast to other dimorphic fungi, the yeast phase of *C. neoformans* is always found in tissues and under normal laboratory conditions.

C. neoformans is saprophytic and is usually associated with avian habitats. The organism is frequently isolated from pigeon droppings and accumulated filth and debris of pigeon roosts. Although the organism passes through the gut of pigeons, spontaneous avian cryptococcosis is extremely rare. The pigeon's high body temperature (42°C) probably protects it from infection because the organism cannot grow at temperatures higher than 39°C. In pigeon droppings, cryptococci may remain viable for at least 2 years, unless exposed to drying or sunlight.

Cryptococcus neoformans occurs commonly in nature, yet the incidence of the disease is low. This suggests that the organism is opportunistic. The predilection for cryptococcal infections in humans with depressed cell-mediated immunity implies that immunologic defense is crucial in resisting infection. In humans, pre-existing immunosuppressive conditions such as lymphoreticular malignancies, sarcoidosis, and acquired immunodeficiency syndrome (AIDS) as well as prolonged corticosteroid treatment are important predisposing factors for cryptococcosis. In cats, infection with feline leukemia virus may increase susceptibility to cryptococcosis, since the virus has immunosuppressive properties, especially on cell-mediated immunity. However, predisposing immunosuppressive disorders have not been found in all cats with cryptococcosis.

The exact mode of infection is unknown. However, it is thought to occur through inhalation of aerosolized organisms. Encapsulated organisms (5 to 20 μm) are too large to enter terminal airways, but shrunken, unencapsulated cryptococci small enough for alveolar deposition (< 2 μm) have been isolated from pigeon droppings and soil. The resultant pulmonary infection may remain localized or may disseminate to other organs. The prominent lesions in the facial region and upper respiratory tract, along with the uncommon finding of pulmonary lesions in cats with naturally occurring cryptococcosis, suggest that direct inoculation of the organisms may result in disease.

CLINICAL SIGNS

Cryptococcosis can be seen at any age but is more common in middle-aged cats (average age 5 years). There does not appear to be a breed or sex predilection for this disease. The infection is usually chronic and may be associated with a variety of signs.

The upper respiratory tract is most commonly affected. Clinical signs may include sneezing, snuffling, unilateral or bilateral serosanguineous to mucopurulent nasal discharge, and respiratory difficulties. Flesh-colored, granulomatous, polyplike masses may protrude from one or both nostrils. Radiographs of the nasal passages may show homogeneous infiltrates and, possibly, destruction of the nasal turbinates. The cervical lymph nodes may be enlarged. Ulcerated or proliferative lesions in the oral cavity are occasionally seen in conjunction with upper respiratory tract infections. Pulmonary involvement is rare.

Cutaneous lesions are also commonly seen in cats with cryptococcosis. Lesions may be single or multiple and most frequently involve the head. These lesions may occur with or without concurrent upper respiratory tract signs. The most common finding is a firm swelling over the bridge of the nose, or planum nasale. These lesions usually involve the subcutaneous tissue. Cutaneous lesions elsewhere on the body are usually characterized by papules and nodules that may fluctuate or feel firm on palpation. Larger lesions tend to ulcerate. Pruritis is usually nonexistent or mild. Generalized skin lesions strongly suggest that the disease is disseminated.

Central nervous system (CNS) signs may occur alone or in association with other signs. Neurologic signs may be mild and progressive or may occur acutely. Neurologic signs associated with CNS cryptococcosis are variable and include depression, changes in temperament, circling, ataxia, convulsions, paresis, apparent loss of smell, and blindness.

Ocular involvement is occasionally seen, and signs include optic neuritis, chorioretinitis, and panophthalmitis. The fundus can be affected, without apparent visual loss. Chorioretinitis is probably a consequence of hematogenous dissemination and suggests that there is systemic involvement, whereas optic neuritis is usually associated with brain involvement.

DIAGNOSIS

A diagnosis of cryptococcosis is made by demonstrating cryptococcal organisms on cytology, in tissue biopsy specimens, or by fungal culture. Serology is also useful in the diagnosis of cryptococcosis.

CYTOLOGY. Smears of spinal fluid, nasal exudate, and exudative skin lesions and aspirates of tissue masses should be examined for the presence of large, round, encapsulated budding yeast. The buds, which are attached to the parent cell by a thin stalk, may break off when quite small, so the yeast tend to vary considerably in size. Useful stains for cytology include Wright's stain, Gram stain, new methylene blue, and India ink. However, India ink preparations can be unreliable, since lymphocytes, fat droplets, aggregated particles of India ink, and yeast contaminants can be confused with cryptococcal organisms. Negative cytologic results do not rule out cryptococcosis because only a small number of the organisms may be present in a sample, making their detection difficult.

BIOPSY. Tissue masses that yield negative or

questionable cytologic results should be biopsied for histopathology. Cryptococcal lesions contain aggregates of encapsulated budding yeasts. On hematoxylin and eosin staining, these organisms stain as faint, round to oval eosinophilic bodies surrounded by a clear halo. Other useful stains include periodic acid–Schiff, methenamine silver, and Masson-Fontana stain. Mayer's mucicarmine is the definitive stain because it colors the cryptococcal capsule rose red but does not stain other fungi that have similar morphologic characteristics.

CULTURE. Swabs of nasal or cutaneous exudate, tissue aspirates, biopsy specimens, cerebrospinal fluid, or any other infected material can be submitted for fungal culture. The best medium for fungal culture is Sabouraud's dextrose agar without cycloheximide, since cycloheximide may inhibit cryptococcal growth. *Cryptococcus neoformans* can grow at 20°C and 36°C but not at 39°C. Opaque, creamy, yeastlike colonies usually appear within 2 to 5 days. Production of the cryptococcal capsule gives the growth a mucoid appearance and consistency. If the submitted sample contains a small number of organisms, growth may be delayed. Thus, it is best to keep cultures for 4 to 6 weeks before discarding them.

SEROLOGY. The detection of cryptococcal capsular antigen using a latex agglutination procedure is the only serologic test useful clinically on a routine basis. This test, which is commercially available, measures the cryptococcal capsular antigen in serum or cerebrospinal fluid of infected cats. The cryptococcal antigen test is also useful for evaluating the animal's progress during therapy. A good prognosis would be indicated by a decrease in antigen titer during therapy, whereas a persistent titer following treatment might suggest the possibility of relapse. In humans, false-negative titers can be seen if the disease is localized, and false-positive titers may be seen in *Klebsiella* infections or if rheumatoid factor is present. The incidence of false-negative and false-positive titers in cats is unknown.

TREATMENT

Although amphotericin B and flucytosine are still the treatments of choice in humans with cryptococcosis, they have been replaced largely by ketoconazole in the treatment of this disease in cats. Ketoconazole, an imidazole derivative, interferes with the synthesis of ergosterol, a sterol that is necessary for fungal cell wall integrity. Because ketoconazole is a fungistatic agent and, therefore, slow-acting, treatment may need to be continued for several months. Ketoconazole can be administered orally, and its absorption from the gastrointestinal tract is enhanced when it is given with food. It is rapidly and extensively distributed throughout the body, with adequate antifungal levels achieved in most tissues except in the testes, brain, and, probably, the eye.

Ketoconazole has been used to successfully treat several cats with cryptococcosis. In general, the dosage ranged from 10 to 20 mg/kg, given orally once daily or divided into two daily doses. One cat required long-term therapy with very high dosages of ketoconazole (72 mg/kg/day) to cure. Treatment should be continued until cryptococcal antigen titers are negative or until 1 or 2 months past resolution of all lesions. For most cats, this means treating for several months.

In cats, the side effects of ketoconazole include anorexia, vomiting, diarrhea, elevated serum liver enzyme levels, and icterus. Giving ketoconazole with food and dividing the dosage two to four times daily may help alleviate signs of anorexia or vomiting. If anorexia persists, ketoconazole therapy should be halted until the cat is eating normally; it should then be reinstituted at a lower dosage, given on an alternate-day basis, or both.

Itraconazole, a triazole antifungal agent, is currently in the investigational stage and is not yet available in the United States. It shares basic principles of activity with ketoconazole and is also administered orally. Unlike ketoconazole, itraconazole may achieve adequate brain levels at therapeutic doses, and it also appears to have less toxic side effects. Itraconazole has been used to successfully treat experimental cryptococcosis in mice, rabbits, and cats. The results in cats spontaneously infected with cryptococcosis are promising but need to be confirmed in future studies.

PUBLIC HEALTH CONSIDERATIONS

Cryptococcosis is not considered a public health hazard because the organism does not aerosolize from culture media or from sites of tissue infection. Transmission of this disease from animal to animal or from animal to human has never been reported. Nevertheless, common sense precautions (i.e., wearing gloves) should be taken when handling infected cats.

References and Supplemental Reading

Barsanti, J. A.: Cryptococcosis. *In* Greene, C. E. (ed.): *Clinical Microbiology and Infectious Diseases of the Dog and Cat.* Philadelphia: W. B. Saunders Co., 1984, pp. 700–709.

Blouin, P., and Conner, M. W.: Cryptococcosis. *In* Holzworth, J. (ed.): *Diseases of the Cat. Medicine and Surgery.* Philadelphia: W. B. Saunders Co., 1987, pp. 332–342.

Davis, C. E.: Cryptococcosis. *In* Braude, A. I., Davis, C. E., and Fierer, J. (eds.): *Infectious Diseases and Medical Microbiology.* Philadelphia: W. B. Saunders Co., 1986, pp. 564–570.

Hansen, B. L.: Successful treatment of severe feline cryptococcosis with long-term high doses of ketoconazole. J. Am. Anim. Hosp. Assoc. 23:193, 1987.

Medleau, L., Hall, E. J., Goldschmidt, M. H., et al.: Cutaneous cryptococcosis in three cats. J.A.V.M.A. 187:169, 1985.

Noxon, J. O., Monroe, W. E., and Chinn, D. R.: Ketoconazole therapy in canine and feline cryptococcosis. J. Am. Anim. Hosp. Assoc. 22:179, 1986.

Pentlarge, V. W., and Martin, R. A.: Treatment of cryptococcosis in three cats, using ketoconazole. J.A.V.M.A. 188:536, 1986.

Schulman, J.: Ketoconazole for successful treatment of cryptococcosis in a cat. J.A.V.M.A. 187:508, 1985.

FELINE TOXOPLASMOSIS

MICHAEL R. LAPPIN, D.V.M.*

Fort Collins, Colorado

ETIOLOGY

The causative agent of feline toxoplasmosis is *Toxoplasma gondii*, an obligate intracellular coccidian parasite. Felidae are the only known definitive hosts. The sexual cycle of *T. gondii* occurs in the small intestine and is completed by oocyst shedding into the environment (enteroepithelial cycle). The organism disseminates throughout the body (extraintestinal cycle) as rapidly dividing forms (tachyzoites) concurrently with the enteroepithelial cycle. Cysts form in most tissues, as the immune response limits replication of the organism. The extraintestinal cycle also takes place in intermediate hosts including fish, amphibians, reptiles, birds, other mammals, and humans after ingestion of sporulated oocysts or tissue cysts.

TRANSMISSION

Cats become infected postnatally, by ingestion of oocysts from fecal contamination or by ingestion of cysts or tachyzoites in the tissues of intermediate hosts. Most cats are infected at weaning age by the ingestion of infected intermediate hosts. After ingestion of tissue cysts, the prepatent period lasts 3 to 10 days, and most previously unexposed cats shed millions of oocysts for approximately 7 days. Oocysts must sporulate under appropriate environmental conditions for 1 to 5 days to become infective. Oocysts ingestion leads to shedding in approximately 50 per cent of previously unexposed cats, with fewer oocysts being passed than with cyst ingestion. The prepatent period is generally longer than 20 days, and a shedding period occurs that can persist for several weeks. Once a cat has recovered from initial infection, it is rare for the cat to reshed oocysts. Occasionally, concurrent parasitism or im-

munosuppression has led to repeat shedding in chronically infected cats, but this is considered to be epidemiologically unimportant.

CLINICAL SIGNS

The enteroepithelial cycle rarely causes clinical signs, although vomiting and diarrhea have been reported occasionally. In kittens, severe enteric disease can result if concurrent illness such as viral respiratory infection occurs just after weaning. When clinical disease develops, it has been associated most frequently with the dissemination and replication of the organism during the extraintestinal cycle. Asexual reproduction occurs intracellularly in all body tissues except non-nucleated red blood cells and results in destruction of the infected cell and development of clinical signs characteristic of the organ system most severely affected. Tissue cysts rarely result in clinical signs but may serve as a source of antigen for immune-complex disease. These cysts occasionally can be reactivated by immunosuppression, which leads to repeat dissemination, clinical signs, and oocyst shedding.

Respiratory tract involvement is common and is manifested by dyspnea and coughing. Anorexia, malaise, lameness, icterus, fever, tonsillar enlargement, lymphadenomegaly, splenomegaly, and evidence of encephalitis often are associated with clinical disease. Muscle discomfort from myositis is frequently detected on direct palpation. Neurologic examination in cats with central nervous system (CNS) signs usually reveals evidence of multifocal inflammatory disease, but focal signs can be present.

Ocular manifestions can include both anterior and posterior chamber changes involving either one or both eyes. Retinochoroiditis caused by organism replication is the primary ocular lesion. Secondary changes include vitreal hemorrhage, vitreal opacity, retinal detachment, iritis, iridocyclitis, hyphema, cataracts, and keratitic precipitates. Whether ante-

*Present address: Dept. of Clinical Sciences, College of Veterinary Medicine and Biomedical Sciences, Colorado State University, Ft. Collins, CO.

rior chamber changes occur only as an extension of retinochoroiditis or whether they are primary lesions is unknown. Histologically, *T. gondii* organisms have not been documented in the tissues of the anterior chamber of cats exhibiting signs of anterior uveitis alone. It is possible that circulating immune-complex deposition leads to the development of pathology in these cases.

RADIOGRAPHIC AND LABORATORY ABNORMALITIES

Radiographic, hematologic, biochemical, and cerebrospinal fluid (CSF) abnormalities often develop as the organism replicates and disseminates.

Thoracic radiographs showing a diffuse interstitial to alveolar pattern with mottled lobar distribution may be strongly suggestive of toxoplasmosis. It is unfortunate that other pulmonary diseases may mimic these radiographic changes, and atypical changes can occur. Ventrodorsal abdominal radiographs may reveal cranial quadrant haziness in the region of the liver and pancreas in individual cases, but this finding is not definitive for *T. gondii*–induced inflammation.

Hematologic changes reported in acute, severe infections include leukopenia characterized by absolute neutropenia, lymphopenia, monocytopenia, eosinopenia, and an inappropriate left shift. The recovery phase of acute illness may be characterized by leukocytosis.

Biochemical abnormalities may include hypoproteinemia and hypoalbuminemia. Muscle necrosis can lead to elevations in serum creatine phosphokinase, lactic dehydrogenase, and aspartate aminotransferase. Hepatic necrosis may be associated with elevated serum alanine aminotransferase, elevated serum bilirubin, and either increased or decreased serum alkaline phosphatase.

Cerebrospinal fluid changes usually consist of increased protein concentration and elevated leukocyte counts. Leukocytes usually are a mixed population of mononuclear cells and neutrophils. Other than actual demonstration of tachyzoites in CSF, these abnormalities can only suggest the diagnosis of toxoplasmosis.

DIAGNOSIS

Fecal Examination

Sugar centrifugation (Table 1) is the preferred technique to demonstrate oocysts. The oocysts are found in the plane of view just under the coverslip. Oocysts are 10 × 12 μ and contain a single central sporoblast immediately after passage (Fig. 1A). After sporulation, the oocyst contains two sporocysts (Fig.

Table 1. *Sheather's Sugar Centrifugal Flotation*

Sheather's sugar solution	
Sugar (regular table sugar)	500 gm
Distilled water	320 ml
Phenol crystals (melt in hot water bath)	6.5 gm

Procedure
1. Soften feces with water to a soft, fluid consistency.
2. Pass aqueous suspension through a tea strainer or two layers of gauze.
3. Thoroughly mix 1 part aqueous fecal suspension with 2 parts Sheather's sugar solution. Pour into a centrifuge tube, and add sufficient solution to bring a meniscus to the tube. Place a coverslip on top. Centrifuge at 1500 rpm for 10 min.
4. Remove coverslip, and place on a slide. Examine at ≥ 200 × magnification.

1B). Oocysts of *Besnoitia darlingi* and *Hammondia hammondi* found in cat feces are indistinguishable from those of *T. gondii*. These coccidians are not pathologic to cats and are rare, so any 10 × 12 μ oocyst detected in cat feces should be considered *T. gondii*.

The short period of oocyst shedding combined with the difficulty in demonstrating oocysts make fecal examination a poor procedure for determining the oocyst shedding status of cats. Fecal examination surveys in the United States usually report less than a 1 per cent incidence of oocyst detection. Oocyst detection usually does not help diagnose clinical disease because signs generally occur after shedding stops.

Serology

This is the most practical diagnostic method to detect infection. Assays detecting circulating antibodies against *T. gondii* and circulating antigens of *T. gondii* have been developed.

Commercially available serologic tests that detect anti–*T. gondii* immunoglobulin G (IgG) include direct hemagglutination, indirect hemagglutination, modified agglutination, latex agglutination, enzyme-linked immunosorbent assay (ELISA), and indirect fluorescent antibody. Positive IgG titers as measured by these assays develop 2 to 4 weeks postinfection (PI), become very high in both clinical disease and subclinical infections, and persist for months to years. A fourfold rise in IgG titer over a 2- to 3-week period is needed to confirm active infection. Commercial assays that give instructions to assess a positive or negative result on a single serum dilution cannot demonstrate rising titers. Although these assays can be used to detect exposure, they cannot diagnose active infection or predict when individual cats may have shed oocysts in the past.

An ELISA recently has been developed that detects anti–*T. gondii* immunoglobulin M (IgM) in

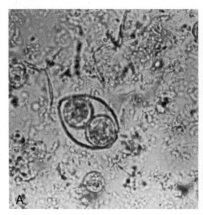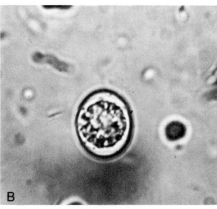

Figure 1. *A*, Sporulated oocyst; *B*, unsporulated oocyst.

the serum of cats (Lappin et al., 1988a). Titers became positive at dilutions of 1:64 or greater in 90 per cent of cats with experimental subclinical infection as soon as 1 week PI and had a duration less than 16 weeks PI. Because of this early rise and short duration, single positive IgM titers are suggestive of active infection and so do not require demonstration of a rising titer. These findings show that IgM measurement also can be used to predict when past oocyst shedding has occurred. Cats with clinical signs referable to toxoplasmosis also develop IgM antibody titers. The combination of typical clinical signs of toxoplasmosis with a positive IgM assay is strongly suggestive of active clinical disease and warrants appropriate therapeutic intervention (Lappin et al., 1988c).

An ELISA has been developed that can detect circulating antigens of *T. gondii* in the serum of cats with experimental subclinical infection (Lappin et al., 1988b). Antigens have been released intermittently from the tissues of these cats for up to 1 year PI. Because of intermittent shedding, antigen detection cannot be used to differentiate infection from clinical disease or predict oocyst shedding. Antigen detection may be most valuable in detecting clinical toxoplasmosis in cats with concurrent immunosuppressive disease (i.e., feline leukemia virus infection) that suppresses antibody production or in peracute infections when antibody levels have not had time to reach measurable quantities.

THERAPY

ENTEROEPITHELIAL CYCLE. Pyrimethamine, sulfonamides, clindamycin, and monensin can reduce levels of oocyst shedding (Table 2). Monensin has been effective experimentally when utilized within 1 to 2 days PI, and its use did not prevent the development of immunity that blocked oocyst shedding in subsequent challenges. Suppression of oocyst shedding could be of benefit in households with pet cats during human pregnancy by decreas-

Table 2. Treatment of Feline Toxoplasmosis (Enteroepithelial Cycle)

Drug	Total Daily Dose (mg/kg)	Frequency	Route
Pyrimethamine	2.0	Daily	PO
Sulfonamides	100	Daily	PO
Clindamycin	25–50	Daily	PO
Monensin	*	Divided b.i.d. to t.i.d.	PO

*0.02% concentration by weight (lb) in dry food.
PO, orally.

ing the risk of exposure to *T. gondii* and subsequent fetal infection.

EXTRAINTESTINAL CYCLE. Pyrimethamine, sulfonamides, trimethoprim, and clindamycin are drugs with known activity against *T. gondii* and can be used to lessen the severity of clinical disease associated with toxoplasmosis in cats (Table 3).

Pyrimethamine (folic acid cycle inhibition) combined with rapid-acting sulfonamides (*p*-aminobenzoic acid cycle inhibition), such as sulfadiazine or triple sulfas, have been the classic treatment for clinical toxoplasmosis because of their synergistic effect. Pyrimethamine inhibits folic acid metabolism in the host as well as in the parasite and so can result in several side effects primarily relating to

Table 3. Treatment of Feline Toxoplasmosis (Extraintestinal Cycle)

Drug	Total Daily Dose (mg/kg)	Frequency	Route
Pyrimethamine	0.5–1	Divided b.i.d. to t.i.d.	PO
Sulfonamides*	60–120	Divided b.i.d. to t.i.d.	PO, IM
Clindamycin	25–50	Divided b.i.d. to t.i.d.	PO, IM

*60 mg/kg can be used when combined with pyrimethamine.
PO, orally; IM, intramuscularly.

Table 4. *Prevention of* T. gondii *Infection*

Keep cats inside, or restrict hunting activities.
Empty cat litterbox daily.
Flush, incinerate, or tightly bag cat feces.
Sterilize litterbox with scalding water.
Never feed raw meat to cats.
Wash hands with hot water after handling raw meat.
Cook meat to 150°F (65.6°C) (medium-well) before eating.
Boil water from outside water supply (e.g., streams) before drinking.
Wear gloves when working in the garden.
Cover children's sandbox when it is not in use.
Control possible paratenic hosts (e.g., cockroaches).

bone marrow suppression. Cats are particularly susceptible to these effects and rapidly develop anemia, leukopenia, and thrombocytopenia. These side effects can be lessened by supplementing with folic acid (50 mg/day PO) baker's yeast (100 mg/kg/day PO), or folinic acid (1 mg/kg/day PO). Other potential problems associated with the use of these drugs in cats include dose-related problems (pyrimethamine is only available in 25-mg tablets) and the difficulty of oral administration in anorectic animals. The efficacy of trimethoprim in the treatment of feline toxoplasmosis is unknown.

Clindamycin, a macrolide antibiotic that inhibits protein synthesis, is well absorbed from the gastrointestinal tract or can be administered parenterally in the anorectic patient. A recent toxicity study in cats documented its safety at dosages up to 50 mg/kg/day administered orally (Greene and Lappin, 1988). Pseudomembranous colitis associated with *Clostridium difficile* overgrowth as described in humans has not been seen in normal cats treated for 6 weeks. Occasional vomiting that is associated with higher dosages early in the treatment period has been adequately controlled by withholding food for 24 hr and reintroducing the drug at increasing

dosages over several days. Diarrhea at cessation of therapy in several cats has resolved without therapy within 3 days and has been felt to be due to normal intestinal flora equilibration.

Clinical signs such as fever, anorexia, and hyperesthesia have resolved as soon as 24 hr after initiation of clindamycin therapy. The minimum duration of treatment should be 14 days. Patients with severe polymyositis, ocular disease, or neurologic deficits may require longer treatment regimens.

PREVENTION

Control of *T. gondii* infection in cats and intermediate hosts including humans revolves around prevention of oocyst shedding and ingestion of tissue cysts (Table 4). Vaccines have been effective in blocking oocyst shedding experimentally but are not currently available.

References and Supplemental Reading

Dubey, J. P.: Toxoplasmosis in cats. Feline Pract. 16:12, 1986.
Feeney, D. A., Sautter, J. H., and Lees, G. E.: An unusual case of acute disseminated toxoplasmosis in a cat. J. Am. Anim. Hosp. Assoc. 17:311, 1981.
Greene, C. E., and Lappin, M. R.: Clinical and biochemical abnormalities associated with oral clindamycin administration in cats. Am. J. Vet. Res. 1988 (in press).
Greene, C. E., and Prestwood, A. K.: Coccidial infections. In Greene, C. E. (ed.): *Clinical Microbiology and Infectious Diseases of the Dog and Cat.* Philadelphia: W. B. Saunders Co., 1984, pp. 826–840.
Lappin, M. R., Greene, C. E., Prestwood, A. K., et al.: Diagnosis of *Toxoplasma gondii* infection in cats utilizing an enzyme-linked immunosorbent assay for immunoglobulin M. Am. J. Vet. Res. 1988a (in press).
Lappin, M. R., Greene, C. E., Prestwood, A. K., et al.: Enzyme-linked immunosorbent assay for the detection of circulating antigens of *Toxoplasma gondii* in the serum of cats. Am. J. Vet. Res. 1988b (in press).
Lappin, M. R., Greene, C. E., Prestwood, A. K., et al.: Clinical toxoplasmosis in 13 cats; serologic diagnosis and management with clindamycin. J. Am. Coll. Vet. Intern. Med. 1988c (in press).

Section

12

URINARY DISORDERS

JEANNE A. BARSANTI, D.V.M.

Consulting Editor

Diagnostic Approach to Canine and Feline Hematuria....................1117
Clinical Evaluation of Renal Function: A Critical Appraisal of
    Procedures and Interpretations 1123
Crystalluria: Causes, Detection, and Interpretation 1127
Spectrum of Clinical and Laboratory Abnormalities in Uremia 1133
Diagnostic Approach to Proteinuria 1139
Positive-Contrast Vaginourethrography for Diagnosis of Lower
    Urinary Tract Disease 1142
Use of Urodynamics in Micturition Disorders in Dogs and Cats..........1145
Urodynamic Abnormalities Associated with Canine Prostatic
    Diseases and Therapeutic Intervention 1151
Feline Vesicourachal Diverticula: Biologic Behavior, Diagnosis, and
    Treatment...1153
Renal Effects of Nonsteroidal Anti-inflammatory Drugs 1158
Infiltrative Urethral Diseases in the Dog..................................1161
Fanconi's Syndrome: Inherited and Acquired............................1163
Renal Failure in Young Dogs 1166
Chronic Renal Disease in Cats 1170
Medical Management of Canine Glomerulonephropathies 1174
Medical Management of Urate Uroliths...................................1178
Canine Calcium Oxalate Urolithiasis: Detection, Treatment,
    and Prevention...1182
Medical Dissolution and Prevention of Cystine Urolithiasis..............1189
Management of Prostatic Neoplasia 1193
Management of Advanced Chronic Renal Failure 1195
Newer Concepts and Controversies on Dietary Management of Renal
    Failure 1198
Use of Drugs to Control Hypertension in Renal Failure 1201
Management of Urinary Tract Infections.................................1204
Feline Perineal Urethrostomy: A Potential Cause of Hematuria,
    Dysuria, and Urethral Obstruction....................................1209
Pharmacologic Management of Urinary Incontinence 1214

DIAGNOSTIC APPROACH TO CANINE AND FELINE HEMATURIA

ARTHUR L. LAGE, D.V.M.

Boston, Massachusetts

Hematuria is the presence of blood in the urine and is certainly cause for alarm, as it may portend serious life-threatening disease. At some stage, nearly every disease of the kidneys or collecting system may be accompanied by hematuria.

> **Axiom One:** Until proved otherwise, one should always consider hematuria a serious symptom of urogenital disease, and even a single episode demands a urologic investigation.

Two considerations are initially important: to recognize that hematuria exists and to localize the source of the blood. Only after these have been accomplished can the clinical significance and implications of hematuria be identified.

CLINICAL DETECTION OF HEMATURIA

When examining a patient with hematuria, practically any disease of the genitourinary tract should be considered as a cause at the outset.

URINE COLLECTION

Urine collection techniques may greatly affect the presence and amount of blood in the urine. In general, a voided urine sample is the best for initial analysis. Of course, in the female, the state of estrogenic stimulus to the uterus and vagina will affect the presence of red blood cells (RBCs). In the male, prostatic changes may contribute to the presence of RBCs. When collecting a voided sample, it is best to collect from midstream urine. The advantage of a voided sample is that no trauma is involved in collection; thus iatrogenic trauma-induced RBCs are not added to the urine, and there is no iatrogenic catheter-induced infection.

A urine sample can be obtained by catheterization directly from the urinary bladder; in general, the hematuria can be shown to originate from the upper urinary tract, the urinary bladder, the ureters, or the kidneys. Blood from the prostate may contaminate bladder urine, especially after the prostate has been palpated; therefore, the findings are not absolutely reliable. The clinician must interpret hematuria from a catheterized sample only after considering how traumatic the catheterization was. A traumatic catheterization or the use of improper equipment may produce significant gross or microscopic hematuria.

A urine sample that is obtained by manually expressing the bladder may be free of iatrogenically produced blood or there can be severe trauma with gross hematuria. In general, the condition of the urinary bladder will determine whether hematuria will be caused by expressing the bladder. If the bladder mucosa is inflamed, infected, or thickened, or if the bladder lumen is occupied by a calculus or neoplasm, the likelihood of adding to or causing hematuria is greatly increased by manually expressing the bladder. Patient cooperation and fullness of the bladder also affect iatrogenic hematuria. A full bladder will usually be easier to express (unless there is partial obstruction). The bladders of males are harder to express than those of females, and thus there is a greater chance for iatrogenic hematuria.

Sterile antepubic cystocentesis is generally safe and does not produce significant iatrogenic hematuria. The previous comments regarding the thickness of the bladder wall and condition of the mucosa may apply.

LABORATORY ANALYSIS

Urinalysis should be performed as soon as possible after the urine has been collected. Formed elements, including RBCs, may begin to deteriorate after their addition to the urine.

Red blood cells and free hemoglobin and myoglobin will produce a positive color reaction with occult blood tests (benzidine, guaiac, or orthotolidine dipsticks). Dipsticks may fail to detect small, but significant, numbers of intact RBCs. Both the sediment and the supernatant should be examined, and only by using both methods can urine be proved to be free of blood. For example

RBCs may lyse in dilute (1.006) or alkaline urine, and the hemoglobin will be liberated. A red supernatant with a negative color reaction with the dipstick is suggestive of pigmentation by porphyrins, beet pigment, pyridium, or other nonorganic iron-containing pigment or red dyes used to color some commercial dog foods. A positive dipstick reaction to the supernatant and negative sediment examination for RBCs usually indicates hemolysis or myolysis; however, red blood cell "ghosts" may be seen. Large amounts of ascorbic acid excreted in the urine or the use of formaldehyde may inhibit or retard the dipstick measurement of hemoglobin.

The presence of red blood cell casts confirms that some or all of the blood is from the renal parenchyma.

Hematuria is called gross or macroscopic when it can be detected by the human eye and microscopic when identified by microscopic examination. The finding of more than two to four RBCs per high-power field is abnormal; however, this figure can vary slightly, depending on the concentration of the urine.

It is important to emphasize that the urine can be contaminated with blood from outside the urinary tract, and the genital tract is always suspect.

Consideration must always be given to the possibility of the presence of a bleeding disorder or disorder of coagulation.

The presence of hematuria, whether macroscopic or microscopic, is an indication for further investigation.

TYPES OF HEMATURIA

Essential, benign essential, or idiopathic hematuria refers to renal hematuria for which no cause can be found. Familial hematuria is essential hematuria that is inherited. False hematuria is redness of the urine due to pigment other than blood. The morphologic location of hematuria is also specified, e.g., renal hematuria originates from the kidneys. Any anatomic locus can be used to describe hematuria, such as urethral and vesical hematuria. Asymptomatic hematuria occurs without any other signs or symptoms.

Hematuria can also be classified according to its timing. Initial hematuria occurs at the beginning of urination. Total hematuria is found throughout urination. Terminal hematuria occurs at the end of urination.

CLINICAL ANALYSIS OF HEMATURIA

Specific Causes

To analyze hematuria, it is best to consider and review the major possible causes (Table 1).

RENAL HEMATURIA

Axiom Two: Asymptomatic hematuria is often of renal origin.

Table 1. *Specific Causes of Hematuria*

Renal Hematuria
  Glomerulonephropathies
  Infections
  Nephrolithiasis
  Neoplasia (tumors)
  Cystic disease of the kidneys
  Infarction
  Trauma
  Recurring macroscopic hematuria of Welsh corgi dogs
  Benign renal bleeding (idiopathic hematuria)
  Parasites
  Strenuous exercise
  Asymptomatic urinary (AU) abnormalities

Collecting and Voiding System Hematuria
  Infections
  Inflammation, structural changes, and malformations
  Calculi
  Neoplasia
  Trauma

Hematuria from Any Site in the Urinary System
  Disorders of bleeding or coagulation

Causes of Hematuria That Are Poorly Understood and Poorly Documented in Dogs and Cats
  Hematuria from exercise or heat stroke
  Acute radiation nephritis
  Drug-induced and nephroallergic hematuria

Hemoglobinuria
  Autoimmune hemolytic anemia
  Disseminated intravascular coagulation
  Transfusion reaction
  Heat stroke
  Splenic torsion
  Postcaval syndrome from dirofilariasis

Moderate to severe hematuria is found in a large variety of renal diseases, and it is of little diagnostic value by itself. When accompanied by red blood cell casts or mixed cellular casts, the presence of acute or subacute inflammatory renal parenchymal disease or violent exercise must be considered.

GLOMERULONEPHROPATHIES. These conditions usually do not occur with isolated hematuria. In almost all cases, the hematuria, whether macroscopic or microscopic, will be accompanied by moderate to severe proteinuria and other signs of glomerular disease. The clinician must use standard methods to determine whether the proteinuria is significant (see *Current Veterinary Therapy IX*, pp. 1111–1114) and further that it is of renal origin (see *Current Veterinary Therapy IX*, pp. 1130–1131). Hypoproteinemia and hypoalbuminemia will give added support to the conclusion that a significant, persistent proteinuria is of glomerular origin. Renal biopsy with evaluation by light, immunofluorescent, and electron microscopic examination of the samples will be needed to classify the type of glomerulonephropathy. Glomerulonephropathy has been diagnosed in the dog and cat as a primary disease and has also been associated with diseases such as canine lupus erythematosus, canine pyometra, canine adenovirus infection, *Dirofilaria immitis* infection, feline infectious peritonitis, and a variety of canine and feline neoplastic diseases such as lymphosarcoma.

INFECTIONS. Acute bacterial pyelonephritis will generally occur with a polymorphonuclear leukocytosis, and the urinalysis usually demonstrates a large number of bacteria, polymorphonuclear leukocytes (PMLs), clumps of white blood cells, and sometimes white blood cell casts. During the early stage of the infection, RBCs may be found, and, on occasion, there may be macroscopic hematuria; however, marked persistent hematuria is not generally a prominent sign of pyelonephritis. In fact, hematuria will usually subside after the acute stage of pyelonephritis, and any persistence of hematuria after the stage of acute infection should prompt the clinician to look for evidence of other disease. Besides a complete blood count (CBC) and urinalysis, the clinician may need urine culture, intravenous pyelography, renal biopsy, and renal function tests to properly approach a case of pyelonephritis. Other clinical features of pyelonephritis may be hyperthermia or pyrexia, painful renal or perirenal area, and vomiting. When pyelonephritis is accompanied by cystitis, the hematuria may be prolonged and more severe, and signs of pollakiuria (unduly frequent passage of urine) and dysuria (painful or difficult urination) will usually be present. RBCs are generally found in small numbers in patients with chronic pyelonephritis.

NEPHROLITHIASIS. Hematuria accompanied by renal or perirenal pain may be suggestive of nephrolithiasis with or without accompanying renal infection; however, signs of nephrolithiasis may be entirely absent. The pain may be elicited only by a careful and subtle examination and may be manifested by a splinting of the abdomen. Hematuria may be either gross or microscopic. Frequently, nephroliths are discovered accidentally when they are radiopaque and radiographic examination of the abdomen is performed for unrelated reasons. Usually signs are related to accompanying urinary tract infection. Radiolucent nephroliths may be diagnosed with the aid of an intravenous pyelogram (IVP). In fact, patients diagnosed as having radiolucent cystic calculi should have an IVP performed to look for radiolucent renal calculi. Pieces of or entire renal calculi may pass into the ureter. Hydronephrosis may develop from renal calculi, and hydronephrosis and hydroureter may result from ureteric calculi.

NEOPLASIA (TUMORS). Good clinical correlation of signs and presence of early renal neoplasia in dogs and cats has been poorly documented.

In renal cell carcinoma, the most common clinical sign is gross hematuria. The blood may be red or coffee colored. Pain and the presence of a compressing or noncompressing mass may also be noted. An interesting finding may be polycythemia caused by an elevated production of renal erythropoietic factor (REF). Spread of renal cell carcinoma is generally by direct invasion of the renal veins, with dissemination through the blood stream, primarily to the lung and skeleton. The diagnosis is generally suggested or established with the use of an IVP or renal arteriogram. The IVP should demonstrate a space-occupying lesion with possible distortion of the normal renal collecting pattern. The arteriogram may show a pattern of local increased vascularity. Of course, biopsy or the finding of neoplastic cells in urine would be confirmatory.

Transitional cell carcinoma may occur in the renal pelvis, the ureter, or the urinary bladder. Hematuria may be seen earlier in this form of tumor than in renal cell carcinoma because of direct contact with the urine flow. Intravenous pyelography and exfoliative cytology are both used to diagnose transitional cell carcinoma of the renal pelvis.

Benign tumors (not cysts) of the kidneys are relatively rare, and therefore all renal masses should be considered malignant until proved otherwise.

CYSTIC DISEASE OF THE KIDNEYS. Small retention cysts occasionally develop in the dog and cat and are of little clinical significance. When a single cyst becomes large, it must be differentiated from a renal tumor. Hematuria is generally not a feature of small retention cysts; however, large solitary cysts may occur with either gross or microscopic hematuria, depending on its junction with the remaining renal parenchyma. Polycystic disease in dogs and cats does occur. Hematuria may or may not be seen with polycystic disease. Pyelonephritis may develop as a result of polycystic disease, in which case the likelihood for hematuria increases. The diagnosis of either a large solitary cyst or polycystic renal disease is aided by an IVP. Arteriography or ultrasonography may also be helpful. Polycystic disease may or may not occur with palpably large kidneys; however, large solitary renal cysts frequently can be palpated.

INFARCTION. Renal infarction, whether a single large infarct or multiple small infarcts, usually produces hematuria. The hematuria is generally gross with a large infarct and either gross or microscopic with multiple small infarcts. Other than the hematuria, signs related to the kidney are generally not seen, as the signs usually reflect the underlying cause of the infarction. On occasion, infarction may be so massive that primary renal failure is the result.

Renal infarction can be highly suspected with an IVP and proved with an arteriogram.

TRAUMA

> **Axiom Three:** Hematuria associated with a history of trauma is an indication for intravenous pyelography (IVp) or other contrast urography.

When difficulty in micturition is also present, the trauma has most likely affected the lower urinary tract. Trauma-associated hematuria may be either gross or microscopic. Hematuria may follow either a wedge or needle biopsy of the kidney. When a needle biopsy is properly taken, the hematuria is usually microscopic.

RECURRING MACROSCOPIC HEMATURIA OF WELSH CORGI DOGS. This is the clinical name given to recurring renal hematuria from renal hemangioectasia, which has been described only in the Welsh corgi breed. The typical presentation is a Welsh corgi dog with hematuria without any apparent signs of illness. Microscopic hematuria may have been present for some time before macroscopic hematuria was noted by the owner. Early middle age has been the usual age of onset; however, the range has been 2 to 10 years. The patient has no stranguria, pollakiuria, or dysuria from this disease. Breed, history, normal physical examination results, urinalysis, IVP, and renal arteriography all help to establish the diagnosis; however, definitive diagnosis is made only by renal biopsy.

BENIGN RENAL BLEEDING (IDIOPATHIC HEMATURIA). A disorder, with some similarities to the hematuria of Welsh corgis, has been seen in young and mature dogs of varying breeds. The bleeding may be so severe that anemia is produced. Urinalysis has shown the presence of frank bleeding, but no inflammatory cells are seen. Arteriograms and IVPs have been unrevealing. At surgery, bleeding from one or both kidneys can be demonstrated by catheterizing the ureters. In unilateral cases, the dogs have responded to removal of the affected kidney with cessation of bleeding. The source of the bleeding in the kidney has not been revealed by histologic examination of removed kidneys. The diagnosis is aided by excluding other possible conditions.

PARASITES. *Dioctophyma renale* infection has been reported to cause gross hematuria. Diagnosis can be made by finding the ova of *D. renale* in the urine of a gravid female. A history of eating uncooked fish may be helpful, as this is the only known means of infection. *Capillaria plica* and *Dirofilaria immitis* may cause renal hematuria.

STRENUOUS EXERCISE. Extreme exercise may lead to temporary microscopic hematuria. Myoglobinuria also may occur.

ASYMPTOMATIC URINARY (AU) ABNORMALITIES. The occurrence of hematuria, proteinuria, and sometimes pyuria without the presence of any other renal syndromes may be called AU. These signs often indicate some type of renal disease but may be present in other urinary tract diseases. The early stages of a number of diseases, including neoplasia, calculi, inflammation, and infection of the kidney, may be represented in AU. The AU may come and go or may progress to the degree that a specific

diagnosis may be established by using appropriate diagnostic aids.

COLLECTING AND VOIDING SYSTEM HEMATURIA

Hematuria originating from the collecting and voiding system is often associated with stranguria (a frequent and painful discharge of urine) or dysuria, pollakiuria, or urinating in abnormal places.

INFECTIONS. Infections of the bladder, prostate, vagina, urethral papilla, or urethra can produce hematuria. Acuteness and severity of infection will dictate the degree of hematuria. In general, chronicity of infection of the prostate, vagina, urethral papilla, and urethra will result in a lessening of the degree of hematuria, with resultant microscopic hematuria. This is more variable in chronic cystitis from infection.

The urinary bladder is usually sensitive in acute cystitis, but with chronicity, bladder wall thickness becomes prominent and palpable sensitivity may decrease. Acute prostatic infection is associated with a palpably painful prostate.

Localizing the source of infection and hematuria may require many diagnostic tests, as infection is frequently found in two or more segments of the urinary system.

INFLAMMATION, STRUCTURAL CHANGES, AND MALFORMATIONS. Inflammatory changes not caused by infection of the bladder, prostate, vagina, urethral papilla, or urethra may produce hematuria. The urinary bladder may have developed or acquired structural damage, with resultant diverticuli or polyps or polypoid changes. Hematuria may be a feature. Diagnosis is made with the use of pneumocystography or positive-contrast cystography.

Benign hypertrophy of the prostate with or without cystic changes may produce hematuria. Frequently, the presenting sign is blood dripping from the tip of the penis between urinations. The prostate is palpably changed and not usually sensitive. A diagnosis may be aided by cytologic evaluation of prostatic fluid.

Vaginitis does not frequently produce hematuria or a bloody discharge. Occasionally, severe vaginitis with pyogranulomatous changes, which may or may not be infected, will produce a small amount of blood in the vaginal discharge. A urine sample collected by cystocentesis will demonstrate that the urine is free of blood.

Urethritis is frequently associated with hematuria, especially if the terminal urethra is primarily involved.

Inflammation and edema of the urethral opeing into the vagina (urethral papillitis) may be accompanied by microscopic hematuria. Usually, the presenting signs are stranguria, dysuria, or pollakiuria.

Diagnosis is made by visual inspection of the urethral papilla or external opening.

In general, hematuria may be found with malformation of the urinary tract.

CALCULI. Cystic calculi of any composition frequently are associated with gross hematuria. Stranguria, pollakiuria, and dysuria are often reported. In general, any dysuria associated with blood at the end of urination is indicative of disease of the lower urinary tract. The diagnosis of cystic calculi will be made by all or a combination of the following: palpation, pneumocystogram, positive-contrast cystogram, double-contrast cystogram, or plain abdominal films.

Ureteric calculi have been diagnosed in dogs as an incidental radiographic finding. Hematuria may be present. The clinician should always investigate the possibility of nephrolithiasis.

Urethral calculi may cause hematuria and severe dysuria in both male and female animals. The possibility of obstruction is present in both sexes but is higher in the male. Diagnosis is made by passing a urethral catheter and feeling the characteristic grating or by radiography using plain films or a positive-contrast retrograde urethrogram.

NEOPLASIA. Persistent, nonresponsive hematuria with or without dysuria is often a sign of neoplasia of the urinary bladder; however, this same finding may be seen in chronic, inadequately treated cystitis or in anatomic defects of the bladder. Diagnosis is supported by pneumocystography and positive-contrast cystography and confirmed by evaluation of exfoliative cytologic and biopsy specimens.

Neoplasia of the prostate is usually associated with hematuria or blood at the end of the penis. The prostate may or may not be sensitive and usually is somewhat enlarged, with firm, irregular nodules in the parenchyma. The prostate gland may be firmly attached to surrounding tissues and may be not freely mobile. Diagnosis is confirmed by biopsy or exfoliative cytologic evaluation of prostatic fluid.

TRAUMA. It is important to repeat that contrast urography is indicated in many cases of hematuria associated with trauma. Pneumocystography is warranted to diagnose trauma to and rupture of the urinary bladder. Retrograde positive-contrast or voiding positive-contrast urethrograms are helpful in diagnosing trauma to and rupture of the urethra.

HEMATURIA FROM ANY SITE IN THE URINARY SYSTEM

Hematuria is not an uncommon finding in patients with disorders of coagulation. Other sites of hemorrhage should be actively sought and, if any doubt exists, bleeding and clotting studies should be done.

CAUSES OF HEMATURIA THAT ARE POORLY UNDERSTOOD AND POORLY DOCUMENTED IN DOGS AND CATS

HEMATURIA FROM EXERCISE OR HEAT STROKE. Proteinuria and hematuria may be seen after strenuous exercise. These abnormalities usually disappear within 1 to 2 days and have little or no clinical significance. Heat stroke, however, can produce longer lasting urinary sediment and functional changes. In heat stroke the essential abnormality in the kidney is acute tubular necrosis (ATN). Other causes of ATN, such as shock, leptospirosis, and some heavy metal poisonings, can be associated with hematuria, usually microscopic. In heat stroke, the hematuria tends to be more severe than in many other causes of ATN.

ACUTE RADIATION NEPHRITIS. With the growing use of radiotherapy, some veterinary clinicians may begin diagnosing microscopic hematuria from acute radiation nephritis. Proteinuria is much more prominent than the hematuria. This condition is usually not present when correct therapeutic doses of radiation are used.

DRUG-INDUCED AND NEPHROALLERGIC HEMATURIA. The potential exists for all drugs that are either metabolized or excreted by the kidneys to cause renal damage and hematuria. As the use of drugs and drug combinations grows, so will the list of drugs that cause hematuria. Some of the more commonly encountered veterinary drugs that can produce nephrotoxicity and hematuria include low-solubility sulfonamides, gentamicin, kanamycin, amphotericin B, penicillin, phenylbutazone, cyclophosphamide (which causes cystitis, not renal damage), penicillamine, and thiacetarsamide. Cephaloridine can produce hematuria in humans, but the dog and cat seem to be resistant.

HEMOGLOBINURIA

Whenever free hemoglobin is detected in the urine, any of the causes of hemolysis should be ruled out. Among the more common causes are autoimmune hemolytic anemia, disseminated intravascular coagulation, transfusion reaction, and heat stroke. Splenic torsion and the postcaval syndrome from dirofilariasis have also been associated with hemolysis.

Problem-Solving Approach

Figure 1 is a modified algorithm that may be useful to determine the cause and significance of hematuria. It is a purely clinical approach and is designed to be direct, with deletion of the obvious. Two points should be considered in using this chart:

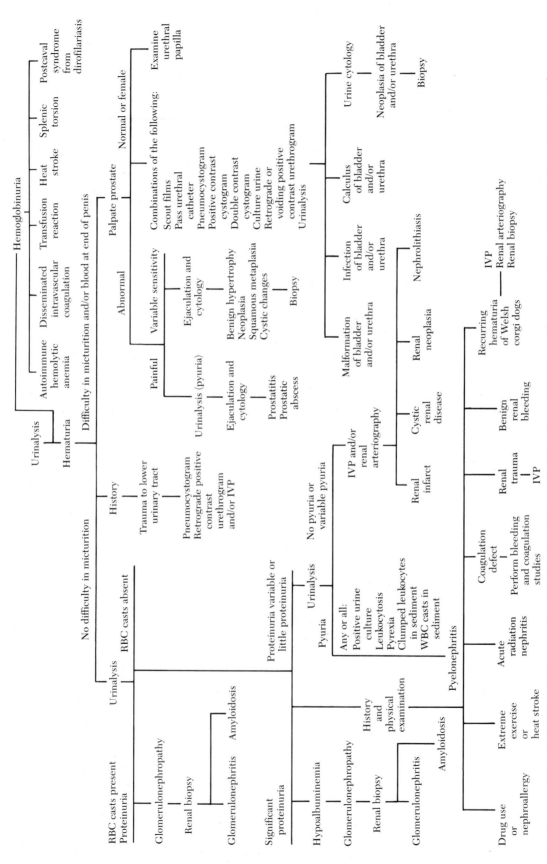

Figure 1. Problem-solving approach to clinical analysis of hematuria. (From Lage, A. L.: *Hematuria, A Clinical Approach: Its Meaning, and Differential Diagnosis in the Dog and Cat.* Small Animal Veterinary Medical Update Series 15. Princeton, NJ: Veterinary Publications, 1978.)

First, difficulty in micturition may be stranguria, dysuria, or pollakiuria (not volume-related polyuria). Second, whenever the chart cannot be followed because a patient has confusing or multiple findings, it is recommended that a culture of the urine, multiple fresh urinalyses, and, most important, an IVP be done early in the case workup.

CONCLUSION

The cause of hematuria can be easy or difficult to identify. It is sometimes obvious, as in the presence of large radiopaque cystic calculi. Some cases of recurring macroscopic hematuria can be difficult to explain; however, almost all cases of hematuria can be diagnosed if a systematic approach to data collection is followed and if the entire spectrum of possible causes is reviewed during the workup.

References and Supplemental Reading

Bovee, K.: *Canine Nephrology.* Philadelphia: Harwal, 1984.
Chew, D. J., and DiBartola, S. P.: *Manual of Small Animal Nephrology and Urology.* New York: Churchill Livingstone, 1986.
Hitt, M. E.: *Hematuria of Renal Origin.* Compendium Cont. Ed. Pract. Vet. 8:14, 1986.
Lage, A. L.: Hematuria, A Clinical Approach: Its Meaning and Differential Diagnosis in the Dog and Cat. *Biweekly Small Animal Veterinary Medical Update—Series 15.* Princeton: Veterinary Publications, 1978, pp. 1–12.

CLINICAL EVALUATION OF RENAL FUNCTION

A Critical Appraisal of Procedures and Interpretations

DELMAR R. FINCO, D.V.M.,
and JEANNE A. BARSANTI, D.V.M.
Athens, Georgia

The increase in sophistication in veterinary practice has led to increased use of diagnostic aids. In nephrology, evaluation of blood urea nitrogen (BUN) and plasma or serum concentration of creatinine (SC) continue to be used for confirming the presence of azotemia. However, other applications of these studies and more specific and more sensitive tests of renal function also are being employed.

Regardless of the test, a knowledge of its proper applications, limitations, and appropriate interpretations is required. This article discusses these points.

GENERALIZED RENAL FAILURE: AZOTEMIC PHASE

Blood Urea Nitrogen and Serum Creatinine Measurement

AZOTEMIA

With generalized renal failure, azotemia usually precedes the development of all clinical signs except polyuria. Determination of BUN or SC is appropriate for establishing that azotemia is present when clinical signs of uremia exist. However, the limitations of BUN and SC must be recognized (see Table 1).

Table 1. *Limitations of Blood Urea Nitrogen and Serum Creatinine as Renal Function Tests*

Limitations of Both
  Insensitive: elevations not detectable until GFR is <25% of normal
  Do not distinguish among prerenal, renal, and postrenal azotemia

Additional Limitations of BUN
  Influenced by dietary protein intake or body protein catabolism
  Urea not handled exclusively by glomerular filtration in the kidney (see text)

Additional Limitations of Creatinine
  Picrate method of analysis is not specific for creatinine and includes a variety of compounds collectively called noncreatinine chromogens
  Intestinal metabolism is induced during uremia, resulting in a nonrenal exit of creatinine from the body

DEGREE OF DYSFUNCTION

BUN and SC, alone or in combination, have been used for purposes beyond documenting azotemia. The magnitude of their elevation has been used as an indicator of the degree of renal dysfunction. To provide a perspective of this use, it is necessary to review how the kidneys excrete each.

Creatinine passes freely through glomerular capillary walls into renal tubules and appears in filtrate in the same concentration as in plasma water. Creatinine is neither reabsorbed nor secreted by renal tubules of the cat and female dog. Thus, all creatinine appearing in the urine of these animals gets there by glomerular filtration. In the male dog, a small amount of additional creatinine is added to the tubule lumen by secretion by the proximal tubules. This tubular secretion is much weaker in the male dog than in some other species (humans and goats). Because tubular action on creatinine is minimal in male dogs, renal excretion of creatinine is nearly all due to glomerular filtration.

Urea also freely passes through glomerular capillaries, but about 40 per cent is reabsorbed by the tubules. This reabsorption is important clinically because the amount reabsorbed is dependent on urine flow rate. A slow rate of urine flow facilitates reabsorption and increases BUN; a high rate of urine flow lessens reabsorption and lowers BUN level. These features of renal excretion of urea and creatinine, together with the limitations listed in Table 1, are the basis for the following statements regarding use of BUN and SC for quantitative measurement of renal function.

1. Both tests are crude indicators of the state of renal function but cannot be interpreted too stringently.

2. BUN values are altered both by the rate of protein catabolism and by urine flow rate. Urine flow rate is influenced by urea generation, water intake, electrolyte intake, and the functioning of the urine-concentrating mechanism. Thus, many factors, including anorexia and dehydration, can cause an animal to retain urea more readily than it retains creatinine and thus to have a disproportionately greater BUN than SC value. Conversely, fluid therapy may enhance urine flow rate, decreasing BUN values without necessarily increasing glomerular filtration rate (GFR).

3. Although not subject to as many influences as BUN, SC still does not precisely reflect GFR. As renal function diminishes, SC does not increase in proportion to the decrease in GFR, apparently because of an increased rate of degradation of creatinine by enteric bacteria.

4. Because levels of both BUN and SC are influenced by prerenal and postrenal factors, in addition to primary renal dysfunction, extrarenal factors must be considered when interpreting values.

In summary, both BUN and SC must be considered crude indicators of renal function. Of the two, SC is probably more reliable for monitoring changes in function.

DIETARY COMPLIANCE

BUN and SC values have been used to monitor compliance with low-protein diets. BUN/SC ratios in patients on low-protein diets should be low because creatinine generation is minimally affected by protein intake, but urea generation is directly related to protein intake and catabolism.

PRERENAL VERSUS PRIMARY RENAL FAILURE

BUN/SC ratios have been advocated for differentiation of prerenal and primary renal failure. With prerenal failure, oliguria and retention of urea should result in a high BUN/SC ratio. Although theoretically sound, a retrospective evaluation of renal failure in dogs indicated that prerenal and primary renal failure could not be differentiated by BUN/SC ratios, apparently because other factors influenced generation or urinary excretion of urea (Finco and Duncan, 1976).

RECIPROCAL OF SC

Serial measurements of the degree of azotemia have been used to evaluate progression of renal dysfunction. Mathematic manipulation of SC values from humans with azotemia led some nephrologists to conclude that the reciprocal of SC, plotted against the date of sampling, gave a linear relationship between 1/SC and time. This manipulation was used to predict the time at which decreased function would require use of dialysis or to note changes in rate of progression of disease. Other nephrologists have harshly criticized this technique because a linear relationship between 1/SC and time is not invariable and because the procedure uses a measurement that is acknowledged to be a crude indicator of renal function. A linear relationship does not exist in many dogs, and the authors find little use for the technique.

GENERALIZED RENAL FAILURE: PREAZOTEMIC PHASE

Urine Concentration Tests

Generalized renal disease may be suspected in some dogs and cats prior to the onset of azotemia because of the existence of proteinuria, polyuria, or other findings. Water deprivation or urine concentration tests have been used to distinguish primary polydipsia from primary polyuria. Although such tests are of value, they often fail to separate generalized renal failure from other causes of primary polyuria in which the kidney is normal except for some functional defect in the concentrating mechanism. Another limitation of these tests is that generalized renal failure causes defects in urine concentration only after two thirds of the renal tissue is nonfunctional.

Clearance Procedures

Of the variety of functions performed by the kidney, no single function perfectly reflects the status of all others. However, it is generally agreed that glomerular filtration rate is the best single measurement to evaluate function when generalized renal disease is suspected. The advantage of GFR measurement is that it is much more sensitive than BUN, SC, or urine concentration tests.

Measurement of renal clearance with inulin is the gold standard for determination of GFR. Textbooks of physiology can be consulted for information on the theory of clearance procedures. The complexity of clearance measurements with inulin makes them unfeasible clinically, and this has led to the use of alternate procedures. The most practical alternate procedure is the determination of endogenous creatinine clearance. Because creatinine concentration in blood remains constant during stable renal function, the need for intravenous infusion of a test substance is obviated. Renal excretion of creatinine is almost exclusively by glomerular filtration in the dog and cat; thus, endogenous creatinine clearance should equal GFR. Unfortunately, the method for creatinine analysis that is generally employed (using picrate) is not specific for creatinine. A variety of other compounds that exist in plasma react as creatinine. These compounds, collectively called noncreatinine chromogens, do not appear in urine. Consequently, they falsely elevate plasma values for creatinine and result in values for clearance that are lower than GFR.

In the authors' hospital laboratory, a kinetic method of analysis that is claimed to be specific for creatinine gives clearance values for endogenous creatinine that are lower than those for inulin clearance. Interpretation of these clearance values using inulin clearance data as the norm would lead to an erroneous diagnosis of renal dysfunction. Although this potential error exists, endogenous creatinine clearance remains a valuable test for renal function if interpreted in the context of its limitations. Because the specificity of plasma creatinine analysis varies among laboratories, and because claims of specificity are questionable, it is necessary to establish individual laboratory values for endogenous creatinine clearance in normal dogs and cats. Unless endogenous creatinine clearance values are proved to be equal to inulin clearance values when both are performed simultaneously, the clearance value for endogenous creatinine should not be referred to as a GFR measurement but merely as endogenous creatinine clearance. An established normal value for endogenous creatinine clearance can be used to interpret endogenous creatinine clearance data from clinical cases with sensitivity nearly equal to that of actual GFR measurements.

Endogenous creatinine clearance procedures have been described for both short-term (20 min) and long-term (24 hr) urine collections (Finco, 1971; Bovee and Joyce, 1979). It is not known whether discrepancies in values from normal dogs in these studies represent differences in analytic methods, diurnal variation in creatinine excretion, or other factors.

Exogenous creatinine clearance measurement refers to the determination of creatinine clearance after additional creatinine has been injected into the patient. The advantage of the exogenous creatinine clearance determination is that interference from noncreatinine chromogens is reduced by dilution to a point at which their effect on creatinine clearance is negligible. Studies have established that exogenous creatinine clearance is the same as inulin clearance when plasma creatinine concentration is increased above 8 mg/dl. Because constant infusion of creatinine is just as laborious as infusing inulin, the traditional method of making exogenous creatinine clearance determinations is not practical clinically. However, reliable results for GFR measurement have still been obtained when the test was simplified by increasing plasma creatinine concentration with a single subcutaneous injection of creatinine (Finco et al., 1981).

Plasma Decay Methods

Renal clearance tests have the disadvantage of requiring urine collections. An alternate approach to evaluation of renal function is to choose a compound that is excreted by the kidney, inject it intravenously, and determine the rate at which it disappears from plasma by analysis of serial samples of plasma. The results may be expressed as the plasma half-life of the substance, and results from patients can be compared with established normal half-life values.

Mathematic manipulation of decay curves has been performed to express results as GFR. However, such manipulation is tenuous because decay curves do not represent urinary excretion exclusively. There may be some nonrenal methods of excretion of substances, and there is loss from plasma into other body compartments. Unless these nonrenal factors are constant under all conditions of use of the test, the single injection method is not valid for estimating GFR. The single injection method must be validated by relating mathematic derivations of GFR to simultaneous measurements of inulin clearance. It also would be advisable to confirm that valid results are obtained under conditions in which nonrenal factors that alter plasma decay have changed. Some single injection methods advocated for measurement of GFR in dogs and cats have been validated, but others have not. Consequently, it is questionable whether some methods claimed to measure GFR actually are doing so. The substances available for the single injection method of measuring renal function are not routinely analyzed by clinical laboratories; these methods are usually available only in teaching hospitals.

"Spot" Clearance or Fractional Excretion Determinations

Because renal excretion of creatinine is exclusively by glomerular filtration in female dogs and in cats, and because in male dogs the tubular secretory mechanism is weak, creatinine can serve as a marker for GFR for tests other than classic clearance procedures. Under conditions of stable renal function, creatinine excretion per 24 hr should not vary. Expressing excretion of any urinary component in terms of amount per unit of creatinine theoretically normalizes values, as is achieved by analysis of 24-hr urine collections.

Creatinine also can serve as a marker for estimation of fractional excretion of any urinary component. Fractional excretion refers to that fraction of filtered material that escapes tubular reabsorption. When a single plasma sample and a random urine sample are obtained for such determinations, it is referred to as a "spot" fractional excretion determination. Measurement of creatinine is performed as a marker of no tubular reabsorption or secretion. The ratio of urine creatinine to plasma creatinine indicates how much water was absorbed as urine traversed the tubules. The ratio of urine concentration to plasma concentration of other substances that are freely filtered (e.g., sodium, potassium, phosphorus, and glucose) reflects both tubular action and water reabsorption. Dividing the plasma-urine ratio of a substance by the creatinine plasma-urine ratio eliminates the water reabsorption factor common to both, and the result is the fraction of the substance filtered that was excreted in the urine (i.e., fractional excretion).

Certain pitfalls exist with the spot method of determination of fractional excretion compared with the classic method, which includes use of clearance procedures and timed urine collections. For spot values to equal classic clearance values, two factors must remain constant: the plasma concentration of the test substance and the homeostatic response of the renal tubule. For many substances, these conditions are often not fulfilled. For example, plasma concentration of several electrolytes (sodium, phosphorus, and potassium) changes during the postprandial state. Some changes also may be related to circadian rhythms. Urinary excretion of sodium and phosphorus increases and urinary excretion of potassium decreases postprandially by large amounts, and circadian rhythms for urine electrolyte excretion may occur as well. Consequently, plasma concentrations at the instant of sampling may have changed from values existing during the pooling of urine in the bladder, and the tubular reabsorption by the kidney may have changed. Another error in the determination is related to measurement of plasma creatinine by the picrate method, as the plasma-urine creatinine ratio is actually greater than what is measured.

Studies comparing spot and classic fractional excretion measurements will be required for each material, under conditions of clinical use, to determine the reliability of the spot procedure.

Care must be taken in interpreting values for fractional excretion, even when the determinations are conducted appropriately. High values for fractional excretion do not necessarily mean that renal dysfunction exists. Fractional excretion values for many substances represent the result of normal renal mechanisms for homeostasis. When dietary intake of many electrolytes is altered, a normal homeostatic response is a change in fractional excretion. Consequently, interpretation of values must include consideration of the animal's intake. "Normal" values for fractional excretion, as well as for daily urinary excretion, can be determined only with recognition of food intake or parenteral therapy. Unusual fractional excretion values may be normal, and an animal's renal function may be normal, in instances when an extreme diet or treatment requires such values for homeostasis.

References and Supplemental Reading

Bovee, K. C., and Joyce, T.: Clinical evaluation of glomerular function: 24-hour creatinine clearance in dogs. J.A.V.M.A. 174:488, 1979.

Finco, D. R.: Simultaneous determination of phenolsulfonthalein excretion and endogenous creatinine clearance in the normal dog. J.A.V.M.A. 159:336, 1971.

Finco, D. R.: Renal functions. In Kaneko, J. J. (ed.): Clinical Biochemistry of Domestic Animals, 4th ed. New York: Academic Press, 1988.

Finco, D. R., and Duncan, J. R.: Evaluation of blood urea nitrogen and serum creatinine concentration as indicators of renal dysfunction. A study of 111 cases and a review of the literature. J.A.V.M.A. 168:593, 1976.

Finco, D. R., Coulter, D. B., and Barsanti, J. A.: Simple, accurate method for clinical estimation of glomerular filtration rate in the dog. Am. J. Vet. Res. 42:1874, 1981.

CRYSTALLURIA: CAUSES, DETECTION, AND INTERPRETATION

CARL A. OSBORNE, D.V.M.,
TIMOTHY D. O'BRIEN, D.V.M.,
St. Paul, Minnesota

MARIAN P. DAVENPORT, M.L.T.,
and CHRIS W. CLINTON, M.T.
Houston, Texas

CLINICAL SIGNIFICANCE AND INSIGNIFICANCE

The advent of effective medical protocols to induce dissolution of struvite uroliths in dogs and cats, and ammonium urate and cystine uroliths in dogs, has focused renewed interest on detection and interpretation of crystalluria. Assessment of urine crystals may aid in detection of underlying metabolic disorders, estimation of the mineral composition of uroliths, and evaluation of medical protocols designed to dissolve them.

Crystals occur only in urine that is, or recently has been, supersaturated with crystallogenic substances. Therefore, crystalluria represents a risk factor for urolithiasis. However, crystalluria (microlithuria) is not synonymous with formation of macrouroliths and the clinical signs associated with them. Nor is it irrefutable evidence of a stone-forming tendency. In fact, crystalluria that occurs in individuals with anatomically and functionally normal urinary tracts is usually harmless because the crystals are eliminated before they grow to sufficient size to cause clinical signs. Likewise, crystals that form following elimination or removal of urine from the urinary tract often are of no clinical importance. Identification of crystals in such patients does not justify therapy.

On the other hand, detection of some types of abnormal crystals in clinically asymptomatic patients (for example, cystine and ammonium urate crystals), detection of large aggregates of crystals frequently observed in normal individuals (for example, struvite or calcium oxalate), or detection of any form of crystals in patients with confirmed urolithiasis may be of diagnostic, prognostic, or therapeutic importance.

In patients with confirmed urolithiasis, microscopic evaluation of urine crystals should not be utilized as the sole criterion of the mineral composition of macroliths. Only quantitative urolith analysis can provide definitive information about the mineral composition of stones. However, interpretation of crystalluria in light of other clinical findings often allows one to establish a tentative identification of the mineral composition of uroliths. Subsequent reduction or elimination of crystalluria by therapy provides a useful index of the efficacy of medical protocols designed to dissolve or prevent uroliths.

FACTORS INFLUENCING CRYSTAL FORMATION

IN VIVO AND IN VITRO VARIABLES. Even though there is not a direct relationship between crystalluria and urolithiasis, detection of crystals in urine is proof that the urine sample is oversaturated with crystallogenic substances. However, oversaturation may occur as a result of *in vitro* events in addition to, or instead of, *in vivo* events. Therefore, care must be used not to overinterpret the significance of crystalluria.

In vivo variables that influence crystalluria include (1) the concentration of crystallogenic substances in urine (which in turn is influenced by their rate of excretion and the volume of water in which they are excreted), (2) urine pH (see Table 1), (3) solubility of crystallogenic substances in urine, and (4) excretion of diagnostic agents (such as radiopaque contrast agents) and medications (such as sulfonamides and ampicillin). *In vitro* variables that influence crystalluria include (1) temperature, (2) evaporation, (3) pH, and (4) the technique of specimen preparation (e.g., centrifugation versus noncentrifugation and volume of urine examined). It is emphasized that *in vitro* changes that occur following urine collection may enhance formation or dissolution of crystals. Although *in vitro* changes may be used to enhance detection of certain types of crystals (e.g., acidification to cause precipitation of cystine), *in vitro* crystal formation may have no clinical relevance to *in vivo* formation and elimina-

Table 1. *Characteristics of Some Urine Crystals*

Type	Appearance	Acid	Neutral	Alkaline
		\<span\>Urine pH\</span\>		
Ammonium urate	Yellow-brown spherulites; thorn apples	+	+	+
Bilirubin	Reddish brown needles or granules	+	–	–
Calcium oxalate dihydrate	Small colorless envelopes (octahedral form)	+	+	±
Calcium oxalate monohydrate	Small spindles, hemp seed or dumbbell shape	+	+	±
Calcium phosphate	Amorphous, or long thin prisms	±	+	+
Cholesterol	Flat colorless plates with corner notch	+	+	–
Cystine	Flat colorless hexagonal plates	+	+	±
Hippuric acid	4- to 6-sided colorless elongated plates or prisms with rounded corners	+	+	±
Leucine	Yellow-brown spheroids with radial and concentric laminations	+	–	–
Magnesium ammonium phosphate	3- to 6-sided colorless prisms	±	+	+
Tyrosine	Fine colorless or yellow needles arranged in sheaves or rosettes	+	–	–
Uric acid	Diamond or rhombic rosettes, or oval plates, structures with pointed ends. Occasionally 6-sided plates	+	–	–

±, Crystals may occur at this pH but not usually.

tion of crystals in urine. When knowledge of *in vivo* urine crystal type is especially important, fresh specimens should be serially examined. The number, size, and structure of crystals should be evaluated, as well as their tendency to aggregate.

URINE pH. The formation and persistence of several types of crystals are influenced by pH. Therefore, it is often useful to consider pH when interpreting crystalluria (Table 1). Different crystals tend to form and persist in certain pH ranges, although there are exceptions. Exceptions may be related to large concentrations of crystallogenic substances in urine or recent *in vivo* or *in vitro* changes in urine pH.

REFRIGERATION. Refrigeration is an excellent method to preserve many physical, chemical, and morphologic properties of urine and urine sediment. However, it must be utilized with caution when evaluating crystalluria from qualitative and quantitative standpoints. Although refrigeration of urine samples is likely to enhance formation of various types of crystals, this phenomemon may have no relationship to events occurring in the patient's body.

DIET. Crystalluria may also be influenced by diet (including water intake). Dietary influence on crystalluria is of diagnostic importance because urine crystal formation that occurs while patients are consuming hospital diets may be dissimilar to urine crystal formation that occurs when patients are consuming diets fed at home.

COMBINATIONS OF CRYSTALS. Crystals form in a complex environment characterized by constant formation of urine of variable composition that traverses different components of the upper and lower urinary tract. In fact, more than one type of crystal may be observed in the same urine sample. Observation of a combination of brushite (calcium hydrogen phosphate dihydrate, a mineral precipitated in acid urine) and calcium apatite (calcium phosphate) crystals in human urine samples supports this hypothesis because brushite would not be expected to form in the alkaline environment required for precipitation of calcium apatite.

Crystals of different composition may also form within the same location. For example, infection-induced magnesium ammonium phosphate crystals may form concomitantly with metabolic crystals (e.g., calcium oxalate, calcium phosphate, and ammonium urate).

IDENTIFICATION OF CRYSTALS

CRYSTAL HABIT

Habit is the term commonly used by mineralogists to refer to characteristic shapes of mineral crystals and is commonly used as an index of crystal composition. However, microscopic evaluation of the habits of urine crystals represents only a tentative indicator of their composition because variable conditions associated with their formation, growth, and dissolution may alter their appearance. Therefore, definitive identification of crystal composition is dependent on optical crystallography, infrared spectrophotometry, thermal analysis, x-ray diffraction, electron microprobe analysis, or a combination of these. If confirmation of the composition of microscopic crystalluria is desirable, it may be of value to attempt to prepare a large pellet of crystals by centrifugation of an appropriate volume of urine in a cone-tipped centrifuge tube. Evaluation of the pellet by quantitative methods designed for urolith analysis may provide meaningful information about crystalluria associated with urolithiasis. However, it is emphasized that the type of crystals identified by this method may only reflect the outer portions of uroliths located in the urinary tract.

The following provides an alphabetic listing of crystals encountered in canine and feline urine, their habits, and their probable significances.

AMMONIUM URATE AND AMORPHOUS URATE CRYSTALLURIA

HABIT. Ammonium urate (also called ammonium biurate) crystals are commonly observed in slightly acid, neutral, and alkaline urine. They are usually brown or yellow-brown in color and may form spherulites or spheric bodies with long irregular protrusions (so-called thorn apple form).

Sodium, potassium, magnesium, and calcium urate salts may precipitate in amorphous form in acid urine (so-called amorphous urates). They may resemble amorphous phosphates but dissolve in an alkaline environment. As the amorphous urate crystals increase in size (Fig. 1), they develop a characteristic yellow or yellow-brown color. Sodium urate may also precipitate as colorless or yellowish needles or as slender prisms occurring in sheaves or clusters.

Ammonium urate and amorphous urate crystals are insoluble in acetic acid. However, addition of 10 per cent acetic acid to urine sediment containing the aforementioned crystals often results in the appearance of uric acid and sometimes sodium urate crystals (see discussion of uric acid crystalluria for details). Addition of acetic acid to amorphous phosphate crystals results in their rapid dissolution, whereas they persist in alkaline urine sediment.

INTERPRETATION. Ammonium urate and amorphous urate may occur in apparently normal dogs and cats, but they are not common. They are frequently observed in dogs with portal vascular anomalies with or without concomitant ammonium urate uroliths. They are also commonly detected in Dalmatians, bulldogs, and other dogs and cats with ammonium urate uroliths caused by disorders other than portal vascular anomalies.

BILIRUBIN CRYSTALLURIA

Bilirubin may crystallize in urine to form yellow-red or reddish brown needles or granules. Bilirubin crystals can be observed in highly concentrated urine from normal dogs. When observed in large numbers in serial samples of urine, they should arouse suspicion of an abnormality in bilirubin metabolism.

CALCIUM OXALATE CRYSTALLURIA

HABIT. Calcium oxalate dihydrate crystals (weddellite) typically are colorless and have a characteristic octahedral or envelope shape. By light microscopy, they resemble small or large squares whose corners are connected by intersecting diagonal lines. Calcium oxalate crystals have been observed in acid, neutral, and alkaline urine samples.

Calcium oxalate monohydrate crystals (whewellite) vary in size and may have a spindle, oval (hemp seed), or dumbbell shape. Calcium oxalate monohydrate crystals with hippuric-acidlike morphologic findings have also been observed in dogs. They are soluble in hydrochloric acid but insoluble in acetic acid. They may occur in combination with calcium oxalate dihydrate and other types of crystals.

Alizarin red S stain has been advocated to presumptively identify calcium oxalate crystals. Calcium oxalate crystals stain with alizarin red S at pH of 7.0 but not at pH 4.2. In contrast, calcium phosphate and calcium carbonate crystals stain at pH of 7.0 *and* 4.2.

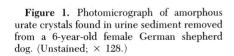

Figure 1. Photomicrograph of amorphous urate crystals found in urine sediment removed from a 6-year-old female German shepherd dog. (Unstained; × 128.)

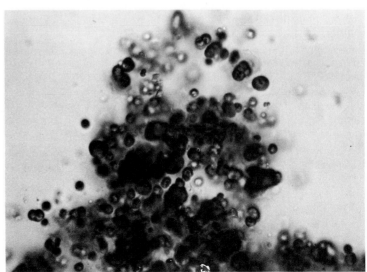

INTERPRETATION. Calcium oxalate dihydrate crystals may occur in apparently normal dogs and cats and in dogs and cats with uroliths primarily composed of calcium oxalate. Although they may be observed in dogs intoxicated with ethylene glycol, they are less common than calcium oxalate monohydrate crystals (ethylene glycol toxicity may also occur without crystalluria).

Calcium oxalate monohydrate crystals may occur alone or in combination with calcium oxalate dihydrate or other types of crystals. Large quantities of calcium oxalate monohydrate (or dihydrate) crystals in fresh urine should prompt consideration of hypercalciuric or hyperoxaluric disorders (such as ethylene glycol toxicity), especially if they occur in aggregates or grow to a large size.

CALCIUM PHOSPHATE CRYSTALLURIA

HABIT. There are many different types of calcium phosphate crystals. They appear to be variously described as amorphous phosphates and calcium phosphates. With the exception of brushite, calcium phosphate crystals tend to form in alkaline urine. Amorphous phosphates resemble amorphous urates. However, amorphous phosphates form in alkaline urine and are soluble in acetic acid. In contrast, amorphous urates often have a yellow granular appearance, and are insoluble in acetic acid, but are soluble in alkali and at 60°C. Scanning electron micrographs of amorphous phosphates found in human urine revealed that they usually have a spheric habit, but may assume doughnut or cast forms. Calcium phosphates may also form long, thin, colorless prisms, sometimes with one pointed end. These crystals may aggregate into rosettes or appear as needles. Calcium phosphate may also precipitate as elongated, lath-shaped brushite crystals in acid urine. It has been suggested that when calcium phosphate is precipitated from an aqueous solution of high supersaturation and pH greater than 7, amorphous phosphates initially appear. The amorphous precipitate may slowly transform into a stable crystalline precipitate by a process of dissolution, renucleation, and crystal growth. The speed of this transformation depends on pH because the stability of amorphous phosphates is enhanced at a high pH.

INTERPRETATION. In the authors' experience, large numbers of crystals presumed to be composed of calcium phosphate have been observed in apparently normal dogs, dogs with persistently alkaline urine, dogs with calcium phosphate uroliths, and dogs with uroliths composed of a mixture of calcium phosphate and calcium oxalate. Small numbers of calcium phosphate crystals may occur in association with infection-induced struvite crystalluria.

CHOLESTEROL CRYSTALLURIA

HABIT. Cholesterol crystals typically appear as large, flat, rectangular plates with a characteristic notch in a corner. By light microscopy, they are colorless and transparent; by polarized light microscopy, they exhibit a variety of brilliant colors.

INTERPRETATION. In people, cholesterol crystals have been reported to be associated with excessive tissue destruction, the nephrotic syndrome, and chyluria. Veterinary experience with them has been too limited to formulate meaningful generalities. However, they have been observed in apparently normal dogs.

CYSTINE CRYSTALLURIA

HABIT. Cystine crystals are colorless and have a characteristic hexagonal (benzene ring) shape with equal or unequal sides (see p. 1190). They may appear singly but commonly aggregate in layers. Their detection may be aided by reduced light intensity because they are thin. Cystine crystals most commonly form in concentrated acid urine. Formation of markedly alkaline urine as a consequence of infection or contamination with urease-producing microbes may cause cystine crystals to dissolve. Addition of glacial acetic acid followed by refrigeration and centrifugation may enhance detection of typical crystals in alkaline urine samples. Cystine crystals are insoluble in acetic acid, alcohol, acetone, ether, and boiling water. They are soluble in ammonia and hydrochloric acid.

INTERPRETATION. Cystine crystalluria is not a normal phenomenon. Cystine uroliths may develop in dogs with the metabolic disorder cystinuria; however, not all patients with cystinuria develop cystine uroliths (see discussion of magnesium ammonium phosphate and uric acid crystalluria for details about differentiation of cystine crystals from struvite or uric acid crystals).

DRUG-ASSOCIATED CRYSTALLURIA

Various drugs excreted in urine may form crystals. Perhaps the most familiar drug-associated crystalluria is that occurring with sulfonamide administration. Sulfonamide drugs may precipitate in urine in characteristic sheaves of clear or brownish needles, usually with eccentric binding. They may also appear as amphorphous crystals with radial striations (Fig. 2). A positive lignin test result supports a diagnosis of sulfonamide crystalluria. Compound uroliths containing varying quantities of sulfonamides have been observed in dogs. Other drug-associated forms of crystalluria have only been documented in people.

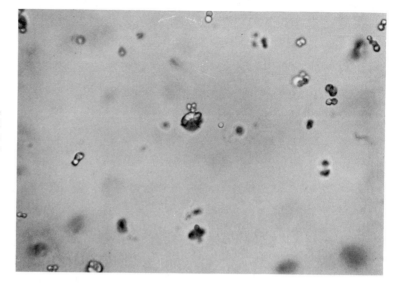

Figure 2. Photomicrograph of sulfonamide crystals in the urine sediment of a 3-year-old female springer spaniel. The dog had been given trimethoprim-sulfamethoxazole tablets orally. (Unstained; × 205.)

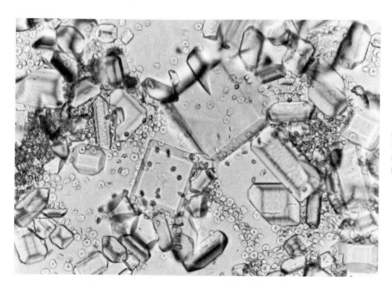

Figure 3. Photomicrograph of magnesium ammonium phosphate crystals in the urine sediment of an adult male cat with urethral obstruction. Note the variation in sizes and shapes. (Unstained; × 128.)

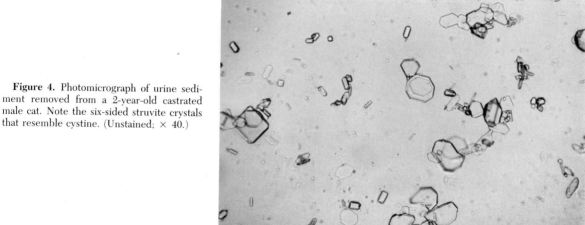

Figure 4. Photomicrograph of urine sediment removed from a 2-year-old castrated male cat. Note the six-sided struvite crystals that resemble cystine. (Unstained; × 40.)

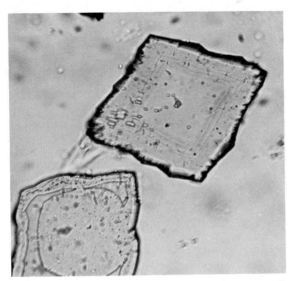

Figure 5. Photomicrograph of uric acid crystal in urine sediment obtained from a 2-year-old male bulldog with urate urocystoliths. Uric acid crystals formed following addition of 10 per cent buffered acetic acid to sediment containing amorphous urates. (Unstained; × 128.)

HIPPURIC ACID CRYSTALLURIA

Hippuric acid crystals are colorless, elongated structures of variable size. They typically have six sides that are connected by rounded corners. They have attracted renewed interest in veterinary medicine because of their apparent association with ethylene glycol toxicity in dogs and cats. However, recent studies of dogs with ethylene glycol toxicity associated with urine crystals presumed to be hippuric acid by light microscopy have revealed that they are calcium oxalate monohydrate. True hippuric acid crystals are apparently rare and of unknown significance.

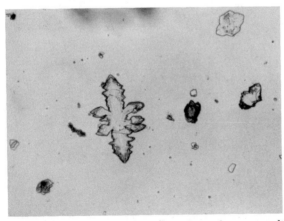

Figure 6. Photomicrograph of uric acid crystal in urine sediment obtained from a 3-year-old male Dalmatian. Uric acid crystals formed following addition of 10 per cent buffered acetic acid to sediment containing amorphous urate cyrstals. (Unstained; × 51.)

LEUCINE CRYSTALLURIA

Leucine crystals typically appear as large yellow or brown spheroids with radial concentric laminations. However, such spheroids may not be pure leucine, because it has been reported that pure leucine forms crystals that resemble hexagonal plates.

In humans, leucine crystals are considered to be indicative of severe liver disease. The significance of leucine crystals in dogs has not been well documented.

MAGNESIUM AMMONIUM PHOSPHATE CRYSTALLURIA

HABIT. Magnesium ammonium phosphate (struvite) crystals typically appear as colorless orthorhombic (having three unequal axes intersecting at right angles) coffinlike prisms. They may have three to six sides and often have oblique ends (Fig. 3). Six-sided struvite crystals in cats (Fig. 4) are sometimes mistaken for cystine crystals. Unlike cystine, however, they occur in association with other forms of struvite and readily dissolve following acidifcation with dilute acetic acid. On occasion, struvite crystals aggregate into fernlike structures. The sharp outlines of struvite crystals characteristically observed in fresh urine may become featherlike or moth eaten in appearance as they dissolve.

INTERPRETATION. Struvite crystals commonly occur in dogs and occasionally in cats in association with free ammonia produced by microbial urease-induced hydrolysis of urea. Struvite crystals commonly occur in cats and occasionally in dogs in the absence of detectable urease. In this instance, the ammonium component of struvite crystals presumably is generated by renal tubules.

In the authors' experience, struvite crystals may be observed in apparently normal dogs and cats; dogs and cats with infection-induced struvite uroliths; dogs and cats with sterile struvite uroliths; dogs and cats with nonstruvite uroliths; dogs and cats with uroliths of mixed composition (for example, nucleus composed of calcium oxalate, shell composed of struvite); and dogs and cats with urinary tract disease without uroliths.

TYROSINE CRYSTALLURIA

Tyrosine crystals appear as fine, highly refractile, colorless or yellow needles aggregated in sheaves or clusters. They have been reported to occur in association with severe liver disease. However, they have not been a common finding with canine or feline liver disorders.

URIC ACID CRYSTALLURIA

HABIT. Uric acid crystals are often yellow or yellow-brown and may occur in a variety of shapes. The most characteristic forms are diamond or rhombic plates, which may contain concentric rings (Fig. 5). They may also appear as rosettes composed of many of the aforementioned crystals aggregated together. Occasionally uric acid crystals form rhomboid plates with paired protrusions from their sides (Fig. 6). Less commonly they appear as six-sided crystals resembling cystine. However, the six-sided crystals occur in association with typical diamond shape or rhomboid forms. Uric acid crystals are soluble in sodium hydroxide but are insoluble in alcohol, hydrochloric acid, and acetic acid.

INTERPRETATION. Although common in humans, naturally occurring uric acid crystalluria is extremely uncommon in dogs and cats. They readily form, however, following addition of 10 per cent acetic acid to canine or feline urine sediment containing amorphous urate or ammonium biurate crystals. Approximately 20 to 30 min are required before the uric acid crystals become visible. They may grow to a large size if preserved overnight in a covered Petri dish humidified with a sponge soaked in water.

References and Supplemental Reading

Foit, F. F., Jr., Cowell, R. L., Brobst, D. F., et al.: X-ray powder diffraction and microscopic analysis of crystalluria in dogs with ethylene glycol toxicity. Am. J. Vet. Res. 46:2404, 1985.

Graff, L.: A Handbook of Routine Urinalysis. Philadelphia: J. B. Lippincott, 1983.

Jones, H. M., and Schrader, W. A.: Ampicillin crystalluria. Am. J. Clin. Pathol. 58:220, 1972.

Kramer, J. W., Bistine, D., Sheridan, P., et al.: Identification of hippuric acid crystals in the urine of ethylene glycol intoxicated dogs and cats. J.A.V.M.A. 184:584, 1984.

Osborne, C. A., O'Brien, T. D., Ghobrial, H. K., et al.: Crystalluria: Observations, interpretations, and misinterpretations. Vet. Clin. North Am. 16:45, 1986.

Proia, A. D., and Brinn, N. T.: Identification of calcium oxalate crystals using alizarin red S stain. Arch. Pathol. Lab. Med. 109:186, 1985.

Thrall, M. A., Dial, S. M., and Winder, D. R.: Identification of calcium oxalate monohydrate crystals by x-ray diffraction in urine of ethylene glycol–intoxicated dogs. Vet. Pathol. 22:625, 1985.

SPECTRUM OF CLINICAL AND LABORATORY ABNORMALITIES IN UREMIA

DAVID J. POLZIN, D.V.M.

St. Paul, Minnesota

DEFINITIONS

RENAL DISEASE. Renal disease indicates the presence of renal lesions of any size, distribution (focal or generalized), or cause (anomalies, infection, endogenous or exogenous toxins, neoplasms, ischemia, immune disorders, hypercalcemia, and trauma) in one or both kidneys. The specific cause or causes of renal lesions may not be known. Renal disease should not be considered synonymous with renal failure, because of the tremendous reserve capacity of the kidneys. Depending on the quantity of renal parenchyma affected and the severity and duration of lesions, renal disease may or may not cause renal failure and uremia.

RENAL FAILURE. Failure is defined as the inability to perform. The kidneys perform multiple functions in maintaining homeostasis, including elimination of waste products of metabolism from the body; regulation of body fluid, acid-base, and electrolyte balance; synthesis of a variety of hormones; and degradation of a variety of hormones and other metabolites. Failure to perform these functions may not be an all-or-none phenomenon. In slowly progressive renal diseases, for example, failure of the ability to concentrate or dilute urine according to body needs typically precedes failure to eliminate waste products of protein metabolism. In turn, laboratory detection of impaired ability to maintain electrolyte and nonelectrolyte solute balance typically precedes onset of polysystemic clinical signs caused by renal dysfunction (uremia). In some situations, renal disease may precede renal failure and, likewise, renal failure may precede uremia. In many instances, however, renal disease does not progress to a state of renal failure.

Chronic Renal Failure. Chronic renal failure (CRF) is defined as primary renal failure that has persisted for an extended period, usually months to years. Regardless of the cause of nephron loss, CRF is characterized by irreversible renal structural lesions. It is typically a progressive condition that culminates in uremia.

Acute Renal Failure. Acute renal failure (ARF) is defined as rapid onset of azotemia or pathologic oliguria over hours to days. Rapid onset of azotemia or oliguria indicates rapid deterioration or loss of renal function. The rapid deterioration characteristic of ARF contrasts with the indolent, inevitable progression of CRF over months to years. The syndrome of ARF encompasses prerenal, postrenal, or primary (intrinsic) renal causes of acute azotemia. Implicit in the diagnosis of ARF is the potential for reversibility as well as the threat of sudden or rapid deterioration in renal function.

AZOTEMIA. Azotemia is defined as abnormal or increased concentrations of urea, creatinine, or other nonprotein nitrogenous substances in blood, plasma, or serum. It is a laboratory finding and may or may not be caused by generalized lesions of the renal parenchyma. Azotemia resulting from generalized lesions of the kidneys is termed primary renal azotemia. Azotemia resulting from decreased renal blood flow or increased urea production is termed prerenal azotemia. Azotemia resulting from abnormal retention of urine in the body as a result of obstruction or rupture of the urinary tract is termed postrenal azotemia. Prerenal or postrenal azotemia may occur in patients with normal or abnormal kidneys.

UREMIA. Uremia is the polysystemic toxic syndrome that occurs as a result of decreased renal function. As opposed to azotemia, which is a laboratory finding, uremia is a clinical syndrome. Although uremia is always accompanied by azotemia and renal failure, azotemia and renal failure may or may not be associated with uremia.

OVERVIEW

Uremia may result from acute or chronic renal failure. The onset and spectrum of clinical signs of uremia may vary depending on the nature, severity, duration (acute or chronic), and rate of progression of the underlying disease; presence or absence of coexistent but unrelated disease; and administration of therapeutic agents (Osborne et al., 1980). In most instances, however, uremia is the clinical result of all progressive, generalized renal diseases, and associated signs are more similar than dissimilar. In addition to manifestations of impaired renal function (azotemia, metabolic acidosis, oliguria or polyuria, and mineral and electrolyte abnormalities), clinical signs and laboratory findings indicative of variable involvement of many organ systems may occur (Tables 1 and 2).

CLINICAL MANIFESTATIONS OF UREMIA

Gastrointestinal System

Gastrointestinal complications are among the most common and prominent clinical signs of uremia and may include anorexia, weight loss, vomiting, diarrhea, and uremic stomatitis. Anorexia and weight loss are common findings that often precede other signs of uremia in dogs and cats. They result in part from the effects of uremic toxins on the medullary emetic chemoreceptor trigger zone but also from uremic gastroenteritis. Weight loss, a finding suggesting CRF rather than ARF, results from inadequate caloric intake, the catabolic effects of uremia, and a low-grade intestinal malabsorption characteristic of uremic gastroenteritis.

Vomiting is a frequent, but inconsistent, finding in uremia. Although often an early manifestation of ARF, vomiting may not occur until the later stages in CRF, particularly when systemic signs have been minimized by properly formulated symptomatic and supportive therapy. The severity of vomiting may not correlate well with the severity of azotemia. Because uremic gastritis may be ulcerative, hematemesis may occur. Vomiting may be a less frequent clinical finding in uremic cats (DiBartola et al., 1987).

Uremic stomatitis may develop in patients with severe uremia. It is characterized by oral ulcerations, brownish discoloration of the dorsal surface of the tongue, necrosis and sloughing of the anterior portion of the tongue, and fetor of breath. The oral mucous membranes may also become dry (xerostomia). These changes occur most often in patients with subacute or chronic uremia but are seen occasionally in patients with acute uremia. Poor oral hygiene may contribute to the onset and severity of uremic stomatitis.

Enterocolitis, manifested as diarrhea, occurs inconsistently in dogs and cats with uremia. It is typically less dramatic than uremic gastritis. Uremic enterocolitis may be hemorrhagic. Gastrointestinal hemorrhage may be present without initial evidence of hematemesis or hemorrhagic diarrhea. Intussusceptions are an occasional complication of uremic enterocolitis.

Urinary System

Altered urine volume is an early sign of renal failure. Polyuria is typical of patients with CRF and occurs in some patients with ARF. Compensatory polydipsia accompanies polyuria. Dehydration will

Table 1. Clinical Manifestations of Uremia

Gastrointestinal System
Uremic gastroenteritis
  Anorexia
  Vomiting
  Diarrhea
  Weight loss (C)*
Uremic stomatitis
  Uremic ulcers on gums and tongue
  Brownish discoloration of dorsal surface of the tongue
  Fetid breath
  Dry mucous membranes (xerostomia)

Urinary System
Altered urine volume
  Polyuria
  Oliguria
  Anuria (urinary obstruction)
Altered kidney size
  Small kidneys (C)
  Renomegaly
Distended urinary bladder (urinary obstruction)

Hemolymphatic System
Anemia (C)
  Pallor of mucous membranes
  Fatigue, listlessness, lethargy, weakness
  Anorexia
Hemorrhagic diathesis
  Hemorrhage from gums
  Bleeding after venipuncture
  Blood in stool or vomitus

Cardiovascular and Pulmonary Systems
Systemic hypertension
Pericarditis, pericardial effusion
Heart disease
Hyperpnea due to metabolic acidosis
Pulmonary edema due to uremic pneumonitis or overhydration
Pneumonia due to immunosuppression

Musculoskeletal System
Renal osteodystrophy (C)
  Decalcification of the mandible—"rubber jaw" and loose teeth
  Skeletal resorption and proliferative fibrosis of the maxilla
  Pathologic fractures, particularly of the mandible
Soft tissue calcifications (C)
Hypokalemic myopathy

Integumentary System
Reduced skin pliability due to dehydration
Increased shedding of hair (C)
Unkempt appearance to hair coat (C)
Loss of normal sheen to hair (C)
Impaired wound healing

Nervous System and Eyes
Uremic encephalopathy and neuropathy
  Dullness
  Drowsiness
  Lethargy
  Tremors
  Tetany
  Gait imbalance
  Myoclonus
  Seizures
  Stupor
  Coma
Scleral and conjunctival injection
Hypertensive retinopathy
  Retinal hemorrhages
  Dilated, tortuous retinal vessels
  Hyphema
  Retinal detachment

*(C), primarily occurs with chronic renal failure.

Table 2. Laboratory Findings in Uremia

Urinary System Abnormalities
Urinalysis
  Urine specific gravity and osmolality inappropriately low
  Mild proteinuria
  Variable urine sediment depending on cause of renal injury; urine sediment most often inactive, but casts, hematuria, pyuria, bacteriuria, or crystalluria occasionally observed
Renal Function Tests
  Elevated serum urea nitrogen and creatinine concentrations
  Inulin and creatinine clearances reduced
  Urine-concentrating ability markedly reduced*
  24-hr urine protein excretion mildly to moderately increased

Electrolyte and Acid-Base Disorders
Sodium
  Hypernatremia
  Hyponatremia
Potassium
  Hypokalemia
  Hyperkalemia
Hyperchloremic or high anion gap metabolic acidosis
Calcium
  Hypocalcemia
  Hypercalcemia
Hyperphosphatemia
Hypermagnesemia

Hematologic Disorders
Anemia
Immunosuppression
Hemorrhagic diathesis

Endocrine Disorders
Increased activities
  Insulin (azotemic pseudodiabetes)
  Parathyroid hormone (renal secondary hyperparathyroidism)
  Glucagon
  Gastrin
Decreased activities
  Erythropoietin
  Triiodothyronine
  Testosterone

Serum Enzyme Activities
Hyperamylasemia
Hyperlipasemia
Elevated serum alkaline phosphatase activity

*Do not perform water deprivation studies on azotemic patients.

occur if fluid consumption fails to compensate for polyuria. Oliguria may be observed with ARF or end-stage CRF. Prerenal factors such as dehydration may cause reversible (physiologic) oliguria to develop in some uremic patients. Administration of adequate quantities of fluids rapidly corrects this physiologic oliguria. Anuria (absence of urine production) suggests urinary obstruction.

Abdominal palpation may reveal small, irregularly shaped kidneys in patients with CRF. However, kidney size may be normal or even increased. In a recent study of feline chronic renal disease, kidney size based on palpation alone was found to be increased in 17 of 68 cats and decreased in 17 of 68 cats (DiBartola et al., 1987). Reduced kidney size typically reflects loss of nephrons and their subsequent replacement with connective tissue. Kidney size may be increased in patients with CRF due to polycystic kidney disease, chronic urinary obstruction, or renal neoplasia. Kidney size is typically normal or increased in patients with ARF; decreased kidney size is unexpected in the absence of pre-existing chronic renal disease.

Abdominal palpation may reveal a grossly distended urinary bladder in dogs and cats that are uremic as a result of lower urinary tract obstruction. Such patients usually have a history of dysuria and/or pollakiuria, suggesting lower urinary tract involvement.

Hemolymphatic System

Nonregenerative anemia is common in patients with CRF. However, onset and severity of anemia do not always correlate well with the degree of renal insufficiency. Anemia may also occur in patients with ARF but is uncommon. Clinical signs of anemia include pallor of the mucous membranes, fatigue, listlessness, lethargy, weakness, and anorexia. That these clinical signs result from anemia is supported by the observation that they improve following transfusion of whole blood or packed red blood cells.

A hemorrhagic diathesis is also characteristic of uremia. It may appear as bleeding from the gums, hemorrhage associated with venipuncture, or gastrointestinal bleeding.

Cardiovascular and Pulmonary Systems

Systemic hypertension is a relatively common complicating factor in dogs with CRF (Cowgill and Kallet, 1983). It tends to be mild in most dogs with CRF but may be more severe in dogs with primary glomerular diseases. Hypertension also occurs in some dogs with ARF. The incidence and severity of hypertension in uremic cats are less well known. Hypertension may be easily overlooked because it is often clinically silent and inconvenient to measure. Hypertensive retinopathy (see below) may provide clinical evidence of systemic hypertension in some patients.

Uremic pericarditis and secondary cardiac disease are rare in uremic dogs and cats. Pericarditis may be characterized by pericardial friction rub, fever, and signs of cardiac tamponade. Cardiac disorders associated with uremia may include tachycardia, cardiac arrhythmias, calcific valvular disease, and left ventricular hypertrophy with consequent heart failure (Brenner et al., 1987; Bovee, 1984; Osborne et al., 1980). Cardiac rhythm disturbances may

result in part from electrolyte imbalances (e.g., hyperkalemia) or uremic cardiomyopathy.

Patients with severe uremia may develop an increased respiratory rate to compensate for anemia, metabolic acidosis, or, uncommonly, pulmonary edema or pneumonia. Pulmonary edema may result from overhydration or, in rare instances, from uremic pneumonitis. Pneumonia occasionally develops in dogs and cats with advanced uremia (Polzin et al., 1984). It may result from uremia-associated immunocompromise or aspiration of vomitus.

Musculoskeletal System

Renal osteodystrophy is unique to CRF. Skeletal lesions do not occur in patients with ARF. Clinically significant renal osteodystrophy occurs most often in immature patients with CRF, presumably because metabolically active, growing bone is more susceptible to the adverse metabolic effects of renal failure (Polzin et al., 1989). For an unexplained reason, bones of the skull are most severely affected and may become so demineralized that the teeth become movable and the jaw can be bent or twisted without fracturing (so-called rubber jaw syndrome). Marked proliferation of connective tissue associated with the maxilla may cause distortion of the face. Pathologic fractures are uncommon in uremic dogs and cats. When they occur, they commonly affect the mandible and seriously impair the animal's ability to eat. Other uncommon clinical manifestations of severe renal osteodystrophy include skeletal decalcification, cystic bone lesions, bone pain, and growth retardation (Finco et al., 1975).

Soft tissue calcification is common in dogs and cats with chronic uremia. Calcification most commonly affects the lungs, kidneys, arteries, stomach, and myocardium.

Hypokalemic polymyopathy has been observed in cats in association with an apparent potassium-losing nephropathy (Dow et al., 1987a,b). Hypokalemia may occur with ARF or CRF. The cardinal sign of hypokalemia, regardless of cause, is generalized muscle weakness. Cats with hypokalemia have been observed to have profound cervical ventroflexion and difficulty ambulating. The author has observed generalized flaccid muscle weakness and mild cardiac rhythm disturbances in hypokalemic uremic dogs. In one dog, muscle weakness was severe enough to cause respiratory failure and death.

Integumentary System

Dehydration is a common finding in patients with uremia and is typically manifested clinically by varying degrees of loss of skin pliability. Hair coats of patients with CRF are typically characterized by increased shedding, an unkempt appearance, and loss of normal sheen. In contrast, patients with acute uremia initially may have healthy-appearing hair coats.

Uremic frost, a crystalline, white material that may accumulate on the skin of uremic human beings, does not occur in uremic dogs and cats.

Nervous System and Eyes

Clinical signs of nervous system dysfunction in uremic dogs and cats may include dullness, drowsiness, lethargy, tremors, gait imbalance, myoclonus, seizures, stupor, and coma (Bovee, 1984). In patients with advanced CRF, these signs may be episodic and vary from day to day. A progressive decline in alertness and awareness typically occurs early in uremia. Patients initially appear depressed, fatigued, and apathetic. In severe, rapidly progressive uremia, these signs may advance to stupor, coma, and seizures. Tremors, myoclonus, and tetany may occur with any form of severe uremia.

Scleral and conjunctival injection are common ocular manifestations of advanced uremia. Hypertensive retinopathy, characterized by dilated, tortuous retinal vessels, retinal hemorrhages, hyphema, and retinal detachments, may develop in patients with renal failure.

LABORATORY FINDINGS IN UREMIA

Urinary System Abnormalities

Typical urinalysis findings for dogs and cats with CRF include inappropriately low urine specific gravity, mild proteinuria, and inactive urine sediment. Pyuria and bacteriuria are relatively uncommon. When present, they may indicate pyelonephritis or secondary urinary tract infection. Other abnormalities in the urinalysis may suggest active urinary tract disease or ARF. For example, hematuria may suggest urolithiasis, neoplasia, infection, or cystic disease. Urinary casts, red blood cells, leukocytes, renal tubular epithelial cells, glucosuria (with normoglycemia), and inappropriately alkaline urine may suggest ARF due to acute tubular necrosis. Urinalysis findings may also provide clues to the cause of renal injury (e.g., glucosuria and alkaline urine pH may suggest proximal tubular disease due to Fanconi's syndrome or acute tubular necrosis) or indicate systemic disease (e.g., glucosuria and ketonuria suggest diabetic ketoacidosis). When uremia results from urinary obstruction, urinalysis may reveal crystalluria, hematuria, or pyuria.

Serum urea nitrogen and creatinine concentrations are consistently increased and creatinine clearance is consistently decreased in uremic patients. Although severity of clinical signs of uremia crudely relates to the magnitude of increase of serum urea nitrogen concentration, renal function tests may not correlate well with clinical signs of uremia. The rate of decrease in renal function and increase in serum urea nitrogen concentration greatly influences the severity of clinical signs of uremia. The more rapid the change, the more profound is the clinical effect. Thus, at similar levels of azotemia, ARF typically results in more severe clinical signs of uremia than CRF.

Electrolyte and Acid-Base Disorders

Because sodium regulatory capacity is retained until advanced stages of renal failure, serum sodium concentrations typically remain normal in patients with uremia. However, hypernatremia or hyponatremia may occur if an imbalance between body water and sodium occurs. Such abnormalities are found most often in oliguric patients or following inappropriate fluid therapy.

Hyperkalemia is uncommon in dogs and cats with polyuric renal failure but is a common finding in patients with oliguric renal failure. In the absence of exogenous sources of potassium, hyperkalemia may result from release of potassium from tissues. It is typically more severe in patients with hypercatabolism caused by trauma, surgery, or sepsis.

Hypokalemia occasionally develops in uremic dogs and cats. Although the precise mechanism has not been determined, it appears to result when urinary loss exceeds dietary intake of potassium. Hypokalemia may result in hypokalemic polymyopathy (see above).

Hyperchloremic or high–anion gap metabolic acidosis commonly occurs in uremic patients. However, it is not a consistent finding, and its occurrence cannot be predicted from the severity of renal dysfunction or urine pH. Mixed acid-base disturbances may occur in patients with pulmonary disease or profuse vomiting.

Serum calcium concentrations are often normal but may be increased or decreased in uremic patients. Interpretation of serum calcium concentration requires knowledge of serum albumin concentration because approximately half of serum calcium is bound to albumin. Thus, hypoalbuminemia may result in hypocalcemia owing to a reduced quantity of albumin-bound calcium. Such hypocalcemia is not clinically significant because plasma ionized calcium concentration remains normal.

Hypercalcemia presents a diagnostic dilemma because hypercalcemia may be the cause or result of renal failure. Because hypercalcemia-induced renal failure may be reversible, it is important to pursue the cause of hypercalcemia to identify patients with calcium-induced renal failure. Hypercalcemia occurring as a result of CRF may not indicate a significant increase in plasma ionized calcium concentration. In two dogs with CRF in which total serum calcium concentrations exceeded 13.5 mg/dl, blood ionized calcium concentrations were within normal limits.

Hyperphosphatemia and hypermagnesemia are common in uremic dogs and cats. Serum phosphate concentrations often roughly parallel serum urea nitrogen concentrations, but marked exceptions occur. Serum magnesium concentrations are usually only mildly to moderately elevated.

Hematologic Disorders

Anemia is common in patients with CRF and is an occasional finding in patients with ARF. It is characterized as a normocytic, normochromic, hypoproliferative anemia. Packed cell volumes are commonly in the range of 15 to 30 volume %. With more severe uremia, the anemia may become progressively worse, and values of 10 ml/100 ml or lower may occur.

Leukocyte numbers are typically normal in renal failure, but uremia may adversely affect leukocyte kinetics and function, leading to enhanced susceptibility to infection. Lymphocyte activity, as measured by lymphocyte stimulation studies, may also be impaired in uremia. However, plasma immunoglobulin concentrations are typically normal.

Uremia is characterized by a defect in platelet function that promotes hemorrhage. Dilute clot retraction values may be reduced. Platelet numbers are usually normal, but mild thrombocytopenia is an occasional finding.

Endocrine Disorders

Uremia results in a variety of endocrine disorders, including increases in plasma parathyroid hormone (renal secondary hyperparathyroidism), insulin (azotemic pseudodiabetes), glucagon, and gastrin activities. Plasma glucose concentrations may be mildly increased owing to insulin resistance characteristic of azotemic pseudodiabetes. Plasma testosterone, erythropoietin, and triiodothyronine activities may be reduced.

Serum Enzyme Activities

Serum amylase and lipase activities are increased in a substantial percentage of patients with CRF. In dogs with CRF, serum amylase activity report-edly increases approximately 2.5-fold over normal values, whereas serum lipase activity increases two- to fourfold. Marked increases in serum amylase or lipase activities rarely develop solely as a result of renal failure. It appears likely that hyperamylasemia and hyperlipasemia of CRF results, at least in part, from reduced renal excretion or degradation of these enzymes. However, the magnitude of enzyme elevation does not appear to correlate well with the severity of renal dysfunction.

Acute pancreatitis occurs in some human patients with CRF, but the incidence of acute pancreatitis in dogs with CRF is unknown. It has been hypothesized that renal failure may promote or induce development of uremic pancreatitis, but evidence supporting this hypothesis is lacking in dogs and cats. Nonetheless, marked elevations in serum amylase and lipase activity should prompt consideration of acute pancreatitis in dogs with CRF. Because of the questionable value of serum pancreatic enzyme activities in patients with CRF, confirmation of acute pancreatitis should be supported by clinical, radiographic, and other laboratory findings.

Serum alkaline phosphatase activity may be increased in patients with severe renal osteodystrophy, particularly young animals, but typically remains within normal limits. Serum alanine aminotransferase (S-ALT), aspartate aminotransferase (S-AST), and creatinine phosphokinase (CPK) activities are usually normal in uremic patients.

References and Supplemental Reading

Bovee, K. C.: Metabolic disturbances of uremia. *In* Bovee, K. C. (ed.): *Canine Nephrology*. Philadelphia: Harwal, 1984, pp. 555–612.

Brenner, B. M., Coe, F. L., and Rector, F. C., Jr.: Systemic consequences of chronic renal failure. *In* Brenner, B. M., Coe, F. L., and Rector, F. C., Jr.: *Clinical Nephrology*. Philadelphia: W. B. Saunders, 1987, pp. 278–292.

Cowgill, L. D., and Kallet, A. J.: Recognition and management of hypertension in the dog. *In* Kirk, R. W. (ed.): *Current Veterinary Therapy VIII*. Philadelphia: W. B. Saunders, 1983, pp. 1025–1028.

DiBartola, S. P., Rutgers, H. C., Zack, P. M., et al.: Clinicopathologic findings associated with chronic renal disease in cats: 74 cases (1973–1984). J.A.V.M.A. 190:1196, 1987.

Dow, S. W., LeCouteur, R. A., Fettman, M. J., et al.: Potassium depletion in cats: Hypokalemic polymyopathy. J.A.V.M.A. 191:1563, 1987a.

Dow, S. W., Fettman, M. J., LeCouteur, R. A., et al.: Potassium depletion in cats: Renal and dietary influences. J.A.V.M.A. 191:1569, 1987b.

Finco, D. R., Osborne, C. A., and Low, D. G.: Physiology and pathophysiology of renal failure. *In* Ettinger, S. J. (ed.): *Textbook of Veterinary Internal Medicine*. Philadelphia: W. B. Saunders, 1975, pp. 1453–1534.

Osborne, C. A., Stevens, J. B., and Polzin, D. J.: Gastrointestinal manifestations of urinary diseases. *In* Anderson, N. V. (ed.): *Veterinary Gastroenterology*. Philadelphia: Lea & Febiger, 1980, pp. 681–704.

Polzin, D. J., Osborne, C. A., Hayden, D. W., et al.: Influence of reduced protein diets on morbidity, mortality, and renal function in dogs with induced chronic renal failure. Am. J. Vet. Res. 45:506, 1984.

Polzin, D. J., Osborne, C. A., and O'Brien, T. D.: Diseases of the kidneys and ureters. *In* Ettinger, S. J. (ed.): *Textbook of Veterinary Internal Medicine*, 3rd ed. Philadelphia: W. B. Saunders, 1989 (in press).

DIAGNOSTIC APPROACH TO PROTEINURIA

JERRY V. WHITE, D.V.M.

Athens, Georgia

GENERAL CONSIDERATIONS

Normal protein excretion values less than 400 mg/day or 30 mg/kg/day have been established for the dog using the trichloroacetic acid–ponceau S method of urinary protein quantitation. Similar values have recently been determined for cats using Coomassie brilliant blue (Russo, 1986). Under normal conditions, low-molecular-weight ($< 10,000$) serum proteins are freely filtered by the renal glomerulus. As serum protein molecular weight increases to that of albumin (approximately 70,000), progressively smaller amounts are filtered owing to size and charge exclusion by the glomerular filtration barrier. Most filtered proteins are resorbed from the glomerular ultrafiltrate and metabolized within the proximal nephron. Proteins that escape total resorption (predominantly albumin) or are secreted by more distal tubule segments (such as Tamm-Horsfall glycoprotein) compose the measurable values in normal urine.

Urinary protein values consistently above normal indicate that at least one of the following pathologic processes is present:

1. Prerenal proteinuria: excessive serum protein, small enough to cross the normal glomerular filter, overwhelms the tubular protein resorptive capability.

2. Renal proteinuria: Selective permeability of the glomerular filter is altered, allowing greater quantities or larger-molecular-weight proteins to enter the glomerular ultrafiltrate; tubular resorptive function is altered, allowing greater quantities of protein to escape into the urine; or renal parenchymal inflammation causes exudation of protein into the tubular lumen.

3. Postrenal proteinuria: inflammation of the lower urinary tract or genital organs allows protein exudation, elevating the normal urine protein content.

The combined presence of several pathologic processes, operating in an additive fashion, often complicates the differential diagnosis and therapy of abnormal proteinuria. Although rarely observed, nonpathologic or functional proteinuria may also occur in dogs during strenuous exercise or with fever. In people, functional proteinuria has also been associated with congestive heart failure and exposure to extreme heat or cold. This proteinuria tends to be mild and transient in nature.

DIAGNOSTIC OBJECTIVES

During management of a suspected proteinuric patient, the clinician's first objective should be to document the consistent presence of an abnormally high urine protein content. Several cleanly collected urine samples should be used. Measurement of protein derived from the genital tract can be avoided by use of samples collected by cystocentesis. Multiple qualitative assays have been developed for urinary protein assessment; however, none are ideal. Tetrabromophenol-impregnated colorimetric reagent strips have become the most commonly used screening method for urine protein. Unfortunately, this dipstick is insensitive to several pathologic urine proteins and is potentially overreactive in the presence of alkaline urine and certain antiseptics. Turbidometric and sulfosalicylic acid screening tests for urinary protein may also give false-positive or false-negative results. Because of these shortcomings, determination of the protein-creatinine ratio (U-P/C) in single urine samples is a more reliable (but time consuming) screening technique for abnormal proteinuria (White et al., 1984; Grauer et al., 1985). Its accuracy depends on the use of a quantitative protein assay (such as the trichloroacetic acid–ponceau S method), which has equal sensitivity for albumin and globulin, and a creatinine assay, which avoids noncreatinine chromogen measurement. A protein-creatinine ratio greater than 1 in serial canine urine samples is indicative of abnormal proteinuria. Determination of this ratio can be used to confirm the results of the previously mentioned qualitative screening methods.

Formulation of a differential diagnosis and investigative plan are the second and third major objectives during management of a confirmed proteinuria. Common conditions that should be considered are listed in Table 1. Postrenal and renal causes of proteinuria are more commonly diagnosed than prerenal causes; however, all origins of potential pathologic changes should be initially considered to prevent formulation of an incomplete or inaccurate diagnosis. An accurate differential diagnosis of proteinuria requires thorough knowledge of the patient's history, physical examination findings, complete blood count (CBC), blood chemistries, urine chemistries, and urinalysis results.

A past medical history of renal disease, edema, hematuria, urinary tract infection, or exposure to

1139

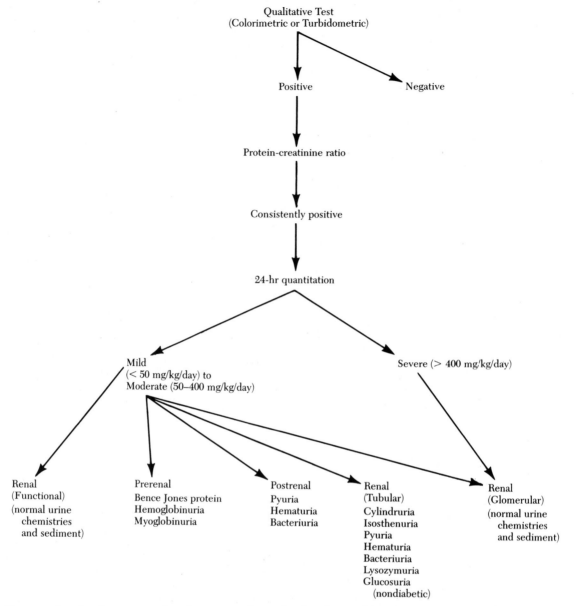

Figure 1. Algorithm for proteinuria based on urine analyses. This algorithm, established with potential results of urine analyses, should be used in conjunction with patient history, physical examination findings, and other laboratory analyses to formulate an appropriate differential diagnosis of the cause of proteinuria.

nephrotoxic drugs and chemicals may be helpful in delineating the underlying cause of proteinuria. The family history of animals from breeds hereditarily predisposed to congenital renal disease should also be investigated. Physical examination may reveal the presence of immune-mediated disease, neoplasia, edema, muscle trauma or weakness, or urinary tract discomfort.

Blood chemistry results and the CBC may be helpful in the identification of prerenal and renal causes of proteinuria. Evidence of hemolysis or leukemia in the CBC warrants investigation of the urine for the presence of hemoglobin or Bence

Jones proteins, respectively. A decreased serum albumin-globulin ratio coupled with hyperglobulinemia is suggestive of multiple myeloma and other causes of macroglobulinemia. Urinary light-chain immunoglobulins (Bence Jones protein) associated with these conditions may be detected by heat precipitation or urine electrophoresis. Glomerular proteinuria due to diabetes mellitus should be considered in the presence of hyperglycemia and ketonemia. Hyperphosphatemia often accompanies severe renal failure, whereas hyperchloremia and hypobicarbonemia may be associated with a renal tubular disorder such as Fanconi's syndrome or

Table 1. *Differential Diagnosis of Proteinuria*

Prerenal
- Hemolytic crisis
- Rhabdomyolysis
- Neoplasia (multiple myeloma, leukemia)

Renal

Glomerular
- Glomerulonephritis
- Amyloidosis
- Glomerular atrophy

Tubular
- Acute renal failure
- Chronic renal failure
- Pyelonephritis
- Renal tubular acidosis
- Fanconi's syndrome

Postrenal
- Lower urinary tract inflammation
- Lower urinary tract infection
- Genital tract inflammation
- Genital tract infection

Functional
- Strenuous exercise
- Pyrexia
- Hypothermia
- Renal passive congestion

renal tubular acidosis. Renal failure indicated by marginal serum creatinine or urea nitrogen elevation or poor urine concentrating ability should be investigated by determination of glomerular filtration rate (Finco et al., 1981).

Urine chemistry and urinalysis results frequently serve as a major aid in the differentiation of renal and postrenal proteinuria. Persistent isosthenuria and granular or cellular casts in urinary sediment may indicate the presence of significant renal disease. Identification of nondiabetic glucosuria or lysozymuria may help to pinpoint abnormal tubular function as the cause of the proteinuria (Biewenga, 1986). The presence of hematuria, pyuria, or bacteriuria does not rule out renal disease; however, these findings are more commonly associated with a postrenal proteinuria.

Unless there is evidence of a pre- or postrenal cause of proteinuria, it becomes diagnostically and therapeutically important to quantitate daily urinary protein loss. Knowledge of this excretory value will help develop a differential diagnosis and aid in future therapeutic assessment. A high correlation ($r^2 = 0.95$) has been established between the U-P/C of single urine samples and the 24-hr excretion of urinary protein. As this ratio increases above the value of 1, its predictive ability becomes progressively less accurate. Therefore, this ratio should be used only as an estimate of daily protein excretion. Accurate determination of daily urinary protein excretion requires measurement of protein in an aliquot of urine collected over a 24-hr period (DiBartola et al., 1980). As indicated in Figure 1, categorization of this value as mild, moderate, or severe proteinuria may be used in conjunction with

laboratory findings to pursue a differential diagnosis. The categories assigned to these values should be interpreted liberally, as they are drawn solely from the author's clinical experience and a limited number of published reports.

Depending on the severity of the condition, most pre- and postrenal proteinurias are associated with a mild (< 50 mg/kg/day) to moderate (50 to 400 mg/kg/day) elevation of urinary protein level. Functional proteinuria is almost always mild and transient, whereas renal proteinuria of tubular origin tends to be moderate but may be mild in the initial stages of cellular damage. Significant glomerular disease rarely causes a mild proteinuria, but this may occur when glomerular filtration rate becomes greatly reduced. Glomerular lesions associated with amyloidosis and membranous glomerulonephritis frequently cause severe (> 400 mg/kg/day) proteinuria. Proteinuric patients often have more than one pathologic process contributing to their urinary protein content. Thus, the categories listed in Figure 1 should not be considered exclusive. For instance, multiple myeloma patients may have both hyperglobulinemia (prerenal proteinuria) and parenchymal renal disease (renal proteinuria), resulting in a severe proteinuria that is not caused by severe glomerular damage.

ADDITIONAL PROCEDURES

A few causes of proteinuria may be particularly difficult to differentiate. Renal proteinurias of either glomerular or tubular origin may occur without significant changes in routine blood chemistries, urine chemistries, or urine sediment composition. Electrophoresis of human urine to determine relative fractions of albumin and alpha-, beta-, and gamma-globulin has been applied to aid in this differentiation. The number of study results available is inadequate to determine the validity of this approach for canine or feline proteinuric patients. Measurement of urinary lysozyme concentration may provide evidence of tubular protein-resorptive dysfunction; however, this test is not routinely available to the private practitioner. Therefore, in the absence of clinical data to support a differential diagnosis of tubular versus glomerular proteinuria, histologic examination of a renal biopsy specimen may be required. The chemical triad often associated with the nephrotic syndrome (proteinuria, hypoalbuminuria, and hypercholesterolemia) is strongly suggestive of glomerular damage. Unfortunately, the amount or type of urinary protein excreted does not reliably predict the amount or type of glomerular damage present (Biewenga, 1986). A renal biopsy should provide both prognostic and diagnostic insight.

References and Supplemental Reading

Biewenga, W. J.: Proteinuria in the dog: A clinicopathological study in 51 proteinuric dogs. Res. Vet. Sci. 41:257, 1986.

DiBartola, S. P., Chew, D. J., and Jacobs, G.: Quantitative urinalysis including 24-hour protein excretion in the dog. J. Am. Anim. Hosp. Assoc. 16:537, 1980.

Finco, D. R., Coulter, D. B., and Barsanti, J. A.: Simple, accurate method for clinical estimation of glomerular filtration rate in the dog. Am. J. Vet. Res. 42:1874, 1981.

Grauer, G. F., Thomas, C. B., and Eicker, S. W.: Estimation of quantitative proteinuria in the dog, using the protein-to-creatinine ratio from a random, voided sample. Am. J. Vet. Res. 46:2116, 1985.

Russo, E. A., Lees, G. E., and Hightower, D.: Evaluation of renal function in cats using quantitative urinalysis. Am. J. Vet. Res. 47:1308, 1986.

White, J. V., Olivier, N. B., Reimann, K., et al.: Use of protein-to-creatinine ratio in a single urine specimen for quantitative estimation of canine proteinuria. J.A.V.M.A. 185:882, 1984.

POSITIVE-CONTRAST VAGINOURETHROGRAPHY FOR DIAGNOSIS OF LOWER URINARY TRACT DISEASE

PETER E. HOLT, B.V.M.S.

Bristol, Great Britain

Even though retrograde vaginourethrography was recommended by Osborne and associates (1972) as an aid to the investigation of cases of ureteral ectopia, its use in small animal veterinary practice has remained limited. It is pertinent therefore to examine the technique in more detail.

INDICATIONS

Positive-contrast vaginourethrography has been particularly valuable in the investigation of animals with urinary incontinence, dysuria, vaginal discharge, and physical vaginal abnormalities (Holt et al., 1982, 1984). The need for urethral catheterization is avoided, and so the entire urethral length can be demonstrated without the obscuration and distortion of the urethra by a catheter. It is particularly useful in those cases in which urethral catheterization is impossible or hazardous (e.g., urethral neoplasia or severe urethritis). By far the most frequent indication (Holt, 1985a) is to assess urethral length and bladder neck position in cases of incontinence due to sphincter mechanism incompetence (Holt, 1985b) to select those suitable for treatment by colposuspension (Holt, 1985c). Retrograde vaginourethrography can be employed in the dog or cat, but, because there are more indications for investigation of the former, the following descriptions apply to the technique in the bitch.

TECHNIQUE

Preparation

Vaginourethrography is performed with the animal under general anesthesia and preferably with an empty large bowel. The latter is achieved by fasting for at least 12 hr, the use of an enema, and exercise to stimulate normal defecation. General anesthesia is induced and then, as with any radio-

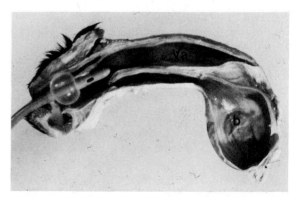

Figure 1. Sagittal section of fixed specimen of the lower urogenital tract of a bitch illustrating the position of the Foley catheter tip and inflated cuff in the vestibule. Va, vagina; u, urethra; b, bladder.

Acknowledgments: Thanks are due to Mrs. J. Latham and Mr. J. Conibear for radiographic and photographic assistance and to Dr. Christine Gibbs for her constructive comments on the manuscript.

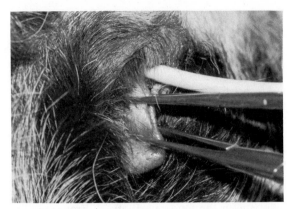

Figure 2. Closure of the vulval lips ventral to the catheter with Allis tissue forceps.

graphic contrast procedure, plain lateral and dorsoventral radiographs are obtained, centered over the area of interest (in this case the caudal abdomen and pelvis), before contrast medium is introduced. An excessively full bladder should be emptied by catheterization or centesis before vaginourethrography is attempted, to avoid the risk of rupture.

Procedure

A 12 French (F) Foley catheter is used to introduce contrast medium. Smaller catheters may be required in small dogs or cats. The examination is routinely performed with the bitch in right lateral recumbency and with the hind limbs extended. Left lateral, oblique, and dorsoventral radiographs may be required later to demonstrate ureteral ectopia (Holt et al., 1982) or vaginal abnormalities (Holt et al., 1984). Although pneumovaginography has been performed in the bitch (Adams et al., 1978; Holt and Sayle, 1981), positive contrast media give the best results. Low-concentration, iodine-based, water-soluble compounds (e.g., Urografin 150, Schering) are most suitable. As with other retrograde techniques, the catheter should be filled with contrast medium before insertion, to prevent the introduction of air bubbles, which may be misinterpreted as significant filling defects in radiographs of the lower urogenital tract.

The catheter tip is inserted into the vestibule, and the cuff is inflated to prevent leakage of contrast medium from the vagina (Fig. 1). The volume of air required to inflate the cuff adequately varies from 3 to 5 ml (in bitches of less than 15 kg of body weight) to 8 ml (in larger bitches). To avoid occlusion of the external urethral orifice by the inflated cuff, the catheter tip should not be passed too far into the vagina. The vulval lips are closed with Allis tissue forceps to prevent the catheter tip from leaving the vestibule (Fig. 2). Contrast medium is introduced through the Foley catheter until the vagina is filled and the medium enters the urethra.

The volume required varies with the size of the bitch (Fig. 3) and can be assessed directly under fluoroscopic observation. If such facilities are not available, the volume required (contrast medium plus catheter cuff air) to fill the vagina until medium enters the urethra is approximately 1 ml/kg of body weight (Holt et al., 1984) (Fig. 3). This volume tends to be slightly lower in spayed than in intact animals and is much higher in bitches under the influence of endogenous or exogenous sex hormones such as estrogens (Fig. 3). To ensure adequate filling and overflow into the bladder, a dosage of 1.5 ml/kg of body weight is recommended, provided the urethra is patent so that there is no risk of overfilling the vagina. A radiograph is taken during injection of the last quarter of the calculated volume to ensure that the urethra is adequately outlined. If there is any resistance to introduction of contrast medium, injection should be stopped and a radiograph should be obtained to investigate the cause of obstruction.

Further radiographs in different positions may be required to demonstrate retrograde filling of ectopic ureters or adjacent lesions; additional boluses of 5

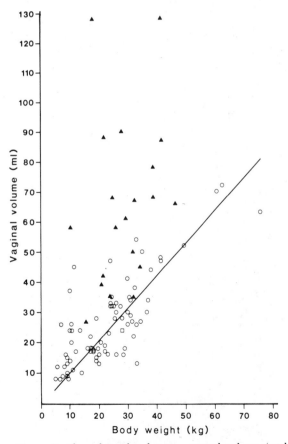

Figure 3. The relationship between vaginal volume (total volume of Foley cuff air and vaginal contrast medium) and body weight in 100 bitches. The line of best fit by regression is shown, excluding 20 bitches under the influence of endogenous or exogenous sex hormones (closed triangles).

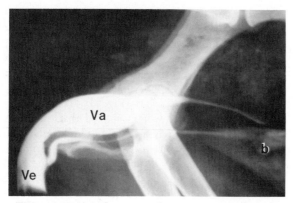

Figure 4. A normal vaginourethrogram. Ve, vestibule; Va, vagina; b, bladder. (With permission from Holt, P., Gibbs, C., and Latham, J. J. Small Anim. Pract. 25:531, 1984.)

to 10 ml of contrast medium are injected during each exposure.

INTERPRETATION

A normal vaginourethrogram is illustrated in Figure 4. The mucosal and urothelial linings of the vagina and urethra are normally smooth. The vagina narrows slightly at its junction with the vestibule and tapers cranially, often with a dorsal filling defect, which represents the dorsal midline fold of the paracervix. Unless the bitch is intact and in estrus, the cervix is not usually patent and contrast medium does not enter the uterus. The urethra is usually seen to be widest at its caudal third, and sometimes longitudinal striations (urethral folds) can be seen.

As far as lower urinary tract disease is concerned, erosions of the urethral mucosa are clearly demonstrated (Fig. 5) and indicate neoplasia (usually carcinoma) or urethritis. Gross spillage of contrast medium is seen in cases of urethral or vaginal rupture. Luminal filling defects such as tumors or calculi, which may prevent insertion of a urethral

catheter, are also outlined. Abnormal communications between lower urogenital tract organs can be shown. These include congenital ectopic ureters opening into the urethra or vagina and acquired uretero- or vesicovaginal fistulas (Fig. 6). If vaginourethrography is performed shortly after intravenous urography, retrograde ureteral filling (e.g., in cases of ureteral ectopia) should not be confused with that arising from intravenous contrast medium excreted through the kidneys. For this reason, vaginourethrography and intravenous urography are ideally done on separate occasions, although it is often more convenient to perform them consecutively under the same anesthetic. Retrograde filling usually results in denser ureteral delineation than intravenous urography.

Vaginal filling defects that may be demonstrated include tumors and congenital septa or vestibulovaginal strictures; these may prevent insertion of a digit or endoscope for examination.

Urethral length and bladder neck position can be assessed and, if necessary, measured directly from the radiographs; an intrapelvic bladder neck in incontinent bitches may be associated with sphincter mechanism incompetence (Holt, 1985b). However, the vaginourethrograms of bitches with excessively large vaginal volumes (e.g., those under the influence of sex hormones) or with large amounts of feces in the rectum should not be used for the assessment of urethral length or bladder neck position. In such cases, the excessive distention of the pelvic viscera results in abnormal cranial displacement of the bladder neck.

COMPLICATIONS

Because contrast medium is being introduced into a closed system, there is a risk that overfilling could cause rupture of lower urogenital tract organs. This risk can be minimized by observing the precautions mentioned above.

Like all retrograde techniques, vaginourethrography has the potential for introducing organisms

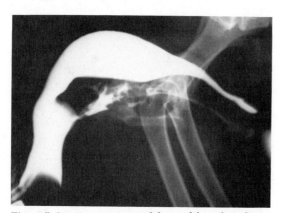

Figure 5. Invasive carcinoma of the caudal urethra of a Cairn terrier. Even if insertion of a catheter into the urethra had been possible, the catheter tip would have obscured part of the lesion during urethrography.

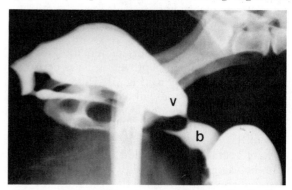

Figure 6. Vaginourethrogram of an incontinent Cavalier King Charles spaniel. Following ovariohysterectomy, a fistula had developed between the caudal bladder (b) and cranial vagina (v) and is clearly demonstrated.

from the vagina or urethra into the bladder or ureter (if ectopic), and sterile instruments and aseptic technique are essential. However, even though prophylactic antimicrobial therapy is not used by the author, vaginourethrography has resulted in no infection in nearly 500 bitches in which it has been employed as a diagnostic aid. It can be confidently recommended as a safe and reliable investigative procedure in animals with possible lower urogenital tract disorders.

References and Supplemental Reading

Adams, W. M., Biery, D. N., and Millar, H. C.: Pneumovaginography in the dog: A case report. J. Am. Vet. Radiol. Soc. 19:80, 1978.

Holt, P. E.: Urinary incontinence in the bitch due to sphincter mechanism incompetence: Prevalence in referred dogs and retrospective analysis of sixty cases. J. Small Anim. Pract. 26:181, 1985a.

Holt, P. E.: Importance of urethral length, bladder neck position and vestibulovaginal stenosis in sphincter mechanism incompetence in the incontinent bitch. Res. Vet. Sci. 39:364, 1985b.

Holt, P. E.: Urinary incontinence in the bitch due to sphincter mechanism incompetence: Surgical treatment. J. Small Anim. Pract. 26:237, 1985c.

Holt, P. E., and Sayle, B.: Congenital vestibulo-vaginal stenosis in the bitch. J. Small Anim. Pract. 22:67, 1981.

Holt, P. E., Gibbs, C., and Pearson, H.: Canine ectopic ureter—a review of twenty-nine cases. J. Small Anim. Pract. 23:195, 1982.

Holt, P. E., Gibbs, C., and Latham, J.: An evaluation of positive contrast vagino-urethrography as a diagnostic aid in the bitch. J. Small Anim. Pract. 25:531, 1984.

Osborne, C. A., Low, D. G., and Finco, D. R.: *Canine and Feline Urology*. Philadelphia: W. B. Saunders, 1972, p. 336.

USE OF URODYNAMICS IN MICTURITION DISORDERS IN DOGS AND CATS

KEITH P. RICHTER, D.V.M.

Rancho Santa Fe, California

In many cases involving abnormal urination patterns, clinical evaluation along with pertinent laboratory tests and radiographic studies yields sufficient information for appropriate management. However, in certain situations, more sophisticated evaluation of urinary bladder and urethral function is necessary. Urodynamic testing yields measurements of pressures and flow rates in the caudal portion of the urinary tract and thus provides an objective evaluation of the functional status of the bladder and urethra. In people, urodynamic testing has been used extensively to define functional disorders of the bladder and urethra and to objectively monitor their treatment. These tests are not frequently performed in veterinary medicine owing to equipment costs, limiting use to the university setting. The most common urodynamic tests performed in veterinary medicine are the urethral pressure profile (UPP) and simultaneous electromyogram (EMG), the cystometrogram (CMG), and voiding uroflowmetry. This article discusses the indications for performing these tests, equipment and techniques, normal findings, and abnormalities encountered with micturition disorders.

URETHRAL PRESSURE PROFILE

The UPP describes the pressures in the bladder neck and urethra as a catheter is moved distally

from the bladder through the entire length of the urethra. The profile represents a perfusion pressure or a minimal distention pressure and is altered by the caliber of the urethra and the compliance of its walls (which is most influenced by smooth muscle tone). This technique can be used as a clinical diagnostic aid or as a research tool to determine urethral function during the storage phase of mic-

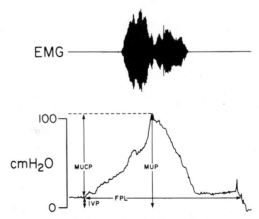

Figure 1. Urethral pressure profile and electromyogram (EMG) recorded simultaneously in a normal female dog. IVP, intravesical pressure (bladder pressure); MUP, maximal urethral pressure (maximum pressure measured); MUCP, maximal urethral closure pressure (MUP − IVP); FPL, functional profile length. (Reprinted with permission from Richter, K. P. and Ling, G. V.: J.A.V.M.A. 187:605, 1985b.)

turition and to identify sites of increased urethral resistance.

Indications for performing a UPP include evaluation of urethral sphincter function in animals with urinary incontinence, identification of the site and extent of a structural urethral obstruction, evaluation of urethral tone in suspected cases of functional urethral obstruction (reflex dyssynergia; see *Current Veterinary Therapy VIII*, p. 1088), and objective evaluation of therapy of these disorders (i.e., measurement of pressure changes following treatment). In addition, intravenous administration of drugs during pressure measurement and observation of pressure changes may allow the clinician to predict the outcome of therapy and therefore to be more selective in choosing the appropriate category of drugs. The UPP can also be combined with simultaneous surface bipolar EMG recording at the site of pressure measurement. Because the EMG records primarily striated muscle activity, it may be useful to evaluate suspected sacral spinal cord or pudendal nerve lesions.

Technique

The UPP is best performed without sedation. A urethral catheter is inserted into the bladder, and all urine is removed. The catheter is perfused with saline at a constant rate (2 ml/min with an infusion pump) and is used to record pressure. Rapid infusion is avoided to keep urethral diameter within the physiologic range and to avoid eventual bladder distention. A three-way stopcock is used to join the catheter, the infusion pump, and a pressure transducer providing input to one channel of a strip-chart recorder through an appropriate amplifier. Commercial monitors are designed for this pur-

pose,* which have additional channels for recording a simultaneous EMG, intra-abdominal pressure (via a rectal catheter), or urine flow rate. After bladder pressure is recorded, the catheter is slowly withdrawn through the entire length of the urethra with a constant speed withdrawal apparatus. If the withdrawal rate equals the paper speed of the strip-chart recorder, direct measurement of urethral length can be made. The resulting tracing plots distance along the urethra on the X axis and urethral pressure on the Y axis. A normal canine UPP and variables measured are depicted in Figures 1 and 2. The reader is referred to the references for normal values. A simultaneous bipolar EMG recording (integrated mode) can be performed at the point of pressure measurement by incorporating two parallel wires exposed at the side hole of the catheter. The wires are then attached to an appropriate integrating amplifier for EMG recording.

Abnormalities Seen in Urethral Pressure Profilometry

Because the UPP indicates the pressure of the urethra during the storage phase of micturition, urethral sphincter abnormalities can be detected by this test. Maximal urethral closure pressure represents the pressure gradient to urine flow from the bladder through the urethra. In dogs with urinary incontinence associated with urethral sphincter incompetence, there is a marked decrease in maximal urethral closure pressure with normal EMG activity (Figs. 3 and 4). These findings are attributable to decreased urethral sphincter smooth muscle tone, as resting smooth muscle tone is the most important component of the urethral sphincter closure mech-

---

*7820 Versatile Uromonitor/Flowmeter, Browne Corp., Carpinteria, CA.

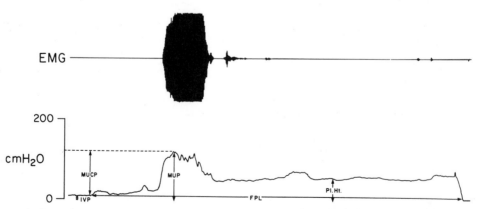

Figure 2. Urethral pressure profile and electromyogram (EMG) recorded simultaneously in a normal male dog. IVP, intravesical pressure (bladder pressure); MUP, maximal urethral pressure (maximum pressure measured); MUCP, maximal urethral closure pressure (MUP − IVP); Pl. Ht., pleateau height (estimated average pressure in penile urethra); FPL, functional profile length. (Reprinted with permission from Richter, K. P. and Ling, G. V.: J.A.V.M.A. 187:605, 1985b.)

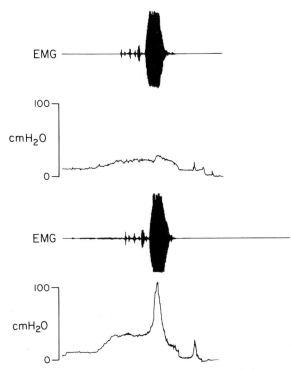

Figure 3. Combined urethral pressure profile and electromyogram (EMG) of an incontinent female dog before (upper tracings) and after (lower tracings) phenylpropanolamine administration. For each set, the EMG is above the simultaneous UPP. (Reprinted with permission from Richter, K. P. and Ling, G. V.: J.A.V.M.A. 187:605, 1985b.)

struction can be assessed by noting the magnitude of the maximal urethral closure pressure. Similarly, the extent of the lesion can be estimated by the distance along which the pressure rise occurs.

The finding of a normal UPP in an animal with inability to urinate is helpful in the diagnosis of functional urethral obstruction (reflex dyssynergia). In this syndrome, there is inability to coordinate urethral relaxation with detrusor contraction. To support the diagnosis, a cystometrogram should document a normal detrusor reflex, and contrast radiography should rule out intraluminal urethral masses. Canine UPPs have been reported in a variety of different structural and functional urethral obstructions (Rosin and Barsanti, 1981).

CYSTOMETROGRAM

The CMG is a recording of changes in intravesical pressure during filling and contraction of the urinary bladder. The recording allows evaluation of the detrusor reflex and function, bladder compliance, bladder capacity, and maximal contraction pressure. The detrusor reflex is a complex multisynaptic pathway. It is initiated from sensory endings of the pelvic nerve, which detect stretching of the bladder wall, resulting in detrusor muscle contraction. Because the detrusor reflex is a prerequisite for normal urination, the CMG allows evaluation of the efficiency of this aspect of micturition, and abnormal results suggest the nature of the problem. Indications for performing a CMG include neurologic disorders in which bladder function is uncertain, bladder wall lesions (for assessment of compliance or elasticity), cases of urinary incontinence (to determine the role of detrusor contractions in the pathogenesis of the problem), and situations in which the effectiveness of detrusor contractions is in doubt (to determine the maximal contraction pressure).

anism. Because alpha-adrenergic sympathetic tone contributes the most to smooth muscle contraction in the urethra, the clinician can rationally select an alpha-adrenergic agonist (such as phenylpropanolamine or ephedrine) as an appropriate drug. Following treatment, there is usually a marked increase in urethral pressures into the normal range associated with the return of continence. The response to therapy can then be objectively assessed by changes in the UPP.

The UPP also has a role in evaluation of animals with urinary incontinence associated with an ectopic ureter. Many of these dogs remain incontinent following surgical correction. In these cases, there is a concurrent abnormality in urethral function. Presurgical evaluation of these patients with a UPP will show decreased maximal urethral closure pressure and allow the clinician to predict which patients will remain incontinent following surgical correction of the ectopic ureter. In these cases, a presurgical trial of an alpha-adrenergic agonist, such as phenylpropanolamine, can be used to evaluate its effect on the UPP. If there is an increase in maximal urethral closure pressure into a range that will maintain continence, postsurgical management with this drug will likely be effective.

In cases of urethral obstruction caused by a structural urethral lesion, the severity of the ob-

Technique

The recording device used in cystometry is similar to that used in urethral pressure profilometry. A transurethral catheter is inserted into the urinary bladder and is used to record intravesical pressure. Alternatively, an antepubic transabdominal catheter can be inserted percutaneously into the bladder; however, this method is considerably more invasive. A carbon dioxide source with a flow control mechanism is attached to the catheter by a three-way stopcock. Commercial units for pressure recording have a built-in carbon dioxide source. Alternatively, saline infusion has been described. A pressure transducer and amplifier calibrated to read intravesical pressure are also attached to the end of

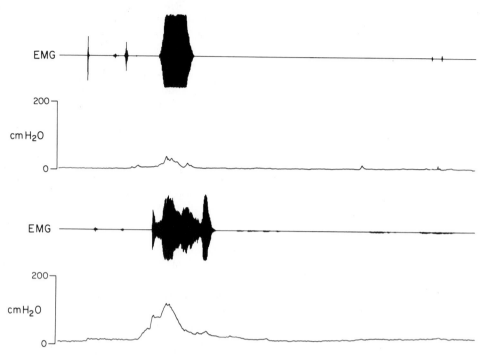

Figure 4. Combined urethral pressure profile and electromyogram (EMG) of an incontinent male dog before (upper tracings) and after (lower tracings) phenylpropanolamine administration. For each set, the EMG is above the simultaneous UPP. (Reprinted with permission from Richter, K. P. and Ling, G. V.: J.A.V.M.A. 187:605, 1985b.)

the catheter. A strip-chart recorder plots volume infused (calculated from the flow rate and paper speed) on the X axis and pressure on the Y axis. Sedation is necessary for adequate restraint and to prevent voluntary suppression of the detrusor reflex. Xylazine is the sedative of choice, yielding the most consistent recording of the detrusor reflex; oxymorphone produces slightly less satisfactory results. General anesthesia abolishes the detrusor reflex and prevents evaluation.

A normal CMG and variables measured are depicted in Figure 5. The storage or filling phase of micturition is designated as the tonus limb of the CMG, whereas the emptying (voiding) phase of micturition constitutes the detrusor reflex. The tonus limb is a record of the compliance of the bladder wall, reflecting the elastic properties of collagen, smooth muscle, and mucopolysaccharide components. Compliance indicates the change in volume for a given change in pressure. Normally, physiologic filling is not accompanied by a significant increase in intravesical pressure (< 12 to 15 cm H_2O) until a detrusor contraction occurs. A detrusor contraction occurs at threshold volume and pressure. Following this, maximal contraction pressure is reached, which is a function of the strength of the detrusor muscle and outflow (urethral) resistance. Normal values in dogs have been reported (Oliver and Young, 1973; Moreau et al., 1983a).

Abnormalities Seen in Cystometry

Abnormal CMG recordings can be seen with disorders of the storage or emptying phases of micturition. Abnormalities of the storage phase can result in changes of the tonus limb. In cases that result in decreased compliance of the bladder wall, there is an increased slope of the tonus limb and a decreased threshold volume (i.e., the threshold pressure is reached sooner). Causes include fibrosis, thickening, inflammation, or neoplastic infiltration of the bladder wall. A rapid infusion rate can give a false-positive increase in the slope of the tonus limb (especially in small bladders). Because of accommodation, a greater bladder capacity is reached with slower infusion rates before stretch receptors initiate a detrusor reflex. On the other hand, an abnormally large bladder capacity, low pressure tonus limb, and a delayed or absent detrusor reflex can be seen. Bladders in this condition are often described as hypotonic, although hypercompliant is a more appropriate description (i.e., the bladder accommodates a greater volume for a given increment in intravesical pressure). Causes include overdistention of the bladder, resulting in alterations in the elastic elements of the bladder wall.

Abnormalities in the emptying phase of urination are seen as abnormalities in the detrusor reflex. In detrusor hyporeflexia or areflexia the ability to elicit a detrusor reflex is diminished or absent owing to neurologic impairment of reflex pathways. This can result from spinal cord lesions or from peripheral neuropathies. This should be distinguished from a hypercompliant bladder as described above, although the CMG appearance is similar. Historical and physical examination findings supplement the CMG and are important for proper diagnosis and management. If a detrusor reflex is initiated, the detrusor contractility can be estimated by the maximal contraction pressure, although this is also influenced by outflow (urethral) resistance.

Detrusor hyperactivity is identified on the CMG as a low detrusor reflex threshold volume. This is characterized by an involuntary detrusor contraction during the storage phase of micturition, usually occurring at low bladder volumes, resulting in a pressure increase of greater than 15 cm H_2O. Clinical signs may include urinary incontinence, nocturia, pollakiuria, and urgency. Causes include sensory abnormalities (such as bladder tumors, infection, inflammation, and calculi) and motor abnormalities. The latter are caused by neuropathies (termed detrusor hyper-reflexia) or by urinary outflow obstruction or idiopathic causes (termed detrusor instability). The latter syndrome has recently been associated with urinary incontinence in the dog and cat (Lappin and Barsanti, 1987). Low threshold volumes are also associated with disorders that decrease bladder wall elasticity (see above). However, in these cases, an increased slope of the tonus limb will be observed, and anticholinergic or smooth muscle antispasmodic treatment will not result in clinical or CMG improvement.

UROFLOWMETRY

Uroflowmetry, the measurement of urine flow, aids in determination of urethral function during the emptying phase of micturition. Often this test is conducted with a simultaneous CMG, which is performed with an antepubic transabdominal percutaneous catheter and saline infusion. This allows determination of urine flow with relation to detrusor contraction, giving an evaluation of both the storage and emptying phases of micturition. Although this method of catheter placement does not interfere with urine flow, it is more invasive than placement of a transurethral catheter. Indications for performing uroflowmetry include abnormal voiding patterns (incontinence or disorders of urine retention) in which urethral function is in doubt or situations in which the relationship of urine flow to detrusor contraction is uncertain.

Technique

To avoid the effect of a transurethral catheter on urine flow, an antepubic transabdominal percutaneous catheter is used to infuse saline into the bladder. This catheter can be used to perform a simultaneous CMG on one channel of a strip-chart recorder as described above. To determine urine flow, urine is collected into a funnel system, which diverts the urine to a flowmeter. The flowmeter provides input to the second channel of the strip-chart recorder. Several types of flowmeters can be used. An electromagnetic transducer can be incorporated into the tubing conducting the urine to record urine flow. A rotating disk–style flowmeter, consisting of a rotating disk maintained at a constant speed, may be used. The energy required to maintain the disk at constant speed when impinged on by the stream of urine is a function of the flow rate. A load cell–style flowmeter measures the differential weight per unit time of a fluid column that urine enters. This is proportional to urine flow.

Uroflowmetry is performed under xylazine sedation to allow adequate restraint without interference with micturition. As the bladder is infused with

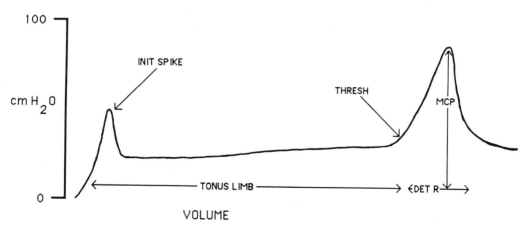

Figure 5. Cystometrogram recorded from a normal dog. Init Spike, initial spike; Thresh, threshold volume and pressure; MCP, maximum contraction pressure; Det R, Detrusor reflex.

saline, intravesical pressure and volume of saline infused are measured (via CMG). When urine flow begins, infusion is stopped. When urine flow ends, the volume infused, the volume urinated, and the residual urine volume are measured. The recording generated is a plot of urine flow versus time. Additional variables determined include mean urine flow rate, maximal instantaneous urine flow rate, flow rate at the instant of maximal intravesical pressure, duration of flow, and delay before onset of flow after detrusor contraction begins. These variables and normal values have been described in the dog (Moreau et al., 1983a).

Abnormalities Seen in Uroflowmetry

One type of abnormality seen with uroflowmetry is increased urethral resistance and decreased urine flow rates during the emptying phase of micturition. Clinically, this is characterized by urine retention, stranguria, and frequent attempts at urination. Causes include structural urethral lesions (such as a neoplastic mass, stricture, or calculus), or functional urethral obstruction (reflex dyssynergia). The latter disorder is characterized by inability to coordinate urethral relaxation with detrusor contractions. This is demonstrated urodynamically by decreased or absent urine flow during detrusor contraction and can have a pattern similar to that of structural urethral lesions (UPP findings may be helpful to distinguish these conditions). There can also be abnormal urine leakage during the storage phase of micturition with reflex dyssynergia if the bladder is overdistended. These findings correlate with the clinical abnormalities of urinary incontinence at rest (during the storage phase) and stranguria with urine retention (during the emptying phase of micturition).

Another abnormal pattern seen with uroflowmetry is decreased urethral resistance during bladder filling, seen clinically as urinary incontinence. When urethral sphincter incompetence is the cause of the incontinence, urine flow will occur prior to a detrusor contraction. To document this, a simultaneous CMG is necessary, allowing this syndrome to be distinguished from detrusor hyperactivity.

References and Supplemental Reading

Gregory, C. R., and Willits, N. H.: Electromyographic and urethral pressure evaluations: Assessment of urethral function in female and ovariohysterectomized female cats. Am. J. Vet. Res. 47:1472, 1986.

Gregory, C. R., Holliday, T. A., Vasseur, P. B., et al.: Electromyographic and urethral pressure profilometry: Assessment of urethral function before and after perineal urethrostomy in cats. Am. J. Vet. Res. 45:2062, 1984.

Lappin, M. R., and Barsanti, J. A.: Urinary incontinence secondary to idiopathic detrusor instability: Cystometrographic diagnosis and pharmacologic management in two dogs and a cat. J.A.V.M.A. 191:1439, 1987.

Moreau, P. M., Lees, G. E., and Gross, D. R.: Simultaneous cystometry and uroflowmetry (micturition study) for evaluation of the caudal part of the urinary tract in dogs: Reference values for healthy animals sedated with xylazine. Am. J. Vet. Res. 44:1774, 1983a.

Moreau, P. M., Lees, G. E., and Hobson, H. P.: Simultaneous cystometry and uroflowmetry for evaluation of micturition in two dogs. J.A.V.M.A. 183:1084, 1983b.

Oliver, J. E., Jr., and Young, W. O.: Air cystometry in dogs under xylazine-induced restraint. Am. J. Vet. Res. 34:1433, 1973.

Richter, K. P., and Ling, G. V.: Effects of xylazine on the urethral pressure profile of healthy dogs. Am. J. Vet. Res. 46:1881, 1985a.

Richter, K. P., and Ling, G. V.: Clinical response and urethral pressure profile changes after phenylpropanolamine in dogs with primary sphincter incompetence. J.A.V.M.A. 187:605, 1985b.

Rosin, A. E., and Barsanti, J. A.: Diagnosis of urinary incontinence in dogs: Role of the urethral pressure profile. J.A.V.M.A. 178:814, 1981.

Rosin, A., Rosin, E., and Oliver, J.: Canine urethral pressure profile. Am. J. Vet. Res. 41:1113, 1980.

URODYNAMIC ABNORMALITIES ASSOCIATED WITH CANINE PROSTATIC DISEASES AND THERAPEUTIC INTERVENTION

R. RANDY BASINGER, D.V.M.,
Columbia, South Carolina

and JEANNE A. BARSANTI, D.V.M.
Athens, Georgia

Because of its intimate anatomic relationship to the bladder and urethra, the diseased prostate gland may interfere with normal storage and voiding of urine. The incidence of urodynamic abnormalities associated with severe prostatic disease is high. Inability to void with urine retention and urinary incontinence with urine dribbling are both seen. Therapeutic surgical interventions can exacerbate these urodynamic abnormalities. Accurate diagnosis and appropriate management of these urodynamic abnormalities are a necessary part of the overall care of the dog with prostatic disease.

HISTORY

One should carefully question owners of all male dogs with suspected prostatic disease about the dog's urination habits. Is stranguria, hematuria, or pollakiuria present? Does the dog initiate a normal full stream without difficulty? Is there normal male "marking" behavior? (Marking behavior implies normal urethral function because of the ability to voluntarily interrupt the urine stream.) Does the dog urinate in inappropriate places or dribble between urinations? If urinary incontinence is present, it is helpful to characterize it as continuous or intermittent.

PHYSICAL EXAMINATION

The prostate gland should be carefully palpated for size, symmetry, contour, and consistency. Whether it is fixed or movable should be determined. The sublumbar lymph nodes should be palpated. The fullness of the bladder should be assessed.

If a urethral discharge is present, it should be compared with urine collected at the same time to determine whether the discharge is due to urinary incontinence or is of prostatic origin.

PRACTICAL ASSESSMENT OF URODYNAMIC FUNCTION

The use of sophisticated urodynamic testing has revolutionized diagnosis of voiding and storage dysfunction and is available at larger referral institutions. However, a great deal of information can be obtained from a thorough integration of historical and physical examination findings.

A complete neurologic examination is the first step in evaluating voiding and storage dysfunction to rule out neurogenic causes of urinary tract dysfunction not attributable to localized pelvic canal disease.

Visual observation of the voiding act in an appropriate environment will allow assessment of the dog's ability to initiate and voluntarily terminate the urine stream.

After the dog has been given ample opportunity to empty its bladder, residual urine volume should be measured. If bladder fullness cannot be accurately assessed by palpation, residual volume should be determined by bladder catheterization. Following proper cleansing of the penis and using aseptic technique, an appropriately sized urinary catheter is passed into the bladder. The resistance to passage of the catheter is evaluated, and urine within the bladder is evacuated and measured. If a high residual volume is present, primary detrusor weakness or inability of a normal detrusor contraction to overcome increased urethral resistance should be suspected. Resistance to manual expression of bladder contents and an estimation of bladder tone should be determined.

If incontinence is present, it is important to determine whether the bladder is distended or

1151

relatively empty when incontinence occurs. Urine dribbling with a distended bladder implies overflow incontinence. An atonic bladder or obstructed urethra is the likely cause of the incontinence. Decompressing the bladder and ensuring urethral patency will be of paramount importance. If the bladder stays relatively empty in an incontinent dog, palpating an absence of resistance to manual expression of the bladder will allow a subjective assessment of poor urethral tone. Eliciting the bulbocavernosus reflex by squeezing the base of the penis and looking for contraction of the anus will determine if the pudendal nerve reflex is present to the anal sphincter, indirectly evaluating external urethral sphincter innervation.

URODYNAMIC ABNORMALITIES OCCURRING WITH PROSTATIC DISEASE AND THEIR PHARMACOLOGIC MANAGEMENT

Three types of urodynamic abnormalities have been reported in association with prostatic disease and surgical intervention.

ATONIC BLADDER DUE TO FUNCTIONAL OR MECHANICAL URETHRAL OBSTRUCTION. These dogs characteristically have overflow incontinence with distended bladders. Usually they can be catheterized, implying some degree of functional urethral obstruction instead of pure mechanical obstruction.

If the bladder is atonic owing to overstretching of the tight junctions within the muscular wall, catheter decompression for several days may be all that is required for the bladder to regain function if the underlying prostatic disease can be resolved.

Bethanecol is a cholinergic agonist that can be used to increase bladder tone and stimulate detrusor contraction. The starting dose of 5 mg orally two to three times daily is increased slowly until a therapeutic level is reached or until signs of toxicity, such as diarrhea or gastrointestinal discomfort, are noted. Urethral obstruction is a contraindication to bethanecol's use. Consequently, if mechanical urethral obstruction is present, it should be relieved by indwelling catheterization or appropriate surgical treatment. If functional urethral obstruction is present, it will be necessary to determine by therapeutic trial whether the smooth or skeletal muscle components of the urethra are causing obstruction. Because bethanecol also stimulates proximal urethral smooth muscle, phenoxybenzamine is often given concurrently to block this effect. The dose for phenoxybenzamine is 2.5 to 15 mg once daily orally. If functional urethral obstruction is still present, diazepam, at dosage of 2 to 10 mg three times daily

orally, or dantrolene, 1.0 to 5.0 mg/kg two to three times per day orally, can be administered to relax the skeletal muscle of the external urethral sphincter.

NORMAL DETRUSOR MUSCLE FUNCTION WITH INCONTINENCE DUE TO DECREASED URETHRAL TONE. These dogs will have incontinence with a small to medium-sized bladder. Urine can be expressed without appreciable resistance.

The resting tone of the smooth muscle internal urethral sphincter can be increased by the alpha-adrenergic agonist phenylpropanolamine administered at a dose of 1.5 mg/kg three times daily orally. This regimen has been effective in treating dogs with incontinence due to primary sphincter incompetence but is only occasionally effective with urethral incompetence due to prostatic disease.

There is no specific medication available to increase the tone of the skeletal muscle external urethral sphincter, so some inability of the patient to rapidly increase urethral pressure in response to excitement and barking should be anticipated.

URINARY INCONTINENCE DUE TO DETRUSOR INSTABILITY. This type of incontinence may be indistinguishable to the owners from incontinence due to decreased urethral pressure. Closer evaluation will reveal closely spaced, involuntary bladder contractions, with short, low-volume spurts of urine.

Involuntary detrusor contractions due to detrusor instability can be effectively controlled with the anticholinergic, antispasmodic drug oxybutynin at a dosage of 0.5 to 5 mg two to three times daily orally.

If these drugs are used without the aid of urodynamic testing to confirm a diagnosis, it is suggested that a 2-week trial be conducted before the treatment is considered a failure. Dosages may be manipulated every 3 days until an optimum level is reached. If any adverse effects are observed, the drug should be discontinued or the dosage reduced (see p. 1214).

References and Supplemental Reading

Basinger, R. R., Rawlings, C. A., and Barsanti, J. A.: Urodynamic alterations after prostatectomy in dogs without clinical prostatic disease. Vet. Surg. 16:405, 1987.
Basinger, R. R., Rawlings, C. A., and Barsanti, J. A.: Urodynamic alterations associated with clinical prostatic diseases and prostatic surgery in 23 dogs. J. Am. Anim. Hosp. Assoc. 1988, (in press).
Hardie, E. M., Barsanti, J. A., and Rawlings, C. A.: Complications of prostatic surgery. J. Am. Anim. Hosp. Assoc. 20:50, 1984.
Lappin, M. R., and Barsanti, J. A.: Urinary incontinence secondary to idiopathic detrusor instability: Clinical signs, diagnosis and pharmacologic management in two dogs and a cat. J.A.V.M.A. 191:1439, 1987.
Moreau, P. M.: Neurogenic disorders of micturition in the dog and cat. Comp. Cont. Ed. Pract. Vet. 4:1, 1982.
Rosin, A. H., and Ross, L.: Diagnosis and pharmacological management of disorders of urinary continence in the dog. Comp. Cont. Ed. Pract. Vet. 3:7, 1981.

FELINE VESICOURACHAL DIVERTICULA

Biologic Behavior, Diagnosis, and Treatment

CARL A. OSBORNE, D.V.M.,
JOHN M. KRUGER, D.V.M.,
and GARY R. JOHNSTON, D.V.M
St. Paul, Minnesota

URACHAL FUNCTION

The urachus is a fetal conduit that provides communication between the urinary bladder and the allantois (a portion of the placenta). This structure allows fetal urine to pass from the urinary bladder to the placenta, where unwanted metabolites are absorbed by maternal circulation and excreted in the mother's urine. During later stages of fetal development, the function of the urachus as a conduit for urine declines, while that of the urethra increases. Urine that passes through the fetal urethra accumulates in the amnionic sac and is processed in a fashion similar to that of urine voided into the allantoic sac. At the time of birth, the urachus is nonfunctional.

The mechanism or mechanisms responsible for atrophy of the urachus have not been defined.

URACHAL DYSFUNCTION

Four variations of urachal anomalies may occur: persistent urachus, urachal cysts, urachal sinus (communication of a partially patent urachus with the exterior via the umbilicus), and vesicourachal diverticula (Fig. 1). These anomalies are encountered uncommonly in immature cats. Persistent urachus, urachal cysts, and urachal sinus have been described (Osborne et al., 1985, 1987).

VESICOURACHAL DIVERTICULA

In contrast to the situation in immature cats, vesicourachal diverticula are commonly encountered in adult male and female cats with hematuria and dysuria (Osborne et al., 1987). Their etiopathogenesis, diagnosis, and treatment are described below.

MICROSCOPIC VESICOURACHAL DIVERTICULA

Even though the urachus is not functional at the time of birth, studies of normal feline urinary blad-

ders have revealed microscopic evidence of urachal remnants in the vertex of the urinary bladder (Osborne et al., 1987; Wilson et al., 1983). From a two-dimensional light microscopic perspective, the structures are characterized by islands of transitional epithelium of varying size that occasionally contain microscopic lumens. It is assumed that the three-dimensional appearance of these structures would be tubular. These microscopic urachal remnants may extend from the level of the submucosa to the subserosa (Fig. 2). Because the mechanism or mechanisms of physiologic atrophy of the urachus are unknown, events that lead to persistence of microscopic urachal remnants in the bladder vertex are also unknown.

ACQUIRED MACROSCOPIC VESICOURACHAL DIVERTICULA

Recent evidence suggests that asymptomatic microscopic urachal remnants persisting at the bladder vertex following birth represent a risk factor for development of acquired macroscopic diverticula later in life (Osborne et al., 1987). Abnormal sustained increase of bladder intraluminal pressure associated with diverse feline lower urinary tract disorders causes tissues of the bladder wall at this site to partially separate. The result is a macroscopic diverticulum of varying size that communicates with the bladder lumen (Osborne et al., 1987). Because feline lower urinary tract disorders frequently occur in adult male and female cats, and yet are uncommon in immature cats, an explanation for the increased occurrence of vesicourachal diverticula in adult cats is apparent.

In one study, radiographically detectable diverticula affecting the vertex of the urinary bladder wall were detected in almost one of four adult cats with hematuria, dysuria, or urethral obstruction (Table 1). The mean age of affected cats was 3.7 yr (range, 1 to 11 yr); clinical signs were not detected when the cats were younger than 1 yr of age. A breed predisposition was not detected. They oc-

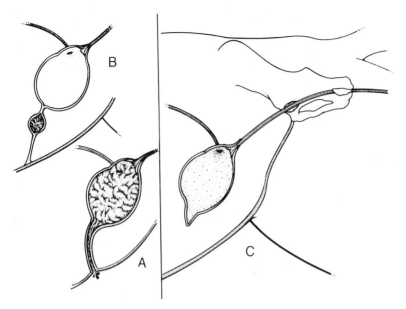

Figure 1. Some congenital urachal anomalies. *A*, Persistent urachus. *B*, Urachal cyst. *C*, Vesicourachal diverticulum. (From Osborne, C. A., Kruger, J. M., and Johnston, G. R.: Vet. Clin. North Am. 17:700, 1987.)

curred twice as often in male (27 per cent) as in female (14 per cent) cats (Osborne et al., 1987) probably because males more commonly developed urethral outflow obstruction due to intraluminal precipitates or swelling or spasm of the urethral wall. The size of the diverticula was approximately four times larger in hematuric, dysuric cats with urethral outflow obstruction than in hematuric, dysuric cats without outflow obstruction.

Factors other than increased bladder intraluminal pressure also are likely to affect the development and size of vesicourachal diverticula. These include the size and length of microscopic lumens within urachal remnants; the type, severity, and duration of the initiating disease; and the severity of inflammation of adjacent tissues.

CONGENITAL MACROSCOPIC VESICOURACHAL DIVERTICULA

Congenital macroscopic vesicourachal diverticula appear to develop prior to or soon after birth and may persist for an indefinite period (Osborne et al., 1987). Because of the infrequency with which they occur, it has been difficult to study their causes. Disorders resulting in abnormally high or sustained pressure within the bladder lumen may be involved. Possibilities include anatomic or functional (reflex dyssynergia) outflow obstruction of the lower urinary tract, disorders associated with detrusor hyperactivity, or abnormal production of a large volume of urine. Further studies are required to investigate these possibilities.

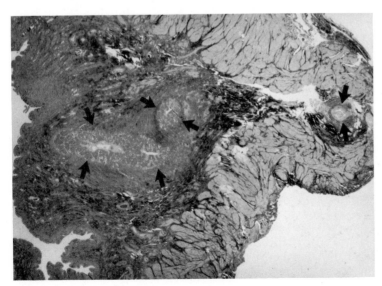

Figure 2. Photomicrograph of a microscopic urachal remnant (arrows) located in the bladder vertex of an adult intact female domestic shorthair pound cat. Lack of connection between submucosal and subserosal urachal segments has probably been caused by the degree of distention of the bladder at the time of fixation with formalin and the plane of transection of the specimen. (Trichrome stain; × 4.) (From Osborne, C. A., Kruger, J. M., and Johnston, G. R.: Vet. Clin. North Am. 17:698, 1987.)

Table 1. *Radiographic Findings in 143 Cats with Naturally Occurring Hematuria and Dysuria*

Finding	Number	%
No abnormalities	14	9.8
Radiodense urethral plug*	5	3.5
Uroliths (31) and sand (1)†	32	21.7
Vesicourachal diverticula	33	23.1
Irregular mucosa	64	44.8
Vesicoureteral reflux	32	22.4

*Detected by survey radiography.

†Excludes material identified by double-contrast cystography that could not be distinguished from blood clots or sand.

Diagnosis

Nonsurgical antemortem confirmation of vesicourachal diverticula requires contrast cystography. In the authors' opinion, positive antegrade cystourethrography and retrograde positive-contrast urethrocystography are the procedures of choice (Johnston et al., 1982). Double-contrast cystography or intravenous urography may also be utilized. Pneumocystography is not recommended because it has not been as consistently reliable as positive-contrast cystography.

Complete distention of the lumen of the urinary bladder with contrast medium is usually recommended to allow meaningful interpretation of the thickness of the bladder wall. However, maximal distention of the lumen of the urinary bladder with contrast medium may obscure small vesicourachal diverticula as a result of stretching of the vertex of the bladder. To minimize this problem, a series of radiographs (at least two) may be obtained with the bladder completely and then partially distended with contrast medium.

The radiographic appearance of extramural vesicourachal diverticula is often characterized by a convex or triangular protrusion from the bladder vertex. Small diverticula may appear as cylindric ductlike structures or saclike abnormalities with a narrow neck that allows communication with the bladder lumen.

Biologic Behavior

Acquired Macroscopic Vesicourachal Diverticula. Spontaneous resolution of acquired macroscopic diverticula has been observed in 15 of 15 adult male cats evaluated by serial radiography. The diverticula were initially identified at the time of radiographic evaluation of these patients for the underlying cause of hematuria, dysuria, or urethral obstruction. When these clinical signs resolved spontaneously or in conjunction with some form of therapy, the vesicourachal diverticula also resolved. Initially the time lapse between initial detection of diverticula and follow-up examination was often more than 1 yr. However, in a 2-year-old intact male with obstructive uropathy caused by a urethral plug, partial resolution of an extramural diverticulum was identified 9 days after initial detection and treatment (Figs. 3 and 4). Complete resolution of the diverticulum occurred 19 days after initial evaluation and treatment (Osborne et al., 1987) (Fig. 5). It is probable that acquired diverticula heal within 2 to 3 weeks following elimination of the underlying cause of increased intraluminal pressure.

Congenital Macroscopic Vesicourachal Diverticula. Diverticula in immature cats as young as 16 weeks of age are presumably congenital. These diverticula may either persist or undergo spontaneous resolution. Persistence of the underlying cause appears to be associated with persistence of diverticula; resolution of the underlying cause appears to be associated with subsequent resolution of the diverticula (Osborne et al., 1987).

Persistent vesicourachal diverticula predispose to bacterial urinary tract infections. Infections caused

Figure 3. Positive contrast retrograde urethrocystogram of a 2-year-old male domestic short-hair cat illustrating a diverticulum protruding from the vertex of the urinary bladder. The cat had a urinary outflow obstruction caused by a urethral plug, which was subsequently removed.

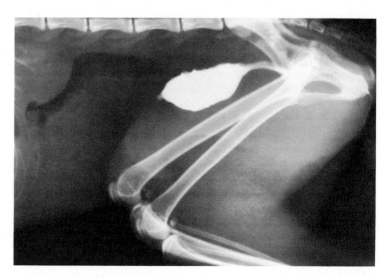

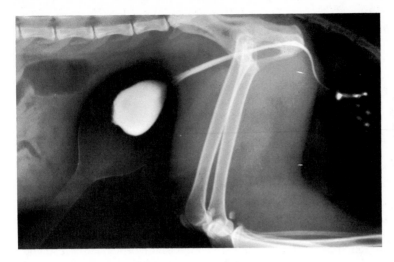

Figure 4. Positive contrast retrograde urethrocystogram of the cat described in Figure 3. This study was performed 9 days after evaluation and treatment. Note reduction in size of the diverticulum. A paddle technique has been used to improve contrast.

by urease-producing calculogenic microbes (especially staphylococci) have resulted in development of infection-induced struvite urocystoliths.

Treatment

Contrary to the widely accepted view that urachal diverticula are a primary factor in development of feline lower urinary tract disease, the authors' studies suggest that most macroscopic diverticula of the bladder vertex are a sequela of lower urinary tract dysfunction. Furthermore, at least some, and probably most, macroscopic diverticula may be self-limiting if the urinary bladder and urethra return to a normal state of function (Osborne et al., 1987).

CATS WITH BACTERIAL URINARY TRACT INFECTION

If bacterial urinary tract infection is confirmed by quantitative culture of urine samples properly collected from a cat with a diverticulum of the bladder vertex, it should be treated with appropriate antimicrobic agents. If present, causes of unrelated disease associated with increased bladder intraluminal pressure should also be eliminated or controlled. If the bladder diverticulum is self-limiting, eradication of the urinary tract infection may result in elimination of lower urinary tract disease.

If bacterial urinary tract infection persists or recurs despite proper antimicrobic therapy, the status of the diverticulum should be re-evaluated by contrast radiography. If a macroscopic diverticulum of the bladder vertex persists in a patient with persistent or recurrent urinary tract infection, diverticulectomy should be considered.

ABACTERIURIC CATS SCHEDULED FOR URETHROSTOMY

If a diverticulum of the bladder vertex is detected by contrast radiography in an abacteriuric male cat

being evaluated for perineal urethrostomy, the client should be informed that removal of the penile urethra (which contributes to local host defenses) combined with the presence of a diverticulum (an abnormality of local host defenses) may result in bacterial urinary tract infection. If the infection is caused by urease-producing bacteria such as staphylococci, infection-induced struvite uroliths may develop. Rather than recommend a perineal urethrostomy or diverticulectomy, one should re-evaluate the indications for urethral surgery and serially evaluate the size of the diverticulum. If the diverticulum subsides, but a confirmed abnormality of the penile urethra predisposing to urethral obstruction persists, the risk of postsurgical urinary tract infection is reduced (but not eliminated). If the diverticulum persists and an abnormality of the penile urethra predisposing to an unacceptable recurrence of urethral obstruction persists, a perineal urethrostomy may be considered. If urethral surgery is performed in a patient with a persistent bladder diverticulum, the cat should be periodically monitored for bacterial urinary tract infection. If frequently recurrent or persistent urinary tract infection occurs after perineal urethrostomy in a cat with a persistent bladder diverticulum, diverticulectomy should then be considered (Osborne et al., 1983).

ABACTERIURIC CATS WITH HEMATURIA AND DYSURIA

The concomitant occurrence of hematuria, dysuria, and urethral obstruction with a diverticulum of the bladder vertex is not an immediate indication for diverticulectomy. The major focus of effort should be directed at detection and elimination of the underlying cause of the lower urinary tract inflammation and the increased pressure within the bladder lumen. If an underlying cause (metabolic

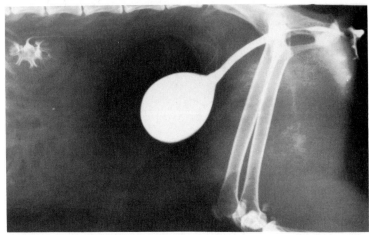

Figure 5. Positive contrast retrograde urethrocystogram of the cat described in Figures 3 and 4. This study was performed 19 days following initial evaluation. A perineal urethrostomy was performed on day 15. There is no evidence of the bladder diverticulum. A paddle technique has been used to improve contrast. Vesicoureteral reflux is evident.

uroliths, urethral plugs, urinary tract infection, infection-induced struvite uroliths, and so on) cannot be identified, the signs of hematuria may spontaneously subside with or without symptomatic therapy (Osborne et al., 1987). Contrast radiography performed 2 to 3 weeks following remission of these signs may reveal partial or complete resolution of the diverticulum.

CATS WITH UROCYSTOLITHS

Cats with acquired diverticula of the bladder vertex and sterile struvite or infection-induced struvite urocystoliths may be successfully managed by medical therapy (Osborne et al., 1983, 1987). Because effective protocols to induce medical dissolution of feline calcium oxalate, calcium phosphate, ammonium urate, and uric acid urocystoliths have not yet been developed, surgery remains the most reliable method for treating patients with metabolic urolithiasis and diverticula of the vertex of the urinary bladder (if present).

References and Supplemental Reading

Johnston, G. R., et al.: Urethrography and cystography in cats. I. Technique, normal radiographic anatomy, and artifacts. Comp. Cont. Ed. Pract. Vet. 4:823, 1982.

Osborne, C. A., Johnston, G. R., Polzin, D. J., et al.: Etiology of feline urologic syndrome: Hypothesis of heterogeneous causes. In Marthens, E. V. (ed.): Proceedings of 7th Annual Kal Kan Symposium, Vernon, CA, 1983. Kal Kan Foods Inc, 1984, pp. 107–124.

Osborne, C. A., et al.: Pathophysiology, diagnosis, and treatment of surgical disorders of the urinary system. In Gourley, I. M., and Vasseur, P. B. (eds.): A Textbook of Small Animal Surgery. Philadelphia: J. B. Lippincott, 1985, pp. 513–516.

Osborne, C. A., Johnston, G. R., Kruger, J. M., et al.: Etiopathogenesis and biological behavior of feline vesicourachal diverticula. Vet. Clin. North Am. [Small Anim. Pract.] 17:697, 1987.

Wilson, G. P., Dill, L. S., and Goodman, R. Z.: The relationship of urachal defects in the feline urinary bladder to feline urologic syndrome. In Marthens, E. V. (ed.): Proceedings of 7th Annual Kal Kan Symposium, Vernon, CA, 1983. Kal Kan Foods Inc, 1984, pp. 125–129.

RENAL EFFECTS OF NONSTEROIDAL ANTI-INFLAMMATORY DRUGS

SCOTT A. BROWN, V.M.D.

Athens, Georgia

EICOSANOIDS

Biochemistry

In 1935 von Euler used the term *prostaglandin* in referring to a compound believed to have been derived from the *prostate gland*, which had potent smooth muscle contractile effects. It is now appreciated that this represented but one example of the ubiquitous biologic functions of arachidonic acid metabolites, collectively termed eicosanoids (prostaglandins, prostacyclin, thromboxanes, leukotrienes, and hydroxy fatty acids). Eicosanoids are derived by enzymatic release and oxidation of the polyunsaturated fatty acid arachidonic acid from cell membranes (Fig. 1). These compounds act as autocoids, i.e., unlike circulating hormones (endocrine), their effects are exerted locally (paracrine), perhaps directly on the cells that produce them (autocrine).

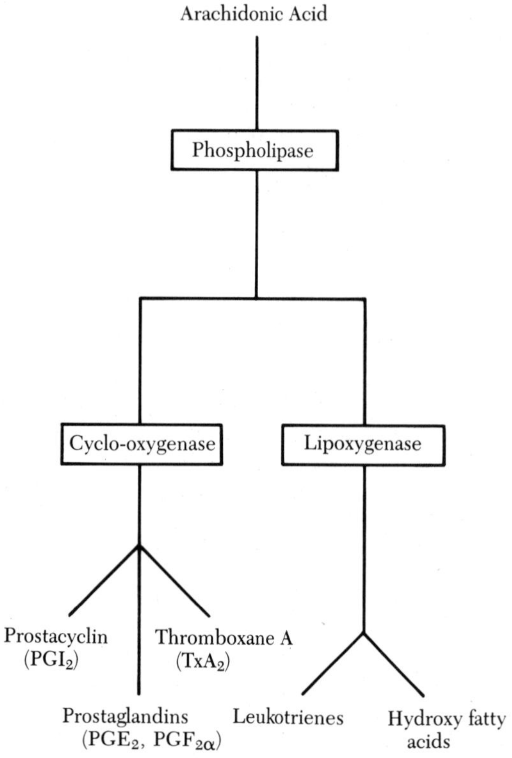

Many stimuli will initiate the arachidonic acid cascade. These include endotoxin, mechanical trauma, thrombin, hypoxia, antigen-antibody reactions, increased intracellular calcium, platelet-derived growth factor, platelet-activating factor, renal nerve stimulation, reduced renal perfusion pressure, furosemide, and a wide variety of vasoactive hormones.

Although all of the biochemical steps in arachidonic acid oxidation are catalyzed by enzymes, three important enzyme activities are central to understanding renal eicosanoid metabolism: phospholipase, cyclo-oxygenase, and lipoxygenase. Phospholipase is responsible for the hydrolytic cleavage of arachidonic acid from membrane phospholipids, which sets the cascade into motion. There are two important renal phospholipase activities, phospholipase A_2 and phospholipase C. Cyclo-oxygenase catalyzes the central pathway (Fig. 1), leading to production of the prostaglandins PGE_2 and $PGF_{2\alpha}$, prostacyclin (PGI_2), and thromboxane A_2 (TXA_2). Lipoxygenase is the central enzyme in the generation of the leukotrienes and hydroxy fatty acids.

Removal of eicosanoids from the kidney is through local enzymatic degradation or outflow in lymph, urine, or venous blood. The half-life of the important metabolites is generally on the order of seconds to a few minutes.

Although referred to as a cascade, it is important to recognize that the production of arachidonic acid

Arachidonic Acid

Figure 1. Overview of arachidonic acid metabolism.

Table 1. *Renal Eicosanoid Production*

Site	Principal Eicosanoid	Effect
Cortex		
Vasculature	PGI_2, PGE_2	Vasodilation
Glomerulus	PGI_2, PGE_2	Maintenance of normal GFR
	TXA_2	Reduction of GFR
Medulla		
Collecting tubule	PGE_2, $PGF_{2\alpha}$	Natriuresis and diuresis
Interstitial cells	PGE_2	Vasodilation/natriuresis/diuresis

metabolites is under considerable control and predominant metabolites will vary as a function of tissue and physiologic state. In the kidney there are marked regional differences in eicosanoid production (Table 1).

Pharmacologic Manipulation

Pharmacologic manipulation of the arachidonic acid cascade may be classified into four general groups:

INHIBITION OF ARACHIDONIC ACID RELEASE BY GLUCOCORTICOIDS. This effect is mediated by induction of a protein, lipocortin, that inhibits phospholipase A_2. The blockade is generally incomplete, and steroid use is associated with many other side effects.

INHIBITION OF CYCLO-OXYGENASE. Nonsteroidal anti-inflammatory drugs (NSAIDs) selectively inhibit production of prostaglandins and thromboxanes. There are more than 20 frequently used medications in this group. This group consists of the *oxicams*, e.g., piroxicam (Feldene, Pfizer); the *pyrazoles*, e.g., phenylbutazone; and the *carboxylic acids*, e.g., acetylsalicylic acid, ibuprofen (Motrin, Upjohn), naproxen (Naprosyn, Syntex), meclofenamic acid (Meclomen, Parke-Davis), indomethacin (Indocin, Merck), sulindac (Clinoril, Merck), fenoprofen, (Nalfon, Eli Lilly), diclofenac, and zomepirac (Zomax, McNeil). These compounds act by a variety of different mechanisms, including competitive antagonism and enzyme inactivation. Acetylsalicylic acid is of particular interest, as it irreversibly acetylates cyclo-oxygenase. This property is useful in the inhibition of platelets, as they are unable to produce new enzyme and remain without cyclo-oxygenase activity until new platelets are produced.

INHIBITION OF LIPOXYGENASE. There are no clinically available compounds that selectively inhibit leukotriene and hydroxy fatty acid production. Benoxaprofen (Oraflex, Eli Lilly) is a carboxylic acid derivative not available in the United States; it has the ability to preferentially inhibit this pathway.

SELECTIVE INHIBITION OF INDIVIDUAL METABOLITES. Phenylbutazone and gold salts appear to act preferentially to lower levels of PGE or $PGF_{2\alpha}$, respectively. Thromboxane synthetase inhibitors have great therapeutic potential in certain renal diseases, although they are not yet readily available for clinical use (e.g., imidazole, substituted imidazole derivatives, and several investigational drugs).

Physiology

Eicosanoids are most well known for their involvement in the mediation of inflammation (and associated pain), fever, and platelet aggregation. It is to control these processes that veterinarians most frequently utilize nonsteroidal anti-inflammatory medications.

Although modulation of intrarenal inflammation and platelet aggregation represents an important effect of eicosanoids in the kidney, most of the deleterious renal effects of NSAIDs occur as a result of interference with renal hemodynamics and excretory function. The principal effects of eicosanoids in the renal cortex are maintenance of normal renal blood flow (RBF) and glomerular filtration rate (GFR) (Patrono and Dunn, 1987) (see Table 1). These cortical effects are critical in counterbalancing circulating and local renal vasoconstrictors. The renal response to any vasoconstrictor (e.g., angiotensin II or norepinephrine) is greatly diminished by the activity of the renal arachidonic acid cascade, in particular PGI_2 and PGE_2. The principal medullary effect of eicosanoids is to promote sodium and water excretion. Prostaglandins are also important in the release of renin, with the subsequent generation of angiotensin II, which stimulates aldosterone release. Aldosterone affects electrolyte balance by enhancing distal tubular sodium reabsorption and potassium secretion.

Lipoxygenase products, hydroxy fatty acids and leukotrienes, are important mediators of inflammation and anaphylaxis. Their production is not inhibited by NSAIDs.

PATHOPHYSIOLOGIC EFFECTS OF NONSTEROIDAL ANTI-INFLAMMATORY DRUGS

For veterinary use, NSAIDs represent a two-edged sword. Although NSAIDs have potent antipyretic and analgesic effects, their prolonged half-life and marked gastrointestinal toxicity in the dog and cat necessitate caution. Gastrointestinal toxicity with mucosal ulceration and marked blood loss may occur with recommended dosages of any NSAID. Renal toxicity, though less commonly recognized, is likely in this setting of volume depletion.

Clinical syndromes associated with NSAID administration in humans include systemic arterial hypertension, hypernatremia, hyponatremia, papillary necrosis, acute renal failure, hyperkalemia, and drug-induced interstitial nephritis (Fig. 2).

The most common renal toxicity in humans and the only reported toxicity in dogs is acute azotemic renal failure with or without electrolyte disorders (hyponatremia, hypernatremia, and hyperkalemia). There is abundant evidence that inhibition of cyclo-oxygenase activity in normal animals and people has negligible effects on renal function. Because renal eicosanoids represent an important system for counterbalancing vasoconstrictor effects, it should be

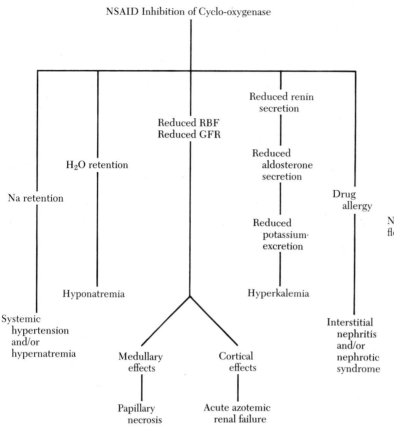

Figure 2. Potential consequences of NSAID administration. RBF, renal blood flow; GFR, glomerular filtration rate.

anticipated that any state with enhanced vasoconstrictor activity or prostaglandin dependency will be sensitive to NSAID administration (Table 2). The result of NSAID use may be reduced GFR and RBF with consequent acute azotemic renal failure.

Sulindac (Clinoril, Merck) has been proposed as a renal-sparing NSAID. The evidence is inconclusive, although the drug may be poorly converted to its active metabolite in the renal cortex. This would theoretically result in selective sparing of cortical eicosanoid production, with the expected result being little effect on renal blood flow and glomerular filtration rate.

Table 2. *Prostaglandin Dependent States**

Congestive heart failure
Liver failure with ascites
Volume/salt depletion
Dehydration
Diarrhea
Dietary sodium restriction
General anesthesia
Diuretic use
Diabetes mellitus
Renal diseases with
Renal insufficiency
Urinary obstruction
Glomerulonephritis
Nephrotic syndrome

*Conditions in which renal function is dependent on prostaglandin synthesis.

DIAGNOSIS AND TREATMENT OF ACUTE AZOTEMIC RENAL FAILURE

This complication should be suspected any time azotemia develops in a patient at risk (Table 2) on NSAID therapy. This toxicity is generally reversible with time (7 to 14 days).

Appropriate therapy would include the following:

1. Withdrawal of NSAID.

2. Intravenous balanced electrolyte fluid therapy to replace deficit and deliver 60 to 100 ml/kg/day. Because NSAIDs interfere with renal excretory ability, these patients will not handle fluid or sodium overload well, and consequently osmotic diuresis or aggressive fluid therapy are not recommended.

3. Assessment of plasma electrolytes and creatinine every 2 to 4 days, with adjustment of therapy accordingly.

4. Because dogs appear to be more susceptible to gastrointestinal than renal NSAID toxicity, the patient should be carefully evaluated for signs of gastrointestinal toxicity and treated appropriately should vomiting, melena, diarrhea, or unexplained anemia occur.

5. Avoidance of diuretics or other nephrotoxins (e.g., aminoglycosides).

6. Avoidance of agents or stimuli that will lead to renal vasoconstriction (e.g., general anesthesia or salt restriction).

References and Supplemental Reading

Bacia, J. J., Spyridakis, L. K., Barsanti, J. A., et al.: Ibuprofen toxicosis in a dog. J.A.V.M.A. 188:918, 1986.
Boothe, D. M.: Prostaglandins: Physiology and clinical implications. Comp. Cont. Ed. Pract. Vet. 6:1010, 1984.
Carmichael, J., and Shankel, S. W.: Effects of nonsteroidal anti-inflammatory drugs on prostaglandins and renal function. Am. J. Med. 78:992, 1985.
Patrono, C., and Dunn, M. J.: The clinical significance of inhibition of renal prostaglandin synthesis. Kidney Int. 32:1, 1987.
Rubin, S. I.: Nonsteroidal antiinflammatory drugs, prostaglandins, and the kidney. J.A.V.M.A. 188:1065, 1986.
Stahl, R. A. K., and Thaiss, F.: Eicosanoids: Biosynthesis and function in the glomerulus. Renal Physiol. 10:1, 1987.

INFILTRATIVE URETHRAL DISEASES IN THE DOG

DAVID T. MATTHIESEN, D.V.M.,
and SCOTT D. MOROFF, V.M.D.
New York, New York

Infiltrative diseases of the canine urethra are relatively uncommon and are caused by neoplasia or granulomatous urethritis. Both entities have been observed predominantly in the female, with neoplasia having a higher prevalence. Clinical signs are similar in both diseases and are characteristic of lower urinary tract disease. Dysuria is caused by obstruction of the urethral lumen and irritation of the urethral mucosa. Hematuria and complete urethral obstruction can also occur. Abdominal palpation may disclose a large, distended urinary bladder if complete urethral obstruction is present. Rectal palpation often discloses thickening and irregularity of the pelvic urethra. If a distal urethral lesion is present, irregularity of the urethral meatus may be revealed by vaginal palpation or inspection. In cases of malignant tumor, the sublumbar lymph nodes may be palpably large because of metastasis.

The most common urethral tumors are of epithelial origin and include squamous cell carcinoma and transitional cell carcinoma. Less commonly reported urethral neoplasms include adenocarcinoma, rhabdomyosarcoma, and hemangiosarcoma (Tarvin et al., 1978; Wilson et al., 1979). Occasionally, a urethral tumor may be an extension of a primary urinary bladder or prostate gland neoplasm. An association between urinary bladder and urethral tumors has been documented in people. One study involving 40 dogs demonstrated a 33 per cent prevalence of synchronous tumors involving both the urethra and urinary bladder (Wilson et al., 1979).

The majority of urethral tumors are seen in old, female, mixed breed dogs. The higher frequency of epithelial tumors as opposed to other histologic types of tumor suggests a higher sensitivity or exposure of the urethral mucosa to carcinogens in the female versus male dog. It has been suggested that male dogs are at less risk because of prostatic secretions into the urethra that dilute carcinogenic compounds within the urethral lumen (Tarvin et al., 1978; Wilson et al., 1979; Crow, 1985). Additionally, the female urethra is lined mainly with squamous epithelium throughout most of its length, whereas the male urethra is lined mainly with transitional epithelium. Squamous epithelium may be more susceptible to the effects of carcinogens. Male dogs have a low prevalence of pelvic or penile urethral tumors, with the majority of urethral tumors involving the prostatic urethra (Tarvin et al., 1978; Wilson et al., 1979). Urethral tumors in the female dog are predominantly found in the distal aspect of the urethra or diffusely throughout the urethra (Tarvin et al., 1978; Wilson et al., 1979). Metastasis can occur, with the regional lymph nodes or lungs being the most common sites.

Granulomatous urethritis is a poorly described disease process in the dog. The disease is clinically indistinguishable from urethral neoplasia. In female dogs with granulomatous urethritis, the most common clinical signs include dysuria, hematuria, and urethral obstruction. As in dogs with neoplasia, a predisposition in older, female, mixed breed dogs is observed. The cause of the disease is unknown. The granulomatous reaction may represent a specific, cell-mediated reaction to one or more antigens or organisms. Whether or not chronic urinary tract infection plays a role in the pathogenesis of the disease is not known.

Histologically, multifocal, nodular to coalescing aggregates of lymphocytes and macrophages with variable numbers of neutrophils are seen within the mucosal and submucosal layers. The urethral epithelial layer is mildly to moderately hyperplastic (Moroff et al., 1988).

DIAGNOSIS

Location of a urethral, infiltrative mass is accomplished by rectal and vaginal palpation, urethral catherization, cystoscopy, voiding or retrograde contrast urethrography, or vaginourethrography. Thoracic and abdominal radiography should be performed to diagnose metastatic disease. Careful radiographic examination of the sublumbar region for lymphadenopathy should be performed. Additionally, examination of the ventral aspect of the lumbosacral vertebral bodies and pelvic bones for evidence of tumor extension is important for staging of the primary urethral tumor.

Contrast radiography of the urethra is important to locate and to determine the extent of the urethral lesion. Multiple filling defects and marked irregularity of the mucosal border are usually apparent (Ticer et al., 1980). Radiographic differentiation of the two diseases on the basis of contrast studies is not possible.

Hematologic and serum biochemical analyses should be performed. Results are usually within normal limits, unless urinary tract obstruction is present. A urinalysis is essential, particularly examination of urine sediment, which will occasionally disclose neoplastic cells in dogs with urethral tumors. Urine collected by cystocentesis should be cultured for bacteria.

After a presumptive diagnosis of urethral mass is made and the mass is located, cytologic and histologic diagnostic procedures should be performed to differentiate the two diseases. Aspiration biopsy (Melhoff and Osborne, 1977) to obtain material for cytologic examination is technically simple to perform. Results have correlated reasonably well with results of histopathologic examination. A 73 per cent agreement between results of cytologic examination and those of histologic examination has been found (Moroff et al., 1988). Cytologic diagnosis of an obstructive urethral lesion can be equivocal, as dogs with neoplasms may have associated inflammation caused by erosion or ulceration of the mucosa.

Briefly, the technique involves use of a flexible, urethral catheter with side ports, which is passed into the urethra just proximal to the lesion. A small volume of normal saline (5 to 10 ml) is flushed into the catheter. Aspiration of a syringe attached to the catheter allows plugs of mucosa to be drawn into the catheter. Digital rectal palpation can be used when necessary to align the catheter within the lesion. Smears of aspirated material are air dried and stained. The aspirates can then be examined and evaluated for differentiation of inflammation versus epithelial neoplasia. Specific identification of the type of epithelial tumor is usually not possible.

Cytologic features of granulomatous urethritis include moderate to high numbers of macrophages and lymphocytes with lesser numbers of neutrophils. The epithelial component generally consists of normal to hyperplastic epithelial cells (Moroff et al., 1988). Cytologic features associated with malignancy include marked to severe cellular pleomorphism and high nuclear-cytoplasmic ratio; nuclei are usually pleomorphic and are occasionally binuclear with prominent, multiple nucleoli and mitotic figures.

Surgical biopsy specimens for histologic examination should be obtained to definitively differentiate neoplastic and inflammatory disease. Abdominal approaches have previously been recommended to obtain biopsy material. In male dogs with prostatic or proximal urethral disease, a caudal abdominal approach is recommended. However, in the majority of female dogs, a less aggressive, perineal approach can be used. A routine episiotomy incision is made. A Gelpi retractor is placed in the edges of the incision, facilitating exposure of the vaginal vault and urethral orifice. In dogs with abnormal urethral tissue extending into the urethral orifice, a specimen of tissue can be obtained by sharp dissection. If the urethral lesion is located further proximally, a specimen can be obtained by gentle placement of a small mosquito hemostat or a small bone curette into the urethra. Because the involved urethra in both diseases consists of friable tissue, retrieval of a small piece of tissue from the urethral lumen can usually be accomplished. Specimens are then submitted for histologic studies.

A Foley catheter should be placed to allow postoperative drainage of urine in dogs with urinary obstruction or severe stranguria. A routine three-layer closure is used for the episiotomy incision.

TREATMENT

Results of surgical treatment of urethral tumors have been uniformly poor because of the advanced stage of disease when first noticed. Most dogs have extensive urethral disease and may have urethrocystic or vulvovaginal extension of the tumor. Ventral midline abdominal approaches with osteotomy of the pubis or splitting of the pelvic symphysis to gain adequate exposure of the urethra have been recommended. If sufficient proximal urethra is free of tumor and there is no vulvovaginal extension, an antepubic urethrostomy can be performed. Urinary continence is maintained if innervation to the bladder neck and proximal urethra is preserved. In dogs with extensive urethral disease and tumor extension into the proximal urethra and trigone, a complete cystectomy-urethrectomy using a urinary diversion procedure (i.e., urethral-colonic or trigonal-colonic anastomosis) can be performed. Little clinical information is available regarding long-term postoperative results.

Radiation therapy or chemotherapeutic protocols to treat a series of dogs with urethral neoplasia have not been described.

Treatment of granulomatous urethritis in dogs should include placement and maintenance of a Foley catheter if complete urethral obstruction or severe stranguria is present. Appropriate antibiotics should be administered, based on results of bacterial culture and sensitivity testing. Anti-inflammatory drugs, prednisolone, or cytoxan alone or in combination have been used. Prednisolone is given in a tapering dosage, beginning at 2 mg/kg/day divided b.i.d. The dosage should be tapered by 50 per cent every 7 to 14 days until the dosage reaches 0.125 mg/kg; corticosteroids are then discontinued. Alkylating drugs (cytoxan) combined with corticosteroids have been administered to dogs with urethral disease with variable results. The current recommendation is to give cytoxan at an initial dosage of 1.5 mg/kg for large dogs, 2.2 mg/kg for medium dogs, and 2.5 mg/kg for small dogs (Scott, 1988). Cytoxan should be given for 4 days each week, followed by 3 days of no administration. It is discontinued after stranguria or urethral obstruction is resolved. Hematologic tests (e.g., complete blood count) should be performed after each cycle of cytoxan adminis-tration because of bone marrow suppression associated with use of this drug.

The Foley catheter should be removed as soon as possible (after 5 to 10 days). Antibiotics should be administered for at least 3 weeks after discontinuation of corticosteroids and cytoxan. Urine should be monitored to be sure any identified infection resolves and does not relapse. Recurrence of urinary obstruction and stranguria should be treated by reinitiating corticosteroid and cytoxan administration.

References and Supplemental Reading

Crow, S. E.: Urinary tract neoplasms in dogs and cats. Comp. Cont. Ed. Pract. Vet. 7:607, 1985.

Melhoff, T., and Osborne, C. A.: Catheter biopsy of the urethra, urinary bladder, and prostate gland. In Kirk, R. W. (ed.): Current Veterinary Therapy VI. Philadelphia: W. B. Saunders, 1977, pp. 1173–1175.

Moroff, S. D., Brown, B. A., Matthiesen, D. T., and Scott, R. C.: Obstructive urethral disease in the female dog: Granulomatous urethritis and neoplastic disease. 1988 (submitted for publication).

Scott, R. C.: Personal communication, 1988.

Tarvin, G., Patnaik, A., and Greene, R.: Primary urethral tumors in dogs. J.A.V.M.A. 172:931, 1978.

Ticer, J. W., Spencer, C. P., and Ackerman, W.: Transitional cell carcinoma of the urethra in four female dogs: Its urethrographic appearance. Vet. Radiol. 21:12, 1980.

Wilson, G. P., Hayes, H. M., and Casey, H. W.: Canine urethral cancer. J. Am. Anim. Hosp. Assoc. 15:741, 1979.

FANCONI'S SYNDROME

Inherited and Acquired

SCOTT A. BROWN, V.M.D.
Athens, Georgia

Fanconi's syndrome refers to metabolic abnormalities caused by a generalized proximal renal tubular disorder, which results in excessive urinary losses of amino acids, glucose, sodium, phosphate, calcium, and other solutes. Fanconi's syndrome has been described in dogs but not, to date, in cats.

ETIOLOGY

The syndrome may be hereditary (primary) or acquired (secondary) (Table 1). Although several heritable diseases are associated with the development of Fanconi's syndrome in humans (e.g., Wilson's disease or hereditary fructose intolerance), similar associations have not been documented in

Table 1. *Potential Causes of Fanconi's Syndrome*

Inherited (Idiopathic)
Basenji
Norwegian elkhound
Shetland sheepdog
Schnauzer

Acquired
Heavy metal poisoning—lead, mercury, cadmium, uranium
Drugs—gentamicin, cephalosporins, outdated tetracycline, cisplatin, streptozotocin
Chemicals—Lysol, maleic acid
Malignancies—multiple myeloma, monoclonal gammopathies
Renal transplantation
Renal cystic disease

dogs. The mechanism of the proximal tubular defect is unknown in most cases. The defect could be caused by abnormal transport proteins in the brush border membrane of the proximal tubular cells, a generalized membrane defect, or a cellular metabolic defect.

CLINICAL SIGNS

Clinical disorders are dependent on the severity of the renal tubular defects and whether concurrent renal failure is present.

In animals without renal failure, the most prominent clinical sign is generally polyuria-polydipsia. Hypokalemia from urinary potassium loss may cause clinical signs of weakness. A defect in proximal tubular bicarbonate reabsorption may result in acidemia, a process referred to as proximal renal tubular acidosis. Phosphaturia may lead to osteomalacia in adult animals or rickets in the young, particularly if there is concurrent urinary calcium loss. Generalized aminoaciduria and glucosuria are considered benign, as they rarely affect plasma concentrations of these solutes.

Concurrent renal failure (reduced glomerular filtration rate) may be present. This is frequently the case with the hereditary form in basenjis and Norwegian elkhounds and the acquired acute renal disease associated with gentamicin administration. In these cases, proximal tubular reabsorptive defects will exacerbate the signs of renal failure. Polyuria, renal tubular acidosis, kaliuresis, and urinary calcium loss as a result of proximal tubular reabsorptive defects will contribute to similar processes of polyuria, uremic acidosis, kaliuresis, and phosphate-calcium imbalance already present in the advanced stages of renal failure. Hypoglycemia would be a theoretic possibility, because glucosuria and reduced renal gluconeogenesis in chronic renal failure may be present. However, hypoglycemia is rarely, if ever, seen.

The syndrome is most well characterized in the basenji breed. Affected basenjis are generally normal until the onset of polyuria, polydipsia, and normoglycemic glucosuria at 2 to 4 yr of age. Renal biopsy results prior to this time may be normal or reveal the presence of megalocytic nuclei in tubular epithelium. The significance of these nuclei is unclear. This disease is present in approximately 30 per cent of adult basenjis in the United States. The clinical course is variable: progressive renal dysfunction leading to uremia and death occurring within a few months of onset of symptoms is found in some dogs, whereas other dogs retain stable renal function for many years. Plasma chemistry profiles are usually normal until azotemia develops. Death is frequently associated with profound proximal renal tubular acidosis and papillary necrosis. The pattern of inheritance is unclear.

DIAGNOSIS

A diagnosis of Fanconi's syndrome should be suspected whenever polyuria and normoglycemic glucosuria are identified, especially in a dog receiving gentamicin therapy or in a basenji or Norwegian elkhound. In cats, transient hyperglycemia is thought to be the most frequent cause of apparent normoglycemic glucosuria.

The presence of acidic urine and a normal anion gap metabolic acidosis is consistent with proximal renal tubular acidosis and supports a diagnosis of Fanconi's syndrome in a dog with normoglycemic glucosuria. The ability to produce acidic urine, despite a proximal tubular bicarbonate reabsorptive defect, is an important feature of Fanconi's syndrome. Bicarbonaturia usually causes alkalinuria. However, in acidemia, the reduced plasma bicarbonate concentration results in less bicarbonate in the glomerular filtrate. Consequently, proximal tubular bicarbonate reabsorption is nearly complete in acidemic animals with Fanconi's syndrome. Because distal tubular hydrogen ion secretion is intact in animals with Fanconi's syndrome, aciduria will be present in states of acidemia. This ability to produce acidic urine is critical in distinguishing between proximal and distal renal tubular acidosis (in which acidic urine is not produced even in states of profound acidemia). Other causes of a normal anion gap metabolic acidosis, such as diarrhea, must be eliminated. Further assessment of bicarbonate reabsorption requires special clearance techniques with infusion of bicarbonate.

Mild proteinuria may be present in cases of Fanconi's syndrome in the dog, with 24-hr urinary protein losses of approximately 300 to 750 mg. Although aminoaciduria is a consistent finding, detection of aminoaciduria requires urine chromatography or amino acid analysis.

It may be difficult to distinguish primary glucosuria in which the tubular transport defect is limited to glucose from the multiple defects of Fanconi's syndrome. The presence of a normal anion gap metabolic acidosis and mild proteinuria may be helpful in some cases. In other cases, renal clearance or chromatography tests may be required. It is important to distinguish Fanconi's syndrome from primary glucosuria, as profound acidemia may develop in animals with Fanconi's syndrome.

Diagnosis of Fanconi's syndrome in a dog with concurrent azotemia is a particularly difficult problem. Increased fractional urinary excretion of sodium and phosphate is a normal homeostatic response in renal failure. However, normoglycemic glucosuria, proximal renal tubular acidosis, and aminoaciduria help to identify the presence of Fanconi's syndrome.

Metabolic screening tests utilizing urine chromatography or measurements of fractional excretions of solutes may be required for accurate diagnosis and characterization of the disease. These measurements, which require timed urine collections and special processing, are done at several referral institutions. Calculation of fractional excretions from a single urine specimen does not aid in the diagnosis of this disease.

THERAPY

The defects appear to be quite variable between individuals and between solutes in the same individual. Consequently, therapeutic management of polyuria, azotemia, acidosis, and hypokalemia should be individualized on the basis of serum chemistry profiles. Because of variable disease expression, the animal should be carefully monitored. Development of severe acidosis, hypokalemia, and progressive decline in renal function is the principal concern. Although there has been no clinical trial to assess appropriate therapy, the following recommendations serve as guidelines:

Serum creatinine, urea nitrogen, electrolyte, and bicarbonate (or total CO_2) levels should be monitored every 10 to 14 days following initial diagnosis and after any alteration in therapy. If stable renal function, acid-base balance, and electrolyte status are achieved, the animal should be frequently re-evaluated (every 2 to 4 months).

Adequate fresh water at all times is the most essential management recommendation for the polyuria. The animal should be maintained on a normal diet unless azotemia is present. At this time, there are few data on which to base recommendations for restriction of dietary intake of protein or phosphate in dogs with concurrent renal failure (see p. 1198). Because marked phosphaturia and calciuria may be present in dogs with Fanconi's syndrome, dietary restriction of phosphate intake in azotemic dogs should be accomplished gradually and attempted only in hyperphosphatemic dogs. Serum calcium and phosphate concentrations should be monitored at the time of diet change, and the new diet withdrawn if hypophosphatemia develops or hypocalcemia worsens.

The presence of a significant bicarbonate reabsorptive defect will cause proximal renal tubular acidosis and may lead to hypokalemia because bicarbonaturia will enhance distal tubular potassium secretion. Sodium bicarbonate or potassium citrate therapy (1 to 9 mEq/kg/day) should be instituted in these cases. However, the proximal tubular bicarbonate reabsorptive defect represents a low transport maximum, i.e., all filtered bicarbonate above a set quantity is spilled into the urine. Consequently, increasing dietary alkali intake will result in increased urinary losses, possibly with little net improvement in plasma bicarbonate level. Consequently, massive doses of alkali may be required to restore acid-base balance. The goal should be a tolerable plasma bicarbonate concentration (e.g., 12 to 18 mEq/L) rather than a normal level. Potassium administration (e.g., potassium chloride or potassium citrate; 1 to 9 mEq/kg/day) may be necessary if hypokalemia develops. The potassium supplementation should be given with a goal of normal plasma potassium concentrations.

Beyond their diagnostic value, urinary glucose, amino acid, and protein losses are not generally of clinical significance. Although theoretically a concern, osteomalacia rarely manifests, and consequently calcium and phosphate dietary therapy or vitamin D supplementation is not indicated without radiographic or clinical data suggesting bone disease. It may be contraindicated with concurrent azotemia.

References and Supplemental Reading

Bovee, K. C., Joyce, T., Blazer-Yost, B., et al.: Characterization of renal defects in dogs with a syndrome similar to Fanconi syndrome in man. J.A.V.M.A. 174:1094, 1979.

Brown, S. A., Rakich, P. M., Barsanti, J. A., et al.: Fanconi syndrome and acute renal failure associated with gentamicin therapy in a dog. J. Am. Anim. Hosp. Assoc. 22:635, 1986.

Easley, J. R., and Breitschwerdt, E. G.: Glucosuria associated with renal tubular dysfunction in three basenji dogs. J.A.V.M.A. 168:938, 1976.

Finco, D. R.: Familial renal disease in Norwegian elkhound dogs: Physiologic and biochemical examinations. Am. J. Vet. Res. 37:87, 1976.

Lee, D. B. N., Drinkard, J. P., Rosen, V. J., et al.: The adult Fanconi syndrome. Medicine 51:107, 1972.

RENAL FAILURE IN YOUNG DOGS

STEPHEN P. DiBARTOLA, D.V.M.,
Columbus, Ohio

DEBORAH J. DAVENPORT, D.V.M.,
Blacksburg, Virginia

and DENNIS J. CHEW, D.V.M.
Columbus, Ohio

When renal failure is diagnosed in a young dog, the clinician must always consider the possibility of underlying familial renal disease. A familial disease is one that occurs in related animals with a higher frequency than would be expected by chance. By comparison, congenital diseases are present at birth and may be genetically determined or result from exposure to adverse environmental factors during development. In juvenile renal diseases (JRDs) of dogs, the kidneys may be normal at birth but undergo structural and functional deterioration during the first few years of life. Some JRDs of dogs probably represent renal dysplasia. The term dysplasia refers to disorganized development of renal parenchyma due to abnormal differentiation and is characterized by the presence of structures in the kidney inappropriate for the stage of development of the animal. In a recent study, the following were considered to be primary lesions suggestive of renal dysplasia: asynchronous differentiation of nephrons, persistent mesenchyme, persistent metanephric ducts, atypical tubular epithelium, and dysontogenic metaplasia (Picut and Lewis, 1987).

The mode of inheritance and specific pathogenesis for JRDs in several breeds of dog are unknown. Polycystic renal and hepatic disease in the Cairn terrier is thought to be inherited as an autosomal recessive trait, whereas hereditary glomerulopathy in the Samoyed is inherited as a sex-linked dominant trait. Many of the JRDs of dogs are variable in severity and rate of progression among individual animals. The clinical and pathologic features of these diseases have been described in the veterinary literature (see supplemental reading) and are reviewed below.

SIGNALMENT

Juvenile renal diseases occur in the cocker spaniel, Norwegian elkhound, Lhasa apso and Shih tzu, basenji, Samoyed, Doberman pinscher, Cairn terrier, standard poodle, Pembroke Welsh corgi, soft-coated wheaten terrier, and bull terrier. They occur sporadically in other breeds as well. In most of these diseases there is no sex predilection. In Samoyeds, however, males are affected early in life and die of renal failure by 15 months of age, whereas females are much less severely affected and develop stable renal disease, which does not progress to renal failure. The age of onset of JRD usually is 6 months to 5 yr, with many dogs presented before 2 yr of age. Renal telangiectasia of the Welsh corgi occurs in older dogs (5 to 13 yr), whereas polycystic renal and hepatic disease in the Cairn terrier is present at birth and affected animals usually are seen at a young age (6 weeks).

HISTORY AND PHYSICAL FINDINGS

The most common historical findings in dogs with JRD are anorexia, lethargy, stunted growth or weight loss, polyuria and polydipsia, and vomiting. Other less common client complaints include poor hair coat, diarrhea, foul breath, and nocturia. In the Pembroke Welsh corgi with renal telangiectasia, the most common client complaints are hematuria, dysuria, and apparent abdominal pain.

Dogs with JRD may be thin and dehydrated. On oral examination, pallor of the mucous membranes, foul odor, and uremic ulceration may be noted. The kidneys usually are small and irregular with the exception of JRD in the Cairn terrier, in which the kidneys are markedly enlarged and abdominal distention is the usual reason for presentation. Renal pain on palpation may be noted in Welsh corgis with renal telangiectasia. Occasionally, Doberman pinschers with JRD are presented for ascites and edema.

Signs of fibrous osteodystrophy such as "rubber jaw" or pathologic fractures usually are more readily detected in young growing dogs with renal failure than in older dogs. Fibrous osteodystrophy may be severe in the Lhasa apso and Shih tzu, cocker spaniel, and standard poodle but usually is not observed in the soft-coated wheaten terrier.

Fundic examination should be performed to evaluate for the presence of systemic hypertension. The observation of retinal detachment, retinal edema, retinal hemorrhage, or tortuosity of retinal vessels should alert the clinician to the possibility of systemic hypertension. Evaluation of blood pressure can be made using Doppler or direct arterial puncture techniques. Hypertension has been documented in cocker spaniels, Lhasa apsos, and Shih tzus with JRD, but it is absent in Norwegian elkhounds. The occurrence of systemic hypertension in other JRD of dogs has not been determined.

LABORATORY FINDINGS

The most common laboratory findings in dogs with JRD are azotemia, hyperphosphatemia, isosthenuria, and nonregenerative anemia. Serum calcium concentrations in dogs with JRD may be normal, decreased, or increased. Hypercalcemia apparently is more common in young dogs with renal failure than in older ones. Compensated metabolic acidosis also may be observed. The presence of hypercholesterolemia and proteinuria should lead the clinician to suspect primary glomerular disease. This may be observed in Doberman pinschers, Samoyeds, standard poodles, and bull terriers with JRD.

Proteinuria may be present in Doberman pinschers, standard poodles, cocker spaniels, Samoyeds, bull terriers, basenjis, Norwegian elkhounds, soft-coated wheaten terriers, Lhasa apsos, and Shih tzus. Only in the Samoyed, bull terrier, and Doberman pinscher, however, is there other evidence of primary glomerular disease. Glucosuria is found in Samoyeds and basenjis, and its presence is variable in the Lhasa apso, Shih tzu, Doberman pinscher, Norwegian elkhound, and cocker spaniel. Urate or uric acid crystals may be seen in the urine sediment of Samoyeds with JRD, and cylindruria is common in Doberman pinschers.

Juvenile renal disease in the basenji is an animal model of Fanconi's syndrome in humans and is characterized by glucosuria, proteinuria, isosthenuria, and aminoaciduria. The loss of amino acids in the urine may be generalized or restricted only to cystine. Affected basenji dogs also demonstrate decreased fractional reabsorption of phosphate, sodium, potassium, and urate. They may have hypokalemia and metabolic acidosis with a normal anion gap (hyperchloremic metabolic acidosis) typical of proximal renal tubular acidosis. Glomerular filtration rate is normal but may decrease later in the course of the disease.

In Welsh corgis with renal telangiectasia, the major laboratory finding is hematuria, but urinary tract infection also may be present. Blood loss anemia is more common than nonregenerative anemia owing to large amounts of blood, which may be lost in the urine. Affected Welsh corgis may develop nephrocalcinosis and calculi, and hydronephrosis may occur if a blood clot or calculus obstructs the ureter.

PATHOLOGIC FINDINGS

Juvenile renal disease may be characterized by the presence of primary dysplastic lesions, compensatory lesions, and degenerative lesions. In many cases, the secondary degenerative lesions overshadow the underlying primary dysplastic lesions, making correct diagnosis difficult. Primary dysplastic lesions that have been observed in some JRD of dogs include immature or "fetal" glomeruli; hyperplasia or adenomatoid proliferation of the medullary tubules, which may represent persistence of metanephric ducts; and persistent mesenchyme in the renal medulla. Such changes are most prominent in the Lhasa apso, Shih tzu, soft-coated wheaten terrier, and standard poodle.

Juvenile renal disease in the Samoyed and bull terrier appears to result from defective basement membranes and may represent animal models of hereditary nephritis in humans. In the Samoyed, a defect in the NC1 domain of type IV collagen results in progressive thickening and splitting of the glomerular basement membranes. In the bull terrier, basement membranes of the glomeruli, Bowman's capsules, and tubules are thickened.

Secondary degenerative lesions that are commonly observed in JRD include interstitial fibrosis, interstitial infiltration by mononuclear inflammatory cells, dystrophic mineralization, and cystic glomerular atrophy. The pathologic features of JRD occurring in several breeds are presented below.

DOBERMAN PINSCHER. In the Doberman pinscher, spheric cysts may be noted in the renal cortex and unilateral renal aplasia has been observed in some affected females. Glomerular lesions are classified as predominantly sclerotic or cystic or a combination of both. Additional glomerular lesions include thickened capillary loops and periglomerular fibrosis. Tubular dilatation and atrophy, interstitial fibrosis, interstitial mineralization, and interstitial infiltration by mononuclear inflammatory cells are common degenerative lesions. Epithelial hyperplasia of the collecting ducts may represent a primary dysplastic or secondary compensatory change. Complement and immunoglobulin deposits in glomeruli have been detected in some dogs, leading to speculation that this JRD may represent a primary familial glomerular disease.

COCKER SPANIEL. Juvenile renal disease in the cocker spaniel has been described as bilateral renal cortical hypoplasia. This disease has not been studied during its early stages and may represent renal dysplasia rather than hypoplasia. Cystic glomerular atrophy and glomerular sclerosis are consistent secondary lesions. Marked tubular changes, including tubular dilatation, tubular atrophy, and mineralization of tubular basement membranes are frequently present. There is medullary interstitial fibrosis but minimal interstitial mononuclear inflammation. Results of immunofluorescence studies to detect complement or immunoglobulins have been negative.

NORWEGIAN ELKHOUND. In the Norwegian elkhound, periglomerular fibrosis is an early histologic lesion that may be detected in some dogs before the onset of azotemia. The number and size of nephrons are normal at this stage. Pathologic findings in dogs with more advanced disease consist of generalized interstitial fibrosis with glomerular sclerosis and atrophy. Tubular changes are mild, except in extremely severe cases, in which tubular atrophy, saccular dilation of the distal tubule and collecting duct, and basement membrane mineralization are noted. Interstitial mononuclear infiltration is recognized only in dogs with advanced disease. Hyperplasia of the collecting ducts also has been observed and may represent a primary dysplastic or secondary compensatory change. Results of immunopathologic studies have been negative.

LHASA APSO AND SHIH TZU. In the Lhasa apso and Shih tzu, affected kidneys may have a so-called dumbbell shape, with most of the cortical tissue present at the renal poles. Microscopic findings include a reduced number of glomeruli; glomerular atrophy; and small, immature, or "fetal" glomeruli, which are hypercellular and have inconspicuous capillary lumens. Tubular changes include atrophy, dilatation, and epithelial hyperplasia. Interstitial fibrosis is particularly severe in the renal medulla, whereas interstitial inflammation is minimal. To a certain extent, increased interstitial medullary tissue may be persistent mesenchyme and may represent a primary dysplastic change. Dystrophic mineralization and hypertrophy of the juxtaglomerular apparatus also may be observed.

BASENJI. Histologic findings in the kidneys of basenjis with Fanconi's syndrome are not consistent. Nonspecific findings include tubular atrophy and interstitial fibrosis. One morphologic marker for this disease may be enlarged, hyperchromatic nuclei in renal tubular cells (renal tubular cell karyomegaly). Affected animals may die of acute renal failure with papillary necrosis or pyelonephritis.

SAMOYED. In the Samoyed, mesangial thickening, glomerular sclerosis, and periglomerular fibrosis are observed by light microscopy. Marked medullary interstitial fibrosis is present, along with tubular basement membrane mineralization. Mononuclear interstitial inflammation is minimal.

Juvenile renal disease in the Samoyed is not a renal dysplasia but a hereditary glomerulopathy characterized by defective regulation of normal glomerular basement membrane structure. At birth, the glomerular basement membranes of affected male Samoyed dogs are normal, but reduplication and bilaminar splitting of the lamina densa is detected by electron microscopic examination at 1 month of age, and this lesion progresses to multilaminar splitting, thickening, and glomerular sclerosis by 8 to 10 months of age. Carrier female dogs have only focal splitting of glomerular basement membranes and do not develop progressive disease. No immune complexes have been observed.

CAIRN TERRIER. Polycystic disease in the Cairn terrier is characterized by the presence of multiple cysts throughout the liver and kidneys. Multiple fusiform to cylindric cysts are present in both the renal cortex and the medulla. These cysts radiate from the capsular surface to the medulla. The renal parenchyma appears normal, except for a decrease in the total number of glomeruli.

STANDARD POODLE. In the standard poodle there is cystic glomerular atrophy and large numbers of immature "fetal" glomeruli, especially in dogs presented at 3 to 4 months of age. Secondary tubular changes consist of focal to diffuse tubular dilatation and atrophy, as well as basement membrane mineralization. The cortical interstitium contains segmental areas of fibrosis, whereas more diffuse lesions occur in the medulla. Interstitial infiltrates of mononuclear cells are minimal in younger dogs and more severe in older dogs.

WELSH CORGI. Welsh corgis with renal telangiectasia have red to black nodules in the kidneys, especially in the renal medulla adjacent to the corticomedullary junction. Clotted blood often is identified in these lesions and in the renal pelvis. Hydronephrosis presumably due to ureteral obstruction occurs in almost half of affected dogs. Similar nodular lesions may be identified in other tissues, including the subcutis, spleen, duodenum, anterior mediastinum, thoracic wall, retroperitoneal space, and central nervous system. Histologically, these lesions are cavernous, blood-filled spaces lined with endothelium, and thrombosis is a frequent finding in the sinuses. These sinuses with their simple endothelial linings may represent vascular malformations rather than benign tumors of vascular origin.

SOFT-COATED WHEATEN TERRIER. Pathologic findings in the soft-coated wheaten terrier suggest a dysplastic disorder of renal maturation. Numerous cystic lesions may be noted grossly in the cortex. Histologically, cortical lesions are segmental, whereas medullary disease is more diffuse. Cortical lesions include interstitial fibrosis, periglomerular fibrosis, cystic glomerular atrophy, decreased numbers of glomeruli, and the presence of immature, "fetal" glomeruli. Medullary changes include tubular atrophy and dilatation, interstitial fibrosis, tubular basement membrane mineralization, and minimal mononuclear inflammatory cell infiltration.

Adenomatous proliferation of the collecting duct epithelium also is a prominent feature. This lesion and the presence of immature, "fetal" glomeruli suggest that JRD in the soft-coated wheaten terrier is a primary renal dysplasia.

BULL TERRIER. In the bull terrier, there is segmental thickening of the basement membranes of the glomerular capillary wall, Bowman's capsule, and the tubules. Glomerular sclerosis and secondary degenerative lesions similar to those observed in other JRD eventually develop. No immune complexes have been detected, and this JRD resembles hereditary glomerulopathy in the Samoyed (Hood, J., Robinson, W. F., and Huxtable, C. R.: Unpublished data, 1987).

TREATMENT

Most JRDs are progressive and ultimately fatal. Therapy is therefore limited to symptomatic measures and conservative medical management of chronic renal failure. The goals of therapy include correction of initial fluid deficits and derangements of acid-base and electrolyte balance, dietary protein restriction, restriction of phosphorus intake, management of metabolic acidosis, management of anemia, control of uremic gastroenteritis, administration of water-soluble vitamins, reduction of stress, and treatment and prevention of urinary tract infection.

At the time of presentation, dogs with chronic renal failure due to JRD often are dehydrated and require appropriate parenteral fluid therapy to correct prerenal azotemia and restore fluid and electrolyte balance. Likewise, the owner should provide unlimited access to fresh water at home as a part of the long-term management of dogs with JRD. Alternate-day administration of water-soluble vitamins is recommended to offset losses that may occur as a result of ongoing polyuria. In animals with severe metabolic acidosis, sodium bicarbonate may be used at a dosage of 25 to 35 mg/kg/day. Adjustment of this dosage is based on repeated blood gas analyses, and an attempt is made to maintain serum bicarbonate concentration above 18 mEq/L.

Dietary protein restriction in patients with chronic renal failure decreases the solute load from protein catabolism, thus ameliorating some clinical signs of uremia. A daily protein intake of approximately 2 gm/kg is recommended for dogs with mild to moderate renal failure. Body weight and serum albumin concentration should be monitored periodically to detect malnutrition. Progressive weight loss and decrease in serum albumin concentration suggest the need to increase protein intake slightly.

Oral phosphorus-binding agents have been used in conjunction with phosphorus-restricted diets to control hyperphosphatemia and blunt secondary renal hyperparathyroidism. Such treatment also may lessen detrimental histologic changes in the kidney, such as interstitial mineralization and fibrosis. Several formulations of phosphorus-binding agents are available, including capsules, tablets, and suspensions of aluminum hydroxide, aluminum carbonate, and calcium carbonate. These products are administered with food to maximize their phosphorus-binding potential, and their dosage is adjusted by frequent monitoring of the serum phosphorus concentration.

Animals with chronic renal failure also may have nonregenerative anemia due primarily to a relative lack of erythropoietin. Occasionally, such anemias are severe enough to necessitate blood transfusion. Often, however, anemia is mild to moderate in severity, and anabolic steroids are used in its management. The effects of anabolic steroids may not be evident for 2 to 3 months after initiation of therapy, and their use has not proved beneficial in dogs with experimentally induced renal failure.

Chronic intermittent vomiting also may be a problem for dogs with JRD. Centrally acting antiemetics such as the phenothiazines or trimethobenzamide may be useful in the control of intractable vomiting. Hypergastrinemia in dogs with renal failure has led to the use of the H_2-receptor blocker cimetidine in the management of uremic gastroenteritis.

Dogs with JRD may be predisposed to urinary tract infection owing to impaired cell-mediated immunity and loss of concentrating ability. As a result, frequent monitoring of the urine sediment is advisable and appropriate antibiotics should be administered whenever urinary tract infection is detected.

References and Supplemental Reading

Davenport, D. J., DiBartola, S. P., and Chew, D. J.: Familial renal disease in the dog and cat. In Breitschwerdt, E. B.: Nephrology and Urology. New York: Churchill Livingstone, 1986, pp. 137–150.

Jansen, B., Thorner, P., Baumal, R., et al.: Samoyed hereditary glomerulopathy: Evolution of splitting of glomerular capillary basement membranes. Am. J. Pathol. 125:536, 1986.

Jansen, B., Thorner, P. S., Singh, A., et al.: Animal model of human disease: Hereditary nephritis in Samoyed dogs. Am. J. Pathol. 116:175, 1984.

Jansen, B., Tryphonas, L., Wong, J., et al.: Mode of inheritance of Samoyed hereditary glomerulopathy: An animal model for hereditary nephritis in humans. J. Lab. Clin. Med. 107:551, 1986.

Lucke, V. M., Kelly, D. F., Darke, P. G. G., and Gaskell, C. J.: Chronic renal failure in young dogs—possible renal dysplasia. J. Small Anim. Pract. 21:169, 1980.

Picut, C. A., and Lewis, R. M.: Microscopic features of canine renal dysplasia. Vet. Pathol. 24:156, 1987.

Robinson, W. S., Shaw, S. E., Huxtable, C. R., et al.: Chronic renal disease in related Bull terriers. Aust. Vet. J. (submitted for publication).

Thorner, P., Jansen, B., Baumal, R., et al.: Samoyed hereditary glomerulopathy: Immunohistochemical staining of basement membranes of kidney for laminin, collagen type IV, fibronectin, and Goodpasture antigen, and correlation with electron microscopy of glomerular capillary basement membranes. Lab. Invest. 56:435, 1987.

CHRONIC RENAL DISEASE
IN CATS

DONALD R. KRAWIEC, D.V.M.,
and HOWARD B. GELBERG, D.V.M.
Urbana, Illinois

Reviews of renal disorders in the cat tend to emphasize general aspects of diagnosis, therapy, and pathophysiology. There are many case reports describing specific feline renal disorders. However, few studies define demographics and intercurrent diseases associated with specific feline renal syndromes. As a result, the risk factors, frequency, and prevalence of different types of feline renal disease are unknown. The authors surveyed all cases of feline renal disease diagnosed at the University of Illinois Teaching Hospital for a 5.5-yr period (July 1981 through December 1986). There were 156 cats diagnosed as having a renal disorder. Of these, 131 had chronic renal disease. Chronic renal disease represents 2.4 per cent of all cats seen during this time period.

Records of cats with chronic renal disease were evaluated for breed, age at onset of renal disease, sex, presenting complaint, clinical diagnosis, necropsy diagnosis, and intercurrent disease. Data on age, sex, and breed were compared with those from all feline admissions during the same time period. Feline admissions data include only information obtained from an animal's first admittance to the hospital. These findings are summarized below and serve as a basis for the discussion in this article.

CHARACTERISTICS OF CATS WITH CHRONIC RENAL DISEASES

AGE, SEX, AND BREED. The average age, at the time of diagnosis, of cats with chronic renal disease was 12.8 yr (median, 14 yr). These ages are higher than those previously reported: 9.2 yr (DiBartola et al., 1987) and 7.42 yr (Cowgill and Spangler, 1981). The majority (72.8 per cent) of cats with chronic renal disease were older than 10 yr (Table 1). Only 13 per cent of the total number of cats seen during this same time period were older than 10 yr of age. Thus, chronic renal failure is much more common in old cats.

Neutered males represented the largest sex group of cats with renal disease, with 48 (40.3 per cent) animals. Forty-three (36.1 per cent) cats were spayed females, 16 (13.5 per cent) were intact males, and 12 (10.1 per cent) were intact females.

More than 94 per cent of cats affected with renal disease were older than 1 yr of age. Of all cats older than 1 yr in the total population seen during the same time period, 1212 (38.6 per cent) were castrated males, 1110 (35.3 per cent) were spayed females, 412 (13.1 per cent) were intact males, and 410 (13 per cent) were intact females. This distribution closely approximates that of cats affected with chronic renal disease. Thus, there does not appear to be a sex preference nor does neutering increase the risk of renal disease.

The majority of cats with renal disease were domestic mix (81.6 per cent). Siamese were the second most frequent breed with renal disease (14.4 per cent), and Persians were third (4 per cent). These breeds were also the three most commonly seen among the 5467 cats admitted during the study: 87.9 per cent of these cats seen were domestic mix, 7.4 per cent were Siamese, and 2.1 per cent were Persian.

PRESENTING COMPLAINT. The most common historical problem of cats with chronic renal disease was anorexia (Table 2). The next most common complaint was polyuria/polydypsia (PU/PD). In only 11 instances was PU/PD the only complaint noted. Because feline excretory habits rarely impact on their owners' lives, PU/PD is an easy abnormality to ignore or overlook.

CLINICAL DIAGNOSIS. Renal failure is usually diagnosed by findings of azotemia and nonconcentrated urine (urine specific gravity between 1.008 and 1.034). Chronic renal failure is additionally

Table 1. *Age at Diagnosis of Cats Having Chronic Renal Disease**

Age in Years	Number of Affected Cats (%)	Total Number of Cats Seen	Percentage of Affected Cats
0–1	6 (4.8)	1934 (38)	0.31
1–2	1 (0.8)	628 (12)	0.16
2–4	7 (5.6)	830 (16)	0.84
4–7	6 (4.8)	644 (13)	0.93
7–10	14 (11.2)	408 (8)	3.43
10–15	42 (33.6)	488 (10)	8.61
>15	49 (39.2)	166 (3)	29.52

*University of Illinois Veterinary Teaching Hospital, July 1981 to December 1986.

Table 2. Presenting Complaint and Intercurrent Diseases in Cats with Chronic Renal Disease*

	Number of Cats (%)
Presenting Complaint	
Anorexia	46 (29.9)
Polyuria/polydypsia	31 (20.1)
Lethargy and depression	17 (11.0)
Vomiting	15 (9.9)
Weight loss	11 (7.1)
Oral cavity problems	8 (5.2)
Neurologic problems	8 (5.2)
Diarrhea	5 (3.2)
Respiratory abnormalities	5 (3.2)
Lower urinary tract problem	4 (2.6)
Blindness	4 (2.6)
Intercurrent Disease	
Neoplasia	27 (30.3)
Hyperthyroidism	16 (18.0)
Liver disease	11 (12.4)
Cardiac disease	11 (12.4)
Lower urinary tract disease	8 (9.0)
Retinal detachment	6 (6.7)
Diabetes mellitus	4 (4.5)
Hypertension	3 (3.4)
Pneumonia	3 (3.4)

*University of Illinois Veterinary Teaching Hospital, July 1981 to December 1986.

characterized by nonregenerative normochromic normocytic anemia, evidence of renal osteodystrophy, bilateral reduction in renal size, and a duration of months to years.

MORPHOLOGIC DESCRIPTION OF THE RENAL LESION. Fifty-four of the cats evaluated either died or were euthanatized, and their kidneys were examined histologically. The most common morphologic lesion was membranous glomerulonephropathy. Membranous glomerulonephropathy was the only histopathologic abnormality in ten cats. It was the primary lesion in an additional five cats. Membranoproliferative glomerulonephropathy was present in three cats. Renal tissue was not assessed by either immunofluorescence or electron microscopy for the presence of immune-mediated glomerulonephritis because significant proteinuria was not identified in any of these cases and, therefore, glomerular disease was not suspected. There was no significant difference between the mean serum albumin levels of cats with severe glomerular lesions (serum albumin, 2.95 gm/dl; n = 10) and those of cats without glomerular lesions (serum albumin, 3.0 gm/dl; n = 9). There was also no significant statistical difference in urine protein determinations. However, the mean urine protein level of cats with severe membranous lesions was 136 mg/dl, whereas the mean urine protein level of cats with no glomerular lesions was 65 mg/dl. Quantitative urine protein determinations were not performed. The average urine specific gravities of the two groups were the same (1.018).

Chronic tubulointerstitial nephritis was the only lesion identified in eight cats, and it was the primary lesion in a single additional cat. Twenty-two cats had a combination of glomerular and tubulointerstitial changes.

Renal neoplasia was identified in three cats. Hydronephrosis and renal hypoxia were each identified in one cat.

INTERCURRENT DISEASES. The most common condition that occurred in association with chronic renal disease was neoplasia (see Table 2). The most common neoplasms identified were thyroid adenoma and adenocarcinoma (n = 7). Squamous cell carcinoma (n = 5) was the second most frequent neoplasm. Other types of neoplasms present were lymphosarcoma, hepatocellular carcinoma, abdominal mesothelioma, mast cell tumor, nasal adenocarcinoma, biliary carcinoma, bronchogenic carcinoma, salivary gland carcinoma, intestinal adenocarcinoma, and pancreatic acinar cell adenoma.

The most common clinical entity that affected cats with chronic renal disease was hyperthyroidism (see Table 2). Neoplasia, hyperthyroidism, and chronic renal failure primarily affect older animals. It is not surprising that they sometimes occur simultaneously. This illustrates the need to evaluate an older animal thoroughly for occult disease even if a primary abnormality has been identified.

Liver disease was present in 11 animals with chronic renal disease (see Table 2). Three cats had hepatic neoplasms, one had hepatic lipidosis, and the rest either had nonspecific hepatocellular degeneration and vacuolization or undefined liver disease.

Lower urinary tract disease was identified in eight cats (see Table 2). Two of these cats had idiopathic lower urinary tract disease, and the rest had bacterial cystitis. Cats are thought to be resistant to bacterial cystitis in part because of their high urine urea content and high urine-concentrating ability. Cats with renal failure have an inability to concentrate their urine, compromising their ability to resist cystitis. Cats with renal failure should, therefore, be carefully evaluated and monitored for bacterial cystitis.

Idiopathic retinal detachment was identified in six cats. Retinal detachment has been associated with renal disease–related hypertension. Three cats with retinal detachment were hypertensive. The other three cats were not evaluated for hypertension. Glomerulonephritis is a common renal disorder associated with hypertension. None of these cats' renal lesions were evaluated histologically, and none were identified clinically as having glomerulonephritis. Any cat with unexplained retinal detachment should be evaluated for renal disease.

Diabetes mellitus was present in four cats with renal disease. Diabetic nephropathy is a human renal disorder characterized by glomerular damage, and it frequently affects diabetic humans. In one study lesions typical of human diabetic nephropathy were found in 12 dogs with spontaneous diabetes (Jeraj et al., 1984). Two of the four cats with diabetes in this study were identified as having glomerular disease on the basis of histopathologic examination of renal tissue. The other two cats' kidneys were not evaluated histologically and were not identified as having a clinical glomerular abnormality. It is worthwhile to periodically evaluate diabetic cats for renal disease.

Cardiac disease was identified in 11 animals. Hypertrophic cardiomyopathy was identified in six of these cats. There is a high association between hypertrophic cardiomyopathy and hyperthyroidism; however, only one of the six cats was hyperthyroid.

CHRONIC RENAL DISEASES THAT AFFECT CATS

Chronic Nephritis

Cats can develop a slow deterioration of renal function that leads to renal failure, end-stage kidney disease, and death. Regardless of the initiating cause, this chronic deterioration is usually characterized histologically by fibrosis and mononuclear cell infiltration, principally of the cortex (chronic interstitial nephritis). Because of the long-standing nature of the disorder and nondistinctive lesions, it is not usually possible to define a precise etiology. However, ischemic abnormalities, such as cardiovascular disease, hypovolemia, shock, and hypoadrenocorticism, may produce an ongoing insult, which is potentially correctable. Infectious agents (bacteria and fungi) and neoplastic processes that may affect renal function should be treated, and the animal should be monitored for recurrence. Likewise, if a renal toxin is identified it should be eliminated from the patient's environment.

Chronic nephritis is considered a self-perpetuating, progressive, irreversible disease. In other species (humans, dogs, and mice), this progression is thought to be due to hypertension, hyperphosphatemia, and an increase in metabolic waste products of protein metabolism that build up in the blood. It is assumed that the same factors play a role in cats.

Therapy is aimed at slowing the progression of the disease and ameliorating the signs of uremia. Typically therapy involves reducing salt intake to control hypertension, restricting dietary protein and phosphorus, providing unlimited access to water, avoiding stress, supplementing the diet with water-soluble vitamins, treating acidosis, giving anabolic agents to promote red blood cell production, and controlling hypocalcemia (see *Current Veterinary Therapy VIII*, pp. 1008–1018).

Glomerulonephritis

Glomerulonephritis is an immune-mediated inflammatory disorder, which has been described in cats (August and Leib, 1984; *Current Veterinary Therapy IX*, p. 1132). Two forms of glomerulonephritis may occur: antiglomerular basement membrane nephritis and immune complex nephritis. Only immune complex glomerulonephritis has been described in cats. It is associated with immune complex deposition in the glomerular capillary network. Immune complex disease is often associated with chronic antigenic stimulation, and numerous chronic inflammatory disorders (e.g., feline leukemia virus and feline infectious peritonitis) have been associated with glomerulonephritis. However, immune complex glomerular nephritis in cats, like its counterpart in humans and dogs, is primarily an idiopathic disorder.

Cats that develop glomerulonephritis may demonstrate renal failure or nephrotic syndrome. The hallmark of glomerular disease is abnormal amounts of urine protein. Increased urine protein concentration can occur as a result of urinary tract infection or hemorrhage; these possibilities must be eliminated before an accurate assessment of glomerular disease–induced proteinuria can be made. Nephrotic syndrome is characterized by proteinuria, hypoalbuminemia, edema, and hypercholesterolemia. Hypoalbuminemia results from loss of protein in the urine in excess of what can be produced by the liver. Decreased oncotic pressure due to hypoalbuminemia produces edema. The cause of hypercholesterolemia is not precisely known, but cholesterol levels are inversely proportional to serum albumin levels.

Specific therapy for glomerulonephritis is aimed at identifying and treating the primary disorder causing chronic antigenic stimulation. Unfortunately, this is often not possible.

Symptomatic therapy for glomerulonephritis is controversial. Anti-inflammatory and immunosuppressive therapies are classically recommended for other types of immune-mediated disease. Some types of human glomerulonephritis (lipoid nephrosis, idiopathic membranous nephropathy, and lupus nephritis) are effectively treated with these types of medications. However, immunosuppressive therapy has not been critically evaluated for use in cats with glomerulonephritis, and glucocorticoids may worsen azotemia.

Antiplatelet and anticoagulant therapies are advocated for treating certain types of human glomerulonephritis. Glomerulonephritis is known to induce hypercoagulation in dogs; however, this has not been noted in cats.

Adding extra protein to a hypoalbuminemic proteinuric animal's diet might help ameliorate the hypoalbuminemia and increase plasma oncotic pressure. However, dietary protein has been known to increase glomerular capillary pressure and worsen the albuminuria associated with some forms of glomerulonephritis (Kaysen et al., 1986). Conversely, decreasing glomerular pressures directly might decrease proteinuria and, therefore, increase serum albumin levels. Converting enzyme inhibitors (captopril and enalapril) have been effectively used in people with glomerulonephritis to reduce glomerular capillary pressures and decrease proteinuria (Heeg et al., 1987). The effects of high- and low-protein diets and converting enzyme inhibitors have not been evaluated in cats with glomerulonephritis.

Moderate restriction of salt intake and administration of diuretics can also be used to treat hypertension and edema that can occur in this disease (Chew et al., 1982; *Current Veterinary Therapy VIII*, p. 1132).

Feline Renal Amyloidosis

Renal amyloidosis has been identified primarily in older cats of both sexes and in numerous breeds (see *Current Veterinary Therapy VIII*, p. 1132). It may have a hereditary tendency in Abyssinian cats. In the dog, renal amyloidosis is primarily a glomerular disorder characterized by proteinuria, renal failure, and uremia. However, in the cat amyloid deposition is located primarily in the medullary interstitium. Amyloid can also be found in feline renal cortical areas and glomeruli. The disease syndrome in the cat is progressive and is characterized by renal failure, uremia, and death. Proteinuria may or may not be present, depending on the degree of glomerular involvement.

Amyloidosis is not an inflammatory disease but may be associated with various inflammatory conditions, neoplasms, and endocrine disorders. It has also been associated with hypervitaminosis A. In most instances an underlying abnormality cannot be identified.

Definitive diagnosis can be made only with histologic evaluation of renal tissue obtained by renal biopsy or at necropsy. Therapy is aimed at identifying and removing underlying disease and treating the animal symptomatically for renal failure. No specific therapy is known to prevent deposition or facilitate the removal of amyloid in cats.

Feline Polycystic Renal Disease

Feline polycystic renal disease is a familial disease principally of kittens. It is characterized by the cystic replacement of substantial amounts of renal tissue. Affected kittens are normal at birth but develop distended abdomens owing to greatly enlarged kidneys. The liver may also be affected by this disease. Animals with polycystic kidneys usually die within the first 2 months of life (Crowell et al., 1979; *Current Veterinary Therapy IX*, p. 1138).

Feline Perirenal Cysts

Perirenal cyst (pseudocyst) is a rare disorder characterized by progressive abdominal enlargement attributable to the accumulation of fluid in a cystlike structure surrounding one or both kidneys (see *Current Veterinary Therapy VIII*, p. 980). These cysts have been reported in intact and neutered male cats. This condition can be differentiated from renal parenchymal enlargement by intravenous urography, which will usually show a normal-sized kidney encased in a fluid-filled sac. The cause of this disorder in cats is unknown, but in humans it has been associated with trauma, urinary tract obstruction, resolving perirenal hematomas, and lymphatic obstruction. Animals generally have progressive abdominal distention. Therapy is aimed at surgically removing the cyst and correcting any identifiable cause.

References and Supplemental Reading

August, J. R., and Leib, M. S.: Primary renal diseases of the cat. Vet. Clin. North Am. 14:1247, 1984.

Brace, J. J.: Perirenal cysts (pseudocysts) in the cat. *In* Kirk, R. W. (ed.): *Current Veterinary Therapy VIII*. Philadelphia: W. B. Saunders, 1983.

Chew, D. J., and DiBartola, S. P.: Feline renal amyloidosis. *In* Kirk, R. W. (ed.): *Current Veterinary Therapy VIII*. Philadelphia: W. B. Saunders, 1983.

Chew, D. J., DiBartola, S. P., Boyce, J. T., and Gaspes, P. W.: Renal amyloidosis in related Abyssinian cats. J.A.V.M.A. 181:139, 1982.

Cowgill, L. D., and Spangler, W. L.: Renal insufficiency in geriatric dogs. Vet. Clin. North Am. 11:727, 1981.

Crowell, W. A.: Polycystic renal disease. *In* Kirk, R. W. (ed.): *Current Veterinary Therapy IX*. Philadelphia: W. B. Saunders, 1986.

Crowell, W. A., Hubbell, J. J., and Riley, J. C.: Polycystic renal disease in related cats. J.A.V.M.A. 175:286, 1979.

DiBartola, S. P., and Chew, D. J.: Glomerular disease in the dog and cat. *In* Kirk, R. W. (ed.): *Current Veterinary Therapy IX*. Philadelphia: W. B. Saunders, 1986.

DiBartola, S. P., Rutgers, H. C., Zack, P. M., and Tarr, M. J.: Clinicopathologic findings associated with chronic renal disease in cats: 74 cases (1973–1984). J.A.V.M.A. 190:1196, 1987.

Heeg, J. E., De Jong, P. E., Van Der Hem, G. K., and De Zeeuw, D.: Reduction of proteinuria by angiotensin converting enzyme inhibition. Kidney Int. 32:78, 1987.

Jeraj, K., Basgen, J., Hardy, R. M., et al.: Immunofluorescence studies of renal basement membranes in dogs with spontaneous diabetes. Am. J. Vet. Res. 45:1162, 1984.

Kaysen, G. A., Gambertoglio, J., Jimenez, I., et al.: Effect of dietary protein intake on albumin homeostasis in nephrotic patients. Kidney Int. 29:572, 1986.

Osborne, C. A., and Polzin, D. J.: Conservative medical management of feline chronic polyuric renal failure. *In* Kirk, R. W. (ed.): *Current Veterinary Therapy VIII*. Philadelphia: W. B. Saunders, 1983.

MEDICAL MANAGEMENT OF CANINE GLOMERULONEPHROPATHIES

JEANNE A. BARSANTI, D.V.M.,
DELMAR R. FINCO, D.V.M.,
Athens, Georgia

and SHELLY L. VADEN, D.V.M.
Raleigh, North Carolina

Glomerulonephropathy is defined as any pathologic process that initially affects the glomerulus and then progresses to secondarily affect the rest of the nephron. Persistent proteinuria is often the first clinical abnormality observed, but eventually signs consistent with generalized renal failure develop. The two major categories of glomerulonephropathies in dogs are renal amyloidosis and glomerulonephritis. The approach to diagnosis of these conditions is reviewed elsewhere (see p. 1139, and *Current Veterinary Therapy IX*, pp. 1111–1114 and 1132–1138).

For the purpose of determining appropriate therapy, patients should be subdivided on the basis of their clinical signs as well as their disease process. Animals with transient proteinuria do not require therapy. Even proteinuria that persists may not require further diagnostic or therapeutic efforts, if it is caused by another illness that may be satisfactorily resolved and if proteinuria is unassociated with any clinical symptoms or other related laboratory abnormalities, such as hypoalbuminemia or azotemia. In these cases, re-evaluation of proteinuria after resolution of the underlying disease process is warranted prior to diagnostic or therapeutic intervention for the proteinuria itself.

This article focuses on treatment of glomerulonephropathies that are the primary reason for the animal's signs of illness. Ideally, therapy should control related abnormal signs (symptomatic therapy), reverse glomerular disease, and prevent further progression of renal injury. At this time, it is unknown whether therapy can prevent progression of naturally occurring canine renal disease (see p. 1195). Symptomatic therapy and specific therapy for amyloidosis and glomerulonephritis are discussed later.

Determination of the value of any therapy must include effects on the natural history of the disease process and what injury or side effects that therapy produces. Only when therapy improves quality or quantity of life over that which occurs without intervention is therapy indicated.

NATURAL HISTORY OF GOMERULONEPHROPATHIES

The natural history of these diseases has not been systematically studied in dogs. However, some insight can be gathered from review of untreated cases and those treated symptomatically.

Renal Amyloidosis

Renal amyloidosis in dogs is thought to result from chronic antigenic stimulation. In some cases, chronic infections or neoplastic conditions are found, but many cases are idiopathic. Review of 26 cases seen at the University of Georgia (UGA) during the period from 1982 to 1987 indicated that the owners had noted related signs for 1 week to 1 yr, with a median of 2 months. Of the 19 dogs that were euthanatized, 8 had an identifiable potential underlying disease (neoplasia, 3; severe chronic skin disease, 3; chronic peritonitis, 1; and chronic urinary tract infections, 1). Two others had pituitary-dependent adrenal hyperplasia. Nine of the dogs had no identifiable predisposing cause for amyloid deposition.

Most of these 26 patients were symptomatic at the time of initial examination. Twelve had azotemia or uremia, 24 had hypoalbuminemia (5 of which were nephrotic), and 5 had evidence of thrombosis. One animal, which was not azotemic initially, was managed symptomatically; disease progressed to end-stage renal failure and death in 10 months. One reported case of renal amyloidosis survived 15 months with symptomatic therapy (Osborne et al., 1970).

In conclusion, renal amyloidosis is a chronic disease process with gradual progression over months to death from end-stage renal failure or from vascular thrombosis.

Glomerulonephritis

Glomerulonephritis is not a single disease entity but includes a wide spectrum of pathologic changes in the glomeruli. The subdivisions include sclerosing, proliferative, membranous, membranoproliferative, and mesangioproliferative glomerulonephritis, each of which can be focal or diffuse. Like amyloidosis, glomerulonephritis is associated with chronic inflammatory or neoplastic diseases. An immune-mediated origin is suspected to be the basis of most cases with antigen-antibody deposition or formation in the glomerulus. Hypertension-related vascular lesions, common in humans, were not noted in dogs (MacDougall et al., 1986). Glomerulonephritis occurs commonly with aging in dogs, but most affected dogs do not have clinical or laboratory evidence of renal disease (Rouse and Lewis, 1975).

The natural history of progressive glomerulonephritis in dogs has not been studied prospectively. Information must be derived from a few retrospective studies and case reports. As with amyloidosis, clients reported their animals to have been ill for 1 to 2 months prior to diagnosis. With membranous glomerulonephritis, a slow progression over months to years has been the general rule in dogs, although some cases have been stable for a year or more (Wright et al., 1981; Osborne and Vernier, 1973). Spontaneous remission of membranous glomerulonephritis with nephrotic syndrome has been reported in a few dogs (Osborne and Vernier, 1973; Osborne et al., 1976; Jaenke and Allen, 1986; DeSchepper et al., 1974). Azotemia indicates a poorer prognosis in dogs and cats, probably because it signifies more advanced disease at time of diagnosis. In one study (Center et al., 1987), dogs that were azotemic at the time of diagnosis survived less than 3 months.

In conclusion, glomerulonephritis is a common lesion in aging dogs and is often unassociated with clinical signs. If clinical signs or laboratory abnormalities are evident, the disease progresses to generalized renal failure in some dogs, whereas in other dogs the disease remains stable or spontaneously resolves. Azotemia indicates a poorer prognosis.

SYMPTOMATIC THERAPY

Dogs with glomerulonephropathies can have proteinuria only or can also have hypoalbuminemia, nephrotic syndrome (proteinuria, hypoalbuminemia, and edema), or azotemia with or without uremia. Dogs with glomerulonephropathies also may be hypertensive, although the relationship of hypertension to severity or progression of disease remains to be determined. Dogs that have severe proteinuria have a tendency to develop thromboembolism. Thus, symptomatic therapy may be required for edema, hypertension, hypercoagulability, or renal failure, depending on the signs in each individual case.

CONTROL OF EDEMA

Dogs with severe proteinuria may develop edema, which is localized or generalized, transudative ascites, or both. One common theory has been that urine protein loss results in hypoalbuminemia, which causes decreased plasma oncotic pressure, transudation of fluid and loss of plasma volume, stimulation of the renin-angiotensin-aldosterone system with sodium retention, worsening fluid retention, and edema. Although this theory is still plausible, some humans with glomerulonephritis have volume expansion rather than contraction, and the renin-angiotensin system is suppressed, not stimulated. A new theory to explain volume expansion is that glomerular disease causes primary sodium retention, leading to edema. Hypoalbuminemia, according to this theory, is produced by dilution from sodium and water retention, as well as loss in urine and decreased intake due to anorexia. Hepatic synthesis may also be impaired.

The importance of plasma volume is related to potential benefits and complications of diuretic therapy. If the patient exhibits volume expansion, natriuretic diuretics such as furosemide are likely to be useful, but osmotic diuretics may worsen the edema if their use results in further expansion of intravascular volume. If the patient has hypovolemia, natriuretic diuretics may further reduce plasma volume, impairing renal perfusion and thus renal function. Judicious use of fluid diuresis may be indicated. Whether dogs with nephrotic syndrome have volume expansion, contraction, or neither (depending on the individual case) is unknown.

With the above reservations, current therapy for edema caused by glomerular disease is use of a sodium-restricted diet and diuretics. A sodium-restricted diet is essential. In the face of azotemia, it is best to institute the change in sodium intake gradually over several weeks. Diuretics should be used cautiously, avoiding side effects of plasma volume contraction and hypokalemia. The drug of choice currently is furosemide at 2.2 mg/kg once or twice a day orally. Because animals usually tolerate edema well, there is no need in most cases to eliminate it rapidly. In fact, treatment may be a detriment if it is accomplished only by inducing dehydration.

The use of plasma transfusions to increase plasma albumin concentrations is unwarranted in most cases, as response is minor and transitory. Plasma transfusions might be useful during short surgical procedures, such as renal biopsy, or during an acute uremic crisis but have little place in long-term management.

CONTROL OF HYPERTENSION

Drug therapy for hypertension is discussed on page 1201. For control of edema, sodium restriction and diuretics are used initially. Other drugs are added as needed.

CONTROL OF THROMBOEMBOLISM

The risk of thromboembolism appears to be directly related to the severity of proteinuria. Although not a common complication (occurring in about 20 per cent of dogs with amyloidosis), pulmonary thromboembolism often results in sudden death, and embolism of other arteries can result in major organ dysfunction. The normal coagulation system is disrupted in glomerular disease by loss of low-molecular-weight clotting factors and antithrombin III in the urine. In addition, hypoalbuminemia and, to a lesser extent, hypercholesterolemia are associated with increased platelet aggregation.

Unfortunately, there is currently no proved (or accepted) method of preventing this complication. Heparin may promote the action of thrombin in the absence of antithrombin III and thus enhance hypercoagulability (Hricik and Smith, 1986). Warfarin has been suggested (Feldman, 1986), but studies of efficacy and complications in dogs are unavailable. Aspirin might be useful, but in people at least, aspirin can suppress renal function, especially if it is used with a sodium-restricted diet (Muther et al., 1981). Thus, at this time no recommendation can be made regarding use of anticoagulants in dogs with severe proteinuria. These drugs are not indicated in dogs that are not hypercoagulable (with normal antithrombin III concentrations or mild to moderate proteinuria).

MANAGEMENT OF ASSOCIATED RENAL FAILURE

The management of generalized renal failure is covered elsewhere (see p. 1195, and *Current Veterinary Therapy IX*, pp. 1167–1173) and will not be reviewed here. However, glomerular diseases have the associated problem of hypoalbuminemia, which is not found in chronic generalized tubulointerstitial diseases. Fluid therapy has the potential to worsen hypoalbuminemia and may worsen or induce edema. Fluid therapy should be used only as needed to correct dehydration or to control uremia.

Previously recommended therapy for canine and feline glomerular disease has been to match dietary protein intake with urine protein output by addition of high-quality protein, such as eggs, to the diet. A similar recommendation was made in human medicine but was questioned because increasing protein intake worsened urine protein loss (Dock, 1974). Currently, restriction of protein intake in glomerulonephritis, as in other chronic renal diseases, is thought to be of benefit in slowing progression of renal injury in humans and laboratory rodents (Oldrizzi et al., 1985; Neugarten et al., 1983; Brenner et al., 1982). The relationship of dietary protein intake to progression of canine glomerulonephritis or renal amyloidosis is not known.

SPECIFIC THERAPY

The first aspect of specific therapy for both amyloidosis and glomerulonephritis should be to identify and eliminate, if possible, any underlying chronic inflammatory or neoplastic disease. If the underlying disease can be controlled prior to the onset of renal failure, the glomerular lesions may regress. If the disease has already resulted in renal failure, progression usually continues even if the underlying disease is successfully treated. Some diseases to consider are pyometra, ehrlichiosis, dirofilariasis, bacterial endocarditis, neoplasia, and systemic lupus erythematosus. If an underlying disease cannot be identified or is not reversible, other specific therapy can be considered.

RENAL AMYLOIDOSIS

Two drugs have recently been studied for specific treatment of renal amyloidosis: dimethyl sulfoxide (DMSO) and colchicine. The mode of action of colchicine is to block further amyloid formation. This drug has been most successfully used in early treatment of familial Mediterranean fever in humans (Zemer et al., 1986). The drug was not effective if people were nephrotic or uremic. The authors have no experience in using this drug for renal amyloidosis.

DMSO was first reported to dissolve amyloid fibrils in laboratory rodents. This effect has since been questioned, and a primary anti-inflammatory action has been proposed. Potential side effects include an unpleasant odor, perivascular inflammation, local thrombosis, and pain on subcutaneous injection of the 90 per cent product.

In people, the drug has usually been given orally

as a 10 per cent solution at 80 mg/kg/day for months to years. One recent review reported improvement in 7 of 23 human patients with AA amyloid (the type of amyloid reported in dogs to date) (Gruys et al., 1981).

Five cases of canine amyloidosis treated with DMSO have been reported. In four cases DMSO was used orally at 300 mg/kg/day (Gruys et al., 1981). One dog was stable for at least 10 months. The other three dogs progressed to uremia in 3 to 9 months, a result indicating no improvement over the natural history of the disease. No decrease in amyloid deposition was found in dogs that died. In another report, a dog lived for 5 yr after diagnosis (Spyridakis et al., 1986). Cause of death at 13 yr of age was unknown. Treatment consisted of 80 mg/kg/day of DMSO injected three times per week for 1 yr subcutaneously and then applied topically for the rest of the dog's life. Serum albumin level increased, urine protein concentration decreased, and the dog appeared normal to its owners. However, urine protein excretion remained greatly increased above normal throughout the follow-up period (2 yr). One reservation about the efficacy of DMSO in this case is that several potential underlying diseases (Sertoli's cell tumor and chronic skin disease) were also controlled at the time DMSO was initiated. The only side effect noted in either study was the unpleasant odor.

DMSO has been used in an additional six patients by the authors and in one patient being treated by a colleague.* Two of these patients had azotemia, all had hypoalbuminemia, and one was nephrotic. All had been sick less than 2 months. None of the animals were uremic at time of treatment. Of these seven patients, two being treated orally developed gastrointestinal disturbances within 2 weeks and DMSO was discontinued. In two patients, the disease continued to progress over 2 to 6 months. The conditions of three patients improved with regard to urine protein excretion, but, to date, none have returned to normalcy (two are still being followed after 14 months and 2 months). In the other dog, the owners discontinued therapy after 1 month because of the odor. The dog that has been followed for 14 months progressed slowly to become azotemic while receiving oral DMSO over 7 months. Route of administration was changed to subcutaneous, and the dog's condition has remained stable for 7 months.

In conclusion, existing experience with DMSO for treatment of canine renal amyloidosis is limited. The drug is apparently not curative and does not benefit all cases. Whether it has any benefit is questionable, although the survival of two treated animals for longer than 1 year and the absence of side effects has prompted continuation of the trial.

*Dr. Paul G. Cavanagh, DACVIM, Westside Veterinary Center, New York, New York.

GLOMERULONEPHRITIS

Specific therapy of glomerulonephritis in humans has focused on use of immunosuppressive drugs and, in particular, glucocorticoids. In recent years, interest has also focused on use of anticoagulants. In people, many retrospective and prospective studies have been done on each subcategory of glomerulonephritis. Results of these studies sometimes differ, and controversies exist. Months of therapy with glucocorticoids, other immunosuppressive therapy, or both are often required before benefit is noted. Specific risks of steroid therapy in renal diseases are aggravation of azotemia and hypertension, in addition to risks associated with steroid use for any purpose.

Unfortunately, no prospective and few retrospective studies of treatment of canine glomerulonephritis are available. A prospective trial of cyclosporine directed by one of the authors (S.V.) is in progress. Retrospective studies of the efficacy of glucocorticoids in dogs and cats have suggested little benefit; however, little information was given concerning dose, duration, or route of therapy, and the number of cases evaluated was small. One study stated that the prevalence of glucocorticoid excess in animals with glomerulonephritis indicated that these drugs would not be effective (Center et al., 1987). However, glucocorticoid excess was usually due to adrenal tumors or therapy for chronic inflammatory diseases. Both neoplasia and chronic inflammation are in themselves causes for glomerulonephritis. In addition, none of the six cases with severe glomerulonephritis (nephrotic syndrome) had a history of glucocorticoid use.

Only four cases of idiopathic glomerulonephritis have been followed by the authors during 5 yr. Three of these were classified as membranous. One was treated symptomatically, recovered, and has remained normal (5-yr follow-up). Two were treated with prednisolone, beginning at 2.2 mg/kg/day for 2 to 3 weeks and then tapered to alternate-day administration at decreasing dosages. In one dog urine protein loss decreased and plasma albumin concentration increased to normal. The dog was euthanatized after 2.5 yr because of other signs of aging, at which time it had mild azotemia and mild hypoalbuminemia. In the other case, serum albumin and BUN levels increased slightly, with no change in serum creatinine concentration. Glucocorticoids were discontinued after 3 months and BUN level returned to normal. The dog's condition continued to improve and was reported to be normal 2 yr after initial diagnosis. The fourth case was due to chronic, cresenteric, proliferative glomerulonephritis. The dog was azotemic when diagnosed, and azotemia worsened with initial steroid therapy. Steroid dose was reduced by 50 per cent, and the dog's condition stabilized temporarily, with death occurring from uremia after 2 months.

In conclusion, although immunosuppressive therapy is generally considered effective for some forms of glomerulonephritis in humans, glucocorticoids have not been shown to have any efficacy over symptomatic therapy in glomerulonephritis in dogs to date. Further prospective trials are needed to determine efficacious therapy for canine glomerulonephritis.

References and Supplemental Reading

Benson, M. D., Dwulet, F. E., and DiBartola, S. P.: Identification and characterization of amyloid protein AA in spontaneous canine amyloidosis. Lab. Invest. 52:448, 1985.

Brenner, B. M., Meyer, T. W., and Hostetter, T. H.: Dietary protein intake and the progressive nature of kidney disease. N. Engl. J. Med. 307:652, 1982.

Center, S. A., Smith, C. A., Wilkinson, E., et al.: Clinicopathologic, renal immunofluorescent, and light microscopic features of glomerulonephritis in the dog: 41 cases (1975–1985). J.A.V.M.A. 190:81, 1987.

DeSchepper, J., Hoorens, J., Mattheeuws, D., et al.: Glomerulonephritis and the nephrotic syndrome in a dog. Vet. Rec. 95:433, 1974.

DiBartola, S. P., and Chew, D. J.: Glomerular disease in the dog and cat. In Kirk, R. W. (ed.): Current Veterinary Therapy IX. Philadelphia: W. B. Saunders, 1986, pp. 1132–1138.

Dock, W.: Proteinuria: The story of 2809 years of trials, errors, and rectifications. Bull. N.Y. Acad. Sci. 50:659, 1974.

Feldman, B. F.: Thrombosis—diagnosis and treatment. In Kirk R. W. (ed.): Current Veterinary Therapy IX. Philadelphia: W. B. Saunders, 1986, pp. 505–509.

Finco, D. R., Barsanti, J. A., and Rawlings, C. A.: Effects of immunosuppressive drug therapy on blood urea nitrogen concentrations of dogs with azotemia. J.A.V.M.A. 185:664, 1984.

Gruys, E., Sijens, R. J., and Biewenga, W. J.: Dubious effect of dimethylsulphoxide on amyloid deposits and amyloidosis. Vet. Res. Commun. 5:21, 1981.

Green, R. A., Russo, E. A., Greene, R. T., et al.: Hypoalbuminemia-related platelet hypersensitivity in two dogs with nephrotic syndrome. J.A.V.M.A. 186:485, 1985.

Hricik, D. E., and Smith, M. C.: Proteinuria and the Nephrotic Syndrome. Chicago: Year Book Medical Publishers, 1986, p. 168.

Jaenke, R. S., and Allen, T. A.: Membranous nephropathy in the dog. Vet. Pathol. 23:718, 1986.

Kaufman, C. E.: Fluid and electrolyte abnormalities in nephrotic syndrome. Postgrad. Med. 76:135, 1984.

MacDougall, D. F., Cook, T., Steward, A. P., et al.: Canine chronic renal disease: Prevalence and types of glomerulonephritis in the dog. Kidney Int. 29:1144, 1986.

Muther, R. S., Potter, D. M., and Bennett, W. M.: Aspirin-induced depression of glomerular filtration rate in normal humans: Role of sodium balance. Ann. Intern. Med. 94:317, 1981.

Neugarten, J., Feiner, H. D., Schacht, R. G., et al.: Amelioration of experimental glomerulonephritis by dietary protein restriction. Kidney Int. 24:595, 1983.

Oldrizzi, L., Rugiu, C., Valvo, E., et al.: Progression of renal failure in patients with renal disease of diverse etiology on a protein restricted diet. Kidney Int. 27:553, 1985.

Osborne, C. A., and Vernier, R. L.: Glomerulonephritis in the dog and cat: A comparative review. J. Am. Anim. Hosp. Assoc. 9:101, 1973.

Osborne, C. A., Johnson, K. H., Perman, V., et al.: Clinicopathologic progression of renal amyloidosis in a dog. J.A.V.M.A. 157:203, 1970.

Osborne, C. A., Hammer, R. F., Resnick, J. S., et al.: Natural remission of nephrotic syndrome in a dog with immune complex glomerular disease. J.A.V.M.A. 168:129, 1976.

Rouse, B. T., and Lewis, R. J.: Canine glomerulonephritis: Prevalence in dogs submitted at random for euthanasia. Can. J. Comp. Med. 39:365, 1975.

Russo, E. A.: Assessment of proteinuria in the dog and cat. In Kirk, R. W. (ed.): Current Veterinary Therapy IX. Philadelphia: W. B. Saunders, 1986, pp. 1111–1114.

Spyridakis, L., Brown, S., Barsanti, J. A., et al.: Amyloidosis in a dog: Treatment with dimethylsulfoxide. J.A.V.M.A. 189:690, 1986.

Wright, N. G., Nash, A. S., Thompson, H., et al.: Membranous nephropathy in the cat and dog. Lab. Invest. 45:269, 1981.

Zemer, D., Pras, M., Sohar, E., et al.: Colchicine in the prevention and treatment of the amyloidosis of familial Mediterranean fever. N. Engl. J. Med. 314:1001, 1986.

MEDICAL MANAGEMENT OF URATE UROLITHS

DAVID F. SENIOR, B.V.Sc.

Gainesville, Florida

Urate salts are a major component of 2 to 8 per cent of urinary stones in dogs. About 60 per cent of urate stones occur in Dalmatian dogs, whereas 40 per cent occur in other breeds. Although urate stones in non-Dalmatian dogs are most often associated with a portosystemic vascular anomaly, other possible causes include Dalmatianlike nucleic acid metabolism, liver failure, or unknown predisposing factors. Most urate stones in dogs are composed of ammonium urate; sodium urate and uric acid stones have been reported rarely. As in all urinary stone formation, the driving force leading to precipitation is supersaturation of urine with the salts of crystals

in the stone. Thus, the presence of excessive urinary ammonium or urate ion, or both, in urine is a major risk factor.

In most dogs, approximately 90 per cent of urate formed from degradation of nucleic acids is converted to allantoin in the liver. In Dalmatian dogs, hepatic uricase activity is diminished so that only 14 to 50 per cent of urate formed from nucleic acid metabolism is converted to allantoin. The 24-hr urinary excretion of urate in Dalmatian dogs is 400 to 600 mg, compared with approximately 60 mg in non-Dalmatian dogs of similar size. When allantoin and urate undergo subsequent urinary excretion, allantoin, being very soluble, remains in solution, whereas urate is relatively insoluble and may precipitate out as uric acid, as sodium urate, or most commonly in the dog as ammonium urate.

Ammonium ion is secreted into the renal tubular lumen as a buffer for secreted hydronium ion (H^+). Ammonium ion excretion is enhanced when an acid load is excreted, as would be typical after an animal protein meal. Thus, Dalmatian dogs fed animal protein excrete increased amounts of both urate and ammonium, which predisposes to urinary ammonium urate precipitation. Although increased ammonium and urate ion are the main risk factors for precipitation, other cations in solution may also interact to a lesser extent. Some dogs with high urate output fail to produce stones, suggesting that stone formation may be enhanced in the absence of a precipitation inhibitor. One candidate for such inhibition is urinary glycosaminoglycan (GAG), which tends to coat urate salt particles with a negatively charged outer layer, thus reducing their tendency to coalesce. However, it is not known if changes of urinary GAGs alter urate stone formation in the dog, and other promoters and inhibitors may be involved.

Yorkshire terrier and miniature schnauzer dogs with portosystemic vascular anomaly are the most common non-Dalmatian dogs with ammonium urate stones. Affected dogs have hyperuricuria and hyperammonuria, presumably because of inadequate hepatic conversion of urate and ammonia to allantoin and urea, respectively. A similar pathogenesis may operate when acquired liver disease leads to extrahepatic shunting of portal blood.

DIAGNOSIS

The mineral content of urinary stones must be established before planning strategies of stone dissolution and prevention. Historical evidence can be valuable. Seventy-five per cent of all stones in adult Dalmatian dogs are composed of urate. A clinical history suggestive of portosystemic vascular anomaly is important, particularly in Yorkshire terriers with stone disease.

If stone material is available, the physical appearance may help. Urate stones are generally smooth, oval to rounded, various shades of green-brown, and often arranged in laminations—hard brittle concentric shells that can be peeled off one after the other. However, all stone material should be submitted to a laboratory capable of performing definitive crystallographic analysis of composition. Dalmatian dogs that form urate stones often void small rounded stone particles that may be seen if a large urine specimen is filtered through a gauze sponge. On examination of the urine sediment, both the

rounded spherulytic and "thorn apple" forms of ammonium urate crystals may be seen.

On radiographic examination, urate stones are relatively radiolucent. However, variable degrees of incorporation of other, more radiodense crystals into the stone, such as struvite or calcium salts, can cause some urate stones to be radiopaque. The radiographic evaluation may need to include intravenous pyelography, double-contrast cystography, and retrograde urethrography, as well as ultrasonography, to completely define the location of urate stones throughout the urinary tract. Patients with portosystemic vascular anomaly frequently have concurrent renal and cystic urate calculi.

MANAGEMENT

Male dogs with urate stones frequently have urethral obstruction, necessitating various emergency procedures such as urethral catheterization, back flushing, urethrohydropropulsion, urethrotomy, and urethrostomy. In patients in stable condition with no urethral outflow obstruction, urate stones can be managed surgically or by nonsurgical dissolution. As urate stones are often small and numerous, complete removal of all stones at surgery may be difficult. A combination of surgical treatment followed by medical dissolution can be used to eliminate all stone material from the urinary tract.

Several factors should be considered in deciding between surgical and nonsurgical treatment, including risk of anesthesia; contraindications to dietary modification and drug administration; owner commitment to prolonged, close dietary management; and the relative expense of either method in the individual hospital setting.

Dissolution of Ammonium Urate Stones in Dalmatian Dogs

To achieve stone dissolution, urine must be undersaturated with respect to stone salts, and the rate of dissolution is dependent on the degree of undersaturation. Dissolution is fastest when the activities* of ammonium and urate ions in urine are reduced to their lowest possible levels. To obtain extreme undersaturation, three strategies are combined: (1) feeding of a low-protein–high-sodium diet, (2) urinary alkalinization, and (3) treatment with allopurinol (Table 1).

The commercial stone dissolution diet (Prescrip-

---

*Activity of an ion refers to the amount of free ion in solution. As many ions tend to bind to a variable extent with one another in a complex solution, such as urine, the activity of ions, such as ammonium and urate, will be less than the chemically measured concentration.

Table 1. *Medical Dissolution of Urate Stones in Dalmatian Dogs*

1. Prescription Diet Canine s/d (Hill's Pet Products) exclusively
   Goal: urine specific gravity, ≤ 1.015; BUN, ≤ 10 mg/dl
2. NaHCO$_3$, 0.5–1 gm (1/8–1/4 tsp)/5 kg t.i.d. PO
   Goal: urine pH of 7.0–7.5
3. Allopurinol, 7–10 mg/kg t.i.d. PO
   Goal: urine urate-creatinine ratio reduced by 50%

tion Diet Canine s/d, Hill's Pet Products) reduces daily urate output while urine volume is increased, resulting in a marked reduction in urinary urate activity. As dogs fed this diet tend to produce acidic urine, an alkalinizing agent should be given to effect so that urinary pH is between 7.0 and 7.5, thereby reducing tubular production of ammonia and diminishing the tendency of ammonium urate to precipitate. The dose of bicarbonate required to achieve such a urine pH must be adjusted for individual animals. A reasonable starting dose, which may require subsequent adjustment, is 0.5 to 1 mg (1/8 to 1/4 tsp)/5 kg every 8 hr orally mixed with food.

The xanthine oxidase inhibitor allopurinol (Zyloprim, Burroughs Wellcome) shifts excretion of nucleic acid metabolites toward hypoxanthine and xanthine from predominantly urate, so that more hypoxanthine and xanthine and less urate are excreted each day. Allopurinol should be given at 7 to 10 mg/kg every 8 hr orally for the duration of the dissolution period.

Several preliminary tests should be performed to determine the safety of a medical approach and to establish baseline information prior to commencing a dissolution protocol. A low-protein–high-sodium diet may cause congestive heart failure patients to decompensate, liver failure patients to develop edema, and renal failure patients to develop hypertension. Cardiac function should be assessed with thoracic radiographs, electrocardiography (ECG), and echocardiography; routine liver and kidney function tests should be performed; and blood pressure should be measured. Reasonable baseline information should include estimation of urinary pH and specific gravity of urine collected in the morning prior to the first meal, examination of the urine sediment for evidence of infection, and estimation of the urinary urate-creatinine ratio (usually about 0.5 to 0.6 before treatment in Dalmatian dogs). Radiographic documentation of stone location, size, and number should be obtained; contrast studies and ultrasonography may be necessary for complete information when the stones are relatively radiolucent.

Patients receiving a dissolution protocol should undergo routine follow-up examinations every 3 to 4 weeks throughout the treatment period to assess adverse effects and determine progress in dissolution. Particular attention should be paid to signs of pulmonary edema, including a moist cough and reduced exercise tolerance, as well as peripheral edema and ascites. Urine should be collected in the morning prior to the first daily meal for determination of pH, specific gravity, composition of urine sediment, and urate-creatinine ratio. If urine pH is outside the desired 7.0 to 7.5 range, adjustment in bicarbonate supplementation should be made. Extremely alkaline urine could be due to infection with a urease-producing organism. Dogs fed a stone dissolution diet (Prescription Diet Canine s/d, Hill's Pet Products) develop a degree of polydipsia and polyuria, and the urine specific gravity should be less than 1.015. Values significantly higher than this may indicate that alternative food is being consumed. The urine sediment should not contain ammonium urate crystals. The urinary urate-creatinine ratio should be at least 50 per cent lower than the pretreatment value. Higher values indicate failure to reduce daily urinary urate excretion owing to failure to maintain the strict diet or failure to give allopurinol at the correct dosage. However, individual animals may not decrease urate output in response to the diet and may not absorb or respond to allopurinol as expected. In such cases, the dosage of allopurinol can be gradually increased until the urate-creatinine ratio is 0.25 to 0.3 or about 50 per cent of the pretreatment value. The possibility that the dog is eating an alternative higher-protein diet can be assessed by measuring the blood urea nitrogen (BUN), which should be less than 10 mg/dl when a low-protein–high-sodium diet (Prescription Diet Canine s/d, Hill's Pet Products) is fed exclusively. When values inconsistent with rapid stone dissolution are found repeatedly, owner compliance may be an insurmountable problem and consideration should be given to a surgical rather than a medical approach to stone disease.

Stone size should be documented radiographically at regular intervals to assess progress in dissolution, and contrast radiography and ultrasonography may be required when the stones are relatively radiolucent. If no dissolution is apparent after 6 to 8 weeks, the stone material may not be composed of ammonium urate. Stone composition should be reassessed for alternative dissolution strategies, or the stone disease can be treated surgically. The full dissolution protocol should be continued for 4 weeks after the first radiographic evidence of complete dissolution.

Dissolution of Urate Stones in Dogs with Portosystemic Vascular Anomaly

A safe, effective method for dissolution of urate stones has yet to be established for dogs with portosystemic vascular anomaly because such patients present special problems. Very-low-protein, high-sodium diets may induce hypoalbuminemia and edema, and alkalinization of the food may cause hepatoencephalopathy, although the latter is less likely when a low-protein diet is fed. Furthermore, impaired hepatic conversion of allopurinol to oxypurinol may alter the effectiveness of allopurinol as a xanthine oxidase inhibitor.

In several instances, dogs with portosystemic vascular anomaly have been reported to spontaneously dissolve urate stones when fed a moderately low-protein–salt-restricted diet (Prescription Diet Canine k/d, Hill's Pet Products) alone with no other medication. The reliability with which this diet may induce urate stone dissolution in this setting is not known.

Surgical correction of portosystemic vascular anomaly may improve liver function and reduce urinary ammonium and urate excretion. If urine becomes undersaturated with respect to ammonium and urate ions, ammonium urate stones should dissolve spontaneously.

Prevention of Ammonium Urate Stones

Urate stones tend to recur frequently after dissolution or surgical resection, and life-long preventive measures may be required in many dogs. The principles of prevention are similar to those of dissolution in that the activity of ammonium and urate ions in urine must be reduced. However, ionic activity in urine need not be reduced to such low levels as those required to induce dissolution, because a more concentrated solution is required to initiate stone formation than to make existing stones grow. The precise degree of reduction required to guarantee prevention is not clear and may vary among individual animals if crystallization and crystal growth inhibitors vary among animals. Thus, recommendations for prevention remain empirical and are based on past effectiveness rather than precise physicochemical data.

Table 2. Prevention of Urate Stones in Dalmatian Dogs

1. Allopurinol, 7–10 mg/kg t.i.d. PO
     Goal: urine urate-creatinine ratio reduced by 50%
2. NaHCO$_3$, 0.5–1 gm (1/8–1/4 tsp)/5 kg t.i.d. PO
     Goal: urine pH, 7.0–7.5
3. Increased urine volume: add salt, 1 gm (1/6 tsp)/5 kg daily, and/or add water to food
     Goal: urine specific gravity, ≤ 1.025

A prevention protocol based on (1) administration of allopurinol, (2) alkalinization of urine, and (3) increased urine volume has been successful in the author's clinic (Table 2). Allopurinol should be given at 7 to 10 mg/kg every 8 hr orally to reduce urinary urate output. The effect of a given dose tends to vary among individual animals, and the aim should be to halve the daily urate output. Progress toward this goal can be monitored by measuring the urate concentration in 24-hr urine specimens or more simply by estimating the urinary urate-creatinine ratio of the morning urine. Ideally, the ratio should decrease by half, and the dose of allopurinol should be adjusted to meet this criterion. Usual values would be a reduction from a pretreatment value of 0.5 to 0.6 to a ratio of about 0.25 to 0.3. Further reduction in urinary urate output with increased doses of allopurinol is possible but not recommended, because several instances of xanthine stone formation have been observed in Dalmatian dogs given excessive allopurinol to prevent urate stones.

Alkalinization of the urine to pH of 7.0 to 7.5 reduces tubular ammonia production. This can be achieved by adding bicarbonate (NaHCO$_3$), 1 mg (1/4 tsp)/5 kg every 8 hr orally with food. Urine volume may be increased by adding salt to the diet, 1 mg (1/6 tsp)/5 kg daily, or more effectively by mixing water with food so that the urine specific gravity is equal to or less than 1.025.

Recently a low-protein–alkaline ash diet (Prescription Diet Canine u/d, Hill's Pet Products) has been formulated to include potassium citrate as an alkalinizing agent. Such a diet may be useful in urate stone prevention, but its effectiveness as a single strategy to control urate stone formation requires validation.

References and Supplemental Reading

Kruger, J. M., and Osborne, C. A.: Etiopathogenesis of uric acid and ammonium urate uroliths in non-Dalmatian dogs. Vet. Clin. North Am. 16:87, 1986.

Ling, G. V., and Ruby, A. L.: Canine uroliths: Analysis of data derived from 813 specimens. Vet. Clin. North Am. 16:303, 1986.

Osborne, C. A., Clinton, C. W., Bamman, L. K., et al.: Prevalence of canine uroliths: Minnesota Urolith Center. Vet. Clin. North Am. 16:27, 1986.

Osborne, C. A., Kruger, J. M., Johnston, G. R., and Polzin, D. J.: Dissolution of canine ammonium urate uroliths. Vet. Clin. North Am. [Small Anim. Pract.] 16:375, 1986.

Schaible, R. H.: Genetic predisposition to purine uroliths in Dalmatian dogs. Vet. Clin. North Am. 16:127, 1986.

Senior, D. F., and Finlayson, B.: Initiation and growth of uroliths. Vet. Clin. North Am. 16:19, 1986.

CANINE CALCIUM OXALATE UROLITHIASIS

Detection, Treatment, and Prevention

JODY P. LULICH, D.V.M.,
CARL A. OSBORNE, D.V.M.,
St. Paul, Minnesota

MARY LOU PARKER, M.B.A., M.T.(A.S.C.P.),
CHRIS W. CLINTON, M.T.,
and MARIAN P. DAVENPORT, M.L.T.
Houston, Texas

MINERAL COMPOSITION

Although different combinations of calcium oxalate salts have been identified in canine uroliths, the predominant form encountered by the authors has been calcium oxalate monohydrate (Table 1). Calcium oxalate dihydrate urolithiasis appears to occur more frequently in humans than in dogs. The significance of this observation has not been determined.

The importance of differentiating calcium oxalate monohydrate from calcium oxalate dihydrate in canine uroliths remains to be established. In humans, it has been suggested that detection of calcium oxalate dihydrate on the outside of a urolith is indicative of recent formation, whereas detection of external layers of calcium oxalate monohydrate indicates lack of recent urolith formation. If valid, this hypothesis would be of clinical significance because it would help to determine the persistence of disorders leading to calcium oxalate urolith formation, and therefore the need for continuous therapy to minimize urolith recurrence. In one study, human patients with calcium oxalate dihydrate uroliths had more urolith recurrences than patients with calcium oxalate monohydrate uroliths, although it has been suggested that calcium oxalate dihydrate may form initially and then be converted to calcium oxalate monohydrate (Schubert, 1981).

APPLIED PHYSICAL CHEMISTRY

Salts are neutral compounds derived from the reversible interaction of a proton donor (such as calcium) and a proton acceptor (such as oxalic acid). The ability of a salt to dissolve in solution is dependent on the concentration of its ions in solution and its interaction with other ions and neutral molecules in the solution.

To illustrate these principles, let pure water represent the solution and calcium oxalate (CaOx) represent the salt. When adding CaOx to water, small amounts dissolve completely because water is *undersaturated* with calcium and oxalate ions (Fig. 1). As more CaOx is added, the water's capacity to dissolve additional CaOx is decreased until the solution becomes *saturated*. In this context, saturation of the solution with calcium and oxalate ions occurs when no additional CaOx can be dissolved at a given pH and temperature of the solution. If additional CaOx is added, it will appear as a solid.

CaOx can also be dissolved in undersaturated urine. However, unlike water, urine is a complex solution containing a unique combination of ionic and nonionic molecules, which may alter solubility. Therefore, addition of CaOx beyond the point of saturation may be associated with further dissolution. Thus, the solution becomes *supersaturated* with calcium and oxalate ions. Supersaturation is conceptually significant because the solution contains enough energy to form solids from dissolved ions (i.e., it is thermodynamically unstable). One method by which the solution returns to thermodynamic stability is by concentrating unwanted calcium and oxalate ions as solids or crystals on preexisting surfaces or templates (e.g., other crystals or foreign material). However, if by addition of more calcium and oxalate ions the solution becomes *oversaturated*, CaOx crystals will form without an existing template. After crystals have formed, available thermodynamic energy favors further crystal growth until the solution again returns to thermodynamic stability (or saturation). Of course, crystal

1182

Table 1. Breed Distribution of Dogs with Calcium Oxalate Urolithiasis

					Calcium Oxalate Uroliths†						
	All Uroliths*				CaOxm		CaOxD		CaOxM/CaOxD		
Number of all Uroliths in Breed	Percentage of all Uroliths in Breed	Number of CaOx Uroliths in Breed	Percentage of CaOx Uroliths in Breed	Breed	100%	70–99%	100%	70–99%	100%	70–99%	Total %
					(Percentage of Breed/Percentage of All Dogs with CaOx Uroliths)						
374	19.7	83	22.2	Miniature schnauzer	14.4/4.8	30/10	6/2	9.6/3.2	24/8	15.7/5.2	100/33.3
174	9.2	22	12.7	Miniature poodle	4.5/0.4	68.2/6	4.5/0.4	9.1/0.8	4.5/0.4	9.1/0.8	100/8.8
66	3.5	17	25.8	Yorkshire	23.5/1.6	17.6/1.2	17.6/1.2	29.4/2	11.8/0.8	0	100/6.8
51	2.7	16	31.4	Lhasa apso	25/1.6	0	31.2/2	25/1.6	0	18.8/1.2	100/6.4
80	4.2	11	13.8	Shih tzu	18.2/0.8	45.4/2	18.2/0.8	9.1/0.4	9.1/0.4	0	100/4.42
14	0.7	7	50	Chihuahua	28.6/0.8	28.6/0.8	14.3/0.4	0	0	28.6/0.8	100/2.81
33	1.7	7	21.2	Pekingese	42.8/1.2	14.3/0.4	14.3/0.4	14.3/0.4	14.3/0.4	0	100/2.81
66	3.5	6	9.1	Daschund	0	50/1.2	0	16.7/0.4	16.7/0.4	16.7/0.4	100/2.41
16	0.8	5	31.2	Pug	0	40/0.8	0	60/1.2	0	0	100/2
63	3.3	4	6.3	Dalmatian	75/1.2	25/0.4	0	0	0	0	100/1.6
14	0.7	4	28.6	Pomeranian	25/0.4	25/0.4	0	0	25/0.4	25/0.4	100/1.6
33	1.7	3	9.1	Bichon frise	0	66.7/0.8	0	0	33.3/0.4	0	100/1.2
4	0.2	3	75	Boston terrier	0	33.3/0.4	0	33.3/0.4	0	33.3/0.4	100/1.2
69	3.6	3	4.3	Cocker spaniel	33.3/0.4	0	0	0	66.7/0.8	0	100/1.2
6	0.3	3	50	Collie	0	66.7/0.8	33.3/0.4	0	0	0	100/1.2
34	1.8	2	59	Beagle	50/0.4	0	0	0	0	50/0.4	100/0.8
6	0.3	2	33.3	Fox terrier	0	50/0.4	0	0	0	50/0.4	100/0.8
21	1.1	2	9.5	Sheltie	50/0.4	50/0.4	0	0	0	0	100/0.8
127	6.7	11	8.7	Eleven breeds‡	18.2/0.8	18.2/0.8	18.2/0.8	18.2/0.8	0	27.3/1.2	100/4.4
310	16.3	30	9.7	Mixed	16.7/2	30/3.6	3.3/0.4	13.3/1.6	16.7/2	20/2.4	100/12
138	7.3	8	5.8	Unknown	12.5/0.4	62.5/2	0	12.5/0.4	0	12.5/0.4	100/3.2
198	10.4	0	0	Unobserved	0	0	0	0	0	0	0
1897	ND	249	13.12	Total	ND/17.2	ND/32.4	ND/9.2	ND/13.2	ND/14	ND/13.6	ND/100

CaOxM, Calcium oxalate monohydrate; CaOxD, calcium oxalate dihydrate; ND, not determined.

*1897 uroliths submitted to the Minnesota Urolith Center, University of Minnesota, College of Veterinary Medicine, St. Paul, MN 55108. All uroliths were analyzed by optical diffraction or x-ray crystallography.

†249 CaOx uroliths evaluated.

‡Only one calcium oxalate urolith observed in each breed.

retention within the urinary tract is a requirement for further crystal growth.

Urine is a complex solution containing "inert" ions (phosphate, sulfate, sodium, potassium, and magnesium) that are unlikely to chemically bond with calcium and oxalate and thereby increase CaOx solubility. The negative ions (phosphate and sulfate) surround positive calcium ions, and the positive ions (sodium, potassium, and magnesium) surround negative oxalate ions. The net effect is a decrease in attraction between calcium and oxalate ions. Because calcium and oxalate ion interaction is required for crystal formation, the solubility of calcium oxalate increases as the concentration of inert ions increases (Fig. 1).

Supersaturation of urine with certain calculogenic ions is also dependent on another group of substances called crystallization inhibitors. These include citrate and pyrophosphates, which chelate calcium. Likewise, certain mucoproteins, glycosoaminoglycans, and other poorly identified substances may interact with calcium. The result is a decrease in the amount of calcium available to bind with oxalate (and phosphate). These inhibitors have been found to be deficient in some calcium oxalate urolith–forming people.

Urine pH also influences crystal formation and growth. Maximal CaOx crystal formation occurs in urine with pH values ranging from 4.5 to 5.5. However, urine pH values greater than 6.5 are associated with a significant decline in CaOx crystal

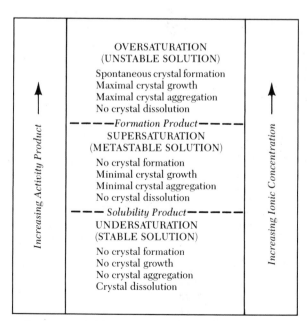

Figure 1. Probable events of calcium oxalate crystallization in relation to increasing activity product and ionic concentration.

formation. In alkaline urine *calcium phosphate* crystal formation is increased. Complexing of available calcium ions with phosphate ions may explain how alkaline urine decreases CaOx crystal formation.

EPIDEMIOLOGY

Canine calcium oxalate uroliths have been encountered in approximately 6 to 10 per cent of the dogs in the United States. Of 1897 uroliths submitted to the Minnesota Urolith Center and analyzed by optical diffraction and x-ray crystallography, 249 (13.1 per cent) contained at least 70 per cent calcium oxalate (see Table 1). Of 249 calcium oxalate uroliths, 124 (50 per cent) were calcium oxalate monohydrate, 55 (22 per cent) were calcium oxalate dihydrate, and 70 (28 per cent) were a mixture of calcium oxalate monohydrate and calcium oxalate dihydrate.

Approximately 70 per cent of calcium oxalate uroliths are encountered in males and approximately 30 per cent in females; most are seen in older dogs (mean age, 8 to 9 yr). They have been most commonly observed in miniature schnauzers, miniature poodles, Yorkshire terriers, Lhasa apsos, Shih tzus, and Dalmatians (see Table 1). Common breeds *not* represented include the boxer, bulldog, golden retriever, Irish setter, Labrador retriever, Samoyed, and springer spaniel. However, lack of data about the popularity of various breeds in areas from which uroliths were obtained precludes formulation of meaningful generalities about the relative risk for calcium oxalate uroliths in these breeds.

ETIOPATHOGENESIS

Current information about the etiopathogenesis of calcium oxalate uroliths has been primarily based on studies in humans and laboratory animals. Factors incriminated in calcium oxalate urolithiasis include hypercalciuria, hyperoxaluria, and hyperuricuria. Although studies in people may serve as valuable models, appropriate caution must be used in extrapolating this information for use in dogs.

Hypercalciuria

In dogs, hypercalciuria is the single most important condition predisposing to calcium oxalate urolith formation. This conclusion is based on the following: (1) As the concentration of ionic calcium increases, urine supersaturation and oversaturation are achieved, promoting calcium oxalate crystal formation and growth. (2) Continued hypercalciuria is associated with urolith recurrence. In people, therapy that decreases the ionic concentration of

calcium in urine is associated with amelioration of urolith recurrence.

Normocalcemic hypercalciuria is thought to result from either intestinal hyperabsorption of calcium (so-called absorptive hypercalciuria) or decreased renal tubular reabsorption of calcium (so-called renal leak hypercalciuria). In contrast, *hypercalcemic hypercalciuria* results from an increased glomerular filtration of calcium, which overwhelms normal renal tubular reabsorptive mechanisms (so-called resorptive hypercalciuria, because excessive bone resorption is associated with elevated serum calcium concentrations).

NORMOCALCEMIC HYPERCALCIURIA

In the authors' series, normocalcemic hypercalciuria has been a much more common finding in dogs with calcium oxalate uroliths than hypercalcemic hypercalciuria. Conceptual understanding of the mechanisms involved in the different types of normocalcemic hypercalciuria is of therapeutic importance. Specific treatment to minimize intestinal absorption of calcium may be of benefit to patients with absorptive hypercalciuria. However, it is potentially deleterious to patients with renal leak hypercalciuria, as it may aggravate negative body calcium balance. Likewise, specific treatment designed to enhance renal tubular reabsorption of calcium could be beneficial to patients with renal leak hypercalciuria but could cause hypercalcemia in patients with absorptive hypercalciuria.

The basic defect in human and presumably canine patients with *absorptive hypercalciuria* is intestinal hyperabsorption of calcium. The result is an increase in the quantity of calcium excreted in urine. Not only is there enhanced filtration of calcium, but decreased renal tubular reabsorption of filtered calcium also occurs as a consequence of decreased parathormone secretion by the parathyroid glands. Hypercalciuria represents an appropriate compensatory response to excessive intestinal absorption of calcium to maintain serum calcium concentration within physiologic limits.

People with absorptive hypercalciuria have a normal or low serum parathormone concentration, normal or low urine cyclic adenosine monophosphate (c-AMP) concentration, and normal fasting urine calcium concentration. Preliminary studies of dogs with apparent absorptive hypercalciuria suggest similar findings. Excessive skeletal mobilization of calcium (resorptive hypercalciuria) and renal leak hypercalciuria are unlikely if fasting urine calcium concentration is normal or low (Table 2).

The specific cause of absorptive hypercalciuria is unknown. Both elevated serum concentrations of 1,25-vitamin D_3 (Kaplan, 1977) and a primary intes-

Table 2. Distinguishing Clinical Manifestations for Different Types of Hypercalciuria

Feature	AH	RH	PHPT
Serum calcium	N	N	↑
Serum PTH	↓/N	↑	↑
Serum phosphorus	N/↓	N	↓/↑*
Urine calcium			
Fasting	N	↑	↑‡
Diagnostic diet†	↑	↑	↑
Urine oxalate	N	N	N
Urine uric acid	N	N	N
Bone density‡	N	↓	↓
Calcium balance‡ (total body)	Positive	Negative	Negative

AH, absorptive hypercalciuria; RH, renal leak hypercalciuria; PHPT, primary hyperparathyroidism; PTH, parathormone; N, normal; ↑, increased; ↓, decreased.

*Standard diet used in the evaluation of normal and calcium oxalate urolith dogs.

†As glomerular filtration rate declines, phosphorus is retained in serum.

‡Based on findings in humans (Zerwekh, 1987).

tinal abnormality (Zewekh, 1987) have been suggested.

The basic defect in patients with renal leak hypercalciuria is impaired tubular reabsorption of calcium. The resulting decline in serum calcium concentration causes secondary hyperparathyroidism, enhanced secretion of parathormone (PTH), and subsequent increased synthesis of 1,25-vitamin D$_3$. A secondary increase in intestinal calcium absorption may further contribute to hypercalciuria.

Human patients with renal leak hypercalciuria have elevated serum parathormone concentrations, elevated urine c-AMP concentrations, normocalcemia, and high fasting urine calcium concentrations (see Table 2). The authors have observed one calcium oxalate–forming miniature schnauzer with this pattern. Other findings in people include hypocitraturia and exaggerated calciuric response to carbohydrate ingestion, an abnormal natriuretic response to thiazides, impaired maximal renal concentrating capacity, and normomagnesemic magnesuria.

HYPERCALCEMIC HYPERCALCIURIA

Hypercalcemic hypercalciuria is characterized by excessive filtration and excretion of calcium in urine as a result of hypercalcemia. Hypercalcemic hypercalciuria is a relatively infrequent cause of calcium-containing uroliths in dogs. When uroliths form, they may be composed primarily of calcium phosphate with lesser quantities of calcium oxalate; calcium oxalate uroliths have also been observed.

Potential causes of hypercalcemia in dogs include primary hyperparathyroidism, pseudohyperparathyroidism, malignant lymphoma, vitamin D intoxication, osteolytic neoplasia, and hyperthyroidism. Although several calcium oxalate (and calcium phos-

phate) uroliths have been noted in dogs with primary hyperparathyroidism, calcium-containing uroliths in dogs caused by pseudohyperparathyroidism, vitamin D intoxication, osteolytic neoplasia, or hyperthyroidism have not been found. A calcium apatite urolith was observed in a dog with malignant lymphoma and normal serum calcium concentration.

Hyperuricuria and Hyperoxaluria

Hyperuricuria and hyperoxaluria are less common causes of calcium oxalate uroliths in people. They have not yet been documented in dogs with calcium oxalate uroliths.

DETECTION

Clinical and Laboratory Findings

Clinical findings associated with calcium oxalate urolithiasis are nonspecific and may be related to urinary tract signs caused by uroliths or the underlying cause of hypercalcemia. Clinical findings directly caused by uroliths are dependent on their anatomic location, duration in specific location, and physical characteristics (size, shape, and number). Signs may also be influenced by secondary urinary tract infection.

Urinalysis results may provide clues in the identification of calcium oxalate urolith–forming patients, but lack of evidence does not imply lack of disease. Calcium oxalate monohydrate and calcium oxalate dihydrate crystals may be present or absent. In some instances, only struvite crystals have been detected; they may be caused by secondary infection with urease-producing bacteria. Urine pH of affected patients is variable. Hematuria and pyuria may or may not occur.

Serum calcium concentrations should be determined. Whether serum calcium concentration is normal or not, determination of serum PTH concentration may help to elucidate the underlying mechanism of disease. In normocalcemic patients, low to normal PTH levels are associated with absorptive hypercalciuria, and elevated PTH levels suggest renal leak hypercalciuria. Hyperparathyroidism is suggested by elevations in both serum calcium and PTH concentrations, in the absence of renal failure.

Radiographic Findings

Calcium oxalate uroliths may be detected anywhere in the urinary tract. They are radiodense compared with soft tissue. Calcium oxalate uroliths may be single or multiple and can vary in size from a millimeter to several centimeters in diameter.

Calcium oxalate monohydrate uroliths are usually round or elliptic and have a smooth polished surface. On occasion, they may develop a jackstone shape. Calcium oxalate dihydrate uroliths, and mixed calcium oxalate monohydrate–calcium oxalate dihydrate uroliths, are usually round to ovoid and have an irregular surface caused by protrusion of sharp-edged crystals.

Urine Chemistries

Understanding the etiopathogenesis of calcium oxalate uroliths in dogs is unavoidably linked to the evaluation of the composition of urine (see Table 2). Timed urine collections were performed in 12 dogs with naturally occurring calcium oxalate urolithiasis. None of the affected dogs were hypercalcemic. Ten were hypercalciuric compared with normal beagle dogs consuming the same standard diet.

Partitioning dogs with similar laboratory findings into three groups revealed more meaningful trends. One group of nine dogs had normal urine calcium excretion while fasting, elevated urine calcium excretion while consuming a standard diet, and low to normal serum parathormone concentrations. These findings are consistent with absorptive hypercalciuria. Two dogs in this group had marginally high fasting urine calcium concentrations. In this group, intestinal hyperabsorption may have been more severe.

One miniature schnauzer dog was hypercalciuric during both fasting and standard diet consumption. This dog also had hyperparathormonemia. A primary defect in tubular reabsorption of calcium was hypothesized (renal leak hypercalciuria).

In the third group, two affected normocalciuric dogs had low levels of urine citrate compared with normal beagle dogs evaluated under identical conditions. These dogs may have formed stones as a result of deficits in crystallization inhibitors, one of which is citrate.

BIOLOGIC BEHAVIOR

Clinical experience with recurrent calcium oxalate uroliths suggests that they may grow from subvisual particles to uroliths of sufficient size to cause clinical signs within 2 to 3 months. It has been suggested that calcium oxalate monohydrate uroliths affecting people grow at a slower rate than calcium oxalate dihydrate uroliths. Comparable data are not available for dogs.

Canine calcium oxalate uroliths tend to recur following surgical removal. In one study of dogs, calcium oxalate uroliths recurred in 25 per cent of the patients treated surgically. It has been suggested that pure calcium oxalate dihydrate uroliths recur more frequently than calcium oxalate monohydrate uroliths in people.

MEDICAL TREATMENT AND PREVENTION

In contrast to dissolution of struvite and urate uroliths, which readily occurs when oversaturation of urine with calculogenic substances is abolished, attempts to dissolve calcium oxalate uroliths in dogs have been unsuccessful. In people, it has been suggested that inability to induce dissolution of calcium oxalate uroliths may be related to inability to effectively reduce urine concentration of calcium and oxalate. Although surgical removal remains the most effective method to remove canine calcium oxalate uroliths, some therapeutic modalities found to be effective in people with calcium oxalate uroliths may be cautiously considered to prevent further growth of calcium oxalate uroliths or to minimize their recurrence following removal.

In general, medical treatment should be formulated in stepwise fashion, with the initial goal of reducing the urine concentration of calculogenic substances. Medications that have the potential to induce a sustained alteration in body composition of metabolites, in addition to urine concentration of metabolites, should be reserved for patients with active or frequently recurrent calcium oxalate uroliths. Caution must be used so that side effects of treatment are not more detrimental than the effects of the uroliths.

Dietary Considerations

Although reduction in dietary oxalate or calcium consumption appears to be a logical approach in formulating therapy for calcium oxalate uroliths, it is not necessarily a harmless maneuver. Reducing consumption of only one of these constituents (such as calcium) may be counterproductive because of an increase in the bioavailability of the other (such as oxalate) for absorption and excretion in urine. In general, therefore, reduction in dietary calcium should be accompanied by an appropriate reduction in dietary oxalate.

People with calcium oxalate uroliths are often cautioned to avoid milk and milk products because their carbohydrate component (lactose) may augment intestinal absorption of calcium from any dietary source. Likewise, they are discouraged from consuming foods containing relatively high quantities of oxalate (usually plant foods).

Although there is agreement that excessive consumption of calcium and oxalate should be avoided, urologists agree that it is not advisable to restrict dietary calcium in calcium oxalate urolith formers unless it has been documented that they have absorptive hypercalciuria. Even then, only moderate restriction is advocated, to prevent negative calcium balances in the body.

Consumption of high levels of sodium may augment renal excretion of calcium in humans and dogs (Walser, 1961). Therefore, moderate dietary restriction of sodium is recommended for active calcium oxalate stone formers.

Studies in laboratory animals, dogs, and people suggest that dietary phosphorus should not be restricted in patients with calcium oxalate urolithiasis, because this action may contribute to urolith formation. Reduction in dietary phosphorus is known to augment hypercalciuria.

Although dietary magnesium may contribute to the formation of magnesium ammonium phosphate uroliths in some species (cats, ruminants, and so on), urine magnesium is thought to inhibit formation of calcium oxalate crystals. Pending further studies, magnesium should not be restricted from the diets of dogs with calcium oxalate uroliths.

Ingestion of foods that contain high quantities of animal protein (meat, poultry, and fish) may contribute to calcium oxalate urolithiasis in people by (1) increasing urine calcium concentration, (2) increasing urine uric acid concentration, and (3) decreasing urine citrate concentration. When dogs were fed a diet containing 47 per cent protein (by dry weight), their 24-hr urine calcium excretion was two times higher than that when consuming a 16 per cent protein diet (by dry weight). Therefore, excessive dietary protein consumption should be avoided in dogs with active calcium oxalate urolithiasis.

The canine calculolytic diet designed to induce struvite urolith dissolution (Canine s/d, Hill's Pet Products) has been evaluated in three dogs with confirmed calcium oxalate uroliths. After periods of treatment ranging from 10 to 24 weeks, there was no formation, growth, or dissolution of urocystoliths. These results are not surprising, because the diet is not restricted in salt but is restricted in phosphorus and magnesium. In addition, consumption of the diet is associated with mild hypercalciuria. Lack of new urolith formation and lack of growth of existing uroliths may have resulted from the marked polyuria caused by consumption of the diet. Pending further studies, a diet moderately restricted in protein, calcium oxalate, and sodium (Prescription Diet New u/d) should be considered to help prevent recurrence of calcium oxalate uroliths in dogs with active urolithiasis.

Thiazide Diuretics

Thiazide diuretics effectively decrease renal excretion of calcium, provided excessive sodium is not present in glomerular filtrate. Thiazides may reduce urine calcium excretion by reducing the filtered load of calcium. However, the primary mechanism is thought to be an indirect augmentation of tubular reabsorption of calcium. Thiazide diuretics cause sodium loss in urine, leading to a mild contraction of extracellular fluid volume. The latter stimulates reabsorption of sodium and calcium (because of closely linked transport mechanisms). Thiazides may also potentiate the action of parathormone in enhancing renal tubular reabsorption of calcium.

Thiazide diuretics have effectively reduced the rate of calcium oxalate urolith recurrence in human patients. Although thiazide diuretic therapy is ideally suited for patients with renal leak hypercalciuria, it apparently has been used in patients with absorptive hypercalciuria without detectable abnormalities associated with excessive body calcium balance. Nonetheless, serum calcium and urine calcium concentration should be monitored during thiazide therapy because the risk of chronic calcium retention exists. Thiazide diuretics should not be given to hypercalcemic patients.

Unwanted side effects that may occur in human patients treated for recurrent calcium oxalate uroliths with thiazides include hypokalemia, hypocitraturia, and chronic calcium retention. Hypokalemia and hypocitraturia are commonly corrected by concomitant oral administration of potassium citrate.

Based on favorable results of thiazide therapy in people with calcium oxalate urolithiasis, it has become popular to recommend thiazides to prevent recurrence of calcium oxalate uroliths in dogs. The authors have had limited clinical experience with use of thiazide diuretics to prevent recurrence of canine calcium oxalate urolithiasis. Oral administration of chlorthiazide at a dosage of 35 mg/kg of body weight per day divided in two equal doses for 4 months to a 3-yr-old male miniature schnauzer with normocalcemic (serum calcium, 10.2 mg/dl) and apparently normocalciuric (24-hr urine calcium, 2.21 mg/kg) calcium oxalate dihydrate urolithiasis resulted in a reduction in urine calcium concentration (24-hr urine calcium, 1.10 mg/kg). However, the serum calcium concentration gradually increased (to 11.2 mg/dl). Although no abnormalities were associated with the change in serum calcium concentration, the possibility of chronic calcium overload exists. This case emphasizes the need to monitor the effects of agents that have the capacity to adversely modify body metabolism.

Citrates

Citrates are calcium oxalate crystal inhibitors because of their ability to complex with calcium to form salts that are more soluble than calcium oxalate. Several investigators have observed that some people with calcium oxalate uroliths have abnormally low quantities of citrate in their urine (Rudman, 1982). Therefore oral administration of citrate has been commonly recommended to prevent recurrence of calcium oxalate uroliths in humans (Pak, 1985). During recent years, the most commonly recommended form of oral citrate has been potassium citrate. This agent is commonly given in conjunction with thiazide diuretics because it tends to minimize thiazide-induced hypokalemia and to enhance citrate excretion in urine.

Recently, wax matrix tablets of potassium citrate (Urocit-K, Mission Pharmacal) have been developed to augment administration and to allow delayed absorption and excretion of citrate throughout the day. A dosage found to be effective in maintaining persistently high urine citrate concentration in people was 60 mEq (3.78 gm) per patient per day divided in two or three equal doses.

There have been no studies of the efficacy of potassium citrate in dogs with calcium oxalate uroliths. Preliminary studies indicate that not all dogs with calcium oxalate urolithiasis have hypocitraturia. Pilot studies suggest that potassium citrate is unlikely to be associated with serious side effects in dogs with calcium oxalate uroliths.

In dogs with hypocitraturia, potassium citrate should be administered to achieve a urine concentration of 70 mg/day (approximately 100–150 mg of potassium citrate per kilogram of body weight per day). Because urine citrate concentrations may be difficult to obtain, urine pH values may be used to assess therapy. Urine pH values greater than 7.0 have been associated with adequate urine citrate concentrations. Because citrates alkalinize urine, excessive potassium citrate might enhance formation or growth of calcium phosphate uroliths.

References and Supplemental Reading

Berlin, T.: Proposed criteria for identifying hyperabsorbers among normocalcemic renal stone formers. Scand. J. Urol. Nephrol. 21:103, 1987.

Bovee, K. C., and McGuire, T.: Qualitative and quantitative analysis of uroliths in dogs: Definitive analysis of uroliths in dogs: Definitive determination of chemical type. J.A.V.M.A. 185:983, 1984.

Finalyson, B., Roth, R., and Du Bois, L.: Calcium oxalate solubility studies. In Urinary Calculi. Madrid, Spain, International Symposium on Renal Stone Research, pp. 1–7, 1972.

Kaplan, R. A., Hausler, M. R., Deftos, L. J., et al.: The role of 1-alpha, 25-dihydroxyvitamin D in the mediation of intestinal hyperabsorption of calcium in primary hyperparathyroidism and absorptive hypercalciuria. J. Clin. Invest. 59:756, 1977.

Klausner, J. S., Fernandez, F. R., O'Leary, T. P., et al.: Canine primary hyperparathyroidism and its association with urolithiasis. Vet. Clin. North Am. 16:227, 1986.

Klausner, J. S., O'Leary, T. P., and Osborne, C. A.: Calcium urolithiasis in two dogs with parathyroid adenomas. J.A.V.M.A. 191:1423, 1987.

Osborne, C. A., Clinton, C. W., Bamman, L. K., et al.: Prevalence of canine uroliths. Vet. Clin. North Am. 16:27, 1986.

Osborne, C. A., Poffenbarger, E. M., Klausner, J. S., et al.: Etiopathogenesis, clinical manifestations, and management of canine calcium oxalate urolithiasis. Vet. Clin. North Am. 16:133, 1986.

Pak, C. Y. C., Fuller, C., Sakhaee, K., et al.: Long-term treatment of calcium nephrolithiasis with potassium citrate. J. Urol. 134:11, 1985.

Rudman, D., Kutner, M., Redd, S. C., et al.: Hypocitraturia in calcium nephrolithiasis. J. Clin. Endocrinol. Metab. 55:1052, 1982.

Schubert, G., and Brian, G.: Crystallographic investigations of urinary calcium oxalate calculi. Int. Urol. Nephrol. 13:249, 1981.

Walser, M.: Calcium clearance as a function of sodium clearance in the dog. Am. J. Physiol. 200:1099, 1961.

Zerwekh, J. E.: Pathogenesis of hypercalciuria. In Pak, C. Y. C. (ed.): Renal Stone Disease. Boston: Martinus Nijhoff Publishing, 1987, pp. 25–45.

MEDICAL DISSOLUTION AND PREVENTION OF CYSTINE UROLITHIASIS

CARL A. OSBORNE, D.V.M.,
St. Paul, Minnesota

ASTRID HOPPE, D.V.M.,
Uppsala, Sweden

and TIMOTHY D. O'BRIEN, D.V.M.
St. Paul, Minnesota

PREVALENCE AND MINERAL COMPOSITION

The prevalence of cystine uroliths in dogs varies with geographic location, being encountered in 2.4 to 3.3 per cent of the stones removed from dogs in the United States (Bovee and McGuire, 1984; Ling and Ruby, 1986; Osborne et al., 1986) and as high as 39 per cent in some European centers (Hicking, 1981). Quantitative analysis of canine cystine uroliths has revealed that most are pure, but a few contain ammonium urate. Ammonium urate uroliths, like cystine uroliths, tend to form in acid urine. Although uncommon, secondary urinary tract infections with urease-producing microbes may result in a nucleus of cystine surrounded by outer layers of struvite.

ETIOPATHOGENESIS

Cystinuria is an inborn error of metabolism characterized by abnormal transport of cystine (a nonessential sulfur-containing amino acid composed of two molecules of cysteine) and other amino acids by the renal tubules. The name cystine was coined because this substance was first identified from urine removed from the urinary bladder (or urocyst) and therefore was thought to have originated from the bladder (Segal and Thier, 1983).

Cystine is normally present in low concentrations in plasma. Normally, circulating cystine is freely filtered at the glomerulus, and most is actively reabsorbed in the proximal tubules. The solubility of cystine in urine is pH dependent. It is relatively insoluble in acid urine but becomes more soluble in alkaline urine.

CANINE CYSTINURIA

Unlike normal dogs, cystinuric dogs reabsorb a much smaller proportion of the amino acid from glomerular filtrate (Bovee, 1984b). Some may even have net cystine secretion.

The exact mechanism of abnormal renal tubular transport of cystine in dogs is unknown. Plasma concentration of cystine in affected dogs is normal, indicating faulty tubular function rather than hyperexcretion (Bovee, 1984a, b). Levels of plasma methionine, a precursor of cystine, have been found to be elevated in cystinuric dogs. Some studies in people suggest that tubular reabsorption of cysteine, the immediate precursor of cystine, may be abnormal (Bartter et al., 1965). In this situation, the increase in urine cystine concentration may result from dimerization of two cysteine molecules in tubular urine.

In dogs with cystinuria, the exact pattern of amino aciduria reported by various investigators has been variable (Bovee, 1984a; Clark and Cuddeford, 1971; Cornelius et al., 1971; Crane and Turner, 1956). Two populations of cystinuric dogs have been reported (Bovee, 1984a). One group had cystinuria without loss of other amino acids. Another group had cystinuria and a lesser degree of lysinuria.

Unless protein intake is severely restricted, cystinuric dogs have no detectable abnormalities associated with amino acid loss, with the exception of formation of cystine uroliths. This occurs because cystine is sparingly soluble at the usual urine pH range of 5.5 to 7.0. Cystinuria would be a medical curiosity if cystine were not the least soluble naturally occurring amino acid. The major causes of morbidity and mortality associated with this disorder are the sequelae of urolith formation.

The exact mechanism of cystine urolith formation

1189

is unknown. Because not all cystinuric dogs form uroliths, cystinuria is a predisposing rather than a primary cause of cystine urolith formation. In one study, 4 of 14 dogs with a history of cystine urolith formation had urine cystine concentrations that fell within the range of those found in control dogs (Bovee, 1984a). Many breeds of dogs have been reported to develop cystine uroliths, especially dachshunds. Empiric clinical observations indicate that English bulldogs also have an unexpectedly high prevalence of cystine uroliths.

With two exceptions, cystine uroliths have been reported only in male dogs (Brown et al., 1977; Ling and Ruby, 1986). However, cystinuria has been observed in female dogs (Bovee, 1984a). This observation suggests that lack of detection of cystine uroliths in females may be related to the passage of small uroliths through their relatively short, wide, and distensible urethras.

Cystine uroliths are usually detected in the bladder or urethra of affected male dogs. Although they are radiodense, they are typically less dense than calcium-containing and struvite uroliths. Pure cystine uroliths are usually multiple, ovoid, and smooth. They have a light-yellow color and vary in size from 0.5 mm to several centimeters in diameter.

Detection of characteristic flat hexagonal cystine crystals provides strong support for a diagnosis of cystinuria (Fig. 1). However, not all dogs with cystine uroliths have concomitant cystine crystalluria. Acidification, refrigeration, and centrifugation of urine may foster cystine crystal formation. If a sufficient quantity of cystine is present in urine (75

to 125 mg/gm of creatinine), the cyanide-nitroprusside test result for cystine will be positive (Kachmar, 1970). Ampicillin and sulfur-containing drugs have been reported to cause false-positive reactions to this test (Pahira, 1987).

BIOLOGIC BEHAVIOR

The precise genetic mode of inheritance of canine cystinuria is unknown; however, both sex-linked and autosomal recessive patterns have been suggested (Bovee, 1986; Brand et al., 1940). Surprisingly, cystine uroliths often are not recognized until affected dogs reach maturity, the average age of detection being approximately 3 to 5 yr (Bovee, 1986). Because cystinuria is an inherited defect, uroliths commonly recur in 6 to 12 months, unless prophylactic therapy has been initiated.

MEDICAL MANAGEMENT

Determination of Urolith Composition

Formulation of effective medical protocols for urolith dissolution is dependent on knowledge of the mineral composition of uroliths. The authors recommend a protocol based on tentative determination of urolith composition (Table 1). Formulation of medical therapy with this approach is usually associated with a high degree of success in dissolving uroliths or arresting their growth. Attempts to induce dissolution of uroliths may be hampered if the uroliths are heterogeneous in composition.

Objectives

Current recommendations for dissolution of cystine uroliths encompass reduction in the urine concentration of cystine and increasing the solubility of cystine in urine. This may be accomplished by (1) dietary modification, (2) alkalinization of urine, and (3) administration of thiol-containing drugs.

DIETARY MODIFICATION

Reduction of dietary protein has the potential of minimizing formation of cystine uroliths. By decreasing intake of methionine, some decrease in urine cystine excretion might occur. An even more important indirect effect would be a reduction in renal medullary urea concentration and associated reduction in urine concentration (Osborne et al., 1985). A protein-restricted alkalinizing diet (Prescription Diet Canine u/d, Hill's Pet Products) was observed to have a beneficial effect in promoting

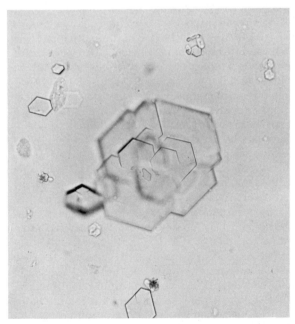

Figure 1. Photomicrograph of urine sediment of a 4-year-old male dachshund illustrating cystine crystals of varying size. (Unstained; × 40.)

Table 1. Factors That May Aid in Determination of Mineral Composition of Canine Uroliths

1. Radiographic density and physical characteristics of uroliths
2. Urine pH
   a. Struvite and calcium apatite uroliths—usually alkaline
   b. Ammonium urate uroliths—acid to neutral
   c. Cystine uroliths—acid*
   d. Calcium oxalate uroliths—variable*
   e. Silica uroliths—acid to neutral*
3. Identification of crystals in uncontaminated fresh urine sediment, preferably at body temperature
4. Type of bacteria, if any, isolated from urine
   a. Urease-producing bacteria, especially staphylococci, and less frequently *Proteus* spp., are typically associated with canine struvite uroliths. Ureaplasmas may cause struvite uroliths
   b. Urinary tract infections often are absent in patients with calcium oxalate, cystine, ammonium urate, and silica uroliths
   c. Calcium oxalate, cystine, ammonium urate, and silica uroliths may predispose patients to urinary tract infections; if infections are caused by urease-producing bacteria, struvite may precipitate around metabolic uroliths
5. Serum chemistry evaluation
   a. Hypercalcemia may be associated with calcium-containing uroliths
   b. Hyperuricemia may be associated with uric acid or urate uroliths
   c. Hyperchloremia, hypokalemia, and acidemia may be associated with distal renal tubular acidosis and calcium phosphate or struvite uroliths
6. Urine chemistry evaluation
   a. Patient should be consuming a standardized diagnostic diet, or the diet consumed when uroliths formed
   b. Excessive quantities of one or more minerals contained in the urolith are expected. The concentration of crystallization inhibitors may be decreased
7. Breed of dog and history of occurrence of uroliths in patient's ancestors or littermates
8. Quantitative analysis of uroliths fortuitously passed during micturition and collected

*Concomitant infection with urease-producing microbes may result in formation of an alkaline urine.

reduction in cystine urocystolith size in a 3-yr-old male dachshund (see discussion of thiol-containing drugs below).

ALKALINIZATION OF URINE

The solubility of cystine is pH dependent. In dogs, the solubility of cystine at a urine pH of 7.8 has been reported to be approximately double that at a urine pH of 5.0 (Treacher, 1966). Changes in urine pH that remain in the acidic range have minimal effect on cystine solubility. Therefore a sufficient quantity of potassium citrate or sodium bicarbonate should be given orally in divided doses to sustain a urine pH of approximately 7.5. Data derived from studies in cystinuric humans suggest that dietary sodium may enhance cystinuria (Cystinuria, 1987; Jaeger et al., 1986). Therefore, potassium citrate may be preferable to sodium bicarbonate as a urine alkalinizer. Further studies are required to evaluate the effect of dietary sodium on urinary excretion of cystine in dogs.

It is of interest that urinary tract infection caused by urease-producing bacteria in an adult male human patient with cystine nephroliths resulted in extreme urine alkalinity and subsequent urolith dissolution (Gutierrez Millet et al., 1985).

THIOL-CONTAINING DRUGS

D-Penicillamine (dimethylcysteine) is a nonmetabolizable degradation product of penicillin that may combine with cysteine to form cysteine–D-penicillamine disulfide (Pahira, 1987). This disulfide exchange reaction is facilitated by an alkaline pH. The resulting compound has been reported to be 50 times more soluble than free cystine (Lotz et al., 1966). The cysteine–D-penicillamine complex does not react with nitroprusside as does cystine, providing a mechanism to titrate dosage of the drug (Pahira, 1987).

The most commonly utilized dosage of D-penicillamine for dogs has been 30 mg/kg/day given in two divided doses (Frimpter et al., 1967). Higher dosages frequently cause vomiting and may cause other undesirable reactions. If nausea and vomiting occur with the aforementioned dosage, the drug may be mixed with food or given at mealtimes. In some instances, it may be necessary to prevent gastrointestinal disturbances by initiating therapy with low dosages and gradually increasing them until full dosage is reached.

D-Penicillamine has been associated with a variety of adverse reactions in people, including immune complex glomerulonephropathy, fever, lymphadenopathy, and skin hypersensitivity (Pahira, 1987). Fever and lymphadenopathy have been found in a dachshund given D-penicillamine at a dosage of 30 mg/kg/day. The signs subsided following withdrawal of the drug and administration of glucocorticoids.

N-(2-Mercaptopropionyl)-glycine (MPG) decreases the concentration of cystine by a thiol disulfide exchange reaction similar to that of D-penicillamine (Pahira, 1987; Pak et al., 1986). Studies in people indicate that the drug is highly effective in reducing urinary cystine concentration and has less toxicity than D-penicillamine (Pak et al., 1986).

Oral administration of MPG at a daily dosage of approximately 30 mg/kg of body weight (divided in two equal doses) was effective in inducing dissolution of multiple cystine urocystoliths in three or four dogs evaluated (Hoppe et al., 1988). Dissolution required 2 to 4 months of therapy. One dog developed nonpruritic vesicular skin lesions following 3 months of therapy. One month following reduction of the daily dosage of MPG from 30 to 25 mg/kg of body weight, the skin lesions healed.

Dissolution of multiple cystine urocystoliths was induced in a 3-yr-old male dachshund by a combination of diet (Prescription Diet Canine u/d, Hill's Pet Products), urine alkalinization (with sodium bicarbonate), and MPG therapy (30 mg/kg/day divided in two equal doses). MPG was utilized because the dog had a history of hypersensitivity to D-penicillamine. Initial therapy with the diet and sodium bicarbonate resulted in reduction of urolith size by 50 per cent over a 10-week period. However, further reduction in urolith size did not occur during the following month. Therefore MPG was added to the regimen. When the dog was evaluated by contrast urethrocystography 1 month later, there was no evidence of uroliths. Cystine urocystoliths recurred approximately 1 yr following dissolution. Treatment of the dog with the identical regimen (Prescription Diet Canine u/d [Hill's Pet Products], sodium bicarbonate, and MPG) resulted in urocystolith dissolution in approximately 1 month. However, the dog developed a Coombs'-positive regenerative spherocytic anemia at that time. Withdrawal of the MPG and oral administration of prednisone was associated with rapid remission of the anemia. These results suggest that dogs with a history of hypersensitivity to D-penicillamine may also have hypersensitivity to MPG. Appropriate evaluations should be performed during use of MPG in dogs with a history of D-penicillamine hypersensitivity.

Summary

Limited clinical studies indicate the feasibility of medical dissolution of cystine uroliths in dogs. Although thiol-containing drugs may induce dissolution when used alone, a combination of dietary, alkalinizing, and thiol drug therapy may be more effective. If convenient, potassium citrate may be substituted for sodium bicarbonate as the alkalinizing agent. Appropriate caution should be used to monitor patients for adverse reactions to this form of therapy.

PREVENTION

Because cystinuria is an inherited metabolic defect, and because cystine uroliths recur in a high percentage of stone-forming dogs within 1 yr following surgical removal (Bovee, 1986), prophylactic therapy should be considered. Dietary therapy combined with urine alkalinization may be initiated with the objective of minimizing cystine crystalluria and promoting a negative cyanide-nitroprusside test result. If necessary, MPG or D-penicillamine may be added to the regimen in sufficient quantity to maintain a urine concentration of cystine below approximately 200 mg/L. If dosage cannot be titrated by measurement of urine cystine concentration, dosages of 30 mg/kg/day of MPG, or 20 to 30 mg/kg/day of D-penicillamine may be considered. Continuous therapy of stone-free cystinuric dogs with MPG has been effective in preventing formation of cystine uroliths in studies performed in Sweden (Hoppe et al., 1988).

References and Supplemental Reading

Bartter, F. C., Lotz, M., Thier, S., et al.: Cystinuria. Ann. Intern. Med. 62:796, 1965.

Bovee, K. C.: Genetic and metabolic diseases of the kidney. In Bovee, K. C. (ed.): Canine Nephrology. Media PA: Harwal, 1984a, p. 339.

Bovee, K. C.: Urolithiasis. In Bovee, K. C. (ed.): Canine Nephrology. Media PA: Harwal, 1984b, p. 335.

Bovee, K. C.: Canine cystine urolithiasis. Vet. Clin. North Am. 16:211, 1986.

Bovee, K. C., and McGuire, T.: Qualitative and quantitative analysis of uroliths in dogs. Definitive determination of chemical type. J.A.V.M.A. 185:983, 1984.

Brand, E., Cahill, G. F., and Kassell, B.: Canine cystinuria. V. Family history of two Irish terriers and cystine determinations in dog urine. J. Biol. Chem. 133:431, 1940.

Brown, N. O., et al.: Canine urolithiasis: Retrospective analysis of 438 cases. J.A.V.M.A. 170:415, 1977.

Clark, W. T., and Cuddeford, D.: A study of amino acids in urine from dogs with cystine urolithiasis. Vet. Rec. 88:414, 1971.

Cornelius, C. E., Bishop, J. A., and Schaffer, M. H.: A quantitative study of amino aciduria in dachshunds with a history of cystine urolithiasis. Cornell Vet. 57:177, 1967.

Crane, C. W., and Turner, A. W.: Amino acid patterns of urine and blood plasma in a cystinuric Labrador dog. Nature 177:237, 1956.

Cystinuria is reduced by low-sodium diets. Nutrition Rev. 45:79, 1987.

Frimpter, G. W., Thouin, P., and Ewalds, B. H.: Penicillamine in canine cystinuria. J.A.V.M.A. 151:1084, 1967.

Gutierrez Millet, V., Praga, M., Miranda, B., et al.: Ureolytic Citrobacter freundii infection of the urine as a cause of dissolution of cystine renal calculi. J. Urol. 133:443, 1985.

Hicking, W., Hesse, A., Gebhardt, M., et al.: Investigation with polarizing microscopy for the classification of urinary stones from humans and dogs. In Smith, L. H., et al.: Urolithiasis: Clinical and Basic Research. New York: Plenum Press, 1981, p. 901.

Hoppe, A., Denneberg, T., and Kagedal, B.: Treatment of normal and cystinuric dogs with 2-mercaptopropionylglycine. Am. J. Vet. Res. 49:923, 1988.

Jaeger, P., Portman, L., Saunders, A., et al.: Anticystinuric effects of glutamine and of dietary sodium restriction. N. Engl. J. Med. 315:1120, 1986.

Kachmar, J. F.: Proteins and amino acids. In Tietz, N. W. (ed.): Fundamentals of Clinical Chemistry. Philadelphia: W. B. Saunders, 1970, p. 248.

Ling, G. V., and Ruby, A. L.: Canine uroliths: Analysis of data derived from 813 specimens. Vet. Clin. North Am. 16:303, 1986.

Lotz, M., Potts, J. T., Jr., Bartter, F.C., et al.: D-Penicillamine therapy in cystinuria. J. Urol. 95:257, 1966.

Osborne, C. A., and Klausner, J. S.: War on urolithiasis: Problems and their solutions. Scientific Proceedings American Animal Hospital Association, Denver CO, 1978, p. 569.

Osborne, C. A., Polzin, D. J., Abdullah, S., et al.: Struvite urolithiasis in animals and man: Formation, detection and dissolution. Adv. Vet. Sci. Comp. Med. 29:1, 1985.

Osborne, C. A., Clinton, C. W., Bamman, L. K., et al.: Prevalence of canine uroliths: Minnesota Urolith Center. Vet. Clin. North Am. 16:27, 1986.

Pahira, J. J.: Management of the patient with cystinuria. Urol. Clin. North Am. 14:339, 1987.

Pak, C. Y. C., Fuller, C., Sakhaee, K., et al.: Management of cystine nephrolithiasis with alpha mercaptopropionyl glycine. J. Urol. 136:1003, 1986.

Segal, S., and Thier, S. O.: Cystinuria. In Stanbury, J. B., and Wyngaarden, J. B. (eds.): The Metabolic Basis for Inherited Disease, 5th ed. New York: McGraw-Hill, 1983, p. 1774.

Treacher, R. J.: Urolithiasis in the dog. II Biochemical aspects. J. Small Anim. Pract. 7:537, 1966.

MANAGEMENT OF PROSTATIC NEOPLASIA

JANE M. TURREL, D.V.M., M.S.

Davis, California

Prostatic carcinoma in the dog is often difficult to diagnose in the early stages of the disease and is even more difficult to manage after the diagnosis is made. These tumors develop in dogs ranging in age from 6 to 12 yr with a mean age of 9 yr. Although most dogs with prostatic carcinoma are intact, many reports exist of dogs with prostatic carcinoma that were castrated at a young age or several years before development of the tumor. Obradovich and associates (1987) showed that castration of dogs at any age had no sparing effect on the risk of development of prostatic carcinoma.

Dogs typically have clinical signs of hematuria, stranguria, rectal tenesmus, and hindlimb weakness. Clinical signs may be either acute or chronic. The prostate gland often is enlarged, is either fixed or freely movable, and may be painful on physical examination. In approximately half the affected dogs, metastatic disease is detected at the time of presentation. The most common metastatic sites are the iliac, lumbar, hypogastric, and sacral lymph nodes; periprostatic tissues; bladder; and lung. Bone metastases are characterized by bony proliferation involving the ventral aspects of the fourth to seventh lumbar vertebrae and the pelvic bones. Prostatic carcinoma must be differentiated from prostatitis, prostatic hyperplasia, and prostatic cyst. Other prostatic tumors (representing less than 10 per cent of all prostatic neoplasms) include adenoma, leiomyoma, fibroma, and sarcomas.

The cause of prostatic carcinoma in dogs in unknown, but several hypotheses have been postulated. The most commonly accepted is that prostatic tissue becomes neoplastic under the influence of androgenic stimulation. The development of prostatic carcinoma in castrated dogs and the apparent failure of dogs with prostatic carcinoma to have palliation of clinical signs when treated by either castration or estrogen therapy suggest that this theory is false. The second hypothesis is that infected, hyperplastic, or cystic prostatic tissues undergo malignant transformation as a result of chronic irritation. However, a review of case histories of dogs with prostatic carcinoma does not uniformly confirm this. The third hypothesis is that adrenal not testicular androgens are responsible for development of prostatic carcinoma. There is some evidence to support this theory, including the development of cancer in castrated dogs.

A complete evaluation of the dog must be made before initiating a treatment plan. The diagnosis should be confirmed from examination of tissue obtained by biopsy. Routine diagnostic procedures include rectal examination to determine local extension and lymph node involvement; survey radiographs of the abdomen followed by pneumocolonic evaluation or urography to determine lymph node, vertebral, bladder, or ureteral involvement; and thoracic radiographs to detect pulmonary metastases. Localized prostatic carcinoma in the absence of detectable metastatic disease indicates that cure should be the goal by using either radiotherapy or prostatectomy. For dogs with locally invasive or metastatic prostatic carcinoma, palliation is the only reasonable goal.

RADIATION THERAPY

Radiation therapy is as effective as prostatectomy for curative treatment of localized prostatic carcinoma in men. The methods of delivering radiation are interstitial brachytherapy, external beam therapy, or a combination of these. In veterinary medicine, intraoperative radiotherapy was developed to deliver a large dose of radiation (20 to 30 Gy) to the neoplastic gland. Briefly, a laparotomy is performed to expose the prostate gland directly to the radiation beam. Tissues dorsal and lateral to the prostate are shielded with sterilized lead sheets and collimation. The radiation beam is directed at the neoplastic tissue using either a high-energy orthovoltage x-ray beam or a high-energy electron beam. Lymph nodes in the sublumbar region that have evidence of metastatic disease can be similarly treated.

Of ten dogs with prostatic carcinoma treated with intraoperative radiotherapy, seven dogs had localized tumor and had mean and median survival times of 8 and 6 months, respectively. Three of those dogs were considered to be cured. Poor survival times were associated with large regional lymph node metastases or extensive surgery before irradiation. The addition of radiation sensitizers, hyperthermia, or further irradiation using either interstitial brachytherapy or external teletherapy may improve these results.

SURGERY

Total prostatectomy is indicated for a malignant tumor confined entirely within the prostate gland. However, it has been associated with high morbidity and mortality in dogs regardless of whether a neoplastic or non-neoplastic condition was being treated. Of nine dogs with prostatic carcinoma treated with prostatectomy, six lived less than 2 months and the remainder died at 7, 8, and 9 months after surgery. Benign tumors and cysts of the prostate can be excised successfully by partial prostatectomy.

HORMONAL TREATMENT

Elimination of all biologically effective circulating androgens is considered the most effective treatment for locally invasive or metastatic prostatic carcinoma in men. Unfortunately, little documentation and no controlled studies exist to support this treatment modality in dogs. Castration is the ultimate procedure for elimination of testicular hormones and has been done therapeutically for canine prostatic cancer either alone or concurrently with other treatment modalities. Obradovich and associates (1987) reported that some dogs with prostatic carcinoma treated with castration or estrogen treatment had palliation of clinical signs, but responses were subjectively evaluated and were not observed

by the authors themselves. Castration may be done on the principle that it will not harm the dog and may help. However, hormonal manipulation cannot be recommended at this time for treatment of prostatic cancer in dogs. The occurrence of this tumor in castrated dogs as well as the poor response to surgical or chemical castration noted by several authors strongly support this conclusion.

CHEMOTHERAPY

The primary indication for treatment of prostatic carcinoma with chemotherapeutic agents is to palliate clinical signs and to prevent progression of metastatic disease. No reports are available that suggest that any chemotherapeutic agent used either singly or in combination is effective in achieving those goals in veterinary medicine. Indeed, no data exist to suggest that these drugs are effective in causing better response rates and longer survival times in men with advanced prostatic carcinoma. Some chemotherapeutic agents that have demonstrated objective response rates in these men are cisplatin, 5-fluorouracil, cyclophosphamide, doxorubicin, and methotrexate. Clearly, clinical trials to study the effectiveness of these drugs in dogs are indicated, but the potential of prolonging life must be weighed against the disadvantages of toxicity, poor quality of life, and expense to the owner.

In summary, no controlled clinical studies are available to identify a superior treatment for prostatic carcinoma. Intraoperative radiotherapy is a promising new technique for treatment of localized prostatic carcinoma, having low morbidity and a 30 per cent likelihood for tumor control. Neither prostatectomy nor castration have been found to give good quality of life or to effectively cure the disease. Finally, chemotherapy should be used only as a last resort for diffuse metastatic disease.

References and Supplemental Reading

Gibbons, R. P.: Prostate cancer—chemotherapy. Cancer 60:586, 1987.

Grayhack, J. T., Keeler, T. C., and Kozlowski, J. M.: Carcinoma of the prostate—hormonal therapy. Cancer 60:589, 1987.

Greiner, T. P., and Johnson, R. G.: Diseases of the prostate gland. In Ettinger, S. J. (ed.): Textbook of Veterinary Internal Medicine, 2nd ed. Philadelphia: W. B. Saunders, 1983.

Hardie, E. M., Barsanti, J. A., and Rawlings, C. A.: Complications of prostatic surgery. J. Am. Anim. Hosp. Assoc. 20:50, 1984.

Hargis, A. M., and Miller, L. M.: Prostatic carcinoma in dogs. Comp. Cont. Ed. Pract. Vet. 5:647, 1983.

Leav, I., and Ling, G. V.: Adenocarcinoma of the canine prostate. Cancer 22:1329, 1968.

Obradovich, J., Walshaw R., and Goullaud E.: The influence of castration on the development of prostatic carcinoma in the dog. J. Vet. Intern. Med. 1:183, 1987.

Turrel, J. M.: Intraoperative radiotherapy of carcinoma of the prostate gland in ten dogs. J.A.V.M.A. 190:48, 1987.

MANAGEMENT OF ADVANCED
CHRONIC RENAL FAILURE

TIMOTHY A. ALLEN, D.V.M.

Topeka, Kansas

Chronic renal failure is defined as a slowly progressive and irreversible impairment of renal function. This slow process allows time for a number of adaptive mechanisms. Some of these adaptive mechanisms are initially beneficial and maintain homeostasis but with time are maladaptive and contribute to the progression of the renal disease. Chronic renal failure may result from a number of processes, including infection or toxic or immunologic injury. Regardless of the inciting cause, after a critical level of dysfunction has been reached there appears to be a common pathway, glomerular hyperfiltration, for progressive renal damage.

Polyuric/uremic chronic renal failure is present when severe reduction in glomerular filtration rate (GFR) results in azotemia (an increase in serum urea nitrogen [SUN] or serum creatinine [SC]). During renal failure a constellation of changes involving multiple organ systems (uremic syndrome) develops. Polyuric/uremic renal failure is recognized clinically by the presence of polyuria, polydipsia, anorexia, vomiting, weight loss, and lethargy.

Creatinine, a metabolite of muscle creatine, is handled almost exclusively by glomerular filtration. The production of creatinine is almost constant each day; therefore, to maintain serum concentrations within reference ranges, renal excretion must also be constant. As GFR is decreased by 50 per cent, the serum concentration of creatinine doubles. This simple inverse relationship between GFR and serum creatinine applies only under steady state conditions with slowly decreasing renal function. Because of the wide normal range for serum creatinine concentrations, it is possible for GFR to be reduced by 50 per cent and the SC to be within the reference range.

Serum urea nitrogen concentration increases with decreasing renal function. In contrast to the constant production of creatinine, urea production will vary, depending on dietary protein and protein catabolism. Gastrointestinal hemorrhage, fever, protein calorie malnutrition, and catabolic drugs, such as steroids and tetracycline, will increase protein breakdown and subsequently increase serum urea concentrations. Renal tubular backdiffusion of urea occurs under conditions of reduced urine flow; therefore dehydration will increase serum urea concentrations without necessarily decreasing GFR. Consequently, increases in urea nitrogen concentration must be interpreted with knowledge of the diet, drugs administered, and clinical status of the patient.

ADAPTIVE MECHANISMS

As renal function decreases, phosphate is retained and its serum concentration increases. A small increase in phosphate concentration will cause a reciprocal change in serum calcium level. A decrease in serum calcium level is a strong stimulus for parathormone (PTH) release. Parathormone has a direct effect on the proximal renal tubule, causing a decrease in phosphate reabsorption. This adaptive process returns phosphate and calcium concentrations to normal but at the price of persistent elevations of PTH. This adaptive mechanism is capable of maintaining calcium and phosphate concentrations within normal limits until more than 80 per cent of GFR is lost. The decrease in phosphate excretion and the adaptations that occur in chronic renal failure illustrate the so-called trade-off hypothesis. Parathormone levels increase progressively and in proportion to the reduction in renal function when phosphate intake is not restricted. Secondary hyperparathyroidism causes increased osteoclast activity and mobilization of bone and may contribute to other manifestations of the uremic syndrome, such as uremic neuropathy.

Some of the clinical signs associated with chronic renal failure are directly related to the adaptive mechanisms that compensate for systemic acidosis. A prime example is the loss of bone mineral, resulting from chronic buffering of acid by bone. Bone buffering mitigates the chronic acidosis but results in demineralization, more extensive osteodystrophy, and increased solute load. Other examples of the consequences of chronic compensation for acidosis are increased work of breathing and reduced respiratory reserve owing to hyperventilation. Ammonium production from glutamine can be markedly increased in chronic renal failure so that marked decreases in blood pH do not occur until late in the progression of renal failure.

Other changes associated with renal failure are

not directly related to adaptive or trade-off mechanisms but rather are due to interference with the normal endocrine functions of the kidney. Erythropoietin is produced by the kidney in response to hypoxia. As renal function deteriorates, there is a decrease in hematocrit. In severe renal failure other factors contribute to the anemia, such as intestinal hemorrhage, shortened red blood cell half-life, and decreased responsiveness of the bone marrow to erythropoietin.

The hydroxylation of 25-hydroxycholecalciferol to the most active metabolite of vitamin D occurs in the renal parenchyma. With nephron loss this reaction is decreased and the concentration of the most active metabolite is reduced. This results in decreased calcium absorption from the gut and decreased serum calcium concentration, which is a potent stimulus for PTH secretion.

PROGRESSIVE RENAL DETERIORATION

People with chronic renal failure often follow a predictable course. In renal failure, the serum creatinine level is inversely proportional to the number of functioning nephrons. Because of glomerular hyperfiltration, nephrons are lost at a constant rate. Consequently the plot of the reciprocal of the serum creatinine versus time is linear. This graphic representation can be used to predict the time until death due to renal failure and to evaluate response to treatment. By projecting the line to the abscissa, it is possible to estimate the age at which terminal renal failure will occur. The effects of treatment can be evaluated by examining changes in the slope of the line.

Most patients with polyuric/uremic renal failure are hypertensive, especially those with glomerulopathies. The estimated incidence of hypertension in dogs with chronic renal failure is between 58 and 93 per cent. Hypertension may cause glomerular changes, which contribute to the deterioration of renal function.

Regardless of the inciting cause, renal failure is associated with interstitial fibrosis and tubular damage. In renal failure the amount of ammonia excreted is increased. Ammonia activates the alternate complement pathway to produce membrane attack complex, which subsequently mediates tubulointerstitial damage. Studies in rats suggest that early institution of bicarbonate supplementation may slow the onset of the tubulointerstitial damage seen in chronic renal failure. By buffering dietary acid load, bicarbonate decreases renal ammonia levels. In addition to bicarbonate treatment, the metabolic acid load can be decreased by dietary protein restriction and prevention of protein catabolism.

CAUSES OF ACUTE DETERIORATION

The usual slow rate of renal functional deterioration in chronic renal failure may be increased by superimposed acute renal failure. These exacerbations may be reversible with prompt recognition and appropriate treatment. All causes of acute renal failure must be considered; however, certain causes seem to occur more commonly in the chronic renal failure patient.

The inability to form maximally concentrated urine and conserve sodium and body water, which occurs in polyuric renal failure, predisposes to volume depletion due to vomiting, diarrhea, prolonged anorexia, or water deprivation. If uncorrected, volume depletion can lead to decreased renal blood flow and an abrupt decrease in GFR.

In the presence of reduced renal function, many drugs given at normally safe doses are nephrotoxic. This is particularly true of aminoglycoside antimicrobials, such as gentamicin, and the nonsteroidal anti-inflammatory drugs, such as ibuprofen and butazolidine.

Because of immunologic dysfunction associated with uremic renal failure, urinary tract infections are more common. These infections may ascend the urinary tract and produce pyelonephritis with rapid deterioration of renal function. Urinary tract infections are particularly common in chronic renal failure patients with concurrent uroliths or anatomic defects.

Electrolyte abnormalities such as hypokalemia or hypercalcemia can lead to an abrupt deterioration in renal function. Hypokalemia causes a concentrating defect and may lead to volume depletion and subsequently decreased GFR. Hypercalcemia is most often associated with neoplasia and causes a concentrating defect and nephrocalcinosis.

The development of congestive heart failure can result in an abrupt deterioration in renal function owing to decreased renal perfusion.

MANAGEMENT RECOMMENDATIONS

All chronic renal failure patients should have levels of serum urea nitrogen, creatinine, electrolytes, calcium, phosphorus, bicarbonate or total carbon dioxide, and hematocrit monitored regularly after the serum creatinine concentration exceeds 2.5 mg/dl. Dietary protein intake should be restricted to control clinical signs associated with the uremic syndrome, when the serum urea nitrogen level is greater than 60 mg/dl. It is recommended that in adult dogs about 8 to 13 per cent of total calories be provided as high-quality protein. This is the equivalent of 1.3 to 2.0 gm of protein per kilogram of body weight per day. Commercially available prescription diets or homemade equivalent diets may be used to provide this degree of protein restriction. Caloric intake should be adjusted to maintain stable weight. The precise caloric requirements for the polyuric/uremic renal failure patient are unknown; however, 70 to 110 kcal/kg/day are recommended. The SUN/SC ratio may be used as a crude indicator of the adequacy of dietary protein restriction. The goal is to reduce the ratio as much as possible while maintaining a stable serum creatinine level. Protein restriction will also limit exogenous acid and phosphate intake. This will delay the onset of problems related to adaptation to acidosis or hyperphosphatemia.

If dietary phosphate restriction does not maintain the serum phosphate below 5.0 mg/dl, phosphate binders such as aluminum hydroxide gel (Amphojel, Wyeth; Alternagel, Stuart), basic aluminum carbonate gel (Basaljel, Wyeth), and calcium carbonate (Tums, Norcliff Thayer; Os-Cal, Marion) are indicated. Aluminum hydroxide gel is administered at an initial dose of 10 to 30 mg/kg every 8 hr with meals. Care should be taken to prevent hypophosphatemia. Constipation occasionally develops as a result of aluminum hydroxide gel treatment. If calcium carbonate is used, serum calcium level should be monitored to ensure that hypercalcemia does not develop.

With severe renal failure, hypocalcemia is frequently present and should be treated after the hyperphosphatemia has been controlled. If the calcium-phosphate product is in excess of 70 (mg/dl), calcium and vitamin D supplementation should be avoided. Each 1-gm tablet of calcium gluconate provides 90 mg of elemental calcium, and each 300-mg tablet of calcium lactate provides 60 mg of elemental calcium. With hypocalcemia and hyperphosphatemia, calcium carbonate is recommended because it will decrease phosphate and increase calcium levels. Each 650-mg tablet of calcium carbonate provides 260 mg of elemental calcium. If the serum calcium concentration is not normalized with calcium supplementation, vitamin D therapy is indicated. Dihydrotachysterol (Hytakerol, Winthrop Labs) contains a hydroxyl group in the pseudo-1 position; therefore this drug does not require renal metabolism to produce the active form of vitamin D. The recommended initial dose of dihydrotachysterol is 125 µg per dog three times per week. Calcitriol (1,25-dihydroxycholecalciferol) (Rocaltrol, Roche Labs) does not require hydroxylation by the kidney either, but it is more expensive. The recommended dose of calcitriol is 0.25 µg per dog three times per week. Regardless of the form of vitamin D used, the initial dose should be low, and the dosage should be adjusted based on serial calcium measurements because hypercalcemia is the major complication of treatment. The maximal effect of dihydrotachysterol may not be achieved for 2 to 4 weeks, and duration of effect after cessation of treatment may be as long as 1 week.

Dietary protein restriction will minimize the clinical signs of the uremic syndrome, such as anorexia and vomiting. It is important that caloric intake be adequate, as the breakdown of endogenous proteins to meet energy requirements is just as undesirable as feeding excess protein.

Anorexia and vomiting associated with uremic gastritis may be treated with H_2 antagonists such as cimetidine or ranitidine. These drugs reduce gastrin secretion and thereby decrease the signs of uremic gastritis. The recommended oral dose of cimetidine is 5 mg/kg every 8 hr, and the recommended oral dose for ranitidine is 2 to 4 mg/kg every 12 hr. Uremia may also cause vomiting by stimulating the chemoreceptor trigger zone; therefore phenothiazine-derivative drugs, such as chlorpromazine, may be helpful in controlling vomiting. The normal sedative dose should be reduced to prevent peripheral vasodilation and subsequently decreased renal perfusion. The recommended antiemetic dose is 0.11 mg/kg given as needed subcutaneously. If it appears that in dogs oral ulcers are contributing to the anorexia, lidocaine (Xylocaine Viscous, Astra) applied to the ulcers may be useful.

To reduce the effects of chronic acidosis, it is necessary to replace bicarbonate lost through tubular wasting or through neutralization of retained nonvolatile acids. Each gram of dietary protein generates 1 mEq of nonvolatile acid, therefore dietary protein should be restricted. If urinary bicarbonate wasting is present, the replacement requirement is much higher. The recommended initial dose of sodium bicarbonate is 8 to 12 mg/kg every 8 hr. Bicarbonate therapy can be given as baking soda: 1 gm of baking soda contains about 12 mEq of sodium bicarbonate. The serum bicarbonate or total carbon dioxide concentration should be monitored, and the dose is adjusted accordingly. The goal of treatment is to maintain the serum bicarbonate and carbon dioxide between 18 and 24 mEq/L. Generally, the risk of overtreating and producing alkalosis is small unless there is severe reduction in renal function or volume contraction. Control of any underlying catabolic process also reduces protein breakdown and acid production. Thus early and successful treatment of systemic infections and gastrointestinal bleeding, feeding adequate calories, and avoidance of catabolic drugs such as tetracycline and glucocorticoids will help minimize acidosis. Some concern has been expressed about the sodium intake associated with sodium bicarbonate treatment and its effect on control of hypertension. The volume expansion associated with sodium bicarbonate is primarily intracellular as compared with vascular volume expansion seen with equimolar amounts of sodium chloride supplementation.

Patients with polyuric/uremic renal failure are likely to experience adverse drug reactions. Many drugs and drug metabolites are excreted by the kidneys and may accumulate in the presence of reduced kidney function. In the presence of renal failure, drugs should only be used if there are clear indications. Nephrotoxic drugs should only be used if there are no safer alternatives. If selected, the dose or dosage interval of the nephrotoxic drug must be adjusted to the level of renal function.

Anabolic steroids may benefit anemic chronic renal failure patients because they promote red blood cell production. Anabolic steroids reputedly stimulate red blood cell precursors in the bone marrow, increase renal production of erythropoietin, and increase red blood cell 2,3,diphosphoglycerate (2,3-DPG) levels, which facilitate oxygen delivery to tissues. Clinical trials establishing the efficacy of anabolic steroids for this use are lacking. Recent advances in molecular biology have resulted in the large-scale synthesis of pure human erythropoietin. Clinical trials using recombinant human erythropoietin have shown that anemia in human chronic renal failure patients can be eliminated.

References and Supplemental Reading

Allen, T. A., Jaenke, R. S., and Fettman, M. J.: A technique for estimating progression of chronic renal failure in the dog. J.A.V.M.A. 190:866, 1987.

Anderson, S., Rennke, H. G., and Brenner, B. M.: Therapeutic advantage of converting enzyme inhibitors in arresting progressive renal disease associated with systemic hypertension in the rat. J. Clin. Invest. 77:1993, 1986.

Brenner, B. M., Meyer, T. W., and Hostetter, T. H.: Dietary protein and the progressive nature of kidney disease: The role of hemodynamically mediated glomerular injury in the pathogenesis of progressive glomerular sclerosis in aging, renal ablation, and intrinsic renal disease. N. Engl. J. Med. 307:652, 1982.

Clive, D. M., Stoff, J. S.: Renal syndromes associated with nonsteroidal anti-inflammatory drugs. N. Engl. J. Med. 310:563, 1984.

Eschbach, J., Egrie, J. C., Downing, M., et al.: Correction of the anemia of end-stage renal disease with recombinant human erythropoietin. N. Engl. J. Med. 316:73, 1987.

Lindeman, R. D., Tobin, J. D., and Shock, N. W.: Association between blood pressure and the rate of decline in renal function with age. Kidney Int. 26:861, 1984.

Lumlertgul, D., Burke, T. J., Gillum, D. M., et al.: Phosphate depletion arrests progression of chronic renal failure independent of protein intake. Kidney Int. 29:658, 1986.

Montgomerie, J. Z., Kalamanson, G. M., and Guze, L. B.: Renal failure and infection. Medicine 47:1, 1968.

Nath, K. A., Hostetter, M. K., and Hostetter, T. H.: Pathophysiology of chronic tubulo-interstitial disease in rats: Interactions of dietary acid load, ammonia, and complement component C3. J. Clin. Invest. 76:667, 1985.

Polzin, D. J., Osborne, C. A., Stevens, J. B., et al.: Influence of modified protein diets on the nutritional status of dogs with induced chronic renal failure. Am. J. Vet. Res. 44:1694, 1983.

Polzin, D. J., Osborne, C. A., Hayden, D. W., et al.: Influence of reduced protein diets, morbidity, mortality, and renal function in dogs with induced chronic renal failure. Am. J. Vet. Res. 45:506, 1984.

Polzin, D. J., and Osborne, C. A.: Diseases of the urinary tract. In Davis, L. E. (ed.): Handbook of Small Animal Therapeutics. New York: Churchill Livingstone, 1985, p. 333.

NEWER CONCEPTS AND CONTROVERSIES ON DIETARY MANAGEMENT OF RENAL FAILURE

DELMAR R. FINCO D.V.M.,
and SCOTT A. BROWN D.V.M.

Athens, Georgia

More than 50 years ago, it was observed that a high-protein diet caused proteinuria and glomerular sclerosis in rats. Interest in this information was rekindled with the recognition that, regardless of the initiating factor in renal disease, its progression might be influenced by dietary factors. In the last 10 years, it has been observed that many forms of renal failure are progressive in rats and that reduction of protein intake decreases mortality and prevents or lessens glomerular sclerosis. Renal micropuncture studies in rats have indicated that

hydraulic pressure in glomerular capillaries is increased with high-protein diets, and many (but not all) investigators incriminate this glomerular hypertension as the cause of the glomerular lesions documented in this species.

Restriction of dietary phosphorus (inorganic phosphate) in rats with compromised renal function also reduces mortality. However, phosphorus deprivation in these studies was severe, and generalized malnutrition, including protein malnutrition, was probably present. The prevailing opinion in current medical literature is that phosphorus is not important in progression of renal failure in the rat.

Because conservative medical management, including dietary management, is the mainstay of therapy for dogs and cats with renal failure, an important question to be answered is whether the findings in rats have any relevance in dogs and cats.

The role of diet in initiation or perpetuation of renal lesions is one issue. Another consideration is the effect of diet on extrarenal manifestations of renal failure. For several decades human beings with renal failure have reported amelioration of symptoms with low-protein diets. Veterinarians have observed benefits in dogs as well. (See discussion of dietary restrictions below.)

PROGRESSION OF RENAL FAILURE

Protein

A few studies have examined the effects of dietary protein on renal function and morphology in the dog. In one study dogs had renal mass reduced to about 25 per cent of normal, then were divided into groups, and were fed diets containing 56, 27, or 19 per cent protein for periods up to 4 yr (Bovee et al., 1979). No deterioration of renal function was found in any of the groups. Some glomerular changes that appeared more severe in the high-protein diet group by light microscopy were not confirmed by electron microscopy (Robertson et al., 1986).

Another study that examined effects of different diets on dogs with surgically reduced renal mass found no decline in function over a period of 40 weeks (Polzin et al., 1984). Dogs in this study had mild azotemia. Mild glomerular lesions and mild proteinuria developed in these dogs, but the lesions were not necessarily related to diet.

Why have dramatic lesions developed in kidneys of rats but not in the kidneys of dogs, when both species have the same reduction in renal mass? One possibility is that the glomerular hypertension that occurs in rats (and is incriminated in the pathogenesis of renal lesions) does not occur or is milder in dogs. Because glomeruli of kidneys of dogs and cats are not accessible for micropuncture, direct measurements of intraglomerular capillary pressure cannot be made to establish if glomerular hypertension exists. Although an increase in single-nephron glomerular filtration rate (GFR) is implied from whole kidney measurements, it has not been established whether this increase is due to intracapillary hypertension or is due to increased capillary surface area associated with hypertrophy. Another possibility is that species vary in the effects of glomerular hypertension. Perhaps carnivores, which routinely ingest large protein meals but eat infrequently, have

adapted to the postprandial response to a protein load. One reviewer suggests that rats have detrimental long-term effects on glomerular function from reduction of renal mass but that dogs, rabbits, and human beings do not (Fine, 1988).

Another possibility is that the studies in dogs previously cited did not allow full expression of effects of protein. The dogs in the first study did not have azotemia (Bovee et al., 1979), and the degree of azotemia was mild in the second study (Polzin et al., 1984). Perhaps the threshold for development of significant renal damage in dogs requires a greater degree of dysfunction than existed in dogs in these studies. Possibly, degree of dysfunction and time are related factors, and the second study did not allow enough time for development of renal dysfunction. Another complicating factor is that the studies cited used diets that varied in components other than protein. Phosphorus and other minerals were present in different concentrations in these diets, and there is no assurance that abnormalities, or lack of them, could be related specifically to protein. Despite the limitations, these studies of dogs are valuable because they refute the myth that high-protein diets cause renal damage in normal dogs. This myth is apparently based on the erroneous assumption that findings in rats apply to dogs.

In conclusion, existing data do not resolve the question of whether the rate of progression of pre-existing renal disease in the dog and cat is accentuated by dietary protein or whether dietary protein restriction in patients with renal failure slows the progression of renal disease. Long-term studies are currently under way that may provide some of this information.

Systemic Hypertension

Experiments by Goldblatt in the 1930's established that partial constriction of a renal artery in the dog led to persistent hypertension. Human patients with systemic hypertension and renal failure may have progression of the renal failure. The cause and effect relationship of renal failure and systemic hypertension has been problematic in human medicine. Studies of naturally occurring renal failure in dogs indicate that many dogs with renal failure have systemic arterial hypertension (Cowgill, 1983). The questions that remain unanswered is whether systemic arterial hypertension is invariably transmitted to renal glomerular capillaries, considering the autoregulatory capacity of the kidney and, if so, whether such hypertension is detrimental to the canine and the feline kidney. The answers to these questions will require careful, controlled studies involving both laboratory models of renal failure and hypertension and naturally occurring diseases.

Phosphorus

The initial studies in rats indicating a beneficial effect of phosphorus restriction on progression of renal failure prompted some investigations in dogs and cats. In a study in cats with surgically reduced renal mass, a diet with inorganic phosphorus salts added to achieve a 1.56 per cent phosphorus content caused obvious renal lesions, typified by mineralization, fibrosis, and mononuclear cell infiltration (Ross et al., 1982). Cats with equal functional impairment fed an identical diet except for the deletion of inorganic phosphorus (diet was 0.42 per cent phosphorus) had few lesions. Differences in renal function between the two groups were not statistically significant, however. This study must be interpreted cautiously because of two points. First, the diet to which the phosphorus was added did not have calcium added to maintain a 1.2:1 calcium-phosphorus ratio, so nutritional secondary hyperparathyroidism may have been superimposed on other factors. Second, inorganic phosphorus may be absorbed from the intestines more avidly than the phosphorus present as a component of natural foods (Finco et al., 1988). This study in cats should be repeated, correcting these detractors.

A study on effects of phosphorus restriction in dogs with azotemia has been done (Brown et al., 1987). Azotemia was induced by surgical reduction of renal mass. One group of dogs received an experimental diet containing 17 per cent protein and 0.44 per cent phosphorus, while another group received the same diet but with 1.5 per cent phosphorus. After 2 yr, mortality from uremia was dramatically lower in the phosphorus-restricted group (25 per cent) than in the phosphorus-replete group (67 per cent). Histologic studies are under way to determine whether phosphorus restriction spares the kidney from development of lesions.

In making species comparisons regarding the role of phosphorus in progression of renal failure, the large differences in phosphorus intake among species should be considered. Dogs and cats normally ingest over 200 mg of phosphorus per kilogram of body weight per day; rats consume over 500 mg/kg/day; and people ingest less than 30 mg/kg/day. In one study in people, the influence of phosphorus restriction on progression of renal failure was assessed by comparing one group of patients getting 6.6 mg/kg/day with another group receiving 12 mg/kg/day. Both groups were ingesting about 2500 kcal per day. For people with a body weight of 70 kg, dietary restriction to 6.6 mg/kg resulted in ingestion of 0.18 mg/kcal and restriction to 12 mg/kg resulted in ingestion of 0.34 mg/kcal. By contrast, dogs consuming 70 kcal/kg ingest phosphorus at a rate of 3.24 mg/kcal on a 1.2 per cent diet, and 1.08 mg/kcal on a 0.4 per cent phosphorus diet. Clearly, as results emerge from clinical trials

on phosphorus restriction in humans, it will be necessary to recognize that phosphorus restriction is a relative term and that results obtained in people may not be applicable to the dog. Likewise, most studies in rats with reduced renal function employed a degree of phosphorus restriction much more profound than that achievable in dogs even with a 0.2 per cent phosphorus diet. Consequently, these studies in rats must be viewed with caution when considering dogs and cats.

Lipids

In rats, some studies indicate that dietary fat intake may influence renal diseases by altering renal eicosanoid production. At this time, some evidence favors a role for prostaglandins, whereas other evidence incriminates thromboxane. The issue is confused because prostaglandins seem protective in some models of renal damage but harmful in others. Further studies will be required to determine if dietary lipids influence renal dysfunction in dogs and cats.

RATIONALE FOR DIETARY RESTRICTIONS DURING RENAL FAILURE IN DOGS AND CATS

The foregoing discussion makes it clear that many issues related to diet and renal failure remain to be resolved. In the future it may become apparent that different causes or types of renal diseases require different dietary approaches. At this time there is no basis for different dietary regimens for differing causes of renal failure.

Protein Restriction

1. No evidence exists to indicate that high-protein levels attained in any commercially available diets are harmful to the kidneys of normal dogs. Dogs without evidence of renal dysfunction need not have protein restriction.

2. Evidence for a beneficial effect from protein restriction on the progression of renal dysfunction in dogs and cats does not exist at present. Dietary protein restriction should not be undertaken with this motive.

3. In renal failure, beneficial effects on uremic signs may be achieved when dietary protein is restricted. If anorexia, weight loss, vomiting, and impaired quality of hair coat are observed, protein restriction may alleviate some or all of these signs.

Phosphorus Restriction

1. Earlier studies in dogs established that dietary restriction of phosphorus prevented renal secondary

hyperparathyroidism (RSH) when phosphorus was restricted in proportion to the reduction in GFR (Slatopolsky et al., 1972). RSH occasionally causes clinical signs in dogs and cats with chronic uremia, and phosphorus restriction is a logical approach to reduce the magnitude of the parathyroid response. Even with diets as low as 0.2 per cent phosphorus, however, it is unlikely that RSH can be prevented completely in dogs with extremely low GFR.

2. One laboratory has hypothesized that parathyroid hormone is a uremic toxin that adversely affects many extrarenal tissues. Unfortunately, others have not been able to confirm these observations. Further research is required to establish whether phosphorus restriction can be justified on this basis.

3. Although the mechanism (renal versus extrarenal) for the difference is not apparent at present, the dramatic difference in mortality between phosphate-replete and phosphate-restricted dogs in the study of Brown and associates (1987) strongly suggests a benefit from phosphorus restriction in dogs. Because dogs in this study had been azotemic for 3 months prior to experimentation, it is apparent that phosphorus restriction need not begin prior to azotemia for a beneficial effect. This study did not address the question of benefits from phosphorus restriction earlier in renal failure.

Other Dietary Adjustments

No data exist to indicate an effect of dietary lipids on renal failure in the dog and cat, in relation to altering either the progression of renal disease or the extrarenal manifestations of uremia. Dietary manipulations to ameliorate systemic hypertension may be indicated to improve extrarenal factors, but no evidence is available to indicate that the natural course of renal deterioration is modified.

References and Supplemental Reading

Bovee, K. C., Kronfeld, D. S., Ramberg C. G., and Goldschmidt, M.: Longterm measurement of renal function in partially nephrectomized dogs fed 56, 27, or 19% protein. Invest. Urol. 16:378, 1979.

Brown, S. A., Finco, D. R., Crowell, W. A., and Barsanti, J. A.: Beneficial effect of moderate phosphate restriction in partially nephrectomized dogs on a low protein diet. Kidney Int. 31:380, 1987.

Cowgill, L. D., and Kallet, A. J.: Recognition and management of hypertension in the dog. In Kirk, R. W. (ed.): Current Veterinary Therapy VIII. Philadelphia: W. B. Saunders, 1983, pp. 1025–1028.

Finco, D. R., Barsanti, J. A., and Brown, S. A.: Influence of dietary source of phosphorus on fecal and urinary excretion of phosphorus and other minerals. Am. J. Vet. Res. (in press).

Fine, L.: Preventing the progresson of human renal disease: Have rational therapeutic principles emerged? Kidney Int. 33:116, 1988.

Polzin, D. J., Osborne, C. A., Hayden, D. W., and Stevens, J. B.: Influence of reduced protein diets on morbidity, mortality, and renal function in dogs with induced chronic renal failure. Am. J. Vet. Res. 45:506, 1984.

Robertson, J. L., Goldschmidt, M., Kronfeld, D. S., et al.: Long-term renal responses to high dietary protein in dogs with 75% nephrectomy. Kidney Int. 29:511, 1986.

Ross, L. A., Finco, D. R., and Crowell, W. A.: Effect of dietary phosphorus restriction on the kidneys of cats with reduced renal mass. Am. J. Vet. Res. 43:1023, 1982.

Slatopolsky, E., Cagler, S., Gradowska, L., et al.: On the prevention of secondary hyperparathyroidism in experimental chronic renal disease using "proportionate reduction" of dietary phosphorus intake. Kidney Int. 2:147, 1972.

USE OF DRUGS TO CONTROL HYPERTENSION IN RENAL FAILURE

LINDA A. ROSS, D.V.M.,
and MARY ANNA LABATO, D.V.M.
North Grafton, Massachusetts

Hypertension has been identified in the majority of dogs and cats with chronic renal failure. The incidence has been reported to range from 50 to 93 per cent in dogs with chronic renal failure (Cowgill and Kallet, 1986); 11 of 17 cats (65 per cent) with varying degrees of renal insufficiency studied by the authors had hypertension. Reduction of blood pressure in these animals is indicated for two reasons. First, sustained hypertension itself results in a variety of pathophysiologic consequences, including left ventricular hypertrophy, characteristic lesions in small arteries and arterioles (hypertrophy and hyperplasia of the tunica media, loss of the internal elastic lamina, and fibrinoid necrosis) (Weiner and Giacomelli, 1983), neurologic abnormalities (most commonly the result of intracerebral hemorrhage), and ocular lesions. The latter range from mere observance of retinal vascular changes (straightening and narrowing of larger retinal vessels with mild hypertension and dilated, tortuous vessels with severe hypertension) to visual disturbances or blindness as the result of retinal hemorrhages, exudates, or detachments (Morgan, 1986). These changes may contribute to the morbidity and mortality of chronic renal failure. Second, hypertension may contribute to the progression of chronic renal failure. Hypertensive renal vascular lesions may initiate further damage to the renal parenchyma. In addition, systemic increases in blood pressure may contribute to glomerular hyperfiltration. There is a growing body of evidence indicating that this phenomenon is involved in the progression of renal failure (Anderson and Brenner, 1987).

Glomerular hyperfiltration occurs when there are increases in the glomerular capillary plasma flow rate and the hydraulic pressure in the glomerular capillary. It occurs as a compensatory phenomenon for the loss of other nephrons (that is, each remaining nephron in the diseased kidney must perform additional work to make up for those that have been lost). Although glomerular hyperfiltration would seem to be beneficial in this regard, it apparently has an adverse effect as well. The sustained increases in pressures and flows are thought to initiate a process (as yet ill-defined) that results in glomerulosclerosis and further loss of nephrons (Anderson and Brenner, 1987). Although systemic hypertension does not cause glomerular hyperfiltration in animals with normal renal function, it does in those with experimentally decreased renal function. It appears that compensatory or protective mechanisms are activated in normal kidneys but are abolished or exhausted in those with decreased nephron numbers.

Clinical studies by the authors in animals with renal disease have not demonstrated significant increases in renal function or survival with antihypertensive therapy. Most of the animals studied, however, had moderate to severe uremia. It is possible that initiation of antihypertensive therapy at an earlier stage of renal failure would be beneficial. Numerous experimental studies have documented that such therapy can prevent progressive deterioration of renal structure and function. Based on these studies, it is recommended that reduction of blood pressure in dogs and cats with renal failure be attempted; however, it should be done judiciously and with careful monitoring of renal function. Antihypertensive therapy (with the exception of dietary sodium restriction) should only be instituted if suitable equipment for direct or indirect measurement of blood pressure is available.

MEDICAL MANAGEMENT OF HYPERTENSION

Hypertension occurs as the result of abnormalities in one or more of the mechanisms involved in the normal control of blood pressure. These abnormalities include increased vascular volume, increased sympathetic tone, and activation of the renin-angiotensin system. If the mechanism associated with a certain disease or in a given animal is known, specific therapy could be instituted. Unfortunately, this is rarely the case. The mechanisms involved in the hypertension associated with chronic renal failure have been poorly characterized and in fact may vary with the type of renal disease. Veterinary clinicians have therefore adopted the human protocol of prescribing drugs with different mechanisms of action in either a stepwise or substitution fashion until blood pressure reduction is achieved (Allen, 1986; Cowgill and Kallet, 1986; Ross, 1987). Following institution of each drug, blood pressure is monitored at 1- to 2-week intervals. If reduction to normal levels is not achieved within 2 to 4 weeks, the drug constituting the next step of therapy is added to or substituted for the drug currently being administered.

Although this therapeutic strategy is usually effective in lowering arterial blood pressure, experimental studies have suggested that not all antihypertensive drugs are equally efficacious in slowing the progression of renal disease. Drugs that fail to normalize glomerular capillary pressure have not protected against glomerulosclerosis in several animal models. Hydralazine and the diuretic hydrochlorothiazide are examples of such drugs. Both stimulate the renin-angiotensin system and increase angiotensin II levels, which result in an increase in glomerular efferent arteriolar tone. Increased glomerular capillary pressure (hyperfiltration) is thus maintained in the face of reduced systemic arterial pressure. Drugs that reduce blood pressure by causing suppression of the renin-angiotensin system (angiotensin-converting enzyme inhibitors) reduce glomerular efferent arteriolar tone, decrease hyperfiltration, and protect against glomerulosclerosis (Anderson and Brenner, 1987). Although these drugs would appear to be the therapy of choice for animals with renal disease, clinical studies are lacking. In addition, they have not consistently reduced blood pressure in these animals, and in fact they have been associated with proteinuria, glomerulopathies, and worsening of renal function in dogs (Knowlen and Kittleson, 1986) and humans. The individual clinician must therefore decide whether to use converting enzyme inhibitors for initial antihypertensive therapy or to follow the traditional stepwise or substitution therapy (see below) in hypertensive animals with renal disease.

Because studies of antihypertensive drugs in dogs and cats with spontaneous renal failure are limited, much of the information on their effect on the kidney has been extrapolated from humans and experimental animal models. More extensive studies are needed to make accurate veterinary recommendations.

SPECIFIC TREATMENT

Dietary Sodium Restriction

Increased extracellular fluid volume may be one of the contributing factors to hypertension. Excess dietary sodium intake, resulting in extracellular fluid volume expansion, has been incriminated in the pathogenesis of primary (essential) hypertension in humans. Most commercial dog foods contain high levels of sodium (up to 1 per cent on a dry weight basis). Reduction of dietary sodium intake has been shown to reduce arterial blood pressure in dogs with renal failure. Although data are lacking for cats, it is assumed that a similar situation exists. Sodium intake should be restricted to 0.1 to 0.3 per cent of the diet (10 to 40 mg/kg of body weight) for dogs and 0.4 per cent of the diet for cats. Because the diseased kidney responds slowly to changes in sodium intake, dietary sodium restriction should be done gradually over a period of several weeks. If dietary sodium restriction fails to produce a decrease in blood pressure, pharmacologic therapy is indicated (Allen, 1986; Cowgill and Kallet, 1986; Ross, 1987).

Diuretics

The rationale for the use of diuretics is similar to that for dietary sodium restriction. Diuretic therapy causes contraction of extracellular fluid volume by inducing natriuresis. Thiazide diuretics are the first therapeutic choice in other forms of hypertension; however, they generally prove ineffective in reducing blood pressure in animals with renal failure. Furosemide (Lasix, Hoechst-Roussel) at a dose of 2 to 4 mg/kg repeated every 12 to 24 hr is the diuretic of choice in these animals. Caution should be used when administering this drug so as to avoid dehydrating the patient and worsening the level of renal function. In addition, some owners may object to the polyuria that may result. The serum potassium concentration should be determined periodically, because furosemide can cause potassium depletion. Oral potassium supplementation is indicated if hypokalemia becomes evident.

Beta-Adrenergic Antagonists

Beta-adrenergic antagonists have become a mainstay in the treatment of humans with hypertension because of their efficacy and relative lack of side effects. Despite this, the precise mechanism by which they reduce blood pressure is still unclear. Several hypotheses have been proposed, including reduction in cardiac output, inhibition of renin secretion, suppression of central sympathetic out-flow, and presynaptic blockade of beta-receptors. The most widely accepted current hypothesis attributes hypotensive activity to a reduction in cardiac output associated with a complex series of adjustments in the balance between beta- and alpha-adrenergic tone.

Beta-blockade can affect the renal vasculature, as well as other peripheral vessels. Administration of propanolol has been associated with decreases in both renal plasma flow (RPF) and glomerular filtration rate in humans, although clinical consequences of this decrease have been minimal. The various beta-blockers appear to vary in this regard; atenolol and pindolol do not change RPF and nadolol may cause it to increase (Textor, 1987).

Propanolol (Inderal, Ayerst) is the beta-blocker most commonly administered to animals. It is given at a dose of 5 to 20 mg repeated every 8 to 12 hr for dogs and 2.5 to 5 mg repeated every 8 to 12 hr for cats (proportional to the size of the animal). It is generally several days before reductions in blood pressure are noted. In the authors' experience, propanolol has been fairly successful in reducing blood pressure in cats with renal disease but has had inconsistent results in dogs. Propanolol may be administered in conjunction with a diuretic or as the sole therapeutic agent.

Vasodilators

Vasodilating drugs are administered if blood pressure fails to decrease with the above therapy (with the exception of the converting enzyme inhibitors, which may be used as initial therapy as discussed above). Hydralazine (Apresoline, Ciba) is a direct arteriolar smooth muscle relaxant. It is associated with stimulation of reflex sympathetic activity to the heart, which causes tachycardia; it also results in activation of the renin-angiotensin system. It is frequently necessary to administer a beta-blocker and a diuretic to maintain reductions in blood pressure. Because other drugs used as single agents are equally or more effective in reducing blood pressure, hydralazine is rarely used in animals with renal failure.

Prazosin (Minipress, Pfizer) is an alpha-receptor antagonist, which causes both arteriolar dilation and venodilation without changes in heart rate and cardiac output. It consistently produces reductions in blood pressure in dogs with minimal side effects. For this reason, it has been used as the first and sole drug in hypertensive dogs with renal disease. Its action appears to be somewhat less predictable in cats, and it is used only if diuretic and beta-blocking therapy fail to lower blood pressure. One side effect can be what has been termed the "first dose" effect (i.e., hypotension and syncope following administration of the first dose). This problem is usually self-limiting, and repeated doses rarely produce the same effect. It may be prudent to hospitalize animals for the first day or two of therapy to monitor this effect. The suggested dose is 1 mg/15 kg repeated every 8 to 12 hr.

The converting enzyme inhibitors prevent the conversion of angiotensin I to angiotensin II. Reductions in blood pressure are primarily the result of this suppression of the renin-angiotensin system (loss of angiotensin II–mediated vasoconstriction and suppression of aldosterone secretion with subsequent natriuresis). Other effects, such as increasing the level of circulating kinins, may play a minor role. As discussed above, these drugs may have an advantage in slowing the progression of renal failure. Captopril (Capoten, Squibb) is the most commonly used drug in this class. The suggested dose is 0.5 to 2.0 mg/kg repeated every 8 to 12 hr for dogs and cats. Because captopril is excreted by the kidneys, the dose must be reduced in proportion to the degree of renal dysfunction. In the authors' experience, anorexia, vomiting, and depression have been common side effects when this drug has been administered to animals with renal failure; this has necessitated discontinuation of therapy in a number of animals. Enalapril (Vasotec, Merck) has the advantage of once daily dosing in humans. Dosage schedules for dogs and cats are not yet available.

Calcium channel blocking drugs, such as verapamil (Isoptin, Knoll; Calan, Searle) and nifedipine (Procardia, Pfizer), cause arteriolar dilation by inhibiting calcium transport through slow channels in smooth muscle cell membranes. They have not been evaluated as antihypertensive agents in animals with renal disease but could be considered in animals that fail to respond to other agents. Verapamil has negative inotropic effects and slows atrioventricular conduction time and therefore should probably not be administered in conjunction with beta-adrenergic antagonists. Nifedipine has a short half-life in the dog, which may limit its clinical usefulness.

References and Supplemental Reading

Allen, T. A.: The treatment of hypertension. *In* Proceedings of the Fourth Annual Veterinary Medical Forum, ACVIM, 1986, pp. 3-105–3-107.
Allen, T. A., Wilke, W. L., and Fettman, M. J.: Captopril and enalapril: Angiotensin-converting enzyme inhibitors. J.A.V.M.A. 190:94, 1987.
Anderson, S., and Brenner, B. M.: Role of intraglomerular hypertension in the initiation and progression of renal disease. *In* Kaplan, N. M., Brenner, B. M., and Laragh, J. H. (eds.): *The Kidney in Hypertension.* New York: Raven Press, 1987, pp. 67–76.
Cowgill, L. D., and Kallet, A. J.: Systemic hypertension. *In* Kirk, R. W. (ed.): *Current Veterinary Therapy IX.* Philadelphia: W. B. Saunders, 1986, pp. 360–364.
Knowlen, G. G., and Kittleson, M. D.: Captopril therapy in dogs with heart failure. *In* Kirk, R. W. (ed.): *Current Veterinary Therapy IX.* Philadelphia: W. B. Saunders, 1986, pp. 334–339.
Morgan, R. V.: Systemic hypertension in four cats: Ocular and medical findings. J. Am. Anim. Hosp. Assoc. 22:615, 1986.
Muther, R. S., Reid, G. M., and Bennett, W. M.: Management of hypertension in the patient with renal insufficiency or renal failure. *In* Kaplan, N. M., Brenner, B. M., and Laragh, J. H. (eds.): *The Kidney in Hypertension.* New York: Raven Press, 1987, pp. 251–268.
Ross, L. A.: Hypertension—pathophysiology and management. *In* Proceedings of the 54th Annual Meeting of the American Animal Hospital Association, 1987, pp. 350–353.
Textor, S. C.: Vasodilators and beta-adrenergic antagonists. *In* Kaplan, N. M., Brenner, B. M., and Laragh, J. H. (eds.): *The Kidney in Hypertension.* New York: Raven Press, 1987, pp. 145–160.
Weiner, J., and Giacomelli, F.: Hypertensive vascular disease. *In* Genest, J., Kuchel, O., Hamet, P., et al. (eds.): *Hypertension.* New York: McGraw-Hill, 1983, pp. 498–524.

MANAGEMENT OF URINARY TRACT INFECTIONS

KENITA S. ROGERS, D.V.M.,
and GEORGE E. LEES, D.V.M.
College Station, Texas

Infection of the urinary tract is a common clinical problem in small animal practice. It is a particularly important disease entity in the dog, with cats being affected much less commonly. Treatment of bacterial urinary tract infection (UTI) with antimicrobial agents often is simple and straightforward. However, successful treatment of UTI in some patients is complex, and the clinician must understand a number of important concepts for the treatment of UTI to be uniformly effective and for the therapeutic outcome to be predictable.

First, the proper use of various diagnostic tests and clinical criteria for diagnosis of UTI must be appreciated. Definitive diagnosis of UTI is based on isolation of organisms from a properly collected urine specimen. Cystocentesis is the specimen collection technique of choice to obtain urine for microbiologic evaluation; urine of healthy dogs and cats is always sterile when it is obtained in this manner. Although clinical signs of cystitis, such as pollakiuria and dysuria, may aid in the detection of UTI, such clinical signs also are associated with numerous noninfectious diseases of the lower urinary tract. Additionally, a substantial proportion of UTI episodes in dogs and cats are subclinical, with the patient exhibiting no clinical signs of urinary disease. Evaluation of urine sediment is another valuable diagnostic aid. Unfortunately, urinalysis results may not reliably indicate therapeutic success or failure. Consequently, the diagnosis of UTI should be based mainly on bacterial isolation, then correlated with carefully interpreted clinical signs and urinalysis results. (A more exhaustive discussion of diagnosis and localization of UTI may be found in *Current Veterinary Therapy IX*, p. 1118).

The role that host defense mechanisms play in the acquisition and the eradication of UTI also must be understood. Normal host defenses against UTI include the resident nonpathogenic flora of the urethra and genitalia, secretory immunoglobulins, and normal micturition and flow of urine, as well as the intrinsic antibacterial properties of urine and of the urinary tract mucosa. Abnormalities that impair one or more of these defenses may render the animal more susceptible to UTI or make existing infection more difficult to eradicate. Examples of abnormalities that impair host defenses include urinary calculi, indwelling urinary catheters, neurologic disorders that inhibit proper voiding, anomalous anatomic structures, diabetes mellitus, and excessive endogenous or exogenous corticosteroids. To optimize the contribution of host defenses to preventing and eradicating UTI, abnormalities such as these must be recognized and corrected whenever possible. The treatment plan should take these abnormalities into account because they may alter the efficacy of antimicrobial drug therapy.

Finally, when the importance of host defense mechanisms is acknowledged, differentiation between uncomplicated and complicated UTI is possible. By definition, UTI is said to be uncomplicated when concomitant abnormalities that might impair defense mechanisms are absent or unrecognized. Uncomplicated infections are more readily eradicated and carry a relatively low risk of producing renal damage. Complicated infections are those associated with additional urinary abnormalities that impair host defense mechanisms. Making a distinction between uncomplicated and complicated infections is always important when formulating therapeutic plans for UTI. When UTI is judged to be complicated, a rational therapeutic plan must include correction or amelioration of the underlying abnormality whenever possible. In general, the duration of treatment needed for complicated infections is longer than that needed for uncomplicated infections. Additionally, distinguishing between un-

complicated and complicated UTI allows the clinician to predict the course of the disease and the outcome of therapy with greater accuracy.

The fundamental principles underlying successful treatment of UTI are that bacterial growth must be controlled and that host defense mechanisms must be optimized, not only to eliminate the current infection, but also to prevent future infection. The most important short-term goal of therapy for UTI is to produce remission of clinical signs, but the long-term goal is to prevent possible sequelae of UTI such as pyelonephritis, bacterial prostatitis, deep-seated infection of the bladder wall, development of urinary calculi, and sepsis. Urinary tract infection is frequently the cause of bacteremia, especially if the kidney and the prostate gland are involved. Prevention of these sequelae is accomplished by prompt recognition and correct treatment of UTI. Additionally, the way that each patient responds to treatment may provide clues about the extent of the infectious disease and the integrity of the animal's defenses against infection.

PRINCIPLES OF ANTIMICROBIAL THERAPY

Besides recognition and correction of impairments of host defenses, treatment of UTI requires administration of appropriate antimicrobial therapy. Formulation of a rational course of therapy involves selection of an appropriate antimicrobial drug, the proper route of administration, and an adequate duration of treatment. The clinician must also judge which patients should be treated, as well as whether ancillary treatment methods are necessary or beneficial. Each of these issues will be discussed separately.

The identity of the infecting organism is the single most important guide to rational selection of the proper antimicrobial agent. The seven genera of organisms that account for most UTI in dogs and cats are *Escherichia, Staphylococcus, Streptococcus, Proteus, Klebsiella, Pseudomonas,* and *Enterobacter*. In most instances, a single strain of bacteria is responsible for the UTI; however, in approximately one fifth of the cases, two or more strains of organisms can be isolated. After the infecting organisms are isolated and identified, an appropriate antimicrobial agent can be selected with considerable accuracy because most urinary pathogens have antimicrobial drug susceptibilities that are highly predictable. Because their efficacy is predictable, certain oral antibiotics become reasonable first choices for therapy when the organism has been identified, even when full susceptibility testing has not been performed. The frequency of occurrence of the common genera of urinary pathogens and their susceptibility to selected antibiotics are provided in Table 1. Recommended dosages and sched-

Table 1. *Frequency of Occurrence and Susceptibility of Common Urinary Pathogens to Selected Oral Antibiotics**

Organism	Frequency of Occurrence	Susceptibility Approaching 100%	Susceptibility Approximately 80%
Escherichia	38%		TMS†
Staphylococcus	15%	Penicillin	
Proteus	14%		Penicillin
Streptococcus	10%	Penicillin	
Klebsiella	8%		Cephalexin
Pseudomonas	3%		Tetracycline
Enterobacter	3%		TMS

*Data from Ling (1986).
†Trimethoprim-sulfa.

ules of administration of these drugs are provided in Table 2.

When mixed infections are present, rational therapy can be based on the identity of the infecting organisms. Combinations of staphylococci, streptococci, and *Proteus* spp. usually can be treated successfully with penicillins. In animals infected with gram-positive cocci and with *E. coli* or with a combination of *E. coli* and *Proteus* spp., trimethoprim-sulfa (TMS) often is effective. When a mixed infection includes any combination of *E. coli* or *Proteus* spp., with *Enterobacter* spp. or *Klebsiella* spp., TMS and cephalexin are the rational antibiotic choices. When a mixed infection includes *Pseudomonas* spp., the other uropathogen should be treated with the most effective agent for that organism, then the *Pseudomonas* spp. should be treated with tetracycline. An alternative method is to use an aminoglycoside that is effective against all the pathogens in a mixed infection that includes *Pseudomonas* spp. However, aminoglycosides generally are not chosen for initial treatment of UTI. These drugs are potentially nephrotoxic and must be administered by injection. The duration of therapy with these drugs often is limited by safety and expense. Thus, use of aminoglycosides usually is reserved for episodes of UTI in which susceptibility

Table 2. *Drug Dosages and Urine Concentrations Achieved in Dogs for Selected Oral Antimicrobial Agents**

Drug	Dosage†	Urine Concentration‡ (μg/dl)
Ampicillin	77 mg/kg	309 ± 55
Penicillin G	110,000 U/kg	294 ± 211
Trimethoprim-sulfa	26 mg/kg	55 ± 19
Cephalexin	55 mg/kg	805 ± 421
Tetracycline	55 mg/kg	138 ± 65

*Data from Ling (1986).
†All drug dosages are to be divided into three daily doses, with the exception of trimethoprim-sulfa, which is given in two daily doses.
‡Values are listed as the mean ± the standard deviation.

testing shows that no other antibiotics are acceptable choices. Except for TMS combinations, simultaneous administration of two or more antimicrobial drugs should be avoided.

Because of the predictable efficacy of certain drugs for treatment of common urinary tract pathogens, antimicrobial drug susceptibility testing is valuable mainly for guiding treatment of UTI caused by microbes with unpredictable susceptibilities and by organisms that did not respond favorably to previous antimicrobial therapy. Microbes with unpredictable susceptibilities are uncommon urinary pathogens. Failure of the common uropathogens to respond to antibiotic therapy as anticipated serves as a reminder that many of these organisms are capable of rapid changes in their drug susceptibilities when they are exposed to antibiotics *in vivo*. Thus, a history of recent antimicrobial drug administration, whether for UTI or some other condition, increases the need to rely on antimicrobial drug susceptibility testing. Many bacteria are capable of changing their susceptibility to antibiotics by transferring extrachromosomal DNA units called R-plasmids among themselves. These genetic pieces are incorporated into the bacterial genome and act in a variety of ways to produce resistance of the bacterial cell to any of several classes of antimicrobial agents. An entire bacterial population can acquire resistance by this method of genetic transfer following even a single dose of an antimicrobial agent. Therefore, urine culture and sensitivity testing is imperative when a patient with UTI has not been cured by treatment with the antibiotic agent of first choice. Results of such testing are required for rational formulation of subsequent antibiotic treatment of this episode of UTI.

The preferred method for evaluation of antimicrobial drug susceptibility requires determination of each drug's minimal inhibitory concentration (MIC) for the organisms. The MIC is the least concentration of a drug sufficient to prevent growth of the bacteria *in vitro*. The efficacy of any therapeutic agent largely depends on attainment of a drug concentration in the *in vivo* environment of the bacteria that exceeds the MIC of the drug for the organisms. Efficacy of agents used to treat UTI correlates with their concentrations in urine better than with their blood concentrations. The peak concentrations that an antimicrobial drug achieves in urine and blood often are markedly different. Indeed, active forms of some antimicrobial drugs used for treatment of UTI attain urine concentrations more than 100 times greater than their peak blood concentrations. The drugs most effective for treatment of UTI are those that are excreted by the kidneys because the mechanism of elimination produces high concentrations of drug in the urine. Therefore, the antimicrobial drug susceptibilities of uropathogens are more appropriately evaluated by comparison of the results of MIC determinations with values for expected urine drug concentration during treatment, rather than by using standardized disk diffusion methods. Results of the latter methods are interpreted on the basis of expected blood concentrations of drugs rather than urine concentrations.

To interpret MIC results, MIC values are compared with urinary concentrations of drugs measured in healthy dogs during treatment with specific regimens (see Table 2). Organisms are highly likely to be susceptible to the drug when their MIC value is less than or equal to one fourth of the mean drug concentration that is obtained in the urine. Although evaluation of the drug susceptibility of uropathogens on the basis of urine rather than blood concentrations is more accurate, some difficulties in interpretation still remain. Available data regarding drug concentrations in urine during treatment were generated by studies of healthy dogs, and these values may not apply to dogs with excessive urine production or impaired renal function. Additionally, unanticipated *in vivo* factors such as the presence of urinary foreign bodies or perturbations of drug metabolism may reduce efficacy of the drug.

Although culture and sensitivity testing with MIC determinations gives the best prediction of drug efficacy, the only definitive method of verifying *in vivo* efficacy of drug therapy is to culture the urine for microbes during and following treatment. Effective antibiotic therapy should eradicate bacteriuria within 1 to 3 days of initiating treatment, and the urine should remain sterile for the duration of the treatment period. Therefore, a sterile culture of urine obtained 3 to 5 days after beginning antibiotic therapy demonstrates that an appropriate antimicrobial agent was selected. When an infection persists despite antibiotic therapy, a more appropriate antimicrobial drug should be selected on the basis of susceptibility test results. Culture of urine obtained 7 to 14 days after cessation of treatment verifies cure of the infection, detects relapse of the infection, or indicates development of a new infection (i.e., reinfection). Prompt relapse of bacteriuria with recrudescence of infection caused by the same organisms as before treatment is usually due to an inadequate duration of treatment for deep-seated infections. Retreatment for a longer time is indicated; however, the susceptibilities of the organisms to drugs may have changed, and MIC determinations should be repeated. Frequent reinfection generally is caused by impairment of host defense mechanisms, rather than by inadequacy of antimicrobial therapy.

In addition to being efficacious, antimicrobial drugs for treatment of UTI need to be safe, convenient, and economical to use. For most episodes of UTI, oral drug administration is preferred. One important exception to this preference is for the initial treatment of acute pyelonephritis. In this circumstance, a parenteral route of administration should be used until systemic clinical signs subside; this usually occurs in 2 to 3 days. Parenteral drug administration also is appropriate whenever UTI is associated with sepsis. Regardless of the route of administration chosen, the therapeutic strategy should ensure that optimal concentrations of the drug persist in the urine as long as possible during each treatment interval. This goal can be achieved in house-trained pets by restricting their opportunity to urinate until just before the time for the next drug treatment. Drug treatments must be given frequently enough to sustain inhibitory concentrations of the drug in the urine. With the exception of TMS, which may be given every 12 hr, antimicrobial agents should be given at least every 8 hr for treatment of UTI.

The appropriate length of antimicrobial therapy will depend on the nature and extent of the UTI. The general goals of therapy are to eradicate the current episode of UTI and to decrease the risk of significant sequelae by using strategies to prevent or suppress clinically important infections associated with irreversible abnormalities. Treatment for 10 to 14 days usually is sufficient to cure uncomplicated urethrocystitis in dogs and cats; however, infections involving the kidney or prostate and deep-seated infections within the bladder wall often require more prolonged courses of therapy. *Bacterial urinary tract infections that occur in noncastrated, adult male dogs should be presumed to involve their prostate glands.* As with any form of bacterial prostatitis, treatment should be continued for at least 4 weeks, and even longer periods of treatment may be required. Acute bacterial prostatitis often responds rapidly to administration of antibiotics, including drugs that do not typically penetrate into normal prostatic secretions. Presumably, the intense inflammatory reaction initiated by acute infections alters the permeability of the prostatic epithelium, allowing the drug to enter the infected prostatic acini. However, the treatment of chronic bacterial prostatitis is often difficult. Such infections usually are caused by aerobic gram-negative rods, and the antibiotics to which these organisms are susceptible often do not cross the blood-prostate barrier without the benefit of a prominent inflammatory response. Because penetration of drug to the site of infection is poor, treatment of chronic bacterial prostatitis may need to be continued for 6 to 8 weeks or longer. *Guidelines for treatment of pyelonephritis are similar to those for prostatitis.* Although episodes of acute, uncomplicated pyelonephritis may be cured by treatment for 2 to 4 weeks, most episodes diagnosed in dogs or cats are complicated, chronic, or both. Consequently, appropriate duration of therapy for pyelonephritis usually is 6 to 8 weeks or longer. Protracted treatment with an appropriate antibiotic also is needed in conjunction with treatment to dissolve urinary calculi associated with UTI.

In some animals, UTI is incurable. If treatment for 2 to 3 months does not produce a cure, subsequent treatment should be limited to that required for adequate control of clinical signs. In animals with incurable UTI and in those that have frequent reinfections, exhaustive diagnostic efforts to discover any potentially treatable abnormalities impairing host defenses must be made. Although necessary, such efforts may not be rewarding. The infection may be incurable because of irreversible impairment of the animal's defense mechanisms against UTI or because the infection is so deep seated that it cannot be eradicated completely.

For animals with frequent reinfections, the alternatives are to treat each episode of UTI as it occurs or to use prophylactic therapy. Treatment of the individual episodes is recommended if they occur less than three times annually. To use prophylactic therapy, the most recent episode of UTI must first be cured. Then, an appropriate antibiotic is given as a single daily (nightly) dose that is approximately one third of the daily dose for conventional therapy. This strategy prevents recolonization of the urinary tract by pathogens and reduces risk of resistant infections. Patients receiving prophylactic therapy should be evaluated at 2- to 4-month intervals to encourage owner compliance, verify sterility of the urine, and measure renal function. The antibiotic of choice for prevention of gram-positive reinfection is amoxicillin. For gram-negative or mixed infections, TMS, cephalexin, or nitrofurantoin is used for prophylactic therapy.

Although episodes of UTI usually are treated when they are diagnosed, the more judicious action in some circumstances is to defer treatment. This is particularly true in patients with temporary impairments of their host defenses, such as those with indwelling urinary catheters, calculi, or disordered micturition. Infection associated with urinary catheterization deserves special mention. For prevention of catheter-induced UTI, intermittent catheterization is superior to indwelling catheterization. When indwelling catheterization is necessary, a closed drainage system should be maintained. Treatment of UTI during indwelling catheterization is not recommended unless the patient becomes symptomatic or septicemic. Treatment during catheterization invites development of a new, more resistant infection and should be avoided if possible. The best time to treat catheter-induced UTI is after the urinary catheter is removed. Another clinical situation in which therapy is temporarily delayed occurs when antibiotics might obscure clinical signs and make correct diagnosis more difficult. One may also choose not to treat an incurable UTI continuously but to provide therapy only when exacerbations of clinical signs occur.

ANCILLARY THERAPY

Antimicrobial drug administration is the mainstay of treatment for UTI, and ancillary therapy is used to complement and amplify the beneficial effects of antimicrobial agents. As discussed previously, the ancillary treatment measures of greatest importance are specific corrections of underlying abnormalities and associated diseases that might impair host defenses. Ancillary treatment considerations include use of urinary pH modifiers, antiseptics, analgesics, and antispasmodics.

Modification of urine pH is not an important or routinely used component of treatment for UTI. In the treatment of UTI, urine pH modifiers usually are meant to cause direct effects on bacterial growth in the urine or to enhance the action of antimicrobial drugs in the urine. Although an acid pH impairs bacterial growth, sufficiently bacteriostatic and bactericidal urine pH values are difficult to sustain. Antimicrobial drug activity in urine is affected by pH, but the efficacy of the antibiotics routinely used to treat UTI does not require pH modification. Canine and feline urine is usually slightly acidic. Only aminoglycosides, which are not preferred for initial therapy, are more active in alkaline urine.

Urinary antiseptics are antibacterial agents that cannot be used to treat systemic infections. These drugs are excreted so rapidly by the kidneys that significant antimicrobial activity occurs only in the urinary tract. Nitrofurantoin is effective against *E. coli*, staphylococci, and streptococci and is well suited for protracted use in animals with normal renal function. It is often satisfactory for prophylactic therapy in animals with frequent reinfection due to impaired defenses. Methenamine is given orally and is excreted in the urine. In the presence of acidic urine, the drug decomposes and liberates formaldehyde, which has an antibacterial activity. Because the action of methenamine depends on an acidic pH, a urinary acidifier is generally given concurrently. Methenamine is one of the few agents that is effective against fungal UTI. Methylene blue and nalidixic acid are other urinary antiseptics, but they should not be used because of their narrow margins of safety. Heinz body hemolytic anemia is associated with the use of methylene blue, particularly in the cat, and nalidixic acid may cause seizures.

Phenazopyridine is a urinary analgesic. This azo dye is given orally and is excreted in the urine, causing an orange discoloration. The drug relieves the discomfort of urethrocystitis in people, but its clinical value in veterinary medicine is not documented. Phenazopyridine also causes a Heinz body hemolytic anemia in the cat. Propantheline is a parasympatholytic drug, which may act as an antispasmodic by reducing spastic detrusor activity. Its usefulness in managing canine and feline cystitis is poorly substantiated.

NEW CONCEPTS

Much of the recent attention in UTI research has been devoted to the most appropriate duration of therapy and to new methods of preventing infection. Single-dose or short-course (3 day) treatment regimens are currently the preferred therapeutic protocol for women with acute urethrocystitis when proper follow-up examinations can be obtained. Women who have concomitant asymptomatic renal infections are identified by discovering that their infections promptly relapse. These individuals may require further diagnostic evaluation, and they need to be treated for their kidney infections. Meanwhile, women with simple urethrocystitis are quickly, safely, and inexpensively cured. Thus, short-course therapy of UTI in women has diagnostic and therapeutic advantages. Preliminary results of similar treatment in dogs has been disappointing. Acceptable efficacy with single-dose therapy has not yet been demonstrated in experimental or naturally induced UTI.

As an understanding of the pathogenesis of UTI has evolved, new approaches to the prevention of infection in susceptible individuals have developed. Those that may have future application include analogues that block molecular sites of attachment on bacterial or mucosal cell walls, suppressing the production of bacterial structures such as fimbriae, and agents that promote development of an immunologic response to the bacterial organisms. Although such measures may alter UTI treatment in the future, current therapeutic goals are to recognize and correct any abnormalities in host defense mechanisms and to administer an appropriate course of antimicrobial therapy. When a rational therapeutic plan is formulated for each patient with UTI, the clinician should be routinely successful in the management of this disease.

References and Supplemental Reading

Lees, G. E., and Rogers, K. S.: Treatment of urinary tract infections in dogs and cats. J.A.V.M.A. 189:648, 1986a.

Lees, G. E., and Rogers, K. S.: Diagnosis and localization of urinary tract infection. In Kirk, R. W. (ed.): Current Veterinary Therapy IX. Philadelphia: W. B. Saunders, 1986, pp. 1118–1123.

Ling, G. V.: Therapeutic strategies involving antimicrobial treatment of the canine urinary tract. J.A.V.M.A. 185:1162, 1984.

Ling, G. V.: Management of urinary tract infections. In Kirk, R. W. (ed.): Current Veterinary Therapy IX. Philadelphia: W. B. Saunders, 1986, pp. 1174–1177.

Ronald, A. R.: Current concepts in the management of urinary tract infections in adults. Med. Clin. North Am. 68:335, 1984.

Senior, D. F.: Bacterial urinary tract infections: Invasion, host defenses, and new approaches to prevention. Comp. Cont. Ed. Small Anim. Pract. 7:334, 1985.

FELINE PERINEAL URETHROSTOMY

A Potential Cause of Hematuria, Dysuria, and Urethral Obstruction

CARL A. OSBORNE, D.V.M.,
DENNIS D. CAYWOOD, D.V.M.,
GARY R. JOHNSTON, D.V.M.,
and JOHN M. KRUGER, D.V.M.

St. Paul, Minnesota

APPLIED ANATOMY AND PHYSIOLOGY

The urethra of male cats may be divided into four segments for descriptive diagnostic and therapeutic purposes (Fig. 1). The *preprostatic urethra* extends from the neck of the urinary bladder to the prostate gland. Because the prostate gland of cats is located several centimeters caudal to the bladder neck, the preprostatic urethra is proportionally longer in male cats than in dogs. The preprostatic urethra is lined by smooth muscle that plays a major role in maintaining urinary continence during the storage phase of micturition.

The prostate gland is proportionately smaller than that in dogs, and the *prostatic urethra* of cats is correspondingly smaller. The prostate gland of male cats does not surround the ventral portion of the prostatic urethra. Although this section of the pros-

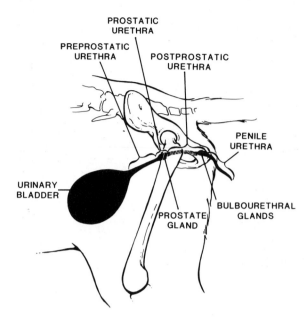

Figure 1. Schematic reproduction of the lower urinary tract of a male cat.

tatic urethra is short, it is occasionally seen as a narrowed region in the midpelvic area of contrast urethrograms (Johnston et al., 1982a).

The *postprostatic (membranous) urethra* extends from the prostate gland to the paired bulbourethral glands, which are located at the caudal aspect of the bony pelvis on the dorsolateral surface of the urethra. This segment of the urethra contains functionally insignificant smooth muscle; it is surrounded by a thick layer of striated muscle (urethralis muscle). The urethralis muscle of male cats is thicker but shorter than the same muscle in dogs (Cullen et al., 1983). The submucosa of the postprostatic urethra contains so-called disseminated prostate glands. Whether these glands have any developmental or functional relationship to the prostate gland is unknown.

The *penile urethra* extends from the bulbourethral glands to the tip of the penis. It lies along the dorsal surface of the penis, embedded in corpus spongiosum penis. The os penis, when present, is not grooved to accommodate the penile urethra. The diameter of the penile urethra becomes progressively smaller toward the external urethral orifice (see Fig. 1).

In addition to its roles during the voiding and storage phases of micturition, the urethra contains an integrated anatomic and functional defense system, which provides resistance to microbial infection. It also impedes retrograde passage of pathogens and semen into more proximal portions of the urinary tract. The predisposition of the narrow penile urethral lumen to obstruction prompts questions about its anatomic configuration. It may be important in reproduction, as male cats produce

only a small volume of ejaculate (less than 1 ml) (Sojka, 1980). It would also facilitate urine spraying, which cats frequently use to mark their domain. The fluid dynamics of the urethra of male cats are similar to those of the garden hose with adjustable nozzle.

CAUSES AND SITES OF URETHRAL OBSTRUCTION

Survey and contrast radiographic evaluation of male cats with lower urinary tract outflow obstruction has revealed a variety of underlying causes (Table 1). Although the penile urethra is a common site of obstruction, other sites may also be involved (Fig. 2). In some instances, more than one site may be affected by etiologically different mechanisms (Osborne et al., 1984). Inability to readily restore urethral patency by flushing the urethral lumen with a sterile physiologic solution should arouse one's suspicion of mural or periurethral lesions at one or more sites in addition to, or instead of, a matrix-crystalline plug lodged in the penile urethra. In this situation, contrast antegrade cystourethrography or retrograde urethrocystography is recommended to further define the site and cause of the abnormality (Johnston et al., 1982b).

COMPLICATIONS OF PERINEAL URETHROSTOMY

The need for, and the type of, medical and surgical procedures designed to treat and prevent feline obstructive uropathy should be based on appropriate diagnosis. Effective therapeutic and preventive medical protocols (Barsanti and Finco, 1986; Osborne et al., 1985a) and surgical techniques (Caywood and Raffe, 1984; Lees et al., 1981; Osborne et al., 1985a) have been reviewed elsewhere.

On occasion, medical procedures designed to correct or prevent recurrent urethral obstruction are ineffective. In these situations, perineal urethrostomies and other surgical procedures designed to bypass the penile urethra are commonly considered, irrespective of underlying cause. Recognizing the symptomatic nature of such treatment, there has been a consensus that nonobstructive signs of lower urinary tract disease (e.g., dysuria, pollakiuria, and hematuria) might persist or recur following surgery. With the exception of complications directly attributable to anesthesia and surgery (anesthetic deaths, postoperative hemorrhage, dehiscence, subcutaneous extravasation of urine, urine scald dermatitis, perineal hernias, strictures, urinary incontinence, urethrorectal fistula, or infection) (Caywood and Raffe, 1984), too little thought was given to the possibility that amputation of the

Table 1. *Possible Causes of Urethral Obstruction in Male Cats*

Primary Causes	Perpetuating Causes	Iatrogenic Causes
Intraluminal	***Intraluminal***	***Tissue Damage***
Urethral plugs (matrix and/or crystals)	White blood cells, red blood cells, and fibrin	Reverse flushing solutions
Urethroliths	Sloughed tissue	Catheter trauma
Tissue sloughed from urinary bladder or urethra	Increased production of mucoprotein	Catheter-induced foreign body reaction
		Catheter-induced infection
Mural or Extramural	***Mural***	***Postsurgical Dysfunction***
Strictures	Inflammatory swelling	Abnormal postprostatic urethral pressure
Prostatic lesions	Muscular spasm (reflex dyssynergia?)	Others?
Urethral neoplasms	Strictures	
Anomalies		
Reflex dyssynergia		
Combinations	***Combinations***	
Others?	***Others?***	

distal urethra might predispose the patient to recurrent signs of lower urinary tract disease owing to mechanisms unrelated to the initial cause of the problem.

Recently, a few pilot studies have been designed to determine the underlying cause of lower urinary tract signs *before* and *after* urethral surgery. The results of these studies suggest that urethrostomies may be associated with significant short-term and long-term complications. They include bacterial urinary tract infections and urolithiasis in addition to urethral strictures.

Bacterial Urinary Tract Infections

Results of several clinical investigations of feline lower urinary tract disease indicate that the initial episode usually occurs in absence of significant numbers of detectable bacteria (Barsanti et al., 1982; Martens et al., 1984). In a prospective study of obstructed and nonobstructed cats at the University of Minnesota, bacterial UTI was identified only in 4 of 143 (2.8 per cent) previously untreated patients. These patients had not been catheterized prior to the time of diagnostic evaluation; none had perineal urethrostomies.

When significant bacteriuria has been confirmed, it frequently (but not invariably) occurred as a secondary or complicating factor rather than a primary etiologic factor. Bacterial UTI is a common sequel to use of indwelling catheters (Lee et al., 1981) and perineal urethrostomy (Gregory and Vasseur, 1983; Gregory et al., 1984a, b).

The authors conducted a prospective clinical trial designed in part to study the complications of medical or surgical treatment in the prevention of male feline intraluminal urethral obstruction. The study consisted of 30 male cats with naturally occurring intraluminal urethral obstruction. Following confirmation of urethral obstruction and collection of baseline information (complete urinalysis, quantitative bacterial culture of urine collected by cystocentesis, hemograms, blood chemistry profiles, and retrograde contrast urethrography), cats were randomly assigned to one of three treatment groups

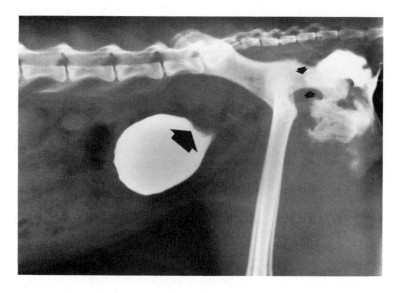

Figure 2. Positive contrast urethrocystogram of the lateral abdomen of a 7-year-old castrated male domestic long-hair cat with urethral obstruction. A perineal urethrostomy was performed 3 days previously. The lumen of the preprostatic urethra has been partially occluded by compression induced by a persistent uterus masculinus (large arrow). The lumen of the postprostatic urethra was completely obstructed by a stricture, presumably inflammatory in origin (small arrows).

(ten cats per group): (1) dietary treatment (Prescription Diet Feline s/d, Hill's Pet Products; formulated to contain reduced quantities of magnesium [0.058 per cent by dry weight] and to promote formation of acid pH [± 6.0]), (2) surgical treatment (perineal urethrostomy by modified Wilson technique), and (3) surgical and dietary treatment (calculolytic diet and perineal urethrostomy). Laboratory data and radiographic studies were obtained 2 weeks and 1 yr following initiation of treatment of all cats. Laboratory and radiographic studies were also determined if signs of lower urinary tract disease recurred at any time following initiation of treatment. In addition, client interviews, physical examinations, complete urinalyses, and quantitative urine cultures were repeated at 1, 3, 6, and 12 months following initiation of treatment. At the conclusion of the study, episodes of bacterial UTI occurred in 17 per cent of the cats treated with perineal urethrostomies, 10 per cent of the cats treated with perineal urethrostomies and dietary therapy, and none of the cats treated with dietary therapy alone (Table 2). Three of the 30 cats developed urocystoliths (see below). There were no recurrences of urethral obstruction in cats treated with dietary therapy, surgery, or both. Likewise, postsurgical strictures were not detected in cats treated by perineal urethrostomy.

In other studies, comparisons of electromyographic and urethral pressure profiles before and after perineal urethrostomies of male cats have revealed a significant decrease of postprostatic urethral pressure and an associated decrease in electromyographic activity (Gregory et al., 1984a). Urinary continence was maintained owing to normal function of the preprostatic urethra. Postsurgical urethral dysfunction was reversible in some cats. However, persistent impairment of postprostatic urethral function was found to enhance the risk of bacterial UTI above that associated with loss of the penile urethra (Gregory et al., 1984b). Whereas urinary tract infection was observed in 18 per cent (2 of 11) of the cats that regained normal urethral pressure and electromyographic activity following perineal urethrostomy, UTI occurred in 57 per cent (4 of 7) of cats with persistently low urethral pressure profiles. This is an explainable association because the midurethral high pressure zone induced by striated muscular activity during the storage phase of micturition has been reported to impede the ascending migration of bacteria in dogs (Mayo and Hinman, 1973).

Urolithiasis

If staphylococcal urinary tract infections develop as a result of surgical removal of the penile urethra and associated local host defense mechanisms, infection-induced struvite urocystoliths may subsequently develop (Osborne et al., 1985b). In the previously described study of surgical or dietary prevention of urethral obstruction, one cat with a perineal urethrostomy (surgery only group) developed a urease-positive staphylococcal urinary tract infection (UTI) 57 days following surgery. The staphylococcal UTI remained asymptomatic until approximately 6 months following surgery, when hematuria and dysuria were observed. Radiography at that time revealed several radiodense urocystoliths. The urocystoliths, presumed to be composed of infection-induced struvite, were subsequently dissolved with combination therapy of the calculolytic diet (Feline s/d, Hill's Pet Products) and therapeutic doses of ampicillin combined with clavulanic acid. A similar phenomenon occurred in another cat with a perineal urethrostomy (surgery only group). The cat developed asymptomatic staphylococcal UTI approximately 30 days following surgery. The staphylococcal UTI remained asymptomatic for 1 yr, at which time hematuria, dysuria, and pollakiuria developed. Multiple, small, radiodense urocystoliths (presumed to be struvite) were identified by radiography at that time. The urocystoliths were

Table 2. *Frequency of Bacterial UTI in Obstructed Male Cats Managed by Surgical or Medical Protocols*

Time of Urinary Tract Infection	Perineal Urethrostomy (n = 10)	Perineal Urethrostomy and Medical Treatment (n = 10)	Medical Treatment (n = 10)
Initial Examination	0/10	0/10	0/10
10–14 days after initiation of treatment	1/10	1/10	0/10
1 month following initiation of treatment	3/10	1/10	0/10
3 months following initiation of treatment	2/10	2/10	0/10
6 months following initiation of treatment	3/10	0/10	0/10
1 year following initiation of treatment	1/9*	2/10	0/10
Frequency of infection	10/59*	6/60	0/60

*One cat dropped from study at 6 months owing to development of urolithiasis.

dissolved by use of the treatment previously described (calculolytic diet and antibiotics).

At the conclusion of the 1-yr study, a slightly radiodense urocystolith (1.5 by 1.0 cm) was identified in a cat assigned to the medical management group. Survey and contrast radiography indicated that the stone was not present at the time of diagnosis, or at the 2 week post-treatment evaluation. Quantitative analysis of the urolith revealed that it was composed of 100 per cent ammonium acid urate. Ammonium urate crystalluria was not present in urine samples evaluated 0.5, 1, 3, or 6 months following initiation of dietary management. Ammonium urate uroliths would not be expected to be prevented by the diet being utilized (Prescription Diet Feline s/d, Hill's Pet Products) because it is not restricted in uric acid precursors (purines) and because it promotes formation of acid urine.

Urethral Strictures

Postoperative urethral strictures have been associated with improper surgical technique, use of postoperative indwelling urethral catheters, and self-trauma (Caywood and Raffe, 1984; Smith, 1985; Smith, et al., 1981). They may be prevented by good surgical technique, avoidance of postoperative urinary catheters, and restraint devices to minimize self-trauma. If postoperative urethral strictures predispose to clinical signs, corrective surgery should be considered, but not before the lower urinary tract has been evaluated by antegrade cystourethrography or retrograde urethrocystography (Caywood and Raffe, 1984; Osborne et al., 1985a).

SUMMARY

Perineal urethrostomies are associated with complications that may mimic primary causes of feline lower urinary tract disorders. Although postoperative urethral strictures may be minimized by proficiency with an effective surgical technique, removal of the distal urethra may result in bacterial urinary tract infections in 25 to 30 per cent of the patients following surgery. Urinary tract infections caused by urease-producing microbes may induce struvite urolith formation. Thus the prophylactic benefits of minimizing recurrent urethral obstruction by urethrostomy must be weighed against a long-term predisposition to recurrent bacterial UTI and urolith formation. Perineal urethrostomies should be avoided unless (1) there are irreversible mural or extramural lesions that cause recurrent or persistent obstruction of the penile urethra, or (2) frequent outflow obstruction of the distal urethra occurs despite properly designed medical management.

References and Supplemental Reading

Barsanti, J. A., and Finco, D. R.: Feline urologic syndrome. In Breitschwerdt, E. B. (ed.): Contemporary Issues in Small Animal Practice: Nephrology and Urology. New York: Churchill Livingstone, 1986, pp. 43–74.

Barsanti, J. A., Finco, D. R., Shotts, E. B., et al.: Feline urologic syndrome. Further investigation into etiology. J. Am. Anim. Hosp. Assoc. 18:391, 1982.

Caywood, D. D., and Raffe, M. R.: Perspectives on surgical management of feline urethral obstruction. Vet. Clin. North Am. 14:677, 1984.

Cullen, W. C., Fletcher, T. F., and Bradley, W. F.: Morphometry of the male feline pelvic urethra. J. Urol. 129:186, 1983.

Gregory, C. R., and Vasseur, P. B.: Long-term examination of cats with perineal urethrostomy. Vet. Surg. 12:210, 1983.

Gregory, C. R., Holliday, T. A., Vasseur, P. B., et al.: Electromyographic and urethral pressure profilometry: Assessment of urethral function before and after perineal urethrostomy in cats. Am. J. Vet. Res. 45:2062, 1984a.

Gregory, C. R., and Vasseur, P. B.: Electromyographic and urethral pressure profilometry: Long-term assessment of urethral function after perineal urethrostomy in cats. Am. J. Vet. Res. 45:1318, 1984b.

Johnston, G. R., Feeney, D. A., and Osborne, C. A.: Urethrography and cystography in cats. Part I. Techniques, normal radiographic anatomy, and artifacts. Comp. Cont. Ed. Pract. Vet. 4:823, 1982a.

Johnston, G. R., Feeney, D. A., and Osborne, C. A.: Urethrography and cystography in cats. Part II. Abnormal radiographic anatomy and complications. Comp. Cont. Ed. Pract. Vet. 4:931, 1982b.

Lees, G. E., Osborne, C. A., Stevens, J. B., et al.: Adverse effects of open indwelling urethral catheterization in normal male cats. Am. J. Vet. Res. 42:825, 1981.

Martens, J. G., McConnell, S., and Swanson, C. L.: The role of infectious agents in naturally occurring feline urologic syndrome. Vet. Clin. North Am. 14:503, 1984.

Mayo, M. E., and Hinman, F.: Role of the midurethral high pressure zone in spontaneous bacterial ascent. J. Urol. 109:268, 1973.

Osborne, C. A., Johnston, G. K., Polzin, D. J., et al.: Redefinition of the feline urologic syndrome: Feline lower urinary tract disease with heterogenous causes. Vet. Clin. North Am. 14:409, 1984.

Osborne, C. A., Polzin, D. J., Feeney, D. A., et al.: The urinary system: Pathophysiology, diagnosis, and treatment. In Gourley, I. M., and Vasseur, P. B. (eds.): General Small Animal Surgery. Philadelphia: J. B. Lippincott, 1985a, pp. 622–624.

Osborne, C. A., Polzin, D. J., Abdullah, S., et al.: Struvite urolithiasis in animal and man: Formation, detection, and dissolution. Adv. Vet. Sci. Comp. Med. 29:1, 1985b.

Osborne, C. A., Polzin, D. J., Johnston, G. R., and Kruger, J. M.: Medical management of feline urologic syndrome. In Kirk, R. W. (ed.): Current Veterinary Therapy IX. Philadelphia: W. B. Saunders, 1986, pp. 1196–1206.

Smith, C. W.: Surgical diseases of the urethra. In Slatter, D. H. (ed.): Textbook of Small Animal Surgery. Vol. 2. Philadelphia: W. B. Saunders, 1985, pp. 1803–1806.

Smith, C. W., Schiller, A. G., Smith, A., et al.: Effects of indwelling catheters in male cats. J. Am. Anim. Hosp. Assoc. 17:427, 1981.

Sojka, N. J.: Feline semen collection, evaluation, and artificial insemination. In Morrow, D. A. (ed.): Current Therapy in Theriogenology. Philadelphia: W. B. Saunders, 1980.

PHARMACOLOGIC MANAGEMENT OF URINARY INCONTINENCE

PHILIPPE M. MOREAU, D.V.M., M.S.,
Limoges, France

and MICHAEL R. LAPPIN, D.V.M., Ph.D.
Fort Collins, Colorado

Urinary incontinence refers to a lack of voluntary control over urine elimination from the body. Urinary incontinence may be due to difficulties in retaining urine (classic incontinence or urethral sphincter incompetence) or eliminating urine (paradoxical incontinence or excessive outlet resistance). Urinary incontinence must be distinguished from abnormal elimination behavior, inadequate house training, and certain clinical conditions such as polyuria, pollakiuria, and dysuria. Finally, any underlying neurologic or urinary tract disease should be identified and appropriate treatment instituted.

When managing patients with urinary incontinence, one should remember two major considerations. First, priority should be given to alterations that require immediate care, such as fluid deficits, electrolyte disturbances, acid-base imbalances, and azotemia. These are often present in cases of urine outflow obstruction. Second, normal micturition should be restored as soon as possible, regardless of the cause. Delays in treating disorders of micturition may lead to complications, such as decubital ulcers and urinary tract infection as a result of urethral incompetence, or postrenal azotemia, electrolyte disturbances, bladder overdistention, bladder atony, hydroureter, and hydronephrosis caused by excessive outlet resistance.

NORMAL MICTURITION

Normal micturition is divided into a storage (filling) phase and an emptying (voiding) phase. During the storage phase, the bladder relaxes and urine accumulates gradually as it is formed. Simultaneously, the urethra contracts to maintain sufficient pressure (outlet resistance), preventing urine flow. During the voiding phase, these pressure relationships are reversed by simultaneous contraction of the bladder and relaxation of the urethra to produce urination. The neuromuscular control of micturition

has been well described (see *Current Veterinary Therapy IX*, pp. 1207–1212).

CAUSES OF URINARY INCONTINENCE

Clinically, storage phase disorders are generally manifested by urinary incontinence, whereas emptying phase disorders are usually manifested by urinary retention and some degree of incomplete bladder emptying, although urinary incontinence may also occur.

Urinary incontinence may have neurogenic or non-neurogenic causes. *Non-neurogenic disorders* should be ruled out first. A variety of *anatomic abnormalities of the lower urinary tract* may cause urinary incontinence. Ectopic ureter is the most common congenital disorder and is usually seen in young female dogs who tend to dribble urine constantly. Other congenital anatomic abnormalities that have been described in dogs and cats with urinary incontinence include exstrophy of urinary bladder, patent urachus, pseudohermaphroditism, ureterocele, urethral diverticulum, urethral fistula (rectal or vaginal), and vestibulovaginal stenosis.

Acquired anatomic anomalies have also been associated with urinary incontinence. Inflammatory or infiltrative diseases of the lower urinary tract, including chronic cystitis and urethritis, neoplasia, urolithiasis, and prostatic disease, may cause damage to muscular components or neuroceptors and impair function of the bladder and urethra. Micturition disorders have also been described following abdominal surgical procedures such as ovariohysterectomies, cystotomy, urethrostomy, and prostatic surgery.

Neurologic disorders are common causes of urinary incontinence in dogs and cats. The pathophysiology of neurogenic incontinence varies with the location and the severity of the lesion. Neurologic lesions disrupting upper motor neurons of the micturition reflex impair voluntary control of urination and produce a spastic neuropathic bladder (also called reflex or automatic bladder). If lower motor neurons are intact, reflex detrusor contraction occurs but is often more frequent and is generally not coordinated with urethral sphincter relaxation. This leads to interrupted, involuntary, and incomplete voiding, with resultant urinary retention due to functional urinary obstruction.

Neurologic lesions that disrupt the lower motor neurons of the micturition reflex abolish detrusor contraction and produce a flaccid neuropathic bladder (also called atonic, nonreflexic, or autonomous bladder). Sensation of fullness and detrusor contraction are no longer present, allowing excessive bladder distention, which may damage tight junctions between smooth muscle fibers, resulting in greatly increased bladder capacity. The bladder fills with urine until intravesical pressure exceeds outlet resistance (urethral sphincter tone), inducing an overflow of urine.

Functional incontinence is present when the bladder and urethra appear to be structurally normal, and no neurologic lesions are identified. Such incontinence might result from sphincter mechanism incompetence, detrusor instability, or both.

CLASSIFICATION BY BLADDER AND SPHINCTER STATES

When selecting drugs for treatment, it is clinically more critical to identify bladder and sphincter states, regardless of the causes and the exact location of the lesions. Categorizing the micturition disorder on the basis of whether it primarily affects the storage or the emptying phase is helpful. However, this classification may be difficult or confusing because in some cases both phases of micturition may be affected simultaneously. Idiopathic incontinence or certain forms of functional disorders of micturition associated with mixed neurogenic lesions may exhibit similar clinical signs. Therefore, it is helpful to classify incontinent patients on the basis of whether the bladder is hypocontractile or hypercontractile, whether the urethral sphincter is hypotonic or hypertonic, and whether the urethral sphincter is acting in synchrony with detrusor activity.

Animals with bladder hypocontractility may have an inability to generate sufficient intravesical pressure caused by loss of bladder innervation. Alternatively, the condition may be caused by impairment of detrusor smooth muscle function, such as occurs when tight junctions are damaged by excessive bladder distention.

Animals with bladder hypercontractility may lack inhibitory control of cholinergic receptors and experience frequent stimulation of the micturition reflex even when intravesical volume is small. Detrusor hyperactivity, detrusor instability, or detrusor hyper-reflexia are terms that have also been used to describe bladder hypercontractile states. Animals with detrusor hyperactivity tend to have involuntary and uncontrolled detrusor muscle contractions during the storage phase. Common symptoms include nocturia, pollakiuria, urgency, and urinary incontinence without a distended urinary bladder. These signs are grouped as the "urge incontinence syndrome" in human medicine. In this condition, the sensation of bladder fullness and need to urinate are increased. Micturition reflex is initiated more frequently and, even though voiding may apparently be normal, the storage phase is shorter than normal. Detrusor hyperactivity can be difficult to differentiate from incontinence due to decreased urethral tone, because in both conditions volumes of urine voided are small and frequent. Urodynamic studies may be required in some cases to differentiate the two. Detrusor instability is a term used to describe detrusor hyperactivity caused by outflow obstruction or unknown causes.

Urethral sphincter dysfunction is an important cause of micturition disorders. *Excessive outlet resistance* is caused by either mechanical or functional (hypertonic) obstructions to urine flow. Mechanical obstructions should be ruled out first by easy passage of a urinary catheter through the urethra. Functional obstructions are caused by failure of the urethra to dilate appropriately as the bladder contracts. Intramural lesions such as edema, fibrosis, hemorrhage, inflammation, or tissue infiltration associated with neoplasia, prostatic enlargement, or urolithiasis may also damage muscular components of the urethra, producing myogenic functional obstruction. Sphincter relaxation failure during detrusor contraction may be caused by neurologic lesions, inducing neurogenic functional obstruction (reflex dyssynergia). Smooth muscle components of the internal sphincter and striated muscle components of the external sphincter can be involved either separately or together. Animals with excessive urethral tone (urethral hyper-reflexia) and excessive outlet resistance may display abnormal urine retention plus a variety of other clinical signs related to lower urinary tract disease, such as dysuria, hematuria, pollakiuria, stranguria, and urinary incontinence.

Urethral incompetence due to *urethral sphincter hypotonicity*, decreased functional urethral length, or both are common features of urinary incontinence. During the storage phase, the urethra normally maintains a resting pressure that exceeds intravesical pressure so that no leakage occurs. Both urethral pressure and length are important for normal continency.

Urethral mechanism incompetence is the most common cause of urinary incontinence in small-animal patients; however, the cause and pathophysiologic mechanisms are still poorly understood. Outlet resistance is not sufficient to prevent urine flow during the storage phase, even when bladder function is apparently adequate and intravesical pressure not excessive. These animals usually have a history of dribbling incontinence, which may be continuous or intermittent, but which is often worse when the animal is recumbent or asleep. Examples of urethral mechanism incompetence are estrogen-responsive urinary incontinence in spayed female dogs and testosterone-responsive urinary incontinence in castrated male dogs.

The urethral sphincter has receptors for reproductive hormones, estrogen and testosterone, in addition to alpha-adrenergic receptors. Incontinence in neutered animals may be partially related to a decreased activity of these receptors. Spontaneous resolution of incontinence in juvenile bitches with onset of the estrus cycle suggests that hormonal influence on urethral sphincter function exists. However, the incidence of urinary incontinence after neutering is low and affected animals may have had marginal urethral function before surgery. Poor response to hormone therapy in some neutered incontinent animals suggests that sphincter mechanism incompetence is not simply an estrogen or testosterone deficiency problem.

Recognition of bladder and urethral status, as well as detrusor-sphincter synergism are based on history, clinical signs, physical and neurologic examination, and ancillary diagnostic tests such as radiography, ultrasonography, endoscopy, and urodynamic studies. Fluoroscopy or ultrasonography may be used to evaluate the bladder, urethra, and surrounding structures. Urodynamic studies measure the relationship of pressure, volume, and flow within the lower urinary tract during various phases of micturition. These tests provide objective data regarding bladder and urethral function for diagnosis, prognosis, and treatment of disorders of micturition. Urodynamic tests that have been performed in dogs and cats include cystometrograms, urethral pressure profiles, and simultaneous cystometry and uroflowmetry studies. Electromyography may also be used to substantiate results of the neurologic examination when lesions of the sacral spinal cord segments are suspected. Electromyography is also used along with various urodynamic studies to evaluate coordination of detrusor contraction with sphincter activities.

PHARMACOLOGIC AGENTS USED FOR LOWER URINARY TRACT CONTROL

Pharmacologic agents are selected for the management of urinary incontinence after urinary tract infection, morphologic abnormalities, and mechanical types of excessive outlet resistance have been ruled out. Various pharmacologic agents may alter bladder and urethral functions. However, their use is often palliative, and they should be administered for as short a period of time as possible. The essential purpose of these drugs is to assist micturition until normal function is restored. General nursing care is often required to avoid bladder overdistention, lower urinary tract infection, and decubital ulcers.

The various pharmacologic agents usually alter urethrovesical function by acting on autonomic or somatic receptors to modify either smooth or striated muscle activity. Knowledge of distribution of the various neuroceptors in the lower urinary tract is important when selecting drugs.

Given the great variety of drugs affecting the lower urinary tract (Table 1), how does one decide which drug to use in an individual case? Drug therapy is the same whether the cause is a neurogenic or a myogenic problem. Therefore, for practical pharmacologic manipulation, it is helpful first to identify the bladder status as being normal, hypercontractile, or hypocontractile; then to determine whether the sphincter status is normal, hypertonic, or hypotonic; and finally to recognize the presence of normal detrusor-sphincter synergism. In cases of bladder-sphincter dyssynergia, drugs that act on sphincter mechanisms (smooth, striated, or both) should be given either alone or in combination with drugs acting on bladder function.

Some general principles apply to most of the drugs used to restore urethrovesical function. Activity and side effects may vary from one patient to another. The effect of a drug may be manifested slowly after treatment has been initiated and may continue after therapy is stopped. (For example, cyclic antidepressor drugs may take several days before demonstrating effect, or the activity of an alpha-blocker may become irreversible with time because of alpha-receptor site destruction.) Most of these drugs also act on other organ systems so that side effects are possible. Generally, drugs should be started at a low dosage, which should gradually be increased every 2 to 3 days until either an adequate response or adverse effects are seen or until the maximum dosage is reached (for dosage regimens, see Table 2). If urethrovesical dysfunction persists after several days of maximum dosage therapy, it is unlikely that normal micturition will return and other drugs should be used either in addition to or in place of the initial treatment.

DRUGS USED FOR BLADDER HYPOCONTRACTILITY

Parasympathicomimetic agents stimulate bladder cholinergic receptors similarly to acetylcholine. Acetylcholine cannot be used clinically because of its dual nicotinic and muscarinic effect and because of its rapid destruction by acetylcholinesterase.

Table 1. *Activity of Pharmacologic Agents on Lower Urinary Tract (LUT) Function*

Class of Drug	General Activity	Activity on LUT	Major Pharmacologic Agents or Class of Drugs
Parasympathetic muscarinic with direct cholinergic activity	Rapid effect on cholinergic receptors	Increase detrusor activity and urethral sphincter smooth muscle contraction	Acetylcholine Bethanechol
Parasympathetic muscarinic with cholinergic activity mediated by cholinesterase inhibition	Slow effect on cholinergic receptors Possible influence on alpha-synapses, CNS, and spinal cord	Increase detrusor activity and urethral sphincter smooth muscle contraction	Distigmine Neostigmine Pyridostigmine
Parasympathetic inhibitors with acetylcholine blocking effects	Acetylcholine inhibition	Detrusor relaxation and inhibition of detrusor contractions	Atropine Oxybutynin Propantheline Flavoxate Dicyclomine
Sympathetic alpha-agonists	Contraction of smooth muscle fibers containing alpha-receptors	Closure of bladder neck and proximal urethra	Ephedrine Norepinephrin Phenylpropanolamine Sexual hormones
Sympathetic alpha-antagonists	Blockage of alpha-adrenergic receptors	Relaxation of bladder neck and of proximal urethra Increase urinary flow	Phenoxybenzamine Nicergoline Moxisylyte
Sympathetic beta-agonist	Relaxation of smooth muscle fibers containing beta-receptors. Favorably influenced by alpha-blockage	Relaxation of bladder body and of urethra	Terbutaline
Sympathetic inhibitors, beta-blocking agents	Inhibition of relaxation of smooth muscle fibers containing beta-receptors. Favorably influenced by alpha-stimulation	Increase urethral pressure	Propanalol
Tricyclic (CNS) depressant agents	Inhibition of norepinephrine reuptake at the synaptic level	Detrusor relaxation. Increase urethral tone	Imipramine
Smooth and striated muscle–stimulating agent	Direct stimulation of smooth or striated muscles	Detrusor and proximal urethra contractions	Prostaglandins
Muscle relaxant (peripheral)	Direct muscle relaxation or indirect by prostaglandin release	Detrusor relaxation. Variable effects on sphincters	Flavoxate Calcium inhibitors Anti-inflammatory drugs
Muscle relaxant (central)	Decrease muscle tone by CNS depressive effect	Striated muscle sphincter relaxation	Baclofen Diazepam

Cholinergic agents should be used with caution in patients with bronchial constriction, cardiac arrythmias, or gastric ulcers and should be avoided if urinary or intestinal obstruction exist.

Bethanechol is a cholinergic agent that resists acetylcholinesterase action and is used in patients with bladder hypocontractility. When used alone, this drug has had disappointing results because it exaggerates bladder-sphincter dyssynergia. If dyssynergia occurs, the drug should be combined with agents leading to internal sphincter relaxation, such as phenoxybenzamine, nicergoline, or moxisylyte.

Anticholinesterasic agents stimulate bladder contraction by blocking acetylcholine degradation enzymes. Agents that have been used include distigmine, neostigmine, and pyridostigmine.

Other agents have been recently advocated for the treatment of hypocontractile bladder. Metoclopramide has been reported to stimulate directly detrusor contractions in humans and dogs. Prosta-

glandins may also modify lower urinary tract function by unknown mechanisms. Prostaglandin E_2 (PGE_2) seems to selectively stimulate detrusor contraction and urethral smooth muscle relaxation. Prostaglandin F_2 seems to induce both detrusor and urethral contraction.

DRUGS USED FOR BLADDER HYPERCONTRACTILITY

Anticholinergic agents inhibit bladder contraction. Side effects are common and include xerostomia, tachycardia, constipation, dilated pupils, and urinary retention. Propantheline is the major parasympatholytic used for its antimuscarinic effect. Oxybutynin has both anticholinergic and antispasmodic effect. Use of oxybutynin in dogs with detrusor hypercontractility and in cats with feline leukemia virus (FeLV)–associated detrusor instability has been beneficial in some cases. Flavoxate has a local

Table 2. Major Pharmacologic Agents Used in Small Animal Patients with Urinary Incontinence

Generic Drug Name	Country Specialty*		Mechanism of Action	Action on LUT†				Use in Humans			Use in Small Animals				Comments and Contraindications
	Country	Proprietary Name		Bladder Body	Neck	Urethral Smooth	Striated Muscle	Dosages	Route	Frequency	Dosages	Rate	Frequency	Utilization§	
Baclofen	B	Lioresal	8, 10, 12	−	−	−	−	10–40 mg; Test: 10–20 mg	PO; IV	q8h	Dog: 1–2 mg/kg Cat: ND	PO	q8h	B	Inhibits medullary interneurons and spinal reflexes; Similar chemical structure to GABA; Acts especially on striated muscle; Potential side effects include vertigo, gastrointestinal disorders, central nervous system disorders, muscle hypotonia, general weakness, pruritus
	CDN	Lioresal													
	CH	Lioresal													
	D	Lioresal													
	F	Lioresal													
	USA	Lioresal (Ciba)													
Diazepam	B	Valium	8, 10	−			−	3–10 mg; Test: 10 mg	PO; IV	q8h	Dog: 0.2 mg/kg Cat: 2.5 mg	PO PO	q8h q8h	B	Prototype of benzodiazepine derivatives with both central and peripheral effects; Potential side effects include asthenia, central depression, vertigo, paradoxical excitability; Contraindications include respiratory insufficiency; Efficacy is questionable
	CDN	Valium	2, 12												
	CH	Valium													
	D	Valium													
	F	Valium Evacalm (Unimed)													
	GB	Valium Euphorbia													
	J	Valium													
	USA	Valium (Roche)													
Imipramine	B	Tofranil	10, 2, 4, 6 (3,5 short action)	−	+	+		25–50 mg; Enuresis: 10–20 mg	PO; PO	q8H; At night	Dog: 5–15 mg Cat: 2.5–5 mg	PO PO	q12h q12h	B	Myorelaxing, anticholinergic, atropinic, alpha and beta sympathetic and local anesthetic effects; Delayed effect (1 week); May induce seizures, tremors, tachycardia, hyperexcitability
	CDN	Impril													
	CH	Tofranil													
	D	Tofranil													
	F	Praminil													
	GB	Tofranil													
	J	Imidol (Yoshitoma)													
	USA	Tofranil (Geigy)													
Prostaglandin E_1	GB	Alprostadil	7, 8	+	−			ND			ND			C	Stimulation or inhibition of smooth muscle activity by acting on norepinephrine release and by modulating its effects on synapses and motor end plate; Only used experimentally
Prostaglandin E_2	D	Minprostin E_2	7, 8	+	−	−	−	ND			ND				
	GB	Arbaprostil													
	J	Prostarmon-E (Ono)													
Nicergoline	CH	Sermion (Fasmitalia)	4, 10	−	−			5–15 mg; Test: 1 mg	PO; IV	q8h; over 1 min	Dog: 1–5 mg Cat: 1–5 mg	PO PO	q8h q8h	B	Used as a cerebral vasodilator; Well tolerated at usual dosage, but effectiveness is questionable
	D	Sermion													
	F	Sermion													

Drug	Country	Trade name	Ref			Dose (human)	Route	Freq	Dose (animal)	Route	Freq	Cat	Comments
Terbutaline	B CDN CH D F GB J USA	Bricanyl Bricanyl Bricanyl Bricanyl Bricanyl Bristurin (Bristol) Bristurin Bricanyl	3, 5, 9	–	–	250–500 µg 2.5–5 mg 0.5 mg	intranasal PO SC	q6h q8–12h q6h	NDE			C	Beta2-effects only Easier to use clinically than other beta-agonists Minimal cardiac effects Effectiveness controversial
Estrogens	B CH D F GB J USA	Ovestin (Organon) Ovocyclin (Ciba) Ovestin Klymoral Ovestin Hormonin Ovestin Holin Diethylstilbestrol Sterandryl	2, 3, 6 6	+	+	1–2 mg NU	PO	q24h	Dog: 0.1–1.0 mg Cat: not recommended	PO	q24h for 3–5 days, then no more than 1 mg/week	D	Potential severe side effect is bone marrow suppression Signs of estrus Exact mechanism of action is unknown
Testosterone cypionate	B, S, D, F, H USA	Depo-testosterone	6		+	NU			Dog: 2.2 mg/kg	IM	q30days	D	Possible recurrence or worsening of prostatic disorders, perianal adenoma, or perineal hernia
Testosterone propionate	B, S, D, F, H USA	Interteston	6	+	+	NU			Dog: 2.2 mg/kg	IM	q2–3days		Potential behavioral adverse effects
Phenylpropanolamine	USA F	Androlan Denoral	2, 3		+	1 capsule	PO	q12h	Dog: 1.5 mg/kg Cat: 1.5 mg/kg	PO	q8–12h	A	Same as ephedrine Present in several nasal decongesting agents
Phenoxybenzamine	B USA CH D GB USA B	Ornade Ornade Dibenzyline Dibenzyline Dibenzyram Blocadren Dibenzyline Buscopan	2, 3 4, 5	–	–	0.3–0.5 mg/kg Test: 1 mg/kg	PO IV	q12–8h slow drip	Dog: 0.25 mg/kg Cat: 0.25 mg/kg	PO	q12h	A	Potential side effects include hypotension, tachycardia, and gastrointestinal irritation
Hyoscine butylbromide	B CDN CH D F J	Buscopan Buscopan Buscopan Buscopan Buscopan Hyospan Butylmido	2, 9	–		20 mg	PO	q6–8h	Dog: 2–5 mg Cat: 1–2 mg	PO PO	q12h q12h	B	Ileus common Contraindicated in glaucoma, mydriasis, tachycardia
Oxybutynin	F USA	Ditropan Ditropan (Marion)	2, 8, 10	–		5 mg	PO	q6–8h	NDE			B	Similar to hyoscine butylbromide
Propantheline	B	Probanthine	2, 8	–		7.5–15 mg, maximum 12 mg/day	PO	q6–8h	Dog: 7.5–15 mg	PO	q8h	A	Similar to hyoscine butylbromide

Table continued on following page

Table 2. Major Pharmacologic Agents Used in Small Animal Patients with Urinary Incontinence Continued

Generic Drug Name	Country Specialty*		Mechanism of Action	Action on LUT†				Use in Humans			Use in Small Animals				Comments and Contraindications
				Bladder		Urethral Muscle									
	Country	Proprietary Name		Body	Neck	Smooth	Striated	Dosages	Route	Frequency	Dosages	Rate	Frequency	Utilization§	
	CDN	Probanthel						Test: 2 mg	IV		Cat: 5–7.5 mg	PO	q4–8h		
	CH	Probanthine													
	DK	Ecoril													
	F	Probanthine													
	GB	Probanthine													
	USA	Probanthine (Searle)													
Ephedrine	B	Ephedrine	3, 5, 9	−	+	+		15–60 mg	PO, SC, IM, IV	q6–8h	Dog: 12.5–50 mg	PO	q8–12h	A	Direct muscle activity. Side effects include anxiety, cardiac arrhythmias, hypertension. Contraindicated in cardiac patients
	D	Ephedrine													
	F	Ephedrine													
	GB	Spaneph Zephrol									Cat: 2–4 mg/kg	PO	q8–12h		
	USA	Ephedrine						Test: 10 mg 10–20 mg	IV PO						
Bethanechol	B	Muscaran	1	+	+	+	+	5–15 mg	IV PO	q6h	Dog: 5–15 mg	PO	q8h	A	May induce nausea, vomiting, dyspnea, arrythmia, abdominal cramps, visual disturbances. Contraindication: pregnancy. Often used with phenoxybenzamine
	CH	Myocholine									Cat: 1.25–5 mg	PO	q8h	A	
	CDN	Duvoid													
	F	Urecholine													
	GB	Mechothane Myotonine													
	USA	Duvoid (NorwichEaton) Bethanechol Urecholine (Merck Sharpe & Dohme)													

Type of Activity	Stimulation	Inhibition
Parasympathetic	1	2
Orthosympathetic alpha	3	4
Orthosympathetic beta	5	6
Somatic	7	8
Encephalic	9	10
Spinal	11	12

*Proprietary names are given according to most common country nomenclature (country letter code corresponds to motor vehicle country code): B, Belgium; CDN, Canada; CH, Switzerland; D, West Germany; DK, Denmark; F, France; GB, Great Britain; H, Hungary; J, Japan; NLN, The Netherlands; S, Sweden.

†This code system gives the site of activity of the drug. Stimulating actions are represented by odd numbers, inhibiting actions by even numbers.

‡Lower urinary tract activity is described by + (contraction or closure) or − (relaxation or opening).

§Utilization code is defined as follows: A, commonly used and accepted in veterinary medicine; B, commonly used in human medicine with little or no experience in veterinary medicine; C, episodic use in human medicine, no use in veterinary medicine; D, episodic use in human medicine, but commonly used in veterinary medicine; NDE, not determined for lower urinary tract function and would require extrapolation from human dosages; NU, not used in humans; ND, not determined.

Many of the drugs included in this table are not approved for use in dogs and cats and pharmacokinetic information for these species is minimal.

anesthetic effect, is an anticholinergic, and has direct smooth muscle–relaxing effect. Experience with this drug in veterinary medicine is limited. Dicyclomine shows both smooth muscle–relaxing and antimuscarinic effects. It has been used successfully in urge incontinence in humans, but clinical evaluation in small animals is lacking.

Beta-adrenergic drugs stimulate beta$_2$-receptors of the bladder body, inducing relaxation. Terbutaline has been used effectively in detrusor hyperreflexia in humans. Experience in veterinary medicine is lacking.

Prostaglandin synthesis inhibitors may be useful to modulate neurotransmission. Aspirin and indomethacin have been used in selected cases in humans. Indomethacin is not recommended for use in the dog or the cat.

Calcium channel inhibitors effect vesical contractility by blocking intra- or extracellular calcium ions, decreasing the availability of calcium ions for detrusor protein (actin and myosin) activities. Studies in small animals with bladder hypercontractility are encouraging.

DRUGS USED TO INCREASE URETHRAL TONE

Alpha-adrenergic agonist agents act on alpha-adrenergic receptors of the bladder neck and proximal urethra (bladder outlet). Smooth muscle is probably the most important component of the urethral sphincter closure mechanism in the resting state. Because alpha-adrenergic stimulation contributes the most to smooth muscle contraction in the urethra, alpha-adrenergic agonists can induce increased urethral tone. Ephedrine and phenylpropanolamine act by inducing norepinephrine release at the synaptic level. Side effects of these drugs include anxious behavior, tremors, dizziness, cardiac arrythmias, hypertension, and urine retention. Phenylpropanolamine, a common respiratory tract decongestant, is often effective in small-animal patients with sphincter mechanism incompetence. This drug is preferred to ephedrine because its side effects (particularly cardiovascular effects) are less severe, and because ephedrine seems to lose effectiveness over time.

Beta-adrenolytic agents theoretically increase the effects of alpha-adrenergic receptors of the bladder outlet. Propanolol has been used successfully for treatment of stress incontinence in women. Cardiac and bronchial side effects can be significant, and the use of this drug in small animals for this purpose is limited.

Tricyclic antidepressor agents such as imipramine increase vesical capacity and urethral sphincter tone. The mechanism for the anticholinergic and alpha-adrenergic effects of these drugs is the inhibition of norephinephrine reuptake at the synaptic

level. Although not uniformly successful, imipramine has been used effectively in dogs with urethral sphincter incompetence and detrusor hyperactivity.

Reproductive hormone replacement therapy is used commonly in animals with urethral sphincter incompetence. Response to estrogens and testosterone can be explained by their effect to enhance the sensitivity of alpha-adrenergic receptors to alpha-agonists. A direct effect of estrogen on smooth muscle fibers of the urethra and the perineal area has also been advocated. In some neutered bitches, alpha-agonists given in conjunction with estrogen were more effective in increasing urethral tone than when given alone.

Diethylstilbestrol administered orally is the drug of choice for estrogen therapy in bitches. Because estrogens can produce several undesirable side effects, including attraction of males, bone marrow suppression, and dermatologic disorders, alpha-agonists may be preferred in some cases.

Testosterone proprionate intramuscularly is the drug of choice for testosterone therapy in incontinent castrated males. If the duration of action is too short, testosterone cypionate can be used. Oral testosterone is usually ineffective because of rapid hepatic degradation of the drug. Side effects include prostatic disorders and behavioral changes such as inappropriate urination, aggression, and sexual excitability.

DRUGS USED TO DECREASE URETHRAL TONE

Urethral tone may be decreased by drug action either on smooth muscle activity (internal sphincter) or on striated muscle activity (external sphincter).

SMOOTH MUSCLE SPHINCTER RELAXATION. The concept of a physiologic urethral internal sphincter is supported by the high number of alpha-adrenergic receptors within the bladder outlet. Alpha-adrenergic blocking agents decrease urethral functional pressure and resistance and are used predominantly in patients with detrusor–urethral internal sphincter dyssynergia and in conjunction with parasympathetic stimulants, such as bethanechol. Phenoxybenzamine is the major alpha-adrenergic antagonist used. Nicergoline or moxisylyte may be selected when phenoxybenzamine is not effective or not available. Prazosin also has a blocking effect on alpha$_1$-receptors of urethral smooth muscle. Side effects of these drugs include hypotension, tachycardia, dizziness, and nasal congestion.

Beta-adrenergic agents may induce smooth muscle relaxation of the urethra by acting on beta-adrenergic receptors. In humans, terbutaline decreases maximal urethral pressure.

STRIATED MUSCLE SPHINCTER RELAXATION. Drugs that relax striated sphincters are used to control urethral spasm but are not specific for the urethra and act on all skeletal muscles of the body. Diazepam is a central myorelaxing agent that has been used in both humans and animals. It is ineffective in treating detrusor-sphincter dyssynergia. Side effects include dizziness, general weakness, and paradoxical excitability.

Baclofen is a mono- and polysynaptic spinal reflex inhibitor that has been used to control muscle spasm. Experience in small animals is limited. Side effects include dizziness, general weakness, and pruritis.

Dantrolene is a calcium antagonist that may be used as a muscle relaxant, especially in diseases related to central nervous system lesions. Its effect on micturition has been reported in humans. Side effects include euphoria, dizziness, and hepatic toxicity after long-term therapy.

References and Supplemental Reading

Barsanti, J. A.: Pharmacology of bladder-urethral function. Proceedings of ACVIM 5th Annual Forum, San Diego, 1987, pp. 161–164.
Barsanti, J. A., and Finco, D. R.: Hormonal responses to urinary incontinence. In Kirk, R. W. (ed.): Current Veterinary Therapy VIII. Philadelphia: W. B. Saunders, 1983, pp. 1086–1087.
Chew, D. J., DiBartola, S. P., and Fenner, W. R.: Pharmacologic manipulation of urination. In Kirk, R. W. (ed.): Current Veterinary Therapy IX. Philadelphia: W. B. Saunders, 1985, pp. 1207–1212.
DiBartola, S. P., and Adams, W. M.: Urinary incontinence associated with malposition of the urinary bladder. In Kirk, R. W. (ed.): Current Veterinary Therapy VIII. Philadelphia, W. B. Saunders, 1983, pp. 1089–1092.
Gotoh, M., Hassoura, M., and Elhilali, M.: Interaction of prostaglandin E_2 and $F_{2\text{-alpha}}$ with calcium on bladder detrusor muscle. J. Urol. 135:431, 1986.
Hackler, R., Broecker, B., et al.: A clinical experience with dantrolene sodium on external urinary hypertonicity in spinal cord injured patients. J. Urol. 124:78, 1986.
Hassouna, M., Nishizawa, O., Miyagawa, I., et al.: Role of calcium ion antagonists on the bladder detrusor muscle: In vitro and in vivo studies. J. Urol. 135:1327, 1986.
Holt, P. E.: Urinary incontinence in the bitch due to sphincter mechanism incompetence: Prevalence in referred dogs and retrospective analysis of sixty cases. J. Small Anim. Pract. 26:181, 1985.
Khanna, O. P.: Disorders of micturition: Neuropharmacologic basis and result of drug therapy. Urology 8:316, 1977.
Lappin, M. R., and Barsanti, J. A.: Urinary incontinence secondary to idiopathic detrusor instability: Cystometrographic diagnosis and pharmacologic management in two dogs and a cat. J.A.V.M.A. 191:1439, 1987.
Lees, G. E., and Moreau, P. M.: Management of hypotonic and atonic urinary bladders in cats. Vet. Clin. North Am. 14:641, 1984.
Mitchell, W. C., and Venable, D. D.: Effects of metoclopramide on detrusor function. J. Urol. 133:791, 1985.
Moreau, P. M.: Neurogenic disorders of micturition in the dog and cat. Comp. Cont. Ed. Pract. Vet. 4:12, 1982.
Moreau, P. M.: Management of neurogenic disorders of micturition. Proceedings of ACVIM 4th Annual Forum, Washington, D.C., 1986, pp. 85–92.
Osborne, C. A., Oliver, J. E., and Polzin, D. E.: Non-neurogenic urinary incontinence. In Kirk, R. W. (ed.): Current Veterinary Therapy VII. Philadelphia: W. B. Saunders, 1980, pp. 1128–1136.
Richter, K. P., and Ling, G. V.: Clinical response and urethral pressure profile changes after phenylpropanolamine in dogs with primary sphincter incompetence. J.A.V.M.A. 6:605, 1985.
Vaidyanathan, S., Rao, M., et al.: Beta adrenergic activity in human proximal urethra: A study with terbutaline. J. Urol. 124:869, 1980.

Section
13

REPRODUCTIVE DISORDERS

PATRICIA N. OLSON, D.V.M.
Consulting Editor

Drugs Affecting Fertility in the Male Dog.................................1224
Ultrasonography and Ultrasound-Guided Biopsy of the Canine
    Prostate 1227
Ultrasonography of the Canine Uterus and Ovary 1239
Chronic Bacterial Prostatitis in the Dog.................................1243
Canine Semen Freezing and Artificial Insemination......................1247
Preputial Discharge in the Dog...1259
Disorders of Sexual Development in Dogs and Cats 1261
Hormonal and Clinical Correlates of Ovarian Cycles, Ovulation,
    Pseudopregnancy, and Pregnancy in Dogs 1269
Dynamic Testing in Reproductive Endocrinology 1282
Induction of Estrus and Ovulation in the Bitch.........................1288
Effects of Drugs on Pregnancy 1291
Drugs That Affect Uterine Motility.....................................1299
Vaginal Prolapse...1302
Diagnosis and Treatment Alternatives for Pyometra in Dogs and Cats ...1305
Vulvar Discharges..1310
Diagnosis of Canine Herpetic Infections 1313
Diagnosis and Treatment of Canine Brucellosis.........................1317
Anesthetic Considerations for Cesarean Section 1321
Care and Diseases of Neonatal Puppies and Kittens.....................1325

DRUGS AFFECTING FERTILITY
IN THE MALE DOG

JONI L. FRESHMAN, D.V.M., M.S.

Fort Collins, Colorado

The sport (breeding, showing, obedience and field trials) of purebred dogs is extremely popular in the United States. Over one million purebred dogs were registered with the American Kennel Club in 1986, and a record was set for number of litters registered (Mandeville, 1987). Owners invest a great deal of time and money in producing and campaigning a champion dog. Such a dog may represent the culmination of years of a planned breeding program. A return on the owner's investment is often planned for by holding the dog at stud. As veterinarians, we need to be aware of adverse effects that medication may have on a dog's semen production and quality.

PHYSIOLOGY

A brief review of the endocrinology involved in canine sperm production is useful in understanding drug effects. Testosterone, secreted by interstitial (Leydig) cells in the testes, promotes spermatogenesis, libido, maintenance of ducts and epididymides, and growth of the prostate gland (Feldman and Nelson, 1987). Testosterone secretion is stimulated by luteinizing hormone (LH) released from the pituitary gland. LH is released as a result of the activity of gonadotropin-releasing hormone (GnRH), produced by the hypothalamus. Negative feedback by testosterone on LH at the pituitary level occurs either directly or after the aromatization of testosterone to an estrogenic compound (Worgul et al., 1981; Winter et al., 1983). Negative feedback by testosterone on GnRH has also been postulated in other species (Caminos-Torres and Snyder, 1977).

Follicle-stimulating hormone (FSH) is also required for sperm production. FSH stimulates development and function of Sertoli's cells. FSH, like LH, is secreted in response to GnRH. FSH secretion may be controlled by inhibin, a substance secreted by Sertoli's cells, acting on the pituitary to depress FSH secretion (Feldman and Nelson, 1987).

In dogs, spermatogenesis takes approximately 62 days, with transport through the epididymis requiring approximately 15 days more (Amann, 1986). Spermatogenesis altered by drugs may not return to normal for several months. Table 1 lists some drugs that have an effect on male reproductive function.

STEROIDAL COMPOUNDS

Steroidal drugs, both sex steroids and glucocorticoids, are commonly used in veterinary practice. Androgenic or anabolic steroids are often used in catabolic disease states or in canine athletes. No anabolic steroid is completely free of androgenic effects (Haupt and Rovere, 1984). Androgens inhibit LH release via negative feedback at the pituitary gland (Falvo et al., 1979). In dogs, androgen administration results in decreased testicular size, daily sperm output, and serum testosterone levels (Freshman et al., 1987).

Estrogenic hormones and drugs may also inhibit LH secretion and, therefore, testosterone and sperm production. Estradiol 17-B and diethylstilbestrol have been shown to prevent LH secretion in dogs (Jones and Boyns, 1974). In dogs, a synthetic estrogenlike compound (KABI 1774) caused inability to ejaculate; decreased sperm count, motility, and volume; and an increase in abnormal spermatozoal morphology (Albanus et al., 1975). After 40 days of administration, complete degeneration of all testicular germ cells had occurred.

Progestagen administration to four dogs resulted in decreased plasma testosterone levels, with no decrease in semen quality (Wright et al., 1979). It is unfortunate that researchers speculating on the effects of progestagens on male reproduction utilized few dogs, with infrequent seminal collections (Olson et al., 1986a; Wright et al., 1979; Jones and Boyns, 1974). Decreased plasma testosterone for a prolonged time period could result in altered sperm production.

Table 1. *Substances Reported to Alter Reproductive Function in Male Dogs*

Methyltestosterone	(Freshman et al., 1987)
Estradiol 17-B	(Jones and Boyns, 1974)
Diethylstilbestrol	(Jones and Boyns, 1974)
KABI 1774	(Albanus et al., 1975)
Betamethasone	(Taha et al., 1981)
Prednisone	(Kemppainen et al., 1983)
Tamoxifen citrate	(Olson et al., 1986b)
Gossypol	(Sang et al., 1986)

Glucocorticoids are among the most commonly administered veterinary drugs. Injections of betamethasone have resulted in decreased semen volume, decreased sperm output, and increased percentages of abnormal sperm (Taha et al., 1981). Plasma concentrations of testosterone were decreased, implying a negative feedback effect on the pituitary or a direct effect on the testes. Plasma LH concentrations were not measured. Alternate-day intramuscular injection of prednisone at a dose of 2.2 mg/kg decreased basal plasma concentrations of LH and testosterone (Kemppainen et al., 1983). Inhibition of LH secretion at the hypothalamic or pituitary level was hypothesized. Caution in using corticosteroids in stud dogs is justified.

CONTRACEPTIVE COMPOUNDS

A review of canine contraception has recently been published. The reader is referred to this publication for details (Olson et al., 1986a). Several compounds are of interest because of their potential effects on spermatogenesis. These agents are being studied for use in pet population control.

Anti-GnRH compounds would function to counteract GnRH and therefore prevent release of LH and FSH, causing inhibition of spermatogenesis. Anti-LH compounds would have a similar effect by directly countering LH (Faulkner et al., 1975).

Powerful GnRH agonists result in infertility by causing downregulation or desensitization of GnRH receptors in the pituitary gland. Resultant decreases in the production of LH and FSH cause inhibition of spermatogenesis (Vickery et al., 1984; Tremblay et al., 1984). Although not critically evaluated in dogs, GnRH antagonists compete with GnRH for binding at pituitary receptor sites but do not stimulate LH and FSH release in humans (Schally, 1981).

Tamoxifen citrate appears to act as an estrogenic compound in dogs, causing a decrease in gonadotropins (Olson et al., 1986b). Although gossypol, a cottonseed pigment, inhibits fertility in male dogs, the side effects can be severe (Sang et al., 1980).

CHEMOTHERAPEUTIC AGENTS

Oncology comprises a significant part of small animal practice. A wide variety of antineoplastic agents are available for the treatment of neoplastic diseases. Owners may desire to breed a dog affected with cancer in order to perpetuate his bloodline. It is unfortunate that information about the effects of many common antineoplastic agents on fertility is lacking even in humans. Canine studies are not available. Antineoplastic agents known to affect

Table 2. Antineoplastic Agents Affecting Spermiogenesis in Men

Busulfan	Cyclophosphamide
Chlorambucil	Methotrexate
Cisplatin	Vincristine

spermiogenesis in humans are listed in Table 2 (McEvoy, 1987).

Several alkylating agents are reported to impair spermiogenesis. Busulfan causes azoospermia and testicular atrophy in men. Chlorambucil has a high incidence of irreversible infertility when used in prepubertal or pubertal males. In adult men, the effect on testicular germinal epithelium appears to be dose dependent and may or may not be reversible. Cyclophosphamide causes azoospermia, which may be permanent, in 10 to 30 per cent of men.

Cisplatin, a platinum-containing antineoplastic agent, causes impairment of spermiogenesis and azoospermia in men. This alteration is generally reversible. Methotrexate, a folic acid antagonist, can cause defective spermatogenesis, oligospermia, and infertility when administered to men. Vincristine, a vinca alkaloid, has been reported to cause azoospermia when used in conjunction with prednisone and cyclophosphamide. No information is available on the effects of vincristine when it is used alone.

The potential for adverse effects on spermatogenesis from other antineoplastic agents certainly exists; the data are simply lacking. In each case, the veterinarian and the owner must weigh the potential benefits and risks to the patient and the desire for propagation of offspring.

MISCELLANEOUS DRUGS

Ketoconazole, an imidazole derivative, is one of the most commonly used antifungal drugs. Its antifungal activity is due to prevention of fungal ergosterol synthesis. In dogs as well as other mammals, ketoconazole inhibits cytochrome P450 17(a)/17,20-lyase, blocking testicular and adrenal androgen biosynthesis as well as cortisol production (DeCoster et al., 1984; Willard et al., 1986; DeCoster et al., 1987). A rebound effect on serum testosterone concentration occurs after cessation of treatment (Willard et al., 1986).

Table 3. Selected Drugs That Cause Sexual Dysfunction in Men

Anticholinergics	Phenytoin
Barbiturates	Primidone
Chlorpromazine	Propranolol
Diazepam	Thiazide diuretics
Digoxin	Verapamil
Levodopa	

Cimetidine, an H_2 receptor antagonist, is used to inhibit gastric acid secretion in conditions predisposing to gastric ulcer formation. Decreased sperm counts, loss of libido, and decreased plasma testosterone levels have been reported in men receiving cimetidine (Lardinois and Mazzaferri, 1985; McEvoy, 1987). Because of a concomitant elevation of LH and FSH, a primary testicular disorder is most probable. A defect in 17-B hydroxysteroid dehydrogenase has been postulated. Of interest, cimetidine, like ketoconazole, has an imidazole ring. Ranitidine, another H_2 receptor antagonist, possesses a furan ring instead and has no apparent adverse effect on reproduction (Zeldis et al., 1983). Ranitidine may be preferred in place of cimetidine in a stud dog.

Spironolactone, a potassium-sparing diuretic, is a synthetic steroid aldosterone antagonist. In men receiving this drug, decreased plasma testosterone concentration, decreased libido, and androgenlike effects have been reported (McEvoy, 1987; Lardinois and Mazzaferri, 1985). No data on sperm production are available; however, a decrease in testosterone concentration could inhibit spermatogenesis.

Diethylcarbamazine (DEC) was reported to cause infertility in dogs in a clinic situation. Several controlled studies were performed using DEC alone and a styrlpyridinium chloride–diethylcarbamazine combination (Herron, 1975; Courtney and Nachreiner, 1976; Alford and Fogleman, 1976). No effect on semen volume, pH, sperm counts, or motility was produced in any study. These data suggest that the infertility observed in clinical patients receiving DEC may have had a different etiology. However, all the controlled studies of the effect of DEC on fertility used relatively low numbers (2 to 4 dogs) in each treatment group, so it is conceivable that an adverse effect could be produced with more subjects. A study evaluating the effect of ivermectin, a recently approved microfilaricide, on male beagles found no adverse effects on spermatogenesis or fertility during 8 months of treatment (Daurio et al., 1987).

DRUGS THAT CAUSE SEXUAL DYSFUNCTION

In humans, a wide array of drugs have been reported to cause decreased libido, impotence, and ejaculatory disturbances (Abramowicz, 1987). Reports of this type are extremely difficult to obtain in the dog. Table 3 lists selected common drugs reported to cause sexual dysfunction in men. Appearance of a similar problem in a stud dog on such medication might indicate trial withdrawal of the drug.

References and Supplemental Reading

Abramowicz, M.: Drugs that cause dysfunction. Med. Let. Drugs Ther. 29:2, 1987.

Albanus, L., BjorKlund, N. E., Gustafsson, B., et al.: Forty days oral toxicity of 2, 6-cis-diphenylhexamethylcyclotetrasiloxane (KABI 1774) in beagle dogs with special reference to effects on the male reproductive system. Acta Pharmacol. Toxicol. 36:93, 1975.

Alford, B. T., and Fogleman, R. W.: Spermatogenesis as a key to interpreting toxicology of parasiticides in the dog. Vet. Toxicol. 18:127, 1976.

Amann, R. P.: Detection of alterations in testicular and epididymal function in laboratory animals. Environ. Health Perspect. 70:149, 1986.

Caminos-Torres, R., Ma, L., and Snyder, P. J.: Testosterone-induced inhibition of the LH and FSH responses to gonadotropin-releasing hormone occurs slowly. J. Clin. Endocrinol. Metab. 44:1142, 1977.

Courtney, C. H., and Nachreiner, R. F.: Effect of diethylcarbamazine on indexes of fertility in the male dog. Am. J. Vet. Res. 37:1095, 1976.

Daurio, C. P., Gilman, M. R., Pulliam, J. D., et al.: Reproductive evaluation of male beagles and the safety of ivermectin. Am. J. Vet. Res. 48:1755, 1987.

DeCoster, R., Beerens, D., Dom, J., et al.: Endocrinological effects of single daily ketoconazole administration in male beagle dogs. Acta Endocrinol. 107:275, 1984.

DeCoster, R., Coene, M. C., Haelterman, C., et al.: Effects of high dose ketoconazole treatment on adrenal mineralocorticoid biosynthesis in dogs and cats. Acta Endocrinol. 115:423, 1987.

Falvo, R. E., Vincent, D. L., Lathrop, J., et al.: Effects of testosterone and testosterone propionate administration on luteinizing-hormone secretion in the male mongrel dog. Biol. Reprod. 21:807, 1979.

Faulkner, L. C., Pineda, M. H., and Reimers, T. J.: Immunizing against gonadotropins in dogs. In Nieschlag, E. (ed.): Immunization with Hormones in Reproduction Research. Amsterdam: North-Holland Pub. Co, 1975, p. 199.

Feldman, E. C., and Nelson, R. W.: Disorders of the canine male reproductive tract. In Feldman, E. C., and Nelson, R. (eds.): Canine and Feline Endocrinology and Reproduction. Philadelphia: W. B. Saunders, 1987, pp. 481–524.

Freshman, J. L., Olson, P. N., Carlson, E. D., et al.: Effects of methyltestosterone on reproductive function in male greyhounds. Proceedings of the Fifth Annual Veterinary Medical Forum, San Diego, CA, 1987, p. 917.

Haupt, H. A., and Rovere, G. D.: Anabolic steroids: A review of the literature. Am. J. Sports Med. 12:469, 1984.

Herron, M. A.: The effect of styrlpyridinium chloride–diethylcarbamazine on spermatogenesis in the dog. Southwest. Vet. 28:197, 1975.

Jones, G. E., and Boyns, A. R.: Effect of gonadal steroids on the pituitary responsiveness to synthetic luteinizing-hormone–releasing hormone in the male dog. J. Endocrinol. 61:123, 1974.

Kemppainen, R. J., Thompson, F. N., Lorenz, M. D., et al.: Effects of prednisone on thyroid and gonadal endocrine function in dogs. J. Endocrinol. 96:293, 1983.

Lardinois, C. K., and Mazzaferri, E. L.: Cimetidine blocks testosterone synthesis. Arch. Intern. Med. 145:920, 1985.

Mandeville, J.: 1986 Registration statistics. AKC Gazette 104:24, 1987.

McEvoy, G. K.: American Hospital Formulary Service Drug Information 1987. Bethesda, MD: American Society of Hospital Pharmacists, Inc., 1987.

Olson, P. N., Nett, T. M., Bowen, R. A., et al.: A need for sterilization, contraceptives, and abortifacients: Abandoned and unwanted pets. Part II. Contraceptives. Comp. Cont. Ed. Pract. Vet. 8:173, 1986a.

Olson, P. N., Nett, T. M., Bowen, R. A., et al.: A need for sterilization, contraceptives, and abortifacients: Abandoned and unwanted pets. Part IV. Potential methods of controlling reproduction. Comp. Cont. Ed. Pract. Vet. 8:303, 1986b.

Sang, G. W., Zhang, P. G., Shi, O. X., et al.: Chronic toxicity of gossypol and the relation to its metabolic fate in dogs and monkeys. Chung-Kuo Yao Li Hsuch Pao 1:39, 1980.

Schally, A. V.: Current status of antagonistic analogs of LH-RH as a contraceptive method in the female. In Zatuchni, G. I., et al. (eds.): Research Frontiers in Fertility Regulation, Vol. 2. Philadelphia: J. B. Lippincott, 1981, p. 5.

Taha, M. B., Noakes, D. E., and Allen, W. E.: The effect of some exogenous hormones on seminal characteristics, libido and peripheral plasma testosterone concentrations in the male beagle. J. Small Anim. Pract. 22:587, 1981.

Tremblay, Y., Belanger, A., Labrie, F., et al.: Characteristics of the inhibitory effect of chronic treatment with an LHRH agonist on testicular steroidogenesis in the dog. Prostate 5:631, 1984.

Vickery, B. H., McRae, G. I., Briones, W., et al.: Effects of an LHRH agonist analog upon sexual function in male dogs. J. Androl. 5:28, 1984.

Willard, M. D., Nachreiner, R., McDonald, R., et al.: Ketoconazole-induced changes in selected canine hormone concentrations. Am. J. Vet. Res. 47:2504, 1986.

Winter, M., Falvo, R. E., Schanbacher, B. D., et al.: Regulations of gonadotropin secretion in the male dog. Role of estradiol. J. Androl. 4:319, 1983.

Worgul, T. J., Santen, R. J., Samojlik, E., et al.: Evidence that brain aromatization regulates LH secretion in the male dog. Am. Physiol. 241:E246, 1981.

Wright, P. J., Stelmasiak, T., Black, D., et al.: Medroxyprogesterone acetate and reproductive processes in male dogs. Aust. Vet. J. 55:437, 1979.

Zeldis, J. B., Friedman, L. S., and Isselbacher, K. J.: Ranitidine: A new H_2-receptor antagonist. N. Engl. J. Med. 309:1368, 1983.

ULTRASONOGRAPHY AND ULTRASOUND-GUIDED BIOPSY OF THE CANINE PROSTATE

SUSAN T. FINN, D.V.M.,
and ROBERT H. WRIGLEY, B.V.Sc.

Fort Collins, Colorado

Disorders of the prostate gland are common in male dogs. Nearly 100 per cent of all glands removed at necropsy from uncastrated dogs older than 7 years of age have histologic evidence of disease (Brendler et al., 1983). Disorders include benign prostatic hypertrophy (BPH), prostatitis, prostatic cysts and abscesses, and neoplasia.

Many therapies exist to treat specific diseases of the canine prostate, including hormones, antimicrobial agents, and surgical procedures. These therapies differ greatly. Therefore, a specific diagnosis is essential for proper therapy and prognosis. An incorrect diagnosis may cause prolonged inappropriate treatment resulting in progression of the disease or possible deterioration of the animal.

However, diagnosis of prostatic disease is difficult; similar signs (i.e., obstipation, locomotor difficulties, fever, coma) are observed in dogs with various types of disease. Current methods for diagnosing prostatic disease (e.g., examining exfoliated prostatic cells, culturing urine and prostatic fluid, and radiography of the prostate) have well-documented limitations (Barsanti and Finco, 1984).

Ultrasonography is the use of high-frequency sound waves in a sonarlike manner to characterize the internal architecture of the prostate. Ultrasonography of the prostate provides an accurate, noninvasive diagnostic technique for evaluating the internal structures of the gland. Ultrasonography also provides a technique to obtain prostatic biopsies representative of the disease process without the trauma of surgery. Ultrasound is the primary means of evaluating human prostatic disease.

INDICATIONS

A clinical evaluation should be performed in every male dog showing signs of prostatic disease. Clinical signs related to the prostate include constipation, dyschezia, hematochezia, "ribbonlike" stools, end-micturition hematuria, persistent urinary tract infection, stranguria, caudal abdominal mass, unexplained fever and leukocytosis, locomotor difficulties, reproductive problems, palpably abnormal prostate, and sublumbar lymph nodes.

However, deficiencies exist in current methods to evaluate canine prostatic disease. Palpation of the prostate gland per rectum and per abdomen is variable and subjective. Palpators cannot distinguish between disease processes. White blood cell count is a poor predictor, with leukocytosis suggesting abscess formation only.

Culturing urine and examining prostatic cells that exfoliate are not always helpful because of lack of specificity. Urine culture results are usually positive with prostatitis but will also be positive with bladder and kidney infections. Abnormalities in an ejaculate are not always due to disorders of the prostate. Other disorders in the urogenital tract (balanoposthitis, orchitis, epididymitis, cystitis, urethritis, bladder tumors, urethral tumors) can result in abnormal semen. Additionally, contamination with gram-positive bacteria from the prepuce and urethra may render interpretation impossible. It may also be difficult to obtain semen from a dog with painful prostatic disease. Routine radiographs can provide only presumptive conclusions on diagnosis by demonstrating size, location, and contour of the prostate.

Therefore, sonography should become an integral part of all diagnostic evaluations of the prostate. This is especially important in situations in which laboratory tests are equivocal or nondiagnostic, response to conservative therapy is inadequate, severe disease is suspected, or a recorded baseline prostatic appearance is desired. Ultrasonography enables the practitioner to evaluate the size, shape, symmetry, and internal architecture of the gland. Solid tissue enlargement can be differentiated from cystic change such as hematocysts, abscesses, and paraprostatic cysts. Localized or diffuse stromal abnormalities may be detected. To a certain extent, disruption of the margins of the prostate can be detected. With this information, the practitioner can formulate an abbreviated differential diagnostic list to develop a therapeutic plan and prognosis. Ultrasound can then be used to monitor disease recurrence and response to therapy.

A biopsy of prostatic tissue is often necessary for a definitive diagnosis of disease. Transperineal or transabdominal percutaneous biopsy, guided by palpation only, results in failure to obtain diagnostic tissue up to 50 per cent of the time. Additionally, serious complications can result if vessels, urethra, occult prostatic abscesses, or bowel are punctured with the "blind" approach. A transrectal prostatic biopsy allows more specificity but may cause bacteremia or urinary tract infection. In the past, surgical laparotomy was the only biopsy technique that allowed visual selection of biopsy sites. With ultrasonic guidance, a biopsy needle can be safely directed by a percutaneous approach into a selected area of the gland. Fine-needle aspirates and drainage of cysts and abscesses can be performed.

SCANNING PROCEDURES

Two routes of imaging the canine prostate have been described; transabdominal (Feeney et al., 1985) and transrectal (Blum et al., 1985). The suprapubic transabdominal approach is most commonly used clinically because of its easy application. For this approach, the animal is placed in comfortable dorsal recumbency in a padded trough (Fig. 1). Restraint of all four legs with nontraumatic ties may enable a single person to perform an examination. With nervous animals or animals in pain, a second person is often required. Chemical restraint can be used but is seldom necessary.

Ultrasonic waves are strongly reflected by an air interface, leaving virtually no sound waves to penetrate to structures below the air interface. Because of the air-filled structure and air-trapping ability of fur, the caudal abdomen must be clipped in a rectangular zone between the cranial aspect of the

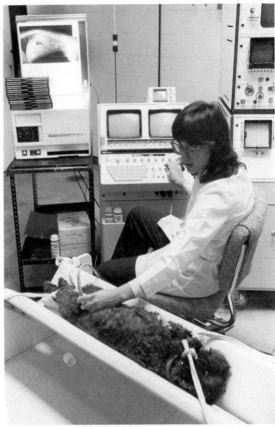

Figure 1. Prostatic ultrasonography of the canine patient. This unsedated dog has been placed in dorsal recumbency in a padded trough. The inguinal region has been clipped from prepuce to pubis and from inguinal fold to inguinal fold.

prepuce to the pubis and from midline to inguinal folds. A manufacturer-approved coupling gel is then applied, and the transducer is placed against the caudal ventral abdominal wall. Gas within an associated section of colon can similarly impede visualization of the prostate. Therefore, a 12-hr fast and a low-volume enema at least 2 hr prior to sonography is beneficial.

Ultrasonic waves easily penetrate fluid-filled structures, with little attenuation or loss of functional diagnostic sound. Therefore, a full urinary bladder is beneficial for improved imaging of the prostate. A readily visible bladder trigone provides a useful landmark for locating the approximate midline of the prostate. A urinary catheter may be placed in the urethra. This will produce an easily visualized bright focal echo, which will assist in identifying the prostatic midline. If the bladder is small, it may be infused with sterile saline (10 ml/kg). A low dose of furosemide has also been used to distend the bladder.

Bone markedly attenuates the ultrasound beam by both absorption and reflection. To avoid this loss of sound waves, the transducer is angled 45° cranially, and the sound beam is directed deep to the pubis into the prostate. The transducer must also be placed lateral to the prepuce and os penis to image the prostate. Small intrapelvic prostates are often difficult to image because of their location under the pubic bone.

Thus far, transrectal endosonography of the dog has been utilized only in research. With the use of compact linear array transducers, this imaging route has become technically feasible for clinical use in the dog. The transrectal approach is the route of choice for evaluating the human prostate, providing the evaluator with superior resolution and the ability to detect prostatic capsule destruction. Clinical trials are necessary before this approach can be utilized by the practicing veterinarian.

Serial scans are made in transverse and sagittal planes through the entire prostate (Fig. 2). Any abnormal-appearing areas should be evaluated in both planes to define the shape and the extent of a lesion and to rule out the possibility of artifact.

An incorrectly set instrument gain can cause artifactual increases or decreases in the echo pattern of the prostate, which may be interpreted as a pathologic condition. Therefore, prior to evaluating the prostate, the gain should be adjusted to make a probably normal spleen, left kidney, and bladder appear correctly. With the mobile skin of the canine, these areas can usually be scanned without additional clipping.

NORMAL PROSTATE

The ultrasonographer should mentally recall the normal anatomy of the caudal abdomen (Fig. 3) and compile a list of criteria to be evaluated when examining the prostate (Table 1). The external dimensions, shape, and location of the prostate should be evaluated first. The normal canine prostate has an ultrasonically established average measurement of 22 mm craniocaudally by 22 mm dorsoventrally, with a range of 13 to 30 mm in each dimension (Fig. 4). However, this size range was established ultrasonographically in a study utilizing dogs 2 to 4 years of age (Carter and Rowles, 1983). In this age

category, 40 to 50 per cent of the dogs probably already had early prostatic changes associated with BPH.

The width (lateral to lateral) of the prostate on the transverse scans is more difficult to assess. The lateral aspects of this circular organ are not perpendicular to the sound beam. Therefore, the echoes that are reflected from these parallel surfaces may not be adequately returned to the receiver to allow visualization. This is known as loss of specular echoes.

The shape of the prostate varies normally from ellipsoid to more circular but should be symmetric (Fig. 4). The symmetry of prostatic tissue is best evaluated on a transverse scan. Although the canine prostate has been described as a bilobed structure, the normal gland may not always appear bilobed sonographically. The only indication of the median raphe may be a slight furrow at midline on transverse scans.

The location of the prostate varies. The normal-sized prostate is usually located to varying degrees within the pelvic canal. The entire normal prostate may not be visualized because of attenuation of the sound beam by the pubic bone.

The margins of the normal prostate should be smooth and continuous (Fig. 4). Unlike the human prostate, the capsule does not appear as an obvious echogenic (echo-producing) structure. This fact, along with the similar transmissibility of sound waves (acoustic impedance) through the prostate and surrounding tissues, makes absolute evaluation of prostatic margins difficult with transabdominal ultrasound. Also, loss of specular echoes from the surfaces of the prostate that are parallel to the sound beam produces difficulty in evaluating the entire perimeter of the prostate. Therefore, obvious disruption of prostatic margins may be visualized only on the dorsal and ventral borders.

Next, the general echogenicity of the prostate should be evaluated (Fig. 4). The normal prostate should have a uniform echogenicity that is coarsely hypoechoic relative to periprostatic fat and surrounding pelvic musculature. The normal prostate

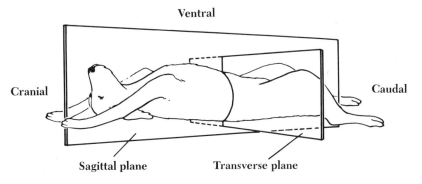

Figure 2. Diagram of the routine scan planes for evaluation of the canine prostate. All ultrasound images are oriented in this manner, with the head to the reader's left, the feet to the right, and the ventral body wall at the top of the image. If possible, the entire prostate should be evaluated with sequential transverse and sagittal scans. Areas of suspected abnormalities should be more thoroughly evaluated with additional oblique views.

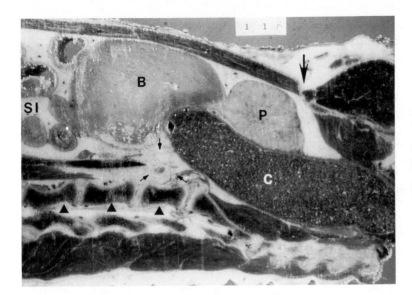

Figure 3. Sagittal section through a frozen canine specimen demonstrating caudal abdominal and pelvic anatomy (B, bladder; P, prostate; SI, small intestine; C, colon, arrowheads, vertebrae). The largest arrow indicates the pubic bone, which often "shadows" the caudal prostate. The small arrows indicate the area of the sublumbar lymph nodes.

should be free of cavitation. Small, circumscribed anechoic areas less than 0.5 cm in size have been described as normal variants in older intact dogs. These probably represent retention cysts or hematocysts, which may be present subclinically in the early BPH complex. No evidence of mineralization should be seen in the normal prostate. A linear area of increased echogenicity has been seen in the area of the prostatic urethra in the normal prostate by some investigators. This is called the hilar echo and is reported to represent the prostatic urethra and confluence of the periurethral ducts. When visualized, the symmetry or asymmetry of the hilar echo has been used as a diagnostic criteria (Feeney et al., 1987).

ABNORMAL PROSTATE

The size of the diseased prostate is usually increased. However, in certain instances of specific disease processes (e.g., uncomplicated BPH, chronic fibrosing prostatitis, and scirrhous carcinoma), the prostate may be within the normal size

Table 1. Ultrasonographic Criteria of the Normal Canine Prostate

Criterion	Evaluation Results
Size	13–30 mm
Shape	Ellipsoid (bilobed)
Location	Intrapelvic
Prostatic margins	Smooth, intact
General echogenicity	Homogeneously coarsely hypoechoic
Focal or multifocal variations	Not seen
Cavitation	Not seen (small retention cysts)
Distal enhancement	Not seen
Mineralization	Not seen

range. The greatest degree of enlargement is seen in cases of abscess formation, paraprostatic cysts, and neoplasia.

No change in shape may be seen in BPH, mild cystic hyperplasia, prostatitis, and early neoplasia. Some nodular change in the shape of the prostate may be seen with cystic hyperplasia and prostatitis, especially on transverse scans. In veterinary medicine, neoplasia is rarely detected so early that the shape of the prostate has not yet changed. The exception is a transitional cell carcinoma of the prostatic urethra. Paraprostatic cysts, abscesses, and neoplasia produce the greatest degree of asymmetry in the shape of the prostate.

As the prostate enlarges, it is usually displaced from the pelvic canal into the abdomen. Without an overlying pubic bone to impede sound waves, the prostate is more easily scanned in this location. The inability to sonographically image the prostate because of its intrapelvic location may indicate lack of enlargement. The only disease process that sonographically demonstrates prostatic margin disruption is neoplasia.

The general echogenicity of the prostate is usually altered by disease. A generalized increased echogenicity of the prostate, which appears as a "whiter" prostate with more internal echoes, may be the result of fibrosis due to chronic inflammation, neoplasia, and the stromal or acinar hypertrophy seen with glandular aging and developing BPH. A generalized decreased echogenicity has been seen by the authors with acute inflammation and edema of the canine prostate. Incorrect instrument gain settings may create an artifactual increase or decrease in the generalized echogenicity of the prostate. Focal or multifocal variations in the normally uniform prostatic parenchyma indicate a pathologic condition. These foci appear as circumscribed areas of increased or decreased echogenicity. The size,

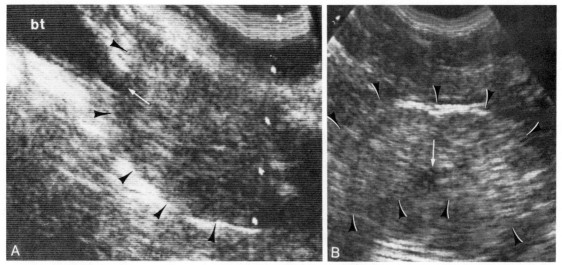

Figure 4. Sagittal *(A)* and transverse *(B)* prostatic ultrasonograms of a normal, 3-year-old male dog. The prostate border (arrowheads) is smooth. The shape is cylindric on the sagittal view and bilobed on the transverse. The parenchyma is homogeneous and coarsely hypoechoic. The size is 3 cm by the 1 cm per division cursor. The bladder trigone (bt) tapers to the prostatic urethra (white arrow) at the center of the prostate. Shadowing from the pubis impedes evaluation of the caudal prostate.

Figure 5. Sagittal *(A)* and transverse *(B)* prostatic ultrasonograms of a 6-year-old male German shepherd dog with prostatic abscess formation. The prostate is approximately 5 cm, using the 1 cm per division cursor. Margins of the gland (arrowheads) are irregular. The shape is asymmetric on the transverse scans. The two abscessed areas (A_1 and A_2) are imaged as cavitations in the left lobe of the prostate with a septation separating them. The borders of the abscesses are irregular. The cavities are still enclosed by a thin rind of prostatic parenchyma. The dorsal abscess (A_2) is anechoic. The ventral abscess (A_1) contains scattered internal echoes that were mobile when visualized with real-time ultrasonography. The echoes probably represent conglomerates of cellular debris. The bright interface and shadowing dorsal and cranial to the prostate on the sagittal scans is colonic gas. Hyperechoic foci that probably represent inflammatory fibrosis are seen in the right lobe of the prostate on the transverse scan (white arrows).

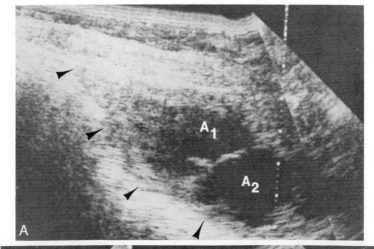

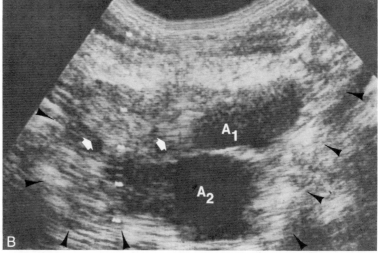

shape, and regularity of the margins and any tendency of the foci to coalesce should be evaluated for any variation in the uniform echo pattern of the prostate.

Cavitation is a specific type of focal or multifocal variation in the prostate. A cavitating lesion is defined as a circumscribed hypoechoic to anechoic structure within the prostatic parenchyma, often showing good through transmission of sound (distal enhancement). Fluid is an example of a very homogeneous substance through which ultrasonic waves pass easily. Because of the lack of echo production within a fluid-filled cavity, it appears black, or anechoic, when scanned. The physical presence of increased sound waves deep to a fluid-filled structure artifactually increases the intensity of echoes from the tissue deep to the fluid, making it brighter, or more hyperechoic. This through transmission artifact of a cavity indicates that the cavity is probably fluid filled. In the case of abscess formation, the purulent fluid usually has through

transmission that decreases as the protein content of the fluid increases. Some accumulations of very similar cells, such as carcinomas, have through transmission of sound. Any cavitations present within the prostatic parenchyma should be observed for size, number, and architecture of the internal surface. The inner margin may be smooth, irregular, or undulant. The cavity can have either a simple structure or multiple septations (Fig. 5).

If the fluid within a cavitation contains cellular debris, such as accumulations of purulent material, echo reflection can occur from these very small nonspecular interfaces. This produces a varying degree of scattered small echoes within a mostly anechoic cavity (Fig. 5). This is most commonly seen with abscess formation. The cellular debris echoes may be fixed in position, as with inspissation, or may be mobile in the fluid matrix. An incorrect high gain setting of the ultrasound machine can artifactually create the appearance of cellular debris within an anechoic cavity.

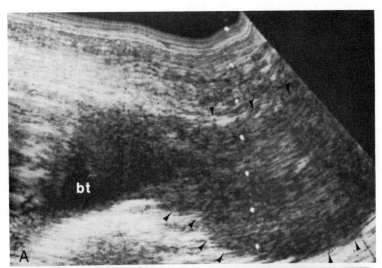

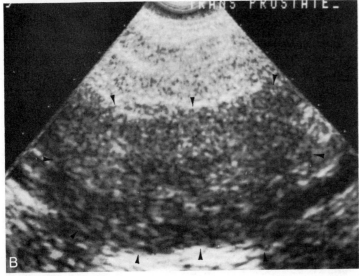

Figure 6. Sagittal *(A)* and transverse *(B)* prostatic ultrasonograms of a 5-year-old male dog with benign prostatic hypertrophy. The prostate is enlarged, measuring approximately 4 cm. The shape (arrowheads), margins, and echogenicity are normal. The bladder trigone (bt) is visualized as an anechoic triangle cranial to the prostate on the sagittal scan.

Table 2. Ultrasonographic Evaluation of the Diseased Prostate*

Evaluation Criterion	Uncomplicated BPH	Complicated BPH	Prostatic Disease			
			Bacterial Prostatitis	*Bacterial Abscesses*	*Paraprostatic Cyst*	*Neoplasia*
Size	(N), ↑	↑	(N), ↑, ↓	↑↑	↑↑	↑↑
Shape	N	N	ABN, SYM	ABN, ASYM	ABN, ASYM	ABN, ASYM
Location	Pelvic inlet, abd.	Pelvic inlet, abd.	Pelvic inlet	(Pelvis), abd.	Ventral abd.	Pelvis, ventral abd.
Prostatic margins	N	N	N, Irregular, intact	Irregular, intact	[N] Smooth	Irregular, disrupted
General parenchymal echogenicity	N, ↑	↑	(↓), ↑	↑	[N, (↑)]	↑
Focal or multifocal variations	−	+	+	+	[(−), +]	+ +
Cavitations	−	+, < 1.5 cm	+	+ +, > 1.5 cm, ~irregular border	+ +, > 1.5 cm, ~smooth border	+, −
Distal enhancement	−	(+ Cystic hyperplasia)	−	+, (−)	+	(+), −
Mineralization	−	−	(+)	(+)	(+) "Egg shell"-like	+

*Findings refer to the majority of the cases, although exceptions exist.

N, Normal; ( ), less common finding; ↑, increased; ↓, decreased; −, not present; +, present; ABN = abnormal; SYM, symmetric; ASYM, asymmetric; [ ], refers to changes observed in the parenchyma of the prostate associated with the paraprostatic cyst.

Another specific focal or multifocal variation in the pathologic prostatic parenchyma is mineralization. Mineralization of prostatic tissue is visualized as hyperechoic areas with variable shadowing if the mineralized area is sufficiently large and dense. Prostatic mineralization may be seen with chronic prostatitis, ductile calculi, neoplasia, and cysts. Prostatic calculi are rare in dogs. Mineralization is a more common characteristic of prostatic adenocarcinoma than of chronic prostatitis. Although uncommon, mineralization associated with prostatic cysts is regular and "egg shell–like" in distribution.

The hilar echo is not a reliable diagnostic sign because of inconsistent visualization. One investigator reports that asymmetry of the hilar echo is seen most commonly with abscesses and neoplasia (Feeney et al., 1987).

SONOGRAPHIC APPEARANCE OF SPECIFIC DISEASES

Benign prostatic hypertrophy in the canine involves a spectrum of disease states with varying degrees of severity. BPH may be complicated or uncomplicated. Uncomplicated BPH (Fig. 6) appears sonographically as an enlarged, noncystic prostate with a symmetric shape and smooth margins. The general echogenicity can be isoechoic (normal) to uniformly hyperechoic. The differential diagnosis includes acute bacterial prostatitis and squamous metaplasia (Table 2).

Complicated BPH may take the form of nonbacterial prostatitis, cystic hyperplasia (Fig. 7), hema-

tocysts, and hematomas. Sonographically, complicated BPH involves some degree of cystic change, ranging from small retention cysts to cavities larger than 1.5 cm. These focal or multifocal cavitations appear as smooth-walled transonic areas with distal enhancement and usually an increased echogenicity to the rest of the prostate resulting from secondary fibrosis and stromal proliferation. There is currently an indication that these purportedly sterile cysts should be cultured for *Mycoplasma* and *Ureaplasma.*

Bacterial prostatitis varies in acoustic appearance with chronicity. As previously mentioned, acute bacterial prostatitis has been seen as a diffusely hypoechoic enlarged prostate. With chronic bacterial prostatitis, the size may be enlarged or actually reduced owing to fibrosis and contracture (Fig. 8). Small cavitations may be recognized as irregular hypoechoic to anechoic foci. The general shape of the prostate is usually symmetric, but the capsular margins may be irregular. The prostatic margins should be intact. With increasing chronicity, prominent irregular hyperechoic foci may develop throughout a coarsely hyperechoic parenchyma (Fig. 9). The major ultrasonic differential diagnosis for chronic bacterial prostatitis is prostatic neoplasia.

Prostatic abscess formation is another prostatic disorder that can create large (greater than 1.5 cm) cavitating lesions (Figs. 5 and 10). These cavitations appear acoustically as hypoechoic to anechoic areas with smooth or irregular internal margins and distal enhancement. The fluid within the cavity may show varying levels of echogenicity, with increasing cellularity of the fluid. In some cases, a fluid-fluid level has been imaged, with dependent sedimen-

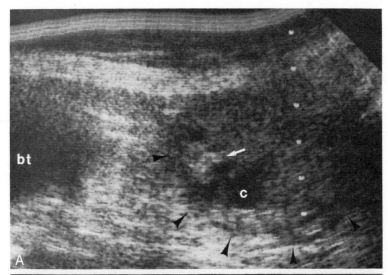

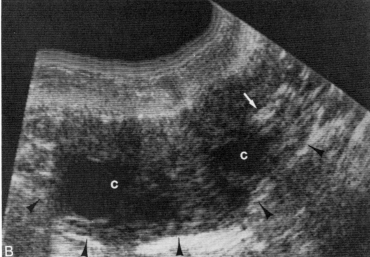

Figure 7. Sagittal *(A)* and transverse *(B)* prostatic ultrasonograms of a 7-year-old male Doberman pinscher with cystic hyperplasia of the prostate. The prostate is over 4 cm in diameter on the sagittal scan, using the 1 cm per division cursor. The shape (arrowheads) on the sagittal scan is normal but is distorted and asymmetric on the transverse scan. Multifocal anechoic cavitations (C) are present, representing cystic change. The largest cyst, measuring approximately 2 cm, is best visualized in the right lobe on the transverse scans. Irregular hyperechoic foci (white arrows) from secondary tissue reaction are associated with the cysts. The trigone of the bladder (bt) is seen on the sagittal scan.

Figure 8. Sagittal prostatic ultrasonogram of an 8-year-old male dog with chronic recurring bacterial prostatitis. The prostate is approximately 3 cm, which is within the normal size range. The shape (arrowheads) and margins appear normal. There is a diffuse hyperechogenicity to the entire prostatic parenchyma. Fibrosis and stromal proliferation may account for this increase in echogenicity. The full bladder (b) is allowing good visualization of the prostate. Dorsal to the prostate, colonic gas is creating a bright interface with shadowing (white arrows).

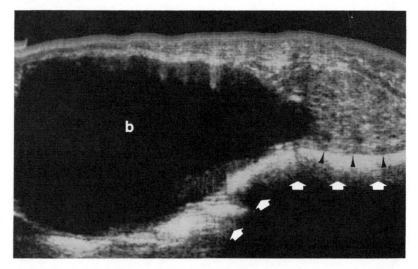

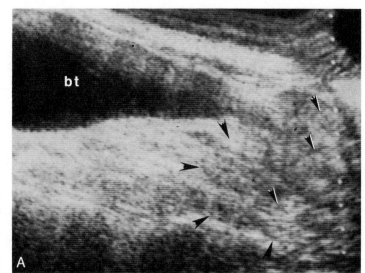

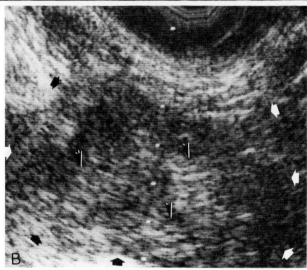

Figure 9. Sagittal *(A)* and transverse *(B)* prostatic ultrasonograms of an 11-year-old male collie with bacterial prostatitis. The prostate is enlarged, measuring approximately 4 cm on the sagittal scan. The borders of the prostate (arrowheads on sagittal, black and white arrows on transverse) are somewhat difficult to define because of the multifocal changes in echogenicity of the prostatic parenchyma. Patchy hyperechoic foci (double arrows) are present throughout the prostate. The foci are most pronounced in the left lobe on the transverse scan. These changes probably represent secondary tissue fibrosis. The bladder trigone (bt) is visualized on the sagittal scan.

tation of the heavier cellular debris (Fig. 11). These cavitations may be lobulated and often contain septations. The general echogenicity of the prostatic parenchyma is usually increased secondary to inflammation and fibrosis. The prostate is enlarged, with an asymmetric shape and intact margins. Aggressive manipulation of the transducer could rupture a thin-walled abscess. Prostatic hematomas and hematocysts may mimic a prostatic abscess.

Paraprostatic cysts are extraparenchymal cystic structures that may have formed from retention cysts that have extended through the prostatic capsule or as remnants of müllerian ducts. Ultrasonically, they are smoothly marginated, anechoic bladderlike structures that extend from the prostate (Fig. 12). If the cyst is very large or extends craniad, it may be difficult to differentiate from the urinary bladder. Urethrocystography can delineate the location of the bladder. A urinary catheter placed within the bladder during an ultrasound examination can also differentiate it from a cyst. The sonogenic nature of a catheter allows it to be visualized

as a linear hyperechoic stripe within the anechoic cavity that is the bladder. The associated prostatic parenchyma may be isoechoic or may demonstrate changes consistent with BPH. The differential diagnosis includes superficially located prostatic cysts or abscesses.

Neoplasia of the prostate may be primary, metastatic, or locally invasive. The most common primary prostatic cancer is adenocarcinoma. Because of the variable behavior of neoplasia, the ultrasonic appearance of a tumor is also variable and often depends on the stage at which the disease is first detected. In veterinary medicine, prostatic neoplasia is often first detected as advanced disease. The majority of neoplastic prostates are enlarged on ultrasonographic examination, although the authors have seen a scirrhous carcinoma that was decreased in size. The enlargement is often asymmetric, with irregular nodular borders, and may demonstrate margin disruption. Characteristic of the internal echo texture of prostatic neoplasia are multifocal, broad, poorly defined hyperechogenic areas that

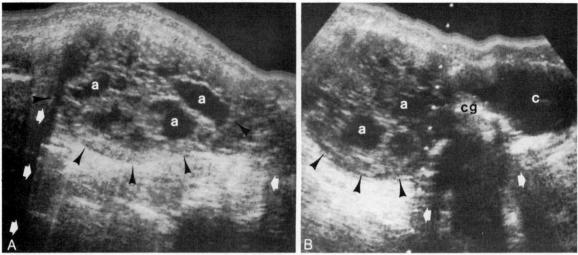

Figure 10. Sagittal *(A)* and transverse *(B)* prostatic ultrasonograms of a 12-year-old male dog with prostatic abscess formation and a paraprostatic cyst. The prostate is markedly enlarged, measuring approximately 7 cm on the sagittal scan. The margins of the gland (arrowheads) surround the internal abscessed area as a thin rind of tissue. The abscesses are anechoic cavitations (a) of varying size, with irregular borders and divided by septae. They are distributed throughout the gland parenchyma. There is a large amount of distal enhancement (white arrows) deep to these fluid-filled structures. A second anechoic structure (c) is seen only on the transverse scans to the left of the midline indicated by the cursor. This paraprostatic cyst is smooth-walled, measures approximately 5 cm in diameter, and extends beyond the borders of the prostate. A small amount of colonic gas (cg) is creating shadowing between the abscessed prostate and the cyst. Linear shadows off of the cranial border of the prostate on the sagittal scan are motional artifacts.

exhibit a tendency to coalesce with an uneven distribution (Fig. 13). It has been reported in ultrasonology of human prostatic carcinoma that many of the tumor foci are hypoechoic. However, secondary tissue reaction with mineralization and fibrosis gives neoplasia a hyperechoic appearance. In dogs, prostatic mineralization is most commonly associated with neoplastic change.

Advanced, secondarily invasive prostatic neoplasia such as transitional cell carcinoma of the prostatic urethra may cause a similar echo appearance. However, the degree of involvement around the urethral region may be more severe than the remainder of the prostate, with hyperechoic foci extending into prostatic tissue from the urethra (Fig. 14). The major ultrasonographic differential diagnosis for prostatic neoplasia is severe chronic prostatitis. Prostatic abscesses may also be seen in association with prostatic neoplasia. Metastatic involvement of sublumbar lymph nodes can be detected with ultrasound. A metastatic sublumbar lymphadenopathy appears sonographically as a variable-sized, ovoid to circular, hypoechoic mass or masses dorsal to the urinary bladder. This ultrasonic appearance of the sublumbar lymph nodes is very indicative of neoplasia. However, sublumbar lymphadenopathy has

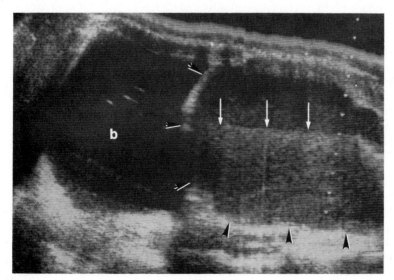

Figure 11. Sagittal prostatic ultrasonogram of a 6-year-old male Great Dane with a prostatic hematoma. *Escherichia coli* was cultured from the hematoma. The prostate is markedly enlarged, measuring approximately 8 cm in diameter. Most of the prostatic parenchyma has been replaced by a large cystic structure (arrowheads). The cyst contained diffuse nonspecular echoes that were seen to move with real-time ultrasonography. This represents cellular debris. The horizontal line (white arrows) is probably a fluid-fluid line created by sedimentation of the heavier particles. Prostatic parenchyma was visualized more caudally but is not seen in this scan. The large circular anechoic area cranial to the hematoma is the bladder (b). Notice the large amount of through transmission deep to both the hematoma and the bladder.

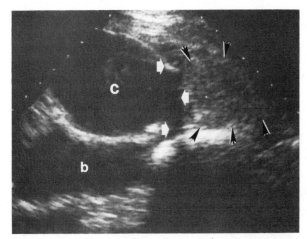

Figure 12. Sagittal prostatic ultrasonogram of a 6-year-old male Malamute with a calcified paraprostatic cyst. The prostate, 4 cm in diameter, is visualized in the caudal ventral portion of the scan (black and white arrowheads). The shape and echogenicity of the gland are fairly normal. Small hyperechoic foci are present along the cranial border adjacent to the cyst. The paraprostatic cyst (c) extends from the prostatic parenchyma as a smooth-walled, anechoic 5 cm cavitation. The walls of the cyst are very echogenic and demonstrate acoustic shadowing, indicating mineralization (white arrows). The anechoic structure deep to the paraprostatic cyst is the bladder (b).

been reported in a case of prostatic abscess formation.

ULTRASOUND-GUIDED BIOPSY

Ultrasound-guided biopsy of the prostate may be obtained either transabdominally or transperineally,

depending on the location of the gland. This technique has not been described in the veterinary literature. Although biopsies may be obtained from the human prostate using local anesthesia only, complete sedation or, preferably, general anesthesia is necessary in the dog. A complete prostatic ultrasound is performed initially to select areas of suspect pathology for biopsy.

Transabdominal biopsy is utilized for enlarged prostates located mostly within the abdomen. After selection of biopsy sites, utilizing transabdominal ultrasound, the caudal abdomen is aseptically prepared as if for abdominal surgery. An assistant may stabilize a large masslike prostate, but this is not required with ultrasonic guidance. A 5-MHz real-time sector transducer is commonly used. Most transducers may be sterilized by following the manufacturer's instructions. More simply, the transducer may be placed within a sterile surgical glove that contains an adequate amount of ultrasonic coupling gel. The sterile encased transducer may now be aseptically controlled by the sonographer. Sterile lubricating gel (Surgilube, E. Fougera & Co., Melville, NY) is then placed between the encased transducer and the abdomen to provide sonic coupling.

The selected biopsy sites are then relocated. The desired biopsy depth is determined using the cursor on the real-time display. The scan plane is identified by the reference mark on the transducer. The biopsy needle is introduced parallel to the scan plane, approximately 1 to 2 cm from the transducer. The angle of introduction varies with the depth of the biopsy site and the distance from the transducer

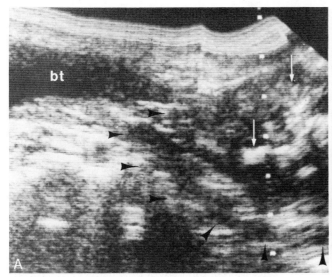
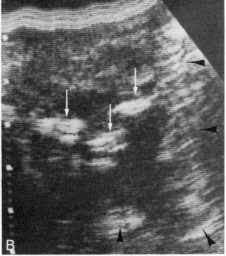

Figure 13. Sagittal (A) and transverse (B) prostatic ultrasonograms of a 12-year-old male dachshund with prostatic adenocarcinoma. The enlarged prostate measures approximately 5 cm. The margins of the prostate (black arrowheads) are difficult to evaluate but appear nodular. The internal architecture of the gland is coarsely complex. Wide, bright coalescing hyperechoic foci (white arrows) are seen throughout the prostate. This probably represents fibrosis and secondary tissue reaction to the infiltrative neoplasia. Some foci are dense enough to create acoustic shadowing. This suggests mineralization. The anechoic areas in the gland probably represent necrosis, hemorrhage, or abscess formation. The bladder trigone (bt) is seen on the sagittal scan.

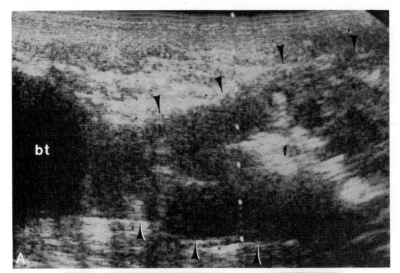

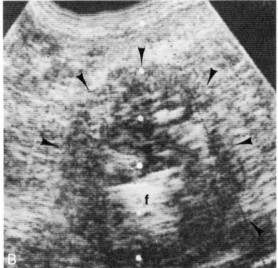

Figure 14. Sagittal *(A)* and *(B)* prostatic ultrasonograms of a 9-year-old castrated male dog with transitional cell carcinoma of the prostatic urethra. The prostate is enlarged, measuring approximately 4 cm, but the shape is fairly normal (arrowheads). The margins are easily evaluated. Within the center of the prostatic parenchyma is a large coalescing very echogenic focus (f). On both the sagittal and the transverse scans, the hyperechoic focus is in the area of the prostatic urethra, as indicated by the bladder trigone (bt). Deep to the focus, the parenchyma appears hypoechoic, owing to sound attenuation by the focus. The remainder of the glandular tissue surrounding the focus appears fairly normal.

that the biopsy needle is introduced. Commercial biopsy guides are available from various manufacturers. However, these devices have been developed to accommodate human, not canine, anatomy. Therefore, the authors usually prefer to manually guide the biopsy needle. The biopsy needle is visualized as it enters the scan plane as a very hyperechoic, mobile, linear echo. Fine adjustments can now be made as the needle is directed into the biopsy site.

Various instruments are utilized for prostatic biopsy and aspiration. For fine-needle aspiration, an 18-gauge aspiration core needle (E-Z-M, Westbury, NY) or a 22-gauge 3½-inch spinal needle is adequate. Inadequate tissue is usually obtained with this instrument for standard histology, but cytology may be performed on the aspirate. A punch biopsy of the prostate is usually required for histologic examination. Tru-cut biopsy needles are used most commonly for prostatic punch biopsies (Disposable biopsy needle 11.4 cm [4½ inch cannula], Travenol

Laboratories, Inc., Deerfield, IL). The use of the aforementioned biopsy instruments requires one individual to manipulate the needle and one individual to orient the ultrasound transducer. A new biopsy device (Biopty, Radioplast, Karlsrogatan, 46, 752 39, Uppsala, Sweden) has been developed for use with ultrasound guidance. The biopsy device contains a spring trigger system that automates needle movement, enabling one operator to retrieve a diagnostic sample.

Human ultrasonologists combine transperineal biopsy with continuous sonographic monitoring using linear array rectal transducers. This combination is unsurpassed in allowing complete visualization of the needle from the perineum into abnormal foci, alteration of the path of the needle to avoid damage to adjoining structures, and exact tissue extraction from nodules as small as 1 cm. Trials of this technique in dogs are required before transperineal ultrasound-guided biopsies can be used in clinical veterinary practice.

CONCLUSION

At this time, veterinary ultrasonography is a practical, sensitive diagnostic modality for imaging the canine prostate gland. An ultrasonographic examination can often be performed by a single technician on the unanesthetized dog. Ultrasonography is indicated in all dogs demonstrating clinical signs of prostatic disease. Ultrasonography is especially indicated in a clinical work-up in which laboratory and radiographic results are nondiagnostic. The ultrasonic appearance of the normal prostate has been well documented. Evidence of prostatic pathology such as enlargement, stromal and acinar hypertrophy, cystic change, fibrosis secondary to inflammation, abscess formation, mineralization, nodular change, and invasive infiltration can be detected with ultrasound. Specific ultrasonographic signs are associated with BPH, bacterial prostatitis, abscess formation, paraprostatic cysts, and neoplasia. If biopsy is indicated for a definitive diagnosis, the biopsy needle may be accurately guided with ultrasound into areas of pathology.

The noninvasive nature and easy application of ultrasound contributes to rapid diagnostic and prognostic results and the ability to monitor response to therapy with repeatable long-term evaluation. A large amount of research remains to be done on the ultrasonographic appearance of various canine prostatic diseases. Canine prostatic ultrasonography can then achieve the state-of-the-art success that it now has in human prostatic evaluation.

References and Suggested Reading

Barsanti, J. A., and Finco, D. R.: Evaluation of techniques for diagnosis of canine prostatic diseases. J.A.V.M.A. 185:198, 1984.

Blum, M. D., Bahnson, R. R., Lee, C., et al.: Estimation of canine prostatic size by in vivo ultrasound and volumetric measurement. J. Urol. 133:1082, 1985.

Brendler, C. B., Berry, L. L., Ewing, A. R., et al.: Spontaneous benign prostatic hyperplasia in the beagle: Age-associated changes in serum hormone levels, and the morphology and secretory function of the canine prostate. J. Clin. Invest. 71:1114, 1983.

Cartee, R., and Rowles, T.: Transabdominal sonographic evaluation of the canine prostate. Vet. Radiol. 24:156, 1983.

Dahnert, W. F., Hamper, U. M., Eggleston, J. C., et al.: Prostatic evaluation by transrectal sonography with histopathologic correlation: The echopenic appearance of early carcinoma. Radiology 158:97, 1986.

Dietze, A.: Use of real-time ultrasound scanning in the diagnosis of small animal reproductive conditions. In Kirk, R. W. (ed.): Current Veterinary Therapy IX. Philadelphia: W. B. Saunders Co., 1986, p. 1258.

Feeney, D. A., Johnston, G. R., and Klausner, J. S.: Two-dimensional gray-scale ultrasonography: Applications in canine prostatic disease. Vet. Clin. North Am. [Small Anim. Pract.] 15:159, 1985.

Feeney, D. A., Johnston, G. R., Klausner, J. S., et al.: Canine prostatic disease: Comparison of ultrasonic appearance with microbiological findings: 30 cases. (1981–1985) J.A.V.M.A. 190:1018, 1987.

Finco, D. R.: Prostatic gland biopsy. Vet. Clin. North Am. [Small Anim. Pract.] 4:367, 1974.

Hoppe, F. E., Hager, D. A., Poulos, P. W., et al.: A comparison of manual and automatic ultrasound-guided biopsy techniques. Vet. Radiol. 27:99, 1986.

McDicken, W. N.: Diagnostic Ultrasonics: Principles and Use of Instruments. New York: John Wiley & Sons, 1976.

Rifkin, M. D., Friedland, G. W., and Shortliffe, L.: Prostatic evaluation by transrectal endosonography: Detection of carcinoma. Radiology 158:85, 1986.

ULTRASONOGRAPHY OF THE CANINE UTERUS AND OVARY

ROBERT H. WRIGLEY, B.V.Sc.
and SUSAN T. FINN, D.V.M.

Fort Collins, Colorado

Ultrasonography is used extensively in medicine to image reproductive and other soft tissue organs. With the advent of less expensive ultrasound machines, this imaging modality is becoming feasible in veterinary medicine. The basic principle of sonographic imaging relies on the observation that a sound pulse may be partially reflected (creating an echo) when it passes through different substances.

The relative strength of the returning echo will be related to the nature of the materials forming this echogenic (echo-producing) interface. Homogeneous liquids, such as water, urine, and blood, reflect few to no echoes and are described as anechoic. A fine, stippled hypoechoic echo pattern is created by parenchymal tissue. High-intensity echoes result from fibrous tissue and areas of mineralization. Gas-filled objects and bone cause marked perturbation of the sound beam, preventing evaluation of underlying structures.

ULTRASOUND MACHINES

Doppler ultrasound instruments detect changes in sound frequency that arise when the beam is reflected by moving surfaces (e.g., fetal heart or pulsating arteries) and blood cells. Frequency changes may be presented as audible sounds (Bartrum and Crow, 1977; Hagen-Ansert, 1978).

A-mode instruments may produce audible sounds whenever the reflected echoes exceed threshold levels of amplitude and depth. Alternatively, the echoes may be displayed as a tracing on an oscilloscope.

B-mode real-time ultrasound machines display a televised two-dimensional cross-sectional image of sound-reflecting objects. B-mode instruments appear to be the most sensitive and accurate for veterinary patients (Rantenen and Ewing, 1982).

PATIENT PREPARATION

Minimal patient preparation is required for ultrasonography of the reproductive tract. A filled urinary bladder aids in visualizing the body of the uterus. Ultrasonography may be performed with the bitch standing or lying down. Air trapped in the haircoat must be eliminated by clipping away sufficient hair, and acoustic gel should be used to couple the ultrasound transducer to the skin. Unlike radiographic techniques, ultrasonography evaluates only a small cross-section of the abdomen at any one time. B-mode evaluation of an organ (e.g., uterus) requires the production of a series of images by moving the transducer over the abdomen in both transverse and sagittal planes.

OVARIAN ULTRASONOGRAPHY

Ovary

The ovary is best evaluated by making sagittal B-mode sonograms of the region adjacent to the caudal pole of the kidneys. Normal anestrous ovaries are rarely detected ultrasonographically. Vesicular follicles may be visualized as 5-mm, anechoic cysts just prior to ovulation (Iraba et al., 1984). Ultrasonic detection of canine corpora lutea has not been reported.

Cystic follicles and luteinized cystic follicles may synthesize and secrete sex steroids, with resultant infertility and persistent estrus (Bloom, 1954; Rowley, 1980). Abnormal ovarian cysts vary greatly in size (up to 19 cm in diameter) and may be unilateral or bilateral (Dow, 1960). Larger ovarian cysts appear ultrasonographically as spherical, anechoic simple cysts lying in the dorsal abdomen just caudal to the kidneys (Fig. 1). Overlying bowel gas may hinder visualization, so serial studies should be made over 1 to 2 days to rule out the presence of ovarian cysts (Olson et al., 1989). Ultrasonographic findings must be interpreted in conjunction with the history and physical findings, as non–hormone-producing ovarian cysts may also develop from the rete ovarii and subsurface epithelial cells (Bloom, 1954).

Functional ovarian tumors may also result in persistent estrus. The tumors may be bilateral or unilateral and are variably sized (4 to 16 cm) (Dow, 1960). Such tumors result in a mixed ultrasonographic appearance because of the presence of fluid-filled, anechoic cysts, hypoechoic or hyperechoic tumor cells, and connective tissue. The larger tumors may drag the ovary ventrally, resulting in loss of proximity to the adjacent kidneys.

Uterus

Transverse and sagittal B-mode ultrasonograms should be made of the caudal abdomen to evaluate the uterus. Overlying gas-filled intestines may prevent ultrasonographic evaluation of the uterine horns. A full urinary bladder displaces the small intestine cranially and provides an acoustic window to the underlying uterus. Normal nongravid uterine horns are rarely detected. The uterine body may be seen as a tubular structure dorsal to the urinary bladder.

UTERINE ULTRASONOGRAPHY

Gravid Uterus

Ultrasonographic detection of early canine pregnancy is confounded by the poor relationship be-

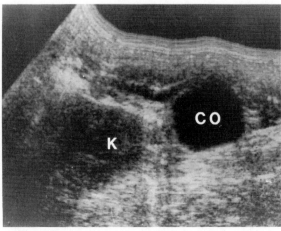

Figure 1. Sagittal sonogram of a bitch in persistent estrus revealed an ovarian cyst (CO) just caudal to the left kidney (K).

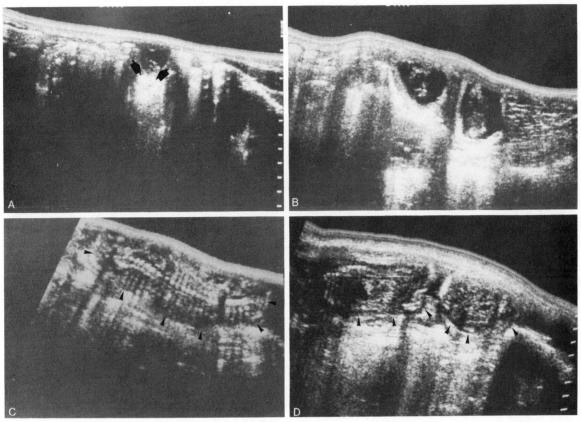

Figure 2. Sagittal sonograms of a normal German shepherd, made during gestation. *A*, Gestational vesicles (arrows) containing fetuses were detected on the 20th day of gestation. *B*, Re-examination at day 30 revealed progressive enlargement of the uterus and fetuses. *C*, Re-examination at day 50 demonstrated a longitudinal image of a fetus (arrowheads). *D* demonstrates transverse images of two fetuses (arrowheads).

tween breeding dates and conception. Estrus may be displayed for 5 to 6 days before, and up to 9 days after, ovulation (Holst and Phemister, 1981). Additional variation results in the survival of ova (up to 3 days) and spermatozoa (up to 11 days) in the canine reproductive tract (Doak et al., 1967). Between conception and day 15 of pregnancy, the uterus may enlarge slightly and become more hypoechoic (Cartee and Rowles, 1984). Placental attachment and growth of the vesicle does not begin until 17 to 21 days after conception. At about this time, the first gestational vesicles are detected by ultrasound (Cartee and Rowles, 1984). The accuracy of B-mode ultrasonographic pregnancy detection

Table 1. *Ultrasonographic Measurements of Normal Canine Uteri and Feti*

Day	$\overline{X}$ Uterine Lumen (mm)	Uterine Lumen Range (mm)	$\overline{X}$ Crown-Rump Length (mm)	Crown-Rump Length Range (mm)	$\overline{X}$ Calvarial Biparietal Diameter (mm)	Calvarial Biparietal Diameter Range (mm)	$\overline{X}$ Body Diameter (mm)	Body Diameter Range (mm)
3–14*	24	23–25	—	—	—	—	—	—
17–23*	20	10–30	10	—	—	—	—	—
27–30*	26	23–30	18	16–21	—	—	6	—
30	—	—	—	—	11	9–18	17	11–40
34–37*	29	25–35	25	23–30	11	—	18	12–22
38–45*	28	25–30	71	22–90	18	13–22	23	17–35
40	—	—	—	—	18	16–22	30	17–48
46–49*	27	25–50	89	86–92	23	19–29	34	25–47
50	—	—	—	90–104	23	20–30	44	24–55
51–60*	—	—	—	—	24	23–27	—	—
55	—	—	146	106–160	26	22–31	52	43–60

*Data from Cartee, R. E., and Rowles, T.: Preliminary study of the ultrasonographic diagnosis of pregnancy and fetal development in the dog. Am. J. Vet. Res. 45:1259, 1984.

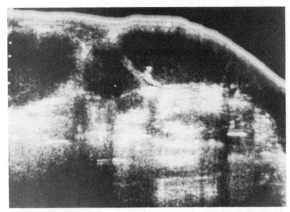

Figure 3. A sagittal sonogram revealed fluid-distended uterine loops resulting from a pyometra.

may not be 100 per cent until 25 days after breeding (Shille and Gontarek, 1985). Ultrasonographic diagnosis of a nongravid uterus should not be made with B-mode instruments until at least 30 days after the last breeding date.

The gestational vesicle appears as an anechoic, fluid-filled cavity containing a semicircular hyperechoic embryo (Fig. 2A through D). Embryonic motion and cardiac activity may be detected as early as the 28th day of gestation. Between days 30 and 40, the head and appendages become visible. After 40 to 45 days, the lumen of the uterus becomes filled by feti. Bony structures and other fetal organs such as the heart, aorta, liver, and stomach become visible in the last trimester (Cartee and Rowles, 1984). Ultrasonography will help estimate litter size but is inaccurate when there are more than four puppies (Shille and Gontarek, 1985).

Uterine diameter, fetal crown-rump length, and calvarial biparietal and body diameters may be measured. Normal canine fetal growth curves are not well established, though preliminary findings provided in Table 1 may be of assistance in estimating gestational age.

A-mode and Doppler equipment may also diagnose canine pregnancy (greater than 32 days gestation). A-mode equipment detected pregnancy in 90 per cent of bitches that subsequently whelped and 83 per cent of nonpregnant bitches (Allen, 1981). Doppler instruments detected bitches that would whelp with an accuracy of 85 per cent between 36 and 42 days after mating and 100 per cent from 43

days to term. The accuracy of detecting nonpregnant bitches was 100 per cent (Allen, 1981).

Uterine Pathology

Fetal death may be detected after approximately day 30 by the absence of heart beat or fetal movements. The feti may be abnormally small or fail to enlarge on subsequent re-examination. Fetal reabsorption may then result in a distorted gestational vesicle containing poorly defined structures.

Endometritis and pyometra are readily distinguished ultrasonographically from a gravid uterus, as the uterus is distended by fluid and no feti are present. The uterus takes on the appearance of an anechoic convoluted tube (Fig. 3). The tortuous convolutions may also appear as anechoic, circular structures when viewed in a transverse plane. Stump pyometras may be detected as hypoechoic to mixed echo lesions located dorsal and caudal to the urinary bladder.

References and Supplemental Reading

Allen, E. W.: Detection of pregnancy in the bitch: A study of abdominal palpation, A-mode ultrasound and doppler ultrasound techniques. J. Small Anim. Pract. 22:609, 1981.

Bartrum, R. J., and Crow, H. C.: *Gray-scale Ultrasound: A Manual for Physicians and Technical Personnel.* Philadelphia: W. B. Saunders Co., 1977.

Bloom, F.: Ovarian cysts. *In* Bloom, F.: *Pathology of the Dog and Cat.* Evanston, IL: American Veterinary Publications, Inc., 1954, p. 390.

Cartee, R. E., and Rowles, T.: Preliminary study of the ultrasonographic diagnosis of pregnancy and fetal development in the dog. Am. J. Vet. Res. 45:1259, 1984.

Doak, R. L., Hall, A., and Dale, H. E.: Longevity of spermatozoa in the reproductive tract of the bitch. J. Reprod. Fertil. 13:51, 1967.

Dow, C.: Ovarian abnormalities in the bitch. J. Comp. Pathol. 70:59, 1960.

Hagen-Ansert, S. L.: *Textbook of Diagnostic Ultrasonography.* St. Louis, MO: C. V. Mosby Co., 1978.

Holst, P. A., and Phemister, R. D.: The prenatal development of the dog: Preimplantation events. Biol. Reprod. 5:194, 1981.

Iraba, T., Matsui, N., Shimizu, R., et al.: Use of echography in bitches for detection of ovulation and pregnancy. Vet. Rec. 115:276, 1984.

Olson, P. N., Wrigley, R. H., Husted, P. W., et al.: Persistent estrus in the bitch. *In* Ettinger, S. J. (ed.): *Textbook of Veterinary Internal Medicine III.* Philadelphia: W. B. Saunders Co., 1989 (in press).

Rantanen, N. W., and Ewing, R. L.: Principles of ultrasound application in animals. Vet. Radiol. 22:196, 1982.

Rowley, J.: Cystic ovary in a dog: A case report. Vet. Med. Small Anim. Clin. December, 1888, 1980.

Shille, V. M., and Gontarek, J.: The use of ultrasonography for pregnancy diagnosis in the bitch. J.A.V.M.A. 187:1021, 1985.

CHRONIC BACTERIAL PROSTATITIS IN THE DOG

LAINE A. COWAN, D.V.M.,
and JEANNE A. BARSANTI, D.V.M.
Athens, Georgia

GENERAL ANATOMY

In the dog, the prostate gland is the sole accessory sex gland. It is a retroperitoneal, bilobed gland that surrounds the urethra at the base of the urinary bladder. At puberty, the prostate gland is located on the floor of the pelvic cavity, but with increased prostatic size or with distension of the urinary bladder, the prostate gland frequently moves cranially into the caudal abdominal cavity. The prostate gland produces seminal fluid and hence plays an important role in sperm transport and function. In addition, the prostate gland may contribute to the defense against bacterial pathogens in the lower urinary tract by secreting an antibacterial factor.

INCIDENCE AND HISTORICAL CLUES

Chronic bacterial prostatitis (CBP) is a common problem in middle-aged and older intact male dogs, with no breed predilection. In one report of dogs referred for signs of prostatic disease, between 5 and 11 per cent had chronic bacterial prostatitis. However, this may underestimate the true incidence of chronic bacterial infections, since dogs with CBP are frequently asymptomatic, and many times only a history of recurrent urinary tract infections suggests the presence of a prostatic problem. Other historical clues that may suggest prostatic disease include a urethral discharge independent of urination, hematuria, tenesmus, or, less commonly, infertility. Most dogs with chronic prostatitis alone do not have systemic signs of disease unless it is complicated by prostatic neoplasia, abscess, or increased estrogen concentrations (exogenous or an estrogen-secreting tumor). The clinical diagnosis is based on historical information, physical examination, and cytologic and microbiologic evaluation of prostatic fluid.

PATHOPHYSIOLOGY

As in most tissues, infection in the prostate gland occurs when numbers or virulence of bacteria overwhelm the host's normal defense mechanisms. Receptors on the uroepithelium and the counterpart bacterial surface structures (adhesins) are thought to play an important role in urogenital bacterial virulence and are currently active areas of investigation.

In humans, increases in antigen-specific secretory IgA and IgG in the prostatic fluid (independent of serum immunoglobulin concentrations) have been documented in patients with bacterial prostatitis. Although prostatic immunoglobulin quantitation has not been examined in dogs, a similiar humoral response is expected. At least two additional mechanisms are thought to protect the prostate from bacterial invasion. The prostate gland secretes a factor (prostatic antibacterial factor, PAF) with bactericidal activity. The antibacterial property of PAF is due primarily to a zinc component that is effective against the majority of common urinary tract pathogens. In addition, the frequent voiding of urine helps to decrease urethral bacteria numbers and, hence, limit contamination of the prostate by urethral organisms.

In 70 per cent of dogs with bacterial prostatitis, a single organism is isolated. *Escherichia coli* is the most common pathogen in canine bacterial prostatitis. Other bacteria frequently cultured include *Pseudomonas*, *Staphylococcus*, *Streptococcus*, and *Proteus*. Although uncommon, *Brucella canis* may cause bacterial prostatitis. *Mycoplasma* species have been considered prostatic pathogens, and anaerobes rarely have been reported to cause prostatitis in humans.

Chronic bacterial prostatitis usually develops insidiously but may occur subsequent to an episode of acute bacterial prostatitis. Any condition that causes an increase in bacterial numbers in the periprostatic urethra or urinary bladder or that decreases the local or systemic host resistance will increase the likelihood of a prostatic infection. Anatomic abnormalities of the urethra, bladder, or prostate, such as calculi, neoplasia, strictures, or congenital abnormalities, may allow urethral bacterial numbers to increase and, hence, predispose the patient to bacterial prostatitis. Neoplasia, squamous metaplasia, and cystic changes may also predispose the prostate to secondary bacterial infections. Reflux of bacteria from the urinary bladder or bacteria that ascend the urethra are considered the most common ways that pathogens colonize the prostate. Microbial pathogens may gain access to the gland via lymphogenous or hematogenous spread, from the epididymis or testes, or via direct extension from the peritoneal or pelvic cavities.

DIAGNOSIS

Chronic bacterial prostatitis must be differentiated from acute bacterial prostatitis, prostatic abscesses, benign prostatic hyperplasia, squamous metaplasia, neoplasia, and periprostatic cysts, since therapy and prognosis differ in each. The diagnosis of chronic bacterial prostatitis is based on the history, physical examination, and cytologic and quantitative microbiologic examination of prostatic fluid. Radiographic and ultrasonographic evaluation of the caudal abdomen, histologic and microbiologic examination of prostatic tissue, and a brucellosis titer also may be helpful.

HISTORY

A history of a recurrent urinary tract infection in an intact male dog and fluid (purulent or sanguineous) dripping from the urethra independent of urination are the most common historical findings. If CBP complicates another prostatic problem, other signs of prostatic abnormalities, such as tenesmus and a stiff or weak hindlimb gait, or systemic signs may be reported by the owner.

PHYSICAL EXAMINATION

Findings of physical examination and rectal palpation alone cannot diagnose CBP, but they do help to rule out different types of prostatic disease. During a complete physical examination, evaluation of the scrotal sac and a digital rectal examination are necessary in a patient with prostatic disease. Scrotal swelling, tenderness, discharge, masses, or abnormal texture may be compatible with brucellosis or testicular neoplasia, which may secondarily involve the prostate gland. Prostatic contour, size, symmetry, texture, mobility, and tenderness should be evaluated by rectal examination. Frequently, simultaneous palpation of the prostate via the caudal abdomen and per rectum is beneficial if the prostate is large or is located abdominally. Chronic bacterial prostatitis in itself does not result in prostatomegaly, nor is the prostate painful on palpation. The contour of the prostatic surface may be irregular secondary to focal or segmental fibrosis.

LABORATORY EVALUATION

When the clinician suspects a prostatic abnormality, the minimum clinical laboratory evaluation should include a complete blood count, a urinalysis, and cytologic and quantitative microbiologic evaluation of the prostatic fluid and any urethral discharge present. Serum chemistries and a screening test for brucellosis may be particularly helpful if reproductive tract or systemic signs are present.

Leukocytosis usually does not occur in dogs with CBP. Hematuria, pyuria, and bacteriuria are commonly present in cystocentesis urine samples from patients with CBP, but a normal urine sediment does not rule out prostatic infection.

Examination of prostatic fluid is the key in the diagnosis of a bacterial prostatic infection. For a diagnosis of bacterial prostatitis, the clinician first must localize the problem to the prostate gland and, second, must compare the prostatic fluid cytology with the microbial culture results to ascertain that an infection is present. Prostatic fluid can be obtained by collecting the third fraction of an ejaculate, by prostatic massage, or, rarely, by fine-needle aspiration of the prostate gland. The problem with obtaining prostatic fluid by either of the first two methods is the difficulty in localizing the infection to the prostate gland, since contamination from the testicle, epididymis, vas deferens, and urethra may contribute to an ejaculate. In addition, bladder and urethral contamination may occur when obtaining prostastic massage fluid. In humans, comparison of first-voided urine, midstream urine, postprostatic massage fluid, and postprostatic massage urine have been used to reliably localize the infection to the prostate gland when higher numbers of organisms are cultured from the postmassage samples. Similarly, comparison of a prostatic massage saline wash with a postprostatic massage wash is reliable in detecting prostatic infections in dogs. To obtain prostatic massage samples, often light sedation helps decrease the amount of physical restraint needed and lessens patient apprehension. After the dog has voided, the remaining urine is removed from the bladder via aseptic catheterization. While the catheter is in the urinary bladder, 5 ml of sterile saline is flushed, aspirated, and saved as prostatic massage sample 1. After retracting the catheter just distal to the prostate (as palpated rectally), the prostate is massaged rectally (or abdominally if the clinician is unable to reach the prostate rectally) for 1 to 2 min. A second 5-ml saline sample is flushed past the prostatic urethra, and the sample is collected by aspirating as the urinary catheter is slowly advanced into the urinary bladder. This sample is saved as prostatic massage sample 2 and is compared to the prostatic massage sample 1 to identify the contribution of extraprostatic contamination. In theory, the advantage of evaluating prostatic massage samples is the ability to more accurately localize the infection to the prostate gland. However, cytology and culture of the ejaculate are more sensitive than prostatic massage in detecting CBP. Also, the prostatic massage technique is unable to identify a bacterial prostatitis when a urinary tract infection is present, since most laboratories will not quantitate bacterial colonies when they are greater than 10^5 per milliliter. In those cases, either prostatic fluid should be collected via ejaculation rather than by prostatic massage, or 24 to 72 hr of systemic antimicrobial therapy that reaches high concentrations in the urine but does not enter the prostate gland (such as ampicillin) may be used in an attempt to clear the urinary tract infection prior to obtaining the prostatic massage samples.

In diagnosing a prostatic bacterial infection, inflammatory cytology and a positive prostatic fluid culture are necessary to decrease the likelihood of mistaking urethral contamination for prostatic infection. Cytologic examination also may be beneficial in detecting concomitant prostatic or urethral neoplasia. A few erythrocytes and occasional leukocytes are normally found in prostatic fluid, and increased numbers of neutrophils and macrophages are indicative of inflammation. Since the normal distal urethral flora consists primarily of gram-positive organisms, gram-positive organisms in prostatic fluid in the absence of inflammatory cytology probably represent contamination rather than bacterial prostatitis. Large numbers (greater than 10^5 colonies per ml) of gram-negative organisms in the presence of inflammatory cytology in an ejaculate, or in the prostatic massage sample 2 (in the absence of significant number of bacteria in prostatic massage sample 1 and with no evidence of abnormalities in the remainder of the reproductive system), is highly suggestive of bacterial prostatitis.

RADIOLOGIC AND ULTRASONOGRAPHIC EXAMINATION

Plain radiographs of the caudal abdomen may help identify or rule out any concomitant prostatic abnormalities. In general, determination of prostatic size, location, and calcification; identification of irregularities in contour; and inspection of the sublumbar lymph nodes, lumbar vertebrae, and pelvis for evidence of metastases may be important clues to help identify prostatic disease. Although prostatomegaly and an irregular prostatic outline have been observed in dogs with bacterial prostatitis, these findings are nonspecific.

Two-dimensional gray-scale ultrasonographic examination of the prostate gland is the best noninvasive technique available to detect alterations in prostatic architecture. Parenchymal focal to multifocal areas of increased echogenicity, shadowing,

and small intraparenchymal anechoic foci have been observed in dogs with bacterial prostatitis. However, none of these changes are diagnostic. The most common benefit of ultrasonographic prostate examination is to help rule out predisposing or secondary prostatic abnormalities (e.g., cystic parenchymal changes that may complicate bacterial prostatitis) or to help identify prostatic abscesses.

HISTOLOGIC EXAMINATION

Rarely is it necessary to obtain histologic confirmation of chronic bacterial prostatitis. Usually, prostatic biopsies are indicated in individual cases to rule out concomitant problems, such as neoplasia. False-negative biopsy results may occur. Usually, only a small section is biopsied; thus, the focal or multifocal lesions of chronic bacterial inflammation may be missed. When representative histologic sections are examined, the presence of neutrophilic inflammation with or without accompanying macrophage and plasma cell infiltration is considered necessary for a diagnosis of active inflammation.

THERAPY

Treatment of bacterial prostatitis in the dog relies on the elimination of any predisposing factors, an appropriate antimicrobial regimen, and adjunctive therapy.

In order for an antimicrobial agent to be useful in the resolution of a bacterial process, the active drug must reach the site of the infection. In CBP, obtaining therapeutic concentrations at the site of infection is problematic because of the blood-prostate barrier. The blood-prostate barrier is the anatomic and functional barrier of the prostatic epithelium's bilipid membrane, which limits the penetration of antimicrobial agents from the plasma into the prostatic secretions. Since antimicrobial agents penetrate this membrane only by passive diffusion, the lipid solubility of the antimicrobial is a major determinant influencing the concentration of the drug obtained in the prostatic fluid. The lipid solubility of a drug at any given time depends on the degree of ionization, which is in turn dependent on the pKa of the drug and the pH of the fluid compartment.

Most antimicrobials are weak acids or weak bases. Weak acids, such as ampicillin and cephalothin, tend to be ionized at plasma pH; conversely, weak bases, such as erythromycin and trimethoprim, tend to be less ionized at a pH of 7.4 and, therefore, are more probably able to enter the prostate gland lumen in therapeutic concentrations.

In dogs with bacterial prostatitis, the prostatic fluid usually remains more acidic than plasma. The decreased pH increases the degree of ionization of the weak bases entering the prostatic secretions. The end result is an ionized, lipid-insoluble drug, which is trapped in the prostatic secretory side of the prostatic epithelium and cannot readily cross the epithelial membrane back into the plasma compartment. So, in CBP, in the presence of acidic prostatic fluid, antimicrobials with basic pKas or antimicrobials that do not ionize to an appreciable extent are the drugs of choice. Prostatic infections with urease-producing organisms, such as *Staphylococcus*, *Proteus*, and *Ureaplasma*, may result in an alkaline pH, thereby altering the effectiveness of the antimicrobial drug.

The degree of protein binding is an additional consideration when planning an antimicrobial therapeutic regimen, since protein-bound drugs are less available for diffusion into the prostate gland. However, the degree of protein binding is not as important as the degree of ionization, and drugs that have a large degree of protein binding, such as clindamycin and chloramphenicol, may still be considered appropriate therapeutic choices. The currently available antibiotics that are known to diffuse into the prostate and attain therapeutic concentrations include erythromycin, clindamycin, oleandomycin, trimethoprim-sulfonamide, chloramphenicol, and carbenicillin. Norfloxacin, an antimicrobial recently approved for use in human medicine, can obtain therapeutic concentrations in the prostatic fluid, and pharmacokinetic studies in the dog are in progress.

The individual antimicrobial agent used in each case should be based on a culture and sensitivity test of the prostatic fluid. (See Table 1 for a list of appropriate antimicrobial choices based on organism isolated.) A minimum of 4 weeks of systemic therapy is considered appropriate for adequate control of the infection, although no objective studies have examined the optimal duration of treatment. Ideally, a second prostatic fluid sample should be cultured 3 to 5 days after initiation of therapy, especially in a patient with a previous history of

bacterial prostatitis, to be certain that the antimicrobial agent chosen is effective in that particular patient. Minimally, prostatic fluid samples should be cultured 5 to 7 days after stopping the antimicrobial, and again in 30 and 60 days. Repeated cultures are essential, since a single negative prostatic fluid culture in a patient with CBP does not rule out the presence of infection and since recurrent infection is common.

If after 4 weeks of appropriate antimicrobial therapy, culture evidence of a bacterial prostatitis persists, several options are available. Continuation or alteration of the antibiotic used depends on the new antimicrobial sensitivities. If no alternative drugs are appropriate, long-term drug therapy may be necessary, and a second 4- to 8-week course of therapy is indicated, with a prostatic fluid culture during the first week of therapy. If no adjunctive therapy has been utilized, it should be instigated at this point.

If the bacteria isolated are not sensitive (*in vitro*) to the antimicrobial agents known to enter the prostate in therapeutic concentrations, usually a therapeutic trial of an antibiotic known to enter the prostate is warranted (a trimethoprim-sulfonamide is usually the drug of choice). Another, less preferred option is to wait a few weeks in hopes that the organism will lose its resistance to the available antibiotics. Prostatectomy, although not recommended for most dogs with CBP, may be necessary with extremely resistant or pathogenic organisms. Prostatectomy is a major procedure that requires surgical expertise and results in urinary incontinence in the majority of patients.

ADJUNCTIVE THERAPY

Only 30 per cent of men with chronic bacterial prostatitis are cured with antimicrobial therapy alone. Similar data are not available for dogs, but a comparable prognosis for cure is expected. The goals of adjunctive therapy are to augment host resistance, decrease the size of the prostate gland, or both.

Hormonal manipulation is the predominant adjuvant therapy utilized to decrease prostatic mass. More specifically, surgical castration, by removing testicular androgens, is the most commonly used method to decrease prostatic size in the canine patient. The reduction in prostatic size in CBP after castration is rapid, with palpably detectable decreased size within 1 week, and a maximum histologic involution by 12 weeks after surgery. Recently, an objective study evaluated the benefits of castration in an experimental model of canine CBP. The castrated dogs had a shorter duration of prostatic infection and had fewer bacteria than the control dogs.

Table 1. *Recommended Antimicrobials for Chronic Bacterial Prostatitis (Based on Culture and Sensitivities) When Prostatic Fluid is Acidic***

	Drug
Gram-positive organism	Chloramphenicol, trimethoprim-sulfa, erythromycin, clindamycin, carbenicillin
Mycoplasma and *Ureaplasma*	Doxycycline, minocycline
Gram-negative organism	Chloramphenicol, trimethoprim-sulfa

*When the prostatic fluid is more alkaline than plasma, trimethoprim-sulfa cannot attain as high a prostatic tissue concentration; carbenicillin and the macrolides may be able to attain higher intraprostatic concentrations; and chloramphenicol should be unaffected, as compared to acidic prostatic fluid.

The negative aspects of castration include the loss of reproductive potential and owner reluctance. Isolated pockets of infection may persist in castrated dogs that have concurrent prostatic abscesses or cysts. Antiandrogens may have a role in therapy of breeding animals or when owner objections persist. Many antiandrogens are currently in the investigational stage in the United States.

The use of estrogens in the treatment of canine prostatic disease is not recommended. The potential side effect of squamous metaplasia of the prostatic epithelium may predispose the dog to bacterial prostatitis, and the potential for life-threatening aplastic anemia, which may occur secondary to estrogen administration, is an unwarranted risk.

Zinc administration has been investigated as an adjunctive therapy in humans, since prostatic fluid zinc is bactericidal and decreased concentration of zinc has been reported in men with bacterial prostatitis. Similar decreases in prostatic fluid or prostatic tissue zinc concentrations do not occur in dogs with bacterial prostatitis. In humans, oral zinc supplementation has not increased prostatic fluid zinc concentrations nor has it altered the course of CBP. At this time, oral zinc therapy has no known therapeutic benefit in the treatment of canine CBP.

COMPLICATIONS AND PROGNOSIS

Clients should be warned of the likelihood of recurrent infection, especially in sexually intact dogs, since only one third of the patients are expected to be cured by antimicrobial therapy alone. With castration and appropriate antibiotics, the majority of patients may be cured. Long-term antimicrobial therapy may have adverse effects. Protracted administration of trimethoprim-sulfonamide may lead to folate deficiency, which may be prevented by folic acid supplementation. Chloramphenicol therapy may cause bone marrow suppression in some patients, which usually resolves with withdrawal of the drug. Long-term administration of chloramphenicol inhibits protein synthesis, which may result in decreased antibody production and impaired wound healing. Potential sequelae to chronic prostatitis include recurrent urinary tract infections, progression to prostatic abscess formation, and pyelonephritis, especially in immunecompromised patients.

References and Supplemental Reading

Barsanti, J. A., and Finco, D. R.: Canine prostatic diseases. Vet. Clin. North Am. 16:587, 1986.

Barsanti, J. A., Prasse, K., Crowell, W., et al.: Evaluation of various techniques for diagnosis of chronic bacterial prostatitis in the dog. J.A.V.M.A. 183:219, 1983.

Branam, J. E., Keen, C., Ling, G., et al.: Selected physical and chemical characteristics of prostatic fluid collected by ejaculation from healthy dogs and from dogs with bacterial prostatitis. Am. J. Vet. Res. 45:825, 1984.

Feeney, D., Johnston, G., Klausner, J., et al.: Canine prostatic disease—comparison of ultrasonographic appearance with morphologic and microbiologic findings: 30 cases (1981–1985). J.A.V.M.A. 190:1027, 1987.

Hornbuckle, W., MacCoy, D., Allan, G., et al.: Prostatic disease in the dog. Cornell Vet. 68:284, 1978.

Winningham, D., Nemoy, N., and Stamey, T.: Diffusion of antibiotics from plasma into prostatic fluid. Nature 219:139, 1968.

CANINE SEMEN FREEZING AND ARTIFICIAL INSEMINATION

P. W. CONCANNON, PH.D.,
and M. BATTISTA, D.V.M.
Ithaca, New York

The first animals reported to become pregnant by artificial insemination were dogs inseminated with fresh semen in studies conducted by Spallanzani around 1780 in Italy. Artificial insemination (AI) of fresh semen is still used instead of natural mating to facilitate breeding when animal transport poses difficulty, to breed more than one bitch with a single ejaculate, or to accomplish a breeding between a pair that will not breed naturally.

COLD STORAGE OF EXTENDED FRESH SEMEN

Properly diluted semen can be refrigerated for several days or longer and still yield fertile sperm when later warmed and used for breeding. Use of undiluted semen is not as successful because of deleterious properties of prostatic fluid or other components of seminal plasma. Common extenders for cold storage of fresh semen are outlined in Table 1. Retention of 50 per cent motility after cooling of dog semen for 2 to 4 days (Province et al., 1984) or 4 to 8 days (Davis et al., 1963; Foote, 1964b) has been reported using 20 per cent egg yolk extenders with or without glycerol, but only for several hours using skim milk (Province et al., 1984). For storage of fresh canine semen, Province and coworkers recommended against the use of glycerol, since in most cases tested, glycerol had a suppressive effect on motility.

Interest in fresh semen cold storage and transport has recently increased among dog breeders because of dissatisfaction with results or reports of results obtained with frozen semen and the availability of overnight air-delivery services to deliver freshly extended semen. Success rates for AI with cooled fresh semen, as with raw fresh semen, are higher than with frozen semen for several reasons. With fresh semen, there is no damage due to freezing, the cervix is less of a barrier, larger numbers of sperm are usually present, fresh sperm live longer in the reproductive tract of the bitch, and timing of inseminations to a particular 1- or 2-day period is not quite so critical. Nevertheless, the long-term storage of frozen semen for use on demand any time in the future would represent a far more useful method for serious breeders, commercial kennels, research colonies, and scientists interested in preserving canine models of inherited diseases.

Table 1. *Name and Composition of Extenders Reported for 1 to 4 Days Cold Storage of Sperm-rich Fraction of Canine Semen**

Citrate–Bicarbonate–Egg Yolk Extender: 100 ml aqueous solution containing citric acid monohydrate (0.07 gm), sodium bicarbonate (0.17 gm), sodium citrate dihydrate (1.16 gm), potassium chloride (0.03 gm), glycine (0.75 gm), glucose (0.24 gm), egg yolk (20 ml); pH 6.8, 308 mOsm/kg (Foote, 1964a; Province et al., 1984)

Caprogen Egg Yolk Extender: 100 ml aqueous solution containing sodium citrate dihydrate (1.56 gm), glycine (0.78 gm), glucose (0.23 gm), N-caproic acid (1.0 ml of 2.5% solution), catalase (1.0 ml of 45 mg% solution), egg yolk (20 ml); pH 7.0, 326 mOsm; bubbled with nitrogen gas immediately before use (Province et al., 1984)

Tris-buffered Egg Yolk Extender: 100 ml aqueous solution containing 2.4 gm tris base (tham), 1.3 g citric acid monohydrate, 1 gm fructose, 3.8 ml glycerol, 20% egg yolk (Gill et al., 1970)

Skim Milk Extender: Skim milk heated at 95° C for 10 min, then cooled; pH 6.5 277 mOsm (Province et al., 1984)

Low-Fat Milk Extender: Sterilized homogenized milk with 2% fat (Christiansen, 1984)

Citrate–Egg Yolk Extender: Sodium citrate, 2.9% solution (80%) and egg yolk (20%) (Christiansen, 1984)

---

*Dilution rates used were 1 part semen to 3 to 10 parts extender at 23–35°C, with subsequent cooling to 5°C over a 2- to 3-hr period.

Antibiotics typically added are 1000 I.U. penicillin and 1 mg dihydrostreptomycin per ml.

Frozen Semen

During the 2 decades since the first reports of AI using frozen semen in dogs, there have apparently been less than 500 pregnancies produced from frozen canine semen worldwide. This estimate includes published reports of 134 research cases and the 101 cases reported for registration of litters with the American Kennel Club (AKC) through the end of 1987. The research cases include 81 that resulted from semen frozen in pellets and approximately 50 cases involving semen frozen in straws. The latter include three cases at Nihon University of Tokyo, five at the University of Minnesota, three at Colorado State University, four at Cornell University, and 36 at the Veterinary College of Norway. Unreported clinical cases are estimated to number 100 in Sweden and other Scandinavian countries, and perhaps 100 in the U.K., Australia, continental Europe, and Africa. These small numbers raise doubts about the efficacy of frozen semen AI in dogs. Therefore, the remainder of this review attempts to summarize the available information, to highlight areas of concern that require further research efforts, and to give background information to veterinarians considering frozen semen AI service in their practices.

Differences among species in sperm shape, size, and biochemical makeup result in variability in the conditions required for successful freezing of sperm. Success in freezing, with resultant fertility, has been greatest with dairy cattle semen; this is due in part to the economic importance of cattle and the large research expenditure. Moreover, bull sperm is more tolerant of freezing than that of most other species, and in cattle transcervical insemination is easily performed. In other species, particularly in dogs, semen freezing has been less successful, but the reasons are not clear. Pregnancy rates after frozen semen AI in cattle, pigs, sheep, and dogs have been about 90 per cent, 70 per cent, 70 per cent, and 40 per cent, respectively, of those obtained with natural mating.

VARIABLES AFFECTING SUCCESS RATES

Artificial insemination utilizing frozen semen involves semen collection, dilution in an extender, equilibration under refrigeration, freezing in convenient volumes, storage, thawing, and insemination of the bitch during the peak of her fertile period. There are many factors that may be critical and require careful attention (Table 2). As alternatives for various steps are combined, the number of possible methods becomes astronomic. Only a few have been tried, and fewer yet compared.

Table 2. *Variables Potentially Affecting Success with Frozen Semen Artificial Insemination in Dogs*

Male:	Fertility of male dog; ability of semen from individual males to be frozen
Semen Collection:	Contamination with presperm, fraction I; prostatic fluid, fraction III; urine or blood; lubricants or detergents. Composition and surface of collection container; contamination with preputial debris; temperature of collecting vessel
Semen Quality:	Sperm number and concentration; sperm motility and progressive motility; percentage of live sperm; percentage of morphologically normal sperm; sperm-agglutination problems
Semen Dilution:	Avoidance of cold shock; composition of extender; time between collection and dilution; temperature of initial dilution; amount of semen dilution (volume); extent of sperm dilution (sperm concentration); number of dilution steps and solutions; force of any centrifugation; amount of light exposure
Equilibration:	Rate of cooling to 5°C; duration of storage at 5°C before freezing.
Freezing:	Freezing form (pellets, ampules, or straws); freezing unit size; freezing method (dry ice; liquid nitrogen vapors); freezing rate(s) from liquid to solid ($-40°C$); freezing rate(s) to final temperature
Thawing:	Thawing medium (original vs. new diluent); thawing rate (i.e., at 23° vs. 37° vs. 45° vs. 75°C); post-thaw storage temperature and time; post-thaw temperature damage; post-thaw motility and vitiality; post-thaw morphology and acrosome integrity; post-thaw thermolability and longevity
Insemination:	Time relative to ovulation; site of insemination (vaginal vs. uterine); volume of insemination; number of live sperm per insemination; genital manipulations

Extenders for Freezing Semen

The terms applied to semen-processing solutions include extender, extending medium, buffer, diluent, or dilution buffer or medium. Semen (or a concentrated preparation of sperm) is diluted in a diluent (i.e., extender) that in most instances includes one or more buffers. A good extender is expected to have nutrient(s) as an energy source, to buffer against harmful changes in pH, to provide a physiologic osmotic pressure and concentration of electrolytes, to prevent growth of bacteria, to protect cells from cold-shock during the cooling process, and to have cryoprotectants that reduce sperm cell damage during freezing and subsequent thaw-

ing. Extenders for freezing semen are based on those initially developed for refrigerating semen at 4°C. The components most often used in the preparation of extenders for freezing dog semen are listed in Table 3. In most published reports on freezing canine semen, extenders have incorporated egg yolk to reduce cold shock and glycerol to reduce freezing damage.

Some of the more frequently utilized types of semen extenders used for freezing dog semen are listed in Table 4. Formulas for the preparation of an unbuffered lactose extender reported to be successful for freezing dog semen in pellets are provided in Table 5. Formulas for preparation of a tris buffer extender often used for freezing dog semen in straws are provided in Table 6. In the preparation of such buffers, a variety of special modifications or added criteria have arisen among laboratories, but only in some instances have they been explicitly stated in reports. Furthermore, much of the freezing of canine semen in recent years has been handled commercially using extenders and protocols that are proprietary and unpublished. Certain peculiarities in extender preparation and semen dilution appear to have developed. Some laboratories have indicated concern about freshness of eggs used; whether and when to centrifuge egg yolk to remove particulate material; using freshly added egg yolk,

Table 3. *Components That Have Been Incorporated Into Some of the Extenders Commonly Used for Freezing Canine Semen*

Aqueous Solutions or Buffers (Physiologic Media)
Sodium citrate (3%)
Skim milk, heat treated
Powdered skim milk (9%)
Unbuffered lactose (11%)
Bicarbonate–sodium phosphate salts solution
Tris buffer, (i.e., tris hydroxymethyl aminomethane, 1–4%)
Tris and citric acid
Tes-N-tris buffer (1–2%)
PIPES (piperazine ethane sulfonic acid) and KOH (potassium hydroxide)

Protein, Fat, or Carbohydrate (Cold-Shock Reducers)
Egg yolk (4–25%)
Egg yolk and skim milk
Isosmotic sugar solution (i.e., 11% lactose)

Cryoprotectant Component (Freeze-Damage Reducers)
None
Glycerol (2–16%)
Dimethylsulfoxide (DMSO)
Isosmotic sugar or starch solution
Lactose and glycerol

Metabolizable Sugar (Nutrient)
None
Glucose
Fructose
Lactose

Antibacterial Antibiotics
Penicillin
Penicillin and streptomycin
Penicillin, streptomycin, and polymyxin

Table 4. Egg Yolk–based Diluents Containing Glycerol as Cryoprotectant That Are Commonly Used for Extending and Freezing Canine Semen and for Which Post-thaw Motility over 40 Per Cent Has Been Reported

Extender	Freeze Form	Reference
Lactose	Pellets	Platz and Seager, 1977
	Straws	Yubi et al., 1987
Tris–glucose–citric acid	Ampules	Foote, 1964a, b
	Straws	Olar, 1984
Tris–fructose–citric acid	Ampules	Gill et al., 1970
	Straws	Andersen, 1975
PIPES-glucose-citrate	Straws	Smith and Graham, 1984

glycerol, or both for each freezing rather than storage of frozen aliquots of entire extender; adding glycerol-containing extender only after a prior extension and equilibration at 5°C; and concentrating semen by centrifugation before or during dilution and thus reducing the effects of raw seminal plasma. Some procedures have shown particular concern for a physiologic osmotic pressure (300 mOsm) and pH (6.9) of the extender (Smith and Graham, 1984), whereas others apparently have not (Seager, 1969; Platz and Seager, 1977).

Semen Collection and Ejaculate Fractionation

Dogs ejaculate semen in three distinct fractions. There is an initial, slightly cloudy to clear-colored and variably sized (0.1–1.0 cc) "pre-sperm emission" (fraction I), then a chalky-white, "sperm-rich fraction" that varies from 0.5 to 6.0 cc in volume (fraction II), and finally a clear "prostatic fluid fraction" that contains relatively little sperm (fraction III) and may be 5 to 30 cc in volume. During a natural mating, fraction I may be released prior to intromission; fractions II and III occur during intromission and the copulatory lock. Following the start of a healthy ejaculation, fractions I, II, and III may be ejaculated over periods of 2 to 20 seconds, 30 seconds to 2 minutes, and 1 to 20 minutes, respectively. For AI, usually little if any of the prostatic fluid fraction (III) is collected in order to save time and gain any advantages of small to moderate volumes. Since prostatic fluid has a harmful effect on sperm survival and freezability in some species, some workers avoid contamination of the sample with fraction III. Some also avoid contamination with the initial pre-sperm fraction I. However, there have been no reports of possible effects of either the pre-sperm fraction or the third fraction on the viability, fertility, or freezability of canine sperm.

Sperm Numbers, Concentration, and Dilution in Extender

Ejaculates from normal dogs contain anywhere from 300 million to 2 billion sperm, in a volume of 0.5 to 6 cc, at concentrations ranging from 100 million to 500 million sperm per cc. A wide range of formulas have been used for dilution of ejaculates before freezing. One method is to dilute at a particular volume ratio, most commonly to a final dilution of 2, 3, or 4 parts extender to 1 part semen. This method is often used under field conditions, allowing the sperm concentration to be determined later.

Alternatively, the sperm concentration is determined initially, and the semen is diluted to a preferred, known concentration, in order to obtain insemination units of a desired number of sperm. Gentle centrifugation has been used to concentrate sperm before or during the dilution procedure (Platz and Seager, 1977; Oettle, 1982). When canine semen is frozen in straws, the semen frequently is diluted with extender to achieve a final sperm concentration between 50 and 200 million sperm per cc such that 1 to 4 of the half-cc straws will

Table 5. Formulas for Preparation of Lactose Extenders Used in Freezing Dog Semen

	Seager, 1969	Olar, 1984	Yubi et al., 1987
Distilled water*	1 L	1 L	1 L
Lactose	110 gm	71 gm	110 gm
Glycerol	4%†	40 ml	40 ml
Egg yolk	200 ml	200 ml	200 ml
Dihydrostreptomycin	1 gm	1 gm	1 gm
Penicillin	10^6 IU	5×10^5 IU‡	10^6 IU
Semen dilution (semen:extender)	1:2	1:2–10	1:1–5
Freezing units	Pellets	Straws	Straws
Postdilution motility	NR	74%	58%

*Start with less than 1 L, and bring up to full volume after addition of other components, using deionized double-distilled water.
†Method, as v/v (40 ml) or w/v (40 gm), not indicated.
‡Centrifuge at 39,000 × gm for 30 min to clarify before use.
NR, not reported.

Table 6. Various Formulas Reported for Preparation of 1-Liter Amounts of Extenders Containing Tris, 15 or 20% Egg Yolk, and 3 to 10 Per Cent Glycerol and Commonly Used for Freezing Dog Semen

Component	Foote,* 1964b	Province et al., 1984	Yubi et al., 1987	Morton, 1987
Tris base	30.3 gm	24.4 gm	29 gm	30 gm
Citric acid	16.9 gm	13.6 gm	13.2 gm	17 gm
Fructose	—	—	12.5 gm	12.5 gm
Glucose	12.5 gm	8.2 gm	—	—
Glycerol	100 ml	30 ml	80 ml	80 ml
Egg yolk	†	200 ml	†	†
Penicillin	10^6 IU	5×10^5 IU	—	—
Streptomycin	1.0 gm	1.0 gm	—	—
Crystamycin	—	—	—	1.6 gm
D.D.D. Water‡	1000 ml (qs)	1000 ml (qs)	1000 ml	1000 ml (qs)
†Egg yolk (replacing buffer volume for volume)	200 ml (v/v) (20%)	—	200 ml (v/) (20%)	150 ml (v/v) (15%)

*Also Olar, 1984; Froman et al., 1984.
‡Double-distilled water.

provide an insemination dose of 100 to 400 million sperm.

Initial dilutions have been done with extender at 37°C to facilitate a physiologic sperm equilibration with extender or at room temperature for simplicity or have been precooled to speed up processing. Extension has been done either stepwise or in a single step. Initial dilutions with one extender have been followed by a further dilution with a second extender. Such sequences have been used to delay the addition of glycerol or other components until after the temperature has been reduced. Such a delayed addition of glycerol until after the semen is cooled has yielded better results in some species but has not been evaluated in dogs.

Equilibration in the Cold

Sperm of most species need to equilibrate with the extender under refrigeration prior to freezing. The best results have usually involved cooling initiated as soon as possible after collection, a slow rate of cooling to reduce "cold shock" damage (i.e., temperature lowered at 6 to 12°C per hour over 2 to 3 hr rather than at 20 to 30°C per hour over ½ to 1 hr), and a storage time at 5°C for longer than 1 hr before freezing. Similar rates and times are probably appropriate for dog semen. However, dog sperm appeared to be rather resistant to cold shock when processed in a tris–egg yolk buffer (Olar, 1984). In that study, dog semen was cooled over 1, 2, or 3 hr and then equilibrated for 1 or 2 hr without any consistent effect on post-thaw results. Nevertheless, very rapid cooling should probably be avoided.

The initial rate of cooling in the refrigerator is affected by sample volume, container size and shape, and the volume of any water jacket. Cooling

times of 1 to 3 hr are obtained in standard 5°C refrigerators by placing the tube of extended semen into a large tube or beaker containing warm or room temperature water. Effects of equilibration times longer than 2 hr after reaching 5°C have not been studied.

Freezing Format

Canine sperm is often frozen in 0.5-cc plastic "French straws," as in the dairy cattle industry. Straws provide a convenient format for handling, labeling, storage and thawing. Alternative formats include bulk semen volumes sealed in ampules, and semen frozen in small spherical pellets on a block of dry ice. However, the current trend towards straws has taken place despite the fact that the greatest number of pregnancies and some of the highest success rates reported for canine frozen semen involved semen frozen as pellets. It is unfortunate that no systematic study comparing sperm motility or fertility after freezing in straws versus pellets has been reported in detail. The research group that developed and most extensively utilized the frozen pellet format for canine semen has indicated that glass vials or variously sized straws can be used instead of pellets with the same extender and dilutions, that motility may then be equal to or worse than that for pellets, and that pellets are preferred (Seager and Fletcher, 1973; Seager et al., 1975).

STRAWS. Cooled, extended semen is drawn into commercial, cotton-plugged 0.5-cc polyvinyl chloride (PVC) straws previously labeled with identification information. The unplugged ends, or both ends, of the straws are packed with powdered polyvinyl pyrrolidone (PVP), which forms a solid seal when the straws are then immersed in cold water. The straws are carefully dried of any moisture and placed on a wire rack suspended in nitrogen vapors above the surface of liquid nitrogen (LN) in a large LN cryostat tank or in a polystyrene box. Alternatively, a commercial programmable freezer that regulates the flow of LN vapors is used. Once frozen in vapors, straws are immersed into liquid nitrogen and are stored in a liquid nitrogen tank until they are used.

PELLETS. The cooled, extended semen is drawn up into a dropper or pipette, and dozens of aliquots of 50 to 100 μl are delivered into rounded depressions previously indented on the flat surface of a piece of solid carbon dioxide. The frozen pellets are then transferred to LN for placement into labeled, perforated nylon vials that are then stored long term under LN (Seager, 1969).

Freezing Rate

The rate of freezing affects post-thaw survival and fertility. Excessively rapid freezing causes quick formation of intracellular ice and damages cells perhaps by disrupting membranes of intracellular organelles. Excessively slow freezing causes cell damage by permitting an excessively abnormal osmotic gradient to develop during the formation of extracellular ice, with cell membrane damage occurring during cell shrinkage and changes in osmotic pressure.

The optimal freezing rate depends on the extender, the cryopreservative, the animal species, and the thawing procedure. Freezing rate is affected by sample volume and the surrounding temperature. With pellets, there is little control over the rapidity of freezing, since it is solely a function of pellet size. Perhaps the extenders most appropriate for rapid freezing of pellets differ from extenders appropriate for slower freezing in straws, where the rate can be more easily controlled.

Semen in straws can be frozen less or more rapidly by placing the freezing rack in a higher or lower position in the LN vapors above the surface of the LN. The rate of freezing can be more precisely controlled and even can be varied during a single freezing, by using a programmable freezer that regulates the flow and temperature of the nitrogen vapors that are pumped through the freezing chamber. Several freezing rates have been reported to yield reasonable motility or fertility for canine semen equilibrated to 5°C in tris–egg yolk or similar extender. These have included a fast rate of 75°C per min in −160°C LN vapors for 10 min using 3 per cent glycerol (Olar, 1984), and an unstated rate for 10 to 15 min at 4 to 6 cm above 8 cm of LN using 8 per cent glycerol in a polystyrene box with 2.5-cm walls (Christiansen, 1984). Using the same 8 per cent glycerol extender, others froze

semen at 6 to 7 cm above the LN for 5 to 10 min and at successively lower positions during the final 2 min before immersion in LN (Morton, 1988). Olar (1984) obtained results better than those with the fast rate of 75°C per min by using slower initial rates of 5°C or 2°C per minute in a programmable freezer. Using a 9 per cent glycerol extender, Smith (1984a, 1984b) froze semen slowly, at an initial rate of 8°C per minute, 8 inches above 2 inches of LN for 30 min.

Thawing Rate and Temperature

Several thawing procedures for dog semen have been reported to yield satisfactory numbers of motile sperm. For pellets of semen in a lactose–egg yolk extender, a 37°C saline or citrate thawing solution is used (Platz and Seager, 1977). For 0.5-ml straws of semen in a tris–egg yolk extender, thawing has been done in a 75°C water bath for 6.5 sec (Andersen, 1975); a 37 to 40°C bath for 1 min (Morton, 1987), and water baths of 35°C for 30 sec, 75°C for 12 sec, or 1°C for 120 sec (Olar, 1984). In the latter study, the best results were obtained with 75°C for 12 sec. In limited studies, motility after rapid thawing at 70°C for 6 sec or 45°C for 30 sec was better than that after slow thawing at 37°C for 50 sec or 23° for several minutes (Battista et al., 1988).

Glycerol Used As a Cryoprotectant

Glycerol is the most commonly used cryoprotectant and apparently yields better results than other cryoprotectants such as dimethylsulfoxide (Christiansen, 1984). Biological polymers such as polysaccharides and starches have been evaluated for freezing sperm of other species (Schmehl et al., 1986) but not for the dog. Freezing dog semen in the absence of a cryoprotectant, as in other species, results in great reduction in the number of surviving motile sperm after thawing. Motility values reported for dog semen frozen without glycerol *versus* with glycerol, were 5 to 11 per cent versus 17 to 23 per cent in varied extenders (Olar, 1984). Concentrations of glycerol have ranged from 2 to 16 per cent. The amount of glycerol used is a matter of concern because in some other species, it depresses fertility of fresh and of thawed sperm. Protocols developed for other species have involved replacement of the glycerol-containing extender with nonglycerolated extender before freezing or after thawing, but these protocols have not been evaluated for dogs. A reasonable balance between sperm survival and fertility for boar sperm was obtained with glycerol concentrations as low as 3 to 4 per cent (Polge, 1985). It is unfortunate that systematic study of dog sperm frozen at varying concentrations below 2 per cent has not been reported.

FERTILITY TESTING OF FROZEN SEMEN

Most controlled studies of variables in freezing dog sperm suffer from the lack of a proven or accepted indicator of fertility and have not involved actual fertility tests. Reports on fertility rates obtained following insemination of bitches with frozen semen are limited, and none have compared fertility for semen frozen by different methods. This is in contrast to such studies in livestock species but is understandable because of peculiarities of dogs. Bitches have only one or two reproductive cycles per year, methods for determining the time of ovulation have only recently been developed, and intrauterine insemination, which is commonly practiced per vagina in other species, is extremely difficult and is rarely performed in dogs.

SUCCESSFUL FROZEN SEMEN PREGNANCIES IN DOGS

Pellets

Many of the frozen-semen AI litters reported were produced from semen frozen in pellets after it was diluted in an extender composed of 11 per cent lactose, 20 per cent egg yolk, and 4 per cent glycerol (Table 5) and was equilibrated for 3 hr. Thawing was done in 3 per cent sodium citrate or saline at 37°C. Insemination was vaginal and yielded fertility rates in seven successive years of 10, 10, 40, 66, 43, 64, and 92 per cent in groups of 21, 29, 20, 38, 37, 11, and 13 bitches, respectively (Seager et al., 1975; Platz and Seager, 1977). The 92 per cent success rate trial involved concentration of semen by centrifugation before extension and vaginal insemination of 200 to 800 million sperm an average of four times per bitch (Platz and Seager, 1977). Earlier success rates of 40 to 60 per cent were obtained by inseminations of 150 to 700 million sperm in 3- to 9-cc volumes twice during estrus (Seager et al., 1975). The only other reported fertility trial using pelleted semen yielded a pregnancy rate of 57 per cent in 14 bitches each inseminated with 150 million sperm three to nine times, daily or every other day (Lees and Castleberry, 1977). Difficulties, if any, in obtaining comparable success rates with this method have not been reported. All other successful fertility testing of frozen canine semen has involved the use of different extenders and freezing in straws.

Straws

For semen frozen in straws, researchers at the Veterinary College of Norway reported a lack of success with intravaginal AI. In contrast, a pregnancy rate of 72 per cent was obtained with intrauterine deposition of 150 to 200 million sperm one to three times during mid or late estrus in 50 bitches. The method involved inserting a metal catheter through the cervix and into the uterus, and massage of the clitoris after insemination (Andersen, 1975; Farstad, 1984). The sperm-rich fraction of semen was extended at 35°C in a tris-fructose-citric acid extender containing 8 per cent glycerol and 20 per cent egg yolk (Table 6) at a sperm concentration of about 150 million per cc, cooled, equilibrated to 5°C over a 3-hr period, frozen in 0.5-ml straws in LN vapors at an unstated rate, and thawed in 75°C water for 6.5 sec.

Using a similar extender and processing technique, thawing at 75°C for 12 sec and alternate-day intravaginal inseminations of 300 million sperm each, researchers at Colorado State University reported a pregnancy rate of only 25 per cent in 12 bitches (Olar, 1984). The low success rate with intravaginal insemination is perhaps not surprising, considering the failures reported by workers in Norway. Similarly, Gill and coworkers (1970) reported failures for all 12 bitches vaginally inseminated with an average of 64 million motile sperm three times during estrus, using semen frozen in straws in a comparable tris–egg yolk extender.

Researchers at the University of Minnesota (Smith and Graham, 1984; Smith, 1984a, b; Smith, 1986) reported higher fertility rates for intrauterine than for intravaginal inseminations performed surgically using semen extended 1:2 in a newly developed zwitterion-buffer extender, equilibrated and cooled over 1 hr, frozen in LN vapors, and later thawed in 37°C water for 50 sec. The pregnancy rates were 46 per cent for intrauterine and 11 per cent for intravaginal insemination in groups of 11 and 9 bitches, respectively, receiving 150 million sperm twice during estrus. The basic extender consisted of 2 parts of a neutral 300 mOsm solution of PIPES acid and KOH, 1 part 0.3 M glucose, and 1 part 0.3 M sodium citrate. The extender was made of 20 per cent egg yolk, clarified by centrifugation, and the supernatant was made of 9 per cent glycerol before use or frozen in aliquots for later use (Smith, 1984a, b). Using the same cryopreservation procedures and a transcervical method of insemination, workers at Cornell obtained only a 30 per cent pregnancy rate in 13 bitches (Battista et al., 1988; unpublished data).

Takeishi and colleagues (1976) reported a 75 per cent pregnancy rate for intracervical inseminations of four bitches in Japan using a less frequently encountered extender (12 per cent skim milk, 4 per cent egg yolk, 1 per cent glucose, 4 per cent glycerol in a sodium citrate–phosphate diluent), and freezing in 1-cc straws.

From the foregoing, it appears that the success

rate depends on the semen-processing technique, the number of motile sperm per insemination, and the site of insemination as well as the correct timing of the insemination. These are considered later.

IN VITRO METHODS TO EVALUATE SEMEN-FREEZING TECHNIQUES

Different extenders, freezing methods, or both for canine semen have not been experimentally compared, based on fertility trials, but some studies have made comparisons based on sperm motility immediately after thawing. The correlation between post-thaw motility and fertility has not been firmly established. It is unfortunate that there have only been limited evaluations of canine semen-freezing techniques employing parameters such as thermostability or extent of acrosome damage.

POST-THAW MOTILITY MEASUREMENTS

Motility estimates are rather subjective and must be standardized or made by the same individuals using the same microscopic magnification and number of sperm when comparing differences due to treatments. Motility can be expressed as the percentage of sperm that are motile or the percentage that are progressively motile, with or without a subjective score of the quality of the motility (Fig. 1). An estimate is made in a 6-μl drop of semen placed on a slide, covered with a 18-mm² coverslip, and examined under a microscope, with all materials heated to 37°C, using either a commercial slide warmer and a heated microscope stage or a chamber heated with incandescent light bulbs. For each sample, several fields are scanned at 450 × magnification, and the percentage of motile sperm is estimated. The percentages of abnormal sperm are also usually noted. Mean percentages of motile sperm reported for normal canine ejaculates vary from 66 to 90 per cent, and ranges within different studies have varied (60 to 90 per cent; 70 to 95 per cent, 80 to 95 per cent). Values for progressive motility, when reported, have ranged from values very slightly to moderately less than those for total motility, or the distinction is not made. Some researchers suggest that only ejaculates with a minimum of 85 to 90 per cent motile sperm, or 75 to 85 per cent progressively motile sperm, should be considered for freezing and that samples with less than 70 per cent motility are poor candidates for freezing.

Post-thaw *versus* prefreeze sperm motility is the most frequently measured index of success in semen-freezing technique, and values have usually been reported along with fertility testing results. Post-thaw motilities reported to result in successful

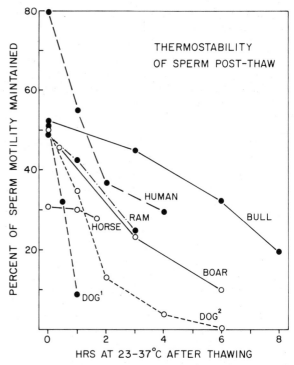

Figure 1. Typical sperm motility percentages for semen of several species, expressed as a percentage of total sperm after freezing and thawing, including semen from bulls (Robbins et al., 1976), humans (Weidel and Prins, 1987), rams (Colas, 1975), boars (Larsson, 1985), and stallions (Cristanelli et al., 1985) during incubation at 37°C, and dog semen during incubation [1] at 37°C (Olar, 1984) and [2] at 23°C (Battista et al., 1988).

pregnancies have included 50 to 70 per cent (Andersen, 1980), 29 to 59 per cent (Platz and Seager, 1977), 34 to 53 per cent (Lees and Castleberry, 1977), and 40 to 60 per cent (Olar, 1984). Most workers strive to obtain at least 50 to 65 per cent motility after thawing, but samples yielding only 30 to 45 per cent often are not discarded, since total numbers of motile sperm desired for insemination can be obtained by increasing the number of total sperm inseminated.

Post-thaw motility has also been used to examine the effects of differing extenders, freezing formats, equilibration times, freezing rates, thaw rates, and the like, some of which have been reviewed earlier. Based on post-thaw motility after freezing in straws, Olar (1984) found that a tris–citric acid–egg yolk buffer was preferable to the lactose–egg yolk buffer normally used for pellets (Tables 5 and 6), that 2 or 4 per cent glycerol was better than higher amounts, that DMSO with or without glycerol failed to yield better results than glycerol alone, and, as reviewed earlier, that a moderate to slow freezing rate and a fast thaw rate were preferable to other approaches. Yubi and coworkers (1987) found no difference in motility for semen extended in lactose versus tris extender, and processed in the same manner, for 12 stud dogs. Battista and colleagues (1988) observed, based on motility, that thawing at 70°C was preferred to 37°C for several extenders, that use of tris extender in straws was better than lactose extender in pellets, and that lactose in pellets was better than lactose in straws.

ACROSOME MORPHOLOGY AFTER THAWING

The absence of reports using acrosome morphology to compare different freezing methods for canine semen is unfortunate. Post-thaw acrosomal integrity may be one of the most reliable criteria for predicting post-thaw fertility. For dog semen, Oettle (1986) demonstrated that acrosome damage occurs in a significant percentage of sperm during each of the three major processing steps when a standard tris–citric acid–egg yolk diluent is used. The decrease in acrosomal morphology was 11 per cent after the initial 3:1 dilution at 32°C, 17 per cent after cold equilibration, and 35 per cent after freezing in straws in LN vapor and thawing at 35°C. At no stage was the acrosome damage found to be significantly correlated to the decrease in motility. Such results question the validity of using only sperm motility immediately after thawing as an index of fertility.

POST-THAW THERMORESISTANCE

Post-thaw thermoresistance, measured as the maintenance of motility during incubation at 37°C, has been suggested as a reasonable indicator of fertility for frozen semen (Larsson, 1985). Post-thaw thermolability may be a major problem for canine sperm, perhaps more so than for other species, and should be used more often for evaluating freezing techniques. The basis of this concern is depicted in Figure 1, using representative data on the post-thaw thermolability of human, bull, ram, boar, and dog sperm. Olar (1984) considered declines in motility over 0.5 or 1 hr at 37°C for several variables in the freezing of dog semen. No treatment effects on thermolability could be demonstrated, and motility after 1 hr was routinely less than 10 per cent and often 0 per cent. Oettle (1982) indicated that post-thaw motility at 32°C was prolonged if concentrated dog semen frozen in a 4 per cent glycerol–tris–egg yolk extender was diluted in a large volume of nonglycerolated extender immediately after thawing, at least in comparison to semen not initially centrifuged and not rediluted after thawing. In one study, thermoresistance during 8 hr at 23°C (using lactose extender) was greater for freezing in pellets than in straws and, for semen frozen in straws and thawed at either 37 or 70°C, thermoresistance was greater with a tris–fructose–citric acid extender than with a PIPES-KOH extender (Battista et al., 1988).

SPERM NUMBERS PER INSEMINATION

Not unexpectedly, success with frozen semen in dogs appears to be related, in general, to the number of sperm per insemination as well as the number of inseminations. The considerable success (40 to 97 per cent) reported for intravaginal deposition of pelleted semen frozen in lactose–egg yolk may be related to inseminations of up to 700 or 800 million sperm (Seager et al., 1975; Platz and Seager, 1977). With the same freezing method but using inseminations of only 150 million sperm, Lees and Castleberry (1977) obtained a generally lower success rate (46 per cent), although they performed more inseminations (three to nine) per bitch. Less success has been reported with vaginal inseminations of smaller numbers of thawed sperm and fewer inseminations per bitch, albeit frozen by a different method. Success rates of 0, 0, 25, and 14 per cent were obtained for intravaginal inseminations of frozen semen using per-insemination sperm doses, respectively, of 60 million (Gill et al., 1970), 150 to 200 million (Andersen, 1975), 300 million (Olar, 1984), and 150 million (Smith and Graham, 1984). These studies apparently involved only two to three inseminations per bitch.

VAGINAL VERSUS UTERINE INSEMINATION

Satisfactory success rates with frozen semen in most other species have been very dependent on bypassing the cervix and inseminating into the uterus. The cervix may likewise present a major barrier for frozen semen in dogs. Andersen (1975) and Farstad (1984) reported success rates in Norway of 78 and 67 per cent following intrauterine deposition, as compared to negligible success following intravaginal deposition. In one controlled study, frozen semen deposited surgically into the uterus versus vaginal insemination yielded pregnancy rates of 46 per cent versus 11 per cent, respectively (Smith and Graham, 1984). For semen extended in a zwitterion buffer containing glycerol and egg yolk and frozen in straws, the apparent advantage of uterine versus vaginal deposition suggests that the processing causes the sperm to become incapable of, or susceptible to, migration through the cervix and uterus.

It is unfortunate that surgical insemination has the associated problems of risk, time, effort, expense, and limited frequency. Intrauterine insemination performed per vagina by passing a catheter through the cervix requires considerable training, skill, experience, and patience on the part of the veterinarian and, in some individual bitches, has simply not been feasible. Scandinavian programs have used a rigid, metal catheter with an offset tip, inserted vaginally inside a plastic sheath, and guided through the cervix by manually fixing the cervix palpated through the abdominal wall. The catheter is then slowly passed through the cervix, using catheter rotation and cervical traction as necessary, and the semen is deposited in the body of the uterus (Andersen, 1975). Intrauterine inseminations have also been conducted by passing flexible catheters through the cervix, using direct endoscopic visualization to monitor and guide the process (Battista et al., 1988).

Intravaginal inseminations are most commonly performed with a 20- to 30-cm plastic infusion pipette attached to a syringe by a length of flexible tubing. The pipette is inserted into the vagina to, and if possible, beyond the posterior tubercle of the vaginal dorsal median fold, and semen is deposited as close to the cervix as possible with the hindquarters of the bitch elevated (Fig. 2). Various manipulations immediately after insemination have been used, including massage of the clitoris (Andersen, 1980), massage of the dorsal surface of the vagina (Gill et al., 1970), and attempts to simulate a copulatory lock, either manually or with the outer case of a syringe (Seager and Fletcher, 1973).

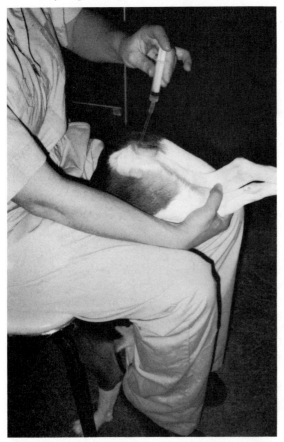

Figure 2. A pipette attached to a syringe is used to inseminate thawed semen into the anterior vagina of a bitch about 3 days after ovulation. Elevation of the hindquarters facilitates retention of the inseminate. (From Concannon, P.W., and Battista, M., in Kal Kan Foods' *Pedigree Forum* 7(1):8–16, 1988.)

TIMING INSEMINATIONS

Obtaining successful pregnancies and reasonable litter sizes with frozen semen is highly dependent upon performing inseminations during the 2 to 3 days in which healthy, fertilizable eggs reside in the oviducts of the bitch. Fresh sperm can remain fertile in the bitch for 6 or 7 days (Concannon et al., 1983). Frozen sperm die rapidly after being thawed and do not survive the long periods that fresh dog sperm do. Routinely performing inseminations at the correct time has become more feasible because of advances in our understanding of the reproductive cycle of the bitch and the time of ovulation, and in methods for estimating the time of ovulation (Concannon, 1986a, b; Concannon et al., 1977). Eggs mature in the oviduct around 2 days after ovulation and live for about 2 more days before they start wasting away. Ovulations occur about 2 days after the surge-release of luteinizing hormone (LH) from the pituitary that triggers ovulation. Therefore, inseminations with frozen semen would ideally occur 4, 5, and 6 days after the LH surge. There are no clinical assays for the LH surge in dogs, but its occurrence can be estimated using criteria of varying accuracy (Concannon, 1986b). Estrus behavior and acceptance of males often begins on the day of the LH surge but may begin 3 or 4 days earlier or 3 or 4 days later, and its onset may not be abrupt and clear. The vaginal mucosa as viewed with an endoscope or proctoscope becomes slightly wrinkled during the LH surge, is more obviously wrinkled 2 days later, and remains wrinkled during the most fertile period, before shedding much of its thickness at the end of the fertile period. At or shortly after the end of the fertile period, the vaginal smear typical of estrus, as well as the wrinkled appearance of the vagina, is quickly lost—just about 8 or 9 days after the LH surge, and 2 to 4 days after the best time for insemination (Concannon and DiGregorio, 1986). In many bitches, the vulva becomes obviously softer between the time of the LH surge and ovulation, about 3 to 4 days before the best time to inseminate with frozen semen. At the same time, the blood levels of progesterone secreted by the ovulating follicles in the ovary rapidly increase, and in some breeding management programs, veterinarians monitor blood levels of progesterone daily or every other day. Frozen semen AI is then performed on the fourth and fifth or sixth day after the first rise in progesterone. Once started, inseminations, if possible, should be repeated on alternate days until the vaginal smear is no longer typical of estrus and has some cells typical of metestrus (i.e., white blood cells and small round epithelial cells). Owners should be told to expect whelping to occur 64 to 66 days after the estimated day of the LH surge, and 60 days after the insemination, if it was properly timed. For the concerned owner, pregnancy diagnosis can be made by ultrasound or palpation at 3 to 4 weeks or by x-ray at 7 to 8 weeks (Concannon, 1986a, c).

REGISTRATION OF FROZEN SEMEN LITTERS

Litters produced by frozen semen artificial insemination have been recognized by the American Kennel Club (AKC) since 1981. They have also been recognized by other registries in the United States and elsewhere, each with its particular requirements and guidelines. The AKC will not recognize litters produced from imported semen. AKC registration of a frozen-semen litter requires submission of the following documentation.

1. Certification by the owner of the semen that its shipment by a specified shipper and its use for the specified insemination were authorized.

2. Certification by the owner of the bitch that the veterinarian performing the insemination was so authorized, indicating the bitch, date, and stud-source of the semen.

3. Certification by the veterinarian as to the specific lots of frozen semen used, the name and address of the person providing the semen, date of receipt of the semen, dates of insemination, and address of the site of insemination.

4. Statement by the owner of the bitch providing the place and date of whelping.

5. Use of units of frozen semen for which the

*Table 7. AKC-approved Collection and Storage Facilities for Frozen Canine Semen**

ANIMAL REPRODUCTIVE SERVICES, INC.
1501 FM 2818
Suite 304
College Station, TX 77840
(409) 693-2842

CANINE CRYOBANK
845 Via de la Paz
Pacific Palisades, CA 90272
(213) 284-4050 or (619) 471-2918

CANINE LIFE LINES
5207 S.W. Barnes Road
Portland, OR 97221
(503) 227-3826

CRYO-GENETIC LABORATORIES
Rt 100 & Blackhorse Road
Ludwigs Corner, Box 256-A
Chester Springs, PA 19425
(215) 458-5888

CRYO TECH INTERNATIONAL, INC.
Rt 1, Box 286
Abbeville, SC 29620
(803) 446-8787

HERDS'S MERCHANT SEMEN
7N330 Dunham Road
Elgin, IL 60120
(312) 741-1444

INTERNATIONAL CANINE GENETICS,
   INC.
527 Hilaire Road
'St. Davids, PA 19087
(215) 688-0836 or (215) 640-4332

INTERNATIONAL CANINE SEMEN BANK,
   INC. NORTHWEST CENTER
P.O. Box 6541
Sandy, OR 97055
(503) 663-7031 or (503) 663-257

INTERNATIONAL CANINE SEMEN BANK
   OF ILLINOIS
Rt 78 North
Virginia, IL 62691
(217) 452-3006

INTERNATIONAL CANINE SEMEN BANK OF OHIO
34910 Center Ridge Road
North Ridgeville, OH 44039
(216) 327-8282

INTERNATIONAL CANINE SEMEN BANK OF TEXAS
1236 Brittmore
Houston, TX 77043
(713) 468-8253

PRESERVATION, INC.
P.O. Box 962
Ocean Shores, WA 98569
(206) 533-6296 or (206) 289-4103

SEAGER CANINE SEMEN BANK, INC.
329 Sioux
Park Forest, IL 60466
(312) 748-0954

SPERMCO, INC.
490 W. Durham Ferry Road
Tracy, VA 95376
(209) 835-3259

SPRING CREEK RANCH & REPRODUCTIVE CENTER
380S Collierville-Arlington Road
Collierville, TN 38017
(901) 853-0550

TRIPLE S. CRYOGENETICS
University of Illinois Trail
Box 217
Philo, IL 61864
(217) 684-2900 or (217) 253-3202

UNITED BREEDERS SERVICE
P.O. Box 211
Lubbock, TX 79408
(806) 745-3419

UNIVERSITY OF GEORGIA
College of Veterinary Medicine
Athens, GA 30602
(404) 542-9368 or (404) 542-3221

*Listed are the names of the facilities whose record keeping practices have been examined and found to be in compliance with AKC's regulations applying to the registration of litters produced artifically using frozen canine semen. AKC does not license, sponsor, or endorse these facilities.

AKC had been previously notified, by an approved collection facility or semen bank, immediately following collection and immediately following any transfer of ownership, relocation or shipment for intended use. Each such notification must include the AKC-registered name and number of the stud, the number of breeding units involved, the dates involved, and names and addresses of all parties, including the storage facility.

AKC-approved facilities are those that the AKC has examined and found to be in compliance with its regulations as regards record keeping ancillary to the collection and storage of semen. For each collection, records must include photographic identification of the stud, owner authorization, number of breeding units, and form of storage (as pellets, ampules, straws, or vials). Records must also indicate the indelible marking of each breeding unit (semen) container with the date and breed and AKC number of the stud, and the dates and circumstances of any shipments or transfers of ownership. Details of all regulations are provided on the special AKC application form for registering a litter from artificial insemination using frozen semen.

The semen collection and storage sites currently approved by the AKC number 18 and are listed in Table 7.

The use of frozen semen was first approved by the AKC in 1981. In the intervening six and a half years, there have been 101 frozen-semen litters registered through December 1987. While the average is only some 16 frozen-semen litters per year, there were 23 in 1987, indicating greater numbers of inseminations, greater success rates, or both. Some semen-collection facilities have been more prominent than others in litter registrations. It is unfortunate that information on actual numbers of frozen-semen inseminations attempted and resulting pregnancy rates are not available. The AKC has separate requirements regarding the use and shipment of cooled, extended fresh semen, which also must be inseminated by a licensed veterinarian.

References and Supplemental Reading

Andersen, K.: Insemination with frozen dog semen based on a new insemination technique. Zuchthygiene 10:1, 1975.

Andersen, K.: Artificial insemination and storage of canine semen. In Morrow, D. A. (ed.): Current Therapy in Theriogenology. Philadelphia: W. B. Saunders Co., 1980, pp. 661–665.

Battista, M., Parks, J., and Concannon, P.: Canine sperm post-thaw survival following freezing in straws or pellets using PIPES, lactose, tris or TEST extenders. Proceedings of the XI International Congress on Animal Reproduction and Artificial Insemination, Dublin, 3:229, 1988.

Christiansen, J.: Artificial breeding and embryo transfer. In Christiansen, J. (ed.): Reproduction in The Dog and Cat. London: Baillière Tindall, 1984, pp. 115–123.

Colas, G.: Effect of initial freezing temperature, addition of glycerol and dilution on the survival and fertilizing ability of deep-frozen ram semen. J. Reprod. Fertil. 42:272, 1975.

Concannon, P. W.: Canine pregnancy and parturition. Vet. Clin. North Am. [Small Anim. Pract.] 16:453, 1986a.

Concannon, P. W.: Clinical and endocrine correlates of canine ovarian cycles and pregnancy. In Kirk, R. W. (ed.): Current Veterinary Therapy, Small Animal Practice, Vol. VIII. Philadelphia: W. B. Saunders Co., 1986b, pp. 1214–1224.

Concannon, P. W.: Physiology and endocrinology of canine pregnancy. In Morrow, D. A. (ed.): Current Therapy in Theriogenology, 2nd ed. Philadelphia: W. B. Saunders Co., 1986c, pp. 491–497.

Concannon, P. W., and DiGregorio, G. B.: Canine vaginal cytology. In Burke, T. (ed.): Small Animal Reproduction and Infertility. Philadelphia: Lea & Febiger, 1986, pp. 96–111.

Concannon, P. W., Hansel, W., and McEntee, F.: Changes in LH, progesterone and sexual behavior associated with preovulatory luteinization in the bitch. Biol. Reprod. 17:604, 1977.

Concannon, P., Whaley, S., Lein, D., et al.: Canine gestation length: Variation related to time of mating and fertile life of sperm. Am. J. Vet. Res. 44:1819, 1983.

Cristanelli, M. J., Amann, R. P., Squires, E. L., et al.: Effects of egg yolk and glycerol levels in lactose-EDTA-egg yolk extender and of freezing rate on the motility of frozen-thawed stallion spermatozoa. Theriogenology 24:681, 1985.

Davis, I. S., Bratton, R. W., and Foote, R. H.: Livability of bovine spermatozoa at 5, −25 and −85°C in tris-buffered and citrate-buffered yolk-glycerol extenders. J. Dairy Sci. 46:333, 1963.

Farstad, W.: Bitch fertility after natural mating and after artificial insemination with fresh or frozen semen. J. Small Anim. Pract. 25:561, 1984.

Foote, R. H.: Extenders for freezing dog semen. Am. J. Vet. Res. 25:37, 1964a.

Foote, R. H.: The effects of electrolytes, sugars, glycerol, and catalase on survival of dog sperm stored in buffered-yolk mediums. Am. J. Vet. Res. 25:32, 1964b.

Foote, R. H., and Leonard, E. P.: The influence of pH, osmotic pressure, glycine and glycerol on the survival of dog sperm in buffered-yolk extenders. Cornell Vet. 54:78, 1964.

Froman, D. P., Amann, R. P., Riek, P. M., et al.: Acrosin activity of canine spermatozoa as an index of cellular damage. J. Reprod. Fertil. 70:301, 1984.

Gill, H. P., Kaufman, C. F., Foote, R. H., et al.: Artificial insemination of beagle bitches with freshly collected, liquid stored and frozen semen. Am. J. Vet. Res. 31:1807, 1970.

Larsson, K.: Boar sperm viability after freezing and thawing. Proceedings of the First International Conference on Deep Freezing of Boar Semen, Uppsala, Sweden, August 1985, pp. 177–187.

Lees, G. E., and Castleberry, M. W.: The use of frozen semen for artificial insemination of German shepherd dogs. J. Am. Anim. Hosp. Assoc. 13:382, 1977.

Morton, D. B.: Artificial insemination with frozen semen in the dog. In James, E. (ed.): Reproductive Clinical Problems in The Dog, 2nd ed. London: Butterworths, 1988 (in press).

Oettle, E. E.: Preliminary report: A pregnancy from frozen centrifuged dog semen. J. S. Afr. Vet. Assoc. 53:269, 1982.

Oettle, E. E.: Changes in acrosome morphology during cooling and freezing of dog semen. Anim. Reprod. Sci. 12:145, 1986.

Olar, T. T.: Cryopreservation of dog spermatozoa. Ph.D. Dissertation, Colorado State University, Fort Collins, CO, 1984.

Platz, C. C., and Seager, S. W. J.: Successful pregnancies with concentrated frozen canine semen. Lab. Anim. Sci. 27:1013, 1977.

Polge, C.: Sperm Freezing: Past, Present, and Future. Proceedings of the First International Conference on Deep Freezing of Boar Semen, Uppsala, Sweden, 1985, pp. 167–173.

Province, C. A., Amann, R. P., Pickett, B. W., et al.: Extenders for preservation of canine and equine spermatozoa at 5°C. Theriogenology 22:409, 1984.

Robbins, R. K., Saacke, R. G., and Chandler, P. T.: Influence of freeze rate, thaw rate and glycerol level on acrosomal retention and survival of bovine spermatozoa frozen in French straws. J. Anim. Sci. 42:145, 1976.

Schmehl, M. K., Vazquez, I. A., and Graham, E. F.: The effects of nonpenetrating cryoprotectants added to TEST-yolk-glycerol extender on the post-thaw motility of ram spermatozoa. Cryobiology 23:512, 1986.

Seager, S. W. J.: Successful pregnancies utilizing frozen dog semen. AI Digest 17:6, 1969.

Seager, S. W. J., and Fletcher, W. S.: Progress on the use of frozen semen in the dog. Vet. Rec. 92:6, 1973.

Seager, S. W. J., and Platz, C. C.: Artificial insemination and frozen semen in the dog. Vet. Clin. North Am. 7:757, 1977.

Seager, S. W. J., Platz, C. C., and Fletcher, W. S.: Conception rates and related data using frozen dog semen. J. Reprod. Fertil. 45:189, 1975.

Smith, F. O.: Update on freezing canine semen. Proceedings of the Annual Meeting of the Society of Theriogenology, Denver, 1984a, pp. 61–73.

Smith, F. O.: Cryopreservation of canine semen: Technique and performance. Ph.D. Dissertation, University of Minnesota, St. Paul, MN, 1984b.

Smith, F. O.: Update on freezing canine semen. *In* Kirk, R. W. (ed.): *Current Veterinary Therapy, Small Animal Practice*, Vol. IX. Philadelphia: W. B. Saunders Co., 1986, pp. 1243–1248.

Smith, F. O., and Graham, E. F.: Cryopreservation of canine semen: Technique and performance. Proceedings of the Xth International Congress on Animal Reproduction and Artificial Insemination, Champaign-Urbana, 1984, Vol. 2, p. 216.

Takeishi, M., Mikami, T., Kodama, Y., et al.: Studies on reproduction in the dog VIII: Artificial insemination using frozen semen. Jpn. J. Anim. Reprod. 22:28, 1976.

Weidel, L., and Prins, G. S.: Cryosurvival of human spermatozoa frozen in eight different buffer systems. J. Androl. 8:41, 1987.

Yubi, A. C., Ferguson, J. M., Renton, J. P., et al.: Some observations on the dilution, cooling and freezing of canine semen. J. Small Anim. Pract. 28:753, 1987.

PREPUTIAL DISCHARGE IN THE DOG

W. E. HORNBUCKLE, D.V.M.,
and M. E. WHITE, D.V.M.
Ithaca, New York

Preputial discharges in dogs are of importance, as they may cause concern among dog owners even when benign and can be signs of serious disorders. The appearance of the discharge is usually the first finding noted by the clinician. Preputial discharges may be broadly categorized as hemorrhagic, purulent, or serous. Each of these types of discharge is associated with a group of diseases, and clinical examination may be used to rule in or out each disease (White et al., 1982). This article will be organized according to the appearance of the discharge. For each type of discharge, the diseases typically associated with it will be outlined, and a step-by-step approach to diagnosis will be presented.

HEMORRHAGIC DISCHARGE

Common causes of hemorrhagic preputial discharge are trauma to the prepuce, penis, urethra, prostate, and bladder; prostatic disease; neoplasia of the prepuce, penis, or urethra; and a foreign body in the prepuce or penis. Less common conditions that can cause bleeding from the prepuce include prolapsed urethra; urolithiasis; primary or secondary urethritis; bleeding disorders (including immune-mediated thrombocytopenia, von Willebrand's disease, and disseminated intravascular coagulation); and ureteral duplication associated with simultaneous incontinence and hematuria (Jones, 1983). Malformations such as a persistent penile frenulum can be associated with small amounts of bleeding from the prepuce (Herron, 1988). Bleeding from the prepuce can be due to renal or ureteral lesions, but for this to occur, there must be associated injury or weakness of the neck of the bladder.

The clinical examination of a patient with hemorrhagic preputial discharge should start with a physical examination to localize the source of the blood. By examination of the prepuce, penis, and urethral orifice the clinician can usually determine the source of the bleeding. The causes of bleeding from the prepuce or external penis that can be detected by physical examination alone include trauma, a foreign body, neoplasia (usually transmissible venereal tumor, papilloma, or carcinoma), urethral prolapse and, rarely, malformations. This portion of the examination is important enough to justify tranquilization or general anesthesia of the dog if necessary.

If the cause of the bleeding is not apparent after physical examination of the prepuce or external penis, the blood must be coming from the urethra, and the remaining differential diagnoses include prostatic disease; trauma to the urethra, prostate, or bladder; urolithiasis; urethritis; bleeding disorders; a foreign body; or neoplasia of the urethra. There is a single case report of ureteral duplication associated with blood coming from the urethra.

The penis, including the os penis, should be palpated to the brim of the pelvis. Swellings in the penis can be caused by urolithiasis, a foreign body such as gunshot or plant awns, hematoma or fracture of the os penis due to trauma, or neoplasia of the urethra such as transitional cell carcimona, squamous cell carcinoma, and rhabdomyosarcoma (Clark et al., 1984). Urethral calculi, when palpated, are most commonly just caudal to the os penis. In rare cases, foreign bodies may be identifiable by palpation.

When a mass is palpated, a catheter should be passed into the urethra. Resistance to passing the catheter may help the clinician differentiate between a focal and a diffuse process involving the urethral mucosa. When a calculus or a small foreign body is suspected, flushing of the urethra with saline should be done. To determine the cause of a swelling in the penis other than a calculus or an obvious foreign body, the catheter should be passed to the lesion, and an aspirate obtained for cytology. Tissue may be aspirated by placing the end of the catheter into the mass and creating negative pressure in the catheter using a syringe; this procedure yields a specimen that is examined using cytology and histology (Rogers et al., 1986). If these procedures do not identify the mass lesion, urethrostomy is indicated for diagnosis.

In cases in which physical examination of the penis and prepuce has not led to a diagnosis, a rectal examination should be done to check for prostatic disease and inflammatory or neoplasic lesions of the urethra. Prostatic diseases include cystic hyperplasia, acute or chronic prostatitis, prostatic abscess, neoplasia (usually adenocarcinoma) (Olson et al., 1987), and calculi. During the rectal examination, paraprostatic cysts may be palpated, often in association with prostatitis or cystic hyperplasia. Paraprostatic cysts that communicate with the urethra may be associated with serous to serosanguineous discharge (see later), but they are rarely primary causes of bleeding from the prepuce. An ejaculate may be collected to determine if the blood is from the prostate. The urethra is a rare site for neoplasia, with squamous cell tumors, transitional cell tumors, or adenocarcinomas in older dogs most common. Urethral rhabdomyosarcoma has been reported in 12- to 18-month-old dogs (Clark et al., 1984). While doing the rectal examination, the clinician should attempt to palpate sublumbar and intrapelvic lymph nodes. During rectal examination of a normal dog, these nodes are not usually palpable, and if they can be easily palpated, a diagnosis of intrapelvic disease is suspected. When a rectal examination does find a mass lesion, an aspirate of the prostatic urethra should be examined for signs of inflammation and neoplasia. Fine-needle biopsy, with or without the assistance of ultrasonography, can be used when confirmation of diagnosis is needed. Radiography may help to determine if metastasis of tumors has occurred.

If the cause of the bleeding was not found during physical examination, the remaining differential diagnoses include prostatic disease not associated with large palpable lesions; trauma to the urethra, prostate, or bladder; urolithiasis; small foreign bodies or neoplasms involving the urethra; urethritis; bleeding disorders; and ureteral duplication. Bleeding disorders such as coagulopathies, disseminated intravascular coagulation, and immune-mediated thyrombocytopenia virtually never present with preputial bleeding as the only clinical sign, and absence of other signs exclude them from the differential diagnosis.

If a diagnosis has not been made at this stage, the cytologic appearance of an aspirate of urethral fluid is compared to that of urine collected by cystocentesis. This, combined with urethrography, should allow the clinician to rule in or out the few remaining differential diagnoses. Ureteral malformation is diagnosed by contrast urography.

PURULENT PREPUTIAL DISCHARGE

The causes of purulent discharge include balanoposthitis, prostatic disease, foreign bodies, primary or secondary urethritis, neoplasia, preputial stenosis, and paraphimosis. Purulent discharge should not be confused with normal smegma. Normal smegma consists of a small amount of yellow-green material that, on cytology, shows variable numbers of epithelial cells, inflammatory cells (primary neutrophils), and extracellular bacteria.

The examination of a dog with purulent discharge would follow the procedure previously outlined for hemorrhagic discharge. Infectious disease may cause visible lesions on the mucosa. Follicular lesions due to lymphoid hyperplasia are sometimes seen in the area of the bulbus glandis and mucosa of the prepuce, but no specific organism has been cultured from these lesions. Culture and cytology of the prepuce, external penis, or urethra should be done to determine the bacterial, viral, or fungal cause of infectious disease. The clinician should be aware that *Escherichia coli, Streptococcus, Staphylococcus, Pseudomonas, Proteus* (Feldman and Nelson, 1987), and *Mycoplasma* are normally cultured from these areas. In cases of prostatic disease associated with hyperestrogenism, there is rarely a visible purulent preputial discharge, but a cytologic evaluation of a tissue imprint of the preputial mucosa may show squamous metaplasia. In such cases, the testes should be palpated for tumors that might be secreting estrogen.

SEROUS PREPUTIAL DISCHARGES

A slight urethral discharge is normal in male dogs. Serous preputial discharge should alert the clinician to the possibility of urinary incontinence, including malformation of the urinary tract such as ectopic ureter. Dogs experimentally infected with herpesvirus developed self-limiting serous preputial discharges 3 to 7 days after inoculation (Hill, 1974). The only other major cause of serous discharge from the prepuce is a prostatic retention cyst or a paraprostatic cyst that communicates with the urethra (Barsanti, 1987).

References and Supplemental Reading

Barsanti, J. A.: Vaginal and preputial discharges. *In* Lorenz, M. D., and Cornelius, L. M. (eds.): *Small Animal Medical Diagnosis.* Philadelphia: J. B. Lippincott Co, 1987, pp. 359–365.

Clark, W. T., Shaw, S. E., and Pass, D. A.: Rhabdomyosarcoma of the urethra in a dog. J. Small Anim. Pract. 25:203, 1984.

Feldman, E. C., and Nelson, R. W.: *Canine and Feline Endocrinology and Reproduction.* Philadelphia: W. B. Saunders Co., 1987, pp. 505–511.

Herron, M. A.: Diseases of the external genitalia. *In* Morgan, R. V. (ed.): *Handbook of Small Animal Practice.* New York: Churchill-Livingstone, 1988, pp. 673–678.

Hill, H., and Mare, C. J.: Genital disease in dogs caused by canine herpsvirus. Am. J. Vet. Res. 35:669, 1974.

Jones, B. R.: Diseases of the ureters. *In* Ettinger, S. J. (ed.): *Textbook of Veterinary Internal Medicine, Diseases of the Dog and Cat.* Philadelphia: W. B. Saunders, 1983.

Olson, P. N., Wrigley, R. H., Thrall, M. A., et al.: Disorders of the canine prostate gland: Pathogenesis, diagnosis, and medical therapy. Comp. Cont. Ed. Pract. Vet. 9:613, 1987.

Rogers, K. S., Wantschek, L., and Lees, G. E.: Diagnostic evaluation of the canine prostate. Comp. Cont. Ed. Pract. Vet. 8:799, 1986.

White, M. E., Lewkowicz, J., and Powers, M.: CONSULTANT, database for computer-assisted diagnosis. Ithaca: New York State College of Veterinary Medicine, 1982 (online).

DISORDERS OF SEXUAL DEVELOPMENT IN DOGS AND CATS

V. N. MEYERS-WALLEN, V.M.D., Ph.D.
and D. F. PATTERSON, D.V.M., D.Ss.
Philadelphia, Pennsylvania

NORMAL SEXUAL DEVELOPMENT

Normal sexual development occurs in three sequential steps, with each step depending upon the successful completion of the previous step: (1) establishment of chromosomal sex, (2) development of gonadal sex, and (3) development of phenotypic sex (Fig. 1). At fertilization, the sex chromosome constitution of the zygote normally becomes either XX or XY and is then maintained by mitotic division in all cell types, including primary germ cells. In early embryonic life, the gonad is undifferentiated. A normal ovary develops if chromosomal sex is XX. Testicular development is dependent upon the presence of a Y chromosome. Development of the internal and external genitalia, exclusive of the gonads, is dependent upon the presence or absence of a testis (Fig. 1). In normal (XY) male embryos, the testis produces two substances necessary for the formation of normal male internal and external structures. Müllerian inhibiting substance (MIS), also known as müllerian inhibiting factor or anti-

müllerian hormone, is a glycoprotein produced by Sertoli's cells that causes the müllerian duct system to regress. The second testicular secretion is testosterone (T), a steroid produced by Leydig's cells, which stabilizes the wolffian duct system so that the vasa deferentia and epididymides are formed. Within cells of the urogenital sinus, genital tubercle, and genital swellings, T is converted by the enzyme 5-alpha-reductase to dihydrotestosterone (DHT), which then stimulates these primordia to form the prostate and male urethra, the penis, and the scrotum. Androgen-dependent masculinization is mediated through the binding of T or DHT to a cytosolic androgen receptor. Testicular descent into the scrotum completes the male external genitalia, but the control of this process is incompletely understood.

In the absence of a testis, a female phenotype develops. Oviducts, uterus, and cranial vagina develop from the müllerian duct system. The wolffian duct system regresses. The urogenital sinus, genital tubercle, and genital swellings become the caudal vagina and vestibule, the clitoris, and the vulva, respectively. Castration of either male or female embryos at the indifferent stage results in development of female ducts and external genitalia, leading to the conclusion that the basic embryonic plan is female. The male phenotype is the result of Y-chromosome–dependent development of the testis,

Original work described in this chapter was supported by the University of Pennsylvania Referral Center for Animal Models of Human Genetic Disease (NIH GRR 02512), the University of Pennsylvania Human Genetics Center (GM 32592), NICHHD National Research Service Award (1F32 HD 06396), NIH grant HD 19393, and a grant from the Mrs. Cheever Porter Foundation.

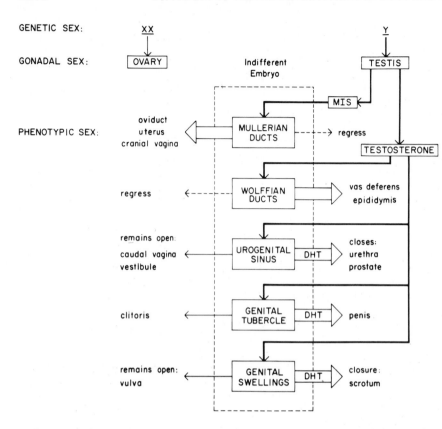

Figure 1. Normal sexual differentiation. (From Morrow, D. A.: *Current Therapy in Theriogenology 2.* Philadelphia: W. B. Saunders Co., 1986.)

Legend:
MIS = Mullerian Inhibiting Substance
DHT = Dihydrotestosterone

which alters the female plan through its hormonal secretions.

DIAGNOSIS OF DISORDERS OF SEXUAL DEVELOPMENT

Intersex animals (animals in which the sex is ambiguous) are usually recognized because their phenotypic sex is abnormal. However, since chromosomal sex determines gonadal sex, which then determines phenotypic sex, an abnormal sexual phenotype can result from a defect occurring at any step. Although various terms have been used to describe these abnormal animals, the most useful terms indicate, as closely as possible, the etiology of the defect. In the following discussion, disorders of sexual development are classified by the initial step at which development differs from normal sexual development. Thus, diagnoses fall into three categories: abnormalities of chromosomal sex, abnormalities of gonadal sex, and abnormalities of phenotypic sex (Table 1).

While examination of buccal smears for sex chromatin bodies does give preliminary information about sex chromosome constitution, definitive diagnosis of chromosomal sex requires direct exami-

nation of the chromosomes and construction of a karyotype. Chromosome preparations from peripheral blood lymphocyte culture are most practical for this purpose (Hare et al., 1966; Meyers-Wallen and Patterson, 1986). Gonadal sex is best determined by histology. Biopsies may be sufficient, but serial sections of the gonad in its entirety may be necessary to identify an ovotestis. A concise description of the internal and external genitalia establishes phenotypic sex. It is necessary to determine which parts of the wolffian and müllerian duct systems are present or absent, and whether the prostate or caudal vagina is present. Histologic examination may be necessary. Regarding the external genitalia, one should determine whether the vulva or prepuce is appropriate in form and position and whether a clitoris or penis is present, and the position of the urinary orifice should be described.

ABNORMALITIES OF CHROMOSOMAL SEX

The dog has 78 chromosomes, including the X and Y chromosomes, which are easily identified by their morphology in a karyotype. The X is the only large metacentric chromosome normally present, and the Y is the smallest metacentric chromosome

Table 1. *Outline of Disorders of Sexual Development*

Abnormalities of Chromosomal Sex
Abnormalities of Chromosome Number

XXY syndrome
XO syndrome
Triple-X syndrome

Chimeras and Mosaics
True hermaphrodite chimeras
XX/XY chimeras with testes
XY/XY chimeras with testes

Abnormalities of Gonadal Sex
XX sex reversal
XX true hermaphroditism
XX male syndrome

Abnormalities of Phenotypic Sex
Female pseudohermaphroditism
Exogenous androgen exposure
Endogenous androgen exposure
Male pseudohermaphroditism
Persistent müllerian duct syndrome
Defects of androgen-dependent masculinization
Hypospadias
Androgen resistance
Cryptorchidism

(Hare et al., 1966). The cat has 38 chromosomes, of which the Y chromosome is the smallest metacentric chromosome identifiable in the karyotype (Hare et al., 1966). The X chromosome is also metacentric but is similar in size to other metacentric chromosomes. Thus, it is difficult to positively identify the feline X chromosome without banding techniques (Bilz et al., 1961). Dogs and cats reported with abnormal sex chromosome constitutions, with the exception of chimeras and mosaics, have been phenotypic males or females with underdeveloped rather than ambiguous genitalia. With few exceptions, these individuals are sterile, and no therapy is indicated.

Abnormalities of Chromosome Number

XXY SYNDROME

The XXY syndrome is likely to be sporadic in occurrence, since it usually arises by nondisjunction of sex chromosomes during meiosis. The reciprocal product of nondisjunction of the sex chromosomes leading to the XXY condition is a gamete containing neither an X nor a Y chromosome; when fertilized by an X-bearing gamete, this zygote becomes XO (discussed later).

In all species in which it has been described, an XXY chromosome constitution gives rise to a phenotypic male with hypoplastic testes devoid of spermatogenesis. This confirms the primary importance of the Y chromosome in the determination of testicular development. However, the presence of two X chromosomes precludes normal spermatogenesis (Gordon and Ruddle, 1981). The testes do produce MIS and testosterone, so a male phenotype results.

The incidence of the XXY syndrome (Klinefelter's syndrome) in humans is approximately 1 in 700 births, making it one of the most frequent chromosomal anomalies (Meyers-Wallen and Patterson, 1986). Good estimates of its frequency in animals are not available, but it is the sex chromosomal defect most often described. The syndrome has been described in the cat (Centerwall and Benirschke, 1975; Moran et al., 1984; Pyle et al., 1971; Thuline and Norby, 1961) and the dog (Meyers-Wallen and Patterson, 1986). Although cats with this syndrome may be of any color, they are most often recognized by a paradoxic coat color pattern: tortoiseshell (or calico) in males. Early in female embryonic development, either the paternal or maternal X chromosome is inactivated in a random fashion within each cell. The inactivated X forms the sex chromatin, or Barr body. Subsequent cell populations derived from these cells bear the same inactivated X. Thus, normal females express paternal and maternal X-linked genes in mosaic pattern (Lyon, 1961). The genes for orange and nonorange coat color in the cat are alleles at the X-linked Orange locus. The O allele produces orange hair color, whereas the O+ allele produces nonorange (black or chocolate brown). The tortoiseshell pattern is seen normally in females heterozygous for these alleles, since only one allele is expressed in each cell population, producing patches of different hair color. Males with this coat color pattern have at least two different X chromosomes, each bearing a different allele at the Orange locus. Commonly, these are XXY males, but other sex chromosome constitutions are possible (see chimeras and mosaics, later).

The XXY syndrome is not recognized as readily in dogs as in tortoiseshell cats, since a coat color paradox does not signal its presence. The one dog reported with a 79,XXY chromosome constitution had a normal male external phenotype, small testes with seminiferous tubular dysgenesis, and no evidence of spermatogenesis (Meyers-Wallen and Patterson, 1986).

XO SYNDROME

In humans, individuals with the XO syndrome (Turner's syndrome) develop as phenotypic females with infantile genitalia and various somatic anomalies including short stature (Engel, 1978). Generally, these individuals show no evidence of a menstrual cycle. Since one X chromosome is absent, Barr bodies do not appear in any cells. Normal development and differentiation of mammalian oocytes require two X chromosomes (Gordon and

Ruddle, 1981). Thus, the ovaries initially develop during fetal life but later degenerate, appearing as fibrous streaks lacking germ cells.

A 6-month-old Doberman pinscher dog with an XO chromosome constitution was recently described (Smith et al., in press). Some physical findings in this dog differed from the classic phenotype of the XO syndrome, leading to the consideration that mosaicism or chimerism may have been present. In general, the XO syndrome should be considered in bitches that have a normal female phenotype but have not cycled by 24 months of age.

Three cats with the XO syndrome have been reported, two of which were kittens living to 3 days of age (Johnston et al., 1983; Long and Berepubo, 1980; Norby et al., 1974), and all were phenotypic females. The adult XO cat described (Johnston et al., 1983) was presented for primary anestrus at 2.5 years of age and was small in stature. Ovarian degeneration apparently occurs postnatally in XO cats, since one kitten described had normal ovarian histology (Norby et al., 1974), and dysgenetic ovaries were described in the adult (Johnston et al., 1983). There is a potential for recognizing XO cats by their coat color pattern when family history is known. For example, matings in which one parent is orange and the other is nonorange should produce female offspring that all have the tortoiseshell pattern. The occurrence of a female that is all orange or all nonorange should suggest the XO condition.

TRIPLE-X SYNDROME

A 79,XXX chromosome constitution was found in an Airedale bitch examined for primary anestrus at 4 years of age (Johnston et al., 1985). Ovaries without follicles, a small uterus, and a female phenotype were present. Resting serum concentrations of LH and FSH were elevated, and serum progesterone was in the normal anestrous range. The etiology is probably meiotic nondisjunction of the sex chromosomes. The incidence of this condition in humans is 1 in 1000 females, but it is apparently rare in the dog (Meyers-Wallen and Patterson, 1986). Although fertile individuals with triple-X syndrome have been described in other species, abnormalities of the estrous cycle and infertility are frequent findings (Johnston et al., 1985).

Chimeras and Mosaics

A *chimera* is an individual composed of two or more cell populations, each population arising from different individuals. Some are caused by the fusion of two zygotes differing in sex chromosome constitution, such that an XX/XY individual is produced.

A *mosaic* is also an individual composed of two or more cell populations having different chromosome constitutions, but the cells originate within the same individual. A mosaic usually arises from mitotic nondisjunction. Four cell populations may arise in this manner (i.e., YO, XXY, XO, XYY), but only one of these populations and the normal cell population need survive to produce a mosaic (e.g., XY/XXY, XY/XYY). The end result, whether chimera or mosaic, is an individual composed of at least two cell populations having different chromosome constitutions. Events producing these animals are usually random; thus, familial aggregation is not expected.

Gonadal sex in chimeras and mosaics depends upon the distribution of the cell populations within the gonadal primordium. If one cell population contains a Y chromosome and the other does not, ovarian and testicular tissue can develop within the same gonad, or the gonad can have some histologic features of both ovary and testis, but the typical appearance of neither. Phenotypic sex is determined by the presence and amount of testicular tissue.

The cat chimera or mosaic can be a tortoiseshell male if at least one cell population contains a Y chromosome that causes male development, and there are at least two X chromosomes, one carrying the orange coat color allele and the other carrying the nonorange allele. There have been reports of tortoiseshell male cats with abnormal sex chromosome constitutions such as XX/XY (Centerwall and Benirschke, 1975; Malouf et al., 1967; Moran et al., 1984), XY/XXY (Centerwall and Benirschke, 1975, 1973; Gregson and Ishmael, 1971; Long et al., 1981; Moran et al., 1984), XY/XYY (Loughman and Frye, 1974), and some multiples of these. Individuals with a significant proportion of XY cells can be fertile males. Those with a significant proportion of XXY cells (Loughman et al., 1970) have a phenotype similar to that of the XXY syndrome (described earlier).

TRUE HERMAPHRODITE CHIMERAS

True hermaphrodites have both ovarian and testicular tissue present in the same individual. One or both gonads may be ovotestes, or one gonad may be an ovary and the other a testis. Of the several canine true hermaphrodites reported with cytogenetic data, chimeras were rare; most have an XX sex chromosome constitution. XX true hermaphrodites will be discussed in the following section, Abnormalities of Gonadal Sex. The three reported cases of canine true hermaphrodite chimeras had either XX/XY or XX/XXY chromosome constitutions, and all had an enlarged clitoris but otherwise were female in external appearance (Meyers-Wallen and Patterson, 1986). The dogs were presented with a history of failure to cycle or chronic vulvar irritation. Internally, testicular and ovarian tissue and a uterus were present in all cases. The ovarian tissue contained follicles and in one case, graafian follicles were present. Testicular tissue consisted of interstitial cells and seminiferous tubules with Sertoli's cells. In only one case, in which the ovotestis was in the inguinal canal, was there evidence of spermatogenesis.

One feline true hermaphrodite with cytogenetic data has been reported (Biggers and McFeely, 1966; Malouf et al., 1967). Although this XX/XY cat had a male phenotype externally, a scrotal testis and an abdominal ovary were found. Müllerian duct derivatives were found adjacent to the ovary.

XX/XY CHIMERAS WITH TESTES

The authors have observed one XX/XY Old English sheepdog that had failed to cycle by 2 years of age (Meyers-Wallen and Patterson, 1986). Chromosome analysis of blood lymphocytes showed approximately 1:1 XX/XY cells. The external genital opening was a cranially displaced vulvalike structure. A hypoplastic penis, classified as such because the urethral opening was at the cranial end, was contained within the vulvalike structure. No scrotum or testis was found on physical examination. Small gonads with the appearance of testes, located near the caudal pole of the kidneys, and a small bicornuate uterus were found during exploratory laparotomy. Dysgenetic testicular tissue lacking spermatogenesis was found in histologic sections.

Several cats with XX/XY chromosome constitutions and male phenotypes have been reported (Centerwall and Benirschke, 1975; Moran et al., 1984). Fertility was variable. One tortoiseshell male cat with XX/XY karyotype had a male phenotype externally and small scrotal testes (Malouf et al., 1967). No müllerian duct derivatives were present. Gonadal histology revealed seminiferous tubules containing only Sertoli's cells, whereas other tubules within the same testis contained apparently normal stages of spermatogenesis. The proportion of aspermatogenic to normal seminiferous tubules (1:1) was the same as the proportion of XX to XY cells in this testis. Spermatozoa were present within the epididymis.

XY/XY CHIMERAS WITH TESTES

Several fertile male cats having normal male external phenotypes and tortoiseshell coat colors have had normal testicular histology, including spermatogenesis (Centerwall and Benirschke, 1973; Ishihara, 1956; Moran et al., 1984). Normal male

chromosome constitutions in the testes have been reported in two of these cats. The most probable explanation is that these individuals had XY/XY chromosome constitutions (Ishihara, 1956).

ABNORMALITIES OF GONADAL SEX

Animals in which chromosomal and gonadal sex do not agree are called *sex reversed*. Although XY sex reversal (XY female) is known in other mammals, only XX sex reversal has been reported in the dog, and neither XX nor XY sex reversal has been described in the cat.

XX Sex Reversal

The following descriptions are based on the authors' studies of inherited XX sex reversal in the cocker spaniel, which is inherited as an autosomal recessive trait (Meyers-Wallen and Patterson, 1986, in press). Similar familial disorders have been described in the beagle, Chinese pug, Kerry blue terrier, and Weimaraner (Meyers-Wallen and Patterson, 1986). The authors have also recently observed a German shorthaired pointer that appears to have this condition. Dogs with XX sex reversal have a 78,XX chromosome constitution and varying amounts of testicular tissue in the gonad, so they have at least one ovotestis or testis. Individuals with this condition are XX true hermaphrodites or XX males. Both phenotypes appear within the same family and are caused by the same genetic defect, which causes mild to severe gonadal masculinization.

XX TRUE HERMAPHRODITISM

A *true hermaphrodite* has both ovarian and testicular tissue. The most common combination of gonads in XX true hermaphrodite dogs is bilateral ovotestes, with ovary and ovotestis being second, and testis and ovotestis being least common. In general, the degree of androgen-dependent masculinization of the internal and external genitalia is positively correlated to the proportion of testicular tissue in the gonads (Meyers-Wallen and Patterson, in press).

If little testicular tissue is present, the wolffian system is usually absent, the oviducts are usually present, and the uterus is always present. Although these dogs usually appear to be normal females externally, they are frequently sterile; some never cycle.

If much testicular tissue is present, testosterone stabilizes the wolffian system, and the epididymides and vasa deferentia develop. The oviducts may be present or absent, but the uterus is always present in its entirety (Meyers-Wallen et al., 1987). Externally, these dogs appear to be masculinized females, having obvious clitoral enlargement or abnormal vulval shape and position.

Some XX true hermaphrodites have reproduced as normal females, despite the presence of testicular tissue and clitoral enlargement. However, it is recommended that these dogs be removed from the breeding population, since they will pass the gene for this defect to all their offspring. The presence of testicular tissue may be detected by measuring peripheral testosterone levels after stimulation with luteinizing hormone (LH) or gonadotropin-releasing hormone (GnRH). However, an inability to demonstrate testosterone elevation after stimulation does not indicate that the dog is a normal female. The presence of testicular tissue in serial histologic sections of the gonad along with a normal female karyotype is diagnostic. Treatment of XX true hermaphrodites and XX males (discussed later) is limited to surgical removal of the gonads and uterus and, if the dog is uncomfortable, excision of the enlarged clitoris.

XX MALE SYNDROME

These dogs have a 78,XX chromosome constitution and bilateral testes that are usually undescended. The entire wolffian duct system is present bilaterally, and the prostate is present. Externally, scrotal development is not evident in bilaterally cryptorchid individuals. The prepuce is present but is usually abnormal in shape or position. All of the XX males that the authors have observed have had penile malformations: hypospadias, hypoplasia, or abnormal curvature. These dogs are invariably sterile; spermatogonia are absent even in testes that are in the scrotum.

Oviducts are absent in all XX males, but a complete uterus is present. Functionally active MIS is produced by testicular tissue of XX males as well as XX true hermaphrodites, and the degree of oviductal regression in each is proportional to MIS production by the ipsilateral gonad (Meyers-Wallen et al., 1987). Failure of regression of the uterine portion of the müllerian duct system implies target organ insensitivity to MIS. Removal of cryptorchid testes and hysterectomy are recommended.

ABNORMALITIES OF PHENOTYPIC SEX

In these animals, chromosomal and gonadal sex are in agreement, but the genitalia are ambiguous. Affected animals are termed either male or female pseudohermaphrodites. A *female pseudohermaphrodite* has an XX chromosome constitution and ovaries, but the internal or external genitalia are masculinized. A *male pseudohermaphrodite* has an

XY chromosome constitution and testes, but the internal or external genitalia are to some degree those of a female. Obviously, this definition excludes XX males, in which chromosomal and gonadal sex do not agree. Male pseudohermaphroditism includes males with hypoandrogenization (varying degrees of hypoplasia of the penis, prepuce, and scrotum) and males with failure of müllerian regression (persistence of müllerian duct derivatives).

Female Pseudohermaphroditism

EXOGENOUS ANDROGEN EXPOSURE

These dogs have a 78,XX chromosome constitution, ovaries, and complete müllerian systems. Masculinization occurs in androgen-responsive tissues, ranging from mild clitoral enlargement to nearly normal male external genitalia with a prostate internally. This condition has not been reported in cats, and rare reports in the dog indicate an iatrogenic etiology (androgen or progestagen administration during gestation) (Meyers-Wallen and Patterson, 1986). Affected dogs are presented as males that show periodic signs of estrus (hematuria, attractivenes to male dogs, swelling of the prepuce or vulva), signs of cystic endometrial hyperplasia-pyometra, or urinary abnormalities such as incontinence from urine pooling in the vagina or uterus. Ovariohysterectomy is recommended. If signs of urinary tract disease are present, contrast studies should be done to establish the diagnosis and treatment of associated urinary tract complications. Prevention may be best achieved by avoidance of sex steroid administration during gestation.

ENDOGENOUS ANDROGEN EXPOSURE

In humans, adrenogenital syndromes are a common cause of female pseudohermaphroditism. In general, these syndromes are due to metabolic errors resulting in decreased cortisol production. Low cortisol levels allow an increase in ACTH production, which leads to an increase in cortisol precursors. Androgens are synthesized from the cortisol precursors because the metabolic error reduces the conversion to cortisol. The excess androgens masculinize the female genitalia. Adrenogenital syndromes have not been described in dogs or cats.

Male Pseudohermaphroditism

PERSISTENT MÜLLERIAN DUCT SYNDROME

Persistent müllerian duct syndrome (PMDS) is a form of inherited male pseudohermaphroditism occurring in miniature schnauzers (Meyers-Wallen and Patterson, 1986). Affected dogs are XY males with bilateral testes and müllerian duct derivatives: oviducts, uterus, and cranial vagina. Externally, affected dogs are normal phenotypic males. The cranial uterine horns are attached to the testes, which may be abdominal, inguinal, or scrotal in location. The entire wolffian duct system and a prostate are present internally. The vasa deferentia are situated in the lateral walls of the uterine horns. Affected miniature schnauzers that are not bilaterally cryptorchid have sired offspring, although semen quality has been subnormal (V. N. Meyers-Wallen, unpublished data). These dogs are usually diagnosed in old age, when they develop signs of pyometra, Sertoli's cell tumor, or both. A similar condition has been reported in an aged poodle in Germany (Niemand et al., 1972) and in a Pekingese in Scandinavia (Svendsen et al., 1985). It is recommended that affected dogs be culled from the breeding population. Treatment consists of gonadectomy and hysterectomy.

DEFECTS OF ANDROGEN-DEPENDENT MASCULINIZATION

Animals in this category are XY males with normal regression of müllerian structures, but subnormal masculinization of internal and external androgen-responsive tissues. The primary defect can be within the hypothalamic-pituitary-testis axis (defects in steroid synthesis, androgen nonproduction or hypoproduction) or in the response of the target organs to androgens (receptor defects or failure of conversion of T to DHT). Inherited defects of this type generally affect prenatal and postnatal male development. In humans, the result is a spectrum of abnormalities, from phenotypically normal but infertile men to individuals with ambiguous genitalia to phenotypic women (Wilson et al., 1983). Only a few defects in this category have been described in dogs and cats. Other categories of inherited male pseudohermaphroditism, reported in mammals other than dogs and cats, will not be discussed here.

Hypospadias

Hypospadias is an abnormality in location of the urinary orifice, being ventral and proximal to the normal site in the glans penis. The urinary orifice may be located in the glans penis (mild hypospadias), the penile shaft (moderate hypospadias), the penoscrotal junction, the scrotum, or the perineum (severe hypospadias) (Hayes and Wilson, 1986). This results from the incomplete fusion of the urethral folds in the formation of the male urethra (urogenital sinus). Although hypospadias may have a multifactorial etiology (Wilson et al., 1983), the common denominator may be inadequate fetal androgen production (T or DHT). One survey of canine hypospadias suggested a familial occurrence in the Boston terrier breed (Hayes and Wilson, 1986). Although teratogen-induced hypospadias has been reported in other species, no similar reports were found in dogs and cats. While other defects may accompany hypospadias, the external genitalia are usually not ambiguous (Ader and Hobson, 1978; Hayes and Wilson, 1986). Cryptorchidism is the most common defect found in association with hypospadias (Hayes and Wilson, 1986), although scrotal abnormalities, persistent müllerian structures, and intersexuality (see section on XX males) have also been reported. Since hypospadias in association with these abnormalities is likely to be an inherited defect, castration at the time of surgical correction is recommended.

Androgen Resistance (Testicular Feminization)

Androgen resistance syndromes have been described in humans, mice, and rats, in which they are inherited as X-linked recessive traits. Individuals with this condition are XY males with (often cryptorchid) testes and a female external phenotype and are invariably sterile. The testicular feminization (Tfm) abnormality is caused by a qualitative or quantitative defect in the cytosolic androgen receptor (Wilson et al., 1983). Although testosterone is produced by the testes, androgen-dependent masculinization fails to occur. Müllerian regression proceeds normally, since MIS action is unimpeded. The authors recently observed a cat with the testicular feminization syndrome that was presented for routine ovariohysterectomy at 6 months of age (Meyers-Wallen et al., submitted). Previous behavior characteristic of estrus had not been observed. The clitoris and vulva were of normal female size and position. Internally, there were two abdominal gonads and no evidence of epididymides, vasa deferentia, uterus, or oviducts. Histologic section of one gonad revealed testicular tissue with no adjacent epididymal tissue. Seminiferous tubules containing Sertoli's cells and few spermatogonia were present, and numerous Leydig's cells were present in the interstitium. Assays of androgen receptors in fibroblast cultures from the vulvar lips showed a deficiency in cytosolic androgen receptors. Castration is recommended in humans with this disorder in order to prevent testicular neoplasia, and may also be the treatment of choice in cats.

The authors have also observed two cats with normal male karyotypes, normal male internal genitalia, scrotal testes, perineal hypospadias, and bifid scrotum. Studies in one cat indicated that dihydrotestosterone and testosterone were not deficient. Androgen receptor studies were not available at the time, but it is likely that this condition is caused by qualitative abnormalities of the androgen receptor, resulting in a form of incomplete testicular feminization.

Cryptorchidism

Although it is an abnormal phenotype of XY males having testes, cryptorchidism is placed here somewhat arbitrarily, since the mechanisms resulting in abnormal testicular descent are incompletely understood. Although cryptorchidism occurs as an isolated defect, it can also occur in association with intersexuality. The following discussion refers only to isolated cryptorchidism. Cryptorchidism has been reported in cats (Hakala, 1984; Sheppard, 1951), but its prevalence is unknown. In dogs, cryptorchidism is the most common disorder of sexual development, occurring in as many as 13 per cent of male dogs presented to small animal clinics (Dunn et al., 1968). Normally, the canine testes descend to the scrotum by 10 days after birth (Gier and Marion, 1969). If both testes are not within the scrotum by 8 weeks of age, a diagnosis of cryptorchidism is warranted. Cryptorchid dogs have been shown to have an increased risk of development of Sertoli's cell tumor (Reif et al., 1979). Isolated cryptorchidism in the dog is likely to have a genetic basis, since

1. It occurs more often in some breeds than others, notably the toy and miniature poodle, Pomeranian, Yorkshire terrier, miniature dachshund, Cairn terrier, Chihuahua, Maltese, boxer, Pekingese, English bulldog, miniature schnauzer, and Shetland sheepdog (Hayes et al., 1985).

2. It has an increased frequency in some lines within breeds, and the frequency increases with inbreeding of those lines (Pullig, 1953).

3. Studies in other mammals (pigs, goats) demonstrate that the incidence of cryptorchidism can be increased by selection of affected or carrier animals for breeding and can be decreased by eliminating those same animals from the breeding population (Warwick, 1961; Willis, 1963).

The exact mode of inheritance of canine cryptorchidism, as in other species, is not known, but the simplest model consistent with available evidence is sex-limited autosomal recessive inheritance. Thus, both males and females can carry the gene for cryptorchidism and pass it to their offspring. Heterozygous males, heterozygous females, and homozygous females will be phenotypically normal carriers. Only the homozygous male will be cryptorchid, since homozygous females cannot express the cryptorchid phenotype, but both will pass the gene to all their offspring. While it is likely that the inheritance of cryptorchidism may be more complicated, the sex-limited autosomal recessive model is useful for genetic counseling. Treatment of affected individuals is limited to castration. If carrier parents

and cryptorchid males are removed from the breeding population, a decrease in the frequency of cryptorchidism should occur within a few generations, as has been shown in other species.

References and Supplemental Reading

Ader, P. L., and Hobson, H. P.: Hypospadias: A review of the veterinary literature and a report of three cases in the dog. J. Am. Anim. Hosp. Assoc. 14:721, 1978.

Biggers, J. D., and McFeely, R. A.: Intersexuality in domestic mammals. In McLaren, A. (ed.): Advances in Reproductive Physiology. London: Logos Press, 1966, pp. 30–58.

Bilz, V. A., Satterthwaite, E. W., and Hare, W. C. D.: Method for the short-term culture of feline lymphocytes for chromosome preparations. Mamm. Chromosome Newsl. 21:161, 1961.

Centerwall, W. R., and Benirschke, K.: Male tortoiseshell and calico (T-C) cats. J. Hered. 64:272, 1973.

Centerwall, W. R., and Benirschke, K.: An animal model for the XXY Klinefelter's syndrome in man: Tortoiseshell and calico male cats. Am. J. Vet. Res. 36:1275, 1975.

Dunn, M. L., Foster, W. J., and Goddard, K. M.: Cryptorchidism in dogs: A clinical survey. Anim. Hosp. 4:180, 1968.

Engel, E.: The chromosomal basis of human heredity. In Stanbury, J. B., Wyngaarden, J. B., and Fredrickson, D. S. (eds.): The Metabolic Basis of Inherited Disease, 4th ed. New York: McGraw-Hill, 1978, pp. 51–78.

Gier, H. T., and Marion, G. B.: Development of mammalian testes and genital ducts. Biol. Reprod. 1:1, 1969.

Gordon, J. W., and Ruddle, F. H.: Mammalian gonadal determination and gametogenesis. Science 211:1265, 1981.

Gregson, N. M., and Ishmael, J.: Diploid-triploid chimerism in 3 tortoiseshell cats. Res. Vet. Sci. 12:275, 1971.

Hakala, J. E.: Reproductive tract anomalies in 2 male cats. Mod. Vet. Pract. 65:629, 1984.

Hare, W. C. D., Weber, W. T., McFeely, R. A., et al.: Cytogenetics in the dog and cat. J. Small Anim. Pract. 7:575, 1966.

Hayes, H. M., and Wilson, G. P.: Hospital incidence of hypospadias in dogs in North America. Vet. Rec. 118:605, 1986.

Hayes, H. M., Wilson, G. P., Pendergrass, T. W., et al.: Canine cryptorchidism and subsequent testicular neoplasia: Case-control study with epidemiologic update. Teratology 32:51, 1985.

Ishihara, T.: Cytological studies on tortoiseshell male cats. Cytologia 21:391, 1956.

Johnston, S. D., Buoen, L. C., Madl, J. E., et al.: X-Chromosome monosomy (37,XO) in a Burmese cat with gonadal dysgenesis. J.A.V.M.A. 182:986, 1983.

Johnston, S. D., Buoen, L. C., Weber, A. F., et al.: X trisomy in an Airedale bitch with ovarian dysplasia and primary anestrus. Theriogenology 24:597, 1985.

Long, S. E., and Berepubo, N. A.: A 37,XO chromosome complement in a kitten. J. Small Anim. Pract. 21:627, 1980.

Long, S. E., Gruffyd-Jones, T., and David, M.: Male tortoiseshell cats: An examination of testicular histology and chromosome complement. Res. Vet. Sci. 30:274, 1981.

Loughman, W. D., and Frye, F. L.: XY/XYY bone marrow karyotype in a male Siamese-crossbred cat. Vet. Med. Small Anim. Clin. 69:1007, 1974.

Loughman, W. D., Frye, F. L., and Condon, T. B.: XY/XXY bone marrow mosaicism in three male tricolor cats. Am. J. Vet. Res. 31:307, 1970.

Lyon, M. F.: Gene action in the X-chromosome of the mouse. Nature 190:372, 1961.

Malouf, N., Benirschke, K., and Hoefnagel, D.: XX/XY chimerism in a tricolored male cat. Cytogenetics 6:228, 1967.

Meyers-Wallen, V. N.: Unpublished data.

Meyers-Wallen, V. N., and Patterson, D. F.: Disorders of sexual development in the dog. In Morrow, D. A. (ed.): Current Therapy in Theriogenology, 2nd ed. Philadelphia: W. B. Saunders Co., 1986, pp. 567–574.

Meyers-Wallen, V. N., and Patterson, D. F.: XX sex reversal in the American cocker spaniel dog: Phenotypic expression and inheritance. Human Genetics (in press).

Meyers-Wallen, V. N., Donahoe, P. K., Manganaro, T., et al.: Mullerian inhibiting substance in sex-reversed dogs. Biol. Reprod. 37:1015, 1987.

Meyers-Wallen, V. N., Wilson, J. D., Fisher, S., et al.: Testicular feminization in a domestic cat, Felis catus (submitted).

Moran, C., Gillies, C. B., and Nicholas, F.: Fertile male tortoiseshell cats. Mosaicism due to gene instability? J. Hered. 75:397, 1984.

Niemand, V. S., Hartig, F., and Hoffman, R.: Klinische, morphologische und zytogenetische Befunde bei einem Pudel mit Pseudohermaphroditismus masculinus internus. Berliner und Munchener Tierarztliche Wochenschrift 12:224, 1972.

Norby, D. E., Hegreberg, G. A., Thuline, H. C., et al.: An XO cat. Cytogenet. Cell Genet. 13:448, 1974.

Pullig, T.: Cryptorchidism in cocker spaniels. J. Hered. 44:250, 1953.

Pyle, R. L., Patterson, D. F., Hare, W. C. D., et al.: XXY sex chromosome constitution in a Himalayan cat with tortoise-shell points. J. Hered. 62:220, 1971.

Reif, J. S., Maguire, T. G., Kenney, R. M., et al.: A cohort study of canine testicular neoplasia. J.A.V.M.A. 175:719, 1979.

Sheppard, M.: Some observations on cat practice. Vet. Rec. 63:685, 1951.

Smith, F. K. W., Buoen, L. C., Weber, A. F., et al.: X-chromosomal monosomy (77,XO) in a Doberman pinscher with gonadal dysgenesis. J. Vet. Int. Med. (in press).

Svendsen, C. K., Thomsen, P. D., and Basse, A.: Two cases of male pseudohermaphroditism in the dog. Nord. Vet. Med. 37:358, 1985.

Thuline, H. C., and Norby, D. E.: Spontaneous occurrence of chromosome abnormality in cats. Science 134:554, 1961.

Warwick, B. L.: Selection against cryptorchidism in Angora goats. J. Anim. Sci. 20:10, 1961.

Willis, M. B.: Abnormalities and defects in pedigree dogs—V. Cryptorchidism. J. Small Anim. Pract. 4:469, 1963.

Wilson, J. D., Griffin, J. E., Leshin, M., et al.: The androgen resistance syndromes: 5-alpha-reductase deficiency, testicular feminization, and related disorders. In Stanbury, J. B., Wyngaarden, J. B., Fredrickson, D. S., et al. (eds.): The Metabolic Basis of Inherited Disease, 5th ed. New York: McGraw-Hill, 1983, pp. 1001–1026.

HORMONAL AND CLINICAL CORRELATES OF OVARIAN CYCLES, OVULATION, PSEUDOPREGNANCY, AND PREGNANCY IN DOGS

P. W. CONCANNON, Ph.D.,
and D.H. LEIN, D.V.M.

Ithaca, New York

This article provides a brief overview of major reproductive events in the bitch and introduces some published and unpublished observations of interest. The emphasis is on variation. There is considerable variation in the extent and timing of the hormonal changes in most clinical and endocrine parameters that must be considered in the course of reproductive evaluations of individual bitches. The major events and hormonal changes of typical nonfertile and fertile cycles are summarized in Figures 1 and 2, respectively.

TIMING AND PHYSIOLOGY OF MAJOR REPRODUCTIVE EVENTS

Stages of the Cycle

In most breeds, the interval from one cycle to the next averages 7 months but can range from 4 to 13 months. Signs of *proestrus* may last from 3 days to 3 weeks; the average is 9 days. *Estrous* behavior likewise may last 3 days to 3 weeks; the average is also around 9 days. The period of peak fertility for natural matings lasts about 5 days, beginning with the day of the preovulatory luteinizing hormone (LH) peak, and usually coincides with behavioral estrus. *Metestrus* (or diestrus), the stage after estrus, usually last 2 to 3 months in the absence of pregnancy, based on progesterone secretion profiles. Pregnancy terminates with parturition 64 to 66 days after the LH peak. *Anestrus*, the period of apparent ovarian inactivity prior to the next proestrus, can range from 1 to 6 months.

THE PREOVULATORY LH SURGE

Reproductive events in the bitch are best timed in relation to the preovulatory LH peak. Maximal release of LH usually occurs within a 1-day period, but levels may be elevated for 1 to 3 days. In evaluating individual cycles, it is often useful to estimate the time of the LH peak from changes in the more readily assessable clinical parameters, as outlined in Figure 3. The behavioral transition from proestrus to estrus often occurs within a day or two of the LH peak. However, first acceptance of a male may occur as early as 4 days before, or as late as 6 days after, the LH peak. A distinct softening

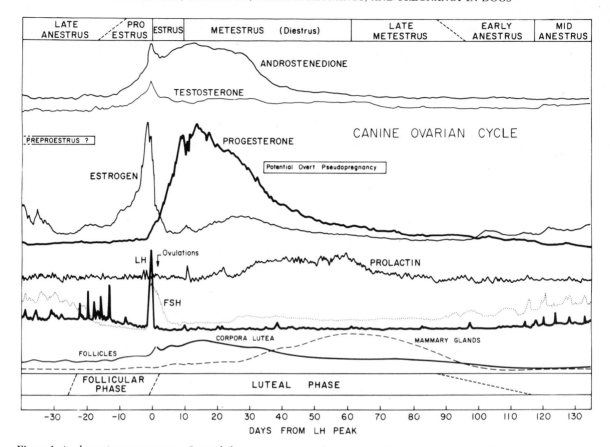

Figure 1. A schematic representation of typical changes in serum or plasma levels of estrogen, **progesterone**, LH, FSH, prolactin, testosterone, and androstenedione reported or presumed to occur during the canine ovarian cycle, and their temporal relation to observable stages and functional phases of the estrous cycle. Basal and peak serum levels of steroids are, respectively, 5–10 and 50 and 100 pg/ml for estradiol, 0.2–0.5 and 15–90 ng/ml for progesterone, 0.1 and 1 ng/ml for testosterone, and 0.2 ng/ml and 2 ng/ml for androstenedione. (Adapted with permission from Concannon, P.: Canine pregnancy and parturition. Vet. Clin. North Am. [Small Anim. Pract.] 16(3):453–475, 1986.)

of the swollen vulva, when observed, usually occurs at 1 to 2 days after the LH peak. A distinct decrease in the abundance of cornified superficial cells in vaginal smears obtained in late estrus usually begins 7 to 9 days after the LH peak but can occur as early as 6 days, or as late as 11 days, after the peak. Earlier changes in the vaginal cytology that might be predictive of the LH peak or ovulation are not consistent in either occurrence or timing. Maximum cornification, as the percentage of epithelial cells that are cornified, may occur as early as 8 or more days before the LH peak or as late as 3 days after the LH peak, when using simple staining methods. An abrupt decrease in red blood cells, noncellular debris, or both may occur around the time of the LH surge. Such changes, while useful, are inconsistent and therefore not reliable. A progressive wrinkling in the vaginal mucosa resulting from loss of edema can be routinely observed around the time of the LH surge and ovulation in normal cycles when they are monitored by vaginoscopic examination. Monitoring of vaginal smears and the endoscopic appearance of the vaginal mucosa are considered in more detail at the end of this section,

along with changes in the electrical resistance of the vaginal mucosa.

PROESTRUS

The onset of proestrus, defined as obvious vulvar swelling, vaginal discharge of uterine blood, or both can occur as early as 3 weeks, or as late as 3 days, before the LH peak. Presumably, the associated follicular phases and rises in estrogen are correspondingly protracted or brief. Vulvar swelling, vaginal edema and cornification, and attractiveness to males become progressively more prominent. Nonsexual behavior gives way to playful behavior, and then proceptive sexual behavior or passive behavior, in response to males' attempts to mount. Estradiol levels rise from 10 to 20 pg/ml at the start of proestrus to reach a peak of 50 to 100 pg/ml by 1 to 2 days before the LH peak, and then decline during and following the LH surge. Progesterone levels rise slowly from less than 0.5 ng/ml to reach around 1 ng/ml at the start of the LH surge and then increase rapidly during and following the LH surge.

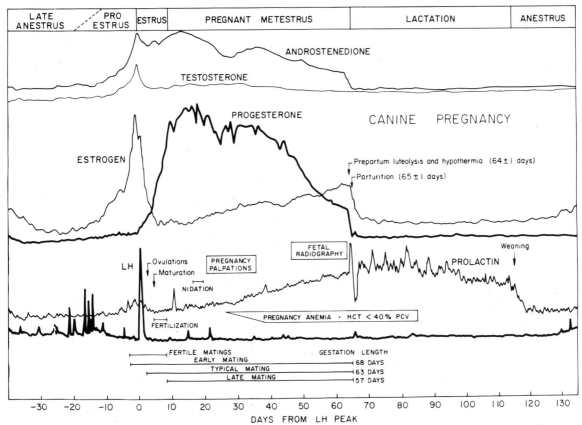

Figure 2. A schematic representation of typical changes in serum or plasma levels of estrogen, progesterone, LH, prolactin, testosterone, and androstenedione reported or presumed to occur during pregnancy and lactation in the bitch, and their relation to indicated events considered important for breeding programs and clinical management of pregnancy. Actual ranges for basal and peak levels of steroids in serum or plasma are the same as those in nonpregnant cycles (see Fig. 1). (Adapted with permission from Concannon, P.: Canine pregnancy and parturition. Vet. Clin. North Am. [Small Anim. Pract.] 16(3):453–475, 1986.)

ESTRUS

Behavioral estrus, characterized by standing firmly for males and by reflex tail-deviation, often begins within 1 or 2 days of the LH surge. The average onset of estrus is the day of the LH peak. The average time of first copulation is 2 days after the LH peak, when the vulva has softened. However, estrus may begin up to 4 days before the LH peak or 6 days after the LH peak. Thus, ovulations, which occur 2 days after the LH surge, may occur early or late in behavioral estrus or may even occur several days before first acceptance of a male. Therefore, for optimal fertility, breedings should occur during early, mid, and late estrus unless there is ample evidence that more restricted matings provide near optimal fertility in a particular breed or line. Progesterone levels increase throughout the 1 to 2 weeks of behavioral estrus, approaching peak levels of 15 to 85 ng/ml, whereas estradiol levels decline. The decline in estrogen is probably critical for normal fertility. Doses of exogenous estrogen that did not prevent pregnancy when administered during proestrus were antinidatory when given during estrus or early metestrus (Bowen et al., 1985).

The duration of behavioral estrus is variable and, at times, unrelated to the period of fertility. Behavioral estrus may last much longer than the fertile period. The latter is better reflected by the period of "vaginal estrus," based on maintenance of vaginal cornification assessed by vaginal cytology or endoscopy.

OVULATION AND FERTILITY. Ovulations usually occur synchronously 2 days after the LH peak. However, the oocytes are ovulated as primary oocytes. They do not mature and become capable of being fertilized until some time later in the distal segments of the uterine tubes. The exact time course has not been determined. Oocyte maturation may not occur until 2 or 3 days after ovulation and, therefore, 4 or 5 days after the LH surge and the average onset of estrus. The fertile life of mature oocytes may be another 2 or 3 days, since matings in late estrus, 7 or 8 days after the LH peak, are often fertile. Pregnancies following matings that do not occur until 9 or 10 days after the LH peak are rare, produce litters of only 1 or 2 pups, and have an apparent gestation length of only 55 to 57 days from mating to parturition. Fortuitous or forced matings more than 2 or 3 days before the LH peak

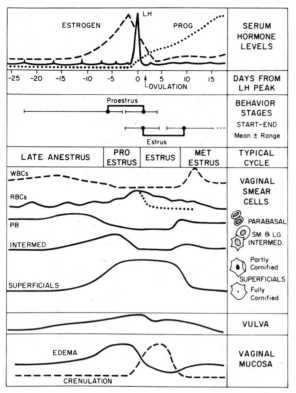

Figure 3. A schematic summary of the temporal relationships among the periovulatory endocrine events, behavioral and vulvar changes, and changes in vaginal smears during proestrus, estrus, and early metestrus in the bitch. (Modified from Concannon P.: Reproductive physiology and endocrine patterns of the bitch. *In* Kirk, R. [ed.]: *Current Veterinary Therapy, Small Animal Practice*, Vol. VIII. Philadelphia: W. B. Saunders, 1983, pp. 886–931.)

Progressive increases in the superficial cell component of vaginal smears and in edema of the vaginal mucosa can be used to monitor the preovulatory rise in estrogen. Crenulation (wrinkling) of the vaginal mucosa is more reflective of the occurrence of the preovulatory LH peak and ovulation than any changes in the vaginal smear at that time, as the latter are inconsistent. The loss of vaginal crenulation and the increase in nonsuperficial cells in the vaginal smear both occur rather abruptly 7 to 9 days after the LH peak, and 5 to 7 days after ovulation, and can be used to retrospectively determine the approximate time of those events. The latter relationship is the basis for considering the occurrence of a physiologically significant transition from "vaginal estrus" to "vaginal metestrus" independent of the termination of "behavioral estrus," which can be extremely variable (see text).

are rarely fertile, but they can result in pregnancies with apparent gestation lengths of 68 to 70 days when they are fertile or followed by subsequent, fertile matings. Canine sperm can remain fertile in the female tract in some instances for 6 to 7 days (Concannon et al., 1983), but the average fertile life may be only 3 or 4 days.

EVENTS OF PREGNANCY

The timing of some of the physiologically important and clinically relevant events of canine pregnancy are outlined in Table 1. Practical aspects to

note include the following. There is considerable variation in the timing of events based on time of breeding versus the time of the preovulatory LH peak. In this review, the cycle and pregnancy are considered to begin with the day of the LH peak (day 0). Vaginal cytology, endoscopy, or both can be used to estimate the time of breeding in relation to the period of fertility. There is a limited period optimal for palpation of uterine implantation swellings between 3 and 5 weeks of pregnancy. Ultrasonography can be used to observe the amnion and embryo by 3 weeks and, starting shortly thereafter, to follow fetal well being, heart beat, and position throughout pregnancy. There is an extensive normochromic anemia during the second half of pregnancy. The use of conventional radiography for pregnancy diagnosis is limited to the last 3 weeks of pregnancy. There is a consistency in gestation length relative to periovulatory endocrine events, such as the LH peak (65 ± 1 days) or the late-estrus shift in the vaginal smear (57 ± 3 days), but not relative to the time of mating (63 ± 7 days).

LUTEAL FUNCTION AND PREGNANCY MAINTENANCE. Maintenance of pregnancy is dependent on ovarian secretion of progesterone throughout gestation and will not tolerate abnormal elevations in estrogen levels. Luteal secretion of progesterone, in both pregnant and nonpregnant cycles, is dependent on pituitary secretion of both LH and prolactin and can be depressed experimentally by administration of anti-LH serum or by prolactin-lowering bromocryptine treatment (Concannon et al., 1987). Progesterone levels, on average, are slightly higher in pregnant than in nonpregnant bitches, but the difference is not significant. Prolactin levels increase throughout the second half of pregnancy, to levels much higher than normally seen at the comparable time in nonpregnant bitches, and may enhance progesterone secretion. The uterus has little or no effect on canine luteal function in nonpregnant bitches, based on studies of the effect of hysterectomy (Olson et al., 1984c). Prostaglandin $F_{2\alpha}$ is luteolytic and, therefore, abortifacient in pregnant dogs from midgestation to term, but repeated injections of 30 to 250 μg/kg twice daily for several days are needed to effect a permanent luteolysis or abortion without excessive side effects (Concannon and Hansel, 1977; Paradis et al., 1983).

POST-IMPLANTATION PREGNANCY. Any pregnancy-specific increases in progesterone and estrogen secretion during the second half of gestation are poorly reflected in blood levels of the hormones because of the hemodilution associated with the normal anemia of pregnancy in the bitch. Total blood volume increases along with body weight increases of 20 to 55 per cent. The maternal hematocrit declines after implantation. The packed cell volume (PCV) normally reaches 40 per cent by

35 days and is usually below 35 per cent at term. The anemia seems to be normochromic and normocytic. There is an associated decrease in hemoglobin and the sedimentation rate. A moderate immunosuppression involving serum immunoglobulin G (IgG) levels below 500 ng/dl has been reported. The extent to which general metabolism and activity of metabolic hormones are altered has not been fully determined. Thyroxine levels and post–adrenocorticotropic hormone (ACTH) cortisol levels may be elevated. Sensitivity to insulin is commonly reduced during late pregnancy (Concannon, 1986a), and pre-existing diabetic or prediabetic states are likely to be aggravated. Fetal skeletons do not become radiopaque until after 44 days of gestation (i.e., 3 weeks before parturition) (Concannon and Rendano, 1983).

PREGNANCY DIAGNOSIS. There are no confirmed methods of pregnancy diagnosis for dogs other than the physical detection of peri-implantation uterine enlargements or the fetoplacental units themselves, using ultrasound or digital palpation starting 3 weeks after ovulation or using conventional radiography during the last 3 weeks of pregnancy (Concannon, 1987). The use of biochemical tests, such as changes in urinary estrogen or in the serum creatinine and immunoglobulin levels, have been suggested but have not been confirmed or put into routine use. There is a distinct increase in relaxin levels, which appears to be pregnancy specific and consistently detectable during the fourth week of pregnancy and thereafter. Relaxin levels may represent a good marker for postimplantation pregnancy, but assays are not readily available. Relaxin levels remain elevated throughout pregnancy, peak at about 7 weeks, decline abruptly to low levels at parturition, and become nondetectable some time during lactation (Steinetz et al., 1987).

PARTURITION

Bitches whelp their litters 64, 65, or 66 days after the preovulatory LH peak, in response to a series of events triggered by maturation of the fetuses. It is probably an increase in fetal cortisol secretion that causes the increase in maternal cortisol levels and increases in maternal prostaglandin $F_{2\alpha}$ to luteolytic levels seen at 1 to 2 days prepartum (Concannon, 1987). The rise in prostaglandin results in a decline in maternal progesterone levels from above 3 ng/ml to below 1 ng/ml during the 24 hr prior to labor. As in other species, progesterone withdrawal most probably causes placental dislocation, further increases in prostaglandin, and increased uterine sensitivity to oxytocin. Prostaglandin also causes uterine contractility because of its direct uterotropic effects. Oxytocin is reflexively released in response to fetal pressure on the cervix and vagina and further enhances uterine contractions. The prepartum decline in progesterone produces a transient hypothermia 6 to 18 hr before the onset of labor. The 2 to 3°F (1 to 1.5°C) fall observed in rectal temperatures obtained two to three times a day can be monitored by owners concerned by an apparent prolonged gestation. There is a prepartum rise in prolactin levels that may be caused by the fall in progesterone; postpartum elevations in prolactin are sucking-dependent.

NONPREGNANT METESTRUS AND MAMMARY GLAND

In the absence of a fertile mating, changes in serum hormone levels are somewhat similar to those that occur during pregnancy, particularly the rise in progesterone for 2 to 3 weeks and maintenance of elevated levels during the 1.5 to 3 months of their protracted decline, analogous to the 2 months of progesterone secretion that supports pregnancy. There may also be either a modest or distinct increase in prolactin during the second half of metestrus, but not as great as that seen in pregnancy. The occurrence of a normal but nonpregnant cycle can be detected, based on careful palpations of the mammary gland chains over time. Following the initial increase in ductal elements, the increased mass of glandular tissue is usually palpable by the fourth week after ovulation. Mammary size becomes maximum at 2 or 3 months after estrus and then subsides (Concannon, 1986c). In older and particularly multiparous bitches, mammary glands may not return to juvenile size during anestrus, but changes in size during nonpregnant cycles are still readily palpable. Increases in overall mammary size can be diagnostic of an otherwise unobserved ovarian cycle.

PSEUDOPREGNANCY

A modest but easily detected mammary development accompanies the extended luteal phase (or so-called physiologic or covert pseudopregnancy) of all nonfertile ovarian cycles in the bitch. In contrast, clinical pseudopregnancy refers to an overt pseudopregnancy, or pseudocyesis, of such an extent that mammary development and body conformation or behavior is not clearly distinguishable from that of late pregnancy or lactation. Many of the symptoms of clinical pseudopregnancy are apparently due to an excessive elevation in prolactin levels caused by an abrupt decline in progesterone (Concannon, 1986c; Smith and McDonald, 1974). Prolactin levels can be suppressed and pseudopregnancy terminated by administration of prolactin-lowering dopamine-agonist compounds such as bromocriptine and related ergot alkaloids, but none are marketed for veterinary rather than human use.

Treatment with an androgen, such as mibolerone (Cheque, Upjohn) at a dose of 16 µg/kg for 5 days, is reported effective in terminating pseudopregnancy (Brown, 1984). Symptoms may also be suppressed by progestin therapy, such as megestrol acetate (Ovaban, Schering), but often recur in response to progestin withdrawal.

INTERESTRUS INTERVALS AND TERMINATION OF ANESTRUS

Termination of anestrus and the onset of proestrus appear to result from an increase in pulsatile GnRH-induced secretion of the gonadotropins LH and follicle-stimulating hormone (FSH). Pulsatile LH release is increased at the end of anestrus (Concannon et al., 1986; Concannon, 1987), and pulsatile administration of GnRH can cause premature termination of anestrus and initiate a follicular phase resulting in proestrus, estrus, and fertile ovulation (Vanderlip et al., 1987). Normal physiologic control over the termination of anestrus at such variable times among individual dogs, after anestrus periods of 1 to 7 months or longer, is not fully understood. Termination of metestrus luteal function and reduced prolactin secretion may be prerequisites for subsequent changes involved in the onset of proestrus (Concannon, 1987). Nadir progesterone levels (< 0.5 ng/ml) occur before the end of anestrus, and the length of anestrus may be reduced by about a month by administration of prostaglandin during metestrus to cause premature luteolysis. In some bitches, suppression of prolactin secretion by chronic administration of bromocriptine not only moderately shortened the luteal phase but also extensively reduced the length of anestrus and resulted in interestrus intervals of less than 4 months (Okkens et al., 1985).

HORMONE LEVELS: PROFILES AND MEASUREMENT

Estrogen

Estradiol levels are at basal values of 5 to 10 pg/ml in very late anestrus, around 10 to 20 pg/ml at the start of proestrus, at peak levels of 50 to 100 pg/ml in late proestrus and 1 to 2 days before the LH surge, reduced during estrus, and variable thereafter; transient elevations to proestrus values with return to baseline have been reported during anestrus (Olson et al., 1982). Levels of estrone tend to parallel those of estradiol (Chakraborty, 1987). Levels of estrogen conjugates have not been reported.

ESTROGEN ASSAYS

Diagnostic radioimmunoassays for estrogen and, more specifically, estradiol are available in many veterinary and human medical service laboratories. However, except in cases of suspected estrogen-secreting tumors, their utility in canine reproduction is doubtful. Postprandial lipid in canine serum may interfere with the assays. Assays intended for human diagnostic methods may not be fully sensitive to the range appropriate for dogs. Interpretation of results is difficult. Peak estradiol levels of 50 to 100 pg/ml are expected in late proestrus, but levels are rapidly reduced during estrus. Furthermore, estradiol levels are variable during metestrus and anestrus. Thus, the finding of either elevated or basal estradiol levels is unlikely to be as informative in evaluating the reproductive status of the bitch as a progesterone measurement viewed in relation to clinical correlates and reproductive history. An ovarian response test involving measurement of increases in estradiol in response to administered gonadotropin might be considered in cases of chronic anestrus or suspected activity of accessory ovarian tissue in spayed bitches. However, in bitches, increases in estradiol levels were inconsistent after administration of one or more injections of FSH (Shille and Stabenfeldt, 1980).

Progesterone

Progesterone levels are normally less than 1 ng/ml during anestrus and until late proestrus. Progesterone levels range from 2 to 4 ng/ml during the LH surge and 4 to 10 ng/ml at ovulation and peak at 15 to 80 ng/ml by days 15 to 30. In the absence of pregnancy, progesterone levels progressively decline and fall below 1 ng/ml sometime between days 50 and 120 of the cycle. In normal pregnancy, also, progesterone levels progressively decline, but they are always maintained at effective levels (3 to 15 ng/ml) until 2 or 3 days before parturition and then fall below 1 to 2 ng/ml during the 24 hr before parturition (Concannon, 1986a, 1986b).

PROGESTERONE ASSAYS

Assay of progesterone in serum or plasma can be used to confirm the occurrence or absence of prior ovulation and the subsequent luteal phase and should be part of any evaluation in which the occurrence or timing of ovarian cycles is in doubt. Progesterone determination can be used to evaluate the occurrence or normal duration of luteal function in a bitch that fails to conceive at an apparently normal estrus, or to detect a missed cycle in a bitch presented for persistent anestrus. Progesterone levels above 5 ng/ml would confirm the occurrence of ovulation within the prior 2 months; above 2 ng/ml, within the prior 3 to 4 months. Levels below 1 ng/ml confirm the absence of ovulation within the prior 2 months and the existence of a true anestrus state. However, isolated instances of progesterone levels of 1 to 3 ng/ml have been observed in single samples from some bitches as late as 80 days postpartum or 120 days of a nonpregnant cycle. Whether the source is follicular or luteal, or possibly adrenal, and its significance are not known.

When progesterone assay results can be obtained rapidly, they can be used to time ovulation and to schedule matings or inseminations for bitches that are difficult to breed and in which behavioral changes associated with normal periovulatory hormone changes are erratic, premature, or delayed. Levels below 1 ng/ml indicate that the LH peak has not yet occurred. Levels of 2 to 5 ng/ml suggest an impending or recent ovulation. Levels of 6 to 10 ng/ml indicate that ovulation has occurred and that the fertile period is nearly over or has ended. Levels higher than 10 ng/ml occur near and after the end of the fertile period. Over the next few years, the use of commercial rapid, colorimetric progesterone assay kits will become commonplace in practices and clinics providing fertility evaluations, and progesterone can then be monitored on a daily basis.

Androgens

Androgen levels have been reported for most reproductive stages (Olson et al., 1984a; Concannon, 1986c). Serum testosterone levels are about 0.1 ng/ml during anestrus, increase during proestrus to reach peak values of about 0.3 to 1.0 ng/ml coincident with the preovulatory LH peak, and then decline and remain below 0.2 ng/ml throughout the luteal phase. Serum androstenedione levels are less than 0.2 ng/ml during anestrus, increase during proestrus to levels of 0.6 to 2.3 ng/ml at the time of the LH peak, and remain elevated during the luteal phase in both pregnant and nonpregnant cycles. Androstenedione follows the pattern of luteal progesterone, reaches peak levels of 0.7 ng/ml around day 20, and declines to 0.5 ng/ml around day 40 and to lower levels during the progression into anestrus. Elevated androgen during proestrus probably reflects production of estrogen precursors by follicles. The significance of luteal production of androstenedione is unknown.

Gonadotropins

Laboratories may report gonadotropin levels in terms of standards of varying potencies, and only relative changes can be reviewed here. Mean levels of FSH are moderately elevated during anestrus and may surpass levels seen during the preovulatory surge; those of LH during anestrus are only slightly elevated (Olson et al., 1982; Shille et al., 1987). LH release is episodic, with pulses of release occurring at intervals of about 1 to 8 hr; reported elevations in mean levels presumably represent increased pulse amplitude, frequency, or both. An increase in the pulse amplitude and frequency of LH occurs in late anestrus and probably causes the onset of proestrous follicle development (Concannon et al., 1986). Levels of FSH and LH are low during most of proestrus. FSH increases along with LH during the preovulatory surge of gonadotropin release at 1 to 2 days after the peak in estrogen (Fig. 1). The surge may involve a 10- to 40-fold increase in LH levels and a 2- to 20-fold increase in FSH levels based on various published and unpublished studies. Following the preovulatory surge, LH levels are low for 2 to 3 weeks apparently because of pituitary depletion (Fernandez et al., 1986). FSH levels appear to be increased slightly during late pregnancy (Reimers et al., 1978). Following ovariectomy, LH and FSH are chronically elevated to levels near or above preovulatory peak levels. A similar situation would be expected in chronic anestrus resulting from primary ovarian failure.

Prolactin and Growth Hormone

Prolactin levels appear to be unaltered by endocrine events of proestrus and estrus. Prolactin levels are moderately increased, about two- or threefold during metestrus, during the period when progesterone levels are declining. Declining progesterone has been suggested as a stimulus for prolactin release in the bitch. Prolactin levels are elevated nine- to tenfold above basal values during late pregnancy, surge acutely to peak levels during the prepartum fall in progesterone, are often reduced shortly postpartum, and then become and remain elevated in response to suckling-induced reflexive release during lactation (Concannon et al., 1978; DeCoster et al., 1983). Hypothalamic control involves thyrotropin-releasing hormone (TRH), which stimulates prolactin release, and dopamine, which inhibits prolactin release. It has been suggested that hyperprolactinemia and resulting galactorrhea occur in bitches with severe hypothyroidism because of increased TRH secretion caused by low levels of thyroxine and loss of negative feedback of TRH secretion (Chastain and Schmidt, 1980).

Hypersecretion of growth hormone (GH) can occur in older bitches in response to luteal-phase progesterone secretion and may result in acromegaly and, possibly, pituitary diabetes (Eigenmann et al., 1981). Similar increases in GH and resulting changes occur in younger dogs given high doses of a contraceptive progestin (McCann et al., 1987).

TIMED BREEDINGS BASED ON VULVAR DETUMESCENCE, VAGINAL SMEARS, VAGINOSCOPY, AND VAGINAL MUCUS ELECTRICAL RESISTANCE

Breeding Management

Standard practice involves bringing the bitch to the location of the male. Such practice is appropriately protective of the male's libido and territoriality, since many males will not perform well in strange surroundings. An obvious recommendation, where possible, is to breed every other day starting when the bitch will first accept the male, until three breedings are obtained. That should guarantee one or two potentially highly fertile matings regardless of whether the bitch started accepting the male 3 days before ovulation, the day of ovulation, or 3 days after ovulation. When breedings are limited to one mating or two closely spaced matings, the likelihood of failure due to breeding too long before the period of peak fertility is enhanced, unless breedings are delayed until after the LH peak has occurred. Restricted matings timed to a particular favored number of days after the first observed vulvar swelling or bloody discharge of proestrus or "heat" (i.e., 9, 11, or 13 days later), are probably a common cause of breeding failures or small litters. Such matings may be occurring well before, or long after, the period of peak fertility. Therefore, good breeding management should, when possible, include spreading of matings over several days of the period of behavioral estrus and an approximation of the period of fertility based on vaginal cytology, vulvar softening, or vaginal wrinkling as well as timing the start of behavioral estrus. The use of rapid progesterone assays to estimate the time of the LH peak and ovulation was reviewed in the preceding section.

Vaginal Cytology

Vaginal smears can be easily and routinely used to monitor the progression of proestrus and estrus (Olson et al., 1984d; Concannon and DiGregorio, 1986; Linde and Karlsson, 1984; Roszel, 1975) and should be part of any breeding management program or fertility examination. Any of several stains permit characterization of the various epithelial cell types, based on size, shape, and nuclear conditions (Fig. 4).

Smears are best obtained from the cranial vagina, using a narrow spreading speculum, a cotton-tipped swab slightly moistened with saline, a deliberate

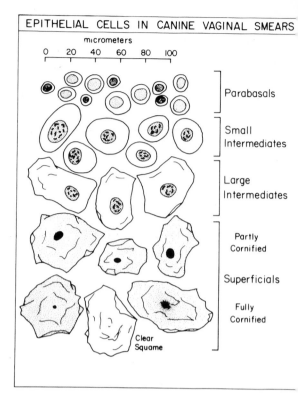

Figure 4. Epithelial cell types commonly observed in canine vaginal smears, drawn to scale. (Adapted from Concannon, P. W., and DiGregorio, G. B.: Canine vaginal cytology. *In* Burke, T. [ed.]): *Small Animal Reproduction and Infertility.* Philadelphia: Lea & Febiger, 1986, pp. 96–111.)

wiping of the mucosa, and transfer to the slide using a gentle, rolling motion. Fixation before drying, with an aerosol or liquid fixative, is preferred but not necessary. Failure to use a speculum to guard the swab results in collection of vestibular epithelial cells in addition to vaginal cells and is likely to result in more variable smears, a less distinct progression of expected changes from one smear to the next, and less than the normal high percentage of superficial cells at the time of peak vaginal cornification. Smears obtained from only the vestibule can be used to monitor the normal endocrine changes, but the typical changes have not been reported in detail and the results are less reliable than with strictly vaginal cytology.

Among useful stains recently reviewed is a modified Wright-Giemsa staining set that is commercially available, rapid, and easy to use (Diff-Quik, American Scientific Products, McGaw Park, IL). Smears should be examined every 1 to 3 days. The normal progression of changes in the relative incidences of different epithelial cell types in the smear is easy to follow (Figs. 5 and 6). Distinguishing between early proestrus and very late estrus or early metestrus can be difficult on the study of only one smear of an unknown cycle. Throughout proestrus, the numbers and average size of epithelial cells progressively increase. Rounded, nonsuperfi-

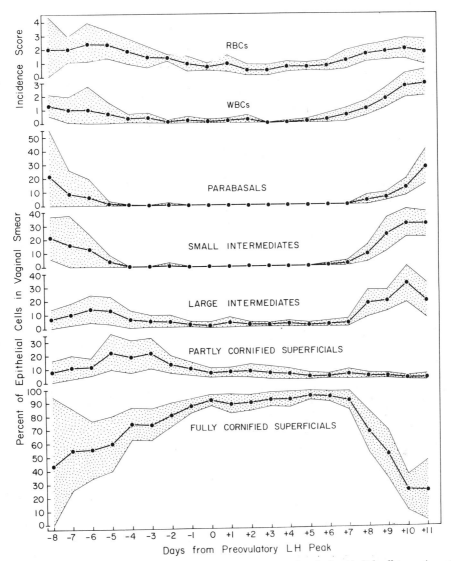

Figure 5. Mean incidence of blood cells (based on relative, subjective scoring) and of epithelial cell types (as actual percentages of epithelial cells counted) observed in vaginal smears obtained at known times relative to the day of preovulatory LH peak. Results are for 18 normal cycles in which the day of the LH peak was determined. (From Concannon, P. W., and DiGregorio, G. B.: Canine vaginal cytology. *In* Burke, T. [ed.]: *Small Animal Reproduction and Infertility.* Philadelphia: Lea & Febiger, 1986, pp. 96–111.)

cial cells (parabasal and small intermediate cells) dominate the early proestrus smear and virtually disappear from the smears by 3 to 4 days before the LH peak, or earlier. Maximum cornification may occur as early as 7 to 8 days before the LH peak or may not occur until 2 to 3 days after the LH peak. Maximum cornification may be represented almost entirely by fully cornified anuclear superficial cells; by a mixture of fully cornified cells and of partly cornified cells containing distinct, condensed nuclei; or, in some cycles, by a retention of some large, well-nucleated intermediate cells along with the superficial epithelial cells (Concannon and Di-Gregorio, 1986). Therefore, there is not much value in considering partly cornified cells separately from

fully cornified cells (Fig. 5). Instead, a more useful parameter is the combination of both cell types in the single category of superficial cells (Fig. 6). Normal, maximal cornification expected in late proestrus and estrus is characterized by the absence of small, round intermediate cells and parabasal cells in the smear. The variation among bitches in the extent and cytologic characteristics of maximal cornification and in its timing precludes any reliable use of changes in epithelial cells to predict the times of the LH surge or ovulation with any immediacy.

Because of the great variation in the relative incidence and progression of large intermediate cells among cycles, this cell type often poses the greatest problems in interpretation of the general

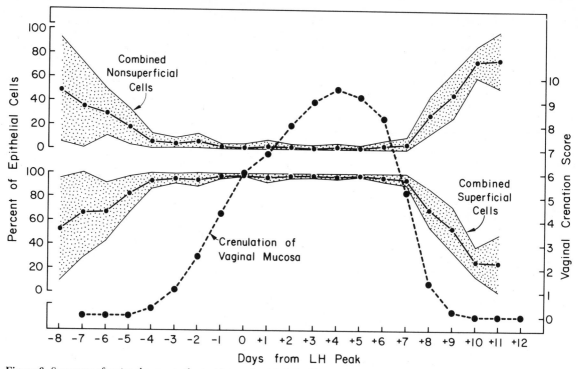

Figure 6. Summary of major changes in the incidence of epithelial cell types in canine vaginal smears considering only superficial cells (partly or fully cornified) versus nonsuperficial cells (including large intermediates) in relation to the day of the LH peak. Mean percentages and their 95 per cent confidence intervals are shown for 18 dogs. Also shown are the mean scores for gross changes in the vaginal surface observed by vaginoscopy of the same dogs. The latter are based on a scoring system for extent of crenulation in mucosal folds, including the following: 0—round and edematous; 4—obvious wrinkling and sacculation; 8—obvious, sharp angulation; 10—maximum angulation; 7—thinner, angulated mucosa; 3—very thin, but wrinkled, shedding epithelium; 0—flattened or small rounded folds with patchy coloration. (From Concannon, P. W., and DiGregorio, G. B.: Canine vaginal cytology. *In* Burke, T. [ed.]: *Small Animal Reproduction and Infertility.* Philadelphia: Lea & Febiger, 1986, pp. 96–111.)

progression of changes in smears during proestrus; for that reason, the large intermediate cell should be recognized and appreciated as a unique cell type. The presence or absence of large intermediate cells is the entire basis of the 0 to 10 per cent values shown for nonsuperficial cells for days −2 to +5 in Figure 6. Large intermediate cells are unique in having large, healthy nuclei characteristic of nonsuperficial cells, combined with the irregular, wrinkled shape characteristic of cornified, squamous superficial cells. They have also been termed transitional or superficial intermediate cells (Concannon and DiGregorio, 1986).

To summarize, there are no acute changes in epithelial cells routinely predictive of the LH peak or of ovulation. In cases in which fully cornified cells completely replace partly cornified cells, the transition usually occurs around the time of ovulation. When there is an abrupt decline in erythrocytes, in the amount of noncellular debris, or in both, the change often occurs between the LH peak and ovulation. More often, red blood cells appear in the smear throughout and beyond estrus. When proestrus is unusually prolonged, there may be concern that behavioral estrus is overdue, and forced mating or artificial insemination may be

warranted. However, no concern should exist until 2 to 3 days after rounded nonsuperficial cells (parabasal and small intermediate cells) have been reduced to fewer than 1 per cent of epithelial cells present.

Smears continue to show near-maximum cornification throughout the fertile period of estrus, and continued collection of smears is important for a more accurate timing of reproductive events, albeit retrospectively. The abrupt, initial reappearance of nonsuperficial cells late in estrus usually begins 7 to 8 days after the LH peak (Figs. 4 and 5). A normal range of 6 to 10 days after the LH peak has been recorded for this shift from vaginal estrus to vaginal metestrus (diestrus). During this period, oocyte fertility rapidly declines, and subsequent matings are unlikely to be fertile. Several studies suggest that the metestrus, or diestrus, "shift" in vaginal cytology can be used with considerable accuracy to time preceding and subsequent events of the fertile cycle (Table 1), based on its occurrence approximately 8 days after the LH peak in the majority of cycles.

The estrus-to-metestrus decline in the percentage of superficial cells in the vaginal smear is usually accompanied by the appearance of moderate or

Table 1. *Timing of Selected Events of the Fertile Ovarian Cycle and Pregnancy of the Domestic Dog in Relation to the Day of the Preovulatory LH Peak and to Potential Times of Fertile Matings*

Selected Reproductive Events	Days Before/After LH Peak*	Days Before/After Fertile Mating†
Onset of proestrus	−25 to −3	
Full vaginal cornification reached	−8 to +3	
Onset of estrus behavior	−4 to +5	
Estradiol peak	−3 to −1	
Decreased vaginal edema	−2 to 0	
OH surge and sharp rise in progesterone	−1 to 0	
LH peak	0	−9 to +3
First fertile mating	−3 to +9	0
Initial crenulation of vaginal mucosa begins	−1 to +1	
Peak vaginal crenulation	2 to 6	
Ovulation of primary oocytes	2	−7 to +5
Oviductal oocytes		
Resumption of meiosis	3	
Extrusion of first polar body	4	−4 to +7
Sperm penetration	3 to 9	0 to 7
Fertilization/pronucleus formation	4 to 9	0 to 7
Loss of unfertilized ova	6 to 9	
Two-cell embryo	6 to 10	1 to 12
Loss of vaginal crenulation	6 to 10	0 to 9
Reduced vaginal cornification	6 to 10	
Return of leukocytes to vaginal smear	5 to 13	
Morulae (8–16 cells) seen in oviduct	8 to 10	
Blastocyst (32–64 cells) entry into uterus	9 to 11	3 to 14
Intracornual migration (1-mm blastocysts)	10 to 13	
Transcornual migration (2-mm blastocysts)	12 to 15	
Attachment sites established, zonae pellucidae shed	16 to 18	9 to 21
Swelling of implantation sites, primitive streak formation	17 to 19	9 to 22
Ultrasound detection of amniotic cavities	19 to 22	10 to 25
Palpable uterine swellings 1 cm in diameter	20 to 25	12 to 28
Ultrasound of fetal heartbeat	22 to 25	13 to 28
Onset of pregnancy anemia	25 to 30	
Uterine swellings detectable by radiography	30 to 32	
Reduced palpability of 3-cm swelling	32 to 34	26 to 38
Hematocrit below 40% PCV	38 to 40	30 to 43
Hematocrit below 35% PCV	48 to 50	40 to 53
Fetal skull and spine radiopaque	44 to 46	36 to 49
Radiographic diagnosis of pregnancy	45 to 48	38 to 50
Fetal pelvis becomes radiopaque	53 to 57	45 to 60
Fetal teeth radiopaque	58 to 61	50 to 64
Prepartum luteolysis and hypothermia	63 to 65	55 to 68
Parturition	64 to 66	57 to 69

*Conservative estimates based on published and unpublished observations.
†Based on fertile single matings from 3 days before to 9 days after the LH peak.

large numbers of neutrophils in the smear. The influx of neutrophils is not as good an indicator as the epithelial cell shift in that the former may occur earlier or much later or may not be particularly prominent or abrupt.

Other epithelial cells may be observed in addition to typical parabasals, small intermediates, large intermediates, and partly or fully cornified superficials. One is the metestrum cell. These are small or large intermediate cells containing one or more neutrophils as inclusions. Metestrum cells are most commonly seen in smears obtained during early metestrus, but may also be seen in anestrus or early proestrus smears, and are therefore not diagnostic of metestrus. Foam cells are epithelial cells with multiple cytoplasmic vacuoles and a foamy appearance. These are also most often encountered during metestrus, but are not specific to metestrus, and may be seen during anestrus.

Individual smears obtained during early or mid-proestrus, without benefit of prior smears, vaginoscopy, or genital examination, can often appear like a smear obtained during the aforementioned late-estrus/early-metestrus transition and, thereby, cause confusion in interpretation. At both times, there can be a similar mixture of superficial and nonsuperficial cells, and moderate numbers of both erythrocytes and white blood cells. Vaginoscopy and vulvar examination usually resolves the confusion.

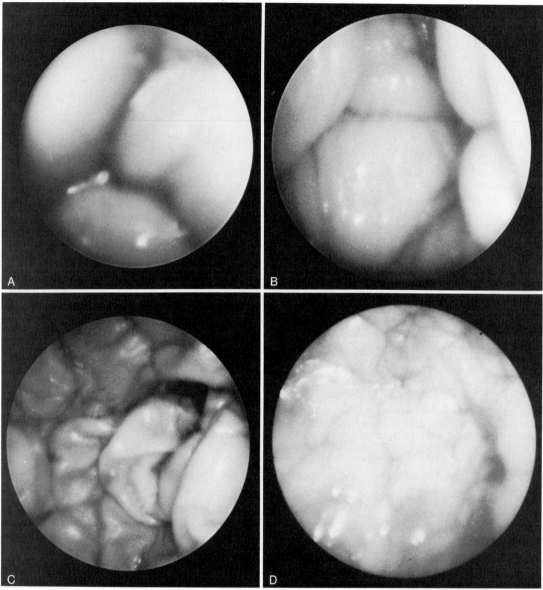

Figure 7. Endoscopic views of canine vaginal mucosal folds. *A*, Large, round, pink to white edematous folds normally seen during proestrus period of increasing estrogen levels; absence of wrinkles; a crenulation score of 0. *B*, Initial wrinkling of surface of large round folds, normally seen shortly before or during the preovulatory LH surge, and prior to ovulation, as estrogen levels decline; score of 2 to 4. *C*, Extensive wrinkling, sacculation, and angulation of mucosa normally observed 2 days after the LH peak, around the time of ovulation; crenulation score of 6. Maximum angulation (score of 8 to 10) and sharpness of peaks, which normally occur during oocyte maturation, about 4 days after the LH peak. *D*, Low, flat mucosa devoid of large wrinkles, with patchy red and white areas on the surface, normally seen at the end of vaginal estrus, 7 to 10 days after the LH peak, during the termination of the period of fertility; crenulation score of 0. (Adapted from Lindsay, F.E.F., and Concannon, P.W.: Normal canine vaginoscopy. *In* Burke, T. [ed.]: *Small Animal Reproduction and Infertility.* Philadelphia: Lea & Febiger, 1986, pp. 112–120.)

Vaginoscopy

During proestrus and estrus, there are obvious and dramatic changes in the gross appearance of the vaginal mucosa, as initially reported by Lindsay (1983). Recent observations demonstrate that the changes can be assessed using either a small-diameter (5-mm) fiberoptic endoscope or a nonoptical pediatric/stricture proctoscope that is 11 mm in diameter (Lindsay and Concannon, 1986). In con-

trast to the situation with vaginal cytology, the gross changes in the vaginal mucosa immediately before and after ovulation are sufficiently consistent in extent and timing to provide a reliable indicator of the onset of the period of fertility. In addition, there is an abrupt change at the end of "vaginal" estrus that corresponds to the late-estrus shift seen in vaginal smears.

The changes observed in the vaginal mucosa surface begin with the enlargement and edema of mucosal folds that occurs during the rise in estrogen throughout most of proestrus. There then begins a progressive loss of edema and concomitant development of an increasingly wrinkled surface during the preovulatory fall in estrogen and the rise in progesterone associated with the LH surge. Maximum wrinkling, or crenulation, and development of angulated folds that have sharp profiles are observed in the interval between ovulation and oocyte maturation. A few days later, around 7 to 8 days after the LH peak and toward the end of the period of fertility, there is an abrupt thinning and flattening of the mucosa over 1 to 3 days, resulting in a low, flaccid mucosa. The mucosa has a patchy, or variegated, appearance characteristic of metestrus, with some of the surface slightly thickened and white, and some thin and red. In contrast, during anestrus, the mucosa is extremely thin, red and fragile. It is during anestrus that the mucosa is most readily traumatized and apt to hemorrhage during a vaginoscopic examination. A typical pattern of edema and wrinkling of vaginal mucosal folds is shown schematically in relation to other periovulatory events in Figure 3. Shown in Figure 6 are the actual mean scores obtained for crenulation of the vaginal mucosa quantitated daily in a group of 18 bitches along with vaginal smears and in relation to the day of the preovulatory LH peak. Examples of the endoscopic appearance of the vaginal mucosa are shown in Figure 7.

Vaginal Electrical Resistance

In cattle, and in arctic foxes bred for fur production, changes in the electrical resistance of the vaginal mucosa in relation to the period of fertility have been extensively studied. The method involves vaginal insertion of a hand-operated, battery-operated resistometer and recording of day-to-day changes in the electrical resistance of the vaginal mucus (VMER) on the surface of the vaginal epithelium. The instrument and the technique originally employed in the application of the method to artificial insemination in foxes have recently been evaluated in bitches in relation to changes in progesterone and vaginal cytology (Gunzel et al., 1986). Those results suggest that, in dogs, the VMER progressively increases throughout the proestrus rise in estrogen levels, and that it stops increasing around the time of the preovulatory LH surge, decline in estrogen, and rise in progesterone. The VMER remains elevated during the fertile period of estrus and rapidly falls at about 7 to 9 days after the LH peak (i.e., at the time of the shift in the vaginal smear from an estrus to a metestrus appearance). When vaginal probes are further developed and marketed for use in dogs, the methodology is likely to become a routine adjunct to other observations in facilities providing breeding management.

References and Supplemental Reading

Bowen, R. A., Olson, P. N., Behrendt, M. D., et al.: The efficacy and toxicity of estrogens commonly used to terminate canine pregnancy. J.A.V.M.A. 186:783, 1985.

Brown, J.: Efficacy and dose titration study of mibolerone for treatment of pseudopregnancy in the bitch. J.A.V.M.A. 184:1467, 1984.

Chakraborty, P.: Reproductive hormone concentrations during estrus, pregnancy and pseudopregnancy in the Labrador bitch. Theriogenology 27:827, 1987.

Chastain, C. B., and Schmidt, B.: Galactorrhea associated with hypothyroidism in intact bitches. J. Am. Anim. Hosp. Assoc. 16:851, 1980.

Concannon, P. W.: Effects of hypophysectomy and of LH administration on luteal phase plasma progesterone levels in the Beagle bitch. J. Reprod. Fertil. 58:407, 1980.

Concannon, P. W.: Canine pregnancy and parturition. Vet. Clin. North Am. [Small Anim. Pract.] 16:453, 1986a.

Concannon, P. W.: Physiology and endocrinology of canine pregnancy. In Morrow, D. (ed.): Current Therapy in Theriogenology, Vol. II. Philadelphia: W. B. Saunders Co., 1986b, pp. 491–497.

Concannon, P. W.: Canine physiology of reproduction. In Burke, T. (ed.): Small Animal Reproduction and Infertility. Philadelphia: Lea & Febiger, 1986c, pp. 23–77.

Concannon, P. W.: The physiology of ovarian cycles, pregnancy and parturition in the domestic dog. Proceedings of the Society of Theriogenology, Austin, Texas, 1987. Hastings, NE: Society for Theriogenology, 1987, pp. 1–39.

Concannon, P. W., and DiGregorio, G. B.: Canine vaginal cytology. In Burke, T. (ed.): Small Animal Reproduction and Infertility. Philadelphia: Lea & Febiger, 1986, pp. 96–111.

Concannon, P. W., and Hansel, W.: Prostaglandin $F_{2\alpha}$-induced leutolysis, hypothermia and abortion in beagle bitches. Prostaglandins 13:533, 1977.

Concannon, P. W., and Rendano, V.: Radiographic diagnosis of pregnancy: The onset of fetal skeletal radiopacity in relation to times of breedings, preovulatory LH release, and parturition. Am. J. Vet. Res. 44:1819, 1983.

Concannon, P. W., Cowan, R. G., and Hansel, W.: LH release in ovariectomized dogs in response to estrogen withdrawal and its facilitation by progesterone. Biol. Reprod. 20:523, 1979.

Concannon, P. W., Hansel, W., and McEntee, K.: Changes in LH, progesterone and sexual behavior associated with preovulatory luteinization in the bitch. Biol. Reprod. 17:604, 1972.

Concannon, P. W., Hansel, W., and Visek, W.: The ovarian cycle of the bitch: Plasma estrogen, LH and progesterone. Biol. Reprod. 12:112, 1975.

Concannon, P. W., Powers, M. E., Holder, W., et al.: Pregnancy and parturition in the bitch. Biol. Reprod. 16:517, 1977.

Concannon, P. W., Weinstein, R., Whaley, S., and Frank, D.: Suppression of luteal function in dogs by luteinizing hormone antiserum and by bromocriptine. J. Reprod. Fertil. 81:175–180, 1987.

Concannon, P. W., Whaley, S., Lein, D., et al.: Canine gestation length: Variation related to time of mating and fertile life of sperm. Am. J. Vet. Res. 44:1819, 1983.

Concannon, P. W., Butler, W. R., Hansel, W., et al.: Parturition and lactation in the bitch: Serum progesterone, cortisol and prolactin. Biol. Reprod. 19:1113, 1978.

Concannon, P. W., Whaley, S., and Anderson, S. P.: Increased LH pulse frequency associated with termination of anestrus during the ovarian cycle of the dog. Biol. Reprod. 34:119, 1986 (abstract).

DeCoster, R., Beckers, J. F., Beerens, D., et al.: A homologous radioimmunoassay for canine prolactin: Plasma levels during the reproductive cycle. Acta Endocrinol. 109:473, 1983.

Eigenmann, J. E.: Diabetes mellitus in elderly female dogs: Recent findings on pathogenesis and clinical implications. J. Am. Anim. Hosp. Assoc. 17:805, 1981.

Fernandez, P., Bowen, R., Nett, T., et al.: Regulation of luteal function in the bitch: Changes in LH and prolactin receptor numbers and in pituitary concentration of LH, FSH and prolactin during diestrus. Biol. Reprod. 34:130, 1986.

Gunzel, A., Koivisto, P., and Fougner, J.: Electrical resistance of vaginal secretion in the bitch. Theriogenology 25:559, 1986.

Holst, P. A., and Phemister, R. D.: Temporal sequence of events in the estrous cycle of the bitch. Am. J. Vet. Res. 36:705, 1975.

Linde, C., and Karlsson, I.: The correlation between the cytology of the vaginal smear and the time of ovulation in the bitch. J. Small Anim. Pract. 25:77, 1984.

Lindsay, F. E. F.: The normal endoscopic appearance of the caudal reproductive tract of the cyclic and non-cyclic bitch: Post-uterine endoscopy. J. Small Anim. Pract. 24:1, 1983.

Lindsay, F. E. F.: Endoscopy of the reproductive tract in the bitch. In Kirk, R. W. (ed.): Current Veterinary Therapy, Small Animal Practice, Vol. VIII. Philadelphia: W. B. Saunders Co., 1983, pp. 912–921.

Lindsay, F. E. F., and Concannon, P. W.: Normal canine vaginoscopy. In Burke, T. (ed.): Small Animal Reproduction and Infertility. Philadelphia: Lea & Febiger, 1986, pp. 112–120.

McCann, J. P., Altszuler, N., Hampshire, J., et al.: Growth hormone, insulin, glucose, cortisol, luteinizing hormone, and diabetes in beagle bitches treated with medroxyprogesterone acetate. Acta Endocrinol. (Copenh.) 116:73, 1987.

Nett, T. M., and Olson, P. N.: Reproductive physiology of dogs and cats. In Ettinger, S. J. (ed.): Textbook of Veterinary Internal Medicine, Vol. 2, 2nd ed. Philadelphia: W. B. Saunders Co., 1983, p. 1698.

Okkens, A. C., Bevers, M. M., Dieleman, S. J., et al.: Shortening of the interoestrous interval and the lifespan of the corpus luteum of the cyclic dog by bromocriptine treatment. Vet. Q. 7:173, 1985.

Olson, P. N., Bowen, R. A., Behrendt, M. D., et al.: Concentrations of reproductive hormones in canine serum throughout late anestrus, proestrus and estrus. Biol. Reprod. 27:1196, 1982.

Olson, P. N., Bowen, R. A., Behrendt, M. D., et al.: Concentrations of testosterone in canine serum during late anestrus, proestrus, estrus and early diestrus. Am. J. Vet. Res. 45:145, 1984a.

Olson, P. N., Bowen, R. A., Behrendt, M. D., et al.: Validation of radioimmunoassays to measure prostaglandins $F_{2\alpha}$ and E_2 in canine endometrium and plasma. Am. J. Vet. Res. 45:119, 1984b.

Olson, P. N., Bowen, R. A., Behrendt, M. D., et al.: Concentrations of progesterone and luteinizing hormone in the serum of diestrous bitches before and after hysterectomy. Am. J. Vet. Res. 45:149, 1984c.

Olson, P. N., Thrall, M. A., Wykes, P. M., et al.: Vaginal cytology. Part 1. A useful tool for staging the canine estrous cycle. Compend. Cont. Ed. 6:288, 1984d.

Paradis, M., Post, K., and Mapletoft, R.: Effects of prostaglandin $F_{2\alpha}$ on corpora lutea formation and function in mated bitches. Can. Vet. J. 24:239, 1983.

Phemister, R. D., Holst, P. A., Spano, J. S., et al.: Time of ovulation in the Beagle bitch. Biol. Reprod. 8:74, 1973.

Reimers, T., Phemister, R., and Niswender, G.: Radioimmunological measurement of follicle-stimulating hormone and prolactin in the dog. Biol. Reprod. 19:673, 1978.

Rendano, V., Lein, D., and Concannon, P. W.: Radiographic evaluation of prenatal development in the beagle: Correlation with times of breeding, LH release and parturition. Vet. Radiol. 25:132, 1978.

Richkind, M.: Possible use of early urine for detection of pregnancy in dogs. Vet. Med. Small Anim. Clin. 78:1067, 1983.

Roszel, J. F.: Genital cytology of the bitch. Vet. Scope 19:3, 1975.

Shille, V. M., and Stabenfeldt, G. H.: Current concepts in reproduction of the dog and cat. Adv. Vet. Sci. Comp. Med. 24:211, 1980.

Shille, V., Thatcher, M., and Lloyd, M.: Concentrations of LH and FSH during selected periods of anestrus in the bitch. Biol. Reprod. 36:184, 1987.

Smith, M. S., and McDonald, L. E.: Serum levels of luteinizing hormone and progesterone during the estrous cycle, pseudopregnancy and pregnancy in the dog. Endocrinology 94:404, 1974.

Steinetz, B., Goldsmith, L., and Lust, G.: Plasma relaxin levels in pregnant and lactating dogs. Biol. Reprod. 37:719, 1987.

Vanderlip, S., Wing, A., Linke, D., et al.: Ovulation induction in anestrous bitches by pulsatile administration of gonadotropin-releasing hormone (GnRH). Lab. Anim. Sci. 37:459, 1987.

Wildt, D., Seager, S., and Chakraborty, P.: Behavioral, ovarian and endocrine relationships in the pubertal bitch. J. Anim. Sci. 53:182, 1981.

DYNAMIC TESTING IN REPRODUCTIVE ENDOCRINOLOGY

VICTOR M. SHILLE, D.V.M., Ph.D.,
Gainesville, Florida

and PATRICIA N. OLSON, D.V.M., Ph.D.
Fort Collins, Colorado

Hormones are frequently measured in the blood of dogs and cats in an attempt to diagnose a variety of reproductive disorders. Measuring a hormone in a single blood sample (usually serum) can be useful. For example, an elevated concentration of progesterone in a single sample following estrus in the bitch or following mating in the cat often indicates ovulation. However, generally, evaluating basal concentrations of hormones in single serum samples is not sufficiently informative to make diagnoses, and repetitive sampling or challenge testing needs to be done. With repetitive sampling, hormones can be measured and the pattern of release (frequency and amplitude of pulses) can be determined. With challenge testing, a substance is administered that causes maximal release or maximal suppression of the hormone being measured.

The hormone concentrations stated in this article are taken from the original research data of several authors, as referenced, and may be used as general guidelines. However, for specific clinical cases, the individual veterinarian should rely on reference values provided by the testing laboratory for the species to be evaluated.

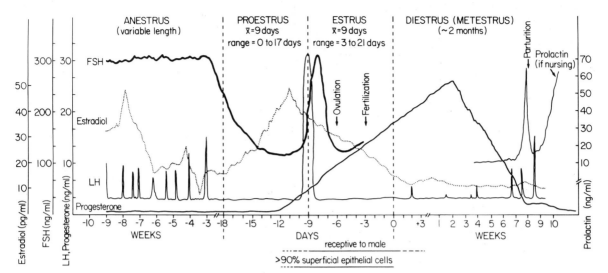

Figure 1. Hormone profiles during the canine estrous cycle. (Reprinted with permission from Morrow D. A. [ed.]: *Current Therapy in Theriogenology*, 2nd ed. Philadelphia: W.B. Saunders Co., 1986, p. 466.)

Gonadal steroids (progesterone, testosterone, estradiol) have the same molecular structure in all species. Therefore, samples from different species may be assayed using an antibody that is specific for the steroid to be measured and does not bind significantly to other steroids with similar structures. However, some species-specific interference with antibody binding may occur, so it is essential to validate the assay with reference samples from the species that is being evaluated. Rapid methods (overnight) for analyzing gonadal steroids are available and reliable but require a laboratory with specialized equipment and trained personnel. Simplified, rapid (less than 2 hr) "animal-side" tests, modified to assay hormones in canine serum, may soon be available for office use by the small animal veterinarian.

The structures of gonadotropins (follicle-stimulating hormone, FSH; luteinizing hormone, LH) are specific for each species. Thus, it is necessary to have antibodies and labeled antigens that accurately measure the FSH and LH of the species that is being evaluated. It is difficult to obtain adequate quantities of purified canine and feline gonadotropins for production of homologous antibody or labeled antigen. It is fortunate that antibodies may occasionally be induced to cross-react with gonadotropins of several species so that heterologous assay systems can be developed. Because of these difficulties, there are only a few laboratories that have validated assays for canine and feline gonadotropins. Techniques to develop monoclonal antibodies against canine or feline gonadotropins may allow specific assays to be developed in the future. As more laboratories are able to measure gonadotropins, patterns of gonadotropin release related to specific infertility syndromes in dogs and cats will

be determined and will provide a framework for diagnosis and therapy.

MEASURING HORMONES IN A SINGLE SERUM SAMPLE

Progesterone

Concentrations of progesterone rapidly increase in the serum of estrous bitches and are elevated above 2 ng/ml for approximately 2 months following estrus in healthy nonpregnant and pregnant bitches (Fig. 1). Concentrations of progesterone during the first 3 weeks following estrus may fluctuate, with concentrations of 10 to 50 ng/ml anticipated on day 15 of diestrus (Olson et al., 1987). Hence, measuring progesterone in a single sample obtained during diestrus may allow one to confirm that ovulation occurred in the bitch, although values may vary greatly among individual animals.

Concentrations of progesterone are also elevated in the serum of diestrous queens following adequate coital stimulation and ovulation. In 12 cats mated to vasectomized males, the first elevation of progesterone above 1 ng/ml was observed about 24 hr after ovulation or 2 days after mating (Shille and Stabenfeldt, 1979). Concentrations rose rapidly, reaching 8 ng/ml on day 5 and peaking at 17 ng/ml on day 18 after coitus. The end of the individual luteal phase was characterized by a gradual decline of progesterone to less than 2 ng/ml. The duration of the nonpregnant luteal phases ranged from 30 to 46 days (Shille and Stabenfeldt, 1979) or 50 days (Verhage et al., 1976) after mating. Levels remain elevated for a longer period in the pregnant queen than in the pseudopregnant queen as a result of the

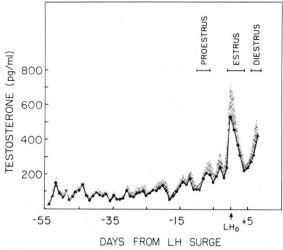

Figure 2. Mean serum concentrations of testosterone in 6 mature bitches during late anestrus, proestrus, estrus, and early diestrus (shaded area = SEM; solid line = range for onset of proestrus, estrus, and diestrus for 6 bitches; LH_0 = day of LH surge). (Reprinted with permission from Olson, P. N., et al.: Am. J. Vet. Res. 45:145–148, 1984.)

production of progesterone by the feline placenta (Malassine and Ferre, 1979).

Testosterone

Concentrations of testosterone in the serum of anestrous bitches and neutered males are generally less than 0.2 ng/ml. Concentrations of serum testosterone in intact males generally range from 0.5 to 9.0 ng/ml (Olson et al., 1987). However, levels in intact males can vary as a result of episodic release of testosterone. Therefore, challenge testing (see later) may be more desirable to determine if Leydig's cells (interstitial cells) are present. Elevated concentrations of testosterone in a "neutered" male may suggest that testicular tissue is present in a nonscrotal location.

Elevated concentrations of testosterone in the serum of infertile bitches may indicate a disorder of sexual development in dogs (e.g., XX true hermaphroditism, male pseudohermaphroditism). Concentrations of testosterone are also elevated in normal bitches during proestrus and estrus (Olson et al., 1984), however, and may approach concentrations found in intact males (Fig. 2).

Estradiol

Although elevated concentrations of estradiol may be present in bitches with follicular cysts or luteinized follicular cysts, in bitches with granulosa cell tumors or in male dogs with functional testicular tumors, caution in overinterpreting a single serum sample assayed for estradiol is in order. Concentra-

tions of estradiol in serum are approximately a thousandfold less than progesterone or testosterone. Therefore, accurately measuring estradiol is more difficult. Even when daily serum samples are obtained from proestrous and estrous bitches, clearly elevated levels may be detected only for a day or two (Fig. 3).

REPETITIVE TESTING

Luteinizing Hormone

Repetitive sampling allows one to determine the magnitude and the frequency of hormone release. For example, blood samples obtained every 20 min from three intact and two castrated mature male dogs were assayed for testosterone and LH (DePalatis et al., 1978). Concentrations of testosterone in the serum of the intact dogs ranged from 0.4 to 6.0 ng/ml over a 24-hr period. LH levels varied from 0.2 to 12.0 ng/ml in the same animals. The interval between peaks of LH (peaks defined as an elevation in which the percentage change from nadir to maximum was at least 25 per cent) was 103.4 ± 14.2 min (n = 17) in the light period and 86.9 ± 8.2 min (n = 23) in the dark period. Corresponding intervals for testosterone peaks were 111.4 ± 12 and 90.0 ± 9.2 min. Although concentrations of testosterone in the serum of the two castrated dogs were below the assay sensitivity, concentrations of LH were high (9.8 ± 2.7 ng/ml), presumably because of lack of negative feedback by gonadal steroids (DePalatis et al., 1978). In another study, concentrations of LH in the serum of nine intact greyhounds bled seven times at 10-min intervals were less than 20 ng/ml in 51 of 63 samples (Freshman et al., 1987). Conversely, serum samples assayed from castrated dogs frequently had concentrations of LH exceeding 30 ng/ml when measured in the same assay system (Olson et al., 1987).

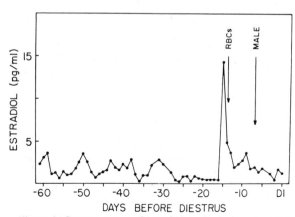

Figure 3. Concentrations of estradiol in the serum of a bitch bled daily during late anestrus, proestrus, estrus, and early diestrus. Note the brief period when levels are elevated.

As demonstrated, concentrations of LH in blood samples from intact and castrated male dogs can overlap. Therefore, obtaining three samples at 20-min intervals may be necessary to differentiate levels found in intact dogs from those in castrated dogs. Such a distinction might prove useful in dogs with no scrotal testes and normal-sized or enlarged prostates (suggesting the presence of androgens) that present with questionable histories concerning castration. Although repetitive sampling is more likely to distinguish between normal intact dogs and castrated dogs than measuring hormones in a single sample, such sampling can be expensive for the client.

Concentrations of LH in the serum of bitches that have been ovariohysterectomized for several months are often above 30 ng/ml. Levels above 30 ng/ml can also be observed in intact bitches during the preovulatory LH surge or occasionally during diestrus (Olson et al., 1984b; Chakraborty et al., 1978), anestrus (Olson et al., 1982; Shille et al., 1987), and early proestrus (Wildt et al., 1978). Elevated concentrations can also be present in intact bitches with ovarian dysplasia (Johnston et al., 1985).

Repetitive sampling for determining concentrations of LH in canine serum may also be useful in male dogs with azoospermia. If peak concentrations or frequency of release is depressed, the infertility may be due to pituitary or hypothalamic malfunction rather than a primary gonadal problem.

Follicle-stimulating Hormone

Elevations in serum concentrations of FSH may correlate with the severity of altered spermatogenesis in dogs (Freshman et al., 1988). Increased levels of FSH in serum may reflect decreased reproduction of germ cells, since production of inhibin by Sertoli's cells decreases when spermatogenesis fails. Hence, as negative feedback by inhibin is reduced, concentrations of FSH increase in serum (Table 1). A second possibility is that the increased levels of FSH in serum are the result of pituitary malfunction. Follicle-stimulating hormone (intact molecule or subunits) is frequently produced by gonadotropin cell adenomas in men with hypogonadism (Snyder, 1987). Because many azoospermic dogs have normal concentrations of testosterone and normal-to-elevated concentrations of LH and FSH in serum, it seems unlikely that treating dogs with either of these gonadotropins will improve their fertility.

Concentrations of FSH are also higher in castrated dogs than in healthy intact dogs. Therefore, measuring FSH may also aid in differentiating healthy intact dogs from castrated dogs. As with LH, concentrations of FSH can vary between individual animals. For example, mean concentrations

Table 1. *Concentrations of Hormones in Serum (ng/ml) from Dogs with Different Percentages of Normal Seminiferous Tubules and from Dogs with Testicular Neoplasia ($\bar{x} \pm SEM$)**

Grade (n = dogs)	FSH	LH	Testosterone
I (n = 17)	73 ± 7	34 ± 9	3 ± 0.5
II (n = 18)	84 ± 9	85 ± 32	3 ± 0.6
III (n = 21)	236 ± 49	96 ± 18	3 ± 0.7
IV (n = 14)	321 ± 58	95 ± 26	3 ± 0.6
ICT (n = 7)	237 ± 104	70 ± 32	5 ± 1.2
SCT (n = 2)	104 ± 23	44 ± 11	2 ± 0.6
or SEM (n = 4)			

Grade I	All tubules show active spermatogenesis.
Grade II	Some or all tubules show depression or arrest of spermatogenesis at various stages or a diminished number of germ cells. No tubules show a complete absence of germ cells.
Grade III	Some but not all tubules show a complete absence of germ cells and contain only Sertoli's cells.
Grade IV	Germ cells are absent from all tubules examined, and they contain only Sertoli's cells.

ICT, interstitial cell tumor; SCT, Sertoli's cell tumor; SEM, seminoma.

*(From Freshman, J. L., Amann, R. P., Bowen, R. A., Soderberg, S. F., et al: Clinical evaluation of infertility in the dog. Comp. Cont. Ed. 10:443, 1988.)

of FSH in nine normal male greyhounds bled at 10-min intervals for 1 hr prior to placement in a research investigation are listed in Table 2 (Freshman et al., 1987).

Concentrations of FSH in the serum of intact bitches vary during the estrous cycle. Mean concentrations were low at 30 days postpartum in seven bitches and increased significantly after 150 days (from 12 to 35 ng/ml) (Shille et al., 1987). In six postpubertal bitches, mean FSH concentrations were also highest in late anestrus (240 to 294 ng/ml) and again near the time of the LH surge (297 ng/ml), whereas lower concentrations were present during proestrus (131 to 200 ng/ml) (Olson et al., 1982). The difference between the absolute values reported by the two investigators are not unusual and illustrate the need for reference values for each laboratory.

Table 2. *Concentrations ($\bar{x} \pm SD$) of FSH (ng/ml) in the Serum of Nine Intact Greyhound Males (Bled at 10-Min Intervals for 1 Hr)*

Dog Number	Mean Concentration (SD)
1	62(4)
2	80(8)
3	293(17)
4	99(3)
5	60(4)
6	109(4)
7	66(3)
8	67(3)
9	99(6)

Progesterone

In the bitch, serum progesterone concentrations rise above 1 ng/ml shortly before, at, or immediately after the preovulatory LH surge that precedes ovulation (Concannon et al., 1977). Thus, it becomes possible to estimate the time of ovulation and relative vigor of luteal activity by repetitive measuring of serum progesterone. A series of blood samples is taken starting when signs of proestrus (serosanguineous vaginal discharge and vulvar edema) are noted. Analysis of progesterone may be done immediately in each sample so that the bitch can be mated at an optimal time. However, assay of many individual samples is expensive. More commonly, blood samples are collected during proestrus and estrus. The serum is stored frozen and analyzed retrospectively only if necessary (i.e., after it is determined that the bitch has failed to become pregnant). Retrospective analysis aids in detection of discrepancies between hormonal events and behavioral or cytologic estrus. It also allows estimation of the activity of corpora lutea and relates time of mating to time of ovulation. In order to rapidly and inexpensively estimate the best time for breeding during the monitored cycle, vaginal smears need to be collected for cytologic evaluation, coincidentally with collection of blood samples (see later).

Luteal competence during pregnancy may be monitored by taking blood samples once weekly until parturition, or for about 9 weeks after mating. Again, the serum samples may be stored and the expense for analysis incurred only if pregnancy does not occur or is interrupted.

Estradiol

Estradiol is the major estrogen produced by the ovarian follicle and, as such, should be suitable for monitoring folliculogenesis. However, it is found in serum concentrations that fluctuate rapidly and are at or below detectable limits for many laboratories. Accurate measurements are therefore difficult, even when repeated sampling is done. In addition, studies in some primate species have shown that patterns of total estrogen metabolites may be more biologically meaningful than patterns of estradiol (Hodges et al., 1979). Until the question of the significance of serum estradiol is resolved in the bitch and the queen, a simple, practical method of estimating estrogen activity is to observe its effects on the vaginal epithelium.

The vaginal epithelium of the bitch and the queen responds to estrogen by proliferation and, as layers accumulate, with cornification. The response is specific and dose-dependent and forms the basis for a reliable bioassay for estrogen. Relative amounts of cornified exfoliated vaginal epithelial cells may be used to estimate amounts of serum estrogen during proestrus and estrus in the healthy cyclic bitch, as well as to diagnose elevated estrogen from abnormal ovarian cysts, granulosa cell tumors, or extraovarian sources. Since the technique is noninvasive and does not require special instrumentation, it lends itself to repetitive sampling and may be used to detect the best time for mating. Techniques and interpretation of findings have been described previously (Olson et al., 1984).

Vaginal Cytology and Serum Progesterone for Staging the Fertile Period

To judge the adequacy of ovarian function and to ascertain that mating is taking place at the appropriate time in the estrous cycle, a series of coincident vaginal smears and blood samples may be collected and evaluated for estrogen and progesterone activity, respectively (Table 3) (Shille and Thatcher, unpublished observations).

Starting with the first few days after proestrus is shown, vaginal smears and venous blood samples are taken three times weekly until noncornified cells reappear on the vaginal smear (diestrus day 1), usually a period of three weeks. Generally, the earliest peak cornification of the vaginal epithelium, as shown by a high proportion of superficial cells (nucleated and anucleated), is related to levels of serum progesterone compatible with ovulation (Table 3) (Shille and Thatcher, unpublished observations; Linde and Karlsson, 1984). Thus, the vaginal cytology data may be used in day-to-day decisions about optimal mating time for the bitch, and serum progesterone values may be used to confirm time of ovulation. Note that serum estradiol values are less informative than cytology or progesterone data (Table 3).

CHALLENGE TESTING

Concentrations of hormones in blood vary throughout the day, depending on the magnitude and the frequency of their release. Therefore, basal concentrations overlap between normal animals and animals with reproductive disorders or between intact animals and castrated animals. Through administering a substance that maximally stimulates an endocrine gland to release the hormone in question, reproductive disorders may be identified or intact animals can be distinguished from castrated ones.

Human Chorionic Gonadotropin Challenge Test

Concentrations of serum testosterone may be measured prior to and following the administration

Table 3. *Progressive Cornification of Exfoliated Vaginal Epithelium Correlated to Serum Progesterone, Estradiol-17beta, and Sexual Behavior in a Bitch**

Estimated Day of Diestrus	Proportion of Epithelial Cell Types (%)				Serum Progesterone (ng/ml)	Serum Estradiol-17beta (pg/ml)	Sexual Behavior
	Parabasal	*Intermediate*	*Superficial*	*Anuclear*			
−17	56	35	9	0	0.1	39	Attractive
−14	7	80	8	5	0.6	48	Attractive
−12	0	21	56	23	0.3	53	Attractive
−10	0	15	63	22	1.4	46	Attractive
−7	0	2	52	46	4.9†	49	Receptive
−5	0	0	42	58	13.4	58	Receptive
−3	0	4	55	41	32.7	27	Receptive
−1	0	5	48	57	51.4	23	Receptive
+2	22	46	27	5	43.1	12	No sexual behavior

*Samples were taken three times weekly. Day 1 is first day of diestrus.

†Progesterone concentration compatible with ovulation (see Wildt, D. E., Chakraborty, P. K., Danko, W. B., et al.: Biol. Reprod. 18:561–570, 1978).

of human chorionic gonadotropin (hCG). An hCG challenge test is indicated in male dogs or cats in which retained testicular tissue is suspected or in females in which a disorder in sexual differentiation is suspected (i.e., presence of ovotestes, testes). Johnston (1987) reported that serum testosterone concentrations were elevated in intact male dogs and cats (Table 4) following the administration of hCG or gonadotropin-releasing hormone (GnRH).

Queens and bitches that demonstrate signs of estrus after ovariohysterectomy may be tested for presence of functional ovarian tissue by inducing the presumed follicles to luteinize in response to hCG. The presence of elevated estrogen should be verified by finding cornified vaginal epithelial cells. Administration of hCG (50 to 100 IU, IM to the queen; 100 to 1000 IU, IM to the bitch) during the apparent estrous episode should result in elevation of progesterone levels above 1.0 ng/ml in 5 to 7 days, if functional ovarian tissue is present.

Lack of response to the hCG challenge in the presence of estrous behavior and cornification of exfoliated vaginal epithelium is compatible with an extraovarian source of estrogen. Such estrogen may come from exogenous administration or from the adrenal cortex. In pony mares that exhibited sexual behavior and elevated serum estrogen within a year

after ovariectomy, the syndrome was reversed by administration of an adrenal-suppressive dose of dexamethasone (Asa et al., 1980). The condition so far has not been proved to occur in ovariectomized dogs and cats. A false-negative response (no progesterone rise in the presence of ovarian tissue) is more likely to occur in the bitch than in the queen, since ovarian follicles in the bitch take longer to mature and may not be able to respond to hCG when the challenge is administered.

Gonadotropin-releasing Hormone Challenge Test

Gonadotropin-releasing hormone can be administered to animals to maximally stimulate maximal release of pituitary gonadotropins. If concentrations of the pituitary hormones increase in serum, concentrations of gonadal hormones will also increase.

Table 4. *Serum Testosterone Concentrations in Intact Male Dogs and Cats**

	Serum Testosterone (ng/ml)	
	Dogs (n = 6)	*Cats (n = 6)*
Resting concentrations	0.5–5.0	<0.05–3.0
4-hr post-hCG (20 μg/lb IM, dogs) (250 μg IM, cats)	4.6–7.5	3.1–9.0
1-hr post-GnRH 1 μg/lb IM, dogs) (25 μg IM, cats)	3.7–6.2	5.0–12.0

*(With permission from Johnston, S. D. AAHA proceedings, 54th Annual Meeting, March 21–27, 1987, Phoenix, Arizona.)

Table 5. *General Responses to Hormonal Stimulation*

Diagnosis	Administration of Hypothalamic Hormone	Administration of Pituitary Hormone
Hypothalamic failure	Pituitary response variable (usually delayed or absent); end-organ response dependent on pituitary and may require priming	End-organ will respond but may require priming
Pituitary failure	No pituitary response; no end-organ response	End-organ will respond but may require priming
End-organ failure	Exaggerated pituitary response; no end-organ response	No end-organ response

(From Schlaff, W. D.: Dynamic testing in reproductive endocrinology. Fertil. Steril. 45:589, 1986. Reproduced with permission of the publisher, The American Fertility Society.)

Falvo and coworkers (1982) demonstrated that administration of GnRH to dogs (50, 125, or 250 ng/kg IV) resulted in a prompt rise (5 to 10 min) in plasma concentrations of LH. Concentrations of LH in blood samples (serum) obtained 10 min after administering 250 ng/kg GnRH IV to four intact greyhounds ranged from 20.8 to 49.5 ng/ml (32 ± 11 ng/ml; n = 8) (Freshman et al., 1987). If repetitive sampling in unstimulated subjects shows no demonstrable release of gonadotropins, GnRH challenge testing may be useful to determine whether gonadotropins can be released after the administration of the hypothalamic hormone. Although not adequately evaluated in dogs or cats, such information has been helpful in identifying potential causes of reproductive failure in humans (Table 5).

Administering GnRH may also be useful in evaluating gonadal status. If pituitary function is optimal, administration of GnRH can replace hCG challenge testing (Table 4).

References and Supplemental Reading

Asa, C. S., Goldfoot, D. A., Garcia, M. C., et al.: Dexamethasone suppression of sexual behavior in the ovariectomized mare. Horm. Behav. 14:55, 1980.
Chakraborty, P. K., Panko, W. B., and Seager, S. W. J.: Hormone levels during the estrous cycle, pregnancy and pseudopregnancy in the Labrador bitch (abstract). Proceedings of the American Society of Animal Science 337:349, 1978.
Concannon, P. W., Hansel, W., and McEntee, K.: Changes in LH, progesterone and sexual behavior associated with preovulatory luteinization in the bitch. Biol. Reprod. 17:604, 1977.
DePalatis, L., Moore, J., and Falvo, R. E.: Plasma concentrations of testosterone and LH in the male dog. J. Reprod. Fertil. 52:201, 1978.
Falvo, R. E., Gerrity, M., Pirmann, J., et al.: Testosterone pretreatment and the response of pituitary LH to gonadotropin-releasing hormone (GnRH) in the male dog. J. Androl. 3:193, 1982.
Freshman, J. L., Amann, R. P., Bowen, R. A., et al.: Clinical evaluation of infertility in the dog. Comp. Cont. Ed. 10:443, 1988.

Freshman, J. L., Olson, P. N., Carlson, E. D., et al.: Effects of methyltestosterone on reproduction in male greyhounds. Proceedings of the ACVIM 5th Annual Forum, San Diego, CA, 1987, p. 917.
Hodges, J. K., Czekala, N. M., and Lasley, B. L.: Estrogen and luteinizing hormone secretion in diverse primate species from simplified urinary analysis. J. Med. Primatol. 8:349, 1979.
Johnston, S. D.: Reproductive disorders: Diagnostic endocrinology. Proceedings of the 54th Annual Meeting of the American Animal Hospital Association, Phoenix, AZ, 1987, p. 184.
Johnston, S. D., Buoen, L. C., Weber, A. F., et al.: X trisomy in an Airedale bitch with ovarian dysplasia and primary anestrus. Theriogenology 24:597, 1985.
Linde, C., and Karlsson, I.: The correlation between the cytology of the vaginal smear and the time of ovulation in the bitch. J. Small Anim. Pract. 25:77, 1984.
Malassine, A., and Ferre, F.: Δ5,3Β Hydroxysteroid dehydrogenase activity in cat placental labyrinth: Evolution during pregnancy, subcellular distribution. Biol. Reprod. 21:965, 1979.
Olson, P. N., Bowen, R. A., Behrendt, M. D., et al.: Concentrations of reproductive hormones in canine serum throughout late anestrus, proestrus and estrus. Biol. Reprod. 27:1196, 1982.
Olson, P. N., Bowen, R. A., Behrendt, M. D., et al.: Concentrations of testosterone in canine serum throughout late anestrus, proestrus, estrus and early diestrus. Am. J. Vet. Res. 45:145, 1984a.
Olson, P. N., Bowen, R. A., Behrendt, M. D., et al.: Concentrations of progesterone and LH in the serum of diestrous bitches before and after hysterectomy. Am. J. Vet. Res. 45:149, 1984b.
Olson, P. N., Nett, T. M., and Crowder, M. E.: Rothgerber Endocrinology Laboratory brochure, May 1987. Department of Physiology, Colorado State University, Fort Collins, CO.
Olson, P. N., Thrall, M. A., Wykes, P. M., et al.: Vaginal cytology. Part 1. A useful tool for staging the canine estrous cycle. Comp. Cont. Ed. Pract. Vet. 6:288, 1984.
Schlaff, W. D.: Dynamic testing in reproductive endocrinology. Fertil. Steril. 45:589, 1986.
Shille, V. M., and Stabenfeldt, G. H.: Luteal function in the domestic cat during pseudopregnancy and after treatment with prostaglandin F_{2alpha}. Biol. Reprod. 21:1217, 1979.
Shille, V. M., and Thatcher, M. J.: Unpublished observations.
Shille, V. M., Thatcher, M. J., and Lloyd, M. L.: Concentrations of LH and FSH during selected periods of anestrus in the bitch (abstract). Biol. Reprod. 36:184, 1987.
Snyder, P. M.: Pituitary adenomas and hypogonadism. In Proceedings of the American Society of Andrology, 12th Annual Meeting, Denver, CO, March 6–9, 1987, pp. 12–16.
Verhage, H. G., Beamer, N. B., and Brenner, R. M.: Plasma levels of estradiol and progesterone in the cat during polyestrus, pregnancy and pseudopregnancy. Biol. Reprod. 14:579, 1976.
Wildt, D. E., Chakraborty, P. K., Danko, W. B., et al.: Relationship of reproductive behavior, serum luteinizing hormone and time of ovulation in the bitch. Biol. Reprod. 18:561, 1978.

INDUCTION OF ESTRUS AND OVULATION IN THE BITCH

JANICE L. CAIN, D.V.M.

Vacaville, California

Methods of estrus induction are readily available for use in large animal medicine, but induction of estrus in bitches has not gained widespread use because of the unreliability of many proposed methods. Estrus may be induced to treat bitches that have a longer than average interestrous interval or are slow in returning to estrus after pharmacologic suppression. Estrus induction may also prove useful as a potential treatment of infertility resulting from prolonged anestrus (i.e., noncycling bitches) or silent heats (i.e., estrus not visibly detected). However, it should be emphasized that prior to utilizing hormonal intervention to treat an apparent problem, steps should be taken to determine the etiology of the infertility (e.g., endocrinologic disease, concurrent drug administration, mismanagement). Many protocols have been devised to induce estrus and ovulation in the bitch, but success has been inconsistent (described later). The unique reproductive physiology of the bitch and the difficulty encountered in attempting to mimic the natural sequence of hormonal events may explain the failure to develop a practical and reliable method of estrus induction. The final section of this article will discuss newer methods being devised to more reliably induce fertile estrus.

Generally, pituitary or hypothalamic hormones are utilized in an attempt to initiate follicular development. The administration of estradiol alone may indeed induce signs of proestrus (e.g., sanguineous vaginal discharge, swollen vulva), and possibly behavioral estrus, but exogenous sources of estradiol alone will not cause ovulation and subsequent pregnancy.

To objectively evaluate methods designed to induce estrus in the bitch, it is necessary to point out a few problems. Over 15 different studies of estrus induction have been reported in the literature—each with differing protocols and experimental designs. Some studies had access to bitches for which the reproductive history and therefore the probable stage of estrous cycle at the time of attempted induction were known. Other studies used prepuberal females or those with an unknown reproductive history. Various criteria were used to judge success, including (1) induction of behavioral estrus only, (2) evidence of ovulation by hormonal evaluation (i.e., serum progesterone concentration > 1 to 2 ng/ml) or visual appearance of ovaries via laparoscopy or necropsy, and (3) outcome of full-term pregnancy. It is also important to realize that some of the bitches used in these studies were presumed to be normal cycling bitches, whereas others were abnormal often because of longer than normal periods of anestrus. Overall, these factors make critical comparison of the different methods described difficult.

GONADOTROPIN INDUCTION OF ESTRUS

Reports recommend the use of pituitary gonadotropins for estrus induction. Some of these protocols have been reviewed (Feldman and Nelson, 1987) and involve the utilization of pregnant mare serum gonadotropin, a product containing both follicle-stimulating hormone (FSH) and luteinizing hormone (LH) bioactivity. Varying dosages and regimens of PMSG were used to induce follicular development and subsequent behavioral estrus. Al-though PMSG is not widely available, its use is of interest.

Most protocols consist of administering PMSG for 9 to 10 days, intramuscularly (IM) or subcutaneously (SC), at doses ranging from 20 to 44 IU/kg/day to 250 to 500 IU/day (Bell and Christie, 1971; Thun et al., 1977; Archbald et al., 1980). Once estrus was observed, or on day 9 or 10, a single IM or SC injection of human chorionic gonadotropin (hCG, Lypho-Med) was used at a dose of 500 IU/dog. Human chorionic gonadotropin also has FSH and LH activity, but the LH activity is greater than that of PMSG and, therefore, stimulates ovulation. Overall ovulation rates ranged from 50 to 83 per cent. All these studies considered ovulation an end point, and either the bitches were euthanized or information was not available on the diestrous phase of the induced cycle. Several subsequent investigations have determined that although ovulation rates may have been high with these methods, few dogs maintained normal corpus luteum (CL) function. It has been determined that bitches require a plasma progesterone concentration greater than 2.5 ng/ml, thus a functional CL, through day 56 of gestation to maintain pregnancy. In one study, bitches were thought to be pregnant by palpation at day 28; however, their progesterone concentrations were less than 1 ng/ml by day 50 postestrus, and they were not pregnant at that time (Renton et al., 1984). Archbald and coworkers (1984) administered megestrol acetate to bitches prior to estrus induction with PMSG/hCG, but all bitches had low (anestrous) plasma progesterone concentrations by 50 days postestrus.

Because of the unavailability of PMSG, some investigators attempted estrus induction by using pituitary origin FSH (F.S.H.-P., Schering) and LH (P.L.H., Burns-Biotec) in regimens designed to mimic endogenous release of the hormones. Overall, results have been disappointing. One study reported folliculogenesis followed by atresia of preovulatory follicles in each of ten bitches (Paisley and Fahning, 1977). Another study used FSH either by single injection of 10 mg IM, or in multiple doses: 1, 2, 4, 8, and 16 mg FSH on days 1 and 2, 3 and 4, 5 and 6, 7 and 8, and 9 and 10, respectively (Shille et al., 1984). Results indicated that four of nine bitches ovulated, but only one conceived and maintained pregnancy (single-injection protocol).

Other investigators attempted to use low-dose estradiol or estrone immediately preceding gonadotropin therapy, since estrogen may induce an increased response by the ovaries to gonadotropins. One study yielded impressive results, with six of seven pregnancies resulting from first a single injection of 30 to 30,000 μg of estrone IM, after which 200 to 400 IU PMSG and 1000 IU hCG were administered on the day of cessation of vaginal bleeding and again on the first day of estrus (Takeishi et al., 1976). Information was not available regarding the reproductive history of the bitches used (i.e., early versus late anestrus). Results were less reliable when diethylstilbestrol (DES, Lilly) was combined with an FSH-LH regimen as follows: (1) 1 mg DES is given PO daily for 4 days, (2) wait 4 days; (3) then administer 2 mg FSH SC b.i.d. until greater than 90 per cent of superficial epithelial cells are seen on vaginal cytology (maximum 10 days of FSH), and (4) 24 hr after maximal stimulation as determined by vaginal cytology, 500 IU hCG are given IV. Breeding was attempted 48 to 72 hr after hCG administration (Olson et al., 1983).

A study provided favorable results also using estrogen treatment prior to gonadotropin administration (Shille, 1987). This method used DES to induce proestrus followed by administration of LH first and then FSH. This protocol was evaluated in seven greyhound bitches that were treated as follows: DES 5 mg/day PO until proestrus was evident and then for 2 days thereafter. If no signs of proestrus were observed by day 7 of DES treatment, the dose was doubled (10 mg/day PO) until a response was elicited (not to exceed 7 additional days of DES therapy). On day 5 of proestrus, 5 mg of LH was injected IM, followed by 10 mg of FSH injected IM on days 9 and 11 of proestrus. Dogs were bred on day 13. This regimen resulted in seven of seven normal pregnancies. This method utilizes gonadotropin administration in a reverse sequence to that of other reported studies. The rationale for this sequence is based on the recognition that in spontaneous early proestrus, plasma LH concentration rises and plasma FSH concentration declines from late anestrus values (Olson et al., 1982). It should be noted that four of seven bitches had received testosterone (to suppress estrus while racing) 12 months prior to inclusion in the study and had remained in anestrus for the 12 months prior to DES treatment. The other three bitches were observed in estrus a minimum of 120 days prior to DES treatment (unknown maximum interval). Whether any of these bitches could have been on the verge of spontaneous estrus is unknown. However, a placebo-treated control group was also evaluated, and no estrous activity was observed. Interestingly, when the study was repeated using bitches that last received testosterone 30 or 150 days prior to attempted induction, none of five and one of three of the bitches responded to DES treatment, respectively. Many questions are raised by this study. For example, the actual biopotency of the gonadotropins used was not determined; therefore, it remains possible that the LH used contained FSH activity (much like PMSG). This method does suggest that a combination of exogenous estrogen followed by gonadotropin administration may succeed in inducing fertile estrus in the bitch; however, P.L.H. is currently unavailable.

GONADOTROPIN-RELEASING HORMONE

As in other endocrinologic systems, the pituitary-ovarian axis requires hypothalamic regulation. Gonadotropin-releasing hormone (GnRH), a decapeptide common to all mammals, is normally released from the hypothalamus in a pulsatile manner at a frequency of one pulse every 70 to 90 min. Many studies have demonstrated the ability of GnRH, administered by pulsatile infusion via a portable pump device, to restore fertility in humans with hypothalamic amenorrhea and hypothalamic hypogonadism. Pulsatile administration of GnRH has also been shown to induce estrus in seasonally anestrous mares. Theoretically, GnRH-induced release of endogenous gonadotropins provides a method of provocative ovarian stimulation that closely simulates normal reproductive endocrine physiology. The unique advantage to the use of exogenous GnRH rather than exogenous gonadotropins is the incorporation of physiologic feedback mechanisms to ensure that precise amounts of FSH and LH are released for folliculogenesis and ovulation.

Studies have been conducted to evaluate the use of GnRH to induce estrus in bitches. These studies utilized portable pump infusion devices (Pulsamat and Zyklomat, Ferring Laboratories, Ridgewood, NJ) to deliver measured amounts of GnRH in saline solution at a pulse frequency of one pulse every 90 min. The pumps were affixed to dogs by a harness and were attached to an aseptically placed jugular catheter. The apparatus was well tolerated by the dogs for the 11- to 12-day treatment period.

One study evaluated the administration of 1.25 µg GnRH every 90 min (0.14 µg/kg/pulse), for 11 to 12 days, to eight bitches (Cain et al., 1988). Seven of eight bitches ovulated, became pregnant, and maintained normal CL function (adequate plasma progesterone concentration) throughout gestation. It is of interest to note that one of the bitches was treated after 730 days of apparent anestrus. Estrus was observed 11 to 16 days after the initiation of GnRH infusion in the seven normal dogs, and after 23 days in the bitch with prolonged anestrus. This method was also successful in shortening the interestrous interval from an expected length of 219 ± 14 days (mean ± standard error of the mean [SEM]) to 148 ± 10 days (mean ± SEM) in six bitches.

Other investigators evaluated the effect of GnRH dose on ovulation and conception (Vanderlip et al., 1987). At a relatively high GnRH dose of 0.40 to 0.68 µg/kg/pulse, three of three bitches ovulated and two conceived. At a medium dose of 0.10 to 0.14 µg/kg/pulse, one of two bitches ovulated and conceived, while at a low dose of 0.04 to 0.08 µg/kg/pulse, two of three bitches ovulated and conceived. Interestingly, one bitch from each of the high-dose and low-dose groups had plasma progesterone concentrations indicative of ovulation 42 and 63 days, respectively, from the start of GnRH administration, whereas the other four bitches had similar rises in plasma progesterone concentration within 15 to 19 days. Whether these two dogs may have demonstrated spontaneous ovulation independent of treatment is unknown. It must be recognized that this study used small numbers of dogs in each treatment group.

A major objection to the utilization of the pulsatile GnRH method as opposed to the injectable gonadotropin methods previously described is the requirement of specialized equipment (i.e., infusion pumps). GnRH can be obtained commercially (GnRH, Ferring Laboratories, Ridgewood, NJ, or Cystorelin, Abbott Laboratories). No adverse reactions to GnRH administration have been observed, and no apparent problems have been recognized in subsequent estrous cycles, natural reproductive ability, or fertility (Cain et al., 1988).

In efforts to continually improve upon results and to seek the most efficient method both in terms of cost and labor, new methods utilizing GnRH are being evaluated. The use of smaller, disposable, less expensive continuous infusion pumps is being investigated. This method shows some indication of response even though it is contrary (continuous infusion) to what is known regarding natural GnRH release (pulsatile). The number of dogs that have been studied is small, but if an optimum successful dose could be determined, the use of an infusion method to induce estrus with GnRH may be widely utilized.

References and Supplemental Reading

Archbald, L. F., Ingraham, R. H., and Godke, R. A.: Inability of progestogen pretreatment to prevent premature luteolysis of induced corpora lutea in the anestrous bitch. Theriogenology 21:419, 1984.

Archbald, L. F., Baker, B. A., Clooney, L. L., et al.: A surgical method for collecting canine embryos after induction of estrus and ovulation with exogenous gonadotropins. Vet. Med. Small Anim. Clin. 75:228, 1980.

Bell, E. T., and Christie, D. W.: Gonadotropin-induced ovulation in the bitch. Proceedings of the VIIth World Congress on Fertility and Sterility, Amsterdam, 1971, pp. 598–599.

Cain, J. L., Cain, G. R., Feldman, E. C., et al.: Induction of fertile estrus in dogs: Use of pulsatile administration of gonadotropin-releasing hormone. A preliminary report. Am. J. Vet. Res. 1988 (in press).

Feldman, E. C., and Nelson, R. W.: Canine and Feline Endocrinology and Reproduction. Philadelphia: W. B. Saunders Co., 1987, pp. 465–466.

Olson, P. N., Nett, T. M., and Soderberg, S. F.: Infertility in the bitch. In Kirk, R. W. (ed.): Current Veterinary Therapy VIII. Philadelphia: W. B. Saunders Co., 1983, pp. 925–931.

Olson, P. N., Bowen, R. A., Behrendt, M. D., et al.: Concentrations of reproductive hormones in canine serum throughout late anestrus, proestrus, and estrus. Biol. Reprod. 27:1196, 1982.

Paisley, L. G., and Fahning, M. L.: Effects of exogenous follicle-stimulating hormone and luteinizing hormone in bitches. J.A.V.M.A. 171:181, 1977.

Renton, J. P., Harvey, M. J. A., and Eckersall, P. D.: Apparent pregnancy failure following mating of bitches at PMSG-induced oestrus. Vet. Rec. 115:383, 1984.

Shille, V. M.: Estrus induction in the bitch. Proceedings: Society of Theriogenology, Annual Meeting, Austin, TX, 1987.

Shille, V. M., Thatcher, M. J., and Simmons, J.: Efforts to induce estrus in the bitch, using pituitary gonadotropins. J.A.V.M.A. 184:1469, 1984.

Takeishi, M., Kodama, Y., Mikami, T., et al.: Studies on reproduction in the dog. XI: Induction of estrus by hormonal treatment and results of the following insemination. Jpn. J. Anim. Reprod. (English abstract). 22:71, 1976.

Thun, R., Watson, P., and Jackson, G. L.: Induction of estrus and ovulation in the bitch using exogenous gonadotropins. Am. J. Vet. Res. 38:483, 1977.

Vanderlip, S. L., Wing, A. E., Felt, P., et al.: Ovulation induction in anestrous bitches by pulsatile administration of gonadotropin-releasing hormone. Lab. Anim. Sci. 37:459, 1987.

EFFECTS OF DRUGS ON PREGNANCY

MARK G. PAPICH, D.V.M.
Saskatoon, Saskatchewan

The author thanks Dr. Patricia M. Blakley for her assistance in collecting material for this manuscript.

Drug administration to a pregnant animal is usually avoided. However, situations often arise that cause us to question the safety of drugs that may be indicated in pregnant patients. This article will investigate the use of drugs in pregnant animals and make recommendations for the use of drugs for specific conditions.

Ethical considerations prevent pharmaceutical companies from performing safety tests in pregnant women, and most drugs intended for use in people carry a disclaimer that states, "Not proven to be safe for use during pregnancy." A similar uncertainty exists for drugs administered to pregnant dogs and cats. If specific studies have demonstrated safety, those results are stated in the comments on Table 1. However, for most drugs, we must extrapolate from studies performed in laboratory animals or from the experience that has been reported in humans.

PHYSIOLOGIC ADAPTATIONS TO PREGNANCY BY THE MOTHER

The majority of research done on physiologic adaptations during pregnancy has been performed in humans, sheep, goats, and laboratory animals. It is unfortunate that there is very little information available in dogs and virtually none in cats. Nevertheless, from information collected in other animals, we have learned that during pregnancy changes in cardiac output, renal clearance, hepatic clearance, and volume of distribution may affect the concentration of a drug in the plasma. Studies in humans have demonstrated that dosages of anticonvulsants, digitalis, and antibiotics occasionally must be increased to provide therapeutic plasma concentrations for the mother (Krauer and Krauer, 1983).

In women, there is an increase in the cardiac output of 40 to 50 per cent and a subsequent increase in renal plasma flow and glomerular filtration rate associated with pregnancy. As a result, drugs eliminated via renal mechanisms are cleared faster. This is particularly true for polar, nonmetabolized antibiotics (e.g., penicillins, cephalosporins, aminoglycosides). There is also increased hepatic clearance for some drugs during pregnancy, probably caused by an increase in activity of the hepatic metabolizing enzymes (Nau et al., 1984). An increased concentration of circulating progesterone during pregnancy is the probable inducer of the hepatic enzymes, but experimental evidence is lacking. We cannot generalize for all drugs, but it has been shown, for example, that for anticonvulsants in women, plasma concentrations were sometimes lower during pregnancy as a result of increased hepatic clearance (Nau et al., 1984; Krauer and Krauer, 1983; Redmond, 1985).

An increase in the volume of distribution for a drug may be caused by decreased protein binding (decreased affinity and lowered albumin concentrations) during pregnancy and an increase in total body water of pregnant animals caused by the addition of fetal and uterine fluids. An increase in the volume of distribution subsequently can lower the plasma concentration of a drug and result in subtherapeutic plasma levels. It may be necessary to monitor the patient carefully to ensure that a therapeutic effect is achieved or to monitor blood concentrations when administering a drug for which a critical minimal therapeutic plasma concentration is defined.

EMBRYO AND FETUS SUSCEPTIBILITY TO DRUG EFFECTS

The developing embryo or fetus becomes an inadvertant recipient of drugs administered to a pregnant animal. Adverse drug effects may be either teratogenic, causing a congenital malformation, or embryotoxic, causing abortion. Most teratogenic studies are performed in rats, mice, or rabbits, and various references have summarized the risks in humans (Briggs et al., 1986; Brendel et al., 1985). However, information in dogs and cats is lacking. It is unfortunate that since the last review of this subject for dogs and cats (Papich and Davis, 1986), there is very little new information.

Embryotoxicity

The conceptus is sensitive to chemical insult early in gestation. In the bitch, a fertilized ova enters the uterus on days 9 to 11, and implantation occurs on days 17 to 21. (For these estimates, day 0 is the time of the LH peak, and it is assumed that the average breeding date is day 1.) Placental development does not occur until day 20. These events take place on days 4 to 5 and 12 to 15, respectively, in the queen (Stabenfeldt and Schille, 1977). During this critical period, the embryo is bathed in uterine fluid, which will attain drug concentrations reflective of maternal extracellular fluid, and all the embryonic cells will be equally susceptible to toxic insult. Exposure to a toxic drug at this time usually results in spontaneous abortion rather than a specific malformation.

The critical time for embryotoxicity is from postconception day 6 to day 20 in dogs, and days 5 to 16 in the cat. Clearly, drug administration should be avoided during this critical time.

Drug Transfer across the Placenta

Once the placenta forms, nutrients and drugs must cross the placenta to reach the fetus. The important factors that govern the transfer of drugs across the placenta are listed in Table 2. There is no true "placental barrier." Differences in the number of tissue layers interposed between mother and fetus have little bearing on the ability of a drug to pass from the mother to the fetus. Even though tremendous placental variability is seen among rodents, carnivores, ungulates, and primates, this difference has not been shown to account for differences in the ability of a drug to cross the placenta of these species (Miller et al., 1976). Virtually all drugs administered to a mother have the capability of entering the fetal circulation. A drug that reaches the fetal circulation in dogs and laboratory animals (there is no information on cats) must be eliminated

Table 1. Safety of Drugs in Pregnancy

Drug	Recommendation	Comments
Antimicrobial Drugs		
Amikacin	C	Aminoglycoside antibiotics easily cross the placenta and may cause 8th nerve toxicity or nephrotoxicity.
Ampicillin	A	Crosses the placenta but has not been shown to be harmful to fetus.
Amoxicillin	A	Crosses the placenta but has not been shown to be harmful to fetus.
Carbenicillin	A	Crosses the placenta but has not been shown to be harmful to fetus.
Cephalosporins	A	Crosses the placenta but has not been shown to be harmful to fetus.
Chloramphenicol	C	May decrease protein synthesis in fetus, particularly in bone marrow.
Ciprofloxacin	D	Do not use during pregnancy; quinolones have been associated with articular cartilage defects.
Clavulanic acid–amoxicillin (Clavamox, Beecham)	A	Crosses the placenta but has not been shown to be harmful to fetus.
Clindamycin	A	Crosses the placenta but has not been shown to be harmful to fetus.
Cloxacillin	A	Crosses the placenta but has not been shown to be harmful to fetus.
Dicloxacillin	A	Crosses the placenta but has not been shown to be harmful to fetus.
Doxycycline	D	Tetracyclines can cause bone and teeth malformations in fetus and may cause toxicity in mother.
Enrofloxacin	D	See ciprofloxacin.
Erythromycin	A	Appears to be safe except for erythromycin estolate, which has been shown to increase the risk of hepatotoxicity in women.
Gentamicin	C	Aminoglycoside antibiotics easily cross the placenta and may cause 8th nerve toxicity or nephrotoxicity. However, specific toxicities from gentamicin have not been reported, and it may be used for a serious infection in place of a suitable alternative.
Hetacillin	A	Crosses the placenta but has not been shown to be harmful to fetus.
Kanamycin	C	Aminoglycoside antibiotics easily cross the placenta and may cause 8th nerve toxicity or nephrotoxicity.
Lincomycin	A	Crosses the placenta but has not been shown to cause problems in fetus.
Metronidazole	C	Teratogenic in laboratory animals, but there is no information for dogs and cats. It should be avoided during the first three weeks of pregnancy.
Neomycin	A	Not absorbed sufficiently to cause systemic effects after oral administration.
Oxacillin	A	Crosses the placenta but has not been shown to be harmful to fetus.
Oxytetracycline	D	Toxic to fetus and may increase risk of hepatitis in mother (see tetracycline).
Penicillin G (benzyl penicillin)	A	Crosses the placenta but has not been shown to be harmful to fetus.
Streptomycin	D	See gentamicin. Streptomycin is associated with higher incidence of 8th nerve toxicity than other aminoglycosides.
Sulfonamides	B	Sulfonamides cross the placenta and have produced congenital malformations in rats and mice, but problems have not been reported in dogs or cats; in people, they have caused neonatal icterus when administered near term. Avoid long-acting sulfonamides.
Tetracycline	D	Tetracyclines can cause bone and teeth malformations in fetus and may cause toxicity in mother.
Trimethoprim-sulfadiazine (Tribrissen, Coopers)	B	Manufacturer states that it is safe during pregnancy in dogs; see also trimethoprim and sulfonamides.
Trimethoprim	B	Teratogenic in rats but probably safe in other species. Folate antagonism and bone marrow depression are possible with prolonged use.
Ticarcillin	A	Crosses the placenta but has not been shown to be harmful to fetus.
Tobramycin	C	Aminoglycoside antibiotics easily cross the placenta and may cause 8th nerve toxicity or nephrotoxicity.
Tylosin	B	No information is available.
Antifungal Drugs		
Amphotericin-B	C	There are no known teratogenic effects, but amphotericin is extremely toxic. Use only if the disease is life threatening, in absence of a suitable alternative.
Griseofulvin	D	Teratogenic in rats; causes multiple skeletal and brain malformations in cats.
Ketoconazole	B	Teratogenic and embryotoxic in rats; antiandrogenic; stillbirths have been reported in dogs.
Miconazole	A	Apparently safe if applied topically.
Antiparasitic Drugs		
Amitraz	C	Manufacturer states that reproduction studies have not been done; no information available.
Diethylcarbamazine	A	Manufacturer states that the drug may be given to dogs throughout gestation.
Dithiazanine iodide (Dizan, TechAmerica)	B	No information is available; iodide salts may cause congenital goiter if administered for prolonged periods during pregnancy.
Fenbendazole	A	Safe. Has been administered to pregnant bitches without producing adverse effects.

Table continued on following page

Table 1. Safety of Drugs in Pregnancy Continued

Drug	Recommendation	Comments
Antiparasitic Drugs Continued		
Dichlorvos (Task, Solvay)	B	Caution is advised when administering cholinesterase inhibitors to pregnant animals; it should not be administered to puppies or kittens, but studies in pregnant dogs and cats suggest that there are no adverse effects during pregnancy.
Ivermectin	A	Safe. Reproduction studies in dogs, cattle, horses, and pigs have not shown adverse effects.
Levamisole	C	No information available.
Mebendazole	A	Safe. In reproduction studies in dogs, it was not teratogenic or embryotoxic.
Piperazine	A	Safe. No known contraindications for the use of piperazine.
Praziquantel	A	Safe. No adverse effects were seen when tested in pregnant dogs and cats.
Thiacetarsamide (Caparsolate sodium, CEVA)	C	No specific information regarding toxicity to fetus is available. It can be hepatotoxic and nephrotoxic, and heartworm adulticide should be postponed until after parturition.
Bunamidine	A	Has been administered to pregnant bitches without problems and is safe in pregnant cats. Slight interference with spermatogenesis has been seen in male dogs.
Pyrantel	A	Safe. Toxicity studies have not shown any adverse effects.
Thenium	A	Safe. Manufacturer states that except in young puppies, there are no known contraindications.
Thiabendazole	B	Thiabendazole is not teratogenic in laboratory animals, but high doses have produced toxemia in ewes.
Trichlorfon	C	Caution is advised when administering organophosphates to pregnant animals. Congenital toxicoses have been reported following administration to pregnant sows. Manufacturer states that trichlorfon should not be administered to pregnant mares, but there are no recommendations for dogs and cats.
Anticancer Drugs		
Doxorubicin hydrochloride (Adriamycin, Adria)	C	May produce malformations in newborn or embryotoxicity.
Azathioprine	C	May produce congenital malformations but has been used in pregnant women safely. It may be a suitable alternative to other drugs when immunosuppressive therapy is required.
Chlorambucil	C	May produce malformations in newborn or embryotoxicity.
Cisplatin	C	May produce congenital malformations, embryotoxicity, or nephrotoxicity.
Cyclophosphamide	C	May produce malformations in newborn or embryotoxicity.
Methotrexate	C	May produce malformations in newborn or embryotoxicity.
Vincristine	C	May produce malformations in newborn or embryotoxicity.
Analgesic Drugs		
Acetaminophen	C	Safety not established in dogs; toxic in cats.
Aspirin	C	Embryotoxicity has been seen in laboratory animals but not in other species. Late in pregnancy, it may produce pulmonary hypertension and bleeding problems (see text).
Flunixin meglumine	C	Safety in pregnancy has not been determined.
Gold (aurothioglucose)	D	Laboratory animal studies clearly show increased congenital malformations.
Ibuprofen	C	Safety in dogs and cats not established.
Indomethacin	C	Can be toxic in adult dogs; can cause premature closure of ductus arteriosus if administered near term.
Phenylbutazone	C	Safety has not been established. Long-term use can depress bone marrow.
Salicylates	C	Embryotoxicity has been seen in laboratory animals but not in other species. Late in pregnancy, it may produce pulmonary hypertension and bleeding disorders.
Anesthetic and Preanesthetic Drugs		
Acepromazine	B	Phenothiazines should be avoided near term; they may produce neonatal CNS depression.
Atropine	B	Crosses the placenta and has been used safely but may cause fetal tachycardia.
Butorphanol	B	Safe for short-term use. Neonatal depression can be treated with naloxone.
Codeine	B	Safe for short-term use. Neonatal depression can be treated with naloxone.
Diazepam	C	See anticonvulsants.
Fentanyl	B	Safe for short-term use. Neonatal depression can be treated with naloxone.
Glycopyrrolate	B	Safe. Does not cross placenta as readily as atropine. Studies in rats and rabbits have not revealed teratogenic effects.
Halothane	C	Decreased learning ability has been reported in rats after *in utero* exposure; depression may be seen in neonates after cesarean section; excessive uterine bleeding may be seen when administered during cesarean section.
Isoflurane	B	Probably safe. Depression may be seen in neonates after cesarean section.

Table 1. *Safety of Drugs in Pregnancy* Continued

Drug	Recommendation	Comments
Anesthetic and Preanesthetic Drugs Continued		
Ketamine	B	Probably safe. Depression may be seen in puppies delivered by cesarean section; may increase intrauterine pressure and induce premature labor.
Lidocaine	A	All local anesthetics appear to be safe when used for a local nerve block or epidural anesthesia.
Meperidine	B	Opiates can produce neonatal sedation and respiratory depression, but the effects can be reversed with the administration of naloxone.
Methoxyflurane	C	Neonatal depression is seen when used for cesarean section.
Morphine	B	Opiates can produce neonatal sedation and respiratory depression, but the effects can be reversed with the administration of naloxone.
Naloxone	A	Has been shown to be safe when administered to newborns within a few minutes after birth.
Nitrous oxide	B	Probably safe. Used frequently for cesarean section without adverse effects.
Oxymorphone	B	Opiates can produce neonatal sedation and respiratory depression, but the effects can be reversed with the administration of naloxone.
Pentobarbital	D	Associated with high incidence of neonatal mortality.
Thiamylal	C	Easily crosses the placenta; all barbiturates produce respiratory depression in fetus; however, thiobarbiturates are not as toxic as pentobarbital.
Thiopental	C	Easily crosses the placenta. All barbiturates produce respiratory depression in fetus; however, thiobarbiturates are not as toxic as pentobarbital.
Gastrointestinal Drugs		
Antacids	A	Safe. Not absorbed systemically.
Antiemetics	B	Probably safe if administered short term.
Cimetidine	B	Safety has not been established, but no reports of toxicity in humans.
Dimenhydrinate	B	Safe if used short term.
Diphenhydramine	B	Safe if used short term.
Diphenoxylate	C	Studies have reported adverse effects in laboratory animals, but no adverse effects have been reported in pregnant dogs, cats, and humans.
Laxatives	B	All laxatives, except Castor Oil (Squibb), are considered safe if they are used short term. Castor Oil causes premature uterine contractions.
Loperamide	C	Same comment as diphenoxylate.
Metoclopramide	B	Safe in laboratory animals, but no studies available for cats or dogs.
Methscopolamine	C	Safety not established.
Misoprostol	D	Synthetic prostaglandin, causes a termination of pregnancy.
Prochlorperazine	B	No reports of toxicity when administered short term.
Ranitidine	B	Safety has not been established, but no reports of toxicity were reported in humans.
Sucralfate	A	Probably safe. Not absorbed systemically.
Sulfasalazine	B	Salicylate component is not absorbed enough to produce adverse effects; sulfonamide may produce neonatal icterus when used near term (see text).
Cardiovascular Drugs		
Atropine	B	Probably safe but may produce fetal tachycardia.
Captopril	C	Has been shown to be embryotoxic in laboratory animals and goats.
Digitalis	A	Probably safe. No adverse effects seen in humans and laboratory animals (see text).
Furosemide	B	No adverse effects have been reported.
Dopamine	B	Probably safe at therapeutic doses.
Heparin	B	Does not appear to cross placenta.
Hydralazine	B	Probably safe. There have been reports of minor toxicity in rats, but it has been administered safely to pregnant women.
Isoproterenol	C	May cause fetal tachycardia; beta-adrenergic drugs inhibit uterine contractions.
Lidocaine	B	Probably safe. May cause fetal bradycardia.
Nitroglycerin	C	No information available.
Nitroprusside	C	There is a risk of fetal cyanide toxicity with prolonged use.
Procainamide	B	Probably safe. May cause fetal bradycardia.
Propranolol	C	May cause fetal bradycardia, respiratory depression, and neonatal hypoglycemia; avoid use near term.
Quinidine	B	Probably safe. May cause fetal bradycardia.
Theophylline	B	No reports of adverse effects.
Thiazide diuretics	C	May cause increased incidence of perinatal mortality.
Warfarin	D	Causes embryotoxicity and congenital malformations, neural tube defects in laboratory animals and humans.
Anticonvulsant Drugs		
Diazepam	C	Has been associated with congenital defects in mice, rats, and people.
Phenobarbital	B	Has been associated with rare congenital defects and bleeding tendencies in newborn but may be safer than other anticonvulsants (see text).

Table continued on following page

Table 1. Safety of Drugs in Pregnancy Continued

Drug	Recommendation	Comments
Anticonvulsant Drugs Continued		
Phenytoin	C	Teratogenic in rats, mice, and people.
Primidone	C	Same risks as phenobarbital and has been associated with increased incidence of hepatitis in adult dogs.
Valproic acid	C	May cause congenital malformations.
Muscle Relaxants		
Dantrolene	C	Safety not established.
Dimethyltubocurarine	B	Quarternary base with negligible placental transfer; it does not affect the fetus unless administered in large doses.
Gallamine	B	Quarternary base with negligible placental transfer; it does not affect the fetus unless administered in large doses.
Methocarbamol	C	Safety not established; manufacturer states that it should not be administered during pregnancy.
Pancuronium	B	Quarternary base with negligible placental transfer; it does not affect the fetus unless administered in large doses.
Succinylcholine	B	Quarternary base with negligible placental transfer; it does not affect the fetus unless administered in large doses.
Endocrine Drugs		
Betamethasone	C	Corticosteroids have been associated with increased incidence of cleft palate and other congenital malformations, and they may induce premature labor and abortion in dogs (see text).
Cortisone	C	Corticosteroids have been associated with increased incidence of cleft palate and other congenital malformations, and they may induce premature labor and abortion in dogs (see text).
Dexamethasone	C	Corticosteroids have been associated with increased incidence of cleft palate and other congenital malformations, and they may induce premature labor (see text). Dexamethasone has caused abortion and fetal death in dogs.
Diethylstilbestrol (DES)	D	Malformation of male and female genitourinary systems.
Estradiolcypionate (ECP)	D	Malformation of male and female genital tracts and bone marrow depression.
Flumethasone	C	Corticosteroids have been associated with increased incidence of cleft palate and other congenital malformations, and they may induce premature labor and abortion in dogs (see text).
Mitotane (o,p-DDD)	D	Adrenocortical necrosis.
Prednisolone	C	Although prednisolone has been administered to pregnant women without adverse effects, caution is advised (see dexamethasone). Prednisolone may be used in serious diseases in absence of a suitable alternative.
Stanozolol	D	Manufacturer states that it should not be administered to pregnant dogs and cats.
Testosterone	D	Causes masculinization of female fetus.
Thyroxine	B	Does not cross placenta easily and has not been associated with any problems.
Miscellaneous Drugs		
Ammonium chloride	B	May cause fetal acidosis; discontinue use during pregnancy.
Aspartame (NutraSweet)	A	No risk.
Dimethylsulfoxide (DMSO)	C	Teratogenic in laboratory animals; manufacturers state that it should not be applied to breeding animals.

A: Probably safe. Although specific studies may not have proved the safety of all drugs in dogs and cats, there are no reports of adverse effects in laboratory animals or in women.
B: Safe for use if used cautiously. Studies in laboratory animals may have uncovered some risk, but these drugs appear to be safe in dogs and cats or these drugs are safe if they are not administered when the animal is near term.
C: These drugs may have potential risks. Studies in people or laboratory animals have uncovered risks, and these drugs should be used cautiously, as a last resort when the benefit of therapy clearly outweighs the risks.
D: Contraindicated. These drugs have been shown to cause congenital malformations or embryotoxicity.

via fetal immature renal mechanisms or diffuse back through the placenta to the mother, because it has been demonstrated that the fetal liver in these animals has no drug-metabolizing capabilities, in contrast to that of the human liver during gestation (humans possess drug-metabolizing capabilities as early as 5 to 6 weeks after conception). Many drugs will not reach appreciable tissue concentrations in the fetus unless the drug has been administered for a duration that is long enough for steady-state concentrations to be achieved. Many of the drugs listed in Table 1 produce no teratogenic effects if they are administered for a short time at relatively moderate doses.

The maternal/fetal pH differential can affect the distribution of drugs in fetal tissues. Fetal tissues are generally 0.1 to 0.2 pH units lower than the mother, and according to the pH-partition hypothesis, drugs that are weak bases (e.g., local anesthetics, aminoglycoside antibiotics) will accumulate in the fetal circulation, and weak acids (e.g., barbiturates, penicillins) will attain low fetal concentrations.

Even though a drug reaches the fetus, it does not necessarily imply that toxicity will occur. Surprisingly, there are very few reports of documented teratogenicity that resulted from drug administration during pregnancy. Recent surveys estimate that 75 to 80 per cent of women take drugs during pregnancy, but obviously, the incidence of adverse effects is much less.

GENERAL RECOMMENDATIONS

Antimicrobial Therapy

All antibiotics that are beta-lactams are considered safe (e.g., penicillin, ampicillin, cephalosporins). These drugs cross the placenta to a moderate extent. However, because their toxicity is limited to the cell wall of bacteria, they are not harmful to the developing fetus at therapeutic doses. As mentioned earlier, because of increased renal clearance or changes in the volume of distribution, a change in dosage regimens may be needed in critically ill patients.

Erythromycin and lincomycin also appear to be safe for use during pregnancy with the exception of the estolate salt of erythromycin, which has been associated with increased concentrations of liver enzymes in women during pregnancy and may be hepatotoxic.

Experience with sulfonamides and trimethoprim-sulfonamide combinations (e.g., Tribrissen, Coopers Animal Health, Kansas City, MO) suggests that these drugs can be used during pregnancy. However, potential problems are possible as a result of folate antagonism due to trimethoprim and neonatal hyperbilirubinemia caused by sulfonamides if they are administered near term. Based on studies with trimethoprim-sulfa in bitches, the manufacturer states that it is safe in pregnant dogs. There have not been problems reported with administration to pregnant women.

The fetus is susceptible to the nephrotoxic effects of aminoglycosides (e.g., gentamicin, tobramycin,

kanamycin), and there is a risk of ototoxicity from aminoglycosides during fetal development. Chloramphenicol should not be administered during pregnancy because it inhibits protein synthesis and can affect fetal bone marrow maturation.

Metronidazole is considered a safe drug during pregnancy. Although it has caused mutagenesis in bacterial experiments and increased carcinogenesis in rodents, there have been no reported adverse effects in other species.

Tetracyclines are definitely contraindicated during pregnancy. They are known to cause teeth and skeletal malformations in the fetus, and in addition, pregnant women are at an increased risk of toxic hepatitis associated with tetracycline therapy (Davis, 1968). It is fortunate that for most infections, a suitable alternative to tetracyclines can usually be selected.

Gastrointestinal Therapy

When a pregnant animal requires treatment for a gastrointestinal disease, specific drugs may be used if the benefits of treatment outweigh the risks (Lewis and Weingold, 1985). Antiemetic drugs are used commonly in pregnant women, and they appear to be safe. There have been no adverse effects reported from the use of antihistamines, phenothiazines, or metoclopramide. However, if phenothiazines are administered near term, neonatal depression or extrapyramidal signs are possible.

Although concern has been expressed regarding the use of sulfasalazine during pregnancy, reports of studies in women suggest that the drug is probably safe. The salicylate component of the drug is apparently absorbed to such a small extent that it does not produce systemic effects. The sulfonamide component can potentially produce neonatal icterus, but this has not been reported. Apparently, the sulfonamide in sulfasalazine does not displace bilirubin from protein-binding sites as easily as do other sulfonamides (Lewis and Weingold, 1985).

Anti-inflammatory Therapy

Nonsteroidal anti-inflammatory drugs (NSAIDs) are commonly prescribed in human medicine, but information regarding their safety is inconclusive. Salicylates have produced teratogenic effects when administered to rats and mice at high doses, but teratogenic effects have not been observed in other species (Lee, 1985).

Veterinarians should be aware of the effects of these drugs in adult animals. Cats are susceptible to toxicity from salicylates and acetaminophen; in dogs, gastrointestinal adverse effects are commonly

Table 2. *Factors That Influence the Transfer of Drugs Across the Placenta*

1. Placental blood supply	7. Duration of drug exposure
2. Age of gestation	8. Maternal/fetal pH differential
3. Placental drug-metabolizing capabilities	9. Maternal/fetal drug protein-binding differences
4. Drug size	10. Species of animal studied
5. Drug's lipid solubility	
6. Drug dose	

reported following administration of ibuprofen, in-domethacin, or naproxen.

The influence of prostaglandins on fetal circula-tion has been the subject of several studies. Pros-taglandins PGE_1, PGE_2, and PGI_2 are direct pul-monary vasodilators, and PGE_2 is responsible for maintaining patency of the ductus arteriosus late in gestation. Although direct proof is lacking, there is a risk of causing pulmonary hypertension if NSAIDs are administered late in pregnancy (Moise et al., 1988; Coceani et al., 1978). NSAIDs have been employed therapeutically in humans, as indometh-acin has been used to close patent ductus arteriosus in infants early after birth.

Other problems reported in humans and labora-tory animals associated with prostaglandin synthesis inhibition are prolonged gestation, and increased bleeding problems at parturition caused by de-creased platelet aggregation.

If mild analgesia is necessary in pregnant dogs and cats, aspirin is probably the best choice, be-cause it is the drug with which we have had the most experience. It has been administered fre-quently, with no reported adverse effects, and phar-macokinetic studies have established safe dosages for dogs and cats.

If more potent anti-inflammatory therapy or im-munosuppressive therapy is necessary during preg-nancy, corticosteroids and other immunosuppres-sants may be administered. Prednisolone and prednisone should be used in preference to the other corticosteroids because they have few miner-alocorticoid effects and are relatively short acting. Longer-acting corticosteroids should be avoided, as dexamethasone has been associated with fetal death and abortion in dogs. It has been difficult to assess the safety of these drugs because they are usually used to treat a severe underlying condition, which may also affect the fetus. Although cortisone has been associated with congenital malformations in laboratory animals, cleft palate in particular, these effects have not been observed in dogs, cats, or humans (Brendel et al., 1985; Pratt and Salomon, 1981). Perhaps the difference can be explained by the fact that the laboratory animal strains used have a high relative number of steroid receptors in com-parison to dogs and cats.

Anticonvulsant Therapy

Anticonvulsant drugs should not be discontinued in a pregnant epileptic animal. The risk of seizures during pregnancy significantly outweighs the risk of fetal effects from anticonvulsant drugs. Neonatal bleeding tendencies have been associated with phe-nobarbital treatment during pregnancy, but other adverse effects have not been observed (Dalessio, 1985).

In humans, teratogenic effects have been ob-served from treatment with phenytoin (Dilantin, Parke-Davis) and valproic acid, but there is no information available on the incidence in dogs and cats. If anticonvulsant therapy is needed during pregnancy, the following recommendations are made: Attempt to maintain the patient on pheno-barbital without the use of other anticonvulsants that might have adverse effects. Because the hepatic clearance may be increased for phenobarbital during pregnancy, dosages may have to be increased based on the results of therapeutic drug monitoring (phe-nobarbital therapeutic plasma concentrations are between 20 and 40 $\mu g/ml$). Administer oral vitamin K to the dam in the last 10 days of gestation. The bleeding tendencies that have been reported in humans are apparently caused by a decrease in vitamin K–dependent clotting factors, and vitamin K administration may minimize this effect in the fetus.

Anesthesia

Information on specific anesthetic agents is listed in Table 1 and has been reviewed recently (Marcella and Short, 1984). Ultrashort-acting barbiturates and inhalant anesthetics can cause neonatal depression. Xylazine and ketamine can increase intrauterine pressure and induce premature labor. Pentobarbital should be completely avoided because it is associ-ated with an unacceptable incidence of fetal mor-tality. Commonly used inhalant anesthetics (e.g., halothane, methoxyflurane, nitrous oxide) appear to be safe, although some transitory depression may be seen in neonates after anesthesia for cesarean section. Possible complications associated with the use of halothane are listed on Table 1.

For the patient requiring anesthesia for cesarean section, epidural anesthesia can be used, with ad-ditional sedation and analgesia by opiates and in-halant anesthetics. The depressant effects of opiates can be reversed in the neonate by instilling 1 to 2 drops of naloxone in the mouth (Marcella and Short, 1984).

SUMMARY

If drugs are administered during pregnancy, cli-nicians should always question the safety of the drugs regarding the fetus and the mother. Because of physiologic changes that occur in pregnancy, dosages for certain drugs (e.g., antibiotics and an-ticonvulsants) may have to be increased. There is no placental barrier to limit drug exposure to the fetus. Although many drugs do not reach tissue concentrations that are as high as those attained in the mother, virtually all drugs have the potential to cross the placenta. Many drugs that are administered are safe if administered cautiously. If a drug listed in Table 1 has a potential for causing adverse effects, the benefit of therapy must clearly outweigh the risk to the fetus when the drug is administered. It is fortunate that the list of drugs known to be toxic to the fetus is short, and in most instances, a suitable alternative to a toxic drug can be selected. Certain treatments (e.g., heartworm adulticide therapy) or surgical procedures should be postponed until after parturition if possible.

References and Supplemental Reading

Brendel, K., Kuhamel, R. C., and Shepard, T. H.: Embryotoxic drugs. Biol. Res. Pregnancy Perinatol 6:1, 1985.

Briggs, G. G., Freeman, R. K., and Yaffe, S. J.: *Drugs in Pregnancy and Lactation*, 2nd ed. Baltimore: Williams and Wilkins, 1986.

Coceani, F., Bodach, E., White, E., et al.: Prostaglandin I-2 is less potent than prostaglandin E-2 on the lamb ductus arteriosus. Prostaglandins 15:551, 1978.

Dalessio, D. J.: Seizure disorders and pregnancy. N. Engl. J. Med. 312:559, 1985.

Davis, J.: Liver damage due to tetracycline and its relationship to pregnancy. *In* Meyler, L. (ed.): *Drug-Induced Diseases*. Amsterdam: Excerpta Medica, 1968.

Juchau, M. R., and Faustman-Watts, E.: Pharmacokinetic considerations in the maternal-placental-fetal unit. Clin. Obstet. Gynecol. 26:379, 1983.

Krauer, B., and Krauer, F.: Pharmacokinetics in pregnancy. *In* Gibaldi, M., and Prescott, L. (eds.): *Handbook of Clinical Pharmacokinetics*. New York: ADIS Health Science Press, 1983, pp. 1–17.

Lee, P.: Anti-inflammatory therapy during pregnancy and lactation. Clin. Invest. Med. 8:328, 1985.

Lewis, J. H., and Weingold, A. B.: The use of gastrointestinal drugs during pregnancy and lactation. Am. J. Gastroenterol. 80:912, 1985.

Marcella, K. L., and Short, C. E.: Anesthetic management of the pregnant animal. Compend. Cont. Ed. 6:942, 1984.

McBride, W. B.: Thalidomide embryopathy. Teratology 16:79, 1977.

Miller, R. K., Koszalka, T. R., and Brent, R. L.: The transport of molecules across placental membranes. *In* Poste, G., and Nicholson, G. L. (eds.): *The Cell Surface in Animal Embryogenesis and Development*. New York: North-Holland Pub. Co., 1976, pp. 145–207.

Moise, K. J., Huhta, J. C., Sharif, D. S., et al.: Indomethacin in the treatment of premature labor. N. Engl. J. Med. 319:327, 1988.

Nau, H., Loock, W., and Schmidt-Gollwitzer, M.: Pregnancy-specific changes in hepatic drug metabolism. *In* Krauer, B., and Krauer, F. (eds.): *Drugs and Pregnancy: Maternal Drug Handling, Fetal Drug Exposure*. Toronto: Academic Press Inc., 1984.

Papich, M. G., and Davis, L. E.: Drug therapy during pregnancy and in the neonate. Vet. Clin. North Am. [Small Anim. Pract.] 16:525, 1986.

Pratt, R. M., and Salomon, D. S.: Biochemical basis for the teratogenic effects of glucocorticoids. *In* Juchau, M. R. (ed.): *The Biochemical Basis of Chemical Teratogenesis*. New York: Elsevier Press, 1981, pp. 179–199.

Redmond, G. P.: Physiologic changes during pregnancy and their implications for pharmacological treatment. Clin. and Invest. Med. 8:317, 1985.

Stabenfeldt, G. H., and Shille, V. M.: Reproduction in the dog and cat. *In* Cole, H. H., and Cupps, P. T., (eds.): *Reproduction in Domestic Animals*, 3rd ed. New York: Academic Press, 1977, pp. 499–527.

DRUGS THAT AFFECT UTERINE MOTILITY

LYNN G. WHEATON, D.V.M.

Urbana, Illinois

The primary function of uterine muscle (myometrium) is to contract and perform work. However, in contrast to the heart, the tasks that the myometrium must perform are so varied that they require the muscle to respond in very different ways at different times. The ova require a motility that moves luminal contents in a cephalocaudal direction, whereas sperm must be propelled in the opposite direction. Intense contractions are needed to expel the fetus and placenta at parturition and to accomplish uterine involution. Also, the canine uterus exhibits active, highly coordinated motility during proestrus and estrus (Wheaton et al., 1988). Yet, the uterus must remain quiescent during pregnancy to protect and nurture the developing fetuses, and it is also quiet during diestrus in the nonpregnant bitch.

HORMONAL REGULATION OF THE UTERUS

Although the uterine muscle is capable of producing massive contractions, it is relaxed until an optimal estrogen:progesterone ratio permits prostaglandin (PG), oxytocin, alpha-adrenergic agents, or all three to stimulate the myometrium. Estrogen maintains the actinomyosin concentration in the myometrial cell and increases the electrical activity of the uterus and cervix (Finn and Porter, 1975). In addition, estrogen can affect uterine motility by stimulating the synthesis and release of prostaglandin and increasing receptor sites for oxytocin and alpha-adrenergic agents. However, although estrogen increases uterine electrical excitability in the ovariectomized or immature animal, in the mature anestrous bitch, exogenous estrogen decreases the frequency of intrauterine pressure cycles and produces periods of prolonged uterine quiescence (Wheaton et al., 1986). It is believed that estrogen exerts this effect on the myometrium via the synthesis of relaxin or a relaxinlike substance (Downing and Porter, 1978). Thus, estrogen can have both a stimulatory and an inhibitory effect on uterine myometrium, and the nature of its effect appears to be determined by sexual maturity and the estrous cycle stage.

Progesterone, "the defense mechanism of pregnancy," blocks the synchrony of contractions between individual myometrial cells so that a contraction wave cannot develop. This effect keeps the uterus quiescent during diestrus or pregnancy. At parturition, propulsive uterine motility cannot proceed until the "blocking" effect of progesterone is withdrawn. Methods by which progesterone exerts its quiescent effect include suppression of oxytocin receptors, inhibition of the release of prostaglandins, and stimulation of the development of beta-adrenergic receptors, since beta-adrenergic agents relax the uterus.

Calcium

Calcium plays an important role in the smooth muscle contraction-relaxation cycle. Calcium is needed for the phosphorylation of myosin light chain, which enhances the ability of the myosin and actin filaments to slide past one another and produce muscle contractions. Calcium concentration is a key factor in effective myometrial contractility, and agents or events that change myometrial calcium concentrations affect myometrial contractility.

It is important to assess the serum calcium concentration in the parturient bitch, particularly when dystocia is suspected. The serum total calcium value must be adjusted for protein or albumin concentration to obtain a correct calcium value (Meuten et al., 1982).

Prostaglandins

Prostaglandin $F_{2\alpha}$ and E_2 are 20-carbon cyclic hydroxyacids formed from arachidonic acid. They are widely distributed in mammalian tissues and are produced by uterine epithelium, myometrium, and cervix. Estrogen stimulates prostaglandin synthesis, particularly from tissue previously exposed to progesterone. In the bitch, prostaglandin $F_{2\alpha}$ is luteolytic and stimulates myometrial contractility. A dose of 5 μg/kg of prostaglandin $F_{2\alpha}$ (Prostin, Upjohn) given intravenously increases intrauterine pressure to greater than 100 mm Hg in the proestrous and estrous bitch and to 60 mm Hg in the diestrous bitch (Fig. 1A) (Wheaton et al., 1988).

Prostaglandin's stimulatory effect on the uterus has been used therapeutically as an abortifacient and as a medical treatment for pyometra. Concannon and Hansel (1977) produced abortion in four of seven bitches receiving intramuscular injections of 20 μg/kg of $PGF_{2\alpha}$ every 8 hr or 30 μg/kg every 12 hr. Abortions occurred 56 to 80 hr after starting $PGF_{2\alpha}$ treatment on days 33 to 53 of the cycle. Abortion has also been produced by giving one intramuscular injection of 20 μg/kg of a synthetic prostaglandin analogue during the middle (30 to 35 days) or late third (53 to 56 days) of gestation (Shille et al., 1984). Bitches aborted 2 days after the single treatment.

Several treatment regimens have been suggested for medical treatment of pyometra. Meyers-Wallen and coworkers (1986) recommend 250 to 500 μg/kg of prostaglandin $F_{2\alpha}$ subcutaneously once daily for 3 to 5 days, although successful evacuation of uterine contents has been achieved with 100 μg/kg given subcutaneously once daily for 3 to 4 days (Nelson et al., 1982). The subcutaneous median lethal dose for prostaglandin in the dog is 5.13 mg/kg (Sokolowski and Geng, 1977).

Prostaglandins induce several side reactions. These include restlessness, hyperventilation, profuse salivation, vomiting, and defecation. Severe hypotension and vascular collapse have also been reported. The frequency and severity of these reactions are dose related, with lower doses producing fewer side effects. Since regimens utilizing higher doses of prostaglandin (250 μg/kg) do not generate greater intrauterine pressures than regimens utilizing lower doses, 50 μg/kg of prostaglandin $F_{2\alpha}$ given every 12 hr should produce uterine contractions comparable to higher doses (250 μg/kg), but with fewer side effects.

Oxytocin

Oxytocin stimulates contraction of the uterine myometrial cells and mammary myoepithelial cells. Estrogen increases the number of oxytocin receptors in the uterus, thereby enhancing its effect. Thus, although the canine diestrous uterus will respond to oxytocin, maximal responses are achieved when the estrogen:progesterone ratio is increased, such as at parturition and during proestrus.

Oxytocin is most commonly used as a therapy for uterine inertia during parturition. Before adminis-

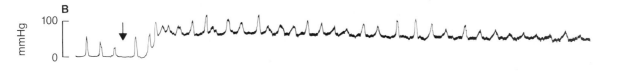

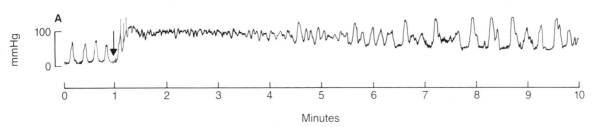

Figure 1. Changes in uterine motility during proestrus induced by the administration of (A) prostaglandin F$_{2\alpha}$ (5 μg/kg, IV) and (B) oxytocin (0.05 USP unit/kg, IV).

tering oxytocin, it is important to diagnose and treat any hypoglycemia or hypocalcemia present. Oxytocin can then be used to augment weak, irregular contractions of the uterus.

The popular dose of oxytocin ranges from 5 to 20 IU in dogs and 3 to 5 IU in cats, given subcutaneously or intramuscularly. The duration of effect is approximately 13 min when given intravenously and 20 min when given intramuscularly or subcutaneously. Therefore, there should be a minimum of 30 min between repeated intramuscular or subcutaneous doses. The recommended dose for a cow is 30 IU, and 10 IU for a pig. Since 1 IU given intravenously can produce an intrauterine pressure of over 100 mm Hg in the proestrous bitch (Fig. 1B), the author believes that *1 to 5 IU of oxytocin given subcutaneously or intramuscularly is a more realistic canine dose*.

Oxytocin produces the greatest increase in intrauterine pressure in the estrogen-primed uterus but also increases intrauterine pressure to 58 mm Hg in the anestrous bitch (Wheaton et al., 1986). Because oxytocin can increase intrauterine pressure even in the presence of low estrogen levels, it may be a useful therapeutic agent in the treatment of postparturient diseases such as metritis and subinvolution of placental sites.

Alpha-Adrenergic and Beta-Adrenergic Agents

The uterus contains both alpha- and beta-adrenergic receptors. Uterine activity is stimulated by alpha-adrenergic agonists, and relaxation of uterine smooth muscle is produced with beta-adrenergic agonists. Estrogen increases the number of myometrial alpha receptors, whereas the progesterone-

treated uterus contains predominantly beta receptors.

The popular sedative-analgesic xylazine (Rompun, Haver) is an alpha-2-adrenergic agent and produces increased intrauterine pressure in the diestrous bitch. This increased intrauterine pressure and the decreased placental perfusion caused by alpha-adrenergic agonists may damage the developing fetus when xylazine is given to the pregnant bitch. In addition, ketamine, often used in combination with xylazine for anesthesia, produces increases in intrauterine pressure during the first trimester in humans but apparently has little effect on uterine activity in the third trimester (James, 1984). Therefore, xylazine and ketamine should be avoided in the pregnant bitch, although they might be useful in the postparturient period to aid in uterine involution.

Beta-adrenergic agents (clenbuterol) have been used to abolish uterine contractions in cattle for the purpose of delaying parturition or for performing obstetric manipulations (Marriner, 1986). They are also used in women to prevent preterm delivery. Epinephrine in low concentrations has beta-adrenergic effects. These effects can decrease uterine contractions and inhibit involution. Thus, epinephrine should not be combined with lidocaine for an epidural block if regional anesthesia is used for a cesarean section.

Inhalation Anesthetic Agents

Halothane anesthesia, at concentrations above 0.8 per cent, has been shown to significantly decrease the force and frequency of uterine contractions (Naftalin et al., 1975). However, low concentrations of other inhalation anesthetic agents apparently do not affect uterine contractions, tone, or responsiveness to oxytocin. Subanesthetic concentrations of methoxyflurane, nitrous oxide, and isoflurane may be used as part of a cesarean section anesthetic regimen without adversely affecting uterine involution.

References and Supplemental Reading

Concannon, P. W., and Hansel, W.: Prostaglandin $F_{2\alpha}$-induced luteolysis, hypothermia, and abortions in Beagle bitches. Prostaglandins 13:533, 1977.

Downing, S. J., and Porter, D. G.: Evidence that inhibition of myometrial activity by oestradiol in the rat is mediated by an RNA-synthetic pathway. J. Endocrinol. 78:119, 1978.

Finn, C. A., and Porter, D. G.: Mechanical activity: Hormonal control. In The Uterus. Acton, MA: Publishing Sciences Group, Inc., 1975, p. 188.

James, F. M.: Non-obstetrical surgery for the pregnant patient. American Society of Anesthesiologists: 35th Annual Refresher Course Lectures, New Orleans, LA, 1984, p. 231.

Marriner, S. E.: How drugs act in the body. Vet. Rec. 119:132, 1986.

Meuten, D. J., Chew, D. J., Capen, C. C., et al.: Relationship of serum total calcium to albumin and total protein in dogs. J.A.V.M.A. 180:63, 1982.

Meyers-Wallen, V. N., Goldschmidt, M. H., and Flickinger, G. L.: Prostaglandin $F_{2\alpha}$ treatment of canine pyometra. J.A.V.M.A. 189:1557, 1986.

Naftalin, N. J., Phear, W. P., and Goldberg, A. H.: Halothane and isometric contractions of isolated pregnant rat myometrium. Anesthesiology 42:458, 1975.

Nelson, R. W., Feldman, E. C., and Stabenfeldt, G. H.: Treatment of canine pyometra and endometritis with prostaglandin $F_{2\alpha}$. J.A.V.M.A. 181:899, 1982.

Shille, V. M., Dorsey, D., and Thatcher, M. J.: Induction of abortion in the bitch with a synthetic prostaglandin analog. Am. J. Vet. Res. 45:1295, 1984.

Sokolowski, S. H., and Geng, S.: Effect of prostaglandin F_2-THAM in the bitch. J.A.V.M.A. 170:536, 1977.

Wheaton, L. G., Pijanowski, G. J., Weston, P. G., et al.: Uterine motility during the estrous cycle: Studies in healthy bitches. Am. J. Vet. Res. 49:82, 1988.

Wheaton, L. G., Rodriquez-Martinez, H., Weston, P. G., et al.: Recording uterine motility in the nonanesthetized bitch. Am. J. Vet. Res. 47:2205, 1986.

VAGINAL PROLAPSE

SHIRLEY D. JOHNSTON, D.V.M.

St. Paul, Minnesota

Vaginal prolapse is protrusion of edematous vaginal tissue into the vaginal lumen and often through the vulva of the intact female dog during time of estrogen stimulation. Affected vaginal tissue arises initially from the ventral midline of the vagina, cranial to the external urethral orifice.

Schutte (1967) defined three types of vaginal prolapse in the bitch, based on severity of the degree of eversion and protrusion of the vaginal tissue. *Type I* is slight to moderate eversion of the vaginal floor cranial to the external urethral orifice. Everted tissue can be detected on digital vaginal examination or on vaginoscopic examination of the affected bitch but does not protrude through the vulvar cleft and therefore is not visible externally except, perhaps, as bulging of the perineum. *Type II* is prolapse of vaginal tissue through the vulvar cleft (Fig. 1A); on vaginal examination, the base of the prolapse can be determined to arise from the cranial vaginal floor (Fig. 1B). *Type III* prolapse refers to prolapse of the entire circumference of the vaginal wall (Fig. 2A); when the ventral part of the prolapse is elevated, the external urethral orifice may be identified (Fig. 2B).

Despite use of the terms "hypertrophy" and "hyperplasia" for vaginal prolapse in the bitch, the histologic change apparent on tissue excised from affected bitches is one of marked edema (Fig. 3), rather than one of histologic hypertrophy or hyperplasia.

CLINICAL FEATURES

Vaginal prolapse occurs primarily in young, intact, large-breed female dogs at time of proestrus or estrus. The age incidence is shown in Table 1, with mean and median ages of first presentation at about 2 years. The disorder has been reported in more than 20 breeds of dogs. Early reports recorded a high incidence in boxers; multiple cases have also been reported in St. Bernards, mastiffs, German shepherd dogs, English bulldogs, Labrador retrievers, Walker· hounds, Chesapeake Bay retrievers, springer spaniels, Weimaraners, and Airedale terriers. In addition, vaginal prolapse has been observed in breeds as small as the beagle and the Lhasa Apsa. There is no information to confirm that this is a hereditary trait, but the condition may be seen in families of purebred dogs, suggesting a hereditary predisposition.

The time of vaginal prolapse with regard to stage of the estrous cycle (Table 2) has been of interest both in understanding the etiopathogenesis of this

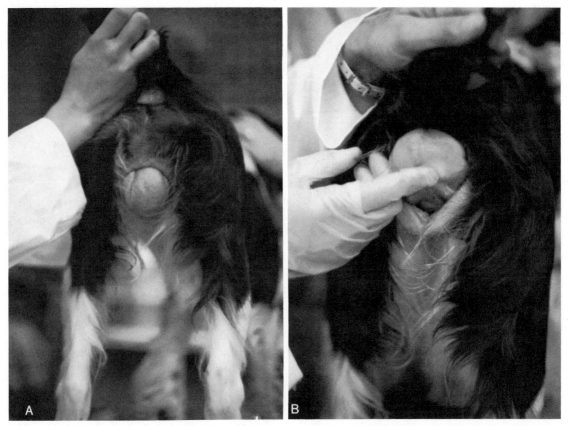

Figure 1. Type II vaginal prolapse in an 8-month-old intact female springer spaniel presented 5 days after onset of proestrus at her first season. *A* shows protrusion of a dome-shaped mass of tissue from the vulva. *B* shows the urethral orifice ventral to the protruding mass, confirming the site of origin of the mass as the cranial ventral vagina.

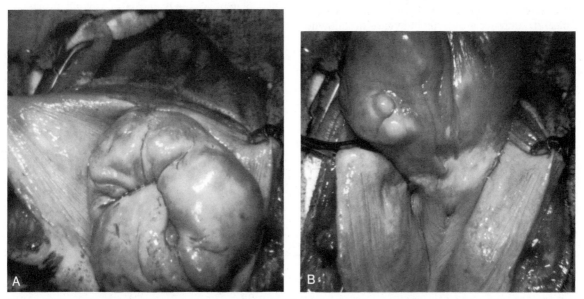

Figure 2. Type III vaginal prolapse in a 5-year-old intact female Walker hound presented in estrus, with a history of recurrent vaginal prolapse at previous seasons and at time of parturition. *A*, The edematous, doughnut-shaped mass of tissue surrounding the cranial vaginal entrance to the cervical os is shown via episiotomy. *B*, The urethral orifice is demonstrated in the floor of the vagina, caudal to the mass of prolapsed tissue.

Table 1. *Age Incidence (Years) of Vaginal Prolapse in the Bitch*

Parameter	Schutte, 1967	Troger, 1970	Johnston, 1988	Total
Age range	0.8–3.3	0.6–3.5	0.6–11	0.6–11
Mean age	1.8	1.5	2.7	2.0
Median age	1.8	NR	1.7	1.75
Number of dogs	21	22	22	65

NR, Not reported.

disorder and in attempting clinical distinction of vaginal prolapse from vaginal neoplasia. The majority of cases reported have shown vaginal prolapse during the follicular (proestrous) or early estrous stage of the cycle, suggesting an influence of estradiol, the major sex steroid secreted during proestrus in this species. Regression of the prolapsed mass begins late in estrus, coincident with decreasing vaginal cornification of the bitch. A few bitches have been observed that show recurrence of vaginal prolapse at time of parturition or at the end of diestrus, when small amounts of estrogen may be secreted.

Presenting signs and symptoms of bitches with vaginal prolapse include the owner's observation of a protruding mass in an otherwise clinically asymptomatic animal, failure to allow normal copulation, and irritation of the vagina or vulva, with licking at the mass and difficulty in urinating. There are no known alterations in the hemogram or serum chemistries profile or in plasma concentrations of reproductive hormones in affected bitches.

If the affected animal is not treated, vaginal prolapse typically regresses and resolves spontaneously at the end of the estrous cycle. The recurrence rate in affected bitches is high. Although clinical data do not always include careful followup, available data suggest recurrence occurs in at least 66 per cent of affected dogs.

DIAGNOSIS

The presence of a vaginal mass is detected by inspection or by digital or vaginoscopic examination of the patient with bulging of the perineum, obstruction to mating or parturition, or vaginal irritation. Differential diagnoses of such a mass include

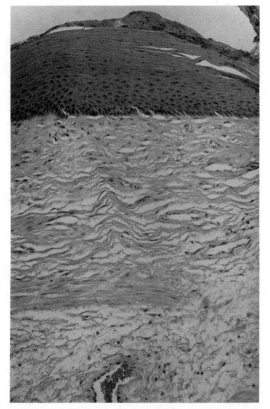

Figure 3. Histologic appearance of prolapsed vaginal tissue surgically removed from the Walker hound bitch shown in Figure 2. The tissue is characterized by a stratified squamous epithelium lining the lumen of the vagina (at right), consistent with the estrous status of the bitch; submucosal tissue is characterized by marked edema (H & E; × 125).

vaginal prolapse, non-neoplastic vaginal polyps, or vaginal neoplasia. Diagnosis of vaginal prolapse is made by assessment of the signalment, history, stage of the estrous cycle, and site of origination of the mass. Prolapse occurs primarily in the young, intact, large-breed dog in proestrus or early estrus or at parturition. Vaginal prolapse is associated with a dome-shaped mass of tissue arising from the cranial floor of the vagina or of a doughnut-shaped mass encircling the cranial vagina. Vaginal neoplasia typically occurs in older, intact, and spayed females and at any location in the vagina, and it does not regress at end of the follicular stage (proestrus or early estrus) of the estrous cycle. Diagnosis may be confirmed histologically in patients that do not exhibit the classic signalment.

Table 2. *Time of Occurrence in the Estrous Cycle of Vaginal Prolapse in the Bitch*

Stage of the Estrous Cycle	Schutte, 1967 (n = 22)	Troger, 1970 (n = 22)	Johnston, 1988 (n = 22)	Total (n = 66)
Proestrus/estrus	18	19	20	57
Diestrus/metestrus	4	0	0	4
Parturition/end diestrus	0	3	2	5
Anestrus	0	0	0	0

TREATMENT

Vaginal prolapse will regress at the end of estrus, so one treatment option is conservative management, topical lubrication of the mass with antibiotic ointment, and application of an Elizabethan collar if the patient chews at the prolapsed tissue. This is appropriate therapy for the puberal bitch scheduled for later ovariohysterectomy or for the puberal bitch intended for breeding when observation of a subsequent season (for recurrence) is planned.

A second treatment option is induction of ovulation at onset of clinical signs when the bitch is still in the follicular phase; this is an attempt to shorten duration of the estrogenic stimulation of the vaginal tissue. Ovulation can be induced in the bitch in the follicular phase with gonadotropin-releasing hormone (Cystorelin, Abbott), 2.2 μg/kg IM, or human chorionic gonadotropin (Pregnyl, Organon), 1000 U IM, given a single time. These regimens should cause elevation in plasma progesterone within a day of their administration. They will not alter the course of the vaginal prolapse if they are given after the bitch has already ovulated or if they are given to bitches suffering vaginal prolapse at parturition or the end of diestrus. There is no information on whether bitches induced to ovulate prematurely release ova capable of undergoing sperm penetration, so this treatment is not advocated for the bitch intended for breeding at the affected cycle. Regression of the prolapse usually follows induction of ovulation by about 1 week.

A third treatment option, and one recommended for purebred bitches intended for breeding purposes that have shown recurrence of vaginal prolapse, is excision of the prolapsed tissue. Such excision has been successful in preventing recurrence of prolapse at later seasons or parturitions. The recommended course is to perform the surgery via an episiotomy late in estrus or following induction of ovulation, when the prolapsed mass is beginning to regress. Following placement of a urethral catheter so as to identify and avoid traumatizing the urethra, an elliptical incision is made in the vaginal mucosa at the base of the mass, which is carefully dissected away and removed. The vaginal mucosa is then sutured with absorbable suture.

Ovariohysterectomy will prevent future estrous cycles and recurrence of vaginal prolapse and is recommended for affected bitches not intended for breeding purposes.

References and Supplemental Reading

Alexander, J. E., and Lennox, J.: Vaginal prolapse in a bitch. Can. Vet. J. 2:428, 1961.
Johnston, S.D.: Personal observation, 1988.
Morgan, R. V.: Urogenital emergencies. Part II. Compend. Contin. Ed. 5:43, 1983.
Pettit, G. D.: Hyperplasia of the vaginal floor. In Bojrab, M. J. (ed.): Current Techniques in Small Animal Surgery. Philadelphia: Lea & Febiger, 1983, p. 352.
Schutte, A. P.: Vaginal prolapse in the bitch. J. S. Afr. Vet. Med. Assoc. 38:197, 1967.
Troger, C. P.: Vaginal prolapse in the bitch. Mod. Vet. Pract. 51:38, 1970.

DIAGNOSIS AND TREATMENT ALTERNATIVES FOR PYOMETRA IN DOGS AND CATS

E. C. FELDMAN, D.V.M.,
Davis, California

and R. W. NELSON, D.V.M.
West Lafayette, Indiana

In the bitch and the queen, pyometra is a hormonally mediated diestrous disorder. The disease results from bacteria infecting an endometrium that has undergone pathologic changes exaggerated by progesterone stimulation. It is possible that bacteria from the vaginal tract contaminate the uterus during proestrus and estrus when the cervix is dilated. This has been demonstrated in as many as 70 per cent of healthy bitches, but these samples were obtained following euthanasia (Baba et al., 1983).

In any case, pyometra is relatively uncommon, suggesting that uterine contamination, if it occurs, is rapidly cleared from the normal bitch. Therefore, intrauterine bacteria cannot solely account for the pathogenesis of pyometra. Significant uterine disease, such as cystic endometrial hyperplasia (CEH), or some other factor (estrogen administration) predisposes some bitches to pyometra (Bowen et al., 1985). Part of the predisposition process is the normal postovulation increase in plasma progesterone concentrations, because pyometra is seen only during or immediately following diestrus, or following exogenous progesterone administration. There is a strong correlation between the incidence of pyometra in dogs younger than 7 years of age that the authors have examined and their receiving estrogen therapy by veterinarians who were attempting to prevent pregnancy. This syndrome is not well understood, since these younger dogs may have normal uterine function for years following successful pyometra therapy. In summary, currently identified factors contributing to the development of pyometra include CEH, bacteria, elevation in serum progesterone concentrations, and exogenous estrogen administration.

The bacteria usually associated with pyometra are *Escherichia coli*. However, staphylococci, streptococci, *Pseudomonas*, *Proteus*, and other organisms have been isolated from the uteri of bitches with pyometra. Not only have these bacteria been recognized in pyometra, but they usually represent common bacteria found in the vaginal vault of the normal bitch (Olson and Mather, 1978; Ling and Kwawer, 1986).

DIAGNOSIS

Signalment, History, and Physical Examination

Pyometra is a disorder recognized in bitches and queens of any age. The signs reported by the owner will depend upon the patency of the cervix. An obvious sign with an open-cervix pyometra is a sanguineous to mucopurulent discharge from the vagina. The discharge is usually first noticed 4 to 8 weeks after standing heat (estrus). Pyometra has been diagnosed as early as the end of standing heat and as late as 12 to 14 weeks after standing heat. Other common signs include lethargy, depression, inappetence, polyuria, polydipsia, and vomiting. Some females with open-cervix pyometra may be recognized quickly by experienced owners. They can be relatively healthy, aside from the abnormal vaginal discharge. The overall health of the bitch or queen with a pyometra is most dependent on how quickly the client recognizes the problem and seeks veterinary assistance. In the queen, pyometra can

be more insidious than in the bitch (Kenney et al., 1987).

Bitches and queens with closed-cervix pyometra may be quite ill at the time of diagnosis. Instead of having an easily recognized sign (vaginal discharge), these animals have an insidious illness consisting initially of depression and inappetence. Untreated females frequently are reported to have polyuria, vomiting, and diarrhea that may result in progressively worsening dehydration. Again, the severity of illness at the time of examination is dependent to a large degree on the ability of an owner to recognize that a significant problem exists and then to seek veterinary care.

Abnormalities on physical examination consistent with pyometra include depression, dehydration, palpable uterine enlargement, and a sanguineous to mucopurulent discharge from the vulva if the cervix is patent ("open"). The rectal temperature can be elevated, normal, or even subnormal, depending on the severity of uterine inflammation, sepsis, and the current status of the patient. Uterine enlargement may be obvious. However, the uterus may be difficult to palpate if it is draining most of its contents or if it is enlarged but flaccid. The size and the weight of the dog or cat and the degree of abdominal relaxation also determine the ease of palpating uterine enlargement. Overzealous palpation should be avoided to prevent rupture of the uterine wall. A palpable uterus is always considered an abnormal finding in the nonpregnant bitch or queen in diestrus.

Clinical Pathology

The total white blood cell count is usually increased in the bitch or queen with closed-cervix pyometra, often exceeding 30,000 cells/mm^3. Many dogs with open-cervix pyometra do not exhibit evidence of the overwhelming infection seen in closed-cervix pyometra. Approximately 50 per cent of bitches with open-cervix pyometra that the authors have examined have had total white blood cell counts within the high normal range or only mildly elevated (fewer than 25,000/mm^3) prior to initiation of any therapy. A mild normocytic, normochromic, nonregenerative anemia (packed cell volume [PCV], 28 to 35) often develops. Concomitant hyperproteinemia (total protein, 7.5 to 10.0 gm/dl) and hyperglobulinemia are less common but result from either or both dehydration and chronic antigenic stimulation of the immune system. The blood urea nitrogen (BUN) may be increased if dehydration and prerenal uremia are present. Urine specific gravities are variable. Proteinuria with or without pyuria and hematuria may be identified. Immune complex deposition in the glomeruli causes a mixed membranoproliferative glomerulonephropathy and leakage of plasma proteins into the glomerular filtrate. The proteinuria gradually resolves with correction of the pyometra.

Radiography, Ultrasonography

It is difficult or impossible to distinguish pregnancy prior to fetal calcification from pyometra on abdominal radiographs. The uterus can be visualized radiographically, beginning with the fourth week of gestation, continuing through pregnancy, and for 2 to 4 weeks after whelping. Radiographic visualization of the uterus at other times is abnormal. Abdominal radiographs should be assessed in a bitch with suspected pyometra to confirm the diagnosis and to identify any unsuspected problems. With pyometra, a fluid-dense tubular structure is often seen in the ventral and caudal abdomen, displacing loops of intestine dorsally and cranially. Two additional primary concerns in a dog with pyometra are the presence or absence of peritonitis from a uterine rupture, and retained nonviable fetal tissue or obvious pregnancy. Abdominal compression may be of value, using a belly band or wooden spoon to displace the intestines away from the uterus. This procedure may enhance radiographic contrast and often allows improved visualization of the uterus. Inability to visualize the uterus radiographically does not rule out pyometra.

Ultrasound has greatly enhanced our ability to ascertain the presence of pyometra and the success of medical treatment. The value of this diagnostic tool is emphasized when abdominal radiographs are inconclusive. Ultrasound allows determination of the size of the uterus, the thickness of the uterine wall, and the presence of fluid within the lumen. If a bitch or queen is pregnant and more than 15 days into gestation, ultrasound will usually identify the presence of fetuses. The fetuses are usually quite obvious by 21 to 25 days of gestation. In some cases, the character of the fluid within the uterus (serous versus viscid) can be determined.

THERAPY

Surgery

OVARIOHYSTERECTOMY. Ovariohysterectomy is the preferred treatment for pyometra unless the owner strongly desires to maintain the reproductive potential of the bitch. The medically stable bitch with pyometra should be a good anesthetic risk. Severely ill bitches should be vigorously treated with intravenous fluids and closely monitored. Appropriate diagnostic tests should be performed to identify abnormalities in hydration, serum electrolytes, acid-base status, and cardiac rhythm. Complications associated with septicemia, bacteremia, and uremia are common. The use of broad-spectrum antibiotics is encouraged, and the veterinarian should realize that bacteremia, when present, is typically an *E. coli* infection (Nelson et al., 1982).

One cannot always wait for "stabilization" of the animal before surgery is performed. In some dogs, surgery should not be postponed more than a few hours. Septicemia and bacteremia originating from the diseased uterus are often responsible for the severe illness, and only surgical removal of that organ will begin to resolve the septic state of the bitch. Supportive therapy should be continued during and after surgery. Antibiotic administration should be continued for 7 to 10 days after removal of the infected uterus.

SURGICAL DRAINAGE. Attempts have been made to treat pyometra surgically while preserving the uterus and ovaries. Dogs and cats have been treated successfully with surgical drainage of the uterus. The authors have utilized this aggressive approach in bitches and queens with retained uterine and extrauterine fetuses. Purulent material should be aspirated, and each uterine horn flushed with an antiseptic solution through in-dwelling tubes daily for several days after surgery (Lagerstedt et al., 1987). Success with this procedure requires both skill and luck. It is not highly recommended. The difficulty of surgical drainage is increased when the pyometra is segmental, and flushing of the horns is not as easy to accomplish.

Medical Treatment (Prostaglandins)

Results of medical therapy, utilizing estrogens, androgens, ergot alkaloids, or oxytocin, have been inconsistent at best and often unsuccessful. Systemic antibiotics are typically ineffective as the sole therapy for canine pyometra. However, treatment with prostaglandin $F_{2\alpha}$ ($PGF_{2\alpha}$) has yielded extremely encouraging results, and prostaglandins offer a consistently reliable medical alternative for therapy.

ACTIONS OF PROSTAGLANDINS. $PGF_{2\alpha}$ has several physiologic effects on the female reproductive system, including contraction of the myometrium and relaxation of the cervix. These effects result in expulsion of uterine contents. Synthesis and secretion of progesterone are the primary functions of the corpora lutea. Lysis of the corpora lutea or transitory inhibition of luteal steroidogenesis also appears to result from administration of $PGF_{2\alpha}$. These actions are partially dependent on the dosage, route, frequency of administration, and timing of $PGF_{2\alpha}$ therapy within the bitch's luteal cycle. Decreased plasma progesterone concentrations eliminate the support for endometrial growth and glandular secretion, which contributes to the pyometra syndrome.

CLINICAL USEFULNESS. Several factors must be considered before initiating $PGF_{2\alpha}$ therapy. The clinician should consider the age of the bitch, the owner's desires to preserve the animal's reproductive potential, the severity of illness at the time of examination, the presence or absence of other concurrent disease, and the patency of the cervix. Medical therapy utilizing prostaglandins should be discouraged in aged bitches (older than 8 years of age) or in bitches whose owners are unsure about, or not interested in, maintaining the reproductive capabilities of their dogs.

Reduction in uterine size and improvement in the patient's clinical signs are not observed for at least 48 hr after beginning prostaglandin therapy. Therefore, this drug is *not* ideal for use in severely ill animals, unless the owner refuses surgery. Concurrent illness or disease may increase the anesthetic risk to an unacceptable level. The effects of $PGF_{2\alpha}$ in these bitches or queens have not been assessed.

$PGF_{2\alpha}$ should be used with caution in bitches and queens with a closed-cervix pyometra because of the relatively poor therapeutic response and the potential for peritonitis. Theoretically, uterine exudate may be expelled into the peritoneal cavity via the fallopian tubes or through a rent in the uterine wall following $PGF_{2\alpha}$-induced myometrial contractions against a cervix that fails to relax or dilate. The use of estrogens to relax the cervix prior to $PGF_{2\alpha}$ therapy is not recommended because of the estrogen enhancement of progesterone effects on the uterus.

$PGF_{2\alpha}$ is not approved for use in the bitch or the queen by the Food and Drug Administration. It is available for use in the cow and the mare. Owners should be so informed, but the authors have not had owners sign a "release" form. (The editors suggest release forms be signed whenever a nonapproved drug is used.)

The bitch or queen to be treated with prostaglandins should first be screened for the presence of fetuses (living or dead) within the uterus. The authors have examined two pregnant bitches referred for $PGF_{2\alpha}$ therapy because of a copious mucopurulent vaginal discharge. Both dogs had severe vaginitis that responded to appropriate nitrofurazone (Furacin, Norden) douche therapy, and both whelped healthy litters. The use of prostaglandin in bitches with mummified fetuses is worrisome because prostaglandin's myotonic effects may lead to tearing of a uterine wall that had previous adhesions and fibrous tissue. Such trauma could result in peritonitis.

THE DRUG USED. Only naturally occurring $PGF_{2\alpha}$ (dinoprost tromethamine [Lutalyse, Upjohn]) should be used, at the dosage recommended later.

Synthetic $PGF_{2\alpha}$ analogues (e.g., cloprostenol, fluprostenol, prostalene) are much more powerful than natural $PGF_{2\alpha}$. *Use of these synthetic products at this recommended dosage could result in shock and possibly death.* The median lethal dose (LD_{50}) for natural $PGF_{2\alpha}$ in the bitch is 5.13 mg/kg. The authors are not aware of comparable LD_{50} information being published for the queen.

PROTOCOL. The authors' recommended $PGF_{2\alpha}$ therapy protocol for the bitch is to administer 0.25 mg $PGF_{2\alpha}$/kg body weight subcutaneously, once daily for 5 days. In addition, concomitant broad-spectrum antibiotics effective against *E. coli* should be administered for 7 to 14 days. Trimethoprim-sulfa or amoxicillin trihydrate–clavulanate potassium (Clavamox, Beecham) have proved to be reliable. A similar protocol is used in the queen; however, the initial dose of $PGF_{2\alpha}$ is 0.1 mg/kg rather than the 0.25 mg/kg used in the bitch.

When treating a bitch or queen with closed- or open-cervix pyometra, a prostaglandin-induced discharge from the vulva is not always obvious. Therefore, the bitch or queen should be closely monitored with several thorough physical examinations per day. One would hope to identify and treat, if necessary, any drug-induced side effects (see following section). Repeated abdominal radiographs may be necessary to be sure that peritonitis is not developing in the bitch or queen being treated for a closed-cervix pyometra.

The bitch or queen should be re-evaluated 2 weeks after completion of the prostaglandin injections. If the sanguineous or mucopurulent vaginal discharge, fever, neutrophilia, or uterine enlargement are still present, treatment with $PGF_{2\alpha}$ should be reinstituted, with an additional 5-day series of injections. If there are no worrisome signs and if the discharge appears clear and serous, further treatment is not required. It is rare for any bitch or queen to require three 5-day series of injections. Such a bitch or queen might have developed pyometra early in diestrus or, more probably, will not respond to $PGF_{2\alpha}$ therapy and will eventually require ovariohysterectomy. However, approximately one third of the bitches successfully treated with prostaglandins have required two 5-day series of injections.

SIDE EFFECTS. Several reactions may be observed after the subcutaneous injection of $PGF_{2\alpha}$. Initially, the bitch may be restless and begin pacing. Hypersalivation and panting commonly occur, followed by some or all of the following: abdominal discomfort, tachycardia, fever, vomiting, and defecation. When present, these reactions can be quite pronounced, causing dramatic signs of illness within 30 to 60 sec of a subcutaneous injection. Usually, reactions last for 20 to 30 min, but they may be observed for as long as 60 min following the injection. The authors have found that walking a dog continuously for 20 to 40 min following prostaglandin administration not only minimizes the signs but also allows for close supervision by a veterinarian or trained technician. The side effects are typically less pronounced with each dose, usually being minor or absent by the fifth injection. Similar reactions are observed in cats following $PGF_{2\alpha}$ administration, with vocalization and intense grooming behavior often seen.

GENERAL RESULTS. One indication of a successful response to $PGF_{2\alpha}$ therapy would be alleviation of clinical signs, such as depression, inappetence, polydipsia, and polyuria. Other indications of treatment success are development of a clear serous vulvar discharge that slowly diminishes before resolving. A decrease in the palpable uterine diameter and a normal leukogram are additional positive changes. The clear serous vaginal discharge is often seen 5 to 14 days after the last $PGF_{2\alpha}$ injection. After a pyometra is surgically extirpated, the peripheral white blood cell count often increases dramatically. This is believed to be due to loss of the "sink" into which white blood cells flood, while the bone marrow continues its response. With medical management of pyometra, the sink remains but the infection clears. Thus, with this form of treatment, the white blood cell count often quickly (within 3 to 10 days) diminishes and becomes a valuable tool for monitoring treatment.

OPEN-CERVIX PYOMETRA. A large majority of the open-cervix pyometra bitches that the authors have treated had complete resolution of their uterine infection. Treatment either failed in a small percentage (fewer than 5 per cent) of dogs or was abandoned because of transient cerebellar signs or acute cardiac tachyarrhythmias (ventricular fibrillation). Two thirds of the successfully treated bitches required one 5-day series of injections, while the remainder required two series. Almost all the bitches that responded favorably to treatment (more than 90 per cent) have whelped litters, and of these bitches, more than 75 per cent have had more than one litter. Redevelopment of pyometra after successfully carrying a litter to term may occur. Results of a recent study (Meyers-Wallen et al., 1986) were less promising, but an explanation for the differences in results is not obvious. Prostaglandin therapy in queens with open-cervix pyometra has been as successful as the treatment in bitches.

Prostaglandin-treated bitches and queens may enter their next estrous cycle early or late. No consistent pattern has been established, and owners are made aware that an early cycle is possible. The authors strongly recommend breeding these animals on the cycle immediately following therapy for several reasons:

1. The bitch or queen may have an abnormal uterus, and recurrence of the pyometra is always possible. Therefore, attempt to obtain a litter while it is possible.

2. Subjectively, pregnant females may be less susceptible to infection than nonpregnant females.

3. There is no apparent benefit to passing or skipping a cycle.

CLOSED-CERVIX PYOMETRA. The results of prostaglandin therapy in bitches with closed-cervix pyometra have not been as positive as with the open-cervix group. There have been fewer dogs treated because the syndrome is less common and because these bitches are often so ill that ovariohysterectomy is immediately chosen. Fewer than half (40 per cent) of the treated bitches had successful results. Those that had a positive response required one or two series of injections, and these did subsequently whelp healthy litters. Of the treatment failures, all were spayed following the lack of response to the prostaglandins or because of prostaglandin-induced side effects. The authors have not yet treated a cat with closed-cervix pyometra.

A guarded prognosis with regard to resolving the pyometra should be given to owners of dogs with closed-cervix pyometra. Nevertheless, medical therapy can be attempted and ovariohysterectomy maintained as an alternative, should the prostaglandin injections fail to resolve the problem. Treatment failure is presumably due to an inability to evacuate the uterus because of the closed cervix. Should a reliable method be developed for dilating the cervix, the ability to help these animals should improve. The authors still attempt medical therapy in closed-cervix pyometra despite one death and the low percentage of successes. No abnormalities, aside from pyometra, were found at necropsy of the bitch that died. This is the only fatality in the bitches that the authors have treated.

Close monitoring is imperative during and immediately after prostaglandin therapy. Monitoring should include daily physical examinations, and periodic hemograms and abdominal radiographs or ultrasonography. Clinically, these dogs should steadily improve, aside from the immediate and transient side effects associated with the prostaglandin injections. Appetite, attitude, and activity quickly return to normal. The development of a uterine discharge, as a result of the injections, is encouraging but is not always obvious. Some fastidious bitches keep themselves extremely clean by licking. Thus, constant licking may be the only evidence of an induced vaginal discharge. In the bitch that is responding to therapy, abdominal radiographs or ultrasound obtained 3 or 4 days after initiating treatment should reveal decreasing uterine size without evidence of peritonitis. Daily or every-other-day hemograms should reveal declining white blood cell counts after the third or fourth day, as the infection clears.

POSTPARTUM ENDOMETRITIS. Although this disease entity is distinct from pyometra, postpartum endometritis can be treated with prostaglandins, using the recommended protocol. The bitches that the authors have treated have responded well to therapy, with clearance of the uterine infection and subsequent successful pregnancy.

LONG-TERM MANAGEMENT

Once a bitch or a queen has been treated medically for pyometra with prostaglandins, it is assumed that a recurrence is always possible. It is suggested that an owner objectively establish a realistic goal of the number of puppies or kittens (litters) to be obtained from that bitch or queen, respectively. The bitch or queen should be bred on each cycle until this goal is met. The bitch or queen should be spayed after whelping the last litter. Owners have complied with these suggestions, and recurrences have perhaps been avoided.

References and Supplemental Reading

Baba, E., Hata, H., Fukata, T., et al.: Vaginal and uterine microflora of adult dogs. Am. J. Vet. Res. 44:606, 1983.

Bowen, R. A., Olson, P. N., Behrendt, M. D., et al.: Efficacy and toxicity of estrogens commonly used to terminate canine pregnancy. J.A.V.M.A. 186:783, 1985.

Feldman, E. C., and Nelson, R. W.: *Canine and Feline Endocrinology and Reproduction.* Philadelphia: W. B. Saunders Co., 1987, pp. 446–454.

Kenney, K. J., Matthiesen, D. T., Brown, N. O., et al.: Pyometra in cats: 183 cases (1979–1984). J.A.V.M.A. 191:1130, 1987.

Lagerstedt, A.-S., Obel, N., and Stavenborn, M.: Uterine drainage in the bitch for treatment of pyometra refractory to prostaglandin $F_{2\alpha}$. J. Small Anim. Pract. 28:215, 1987.

Ling, G., and Kwawer, J.: Unpublished data, 1986.

Meyers-Wallen, V. N., Goldschmidt, M. H., and Flickinger, G. L.: Prostaglandin $F_{2\alpha}$ treatment of canine pyometra. J.A.V.M.A. 189:1557, 1986.

Nelson, R. W., Feldman, E. C., and Stabenfeldt, G. H.: Treatment of canine pyometra and endometritis with prostaglandin $F_{2\alpha}$. J.A.V.M.A. 181:899, 1982.

Olson, P. N., and Mather, E. C.: Canine vaginal and uterine bacterial flora. J.A.V.M.A. 172:708, 1978.

VULVAR DISCHARGES

CHERI A. JOHNSON, D.V.M., M.S.

E. Lansing, Michigan

Discharges from the vulva are relatively common in bitches but unusual in queens. The clinician must determine the nature and the source of the discharge and whether or not it is normal. A sensible therapeutic plan can then be formulated. History, physical examination, vaginal cytology, and vaginoscopy are the most important diagnostic tools. The history should include a description of the amount, the duration, and the appearance of the discharge. The temporal relationship between the onset of the discharge and the stage of the estrous cycle should be investigated. The administration of medicaments, especially hormonal drugs, should be noted. The owner should be asked about changes in the animal's micturition, water consumption, appetite, and attitude or other signs of systemic illness.

A complete physical examination is done to determine the general health of the animal. The presence of any historical or physical abnormalities in systems other than the reproductive tract will dictate a more thorough and aggressive approach. Historical or physical findings such as polydipsia-polyuria, vomiting, dehydration, fever, lethargy, abdominal pain, abdominal distention or stranguria in a bitch or a queen with a vulvar discharge should cause the clinician to include such things as a complete blood count (CBC), biochemical profile, urinalysis, and abdominal radiographs in the initial data base.

The nature of the discharge can be determined best by cytologic examination. The techniques for obtaining, staining, and interpreting the samples have been described (Olson et al., 1984a, 1984b). The vestibule, clitoris, clitoral fossa, and vulvar skin should be avoided because samples contaminated with cells from those areas are difficult to interpret. The cytologic examination should be systematic. The morphologic characteristics and the numbers of the vaginal epithelial cells, red blood cells, white blood cells, and bacteria are noted during each examination. The slides are then scrutinized for the presence of other elements such as neoplastic cells, mucus, debris, uteroverdin (biliverdin), endometrial cells, or macrophages.

Estrogen causes proliferation and maturation (cornification) of the vaginal epithelium. The effects of estrogen are easily monitored with vaginal cytology. Significant numbers of mature or cornified epithelial cells are found only when estrogenic stimulation is present or in samples contaminated with the normal, keratinized cells from the skin or clitoral fossa. Abnormal estrogenic stimulation can occur because of cystic ovarian follicles, functional ovarian tumors, or inappropriate administration of exogenous estrogens. Evidence of estrogenic stimulation is normal during proestrus, estrus, and early diestrus.

Red blood cells (RBCs) are common in normal and abnormal vulvar discharges. Their significance is determined by the other cells that accompany them. Estrogen causes diapedesis of RBCs. Therefore, RBCs with mature (cornified) epithelial cells are expected cytologic findings during normal proestrus and estrus. They could also be present because of exogenous estrogenic stimulation or ovarian pathology. Red blood cells mixed with mucus are normally found in the postpartum vaginal discharge, lochia. When the cytologic appearance is essentially that of peripheral blood, with noncornified epithelial cells, the cause of hemorrhage should be sought. The causes of hemorrhage include subinvolution of placental sites, vaginal laceration, uterine and vaginal neoplasia, uterine torsion, and coagulopathies. Bleeding can accompany any inflammatory process. When the number of white blood cells exceeds that of peripheral blood, the cause of the inflammation (rather than the cause of RBCs per se) should be determined. The presence of a bloody vulvar discharge, even with attraction of male dogs, does not always indicate proestrus or estrus.

White blood cells, with or without bacteria, are the predominant cells found during inflammation. They are also normally found in large numbers during the first 1 to 2 days of diestrus, and in lesser numbers in normal lochia. Septic or purulent vulvar discharges may originate from the vulva, vestibule, vagina, or uterus. Because of markedly different prognoses, the source of a septic or purulent discharge should be investigated immediately. If vulvitis or vaginitis is the cause, physical evidence of inflammation (e.g., hyperemia, edema, pain, mucosal lesions) should be present. These findings would not exclude the possibility of concurrent uterine pathology.

Endometrial cells may be found on cytologic preparations of vulvar discharges. The presence of endometrial cells indicates uterine involvement. Endoscopic examination of the cervix and cranial vagina may establish a uterine source of the discharge. Abdominal radiography, ultrasonography, or both are helpful in evaluation of the uterus. Knowledge of the stage of the estrous cycle is also essential for the evaluation of uterine pathology. During the luteal phase (diestrus), a septic or purulent discharge can occur because of cystic endometrial hyperplasia-pyometra, pregnancy with concurrent uterine or vaginal infection, or impending abortion. If the discharge occurs postpartum, after abortion, or otherwise during anestrus, consider metritis or uterine stump granuloma or abscess. Predisposing causes of metritis include retained placenta, retained fetus, abortion, and obstetric procedures.

Leiomyoma is the most common neoplasm of the uterus and vagina in both the bitch and the queen. This neoplasm does not exfoliate readily, and therefore, neoplastic cells are not usually found in cytologic preparations. Uterine and vaginal leiomyomas often cause a hemorrhagic vulvar discharge. Transmissible veneral tumors (TVTs) may or may not cause a vulvar discharge. Most often, bitches with TVT are examined because of a mass protruding from the vulva. Neoplastic cells exfoliate easily from TVTs. Transitional cell carcinomas of the urethra cause stanguria, with or without a bloody vulvar discharge. Cytologic and biopsy specimens of the external urethral orifice can often be obtained through the endoscope. Urethral transitional cell carcinomas and vaginal squamous cell carcinomas have been identified by vaginal cytology.

Mucus is the predominant component of lochia. It may also be seen during normal late pregnancy and possibly in scanty amounts during the nonpregnant, luteal phase (diestrus). Mibolerone and testosterone administration in intersex animals may produce a slight, mucoid discharge apparently because of androgenic stimulation. Cervicitis and mucometra could also be associated with a mucoid discharge. Some bitches with scanty, mucoid vulvar discharge are apparently normal.

Positional urinary incontinence (pooling of urine in the vagina) occurs in some bitches. These animals are usually examined because of apparent urinary incontinence. However, they may be presented because of a watery vaginal discharge or because of urine-induced vaginitis. Pooling of urine can usually be identified during vaginoscopy. Vaginal, ureteral, or urethral anomalies could cause urine accumulation in the vagina. Vaginal and urethral lesions may be identified during vaginoscopy. The ureters are best evaluated by excretory urography.

Biliverdin, a dark-green blood pigment, is normally found in the placenta. The presence of uteroverdin in a vulvar discharge indicates placental separation. This is normal during labor. In the absence of labor, uteroverdin may be found in bitches with dystocia. It may also be seen during or after abortion.

The source of the discharge can be determined best by physical examination of the vulva and clitoris and by endoscopic examination of the vestibule, urethral orifice, and vagina. Vulvar discharge caused by perivulvar and vulvar dermatitis is easily recognized. The only important diagnostic consideration is whether the inflammatory process is confined to the vulva.

The technique and equipment used for vaginoscopy and the endoscopic appearance of the canine vagina have been described (Christensen, 1979; Lindsay, 1983a, 1983b; Pineda et al., 1973; Wykes and Soderberg, 1983). Vaginoscopy is used to evaluate the source of vulvar discharges; to identify the nature and extent of vaginal abnormalities; to obtain specimens for biopsy, culture, or both; and to assess cervical patency. The canine vagina is quite long. In beagles, it is 10 to 14 cm in length and 1.5 cm in diameter. Therefore, endoscopy equipment should be at least 10 cm long. The diameter of the endoscope will be dictated by the individual bitch. Proctoscopes or anoscopes made for use in children or adults work well for vaginoscopy. The anoscopes are usually too short for viewing the cranial vagina, even in small bitches. Flexible fiberoptic equipment can be passed through a speculum if additional length or a smaller diameter is needed. Insufflation of the vagina with air is helpful for thorough inspection.

Vaginoscopy is performed in the awake, standing bitch. Sedation is rarely necessary unless a biopsy is planned. The perineum is inspected and cleansed. The endoscope is lubricated with warm saline or a sterile, water-soluble lubricant. The clitoris and clitoral fossa must be avoided. Therefore, the speculum is passed through the dorsal commissure of the vulva, in a dorsal direction. There is normally slight resistance near the vestibulovaginal junction. This is especially true for prepuberal and oophorectomized bitches, in which the diameter of that area is sometimes surprisingly narrow. The angle of the speculum is adjusted to a more horizontal direction after passing through the vestibulovaginal junction.

During proestrus, the longitudinal folds of the vagina are edematous, round, and smooth. New folds develop, and often the entire vaginal lumen is filled with folds. There is bright-red, clear fluid in the vaginal lumen, often in large amounts. As estrus approaches, the vaginal folds become lower and wrinkled. During estrus, the vaginal folds have a sharp, angular, crinkled appearance. The mucosa is pale. The vaginal lumen is wide. There is a lesser amount of luminal fluid than during proestrus. This fluid is clear and usually straw-colored; however, it may continue to be bright red throughout estrus.

During the luteal phase of the cycle (diestrus), the vaginal folds are low, round, and soft. The folds in the cranial vagina have a characteristic rosette appearance and may be mistaken for the cervix. Vaginal mucus, which is clear or opalescent, is present in the lumen. The mucous membranes have streaks of hyperemia. During anestrus and in oophorectomized bitches, the vaginal folds are low and round and do not fill the vaginal lumen. There is a scant, thin mucous coating, which gives the mucous membranes a translucent, pink-red appearance. The mucous membranes are thin and easily traumatized. Submucosal hemorrhages occur from seemingly gentle contact with the endoscope. There is usually some resistance to the passage of the endoscope, especially in neutered animals, so the instrument must be well-lubricated.

The appearance of the cranial vagina of the bitch deserves mention because it is sometimes confusing. One of the vaginal folds, known as the dorsal median postcervical fold, is often mistaken for the cervix. This fold extends from the caudal edge of the vaginal portion of the cervix, along the dorsal midline, and eventually blends into lesser folds of the vagina. It is composed of longitudinal and oblique smooth muscle bundles and irregularly arranged collagen. Unlike other folds of the vagina, the dorsal median postcervical fold has no elastic fibers. In beagle-sized bitches, this fold is 15 to 42 mm in length and 2 to 10 mm in width, compared with the average vaginal length in the same group of bitches of 158 ± 30 mm. Because of its length, location, and inelastic nature, the dorsal median postcervical fold prevents visualization and catheterization of the canine cervix, except on rare occasions.

The vaginal portion of the cervix is tubular. Small furrows radiate from the os, giving it the appearance of a star. The cervical os is not obviously patent, even when uterine fluid is seen flowing from it, except during the puerperium. The vaginal lumen around the cervix and cranial aspect of the dorsal median postcervical fold is quite narrow, and instruments of small diameter (0.5 cm) are usually necessary to visualize the cervix. The narrow paracervical vaginal lumen, the dorsal median postcervical fold, or the rosette appearance of the cranial vagina during diestrus is often confused with the cervix.

The significance of a vulvar discharge is determined by its cellular composition, its source, and the stage of the reproductive cycle. These are evaluated by history, physical examination, vaginal cytology, and vaginoscopy. In bitches, certain vulvar discharges are normal for some stages of the estrous cycle. Because it is so uncommon in queens, any vulvar discharge should be considered abnormal until proven otherwise.

References and Supplemental Reading

Christensen, G. C.: The urogenital apparatus. In Evans, H. E., and Christensen, G. C. (eds.): Miller's Anatomy of the Dog. Philadelphia: W. B. Saunders Co., 1979, p. 590.

Lindsay, F. E. F.: Endoscopy of the reproductive tract in the bitch. In Kirk, R. W. (ed.): Current Veterinary Therapy VIII. Philadelphia: W. B. Saunders Co., 1983a, p. 912.

Lindsay, F. E. F.: The normal endoscopic appearance of the caudal reproductive tract of the cyclic and noncyclic bitch: Post-uterine endoscopy. J. Small Anim. Pract. 24:1, 1983b.

Olson, P. N., Thrall, M. A., Wykes, P. M., et al.: Vaginal cytology. Part I. A useful tool for staging the canine estrous cycle. Compend. Cont. Ed. 6:288, 1984a.

Olson, P. N., Thrall, M. A., Wykes, P. M., et al.: Vaginal cytology. Part II. Its use in diagnosing canine reproductive disorders. Compend. Cont. Ed. 6:385, 1984b.

Pineda, M. H., Kainer, R. A., and Faulkner, L. C.: Dorsal median postcervical fold in the canine vagina. Am. J. Vet. Res. 34:1487, 1973.

Wykes, P. M., and Soderberg, S. F.: Congenital abnormalities of the canine vagina and vulva. J. Am. Anim. Hosp. Assoc. 19:995, 1983.

DIAGNOSIS OF CANINE HERPETIC INFECTIONS

JAMES F. EVERMANN, PH.D.

Pullman, Washington

There has been a resurgence of interest in canine herpesvirus (CHV) infection and disease over the past few years as a result of the convergence of several independent lines of investigation. Although the pathogenesis of CHV was described over 20 years ago (Carmichael et al., 1965; Stewart et al., 1965), an in-depth analysis of the *in utero* infection was not well delineated until more recently (Hashimoto and Hirai, 1986). This newer information has added to our knowledge of the maternal-fetal pathogenesis of CHV and has allowed for a more accurate time-frame in which to diagnose CHV (Hashimoto and Hirai, 1986). Coincident with the studies on CHV, there have been major advances in the biology of herpesviruses affecting other animals, as well as those affecting humans (Corey, 1985; Percy, 1982). These studies have increased our understanding about the immune responsiveness to herpetic infections and the state of latency that appears to occur universally in all species infected with herpesviruses (Rouse, 1985; Werner and Zerial, 1985).

Despite the increase in scientific knowledge regarding CHV, it still remains one of the few viruses of dogs that is capable of causing fatal infection. There is no vaccine available for the prevention of disease (Greene and Kakuk, 1984; Kraft et al., 1986). It is, perhaps, for this reason that our understanding of CHV should be of utmost concern, so an accurate and prompt diagnosis can be made and so clients can be advised on the best ways to prevent (control) CHV infection in their dogs. The objectives of this review are to present some thoughts on the laboratory diagnosis and clinical management of CHV infections. However, as a prelude to this, aspects of the infection and the disease processes will be presented so that the full clinical perspective can be realized.

INFECTION PROCESS

Canine herpesvirus is an enveloped, double-stranded DNA virus that is highly labile in the environment and is readily inactivated by such factors as sunlight, drying, and heat. It is for these reasons that CHV is predominantly spread directly by secretions from dog to dog in close contact. The spread is primarily horizontal as a result of licking (saliva and nasal mucus) or by coughing (aerosol) (Carmichael, 1970; Kraft et al., 1986). Other modes of virus spread include vertical (*in utero*) transmission and, in rare circumstances, venereal spread (Greene and Kakuk, 1984; Hashimoto and Hirai, 1986).

As with other members of the herpesvirus family, CHV is primarily an opportunistic pathogen in the immunocompromised dog. The two periods of *extreme susceptibility* to CHV infection are during pregnancy and the neonatal period (Carmichael, 1970; Hashimoto and Hirai, 1986). Other periods of susceptibility include times of stress (during stays in humane facilities and boarding kennels and during dog shows) and the period of immunosuppressive therapy (i.e., dogs being treated for dermatomyositis or on a treatment regimen for neoplasia [Kraft et al., 1986]). Wild canids being held in captivity should also be considered at high risk for infection and disease associated with CHV (Evermann et al., 1984).

Infection with CHV results in both B-cell (humoral) and T-cell (cell-mediated) immune responsiveness. However, the immunogenicity of the herpesvirus is weak, and, therefore, the antibody response following infection is usually low and rarely persists for periods longer than 60 days. The T-cell response is essential for controlling CHV infection as determined by experiments using anti-thymocyte serum. Therefore, conditions that perturb T-cell function in the dog could be expected to enhance the infectious process of CHV, that is, concurrent canine parvovirus infection, drug-induced T-cell suppression (cytoxan), and stress-induced release of T-cell modulators (Kraft et al., 1986).

Another factor that needs to be considered in the pathogenesis of CHV is the establishment of latency. Although there is a paucity of data on CHV latency, it is known that herpetic infections usually result in latency being established at the site of initial infection, which in the majority of cases of CHV would be the ganglion innervating the oropharyngeal region (Corey, 1985; Rouse, 1985). It

The author wishes to express his appreciation to Tony Gallina, Alison McKeirnan, Dick Ott, John Gorham, and Susan Kraft-Basaraba for their generous support of time and facilities for diagnostic and research efforts in small animal infectious diseases.

1313

should be understood that once a dog has been infected by CHV, it is more than likely infected for life. The infection may take the form of either a latent infection or an active infection. During the latent period, the dog would appear clinically normal (inapparent infection), and the CHV would not be detected in secretions. However, under the appropriate stress (e.g., hormonal, infectious, physiologic), CHV could be shed (stress-related shedding from carrier dog) with or *without* clinical signs (Kraft et al., 1986).

DISEASE PROCESS

The clinical signs manifested by dogs with CHV infection vary from mild to severe, depending upon the age, the presence of maternal CHV antibody, stress, and concurrent microbial infections (Hashimoto and Hirai, 1986; Kraft et al., 1986). Diseases induced by CHV are closely related to the two periods of extreme susceptibility to CHV (i.e., pregnancy and neonatal period) and, to a lesser extent, to temporary periods of immunosuppression due to stress.

Of the diseases caused by CHV, acute hemorrhagic neonatal septicemia is considered to be the most severe because of the high mortality rate in affected puppies and the pathologic features that are comparable to herpetic infections in the human neonate (Carmichael, 1970; Martin et al., 1985; Percy, 1982). The acquisition of CHV infection by puppies during the pre- and postnatal periods may occur by one of three routes. These include vertical infection *in utero* just prior to whelping; infection via vaginal-cervical secretions during passage through the birth canal; and infection after birth by secretions from the *recently* infected bitch (prior to onset of natural immunity) or secretions from other dogs allowed to commingle with puppies. Since the neonatal form of CHV infection is considered so fatal, it is important to emphasize that the pregnant bitch and puppies are unusually susceptible 3 weeks prior to and 3 weeks after whelping. This constitutes a "6-week danger period" for CHV-induced disease (Fig. 1).

Of emerging importance is the role of CHV infection of the bitch, especially during pregnancy. Studies have revealed that CHV is capable of a systemic infection of the pregnant bitch, thereby allowing for placental infection and placentitis (Hashimoto and Hirai, 1986). Abortion and the birth of premature puppies may occur during the second trimester of gestation after experimental inoculation of CHV. These results have also suggested that CHV-induced abortions or reproductive failure may occur during a limited period of gestation, similar to that occurring with *Brucella canis* infection. It is now apparent that fetal death, mummification, abor-

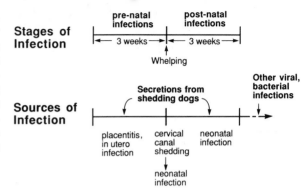

Figure 1. The 6-week danger period for susceptible dogs to become infected with canine herpesvirus.

tion, premature birth, or abnormal parturition can be associated with prenatal CHV infection of bitches (Hashimoto and Hirai, 1986; Olson et al., 1987).

The third disease period to be considered with CHV may occur in older puppies or adult dogs. During this period, the disease is generally regarded as mild, limited to the mucosal surfaces of the upper respiratory and genital tracts and the conjunctiva (Kraft et al., 1986). The localization of CHV to the mucosal cells is important in the pathogenesis of the disease, since such localization offers a unique way of maintaining virus infection but still allows for virus to be shed to susceptible dogs in the population (e.g., pregnant bitches, neonatal puppies).

LABORATORY DIAGNOSIS AND CLINICAL MANAGEMENT

Rationale

The laboratory diagnosis of CHV infection should be used to confirm the presence of CHV in a single dog or a population of dogs, so appropriate management steps can be instituted. Table 1 lists the samples to be collected in order to confirm a diagnosis of CHV infection. The importance of the diagnosis would be related directly to the type of disease manifestation that is reported by the client and observed by the clinician. The occurrence of neonatal deaths or reproductive failure should include CHV in the differential diagnosis (Table 2). Diagnostic pursuit of CHV as a possible cause of upper respiratory or genital tract disease and conjunctivitis would be advised, particularly if breeding-age dogs are in the vicinity or if the chances for commingling of dogs and, therefore, virus spread were determined to be high. Similar samples may be collected from dogs suspected of being inapparent carriers of CHV or as part of a reproductive fitness (pre-breeding) examination (Table 1).

Since there is no vaccine available for prevention of CHV-related diseases, management of the infec-

Table 1. *Collection of Clinical Samples for Confirmation of Canine Herpesvirus Infection*

Types of Infection	Organs and Tissues Affected	Samples to Collect
Neonatal (systemic) infection	Systemic infection involving all body organs	Liver, kidney, spleen chilled for virology; fixed in buffered formalin for histopathology Serum from bitch*
Abortion, pregnancy failure	Systemic infection of bitch	Fetal liver, kidney, spleen or whole puppy chilled for virology Placenta chilled for virology Serum from bitch*
Upper respiratory, conjunctival, urogenital infections	Localized infection	Nasal swabs, transtracheal wash, conjunctival swab, vaginal swab (vaginitis), preputial swab (balano-posthitis) Serum from bitch*, stud
Inapparent carrier ("shedder") condition	Localized infection	As for preceding entry

*Serum should also be checked for *Brucella canis* antibodies.

tion is essential for control. The most severe forms of CHV disease involve infections of pregnant bitches and neonatal puppies. The time of highest susceptibility (the "6-week danger period") should be a time of isolation for the pregnant bitch and the bitch and her puppies 3 weeks after whelping (Fig. 1).

Interpretation of Results

The diagnosis of a presumptive CHV infection may be made on the basis of history and clinical signs for the neonatal form only. This form has been well documented and usually results in a number of puppies in the same litter being affected, producing incessant crying and, upon necropsy, hemorrhagic spots on the kidneys and other internal organs (Greene and Kakuk, 1984; Hashimoto and Hirai, 1986). The other forms of CHV infection are more difficult to diagnose and, for this reason,

should be added to the list for a differential diagnosis in the event of abortion or pregnancy failure (Table 2) and acute upper respiratory distress, conjunctivitis, and urogenital infections of both sexes (Burke, 1986; Feldman et al., 1987; Lein, 1986; Olson et al., 1987).

Swab samples (Culturettes, Marion Scientific, Kansas City, MO) and tissue samples (Table 1) collected aseptically coincident with clinical signs will allow for a high percentage of CHV isolation (Greene and Kakuk, 1984; Evermann et al., 1984). The samples must be kept refrigerated while en route to the laboratory and should *not* be frozen. Virus isolation requires a 7- to 10-day period in canine cells (MDCK or A-72 cells, American Type Culture Collection, Rockville, MD) and subsequent identification by virus neutralization with specific antiserum.

Serum samples should be collected at the time clinical signs are manifested or as soon after as possible. The serum neutralization test is used to

Table 2. *Diagnosing Reproductive Problems in the Bitch*

Normal Interestrous Intervals and Normal Estrous Periods		Prolonged Interestrous Intervals (Twice Normal Length)	Failure to Cycle	Shortened Interestrous Intervals	Prolonged Estrus (> 21 Days)
Refuses to be Mated	**Accepts Male**				
a) Atypical cycles	a) Atypical cycles	a) Thyroid or adrenal disorders	a) Young age	a) Uterine disease	a) Cystic ovaries
b) Vaginal/vulvar abnormalities	b) Uterine or oviduct anomalies	b) Aging	b) Genetic causes of gonadal dysfunction	b) "Split" estrous period	b) Granulosa cell tumor
c) Psychological	c) Infectious causes of pregnancy failure	c) "Silent" estrous periods	c) Pituitary dysfunction	c) Cystic ovaries	c) Liver disease
	d) Hormonal causes of pregnancy failure		d) Previously neutered	d) Ovulation failure	d) Estrogen therapy
	e) Genetic causes of gonadal malfunction or pregnancy failure		e) Thyroid or adrenal gland disorders	e) Premature luteal regression	
			f) Aging		
			g) "Silent" estrous periods		
			h) Drug therapy		

(Data from Olson, P. N., Behrendt, M. D., and Weiss, D. E.: Reproductive problems in the bitch: Formulating your diagnostic plan. Vet. Med. May, 1987, pp. 482–496.)

detect serum antibodies to CHV (test availability varies from laboratory to laboratory). The test requires a 5- to 8-day period for final antibody determination. Since CHV, and herpesviruses in general, induce such a weak humoral immune response, the serum antibody titer will rise and fall quickly (4 to 8 weeks) following exposure. The CHV antibody titer will be relatively low (1:2 up to 1:32), especially when compared with the more potent canine viral immunogens, such as canine distemper virus and canine adenovirus, which induce serum-neutralizing antibodies as high as 1:320 to 1:1280. The occurrence of *any* serum-neutralizing antibody titer to CHV ($\geq$ 1:2), coincident with clinical signs, is considered of diagnostic significance.

Treatment and Prognosis

Therapy for dogs suspected of or diagnosed as being infected with CHV is for the most part supportive, since there is no vaccine available (Hashimoto and Hirai, 1986; Kraft et al., 1986). Therapy for suspected neonatal CHV infection should begin by placement of the litter beneath a heat lamp to obtain an ambient temperature of 102.2°F (39°C). The puppies should be maintained by tube feeding at least four times a day with a commercial milk replacer. Antiviral chemotherapy with drugs designed to lessen the severity of human herpetic infections (acyclovir) may be used in an attempt to control CHV. However, the regimen is somewhat empiric, since controlled clinical studies of the effects of this drug on CHV have not yet been reported.

The prognosis for puppies infected *in utero* or as neonates with CHV is not good. The possibility of permanent nervous, renal, or lymphoid tissue damage in survivors should also be considered (Kraft et al., 1986). Bitches that have aborted or have had confirmed CHV-associated reproductive failure should be monitored closely for the recurrence of CHV disease. Although recurrent herpetic infection has been reported in subsequent litters, the majority of reports and clinical impressions have indicated that subsequent litters were normal. Measurable colostral antibody apparently protects suckling neonates from disease but not from inapparent infection (Kraft et al., 1986). When taken together, the best treatment for CHV is prevention from infection, especially during the 6-week danger period.

References and Supplemental Reading

Burke, T. J.: *Small Animal Reproduction and Infertility. A Clinical Approach to Diagnosis and Treatment.* Philadelphia: Lea & Febiger, 1986.

Carmichael, L. E.: *Herpesvirus canis*: Aspects of pathogenesis and immune response. J.A.V.M.A. 156:1714, 1970.

Carmichael, L. E., Squire, R. A., and Krook, L.: Clinical and pathologic features of a fatal viral disease of newborn pups. Am. J. Vet. Res. 26:803, 1965.

Corey, L.: The natural history of genital herpes simplex virus: Perspectives on an increasing problem. *In* Roizman, B., and Lopez, C. (eds.): *The Herpesviruses*, Vol. 4. New York: Plenum Press, 1985, pp. 1–36.

Evermann, J. F., LeaMaster, B. R., McElwain, T. F., et al.: Natural infection of captive coyote pups with a herpesvirus antigenically related to canine herpesvirus. J.A.V.M.A. 185:1288, 1984.

Feldman, E. C., and Nelson, R. W.: Canine female reproduction. *In* Feldman, E. C., and Nelson, R. W. (eds.): *Canine and Feline Endocrinology and Reproduction.* Philadelphia: W. B. Saunders Co., 1987, pp. 399–480.

Greene, C. E., and Kakuk, T. J.: Canine herpesvirus infection. *In* Greene, C. E. (ed.): *Clinical Microbiology and Infectious Diseases of the Dog and Cat.* Philadelphia: W. B. Saunders Co., 1984, pp. 419–429.

Hashimoto, A., and Hirai, K.: Canine herpesvirus infection. *In* Morrow, D. A. (ed.): *Current Therapy in Theriogenology*, Vol. 2. *Diagnosis, Treatment and Prevention of Reproductive Diseases in Small and Large Animals.* Philadelphia: W. B. Saunders Co., 1986, pp. 516–520.

Kraft, S., Evermann, J. F., McKeirnan, A. J., et al.: The role of neonatal canine herpesvirus infection in mixed infections in older dogs. Comp. Cont. Ed. Pract. Vet. 8:688, 1986.

Lein, D. H.: Infertility and reproductive diseases in bitches and queens. *In* Roberts, S. J. (ed.): *Veterinary Obstetrics and Genital Diseases* (Theriogenology). Woodstock, VT: S. J. Roberts Publisher, 1986, pp. 675–698.

Martin, J. R., Reed, E. V., and Striegl, L. C.: Acute thymic atrophy in severe herpes simplex virus type 2 infection. *In* Gilmore, N., and Wainberg, M. A. (eds.): *Viral Mechanisms of Immunosuppression.* New York: Alan R. Liss, Inc., 1985, pp. 185–190.

Olson, P. N., Behrendt, M. D., and Weiss, D. E.: Reproductive problems in the bitch: Formulating your diagnostic plan. Vet. Med. 81:482–496, 1987.

Percy, D. H.: Animal models of human disease. Type 2 herpes simplex infection and neonatal canine herpes infection. Comp. Pathol. Bull. 14:2, 1982.

Rouse, B. T.: Immunopathology of herpesvirus infections. *In* Roizman, B., and Lopez, C. (eds.): *The Herpesviruses*, Vol. 4. New York: Plenum Press, 1985, pp. 103–120.

Stewart, S. E., David-Ferreira, J., Lovelace, E., et al.: Herpes-like virus isolated from neonatal and fetal dogs. Science 148:1341, 1965.

Werner, G. H., and Zerial, A.: Effects of immunopotentiating and immunomodulating agents on experimental and clinical herpesvirus infections. *In* Roizman, B., and Lopez, C. (eds.): *The Herpesviruses*, Vol. 4. New York: Plenum Press, 1985, pp. 395–416.

DIAGNOSIS AND TREATMENT OF CANINE BRUCELLOSIS

PAUL NICOLETTI, D.V.M.

Gainesville, Florida

Dogs may become infected with four of the six species of the genus *Brucella: B. melitensis, B. suis, B. abortus*, and *B. canis*. They may occasionally be mechanical or biologic vectors for transmission to other animals or humans. In general, infections with *Brucella* species, except *B. canis*, are self-limiting.

INFECTIONS WITH B. MELITENSIS, B. SUIS, AND B. ABORTUS. Apparently, the first reported isolation of any *Brucella* species from a dog in the United States was in 1931 (Planz, 1931). *B. suis* was isolated from a dog with fever and an abscess in a testicle. There were several previously reported cases in other countries.

Natural and experimental infections of the three classic species of *Brucella* have been reported by many workers. Natural infections occur through ingestion of contaminated milk or meat, fetal membranes, or aborted fetuses of livestock. Dogs appear to be quite resistant to brucellosis, as infections often produce no clinical evidence of disease and persist for varying time periods (Feldman et al., 1935; Kerby et al., 1943; Pidgeon et al., 1987). However, many signs of infection have been reported. These include abortion, orchitis and epididymitis, diskospondylitis, polyarthritis, posterior paresis, fever, and uveitis. The bacteria may be shed from semen, uterine and vaginal discharges, urine, and feces. In addition, they may be cultured from many body tissues, especially lymph nodes.

Infected dogs usually have positive results on conventional serologic methods used to diagnose brucellosis in livestock, such as the card or tube agglutination tests (Barr et al., 1986; Love et al., 1952; Morse et al., 1951; Pidgeon et al., 1987; Taylor et al., 1975). Natural or experimentally induced infections have been transmitted to livestock (Kiok et al., 1978; Kormendy and Nagy, 1982).

Apparently, no studies have been reported on the effectiveness of treatment of brucellosis in dogs caused by *B. melitensis* or *B. suis*. A dog infected with *B. abortus* was successfully treated following surgical removal of an abnormal testicle (Love et al., 1952).

INFECTIONS WITH B. CANIS. Natural infections with *B. canis* appear to be limited to the Canidae. Other animals such as livestock, cats, rabbits, and primates have been found to be quite resistant to experimental infection. Humans are accidental hosts, and infections are relatively mild compared with those caused by other *Brucella* species (Greene and George, 1984).

The means of transmission, clinical signs and pathogenesis, epizootiology, public health considerations, diagnosis, and treatment of *B. canis* infections have been reviewed (Greene and George, 1984; Meyer, 1983; Pollock, 1979). Therefore, the remainder of this article will be largely limited to the latter two aspects.

DIAGNOSIS

Brucellosis in dogs should be considered in the differential diagnosis when there are signs such as infertility, abortion or neonatal mortality, epididymitis, testicular abnormalities, scrotal dermatitis, or lymphadenopathy. Cases of diskospondylitis (Henderson et al., 1974; Smeak et al., 1987) and uveitis (Saegusa et al., 1977) caused by *B. canis* have also been reported. Many infected dogs have no overt signs of infection. It is necessary to diagnose the disease by either or both bacteriologic and serologic methods.

Bacteriology

The bacteriologic confirmation of infection with *B. canis* may be difficult in some cases, especially in chronic cases and in live animals. Nevertheless, isolation of the organisms is proof of infection and very important in confirming the disease in kennels.

There are many specimens for potential recovery of *B. canis*. In the live animal, blood cultures are often the most practical and rewarding. A bacteremia is detected 2 to 4 weeks following oral exposure and persists generally more than 1 to 2 years (Carmichael and George, 1976). The bacteria are found mostly in the leukocytes. Because of the low numbers of circulating organisms, direct plating onto solid medium is not reliable.

In the author's laboratory, 5 ml of peripheral blood is added to 50 ml of tryptose broth, which is incubated at 37°C for approximately 9 days. Subcultures are made onto tryptose agar at days 3, 6,

1317

and 9 of incubation. Negative cultures are then discarded.

Colonies of *B. canis* are naturally rough or mucoid and translucent. The organisms are usually identified by colonial morphology and agglutination, using specific antiserum. They do not require carbon dioxide for growth and are resistant to bacteriophage.

Other fluid specimens that may be cultured on solid media are urine, uterine or vaginal discharges, and semen ejaculates. *B. canis* may also be isolated from placental or fetal tissues. It is usually necessary to use antibiotics such as bacitracin and polymyxin in the medium to avoid overgrowth with contaminants.

A large number of tissues may be cultured at necropsy. These include the spleen, lymph nodes, prostate gland and epididymides, testes, bone marrow, and the gravid uterus. The nongravid uterus may also be infected (Nicoletti and Chase, 1987). Diskospondylitic or ocular lesions may also be cultured. The spleen and lymph nodes are the most probable sites of isolation in nonbacteremic dogs (Greene and George, 1984).

Serology

Serologic procedures are the most common and practical methods available for diagnosing canine brucellosis, because of the limitations of bacteriologic procedures, such as time and failure to isolate the organisms. However, it is very important that the sera be free of hemolysis and that results of tests be carefully interpreted. Case histories, physical findings, and laboratory test data should be compared.

B. canis differs from the three classic species of *Brucella* and lacks the lipopolysaccharide-endotoxin antigens that form smooth colonies. Therefore, it does not cross-react serologically with the classic species, and this causes some difficulties in preparing diagnostic antigens (Meyer, 1983).

One or more of three general serologic procedures are currently used. These are the rapid slide agglutination test (RSAT) with or without mercaptoethanol (ME), the tube agglutination test (TAT) with or without ME, and the agar gel immunodiffusion test (AGID).

The RSAT was developed in 1974 as a rapid procedure (George and Carmichael, 1974). It is a valuable method because it is simple and sensitive, and a negative result is nearly conclusive that the dog is not infected. Therefore, it is an excellent screening procedure. However, there may be many false-positive results because of cross-reactions caused by antibodies to other bacteria such as *Bordetella bronchiseptica*, *Pseudomonas*, and a *Moraxella*-like organism (Carmichael, 1976). Up to

65 per cent of the positive results with RSAT may be false, so further serologic tests must be performed (Greene and George, 1984). A commercial kit is available (Fig. 1).

A modification of the RSAT has been developed that uses 2-mercaptoethanol to reduce heterologous immunoglobulin M (IgM) agglutination (Badakhsh et al., 1982). The author found that the modified test eliminated false-positive reactions in 27 sera studied, but sera of all 12 infected dogs were positive. In recent infections, the modified test could be falsely negative for 1 to 2 weeks in RSAT-positive sera (Greene and George, 1984). An improved antigen was recently described for the slide agglutination test (Carmichael and Joubert, 1987). Replacement of *B. ovis* antigen with *B. canis* (M −) cells significantly reduced false-positive results. The tube agglutination test (TAT) is a widely used procedure in laboratories following a positive RSAT. Most laboratories use antigens furnished by the United States Department of Agriculture (USDA). Some diagnostic laboratories produce TAT antigen using a stock culture and procedures furnished by the USDA. While no criteria for classification of dogs are universal, a titer of 1:200 or greater is generally considered presumptive evidence of infection. Good correlations have been found between titers greater than or equal to 1:200 and recovery of the organism by blood cultures (Nicoletti and Chase, 1987; Pollock, 1979).

Some authors have reported that infected male dogs may be seronegative and have localized organisms in epididymides or the prostate gland (Flores-Castro et al., 1977; Moore and Kakuk, 1969).

The TAT usually becomes positive by 2 to 4

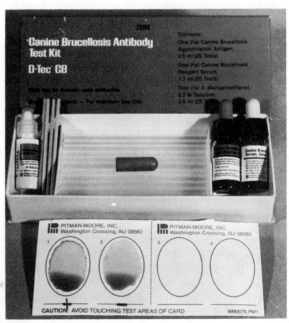

Figure 1. A commercial kit for the rapid detection of antibodies to *Brucella canis*.

weeks following exposure and concurrent with bacteremia (Carmichael and Kenney, 1968). A titer below 1:200 should be considered suspicious, and retests at least 2 weeks later should be conducted. Additional problems of interpretation may result from autoagglutination of hemolyzed serum samples and heterospecific reactions caused by antibodies to other bacteria.

Mercaptoethanol has been used to increase the specificity of the TAT similar to that of the RSAT. The titers of the TAT when ME is added may be delayed 1 to 2 weeks, but there are fewer false-positive reactions (Greene and George, 1984).

An agar gel immunodiffusion test (AGID) using one or more antigens prepared by differing methods is available in some laboratories. The AGID test is recommended to retest sera that are positive to the RSAT or TAT. The most specific but least sensitive AGID test used a protein antigen extracted from the cytoplasm of B. canis (Zoha and Carmichael, 1982). It was sensitive within 4 to 8 weeks after onset of bacteremia and was positive for at least 12 months after the end of bacteremia, when other test results were equivocal. A recent study confirmed that the AGID test may be negative in early infection and when other tests are positive (Nicoletti and Chase, 1987). An advantage of the test is the rapid seroconversion from positive to negative following apparent successful therapy. It is unfortunate that AGID antigens are not readily prepared free from cross-reacting lipopolysaccharide and that immunodiffusion procedures are generally limited to laboratories with specialized facilities and specially trained personnel (Moore and Kakuk, 1969).

Several other serologic procedures have been described. These include a counterimmunoelectrophoresis, indirect immunofluorescence, and complement fixation. None of these has been used except for research purposes.

None of the serologic methods available are conclusive in diagnosing canine brucellosis. The sensitivity and specificity vary as a result of differences in procedures, time of infection, and interpretation of results.

Other Procedures

Hematologic and biochemical values are nonspecific in canine brucellosis (Greene and George, 1984). Urinalysis is usually normal. Radiographic examinations of diskospondylitis or other abnormalities should be further studied by serologic and bacteriologic procedures.

Semen morphology should always be evaluated in dogs with suspected brucellosis. Abnormalities include immature sperm and head-to-head agglutination with inflammatory cells (Greene and George, 1984).

TREATMENT

Since the discovery of B. canis in the 1960s, several workers have considered chemotherapy as an alternative to euthanasia of infected dogs. As with other Brucella infections, the success of treatment has varied. The antibiotic regimens have not been consistent. Most clinicians have not been optimistic about permanent cures. The failures have generally been attributed to the intracellular localization of Brucella organisms, especially those of the reticuloendothelial system, and the failure of antibiotics to gain access to the intracellular environment (Nicoletti and Chase, 1987).

B. canis is susceptible to a large number of antibiotics, but therapy for cases of brucellosis has resulted in failures or relapses in both natural and experimental infections. Bacteremia may recur, or localization of organisms may occur in some tissues following treatment. Aborting females may subsequently produce normal litters with or without therapy, but they may transmit infection to their surviving offspring; treated males may develop irreversible sterility and have localized infection in the prostate gland, with continued shedding of the organisms (Greene and George, 1984). Because of the limited successes of chemotherapy, most workers recommend that infected dogs be excluded from further breeding.

A review of the use of antibiotics to control or eliminate canine brucellosis was recently published (Nicoletti and Chase, 1987). The report summarized studies on antibiotic usage in experimental and natural infections. A case documentation was presented when 20 infected and 28 uninfected dogs were simultaneously treated to control an outbreak. The treatment regimen was oral tetracycline, 500 mg three times daily (10 mg/kg/day for 30 days), along with streptomycin, 15 mg/kg intramuscularly on days 1 to 7 and 24 to 30. Of 20 infected dogs, 15 were considered to be cured with one treatment regimen, and two of four dogs that were re-treated were also cured. The authors felt that there is justification for simultaneously treating seronegative and seropositive dogs in kennel outbreaks. Serologic tests were very useful in evaluating treatment successes. Titers receded rapidly following successful therapy but soon became elevated in dogs with relapsing infection.

At least three additional studies have reported on chemotherapy of naturally infected dogs. In a study of 24 infected dogs, investigators gave four weekly intramuscular injections of oxytetracycline (20 mg/kg) (Liquamycin La-200, Pfizer) and daily intramuscular injections of streptomycin (15 mg/kg) for the initial 7-day period (Zoha and Walsh, 1982). Six months after the final treatment, 19 of the 24 dogs (79 per cent) were serologically and culturally negative. In another study, 6 of 12 naturally infected bitches were treated with oral tetracycline followed by dihydrostreptomycin and then by oral trimethoprim-sulfadiazine (Johnson et al., 1982). None of the six was cured. There was a statistical difference in the reproductive performance of treated dogs and the six untreated control subjects. Six seropositive dogs were treated with various regimens in another study (Hubbert et al., 1980). Based upon serologic findings, two dogs that received tetracycline and streptomycin were apparently cured, whereas four dogs that received other drugs did not respond favorably to treatment.

The most extensive studies on experimentally infected dogs used 13 different regimens in 80 dogs in groups of three or more (Flores-Castro and Carmichael, 1981). The best results were obtained with a total daily dose of 10 mg/kg of minocycline hydrochloride (Minocin, Lederle) administered for 14 days, and a total daily dose of 4.5 mg/kg of streptomycin given twice a day for 7 days. Fifteen of 18 dogs (83 per cent) were considered cured on the basis of cultures of blood and tissues at the time of euthanasia, 6 to 28 weeks after treatment. Minocycline alone was not effective in 8 of 11 dogs.

An evaluation of reported studies on treatment of natural and experimental cases of canine brucellosis leads to the conclusion that long-term therapy is necessary. As with *Brucella* infections in other animal species, a combination of tetracycline and streptomycin is superior to other regimens. In general, use of these antibiotics has led to approximately 80 per cent successful therapy when subsequent serologic and, in some cases, bacteriologic criteria are used for evaluations. Repeated therapy, neutering, artificial insemination, and euthanasia are options for consideration following a review of the individual cases of canine brucellosis.

References and Supplemental Reading

Badakhsh, F. F., Carmichael, L. E., and Douglass, J. A.: Improved rapid slide agglutination test for presumptive diagnosis of canine brucellosis. J. Clin. Microbiol. 15:286, 1982.

Barr, S. C., Eilts, B. E., Roy, A. F., et al.: *Brucella suis* biotype 1 infection in a dog. J.A.V.M.A. 189:686, 1986.

Carmichael, L. E.: Canine brucellosis: An annotated review with selected cautionary comments. Theriogenology 6:105, 1976.

Carmichael, L. E., and George, L. W.: Canine brucellosis: New knowledge. Dev. Biol. Stand. 31:237, 1976.

Carmichael, L. E., and Joubert, J. C.: A rapid slide agglutination test for the serodiagnosis of *Brucella canis* infection that employs a variant (M−) organism as antigen. Cornell Vet. 77:3, 1987.

Carmichael, L. E., and Kenney, R. M.: Canine abortion caused by *Brucella canis*. J.A.V.M.A. 152:605, 1968.

Feldman, W. H., Bollman, J. L., Olson, C., Jr.: Experimental brucellosis in dogs. J. Infect. Dis. 56:321, 1935.

Flores-Castro, R., and Carmichael, L. E.: *Brucella canis* infection in dogs. Rev. Latinoam. Microbiol. 23:75, 1981.

Flores-Castro, R., Suarez, F., Ramirez-Pfeiffer, C., et al.: Canine brucellosis: Bacteriological and serological investigation of naturally infected dogs in Mexico City. J. Clin. Microbiol. 6:591, 1977.

George, L. W., and Carmichael, L. E.: A plate agglutination test for the rapid diagnosis of canine brucellosis. Am. J. Vet. Res. 35:905, 1974.

Greene, C. E., and George, L. W.: Canine brucellosis. In Greene, C. E. (ed.): *Clinical Microbiology and Infectious Diseases of the Dog and Cat.* Philadelphia: W. B. Saunders Co., 1984, pp. 646–662.

Henderson, R. A., Hoerlein, B. F., Kramer, T. T., et al.: Discospondylitis in three dogs infected with *Brucella canis*. J.A.V.M.A. 165:451, 1974.

Hubbert, N. L., Bech-Nielsen, S., and Barta, O.: Canine brucellosis: Comparison of clinical manifestations with serologic test results. J.A.V.M.A. 177:168, 1980.

Johnson, C. A., Bennett, M., Jensen, R. K., et al.: Effect of a combined antibiotic therapy on fertility in brood bitches infected with *Brucella canis*. J.A.V.M.A. 180:1330, 1982.

Kerby, G. P., Brown, I. W., Jr., Margolis, G., et al.: Bacteriological observations on experimental brucellosis in dogs and swine. Am. J. Pathol. 19:1009, 1943.

Kimberling, C. V., Luchsinger, D. W., and Anderson, R. K.: Three cases of canine brucellosis. J.A.V.M.A. 148:900, 1966.

Kiok, P., Grunbaum, E. G., Letz, W., et al.: Der hund als reinfektion seuelle für brucellose freie rinderbestände. Mht. Vet. Med. 33:700, 1978.

Kormendy, B., and Nagy, G. Y.: The supposed involvement of dogs carrying *Brucella suis* in the spread of swine brucellosis. Acta Vet. Acad. Sci. Hung. 30:3, 1982.

Love, R. J., Hemphill, J., Jr., Cooper, M. S., et al.: Epididymitis in a dog caused by *Brucella abortus* and treatment with aureomycin. Cornell Vet. 42:36, 1952.

Meyer, M. E.: Update on canine brucellosis. Mod. Vet. Pract. 64:987, 1983.

Moore, J. A., and Kakuk, T. J.: Male dogs naturally infected with *Brucella canis*. J.A.V.M.A. 155:1352, 1969.

Morse, E. V., Kowalczyk, T., and Beach, B. A.: The bacteriologic aspects of experimental brucellosis in dogs following exposure. I. Effects of feeding aborted fetuses and placentas to adult dogs. Am. J. Vet. Res. 12:219, 1951.

Nicoletti, P., and Chase, A.: The use of antibiotics to control canine brucellosis. Compend. Cont. Ed. Pract. Vet. 9:1063, 1987.

Nicoletti, P., and Chase, A.: An evaluation of methods to diagnose *Brucella canis* infection in dogs. Compend. Cont. Ed. Pract. Vet. 9:1071, 1987.

Nicoletti, P. L., Quinn, B. R., and Minor, P. W.: Canine to human transmission of brucellosis. NY State J. Med. 67:2886, 1967.

Pidgeon, G. L., Scanlan, C. M., Miller, W. R., et al.: Experimental infection of dogs with *Brucella abortus*. Cornell Vet. 77:339, 1987.

Planz, J. F.: *Brucella* infection in a dog. J.A.V.M.A. 79:251, 1931.

Pollock, R. V. H.: Canine brucellosis: Current status. Compend. Cont. Ed. Pract. Vet. 1:255, 1979.

Saegusa, J., Ueda, K., Goto, Y., et al.: Ocular lesions in experimental canine brucellosis. Jpn. J. Vet. Sci. 39:181, 1977.

Smeak, D. D., Olmstead, M. L., and Hohn, R. B.: *Brucella canis* osteomyelitis in two dogs with total hip replacements. J.A.V.M.A. 191:986, 1987.

Taylor, D. J., Renton, J. P., and McGregor, A. B.: Case report: *Brucella abortus* biotype 1 as a cause of abortion in a bitch. Vet. Rec. 96:428, 1975.

Zoha, S. J., and Carmichael, L. E.: Serological responses of dogs to cell wall and internal antigens of *Brucella canis*. Vet. Microbiol. 17:35, 1982.

Zoha, S. J., and Walsh, R.: Effect of a two-stage antibiotic regimen on dogs naturally infected with *Brucella canis*. J.A.V.M.A. 180:1474, 1982.

ANESTHETIC CONSIDERATIONS
FOR CESAREAN SECTION

J. L. GRANDY, D.V.M.

Fort Collins, Colorado

There are many factors to consider in anesthetizing small animal patients for a cesarean section. This article will review the physiologic and pharmacologic considerations involved and offer some rational drug regimens for this surgery.

PHYSIOLOGIC CHANGES DURING PREGNANCY

To provide the best anesthesia for cesarean section, the clinician must understand some of the maternal physiologic changes that take place during pregnancy and how these may affect the course of anesthesia.

Respiratory Changes

In pregnant women, there is an upward shift of the diaphragm and, as a result, a decrease in functional residual capacity (FRC). Functional residual capacity is the volume of air left in the lung at the end of normal expiration, and a reduction in this results in a decrease in the patient's oxygen reserves. Oxygen (O_2) uptake increases during pregnancy and labor because of increased maternal metabolism and the work of breathing. As a result of the reduced O_2 reserves, at a time when O_2 requirements may be increased, maternal respiratory depression without supplemental O_2 can easily result in fetal hypoxemia (Schnider and Gershon, 1986).

An increase in minute ventilation and a resultant decrease in arterial carbon dioxide pressure (Pa_{CO_2}) have been shown to occur during pregnancy. Despite a lower Pa_{CO_2}, normal pH is maintained as a result of renal compensation and a decrease in serum bicarbonate. This increase in ventilation is in excess of the elevation in basal metabolic rate that occurs during pregnancy and, in women, is thought to be due to respiratory stimulating properties of progesterone. The decrease in FRC combined with the increased minute ventilation also increases the speed of induction of anesthesia when inhalant anesthetics are used (Schnider and Gershon, 1986).

Cardiovascular Changes

The cardiovascular system of the pregnant animal is significantly stressed during pregnancy and parturition. In pregnant women, cardiac output increases 30 to 40 per cent during the first trimester of pregnancy (Schnider and Gershon, 1986). During labor, uterine contractions increase central blood volume and cardiac output by an additional 10 to 25 per cent. Blood pressure does not increase during a normal pregnancy, as peripheral vascular resistance is decreased, but arterial blood pressure does rise with uterine contractions during labor.

The total blood volume increase in dogs during pregnancy is primarily due to a rise in plasma volume, resulting in a decreased packed cell volume (PCV). In dogs, PCV is 32 per cent lower at term than at the start of pregnancy (Concannon et al., 1977). Although this dilutional anemia reduces the O_2-carrying capacity of blood, O_2 transport to important organs increases during pregnancy because of increased cardiac output, decreased blood viscosity, and increased maternal arterial oxygen pressure (Pa_{O_2}) as a result of hyperventilation and vasodilation (Schnider and Gershon, 1986).

The circulating activity of coagulation factors VII, VIII, IX, and XI is significantly increased in pregnant dogs (Gentry and Liptrap, 1977).

Central Nervous System Changes

During pregnancy, less local anesthetic is required to produce a given level of epidural analgesia. Although this has been attributed to a decrease in the volume of the epidural space resulting from venous engorgement of the vessels because of increased abdominal pressure, it now appears that other factors may be more important. Studies indicate that nerve fibers may have an increased sensitivity to local anesthetics during pregnancy (Schnider and Gershon, 1986).

Maternal requirements for inhalant anesthetics are also reduced during pregnancy as much as 40 per cent (Palahniuk et al., 1974). Although the mechanism for this is not completely understood, it appears from studies in rabbits that there is a pregnancy-induced activation of the endorphin system. There is no correlation between the reduction in anesthetic requirements and changes in serum progesterone levels.

Gastrointestinal Changes

The risk of regurgitation in the pregnant patient is increased as a result of the cranial displacement of the stomach, decreased lower esophageal sphincter tone, and slower gastric emptying time.

Fetal Anatomy and Physiology

Drug metabolism by the fetus is limited. Hepatic biotransformation pathways associated with microsomal enzyme systems are deficient, and in addition, only a portion of the blood returning to the fetus from the placenta enters the liver. The rest bypasses the liver via the ductus venosus and enters the inferior vena cava. From 34 to 91 per cent of umbilical vein blood has been reported to bypass the liver (Welsch, 1982). Mixing of blood from the placenta with that from the lower fetal body does help dilute drugs that have crossed the placenta.

PLACENTAL DRUG TRANSFER

All drugs cross the placenta, primarily by diffusion, and reach the fetus. The rate and the extent of transfer differ among various compounds (Welsch, 1982). The rate of diffusion is determined by the maternal-fetal drug gradient, uterine and umbilical blood flow, and drug molecular weight, protein binding, lipid solubility, and degree of ionization. Maternal drug concentration is increased by high total dose, use of slowly metabolized drugs, and administration of drugs into highly vascular areas. Increasing the degree of ionization and lipid solubility and decreasing molecular weight favor placental drug transfer. Only free drug (i.e., not bound to albumin) can cross the placenta. Almost all anesthetic drugs have a low molecular weight, are partially nonionized at physiologic pH, are highly lipid soluble and are at least partly nonprotein bound, and will rapidly cross the placenta. Once the drug crosses the placenta, the effects on the fetus depend on the fetal drug uptake, distribution, metabolism, and elimination.

ANESTHETIC TECHNIQUES

Prior to anesthesia, the patient should be in the best condition possible. Fluid deficits should be corrected as much as possible beforehand and fluid therapy continued intraoperatively. Placental blood flow may be reduced by dehydration, reduced cardiac output, and hypotension. Decreased placental perfusion will adversely affect the fetuses.

Regional Anesthesia

Injection of the appropriate amount of local anesthetic into the maternal epidural space will provide sufficient analgesia for surgery. When properly performed, this type of anesthesia is the least depressing to the fetus of all anesthetic techniques and usually results in the delivery of vigorous neonates. Proper administration of epidural analgesia does require skill and practice on the part of the clinician. The usual site of epidural injection of local anesthetic in dogs is the lumbosacral intervertebral space. The technique has been well described elsewhere (Klide, 1968), and prior to attempting an epidural injection, this review should be read.

Lidocaine and mepivacaine are local anesthetics commonly used for epidural analgesia for cesarean sections. These drugs have a duration of 90 to 120 min. A dose rate of 1 ml/3.5 kg of 2 per cent lidocaine or mepivacaine is appropriate for a cesarean section.

Local anesthetics administered by any route will cross the placenta, and lidocaine administered intravenously to the dam appears in umbilical venous blood in 2 to 3 min (Welsch, 1982). The amount of local anesthetic that crosses the placenta and the rate of passage depend in part upon the route of administration and the total dose used. Epidural administration of the recommended doses does not result in levels of local anesthetic sufficient to depress the fetus.

The majority of small animal patients presented for cesarean section that are candidates for an epidural block will require some degree of sedation. A low dose of either oxymorphone (see Table 1) or meperidine is usually appropriate. If oxymorphone is used, atropine should also be administered. Excessive sedation should be avoided, as it will predispose the mother to aspiration pneumonia,

Table 1. *Dosages of Anesthetic Drugs*

Atropine	0.04 mg/kg sc
Oxymorphone	0.05 to 0.1 mg/kg sc, IV (maximum 3 mg)
Diazepam	0.2 mg/kg IV
Meperidine	4 mg/kg sc only
Ketamine	3 to 6 mg/kg IV
Fentanyl-droperidol	1 ml/25 kg
Naloxone	0.04 mg/kg; 1/2 IV, 1/2 IM
Doxapram	0.25 mg total in neonate
Dopamine	5 μg/kg/min (e.g., in a 20-kg dog, 40 mg of dopamine in 100 ml administered at a rate of 15 drops/min, using a dripset with 60 drops/ml)

hypotension, and hypoxemia. Furthermore, hypoxemia and drug-induced depression in the fetus may result. If airway reflexes are impaired, the patient should be intubated and allowed to inspire oxygen. Supplemental oxygen administration via face mask should be given to all pregnant patients in dorsal recumbency.

Complications and Contraindications of Regional Anesthesia

In addition to blocking pain fibers, epidural analgesia also blocks the sympathetic fibers that innervate blood vessels. As a result, vasodilation will occur in the area of analgesia and contribute to any preexisting maternal hypotension. Blood pressure should be monitored using a Doppler ultrasound flow detector (Park Electronics Inc., Beaverton, OR), and intravenous fluid administration should be started prior to local anesthetic injection and continued throughout surgery.

Central nervous system toxicity resulting in convulsions occurs when the amount of local anesthetic in the arterial blood exceeds a critical level. High blood levels occur with accidental intravascular injection or repeated injections of local anesthetic resulting in high total dose of drug. Convulsions due to local anesthetic toxicity should be controlled with diazepam or a thiobarbiturate, and the patient should be intubated and ventilated, as the convulsion threshold is inversely proportionate to Pa_{CO_2}. High circulating levels of local anesthetic also result in myocardial depression, reduced cardiac output, and hypotension.

Excessive cranial migration of local anesthetic in the epidural space occurs if too large a volume of local anesthetic has been injected relative to the patient's size or if a higher than recommended concentration of drug has been used. Too rapid an epidural injection of local anesthetic and placing the patient in a head-down position after injection will also result in too cranial a block. Respiratory muscle paralysis and significant circulatory compromise will occur if the block reaches the high thoracic vertebral segments. Epidural analgesia is contraindicated with hypovolemic shock, septicemia, and spinal cord disease.

GENERAL ANESTHESIA

The duration of general anesthesia prior to delivery should be as short as possible in order to minimize fetal depression. To accomplish this, the animal should be clipped and prepped for surgery beforehand, and the surgeon should be ready to start surgery immediately after induction.

Preanesthetic Medication

Preanesthetic drugs are administered to sedate the patient before an epidural block or to reduce the amount of drug needed for induction and maintenance of anesthesia. In addition, anticholinergic drugs such as atropine are used to decrease salivary and bronchial secretions. Although atropine easily crosses the placenta and increases fetal heart rate, it is still usually administered if oxymorphone or fentanyl is being used, since both these drugs decrease heart rate. Glycopyrrolate is an anticholinergic drug that crosses the placenta less than atropine, but it may not be as effective as atropine in preventing bradycardia due to oxymorphone or fentanyl.

Tranquilizers such as acepromazine and droperidol rapidly cross the placenta and appear in fetal blood. While low doses of these drugs may only minimally depress the neonate, the alpha-adrenergic blockade produced may potentiate maternal hypotension and result in decreased uterine blood flow and fetal hypoxemia. Xylazine is generally avoided in small animal patients, since respiratory depression in the fetus may be severe (Muir, 1984). Xylazine may also increase intrauterine pressure (see p. 1301).

Narcotics such as oxymorphone, fentayl, and meperidine are analgesics that will also sedate the patient. Meperidine is the least potent of these narcotics and has the least amount of sedation associated with it. Although narcotics do cross the placenta, respiratory depression in the newborn can be reversed with a narcotic antagonist.

Induction Drugs

Following appropriate premedication, anesthesia may be induced in a number of ways. The combination of oxymorphone and diazepam (Table 1) can be used intravenously for induction following premedication with atropine. Approximately one fourth to one third of the total oxymorphone dose should be administered slowly, usually in conjunction with intravenous fluids. This is followed by one fourth to one third of the diazepam dose, again administered slowly. Since narcotics are potent respiratory depressants, it is advisable to have the animal breathe O_2 through a face mask during induction to prevent hypoxemia. Induction with this drug combination is slower than with a thiobarbiturate and frequently results in tachypnea, which may necessitate positive-pressure ventilation following intubation. Diazepam does cross the placenta rapidly, and maternal and fetal blood levels are approximately equal within minutes of an intravenous dose. The human neonate is capable of metabolizing small doses of diazepam, but when the total dose exceeds 30 mg, lethargy, hypothermia, and decreased feeding may result.

Since oxymorphone is a potent analgesic, only low amounts of volatile anesthetic should be needed for maintenance of anesthesia. Narcotic-induced respiratory depression in the dam or the offspring may be reversed using naloxone. Narcotic antagonists have a shorter duration of action than the narcotic, and therefore, the neonate should be observed for several hours and redosed with an antagonist if needed.

The combination of fentanyl-droperiodol can be used for induction. The same considerations apply as with oxymorphone. In addition, hypotension due to droperidol may be a problem.

Meperidine may be useful as a premedication drug, given subcutaneously, but should not be administered intravenously to dogs, as this route is associated with hypotension.

Thiopental rapidly crosses the placenta and is present in the fetal circulation in less than 2 min following a single intravenous dose of 4 mg/kg. In humans, it appears that the fetal brain will not be exposed to high concentrations of barbiturate if the induction dose is less than 4 mg/kg (Schnider and Gershon, 1986). In veterinary anesthesia reviews, it has been recommended that the dose be less than 8 mg/kg (Muir, 1984). Obviously, the lowest dose possible is desirable, and premedication of the patient with a narcotic will facilitate thiobarbiturate induction. There is no advantage in delaying delivery until the thiopental has been redistributed in the mother or the fetus (Schnider and Gershon, 1986). Pentobarbital or intermittent doses of a thiobarbiturate to maintain general anesthesia will markedly decrease the chances of delivery of live neonates.

Ketamine crosses the placenta of dogs and cats, causing depression of the neonate. Ketamine may increase uterine tone to the point of reducing blood flow and potentially contributing to neonatal hypoxemia.

Induction of anesthesia may also be accomplished with a volatile anesthetic. This type of induction is usually preferable to using ketamine or thiopental. Following suitable premedication, an appropriate-size mask is placed over the dog's muzzle, and the concentration of volatile anesthetic is gradually increased until tracheal intubation is possible. Any struggling by the patient during the later stages of this type of induction can be overcome by the intravenous administration of a small amount of either diazepam or oxymorphone at that time.

Inhalational anesthetics cross the placenta rapidly, and neonatal depression is proportional to the depth and duration of anesthesia. Drugs that are less soluble in blood and tissues, such as halothane, isoflurane, or enflurane, are preferable to a highly soluble drug such as methoxyflurane. With rela-

tively insoluble drugs, induction, changes in planes of anesthesia, and recovery will be faster. In addition, these drugs undergo far less metabolism than methoxyflurane. Neonatal depression due to methoxyflurane may resolve very slowly because of its high solubility in blood and tissues. Nitrous oxide may be used to supplement other inhalational anesthetics, but its potency in domestic animals is significantly less than in humans. It should not be administered in concentrations greater than 50 per cent. Nitrous oxide is rapidly transferred across the placenta, and administration for longer than approximately 15 min may result in fetal depression. Diffusion hypoxia may occur in neonates as a result of nitrous oxide administration, and supplemental O_2 for 5 to 10 min following delivery may be necessary.

Neuromuscular-blocking drugs do not readily cross the placenta. The administration of any of these drugs requires prompt endotracheal intubation and positive-pressure ventilation. These drugs should be used only by personnel skilled in their administration and reversal, and with access to appropriate patient support. Neuromuscular-blocking drugs do not produce any anesthesia and must be used with sufficient amounts of anesthetic drugs.

Maintenance of Anesthesia

Since the risk of aspiration pneumonia is increased in pregnant patients, as soon as possible the animal should be intubated with a cuffed endotracheal tube. While induction of general anesthesia for cesarean section may be achieved with a number of different drugs, anesthesia is best maintained using the lowest possible dose of volatile anesthetic. Since the MAC (minimal alveolar concentration needed to prevent purposeful patient movement in response to a painful stimulus in 50 per cent of animals) value of inhalation anesthetics is reduced by up to 40 per cent during pregnancy, vaporizer dial settings should be lower than usual (Palahniuk et al., 1974). The use of a narcotic for premedication or induction may also help reduce the amount of volatile anesthetic required.

MONITORING AND SUPPORT

Maternal respiratory depression due to anesthetic drugs, abdominal distention, or positioning may result in respiratory acidosis. Positive-pressure ventilation may be necessary to prevent or correct respiratory acidosis. Fetal hypoxemia and acidosis markedly alter the distribution of fetal cardiac output, and as a result, blood flow to the fetal heart, placenta, brain, and adrenals is increased at the expense of flow to the kidneys, lungs, spleen, gastrointestinal tract, and muscle (Welsch, 1982). The administration of volatile anesthetic drugs in O_2 should help correct any maternal hypoxemia.

In order to maintain good organ perfusion, the systolic arterial blood pressure should be greater than 100 mm Hg. Systolic arterial blood pressure can be easily measured using a Doppler ultrasound flow detector. A pressure between 80 and 100 mm Hg will usually respond favorably to a small increase in fluids and a decrease in anesthetic vaporizer dial settings. A systolic blood pressure less than 80 mm Hg should be treated more aggressively with intravenous fluids and reduction in the amount of anesthetic; if the patient fails to respond, a positive inotropic drug such as dopamine or dobutamine may need to be administered. Dopamine and dobutamine are potent sympathomimetic drugs that must be diluted and then administered as a constant intravenous infusion.

Aortocaval compression is an important cause of hypotension, decreased cardiac output, and neonatal depression in pregnant women. In order to minimize these effects, women undergoing cesarean sections are placed in a lateral tilt position. In one study of pregnant anesthetized dogs, maternal posture had no effect on arterial blood pressure, but cardiac output was not measured in these animals (Probst and Webb, 1983). The dogs in this same study were anesthetized close to the end of pregnancy and then again at 2 to 3 months after parturition, using the same anesthetic drugs both times. Arterial blood pressure and Pa_{O_2} were significantly lower and Pa_{CO_2} significantly higher during the pregnant anesthesia than during the second anesthesia.

CARE OF THE NEWBORN

The nasal passages and oropharynx should be cleared of fluid and mucus immediately upon delivery, and the neonate should be dried and kept warm. If respiratory depression is apparent and narcotics have been used, naloxone may be administered intravenously, sublingually, or subcutaneously. Gentle massage of the thorax may assist ventilation, and oxygen should also be administered. In unresponsive patients, the respiratory stimulant doxapram may be administered either sublingually or into the umbilical vein. Those whose respiratory system is still depressed should be intubated (using a 16- or 18-gauge catheter) and ventilated at the rate of 12 breaths/min using a bulb syringe.

References and Supplemental Reading

Concannon, P. W., Powers, M. E., Holder, W., et al.: Pregnancy and parturition in the bitch. Biol. Reprod. 16:517, 1977.

Finster, M., and Pedersen, H.: Placental transfer and fetal uptake of drugs. Br. J. Anaesth. 51:25S, 1979.

Gentry, P. A., and Liptrap, R. M.: Plasma levels of specific coagulation factors and oestrogens in the bitch during pregnancy. J. Small Anim. Pract. 18:267, 1977.

Klide, A.: Epidural analgesia in the dog and cat. J.A.V.M.A. 153:165, 1968.

Muir, W. W.: An Outline of Veterinary Anesthesia. Columbus: The Ohio State University Press, 1984.

Palahniuk, R. J., Schnider, S. M., and Eger, E. I., II: Pregnancy decreases the requirements for inhaled anesthetic agents. Anesthesiology 41:82, 1974.

Probst, C. W., and Webb, A. I.: Postural influence on systemic blood pressure, gas exchange and acid/base status in the term-pregnant bitch during general anesthesia. Am. J. Vet. Res. 44:1963, 1983.

Schnider, S. M., and Gershon, L.: Anesthesia, 2nd ed. New York: Churchill Livingstone, 1986.

Welsch, F.: Placental transfer and fetal uptake of drugs. J. Vet. Pharmacol. Ther. 5:91, 1982.

CARE AND DISEASES OF NEONATAL PUPPIES AND KITTENS

DENNIS F. LAWLER, D.V.M.

St. Louis, Missouri

Veterinarians treating very young puppies and kittens often face medical limitations, because of the patients' small size, as well as nonmedical limitations, especially financial concerns. The history provided may be vague or difficult to interpret, owing to the neonate's narrow response range. Further, it may be impractical or impossible to obtain samples such as blood for laboratory evaluation.

However, this does not mean that neonatal medicine is not rewarding. Unquestionably, there are situations, such as genetic or accidentally occurring abnormalities of anatomy and physiology, that lead inevitably to death. In other instances, therapy is possible with early diagnosis. The veterinarian may be able to provide more accurate prognostic information, thus allowing for a better informed and more satisfying decision on the part of the client. Finally, guidance in terms of genetic counseling or solving management problems may be offered.

The key to successful neonatal and pediatric practice is prevention. Understanding that preventive medicine has both individual and population bases will enable the veterinarian to make positive contributions to neonatal medicine.

GENERAL CARE

The attitude and activity of the young should be noted prior to their being handled. Normal neonates usually huddle together, especially during periods of inactivity. Abnormal litters may be spread about, not seeking one another or the dam. Hungry puppies and kittens may be restless and may cry, but should quiet down and sleep when they are full. Those that are constantly restless or vocal, remain separate from the group, or seem to lack vigor should be examined carefully (Table 1), as should their dam. Frequent, gentle handling of young puppies and kittens seems to improve both physical and social development.

The muscle tone of the neonate should be noted. The muscle tone of the normal neonatal kitten is less impressive than that of the normal neonatal puppy, and one species should not be used as a standard for the other. Likewise, there is considerable variation in vigor at birth among dog breeds. Decreased muscle tone and activity often precede the onset of other outward signs of illness in neonates. These individuals can rapidly lose the ability to nurse effectively and may be neglected by the dam. Small or weak puppies and kittens may appear to nurse and develop abdominal fullness, yet remain restless, become weak, and die. Postmortem examination reveals air, but no milk in the stomach, indicating ineffective nursing. If weak but apparently nursing puppies and kittens do not improve within a few hours, supplemental tube feeding and other supportive therapy should be initiated.

The body temperature of the neonate should be noted. With a little experience, hypothermia can be readily recognized by handling. The normal rectal temperature of puppies and kittens at birth has been reported to be as low as 36°C (96.8°F), reaching adult levels by week 4. Neonates are essentially poikilothermic animals for about 2 weeks.

For bitches or queens with long hair, dense hair coats, or weak young, it may be necessary to clip sufficient hair to allow easier access to the nipples. Caution should be exercised to avoid injury to nipples when this is done. The clinician should ensure that the dam has sufficient milk and is nursing and caring for her young. Hyperplastic nipples on older bitches may encumber nursing by small or weak puppies.

For weak, small kittens and puppies and in situations of maternal neglect, inadequate lactation, or lactation failure, supplemental tube feeding should be initiated with milk replacer as appropriate to the species. If a lactating dam is available, cross-fostering often is desirable. Most bitches and queens will readily accept fostered young, but smaller neonates should not be placed with those that are larger or more mature, even if their ages are similar.

Normal kittens and puppies should be weighed about once weekly. If birth weight is low or if progress is slow, body weight should be monitored more frequently, perhaps every 48 to 72 hr. Where more extensive intervention is needed, such as orphan-rearing, daily weight measurement is most helpful. The normal birth weight for kittens is 100 gm $\pm$ 10 gm. The very minimal acceptable weight gain for nursing kittens is 7 to 10 gm daily. Corresponding values for puppies vary with the breed, but healthy puppies should double their birth weight by about 7 to 10 days of age.

MORBIDITY AND MORTALITY

For both dogs and cats, birth weight has been shown to be an important predictor of survival. It has been suggested that immaturity of a variety of physiologic processes, especially cardiopulmonary function, accompanies low birth weight. Suggested causes of neonatal morbidity and mortality include environmental factors (i.e., extremes of temperature and humidity, sudden weather changes, sanitation problems), nutrition, inadequate thermoregulation, trauma, cannibalism, anatomic birth defects, inborn errors of metabolism, dystocia or prolonged labor and the associated hypoxia or anoxia, and infections. In particular, dystocia and prolonged labor are very significant causes of early death in dogs and cats.

Depending upon the breed, methods of breeding stock selection, husbandry, and sanitation practices, puppy and kitten losses by weaning may vary from 10 to 30 per cent or more of all full-term neonates. Typically, about 65 per cent of puppy and kitten losses occur during the first week of life, and about one half of these losses are stillbirths. By contrast, postweaning losses normally should not exceed 1 to 1.5 per cent. In the neonatal period, most losses are probably due to noninfectious causes.

Table 1. Outline of Physical Examination of Neonates

Tail: Check for length, mobility, deformities.

Limbs: Check for deformities or absence of long bones; number and position of toes and pads; position of limbs at rest and during movement; tendon contracture; soft tissue (bruises, swellings, wounds); and joints (deformities, range of mobility).

Anus: Check for patency, redness, swelling, signs of diarrhea (overeating, infection, environment). Persistent inflammation may result from diarrhea, excessive maternal attention, or both. Pain may be present.

Perineum: Check for inflammation, fecal staining.

External Genitalia: Check position and appearance; inflammation due to inappropriate nursing by siblings or excessive bitch attention, especially with small litters; stimulate urination; urine flow (hematuria usually due to trauma or infection).

Spine: Check body length as appropriate for size and breed; deformities such as lordosis, kyphosis, and scoliosis.

Thoracic Cage: Check whether symmetric or deformed. If wounds are present, that is, due to bitch trauma, observe respiration, and palpate for rib fractures. With deformities, respiratory compromise can be increasingly severe as growth proceeds; associated spinal deformities may be present.

Ventral Abdomen: Pink skin color is normal. Pallor can indicate anemia (which is common in kittens but less common in puppies) or internal hemorrhaging due to birth trauma, torn umbilical vessels, clotting disorder. Check for cyanosis due to cardiovascular or respiratory problem; often lungs will have a fetal appearance. Check umbilicus for inflammation, swelling, drainage. The umbilicus normally falls off by 2 to 3 days of age. Occasionally, the bitch will remove viscera through congenital or traumatic opening.

Abdomen: Should be enlarged after nursing, with the puppy quieted into a restful state. An enlarged abdomen with weakness or continued restlessness may indicate that the puppy is swallowing air or has an infection; an enlarged abdomen may be accompanied by cyanosis, crying, pain, dehydration, and deterioration. This set of signs and symptoms indicates a poor prognosis.

Chest: One may attempt auscultation, but this is often unrewarding in neonates unless it is done serially. In the evaluation of puppies, it is more useful to evaluate rate and depth of respirations, heart rate, activity level, muscle tone, and nursing ability. Dyspnea or cyanosis is usually subtle unless the condition is extremely serious.

Skin: Check for wounds, most often caused by an overzealous bitch; state of hydration (the skin wrinkles and loses turgor with dehydration); completeness of hair cover, along with birth weight, which can indicate state of maturity. Foot pads should be examined for anatomic abnormalities or irritation from bedding.

Head and Neck: Check for mobility; rooting reflex; position at rest and during movement.

Skull: check shape, size, and fontanelle.

Ears: Check size and position.

Eyes and Eyelids: Check for neonatal ophthalmia. Eyelids may open early naturally; if so, watch for signs of inadequate tear production.

Nose: Check appearance of patency of nostrils; presence of fluids (mucus, pus, blood, milk, clear discharge).

Mouth: Check color of mucous membranes (dehydration is often accompanied by a bright pink to reddish color); presence of cyanosis; suckling reflex; moistness (hydration); temperature to digital palpation; bedding material in mouth, which can interfere with nursing; cleft palate. Puppies with cleft palate cannot nurse effectively, and milk usually exudes from mouth and nostrils. Aspiration pneumonia and starvation are common causes of death when cleft palate is undetected.

Nervous System: Responses are difficult or impossible to evaluate in weak puppies. Evaluate alertness and response to stimulus (such as handling); voluntary and involuntary motor function; posture and movement; cranial nerves. Adequate rooting and suckling reflexes, along with normal vestibular function, are critical to the neonate. With puppies, serial evaluations are usually necessary to define suspected nervous dysfunctions.

It should also be remembered that, in puppies and kittens, flexor dominance exists through about day 4, followed by extensor dominance through about day 21. After this time, normotonia is achieved.

Noninfectious Causes

Environmental factors, nutritional inadequacy, trauma, and cannibalism are manageable problems, although careful interview of the client may be necessary to discern their existence and severity. Careful attention should be given to environmental conditions such as fluctuations in temperature and humidity, ventilation, air changes, drafts, and moisture, especially during seasons of the year when the weather is more variable. Wind barriers, improved sanitation, insect and rodent control, supplemental heat, humidity control, increased or decreased air movement, and attention to air handling systems are examples of practical recommendations that may be appropriate. The type of construction and housing provided in the kennel or cattery may also play a role in management problems, especially relative to sanitation.

Nutritional or genetic counseling likewise may be indicated. Popular fads, emotion, and financial considerations are commonly found to be factors influencing clients in these areas. Thus, thorough evaluation and good communication are necessary skills for the clinician.

Older dams and those that are very nervous are more likely to cannibalize their young, but if this becomes a kennel or cattery problem, careful review of reproduction and general management techniques is in order. Crowding, excessive noise, methods of breeding stock selection, or other possible disruptive influences should be considered.

Experience has shown that choice of breeding stock according to objective performance standards (Table 2) helps minimize many compromising situations that result from poor reproductive capacity. Poor reproductive performance seems to be familial in many instances, although it is debatable whether many of these observations represent genetic problems or whether inadequate management of repro-

Table 2. *Commonly Measured Parameters of Reproductive Performance*

1. Reproductive performance of ancestors, siblings, offspring.
2. Comparative performance on parity basis (requires accurate records).
3. State of health of sire and dam.
4. Age of sire and dam (decline in production after approximately 6 years of age in females; later in normal males).
5. Estrous cyclic activity and mating behavior.
6. Dam's body condition during gestation and lactation (consider with food intake).
7. Conception failure, resorption, abortion (documentation?).
8. Parturition (time? difficulty? assisted? dystocia?).
9. Postpartum complications.
10. Cannibalism (dam's temperament and age; offspring quality).
11. Trauma to offspring (overmothering, dam's temperament).
12. Birth defects (gross, subgross, metabolic; genetic versus environmental). Some defects are not detectable in neonatal period.
13. Litter size.
14. Birth weight.
15. Mortality (liveborn, stillborn, identifiable causes).
16. Rate of weight gain through lactation (vigor, complicating illnesses, quality of lactation).
17. Temperament of offspring.
18. Temperament of dam (changes?)
19. Mothering instinct of dam (consider along with offspring quality).
20. Lactation ability (initiation–first week; maintenance over subsequent weeks). Consider along with food intake.
21. Weaning weight of offspring.
22. Postweaning adjustment of offspring (food intake, weight gain, activity, and attitude are accurate reflections of health and maturity).

duction or other aspects of husbandry are the important factors.

Most inborn errors of metabolism are autosomal recessive traits, and most involve defects in enzymes. Partial loss of enzyme activity may occur and may become evident only in times of increased stress or greater use of the involved metabolic pathway(s). Specific groups of clinical signs are produced by most such defects, but the signs themselves are usually nonspecific. Gross anatomic defects are often absent. That such a disorder might be present must therefore be suspected by the clinician. Often, the basis for this suspicion is epidemiologic in nature, such as repeated losses from successive litters by the same bitch or unusual patterns of puppy mortality in related bitches. While therapy may or may not be feasible in individual cases, the importance of pursuing diagnosis to establish direction for expensive and time-consuming breeding programs is clear. The clinical manifestations of inborn errors of metabolism that have been documented in dogs and cats have been described by Jezyk (1983).

In addition to hypoxia and anoxia, hypoglycemia, hypothermia, and dehydration are common neonatal problems that can result from a variety of initiating events. Normoglycemic and hyperglycemic responses may not be optimally functional in compromised neonates. A poor epinephrine-stimulated hyperglycemic response to hypothermia and hypoglycemia exists, as does poor thermoregulation (shivering and peripheral vasoconstriction). The increased metabolic rate that results from the body's attempt to maintain temperature increases glucose utilization and can lead to hypoglycemia.

Sepsis can lead to hypoglycemia, possibly owing to impaired glycogenolysis and gluconeogenesis (resulting from liver dysfunction, decreased liver perfusion, or both), depletion of liver and muscle glycogen, excessive glucose consumption in peripheral tissues or by bacteria and leukocytes, compounds with insulinlike activity, salicylates (with metabolic acidosis), or disrupted intermediary metabolism of glucose.

Endocrine activity differs somewhat in human neonates, compared to adults. Insulin is probably more important in protein synthesis. Glucagon promotes both glycogenolysis and gluconeogenesis. Cortisol induces liver glycogen storage near term but not postnatally. Corticoids do not appreciably stimulate gluconeogenesis in neonates.

Transfer from the human maternal environment to self-sufficiency, and withdrawal of umbilical circulation, can lead to a significant decline of blood glucose if hypoxia has occurred. Liver glycogen stores that may be present decline in the fasting infant. After 24 hr, gluconeogenesis is the primary support of the infant's blood glucose levels. Kliegman and Morton's study (1987) of apparently normal neonatal beagles compared fasted states of 3 hr versus 24 hr duration. Puppies fasted for the longer period of time had reduced circulating levels of free fatty acids, glycerol, and triglycerides. The turnover rate of fat-related fuels was also lower. Glucose, alanine, and lactate turnover rates were not different between the two groups. However, the main source of glucose production changed from glycogenolysis at 3 hr to gluconeogenesis *and* glycogenolysis at 24 hr, accompanied by a decline in hepatic glycogen, but not a total depletion.

By contrast, unhealthy or abnormal neonates may have fewer gluconeogenic precursors and decreased ability to generate or utilize other energy sources because of immature enzyme function, small muscle mass (amino acids), lack of fat stores (glycerol and fatty acids), and less hepatic glycogen. Thus, hypoglycemia might be expected to develop more quickly, with an increased likelihood of clinically significant signs. Immature feedback mechanisms between plasma and liver relative to glucose concentration and production may also be contributory, and anorexia worsens the situation.

In addition, some of the inborn errors of enzyme metabolism are also associated with hypoglycemia, in which case hypoglycemia can be the event that initiates clinically evident disease, followed by hypothermia and then cardiovascular collapse.

Regardless, the net result of prolonged lack of substrate is likely to be a reduction of available oxidizable fuels, a problem that may be compounded by pre-existing metabolic compromise. While normal neonates do have some adaptive mechanisms to deal with hypoglycemia, the lack of appropriate cardiovascular and other physiologic responses can result in serious and perhaps irreversible injury in hypoglycemic, hypothermic, hypoxic, and dehydrated neonates.

Despite this poor regulation of blood glucose, the large brain:body mass ratio of the neonate contributes to a high glucose requirement (i.e., in humans, two to four times that of adults). Increases in glucose demands or reduction of intake may therefore precipitate hypoglycemia much more easily than in older patients.

Clinical signs of hypoglycemia include weakness, hypothermia, crying, bradycardia, respiratory distress, convulsions, and coma. Diagnostic blood samples are often difficult to obtain from puppies and kittens exhibiting these signs. Since hypoglycemia, hypothermia, and dehydration often occur together and can be complicated (perhaps irreversibly) by hypoxia in neonates, therapy should be initiated empirically and early.

Useful steps in general preventive medicine and supportive care of compromised neonates can be summarized as follows (Atkins, 1984; Lawler and Bebiak, 1986):

1. Prevention via optimal breeding selection and bitch care is most important.

2. Hypothermic neonatal patients should be warmed slowly (1 to 3 hr) to rectal temperature of 97 to 98°F (36.1 to 36.7°C). Normothermia should be maintained.

3. Encourage nursing to provide colostrum and to spare hepatic glycogen.

4. Monitor daily weight change (5 to 10 per cent gain per day).

5. Watch for overcompetition, rejection, or impaired nursing ability.

6. Consider intravenous fluid therapy, especially with isotonic glucose solutions.

7. Warm neonates before oral administration of milk replacer. A rectal temperature lower than 94°F (34.4°C) is accompanied by lack of digestive function.

8. Subcutaneous administration of warmed lactated Ringer's solution may be given at the rate of 1 ml/30 gm body weight. This may be followed by warmed 5 to 10 per cent glucose solution by stomach tube, at 0.25 ml/30 gm body weight.

9. Shield heating pads to prevent burning of the weak neonate, which may be unable to move away from excessive heat. Maintain ambient temperature at 85 to 95°F (29.4 to 35°C) (week 1), with a relative humidity of 55 to 65 per cent. Provide a 30 to 40 per cent oxygen environment if possible, until stabilization occurs. Retinopathies can result from prolonged excessive oxygen exposure.

10. Maintain caloric intake via oral milk replacer when normothermia is achieved.

11. Vitamin K may be given intramuscularly or subcutaneously, .01 to .1 mg, to help avoid bleeding.

ORPHANS. Orphaned puppies should be kept together and provided with colostrum if possible. Puppies may be fed about four times daily if they are normal. Normal kittens may do better with four to six daily feedings. Fewer feedings will be required if a lactating dam is available to provide at least some milk. Smaller or weak puppies and kittens require more frequent feeding (i.e., every 2 to 3 hr), with smaller amounts given at each feeding. The milk replacer concentration may be gradually strengthened with growth. However, caution must be exercised to avoid osmotic diarrhea. It is also important to shake canned formulas prior to use, to avoid osmotic diarrhea because of feeding of settled contents. In some instances, particularly with severe or prolonged diarrhea, subcutaneous lactated Ringer's solution should be administered (1 ml/30 gm body weight).

Infections

In general, infections are involved in relatively few neonatal deaths when compared with other causes. However, in certain instances or geographic areas, they may present extremely serious problems. Krakowka (1977) reported that the following canine infectious diseases can be acquired transplacentally: herpesvirus, adenovirus-1, canine distemper virus, *Brucella canis*, *Streptococcus*, *Haemobartonella canis*, *Toxoplasma gondii*, *Toxocara canis*, *Ancylostoma caninum*, and *Dirofilaria immitis*.

CANINE HERPESVIRUS

Canine herpesvirus (CHV) is thought to be a more common cause of neonatal deaths than are other viruses. The infection can be acquired *in utero* or in the birth canal. Postnatal contact with virus-containing saliva or vaginal discharges of affected dams and contact with other puppies are possible means of infection. The virus is ubiquitous, but clinically affected litters are more likely to be produced by younger dams. If infection is acquired *in utero*, fetal death, mummification, abortion, or neonatal death can result. Most deaths occur between approximately the ninth and fourteenth days of life. Severe clinical disease in a puppy older than 4 weeks, coincident with the attainment of adult body temperature ranges, is unlikely. However, mild or inapparent infection of the respiratory or genital tract may occur in older dogs. Stress may induce recrudescent shedding of the virus from the respiratory or genital tract.

Clinically, affected young puppies present with an acute, severe illness characterized by listlessness, anorexia, persistent crying, abdominal pain, bloating, rapid and shallow respiration, hypothermia, paddling of limbs, and opisthotonos. Commonly, the clinical course of the disease ends in death in 18 to 24 hr.

Postmortem pathology consists of multiple areas of hemorrhage and necrosis in the liver and kidneys. Pulmonary and intestinal hemorrhages, bronchopneumonia, splenomegaly, and encephalitis have also been reported. Histopathology, virus isolation, and immunofluorescence all contribute to laboratory confirmation. While no commercially available vaccines exist, serum antibodies are protective. Thus, sera from dogs with antibody titers to CHV can be given at birth to puppies at high risk, such as those in a breeding kennel where recent losses of neonates to CHV have occurred. Elevation of ambient temperature to 100°F (37.8°C) for 1 to 2 hr, with fluid administration every 15 to 20 min, may also be helpful. Losses of successive litters from the same bitch may occur but seem to be uncommon.

In the presence of an outbreak of CHV in a breeding kennel, it is advisable to observe stringent sanitation and to limit introduction of new animals. Separation of infected litters or dams from those with no history suggestive of CHV and careful attention to traffic patterns and possible fomite transmission are recommended. Bitches with suspected genital lesions should not be bred, and separation of all neonates from such bitches should be stressed.

CANINE DISTEMPER

Improved products for vaccination have reduced puppy mortality from canine distemper (CD). However, canine distemper is still a commonly reported clinical and pathologic diagnosis in the dog. While the role of CD in puppy mortality has diminished,

it is known that infection of the dam during pregnancy can cause fetal death, abortion, or the birth of weak puppies that survive only a short time. Significant laboratory findings include lymphopenia and anemia. Immunofluorescence of bone marrow specimens may demonstrate infection. In young puppies, thymic atrophy and focal interstitial pneumonia may be observed at necropsy.

INFECTIOUS CANINE HEPATITIS (CAV-1)

Dogs recovering from infectious canine hepatitis (CAV-1) may shed virus in the urine for extended periods of time. In pregnant bitches, this provides a favorable environment for acquisition of the virus by puppies during parturition. CAV-1 may also infect puppies *in utero*, although this is considered to be uncommon. *In utero* infection may result in weak puppies at birth, with death occurring within a few days. While effective vaccines and vaccination strategies have greatly reduced deaths from neonatal CAV-1, the possibilities of carrier bitches and persistent postinfection virus shedding in the urine in isolated situations should not be overlooked.

Postmortem findings in naturally occurring cases include peritoneal effusion and hemorrhage, generalized organ congestion, pulmonary edema, and intestinal hemorrhages in addition to liver pathology. Fibrinous peritonitis, thymic and pulmonary hemorrhage, meningeal congestion, and edema of the gallbladder wall have also been reported in investigative settings. If laboratory confirmation of CAV-1 is required, histopathology, immunofluorescence, and virus isolation all are helpful. When dealing with occasional kennel outbreaks of CD or CAV-1, general management considerations are similar to those described for CHV.

FELINE PANLEUKOPENIA

The cause of feline panleukopenia (FPL) is a parvovirus that is closely related to canine parvovirus (CPV). Maternally derived antibodies can interfere with immunization, just as with CPV in puppies. Extreme leukopenia is accompanied by a poor prognosis in cats suffering from FPL. If susceptible kittens are infected with feline parvovirus (FPV) *in utero* or shortly after birth, cerebellar ataxia syndrome can occur. This condition is characterized by a wide stance and hypermetria. As with CPV-induced myocarditis in puppies, cerebellar ataxia syndrome is uncommon today because of the presence of adequate maternally derived antibody in most neonatal kittens. The presence of severe leukopenia as well as necropsy and histopathology and various serologic methods can be used to confirm the diagnosis of feline panleukopenia when necessary. Effective vaccines and sound management procedures have resulted in a generally lower incidence of FPL, even in catteries. However, the clinician should be alert to the possibility of isolated occurrences. Modified live virus FPL vaccines should not be administered during pregnancy. Administration of required vaccines prior to mating should be a high priority in breeding catteries and kennels. The author prefers killed FPL virus vaccines.

CORONAVIRUSES AND ROTAVIRUSES

The relationship (if any) of canine and feline enteric coronaviruses to neonatal disease has not been defined. Earlier suggestions that the feline infectious peritonitis (FIP) coronavirus might be responsible for considerable feline neonatal mortality have not yet been confirmed. Additional research will be required to elucidate the relationship of coronaviruses to canine and feline neonatal problems. The same is true for canine and feline rotaviruses. Although rotaviruses are known to cause neonatal diarrhea in many mammals, including humans, their role in neonatal puppies and kittens is not fully understood. Reported cases have usually involved animals younger than 6 weeks old. An enzyme-linked immunoassay system is commercially available and is an accurate and rapid means of diagnosis.

FELINE UPPER RESPIRATORY DISEASE

Feline viral rhinotracheitis (FVR) and feline calicivirus (FCV) are reportedly responsible for some 90 per cent of feline upper respiratory disease. Carrier states exist for both viruses, with continuous (FCV) or intermittent (FVR) viral shedding. Complicating bacterial infections are common. In problem catteries, early weaning programs, strict age segregation and sanitation, and more intensive vaccination schedules are frequently needed.

FELINE LEUKEMIA VIRUS

Feline leukemia virus (FeLV) can cause a range of neoplastic and degenerative diseases in cats. Cats infected with FeLV have a high incidence of reproductive problems, including abortion, fetal resorption, and the birth of weak kittens that survive only a few weeks. FeLV-infected queens can give birth to kittens that appear healthy but that carry transplacentally acquired FeLV. This may be one means by which the disease is perpetuated.

BACTERIAL DISEASES

Bacterial infections can be acquired transplacentally, via the umbilicus, orally, or in the birth canal. The following suggestions concerning antibiotic therapy in the neonate should be interpreted as guidelines only and are not intended to be a substitute for thorough clinical and laboratory evaluation. Jones (1987) summarized information on common bacterial diseases of neonates.

Septicemias are caused mainly by *Escherichia coli* and beta-hemolytic streptococci, and less commonly by staphylococci or gram-negative enteric organisms other than *E. coli*. Broad-spectrum antibiotics are indicated, and cephalosporins are less potentially toxic to neonates than some other antibiotics. Penicillin or ampicillin, with an aminoglycoside, is an alternative, but aminoglycosides should be used very cautiously in neonates. Bacterial meningitis is caused by a similar range of organisms, often being secondary to septicemia. Preferred antibiotics include ampicillin or cephalosporins. Chloramphenicol and trimethoprim are potentially more toxic alternatives.

While respiratory infections in neonates are common, they are often viral in origin. Bacterial pathogens include *Bordetella* in puppies and *Pasteurella* in kittens, and neonatal death from pneumonia is not unusual. For *Pasteurella* infections, ampicillin or amoxacillin is preferred, whereas *Bordetella* infections may respond to tetracyclines, trimethoprim-sulfa, or aminoglycosides. However, since all these antibiotics are potentially toxic to the neonate, attention to the environment and sanitation is a very important preventive measure.

Aspiration pneumonias are usually mixed floral infections. These can result from esophageal dysfunction or from errors in tube or bottle feeding. Broad-spectrum antibiotics should be used.

Enteritis in neonates is often associated with *E. coli*, for which oral polymyxin, neomycin, or trimethoprim-sulfa is suggested. The drug of choice for *Salmonella* infections is trimethoprim-sulfa. *Campylobacter* infections are being diagnosed more frequently, and erythromycin is the drug of choice.

Urinary infections should be differentiated initially by gram-staining. Gram-positive infections are frequently due to beta-lactamase–positive staphylococci, for which amoxacillin–clavulanic acid is appropriate. This drug may also be preferable against gram-negative urinary infections (pending culture sensitivity testing) because of lower potential toxicity than the alternative trimethoprim-sulfa.

Jones (1987) suggested minimal dose adjustment (compared with adult-dose schedules), with lengthened dose intervals for penicillins and cephalosporins, and minimal adjustment for tetracyclines, macrolides, lincosamides, and metronidazole. Longer dose intervals should be used for aminoglycosides.

Reduced doses are appropriate for chloramphenicol and sulfonamides, while trimethoprim should be given at a reduced dose and at longer dose intervals. However, in very young patients, it is probably better to avoid administration of tetracyclines, aminoglycosides, chloramphenicol (especially in kittens), sulfonamides, and trimethoprim when possible. Tetracyclines bond to calcium, depositing in newly formed bones and teeth. This can lead to bone deformity and teeth discoloration, with enamel dysplasia. Renal and hepatic toxicity may also occur. Chloramphenicol can be retained for excessive lengths of time because of the relative lack of ability in the neonate to conjugate this drug with glucuronide for excretion (especially in kittens). Also, inhibition of protein synthesis by chloramphenicol can lead to maturation abnormalities of rapidly growing cells, such as in bone marrow. All aminoglycosides are potentially ototoxic and nephrotoxic. The necessity for excretion by immature kidneys can lead to inappropriate retention of these drugs in the neonate. Trimethoprim can lead to hematologic abnormalities similar to those that can be caused by antifolate drugs (anemia, leukopenia, thrombocytopenia). Hepatic cholestasis can also result.

The terms "toxic milk syndrome" and "acid milk" are applied to a syndrome in neonates characterized by bloating, crying, redness and edema of the anus, green diarrhea, and dehydration. Although commonly ascribed to metritis or subinvolution of the uterus, the actual causes(s) is (are) not known, and puppies of bitches with uterine subinvolution usually remain healthy. Supportive treatment includes removal from the bitch, at least temporarily, and glucose/fluid support, use of an incubator, and antibiotics.

Although "fading" neonatal puppies and kittens are often considered to be the victims of bacterial infection, it is more probable that this term is representative of a variety of diverse disorders, and thus the term itself has relatively little meaning.

BRUCELLOSIS

Brucella canis is the cause of an extremely serious, contagious disease in dogs. In one study, 85 per cent of *Brucella canis*–associated canine abortions occurred between days 45 and 55 of gestation. Puppies either were dead at birth or died within a few hours. Partial autolysis was common. If the litter is carried to term, both live and dead puppies may be born. Surviving puppies are often bacteremic for at least 2 months after birth and may remain infected for long periods of time. *Brucella canis* is a kennel disaster and a human health hazard. Many veterinarians recommend euthanasia for proven infected animals because of the difficulty

of effecting a complete cure, the zoonotic potential of the disease, and the devastating reproductive implications.

Other than abortion in females and epididymitis in males, the clinical findings are usually nonspecific. Definitive diagnosis is by serologic and bacteriologic methods. An active and ongoing testing program for brucellosis is an absolute necessity in any canine breeding facility.

Parasites

Several parasitic diseases of neonatal puppies and kittens also merit attention. Most puppies are infected with roundworms early in life, having acquired the infection mainly by parasite migration prenatally. Lactogenous spread may occur also but is not considered to be the most important route by which the disease is acquired by dogs. The symptoms depend on the age of the puppy, how the infection was acquired, and the species of roundworm present.

Toxocara canis larvae encysted in the tissues of the pregnant bitch are reactivated during the last trimester. They migrate across the placenta to the fetus *in utero*. They remain in the liver and lungs of the fetus until after birth, when they move to the gut. The bitch also can pass infective larvae to puppies in her milk. If the ascarid burden acquired prenatally is very heavy, or if an extremely heavy transmammary infection is acquired shortly after birth, puppies may die very early in life, during the roundworms' migratory stages.

Intestinal stages of the parasite can interfere with digestion, resulting in enteritis, poor growth, and poor nutrient utilization. In puppies younger than age 5 weeks of age, most *Toxocara canis* larvae take the migratory route through the liver and lungs after release into the upper intestine. Following migration, the parasites mature in the gut. If the puppies are older than about 5 weeks, larvae tend to be distributed from the lungs to the somatic tissues of the body, where they encyst. After about age 12 weeks, many larvae encyst rather than reentering the gut.

While prenatal infection occurs only with *Toxocara canis*, transmammary infection occurs with both *Toxocara canis* and *Toxocara cati*. *Toxascaris leonina*, *T. canis*, and *T. cati* all undergo mucosal migration in the intestine, while liver-to-lung and somatic migration are characteristic only of *T. canis* and *T. cati*. Somatic migration of *T. cati* is the main source of transmammary ascarid infection in kittens.

Another common and potentially severe parasite problem in neonates is hookworm infection. The parasite load and the virulence of the hookworms, and the resistance of the host, dictate the severity of the infection. *Ancylostoma caninum* sucks more blood than do other hookworms of dogs and is therefore more pathogenic. *Ancylostoma tubaeforme* is more pathogenic to cats. The adult dog is the main source of infection for puppies, although infective larvae do persist in warm, moist environments for several weeks. Ingestion and cutaneous penetration by larvae are the main routes by which infection is acquired in older puppies. The two principal routes by which neonates may become infected are the transplacental and the transmammary. In dogs and cats, the transmammary route is currently considered to be more important.

As with roundworms, there are numerous effective anthelmintics available for the control of hookworms. The author prefers pyrantel pamoate (Nemex, Pfizer) in young animals. In severe cases in young puppies, blood transfusion may be necessary so that the animal will live long enough for the anthelmintic to have a positive effect, and hookworms may cause death before eggs can be identified in feces.

Treatment of pregnant bitches with a prolonged course of fenbendazole, extending from day 40 of pregnancy through the second week of lactation, has been reported to reduce the roundworm and hookworm burdens. This extended course of medication is expensive and is usually reserved for problem situations.

Coccidian oocysts are commonly found on routine fecal flotation examinations of young puppies and kittens. Ordinarily, this is a self-limiting disease, and therapy is frequently not required. The disease can be a problem in large kennels where other enteric diseases are seen in young puppies. If young puppies and kittens are unthrifty, are growing poorly, and have associated signs of enteritis, treatment is warranted. Dehydration, depression, and anemia may occur in severe cases.

Cryptosporidium is a coccidian parasite that has recently received attention because of its potential public health implications. Young animals may be more prone to infection and appear more likely to become clinically ill. Immunity is not passively transferred to the young through the colostrum. Cryptosporidiosis is characterized by a watery diarrhea, loss of weight, and loss of appetite. Often, this disease occurs secondary to immune compromise.

As part of the control of coccidiosis, good hygiene, adequate nutrition and control of concurrent parasitic and viral intestinal disorders all are important. In extremely severe cases, prophylactic use of coccidiostats may be necessary. *Cryptosporidium* oocysts are quite resistant to disinfection, and control is therefore difficult. *Cryptosporidium* should be carefully searched for by clinicians dealing with problem situations, since it bears the potential for zoonotic transmission.

Giardia is no longer considered to be exclusively host-specific and is a very common small animal parasite. Therefore, the diagnosis of giardiasis in pets is important in terms of public health. *Giardia* is a normal inhabitant of the bowel, but the presence of large numbers of trophozoites in the small intestine is usually associated with clinical signs. Freshly passed cysts are immediately infective and remain so for several weeks under conditions of warmth and humidity, but the trophozoites are labile once outside the host. The infective cysts are ingested by a new host, constituting the main form of transmission of the disease. Preliminary data have suggested that quarternary ammonium compounds can be effective in destroying *Giardia* cysts. Therefore, the routine use of these compounds for therapy should be considered in problem situations.

CONCLUSION

Veterinarians are often called upon for advice and assistance in situations of impending neonatal mortality. However, careful attention to epidemiologic data and preventive medicine are perhaps the most important functions of the veterinarian in canine and feline neonatology today.

References and Supplemental Reading

Atkins, C. E.: Disorders of glucose homeostasis in neonatal and juvenile dogs: Hypoglycemia. Part I. Compend. Contin. Ed. 6:197, 1984.
Bebiak, D. M., Lawler, D. F., and Reutzel, L. F.: Nutrition and management of the dog. Vet. Clin. North Am. 17:505, 1987.
Essex, M.: Feline leukemia: A naturally occurring cancer of infectious origin. Epidemiology 4:189, 1982.
Gerstman, B. B.: The epizootiology of feline leukemia virus infection and its associated diseases. Compend. Contin. Ed. 7:766, 1985.
Jezyk, P. F.: Metabolic diseases: An emerging area of veterinary pediatrics. Compend. Contin. Ed. Pract. Vet. 5:1026, 1983.
Jones, R. L.: Special considerations for appropriate antimicrobial therapy in neonates. Vet. Clin. North Am. 17:577, 1987.
Kliegman, R. M., and Morton, S.: The metabolic response of the canine neonate to twenty-four hours of fasting. Metabolism 36:521, 1987.
Krakowka, S.: Transplacentally acquired microbial and parasitic disease of dogs. J.A.V.M.A. 171:750, 1977.
Lawler, D. F., and Bebiak, D. M.: Nutrition and management of reproduction in the cat. Vet. Clin. North Am. 16:495, 1986.
Lawler, D. F., and Monti, K. L.: Morbidity and mortality in neonatal kittens. Am. J. Vet. Res. 45:1455, 1984.
Monson, W. J.: Orphan rearing of puppies and kittens. Vet. Clin. North Am. 17:567, 1987.
Phelps, D. L., and Rosenbaum, A. L.: Effects of variable oxygenation and gradual withdrawal of oxygen during the recovery phase in oxygen-induced retinopathy: Kitten model. Pediatr. Res. 22:297, 1987.
Pollock, R. V. H.: Canine brucellosis: Current status. Compend. Cont. Ed. Pract. Vet. 1:255, 1979.
Sherding, R. G.: Diseases of the Small Bowel. *In* Ettinger, S. J. (ed.): *Textbook of Veterinary Internal Medicine*, 2nd ed. Philadelphia: W. B. Saunders Co., 1983.
Zimmer, J. F., and Pollock, R. V. H.: Esophageal, gastric, and intestinal disorders of young dogs and cats. Vet. Clin. North Am. 17:641, 1987.

APPENDICES

ROBERT W. KIRK, D.V.M.
and JOHN D. BONAGURA, D.V.M.
Consulting Editors

A ROSTER OF NORMAL VALUES FOR DOGS AND CATS 1335

TABLES OF NORMAL PHYSIOLOGIC DATA 1346

63-DAY PERPETUAL GESTATION CHART 1347

RECOMMENDED NUTRIENT ALLOWANCES FOR DOGS
(PER LB OR KG OF BODY WEIGHT PER DAY) 1348

CALORIC REQUIREMENTS FOR ADULT DOGS BASED ON
PHYSICAL ACTIVITY AND BREED SIZE 1349

RECOMMENDED DAILY CALORIC INTAKE DURING
FIRST FOUR WEEKS OF LIFE 1350

COMPOSITION OF MATERNAL MILK AND SUBSTITUTES 1351

NUTRITIONAL REQUIREMENTS (AMOUNTS PER POUND
OF BODY WEIGHT PER DAY) OF ADULT CATS
AND 10-WEEK-OLD KITTENS 1352

RECOMMENDED DAILY METABOLIZABLE ENERGY
ALLOWANCES FOR CATS 1353

COMPENDIUM OF CANINE VACCINES, 1988 1354

COMPENDIUM OF FELINE VACCINES, 1988 1356

COMPENDIUM OF ANIMAL RABIES CONTROL, 1989 1357

IMMUNIZATION PROCEDURES 1361

USE OF ANTIMICROBIAL AGENTS FOR TREATMENT
OF INFECTIONS 1363

CONVERSION TABLE OF WEIGHT TO BODY SURFACE
AREA (IN SQUARE METERS) FOR DOGS 1365

EQUIVALENTS AND CONVERSION FACTORS 1366

ANTINEOPLASTIC AGENTS IN CANCER THERAPY 1367

TABLE OF COMMON DRUGS: APPROXIMATE DOSES 1370

A ROSTER OF NORMAL VALUES FOR DOGS AND CATS

JOHN BENTINCK-SMITH, D.V.M.,
Mississippi State, Mississippi

and TRACY W. FRENCH, D.V.M.
Ithaca, New York

Age, sex, breed, diurnal periodicity, and emotional stress at the time of sampling can cause variation in normal values. The methodology also affects the biologic measurements. For these reasons practitioners are well advised to use the normal values supplied by the laboratory they patronize. However, this laboratory must have determined their normal ranges and means by a sufficient number of normal samples to provide statistical validity. The laboratory should run control serum samples and provide other means of quality control.

Since biochemical results are most frequently determined on Technicon SMA, equipment values for this method are provided (through the courtesy of Dr. A. I. Hurvitz and Dr. Robert J. Wilkins of the Animal Medical Center, New York). Other data are derived from the New York State College of Veterinary Medicine, the Ralston Purina Corp., Biozyme Veterinary Laboratory (a division of Biozyme Medical Laboratories, Inc.), standard texts, and the literature. References are cited as footnotes within the tables and appear in full at the end of this appendix. Values for reptiles and exotic animals can be found in *Current Veterinary Therapy VII* (pp. 748 and 749) and *Current Veterinary Therapy VI* (p. 795). Values for small laboratory animals (pp. 743–746), llamas (p. 738), and ferrets (pp. 766–767) are found in this volume.

Inappropriate collection and preparation, prolonged storage, hemolysis, lipemia, and hyperbilirubinemia may invalidate the laboratory results.

*Normal Blood Values**

Erythrocytes	Adult Dog	Average	Adult Cat	Average
Erythrocytes (millions/μl)	5.5–8.5	6.8	5.5–10.0	7.5
Hemoglobin (gm/dl)	12.0–18.0	14.9	8.0–14.0	12.0
Packed cell volume (vol. %)	37.0–55.0	45.5	24.0–45.0	37.0
Mean corpuscular volume (femtoliters)	66.0–77.0	69.8	40.0–55.0	45.0
Mean corpuscular hemoglobin (picograms)	19.9–24.5	22.8	13.0–17.0	15.0
Mean corpuscular hemoglobin concentration (gm/dl)				
Wintrobe	31.0–34.0	33.0	31.0–35.0	33.0
Microhematocrit	32.0–36.0	34.0	30.0–36.0	33.2
Reticulocytes (%) (excludes punctate retics.)	0.0–1.5	0.8	0.2–1.6	0.6
Resistance to hypotonic saline (% saline solution producing)				
Minimum	0.40–0.50	0.46	0.66–0.72	0.69
Initial and complete hemolysis				
Maximum	0.32–0.42	0.33	0.46–0.54	0.50
Erythrocyte sedimentation rate	PCV 37	13	PCV 35–40	7–27
(mm at 60 min)	PCV 50	0		
RBC life span (days)	100–120		66–78	
RBC diameter (μm)	6.7–7.2	7.0	5.5–6.3	5.8

Leukocytes	Adult Dog	Average	Adult Cat	Average
Leukocytes (no/μl)	6,000–17,000	11,500	5,500–19,500	12,500
Neutrophils-Bands (%)	0–3	0.8	0–3	0.5
Neutrophils-Mature (%)	60–77	70.0	35–75	59.0
Lymphocyte (%)	12–30	20.0	20–55	32.0
Monocyte (%)	3–10	5.2	1–4	3.0
Eosinophil (%)	2–10	4.0	2–12	5.5
Basophil (%)	Rare	0.0	Rare	0.0
Neutrophils-Bands (no/μl)	0–300	70	0–300	100
Neutrophils-Mature (no/μl)	3,000–11,500	7,000	2,500–12,500	7,500
Lymphocytes (no/μl)	1,000–4,800	2,800	1,500–7,000	4,000
Monocytes (no/μl)	150–1,350	750	0–850	350
Eosinophils (no/μl)	100–1,250	550	0–1,500	650
Basophils	Rare	0	Rare	0

*From Schalm et al., 1975.

1335

Canine Blood Values at Different Ages—Average Values*

Age	RBC Millions/µl	Retic. %†	Nucl. RBC/ 100 WBC†	Hb gm/dl	PCV Vol. %	WBC/µl	Neut./µl	Bands/µl	Lymph./µl	Eos./µl
Birth	5.75	7.1	1.8	16.70	50	16,500	1,300	400	2,500	600
2 weeks	3.92	7.1	1.8	9.76	32	11,000	6,500	100	3,000	300
4 weeks	4.20	7.1	1.8	9.60	33	13,000	8,600	0	4,000	40
6 weeks	4.91	3.6	1.8	9.59	34	15,000	10,000	0	4,500	100
8 weeks	5.13	3.9	0.3	11.00	37	18,000	11,000	234	6,000	270
12 weeks	5.27	3.9	Rare	11.60	36	15,300	9,400	115	4,600	322

*From Andersen and Gee, 1958.
†See Ewing et al., 1972.

Canine Blood Values at Different Ages*

	Sex	Birth to 12 Mo.	Average	1–7 Yr.	Average	7 Yr. and Older	Average
Erythrocytes (million/µl)	Male	2.99–8.52	5.09	5.26–6.57	5.92	3.33–7.76	5.28
	Female	2.76–8.42	5.06	5.13–8.6	6.47	3.34–9.19	5.17
Hemoglobin (gm/dl)	Male	6.9–16.5	10.7	12.7–16.3	15.5	14.7–21.2	17.9
	Female	6.4–18.9	11.2	11.5–17.9	14.7	11.0–22.5	16.1
Packed Cell Volume (vol. %)	Male	22.0–45.0	33.9	35.2–52.8	44.0	44.2–62.8	52.3
	Female	25.8–55.2	36.0	34.8–52.4	43.6	35.8–67.0	49.8
Leukocytes (thousands/µl)	Male	9.9–27.7	17.1	8.3–19.5	11.9	7.9–35.3	15.5
	Female	8.8–26.8	15.9	7.5–17.5	11.5	5.2–34.0	13.4
Neutrophils Mature (%)	Male	63–73	68	65–73	69	55–80	66
	Female	64–74	69	58–76	67	40–80	64
Lymphocytes (%)	Male	18–30	24	9–26	18	15–40	29
	Female	13–28	21	11–29	20	13–45	29
Monocytes (%)	Male	1–10	6	2–10	6	0–4	1
	Female	1–10	7	0–10	5	0–4	1
Eosinophils (%)	Male	2–11	3	1–8	4	1–11	4
	Female	1–9	5	1–10	6	0–19	6

*From 1975 Normal Blood Values for Dogs.

Feline Blood Values at Different Ages*

Age	RBC Millions/µl		Hb gm/dl	PCV Vol. %	WBC/µl	Neut./µl	Lymph./µl
Birth	4.95	12.2	44.7	7,500			
2 weeks	4.76	9.7	31.1	8,080			
5 weeks	5.84	8.4	29.9	8,550			
Average†	4.80	7.5	26.2	11,770	4,600	6,970	
Range†	3.90–5.70	6.6–8.4	21.0–33.5	7,500–14,500		4,500–9,400	
6 weeks	6.75	9.0	35.4	8,420			
8 weeks	7.10	9.4	35.6	8,420		4,900	
Average†	5.90	7.5	26.2	12,400	7,500	1,925–10,100	
Range	3.30–7.30	7.6–15.0	22–38	6,900–23,100			

*From Schalm et al., 1975.
†See Anderson et al., 1971.

Feline Blood Values at Different Ages*

	Sex	Birth to 12 Mo.	Average	1–5 Yr.	Average	6 Yr. and Older	Average
Erythrocytes (millions/μl)	Male	5.43–10.22	6.96	4.48–10.27	7.34	5.26–8.89	6.79
	Female	4.46–11.34	6.90	4.45–9.42	6.17	4.10–7.38	5.84
Hemoglobin (gm/dl)	Male	6.0–12.9	9.9	8.9–17.0	12.9	9.0–14.5	11.8
	Female	6.0–15.0	9.9	7.9–15.5	10.3	7.5–13.7	10.3
Packed cell volume (vol. %)	Male	24.0–37.5	31	26.9–48.2	37.6	28.0–43.8	34.6
	Female	23.0–46.8	31.5	25.3–37.5	31.4	22.5–40.5	30.8
Leukocytes (thousands/μl)	Male	7.8–25.0	15.8	9.1–28.2	15.1	6.4–30.4	17.6
	Female	11.0–26.9	17.7	13.7–23.7	19.9	5.2–30.1	14.8
Neutrophils Mature (%)	Male	16–75	60	37–92	65	33–75	61
	Female	51–83	69	42–93	69	25–89	71
Lymphocytes (%)	Male	10–81	30	7–48	23	16–54	30
	Female	8–37	23	12–58	30	9–63	22
Monocytes (%)	Male	1–5	2	1–5	2	0–2	1
	Female	0–7	2	0–5	2	0–4	1
Eosinophils (%)	Male	2–21	8	1–22	7	1–15	8
	Female	0–15	6	0–13	5	0–15	6

*From 1975 Normal Blood Values for Cats.

Effect of Pregnancy and Lactation on Blood Values of the Dog*

	Gestation				Term	Lactation		
	2 Weeks	4 Weeks	6 Weeks	8 Weeks	0 Weeks	2 Weeks	4 Weeks	6 Weeks
RBC (millions/dl)	8.85	7.48	6.73	6.26	4.53	5.13	5.65	6.15
PCV (Vol. %)	53	47	44	37	32	34	38	42
Hb (gm/dl)	19.6	16.4	14.7	13.8	11.0	11.7	12.8	13.4
Sedimentation rate (mm at 60 min)	0.6	11.0	31.0	14.0	12.0	14.0	14.0	13.0
WBC (thousands/dl)	12.0	12.2	15.7	19.0	18.9	16.9	17.1	15.9

*From Andersen and Gee, 1958.

Effect of Pregnancy and Lactation on Blood Values of the Cat*

	Gestation					Term	Lactation	
	1 Day Past Conception	2 Weeks	4 Weeks	6 Weeks	8 Weeks	0 Weeks	2 Weeks	4 Weeks
RBC (millions/dl)	8.0	7.9	7.1	6.7	6.2	6.2	7.4	7.4
PCV (Vol. %)	36.1	37.0	33.0	32.0	28.0	29.0	33.0	33.0
Hb (gm/100 ml)	12.5	12.0	11.0	10.8	9.5	10.0	11.5	11.2
Reticulocytes (%) (includes punctate retics.)	9	11	9	10	20.1	15	9	6

	Adult Dog	Average	Adult Cat	Average†
Thrombocytes × 10⁵/μl	2–5	3–4	3–8	4.5
Icterus index	2–5 units		2–5 units	
Plasma fibrinogen (gm/L)	2.0–4.0		0.50–3.00	

*From Berman, 1974.
†From Schalm et al., 1975.

Normal Bone Marrow (Percentage)

Erythrocytic Cells	Dog*	Cat†
Rubriblasts	0.2	1.71
Prorubricytes	3.9	12.50
Rubricytes	27.0	
Metarubricytes	15.3	11.68
Total erythrocytic cells	46.4	25.89
Granulocytic Cells		
Myeloblasts	0.0	1.74
Progranulocytes	1.3	0.88
Neutrophilic myelocytes	9.0	9.76
Eosinophilic myelocytes	0.0	1.47
Neutrophilic metamyelocytes	7.5	7.32
Eosinophilic metamyelocytes	2.4	1.52
Band neutrophils	13.6	25.80
Band eosinophils	0.9	—
Neutrophils	18.4	9.24
Eosinophils	0.3	0.81
Basophils	0.0	0.002
Total granulocytic cells	53.4	58.542
M:E Ratio—Average	1.15:1.0	2.47:1.0
M:E Ratio—Range (Schalm)	0.75–2.50:1.0	0.60–3.90:1.0
Other Cells		
Lymphocytes	0.2	7.63
Plasma cells	0	1.61
Reticulum cells	0	0.13
Mitotic cells	0	0.61
Unclassified	0	1.62
Disintegrated cells	0	4.60

*From Schalm et al., 1975.
†From Penny et al., 1970.

Hematology Reference Ranges (Coulter Model S + IV)*

Parameter	Adult Dog	Adult Cat
Erythrocytes (millions/μl)	5.6–8.5	5.5–10.3
Hemoglobin (gm/dl)	13.7–19.6	8.4–15.0
Hematocrit (%)	39–56	25–45
Mean cell volume (fl)	65–72	41–51
Mean cell hemoglobin conc. (gm/dl)	32–37	32–36
Mean cell hemoglobin (pg)	21–26	14–17
Red cell distribution width (RDW)	12–15	15–20
Leukocytes (thousands/μl)	7.5–19.9	6.1–21.1
Platelets (thousands/μl)	179–510	215–760
Mean platelet volume (fl)	8–12	11–15

*Based on results from 50 clinically normal individuals of each species as determined at the New York State College of Veterinary Medicine. The results obtained from this model may vary with the exact instrument settings employed.

Système International (S.I.) is the system for reporting clinical laboratory data currently used in most countries worldwide. A transition to this method now is under way in the United States. The following table gives arbitrary examples of common hematology and clinical chemistry test results, expressed in both conventional (old) and S.I. units, and supplies the multiplication factors for converting results between the two systems.

Système International (S.I.) Conversion Factors for Common Hematology and Clinical Chemistry Tests

| Analyte | Example Values Expressed in | | Conversion Factors (×) | |
	Old Units	S.I. Units	Old Units to S.I. Units	S.I. Units to Old Units
Hematology				
RBC	$6.0 \times 10^6/mm^3$	$6.0 \times 10^{12}/L$	10^6	10^{-6}
PCV	45%	0.45L/L	0.01	100
Hemoglobin	15.0 gm/dl (%)	150 gm/L	10	0.1
MCV	$75 \mu^3$	75 fl	No change	No change
MCHC	33 gm/dl (%)	330 gm/L	10	0.1
MCH	$25 \mu\mu g$	25 pg	No change	No change
WBC	$15.0 \times 10^3/mm^3$	$15.0 \times 10^9/L$	10^6	10^{-6}
Platelets	$250 \times 10^3/mm^3$	$250 \times 10^9/L$	10^6	10^{-6}
Clinical Chemistry				
Albumin	3.0 gm/dl	30 gm/L	10.0	0.10
Ammonia (NH_3)	20.0 μg/dl	12 μmol/L	0.5871	1.7
Bicarbonate	25 mEq/L	25 mmol/L	No change	No change
Bile acids (total)	1.0 mg/L	2.5 μmol/L	2.547	0.3926
Bilirubin (total)	0.2 mg/dl	3 μmol/L	17.1	0.0585
Bilirubin (direct)	0.1 mg/dl	2 μmol/L	17.1	0.0585
Calcium	10.0 mg/dl	2.5 mmol/L	0.250	4.008
Chloride	100 mEq/L	100 mmol/L	No change	No change
Cholesterol	200 mg/dl	5.17 mmol/L	0.02586	38.7
Creatinine	1.0 mg/dl	90 μmol/L	88.40	0.0113
Globulins (total)	3.0 gm/dl	30 gm/L	10.0	0.10
Glucose	100 mg/dl	5.6 mmol/L	0.05551	18.02
Iron	100 μg/dl	18 μmol/L	0.1791	5.59
Iron-binding capacity	300 μg/dl	54 μmol/L	0.1791	5.59
Lead	25 μg/dl	1.21 μmol/L	0.04826	20.7
Magnesium	2.0 mg/dl	0.82 mmol/L	0.4114	2.43
Phosphate (P_i)	4.0 mg/dl	1.29 mmol/L	0.3229	3.10
Potassium	4.0 mEq/L	4.0 mmol/L	No change	No change
Protein (total)	7.0 gm/dl	70 gm/L	10.0	0.1
Sodium	145 mEq/L	145 mmol/L	No change	No change
Triglycerides	50 mg/dl	0.56 mmol/L	0.01129	88.5
Urea nitrogen	15 mg/dl	5.4 mmol/L	0.3570	2.8

Key: mmol/L, millimoles/liter; μmol/L, micromoles/liter; pg, picograms; fl, femtoliters.

Blood, Plasma, or Serum Chemical Constituents: Part I
(B) = Blood, (P) = Plasma, (S) = Serum

Chemical constituents are liable to show markedly different values, depending on the method employed.

Constituent	Adult Dog — Coulter Chemistry*	Adult Dog — Technicon SMA†	Adult Cat — Coulter Chemistry*	Adult Cat — Technicon SMA†
Urea N(s) (mg/dl)	8–23	10–22	18–32	5–30
Glucose (S) (mg/dl)	71–115	50–120	66–95	70–150
Total bilirubin (S) (mg/dl)	0.1–0.6	0–0.6	0.15–0.3	0–0.8
Total protein (S) (gm/dl)	5.2–7.0	5.4–7.8	5.9–7.3	5.5–7.5
Albumin (S) (gm/dl)	2.7–3.8	2.2–3.4	2.2–3.0	2.2–3.5
Alkaline phosphatase (S) (IU/L)	10–82	20–120	7–30	10–80
Calcium (S) (mg/dl)	9.8–11.4	9–11.6	8.9–10.6	7.6–11.0
Inorganic phosphorus (S) (mg/dl)	2.8–5.1	3.9–6.3	4.3–6.6	3.2–6.3
LDH (S) (IU/L)	8–89	40–200	33–99	10–200
AST or SGOT (S)	13–93‡	5–80§	32–58‡	10–60§
ALT or SGPT (S) (IU/L)	15–70	5–25	10–50	10–60
Total CO_2 (S) (mEq/L)	18–25	17–25‖	18–25	16–25‖
Creatinine (S) (mg/dl)	0.5–1.2	0.4–1.5‖	0.5–1.7	1.3–2.1‖
Uric acid (S) (mg/dl)		0.2–0.8‖		0.1–0.7‖
Total cholesterol (S) (mg/dl)	82–282	156–294‖	41–225	116–126‖
Triglycerides (S) (mg/dl)		10–42‖		6–58‖
CPK (S) (IU/L)	12–84	27–93‖	6–130	62–262‖
GGT (S) (IU/L) (Centrifugal analysis**)	1.4–11.5		1.8–18.3	

Chemical Values Affected by Age	Dog < 6 Mo–SMA†	Cat < 6 Mo–SMA†
Inorganic phosphorus (S) (mg/dl)	3.9–9.0	3.9–8.1
Calcium (S) (mg/dl)	7.0–11.6	7.0–11.0
Alkaline phosphatase (S) (IU/L)	20–200	10–120
LDH (S) (IU/L)	40–400	10–300

	Sex	Dogs‡‡ and Cats‡‡ — Birth to 12 mo.	Average	1–5 yr.	Average	6 yr. and Older	Average
Total Protein (S) (gm/dl) (Dogs)	Male	3.90–5.90	5.15	4.90–9.60	6.33	5.5–7.3	6.4
	Female	4.00–6.40	5.58	5.50–7.80	6.34	4.7–7.5	6.2
Total Protein (S) (gm/dl) (Cats)	Male	4.3–10.0	6.4	6.8–10.0	8.1	6.2–8.5	7.2
	Female	4.8–9.1	6.4	6.6–8.9	7.4	6.0–9.0	7.3

Electrophoresis	Dog	Cat
Albumin (S) (gm/dl)	2.3–3.4	2.3–3.5
Globulin (S) (gm/dl)	3.0–4.7	2.6–5.0
Alpha 1 (S) (gm/dl)	0.3–0.8	0.3–0.5
Alpha 2 (S) (gm/dl)	0.5–1.3	0.4–1.0
Beta (S) (gm/dl)	0.7–1.8	0.6–1.9
Gamma (S) (gm/dl)	0.4–1.0	0.5–1.5
Albumin/globulin ratio, A/G (S)	0.7–1.1	0.5–1.0

*From Tasker, 1978.
†From Wilkins and Hurvitz, 1978.
‡Trans Act Units/liter (General Diagnostics). 1 Trans Act Unit of SGOT activity is the amount of enzyme in 1 liter of sample that will form 1 mM of oxalic acid in 1 minute under specified conditions.
§U/liter.
‖See Biozyme Veterinary Laboratory, 1978.
**From Boyd, 1984.
††From *1975 Normal Blood Values for Dogs*
‡‡From *1975 Normal Blood Values for Cats*.

Blood, Plasma, or Serum Chemical Constituents: Part II
(B) = Blood, (P) = Plasma, (S) = Serum

Chemical constituents are liable to show markedly different values depending on the method employed.

Other Constituents	Adult Dog	Adult Cat
Lipase (S)		
(Sigma Tietz Units/ml)	0–1	0–1
Roe Byler Units (S)	0.8–12	0–5
IU (S)	13–200	0–83
Amylase (S)		
Harleco Units/dl	0–800	0–800
Harding Units/dl	1600–2400	0–2700**
Dy Amyl (General Diagnostics)	<3200**	0–2600**
Caraway Units/dl*	330–1530	170–1170
Lactic acid (S) (mg/dl)	3–15	
Pyruvate (B) (mEq/L)	0.1–0.2	
Cholesterol esters (S) (mg/dl)	84–168	45–120
Free cholesterol (S) (mg/dl)	28–84	15–60
Total lipid (P) (mg/dl)	47–725	145–607
Free glycerol (S) 24-hr fast (mg/dl)†	14.2–23.2	145–607
Bromsulfalein retention test (P) (%)	<5	
Iron (S) (μg/dl)	94–122	68–215
Total iron-binding capacity (S) (μg/dl)	280–340	170–400
Lead (B) (μg/dl)	0–35	0–35

	Dogs		Cats	
Electrolytes	Coulter‡	Technicon§	Coulter‡	Technicon§
Sodium (S) (mEq/L)	143–151	144–154	150–162	147–161
Potassium (S) (mEq/L)	4.1–5.7	3.8–5.8	3.7–5.5	3.7–4.9
Magnesium (S) (mEq/L)	1.4–2.4	1.07–1.73	2.2	1.92–2.28
Chloride (S) (mEq/L)	103–115	93–121	114–124	80–158
Sulfate (S) (mEq/L)	2.0			
Osmolality (S) (mOsm/kg)	280–310		280–310	
pH (Corning)	7.31–7.42		7.24–7.40	

Blood Gases	Adult Dog	Adult Cat
P_{O_2} (B) mm Hg (arterial)‖	85–95	—
(B) mm Hg (venous)‖	40–60	—
P_{CO_2} (B) mm Hg (arterial)‖	29–36	—
(B) mm Hg (venous)‖	29–42	—
Base excess (B) (mEq/L)	±2.5	±2.5
Bicarbonate (P) (mEq/L)	17–24	17–24

*From *Chemassay Amylase.*
†From Rogers et al., 1975.
‡From Tasker, 1978.
§From Biozyme Veterinary Laboratory, 1978.
‖Standard temperature and pressure.
**From Benjamin, 1978.

Blood, Plasma, or Serum Chemical Constituents: Part III
(B) = Blood, (P) = Plasma, (S) = Serum

Chemical constituents are liable to show markedly different values depending on the method employed.

Endocrine Secretions	Adult Dog		Adult Cat	
	Resting Level	*Post-ACTH**	*Resting Level*	*Post-ACTH**
Cortisol (S) (RIA) (mg/dl)†	1.8–4	3–4 × Pretreatment	1–3	3–4 × Pretreatment
Cortisol (S) (CPB) (mg/dl)‡	2–6	3–4 × Pretreatment§	2–5	3–4 × Pretreatment§
Cortisol (S) (fluorometric) (μg/dl)	5–10	10–20		

	Resting Level	*Post-TSH‖*	*Resting Level*	*Post-TSH*
T_4 (P) (RIA) (μg/dl)**	1.52–3.60	At least 3- to 4-fold	1.2–3.8	
T_3 (P) (RIA) (ng/dl)**	48–154	More than 10 ng increase		
Protein-bound iodine (μg/dl)‡‡	1.6–3.0	Increase of 3 μg/dl (mean)		

T_4 Changes With Age	Dog	Cat
T_4 (S) (RIA)	Decrease of 0.07 μg/dl per year of age**	No values for cat
T_4 (S) (CPB) (μg/dl)		
10–12 wk‡‡	3.24 ± 0.51	2.82 ± 0.73
1 hr‡‡	2.25 ± 0.33	2.43 ± 0.55

	Adult Dog	Adult Cat
Thyroid uptake of radioiodine (^{131}I)(%)‡‡	17–30	
Insulin (S) (RIA) (μU/ml)§§	0–30	0–50

Plasma Proteins			
Basenji Dogs‖		Cats***	
Age	*Plasma Proteins (gm/dl)*	*Age*	*Plasma Proteins (gm/dl)*
6–8 weeks	5.33 ± 0.29	Adults (younger animals have lower values)	6–8
9–12 weeks	5.87 ± 0.46		
4–6 months	6.6 ± 0.25		
1–2 years	7.03 ± 0.33		

*Two μg ACTH gel IM 2 hours after injection.

†Data from Thomas J. Reimers, Assistant Professor and Director of the Endocrinology Laboratory, New York State College of Veterinary Medicine, Cornell University, Ithaca, New York.

‡Data from R. Wallace, Research Support Specialist, New York State College of Veterinary Medicine, Cornell University, Ithaca, New York.

§Data from D. W. Scott, Assistant Professor of Medicine, Department of Clinical Sciences, New York State College of Veterinary Medicine, Cornell University, Ithaca, New York.

‖Five μg TSH IV 4–6 hours after injection.

**From Belshaw and Rijnberk, 1979.

††From Benjamin, 1978.

‡‡From Kallfelz and Erali, 1973; personal communication from R. A. Kallfelz, Associate Professor of Clinical Nutrition, Department of Large Animal Medicine, Obstetrics, and Surgery, New York State College of Veterinary Medicine, Cornell University, Ithaca, New York.

§§Data from R. J. Wilkins, Animal Medical Center, New York, New York.

‖‖From Ewing et al., 1972.

***From Schalm et al., 1975.

Hemostatic Values*

	Adult Dog	Adult Cat
Bleeding time	2–4	1–5†
Dorsum of nose (min)	85–110	
Lip (sec)	2.5–3	
Ear (min)	1–2	
Abdomen (min)		
Whole blood coagulation time		
Glass (Lee and White) (min)	6–7.5	8†
Silicone (Lee and White) (min)	12–15	
Capillary tube (min)‡	3–4	5.2 ± 0.2§
Activated coagulation time of whole blood		
Room temp. (sec)	60–125‖	A limited number of cats have shown a
	83–129**	range similar to that of the dog.
37°C (sec)	64–95**	
Prothrombin time (sec)‡	6–10	8.6 ± 0.5§
Puppies 1–4 hours old (sec)††	42.2	
6–12 hours old (sec)	49.1	
16–48 hours old (sec)	36.8	
48 hours old (sec)	24.5	
Russell's viper venom time (sec)‡‡	11	9
Partial thromboplastin time (sec)	15–25	
Prothrombin consumption (sec)‡‡	20.5	20
Fibrin degradation products (μg/ml)	<10	

*No test should be interpreted without an accompanying normal control.
†From Seager and Fletcher, 1972.
‡From Coles, 1974.
§From Osbaldiston et al., 1970.
‖From Byars et al., 1976.
**From Middleton and Watson, 1978.
††From Benjamin, 1978.
‡‡From Rowsell, 1969.

Normal Renal Function and Urine Values

Urine*	Adult Dog	Adult Cat
Specific gravity		
Minimum	1.001	1.001
Maximum	1.060	1.080
Usual limits (normal water and food intake)	1.018–1.050	1.018–1.050
Volume (ml/kg body weight/day)	24–41	22–30
Osmolality urine (mOsm/kg)		
Usual range	500–1200	
Maximal limits	2000–2400	
Osmolality plasma	300	

Urine Constituents†	Adult Dog	Adult Cat
Creatinine (mg/dl)	100–300	110–280
Urea (gm/dl)	1.0–2.5	1.0–3.0
Protein (mg/dl)	0–30	0–20
Amylase (Somogyi units)	50–150	30–120
Sodium (mEq/L)	20–165	
Potassium (mEq/L)	20–120	
Calcium (mEq/L)	2–10	
Inorganic phosphorus (mEq/L)	50–180	

Urinalysis—Semiquantitative Values	Adult Dog	Adult Cat
Protein sulfosalicylic acid	0–trace	0–trace
Protein Multistix (Miles Laboratories)‡	0–1+	0–1+
Glucose	0	0
Ketones	0	0
Bilirubin	0	0
10–20% Dogs—high specific gravity	1+	
5% Cats—high specific gravity		1+
Urobilinogen (Ehrlich unit)	0–1	0–1
(Wallace-Diamond)	<1:32	<1:32

Normal Renal Function and Urine Values Continued

Urine Total Protein Excretion (24 hr) in the Dog (Trichloroacetic Acid Ponceau Method)			
N	Range (mg)	X̄	SD
17†	48–1040	333 mg	± 309 mg
10§	8–151	38 mg	

Renal Function—Dog*	
Effective renal plasma flow	266 ± 66 ml/min/m² body surface
	13.5 ± 3.3 ml/min/kg body weight
Glomerular filtration rate	84.4 ± 19 ml/min/m² body surface
	4 ml/min/kg body weight

Renal Function Tests—Dog	
Phenolsulfonphthalein	
Excretion in urine at 20 min, 6-mg dose‖	21–66%
Clearance (P) 1 mg/kg at 60 min**	<80 μ/ml
T$_{1/2}$ clearance 5 mg/kg††	19.6 min
Creatinine, endogenous clearance*	60 ± 22 ml/min/m² body surface
	2.98 ± 0.96 ml/min/kg body weight

*From Osborne et al., 1972.
†Data from R. J. Wilkins, Animal Medical Center, New York, New York. Values are markedly affected by degree of concentration.
‡From DiBartola et al., 1980.
§From Barsanti and Finco, 1979.
‖From Coles, 1974.
**From Kaufman and Kirk, 1973.
††From Brobst et al., 1967.

Cerebrospinal Fluid and Synovial Fluid

Cerebrospinal Fluid*	Adult Dog	Adult Cat
Color	Clear, colorless	Clear, colorless
Pressure (mm H$_2$O)	<170	<100
Cells/μl	<5 lymphocytes	<5 lymphocytes
Protein (ml/dl)	<25	<20
Glucose (mg/dl)	61–116	85

Normal Synovial Fluid— Carpal, Elbow, Shoulder, Hip, Stifle, and Hock Joints†	Adult Dog	
	Range	Mean
Amount (ml)	0.01–1.00	0.24
pH	7–7.8	7.33
Leukocytes (× 10³/μl)	0–2.9	0.43
Erythrocytes (× 10³/μl)	0–320.0	12.15
Neutrophils/μl	0–32	3.63
Neutrophils (%)‡	10	
Monocytes/μl	0–838	230.77
Lymphocytes/μl	0–2436	245.6
Clasmatocytes/μl	0–166	14.69
Mononuclear cells (%)‡	90	
Mucin clot	Tight, ropy clump; clear supernatant	

*Data from A. de Lahunta, Professor of Anatomy, Department of Clinical Sciences, New York, State College of Veterinary Medicine, Cornell University, Ithaca, New York.
†From Sawyer, 1963.
‡From Miller et al., 1974.

Canine Semen*

Regular Collection by Hand Manipulation With a Teaser (125 Ejaculates From Small Dogs, Mostly Beagles)†	Mean	Standard Deviation	Range
Volume	−5	4.3	0.5–20.4
% Motile sperm	75	7.5	30–90
% Normal sperm	86	14.7	34–97
pH	6.72	0.19	6.49–7.10
Concentration/mm³ (10^3)	148	84.6	27.2–388.8
Total sperm per ejaculate (10^6)	528	321.0	94–1428

Fractionated Ejaculates (Based on 65 Ejaculates)	Mean	Range	pH
First fraction	0.8 ml	0.25–2.00	6.37
Second fraction	0.6 ml	0.40–2.00	6.10
Third fraction	0.4 ml	1.0–16.3	7.20

Ejaculates From Purebred Labrador Retrievers, 18 to 48 Months Old‡	Mean	Range
Volume (ml)	2.2§	0.5–6.5
% Motile sperm	93	75–99
% Unstained sperm (eosin-nigrosin)	84	61–99
Concentration/mm³ (10^3)	564	103–708

*Revisions and corrections courtesy of R. H. Foote, Professor of Animal Physiology, Department of Animal Science, New York State College of Life Sciences, Cornell University, Ithaca, New York.

†From Boucher, 1957.

‡From Seager and Fletcher, 1972.

§Only the first two fractions were collected, resulting in smaller volume and higher concentration of sperm/mm³ than would result if all the prostatic fluid (third fraction) were obtained.

References and Supplemental Reading

Andersen, A. C., and Gee, W.: Normal values in the beagle. Vet. Med. 53:135, 156; 1958.

Anderson, L., Wilson, R., and Hay, D.: Haematological values in normal cats from four weeks to one year of age. Res. Vet. Sci. 12:579, 1971.

Baker, H. J.: Laboratory evaluation of thyroid function. In Kirk, R. W. (ed.): Current Veterinary Therapy IV. Philadelphia: W. B. Saunders, 1971.

Barsanti, J. A., and Finco, D. R.: Protein concentration in urine of normal dogs. Am. J. Vet. Res. 40:1583, 1979.

Belshaw, B. E., and Rijnberk, A.: Radioimmunoassay of plasma T₄ and T₃ in the diagnosis of primary hypothyroidism in dogs. J. Am. Anim. Hosp. Assoc. 15:17, 1979.

Benjamin, M.: An Outline of Veterinary Clinical Pathology, 3rd ed. Ames, IA: Iowa State University Press, 1978.

Berman, E.: Hemogram of the cat during pregnancy and lactation and after lactation. Am. J. Vet. Res. 35:457, 1974.

Biozyme Veterinary Laboratory (a division of Biozyme Medical Laboratories, Inc.): Normal Ranges Chemistry. Olean, NY: Biozyme Veterinary Laboratory, 1978.

Boucher, J. H.: Evaluation of semen quality in the dog and the effects of frequency of ejaculation upon semen quality, libido and restoration of sperm reserves. M. S. Thesis, Cornell University, Ithaca, N.Y., 1957.

Boyd, J. W.: The interpretation of serum biochemistry test results in domestic animals. Vet. Clin. Pathol 13(2):7, 1984.

Brobst, D. F., Carter, J. M., and Horron, M.: Plasma phenolsulfonphthalein determination as a measure of renal function in the dog. 17th Gaines Veterinary Symposium, University of Minnesota, 1967, p. 15.

Byars, T. D., Ling, G. V., Ferris, N. A., and Keeton, K. S.: Activated coagulation time (ACT) of whole blood in normal dogs. Am. J. Vet. Res. 37:1359, 1976.

Chemassay Amylase. Pitman-Moore, Inc., Washington Crossing, N.J. 08560.

Coles, E. H.: Veterinary Clinical Pathology, 2nd ed. Philadelphia: W. B. Saunders, 1974.

DiBartola, S. P., Chew, D. J., and Jacobs, G.: Quantitative urinalysis including 24-hour protein excretion in the dog. J. Am. Anim. Hosp. Assoc. 16:537, 1960.

Ewing, G. O., Schalm, O. W., and Smith, R. S.: Hematologic values of normal Basenji dogs. J.A.V.M.A. 161:1661, 1972.

Kallfelz, F. A., and Erali, R. P.: Thyroid function tests on domesticated animals. Am. J. Vet. Res. 34:1449, 1973.

Kaufman, C. F., and Kirk, R. W.: The 60-minute plasma phenolsulfonphthalein concentration as a test of renal function in the dog. J. Am. Anim. Hosp. Assoc. 9:66, 1973.

Kraft, W.: Schielddrusenfunktionsstörunge. beim Hund. (Thyroid function disturbances in the dog). Thesis, Justus Liebig University, Giessen, West Germany, 1964. (Cited by Belshaw.)

Lundberg, G. D., Iverson, C., and Radulescu, G.: Now read this: The SI units are here. J.A.M.A. 255:2329, 1986.

Middleton, D. J., and Watson, A. D. J.: Activated coagulation times of whole blood in normal dogs and dogs with coagulopathies. J. Small Anim. Pract. 19:417, 1978.

Miller, J. B., Perman, V., Osborne, C. A., Hammer, R. F., and Gambardella, P. C.: Synovial fluid analysis in canine arthritis. J. Am. Anim. Hosp. Assoc. 10:392, 1974.

1975 Normal Blood Values for Cats. Ralston Purina Co., Professional Marketing Services, Checkerboard Square, St. Louis, Missouri 63188.

1975 Normal Blood Values for Dogs. Ralston Purina Co., Professional Marketing Services, Checkerboard Square, St. Louis, Missouri 63188.

Osbaldiston, G. W., Stowe, E. C., and Griffith, P. R.: Blood coagulation: Comparative studies in dogs, cats, horses and cattle. Br. Vet. J. 126:512, 1970.

Osborne, C. A., Low, D. G., and Finco, D. R.: Canine and Feline Urology. Philadelphia: W. B. Saunders, 1972.

Penny, R. H. C., Carlisle, C. H., and Davidson, H. A.: The blood and marrow picture of the cat. Br. Vet. J. 126:459, 1970.

Rogers, U. A., Donovan, E. F., and Kociba, G. J.: Lipids and lipoproteins in normal dogs and dogs with secondary hyperlipoproteinemia. J.A.V.M.A. 166:1092, 1975.

Rowsell, H. C.: Blood coagulation and hemorrhage disorders. In Medway, W., Prier, J. E., and Wilkinson, J. S. (eds.): Textbook of Veterinary Clinical Pathology. Baltimore: Williams & Wilkins, 1969, p. 247.

Sawyer, D. C.: Synovial fluid analysis of canine joints. J.A.V.M.A. 143:609, 1963.

Schlam, O. W., Jain, N. C., and Carroll, E. J.: Veterinary Hematology. 3rd ed. Philadelphia: Lea & Febiger, 1975.

Seager, S. W. J., and Fletcher, W. S.: Collection, storage, and insemination of canine semen. Lab. Anim. Sci. 22:177, 1972.

Tasker, J. B.: Reference values for clinical chemistry using the Coulter Chemistry System. Cornell Vet. 68:460, 1978.

Wilkins, R. J., and Hurvitz, A. L.: Profiling in Veterinary Clinical Pathology. Tarrytown, NY: Technicon Instruments Corp., 1978, pp. 17, 19.

TABLES OF NORMAL PHYSIOLOGIC DATA

Electrocardiography*

It is recognized that normal and abnormal electrocardiographic measurements overlap and that the criteria for the normal electrocardiogram serve only as a guide for the clinician. Deviatons from normal in an individual electrocardiogram suggest but are not always diagnostic of heart disease. As additional statistical data become available for the electrocardiograms of dogs of each breed, body type, age, and sex, the data herein may require revision and "normal" may be more precisely defined. The *value of serial electrocardiograms* from an individual cannot be overemphasized, since serial changes best demonstrate electrocardiographic abnormalities.

Criteria for the Normal Canine Electrocardiogram†

Heart rate—60 to 160 beats per minute for adult dogs; up to 180 beats per minute in toy breeds, and 220 beats per minute for puppies.

Heart rhythm—Normal sinus rhythm; sinus arrhythmia; and wandering sinoatrial pacemaker.

P wave—Up to 0.4 millivolt in amplitude; up to 0.04 second in duration (may be longer in giant breeds); always positive in leads II and aVF; positive or isoelectric in lead I.

P-R interval—0.06 to 0.14 second duration.

QRS complex—Mean electric axis, frontal plane, 40 to 100 degrees.

Amplitude—Maximum amplitude of R wave 2.5 to 3.0 millivolts in leads II, III, and aVF. Complex positive in leads II, III, and aVF; negative in lead V_{10}.

Duration—To 0.05 second (0.06/second in dogs over 40 lbs).

Q-T segment—0.15 to 0.22 second duration.

ST segment and T wave—ST segment free of marked coving (repolarization changes).

ST segment depression not greater than 0.2 millivolt.

ST segment elevation not greater than 0.15 millivolt.

T wave negative in lead V_{10}.

T wave amplitude not greater than 25 per cent of amplitude of R wave.

Criteria for the Normal Feline Electrocardiogram†

Heart rate—240 beats per minute maximum.

Heart rhythm—Normal sinus rhythm or, infrequently, sinus arrhythmia.

P wave—Positive in leads II and aVF: may be isoelectric or positive in lead I; should not exceed 0.03 second in duration.

P-R interval—0.04 to 0.08 second duration (inversely related to the heart rate).

QRS complex—More variable than in the canine; the mean electric axis in the frontal plane is often insignificant. Often the QRS complex is nearly isoelectric in all frontal plane limb leads (so-called horizontal heart).

Amplitude—The amplitude of the R wave is usually low; marked amplitude of R waves (over 0.8 millivolt) in the frontal plane leads may suggest ventricular hypertrophy.

Duration—Less than 0.04 second.

Q-T segment—0.16 to 0.18 second duration.

ST segment and T wave—ST segment and T wave should be small and free of repolarization changes as well as marked depression of elevation

---

*From Ettinger, S. J., and Suter, P. F.: *Canine Cardiology*. Philadelphia: W. B. Saunders, 1970, pp. 102–169.

†From Ettinger, S. J.: *Textbook of Veterinary Internal Medicine*, 2nd ed. Vol. I. Philadelphia: W. B. Saunders, 1983, p. 984.

63-DAY PERPETUAL GESTATION CHART

Conception—Jan.	1 2 3 4 5 6 7 8 9 10 11 12 13 14 15 16 17 18 19 20 21 22 23 24 25 26 27		28 29 30 31
Due—March	5 6 7 8 9 10 11 12 13 14 15 16 17 18 19 20 21 22 23 24 25 26 27 28 29 30 31	April	1 2 3 4
Conception—Feb.	1 2 3 4 5 6 7 8 9 10 11 12 13 14 15 16 17 18 19 20 21 22 23 24 25 26		27 28
Due—April	5 6 7 8 9 10 11 12 13 14 15 16 17 18 19 20 21 22 23 24 25 26 27 28 29 30	May	1 2
Conception—Mar.	1 2 3 4 5 6 7 8 9 10 11 12 13 14 15 16 17 18 19 20 21 22 23 24 25 26 27 28 29		30 31
Due—May	3 4 5 6 7 8 9 10 11 12 13 14 15 16 17 18 19 20 21 22 23 24 25 26 27 28 29 30 31	June	1 2
Conception—Apr.	1 2 3 4 5 6 7 8 9 10 11 12 13 14 15 16 17 18 19 20 21 22 23 24 25 26 27 28		29 30
Due—June	3 4 5 6 7 8 9 10 11 12 13 14 15 16 17 18 19 20 21 22 23 24 25 26 27 28 29 30	July	1 2
Conception–May	1 2 3 4 5 6 7 8 9 10 11 12 13 14 15 16 17 18 19 20 21 22 23 24 25 26 27 28 29		30 31
Due–July	3 4 5 6 7 8 9 10 11 12 13 14 15 16 17 18 19 20 21 22 23 24 25 26 27 28 29 30 31	August	1 2
Conception—June	1 2 3 4 5 6 7 8 9 10 11 12 13 14 15 16 17 18 19 20 21 22 23 24 25 26 27 28 29		30
Due—August	3 4 5 6 7 8 9 10 11 12 13 14 15 16 17 18 19 20 21 22 23 24 25 25 27 28 29 30 31	Sept.	1
Conception—July	1 2 3 4 5 6 7 8 9 10 11 12 13 14 15 16 17 18 19 20 21 22 23 24 25 26 27 28 29		30 31
Due—September	2 3 4 5 6 7 8 9 10 11 12 13 14 15 16 17 18 19 20 21 22 23 24 25 26 27 28 29 30	Oct.	1 2
Conception—Aug.	1 2 3 4 5 6 7 8 9 10 11 12 13 14 15 16 17 18 19 20 21 22 23 24 25 26 27 28 29		30 31
Due—October	2 3 4 5 6 7 8 9 10 11 12 13 14 15 16 17 18 19 20 21 22 23 24 25 26 27 28 29 30	Nov.	1 2
Conception—Sept.	1 2 3 4 5 6 7 8 9 10 11 12 13 14 15 16 17 18 19 20 21 22 23 24 25 26 27 28		29 30
Due—November	3 4 5 6 7 8 9 10 11 12 13 14 15 16 17 18 19 20 21 22 23 24 25 26 27 28 29 30	Dec.	1 2
Conception–Oct.	1 2 3 4 5 6 7 8 9 10 11 12 13 14 15 16 17 18 19 20 21 22 23 24 25 26 27 28 29		30 31
Due—December	3 4 5 6 7 8 9 10 11 12 13 14 15 16 17 18 19 20 21 22 23 24 25 26 27 28 29 30 31	Jan.	1 2
Conception—Nov.	1 2 3 4 5 6 7 8 9 10 11 12 13 14 15 16 17 18 19 20 21 22 23 24 25 26 27 28 29		30
Due—January	3 4 5 6 7 8 9 10 11 12 13 14 15 16 17 18 19 20 21 22 23 24 25 26 27 28 29 30 31	Feb.	1
Conception—Dec.	1 2 3 4 5 6 7 8 9 10 11 12 13 14 15 16 17 18 19 20 21 22 23 24 25 26 27		28 29 30 31
Due—February	2 3 4 5 6 7 8 9 10 11 12 13 14 15 16 17 18 19 20 21 22 23 24 25 26 27 28	March	1 2 3 4

From Kirk, R. W., and Bistner, S. I.: *Handbook of Veterinary Procedures and Emergency Treatment*, 4th ed. Philadelphia: W. B. Saunders, 1985.

RECOMMENDED NUTRIENT ALLOWANCES FOR DOGS (PER LB OR KG OF BODY WEIGHT PER DAY)*

Nutrient	Per Lb	Per Kg	Nutrient	Per Lb	Per Kg
Protein (gm)	2.25	5.0	Vitamins		
Fat (gm)	0.70	1.5	Vitamin A (IU)	50	110
Linoleic acid (gm)	0.1	0.22	Vitamin D (IU)	5	11
Carbohydrate†	–	—	Vitamin E (μg)	0.55	1.2
			Thiamine (μg)	11.0	24
Minerals			Riboflavin (μg)	22.0	48
Calcium (mg)	120	265	Pyridoxine (μg)	11.0	24
Phosphorus (mg)	100	220	Pantothenic acid (μg)	100	220
Potassium (mg)	65	144	Niacin (μg)	114	250
Sodium chloride (mg)	91	200	Folic acid (μg)	1.8	4
Magnesium (mg)	6.4	14	Vitamin B_{12} (μg)	0.5	1.1
Iron (mg)	0.6	1.32	Biotin (μg)	1.0	2.2
Copper (mg)	0.07	0.16	Choline (mg)	11.8	26
Manganese (mg)	0.05	0.11			
Zinc (mg)	1.0	2.2			
Iodine (mg)	0.015	0.033			
Selenium (mg)	1.1	2.42			

*1977 modification by Cornell Research Laboratory for Diseases of Dogs; data taken from NAS-NRC Publication No. 8, Nutrient Requirements of Dogs, 1974.

†Carbohydrate as such has not been shown to be required. As a common ingredient of most dog foods, it serves as an excellent source of energy and may be required for reproduction.

From Sheffy, B. E.: Nutrition and nutritional disorders. Vet. Clin. North Am. 8:10, 1978.

CALORIC REQUIREMENTS FOR ADULT DOGS BASED ON PHYSICAL ACTIVITY AND BREED SIZE*

	Mature Weight		House Dog†	Active Dog‡	Working Dog§
	Kg	*Lb*	*Calories*	*Calories*	*Calories*
Small Breeds	2.3	5	200	250	300
	4.5	10	400	500	600
	6.8	15	600	750	900
	9.1	20	800	1000	1200
Medium Breeds	9.1	20	560	700	840
	11.4	25	700	875	1050
	13.6	30	840	1050	1260
	15.9	35	930	1225	1470
	18.2	40	1120	1400	1680
	20.5	45	1260	1575	1890
	22.7	50	1400	1750	2100
	25.0	55	1540	1925	2310
	27.3	60	1680	2100	2520
	29.5	65	1820	2275	2730
	31.8	70	1980	2450	2940
	34.1	75	2100	2625	3150
Large Breeds	34.1	75	1800	2250	2700
	36.4	80	1980	2400	2880
	38.6	85	2040	2550	3060
	40.9	90	2160	2700	3240
	43.2	95	2280	2850	3420
	45.5	100	2400	3000	3600
	47.7	105	2520	3150	3780
	50.0	110	2640	3300	3960
	52.3	115	2760	3450	4140
	54.5	120	2880	3600	4320
	56.8	125	3000	3750	4500
	59.1	130	3120	3900	4680
	61.4	135	3240	4050	4860
	63.6	140	3360	4200	5040
	65.9	145	3480	4350	5220
	68.2	150	3600	4500	5400

*These are average daily requirements. Animal requirements may vary according to age, breed, body and environmental temperature, temperament, and degree of activity. Owing to temperament, there is some overlap between the largest animals of some breeds and the smallest of others.

†Caloric requirements of house dogs = adult dogs maintained in laboratory cages.

‡Active dogs = adult dogs allowed to free run in outside pens, 125 to 480 square feet in size.

§Working dogs = adult dogs running at 5 mph on a 6 per cent incline for 4 hours each day.

Data courtesy of Ralston Purina Company, St. Louis, Missouri.

From Kirk, R. W., and Bistner, S. I.: *Handbook of Veterinary Procedures and Emergency Treatment,* 4th ed. Philadelphia: W. B. Saunders, 1985.

RECOMMENDED DAILY CALORIC INTAKE DURING FIRST FOUR WEEKS OF LIFE

Dog			Cat (Estimated)	
Kcal/oz BW	*Kcal/gm BW*	*Week*	*Kcal/gm BW*	*Kcal/oz BW*
3.8	0.133	1	0.20	5.7
4.4	0.155	2	0.22	6.3
5.0–5.7	0.175–0.20	3	0.27	7.7
5.7+	0.20+	4	0.29	8.3

*Amount of formula per day (ml) = weight of young (in gm) kcal factor (per gm BW) for age.

From Kirk, R. W., and Bistner, S. I.: *Handbook of Veterinary Procedures and Emergency Treatment*, 4th ed. Philadelphia: W. B. Saunders, 1985.

COMPOSITION OF MATERNAL MILK AND SUBSTITUTES

	Kcal Per ml	% Solids	Fat	Protein	Carbohydrate
Bitch milk	1.5	24.0	44.1	33.2	15.8
Esbilac powder*†	1.0	98.4	44.1	33.2	15.8
Esbilac liquid*	0.9	15.3	44.1	33.2	15.8
Cow milk	0.7	12.0	30.0	25.6	38.5
Evaporated milk‡	1.2	14.0	15.8	13.9	19.5
Cat milk	0.9	18.2	25.0	42.2	26.1
KMR*	0.9	18.2	25.0	42.2	26.1

*Manufactured by Pet-Vet Products, Borden Chemical Company, Borden, Inc., Norfolk, Virginia 23501.
†1 volume to 3 volumes water.
‡4 volumes to 1 volumes water.
From Kirk, R. W., and Bistner, S. I.: *Handbook of Veterinary Procedures and Emergency Treatment*, 4th ed. Philadelphia: W. B. Saunders, 1985.

NUTRITIONAL REQUIREMENTS (AMOUNTS PER POUND OF BODY WEIGHT PER DAY) OF ADULT CATS AND 10-WEEK-OLD KITTENS*

Nutrients	Adult	Kittens
Protein (gm)†	2.9	8.6
Energy (kcal)	40.0	115.0
Fat (gm)‡	1.5	3.2
Minerals		
Calcium (mg)	90	290
Phosphorus (mg)	80	230
Magnesium (mg)	5	14
Potassium (mg)	30	90
Sodium chloride (mg)	50	140
Iron (μg)	10	30
Copper (μg)	0.5	1.4
Manganese (μg)	0.9	2.8
Zinc (μg)	3.2	8.6
Iodine (μg)	0.1	0.3
Sodium (μg)	0.01	0.03
Vitamins		
Vitamin A (IU)§	100	290
Vitamin D (IU)	10	29
Vitamin E (IU)	1	3
Thiamine (mg)	0.05	0.14
Riboflavin (mg)	0.05	0.14
Pantothenic acid (mg)	0.10	0.28
Niacin (mg)‖	0.50	1.0
Pyridoxine (μg)	45	140
Folic acid (μg)	9	30
Biotin (μg)	0.5	1
Vitamin B_{12} (μg)	0.2	0.6
Choline (mg)	20	57

*Modified by F. A. Kallfelz from Nutrient Requirements of Cats. Publication No. 13. Washington, D.C., National Academy of Sciences–National Research Council, 1978.

†In addition to the essential amino acids, the cat (particularly the growing kitten) has a requirement for the amino-sulfonic acid taurine, which is found in highest concentrations in certain seafoods. Cat foods should contain at least 0.02 per cent taurine on a dry basis.

‡Although this may represent basal fat requirements, fat enhances palatability and is found at high levels in many cat foods. The cat has an absolute requirement for arachidonic acid, which should compose 0.02–0.05 per cent of the diet on a dry basis.

§The cat cannot convert beta-carotene to vitamin A and thus has an absolute requirement for this vitamin.

‖The cat cannot use tryptophan as an adequate source of niacin and must have niacin in the diet.

RECOMMENDED DAILY METABOLIZABLE ENERGY ALLOWANCES FOR CATS*

Kitten (wk of age)	Kcal/kg BW†	Adult‡	Kcal/kg BW
10	250	Inactive	70
20	130	Active	85
30	100	Gestation	100
40	80	Lactation	250

*Metabolizable energy allowances based on 4 kcal/gm of dietary protein and carbohydrate (nitrogen-free extract), and 9 kcal/gm of dietary fat. These allowances are presumed to apply in a thermoneutral environment (approximately 22°C).

†Body weight.

‡Fifty weeks of age and older.

From Nutrient Requirements of Cats. Publication No. 13 Washington, D.C., National Academy of Sciences–National Research Council, 1978.

COMPENDIUM OF CANINE VACCINES, 1988*

FREDERIC W. SCOTT, D.V.M.

Ithaca, New York

Vaccine Name	Marketed by	Type	CDV	CA1	CA2	CPI	Lep	Bor	Rab	MV	CPV	FPV	CCV
Adenomune-7	TechAmerica	A/I	x	x	x(i)	x	x(i)					x(i)	
Adenomune-7-L	TechAmerica	A/I	x	x	x(i)	x	x(i)					x	
Annumune	Fort Dodge	I							x				
Biorab-1	Biologics Corp.	I							x				
Biorab-3	Biologics Corp.	I(3)							x				
Bronchicine	TeachAmerica	I						x					
Canine Distemper Hepatitis	Colorado Serum	A	x	x									
Canine Distemper-Hepatitis-Leptospira	Colorado Serum	A/I	x	x			x(i)						
CoughGuard-B	Norden	I						x					
CoughGuard-BP	Norden	A/I				x		x(i)					
Cytorab	Coopers	I							x				
D-Vac-7	Bio-Ceutic	A/I	x	x	x	x	x(i)				x(i)	x	
Duramune Cv-K	Fort Dodge	I											x
Duramune DA₂LP + Pv	Fort Dodge	A/I	x		x	x	x(i)				x		
Duramune DA₂P + Pv	Fort Dodge	A	x		x	x					x		
Duramune-Pv	Fort Dodge	A									x		
Dura-Rab 1	ImmunoVet/Vedco	I							x				
Dura-Rab 3	ImmunoVet/Vedco	I(3)							x				
Endurall-K	Norden	I							x				
Endurall-R	Norden	A(3)							x				
Epivaxine DA₂P	Coopers	A	x		x	x							
Epivaxine DA₂PPv	Coopers	A/I	x		x	x					x(i)		
Epivaxine DA₂PL	Coopers	A/I	x		x	x	x(i)						
Epivaxine DA₂PPvL	Coopers	A/I	x		x	x	x(i)				x(i)		
FirstDose CPV	Norden	A									x		
Fromm D	Solvay	A	x										
Galaxy DA₂L	Solvay	A/I	x		x	x	x(i)						
Galaxy DA₂PL	Solvay	A/I	x		x	x	x(i)						
Galaxy 6 MHP	Solvay	A	x		x	x	x(i)				x		
Galaxy 6 MHP-L	Solvay	A/I	x		x	x	x(i)				x		
Galaxy 6 MP-L	Solvay	A/I	x		x	x	x(i)					x	
Imrab	Pitman-Moore	I(3)							x				
Imrab-1	Pitman-Moore	I							x				

Product	Source	Type	CDV	MV	CA1	CA2	CPI	CPV	CCV	Lep	Bor	Rab
Intra-Trac-II	Schering	A(1)					x				x	
Naramune-2	Bio-Ceutic	A(1)					x				x	
Neurogen-TC	Bio-Ceutic	A(3)										x
Paramune-5	TechAmerica	A/I	x		x		x	x	x	x(i)		
Parvocine	TechAmerica	I						x				
Parvocine-MLV	TechAmerica	A						x				
Parvoid 2	Solvay	A						x				
Puppyshot	Fort Dodge	A/I	x		x		x	x		x(i)		
Quantum	Pitman-Moore	A	x		x		x					
Quantum 4	Pitman-Moore	A	x		x		x	x				
Quantum 6	Pitman-Moore	A/I	x		x		x	x		x(i)		
Rabvac 3	Solvay	I(3)										x
Sentrypar	Beecham	A					x					
Sentrypar DHP	Beecham	A	x		x		x	x				
Sentrypar DHP/L	Beecham	A/I	x		x		x	x		x(i)		
Sentryvac-DHP	Beecham	A	x		x		x	x				
Sentryvac-DHP/L	Beecham	A/I	x		x		x	x		x(i)		
Tissuvax 5	Pitman-Moore	A/I	x		x		x	x		x(i)		
Tissuvax 6	Pitman-Moore	A/I	x		x		x	x	x	x(i)		
Trimune	Fort Dodge	I(3)										x
Trirab	Coopers	I(3)										x
Vanguard CPV (ML)	Norden	A						x				
Vanguard CPV	Norden	I						x				
Vanguard DA2L	Norden	A/I	x			x				x(i)		
Vanguard DA2MP	Norden	A	x	x		x	x					
Vanguard DA2P	Norden	A	x			x	x					
Vanguard DA2P + CPV	Norden	A	x			x	x	x				
Vanguard DA2PL	Norden	A/I	x			x	x			x(i)		
Vanguard DA2PL + CPV	Norden	A/I	x			x	x	x		x(i)		
Vanguard D-M	Norden	A	x	x								
Vanguard DMP	Norden	A	x	x			x					
Vovax	Coopers	I							x			

A, Attenuated (modified live virus, or MLV); I, inactivated (killed); A/I, combination of attenuated and inactivated; (i), inactivated components of mixed attenuated and inactivated vaccine; Bor, *Bordetella bronchiseptica*; CA1, canine adenovirus-1 (infectious canine hepatitis); CA2, canine adenovirus-2; CCV, canine coronavirus; CDV, canine distemper virus; CPI, canine parainfluenza; CPV, canine parvovirus; FPV, feline parvovirus (feline panleukopenia virus); Lep, leptospirosis (usually *L. canicola* plus *L. icterohaemorrhagiae*); MV, measles virus; Rab, rabies virus; (1), intranasal administration; (3), triennial booster after primary vaccination at 3 months and 1 year later.

*Canine vaccines licensed by the USDA and marketed in the United States. Modified from *Veterinary Pharmaceuticals and Biologicals*, 5th ed. Veterinary Medicine Publishing Co., Lenexa, KS, 1987/1988; and *Compendium of Animal Rabies Vaccines*, 1988, J.A.V.M.A. 192:18–22, 1988.

COMPENDIUM OF FELINE VACCINES, 1988*

FREDERIC W. SCOTT, D.V.M.

Ithaca, New York

Vaccine Name	Marketed by	Type	Vaccine Components					
			FPV	FVR	FCV	FP$_n$	Rabies	FeLV
Annumune	Fort Dodge	I					x	
Biorab-1	Biologics Corp.	I					x	
Biorab-3	Biologics Corp.	I					x	
Cytorab	Coopers	I					x	
Cytorab RCP	Coopers	A/I	x	x	x		x(i)	
Dura-Rab I	ImmunoVet/Vedco	I					x	
Dura-Rab 3	ImmunoVet/Vedco	I(3)					x	
Eclipse 1	Solvay	A	x					
Eclipse 1KP	Solvay	I	x					
Eclipse 3	Solvay	A	x	x	x			
Eclipse 3KP	Solvay	A/I	x(i)	x	x			
Eclipse 3KP-R	Solvay	A/I	x(i)	x	x		x(i)	
Eclipse 4	Solvay	A	x	x	x	x		
Eclipse 4KP	Solvay	A/I	x(i)	x	x	x		
Eclipse 4KP-R	Solvay	A/I	x(i)	x	x	x	x(i)	
Eclipse 4-R	Solvay	A/I	x	x	x	x	x(i)	
Endurall-K	Norden	I					x	
Endurall-R	Norden	A					x	
Epifel RCP	Coopers	A/I	x(i)	x	x			
Felocell CVR	Norden	A	x	x	x			
Felocine	Norden	I	x					
Felomune CVR	Norden	A/I		x	x			
Fel-O-Vax PCT	Fort Dodge	I	x	x	x			
Fel-O-Vax PCT-R	Fort Dodge	I(3)	x	x	x		x	
FVR-C-P	Pitman-Moore	A/I	x(i)	x	x			
FVR-C-P (MLV)	Pitman-Moore	A	x	x	x			
Imrab	Pitman-Moore	I(3)					x	
Imrab-1	Pitman-Moore	I					x	
Leukocell	Norden	I						x
Panacine RC	Beecham	A	x	x	x			
Panavac	Beecham	I	x					
Panavac RC	Beecham	A/I	x(i)	x	x			
Psittacoid	Solvay	A				x		
Rabcine	Beecham	I					x	
Rabcine-3	Beecham	I(3)					x	
Rabguard-TC	Norden	I(3)					x	
Rabmune-3	Beecham	I(3)					x	
Rabvac 1	Solvay	I					x	
Rabvac 3	Solvay	I(3)					x	
Respomune-CP	TechAmerica	A/I	x(i)	x	x			
Rhinolin-CP	Bio-Ceutic	A(I)	x	x	x			
Rhinopan-MLV	Tech-America	A	x	x	x			
Trimune	Fort Dodge	I(3)					x	
Trirab	Coopers	I					x	

A, Attenuated (modified live virus, or MLV); I, inactivated (killed); A/I; combination of attenuated and inactivated; (i), inactivated component of mixed attenuated and inactivated vaccine; FPV, feline parvovirus (panleukopenia); FVR, feline viral rhinotracheitis (feline herpesvirus-1); FCV, feline calicivirus; FeLV, feline leukemia virus; FP, feline pneumonitis (*Chylamydia*); (1), intranasal administration; (3), triennial booster after primary vaccination at 3 months and 1 year later.

*Feline vaccines licensed by the USDA and marketed in the United States. Modified from *Veterinary Pharmaceuticals and Biologicals*, 5th ed. Lenexa, KS, Veterinary Medicine Publishing Co., 1987/1988; and *Compendium of Animal Rabies Control*, 1988, J.A.V.M.A. 192:18–22, 1988.

Compendium of Animal Rabies Control, 1989

Prepared by: The National Association of State Public Health Veterinarians, Inc.

Part I: <u>Recommendations for Immunization Procedures</u>

The purpose of these recommendations is to provide information on rabies vaccines to practicing veterinarians, public health officials, and others concerned with rabies control. This document serves as the basis for animal rabies vaccination programs throughout the United States. Its adoption will result in standardization of procedures among jurisdictions, which is necessary for an effective national rabies control program. These recommendations are reviewed and revised as necessary prior to the beginning of each calendar year. All animal rabies vaccines licensed by the USDA and marketed in the United States are listed in Part II of the Compendium, and Part III describes the principles of rabies control.

A. <u>VACCINE ADMINISTRATION:</u> It is recommended that all animal rabies vaccines be restricted to use by or under the supervision of a veterinarian.

B. <u>VACCINE SELECTION:</u> In comprehensive rabies control programs, it is recommended that only vaccines with 3-year duration of immunity be used. This eliminates the need for annual vaccination and constitutes the most effective method of increasing the proportion of immunized dogs and cats (See Part II).

C. <u>ROUTE OF INOCULATION:</u> Unless otherwise specified by the product label or package insert, all vaccines must be administered intramuscularly at one site in the thigh.

D. <u>WILDLIFE VACCINATION:</u> Vaccination is not recommended since no rabies vaccine is licensed for use in wild animals. It is recommended that wild or exotic animals susceptible to rabies should not be kept as pets. Offspring born to wild animals bred with domestic dogs or cats will be considered as wild animals.

E. <u>ACCIDENTAL HUMAN EXPOSURE TO VACCINE:</u> Accidental inoculation may occur in individuals during administration of animal rabies vaccine. Such exposure to inactivated vaccines constitutes no rabies hazard. There have been no human cases of rabies resulting from needle or other exposure to a licensed modified-live-virus vaccine in the United States.

F. <u>IDENTIFICATION OF VACCINATED DOGS:</u> It is recommended that all agencies and veterinarians adopt the standard tag system. This will aid the administration of local, state, national and international procedures. Dog license tags should not conflict in shape and color with rabies tags. It is recommended that anodized aluminum rabies tags should be less than 0.064″ in thickness.

1. *RABIES TAGS*

CALENDAR YEAR	COLOR	SHAPE
1989	Blue	Rosette
1990	Orange	Fireplug
1991	Green	Bell
1992	Red	Heart

2. *RABIES CERTIFICATE:* All agencies and veterinarians should use the NASPHV form #50 Rabies Vaccination Certificate, which can be obtained from vaccine manufacturers.

THE NASPHV COMPENDIUM COMMITTEE
Suzanne R. Jenkins, VMD, MPH, Chair
Keith A. Clark, DVM, PhD
Russell W. Currier, DVM, MPH
Russell J. Martin, DVM, MPH
Grayson B. Miller, Jr., MD
F.T. Satalowich, DVM, MSPH
R. Keith Sikes, DVM, MPH

Address all correspondence to:
Suzanne R. Jenkins, VMD, MPH
Virginia Department of Health
Office of Epidemiology
109 Governor Street
Richmond, Virginia 23219

CONSULTANTS TO THE COMMITTEE
Melvin K. Abelseth, DVM, PhD
Kenneth L. Crawford, DVM, MPH
David W. Dreesen, DVM, MPVM, AVMA Council on Public Health and Regulatory Veterinary Medicine
Thomas R. Eng, VMD, MPH, Centers for Disease Control
David A. Espeseth, DVM, APHIS, USDA
Paul Waters, Representative, Veterinary Biologics Section, Animal Health Institute
William G. Winkler, DVM, MS

ENDORSED BY:
American Veterinary Medical Association (AVMA)
Council of State and Territorial Epidemiologists

Part II: Vaccines Marketed in the United States, and NASPHV Recommendations

PRODUCT NAME	PRODUCED BY	MARKETED BY	FOR USE IN[1]	DOSAGE[2]	AGE AT PRIMARY VACCINATION[3]	BOOSTER RECOMMENDED
A) MODIFIED LIVE VIRUS						
ENDURALL-R	NORDEN License No. 189	Norden	Dogs Cats	1 ml 1 ml	3 mos. & 1 yr. later 3 months	Triennially Annually
B) INACTIVATED						
TRIMUNE	FORT DODGE License No. 112	Ft. Dodge	Dogs Cats	1 ml 1 ml	3 mos. & 1 yr. later	Triennially Triennially
ANNUMUNE	FORT DODGE License No. 112	Ft. Dodge	Dogs Cats	1 ml 1 ml	3 months 3 months	Annually Annually
BIORAB-1	SCHERING License No. 165-A	Biologics Corp.	Dogs Cats	1 ml 1 ml	3 months 3 months	Annually Annually
BIORAB-3	SCHERING License No. 165-B	Biologics Corp.	Dogs Cats	1 ml 1 ml	3 mos. & 1 yr. later 3 months	Triennially Annually
RABMUNE 3	SCHERING License No. 165-A	Beecham	Dogs Cats	1 ml 1 ml	3 mos. & 1 yr. later 3 months	Triennially Annually
DURA-RAB 1	IMMUNOVET License No. 302-A	ImmunoVet & Vedco, Inc. Fermenta Animal Health	Dogs Cats	1 ml 1 ml	3 months 3 months	Annually Annually
DURA-RAB 3	IMMUNOVET License No. 302-A	ImmunoVet & Vedco, Inc. Fermenta Animal Health	Dogs Cats	1 ml 1 ml	3 mos. & 1 yr. later 3 mos. & 1 yr. later	Triennially Triennially
RABCINE 3	IMMUNOVET License No. 302-A	Beecham	Dogs Cats	1 ml 1 ml	3 mos. & 1 yr. later 3 mos. & 1 yr. later	Triennially Triennially
RABCINE	BEECHAM License No. 225	Beecham	Dogs Cats	1 ml 1 ml	3 months 3 months	Annually Annually
ENDURALL-K	NORDEN License No. 189	Norden	Dogs Cats	1 ml 1 ml	3 months 3 months	Annually Annually
RABGUARD-TC	NORDEN License No. 189	Norden	Dogs Cats Sheep Cattle Horses	1 ml 1 ml 1 ml 1 ml 1 ml	3 mos. & 1 yr. later 3 months 3 months 3 months	Triennially Triennially Annually Annually Annually
CYTORAB	COOPERS ANIMAL HEALTH INC. License No. 107	Coopers	Dogs Cats	1 ml 1 ml	3 months 3 months	Annually Annually
TRIRAB	COOPERS ANIMAL HEALTH INC. License No. 107	Coopers	Dogs Cats	1 ml 1 ml	3 mos. & 1 yr. later 3 months	Triennially Annually
RABVAC 1	SALSBURY License No. 195-A	Solvay Veterinary	Dogs Cats	1 ml 1 ml	3 months 3 months	Annually Annually
RABVAC 3	SALSBURY License No. 195-A	Solvay Veterinary	Dogs Cats Horses	1 ml 1 ml 2 ml	3 mos. 1 yr. later 3 months	Triennially Triennially Annually
IMRAB	RHONE MERIEUX, INC. License No. 298	Pitman-Moore	Dogs Cats Sheep Cattle Horses	1 ml 1 ml 2 ml 2 ml 2 ml	3 mos. & 1 yr. later 3 months 3 months	Triennially Triennially Triennially Annually Annually
IMRAB-1	RHONE MERIEUX, INC. License No. 298	Pitman-Moore	Dogs Cats	1 ml 1 ml	3 months 3 months	Annually Annually
C) COMBINATION						
ECLIPSE 3 KP-R	SALSBURY License No. 195-A	Solvay Veterinary	Cats	1 ml	3 months	Annually
ECLIPSE 4 KP-R	SALSBURY License No. 195-A	Solvay Veterinary	Cats	1 ml	3 months	Annually
CYTORAB RCP	COOPERS ANIMAL HEALTH INC. License No. 107	Coopers	Cats	1 ml	3 months	Annually
FEL-O-VAX PCT-R	FORT DODGE License No. 112	Fort Dodge	Cats	1 ml	3 mos. & 1 yr. later	Triennially
ECLIPSE 4-R	SALSBURY License No. 195-A	Solvay Veterinary	Cats	1 ml	3 months	Annually

1. Refers only to domestic species of this class of animals.
2. All vaccines must be administered <u>intramuscularly</u> at one site in the thigh unless otherwise specified by the label.
3. Three months of age (or older) and revaccinated one year later.

1358

Part III: Rabies Control

A. PRINCIPLES OF RABIES CONTROL

1. *HUMAN RABIES PREVENTION:* Rabies in humans can be prevented either by eliminating exposures to rabid animals or, in exposed persons, by prompt local wound treatment combined with appropriate passive and active immunization. The rationale for recommending preexposure and postexposure rabies prophylaxis and details of their administration can be found in the current recommendations of the Immunization Practices Advisory Committee (ACIP) of the U.S. Public Health Service. These recommendations, along with information concerning the current local and regional status of animal rabies and the availability of human rabies biologics, are available from state health departments.

2. *DOMESTIC ANIMALS:* Local governments should initiate and maintain effective programs to remove stray and unwanted animals and ensure vaccination of all dogs and cats. Since cat rabies cases frequently exceed the annually reported cases in dogs, immunization of cats should be required. Such procedures in the U.S. have reduced laboratory confirmed rabies cases in dogs from 6,949 in 1947 to 170 in 1987. The recommended vaccination procedures and the licensed animal vaccines are specified in Parts I and II of the NASPHV's annually released compendium.

3. *RABIES IN WILDLIFE:* The control of rabies in foxes, skunks, raccoons and other terrestrial animals is very difficult. Selective reduction of these populations when indicated may be useful, but the utility of this procedure depends heavily upon the circumstances surrounding each rabies outbreak (See C. Control Methods in Wild Animals).

B. CONTROL METHODS IN DOMESTIC AND CONFINED ANIMALS

1. *PREEXPOSURE VACCINATION AND MANAGEMENT*

Animal rabies vaccines should be administered only by or under the direct supervision of a veterinarian. This is the only way to assure the public that the animal has been properly immunized. Within one month after vaccination, a peak rabies antibody titer is reached and the animal can be considered to be immunized (See Parts I and II of the compendium for recommended vaccines and procedures).

(a) DOGS AND CATS

All dogs and cats should be vaccinated against rabies commencing at three months of age and revaccinated in accordance with Part II of this Compendium.

(b) LIVESTOCK

It is not economically feasible, nor is it justified from a public health standpoint, to vaccinate all livestock against rabies. Owners and veterinary clinicians may consider immunizing certain livestock, especially those which are valuable and/or may have high contact with humans, located in areas where wildlife rabies is epizootic.

(c) OTHER ANIMALS

(1) *ANIMALS MAINTAINED IN EXHIBITS AND IN ZOOLOGICAL PARKS*

Captive animals not completely excluded from all contact with local vectors of rabies can become infected with rabies. Moreover, such animals may be incubating rabies when captured. Exhibit animals susceptible to rabies should be quarantined for a minimum of 180 days. Since there is no rabies vaccine licensed for use in wild animals, vaccination even with inactivated vaccine is not recommended. Preexposure rabies immunization of animal workers at such facilities is recommended. This may reduce the need for euthanasia of valuable animals for rabies testing after they have bitten a handler.

(2) *WILD ANIMALS*

Because of the existing risk of rabies in wild animals (especially raccoons, skunks and foxes), the AVMA, the NASPHV and the Council of State and Territorial Epidemiologists (CSTE) strongly recommend the enactment of state laws prohibiting the importation, distribution and relocation of wild animals and wild animals crossbred to domestic dogs and cats. These same organizations continue to recommend the enactment of laws prohibiting the distribution or keeping of wild animals as pets. Moreover, the NASPHV and CSTE recommend that ferrets not be kept as pets, since they have severely bitten many people, especially inflicting mutilating bites to infants. Ferrets are susceptible to and could transmit rabies. Because the period of rabies virus shedding in infected ferrets is unknown, confinement and observation of ferrets that bite people are not appropriate.

2. *STRAY ANIMAL CONTROL*

Stray dogs or cats should be removed from the community, especially in rabies epizootic areas. Local health department and animal control officials can enforce the pickup of strays more efficiently if owned animals are confined or kept on leash. Strays should be impounded for at least three days to give owners sufficient time to reclaim animals apprehended as strays and to determine if human exposure has occurred.

3. *QUARANTINE*

(a) *INTERNATIONAL.* Present USPHS regulations (42 CFR No. 71.51) governing the importation of dogs and cats are minimal for preventing the introduction of rabid animals into the United States. All dogs and cats imported from countries with endemic rabies should be vaccinated against rabies at least 30 days prior to entry into the United States. The Centers for Disease Control (CDC) are responsible for these animals imported into the United States. Their requirements should be coordinated with interstate shipment requirements. The health authority of the state of destination should be notified within 72 hours of any animal conditionally admitted into its jurisdiction.

The conditional admission into the United States of such animals must be subject to state and local laws governing rabies. Failure to comply with these requirements should be promptly reported to the director of the CDC.

(b) <u>INTERSTATE</u>. Prior to interstate movement, dogs and cats should be vaccinated against rabies according to the compendium's recommendations at least 30 days prior to movement. While in transit they should be accompanied by a currently valid NASPHV Form #50 Rabies Vaccination Certificate. One copy of the certificate should be mailed to the appropriate Public Health Veterinarian or State Veterinarian of the state of destination.

(c) *HEALTH CERTIFICATES*. *If a certificate is required for dogs and cats in transit, it must not replace the NASPHV rabies vaccination certificate.*

4. *ADJUNCT PROCEDURES*

Methods or procedures which enhance rabies control include:

(a) <u>LICENSURE</u>. Registration or licensure of all dogs and cats may be used as a means of rabies control by controlling the stray animal population. Frequently a fee is charged for such licensure and revenues collected are used to maintain rabies or animal control programs. Vaccination is an essential prerequisite to licensure.

(b) <u>CANVASSING OF AREA</u>. This includes house-to-house calls by members of the animal control program to enforce vaccination and licensure requirements.

(c) <u>CITATIONS</u>. These are legal summonses issued to owners for violations including the failure to vaccinate or license their animals. The authority for officers to issue citations should be an integral part of each animal control program.

(d) <u>LEASH LAWS</u>. All communities should adopt leash laws which can be incorporated in their animal control ordinances.

5. *POSTEXPOSURE MANAGEMENT*

ANY DOMESTIC ANIMAL THAT IS BITTEN OR SCRATCHED BY A BAT OR BY A WILD, CARNIVOROUS MAMMAL WHICH IS NOT AVAILABLE FOR TESTING SHOULD BE REGARDED AS HAVING BEEN EXPOSED TO A RABID ANIMAL.

(a) <u>DOGS AND CATS</u>. When bitten by a rabid animal, unvaccinated dogs and cats should be destroyed immediately. If the owner is unwilling to have this done, the animal should be placed in strict isolation for six months and vaccinated one month before being released. Dogs and cats that are currently vaccinated should be revaccinated immediately and observed by the owner for 90 days.

(b) <u>LIVESTOCK</u>. All species of livestock are susceptible to rabies; cattle are among the most susceptible of all domestic animals. Livestock bitten by rabid animals should be destroyed (slaughtered) immediately. If the owner is unwilling to have this done, the animal should be kept under very close observation for six months.

The following are recommendations for owners of livestock exposed to rabid animals:

(1) If livestock is slaughtered within seven days of being bitten, tissues may be eaten without risk of infection, provided that liberal portions of the exposed area are discarded. Federal meat inspectors will reject for slaughter any animal known to have been exposed to rabies within eight months.

(2) Neither tissues nor milk from a rabid animal should be used for human or animal consumption. However, as pasteurization temperatures will inactivate rabies virus, the drinking of pasteurized milk or eating of completely cooked meat does not constitute a rabies exposure.

6. *MANAGEMENT OF ANIMALS THAT BITE HUMANS*

A healthy dog or cat that bites a person should be confined and observed for 10 days and evaluated by a veterinarian at the first sign of illness during confinement or before release. Any illness in the animal should be reported immediately to the local health department. If signs suggestive of rabies develop, the animal should be humanely killed and its head removed and shipped, under refrigeration, for examination by a qualified laboratory designated by the local or state health department. Any stray or unwanted dog or cat that bites a person may be killed immediately and the head submitted, as described above, for rabies examination.

C. <u>CONTROL METHODS IN WILD ANIMALS</u>

The public should be warned not to handle wild animals. Bats and wild carnivorous mammals, as well as wild animals cross-bred with domestic dogs and cats, that bite people should be killed and appropriate tissues should be sent to the laboratory for examination for rabies. A person bitten by any wild animal should immediately report the incident to a physician who can evaluate the need for antirabies treatment (see current Rabies Prophylaxis Recommendations of the Immunization Practices Advisory Committee: Rabies).

1. *TERRESTRIAL MAMMALS*

Continuous and persistent government-funded programs for trapping or poisoning wildlife as a means of rabies control are not cost effective in reducing wildlife reservoirs or rabies incidence on a statewide basis. However, limited control in high-contact areas (picinic grounds, camps, suburban areas) may be indicated for the removal of selected high-risk species of wild animals. The state wildlife agency should be consulted early to manage any elimination programs in coordination with the state health department.

2. *BATS*

(a) Rabid bats have been reported from every state except Hawaii, and have caused human rabies in the United States. It is neither feasible nor desirable, however, to control rabies in bats by areawide bat population reduction programs.

(b) Bats should be excluded from houses and surrounding structures to prevent direct association with people. Such structures should then be made bat-proof by sealing entrances.

(Reprinted with permission from J.A.V.M.A., Vol. 194, No. 2, January 15, 1989, pp. 188–192.)

IMMUNIZATION PROCEDURES*

IMMUNIZATION OF WILD ANIMAL SPECIES AGAINST COMMON DISEASES

As with domestic animals, there is no unanimous opinion as to the proper methods that should be used in immunizing wild animals. The following information represents current approaches to vaccination in managing wild species maintained in zoos or game parks. *Private ownership of wild animal species as pets is strongly discouraged! No rabies vaccine is approved for any wild species.*

FAMILY CANIDAE. Coyote, fox, jackal, wolf, dingo, cape hunting dog, and so on.

Canine Distemper—Infectious Canine Hepatitis (ICH). Administer modified live virus (MLV) vaccine as for domestic dogs. Revaccinate annually and prior to anticipated possible exposure if 6 months have elapsed since last vaccination.

Parvovirus. Canine parvovirus vaccines are being used on wild canids, but there are no data to support statements on efficacy or safety.

Rabies. No rabies vaccine is licensed for use. Limited testing indicates that wild animals have unpredictable responses to rabies vaccinations. If vaccination *must* be used in animals confined in zoos or game parks, administer only inactivated rabies vaccine.

FAMILY FELIDAE. Tiger, leopard, lion, cheetah, jaguar, lynx, ocelot, margay, bobcat, mountain lion, jungle cat, golden cat, and so on.

Feline Panleukopenia. Wild felids appear to be exquisitely susceptible to the feline panleukopenia virus. Proper and adequate vaccination is a *must!* Vaccinate with MLV vaccine containing rhinotracheitis and calicivirus vaccines. Begin vaccination when the animal is 6 to 8 weeks of age, and repeat two or three times at 4-week intervals. Revaccinate adults at 12-month intervals. Use manufacturers' recommendations.

Pneumonitis. The use of MLV pneumonitis vaccine is definitely an *elective procedure* and cannot be recommended as a routine procedure for the individual cat. Pneumonitis vaccine might best be administered to wild felids with anticipated exposure to other domestic or wild felids (such as at cat shows). In this situation, the vaccine should be administered 10 to 14 days prior to anticipated exposure.

Rabies. No rabies vaccine is licensed for use.

Limited testing indicates that wild animals have unpredictable responses to rabies vaccinations. If vaccination *must* be used in animals confined in zoos or game parks, administer only inactivated rabies vaccine.

FAMILY PROCYONIDAE. Lesser panda, raccoon, coatimundi, and kinkajou.

Canine Distempter. MLV vaccine may be administered according to the manufacturers' recommendations. Adults should be revaccinated annually.

Infectious Canine Hepatitis. Limited data available; inapparent infection may occur in raccoons. No recommendations.

Feline Panleukopenia. Although proven cases have been reported only in the raccoon and the coatimundi, the current trend is to vaccinate all captive members of the family Procyonidae. MLV vaccine may be used according to the manufacturers' recommendations. Adults should be revaccinated every 12 months.

Pneumonitis. Elective procedure as per family Felidae.

Rabies. No rabies vaccine is licensed for use. Limited testing indicates that wild animals have unpredictable responses to rabies vaccinations. If vaccination *must* be used in animals confined in zoos or game parks, administer only inactivated rabies vaccine.

FAMILY VIVERRIDAE. Binturong, fossa, linsang, mongoose, and civet.

Canine Distemper. Cases of proven canine distemper have been reported in the binturong and civet. It is suggested that all captive viverrids be vaccinated for canine distemper as per the family Canidae.

Infectious Canine Hepatitis. No data available.

Feline Panleukopenia. Cases are poorly documented, but it has been recommended that at least the binturong if not all captive viverrids be vaccinated for feline panleukopenia as per the family Felidae.

Rabies. No rabies vaccine is licensed for use. Limited testing indicates that wild animals have unpredictable responses to rabies vaccinations. If vaccination *must* be used in animals confined in zoos or game parks, administer only inactivated rabies vaccine.

FAMILY URSIDAE. Bears

Canine Distemper. Although several species of bears are reported to be susceptible to canine distemper, bears are not routinely vaccinated at zoos. In some cases, it may be advisable to use MLV vaccine as per family Canidae.

Infectious Canine Hepatitis. Infection of bears

---

*See also compendia on rabies (p. 1357), canine (p. 1354), and feline vaccines (p. 1356).

From Kirk, R. W., and Bistner, S. I.: *Handbook of Veterinary Procedures and Emergency Treatment,* 4th ed. Philadelphia: W. B. Saunders, 1985.

1361

with ICH has been described but not confirmed. No recommendations.

Feline Panleukopenia. Cases of panleukopenia (not verified by virus isolation) have been reported in young bear cubs. No recommendations can be given at this time as to the advisability of vaccinating bears for feline panleukopenia.

Rabies. No rabies vaccine is licensed for use. Limited testing indicates that wild animals have unpredictable responses to rabies vaccinations. If vaccination *must* be used in animals confined in zoos or game parks, administer only inactivated rabies vaccine.

FAMILY HYAENIDAE. Hyenas.

Canine Distemper. All species of hyena are susceptible and should be vaccinated for canine distemper as per family Canidae.

Infectious Canine Hepatitis. No data available.

Rabies. No rabies vaccine is licensed for use. Limited testing indicates that wild animals have unpredictable responses to rabies vaccinations. If vaccination *must* be used in animals confined in zoos or game parks, administer only inactivated rabies vaccine.

FAMILY MUSTELIDAE. Ferret, mink, otter, skunk, weasel, wolverine, badger, marten, sable, grison, and fisher.

Canine Distemper. The mink, ferret, and skunk are susceptible, and probably all captive mustelids should be vaccinated for canine distemper using an MLV vaccine as per family Canidae.

Infectious Canine Hepatitis. Limited data available. No recommendations.

Viral Enteritis (may be variant of feline panleukopenia). Mink only. Administer autogenous or commercial mink enteritis formalized vaccine or killed feline panleukopenia virus vaccine. Kits, 6 to 8 weeks of age; adults should be revaccinated annually. Follow manufacturers' recommendations.

Feline Panleukopenia. It has been suggested that all mustelids except the ferret are susceptible to feline panleukopenia and should receive vaccine as per the family Felidae. Mink should receive either killed panleukopenia vaccine or formalized mink enteritis vaccine. They need not receive both.

Botulism (mink and ferret). (*Clostridium botulinum*) type C toxoid. Kits can be vaccinated at 10 to 12 weeks of age; adults should be revaccinated yearly.

Rabies. No rabies vaccine is licensed for use. Limited testing indicates that wild animals have unpredictable responses to rabies vaccinations. If vaccination *must* be used in animals confined in

zoos or game parks, administer only inactivated rabies vaccine.

ORDER MARSUPIALIA, FAMILY DIDELPHIDAE. Opossum.

The opossum is highly resistant to infection by canine distemper and rabies and probably does not need to be vaccinated for these diseases.

ORDER PRIMATES. Subhuman.

Poliomyelitis (apes only–gorilla, orangutan, chimpanzee, and gibbon.) Live oral polio virus vaccine. Adults, one 12-month booster with trivalent vaccine. Initial dose, a child's dose of trivalent vaccine administered twice at 6- to 8-week intervals.

Rabies. No rabies vaccine is licensed for use. Limited testing indicates that wild animals have unpredictable responses to rabies vaccinations. If vaccination *must* be used in animals confined in zoos or game parks, administer only inactivated rabies vaccine.

Tuberculosis (immunization not recommended). Susceptible nonhuman primates should be subjected to periodic tuberculin tests and either eliminated or vigorously treated with appropriate medication if found to be positive. Test procedure (WHO recommendations): Koch's Old Tuberculin (full strength) 0.1 cc *intradermally* in the upper eyelid. Read test at 24, 48, and 72 hours postinjection; positive test is characterized by swelling and erythema with closure of the eye. Should have three successive negative tests at 2-week intervals.

Measles, Smallpox, and Similar Diseases. Vaccination of primates (especially apes) against the common childhood diseases is an elective procedure and depends on the degree of exposure to which the primate may be subjected. Consult with a pediatrician on the choice of immunizing agent(s).

Hepatitis. Where the possibility of disease exists or where there is known exposure to a hepatitis patient, gamma globulin IM may be administered prophylactically.

ORDER RODENTIA. Mouse, rat, hamster, gerbil, guinea pig, and squirrel.

Rabies. Vaccination is not recommended for these animals if they remain caged.

ORDER LOGAMORPHA. Rabbit and hare.

See order *Rodentia.*

References and Supplemental Readings

Fowler, M. E.: Immunoprophylaxis in nondomestic carnivors. *In* Kirk, R. W. (ed.): *Current Veterinary Therapy VIII.* Philadelphia: W. B. Saunders Company, 1983, p. 1129.

USE OF ANTIMICROBIAL AGENTS FOR TREATMENT OF INFECTIONS

Organism	Disease	Drugs of Choice	Alternative Drugs
Actinomyces	Actinomycosis	Penicillin G*	Tetracyclines
Anaerobic organisms *Peptococcus, Peptostreptococcus, Lactobacillus*	Soft tissue infections, granulomas, wound infections after GI surgery	Chloramphenicol, ampicillin, clindamycin/lincomycin	Penicillin, cephaloridine, erythromycin
Bacillus anthracis	Anthrax	Penicillin G	Erythromycin, cephalosporin, tetracyclines
Bacteroides	Wound infections	Chloramphenicol, clindamycin	Tetracycline, cephalosporin
Blastomyces, Candida, Coccidioides, Cryptococcus, Mucor, Aspergillus	Pneumonia, skin and soft-tissue lesions, bone lesions, disseminated disease	Amphotericin B	2 hydroxystilbamide† *(Blastomyces)*, flucytosine† *(Candida, Cryptococcus)*
Bordetella bronchiseptica	Respiratory infections	Tetracyclines	Chloramphenicol
Brucella canis	Abortions	Tetracyclines with streptomycin	Chloramphenicol with streptomycin
Chlamydia psittaci	Respiratory infections, conjunctivitis	Tetracyclines	Chloramphenicol
Clostridium tetani	Tetanus	Penicillin G*	Erythromycin
Clostridia (other)	Gas gangrene	Penicillin G*	Tetracyclines
Coccidia	Coccidiosis	Sulfonamides	Nitrofurazone
Escherichia coli	Urinary tract infections	Gentamicin, ampicillin	Cephalosporins, nitrofurantoin, chloramphenicol, tetracyclines, sulfonamides, Tribrissen (trimethoprim-sulfadiazine)
	Other infections	Ampicillin, chloramphenicol, tetracyclines	Aminoglycosides, polymyxins
Fusobacterium	Ulcerative stomatitis	Penicillin G	Tetracyclines, metronidazole
Giardia	Enteritis	Penicillin G	Quinacrine, glycobiarsol
Haemobartonella	Infectious anemia	Tetracycline‡	Chloramphenicol‡
Klebsiella, Enterobacter	Respiratory, urinary tract infections	Kanamycin, gentamicin	Cephalosporins, chloramphenicol
Leptospira	Leptospirosis	Penicillin G with streptomycin	Tetracyclines
Microsporum, Trichophyton, Epidermophyton	Skin, hair, and nail bed infections	Griseofulvin	—
Mycobacterium	Tuberculosis	Isoniazid with streptomycin or *p*-aminosalicylic acid	—
Mycoplasma	Respiratory infection (?), conjunctivitis	Erythromycin Chloramphenicol, tetracycline	—
Neorickettsia	Salmon disease	Tetracyclines	Chloramphenicol
Nocardia	Nocardiosis	Sulfonamides with ampicillin or Tribrissen	Ampicillin with erythromycin
Pasteurella multocida	Abscesses, respiratory infections	Penicillin G*	Tetracyclines, ampicillin
Pentatrichomonas	Trichomonal enteritis	Metronidazole	Glycobiarsol
Pityrosporum	Skin and ear infections	2% "tame" iodine or 25% glyceryl triacetate topically	—
Proteus mirabilis	Urinary tract and soft-tissue infections	Ampicillin, cephalosporin, nitrofurantoin§	Chloramphenicol, aminoglycosides
Pseudomonas	Urinary tract and soft-tissue infections, burns	Gentamicin, tobramycin	Carbenicillin with amikacin
Salmonella	Gastroenteritis	Chloramphenicol	Ampicillin, nitrofurantoin

Table continued on following page

Organism	Disease	Drugs of Choice	Alternative Drugs
Staphylococcus aureus	Pyoderma, endocarditis, osteomyelitis, soft-tissue infections	Penicillin G–sensitive: penicillin G Pencillin G-resistant: cloxacillin, erythromycin	Ampicillin, macrolides, lincomycin Cephalosporins, chloramphenicol, lincomycin
Streptococcus	Urinary tract infections, otitis, soft-tissue infections, upper respiratory infections	Penicillin G	Ampicillin, cephalosporins, erythromicin
Toxoplasma	Toxoplasmosis	Pyrimethamine with sulfonamide	—

*Large dosage.

†Used to treat these infections in humans; efficacy in dogs and cats uncertain.

‡Efficacy questionable.

§Urinary tract infections only.

Modified from Aronson, A. L., and Kirk, R. W.: Antimicrobial drugs. *In* Ettinger, S. J. (ed.): *Textbook of Veterinary Internal Medicine*. Philadelphia, W. B. Saunders Company, 1975, pp. 338–366.

CONVERSION TABLE OF WEIGHT TO BODY SURFACE AREA (IN SQUARE METERS) FOR DOGS*

Kg	M²	Kg	M²
0.5	0.06	26.0	0.88
1.0	0.10	27.0	0.90
2.0	0.15	28.0	0.92
3.0	0.20	29.0	0.94
4.0	0.25	30.0	0.96
5.0	0.29	31.0	0.99
6.0	0.33	32.0	1.01
7.0	0.36	33.0	1.03
8.0	0.40	34.0	1.05
9.0	0.43	35.0	1.07
10.0	0.46	36.0	1.09
11.0	0.49	37.0	1.11
12.0	0.52	38.0	1.13
13.0	0.55	39.0	1.15
14.0	0.58	40.0	1.17
15.0	0.60	41.0	1.19
16.0	0.63	42.0	1.21
17.0	0.66	43.0	1.23
18.0	0.69	44.0	1.25
19.0	0.71	45.0	1.26
20.0	0.74	46.0	1.28
21.0	0.76	47.0	1.30
22.0	0.78	48.0	1.32
23.0	0.81	49.0	1.34
24.0	0.83	50.0	1.36
25.0	0.85		

*Although the above chart was compiled for dogs, it can also be used for cats. A formula for more precise values follows:

$$\text{BSA in M}^2 \quad \frac{K \times W^{2/3}}{10^4} \quad \textit{Given that}$$

BSA = body surface area
M² = sq meters
W = weight in gm
K = 10.1 (dogs), 10.0 (cats)

From Ettinger, S. J.: *Textbook of Veterinary Internal Medicine.* Vol. I. Philadelphia, W. B. Saunders, 1975, p. 146.

EQUIVALENTS AND CONVERSION FACTORS

Weight Equivalents

1 lb = 453.6 gm = 0.4536 kg = 16 oz
1 oz = 28.35 gm
1 kg = 1,000 gm = 2.2046 lb
1 gm = 1,000 mg
1 mg = 1,000 μg = 0.001 gm
1 μg = 0.001 mg = 0.000001 gm
1 μg per gm or 1 mg per kg is the same as ppm

METRIC	APOTHECARY
0.1 milligram (mg) =	$\frac{1}{600}$ grain (gr)
0.15 mg =	$\frac{1}{400}$ gr
0.2 mg =	$\frac{1}{300}$ gr
0.25 mg =	$\frac{1}{250}$ gr
0.3 mg =	$\frac{1}{200}$ gr
0.4 mg =	$\frac{1}{150}$ gr
0.5 mg =	$\frac{1}{120}$ gr
1.0 mg =	$\frac{1}{60}$ gr
15.0 mg =	$\frac{1}{4}$ gr
30.0 mg =	$\frac{1}{2}$ gr
40.0 mg =	$\frac{2}{3}$ gr
50.0 mg =	$\frac{3}{4}$ gr
60.0 mg =	1 gr (0.06 gm)
1.0 gm =	15 gr

Volume Equivalents

Household	Metric
1 drop (gt)	= 0.06 milliliter (ml)
15 drops (gtt)	= 1 ml (1 cc)
1 teaspoon (tsp)	= 5 (4) ml
1 tablespoon (tbs)	= 15 ml
2 tablespoons	= 30 ml
1 ounce (oz)	= 30 ml
1 teacup	= 180 ml (6 oz)
1 glass	= 240 ml (8 oz)
1 measuring cup	= 240 ml (1/2 pint)
2 measuring cups	= 500 ml (1 pint)

Weight–Unit Conversion Factors

Units Given	Units Wanted	For Conversion Multiply by
lb	gm	453.6
lb	kg	0.4536
oz	gm	28.35
kg	lb	2.2046
kg	mg	1,000,000.
kg	gm	1,000.
gm	mg	1,000.
gm	μg	1,000,000.
mg	μg	1,000.
mg/gm	mg/lb	453.6
mg/kg	mg/lb	0.4536
μg/kg	μg/lb	0.4536
Mcal	kcal	1,000.
kcal/kg	kcal/lb	0.4536
kcal/lb	kcal/kg	2.2046
ppm	μg/gm	1.
ppm	mg/kg	1.
ppm	mg/lb	0.4536
mg/kg	%	0.0001
ppm	%	0.0001
mg/gm	%	0.1
gm/kg	%	0.1

Temperature Conversion

°Celsius to °Fahrenheit: (°C) $\left(\frac{9}{5}\right) + 32°$

°Fahrenheit to °Celsius: (°F − 32°) $\left(\frac{5}{9}\right)$

Conversion Factors

1 milligram	=	1/65	grain	(1/60)
1 gram	=	15.43	grains	(15)
1 kilogram	=	2.20	pounds	(avoirdupois)
		2.65	pounds	(Troy)
1 milliliter	=	16.23	minims	(15)
1 liter	=	1.06	quarts	(1 +)
		33.80	fluid ounces	(34)
1 grain	=	0.065	gm	(60 mg)
1 dram	=	3.9	gm	(4)
1 ounce	=	31.1	gm	(30 +)
1 minim	=	0.062	ml	(0.06)
1 fluid dram	=	3.7	ml	(4)
1 fluid ounce	=	29.57	ml	(30)
1 pint	=	473.2	ml	(500 −)
1 quart	=	946.4	ml	(1000 −)

Figures in parentheses are commonly employed approximate values.

ANTINEOPLASTIC AGENTS IN CANCER THERAPY

Agent (Brand Name, Supplier)	Action and Cell Cycle Specificity	Indication	Dosage and Administration	Toxicities	Comments
Alkylating Agents					
Cyclophosphamide (Cytoxan, Mead Johnson; Neosar, Adria) Tabs: 25 and 50 mg Inj: 100-, 200-, and 500-mg vials; 1- and 2-gm vials	Alkylating activity by metabolite phosphoramide mustard. Believed to cross-link DNA. Cell cycle nonspecific.	Primarily lymphoreticular neoplasms. Also mast cell, hemangiosarcoma, mammary carcinoma.	1. 50 mg/m² PO q 48 hr. 2. 50 mg/m² PO q 24 hr × 4d; repeat weekly. 3. 100-200 mg/m² IV q 21 d.	Leukopenia, gastroenteritis, hemorrhagic cystitis. May induce transitional cell carcinoma of bladder.	Must be activated by liver. Excreted primarily by kidney. Metabolites protein bound.
Chlorambucil (Leukeran, Burroughs Wellcome) Tabs: 2 mg	Bifunctional alkylation of DNA. Creates intra- and interstrand cross-links. Cell cycle nonspecific.	Lymphoreticular neoplasms, macroglobulinemia, polycythemia vera.	2-4 mg/m² PO q 48 hr.	Leukopenia.	Relatively free of gastrointestinal effects.
Busulfan (Myleran, Burroughs Wellcome) Tabs: 2 mg	Bifunctional alkylating agent. Interacts with cellular thiol groups. Little DNA cross-linking. Cell cycle nonspecific.	Chronic granulocytic leukemia; of no benefit in "blastic" phase.	3-4 mg/m² PO q 24 hr. Discontinue when total WBC approx. 15,000. Repeat p.r.n.	Leukopenia. Rare bronchopulmonary dysplasia with pulmonary fibrosis.	May require 2 weeks to observe response. If rapid decline in total leukocytes; discontinue drug.
Melphalan (Alkeran, Burroughs Wellcome) Tabs: 2 mg	Bifunctional alkylating agent. Phenylalanine derivative of nitrogen mustard. Cell cycle nonspecific.	Multiple myeloma; some lymphoreticular neoplasms, osteosarcomas, mammary and lung tumors.	2-4 mg/m² PO q 48 hr.	Infrequent leukopenia.	Response may be gradual over many months.
Triethylenethiophosphoramide (Thiotepa, Lederle) Inj: 15 mg vial	Radiomimetic. Believed to disrupt DNA bonds by release of ethyleneamine radicals. Cell cycle nonspecific.	Systemic use for carcinomas. Intravesical use for transitional cell. Intracavitary use for neoplastic effusions.	9 mg/m² IV q 7-28 d. 0.6-0.8 mg/kg intracavitary. 60 mg intravesicular in 30-60 ml water for 2 hr.	Leukopenia.	Not a vesicant. May be given intralesionally.
Mechlorethamine HCl (Mustargen, Merck) Inj: 10-mg vial	Cytoxic, mutagenic and radiomimetic. Exact mechanism of action unknown. Cell cycle nonspecific.	Lymphoreticular neoplasms, pleural and peritoneal effusions.	5 mg/m² PO, IV, or intracavitary; repeat p.r.n.	Leukopenia. Nausea and vomiting dose-limiting side effects.	Severe vesicant. Sloughing may occur if extravasated.
Cisplatin (Platinol, Bristol-Myers) Inj: 10- and 50-mg vials	Action similar to bifunctional alkylating agents. Produces DNA cross-links. Cell cycle nonspecific.	Osteosarcoma, transitional cell carcinoma, squamous cell carcinoma.	50-70 mg/m² IV over 20 min. Administer 0.9% saline IV for 4 hr pre- and 2 hr post-infusion.	Nausea, vomiting, renal toxicity, bone marrow depression. Dose-related pulmonary toxicity in cat.	Do not use aluminum-containing needles; precipitates on contact. Eliminated through kidney.

Table continued on following page

1367

Antimetabolites

Drug	Action	Indications	Dosage	Toxicity	Comments
Mercaptopurine (Purinethol, Burroughs Wellcome) Tabs: 50 mg	Feedback enzyme inhibitor of DNA synthesis. S-phase specific.	Acute lymphocytic and granulocytic leukemia, immune-mediated disease.	50 mg/m² PO q 24 hr to effect, then q 48 hr or p.r.n.	Infrequent leukopenia.	Must be activated within tumor cells; "lethal" synthesis.
Thioguanine (Thioguanine, Burroughs Wellcome) Tabs: 40 mg	Feedback enzyme inhibitor of DNA synthesis. S-phase specific.	Acute lymphocytic and granulocytic leukemia.	Dogs: 40 mg/m² PO q 24 hr × 4–5 d, then q 3 d thereafter. Cats: 25 mg/m² PO q 24 hr × 1–5 d, then repeat cycle q 30 d p.r.n.	Leukopenia, thrombocytopenia may be severe in cats. Hepatotoxicity.	As for mercaptopurine. Cross-resistance between thioguanine and mercaptopurine is extensive.
Fluorouracil (Fluorouracil, Roche; Adrucil, Adria) Inj: 500-mg vial	Inhibits enzyme thymidylate synthetase. Results in thymidine deficiency leading to inhibition of DNA synthesis. S-phase specific.	Mammary, gastrointestinal, liver, and lung carcinomas, and carcinomatosis.	150 mg/m² IV or intracavitary q 7 d.	Dogs: cerebellar ataxia. Cats: neurotoxicity precludes usage.	Cleared by hepatic degradation.
Cytosine arabinoside (Cytosar-U, Upjohn) Inj: 100- and 500-mg vials	Appears to inhibit DNA polymerase activity; mechanism incompletely understood. S-phase specific.	Lymphoreticular neoplasms, myeloproliferative disease, and CNS lymphoma.	100 mg/m² IV or SC q 24 hr × 2–4 d; repeat p.r.n. 20 mg/m² intrathecally × 1–5 d.	Leukopenia.	May be given intrathecally.
Methotrexate (Methotrexate, Lederle; Folex, Adria; Mexate, Bristol) Tabs: 2.5 mg Inj: 5-, 20-, 25-, 50-, 100-, 200-, and 250-mg vials	Competitive enzyme inhibitor of folic acid reductase. S-phase specific.	Lymphoreticular neoplasms, myeloproliferative disorders, transmissible venereal and Sertoli's cell tumors, osteosarcoma.	"High dose": 5–10 mg/m² PO, IV, IM, or intrathecally followed 2–4 hr later with leucovorin 3 mg/m². "Normal dose": 2.5 mg/m² q 24 hr. Adjust dose/frequency according to toxicity.	Leukopenia, vomiting, renal tubular necrosis with "high dose" regimen.	May be given intrathecally. Primarily excreted by kidney.

Vinca Alkaloids

Drug	Action	Indications	Dosage	Toxicity	Comments
Vincristine (Oncovin, Lilly) Inj: 1-, 2-, and 5-mg vials	Appears to arrest mitotic division in metaphase; mechanism incompletely understood. M-phase specific.	Lymphoreticular neoplasms, carcinomas, sarcomas, and transmissible venereal tumor.	0.5–0.75 mg/m² IV q 7–14 d.	Constipation, diarrhea, and peripheral neuropathies.	Severe vesicant. Primarily excreted by liver.
Vinblastine (Velban, Lilly) Inj: 10-mg vial	Affects cell energy production. Exhibits antimitotic activity. Primarily M-phase specific.	Lymphoreticular neoplasms, some carcinomas.	2 mg/m² IV q 7–14 d.	Leukopenia, epilation, peripheral neuritis.	Severe vesicant. Primarily excreted by liver.

Antitumor Antibiotics

Drug	Action	Indications	Dosage	Toxicity	Comments
Bleomycin (Blenoxane, Bristol-Myers) Inj: 15-IU vial	Appears to inhibit DNA synthesis. Lesser inhibition of RNA and protein synthesis. Cell cycle nonspecific.	Squamous cell carcinoma, lymphoma, other carcinomas.	10 U/m² IV or SC q 24 hr × 3–4 d, then 10 U/m² q 7 d. Max. accumulative dose 200 U/m².	Rare interstitial pneumonia leading to pulmonary fibrosis.	Has no toxic effects on the blood-forming elements.

Agent (Brand Name, Supplier)	Action and Cell Cycle Specificity	Indication	Dosage and Administration	Toxicities	Comments
Doxorubicin (Adriamycin, Adrial) Inj: 10- and 50-mg vials	Intercalates between DNA base pairs. Inhibits DNA, RNA, and protein synthesis. Cell cycle nonspecific.	Lymphoreticular neoplasms, soft tissue and bone sarcomas, thyroid and mammary carcinomas, other carcinomas.	30 mg/m² IV or intracavitary q 21 d or 10 mg/m² IV q 7 d. Max. accumulative dose 240 mg/m². Pretreat with antihistamine.	Leukopenia, thrombocytopenia, vomiting, diarrhea, epilation, cardiomyopathy, and urticaria.	Severe vesicant. Does not cross blood-brain barrier. Primarily excreted by liver.
Dactinomycin (Cosmegen, Merck) Inj: 0.5-mg vial	Intercalates between DNA bases. Inhibits mRNA synthesis. Cell cycle nonspecific.	Lymphoreticular neoplasms, some carcinomas and sarcomas.	1.5 mg/m² IV q 7 d.	Leukopenia.	Severe vesicant. Use "two-needle" technique.
Plicamycin (Mithracin, Miles) Inj: 2.5-mg vial	Binds DNA and inhibits mRNA and protein synthesis; exact mechanism unknown. Cell cycle nonspecific.	Malignant testicular neoplasia and hypercalcemia.	0.025 mg/kg IV q 24 hr × 8–10 d; repeat q 30 d or p.r.n. Give over 4–6 hr. Dilute in saline.	Hemorrhagic syndrome and gastroenteritis.	Demonstrates calcium-lowering effect unrelated to tumoricidal activity.
Hormonal Agents					
Prednisone and prednisolone (various suppliers) Tabs: 1, 2.5, 5, 10, 20, 25, and 50 mg	Penetrates to nucleus and affects RNA production. Mechanism not well understood. Cell cycle nonspecific.	Lymphoreticular neoplasms, mast cell tumors, brain tumors.	10–40 mg/m² PO q 24 hr × 7 d, then 10–20 mg/m² q 24–48 hr.	Pancreatitis, diarrhea, cushingoid state.	Prednisone must be activated to prednisolone by the liver.
Diethylstilbestrol (Diethylstilbestrol, Lilly) Tabs: 0.1, 0.25, 0.5, 1, and 5 mg	Enters cytoplasm and is transported to nucleus, where drug affects mRNA and protein synthesis. Cell cycle nonspecific.	Perianal gland adenoma and prostatic hyperplasia.	0.1–1 mg/dog PO q 24–48 hr.	Feminization, occasional bone marrow aplasia.	May cause irreversible bone marrow suppression and aplastic anemia.
Miscellaneous Agents					
Mitotane (Lysodren, Bristol-Myers) Tabs: 500 mg	Adrenal cytotoxic. Primary action on adrenal cortex; biochemical mechanism unknown.	Adrenal cortical carcinoma (functional and nonfunctional).	50 mg/kg PO q 24 hr to effect, then 25 mg/kg PO q 3 d.	Vomiting, anorexia, diarrhea, nausea, weakness, and adrenocorticosuppression.	Discontinue temporarily in shock or severe traumatic conditions.
Asparaginase (Elspar, Merck) Inj: 10,000-IU vial	Enzyme that hydrolyzes serum asparagine to aspartate and ammonia. Deprives tumor cells of asparagine. G₁-phase specific.	Lymphoreticular neoplasia, acute lymphocytic leukemia.	10,000–30,000 IU/m² SC, IM, IP, or IV q 7 d or p.r.n. Pretreat with antihistamine.	Pancreatitis, anaphylaxis.	Increased risk of anaphylaxis with retreatments. Only inhibits tumor cells; no effect on normal cells.
Dacarbazine (DTIC-Dome, Miles) Inj: 100- and 200-mg vials	Exhibits alkylating and antimetabolite activity; exact mechanism unknown. Cell cycle nonspecific.	Lymphoreticular neoplasia. Minimal activity in malignant melanoma and osteosarcoma.	200–250 mg/m² IV q 24 hr × 5 d; repeat q 21 d.	Anorexia, vomiting, diarrhea, cytopenia.	Drug extravasation may result in tissue damage and severe pain.
Hydroxyurea (Hydrea, Squibb) Caps: 500 mg	Inhibits DNA synthesis without interfering with mRNA and protein synthesis. S-phase specific.	Polycythemia vera, chronic granulocytic leukemia.	500 mg/m² PO q 12 hr × 7–10 d to effect, then decrease to 500 mg/m² PO q 24 hr or p.r.n.	Leukopenia, anemia, occasional thrombocytopenia, vomiting, and nail slough.	Primarily excreted by kidney.

Table courtesy of James P. Thompson, D. V. M. Discussion of these agents can be found in the article "Antineoplastic Agents in Cancer Therapy" (p. 472).

TABLE OF COMMON DRUGS: APPROXIMATE DOSES

Drug Name	Dog	Cat	Additional Information
Acetazolamide	10 mg/kg q6h PO	None	
Acetylcysteine (Mucomyst)	*Eye:* Dilute to 2% of soln with artificial tears and apply topically q2h to eye for maximum of 48 h	Same	
	Respiratory: 50 ml/h for 30–60 min q12h by nebulization		
	Acetaminophen Poisoning: 140 mg/kg PO, IV (loading dose), then 70 mg/kg q4h for 4–5 treatments	Same	
Acetylpromazine (acepromazine)	0.055–0.11 mg/kg IV, IM, SC	0.055–0.11 mg/kg IM, SC	
	0.55–2.2 mg/kg PO	1.1–2.2 mg/kg PO	
Acetylsalicylic acid (aspirin)	*Analgesia:* 10 mg/kg q12h PO	*Analgesia:* 10 mg/kg q52h PO	IX-415, X-50, X-567
	Antirheumatic: 40 mg/kg q18h PO or 25 mg/ kg q8h	*Antirheumatic:* 40 mg/kg q72h	
ACTH	2 units/kg/day IM (therapeutic) or		
	20 units/dog IM (response test; take post sample in 2 hr)	10 units/cat IM (response test)	
Actinomycin D (Cosmegen)	0.015 mg/kg q3–5 days IV, wait 3 weeks for marrow recovery; 1.5 mg/m² once weekly	Same	
Activated charcoal			IX-137
Aldactone (spironolactone)	1–2 mg/kg q12h	Same	
Allopurinol (Zyloprim)	10 mg/kg q8h PO, then reduce to 10 mg/kg PO daily	None	
Amforol	2–6 tablets/9 kg initially	None	
	Maintenance: 1–3 tabs/9 kg q8h		
Amikacin	11 mg/kg q12h IM, SC	None	
Amitraz (Mitaban)	10.6 ml in 2 gallons water, dip q2wk for 3 treatments, let dry on	None	IX-534
Aminophylline	10 mg/kg q8h PO, IM, IV	6.6 mg/kg q12h PO	IX-281
Ammonium chloride	100 mg/kg q12h PO	¼ tsp powder/feeding	
Amoxicillin	22 mg/kg q12h PO	Same	
Amphetamine	4.4 mg/kg IV, IM	Same	
Amphotericin B	0.15–1.0 mg/kg dissolved in 5–20 ml 5% dextrose and water given rapidly IV 3 times weekly for 2–4 mo; do not exceed 2.0 ml/kg; pretreat with antiemetics if needed; monitor BUN	Same	IX-536, IX-1143, X-1100
Ampicillin (Polyflex, Princillin)	10–20 mg/kg q6h PO; 5–10 mg/kg q6h IV, IM, SC	Same	
Amprolium	100–200 mg/kg/day in food or water for 7–10 days	None	
Amrinone			IX-327
Antacid drugs			IX-867, X-247, X-911
Anterior pituitary gonadotropin	*Bitches:* 100–500 units once daily to effect	None	
Anthelmintics			IX-921–923, X-879
Antiarrhythmic drugs			IX-346, X-284
Anticonvulsant drugs			IX-836, X-881
Antidiarrheal drugs			IX-868
Antidotes (poisoning)			IX-138, X-117
Antiemetic drugs			IX-884
Antifungal drugs			X-1100
Antihypertensive drugs			IX-360, X-1201
Antineoplastic drugs			X-402, X-472, X-475, X-494, Appendix
Apomorphine	0.02 mg/kg IV or 0.04 mg/kg SC; ¼–½ tablet in conjunctival sac, flush once emesis begins	None	

Drug Name	Dog	Cat	Additional Information
Ascorbic acid (vitamin C)	100–500 mg/day (maintenance) or 100—500 mg q8h (urine acidifier)	100 mg/day (maintenance) or 100 mg q8h (urine acidifier)	
L-Asparaginase	400 IU/kg IP weekly, maximum dose is 10,000 IU	Same	
Atropine	0.05 mg/kg q6h IV, SC, IM or 1% soln in eye *Organophosphate poisoning:* 0.2–2.0 mg/kg IV, SC, IM. Give ¼ dose IV and remainder IM or SC as needed	Same	
Aurothioglucose (Solganol)	First wk 5 mg IM; second wk 10 mg IM; then 1 mg/kg once/wk IM, decreasing to once/mo	First wk, 1 mg IM; second wk, 2 mg IM; then 1 mg/kg once/wk IM, decreasing to once/mo	
Azathioprine	2 mg/kg q24h PO	None	X-571
BAL	4 mg/kg q4h IM until recovered	None	
Beta-adrenergic blockers			IX-343
Betamethasone (Betasone)	0.028–0.055 ml/kg IM; give only once	None	
Bethanechol (Urecholine)	5–25 mg q8h PO	2.5–5.0 mg q8h PO	
Bismuth, milk of	10–30 ml q4h PO	Same	
Bismuth (subnitrate, subgallate, or subcarbonate)	0.3–3.0 gm q4h PO	Same	
Bleomycin (Blenoxane)	10 mg/m² daily IV or SC for 4 days, then 10 mg/m² weekly to a maximum total dose of 200 mg/m²	Same	
Blood	20 ml/kg IV or IP or to effect	Same	
Brewer's yeast	0.2 gm/kg once daily PO	Same	
Bromsulphalein (BSP) (5% solution)	*Test only:* 5 mg/kg IV; post sample in 30 min	None	
Bronchodilator drugs			IX-278
Bunamidine (Scolaban)	25–50 mg/kg PO. Fast 3 hr before and after administration.	Same	
Busulfan (Myleran)	4.0 mg/m² daily PO; 0.1 mg/kg daily	None	
Butorphanol	0.055–0.11 mg/kg q6–12h SC up to 7 days; 0.55 mg/kg q6–12h PO	None	
Caffeine	0.1–0.5 gm IM	None	
Calcitonin			IX-86
Calcium carbonate	1–4 gm/day PO	Same	
Calcium chloride (10% solution)	1–2 ml IV, IC	0.05–0.1 mg/kg IV, IC	
Calcium EDTA	100 mg/kg diluted to 10 mg/ml in 5% dextrose and given SC in 4 divided doses; continue for 5 days	Same	IX-148
Calcium gluconate (10% solution)	10–30 ml IV (slowly)	5–15 ml IV (slowly)	
Calcium lactate	0.5–2.0 gm PO	0.2–0.5 gm PO	
Calcium Na₂ EDTA	100 mg/kg body weight per day, SC, for 2–5 days—daily dose divided into 4 equal portions after dilution to approx. 10 mg CaNa₂ EDTA/ml 5% dextrose solution		X-157
Calcium salts			IX-1042
Canine DA₂P vaccine	1 vial SC at 8, 12, and 16 wk of age; annual booster	None	
Canine parvovirus vaccine (MLV)	1 ml SC 8, 12, 16, and 20 wk; annual revaccination	None	
Captan	0.2–0.25% soln topically, 2 to 3 times weekly	Same	
Captopril	0.5–2 mg/kg q8–12h PO	2 mg q8–12h PO	IX-334
Carbamazepine			IX-841
Carbenicillin	15 mg/kg q8h IV	Same	
Castor oil	8–30 ml PO	4–10 ml PO	
Cefadroxil	22 mg/kg q12h PO	22 mg/kg once daily PO	
Cefazolin	11–22 mg/kg q6–8h IM, IV	Same	
Cefoxitin	22 mg/kg q8h IV, IM		
Cephalexin	22 mg/kg q8h PO	Same	X-74
Cephalosporins			
Cephalothin sodium	22–44 mg/kg q6–8h IM, IV	Same	
Cephapirin	10–20 mg/kg q6h IM, IV	Same	

Table continued on following page

Drug Name	Dog	Cat	Additional Information
Charcoal, activated (Requa)	0.3–5 gm q8–12h PO *Poisoning:* 1–2 tsp/10–15 kg in 200 ml tap water; administer by stomach tube	Half the canine dose	
Chemotherapeutic drugs See *Antineoplastic drugs*			
Cheracol	5 ml q4h PO	3 ml q4h PO	
Chlorambucil (Leukeran)	0.1–0.2 mg/kg PO once daily	2 mg every other day PO	X-571
Chloramphenicol	50 mg/kg q8h PO, IV, IM, SC	Same, except q12h	
Chlordane	0.5% solution on dog or premises	None	
Chlorethamine	0.2–1.0 gm q8h PO	100 mg q8h PO	
Chlorpheniramine	4–8 mg q12h PO	2 mg q12h PO	
Chlorpromazine (Thorazine)	3.3 mg/kg PO once to 4 times daily 1.1–6.6 mg/kg IM once to 4 times daily 0.55–4.4 mg/kg IV once to 4 times daily	Same	
Chlortetracycline	20 mg/kg q8h PO	Same	
Chlorthiazide (Diuril)	20–40 mg/kg q12h PO	Same	
Chrysotherapy See *Gold therapy*			
Cimetidine (Tagamet)	5–10 mg/kg q6–12h	None	X-575, X-913
Cisplatin			X-491, X-497
Clavamox	13.75 mg/kg q12h PO		
Clavulanate antibiotics			X-78
Cloxacillin	10 mg/kg q6h PO, IV, IM	Same	
Cod liver oil	1 tsp/10 kg once daily PO	Same	
Codeine	*Pain:* 2 mg/kg q6h SC *Cough:* 5 mg/dose q6h PO	None	
Colistimethate (Coly-Mycin)	1.1 mg/kg q6h IM	Same	
Cromolyn sodium			IX-283
Cyclophosphamide	6.6 mg/kg PO for 3 days, then 2.2 mg/kg PO once daily; 200 mg/m² IV weekly, maximum dose is 250 mg	10 mg/kg IV weekly	X-570
Cyclosporine			X-513, X-572
Cyclothiazide	0.5–1.0 mg/PO once daily	None	
Cytarabine (Cytosar)	5–10 mg/kg once daily for 2 wk, or 30–50 mg/kg IV, IM, SC once/wk; 100 mg/m² once daily IV, IM for 4 days, then 150 mg/m²	Same	
Dacarbazine (DTIC)	100 mg/m² IV days 1–5, q3weeks in combination therapy; 200 mg/m² × 5 days, q3 weeks IV; 300 mg/m², q3 weeks IV	Same	
Dapsone	1.1 mg/kg q8h PO	None	
Darbazine	0.14–0.2 ml/kg q12h SC: 2–7 kg: 1 #1 capsule q12h PO; 7–14 kg: 1–2 #1 capsules q12h PO; Over 14 kg: 1 #3 capsule q12h PO	0.14–0.22 ml/kg q12h SC	
Delta Albaplex	3–7 kg: 1–2 tablets/day PO; 7–14 kg: 2–4 tablets/day PO; 14–27 kg: 4–6 tablets/day PO; Over 27 kg: 6–8 tablets/day PO	1 tablet q12h PO	
Depo-penicillin	15,000–30,000 U/kg q48h IM, SC	Same	
Desmopressin acetate (DDAVP)	2 to 4 drops once or twice daily, intranasally or in the conjunctival sac	Same	X-975
Desoxycorticosterone acetate (Doca)	1–5 mg q24h IM	0.5–1.0 mg q24h IM	
Desoxycorticosterone pivalate	Each 25 mg releases 1 mg Doca/day for 1 mo IM dose: 5–10 mg once/mo to effect	Same	
Dexamethasone (Azium)	0.25–1.0 mg IV, IM once daily; 0.25–1.25 mg PO once daily *Shock:* 5 mg/kg IV	0.125–0.5 mg once daily PO, IV, IM *Shock:* same	
Dextran	20 ml/kg IV to effect	Same	
Dextrose solutions (5% in water, saline, or Ringer's)	40–50 mg/kg q24h IV, SC, IP	Same	
Diazepam (Valium)	2.5–20 mg IV, PO; 10-mg bolus IV (slowly) if in status epilepticus; repeat if no effect	2.5–5.0 mg IV, PO	X-63
Diazoxide	10–40 mg/kg/day divided PO	None	
Dichlorphenamide	2–4 mg/kg q8h PO	10–25 mg q8h PO	

Drug Name	Dog	Cat	Additional Information
Dichlorvos (Task)	26.4–33 mg/kg PO; in risk animals divided dose, give remaining half 8–24 h later	None	
Dicloxacillin (Dicloxin)	11–55 mg/kg q8h PO	Same	
Diethylcarbamazine (Caricide, Cypip, Filaribits)	*Treatment of ascarids:* 55–110 mg/kg PO *Prevention of ascarids:* (Cypip) 3.3 mg/kg PO once daily *Prevention of heartworms:* (Caricide, Filaribits) 6.6 mg/kg PO once daily	*Treatment of ascarids:* 55–110 mg/kg PO	IX-418
Diethylstilbestrol (DES)	0.1–1.0 mg/day PO	0.05–0.10 mg/day PO (caution)	
Di-Gel (liquid)	30–60 ml PO	Half the canine dose	
Digitoxin (Foxalin-Vet)	0.033–0.11 mg/kg PO, divided twice daily	None	
Digoxin (Lanoxin, Cardoxin)	*Maintenance:* 0.0055–0.011 mg/kg q12h PO; or 0.22 mg/m² BSA q12h PO *Rapid digitalization:* Twice the oral maintenance dose for 24–48 h, then begin oral maintenance dose 12 h later; or 0.011 mg/kg IV q1h to effect, to a maximum *total* dose of 0.044 mg/kg. Begin oral maintenance dose 12–24 h later.	*Maintenance:* 0.0035–0.0055 mg/kg once or twice daily, PO (with caution)	IX-326, IX-384
Dihydrocodeinone	5 mg q6h PO	None	
Dihydrostreptomycin	10 mg/kg q8h IM, SC	Same	
Dihydrotachysterol	0.01 mg/kg/day	1–2 drops q12–24 h PO	IX-93, IX-1042
Diltiazem	0.5–1.3 mg/kg PO q8h		IX-342, X-276
Dimenhydrinate (Dramamine)	25–50 mg q8h PO	12.5 mg q8h PO	
Dimercaprol (BAL)	2.5–5 mg/kg b.w. IM as 10% soln. in oil. (Dose of 5 mg/kg used only in acute cases and only on first day.) *Injections:* q4h on days 1 and 2; q8h on day 3; b.i.d. for next 10 days	Same	X-161
Dioctyl sulfosuccinate (Surfak)	One or two 50-mg capsules q12–24h PO	1 50-mg capsule q12–24h PO	
Diphenhydramine (Benadryl)	2–4 mg/kg q8h PO; 5–50 mg q12h IV	Same	
Diphenylhydantoin (Dilantin) See *Phenytoin*			
Diphenylthiocarbazone	60 mg/kg q8h PO for 5 days beyond recovery	None	
Dipyrone	25 mg/kg SC, IM, IV, may repeat q8h	Same	
Disinfectants			X-90
Disophenol (DNP)	10 mg/kg SC; may be repeated in 2–3 wk	None	
Disopyramide	6–15 mg/kg q8h PO	None	
Dithiazanine (Dizan)	6.6–11 mg/kg PO once daily for 7–10 days	None	
Dobutamine HCl (Dobutrex)	250 mg in 1,000 ml 5% dextrose, IV at a rate of 2.5 μg/kg/min	None	IX-325
Docusate calcium	1 or 2 50-mg capsules q12–24h PO; *Enema:* 60–120 ml rectally	1 50-mg capsule q12–24h PO; *Enema:* 60 ml rectally	
Docusate sodium	50–300 mg q12h PO	50–100 mg q12–24h PO	
Domeboro's solution	1–2 tablets/pint water; apply topically q8h; store soln no longer than 7 days	Same	
Dopamine HCl (Intropin)	40 mg in 500 ml lactated Ringer's, IV at a rate of 2–8 μg/kg/min	Same	IX-325
Doxapram (Dopram)	5–10 mg/kg IV *Neonate:* 1–5 mg SC, sublingual or umbilical vein	5–10 mg/kg IV *Neonate:* 1–2 mg SC, sublingual vein	
Doxorubicin (Adriamycin)	30 mg/m² IV weekly	20 mg/m² IV weekly	X-490
Doxycycline	5 mg/kg (loading dose) PO, 2.5 mg/kg in 12h, then 2.5 mg/kg q24 h	Same	
Doxylamine succinate	1–2 mg/kg q8h IM	Same	
Edrophonium	0.11–0.22 mg/kg IV	None	
Emetrol	4–12 ml q15min PO until emesis ceases	Same	

Table continued on following page

Drug Name	Dog	Cat	Additional Information
Enflurane (Ethrane)	*Induction:* 2–3% *Maintenance:* 1.5–3%	Same	
Enilconazole	*Penicillium* infection: Dip patient in solution of 2000 ppm. *Nasal aspergillosis:* 20 mg/kg divided into 2 treatments per day and flushed through the sinuses and nostrils every day for 7–10 days		X-84, X-1107
Ephedrine	12.5–50 mg PO q8–12h	2–4 mg/kg PO q8–12h	X-1221
Epinephrine (1:1000 soln)	0.1–0.5 ml SC, IM, IV, or intracardiac	0.1–0.2 ml SC, IM, IV, or intracardiac	IX-325, X-331
Erythromycin	10 mg/kg q8h PO	Same	
Estradiol cyclopentaneo-propionate (ECP)	0.25–2.0 mg IM *once* *Abortifacient:* 22 μg/kg IM to maximum 1.0 mg at time of estrus; never repeat in same estrus	0.25–0.5 mg IM *once* *Abortifacient:* 250 μg IM 40 hr after copulation	
Estradiol cypionate			IX-1237
Ether	0.5–4.0 ml (*Induction:* 8%; *Maintenance:* 4%; inhalant to effect)	Same	
Ethoxzolamide (Cardrase)	4 mg/kg q12h PO	Same	
Ethyl alcohol			IX-211
Feline leukemia vaccine	—	1 ml SC at 9 wk or older; repeat in 2–3 wk; booster dose in 2–4 mo; annual revaccination	
Feline panleukopenia vaccine	—	1 vial SC at 8, 12, and 16 wk of age; annual booster	
Fenbendazole	50 mg/kg/day for 3 days	*Lungworms:* 50 mg/kg PO once	
Fentanyl (Sublimaze)	0.02–0.04 mg/kg (preanesthetic) IM, IV, SC	Same, but use with tranquilizer to prevent excitation	
Ferrous sulfate	100–300 mg/kg q24h PO	50–100 mg q24h PO	IX-523
Festal	1–2 tablets PO with or immediately after feeding	1 tablet PO with or immediately after feeding	
Flucytosine (Ancobon)	100 mg/kg q12h PO	Same	IX-562, X-1102
Fludrocortisone (Florinef)	0.2–0.8 mg once daily PO	0.1–0.2 mg once daily PO	IX-976
Flumethasone (Flucort)	0.06–0.25 mg once daily PO, IV, IM, SC	0.03–0.125 mg once daily PO, IV, IM, SC	
Flunixin	0.3 mg/kg IM, IV	None	X-51
5-Fluorouracil	100–200 mg/m² IV weekly; 2–5 mg/kg IV weekly	Do not use	
Folic acid	5 mg/day PO	2.5 mg/day PO	
Furosemide (Lasix)	2.5–5.0 mg/kg once or twice daily at 6- to 8-h intervals PO, IM, IV	2.5 mg/kg once or twice daily at 6- to 8-h intervals PO, IM, IV	
Gentamicin	2 mg/kg q8h IM, SC	Same	IX-1146
Glucagon	*Tolerance test:* 0.03 mg/kg IV	None	
Glucocorticoid therapy			IX-944–962, X-54, X-896
Glycerin	0.6 ml/kg q8h PO	Same	
Glycopyrrolate	0.01 mg/kg IM or SC	None	
Gold Therapy			X-573
Griseofulvin	50 mg/kg PO once daily with fat for 6 wk	Same	IX-562
Growth hormone	0.1 U/kg, three times per week for 4–6 wk; alternative dosage: 2–5 U (<14 kg b.w.) or 5 U (>14 kg b.w.) every other day for 10 treatments		X-979
Halothane (Fluothane)	*Induction:* 3% *Maintenance:* 0.5–1.5%	Same	
Heparin	Initial IV dose: 200 units/kg; continue by SC administration q8h	Same	IX-507, X-297
Hetacillin (Hetacin)	10–20 mg/kg q8h PO	Same	
Hydralazine	1 mg/kg q8h PO	None	IX-333
Hydrochlorothiazide (Hydrodiuril)	2–4 mg/kg q12h PO	Same	
Hydrochloric acid			IX-71
Hydrocortisone (Solu-Cortef)	4.4 mg/kg q12h PO *Shock:* 50 mg/kg IV	Same Same	
Hydrogen peroxide (3%)	5–10 ml q 15 min PO until emesis occurs	Same	

Drug Name	Dog	Cat	Additional Information
Hydroxyurea (Hydrea)	80 mg/kg q 3 days PO; 40–50 mg/kg divided twice daily PO; 20–30 mg/kg PO as a single daily dose	Same	
Hydroxyzine	10–50 mg q8h PO	10 mg q12h PO	
Innovar-Vet	0.1–0.14 ml/kg IM; 0.04–0.09 ml/kg IV; Administer with atropine to minimize bradycardia and salivation	CNS excitation—do not use.	
Insulin (regular crystalline)	2 units/kg q2–6h IV (ketoacidosis), modified to effect *Hyperkalemia:* 0.5–1.0 units/kg with 2 gm dextrose per unit of insulin	3–5 units SC q6h, modified to effect	IX-993, IX-1003, X-1011
Insulin (intermediate)	0.5–1.0 units/kg q24h SC, modified as needed	3–5 units q24h SC, modified as needed	
Insulin (NPH isophane)			IX-994
Insulin (PZI)			IX-994
Iron (see ferrous sulfate)			
Isoproterenol (Isuprel)	0.1–0.2 mg q6h IM, SC; 15–30 mg q4h PO 1 mg in 250 ml 5% dextrose, IV at a rate of 0.01 μg/kg/min	Same 0.5 mg in 250 ml 5% dextrose, IV to effect	
Isosorbide dinitrate	0.5–2.0 mg/kg PO q 8h		IX-332
Isuprel	Elixir: 0.44 ml/kg q8h PO		
Ivermectin	*Microfilaricide:* 0.25 mg/kg PO 2 wk after adulticide therapy. *Preventive:* 6 μg/kg once per month PO	None	IX-418, IX-743, X-141, X-266, X-560
Jenotone (aminoproprazine fumarate)	2 mg/kg q12h IM, SC	Same	
Kanamycin (Kantrim)	10 mg/kg q6h PO; 7 mg/kg q6h IM, SC	Same	
Kaopectate	1–2 ml/kg q2–6h	Same	
Ketamine (Vetalar)	None	*Restraint:* 11 mg/kg IM *Anesthesia:* 22–33 mg/kg IM; 2.2–4.4 mg/kg IV	
Ketoconazole	10 mg/kg/day PO with acid food	Same	IX-564, IX-1079, X-82, X-577, X-1027, X-1106
Lactated Ringer's solution	40–50 ml/kg/day IV, SC, IP	Same	
Lactulose	*Constipation:* 1 ml/4.5 kg q8h PO to start, then adjust *Hepatic encephalopathy:* 30–45 ml q8h PO	Same	
Laxatives			IX-907
Laxatone	*Laxative:* 2–4 ml PO 2–3 days/wk	*Laxative:* 1–2 ml PO 2–3 days/wk *Hairballs:* 2–4 ml/day PO for 2–3 days; then 1–2 ml 2–3 days/wk	
Leucovorin	3 mg/m² within 3h of methotrexate administration	None	
Levamisole (L-tetramisole)	*Microfilariae:* 10 mg/kg once daily PO for 6–10 days *Immunostimulant:* 0.5–2 mg/kg 3 times weekly PO	*Lungworms:* 20–40 mg/kg PO every other day for 5 or 6 treatments None	IX-1093, X-576
Levarterenol (norepinephrine)	1–2 ml in 250 ml of drip, IV to effect	None	
Lidocaine (without epinephrine) (Xylocaine)	1–2 mg/kg IV bolus, followed by IV drip, 0.1% soln at 30–50 μg/kg/min	Do *not* use as antiarrhythmic	
Lime sulfur	3% solution, dip once a week for 4–6 wk, let dry on	Same	
Lincomycin	15 mg/kg q8h PO; 10 mg/kg q12h IV, IM	Same	
Liothyronine	4 μg/kg q8h PO	None	
Lomotil	2.5 mg q8h PO	None	
Magnesium hydroxide (milk of magnesia)	*Antacid:* 5–30 ml PO *Cathartic:* 3–5 times the antacid dose	*Antacid:* 5–15 ml PO	
Magnesium sulfate (Epsom salts)	8–25 gm PO	2–4 gm PO	
Mannitol (20% soln)	1.0–2.0 gm/kg q6h IV	Same	
MCT OIL (Mead Johnson, 8.3 kcal/gm) (MCTs, medium-chain triglycerides)	1–2 ml/kg body weight daily in food		IX-888, IX-913

Table continued on following page

Drug Name	Dog	Cat	Additional Information
Measles vaccine	1 vial SC to dogs between 6 and 8 wk of age	None	
Mebendazole (Telmintic)	22 mg/kg with food q24h for 3 days	None	
Meclizine (Bonnie)	25 mg once daily PO	12.5 mg once daily PO	
Megestrol acetate (Ovaban)	*Skin:* 1 mg/kg/day PO	*Skin:* 5 mg/day PO for 1 wk, then twice weekly	
	Behavior: 2–4 mg/kg once daily; reduce to half dose at 8 days for maintenance	*Behavior:* 2–4 mg/kg once daily; reduce to half dose at 8 days for maintenance	
	To postpone estrus: In proestrus: 2 mg/kg PO daily for 8 days In anestrus: 0.5 mg/kg PO daily for 32 days False pregnancy: 2.0 mg/kg PO daily for 8 days	None	
Melatonin	1–2 mg once daily SC for 3 days; repeat monthly as needed	None	
Melphalan (Alkeran)	0.05–0.1 mg/kg PO once daily; 1.5 mg/m² PO once daily for 7–10 days, then no therapy for 2–3 wk	Same	
Meperidine (Demerol)	10 mg/kg IM as needed	3 mg/kg IM as needed	
6-Mercaptopurine (6-MP)	50 mg/m² daily PO or 2 mg/kg daily	None	
Metamucil	2–10 gm q12–24h in wetted or liquid food	2–4 gm q12–24h in wetted or liquid food	
Metaraminol (Aramine)	2–10 mg SC, IM; 10–50 mg/500 ml saline infused IV to effect	None	
Methenamine mandelate (Mandelamine)	10 mg/kg q6h PO to effect	None	
Methicillin	20 mg/kg q6h IV, IM	Same	
Methimazole (Tapazole)		10–15 mg/day, modified as necessary	IX-1028, X-1001
DL-Methionine	0.2–1.0 gm q8h PO	0.2 gm q8h PO	
Methischol	1 capsule/15 kg q8h PO	1 capsule q12h PO	
Methocarbamol	44.4–222.2 mg/kg IV 44.4 mg/kg q8h PO first day, then 22.2–44.4 mg/kg q8h	Same	
Methohexital (Brevital)	11 mg/kg IV (2.5% soln)	Same	
Methotrexate	0.06 mg/kg once daily PO (may vomit); 0.5 mg/kg IV, maximum dose is 25 mg	0.06 mg/kg once daily PO (may vomit); 0.8 mg/kg IV	
Methoxamine	0.2 mg/kg IV	Same	
Methoxyflurane (Metofane)	*Induction:* 3% *Maintenance:* 0.5–1.5%	Same	
Methylprednisolone (Medrol, Depomedrol)	See *Prednisolone* 1.0 mg/kg IM every 2 wk	Same 20 mg/cat IM once	
Methyltestosterone	0.5 mg/kg q24h PO	Same	
Metoclopramide	0.2–0.4 mg/kg q6–8h PO, SC 1.0–2.0 mg/kg/24 hr in IV continuous infusion	Same	IX-865
Metronidazole	25 mg/kg q12h PO for 5 days	Same	
Mibolerone	30 mcg/0.45–11.3 kg, 60 mcg/11.8–22.7 kg, 120 mcg/23–45.3 kg, 180 mcg/45.8 kg and over daily PO German shepherd and German shepherd mix: 180 μg all weights daily PO	None	
Milk of Magnesia. See *Magnesium hydroxide*			
Milrinone	0.5–1.0 mg/kg PO q12h		IX-329
Mineral oil	2–60 ml PO	2–10 ml PO	
Mithramycin	2 μg/kg IV once daily for 2 days	Same	IX-86
Mitotane (*o,p'*-DDD)	50 mg/kg once daily PO to effect (approx. 5–10 days), then once every 2 wk	None	IX-968, X-1024, X-1033
Morphine	1 mg/kg SC, IM as needed	0.1 mg/kg SC, IM as needed	
Nafcillin	10 mg/kg q6h PO, IM	Same	
Nalorphine	1.0 mg/kg IV, IM, SC	None	
Naloxone (Narcan)	0.04 mg/kg IV, IM, SC	None	
Nandrolone decanoate	1.0–1.5 mg/kg/wk IM	1 mg/kg per week IM	X-24
Natamycin	*Nasal flush:* 0.1% soln infused over 15- to 25-min period twice weekly for 2–3 wk		

Drug Name	Dog	Cat	Additional Information
Neo-Darbazine	1 #1 capsule q12h PO (4.5–9 kg) 2 #1 capsules q12h PO (9–13.6 kg) 3 #1 capsules or 1 #3 capsule q12h PO (13.6–27.3 kg) 1 or 2 #3 capsules q12h PO (over 27.3 kg)	None	
Neomycin (Biosol)	20 mg/kg q6h PO; 3.5 mg/kg q8h IV, IM, SC	Same	
Neostigmine (Stiglyn)	1–2 mg IM as needed; 5–15 mg PO as needed	None	
Nifedipine			IX-341
Nikethimide (Coramine)	7.8–31.2 mg/kg IV, IM, SC	Same	
Nitrofurantoin	4 mg/kg q8h PO; 3 mg/kg q12h IM	Same	
Nitroglycerin			IX-332
Nonsteroidal anti-inflammatory drugs			X-47, X-566, X-642, X-1158
Norfloxacin	3–7 mg/kg q12h PO		
Novobiocin	10 mg/kg q8h PO	Same	
Nystatin	100,000 units q6h PO	Same	
Octin (Isometheptene)	0.5–1.0 ml IM; 1 tablet q8–12h PO	0.25–0.5 ml IM; ½–1 tablet q12h PO	
o,p'-DDD See mitotane			
Ophthalmic drugs			IX-684
Orgotein	5 mg once weekly SC	None	
Ouabain	0.02–0.04 mg/kg total dose IV, ¼–½ dose initially, then ¼ dose q30min *Maintenance dose:* ¼ of total dose q3h	None	
Oxacillin	11–22 mg/kg q8h PO	Same	
Oxazepam		2.5 mg b.i.d.	X-23
Oxymetholone	1 mg/kg q8–24h PO	Same	
Oxymorphone (Numorphan)	0.1–0.2 mg/kg SC, IM, IV as needed	Same	
Oxytetracycline	20 mg/kg q8h PO; 7 mg/kg q12h IV, IM	Same	
Oxytocin	5–10 units IM, IV; repeat q15–30 min	0.5–3.0 units IM, IV	X-1300
2-PAM	40 mg/kg IV over 2-min period, q12h as needed (may be given IM or SC)	20 mg/kg	
Pancreatic enzyme replacement (therapy)	2 tsp powdered non–enteric-coated pancreatic extract per 20 kg body weight with each meal		X-930
Pancreatin	2–10 tablets with food	1–2 tablets with food	
Pancuronium	0.1 mg/kg IV	None	
Paregoric	3–5 ml q6h PO	None	
D-Penicillamine (Cuprimine)	10–15 mg/kg q12h	None	IX-148, X-891, X-1191
Penicillin G, benzathine	40,000 U/kg q 5 days IM	Same	
Penicillin G (Na or K)	40,000 U/kg q6h PO (not with food), 20,000 U/kg q4h IV, IM, SC	Same	
Penicillin G, procaine	20,000 U/kg q12–24h IM, SC	Same	
Penicillin V	10 mg/kg q8h PO	Same	
Pentazocine (Talwin)	0.5–1.0 mg/kg IM maximum. **Never IV.** *Sedation:* 2–4 mg/kg IV *Anesthesia:* 30 mg/kg IV to effect	None Same	
Pepto-Bismol	2.2 ml/kg PO	None	
Phenobarbital	*Status epilepticus:* 6 mg/kg q6–24h IM, IV as needed *Less severe conditions:* 2 mg/kg PO twice daily	Same	IX-839
Phenoxybenzamine	0.25–0.5 mg/kg q6–8h PO	Same	
Phenylbutazone (Butazolidin)	22 mg/kg q8h IV; 10–15 mg/kg q 8h PO; total dose not to exceed 0.8 gm/day	None	Use with *great* caution
Phenylephrine (Neo-Synephrine)	0.15 mg/kg IV; 10% soln topically in eye	Same	
Phenylpropanolamine	1.5 mg/kg PO q12h	1.5 mg/kg PO q8–12h	X-1221
Phenytoin (Dilantin)	*Antiepileptic:* 50–80 mg/kg q8h PO *Antiarrhythmic:* 50–100 mg IV over 5-min period, maximum total dose 24 mg/kg, 8–15 mg/kg q8h PO	*Antiepileptic:* 2–3 mg/kg/day; 20 mg/kg/wk *Antiarrhythmic:* None	IX-840

Table continued on following page

Drug Name	Dog	Cat	Additional Information
Phthalylsulfathiazole (Sulfathalidine)	50 mg/kg q6h PO; 100 mg/kg q12h PO	Same	
Phytonadione (vitamin K₁)	5–20 mg q12h IV, IM, SC following IV therapy 5 mg q12h PO for 7 days; *Long-acting anticoagulant poisoning:* 5 mg/kg SC in several sites, followed in 8–12h with 5 mg/kg q8–12h for 2–3 wks PO	1–5 mg q12h IV, IM, SC	
Piperazine	110 mg/kg PO, repeat in 21 days	Same	
Pitressin (ADH)	10 U IV, IM (aqueous) or 0.5–1.0 ml IM every other day (oil)	Same	
Polymyxin B	2 mg/kg q12h IM; *Aerosol:* Nebulize 300,000 units in 2.5 ml saline q8–12h	Same	
Potassium chloride	1–3 gm/day PO IV: maximum 10 mEq/hr and 40 mEq/day/dog	0.2 gm/day PO	IX-105, IX-950, X-814
Praziquantel (Droncit)	½ tablet/2.3 kg and under 1 tablet/2.7–4.5 kg 1½ tablets/5–6.8 kg 2 tablets/7.3–13.6 kg 3 tablets/14–20.5 kg 4 tablets/20.9–27.3 kg 5 tablets/maximum over 27.3 kg	½ tablet/1.8 kg and under 1 tablet/2.3–5.0 kg 1½ tablets/5 kg and over	
Prazosin	1–2 mg q8–12h PO	None	IX-333
Prednisolone (Solu-Delta-Cortel)	*Allergy:* 0.5 mg/kg twice daily PO or IM *Immune suppression:* 2.0 mg/kg twice daily PO or IM *Prolonged use:* 0.5–2.0 mg/kg every other morning *Shock:* 5.5–11 mg/kg IV, then q 1, 3, 6, or 10 h as needed	1.0 mg/kg twice daily PO or IM 3.0 mg/kg twice daily PO or IM 2.0–4.0 mg/kg every other evening PO Same	
Primidone	55 mg/kg PO once daily	None	IX-839
Procainamide (Pronestyl)	10–12 mg/kg q8h PO sustained-release (SR) 10–12 mg/kg q6h PO 11–22 mg/kg IM q3–6h; 100-mg bolus IV, followed by IV drip at 10-40 µg/kg/min	None	
Promazine (Sparine)	2.2–4.4 mg/kg IV, IM	Same	
Promethazine (Phenergan)	0.2–1.0 mg/kg q8–12h PO, SC	None	
Propantheline (Pro-Banthine)	Small: 7.5 mg q8h PO Medium: 15 mg q8h PO Large: 30 mg q8h PO	7.5 mg q8h PO	
Propiopromazine (Tranvet)	1.1–4.4 mg/kg PO once or twice daily	None	
Propranolol (Inderal)	0.2–1.0 mg/kg q8h PO 0.04–0.06 mg/kg IV slowly	Same 0.25 mg diluted in 1 ml saline, 0.2 ml IV boluses to effect	IX-344, IX-378
Propylthiouracil	11 mg/kg q12h PO	Same	IX-1029
Prostaglandin F₂α			IX-1233, IX-1239, X-1107
Pyrantel pamoate	5 mg/kg PO, repeat in 3 wk	10 mg/kg PO, repeat in 3 wk	IX-1233, IX-1239
Pyrethrin			IX-579
Pyridostigmine	2 mg/kg q12h PO		
Pyrimethamine	1 mg/kg q24h PO for 3 days, then 0.5 mg/kg q24h PO	Same	
Quadrinal	¼ to ½ tablet q4–6h PO	¼ tablet q4–6h PO	
Quibron	1–3 capsules q8h PO *Elixir:* 5 ml/15 kg q8h PO	½ capsule q8h PO *Elixir:* 2 ml q8h PO	
Quinacrine (Atabrine)	50–100 mg q12h PO for 3 days, repeat in 3 days	None	
Quinidine gluconate (Quinaglute)	8–20 mg/kg q8–12h PO 8–20 mg/kg IM or slow IV q8h	None	
Quinidine polygalacturonate (Cardioquin)	8–20 mg/kg q8–12h PO	None	
Quinidine sulfate	8–20 mg/kg q6–8h PO	None	
Rabies vaccine (CEO)	1 vial IM (as per state regulations)	Same	
Rabies vaccine (TCO)	1 vial IM (as per state regulations)	Same	
Ranitidine	2.2–4.4 mg/kg q12h PO	None	X-914
Riboflavin	10–20 mg/day PO	5–10 mg/day PO	
Ringer's solution	40–50 ml/kg day IV, IP, SC	Same	

Drug Name	Dog	Cat	Additional Information
Rompum. See *Xylazine*			
Septra	30 mg (combined) kg q24h PO or 15 mg/kg q12h	None	
Sodium bicarbonate	50 mg/kg q8–12h PO (1 tsp powder equals 2 gm)	Same	IX-61, X-333
	1 mEq/kg IV immediately, add 3 mEq/kg to drip	Same	
Sodium chloride (0.9% soln)	40—50 ml/kg/day IV, IP, SC	Same	
Sodium iodine (20% soln)	1 ml/5 kg q8–12h PO, IV	Same	X-1103
Sodium nitroprusside	1–10 μg/mg/min		IX-332
Sodium sulfate (Glauber's salt)	*Purgative:* 10–25 mg PO *Laxative:* 1/5 the purgative dose	*Purgative:* 2–4 gm PO	
Somatostatin			X-1019
Spectinomycin	5.5–11 mg/kg q12h IM; 22 mg/kg q12h PO	None	
Stanozolol (Winstrol-V)	½–2 tablets q12h PO 25–50 mg IM weekly	½ tablet q12h PO 25 mg IM weekly	
Styrid Caricide	1 ml/10 kg once daily PO for heartworm prevention	None	
Sucralfate	½–1 tablet q6–8 PO		X-914
Sulfonamides:			IX-606, X-572
Phthalylsulfathiazole	100 mg/kg q12h PO (not absorbed)	Same	
Sulfadiazine	220 mg/kg initial dose, then 110 mg/kg q12h	Same	
Sulfadimethoxine	25 mg/kg q24h PO, IV, IM	Same	
Sulfamethazine, sulfamerazine, sulfadiazine (Triple sulfa)	50 mg/kg q12h PO, IV	Same	
Sulfasalazine (Azulfidine)	10–15 mg/kg q6h PO	None	
Sulfathalidine	100 mg/kg q12h PO (not absorbed)	Same	
Sulfisoxazole, sulfamethizole	50 mg/kg q8h PO	Same	
Tannic acid (Tannalbin)	1 tablet/5 kg q12h PO; decrease dose for several days after diarrhea is under control	Same	
Tan-Sal (5% tannic acid, 5% salicylic acid, and 70% ethyl alcohol)	Topical, q8h; no more than two treatments	Same	
Taurine		250–500 mg q12h PO	X-251
Temaril-P	1 capsule PO q24h (up to 5 kg) 2 capsules PO q24h (5–10 kg) 4 capsules PO q24h (10–20 kg) 6 capsules PO q24h (over 20 kg)	Same	
Terbutaline	1.25–5 mg q8–12h PO	1.25 mg q8–12h PO	
Testosterone	2 mg/kg once daily q 2–3 days PO up to 30 mg total; 2 mg/kg (up to 30 mg total) IM (repositol) q 10 days	Same	
Tetanus antitoxin	100–500 U/kg, maximum 20,000 U (initial test of 0.1–0.2 ml SC 15–30 min prior to IV dose)	Same	
Tetracycline	20 mg/kg q8h PO; 7 mg/kg q12h IV, IM	Same	
Thenium closylate	500 mg PO for dogs heavier than 4.55 kg; 250 mg twice daily for those 2.27–4.55 kg; repeat in 2–3 wk	None	
Theophylline	9 mg/kg q6–8h PO	4 mg/kg q8–12h PO	IX-281
Thiabendazole	50 mg/kg once daily PO for 3 days; repeat in 1 mo	None	
Thiacetarsamide (Caparsolate)	2.2 mg/kg IV twice daily for 2 days	None	IX-414, IX-424, X-132, X-265
Thiamine	10–100 mg/day PO	5–30 mg/day PO	
Thiamylal (Surital, Bio-Tal)	17.5 mg/kg IV (4% soln)	Same, but use 2% soln	
6-Thioguanine (6-TG)	1 mg/kg/day PO	Same	
ThioTEPA	0.2–0.5 mg/m² as single dose separated weekly, IV or intracavitary; 0.2–0.5 mg/kg daily × 5 or 10 days IV, repeat q3 weeks; 9 mg/m² as single dose or in 2–4 divided doses or successive days IV or intracavitary	Same	

Table continued on following page

Drug Name	Dog	Cat	Additional Information
Thyroid (desiccated)	10 mg/kg/day PO	Same	
L-Thyroxine	22 μg/kg q12h PO	0.05–0.1 mg PO once daily	IX-1021, X-283, X-602, X-992, X-1000
Timolol	1 drop in the eye q12–24h		
Toluene (methylbenzene)	200 mg/kg PO	Same	
Tranquilizers			X-63
Tresaderm	Topically, q12h; maximum duration of treatment 7 days	Same *for ear mites – 7 days, stop for a wk, 7 days again*	
Triamcinolone (Vetalog)	0.25–2 mg once daily PO for 7 days; 0.11–0.22 mg/kg IM, SC 0.11–0.22 mg/kg IM, SC	0.25–0.5 mg once daily PO for 7 days	
Trichlorfon (Neguvon)	3% solution to whole body q 3 days	None	
L-Triiodothyronine			IX-1023, X-602, X-994
Trimethobenzamide (Tigan)	3 mg/kg q8h IM	None	
Trimethoprim and sulfadiazine (Tribrissen)	15 mg (combined) kg q12h, or 30 mg (combined)/kg q24h PO, SC	None	
Tripelennamine	1.0 mg/kg q12h PO; 1 ml/20 kg IM	Same	
Trisulfapyrimidine	50 mg/kg q12h PO	None	
TSH (thyroid-stimulating hormone)	1 unit IV (response test); post sample in 4 h	5 units SC	
Tylosin	10 mg/kg q8h PO; 5 mg/kg q12h IV, IM	Same	
Valproic acid			IX-841
Vasodilator drugs			IX-329, X-1203
Vasopressin tannate	1–5 units SC or IM q24 to 72h	1–2 units SC or IM q24 to 72h	X-975
Verapamil	0.1–0.3 mg/kg IV slowly, not to exceed 5 mg total dose 1–3 mg/kg q6–8h PO	None	IX-341
Vermiplex	*Single-dose method:* 1 #000 capsule/0.23 kg 1 #00 capsule/0.57 kg 1 #0 capsule/1.14 kg 1 #1 capsule/2.27 kg 1 #2 capsule/4.55 kg 1 #3 capsule/9.1 kg 1 #4 capsule/18.2 kg Can be repeated in 2–4 wk *Divided-dose method:* Divide body weight by 5 and administer appropriate size capsule once daily for 5 days; can be repeated in 2–4 wk	Same	
Vinblastine (Velban)	2 mg/m² weekly or biweekly IV; 0.05–0.1 mg/kg q7–10 days IV	Same	
Vincristine (Oncovin)	0.7 mg/m² weekly IV; 0.025 mg/kg weekly IV	Same	
Viokase	Mix into food 20 min prior to feeding; 1–3 tsp/lb of food	Same	
Vi-Sorbin	1–3 tsp/day PO	½ tsp/day PO	
Vitamins			IX-40
Vitamin A (Retinoids)	400 units/kg/day PO for 10 days	Same	IX-593, X-553, X-791
Vitamin B complex	0.5–2.0 ml q24h IV, IM, SC	0.5–1.0 ml q24h IV, IM, SC	
Vitamin B₁₂	100–200 μg/day	50–100 μg/day	
Vitamin D	30 units/kg/day PO for 10 days	Same	
Vitamin E	500 mg/day PO	100 mg/day PO	IX-595, X-574
Vitamin K₁			IX-162
Xylazine (Rompun)	1.1 mg/kg IV; 1.1–2.2 mg/kg IM, SC	Same	

Compiled by Richard Johnson, Reg. Ph.

INDEX

Note: Page numbers in *italics* refer to illustrations; page numbers followed by the letter t refer to tables. Page numbers following roman numerals VIII and IX refer to pages in earlier editions.

Abdominocentesis, in llama, 736
Abiotrophy, cerebellar, 840
Abortifacients, VIII:945
Abortion, in feline leukemia virus infection, 1073
Abscess, of orbit, 639
of prostate, *1231*, 1233–1235, 1233t, *1236*
periapical, 954–955. See also *Root canal.*
Acantholytic cells, 617
Acanthomatous epulis, 504
Acanthosis nigricans, 632, 632t
Acepromazine, in chemical restraint, butorphanol with, 63, 68
morphine with, 68
oxymorphone with, 68
in pregnancy, 1294t
Acepromazine maleate, in aortic thromboembolism, in cats, 297–298
Acetaminophen, IX:188
antidote for, 121t, 883
hepatic toxicity due to, 881–882
in pregnancy, 1294t
pharmacology of, 51
poisoning due to, 108
Acetazolamide, approximate doses of, 1370
in glaucoma, 649
in hydrocephalus, 846
Acetylcysteine, approximate doses of, 1370
Acetylpromazine, approximate doses of, 1370
Acetylsalicylic acid. See *Aspirin.*
Achlorhydria, in intestinal bacterial overgrowth, 933
Acid, corrosive, antidote for, 120t
Acid ingestion toxicosis, 169–170
Acid milk syndrome, 1332
Acid-base balance, in poisoning, 124–125
in shock, 327
in uremia, 1137–1138
Acidosis, in chronic renal failure, 1195
metabolic, diagnosis and treatment of, IX:59
in acute toxicant-induced renal failure, 129
in poisoning, 124

Acidosis *(Continued)*
respiratory, diagnosis and treatment of, IX:59
Acoustic reflex, 807–809, *808*
Acquired immunodeficiency syndrome, feline, IX:436
Acromegaly, diabetes mellitus and, IX:1006
in cats, 981–984
clinical features of, 981–982, 982t
diagnosis in, 983
etiology of, 981
prognosis in, 984
screening laboratory tests in, 983
treatment in, 983–984
insulin resistance in, 1015–1016
Acromelanism, 632
ACTH, approximate doses of, 1370
endogenous, in cats, 1040
measurement of, 964
ACTH stimulation test, 961–962
dexamethasone suppression test and, in cats, 1040
in dogs, 963–964
in cats, 1039–1040
in hypoadrenocorticism, in cats, 1044
Actinic lesions, of nose and footpads, 620
Actinomyces, antimicrobial agents for, 1363
Actinomycin, approximate dose of, 1370
Actinomycosis, VIII:1184
Activated clotting time, 440
Acupuncture, IX:36
Acute phase proteins, 468–471
characteristics of, 468, 469t
conditions associated with increased, 469, 470t
in veterinary medicine, 470–471
synthesis of, 468–469, 469–470, *470*
Acute phase reactants, negative, 468
Addison's disease. See *Hypoadrenocorticism.*
Adenitis, sebaceous, 558
Adenocarcinoma, of anal sac, 989
of colon, 940
Adenoma, pituitary, in hyperparathyroidism, 986
Adenopathy, hilar, 193
Adnexal tumors, IX:679, 692–695

Adrenal feminization or masculinization, alopecia in, 599–600
Adrenal suppression, in glucocorticoid therapy, 55
Adrenalectomy, in hyperadrenocorticism, 1029–1030
Adrenocortical neoplasia, diagnosis of, 1035
hyperadrenocorticism due to, 1024–1025
in cats, 1041
o,p'-DDD therapy in, 1034–1037
initial therapy in, 1036
maintenance therapy in, 1036
prognosis in, 1037
side effects in, 1036–1037
Adrenocorticotropic hormone. See *ACTH.*
Aeromonas hydrophila, in fish, 718
Afghans, chylothorax in, 393
Afterload, ventricular, drug therapy effects on, 309, *309*
in dilated cardiomyopathy, 244–245, 245t
Agar dilution, for anaerobes, 72
Aguirre syndrome, 630
Air space disease, 193
Airway, in cardiopulmonary resuscitation, 330–331
in pulmonary edema, 389
in tracheal collapse, 354
obstruction, evaluation of, 196
small, obstruction of, 197–198
Albinism, melanin disorder in, 628
ocular dysgenesis in, 664–665
Albuterol toxicosis, 109
Aldactone, approximate doses of, 1370
Aldicarb toxicosis, 103
Aleutian disease, of ferret, 774
Algorithms, clinical, IX:26
Alkali, caustic, antidote for, 120t
Alkali ingestion toxicosis, 170
Alkaline phosphatase activity, in blood and bone marrow cells, 465, 466t
in leukemia, 466, 467t
Alkaloids, antidote for, 120t
Alkalosis, metabolic, in poisoning, 124–125
treatment of, IX:59

Alkylamine, in pruritus, 567t
Alkylating agents, 472–473, 473t
Allergen test, intradermal, 542
Allergic alveolitis, extrinsic, 375–376, 375t
Allergic conjunctivitis, 675
Allergic dermatitis, of pinnae, 624
Allergic drug reactions, IX:444
Allergic pruritus, fatty acid supplements in, 564
Allergy. See also *Hypersensitivity reactions.*
  drug, 542, 542t
  in cats, 583–585
  periocular pruritus in, 679
Allethrin toxicosis, 104
Allopurinol, approximate doses of, 1370
Alopecia, estrogen-responsive, 605
  flank, in intact female dogs, 597
    seasonal, 600
  growth hormone deficiency and, IX:1015
  in adrenal feminization or masculinization, 599–600
  in growth-hormone responsive dermatosis, 978–980, 980t
  in intact female dogs, 597
  in male feminizing syndrome, 599
  in neutered female dogs, 596–597
  in neutered male dogs, 597–598
  in testicular neoplasia, 598
  of pinnae, 623
  periocular, 680
  symmetric, in cats, IX:545
    thyroid hormones in, 603
Alpha-adrenergic agents, uterine effects of, 1301
Alpha-adrenergic agonists, in cardiopulmonary resuscitation, 332, 332t
Aluminum hydroxide, as antacid, 912, 913t
  in chronic advanced renal failure, 1197
Alveolar membrane permeability, in pulmonary edema, 391–392
Alveolitis, extrinsic allergic, 375–376, 375t
Alveolocapillary membrane, in pulmonary edema, 386
Amelanosis, 628–630
  genetic, 628–630
  pathogenesis of, 629t
Amforol, approximate doses of, 1370
Amikacin, approximate doses of, 1370
  in pregnancy, 1293t
Amino acids, food intake effects of, 19
  in parenteral nutrition, 26–27
Aminocaproic acid, in degenerative myelopathy, 832–833
Aminophylline, approximate doses of, 1370
  in bronchitic pulmonary eosinophilia, 373
4-Aminopyridine toxicity, 101
Amiodarone, adverse effects of, 313t
Amitraz, approximate doses of, 1370
  in pregnancy, 1293t
  toxicity of, 110
Amitriptyline, in pruritus, 567
Ammonia tolerance testing, in hepatic disease, 874

Ammonium chloride, approximate doses of, 1370
  in pregnancy, 1296t
Ammonium urate crystaluria, 1129
Amoxicillin, approximate doses of, 1370
  in pregnancy, 1293t
Amoxicillin/calvulanic acid, 79–80, 80t
Amphetamine, approximate doses of, 1370
Amphibians, 697
Amphotericin B, approximate doses of, 1370
  in pregnancy, 1293t
  ketoconazole and, 83
  nephrotoxicity of, IX:1142
  systemic, 1101–1102, 1102t
Ampicillin, approximate doses of, 1370
  in pregnancy, 1293t
  in urinary tract infection, 1206t
Amprolium, approximate doses of, 1370
Amrinone, adverse effects of, 313t
  approximate doses of, 1370
  in dilated cardiomyopathy, 247, 249t
Amyloidosis, renal, in cats, 1173
  medical management of, 1176–1177
  natural history of, 1174–1175
Amyloodinium, of fish, 713, 716
Anaerobic infection, 1082–1085
  antimicrobial susceptibility testing in, 72–73, 1084t
  bacteriology in, 1082
  clinical features of, 1082–1083, 1083t
  diagnosis of, 1083
  pathogenesis of, 1082
  treatment of, 1083–1084, 1084t
    antimicrobial, 1083–1084, 1084t
    surgical, 1083
Anal sac, apocrine cell adenocarcinoma of, 989
Analysis of variance (ANOVA), 14t
Anaphylactoid reactions, 539–540, 539t
Anaphylaxis, 538–539, 539t
Ancylostoma caninum, in neonate, 1332–1333
Ancylostoma tubaeforme, in neonate, 1333
Androgen, effects of, on male dog fertility, 1224
  endogenous exposure to, 1266
  exogenous exposure to, 1266
Androgen resistance, 1267–1268
Androgen-dependent masculinization, defects of, 1267–1268
Androgens, cyclic levels of, 1275
  in dermatology, 605–606
Anemia, aplastic, in feline leukemia virus infection, 1072–1073
  crystalloid fluid therapy and, 325
  hemolytic, in feline leukemia virus infection, 1072–1073
    in hypophosphatemia, 44–45, 45t
    nonspherocytic, 433, 435
  in cats, 425–429
    aplastic, 427–428
    bone marrow biopsy in, 428
    classification of, 425–428
    clinical signs of, 425
    laboratory tests in, 425
    nonregenerative, 427–428
    regenerative, 426–427
    reticulocyte count in, 425–426

Anemia *(Continued)*
  in cats, transfusion in, 428
    treatment of, 428–429
  in hereditary erythrocyte disorders, 431
  in myxedema, 999
  in uremia, 1136, 1138
Anesthesia, emergency, aspiration pneumonia prevention in, 382
  hepatic toxicity due to, 881
  in birds, 776–779
    anesthetic protocol in, 776–777
    inhalation agents in, 777–779
    injectable agents in, 777, 777t
    monitoring in, 779
    preanesthetic considerations in, 776
    recovery in, 779
  in bronchoscopy, 221
  in cesarean section, 1322–1325
    dosages for, 1322t
    general techniques for, 1323–1324
      induction drugs for, 1323–1324
      maintenance in, 1324
      preanesthetic medications in, 1323
    monitoring and support in, 1324–1325
    newborn care after, 1325
    regional techniques for, 1322–1323
  in ferret, 771, 771t
  in fish, 707
  in hyperthyroidism, 1005–1006
  in laboratory animals, 761, 765t
  in llama, 735
  in nondomestic carnivores, 733
  in pregnancy, 1298
  inhalation, uterine effects of, 1301–1302
  reflux esophagitis due to, 908
Anestrus, termination of, 1274
Angiitis, in pulmonary eosinophilia, 374–375
Angioedema, 540
Animals, wild, immunization of, against common diseases, 1361–1362
Anion gap, diagnostic and therapeutic applications of, IX:52
Anisocoria, 688–690
  afferent lesions in, 689
  causes of, 689–690
  differentiating features of, 690t
  efferent lesions in, 689
  pupillary light reflex in, 689
  treatment of, 690
Anorexia, 18–24. See also *Appetite.*
  immunodeficiency in, 18
  in cats, detrimental effects of, 18–19
  in uremia, 1134
  interleukin-1 in, 20
  tryptophan in, 21
Ant sting, 184–185
Antacids, in gastrointestinal ulcer, 912–913, 913t
  in pregnancy, 1295t
  in reflux esophagitis, 909
Anterior cleavage syndrome, 665
Antiarrhythmic drugs, IX:346
  adverse effects of, 313t
Antibiotics. See *Antimicrobials;* individual drugs.

Anticholinergic drugs, adverse effects of, 313t
in gastrointestinal ulcer, 916–917
toxicities of, 314
Anticoagulant therapy, effect of, on blood samples for endocrinology, 969
for laboratory samples, 412t
in aortic thromboembolism, in cats, 300–301
rodenticide, 143–146. See also *Rodenticides.*
Anticoagulation studies, blood samples for, 415
Anticonvulsant therapy, IX:836
in pregnancy, 1298
Antidepressants, tricyclic, in pruritus, 567
Antidiuretic hormone, in diabetes insipidus, 975–976
in fluid balance, 37
physiology of, 973
Antiemetics, in pregnancy, 1295t
Anti-FOCMA antibody, FeLV vaccination and, 1053–1054, 1057–1058
Antifreeze poisoning, IX:206
Antifungal chemotherapy, in dermatology, IX:560
systemic, 1101–1105
amphotericin B in, 1101–1102
combination, 1104
flucytosine in, 1103–1104
guidelines for, 1105
imidazole in, 1102–1103
iodides in, 1104
monitoring, 1104–1105
Antigens, as soft tissue markers, 411t, 412
in hypersensitivity reactions, 541–542
Anti-GP70 antibody, FeLV vaccination and, 1053, 1054
Antihistamines, in pruritus, 566–567
Anti-idiotype vaccines, 512
Anti-insulin antibodies, 1018
Antimicrobial sensitivity tests, of calvulanate-potentiated antibiotics, 80t
Antimicrobial susceptibility tests, 70–74
dilution tests as, 70–71
disk diffusion assay as, 71–72
in urinary tract infection, 1206–1207
interpretation of, 73–74
of anaerobes, 72–73, 1084t
agar dilution in, 72
broth dilution in, 72
disk elution in, 72
of enteric bacteria, 1096–1098
quality control of, 73
types of, 70–72
Antimicrobials. See also individual drugs.
bacterial resistance to, IX:1084
beta-lactam, bacterial resistance to, 78
calvulanate-potentiated, 78–81
for specific microorganisms, 1363–1364
in birds, IX:733
in chemotherapy-induced myelosuppression, 496
in dermatology, IX:566
in pregnancy, 1297
minimal bactericidal concentration (MBC) of, 70–72

Antimicrobials *(Continued)*
minimal inhibitory concentration (MIC) of, 70–72
principles of, VIII:41
prophylactic, in surgery, IX:24
Antineoplastic drugs, 472–475. See also *Chemotherapy.*
Antinuclear antibodies, methimazole-induced, 1004
Antiplatelet antibody, in thrombocytopenia, 441
Antiplatelet therapy, in aortic thromboembolism, in cats, 300
nonsteroidal anti-inflammatory drugs in, 51–52
Antiseborrheic agents, in dermatology, IX:596
Antiseptic toxicosis, 166–169
Antiseptics, phenolic, 162t
Antishock trousers, in cardiopulmonary resuscitation, 332–333
Antithrombin-III, in disseminated intravascular coagulation, 452–453, 455–456
Antithyroid hormone antibody, in hypothyroidism, 997
Antitussive drugs, toxicities of, 314–315
Antral pyloric hypertrophy syndrome, 918–921
clinical presentation in, 919–920
diagnosis of, 920–921
barium studies in, 920
histologic, 920–921
etiopathogenesis of, 919
prognosis in, 921
treatment of, 921
Anus, disease of, IX:916
Aortic stenosis, echocardiography in, 204, 208, *208–209*
Aortic thromboembolism, in cats, 295–302
clinical presentation in, 295–296
collateral vascularization failure in, 295, *296*
due to cardiomyopathy, 295, *295–296*
medical therapy in, 297–298
predisposing factors in, 300
prognosis in, 297
prophylaxis in, 299–301
anticoagulant therapy in, 300–301
antiplatelet therapy: aspirin in, 300
surgical therapy in, 297
thrombolytic therapy in, *298,* 298–299
Apocrine cell adenocarcinoma, of anal sac, 989
Apomorphine, 117
approximate doses of, 1370
Appetite, 18–24. See also *Anorexia.*
central nervous system loci in control of, 21, 21t
neural pathways and substances in control of, 19t, 20–21
regulation of, 19–21, *20*
stimulation of, 21–23
chemical, 23–24
in cats, 21–22
in dogs, 22–23
APUD cells, 1020

Aquarium, equipment for, 703–704
water quality in, 704–706
Arachidonic acid metabolism, *48,* 48–49, 49t, *1158,* 1158–1159
glucocorticoid therapy effects on, 57
pharmacologic manipulation of, 1159
Argulus, in fish, *713,* 716
Arrhythmia, atrial, 271–278. See also *Atrial tachyarrhythmia.*
drug therapy in, IX:346
in bronchoscopy, 221
in congenital heart disease, 229–230
in shock, 326
ventricular, 278–286. See also *Ventricular arrhythmia.*
Arsenic poisoning, 104–105, 159–161
antidote for, 120t, 121t
clinical signs of, 159–160
diagnosis of, 160
prognosis and treatment of, 160–161
source of, 159
Arterial blood gas analysis, in chronic bronchitis, 365
in pulmonary edema, 390
in respiratory emergencies, 200
Arterial catheterization, in shock, 321–322
Arterial O_2 content (CaO_2), 321t
Arterial pulse, in diagnosis of congenital heart disease, 227–228
physical examination of, 190
Arterial-venous O_2 content difference (Ca-v_{O_2}), 321t
Arthritis, enteropathic, 549
fatty acid supplements in, 564–565
hepatopathic, 549
immune-mediated nonerosive, 543–551
blood chemistry and urinalysis in, 546
causes of, 543, 544t
clinical features in, 544
clinicopathologic findings in, 546–548
diagnosis of, 548–549
differential diagnosis of, 545–546
hemogram in, 546
history and physical examination in, 543–544
microbiologic findings in, 548
radiographic findings in, 548
serologic findings in, 547–548
synovial fluid analysis in, 546–547
treatment of, 549–551
in Lyme borreliosis, 1086
infectious, differential diagnosis of, 545
Arthropathy, acromegalic, 982
classification of, 544t
Arytenoid cartilage, anatomy of, 344, *344*
Ascites, in tricuspid regurgitation, 237
Ascorbic acid, approximate doses of, 1371
Asparaginase, 474
for cancer therapy, 1369
in lymphoma, 485–486, 485t
L-Asparaginase, approximate doses of, 1371
preparation and administration of, 478t
Aspartame, in pregnancy, 1296t

Aspergillosis, in birds, VIII:611
  of nasal cavity, 1106–1109
    clinical management of, 1107–1109
      surgery in, 1107
      systemic therapy in, 1107
      topical therapy in, 1107–1109, 1108
    clinical signs of, 1106–1107
    diagnosis of, 1107
    etiology of, 1106
    in cats, 1109
    ketoconazole in, 83
  rhinosinusitis in, 338
Aspergillus, antimicrobial agents for, 1363
Aspiration pneumonia, 379–382
Aspirin, IX:188
  approximate doses of, 1370
  in aortic thromboembolism, in cats, 300
  in chemotherapy-induced myelo-suppression, 497
  in disseminated intravascular coagulation, 457
  in heartworm disease in dogs, 265
  in hypertrophic cardiomyopathy in cats, 253
  in ophthalmology, 643t–644t
  in pregnancy, 1294t
  in pruritus, 567–568
  in uveitis, 655
  pharmacology of, 50
  platelet effects of, 464
  toxicosis of, 108
Asthma, in cats, small airway obstruction in, 197–198
Atenolol, in atrial tachyarrhythmia, 276
  in dilated cardiomyopathy, 246, 249t
  in ventricular tachyarrhythmias, 284t
Atopy, fatty acid supplements in, 563–564
  in cats, 583–584
  periocular pruritus in, 679
  RAST and ELISA testing in, 592–595
Atria, normal activation of, 271
Atrial arrhythmias, in congenital heart disease, 229–230
Atrial contraction, premature, 271, 272
  drug therapy in, 276
Atrial fibrillation, 271, 272–273, 273–274
  drug therapy in, 277
Atrial flutter, 272
Atrial pacemaker, wandering, 271
Atrial rupture, left, in mitral regurgitation, 233
Atrial septal defect, breed and sex predilections for, 225t
  Doppler echocardiographic features of, 230t
  murmur in, 225, 227
  surgical correction of, 230
Atrial standstill, 288–289
Atrial tachyarrhythmia, 271–278
  clinical assessment of, 271–275
  clinical causes of, 275–276
  differential diagnosis of, 275
  drugs and methods for treatment of, 276–278
  recurrent or sustained, 276–277
  types of, 271–273, 272–273
  vagal maneuvers and, 275
  ventricular response to, 273, 273–275

Atrial tachyarrhythmia (Continued)
  with congestive heart failure, 277
  without congestive heart failure, 277
Atrial tachycardia, 271–272, 273
Atrioventricular block, 287–288
Atrioventricular conduction, in atrial tachyarrhythmia, 273, 273–275
Atrioventricular insufficiency, echocardiography in, 201–208, 202–209
  in cats, 212
Atropine, adverse effects of, 313t
  antidote for, 121t
  approximate doses of, 1371
  in cardiopulmonary resuscitation, 333
  in cesarean section, 1322t
  in pregnancy, 1294t–1295t
  in uveitis, 655
Attributable risk, 14t
Audiometry, electroencephalographic, 810–811
  impedance, 807–809, 808
Auditory evoked response, 809–810
  cochlear microphonics in, 810, 811
  early latency components of, 809–810, 809–810
  middle latency components of, 810, 811
Auranofin, in dermatology, 574
Aurothioglucose, approximate doses of, 1371
  in dermatology, 573–574
Aurothiomalate, in dermatology, 573–574
Auscultation, in chronic bronchitis, 362–364
  in congenital heart disease, 225–227, 226
  in dilated cardiomyopathy, 242–243
  in mitral and tricuspid regurgitation, 234
  of chest, 190
  of heart, 190
Autoimmune dermatosis, periocular lesions in, 680
Autoimmune disorders, laboratory detection of, 418–419, 418t
Avicides, 101
Axonopathy, progressive, in boxers, 825, 828–829
Azathioprine, approximate doses of, 1371
  in dermatology, 571–572
  in lymphocytic-plasmacytic enteritis, 925
  in pregnancy, 1294t
  in pruritus, 568–569
  in uveitis, 655
Azotemia, 1123–1124
  definition of, 1134
  in acute toxicant–induced renal failure, 127
AZT, in feline leukemia virus infection, 1071

B cells, glucocorticoid therapy effects on, 56–57
Babesiosis, IX:1096, 419–420
Bacille Calmette-Guérin, 508
  preparation and administration of, 478t
Bacillus anthracis, antimicrobial agents for, 1363

Baclofen, in urinary incontinence, 1218
Bacteremia, 1077–1081
  blood culture in, 1079, 1080t
  continuous, 1079
  diagnosis of, 1079
  etiology of, 1078
  from urinary tract, IX:1150
  intermittent, 1079
  pathogenesis of, 1078–1079
  Pseudomonas, 1081
  Staphylococcus intermedius, 1081
  therapy in, 1079–1080, 1080t
  transient, 1079
Bacteria. See also individual types.
  disinfectants and, 92
Bacterial infection, diagnosis of, VIII:1148
Bacterial infertility, IX:1240
Bacterial overgrowth, intestinal, 933–938. See also Intestinal bacterial overgrowth.
Bacterial resistance, to antimicrobials, IX:1084
Bacteroides, antimicrobial agents for, 1363
BAL, approximate doses of, 1371
  in arsenic poisoning, 160–161
Barbiturates, antidote for, 121t
  in chemical restraint, of cats, 69
    of dogs, 64–65
  in dogs, 68
Barium salts, antidote for, 120t
Basal energy requirement, 34–35, 35t
Basenji, Fanconi's syndrome in, 1164
  juvenile renal disease in, 1168
  pyruvate kinase deficiency in, 434, 435
Bee sting, 184–185
Behavior control, progestins and, VIII:62
Behavior problems, prevention of, VIII:52
  therapy for, VIII:58
Belladonna alkaloids, antidote for, 121t
Bendiocarb toxicosis, 103
Bentiromide absorption test, 929, 929–930
Benzocaine toxicity, 110
Benzodiazepines, in chemical restraint, 63–64
  toxicity of, 108
Bernese mountain dog, hypomyelination in, 836–837
Beta-adrenergic agents, uterine effects of, 1301
Beta-adrenergic agonists, toxicities of, 312
Beta-adrenergic blockers, drug interactions with, 311t
  in dogs and cats, IX:343
  in hypertension in renal failure, 1203
Beta-cell tumors, somatostatin analogue treatment of, 1021–1022, 1023t
Beta-lactam antibiotics, bacterial resistance to, 78
Beta-lactamases, 78, 79
Betamethasone, approximate doses of, 1371
  effects on male dog fertility of, 1225
  in pregnancy, 1296t
Betaxolol, in glaucoma, 650
Bethanechol, approximate doses of, 1371
  in urinary incontinence, 1220t
Bias, in clinical studies, 10

Bicarbonate, in maintenance fluid therapy, 42
Biguanide disinfectant, 92
Bile acids, enterohepatic circulation of, 875, 876
  metabolism of, 875–878
  postprandial values of, 876
  serum, determinants of concentration of, 876–877
    disease applications of, 877, 877–878
    in hepatobiliary function testing, 875
    normal vs abnormal, 877
    technique for measurement of, 876
Bile salts, in reflux esophagitis, 907–908
Bile sludge, in cholelithiasis, 885
Bilirubin crystaluria, 1129
Biliverdin, in vulvar discharge, 1311
Biologic response modifiers, 507–513
  bacterial agents as, 508–509
  bone marrow transplantation as, 512–513
  chemical agents as, 509–510
  cytokines and lymphokines as, 511
  interferons as, 510
  mechanism of action of, 508
  monoclonal antibodies as, 512
  thymosins as, 510–511
  types of, 508t
Biopsy, bone marrow, in anemia, 428
  bronchoscopic, 223
  endomyocardial, in dilated cardiomyopathy, 244
  for fish, 707–708
  in cryptococcosis, 1110–1111
  in gastritis, 867
  liver, VIII:813
  muscle, in dermatomyositis, 608
  prostate, ultrasonography in, 1237–1238
Birds, anesthesia in, 776–779
  antibiotic therapy in, IX:733
  aspergillosis in, VIII:611
  bacterial infections in, VIII:637
  cytology in diagnostics for, IX:725
  egg-bound, IX:746
  endocrinology of, IX:702
  feather-picking in, VIII:646
  fractures in, VIII:630
  giardiasis in, IX:723
  gout in, VIII:635
  imaging for, 786–789
    chemical restraint for, 786–787
    film-screen combinations for, 787
    magnetic resonance imaging for, 789
    mechanical restraint for, 787
    radiography in, 787–788, 787–788
    ultrasonography for, 788
  ivermectin in, IX:743
  microbiologic techniques for, 780–786
    direct examination in, 783
    fungi and yeast in, 783
    gram-negative bacteria in, 782–783
    gram-positive bacteria in, 782
    importance of, 780
    in-house vs professional lab in, 781–782
    interpretation of, 784–785
    normal intestinal microflora in, 783–784
    processing sample in, 782–783
    reporting in, 783

Birds (Continued)
  microbiologic techniques for, sample collection in, 780–781
    environmental, 781
    gastrointestinal, 780
    respiratory, 780–781
    therapy and, 785–786
  oil-contaminated, rehabilitation of, IX:719
  ophthalmology for, IX:616
  oropharyngeal diseases of, IX:699
  orphaned, care and feeding of, IX:775
  parasites of, VIII:641
  poison control center calls about, 100t–101t
  poisonings in, 113
    plant, IX:737
  pox in, VIII:633
  psittacine, lead poisoning in, IX:713
    viral disease of, IX:705
  psittacosis due to, 698–699
  raptorial, bumblefoot in, VIII:614
  salmonellosis in, VIII:637
  scaly face in, VIII:626
  toxic chemicals and, VIII:606
  toxicants of, IX:165
  trichomoniasis in, VIII:619
Bismuth, approximate doses of, 1371
Bismuth salts, antidote for, 120t
Bitch, fertility examination in, VIII:909
  intact, alopecia in, 597
  neutered, alopecia in, 596–597
  pseudohermaphroditism in, 1266
Bite, centipede, 185
  gila monster, 181–182
  snake, 123t, 177–181. See also Snake bite.
  spider, 182–183
  tick, 185
  types of, 951–952, 952–953
  wry, 952–953, 953
  wounds, respiratory emergencies due to, 199
Blastomycosis, antimicrobial agents for, 1363
  ketoconazole in, 82
  of nose and footpads, 618
Bleach toxicosis, 165–166
Bleeding, in disseminated intravascular coagulation, 452
  renal, benign, 1120
Bleeding disorders, 436–441
  acute, increasing degrees of, 319t
  age of onset of, 437
  anemia due to, 426
  breeds with, 438
  clinical assessment in, 437–439
  drug and vaccination history and, 437
  family history of, 438
  genetics of, 438
  intracranial, traumatic, 847
  laboratory assessment of, 439–441
    sample handling in, 439
    screening tests in, 439–441
    specific tests for, 441
  mucosal, tracheobronchial, 222
  nonsteroidal anti-inflammatory drug toxicity in, 53
  patient history in, 437–438
  physical examination in, 438–439
  trauma and, 437

Bleeding time, 440
  buccal mucosal, 447–448, 448
Bleomycin, approximate doses of, 1371
  doxorubicin, cyclophosphamide protocol, for soft tissue tumors, 492
  for cancer therapy, 1368
Bleomycin sulfate, preparation and administration of, 477t
Blepharoconjunctivitis, in rabbits, 682
Blindness, diagnosis of, 690–691
  sudden, 639, 644–647
Blood, parasites of, 419–424
  volume expansion of, 324–325, 326t
Blood cells, cytochemistry of, 465–466, 466t
Blood chemistry, in dogs and cats, 1340–1342
  in ferret, 766t
  in laboratory animals, 743t–744t
  in mitral and tricuspid regurgitation, 234–235
Blood culture, in bacteremia, 1079, 1080t
Blood disease, immune-mediated, IX:498
Blood film examination, 439–440
Blood flow, in cardiopulmonary resuscitation, 332
Blood gas analysis, arterial, in chronic bronchitis, 365
  in pulmonary edema, 390
  in respiratory emergencies, 200
Blood ocular barrier, 652
Blood pressure, in shock, 325–326
Blood samples, for anticoagulation studies, 415
  for endocrinology testing, 968–970
    anticoagulants, hemolysis, lipemia and, 968–969, 970
    fasting, reproductive state, stress, pulsatile secretion and, 969–970
  for fish, 708–709
Blood smear, in disseminated intravascular coagulation, 454
  stains for, 413t, 415
Blood substitute therapy, IX:107
Blood transfusion, VIII:408
  granulocyte, in chemotheapy-induced myelosuppression, 497
  in anemia, 428
  reactions to, in cats, IX:515
Blood typing, in cats, 428
Blood urea nitrogen (BUN), in azotemia, 1123–1124, 1123t
  in renal failure, 1195
  in total parenteral nutrition, 29
Blood values, for dogs and cats, 1335–1337
Blown coat, in intact female dogs, 597
Body odor, of ferret, 772
Body surface area, in chemotherapy calculations, 485
  to weight conversion table, 1365
Bone, in radiation therapy complications, 506–507
  infection of, anaerobic, 1083
Bone marrow, biopsy of, in anemia, 428
  cellular development in, 494–495
  chemotherapy effects on, 495–497
  cytochemistry of, 465–466, 466t
  hypoplasia of, estrous, in ferret, 769–770

Bone marrow *(Continued)*
  normal, in dogs and cats, 1338
  toxicity, estrogen-induced, IX:495
Bone marrow transplantation, 512–513, 515–521
  chemotherapy for recipient in, 520
  diseases treatable with, *516*
  donor selection in, 518–519
  graft-vs-host disease and, 520–521
  hematologic changes after, *518*
  hematologic engraftment and, 520
  high-dose radiotherapy for recipient in, 519–520
  in malignant disease, 517
  in nonmalignant disease, 517
  methodology for, 517–518, *518*
  recipient preparation in, 519–520, 519t
  types of, 517
Borate, toxicosis of, 168
  trade names of products with, 163t
Bordetella bronchiseptica, antimicrobial agents for, 1363
  infection with, 367–368
Boric acid toxicosis, 105, 168
Borreliosis, Lyme, 1086–1087
Botulin, antidote for, 123t
Bouvier de Flandres, laryngeal paralysis in, 346
Boxer, cardiomyopathy in, 241
  progressive axonopathy in, 825, 828–829
Brachygnathia, 951, *952*
Bradycardia, 286–289. See also *Cardiac pacemakers.*
  causes of, 286–289
  electrocardiography in, *287*
  in myxedema, 998
  medical treatment of, 289
  sinus, 286–287
Brain trauma, 847
  glucocorticoid therapy for, 60
Brain stem auditory evoked response, 809–810, *809–810*
Brain stem reflexes, in trauma, 849–850
Brain tumors, in dogs and cats, IX:820
  radiation therapy for, 504
Breathing. See also *Respiratory; Ventilation.*
  in cardiopulmonary resuscitation, 330–331
  in pulmonary edema, 389–390
  normal vs abnormal, 189
  stertorous, 342, 342t
  stridorous, 342t, 343
Breeding management, 1276–1281. See also *Reproduction; Reproductive.*
  timing of, 1276
  vaginal cytology in, *1276–1278*, 1276–1279
  vaginal electrical resistance in, 1281
  vaginoscopy in, *1280*, 1280–1281
Bretylium, adverse effects of, 313t
  in cardiopulmonary resuscitation, 334
Brewer's yeast, approximate doses of, 1371
Brittany spaniels, complement deficiency in, 524
Brodifacoum rodenticide toxicosis, 106
Bromadiolone rodenticide toxicosis, 106

Bromethalin, poisoning due to, 106–107, 147–148, 147t
Bromides, antidote for, 121t
Bromsulphalein, approximate doses of, 1371
Bronchial tree, of dog, nomenclature for, *223*
Bronchitis, chronic, IX:306, 361–365
  auscultation in, 362–364
  bacterial infection in, 367–368
  bronchoscopy in, 364
  clinical findings in, 362–365
  eosinophilic, 368
  etiopathogenesis of, 361–362
  lesions and clinical signs in, *363*
  nonspecific, 368
  physical examination in, 362
  sputum analysis in, 362, 364
  therapy in, 366–368
  thoracic radiography in, *363*, 364
Bronchoalveolar lavage, bronchoscopic, 223–224
Bronchodilator therapy, IX:278
  adverse effects of, 313t
Bronchogenic carcinoma, 192
Bronchoscope, rigid, 219
Bronchoscopy, 219–224
  anesthesia, monitoring, patient positioning in, 220–221
  complications of, 224
  equipment for, 219–220
    care and cleaning of, 220
    flexible endoscopes in, 219–220
    rigid bronchoscopes in, 219
    sources of, 220
  indications and contraindications for, 220, 220t
  normal and abnormal findings in, 221–222
  sample procurement and handling in, 223–224
  technique in, 222–224
  terminology for, 221, *223*
Bronchus, bronchoscopic anatomy of, *222*
Broth dilution, for anaerobes, 73
Brucellosis, 1317–1320
  antimicrobial agents for, 1363t
  bacteriology in, 1317–1318
  diagnosis of, 1317–1319
  in neonate, 1332
  serology in, *1318*, 1318–1319
  species in, 1317
  treatment of, 1319–1320
Brucine, antidote for, 123t
Budgerigars, scaly face in, VIII:626
Bufo toads, antidote for, 121t
Bull terrier, juvenile renal disease in, 1169
Bumblefoot, in raptorial birds, VIII:614
BUN. See *Blood urea nitrogen (BUN).*
Bunamidine, approximate doses of, 1371
  in pregnancy, 1294t
Busulfan, 473
  approximate doses of, 1371
  effects on male dog fertility of, 1225
  for cancer therapy, 1367
Butorphanol, acepromazine and, in chemical restraint of dogs, 68
  approximate doses of, 1371
  for nausea in chemotherapy, 481

Butorphanol *(Continued)*
  in chemical restraint, 66–67
  in pregnancy, 1294t
  in tracheal collapse, 355
  xylazine and, in chemical restraint of dogs, 68–69
Butyrophenones, in chemical restraint, 63

Cachexia, cardiac, 302–303
  in feline leukemia virus infection, 1071
Caffeine, approximate doses of, 1371
  toxicity of, IX:191, 112
Cairn terrier, juvenile renal disease in, 1168
Calcification, of pulmonary nodule, 191
Calcitonin, approximate doses of, 1371
  in cholecalciferol toxicosis, 150–151
Calcium, antagonists of, IX:340
  homeostatic control of, 148–149
  in cardiopulmonary resuscitation, 334
  uterine effects of, 1300
Calcium carbonate, approximate doses of, 1371
  in chronic advanced renal failure, 1197
Calcium chloride, approximate doses of, 1371
Calcium EDTA, approximate doses of, 1371
Calcium gluconate, approximate doses of, 1371
  in chronic advanced renal failure, 1197
Calcium lactate, approximate doses of, 1371
Calcium oxalate crystalluria, 1129–1130
Calcium phosphate crystalluria, 1130
Calcium salts, approximate doses of, 1371
Calciuresis, in cholecalciferol toxicosis, 150
Calculi, renal, hematuria due to, 1119, 1121. See also *Urolithiasis.*
Calicivirus infection, feline neonatal, 1331
  in small animals, IX:1062
Caloric requirements. See also *Food; Nutrition.*
  based on breed, 1349
  for cats, 1353
  for neonates, 1350
  ideal daily intake of, 1008
Calories, in congestive heart failure, 305
  in enteral nutrition, 35, 35t
  in maintenance fluid therapy, 40, *41*
  in malnutrition, 30
Camel, hemogram of, 737t
Campylobacter, 943
Campylobacter enteritis, 943–946. See also *Enteritis.*
Campylobacter jejuni, 943–944
Campylobacteriosis, in dogs and cats, IX:1073
CaNa$_2$EDTA, in lead poisoning, 157–158
Cancer. See also *Neoplasia.*
  hyperthermia in, VIII:423
  infectious complications of, IX:464
  radiation therapy for, VIII:428
Candida, antimicrobial agents for, 1363
  ketoconazole in, 82

Canine DA2P vaccine, approximate doses of, 1371

Canine herpesvirus infection. See *Herpesvirus infection.*

Canine parvovirus, antigenic variation in, 1075–1076
enteritis, nonsteroidal anti-inflammatory drugs in, 53
vaccine, approximate doses of, 1371

Capillary permeability, in pulmonary edema, 391–392

Capillary refill time, in congenital heart disease, 227

Captan, approximate doses of, 1371

Captopril, adverse effects of, 313t
approximate doses of, 1371
in dilated cardiomyopathy, 247–248, 249t
in heart failure, IX:334
in hypertension in renal failure, 1204
in hypertrophic cardiomyopathy in cats, 253
in mitral regurgitation, 236t, 237
in pregnancy, 1295t
nutritional concerns with, 304

Carapace, anatomy of, 789
repair of injuries to, 790

Carbamate insecticides, 103, 135–137
toxic reaction to, IX:150, 135–137
clinical signs of, 136
diagnosis of, 136
mechanism of action of, 135
treatment of, 136–137

Carbamazepine, approximate doses of, 1371

Carbaryl toxicosis, 103

Carbenicillin, approximate doses of, 1371
in pregnancy, 1293t

Carbenoxolone, in gastrointestinal ulcer, 916

Carbofuran toxicosis, 103

Carbohydrate malassimilation, IX:889

Carbon monoxide, antidote for, 121t
toxicity of, 383

Carbon tetrachloride, antidote for, 120t

Carbonic anhydrase inhibitors, in glaucoma, 649

Carcinogenesis, VIII:152. See also *Neoplasia.*

Carcinoma, bronchogenic, 192
squamous cell, of nose and footpads, 620

Cardiac arrest, types of, 335t

Cardiac cachexia, 302–303

Cardiac catheterization, in congenital heart disease, 229

Cardiac compression, external, 332, 333
internal, 332, 333

Cardiac disorders. See *Heart disease; Heart failure.*

Cardiac output, in dilated cardiomyopathy, 244–245, 245t

Cardiac pacemakers, VIII:373, 289–294
equipment for, 289–290, 290
implantation of, 291, 292
patient aftercare and follow-up in, 291–294, 293–294
patient preparation for, 290–291
wandering atrial, 271

Cardiac tamponade, echocardiography in, 217, 218
in mitral regurgitation, 237

Cardiac tumor, echocardiography in, 218

Cardiogenic shock, 318

Cardiomegaly, in dilated cardiomyopathy, 243

Cardiomyopathy, acromegalic, 981
dilated, echocardiography in, 212, 213
in boxers, 241
in cats, 251, 254–262
aortic thromboembolism due to, 295, 296
aspirin therapy in, 52
clinical presentation in, 252
definitive diagnosis of, 256
diet history in, 257–258
dietary recommendations in, 261–262
due to taurine deficiency, 255–256, 257–259
etiology and pathophysiology of, 254
plasma taurine concentrations in, 258
prognosis in, 261
traditional heart failure therapy in, 259–260
treatment of taurine deficiency in, 260–261
in Doberman pinschers, 242
in dogs, 241–250
diagnosis of, 242
diagnostic studies in, 243–244
hemodynamic assessment and patient monitoring in, 244–245, 245t
history and signalment in, 242
pharmacotherapy in, 245–248, 249t
physical examination in, 242–243
secondary, 248–250
in hypophosphatemia, 46
hypertrophic, echocardiography in, 212
in cats, 251, 252–254
aortic thromboembolism due to, 295, 295
aspirin therapy in, 52
clinical presentation in, 252
definitive diagnosis of, 253
etiology and pathophysiology of, 252–253
prognosis in, 253–254
therapy in, 253
in dogs, 250–251

Cardiopulmonary disease, clinical signs in, 188–189
diagnostic approach to, 188
history in, 188–191
management of specific types of, 191–194. See also specific types.
physical examination in, 189–190
thoracic radiography in, 190–191

Cardiopulmonary drug therapy, 308–315. See also individual drugs.
deleterious systemic effects of, 308–310, 309
harmful drug-drug interactions in, 310–312, 310t–311t
individual toxicities of, 312, 313t
pharmacokinetic interactions in, 310t
therapeutic drug strategies in, 308

Cardiopulmonary resuscitation, 330–336
airway and breathing in, 330–331

Cardiopulmonary resuscitation (*Continued*)
alpha-agonist drugs in, 332, 332t
antishock trousers in, 332–333
blood flow in, 332
checklist for, 331t
circulation in, 331–333, 332t
defibrillation in, 334, 335t
drug therapy in, 333–334
external cardiac compression in, 332, 333
fluid therapy in, 332
intermittent abdominal compression in, 333
internal cardiac compression in, 332, 333
postresuscitation cerebral failure in, 335
postresuscitation monitoring and support in, 334–336
thoracotomy in, 332, 333

Cardiovascular system, in pregnancy, 1321

Carditis, Lyme, 248–250

Carnitine deficiency, hepatic lipidosis in, 869
cardiomyopathy in, 241

Carnivores, echinococcosis due to, 701–702
immunoprophylaxis in, VIII:1129
nondomestic, immobilization of, 733
immunization for, 729t
infectious diseases of, 728–730
management of, 732
nutrition for, 730
parasitism of, 731–732
pest control for, 730–731
physical examination of, 732–733
preventive medicine for, 727–733
quarantine for, 732–733
rabies immunization for, 729
recordkeeping for, 733
toxicities of, 732
rabies due to, 702
ringworm due to, 702
toxoplasmosis due to, 702
trypanosomiasis due to, 702–703
visceral larva migrans due to, 701

Case control studies, 10–11

Castor oil, approximate doses of, 1371

Castration, in rabbits, 761, 765

Cataract, congenital/neonatal, 669–671
nutritional, 670–671
suspected, 670
in ferret, 685
in guinea pig, 684
in mouse, 684
in rabbits, 682
in rats, 683
microphthalmia with, 665–666

Cathartics, in poisoning, 118

Catheter, in maintenance fluid therapy, 41–42
in total parenteral nutrition, 27, 29

Catheterization, arterial, in shock, 321–322
cardiac, in congenital heart disease, 229
urinary, IX:1127
venous, in shock, 321–322

Cats. See also individual topics.
acromegaly in, 981–984

Cats (Continued)
  allergy in, 583–585
  alopecia in, IX:545
  anemia in, 425–429
  anorexia in, 18–19
  aortic thromboembolism in, 295–302
  appetite stimulation in, 21–22
  approximate dosages of common drugs
    for, 1370–1380
  asthma in, 197–198
  atrioventricular insufficiency in, 212
  bacteremia in, 1078
  bacterial pneumonia in, 377
  beta-adrenergic blockers in, IX:343
  blood, plasma, serum chemical constit-
    uents in, 1340–1342
  blood transfusion reactions in, IX:515
  blood typing in, 428
  blood values in, 1335–1337
    at different ages, 1336–1337
    normal, 1335
    pregnancy and lactation and, 1337
  bone marrow values in, 1338
  brain tumors in, IX:820
  calculation of TPN nutrients for, 26
  caloric allowances for, 1353
  caloric intake of, 19
  campylobacteriosis in, IX:1073
  cardiomyopathy in, 251–262
  cerebellar diseases of, 838–840
  cerebrospinal fluid values in, 1344
  chemical restraint for, 69
  chemotherapy for lymphoma in, 485t
  chimeric, 1264–1265
  cisplatin in, 499
  colitis in, IX:896
  congenital birth defects in, IX:1248
  conjunctivitis in, 661
  cryptococcosis in, 1109–1111
  cytauxzoonosis in, 423
  diabetes mellitus in, IX:1000
  dysautonomia in, IX:802
  eosinophilic pneumonia in, 370
  electrocardiography in, 1346
  eyelid tumors in, 693t
  fertility disorders in, VIII:936
  food preferences in, 19
  glaucoma in, IX:656
  glomerular disease in, IX:1132
  haemobartonellosis in, 423–424
  heartworm disease in, IX:420, 269–270
  hematology reference ranges in, 1338
  hemostatic values in, 1343
  hepatic disease in, 873–878
  hepatic function in, IX:924
  hepatic lipidosis in, 869–873
  herpes keratitis in, 657
  herpesvirus infection in, 662–663
  hyperadrenocorticism in, 1038–1042
  hyperchylomicronemia in, 1048
  hyperthyroid heart disease in, IX:399
  hyperthyroidism in, IX:1026, 212–214,
    214, 1002–1007, 1016, 1171
  hypoadrenocorticism in, 1043–1045
  hypokalemic polymyopathy of, 812–
    815
  hypothyroidism in, 1000–1001
  infectious peritonitis and coronaviruses
    of, IX:1059
  inflammatory bowel disease in, IX:881
  ivermectin in, 562

Cats (Continued)
  laryngeal disease of, IX:265
  Latrodectus (black and red widow spi-
    der) bite of, 182
  lead poisoning in, 159
  leukemia virus infection in. See Feline
    leukemia virus infection.
  lymphoid hyperplasia in, 535–537
  mammary hypertrophy-fibroadenoma
    complex in, IX:477
  mast cell tumors of, 627–628
  miliary dermatitis of, IX:538
  myocardial disease in, IX:380
  nasal aspergillosis in, 1109
  nasogastric tube fixation in, 33
  normal development of, IX:1248
  nutritional requirements of, 1352
  pancreatitis in, 893–896
  perirenal cyst in, 1173
  plague and, 1088–1089
  poison control center calls about,
    100t–101t
  polycystic renal disease in, 1173
  polyuric renal failure in, VIII:1008
  portosystemic shunt in, IX:825
  poxvirus infection in, IX:605
  pregnancy termination in, IX:1236
  proteinuria in, IX:1111
  pseudorabies in, IX:1071
  renal amyloidosis in, 1173
  renal disease in, chronic, 1170–1173
  renal function in, IX:1103, 1343–1344
  reproduction in, VIII:932
  reproductive disorders of, IX:1225
  streptococcus A infection in, 1094–
    1095
  stress-induced hyperglycemia in, 29
  struvite urolithiosis in, IX:1188
  synovial fluid values in, 1344
  taurine and, 255, 255t
  thiamine deficiency in, 813
  thoracic duct ligation in, 397–398
  tissue plasminogen activator (t-PA) in,
    299
  toxoplasmosis in, 1112–1115
  urethra in, 1208–1209, 1209
  urethrostomy in, 1208–1213
  urinary incontinence in, IX:1159
  urine values in, 1343–1344
  urologic syndrome in, IX:1196
  vaccines for, 1356
  ventricular premature contractions in,
    283–285
  vesicourachal diverticula in, 1153–
    1157
  viral enteritis in, VIII:1168
  whiskers of, sensitivity of, 22
  XO syndrome in, 1264
  XXY syndrome in, 1263
Cat-scratch fever, 1099–1101
  clinical signs of, 1099
  etiology of, 1099–1100
  in humans, 1100–1101
    cat in, 1100
    diagnosis of, 1100
    treatment and prevention of, 1100–
      1101
Caval syndrome, in heartworm disease,
    267–268
Cavitation, pulmonary, 193
Cefadroxil, approximate doses of, 1371

Cefazolin, approximate doses of, 1371
Cefoxitin, approximate doses of, 1371
Cell culture, sample preparation for, 413
Cellular immunology, sample prepara-
    tion for, 418, 418t
Cellulitis, juvenile, periocular, 679–680
  orbital, 639
Centipede bite, 185
Central nervous system, depression of,
    in poisoning, 125
  glucocorticoid therapy for, 59–60
  hyperactivity of, in poisoning, 125
  in appetite control, 21, 21t
  in pregnancy, 1321–1322
  in uremia, 1137
  infection of, treatment of, IX:818, 1085
  necrotizing vasculitis of, glucocorticoid
    therapy in, 60
  neoplasia of, visual deterioration in,
    646
  reticulosis in, VIII:732
Central venous pressure, in maintenance
    fluid therapy, 40–41
  in shock, 321
  measurement of, 190
Cephalexin, approximate doses of, 1371
  in urinary tract infection, 1206t
Cephalosporins, 74–77
  generations of, 75, 75t
  in anaerobic infection, 1084–1085,
    1084t
  in pregnancy, 1293t
  mechanism of action of, 74–75
  pharmacology of, 75–76
  therapeutic uses of, 76–77
  toxicology of, 76
Cephalothin sodium, approximate doses
    of, 1371
Cephapirin, approximate doses of, 1371
Cerebellar abiotrophies, 840
Cerebellar disease, congenital, 838–841
  in cats, 838–840, 839
  in dogs, 840, 840–841
Cerebellum, functional anatomy of, 838
Cerebral edema, traumatic, 847
Cerebral failure, postresuscitation, 335
Cerebrospinal fluid values, 1344
Ceruloplasmin, as acute phase proteins,
    471
Cervical spondylopathy, 858
Cervix, vaginoscopic appearance of, 1312
Cesarean section, anesthesia in, 1322–
    1325. See also Anesthesia.
  neonatal care after, 1325
Cestodes, in fish disease, 713, 717
Chalazion, 692
Charcoal, activated, 117, 118, 119t
  approximate doses of, 1372
Chediak-Higashi syndrome, melanin dis-
    order in, 629
  ocular signs of, 664
Chemical hypomelanosis, 630
Chemical pneumonitis, 379–380
Chemical restraint, 63–70. See also Re-
    straint, chemical.
Chemotherapy, 472–475. See also indi-
    vidual drugs.
  acute reactions to, 480–481
  administration of, 480–481
  adverse effects of, VIII:419
  agents in, 1367–1369

Chemotherapy (Continued)
  alkylating agents in, 472–473, 473t
  antifungal, amphotericin B in, 1101–
    1102, 1102t
    combination, 1104
    flucytosine in, 1103–1104
    guidelines for, 1105t
    imidazole in, 1102–1103
    iodides in, 1104
    monitoring, 1104–1105
    systemic, 1101–1105
  antimetabolites in, 473
  antitumor antibiotics in, 474
  body surface area for calculation of,
    485
  effects on bone marrow of, 495–497
  effects on male dog fertility of, 1225
  extravasation in, 474–475, 480
  hormonal agents in, 474
  in acute lymphoblastic leukemia, 1366
  in bone marrow transplantation, 520
  in cancer treatment, IX:467
    resistance in, IX:471
  in creatinemia, 472t
  in hyperbilirubinemia, 472t
  in lymphoma, 1366
  in neutropenia, 472t
  in solid tumors, 489–493
  in thrombocytopenia, 472t
  information for owner in, 479
  painful infusions in, 480
  plant alkaloids in, 473–474
  precautions for drug handling in, 479–
    480
  toxicity of, 494
  vomiting and antiemetic therapy in, 481
Cheracol, approximate doses of, 1372
Chest, auscultation of, 190
  external, physical examination of, 189
  flail, traumatic, 198
  percussion of, 190
Cheyletiellosis, ivermectin in, 562
Chilodonella, 712, 713–714
Chimera, 1264–1265
  true hermaphrodite, 1264–1265
Chinchilla, ocular disorders in, 685
Chlamydia psittaci, antimicrobial agents
    for, 1363t
Chlamydiosis, serologic test results for,
    IX:731
Chlorambucil, 473
  approximate dose for, 1372
  effects of, on male dog fertility, 1225
  in cancer therapy, 1367
  in dermatology, 571
  in immune-mediated nonerosive ar-
    thritis, 550–551
  in pregnancy, 1294t
  preparation and administration of,
    476t
Chloramphenicol, approximate doses of,
    1372
  in anaerobic infection, 1084, 1084t
  in pregnancy, 1293t
Chlordane, approximate doses of, 1372
  toxicosis of, 103–104
Chlorethamine, approximate doses of,
    1372
Chlorfenvinphos toxicosis, 102
Chlorhexidine, 92
  toxicosis of, 166 .

Chlorine-containing disinfectants, 91
Chloroacetate esterase, in blood and
    bone marrow cells, 465–466, 466t
  in leukemia, 466–467, 467t
Chlorpheniramine, approximate doses of,
    1372
Chlorpromazine, approximate doses of,
    1372
Chlorpropamide, in diabetes insipidus,
    977
Chlorpyrifos toxicosis, 102
Chlortetracycline, approximate doses of,
    1372
Chlorthiazide, approximate doses of,
    1372
Chocolate toxicosis, IX:191, 112
Cholangiohepatitis complex, 885
Cholangitis, 885, 885
Cholecalciferol, toxicosis due to, 107,
    148–152
  clinical signs of, 149
  diagnosis of, 140–150
  median lethal dose in, 148
  treatment of, 150–152
Cholecystitis, 885, 885
Cholecystotomy, 888
Cholelithiasis, 884–889
  clinical manifestations of, 885–886
  diagnosis of, 886–887
  etiology of, 884, 885
  recurrence of, 888–889
  treatment of, 886–889
    cholecystotomy in, 888
    fluid therapy in, 887
    systemic antibiotics in, 887–888
Cholestasis, bile acid concentrations in,
    877, 878
Cholesterol crystalluria, 1130
Cholinergic agents, antidote for, 121t
Cholinesterase inhibitors, antidote for,
    121t
Chordae tendineae, myxomatous degen-
    eration in, 232
  rupture of, echocardiography in, 204,
    206
  in mitral regurgitation, 233
Chorionic gonadotropin challenge test,
    human, 1286–1287
Chorioretinitis, nonsteroidal anti-inflam-
    matory agents in, 643t
Choristoma, of conjunctiva, 694
Chow chows, dysmyelination in, 835–
    836
  tyrosinase deficiency in, melanin dis-
    order in, 629
Chromosomal sex, abnormalities of,
    1262–1265
Chrysotherapy, in dermatology, 573–
    574
  in immune diseases, VIII:448
  in pruritus, 569
Chylothorax, IX:295, 393–399
  chylous fluid characteristics in, 394,
    395, 395t
  diagnosis of, 393–394, 395, 395t
  ether clearance test in, 394
  etiology of, 393, 394
  in cardiomyopathy in cats, 252
  management of, 396
  medical therapy in, 394–395, 397t
  pleurodesis in, 406

Chylothorax (Continued)
  surgical management of, 395–399
    pleuroperitoneal shunt in, 398–399
    pleurovenous shunt in, 399
    postoperative care in, 398
    thoracic duct ligation in, in cat,
      397–398
    in dog, 396–397, 397–398
Ciliary dyskinesia, primary, 338
  neutrophil abnormality in, 524
Cimetidine, 509
  approximate dose for, 1372
  drug interactions with, 916t
  effects of, on male dog fertility, 1226
  in chronic advanced renal failure, 1197
  in dermatology, 575
  in gastrinoma, 1023
  in gastrointestinal ulcer, 914, 914–915,
    915t–916t
  in pregnancy, 1295t
  in pruritus, 567
  in reflux esophagitis, 909
  ranitidine vs, 915t
Ciprofloxacin, in pregnancy, 1293t
Circadian rhythm, effect on blood sam-
    ples for endocrinology of, 969–970
Circulation, in cardiopulmonary resusci-
    tation, 331–333
  in shock, 316, 317t
Cirrhosis, bile acid concentrations in,
    877, 877–878
Cisplatin, 497–501
  approximate dose for, 1372
  clinical trials in cats with, 499
  clinical trials in dogs with, 498–499,
    499
  effects of, on male dog fertility, 1225
  in cancer therapy, 1367
  in pregnancy, 1294t
  in soft tissue tumors, 491–492
  in systemic chemotherapy, 499–501,
    500t
  intracavitary, 501
  intralesional, 501
  intravesicular, 501
  pharmacology of, 498, 498
  preparation and administration of, 478t
  toxicity of, 498
Clavamox, approximate doses of, 1372
Clavulanate-potentiated antibiotics, 78–
    81
Clavulanic acid, 78–79, 79
Clavulanic acid-amoxicillin, in preg-
    nancy, 1293t
Cleaning agent toxicosis, 163–164
Cleft palate, 338
Clenbutarol, uterine effects of, 1301
Clindamycin, in anaerobic infection,
    1084, 1084t
  in pregnancy, 1293t
  in toxoplasmosis, 1115
Clinical algorithms, IX:26
Clinical chemistry tests, S.I. conversion
    factors for, 1339
Clinical studies, 8–18. See also Statis-
    tics.
  case control, 10–11
  characteristics of, 10t
  cohort, 11
  definitions of, 9
  descriptive, 9, 10t

Clinical studies (Continued)
  experimental, 11
  explanatory, 10–11
  observational, 10–11
Clinical trials, 11
Clonidine stimulation test, 967
Clostridium perfringens infection, clinical features of, 1082
  treatment of, 1085
Clostridium tetani, antimicrobial agents for, 1363t
Clot lysis, 441
Clot retraction, 440
Clotrimazole, 578
Clotting factors, assay for, 441
  snake venom effects on, 179
  vitamin K and, 143
Clotting studies, in disseminated intravascular coagulation, 454, 455
Clotting time, activated, 440
  thrombin, 440–441
  whole blood, 440
Cloxacillin, approximate dose for, 1372
  in pregnancy, 1293t
Coagulation, disseminated intravascular, 451–457. See also Disseminated intravascular coagulation.
  vitamin K in, 143
Coal tar derivative toxicosis, 166–167
Cobalamin malabsorption, selective, 435
Cocaine intoxication, 176–177, 176t
Coccidia, antimicrobial agents for, 1363t
Coccidioides, antimicrobial agents for, 1363
Coccidioidomycosis, IX:1076
Cochlear microphonics, 810, 811
Cockatoo beak and feather disease syndrome, IX:710
Cocker spaniel, juvenile renal disease in, 1167–1168
  vitamin A–responsive dermatosis of, retinoids in, 554–556
Cod liver oil, approximate doses of, 1372
Codeine, approximate doses of, 1372
  in pregnancy, 1294t
Coefficient of confidence, 14
Coefficient of correlation, 14t
Coefficient of determination, 14t
Cohort studies, 11
Cold agglutinin disease, nose and footpad in, 620
Colistimethate, approximate dose for, 1372
Colitis, chronic, in dog and cat, IX:896
  colonoscopy in, 868
  plasmacytic-lymphocytic, 938–943
    colonoscopy in, 941–942, 941–942
    diet therapy in, 942
    differential diagnosis and diagnostic plan in, 939–941, 939t–940t
    history and clinical signs of, 939
    therapeutic plan in, 942–944, 943t
  proliferative, in ferret, 774
  ulcerative, histiocytic, 940
Collateral vascularization, in aortic thromboembolism, 295, 296
Collie, gray, syndrome of, 629
  ivermectin in, 561
Coloboma, eyelid, 659
Colon, malignant tumors of, 940
  mucosa of, normal, 942, 942
  polyps of, 940

Colonoscopy, 868
  in plasmacytic-lymphocytic colitis, 941–942, 941–942
Columnaris disease, in fish, 718
Coma, myxedema in, 998–1000
Coma scale, small animal, 848, 849
Complement deficiency, in Brittany spaniels, 524
Computer-aided diagnosis, 2–7
  advantages of, 3
  clinical judgment and, 6–7
  components of, 4
  continuing education and, 6–7
  data base in, 4–5, 5
  inference engine in, 5–6, 7
  kinds of systems for, 3–6
  menu-driven system in, 3–4
  open-entry system in, 4
  user interface in, 3–4
Concussion, 847
Confidence coefficient, statistical, 14
Confidence interval, statistical, 14
Congenital birth defects, in cats, IX:1248
Congenital heart disease, 224–231. See also individual types; Heart disease, congenital.
Congestive heart failure. See Heart failure, congestive.
Conjunctiva, acquired melanosis of, 676
  developmental disorders of, 675
  disorders of, IX:624
  epithelial hyperplasia of, 676
  fibrous histiocytoma of, 676–677, 694
  neoplasia of, 677, 694–695
  non-neoplastic lesions of, 694
  symblepharon of, 675
  trauma to, 674–675
Conjunctivitis, 673–678
  allergic, 675–676
  bacterial, 673–674
  chlamydial, 674
  examination in, 673
  follicular, 676
  frictional irritants in, 676
  fungal, 674
  herpetic, in neonatal cats, 662
  immune-mediated, 675–676
  in ferret, 685
  in guinea pig, 684
  in rabbits, 682
  in rats, 683
  in systemic infection, 674
  infectious, 673–674
  neonatal, 661
  non-neoplastic proliferative diseases of, 676–677
  nonsteroidal anti-inflammatory agents in, 643t
  parasitic, 674
  signs of, 673
  symptomatic treatment of, 677–678
  toxic, 676
  viral, 674
Consciousness, level of, 848, 849t
Constipation, IX:904
Contact dermatitis, allergic, 541
  of nose and footpads, 619
Contact lenses, hydrophilic, 640–641
  characteristics and advantages of, 640
  cleaning and disinfecting, 641

Contact lenses (Continued)
  hydrophilic, contraindications and complications of, 641
    fitting, 640
    indications for, 640–641
Continuous data, 12t
Contraceptives, effects of, on male dog fertility, 1225
Contrast agents, radiopaque, adverse reactions to, IX:47
  urinalysis and, IX:1115
Control groups, external, 9
  internal, 9
Contusion, pulmonary, traumatic, 198–199
Copepods, in fish disease, 713, 716–717
Copper, antidote for, 120t, 121t
Copper metabolism, 891
  in West Highland white terriers, 889–890
Copper toxicity, hepatic, 889–893
  copper chelators in, 890–891
  dietary restriction in, 892
  reducing copper absorption in, 892
Cor pulmonale, IX:313
Cornea, disorders of, IX:642, 643t
  laceration of, 637
Corneal ulceration, 637–638, 656–658
  causes of, 656
  deep, treatment of, 657
  herpetic, in cats, 657
  initial assessment in, 656
  superficial, nonhealing, 656–657
Coronary perfusion pressure, 321t
Coronaviruses, in cats, IX:1059
  in dogs, neonatal, 1331
Corpuscular volume, mean, IX:509
Correlation, coefficient of, 14t
Corticosteroids, in chemotherapy-induced myelosuppression, 496–497
  in latent feline leukemia virus infection, 528–529
  in lymphocytic-plasmacytic enteritis, 923
  in nausea in chemotherapy, 481
  in plasmacytic-lymphocytic colitis, 943
  in shock, 327–328
  in tracheal collapse, 356
  in uveitis, 654–655
Cortisol concentration, basal, in cats, 1039
  plasma or serum, 961
Cortisone, in pregnancy, 1296t
Corynebacterium parvum, 508–509
Cough, "goose honk," 354
  in diagnosis of cardiopulmonary disease, 189
  in heart failure, 234
  paroxysmal, 195
  without pulmonary opacification, 191
Cough suppressants, in chronic bronchitis, 367
Coumarin, in aortic thromboembolism, in cats, 300–301
Coumarin-derivative anticoagulants, antidote for, 121t
Cow, hemogram of, 737t
Crackles, 190
Cranial nerves, ophthalmic, 689t
Craniocerebral trauma, 847–853
  ancillary diagnostic methods in, 850–851

Craniocerebral trauma *(Continued)*
  anticonvulsant therapy in, *851,* 853
  brain injury in, 847
  brainstem reflexes in, 849–850
  emergency management and therapy
    in, *850*
  initial evaluation in, 848, 848t
  level of consciousness in, 848, 849t
  management of, 848–853
  motor activity in, 848–849, *849*
  neurologic evaluation in, 848–850,
    848t–849t, *849*
  neurologic history in, 848, 848t
  pathogenesis of, 847–848
  patient monitoring and continued
    therapy in, *851,* 853
  respiratory pattern in, 848, 848t
  skull fracture in, 847–848
  small animal coma scale in, 848, *849*
  surgical management of, *851,* 853
  therapy in, *851–852,* 851–853
C-reactive protein, as acute phase pro-
    tein, 470–471
Creatine kinase, serum, in hypophospha-
    temia, 46
Creatinemia, chemotherapy modifica-
    tions in, 472t
Creatinine, in azotemia, 1123–1124,
    1123t
  in renal failure, 1195
Creatinine clearance, endogenous, 1125
  exogenous, 1125
  spot or fractional, 1126
Cresol, antidote for, 120t
Cricoid cartilage, anatomy of, 343, *344*
Cricothyroid muscles, anatomy of, 344,
    345
Crocodiles, sexual identification in, 801–
    802, *802*
Cromolyn sodium, approximate dose for,
    1372
Cruelty, 89–90
  by ignorance, 90
  by neglect, 89–90
  intentional, 89
Cryptococcosis, in cats, 1109–1111
    clinical signs of, 1110
    diagnosis of, 1110–1111
    etiology of, 1109–1110
    public health considerations in, 1111
    treatment of, 1111
  in feline leukemia virus infection, 1071
  ketoconazole in, 82–83
  of nose and footpads, 618
  rhinosinusitis in, 340
Cryptococcus, antimicrobial agents for,
    1363
Cryptococcus neoformans, 1109–1110
Cryptorchidism, 1268
  alopecia in, 597–598
Cryptosporidiosis, in reptiles, IX:748
Cryptosporidium, in neonate, 1333
Crystalloid, in parenteral nutrition, 27
Crystalluria, 1127–1133. See also *Uroli-
    thiasis.*
  ammonium urate and amorphous
    urate, 1129, *1129*
  bilirubin, 1129
  calcium oxalate, 1129–1130
  calcium phosphate, 1130
  cholesterol, 1130

Crystalluria *(Continued)*
  clinical significance and insignificance
    of, 1127
  crystal characteristics in, 1128t
  crystal habit in, 1128–1129
  cystine, 1130
  drug-associated, 1130, *1131*
  factors influencing, 1127–1128
  hippuric acid, 1132
  leucine, 1132
  magnesium ammonium phosphate,
    1131, 1132
  tyrosine, 1132
  uric acid, 1133
Culture, blood, in bacteremia, 1079,
    1080t
  duodenal fluid, in intestinal bacterial
    overgrowth, 935
Curare, antidote for, 121t
Cushing's syndrome. See also *Hyper-
    adrenocorticism.*
Cutaneous conditions. See *Dermatitis;
    Dermatology; Skin.*
Cutaneous horns, of footpads, 620–621
Cuticle bleeding time, 440
Cyanide, antidote for, 121t
Cyanoacrylate toxicity, 111
Cyanosis, respiratory causes of, 196, 196t
Cyclo-oxygenase, in arachidonic acid me-
    tabolism, *1158,* 1158–1159
Cyclophosphamide, 473
  approximate doses of, 1372
  bleomycin, doxorubicin and protocol,
    for soft tissue tumors, 492
  doxorubicin and protocol, for soft tis-
    sue tumors, 490t, 491
  effects of, on male dog fertility, 1225
  in cancer therapy, 1367
  in dermatology, 570–571
  in immune-mediated nonerosive ar-
    thritis, 550–551
  in lymphocytic-plasmacytic enteritis,
    925
  in lymphoma, 485–486, 485t
  in pregnancy, 1294t
  in pruritus, 568–569
  in uveitis, 655
  preparation and administration of, 476t
  vincristine, doxorubicin and protocol,
    for soft tissue tumors, 490t, 491
Cyclosporine, 513–515
  adverse effects of, 515
  approximate dose for, 1372
  dosages for, 514
  in dermatology, 572
  in uveitis, 655
  mechanism of action of, *514*
  pharmacologic properties of, 513–514
Cyclothiazide, approximate doses of,
    1372
Cyproheptadine, in appetite stimulation,
    23
Cyst, epidermal inclusion, retinoids in,
    558
  paraprostatic, 1235, *1237*
  perirenal, of cats, 1173
  pulmonary, differential diagnosis of,
    193
Cystic calculi, hematuria due to, 1121
Cystic disease of kidneys, hematuria due
    to, 1119

Cystine crystalluria, 1130
Cystine urolithiasis, 1189–1192
Cystography, IX:1124
Cystometrogram, 1147–1149, *1149*
Cytarabine, approximate doses of, 1372
Cytauxzoonosis, in cats, 423
  anemia due to, 427
Cythioate toxicosis, 102
Cytokine, as biologic response modifier,
    511
Cytology, exfoliative, sample preparation
    for, 410
  for birds, IX:725
Cytosine arabinoside, for cancer therapy,
    1368
  preparation and administration of, 476t

2,4-D toxicosis, 107
Dacarbazine, approximate doses of, 1372
  doxorubicin and, protocol for soft tis-
    sue tumors, 490t, 491
  for cancer therapy, 1369
  preparation and administration of, 476t
Dachshund, long-haired, sensory neu-
    ropathy in, 824–825
Dacryoadenitis, in rats, 683
Dactinomycin, for cancer therapy, 1369
Dactylogyrids, in fish disease, *713,* 717
Dalmatian, medical management of uro-
    lithiasis in, 1179–1180, 1180t
Dantrolene, in pregnancy, 1296t
Dapsone, approximate doses of, 1372
  in dermatology, 572–573
Darbazine, approximate doses of, 1372
Data, in statistical analysis, 12, 12t
o,p'-DDD treatment protocol. See also
    Mitotane.
  in adrenocortical neoplasia, 1034–1037
    initial therapy in, 1036
    maintenance therapy in, 1036
    prognosis in, 1037
    side effects of, 1036–1037
  in hyperadrenocorticism, 1025–1028
    adverse reactions to, 1027–1028
    failure to respond to, 1028
    maintenance therapy with, 1027
    time sequence for improvement in,
      1028
    with diabetes mellitus, 1026–1027
    with overt polydipsia, 1025–1026
    without overt polydipsia, 1026
Deafness, 805–811
  auditory evoked response in, 809–810
  cochlear microphonics in, 810, *811*
  early latency components of, 809–
    810, *809–810*
  middle latency components of, 810,
    811
  behavioral evaluation in, 806
  classification and occurrence of, 805–
    806
  clinical evaluation of, 806–811
  conductive, 805–806
  electrodiagnostic evaluation in, 806–
    811
  electroencephalographic audiometry
    in, 810–811
  hearing aid in, 806
  hereditary, 806

Deafness (Continued)
  impedance audiometry in, 807–809, 808
    acoustic reflex in, 807–809, 808
    tympanometry in, 807, 808
  ocular dysgenesis and, 664–665
  sensorineural, 806
Death of pet, coping strategies for, VIII:72
Decerebrate rigidity, 849, 849
Defibrillation, in cardiopulmonary resuscitation, 334, 335t
Degenerative myelopathy, 830–833
Degenerative radiculomyelopathy, 830
Degus, ocular disorders in, 685
Delta Albaplex, approximate doses of, 1372
Demodicosis, IX:531
  ivermectin in, 562
  periocular, 678–679
Demyelination, 834
Dental disease. See also Exodontia.
  in rabbits and rodents, IX:759
  rhinitis and, 341
Dependent variable, 14t
Depo-penicillin, approximate doses of, 1372
Dermatitis. See also Skin.
  allergic, of pinnae, 624
  atopic, fatty acid supplements in, 563–564
  contact, allergic, 541
    of nose and footpads, 619
  flea-bite, in cats, 584–585
    in dogs, 587
  miliary, in cats, IX:538, 585
  solar, of pinnae, 623
Dermatology. See also Skin.
  antibacterial agents in, IX:566
  antifungal agents in, IX:560
  antiseborrheic agents in, IX:596
  hormonal replacement therapy in, 602–606
    androgens in, 605–606
    estrogens in, 604–605
    growth hormone in, 604
    thyroid hormone in, 602–603
  immunomodulating drugs in, 570–576
  nutritional therapy in, IX:591
  parasiticide therapy in, IX:571
  progestagens in, IX:601
  retinoids in, 553–559
  sulfones and sulfonamides in, IX:606
Dermatomyositis, familial canine, 606–609
  cause and pathogenesis of, 608
  clinical features of, 606–607
  diagnosis of, 607–608
  muscle biopsy in, 608
  treatment and management of, 608–609
  periocular lesions in, 680
Dermatophilosis, VIII:1184
Dermatophytosis, of pinnae, 625
  periocular, 678–679
Dermatosis, autoimmune, periocular lesions in, 680
  growth-hormone responsive, 978–980, 980t
  lichenoid, 614–615
  lichenoid-psoriasiform, 614–615
  of eyelid, 678–681, 678t

Dermatosis (Continued)
  of nose and foot pads, 616–621, 617t. See also individual types.
  of pinnae, 621–625, 621t–622t
  periocular, 678–681, 678t
  pustular, sterile, IX:554
  sex hormone-related, 595–601
    clinical evaluation of, 596
    diagnosis and therapy of, 601
    in adrenal feminization or masculinization, 599–600
    in flank alopecia, 600
    in hormonal hypersensitivity, 600–601
    in intact females, 597
    in intact males, 598
    in male feminizing syndrome, 599
    in males with palpably normal testes, 599
    in neutered female dogs, 596–597
    in neutered males, 597–598
    in pruritus, 601
    in testicular neoplasia, 598
  testosterone-responsive, 605–606
  vitamin A–responsive, in cocker spaniels, 554–556
  zinc-responsive, 619
    periocular, 679
Dermoid, of conjunctiva, 694
  ophthalmologic, 660–661
Desmopressin acetate, in diabetes insipidus, 976–977
Desoxycorticosterone acetate, approximate doses of, 1372
  in hypoadrenocorticism, in cats, 1045
Desoxycorticosterone pivalate, approximate doses of, 1372
Desquamation, in radiation therapy complications, 505–506
Detergent toxicosis, 164–165
  anionic (surfactant) products in, 164
  antidote for, 120t
  builder products in, 165
  cationic (quaternary ammonium) products in, 164–165
  nonionic products in, 165
Determination, coefficient of, 14t
Detrusor muscle function, urinary incontinence and, 1152
Dexamethasone, approximate doses of, 1372
  gastrointestinal complications of, 902
  in hydrocephalus, 846
  in pregnancy, 1296t
  structure of, 58
Dexamethasone suppression test, ACTH stimulation test and, in cats, 1040
  in dogs, 963–964
Dextran, approximate doses of, 1372
  for blood volume expansion, 325
  hypertonic saline and, in shock, 328–329
Diabetes insipidus, 973–978
  clinical features of, 974
  diagnostic tests of, 974–976
    ADH trial as, 975–976
    gradual water deprivation test as, 975
    Hickey-Hare test as, 976
    modified water deprivation test as, 974–975
    plasma ADH concentration as, 976
    random plasma osmolality as, 974

Diabetes insipidus (Continued)
  differential diagnosis of, 974
  etiology of, 973–974
  laboratory findings in, 974
  nephrogenic, IX:1140
  prognosis in, 978
  treatment of, 976–977
Diabetes mellitus, IX:991
  acromegaly in, IX:1006, 982
  classification of, 1012, 1012t
  dietary therapy in, 1008–1011
    composition of diet for, 1009–1010
    feeding schedule for, 1009
    fiber in, 1010–1011
    pancreatitis and, 1011
  hepatic lipidosis in, 869
  hyperadrenocorticism and, 1026–1027
  hypercholesterolemia and, 1049
  hyperlipidemia in, 1048–1049
  in cats, IX:1000
  insulin-resistant, 1012–1019
    acromegaly and, 1015–1016
    Cushing's syndrome and, 1015
    disease associations in, 1012–1013, 1013t
    flow chart for ruling out causes of, 1014
    hyperthyroidism and, 1016
    insulin antibodies and, 1018
    liver disease and, 1018
    obesity and, 1016–1017
    pregnancy and, 1018
    renal failure and, 1017–1018
    sepsis and, 1018
    type I vs type II diabetes and, 1013–1014
  maintenance fluid therapy in, 42
  neutrophil abnormality in, 525
  obesity and caloric intake in, 1008–1009
  with chronic renal disease in cats, 1171–1172
Diabetic ketoacidosis, IX:987
  hypophosphatemia in, 44, 45t
Diagnostic errors, drug-related, IX:183
Diagnostic process, 2–3
  computers in, 3
  hypothetical-deductive process in, 2
  pitfalls in, 2
Dialysis, peritoneal, in poisoning, 123–124
Diaphragm, hernia of, traumatic, 199
Diarrhea, in Campylobacter enteritis, 945
  in intestinal bacterial overgrowth, 935
  secretory, nonsteroidal anti-inflammatory drugs in, 53
  small bowel vs large bowel, 939–940, 939t–940t
Diazepam, approximate doses of, 1372
  in appetite stimulation, 23
  in cesarean section, 1322t
  in chemical restraint, 63–64
  in pregnancy, 1294t, 1295t
  in urinary incontinence, 1218
  oxymorphone and, in chemical restraint of dogs, 68
Diazoxide, approximate doses of, 1372
  in beta-cell tumors, 1022
p-Dichlorobenzene toxicosis, 104
Dichloromethylene diphosphonate, in hypercalcemia of malignancy, 991–992

Dichlorphenamide, approximate doses of, 1372
  in glaucoma, 649
Dichlorvos, approximate doses of, 1373
  in pregnancy, 1294t
  toxicosis due to, 102
Dicloxacillin, approximate doses of, 1373
  in pregnancy, 1293t
Dieffenbachia toxicity, 113
Diet. See also *Caloric requirements; Calories; Food; Nutrition.*
  homemade, in mineral and sodium restriction, 304t
    in protein/phosphorus restriction, 304t
    in sodium restriction, 304t
    low-fat, 397t
  supplements to, liquid, 306t
Diethylcarbamazine, approximate doses of, 1373
  effects of, on male dog fertility, 1226
  for heartworm preventive therapy, 266
  hepatic toxicity due to, 880
  in pregnancy, 1293t
  toxicity due to, 109–110
Diethylstilbestrol, approximate doses of, 1373
  in cancer therapy, 1369
  in pregnancy, 1296t
  preparation and administration of, 478t
Di-Gel, approximate doses of, 1373
Digitalis, in pregnancy, 1295t
Digitalis glycosides, adverse effects of, 313t
  antidote for, 121t
Digitalis intoxication, in Doberman pinschers, 245
Digitoxin, approximate doses of, 1373
Digoxin, approximate doses of, 1373
  drug interactions or adverse conditions with, 311t
  in atrial tachyarrhythmia, 276
  in dilated cardiomyopathy, 245, 249t
  in mitral and tricuspid regurgitation, 235–236
Dihydrocodeinone, approximate doses of, 1373
Dihydrostreptomycin, approximate doses of, 1373
Dihydrotachysterol, approximate doses of, 1373
  in chronic advanced renal failure, 1197
Diltiazem, adverse effects of, 313t
  approximate doses of, 1373
  in atrial tachyarrhythmia, 276
  in dilated cardiomyopathy, 246, 249t
Dimenhydrinate, approximate doses of, 1373
  in pregnancy, 1295t
Dimercaprol, in arsenic poisoning, 160–161
2,3-Dimercaptosuccinic acid, in lead poisoning, 157
Dimethyl sulfoxide, in pregnancy, 1296t
  in renal amyloidosis, 1176–1177
Dimethyl tubocurarine, in pregnancy, 1296t
Dimpylate toxicosis, 102
Dioctophyma renale infection, hematuria due to, 1120
Dioctyl sulfosuccinate, approximate doses of, 1373

Diphacinone, coagulopathy of, VIII:399
  toxicosis due to, 106
Diphenhydramine, approximate doses of, 1373
  in pregnancy, 1295t
Diphenoxylate, in pregnancy, 1295t
Diphenylhydantoin, approximate doses of, 1373
Diphenylthiocarbazone, approximate doses of, 1373
Dipyrone, approximate doses of, 1373
Dirofilariasis. See *Heartworm disease.*
Dishwasher detergent toxicosis, 166
Disinfection, 90–95
  additives in, 92
  biguanides for, 92
  birds and reptiles and, VIII:606
  definitions in, 91t
  environmental considerations in, 93–94
  halogens for, 91
  ideal agent for, 90–91
  in zoonotic disease, 93
  microorganism susceptibility to, 92–93
  phenolics for, 91, 162t
  principles of, 94–95
  quaternary ammonium compounds for, 91–92
  toxicosis due to, 166–169
Disk diffusion assay, antimicrobial, 71–72
Disk elution, for anaerobes, 73
Diskospondylitis, IX:810, 545
Disophenol, approximate doses of, 1373
Disopyramide, adverse effects of, 313t
  approximate doses of, 1373
Disseminated intravascular coagulation, 451–457
  associated diseases and conditions in, 452t
  bleeding in, 452
  clinical features of, 454, 455
  hemolysis in, 453, 454
  laboratory diagnosis of, 454–456
  pathogenesis of, 451–454, 453–454
  shock and, 453, 454
  therapy in, 456–457
Dissociative agents, in chemical restraint, 67
Distemper, 342
  footpad disorders in, 619
  in ferret, 767–768, 768t
  neonatal, 1330
  treatment of, 86
Distribution, normal, definition of, 10t
Disulfoton toxicosis, 103
Dithiazanine, approximate doses of, 1373
Dithiazanine iodide, in pregnancy, 1293t
Diuretics, adverse effects of, 313t
  in calcium oxalate urolithiasis, 1187
  in hypertension in renal failure, 1203
  in mitral and tricuspid regurgitation, 235
  in poisoning, 123
  in pregnancy, 1295t
Diverticula, vesicourachal, 1153–1157
Doberman pinscher, cardiomyopathy in, 242
  chronic hepatitis in, IX:937
  digitalis intoxication in, 245
  juvenile renal disease in, 1167
  neutrophil defect in, 524

Doberman pinscher (Continued)
  renal disease in, VIII:975
  wobbler syndrome in, 858–862
Dobutamine, adverse effects of, 313t
  approximate doses of, 1373
  for blood pressure, in shock, 326
  in dilated cardiomyopathy, 247, 249t
Docusate calcium, approximate doses of, 1373
Docusate sodium, approximate doses of, 1373
Dogs. NB: All index entries refer to dogs unless otherwise noted.
  approximate dosages of common drugs for, 1370–1380
  blood, plasma, serum chemical constituents in, 1340–1342
  blood values for, 1335–1337
    at different ages, 1336
    normal, 1335
    pregnancy and lactation and, 1337
  bone marrow values in, 1338
  caloric requirements based on breed for, 1349
  cerebrospinal fluid values in, 1344
  electrocardiography in, normal criteria for, 1346
  hematology reference ranges in, 1338
  hemostatic values in, 1343
  nutrient allowances for, 1348
  renal function values in, 1343–1344
  semen values in, 1345
  synovial fluid values in, 1344
  urine values in, 1343–1344
  vaccines for, 1354–1355
Domeboro's solution, approximate doses of, 1373
Dopamine, adverse effects of, 313t
  approximate doses of, 1373
  for blood pressure, in shock, 326
  in acute toxicant-induced renal failure, 128–129
  in cesarean section, 1322t
  in dilated cardiomyopathy, 247, 249t
  in mitral and tricuspid regurgitation, 236
  in pregnancy, 1295t
Doxapram, approximate doses of, 1373
  in cesarean section, 1322t
Doxepin, in pruritus, 567
Doxorubicin, 474
  approximate doses of, 1373
  cyclophosphamide and, protocol for soft tissue tumors, 490t, 491
  cyclophosphamide, bleomycin and, protocol for soft tissue tumors, 492
  cyclophosphamide, vincristine and, protocol for soft tissue tumors, 490t, 491
  dacarbazine and, protocol for soft tissue tumors, 490t, 491
  in cancer therapy, 1369
  in lymphoma, 485–486, 485t
  in pregnancy, 1294t
  in soft tissue tumors, 490–491, 490t
  preparation and administration of, 477t
Doxycycline, approximate doses of, 1373
  in pregnancy, 1293t
Doxylamine succinate, approximate doses of, 1373
Droperidol, in chemical restraint, 63

Drug abuse, VIII:139
    small animals and, 171–177. See also
        specific illicit drugs.
Drug effects, on embryo and fetus, 1292,
        1296–1297
    on fertility in male dog, 1224–1226
    on pregnancy, 1291–1299
Drug eruptions, nose and footpad in,
        619–620
Drug metabolism, fetal, 1322
Drug reactions, adverse, IX:169, IX:176
    allergic, IX:444, 542, 542t
    crystalluria as, 1130, 1131
    in chronic advanced renal failure,
        1197–1198
    hematuria as, 1121
    hepatotoxic, 878–884. See also Hepatic
        disease, drug-induced.
    polyarthritis as, 545
Drug transfer, placental, 1322
Drug-related diagnostic errors, IX:183
Drugs, effect of, on blood samples for
        endocrinology, 969–970
    poisoning due to, 107–109
    safety of, in pregnancy, 1293t–1296t
    veterinary, poisoning due to, 109–111
Ductus arteriosus, patent, breed and sex
        predilections for, 225t
    Doppler echocardiographic features
        of, 230t
    echocardiography in, 208–212, 210–
        211
    murmur in, 227
    surgical correction of, 230
Duodenal fluid culture, in intestinal bac-
        terial overgrowth, 936
Duodenogastric reflux, 908
Duodenum, endoscopy of, 867–868
Dwarfism, pituitary, 604
Dysautonomia, in cats, IX:802
Dysmyelination, 834
    in chow chows, 835–836
Dyspnea, in diagnosis of cardiopulmo-
        nary disease, 189
    in tracheal collapse, 354
    without pulmonary opacification, 191
Dysproteinemia, platelet disorders in,
        463
Dysuria, vesicourachal diverticula and,
        1156–1157

Ear, allergic dermatitis of, 624
    alopecia of, 623
    dermatophytosis of, 625
    dermatosis of, 621–625, 621t–622t
    diseases of, VIII:47
    flystrike of, 622
    frostbite of, 622
    marginal seborrhea of, 623
    mites, of ferret, 770–771
    odontic mange of, 624
    scabies of, 623–624
    seborrhea of, 623
    solar dermatitis of, 623
    structure and function of, 805
    trauma to, 624
Echinococcosis, due to carnivores, 701–
        702

Echocardiography, 201–218
    Doppler, 208, 209
    in bacterial endocarditis, 239
    in congenital heart disease, 229, 230t
    in dilated cardiomyopathy, 243–244
    in heartworm disease, 216, 216–218,
        264
    in mitral and tricuspid regurgitation,
        234
    in myocardial disease, 212–216, 213–
        216
    in pericardial effusion, 217–218, 218
    in shunts, 208–212, 210–212
    in valvular and subvalvular lesions,
        201–208, 202–209
    interpretation of, 205t
    M-mode and two-dimensional, 204t
Echothiophate, in glaucoma, 650
Econazole, 578
Ectoparasite monitoring, for laboratory
        animals, 746–747
Edema, cerebral, traumatic, 847
    in glomerulonephropathy, 1175–1176
    in myxedema, 998
    laryngeal, 197
    mucosal, tracheobronchial, 222
    pulmonary, 385–392. See also Pulmo-
        nary edema.
Edrophonium, approximate doses of,
        1373
EDTA, in cholecalciferol toxicosis, 151
Efferent sympathetic pathway, ocular,
        688
Effusion, pericardial, echocardiography
        in, 218, 218
    pleural, differential diagnosis of, 192,
        194
    respiratory emergencies due to, 199
Ehrlichiosis, IX:1080, 420–421
    platelet disorders in, 464
Eicosanoids, 1158, 1158–1159, 1158t
    physiology of, 1159
Eimeria, of fish, 715
Electrocardiography, for ferret, 767t
    Holter, in dilated cardiomyopathy, 246
    in chronic bronchitis, 365
    in congenital heart disease, 228
    in dilated cardiomyopathy, 243
    in heartworm disease, 264
    in mitral and tricuspid regurgitation,
        234
    normal criteria for, in dogs and cats,
        1346
Electroencephalography, in audiometry,
        810–811
    in hydrocephalus, 844, 845
Electrolyte balance, glucocorticoid ef-
        fects on, 54–55
    in parenteral nutrition, 27, 27t
    in uremia, 1137–1138
Electron microscopy, fixatives for, 412–
        413, 412t
ELISA testing, in atopy, in dogs, 592–
        595
Embden-Meyerhof pathway, 430, 430
Embryo, drug effects on, 1292, 1296–
        1297
Emergencies, ocular, 636–639. See also
        Ocular emergencies.
    respiratory, 195–201. See also Respi-
        ratory emergencies.

Emergency kit, for poisoning, VIII:92
Emesis. See Vomiting.
Emetrol, approximate doses of, 1373
Emphysema, subcutaneous, in traumatic
        pneumothorax, 198
Enalapril, adverse effects of, 313t
Endocarditis, bacterial, IX:402, 237–240
    clinical signs of, 238
    diagnosis of, 238–239
    differential diagnosis of, 545
    medical management of, 239–240
    pathology and pathogenesis of, 237–
        238
    vegetative, echocardiography in, 204,
        207
Endocrine diagnostic tests, 961–967
    of gonadal function, 966–967
    of growth hormone, 967
    sources of substances for, 962t
    of hypothalamic-pituitary-adrenocorti-
        cal axis, 961–965
    of pancreatic endocrine function, 966
    of thyroid function, 965–966
Endocrine disorders, ketoconazole for,
        83–84
Endocrine hypermelanosis, 631
Endocrine neoplasia, of gastroenteropan-
        creatic system, 1020–1023, 1020t
Endocrinology, of birds, IX:702
    reproductive, 1282–1288. See also in-
        dividual hormones.
Endodontics, 954–959
    files for, 956–957
    pathogenesis and diagnosis in, 954–
        956
    radiography in, 955
    root canal in, 956–959. See also Root
        canal.
Endometrial cells, in vulvar discharge,
        1311
Endometritis, postpartum, prostaglan-
        dins in, 1309–1310
    ultrasonography of, 1242, 1242
Endomyocardial biopsy, in dilated car-
        diomyopathy, 244
Endophthalmitis, nonsteroidal anti-in-
        flammatory agents in, 643t
Endoscope, flexible, 219–220
Endoscopy, 864–868
    equipment selection for, 865
    gastrointestinal, 865–868
    in duodenal abnormalities, 867–868
    in esophageal disorders, 866–867
    in gastric abnormalities, 867
    in intestinal bacterial overgrowth, 936
    in large intestinal disorders, 868
    in lymphocytic-plasmacytic enteritis,
        924
    instrumentation in, 864–865
Endosulfan toxicosis, 104
Endotoxic shock, nonsteroidal anti-in-
        flammatory drugs in, 52–53
Enema, hypertonic sodium phosphate,
        intoxication by, IX:212
    retention, in plasmacytic-lymphocytic
        colitis, 943
Enflurane, approximate doses of, 1374
English pointers, sensory neuropathy in,
        824
English springer spaniels, phosphofruc-
        tokinase deficiency in, 434, 434–435

Enilconazole, 84, 579
    approximate doses of, 1374
    in aspergillosis of nasal cavity, 1108
Enrofloxacin, in pregnancy, 1293t
Enteral nutrition, in hepatic lipidosis,
    871–872
Enteric bacteria, antimicrobial-resistant,
    1096–1098
    communicability of, 1097–1098
    R plasmids in, 1096–1097, 1096t
Enteritis, bacterial, IX:872
    Campylobacter, 944–947
        clinical signs of, 945
        diagnosis of, 946
        epidemiology of, 944–945
        etiologic agent in, 944
        histopathology in, 946
        laboratory findings in, 945–946
        pathogenesis of, 945
        prevention of, 947
        therapy in, 946–947
        zoonotic potential in, 947
    eosinophilic-plasmacytic, glucocorti-
        coids in, 902
    lymphocytic-plasmacytic, 922–926
        diagnosis of, 923–925
        dietary management of, 926
        endoscopic biopsy in, 924
        histologic findings in, 925
        history and clinical signs of, 923
        pathogenesis of, 922–923
        therapy in, 925–926
    neonatal, 1331
    parvovirus, nonsteroidal anti-inflam-
        matory drugs in, 53
    viral, in cats, VIII:1168
        in dogs, VIII:1164
Enterobacter, antimicrobial agents for,
    1363t
Enterocolitis, in uremia, 1134
Enteropathic arthritis, 549
Enteropathy, wheat-sensitive, in Irish
    setters, IX:893
Entropion, neonatal, 659–660
Environment, culture of, for birds,
    781
    disinfection of, 93–94
Eosinophilia, pulmonary, 369–375. See
    also *Pulmonary eosinophilia*.
Eosinophilic granuloma complex, in cats,
    585
Ephedrine, adverse effects of, 313t
    approximate doses of, 1374
    in urinary incontinence, 1220t
Epibulbar melanoma, 695
Epidermal inclusion cyst, retinoids in,
    558
Epidermal necrolysis, toxic, nose and
    footpad in, 619–620
Epidermophyton, antimicrobial agents
    for, 1363t
Epidermotropic lymphoma, IX:609
Epiglottic cartilage, anatomy of, 343–
    344, *344*
Epilation, in radiation therapy complica-
    tions, 505
Epinephrine, adverse effects of, 313t
    approximate doses of, 1374
    in bronchitic pulmonary eosinophilia,
        373
    in glaucoma, 650

Epiphora, in mice, 683–684
    in rabbits, 682
    in rats, 683
Epistaxis, 337
    emergency, 195
    recurrent, 436
Epistylis, *712*, 714
Epulis, acanthomatous, radiation therapy
    for, 504
Erythema, necrolytic migratory, 680
    nose and footpads in, 620
Erythema chronicum migrans, in Lyme
    borreliosis, 1086
Erythrocytes, 429–430, *430*
    clinical signs of, 431–433
    cobalamin malabsorption, 435
    electronic sizing of, IX:509
    hereditary disorders of, 429–436
    in hypophosphatemia, 44–45, 45t
    in vulvar discharge, 1311
    laboratory diagnosis of, 433, *434*
    nonspherocytic hemolytic anemia, 435
    osmotic fragility test in, 433, *434*
    phosphofructokinase deficiency, 434–
        435
    pyruvate kinase deficiency, 435
    sample preparation for, 413t–414t,
        415–416
    therapy and prevention of, 433–434
    types of, 431, 432t
Erythromycin, approximate doses of,
    1374
    in pregnancy, 1293t
    in pruritus, 568
Erythropoiesis disorders, therapy for,
    IX:490
Escherichia coli, antimicrobial agents for,
    1363t
Esophageal disease, endoscopy in, 866–
    867
Esophageal sphincter, lower, 906
Esophageal stricture, 904–906
    clinical signs of, 905
    diagnosis of, 905
    pathogenesis of, 904–905
    treatment of, 905–906
Esophagitis, esophageal stricture due to,
    904–905
    reflux, 906–910
        diagnosis of, 908–909
        endoscopy in, 867
        factors that promote, 908
        mechanism of mucosal damage in,
            907–908
        mechanism of reflux in, 907
        treatment of, 909–910
Esterase, in blood and bone marrow
    cells, 465, 466t
    in leukemia, 466–467, 467t
Estradiol, repetitive testing of, 1286
    single serum samples of, 1284, *1284*
Estradiol cyclopentaneopropionate, ap-
    proximate doses of, 1374
Estradiol cypionate, approximate doses
    of, 1374
    in pregnancy, 1296t
Estrogen, cyclic levels of, 1274
    effects of, on male dog fertility, 1224
    in dermatology, 604–605
    in urinary incontinence, 1219t
    serum or plasma, measurement of, 967

Estrogen-induced bone marrow toxicity,
    IX:495
Estrogen-induced pancytopenia, in fer-
    ret, IX:762
Estrogen-responsive alopecia, 605
Estrous bone marrow hypoplasia, in fer-
    ret, 769–770
Estrus, 1270–1272
Estrus induction, 1287–1291
    gonadotropin in, 1289–1290
    gonadotropin-releasing hormone in,
        1290–1291
Ethanol ingestion, 172–173, 172t
    clinical features of, 173
    denaturing compounds and, 172t
    toxicity of, 112
    toxicology of, 172–173
    treatment of, 173
Ethanolamine, in pruritus, 567t
Ether, approximate doses of, 1374
Ether clearance test, in chylothorax, 394
Ethoxzolamide, approximate doses of,
    1374
Ethyl alcohol, approximate doses of,
    1374
Ethylene glycol, antidote for, 122t
    toxicity of, IX:206, 111
Ethylenediamine, in pruritus, 567t
Etoposide, preparation and administra-
    tion of, 477t
Etretinate, reports of usage of, 556t
Euthanasia, of whales, 725–726
Exercise, strenuous, hematuria due to,
    1120, 1121
Exfoliative cytology, sample preparation
    for, 410
Exodontia, 948–950
    in dogs, 949–950
    in multi-rooted teeth, 948–949
    in single-rooted teeth, 948
    indications for, 948
    oral-nasal fistula in, 949–950, 950–951
Exotic animals, carnivorous, immunopro-
    phylaxis in, VIII:1129
    total parenteral nutrition in, VIII:657
Exotic pets, flea control and, 591
Extracorporeal immunoadsorption, 509
Extravasation, of antineoplastic agents,
    474–475, 480
Eye. See under *Ocular; Ophthalmic*.
Eyelid, agenesis of, 659
    coloboma of, 659
    delayed separation of, 660
    dermatosis of, 678–681, 678t
    disorders of, IX:624
    histiocytoma of, 692
    laceration of, 636–637
    premature or delayed opening of, 660
    tumors of, 692–694
        cryosurgery for, 693
        immunotherapy for, 693
        in cats, 693t
        in dogs, 692t
        radiation therapy for, 693–694
        surgery for, 693

Facial fold pyoderma, 679
Factor VIII, biochemistry of, 442–443

Factor VIII deficiency, 442–445
  breeds affected in, 443
  clinical symptoms in, 443–444
  diagnosis of, 444
  genetic model of, 445
  inheritance of, 443
  therapy in, 444–445, 444t–445t
Factor IX, biochemistry of, 442–443
Factor IX deficiency, 442–445
  breeds affected in, 443
  clinical symptoms in, 443–444
  diagnosis of, 444
  genetic model of, 445
  inheritance of, 443
  therapy in, 444–445, 444t–445t
Fading kitten syndrome, 1074
Famotidine, in gastrointestinal ulcer, 915
Fanconi's syndrome, 1163–1165
  clinical signs of, 1164
  diagnosis of, 1164–1165
  etiology of, 1163–1164, 1163t
  therapy in, 1165
Fasting, effect on blood samples for endocrinology of, 969–970
  pathophysiology of, 30–31
Fat, food intake effects of, 19
Fat metabolism, in liver, 869
Fatty acid metabolism, 563, 564
Fatty acid supplements, in arthritis, 564–565
  in atopy, 563–564
  in idiopathic seborrhea, 564
Fatty liver. See Hepatic lipidosis.
Feather-picking, in birds, VIII:646
Fecal analysis, for birds, 780
  for laboratory animals, 747
  in pancreatic insufficiency, 930, 930
  in toxoplasmosis, 1113, 1113t
Feline acquired immunodeficiency syndrome, IX:436
Feline immunodeficiency virus, lymphadenopathy in, 536
Feline leukemia virus infection, abortion and infertility in, 1073
  anemia in, 427, 1072–1073
  antigen tests for, 1065–1068
    clinical applications of, 1068
    comparisons of, 1067–1068
    saliva in, 1066
    serum in, 1065–1066
    stage of disease and, 1065–1066
    tears in, 1066–1067
  cachexia in, 1072
  confirmation of, 1069–1070
    ELISA tests for, 1069–1070
    IFA tests for, 1069–1070
  fading kitten syndrome in, 1074
  feline acquired immunodeficiency syndrome and, IX:436
  fever in, 1072
  glomerulonephritis in, 1073
  hematologic consequences of, IX:488
  immunodiagnosis of, IX:448
  in ferret, 775
  infections associated with, 1071–1072
  latent, 526–529
    clinical significance of, 527
    corticosteroid therapy and, 528–529
    diagnosis of, 526–527
    epidemiologic significance of, 527–528
    horizontal transmission of, 527–528

Feline leukemia virus infection (Continued)
  latent, milk transmission of, 528
    prenatal infection with, 528
    prevalence and duration of, 527
  lymphadenopathy in, 535, 1074
  lymphoid leukemia in, 1074
  lymphosarcoma in, 1074
  neonatal, 1331
  neurologic disease in, 1073–1074
  neutropenia in, 1073
  osteochondromatosis in, 1074
  patient management in, 1069–1076
  polyarthritis in, 1073
  prevention of, 1075
  prognosis in, 1074–1075
  public health considerations in, 1075–1076
  sequential pathogenesis of, 1065
  therapy in, 1070–1071
    antiviral drugs in, 1070–1071
    biologic response modifiers, immunoabsorption, transplantation in, 1070
    passive immunotherapy in, 1070
  thrombocytopenia in, 1073
  transmission of, 526
  types of, 1069
  unifying concepts of, IX:1055
  vaccination for, 1052–1064, 1075
    adverse postvaccination reactions to, 1058
    age considerations in, 1055
    anti-FOCMA antibody production and, 1053–1054
    anti-FOCMA antibody testing in, 1057–1058
    anti-GP70 antibody production and, 1053, 1054
    antibody responses to yearly revaccination in, 1054
    approximate dose for, 1374
    complement-dependent cytotoxic antibody response in, 1064
    diagnostic testing prior to, 1060
    efficacy of, 1052–1053
    evaluation of antibody concentrations in, 1055–1056
    FeLV testing before, 1054
    in FeLV-positive cats, 1060–1061
    in high intensity exposure situations, 1055
    in maintaining FeLV-free colony, 1061
    in viremic cats, 1054–1055
    indications for, 1059
    interrupted series of, 1056–1057
    postvaccination antibody testing in, 1057–1058
    postvaccination reactions to, 1063–1064
    prevaccination antigen testing in, 1057
    prevention of latency in, 1062, 1062t
    prevention of neoplasia in, 1063
    prevention of viremia in, 1061–1062
    recommended schedule for, 1063
    results of, after 3 IM vaccine doses, 1062t
    safety and efficacy of, 1058–1059
Feline panleukopenia virus infection, in utero, 839, 839
  neonatal, 1330–1331

Feline panleukopenia virus infection (Continued)
  vaccine for, approximate doses of, 1374
Feline poxvirus infection, IX:605
Feline T-lymphotropic virus infection, 530–534
  cytopathic effects of, 530–531
  diagnosis of, 531
  etiology of, 530–531
  lymphadenopathy in, 536
  pathogenesis and clinical signs of, 531–533, 532t
  pathology in, 533
  seroepidemiology and transmission of, 533–534
  treatment and prevention of, 534
Female dogs, fertility examination in, VIII:909
  intact, alopecia in, 597
  neutered, alopecia in, 596–597
  pseudohermaphroditism in, 1266
Feminization, adrenal, alopecia in, 599–600
  hypermelanosis in, 631
  testicular, 1267–1268
Fenbendazole, approximate doses of, 1374
  in pregnancy, 1293t
Fenoxycarb, 592
Fentanyl, approximate doses of, 1374
  in chemical restraint, 66
  in pregnancy, 1294t
Fentanyl-droperidol, in cesarean section, 1322t
Fenthion toxicosis, 102–103
Fenvalerate toxicosis, 104
Ferret, 765–775
  anesthesia for, 771, 771t
  attacks on human infants by, 772
  body odor of, 772
  diet of, 773–774
  electrocardiography for, 767t
  estrogen-induced pancytopenia in, IX:762
  estrous bone marrow hypoplasia in, 769–770
  flea control for, 591
  hematologic values for, 766t
  history, physical examination, restraint for, 767
  housing for, 773
  immunization for, 767–768, 768t
  medical conditions of, 774–775
  ocular disorders in, 685
  parasites of, 770–771
  physical care of, 774
  preventive medical care for, IX:772
  reproductive physiology in, 768–769
    female and, 769
    male and, 768–769
  serum chemistry for, 767t
  species characteristics of, 766, 766t–767t
  surgery in, 771–772
  urinalysis for, 767t
Ferritin, as acute phase protein, 471
Ferrous sulfate, approximate doses of, 1375
Fertility. See Breeding management; Reproduction; Reproductive.
Fertilizers, 107

Festal, approximate doses of, 1374
Fetus, development of, radiographic
    monitoring in, VIII:947
    drug effects on, 1292, 1296–1297
    drug metabolism in, 1322
    ultrasonography of, 1241t
Fever, beneficial effects of, 50
    cat-scratch, 1099–1101
    in chemotherapy-induced myelo-
        suppression, 496
    in feline leukemia virus infection, 1072
    in neutrophil dysfunction, 523
Fiber, dietary, in diabetes mellitus,
    1010–1011
Fiberglass insulation toxicity, 112
Fibrillation, atrial, 271, 272–273, 273–
    274
    drug therapy in, 277
    ventricular, 280
Fibrin degradation product test, 455
Fibrin monomer test, 455
Fibrin/fibrinogen degradation products,
    441
Fibrinogen, as acute phase protein, 470
Fibrinogen assay, in disseminated intra-
    vascular coagulation, 454
Fibrinolytic system, 298, 298
Fibrosis, as radiation therapy complica-
    tion, 507
    pulmonary, 365–366, 368
Fibrous histiocytoma, of conjunctiva,
    676–677, 694
Fish disease, 703–720
    anesthesia for examination in, 707
    antemortem diagnostics in, 707–709
    aquarium in, 703–704
    bacterial, 717–718
        Aeromonas-Pseudomonas complex
            in, 718
        columnaris, 718
        mycobacteriosis in, 718
    behavioral signs of, 708t
    biopsy in, 707–708
    blood sampling in, 708–709
    cultures in, 708
    diagnostic approach to, 703–711
    external signs of, 709t
    fish in, 706–707
    history taking and physical examina-
        tion in, 703, 704
    mycotic, 718–719
    new tank syndrome in, 705–706
    nutrition in, 706
    parasitic, 711–717
        Amyloodinium in, 713, 716
        cestodes in, 713, 717
        Chilodonella in, 712, 713–714
        copepods in, 713, 716–717
        digenetic trematodes in, 713, 717
        Epistylis in, 712, 714
        Hexamita in, 712, 715
        Ichthyobodo necatrix in, 712, 714–
            715
        Ichthyophthirius multifiliis in, 711–
            713, 712
        monogenetic trematodes in, 713,
            717
        nematodes in, 713, 717
        Scyphidia and Glossatella in, 712,
            714
        sporozoans in, 713, 715–716
        Tetrahymena pyriformis in, 712, 714
        Trichodinids in, 712, 714

Fish disease (Continued)
    parasitic, postmortem examination in,
        709–711
    stress and, 706
    treatment of, 719–720, 720t
    viral, 719
    water quality and aquarium mainte-
        nance in, 704–706
Fistula, oral, root canal and, 955
    oral-nasal, 341, 949–950, 950–951
Fixatives, for electron microscopy, 412–
    413, 412t
Flail chest, traumatic, 198
Flank alopecia, in intact female dogs,
    597
    seasonal, 600
Flea control, 588–592
    alternative methods for, 591
    exotic pets and, 591
    for animals not on systemic organo-
        phosphates, 589t
    for animals on systemic organophos-
        phates or special needs households,
        588t
    future of products for, 591–592
    pest control operators vs veterinarians
        in, 588
    product choices for, 590t
    recommended program for, 588–591
Flea-bite allergic dermatitis, in cats,
    584–585
    in dogs, 587
    in German shepherd pyoderma, 612
Fleas, 586–588
    ivermectin in, 562
    life cycle of, 587–588
    of ferret, 771
    species of, 587
Flexibacter columnaris, in fish, 718
Fluconazole, 1103
    in aspergillosis of nasal cavity, 1107
Flucytosine, 1103–1104
    approximate doses of, 1374
Fludrocortisone, approximate doses of,
    1374
Fluid, VIII:28
    extracellular, 37
    intracellular, 37
Fluid balance, electrolyte and, glucocor-
    ticoid effects on, 54–55
    mechanisms of, 37–38
Fluid order–flow sheet, 38, 39
Fluid therapy, in blood volume expan-
    sion, 324–325, 326t
    in cardiopulmonary resuscitation, 332
    in cholelithiasis, 887
    in craniocerebral trauma, 851
    in hypoadrenocorticism, in cats, 1044–
        1045
    in pancreatitis, 896
    in poisoning, 124
    in uremia, VIII:989
    maintenance, 37–43
        additives in, 42, 42t
        caloric requirements in, 40, 41
        cessation of, 43
        equipment for, 41–42
        fluid order–flow sheet in, 38, 39
        fluid types in, 38, 40t
        fluid volume in, 38–40, 41
        in disease states, 42–43
        monitoring in, 40–41
        therapeutic plan in, 38–42

Flumethasone, approximate doses of,
    1374
    in pregnancy, 1296t
Flunixin meglumine, approximate doses
    of, 1374
    in ophthalmology, 643t–644t
    in pregnancy, 1294t
    in uveitis, 655
    pharmacology of, 51
Fluoride, antidote for, 120t, 122t
Fluoroacetate, antidotes for, 122t
5-Fluorouracil, 473
    approximate doses of, 1374
    doxorubicin, cyclophosphamide and,
        protocol, 402t
    in cancer therapy, 1368
    in soft tissue tumor, 492–493
    preparation and administration of, 477t
    toxicity of, 109
Flutter, atrial, 272
Flystrike, of pinnae, 622
Folic acid, approximate doses of, 1374
Follicle-stimulating hormone, cyclic lev-
    els of, 1275
    in sperm production, 1224
    repetitive testing of, 1285, 1285t
Follicular conjunctivitis, 676
Folliculitis, bacterial, periocular, 679
Food. See also Caloric requirements;
    Calories; Diet; Nutrition.
    canned pet, nutritional content of, 36t
    contaminated, IX:221
    human, nutrient content of, 305t
    pet, sodium content of, 307t
Food allergy, in cats, 584
    periocular pruritus in, 679
Food intake, 19–21
    central nervous system loci in control
        of, 21, 21t
    neural pathways and substances in
        control of, 19t, 20–21
Footpad, dermatosis of, 616–621, 617t
Foramen ovale, patent, echocardiogra-
    phy in, 212, 212
Foreign bodies, in aspiration pneumonia,
    381
    in larynx, 197
    in nose, 195, 340–341
    in trachea, 197
Forensic toxicology, 114–115
Formaldehyde, antidote for, 120t
Fractional shortening, formula for, 256
Fracture, in birds, VIII:630
    skull, 847–848
Fragmentocyte, in disseminated intravas-
    cular coagulation, 453, 454
Frank-Starling mechanism, 232–233,
    233
Frostbite, of pinnae, 622
Fundus, optic, congenital/neonatal disor-
    ders of, 671–672
Fungal infection, diagnosis of, VIII:1157
    ketoconazole for, 82–83
    subcutaneous and opportunistic,
        VIII:1177
    systemic, VIII:1180
Furosemide, adverse effects of, 313t
    approximate doses of, 1374
    in acute toxicant-induced renal failure,
        128
    in dilated cardiomyopathy, 247, 249t
    in hypertrophic cardiomyopathy in
        cats, 253

Furosemide (Continued)
in mitral and tricuspid regurgitation, 235
in pregnancy, 1295t
nutritional concerns with, 303
Fusobacterium, antimicrobial agents for, 1363t
antimicrobial susceptibility testing of, 73

Gallamine, in pregnancy, 1296t
Gallop rhythm, in dilated cardiomyopathy, 242–243
Gamma rays, 503
Garbage, contaminated, IX:221
Gases, toxic, IX:203
Gasoline toxicity, 111
Gastric acid hyposecretion, in intestinal bacterial overgrowth, 933
Gastric dilatation-volvulus, IX:856
Gastric intubation, in laboratory animals, 760
in llama, 735
Gastric lavage, in poisoning, 117–118
Gastric motility, reflux esophagitis due to, 908
Gastrinoma, medical treatment of, 1022–1024
Gastritis, chronic, IX:852
endoscopic biopsy in, 867
Gastroenteropancreatic system, endocrine neoplasia of, 1020–1023, 1020t
Gastrointestinal disorders, in rabbits, VIII:654
nutrition in, IX:909
parasitic, IX:921
therapeutics of, IX:862
Gastrointestinal endoscopy, 865–867
in duodenal abnormalities, 867–868
in gastric abnormalities, 867
in large intestinal disorders, 868
indications for, 867
Gastrointestinal tract, atrophy of, in total parenteral nutrition, 25
blind loop of, 933, 933
chronic bacterial overgrowth of, 933–938. See also Intestinal bacterial overgrowth.
epithelial cell turnover in, 911
glucocorticoid effects on, 60, 897–903
immune system of, 922–923
in birds, microflora of, 783–784
in llama, 735
in radiation therapy complications, 506
in stressed starvation, 31
mucosal blood flow in, 911
mucus-bicarbonate barrier of, 911
nonsteroidal anti-inflammatory drug toxicity in, 53
prostaglandins in mucosal protection in, 911–912
stagnant loop of, 933, 934
villous atrophy in, 927, 928
Gastrointestinal ulcer, 911–918
acid rebound in, 913
acid suppression in, 912
antacid drugs in, 912–913, 913t
anticholinergic drugs in, 916–917
cytoprotective drugs in, 917
due to glucocorticoid therapy, 60

Gastrointestinal ulcer (Continued)
due to nonsteroidal anti-inflammatory drugs, 53
histamine H$_2$-receptor antagonists in, 914, 914–915, 915t–916t
licorice products in, 917
proton pump inhibitors: omeprazole, 917
synthetic prostaglandins in, 917
Gastrostomy tube feeding, 33–34
percutaneous placement in, 34
surgical placement in, 33–34
Genes, resistance, in antimicrobial-resistant enteric bacteria, 1096–1097, 1096t
Genetics, of bleeding disorders, 438
Gentamicin, approximate doses of, 1374
in pregnancy, 1293t
nephrotoxicity of, IX:1146
Gerbils, diseases of, 759t
ocular disorders in, 685
sex determination in, 740t, 741
German shepherd, intestinal bacterial overgrowth in, 934
German shepherd pyoderma, 610–613
clinical features of, 610–611
diagnosis of, 611
flea-bite hypersensitivity in, 612
hypothyroidism in, 612
immune system evaluation in, 613
management of, 611–613
physical examination in, 612
pruritus in, 612
recurrent, 612–613
Gestation chart, perpetual 63–day, 1347
Giardia, antimicrobial agents for, 1363t
in birds, IX:723
in colitis, 940
in neonate, 1333
Gila monster bite, 181–182
Gingivitis, in feline leukemia virus infection, 1071–1072
Glaucoma, acute, 638
congenital/neonatal, 667
in dogs and cats, IX:656
in rabbits, 682
medical therapy in, 647–651
emergency, 648–649, 648t
lens luxation and, 647–648
maintenance, 648t, 649–650
adrenergic agonists in, 650
adrenergic antagonists in, 650
carbonic anhydrase inhibitors in, 649
miotics in, 649–650
prophylactic, 650–651
salvage, 651
Globe, proptosis of, 636
trauma to, nonsteroidal anti-inflammatory agents in, 643t
Glomerular disease, in dog and cat, IX:1132
Glomerular filtration rate, 1125
creatinine clearance for, 1125
in acute toxicant-induced renal failure, 127, 128–129
plasma decay methods for, 1125–1126
spot clearance or fractional excretion determinations in, 1126
Glomerulonephritis, hematuria due to, 1118–1119
in cats, 1172–1173

Glomerulonephritis (Continued)
in feline leukemia virus infection, 1073
medical management of, 1177–1178
natural history of, 1175
Glomerulonephropathy, associated renal failure in, 1176
control of edema in, 1175–1176
medical management of, 1174–1178
natural history of, 1174–1175
specific therapy in, 1176–1178
symptomatic therapy in, 1175–1176
thromboembolism in, 1176
Glossatella, 712, 714
Glucagon, approximate doses of, 1374
Glucocorticoids, 54–62
adrenal suppression in, 55
adverse effects of, 59t
anti-inflammatory and immunosuppressive effects of, 55–57, 897
approximate doses of, 1374
arachidonic acid release inhibition by, 1159
bases in, 54t
biologic effects of, 898–899
clinical uses of, 59–62
in central nervous disease, 59–60
in immune-mediated disease, 60–61
in shock, 61–62
comparison of agents of, 899t
gastrointestinal complications of, 902–903
gastrointestinal effects of, 897–903
hepatic toxicity due to, 882
hepatopathy due to, 900–901
in appetite stimulation, 23
in cholecalciferol toxicosis, 150
in degenerative myelopathy, 832
in glomerulonephritis, 1177
in hepatic disease, 900
in hypercalcemia of malignancy, 991
in hypoadrenocorticism, in cats, 1045
in immune-mediated nonerosive arthritis, 549–550
in inflammatory bowel disease, 901–902
in nonendocrine disease, IX:954
in pancreatic insufficiency, 932
in pancreatitis, 896, 903
initiation and maintenance of therapy with, 899t
liver and, 900–901
metabolic effects of, 54
metabolism of, 898
plasma binding and biologic effects of, 897–898
preparation types in, 899t
preparations for, 57–59, 58
comparison of, 55t, 58
injectable, 58–59, 58t
steroid esters as, 58–59, 58t, 59
structure-activity relationships in, 57–58, 58
receptors for, 899–900
water and electrolyte balance in, 54–55
Glucose, blood, in fasting, 30–31
food intake and, 19–20
in shock, 328
Glucose intolerance, in Cushing's syndrome, 1015

Glucosuria, in juvenile renal disease, 1167
in total parenteral nutrition, 29
Glycerin, approximate doses of, 1374
Glycerol, as cryoprotectant, 1252–1253
Glycopyrrolate, approximate doses of, 1374
in pregnancy, 1294t
Glyphosate toxicosis, 107
Gold therapy, in dermatology, 573–574
in immune diseases, VIII:448
in pregnancy, 1294t
in pruritus, 569
Golden retriever myopathy, IX:792
Gonadal function, tests of, 966–967
Gonadal sex, abnormalities of, 1265–1266
Gonadotropin, cyclic levels of, 1275
in estrus induction, 1289–1290
Gonadotropin-releasing hormone, in estrus induction, 1290–1291
Gonadotropin-releasing hormone challenge test, 1287–1288
Gout, in birds, VIII:635
Graft-vs-host disease, in bone marrow transplantation, 520–521
Granulocyte transfusion, in chemotherapy-induced myelosuppression, 497
Granulocyte-macrophage colony stimulating factor, in chemotherapy-induced myelosuppression, 496–497
Granulocytopenia, in chemotherapy-induced myelosuppression, 495
Granuloma, of conjunctiva, 694
Granulomatosis, in pulmonary eosinophilia, 374–375
Granulomatous meningoencephalitis, VIII:732, 854–858. See also Meningoencephalitis, granulomatous.
Gray collie syndrome, 629
Griseofulvin, approximate doses of, 1374
hepatic toxicity due to, 881
in pregnancy, 1293t
Growth hormone, basal, measurement of, 967
cyclic levels of, 1275–1276
deficiency, alopecia and, IX:1015
diagnosis of, 979
hypermelanosis in, 631
excess. See Acromegaly.
in dermatology, 604
oversecretion of, IX:1006
Growth hormone-responsive dermatosis, 978–980, 980t
Guinea pigs, diseases of, 751t–753t
ocular disorders of, 684
sex determination in, 740t, 741
Gut-associated lymphoid tissue (GALT), 922
Gyrodactylids, in fish disease, 713, 717

H₁ antagonists, in pruritus, 566–567
H₂ antagonists, in pruritus, 567
Haemobartonella infection, antimicrobial agents for, 1363t
in cats, 423–424
anemia due to, 426–427
in feline leukemia virus infection, 1072

Hair, senile graying of, 630
Hair loss. See Alopecia.
Hair pattern, sex steroid influence on, 596
Hallucinogens, antidotes for, 122t
Halogen disinfectants, 91
Halothane, approximate doses of, 1374
hepatic toxicity due to, 881
in birds, 778
in chemical restraint, 67
in pregnancy, 1294t
uterine effects of, 1301
Hamster, diseases of, 754t–755t
ocular disorders in, 684–685
sex determination in, 740t, 741
Haptoglobin, as acute phase proteins, 471
Hard pad disease, 619
Head trauma, nervous system injury and, IX:830
Hearing, structure and function of ear in, 805
Hearing aid, 806
Hearing loss. See Deafness.
Heart, auscultation of, 190
taurine and, 255
Heart block, 287–288
Heart disease, acquired, 231–240. See also individual types.
bacterial endocarditis as, 237–240
mitral and tricuspid regurgitation as, 232–237
congenital, 224–231. See also individual types.
diagnosis of, 225–229
physical examination in, 225–228, 227
signalment and history in, 225, 225t
therapy in, 229–231
hyperthyroid, in cats, IX:399
in ferret, 775
overview of treatment of, IX:319
Heart failure, captopril in, IX:334
congestive, cardiac cachexia in, 302–303
differential diagnosis of, 193
drug therapy in, nutrition and, 303–304
foods to avoid in, 306t
in atrial tachyarrhythmia, 277
in congenital heart disease, 229
in mitral regurgitation, 237
nutrition in, 302–307. See also Nutrition.
obesity and overfeeding in, 304
recipes for homemade diets in, 304t
renal and hepatic dysfunction in, 303
sodium and water retention in, 302
vasodilators in, 236–237, 237t, 309, 309
cough in, 234
maintenance fluid therapy in, 43
positive inotropic drugs in, IX:323
right-sided, in heartworm disease, 268–269
Heartworm disease, in cats, IX:420, 269–270
respiratory emergencies due to, 200
in dogs, 263–269
adulticide therapy in, 265–266

Heartworm disease (Continued)
in dogs, aspirin in, 52
caval syndrome due to, 267–268
echocardiography in, 216, 216–218
microfilaricide therapy in, 266
occult, 264–265
persistent post-therapeutic, 266
preadulticide evaluation in, 263–264
preventive therapy in, 266
pulmonary thromboembolism due to, 266–267
respiratory emergencies due to, 200
right-sided heart failure due to, 268–269
therapy in, IX:406
thiacetarsamide in, 131–134
in ferret, 770
in nondomestic carnivores, 731
Heat stroke, hematuria due to, 1121
Heinz bodies, in anemia, 426
Hemarthrosis, causes of, 436
Hematocrit, in shock, 327
Hematology, S.I. conversion factors for, 1339
Hematology laboratory, sample preparation for, 412t–417t, 413–417, 439
Hematology reference ranges, in dogs and cats, 1338
Hematopoiesis, canine cyclic, melanin disorder in, 629
extramedullary, in cats, 535
Hematoxylin and eosin stain, 410
Hematuria, 1117–1123
clinical detection of, 1117–1118
collecting and voiding system in, 1120–1121
drug-induced, 1121
idiopathic, 1120
nephroallergic, 1121
problem solving approach to, 1121–1123, 1122
recurring macroscopic, in Welsh Corgi dogs, 1120
renal, IX:1130, 1118–1119
specific causes of, 1118–1123, 1118t
trauma in, 1119–1120
types of, 1118
vesicourachal diverticula and, 1156–1157
Hemoglobinopathy, in dogs, 431
Hemoglobinuria, 1121
Hemogram, in chronic bronchitis, 365
of llama, camel, cow, horse, 737t
Hemolysis, in blood samples for endocrinology, 969, 970
in disseminated intravascular coagulation, 453, 454
in hypophosphatemia, 44–45, 45t
in laboratory samples, 412t, 415
Hemophilia A, 442–445. See also Factor VIII deficiency.
Hemophilia B, 442–445. See also Factor IX deficiency.
Hemorrhage. See Bleeding.
Hemorrhagic septicemia, acute neonatal, herpesvirus, 1314
Hemorrhagic shock, 318, 319t
glucocorticoid therapy in, 61
Hemostasis, laboratory assessment of, 439–441
sample handling in, 439

Hemostasis *(Continued)*
  laboratory assessment of, sample preparation for, 416–417, 416t–417t
    screening tests in, 439–441
    specific tests for, 441
    sequence of, 458t
Hemostatic values, in dogs and cats, 1343
Hemothorax, differential diagnosis of, 194
Henneguya, of fish, 716
Heparin, antidotes for, 122t
  approximate doses of, 1374
  effect of, on blood samples for endocrinology, 969
  in aortic thromboembolism, in cats, 297
  in disseminated intravascular coagulation, 456–457
  in pregnancy, 1295t
Hepatic disease, ammonia tolerance testing in, 874
  bile acid concentrations in, 877, 877–878
  chronic, IX:939
  copper toxicity in, 891–893
    in West Highland white terriers, 889–890
  diet therapy in, VIII:817
  drug use in, 883–884
  drug-induced, 878–884
    acute injury in, 880–882
    analgesics in, 881–882
    anthelmintics in, 880–881
    anticonvulsants in, 882–883
    antimicrobials in, 881
    chronic injury in, 882–883
    diagnosis of, 883
    human vs animal, 879–880, 880t
    idiosyncratic, 879, 879t
    inhalation anesthetics in, 881
    intrinsic, 879, 879t
    mechanisms of, 878–879, 879t
    steroids in, 882
    treatment of, 883
  glucocorticoids in, 900
  in cats, 873–878
    bile acid metabolism in, 875–878
    liver function tests in, 874
    routine laboratory testing in, 873–874
    serum bile acids in, 875
  insulin resistance in, 1018
  methimazole-induced, 1004
  platelet disorders in, 463
  pulmonary edema and, 387
  with chronic renal disease in cats, 1171
Hepatic failure, acute, IX:945
Hepatic function, biochemical evaluation of, in dog and cat, IX:924
Hepatic lipidosis, in cats, 869–873
  carnitine deficiency and, 869
  clinical description of, 870
  diabetes mellitus and, 869
  diagnosis of, 870–871
  obesity and, 869
  pathophysiologic mechanisms of, 871
  prognosis in, 873
  starvation and, 869–870
  treatment of, 871–873
Hepatic metabolism, of glucocorticoids, 900

Hepatitis, chronic, in Doberman pinschers, IX:937
  neonatal, 1330
Hepatobiliary function testing, 874
Hepatocyte-stimulating factor, acute phase proteins and, 470
  quantitation of, 470
Hepatopathic arthritis, 549
Hepatopathy, steroid-induced, 900–901
Hepatozoonosis, IX:1099
  in dogs, 421
Herbicides, IX:153, 107
Hereditary myopathy of Labrador retrievers, 820–822
  clinical signs of, 820
  control of, 822
  diagnosis of, 821
  differential diagnosis of, 821
  neurologic examination in, 820–821
  nomenclature in, 820
  prognosis in, 821
  treatment of, 821–822
Hermaphrodite, true, 1264–1265
  XX true, 1265–1266
Hernia, diaphragmatic, traumatic, 199
  hiatal, reflux esophagitis due to, 908
Herpes keratitis, in cats, 657
Herpesvirus infection, 1313–1316
  clinical samples for confirmation of, 1315t
  disease process in, 1314, *1314*
  extreme susceptibility to, 1313
  infection process in, 1313–1314
  laboratory diagnosis of, 1314–1316, 1315t
  latent, 1313–1314
  neonatal, 1329–1330
  ophthalmic, in neonatal cats, 662–663
  treatment and prognosis in, 1316
Hetacillin, approximate dose for, 1374
  in pregnancy, 1293t
Hexamita, 712, 715
Hickey-Hare test, in diabetes insipidus, 976
High-altitude, pulmonary edema due to, 387
Hilar adenopathy, 193
Hilar mass lesions, 193
Hip dysplasia, fatty acid supplements in, 565
Hippuric acid crystalluria, 1132
Histamine H_2–receptor antagonists, in gastrointestinal ulcer, *914*, 914–915, 915t–916t
Histiocytic ulcerative colitis, 940
Histiocytoma, 625–626
  fibrous, of conjunctiva, 676–677, 694
  of eyelid, 692
Histiocytosis, cutaneous, 626
  malignant, 626
  systemic, 626
Histology, sample preparation for, 410–411, 411t
Hives, 540
Hoarseness, in cardiopulmonary disease, 189
Holter electrocardiography, in dilated cardiomyopathy, 246
Hookworm infection, in neonate, 1332–1333
Hormonal hypersensitivity, 600–601
Hormonal hypomelanosis, 630

Hornet sting, 184–185
Horse, hemogram of, 737t
Household and commercial products, IX:193
Human foods, nutrient content of, 305t
Humane society veterinary practice, 85–90
  administrative aspects of, 89–90
  animal patients of, 85–87
  animal stresses in, 87
  clients of, 85
  cruelty investigations in, 89–90
  distemper in, 86
  flow chart for animal control in, 86, *86*
  food and water management in, 87
  food purchasing in, 88
  management aspects of, 88
  media and public service announcements in, 89
  medical aspects of, 85–87
  police assistance in, 89
  preventive medicine in, 86
  record keeping in, 87
  staff training program in, 88
  unadoptable animals in, 87
  vaccination in, 87
Hydralazine, adverse effects of, 313t
  approximate dose for, 1374
  in aortic thromboembolism, in cats, 298
  in dilated cardiomyopathy, 248, 249t
  in hypertension in renal failure, 1203
  in mitral regurgitation, 236, 237t
  in pregnancy, 1295t
  nutritional concerns with, 304
Hydramethylnon toxicosis, 105
Hydrocarbons, volatile, IX:197
Hydrocephalus, 842–847
  clinical findings in, 844
  diagnosis of, 844, *845*
  hereditary, 842–843
  pathogenesis of, 842–844, *843*
  perinatally acquired, 843
  terminology in, 842, *842*
  treatment of, 844–847
Hydrochloric acid, approximate doses for, 1374
Hydrochlorothiazide, approximate doses for, 1374
Hydrocodone, in tracheal collapse, 355
Hydrocortisone, approximate doses for, 1374
Hydrogen peroxide, approximate doses for, 1374
Hydroxyurea, approximate doses for, 1375
  for cancer therapy, 1369
Hydroxyzine, approximate doses for, 1375
Hyoscine butylbromide, in urinary incontinence, 1219t
Hyperadrenocorticism, IX:963
  adrenocortical neoplasia in, o,p'-DDD therapy in, 1034–1037
  diabetes mellitus and, 1026–1027
  in cats, 1038–1042
    clinical features of, 1038, 1038t
    laboratory findings in, 1039, 1039t
    pituitary adrenal function in, 1039–1041
    prognosis in, 1041–1042
    treatment of, 1041

Hyperadrenocorticism (Continued)
  insulin resistance and glucose intolerance in, 1015
  ketoconazole in, 83
  pituitary-dependent, 1024–1031
    adrenalectomy in, 1029–1030
    adrenocortical tumor vs, 1024–1025
    differential diagnosis of, 1024–1025
    hypophysectomy in, 1030
    in cats, 1041
    ketoconazole therapy in, 1028–1029
    o,p'-DDD therapy in, 1025–1028
    radiation therapy in, 1030–1031
Hyperalimentation, intravenous, 25
Hyperandrogenism, insulin resistance in, 1018
Hyperbilirubinemia, chemotherapy modifications in, 472t
Hypercalcemia, cholecalciferol-induced, 148–152. See also Cholecalciferol, toxicosis due to.
  clinical signs of, 149
  humeral, of malignancy, 988–989
  in hyperparathyroidism, 985
  malignancy-associated, 988–992
    approach to diagnosis and treatment of, 990
    diagnosis of, 990–991
    differential diagnosis of, 991
    in lymphosarcoma and apocrine cell adenocarcinoma of anal sac, 989
    pathogenic mechanisms in, 988–989
    pathophysiology of, 989–990
    prognosis after treatment of primary malignancy in, 992
    supportive management in, 991–992
  osteolytic, 988
  treatment of, IX:75
Hypercalciuria, in urolithiasis, 1184–1185, 1185t
Hypercholesterolemia, 1049
  in myxedema, 999
Hyperchylomicronemia, in cats, 1048
Hypereosinophilic syndrome, pulmonary manifestations of, 375
Hyperglycemia, food intake and, 19–20
  in total parenteral nutrition, 29
Hyperinsulinemia, endogenous, 1013
Hyperkalemia, in acute toxicant–induced renal failure, 129
  in maintenance fluid therapy, 42, 42t
  treatment of, IX:94
Hyperkeratosis, idiopathic, 619
Hyperlipemia, IX:1045
Hyperlipidemia, 1046–1050
  combined forms of, 1049
  diagnosis of, 1047–1048
  hypercholesterolemia in, 1049
  hypertriglyceridemia in, 1048–1049
  in diabetes mellitus, 1048–1049
  in miniature schnauzers, 1048
  laboratory tests in, 1047–1048
  lipoproteins in, 1046–1047
  terminology in, 1046
  treatment of, 1049–1050
Hyperlipoproteinemia, combined, 1049
Hypermelanosis, 630–632
  acquired, 631–632
  genetic, 631
  of difficult classification, 632t
  pathogenetic mechanisms of, 631t

Hypernatremia, fluid balance effects of, 37
Hyperparathyroidism, in chronic renal failure, 1195
  primary, 985–987
    clinical signs in, 986
    diagnostic aids in, 985–986
    differential diagnosis and diagnostic plan in, 985
    surgical treatment of, 986–987
Hypersensitivity, pulmonary, IX:285, 369–376
    extrinsic allergic alveolitis as, 375–376
    pulmonary eosinophilia as, 369–375
Hypersensitivity reactions, 537–543
  antigen factors in, 541–542
  diagnosis of, 542–543, 542t
  exposure factors in, 542
  host factors in, 541
  to drugs, 542, 542t
  type I, 537–540
    anaphylactoid reactions in, 539–540, 539t
    anaphylaxis in, 538–539, 539t
    mediators of, 538t
    urticaria and angioedema in, 540
  type II, 540
  type III, 540–541
  type IV, 541
Hypertension, in renal failure, beta-adrenergic agonists in, 1203
    dietary sodium restriction in, 1203
    diuretics in, 1203
    medical management of, 1201–1204
    vasodilators in, 1203–1204
  in uremia, 1136
  pulmonary, 191
    Doppler echocardiographic features of, 230t
  systemic, IX:360
    renal failure and, 1199
Hypertensive retinopathy, 690
Hyperthermia, in cancer, VIII:423
  in poisoning, 124
Hyperthyroid heart disease, in cats, IX:399
Hyperthyroidism, in cats, IX:1026
    antithyroid drugs in, 1002–1004, 1003t
    echocardiography in, 212–214, 214
    insulin resistance in, 1016
    radioactive iodine therapy in, 1007–1008
    surgical therapy in, 1005–1007
    treatment modality advantages and disadvantages in, 1003t
    with chronic renal disease, 1171
Hypertriglyceridemia, 1048–1049
Hypervitaminosis A, in turtles, 793–794, 795
Hyphema, 639
Hypoadrenocorticism, IX:972
  in cats, 1042–1045
    clinical features of, 1043t
    diagnosis of, 1044
    laboratory findings in, 1044
    pathophysiology of, 1042–1043
    primary, 1043
    secondary, 1043
    treatment of, 1044–1045
  in glucocorticoid therapy, 55

Hypoalbuminemia, corticosteroid dosage in, 898
Hypocalcemia, due to thyroidectomy, 1006
  treatment of, IX:91
Hypochlorite toxicity, 112
Hypoglycemia, IX:982
  in neonate, 1328–1329
Hypogonadism, dermatosis in, 598
Hypokalemia, in maintenance fluid therapy, 42, 42t
  in total parenteral nutrition, 29
  treatment of, IX:101
Hypokalemic polymyopathy, in uremia, 1136
  of cats, 812–815
    biochemical findings in, 812–813
    causes of, 813–814
    clinical signs of, 812, 812
    diagnostic criteria in, 813
    differential diagnosis of, 813
    neuromuscular evaluation in, 813
    nutrition and, 814
    treatment of, 814–815
    treatment response in, 815
Hypomelanosis, 628–630
  acquired, 630
  genetic, 628–630
  pathogenesis of, 629t
  primary, of difficult classification, 630
Hypomyelination, 834–837
  in Bernese mountain dog, 836–837
  in Lurcher puppies, 837
  in Samoyeds, 836
  in Springer spaniels, 834–835, 835
  in Weimaraners, 836
Hyponatremia, fluid balance effects of, 37
  in myxedema, 999
Hypoparathyroidism, IX:1039
Hypophosphatemia, 43–47
  clinical signs of, 44–46, 45t
  conditions associated with and mechanisms of, 44, 45t
  etiopathogenesis of, 44, 45t
  in maintenance fluid therapy, 42
  therapy in, 46–47, 46t
Hypophysectomy, in hyperadrenocorticism, 1030
  in pituitary macroadenoma, 1032
Hypoproteinemia, crystalloid fluid therapy and, 325
  in pulmonary edema, 385–386
Hyposomatotropism, adult onset, 604
Hypospadias, 1267
Hypothalamic-pituitary-adrenal axis, in glucocorticoid therapy, 55
  tests of, 961–965
Hypothalamus, in appetite control, 21
Hypothermia, in poisoning, 124
Hypothesis, null, 16t
  research, 16t
Hypothesis test, 15–18
  level of significance in, 16–17
  outcome of, 17
  reliability measure in, 17–18
  terminology in, 16t
  test statistic in, 17
Hypothyroidism, 602–603, 993–997
  anemia in, 428
  antithyroid hormone antibodies in, 997
  diagnosis of, 602–603

Hypothyroidism *(Continued)*
hypercholesterolemia and, 1049
in cats, 1000–1001
in German shepherd pyoderma, 612
primary and secondary, 602
severe, stupor and coma in, 998–1000
skin effects of, 602
sodium levothyroxine therapy in, 993–995
monitoring in, 994–995
response to, 994
sodium liothyronine therapy in, 995–997
therapeutic recommendations based on serum thyroid hormone levels in, 996t
therapeutic response and monitoring in, 603
thyroid hormone preparations and dosage in, 603
thyroid hormone replacement products in, 994t
Hypotrichosis, symmetric, in cats, 585–586
Hypovitaminosis A, in turtles, 791–795
Hypovolemia, in poisoning, 124

Ibuprofen, in pregnancy, 1294t
pharmacology of, 50–51
toxicity of, 108
Ichthyobodo necatrix, 712, 714–715
Ichthyophthirius multifiliis, 711–713, 712
Ichthyosis, lamellar, retinoids in, 557–558
Idioventricular rhythm, 280
Ileus, enteral nutrition in, 31–32
Illinois Animal Poison Information Center (IAPIC), 97
Illness/injury/infection energy requirement (IER), 26
Imidazole, 577–579
clinical uses of, 578
derivatives of, 82–84
mechanism of action of, 577
metabolism of, 577–578
newer, 579
side effects of, 578–579
systemic, 1102–1103
types of, 578t
Imipramine, in urinary incontinence, 1218
Immune complexes, in degenerative myelopathy, 832
in dermatomyositis, 608
in lymphocytic-plasmacytic enteritis, 923
Immune system, of gastrointestinal tract, 922–923
Immune-mediated disease, diagnosis of, IX:427
glucocorticoid therapy in, 60–61
gold therapy for, VIII:448
of blood, test interpretation in, IX:498
therapy for, VIII:443
Immune-mediated nonerosive arthritis. See *Arthritis, immune-mediated nonerosive.*
Immunization. See *Vaccination.*
Immunoadsorption, extracorporeal, 509

Immunochemical studies, sample preparation for, 417t, 418
Immunodeficiency, IX:439
feline acquired, IX:436
in anorexia, 18
in stressed starvation, 31
in Weimaraners, 524
virus, feline, 536
Immunohistochemistry, sample preparation for, 411–412, 411t
Immunologic tests, interpretation of, IX:427
Immunology, respiratory, IX:228
Immunology laboratory, sample preparation for, 417–419, 417t–418t
Immunomodulators, IX:1091
in dermatology, 570–576
Immunoprophylaxis, in nondomestic carnivores, VIII:1129
Immunoregulin, 509
in dermatology, 576
Immunostimulation, 570
Immunosuppression, glucocorticoid, 55–57
Impedance audiometry, 807–809, *808*
Incontinence, urinary, 1214–1222. See also *Urinary incontinence.*
Independent variable, 14t
Indomethacin, in pregnancy, 1294t
pharmacology of, 50
Infarction, renal, hematuria due to, 1119
Infection. See also individual organisms and disorders.
anaerobic, 1082–1085
in chemotherapy-induced myelosuppression, 496
in diabetes mellitus, 525
in neutrophil dysfunction, 522
Infectious hypomelanosis, 630
Infertility. See *Reproductive disorders.*
Inflammatory bowel disease, glucocorticoids in, 901–902
idiopathic. See *Enteritis, lymphocytic-plasmacytic.*
in cats, IX:881
Inflammatory response, *48,* 48–49
glucocorticoid effects on, 55–57, 897
Influenza, in ferret, 775
Innovar-Vet, approximate dose for, 1375
in chemical restraint, 67
Inotropic drugs, positive, in heart failure, IX:323
Insecticides, 101–106
birds and reptiles and, VIII:606
carbamate, IX:150, 103, 135–137
miscellaneous, 104–106
organochlorine, 103–104
organophosphorus, IX:150, 101–103, 135–137
pyrethrin and pyrethroid, 104, 137–140
Insemination, timing of, 1256–1257
vaginal vs uterine, with frozen semen, 1255–1256, *1256*
Insulin, approximate dose for, 1375
food intake effects of, 19
glucocorticoid effects on, 54
hypophosphatemia due to, 44, 45t
in stress-induced hyperglycemia, in cats, 29
serum, fasting, tests of, 966

Insulin resistance, 1012–1019. See also *Diabetes mellitus, insulin-resistant.*
antiinsulin antibodies in, 1018
in acromegaly, 1015–1016
in Cushing's syndrome, 1015
in hepatic disease, 1018
in hyperandrogenism, 1018
in hyperthyroidism, 1016
in obesity, 1016–1017
in pheochromocytoma, 1018
in pregnancy, 1018
in renal failure, 1017–1018
in sepsis, 1018
Insulinoma, medical treatment of, 1021–1022
Interestrus, intervals of, 1274
Interferon, as biologic response modifier, 510
in degenerative myelopathy, 833
Interleukin-1, acute phase proteins and, 470
in anorexia, 20
Interleukin-2, as biologic response modifier, 511
Intestinal bacterial overgrowth, 933–938
causes of, 933–933, *933–934*
diagnosis of, 935–936, 936t
duodenal fluid culture in, 936
pathophysiology of, 934–935
treatment of, 937–938, 938t
vitamin B12 deficiency in, 935
D-xylose absorption test in, 936
Intestinal hypomotility, enteral nutrition in, 31–32
Intestinal lymphangiectasia, IX:885
Intracardiac thrombus, echocardiography in, 212, *214*
Intracranial hemorrhage, traumatic, 847
Intradermal allergen test, 542
Intravenous infusion pump, in total parenteral nutrition, 28
Iodine, radioactive, in hyperthyroidism, 1007–1008
Iodophors, 91
Ipecac syrup, 117
Irish setters, wheat-sensitive enteropathy in, IX:893
Iron, antidote for, 120t
Iron metabolism, disorders of, IX:521
laboratory studies for, 413t, 415–416
Iron salts, antidotes for, 122t
approximate doses of, 1375
Isoflurane, in birds, 778–779
in chemical restraint, 67
in pregnancy, 1294t
Isopropanol toxicosis, 167–168
Isoproterenol, adverse effects of, 313t
approximate doses of, 1375
in pregnancy, 1295t
Isosorbide dinitrate, approximate doses of, 1375
in mitral regurgitation, 236–237
Isotretinoin, reports of usage of, 555t–556t
Isuprel, approximate doses of, 1375
Itraconazole, 84, 579, 1103
in aspergillosis of nasal cavity, 1107
in cryptococcosis, 1111
Ivermectin, 560–562
approximate doses of, 1375
clinical applications of, 561–562

Ivermectin (Continued)
  for ectoparasites in cats, 562
  for ectoparasites in dogs, 561–562
  for heartworm disease in dogs, 266
  for heartworm preventive therapy, 266
  in birds, reptiles, small mammals,
    IX:743
  in pregnancy, 1294t
  pharmacology of, 560
  safety of, 560–561
  toxic reaction to, 110, 140–142
    acute signs of, 141
    susceptibility to, 141
    treatment of, 141–142

Jejunostomy feeding, needle catheter, 34
Jenotone, approximate doses of, 1375
Jugular vein, physical examination of,
    190
  in congenital heart disease, 227

Kanamycin, approximate doses of, 1375
  in pregnancy, 1293t
Kaopectate, approximate doses of, 1375
Keratinization defects, of nose and foot-
    pads, 619
  retinoids in, 557
Keratitis, herpetic, in neonatal cats, 662
  ulcerative, 637–638, 656–658. See also
    Corneal ulceration.
Keratoconjunctivitis, herpetic, in neona-
    tal cats, 662
Keratoconjunctivitis sicca, 676
  herpetic, in neonatal cats, 662
  in radiation therapy complications, 506
  neonatal, 663–664
Keratosis, lichenoid, 615
Ketamine, approximate dose for, 1375
  in birds, 777t
  in cesarean section, 1322t
  in chemical restraint of cats, 69
  in chemical restraint of dogs, 67, 69
  in pregnancy, 1295t
Ketoacidosis, diabetic, IX:987
  hypophosphatemia in, 44, 45t
Ketoconazole, 82–84, 1103
  amphotericin B and, 83
  approximate doses of, 1375
  clinical uses of, 578
  effects of, on male dog fertility, 1225
  in aspergillosis, of nasal cavity, 1107
  in cryptococcosis, 1111
  in endocrine disorders, 83–84
  in fungal disorders, 82–83
  in hyperadrenocorticism, 1028–1029
  in pregnancy, 1293t
  metabolism of, 577–578
  pharmacology of, 82
  side effects of, 83–84, 578–579
Key-Gaskell syndrome, 689
Kidneys, disorders of. See under Renal.
  in fluid balance, 37
  in uremia, 1135–1136
Kitten, fading, in feline leukemia virus
    infection, 1074
  in group G streptococcal infection,
    1091–1093

Klebsiella, antimicrobial agents for, 1363t
Kleinfelter's syndrome, 1263

Laboratory, endocrine, sample prepara-
    tion for, 961, 968–972
  blood samples and, 968–970
  serum and plasma samples in,
    970–971
  sample transportation for, 971–972
  hematology, sample preparation for,
    412t–417t, 413–417, 439
  immunology, sample preparation for,
    417–419, 417t–418t
  oncology, sample preparation for, 410–
    413, 411t–412t
Laboratory animals, 738–765. See also
    individual species.
  blood and serum collection techniques
    for, 742–746, 743t–746t
  complete blood count and plasma
    and serum in, 744, 746
  needle-hub venipuncture technique
    in, 742
  orbital bleeding technique in, 742,
    744
  communicable diseases in, 765
  diseases of, 747, 748t–759t
  drug dosages for, 760, 762t–764t
  ectoparasite monitoring for, 746–747
  fecal analysis in, 747
  gastric intubation and artificial alimen-
    tation in, 760, 761t
  manual restraint of, 741–742
  physical examination of, 738–740, 739t
  radiography for, 747, 760t
  sex determination in, 740t, 741, 741
  surgery and anesthesia in, 761, 765t
  urinalysis for, 746
  urine collection for, 746
  virus diagnostic testing for, 746t, 747
Laboratory studies, 11
Labrador retrievers, hereditary myopa-
    thy of, 820–822
Lacrimal punctum, imperforate, neona-
    tal/congenital, 663
Lacrimal system, disorders of, IX:634
Lactated Ringer's solution, approximate
    dose for, 1375
Lactation, blood values in, for dog and
    cat, 1337
  hormonal events of, 1271
Lactobacillus, antimicrobial agents for,
    1363
Lactulose, approximate dose for, 1375
Lamellar ichthyosis, retinoids in, 557–
    558
Larva migrans, visceral, due to carni-
    vores, 701
Laryngeal disease, of dogs and cats,
    IX:265
Laryngeal muscles, function of, 345
Laryngeal nerve, anatomy of, 344–345
Laryngeal paralysis, IX:789, 343–353
  acquired, 347
  congenital, 346
  diagnosis and management of, 348–349
  history and clinical signs of, 348
  pathogenesis of, 345

Laryngeal paralysis (Continued)
  postoperative care in, 352–353
  signalment and cause of, 345–347
  treatment of, 349–352
    arytenoid lateralization and conser-
      vative partial laryngectomy in,
      352
    arytenoid lateralization in, 349–352,
      351–352
    partial laryngectomy in, 349, 350
Laryngectomy, 197
Larynx, anatomy of, 343–345, 344–345
  function of, 345
  in airway obstruction, 197
  neoplasms of, 402–403
  physical examination of, 189
Lasalocid toxicity, 111
Lasers in dermatology, 580–582
  argon dye, 581–582
    advantages of, 581–582
    application of, 582
    disadvantages of, 582
  carbon dioxide, 580–581
    advantages of, 580
    applications of, 581
    disadvantages of, 580–581
    equipment for, 581
Lavage, bronchoalveolar, bronchoscopic,
    223–224
  gastric, in poisoning, 117–118
  peritoneal, diagnostic, IX:3
Laxatives, in pregnancy, 1295t
Laxatone, approximate dose for, 1375
Lead poisoning, IX:145, 111, 152–159
  absorption, distribution, retention, ex-
    cretion in, 152–153
  age and, 153
  antidote for, 120t, 122t
  clinical signs of, 154
  diagnosis of, 155
  in cats, anemia due to, 427
  in pets other than dogs, 158
  in psittacine birds, IX:713
  laboratory findings in, 154
  pathologic findings in, 158
  prognosis in, 158
  radiographic findings in, 155
  season for, 153–154
  sources of, 153
  supportive treatment in, 158
  treatment of, 155–157
    CaNa$_2$EDTA in, 156–157
    D-penicillamine in, 157
    2,3–dimercaptosuccinic acid in, 157
    veterinarian's obligation in, 158
Lenperone, in chemical restraint, 63
Lens, contact, hydrophilic, 640–641
  diseases of, IX:660
Lentigines, melanin disorders in, 631
Leptospirosis, antimicrobial agents for,
    1363t
  due to rodents, 700
Lernaea, in fish, 713, 716–717
Leucine crystalluria, 1132
Leucovorin, approximate dose for, 1375
Leukemia, acute lymphoblastic, chemo-
    therapy and prognosis in, 487,
    488t, 1366
  clinical evaluation in, 482–483
  diagnosis of, 484
  lymphoma vs, 484t

Leukemia (Continued)
  chronic lymphocytic, clinical evalua-
      tion in, 482–483
    diagnosis of, 484
    lymphoma vs, 484t
    prognosis and treatment in, 487–488
  cytochemical markers of, 466–468,
      467t
  lymphoid, in feline leukemia virus in-
      fection, 1074
Leukemia virus infection, feline. See Fe-
    line leukemia virus infection.
Leukocyte adhesion protein deficiency,
    523–524
Leukocyte count, in chemotherapy-in-
    duced myelosuppression, 495
  in vulvar discharge, 1311
Leukocyte studies, sample preparation
    for, 415t, 416
Leukoencephalomyelopathy, in Rott-
    weiler dogs, IX:805
Levamisole, 509–510
  approximate doses of, 1375
  in dermatology, 576
  in pregnancy, 1294t
Levarterenol, approximate dose for, 1375
Levothyroxine sodium, approximate
    doses of, 1375
  in hypothyroidism, 993–995
  in myxedema, 1000
Lhasa Apso, juvenile renal disease in,
    1168
Lichenoid dermatosis, 614–615
Lichenoid keratosis, 615
Lichenoid-psoriasiform dermatosis, 614–
    615
Licorice compounds, in gastrointestinal
    ulcer, 917
Lidocaine, adverse effects of, 313t
  approximate dose for, 1375
  in cardiopulmonary resuscitation, 334
  in cesarean section, 1322
  in dilated cardiomyopathy, 246, 249t
  in pregnancy, 1295t
  in ventricular tachyarrhythmias, 284t
Lime sulfur, approximate doses of, 1375
d-Limonene toxicosis, 105
Lincomycin, approximate doses of, 1375
  in pregnancy, 1293t
Lindane toxicosis, 103
Linear association, statistical, 12, 13t
Linear regression, 14t
Liothyronine, approximate doses of, 1375
  in hypothyroidism, 995–997
Lipemia, in total parenteral nutrition, 29
Lipidosis, hepatic, 869–873. See also He-
    patic lipidosis.
Lipids, in parenteral nutrition, 27
  renal failure and, 1200
Lipocortin, 899
Lipoid pneumonia, 380–381
Lipoproteins, 1046–1047
Lipoxygenase, in arachidonic acid metab-
    olism, 1158, 1158–1159
Liquid diet supplements, 306t
Lithium, in chemotherapy-induced mye-
    losuppression, 496
Litter, frozen semen, registration of,
    1257–1258
Liver, biopsy of, VIII:813
  disease of. See Hepatic disease.
  fat metabolism in, 869

Lizards, sexual identification in, 798,
    798–801, 800–801
Llama, 734–737
  abdominocentesis in, 736
  congenital and hereditary conditions
      of, 737t
  digestive system in, 735
  examination of, 734
  gastric intubation in, 735
  hematology and clinical pathology for,
      736–737, 737t
  infectious diseases of, 736
  musculoskeletal system of, 736
  noninfectious diseases of, 737
  parasitic diseases of, 736
  preventive medicine for, 736
  restraint and handling of, 734
  sedation and anesthesia in, 735
  urogenital system in, 735–736
  venipuncture in, 734–735
Loffler's syndrome, 369–370
Lomotil, approximate doses of, 1375
Loperamide, in pregnancy, 1295t
Lung, disease of. See under Pulmonary.
  injury of, response to, IX:235
Lung compliance, in pulmonary edema,
    389
Lupus erythematosus, discoid, 618
  systemic, blood chemistry in, 546
    cutaneous involvement in, 618
    hemography in, 546
    history and physical examination in,
      543–545
    serologic findings in, 548
    treatment of, 549–551
    urinalysis in, 546
Lurcher puppies, hypomyelination in,
    837
Luteinizing hormone, cyclic levels of,
    1275
  preovulatory surge of, 1269–1270
  repetitive testing of, 1284–1285
Lyme borreliosis, 1086–1087
Lyme carditis, 248–250
Lyme disease, IX:1100
Lymph node hyperplasia, distinctive pe-
    ripheral, in cats, 536
  in feline leukemia virus infection,
      1074
Lymphadenitis, in streptococcus G infec-
    tion of kittens, 1092, 1093
Lymphadenopathy, in cats, 535–537
  in feline leukemia virus infection, 1074
Lymphangiectasia, intestinal, IX:885
  thoracic, 393, 394
Lymphocystis disease, in fish, 719
Lymphocytes, glucocorticoid effects on,
    56–57, 897
Lymphocytic-plasmacytic enteritis, 922–
    926. See also Enteritis.
Lymphoid hyperplasia, in cats, 535–537
Lymphokine, as biologic response modi-
    fier, 511
Lymphoma, 482–487
  acute lymphoblastic leukemia vs, 484t
  chemotherapy and prognosis in, 484–
      487, 485t, 1366
  chronic lymphocytic leukemia vs, 484t
  clinical evaluation of, 482–483
  clinical staging of, 483–484, 483t
  cutaneous, retinoids in, 558
  diagnosis of, 484

Lymphoma (Continued)
  epidermotropic, IX:609
  extranodal, IX:473
  hypercalcemia of malignancy in, 990
  lymphadenopathy in, 535
Lymphomatoid granulomatosis, pulmo-
    nary, 404
Lymphosarcoma, hypercalcemia of ma-
    lignancy in, 989
  in feline leukemia virus infection, 1074
  of colon, 940
  pulmonary, 192

Macroadenoma, pituitary, 1031–1034
Macrocytosis, familial, of poodles, 431
Macrophages, glucocorticoid therapy ef-
    fects on, 57
Magnesium ammonium phosphate crys-
    talluria, 1132
Magnesium hydroxide, approximate dose
    for, 1375
  as antacid, 912, 913t
Magnesium sulfate, approximate doses
    of, 1375
Magnetic resonance imaging, in birds,
    789
  in reptiles, 789
Maintenance energy expenditure, 34–35,
    35t
Malathion toxicosis, 102
Male dog, fertility in, drugs affecting,
    1224–1226
  intact, alopecia in, 598
  neutered, 597–598
  sexual dysfunction in, drugs causing,
    1226
  with palpably normal testes, alopecia
    in, 599
Male feminizing syndrome, alopecia in,
    599
Malignancy-associated hypercalcemia,
    988–992. See also Hypercalcemia,
    malignancy-associated.
Malnutrition, protein and caloric, 30
Mammals, orphaned, care and feeding
    of, IX:775
  small, calicivirus infection in, IX:1062
    ivermectin in, IX:743
    peripheral vestibular disease in,
      IX:794
    physical restraint and sexing in,
      IX:764
Mammary gland, metestrus and, 1273
Mammary hypertrophy-fibroadenoma
    complex, in cats, IX:477
Mammary tumors, in dogs, IX:480
Mange, otodetic, of pinnae, 624
Mannitol, approximate dose for, 1375
  in acute toxicant–induced renal fail-
    ure, 128
  in craniocerebral trauma, 851–852
Marihuana intoxication, 109, 175–176,
    175t
Masculinization, adrenal, alopecia in,
    599–600
  androgen-dependent, 1267–1268
Mast cell tumors, of skin, in cats, 627–
    628
Masticatory muscle disorders, 816–819
  clinical findings in, 817
  diagnostic approach in, 817, 819

Masticatory muscle disorders (*Continued*)
  histopathologic findings in, 816
  immunocytochemical findings in, 817, 818
  myositis in, 817–819
  treatment of, 817–819
Matching, statistical, 14t
MCT OIL, approximate dose for, 1375
Mean, definition of, 10t
Measles vaccine, approximate doses of, 1376
Mebendazole, approximate doses of, 1376
  hepatic toxicity due to, 880
  in pregnancy, 1294t
Mechlorethamine HCl, for cancer therapy, 1367
Meclizine, approximate doses of, 1376
Median, definition of, 10t
Megaesophagus, IX:848
  endoscopy in, 867
Megakaryocytes, hypoplasia of, 458–459
Megestrol acetate, approximate doses of, 1376
  hepatic toxicity due to, 882
  in appetite stimulation, 24
Melanin pigmentation disorders, 628–632. See also *Hypermelanosis; Hypomelanosis.*
Melanoma, epibulbar, 695
Melanosis, of conjunctiva, 676
Melatonin, approximate doses of, 1376
Melphalan, approximate doses of, 1376
  for cancer therapy, 1367
  for soft tissue tumors, 492
  preparation and administration of, 476t
Meningitis, IX:814
  aseptic, in dogs, glucocorticoid therapy in, 60
  suppurative, steroid-responsive, 60
Meningoencephalitis, granulomatous, VIII:732, 854–858
  clinical course of, 856
  clinical signs of, 856–857
  diagnosis of, 857
  differential diagnosis of, 857
  disseminated vs focal, 854
  distribution in, 854, 856
  etiology and pathogenesis of, 854–855
  glucocorticoid therapy in, 60
  incidence of, 856
  pathology in, 854, 855
  prognosis and treatment in, 857–858
Meperidine, approximate doses of, 1376
  in cesarean section, 1322t
  in chemical restraint, 66
  in pregnancy, 1295t
Mepivacaine, in cesarean section, 1322
6–Mercaptopurine, approximate doses of, 1376
  for cancer therapy, 1368
Mercury, antidote for, 120t, 121t
Metabolic acidosis, diagnosis and treatment of, IX:59
  in acute toxicant–induced renal failure, 129
  in poisoning, 124
Metabolic alkalosis, in poisoning, 124–125
Metabolic toxic retinopathy, 644–645

Metacercaria, in fish disease, 713, 717
Metaldehyde, antidote for, 122t
  poisoning, VIII:106, 106
Metamucil, approximate doses of, 1376
Metaraminol, approximate doses of, 1376
Metestrus, 1273
Methanol, antidote for, 122t
Methemoglobinemia-producing agents, antidote for, 122t
Methenamine mandelate, approximate doses of, 1376
  in urinary tract infection, 1208
Methicillin, approximate doses of, 1376
Methimazole, 1002–1005
  advantages of, 1002, 1003t
  adverse effects of, 1003t, 1004–1005
  approximate doses of, 1376
  initial treatment with, 1002–1003
  long-term treatment with, 1003–1004
DL-Methionine, approximate doses of, 1376
  toxicity of, 110–111
Methischol, approximate doses of, 1376
Methocarbamol, approximate doses of, 1376
  in pregnancy, 1296t
Methohexital, approximate doses of, 1376
  in chemical restraint, 64–65
Methomyl toxicosis, 103
Methoprene, 591–592
  toxicosis, 105–106
Methotrexate, approximate doses of, 1376
  effects of, on male dog fertility, 1225
  in cancer therapy, 1368
  in lymphoma, 485–486, 485t
  in pregnancy, 1294t
  preparation and administration of, 476t
Methoxamine, approximate doses of, 1376
Methoxyflurane, approximate doses of, 1376
  hepatic toxicity due to, 881
  in birds, 778
  in pregnancy, 1295t
Methscopolamine, in pregnancy, 1295t
Methylprednisolone, approximate doses of, 1376
Methyltestosterone, approximate doses of, 1376
Methylxanthine toxicity, IX:191, 112, 313t, 314
Metoclopramide, approximate doses of, 1376
  for nausea in chemotherapy, 481
  in aspiration pneumonia prevention, 382
  in pregnancy, 1295t
  in reflux esophagitis, 909
Metronidazole, approximate doses of, 1376
  in anaerobic infection, 1084, 1084t
  in lymphocytic-plasmacytic enteritis, 925
  in plasmacytic-lymphocytic colitis, 943
  in pregnancy, 1293t
  toxicity, 110
Metyrapone suppression test, 964–965
Mexilitine, adverse effects of, 313t
Mibolerone, approximate doses of, 1376
  hepatic toxicity due to, 882

Mice, diseases of, 756t–758t
  sex determination in, 740t, 741
Miconazole, 578, 1103
  in pregnancy, 1293t
Microbiologic techniques, for birds, 780–786. See also under *Birds.*
Microorganisms, disinfectants and, 92–93
Microphthalmia, 665–667
  in anterior cleavage syndrome, 665
  in cataract, 665–666
  in ocular dysgenesis and white coat color, 666–667
Microsporum, antimicrobial agents for, 1363t
Micturition, disorders of, 1145–1150. See also *Urination disorders.*
  normal, 1214
  spinal lesions and, VIII:722
Midazolam, in chemical restraint, 63–64
  oxymorphone and, in chemical restraint of dogs, 68
Migratory erythema, necrolytic, 680
  nose and footpads in, 620
Miliary dermatitis, in cats, IX:538, 585
Milk, maternal and substitute, composition of, 1351
  toxic or acid, syndrome of, 1332
Milrinone, approximate doses of, 1376
  in dilated cardiomyopathy, 247
Mineral and sodium restriction, homemade recipes for diet in, 304t
Mineral oil, approximate dose for, 1376
  in lipoid pneumonia, 380–381
Minimal bactericidal concentration (MBC), of antibiotic, 70–72
Minimal inhibitory concentration (MIC), of antibiotic, 70–72
  in urinary tract infection, 1206–1207
Minocycline HCl, in brucellosis, 1320
Miotics, in glaucoma, 649–650
Misoprostol, in pregnancy, 1295t
Mites, ear, of ferret, 770–771
Mithramycin, approximate doses of, 1376
  in cholecalciferol toxicosis, 151
  in hypercalcemia of malignancy, 992
Mitotane, approximate doses of, 1376
  in cancer therapy, 1369
  in pregnancy, 1296t
Mitral dysplasia, breed and sex predilections for, 225t
  Doppler echocardiographic features of, 230t
  murmur in, 225
Mitral insufficiency, echocardiography in, 201–204, 202–206
Mitral regurgitation, cardiac tamponade in, 237
  clinical signs of, 233–234
  congestive heart failure in, 237
  diagnosis of, 234–235
  differential diagnosis of, 235
  in dogs, 232–237
  incidence and pathology of, 232
  medical management of, 235–237
    initial therapy in, 235
    inotropic drugs in, 235–236
    vasodilators in, 236–237, 236t
  myxomatous degeneration in, 232
  pathophysiology of, 232–233, 233
Mitral valve, anatomy and function of, 232
  components in closure of, 232

Mixed venous O_2 content (C$v o_2$), 321t
Mode, definition of, 10t
Molluscacides, 106
Monoclonal antibodies, as biologic response modifier, 512
Morphine, acepromazine and, in chemical restraint of dogs, 68
   antidote for, 122t
   approximate dose for, 1376
   in chemical restraint, 66
   in pregnancy, 1295t
Mosaic, 1264–1265
Mouse, ocular disorders of, 683–684
N-MPG, in cystine urolithiasis, 1191–1192
Mucor, antimicrobial agents for, 1363
Mucositis, in radiation therapy complications, 506
Mucous membranes, in diagnosis of congenital heart disease, 227
   tracheobronchial, 222
Mucus-bicarbonate barrier, of gastrointestinal tract, 911
Mullerian duct syndrome, persistent, 1266–1267
Mullerian inhibiting substance, 1261
Muramyl dipeptide, 509
Murmur, in bacterial endocarditis, 238
   in mitral regurgitation, 234
   in tricuspid regurgitation, 234
   systolic, in diagnosis of congenital heart disease, 225–227, *226*
   physiologic, 227
Muscle biopsy, in dermatomyositis, 608
Muscle cramping, in Scottish terriers, VIII:702
Musculoskeletal system, of llama, 736
Mutagenesis, VIII:128
Mycobacteriosis, cutaneous, IX:529
   in fish, 718
Mycobacterium, antimicrobial agents for, 1363t
Mycoplasma, antimicrobial agents for, 1363t
Mycoplasma infertility, IX:1240
Mycosis, deep, of nose and footpads, 618
   diagnosis of, VIII:1157
   subcutaneous and opportunistic, VIII:1177
   systemic, VIII:1180
Mycosis fungoides, 618
   retinoids in, 558
Mycotoxicosis, IX:225
Myelination, 834. See also *Hypomyelination.*
Myeloid metaplasia, in cats, 535
Myeloma, hypercalcemia of malignancy in, 990–991
Myelopathy, degenerative, 830–833
   clinical signs of, 830–831
   diagnosis of, 831
   etiology of, 831–832
   pathologic findings in, 831
   treatment of, 832–833
Myeloproliferative disease, platelet disorders in, 463
Myelosuppression, chemotherapy-induced, 495–497
Myelotoxicity, due to phenylbutazone, 53
Myocardial carnitine deficiency, in cardiomyopathy, 241

Myocardial contractility, in dilated cardiomyopathy, 244, 245t
   in mitral regurgitation, 233
   in poisoning, 124
Myocardial disease, in cats, IX:380
   in dogs, IX:370
Myocarditis, pyogranulomatous, echocardiography in, 214–216, *215–216*
Myopathy, of golden retriever, IX:792
   of Labrador retrievers, hereditary, 820–822
Myositis, VIII:681
   masticatory, 817–819
Myotonia, VIII:686
Myxedema, stupor and coma in, 998–1000

Nadolol, in atrial tachyarrhythmia, 276
Nafcillin, approximate dose for, 1376
Nalbuphine, in chemical restraint, 67
Nalorphine, approximate doses of, 1376
Naloxone, approximate doses of, 1376
   in cesarean section, 1322t
   in chemical restraint, 67
   in pregnancy, 1295t
Nandrolone decanoate, approximate doses of, 1376
   in appetite stimulation, 24
Naphthalene toxicosis, 104
Naproxen, pharmacology of, 51
Narcolepsy, VIII:755
Nasal cavity, aspergillosis of, 1106–1109
   ketoconazole in, 83
   foreign body in, 195
   in airway obstruction, 196–197
   neoplasms of, 399–402
      histopathology of, 400
      prevalence of, 400t
      radiation therapy for, 504
      radiography in, 400–401
      therapy in, 401–402, 401t–402t
      tumor staging in, 403t
Nasal discharge, 337–342
   in congenital disease, 338
Nasal sinus culture, from birds, 780–781
Nasal-digital hyperkeratosis, 619
Nasal-oral fistula, *949–950*, 950–951
Nasogastric tube feeding, 32–33
Nasolacrimal system, neonatal disorders of, 663–664
Nasopharyngeal polyps, 341
Natamycin, approximate dose for, 1376
National Animal Poison Information Network (NAPINet), 97
Nausea, due to chemotherapy, 481
   food aversion in cats and, 22
   food aversion in dogs and, 22
Neck veins, physical examination of, 190
Necrolysis, toxic epidermal, nose and footpad in, 619–620
Necrolytic migratory erythema, 680
   nose and footpads in, 620
Necrotizing skin disease, VIII:473
Necrotizing vasculitis, of central nervous system, glucocorticoid therapy in, 60
Nematodes, in fish disease, *713*, 717
Neo-Darbazine, approximate doses of, 1377

Neomycin, approximate doses of, 1377
   in pregnancy, 1293t
Neonatal disease, 1325–1333
Neonatal hemorrhagic septicemia, acute, herpesvirus, 1314
Neonatal infection, bacterial, 1331–1332
   brucellosis, 1332
   canine distemper, 1330
   canine herpesvirus, 1329–1330
   coronavirus and rotavirus, 1331
   feline leukemia virus, 1331
   feline panleukopenia, 1330–1331
   feline upper respiratory disease, 1331
   infectious canine hepatitis, 1330
   parasitic, 1332–1333
Neonate, caloric requirements of, 1350
   compromised, management of, 1329
   enteral nutrition in, 31
   general care of, 1326
   in cesarean section, 1325
   morbidity and mortality in, noninfectious causes of, 1326–1329
      breeding stock in, 1327–1328, 1328t
      environmental, 1327
      hypoglycemia in, 1328–1329
   ophthalmic disorders of, 658–672. See also individual disorders.
   orphaned, 1329
   physical examination of, 1327t
Neoplasia, brain, in dogs and cats, IX:820
   cardiac, echocardiography in, 218
   central nervous system, visual deterioration in, 646
   conjunctiva, 677, 694–695
   cutaneous, retinoids in, 558–559
   endocrine, of gastroenteropancreatic system, 1020–1023, 1020t
   eye and adnexa, IX:679, 692–695
   eyelid or periocular region, 680–681, 680t, 692–694,
   hypermelanosis in, 631–632
   hyperthermia in, VIII:423
   hypomelanosis due to, 630
   infectious complications of, IX:464
   larynx and trachea, 402–403
   lung, 403–404
   mast cell, in cats, 627–628
   nasal, 340
      and footpads, 620
      nasal passages and paranasal sinuses, 399–402
   nictitating membrane, 694–695
   prostatic, 1193–1194, 1235–1237, *1237–1238*
      hematuria due to, 1121
   radiation therapy for, VIII:428
   renal, hematuria due to, 1119
   respiratory, 399–405
   testicular, alopecia in, 598
   thyroid, IX:1033
   urethral, 1161–1163
   urinary bladder, 1121
   vulvar discharge due to, 1311
   with chronic renal disease in cats, 1171
Neorickettsia, antimicrobial agents for, 1363t
Neostigmine, approximate doses of, 1377
Nephritis, chronic, in cats, 1172
   radiation, hematuria due to, 1121

Nephroallergic hematuria, 1121
Nephrolithiasis, hematuria due to, 1119, 1121. See also *Urolithiasis.*
Nephrotic syndrome, hypercholesterolemia and, 1049
Nephrotoxicity, amphotericin B in, IX:1142
  cephalosporins in, 76
  gentamicin in, IX:1146
  mechanisms of, 126–127, 126t. See also *Renal failure, acute, toxicant-induced.*
Nervous system, central. See *Central nervous system.*
  peripheral, anatomy of, *823*
Neuritis, optic, 646
Neuro-ophthalmology, 687–691
  anatomy in, 687–688, *688*
  disorders of, 688–691, 688t–690t
Neuroaxonal dystrophy, in Rottweiler dogs, IX:805
Neuroleptanalgesia, in chemical restraint of cats, 69
  in dogs, 68–69
Neurologic disease, in feline leukemia virus infection, 1073–1074
Neuromuscular system, in hypophosphatemia, 46
Neuropathy, peripheral, acromegalic, 982
  sensory, 822–827
Neutropenia, chemotherapy modifications in, 472t
  cyclic, melanin disorder in, 629
  in feline leukemia virus infection, 1073
Neutrophil, in chemotherapy-induced myelosuppression, 496
  in hypophosphatemia, 45
  morphology and physiology of, 521–522
  polymorphonuclear, glucocorticoid therapy effects on, 56
Neutrophil dysfunction, 521–525
  acquired, 525
  clinical abnormalities in, 522
  clinical management of, 523
  congenital, 523–525
  laboratory evaluation in, 522–523, 523t
  types of, 522t
Nicergoline, in urinary incontinence, 1218t
Nictitating membrane, neoplasia of, 694–695
Nifedipine, approximate doses of, 1377
Nikethimide, approximate doses of, 1377
Nitrofurantoin, approximate doses of, 1377
  in urinary tract infection, 1208
Nitroglycerin, approximate doses of, 1377
  in dilated cardiomyopathy, 247, 249t
  in mitral regurgitation, 236–237, 237t
  in pregnancy, 1295t
Nitroprusside, in mitral and tricuspid regurgitation, 236
  in mitral regurgitation, 236t, 237
  in pregnancy, 1295t
Nitrous oxide, in pregnancy, 1295t
Nizatidine, in gastrointestinal ulcer, 915
Nocardia, antimicrobial agents for, 1363t
Nocardiosis, VIII:1184
Nociception, 822, 823

Nodule, pulmonary, 191
Nominal data, 12t
Nonsteroidal anti-inflammatory drugs, 47–53
  adverse effects of, 53
  analgesic effects of, 49
  anti-inflammatory effects of, 49
  antipyretic effects of, 49–50
  azotemic renal failure due to, 1159–1160
  classes of, 50–51
  classification of, 48, 48t
  cyclo-oxygenase inhibition by, 1159
  in ophthalmology, 642–644, 643t–644t
  in pregnancy, 1297–1298
  in pruritus, 566–569
  in uveitis, 655
  mechanism of action of, 49–50, 642
  pathophysiologic effects of, 1159–1160, *1160*
  platelet effects of, 464
  therapeutic uses of, 51–53
  toxicities of, 108, 315
Norfloxacin, approximate doses of, 1377
Norwegian elkhound, juvenile renal disease in, 1168
Nose. See also *Nasal cavity.*
  dermatosis of, 616–621, 617t
  foreign bodies in, 340–341
  neoplasia of, 340
Nosocomial infection, control of, IX:19
Novobiocin, approximate doses of, 1377
N–P–K toxicosis, 107
Nuclear imaging, applications and availability of, IX:11
Null hypothesis, 16t
Nutrition. See also *Caloric requirements; Calories; Diet; Food.*
  cataract due to, congenital/neonatal, 670–671
  enteral, 30–37
    calculation of nutrient requirements in, 34–35, 35t
    definition of, 30
    flow diagram for choosing, *35*
    forced oral, 32
    gastrostomy tube, 33–34
    human products for, 36t
    in laboratory animals, 760, 761t
    indications for, 31–32
    monitoring in, 36–37
    nasogastric tube, 32–33
    needle catheter jejunostomy, 34
    orogastric tube, 32
    parenteral vs, 31
    parenteral with, 32
    pharyngostomy tube, 32
    products and methods for, 35–36, 36t
    routes of, 32–34
    for cats, 1352
    for dogs, 1348
    for ferret, 773–774
    for nondomestic carnivores, 730
    for turtles, 791, 792t–793t
  in calcium oxalate urolithiasis, 1186–1187
  in chronic advanced renal failure, 1196–1197
  in chronic hepatic insufficiency, VIII:817
  in chylothorax, 395, 397t

Nutrition *(Continued)*
  in congestive heart failure, 302–307
    dietary management in, 304–307, 304t–307t
    drug therapy and, 303–304
    foods to avoid in, 306t
    goals of, 302t
    liquid diet supplements in, 306t
    obesity and overfeeding in, 304
    pathophysiology of, 302–303
    recipes for homemade foods in, 304t
  in cystine urolithiasis, 1190–1191
  in dermatology, IX:591
  in diabetes mellitus, 1008–1011
  in fish disease, 706
  in gastrointestinal disease, IX:909
  in hepatic copper toxicosis, 892
  in hepatic lipidosis, 871–872
  in hypokalemic polymyopathy, 814
  in lymphocytic-plasmacytic enteritis, 926
  in obesity with insulin resistance, 1017
  in pancreatic insufficiency, 931
  in pancreatitis, 895–896
  in plasmacytic-lymphocytic colitis, 942
  in shock, 328
  in taurine deficiency, 261–262
  nutrient content of human foods, 305t
  parenteral, 25–29
    enteral vs, 31
    enteral with, 32
    flow diagram for choosing, *35*
    in uremic crisis, VIII:994
    indications for, 25
    manufacturers of, 28t
    partial, 25, 28, 28t
    total, 25
      administration of, 27–29, 28t
      calculation of nutrients in, 25–26, *25–26,* 25–26
      complications of, 28–29
      components of, 26–27, 27t
      compounding, 27
      cost of, 27
      discontinuation of, 28
      in exotic animals, VIII:657
      monitoring in, 28, 28t
Nutritional hypomelanosis, 630
Nystagmus, 691
Nystatin, approximate doses of, 1377

Obesity, enteral nutrition in, 31
  in congestive heart failure, 304
  in diabetes mellitus, 1008–1009
  in hepatic lipidosis, 869
  insulin resistance in, 1016–1017
Octin, approximate doses of, 1377
Ocular disorders, of ferrets, 685
  of gerbils, 685
  of guinea pig, 684
  of hamster, 684–685
  of mouse, 683–684
  of rabbits, 681–682
  of rats, 682–683
Ocular dysgenesis, anterior, 665
  microphthalmia with, 666–667
  with albinism and deafness, 664–665
Ocular emergencies, 636–639
  acute glaucoma as, 638
  acute vision loss as, 639

Ocular emergencies *(Continued)*
  corneal laceration as, 637
  corneal ulceration as, 637–638
  eyelid laceration as, 636–637
  hyphema as, 639
  orbital cellulitis/abscess as, 639
  proptosis of globe as, 636
  uveitis as, 638–639
Ocular infectious disease, IX:673
Ocular position/movement, 688
Ocular therapeutics, IX:684
Oleander, antidote for, 121t
Oliguria, in maintenance fluid therapy, 40
  in uremia, 1135
Olsalazine, in plasmacytic-lymphocytic colitis, 943
Omeprazole, in gastrinoma, 1023
  in gastrointestinal ulcer, 917
Omphalophlebitis, in streptococcus G infection of kittens, 1092
Oncologic emergencies, IX:452
Oncology laboratory, sample preparation for, 410–413, 411t–412t
Ophthalmic disorders, as radiation therapy complication, 506
  neonatal, 658–672. See also individual disorders.
  of reptiles, IX:621
  tumors of eye as, IX:679
Ophthalmology, in caged birds, IX:616
  nonsteroidal anti-inflammatory agents in, 642–644, 643t–644t
  referral in, 686–687
Opioids, in chemical restraint, 66–67, 66t
Optic fundus, congenital/neonatal disorders of, 671–672
Optic nerve, diseases of, IX:669
  hypoplasia and aplasia of, 672
Optic neuritis, 646
Oral diagnosis, 951–954
  developmental evaluation in, 951–952, 952–953
  endodontic evaluation in, 954
  interceptive orthodontics in, 953–954
Oral feeding, forced, 32
Oral fistula, root canal and, 955
Oral-nasal fistula, 341, 949–950, 950–951
Orbit, cellulitis/abscess, 639
  diseases of, VIII:577
Orbital bleeding technique, for laboratory animals, 742, 744
Ordinal data, 12t
Organ transplantation, IX:114
Organochlorine insecticides, 103–104
Organophosphorus insecticides, 101–103, 135–137
  toxicity of, IX:150, 135–137
    clinical signs of, 136
    diagnosis of, 136
    mechanism of action of, 135
    treatment of, 136–137
Orgotein, approximate doses of, 1377
  in pruritus, 568
Ornithosis, 698–699
Orogastric tube feeding, 32
Oropharyngeal diseases, of birds, IX:699
Oropharyngeal infection, anaerobic, 1082–1083
Orphans, care and feeding of, IX:775

Orthodontics, 953–954
Osmotic fragility test, in hereditary erythrocyte disorders, 433, 434
Osteochondromatosis, in feline leukemia virus infection, 1074
Osteodystrophy, renal, in uremia, 1136
Osteoradionecrosis, 506–507
Osteosarcoma, radiation therapy for, 505
Otodetic mange, of pinnae, 624
Ouabain, approximate doses of, 1377
Ovarian cycle, clinical and endocrine correlates of, IX:1214
  estrus in, 1270–1272
  hormonal events of, 1270
  interestrus and anestrus in, 1274
  metestrus in, 1273
  preovulatory LH surge in, 1269–1270
  proestrus in, 1270
  pseudopregnancy in, 1273–1274
  stages of, 1269–1274
Ovarian imbalance type I, 631
Ovarian imbalance type II, 605
Ovariohysterectomy, alopecia in, 596–597
  in pyometra, 1307
Ovary, ultrasonography of, 1240, 1240
Overfeeding, in congestive heart failure, 304
Ovulation, 1270–1272
Oxacillin, approximate doses of, 1377
  in pregnancy, 1293t
Oxalates, antidote for, 122t
Oxalic acid, antidote for, 120t
Oxazepam, approximate doses of, 1377
  in appetite stimulation, 23
Oxibendazole, hepatic toxicity due to, 880–881
Oxybutynin, in urinary incontinence, 1219t
Oxygen delivery, in shock, 326–327
Oxygen therapy, in aspiration pneumonia, 381
Oxygen transport, in shock, 320, 321t
Oxymetazoline toxicosis, 109
Oxymetholone, approximate doses of, 1377
Oxymorphone, acepromazine and, in chemical restraint of dogs, 68
  approximate doses of, 1377
  diazepam and, in chemical restraint of dogs, 68
  in cesarean section, 1322t
  in chemical restraint, 66
  in pregnancy, 1295t
  midazolam and, in chemical restraint of dogs, 68
Oxytetracycline, approximate doses of, 1377
  in brucellosis, 1319
  in pregnancy, 1293t
Oxytocin, approximate doses of, 1377
  uterine effects of, 1300–1301

P wave, normal, 271
Pacemaker. See *Cardiac pacemakers.*
Pain control, in poisoning, 125
Palate, cleft, 338
2–PAM, approximate doses of, 1377

Pancreas, endocrine, tests of function of, 966
Pancreatic acinar atrophy, 927, 928–929, 929
Pancreatic insufficiency, exocrine, 927–932
  clinical signs of, 927–928
  diagnosis of, 928–931
    bentiromide absorption test in, 929, 929–930
    fecal proteolytic activity in, 930, 930
    serum trypsinlike immunoreactivity in, 928–929, 929
  etiology of, 927
  in intestinal bacterial overgrowth, 933–934
  pathophysiology of, 927
  treatment of, 931–932
    antibiotic therapy in, 931–932
    dietary modification in, 931
    enzyme replacement of, 931
    glucocorticoid therapy in, 932
    vitamin supplementation in, 931
Pancreatin, approximate doses of, 1377
Pancreatitis, acute, VIII:810
  chronic, end-stage, 927
  glucocorticoids in, 903
  in cats, 893–896
    clinical manifestations of, 894
    etiology of, 894
    laboratory findings in, 894–895
    pathology in, 893–894
    prognosis in, 896
    treatment of, 895–896
  in diabetes mellitus, 101
  in uremia, 1138
  parenteral nutrition in, 32
  platelet disorders in, 464
Pancuronium, approximate doses of, 1377
  in pregnancy, 1296t
Pancytopenia, estrogen-induced, in ferret, IX:762
Panleukopenia virus infection, feline, in utero, 839, 839
  neonatal, 1330–1331
  vaccine for, approximate doses of, 1374
Panniculitis, VIII:471
Papanicolaou preparations, 410
Paralysis, posterior, in cardiomyopathy in cats, 252
Paranasal sinuses, neoplasms of, 399–402
  histopathology of, 400
  prevalence of, 400t
  radiography in, 400–401
  therapy in, 401–402, 401t–402t
  tumor staging in, 403t
Paraprostatic cyst, 1235, 1237
Paraquat toxicosis, 107
Parasites, in conjunctivitis, 674
  in hematuria, 1120
  in hypomelanosis, 630
  in neonate, 1332–1333
  in pulmonary eosinophilia, 374
  in reptiles, VIII:599
  of birds, VIII:641
  of blood, 419–424
  of ferret, 770–771
  of gastrointestinal tract, IX:921

Parasites (*Continued*)
  of llama, 736
  of nondomestic carnivores, 731–732
  of urinary tract, IX:1153
  therapy for, in dermatology, IX:571
Paregoric, approximates doses of, 1377
Parenteral medicine, for laboratory animals, 747, 760, 760t
Parrots, lead poisoning in, 158
Partial thromboplastin time, 440
Parturition, hormonal events of, 1273
Parvovirus, canine, antigenic variation in, 1076–1077
  enteritis, nonsteroidal anti-inflammatory drugs in, 53
  vaccine, approximate doses for. 1371
Pasteurella multocida, antimicrobial agents for, 1363t
Pasteurellosis, in rabbits, VIII:669
Patent ductus arteriosus, breed and sex predilections for, 225t
  Doppler echocardiographic features of, 230t
  echocardiography in, 208–212, *210–211*
  murmur in, 227
  surgical correction of, 230
Patent foramen ovale, echocardiography in, 212, *212*
Pea eye, in guinea pig, 684
Pelger-Huët anomaly, neutrophil abnormality in, 524–525
Pemphigus erythematosus, 618
Pemphigus foliaceus, 617–618
Penicillamine, in copper toxicity, 892–893
D-Penicillamine, approximate doses of, 1377
  in cystine urolithiasis, 1191
  in lead poisoning, 157
Penicillin, development of resistance to, 75
  in anaerobic infection, 1083, 1083t
Penicillin G, approximate doses of, 1377
  in pregnancy, 1293t
  in urinary tract infection, 1206t
Penicillin V, approximate doses of, 1377
Pentatrichomonas, antimicrobial agents for, 1363t
Pentazocine, approximate doses of, 1377
Pentobarbital, in pregnancy, 1295t
  toxicity of, 110
Pepsin, in reflux esophagitis, 907
Pepto-Bismol, approximate doses of, 1377
Peptococcus, antimicrobial agents for, 1363
Peptostreptococcus, antimicrobial agents for, 1363
Percussion, chest, 190
Perfusion, tissue, in shock, 320, 321t
Periapical abscess, 954–955. See also *Root canal.*
Pericardial disease, IX:364
Pericardial effusion, echocardiography in, 218, *218*
Pericarditis, in uremia, 1136
Periocular dermatosis, 678–681, 678t
Periodic acid–Schiff reaction, in blood and bone marrow cells, 466, 466t
  in leukemia, 467, 467t

Peripheral nervous system, anatomy of, *823*
Peripheral neuropathy, acromegalic, 982
Perirenal cyst, of cats, 1173
Peritoneal dialysis, in poisoning, 123–124
Peritoneal infection, anaerobic, 1083
Peritoneal lavage, diagnostic, IX:3
Peritonitis, anaerobic, treatment of, 1085
  infectious, in cats, IX:1059
Peritumoral halo, 630
Peroxidase activity, in blood and bone marrow cells, 465, 466t
  in leukemia, 466, 467t
Persistent hyperplastic primary vitreous, 667–668
Persistent hyperplastic tunica vasculosa lentis, 667–668
Persistent pupillary membrane, 668–669
Pest control, for nondomestic carnivores, 730–731
Petrochemicals, IX:197
Petroleum distillates, antidote for, 120t
  toxicity of, 111
Peyer's patches, 922
pH, of urine, in poisoning, 123
  in urinary tract infections, 1208
Phagocytosis, glucocorticoid therapy effects on, 56
Pharmacogenetics, 541
Pharyngostomy tube feeding, 32
Phenazopyridine, in urinary tract infection, 1208
Phencyclidine intoxication, 173–174
  clinical features of, 174
  street nomenclature for, 173t
  toxicology of, 173–174
  treatment of, 174
Phenobarbital, approximate doses of, 1377
  in hydrocephalus, 846
  in pregnancy, 1295t
Phenol, antidote for, 120t
  toxicosis of, 166–167
Phenolic compound toxicosis, 166–167
Phenolic disinfectants, 91
Phenothiazine, antidote for, 123t
  in chemical restraint, 63
  in nausea in chemotherapy, 481
  in pruritus, 567t
Phenotypic sex, abnormalities of, 1266–1268
Phenoxybenzamine, approximate doses of, 1377
  in urinary incontinence, 1219t
Phenylbutazone, approximate doses of, 1377
  in ophthalmology, 643t–644t
  in pregnancy, 1294t
  in uveitis, 655
  pharmacology of, 50
Phenylephrine, approximate doses of, 1377
Phenylpropanolamine, in urinary incontinence, 1219t
  toxicosis of, 109
Phenytoin, adverse effects of, 313t
  approximate doses of, 1377
  hepatic toxicity due to, 882–883
  in pregnancy, 1296t
  in ventricular tachyarrhythmias, 284t

Pheochromocytoma, IX:977
  insulin resistance in, 1017
Philodendron toxicity, 112
Phosmet toxicosis, 102
Phosphofructokinase deficiency, in English springer spaniels, *434*, 434–435
Phospholipase, in arachidonic acid metabolism, *1158*, 1158–1159
Phosphorus, antidote for, 120t
  in applied physiology and biochemistry, 43–44
  in maintenance fluid therapy, 42
  oral and parenteral sources of, 46, 46t
  restricted, in renal failure, 1200–1201
Photodynamic therapy, 581–582
Phthalylsulfathiazole, approximate doses of, *1378*, 1379
Physical hypomelanosis, 630
Physical restraint, for small mammals and reptiles, IX:764
Physostigmine, in ivermectin toxicity, 141–142
Phytonadione, approximate doses of, 1378
Phytotoxin, antidote for, 123t
Pigmentation disorders, melanin, 628–632. See also *Hypermelanosis; Hypomelanosis.*
Pilocarpine, in glaucoma, 649–650
Pine oil, trade names of products with, 163t
  toxicity of, 112, 168–169
Pinnae. See *Ear.*
Piperazine, approximate doses of, 1378
  in pregnancy, 1294t
  in pruritus, 567t
  toxicity of, 110
Piperidine, in pruritus, 567t
Piroxicam, pharmacology of, 51
Pitressin, approximate doses of, 1378
Pituitary adenoma, in hyperparathyroidism, 986
Pituitary dwarfism, 604
Pituitary macroadenoma, 1031–1034
  diagnosis of, 1031–1032, *1032*
  hypophysectomy in, 1032
  radiation therapy in, 1030–1031, 1032–1034
  treatment options in, 1032–1034
  treatment recommendations in, 1034
Pityrosporum, antimicrobial agents for, 1363t
Pizotyline, in appetite stimulation, 23
Placenta, drug transfer across, 1292, 1296–1297, 1322
  subinvolution of, IX:1231
Plague, 1088–1091
  animal-to-human transmission of, 1088
  bubonic, 1089
  control of, 1090–1091
  diagnosis of, 1089–1090
  due to rodents, 700–701
  historical, 1088
  in dogs and cats, 1089
  in humans, 1089
  occurrence in animals, 1088
  pneumonic, 1089
  rodent-to-dog and rodent-to-cat transmission of, 1088–1089
  septicemic, 1089
  treatment of, 1090

Plant poisoning, VIII:145, 112
　in birds and reptiles, IX:737
　ornamental, IX:216
Plasma cell pododermatitis, 620
Plasma chemical constituents, in dogs
　　and cats, 1340–1342
Plasma colloid oncotic pressure, in pul-
　　monary edema, 385–386
Plasma fibrinogen assay, in disseminated
　　intravascular coagulation, 454
Plasma samples, for endocrinology test-
　　ing, 970–971, 971
Plasmacytic-lymphocytic colitis, 939–944.
　　See also Colitis.
Plasmacytic-lymphocytic synovitis, diag-
　　nosis of, 549
　history and physical examination in,
　　544–545
　treatment of, 549–551
Plasmid, R, in antimicrobial-resistant en-
　　teric bacteria, 1097–1098, 1097t
Plastic dish syndrome, 619
Plastron, anatomy of, 789
　repair of injuries to, 790
Platelet count, 439–440
Platelet function testing, 441
Platelets, 439–440, 457–464
　acquired disorders of, 463–464, 463t–
　　464t
　drug-induced disorders of, 464, 464t
　in chemotherapy-induced myelo-
　　suppression, 495
　in disseminated intravascular coagula-
　　tion, 454
　in hypophosphatemia, 46
　increased numbers of, 461–462, 462t
　inherited disorders of, 462–463, 462t
　laboratory evaluation of, 417t
　nonsteroidal anti-inflammatory drug
　　effects on, 51–52
　normal physiology of, 457–458, 458t
　thrombocytopenia of, 458–461. See
　　also Thrombocytopenia.
Pleural effusion, differential diagnosis of,
　　192, 194
　respiratory emergencies due to, 199
Pleural infection, anaerobic, 1083
Pleural mass lesion, 191–192
Pleurectomy, in pleurodesis, 408
Pleurodesis, 405–408
　chemotherapeutic agents in, 407
　indications for, 406
　mechanism of action in, 405–406
　pleurectomy in, 408
　quinacrine in, 407
　talc in, 407–408
　tetracycline in, 406–407
Pleuroperitoneal shunt, in chylothorax,
　　398–399
Pleurovenous shunt, in chylothorax, 399
Plicamycin, for cancer therapy, 1369
Plistophora, of fish, 715
Pneumomediastinum, in traumatic pneu-
　　mothorax, 198
Pneumonia, 376–384
　aspiration, 379–382
　　chemical, 379–380
　　conditions predisposing to, 379t
　　inert substances in, 380
　　lipoid substances in, 380–381
　　particulate matter in, 380
　　prevention of, 382

Pneumonia (Continued)
　　treatment of, 381–382
　bacterial, 376–379
　　clinical findings in, 377
　　diagnosis of, 377–378
　　treatment of, 378–379
　eosinophilic, chronic, 370
　lobar, differential diagnosis of, 192
　smoke inhalation, 382–384
　　complicating factors in, 384
　　diagnosis of, 383–384
　　pathophysiology of, 382–383
　　stages of, 383t
　　treatment of, 384
Pneumonitis, chemical, 379–380
　noninfectious, differential diagnosis of,
　　192
Pneumothorax, closed chest, traumatic,
　　198
　open chest, traumatic, 198
　pleurodesis in, 406
Pododermatitis, plasma cell, 620
Poinsettia toxicity, 112
Point estimate, statistical, 14
Poisoning, 97–113. See also individual
　　toxins.
　antidotes in, 118–119, 120t–123t
　antifreeze, IX:206
　avicides in, 101
　calls to poison control center for, 98t–
　　101t
　　birds and, 100t–101t
　　cats and, 99t–100t
　　dogs and, 98t–99t
　chocolate and caffeine, IX:191
　clinical signs of, IX:132
　diphacinone, VIII:399
　elimination of absorbed toxicants in,
　　119–124
　emergency and general treatment of,
　　IX:135
　emergency intervention in, 116–117
　emergency kit for, VIII:92
　ethanol in, 112
　ethylene glycol, IX:206
　fertilizers in, 107
　forensic toxicology in, 114–115
　herbicides in, 107
　human medicines in, 107–109
　in caged birds, 113
　in nondomestic carnivores, 732
　incidence of, 97–101, 98t–101t
　insecticide. See Insecticides.
　lead. See Lead poisoning.
　metaldehyde, VIII:106
　methylxanthine, IX:191, 112
　miscellaneous chemicals in, 111–112
　molluscacides in, 106
　physical agents in, 112
　plant, VIII:145, 112
　　in birds and reptiles, IX:737
　　ornamental, IX:216
　poison control centers and diagnostic
　　labs in, 125
　preliminary client instructions in, 116
　prevalence of, IX:120
　preventing further absorption in, 117–
　　118
　　adsorbents in, 118
　　cathartics in, 118
　　emesis in, 117
　　gastric lavage in, 117–119

Poisoning (Continued)
　rodenticides in, 106–107, 143–146.
　　See also Rodenticides.
　strychnine, VIII:98
　supportive measures in, 124–125
　toad, VIII:160
　treatment of, 116–125
　veterinary medicines in, 109–111
Poliosis, idiopathic, 619
Polyarthritis, drug-induced, 545
　idiopathic, diagnosis of, 549
　　history and physical examination in,
　　543–545
　　treatment of, 549–551
　in feline leukemia virus infection, 1073
Polycystic renal disease, IX:1138
　hematuria due to, 1119
　in cats, 1173
Polycythemia, VIII:406
Polydipsia, due to glucocorticoid ther-
　　apy, 55
　in uremia, 1134–1135
　water intake monitoring in, 1025
Polymorphonuclear neutrophil, glucocor-
　　ticoid therapy effects on, 56
Polymyopathy, hypokalemia, 812–815,
　　1136. See also Hypokalemic polymy-
　　opathy.
Polymyxin B, approximate doses of, 1378
Polyps, of colon, 940
　of nasopharyngeal, 341
Polyuria, due to glucocorticoid therapy,
　　55
　in uremia, 1134–1135
Poodle, familial macrocytosis of, 431
　standard, juvenile renal disease in,
　　1168
Population, statistical, 11
Portosystemic shunt, bile acid concentra-
　　tions in, 877, 877–878
　in cats, IX:825
Portosystemic vascular anomaly, urolithi-
　　asis in, 1180–1181
Posterior paralysis, in cardiomyopathy in
　　cats, 252
Post-inflammatory hypermelanosis, 631
Post-inflammatory hypomelanosis, 630
Postmortem examination, for fish, 709–
　　711
Postpartum endometritis, prostaglandins
　　in, 1309–1310
Postpartum period, VIII:959
Potassium, in hypokalemic polymyopa-
　　thy, 812
　in maintenance fluid therapy, 42, 42t
Potassium chloride, approximate doses
　　of, 1378
Potassium citrate, in calcium oxalate uro-
　　lithiasis, 1187–1188
　in Fanconi's syndrome, 1165
Potassium iodide, antifungal, 1104
Pox, avian, VIII:633
Poxvirus infection, feline, IX:605
Prausnitz-Küstner test, 542
Praziquantel, approximate doses of, 1378
　in pregnancy, 1294t
Prazosin, adverse effects of, 313t
　approximate doses of, 1378
　in hypertension in renal failure, 1203–
　　1204
　in mitral regurgitation, 236t, 237
Precancer, IX:460

Precordial palpation, in diagnosis of congenital heart disease, 227
Prednisolone, 474
  approximate doses of, 1378
  in appetite stimulation, 23
  in beta-cell tumors, 1021–1022
  in cancer therapy, 1369
  in eosinophilic-plasmacytic enteritis, 902
  in inflammatory bowel disease, 901–902
  in pancreatitis, 903
  in pregnancy, 1296t
  in uveitis, 655
  structure of, 58
Prednisone, 474
  effects of, on male dog fertility, 1225
  in cancer therapy, 1369
  in hydrocephalus, 846
  in lymphoma, 485–486, 485t
  in tracheal collapse, 356
  in uveitis, 655
  preparation and administration of, 478t
Pregnancy, anesthesia in, 1298
  anticonvulsant therapy in, 1298
  anti-inflammatory therapy in, 1297–1298
  antimicrobial therapy in, 1297
  blood values in, for dog and cat, 1337
  clinical and endocrine correlates of, IX:1214
  diagnosis of, 1273
  drug effects on, 1291–1299
  gastrointestinal therapy in, 1297
  herpesvirus infection in, 1314, 1314
  hormonal events of, 1272–1273
  insulin resistance in, 1018
  maintenance of, luteal function and, 1272
  physiologic changes in, 1292, 1321–1322
    cardiovascular, 1321
    central nervous system, 1321–1322
    gastrointestinal, 1322
    respiratory, 1321
  post-implantation, 1272–1273
  reflux esophagitis in, 908
  safety of drugs on, 1293t–1296t
  termination of, in dogs and cats, IX:1236
  timing in relation to LH surge of, 1279t
  ultrasonography in, 1240–1242, 1241, 1241t
Preload, drug therapy effects on, 309, 309
  ventricular, in dilated cardiomyopathy, 244–245, 245t
Premature atrial contraction, 271, 272
  drug therapy in, 276
Premature ventricular contraction, 278, 279
  drug therapy in, 283–285
  in bronchoscopy, 221
Preovulatory LH surge, 1269–1270
Preputial discharge, 1257–1261
  hemorrhagic, 1259–1260
  purulent, 1260
  serous, 1260–1261
Preventive medicine, in humane society veterinary practice, 86

Primidone, approximate doses of, 1378
  hepatic toxicity due to, 882–883
  in pregnancy, 1296t
Probability, statistical, 16t
Procainamide, adverse effects of, 313t
  approximate doses of, 1378
  in dilated cardiomyopathy, 246, 249t
  in pregnancy, 1295t
  in ventricular tachyarrhythmias, 284t
Prochlorperazine, in pregnancy, 1295t
Proestrus, 1270
Progestagen, effects of, on male dog fertility, 1224
  in dermatology, IX:601
Progesterone, cyclic levels of, 1274–1275
  repetitive testing of, 1286
  serum, in estrous cycle, 1283, 1283–1284
    in fertility staging, 1286, 1287t
    measurement of, 966–967
Progestins, behavior control and, VIII:62
Prognathia, 951, 952
Prolactin, cyclic levels of, 1275–1276
Prolate toxicosis, 102
Promazine, approximate doses of, 1378
  in chemical restraint, 63
Promethazine, approximate doses of, 1378
Propantheline, approximate doses of, 1378
  in urinary incontinence, 1218t–1219t
Propetamphos toxicosis, 102
Propionibacterium acnes, 509
Propiopromazine, approximate doses of, 1378
Propoxur toxicosis, 103
Propranolol, adverse effects of, 313t
  approximate doses of, 1378
  in atrial tachyarrhythmia, 276
  in dilated cardiomyopathy, 246, 249t
  in hypertension in renal failure, 1203
  in hypertrophic cardiomyopathy in cats, 253
  in pregnancy, 1295t
  in ventricular tachyarrhythmias, 284t
Proprioception, 822, 823
Proprionic acid derivatives, pharmacology of, 50–51
Proptosis, of globe, 636
Propylthiouracil, 1002
  approximate doses of, 1378
Prostaglandins, approximate doses of, 1378
  in gastrointestinal mucosal protection, 911–912
  in postpartum endometritis, 1309
  in pyometra, 1307–1310
  in reproduction, IX:1233
  in urinary incontinence, 1218t
  renal function dependence on, 1160t
  synthetic, in gastrointestinal ulcer, 917
  uterine effects of, 1300, 1301
Prostate, abscess of, 1231, 1233–1235, 1233t, 1236
  anatomy of, 1243
  benign hypertrophy of, 1232, 1233, 1233t, 1234
  diagnosing disease of, 1227–1228
  hypertrophy of, hematuria due to, 1120
  massage of, for fluid sample, 1244–1245

Prostate (Continued)
  neoplasia of, 1193–1194
    chemotherapy in, 1194
    clinical signs of, 1193
    hematuria due to, 1121
    hormonal therapy in, 1194
    radiation therapy in, 1193–1194
    surgery in, 1194
    ultrasonography in, 1231, 1237–1238, 1237–1238
  ultrasonography of, 1227–1239
    abnormal anatomy in, 1230–1233, 1231
    biopsy in, 1237–1238
    in abscess formation, 1231, 1233, 1236
    in bacterial infection, 1233, 1234–1235
    in benign hypertrophy, 1233, 1234
    in cavitation, 1231, 1232
    in mineralization, 1233
    in neoplasia, 1231, 1237–1238, 1237–1238
    in paraprostatic cysts, 1231, 1235, 1237
    normal anatomy in, 1229–1230, 1230–1231, 1230t
    scanning procedures in, 1228–1229, 1228–1229
  urodynamics in disease of, 1151–1152
Prostatitis, bacterial, 1243–1247
  adjunctive therapy in, 1246–1247
  antimicrobial therapy in, 1207
  complications and prognosis in, 1247
  diagnosis of, 1244
  histologic examination in, 1245
  history in, 1244
  incidence and historical clues in, 1243
  laboratory evaluation in, 1244–1245
  pathophysiology of, 1243–1244
  physical examination in, 1244
  radiologic and ultrasonographic examination in, 1245
  therapy in, 1245–1246, 1246t
  ultrasonography of, 1233, 1233t, 1234–1235
Protein, acute phase, 468–471. See also Acute phase proteins.
  C-reactive, as acute phase proteins, 470–471
  catabolism of, in stressed starvation, 31
  glucocorticoid effects on, 54
  in congestive heart failure, 305–306
  in enteral nutrition, 35, 35t
  in malnutrition, 30
  in parenteral nutrition, 26–27
  induced by vitamin K absence or antagonists, IX:513
  renal failure effects of, 1199
  restricted, in renal failure, 1200
Protein A (SpA), 509
  staphylococcal production of, 610
Protein/phosphorus restriction, home-made recipes for diet in, 304t
Proteinuria, 1139–1141
  additional procedures in, 1141
  diagnostic objectives in, 1139–1141, 1140
  differential diagnosis of, 1141t

Proteinuria *(Continued)*
  in dog and cat, IX:1111
  in juvenile renal disease, 1167
  pathologic processes in, 1139
  postrenal, 1139
  prerenal, 1139
  renal, 1139
Proteus mirabilis, antimicrobial agents
    for, 1363t
Prothrombin time, 440
Proton pump inhibitors, in gastrointes-
    tinal ulcer, 917
Pruritus, VIII:499
  allergic, fatty acid supplements in, 564
  antibiotics in, 568
  antihistamines in, 566–567
  aspirin in, 567–568
  cytotoxic immunosuppressants in, 568–
    569
  gold salt therapy in, 569
  in German shepherd pyoderma, 612
  nonsteroidal anti-inflammatory agents
    in, 566–569
  orgotein in, 568
  periocular, allergic, 679
  sex hormone-responsive, 601
  tricyclic antidepressants in, 567
  vitamin E in, 568
  zinc in, 568
Pryor's reflex, 806
Pseudo-Cushing's syndrome, 978
Pseudoephedrine toxicity, 109
Pseudohermaphroditism, female, 1266
  male, 1266–1268
Pseudomonas, antimicrobial agents for,
    1363t
  bacteremia due to, 1081
  in fish, 718
Pseudopregnancy, 1273–1274
Pseudorabies, in dogs and cats, IX:1071
Psittacosis, 698–699
Psychodermatosis, IX:557
Public health considerations, antimicro-
    bial-resistant enteric bacteria and,
    1097
  in cryptococcosis, 1111
  in feline leukemia virus infection,
    1075–1076
  in sporotrichosis, 634
  streptococcus G infection of kittens
    and, 1092, 1093
Pulmonary capillary pressure, in pulmo-
    nary edema, 385
  in shock, 321–322
Pulmonary cavitation, 193
Pulmonary contusion, traumatic, 198–
    199
Pulmonary cysts, 193
Pulmonary drugs, toxicities of, 312–315
Pulmonary edema, 385–392
  acute cardiogenic, 390–391
  alveolocapillary membrane permeabil-
    ity in, 386
  capillary permeability in, 391–392
  clinical manifestations of, 387–389,
    388, 388t
  decreased plasma colloid oncotic pres-
    sure in, 385–386
  etiologic factors in, 386–387
  fulminating cardiogenic, pharmaco-
    therapy in, 244
  high-altitude, 387

Pulmonary edema *(Continued)*
  in congestive heart failure, 193
  in dilated cardiomyopathy, 243
  in liver disease and, 387
  in mitral regurgitation, 233
  in pulmonary thromboembolism, 387
  increased hydrostatic pressure in, 385
  lung function effects of, 389–390
  management of, 390–392, 391t
  neurogenic, 387
  pathophysiologic mechanisms of, 385–
    386, 385t
  pulmonary lymphatic insufficiency in,
    386
Pulmonary eosinophilia, 369–375
  bronchitic or asthmatic, 370–374
    clinical signs of, 371
    histopathology of, 370–371
    inpatient management of, 372–373
    outpatient therapy in, 372
    physical findings in, 371
    radiographic and laboratory exami-
      nation in, 371
    refractory, 373–374
    treatment in, 371–372
  chronic or prolonged, 370
  differential diagnosis of, 192–193
  occasional, 375
  parasitic, 374
  transitory or simple (Löffler's syn-
    drome), 369–370
  with angiitis and granulomatosis, 374–
    375
  with hypereosinophilic syndrome, 375
Pulmonary fibrosis, 365–366, 368
Pulmonary hypersensitivity, IX:285,
    369–376
  extrinsic allergic alveolitis as, 375–376
  pulmonary eosinophilia as, 369–375
Pulmonary hypertension, 191
  Doppler echocardiographic features of,
    230t
Pulmonary interstitial disease, 365–366
Pulmonary lymphatic system, in pulmo-
    nary edema, 386
Pulmonary lymphosarcoma, 192
Pulmonary mass lesion, 191–192
Pulmonary neoplasms, 403–404
Pulmonary nodule, 191
Pulmonary opacification, cough or dys-
    pnea without, 191
Pulmonary thromboembolism, VIII:257
  in heartworm disease, 266–267
  pulmonary edema and, 387
Pulmonary vascular resistance, 321t
Pulmonic stenosis, breed and sex predi-
    lections for, 225t
  Doppler echocardiographic features of,
    230t
  echocardiography in, 204, 207
  murmur in, 225
  surgical correction of, 231
Pulse, arterial, in diagnosis of congenital
    heart disease, 227–228
  physical examination of, 190
  venous, in diagnosis of congenital
    heart disease, 227
Pupillary light reflex, in anisocoria, 689
Pupillary membrane, persistent, 668–
    669
Pupillomotor pathway, 687–688, *688*
  lesions of, ocular signs of, 688t

Puppy. See also *Neonate.*
  shaking, 834–835, *835*
Pustular dermatoses, sterile, IX:554
P-value, 16t
Pyelonephritis, bacterial, hematuria due
    to, 1119
Pyloric hypertrophy syndrome, antral,
    918–921. See also *Antral pyloric hy-
    pertrophy syndrome.*
Pyoderma, facial fold, 679
  German Shepherd, 610–613
Pyometra, 1305–1310
  anaerobic, treatment of, 1085
  clinical pathology in, 1306–1307
  diagnosis of, 1306–1307
  long-term management of, 1310
  radiography and ultrasonography in,
    1307
  signalment, history, physical examina-
    tion in, 1306
  therapy in, 1307–1309
    in closed-cervix disease, 1309
    in open-cervix disease, 1309
    ovariohysterectomy in, 1307
    prostaglandins in, 1307–1310
      actions of, 1307
      clinical usefulness of, 1308
      drug used in, 1308
      general results of, 1309
      protocol in, 1308
      side effects of, 1308–1309
    surgical drainage in, 1307
  ultrasonography of, 1242, *1242*
Pyothorax, IX:292
  anaerobic, 1083, 1085
Pyrantel pamoate, approximate doses of,
    1378
  in pregnancy, 1294t
Pyrazolone derivatives, pharmacology of,
    50
Pyrethrin, approximate doses of, 1378
  toxic reaction to, 104, 137–140. See
    also *Pyrethroid.*
Pyrethroid, toxic reaction to, 137–140
  clinical signs of, 139
  diagnosis of, 139
  GABA and cyclic GMP effects of,
    139
  ion-channel effects of, 138–139
  mechanism of action of, 138–139
  syndromes of, 138
  toxic levels in, 137–138, 138t
  treatment of, 139–140
Pyridostigmine, approximate doses of,
    1378
Pyrimethamine, approximate doses of,
    1378
  in toxoplasmosis, 1114–1115, 1114t
Pyruvate kinase deficiency, in basenjis,
    434, 435

Quadrinal, approximate doses of, 1378
Quaternary ammonium compounds, 91–
    92
  toxicosis of, 164–165
Quibron, approximate doses of, 1378
Quinacrine, approximate doses of, 1378
  in pleurodesis, 407
Quinidine, adverse effects of, 313t
  in atrial tachyarrhythmia, 276

Quinidine (*Continued*)
in pregnancy, 1295t
in ventricular tachyarrhythmias, 284t
Quinidine gluconate, approximate doses of, 1378
Quinidine polygalacturonate, approximate doses of, 1378
Quinidine sulfate, approximate doses of, 1378

R plasmids, in antimicrobial-resistant enteric bacteria, 1096–1097, 1096t
Rabbits, castration in, 761, 765
dental problems in, IX:759
diseases of, 748t–750t
gastrointestinal disorders of, VIII:654
manual restraint of, 742
ocular disorders of, 681–682
pasteurellosis in, VIII:669
sex determination in, 740t, 741, *741*
tularemia due to, 699–700
Rabies, IX:1066
control of, 1357–1360
due to carnivores, 702
in ferret, 768
Rabies vaccine, 1357
approximate doses of, 1378
for nondomestic carnivores, 729
Radiation nephritis, hematuria due to, 1121
Radiation therapy, 502–507
as alternative therapy, 505
as optimal therapy, 504
as palliative therapy, 505
case selection in, 504–505
complications of, 505–507
early, 505–506
late, 506–507
equipment for, 502–503
in bone marrow transplantation, 519–520
in cancer, VIII:428
in multimodality therapy, 504–505
in pituitary macroadenoma, 1030–1031, 1033–1034
in prostatic neoplasia, 1193–1194
outcome in, 503–504, 503t
total dose for 50% control probability in, 503, 503t
Radiculomyelopathy, degenerative, 830
Radiographic contrast media, urinalysis and, IX:1115
Radiography, in birds, 787–788, *787–788*
in calcium oxalate urolithiasis, 1185–1186
in endodontics, 955
in fetal development, VIII:947
in laboratory animals, 747, 760t
in pyometra, 1307
in reptiles, 788–789
thoracic, IX:250, 190–191
in bacterial pneumonia, 377
in chronic bronchitis, *363*, 364
in congenital heart disease, 228–229
in dilated cardiomyopathy, 243
in heartworm disease, 264, 265
in mitral and tricuspid regurgitation, 234
in pulmonary edema, 389

Radiopaque contrast agents, adverse reactions to, IX:47
Rales, 190
Range, definition of, 10t
Ranitidine, approximate dose of, 1378
cimetidine vs, 915t
effects of, on male dog fertility, 1226
in gastrinoma, 1023
in gastrointestinal ulcer, *914*, 914–915, 915t–916t
in pregnancy, 1295t
RAST testing, in atopy, in dogs, 592–595
Rats, diseases of, 756t–758t
ocular disorders of, 682–683
sex determination in, 740t, *741*
Re-entrant supraventricular tachycardia, 273, *273*
Rectal cytology, in colitis, 940–941
Rectum, disease of, IX:916
Red cells. See *Erythrocytes.*
Red squill, antidote for, 123t
Referral, in ophthalmology, 686–687
therapy by, IX:34
Reflux esophagitis, 906–910. See also *Esophagitis, reflux.*
endoscopy in, 867
Regurgitation, in snakes, IX:749
Relative risk, 14t
Renal amyloidosis, in cats, 1173
medical management of, 1176–1177
natural history of, 1174–1175
Renal calculi, hematuria due to, 1119, 1121. See also *Urolithiasis.*
Renal cell carcinoma, hematuria due to, 1119
Renal disease, chronic, anemia in, 428
in cats, 1170–1173
age, sex, breed in, 1170, 1170t
chronic nephritis as, 1172
clinical diagnosis in, 1170–1171
glomerulonephritis as, 1172–1173
intercurrent disease in, 1171–1172, 1171t
lesion morphology in, 1171
perirenal cysts in, 1173
polycystic renal disease as, 1173
presenting complaint in, 1170, 1171t
renal amyloidosis as, 1173
definition of, 1133
in Doberman pinschers, VIII:975
in hypokalemic polymyopathy, 812–813
juvenile, 1166–1169
history and physical findings in, 1166–1167
laboratory findings in, 1167
pathologic findings in, 1167–1169
signalment in, 1166
treatment of, 1169
polycystic, IX:1138
hematuria due to, 1119
in cats, 1173
Renal dysplasia, primary lesions in, 1166
Renal failure, acute, toxicant-induced, 126–130
clinical pathology and diagnosis in, 127
glomerular filtration rate and urine production in, 128–129
management of, 127–128
mechanisms of, 126–127, 126t

Renal failure (*Continued*)
acute, toxicant-induced, treatment guidelines in, 129–130, 129t
azotemic, 1123–1124
blood urea nitrogen and serum creatinine in, 1123–1124, 1123t
due to nonsteroidal anti-inflammatory drugs, 1159–1160
cephalosporins in, 76
chronic, conservative medical management of, IX:1167
insulin resistance in, 1017–1018
chronic advanced, 1195–1198
acute deterioration in, 1196
adaptive mechanisms in, 1195–1196
management recommendations in, 1196–1198
nutrition in, 1196–1197
progressive deterioration in, 1196
chronic polyuric, in cats, VIII:1008
definition of, 1133–1134
dietary management of, 1198–1201
due to hypercalcemia, 149
hypertension in, medical management of, 1201–1204
in Fanconi's syndrome, 1164
in glomerulonephropathy, 1176
in young dogs, 1166–1169. See also *Renal disease, juvenile.*
lipids and, 1200
maintenance fluid therapy in, 40
phosphorus restriction in, 1200, 1200–1201
preazotemic phase of, 1124–1126
clearance procedures in, 1125
plasma decay methods in, 1125–1126
spot clearance or fractional excretion determinations in, 1126
urine concentration tests in, 1124–1125
protein effects on, 1199
protein restriction in, 1200
systemic hypertension and, 1199
Renal function, in dog and cat, IX:1103, 1343–1344
prostaglandin synthesis and, 1160t
Renal hematuria, IX:1130, 1118–1119
Renal hemorrhage, benign, 1120
Renal infarction, hematuria due to, 1119
Renal neoplasia, hematuria due to, 1119
Renal osteodystrophy, in uremia, 1136
Renal scintigraphy, IX:1108
Renal system, nonsteroidal anti-inflammatory drug toxicity in, 53
Reproduction. See also *Breeding management.*
drugs affecting, in male dog, 1224–1226
examination, in female dogs, VIII:909
in male dogs, VIII:956
fertility regulation in, VIII:901
in cat, VIII:932
performance, parameters of, 1328t
postpartum period of, VIII:959
prostaglandin therapy in, IX:1233
timing and physiology of, in female dog, 1269–1274, *1270–1272*
in ferret, 768–769
Reproductive disorders, diagnosis of, 1315t
in cats, VIII:936, IX:1225

Reproductive disorders (*Continued*)
  in dogs, VIII:962, IX:1225
  in feline leukemia virus infection, 1073
  mycoplasma, ureaplasma, bacterial
    causes of, IX:1240
  real-time ultrasound in, IX:1258
Reproductive endocrinology, 1282–1288.
    See also individual hormones.
  challenge testing in, 1286–1288, 1287t
  hormone levels in, 1274–1276
  repetitive testing in, 1284–1286, 1285t
  single serum sample testing in, 1283–
    1284, *1283–1284*
Reptiles, 697–698
  cryptosporidiosis in, IX:748
  imaging for, 786–789
    chemical restraint for, 786–787
    film-screen combinations for, 787
    magnetic resonance imaging for, 789
    mechanical restraint for, 787
    radiography for, 788–789
  ivermectin in, IX:743
  ophthalmic disease of, IX:621
  parasites in, VIII:599
  physical restraint and sexing in, IX:764
  plant poisoning in, IX:737
  toxic chemicals and, VIII:606
Research hypothesis, 16t
Resistance genes, in antimicrobial-resis-
    tant enteric bacteria, 1096–1097,
    1096t
Respiration. See also *Breathing; Ventila-
    tion.*
Respiratory acidosis, IX:59
Respiratory distress, 196–198
  clinical signs of, 196
  larynx in, 197
  nasal cavity in, 196–197
  nonrespiratory disorders vs, 196
  small airways in, 197–198
  trachea in, 197
Respiratory emergencies, 195–201
  life-threatening, 196–200
    arterial blood gas evaluation in, 200
    cyanosis as, 196, 196t
    heartworm disease as, 200
    pleural effusion as, 199
    pulmonary parenchymal disease as,
      200
    respiratory distress as, 196–198
    tracheostomy in, 200
    trauma as, 198–199
  non–life-threatening, 195
Respiratory immunology, IX:228
Respiratory infection, neonatal, 1331
Respiratory neoplasia, 399–404
  of larynx and trachea, 402–403
  of lung, 403–404
  of nasal passages and paranasal si-
    nuses, 399–402
Respiratory pattern, in craniocerebral
    trauma, 848, 848t
Respiratory sounds, in diagnosis of car-
    diopulmonary disease, 189
Respiratory system, in pregnancy, 1321
  physiology of, VIII:191
Respiratory tract, lower, bacteriology of,
    IX:247
Respiratory tract disease, chronic, 361–
    368
  bronchitis as, 361–365. See also
    Bronchitis.

Respiratory tract disease (*Continued*)
  differential diagnosis of, 366
  pulmonary interstitial diaease as,
    365–366
  therapy in, 366–368
  upper, in cats, 341–342
    medical management of, 337–343.
      See also individual types.
  viral, nasal cavity in, 197
Restraint, chemical, 63–70
  agents for, 63–68, 64t–66t
  dissociative agents as, 67
  drawbacks to, 69–70
  drug combinations as, 67–68
  in cats, 69
  in dogs, 68–69
  inhalants as, 67
  manufacturers and formulations of,
    64t
  opioids as, 66–67, 66t
  sedative-hypnotics as, 64–66
  time duration of techniques in, 68t
  tranquilizers as, 63–64
Reticulocyte count, in anemia, 425–426
Reticulosis, in central nervous system,
    VIII:732
Retina, diseases of, IX:669
Retina syndrome, silent, 644–645
Retinal degeneration, in rats, 683
  sudden acquired, 644–645
Retinal detachment, 645–646
  with chronic renal disease in cats,
    1171
Retinal dysplasia, 671–672
Retinoids, 553–559
  clinical applications of, 554–559
  in cutaneous neoplastic disorders,
    558–559
  in epidermal inclusion cysts, 558
  in keratinization abnormalities, 557
  in lamellar ichthyosis, 557–558
  in schnauzer comedo syndrome, 558
  in sebaceous adenitis, 558
  in seborrheic syndromes, 556–557
  in vitamin A–responsive dermatosis in
    cocker spaniels, 554–556
  mechanisms of action of, 553–554
  pharmacokinetics of, 553
  reports on usage of, 555t–556t
  side effects of, 559
Retinol, reports of usage of, 555t
Retinopathy, hypertensive, 690
  metabolic toxic, 644–645
Retrovirus, 530
Rheumatoid arthritis, differential diagno-
    sis of, 545–546
Rheumatoid factor, 547–548
Rhinitis, chronic, in feline leukemia vi-
    rus infection, 1071
  dental disease and, 341
Rhinorrhea, 337–342
Rhinosinusitis, mycotic, 338–340
Rhinosporidiosis, rhinosinusitis in, 338–
    340
Rhinotracheitis, feline viral, neonatal,
    1331
  in feline leukemia virus infection, 1071
Rhonchi, 190
Riboflavin, approximate doses of, 1378
Rima glottidis, anatomy of, 344, *344*
Ringer's solution, approximate doses of,
    1378

Ringer's solution (*Continued*)
  lactated, approximate doses of, 1375
Ringworm, due to carnivores, 702
Risk, statistical, 14t
Rocky Mountain spotted fever, IX:1080
  due to rodents, 700
  in dogs, 421–422
Rodenticides, 106–107, 143–146
  anticogulant, IX:156
  mechanism of action of, 143
  toxicity due to, 143–144, 144t
    clinical signs of, 144
    diagnosis of, 144–145
    treatment of, 144t, 145–146
  toxicology of, IX:165
  trade names of, 145t
Rodents, dental problems in, IX:759
  in transmission of plague, 700–701,
    1088–1089
  leptospirosis due to, 700
  Rocky Mountain spotted fever due to,
    700
Rompum, approximate doses of, 1379
Root canal, 956–959
  access for, 956
  apical diameter in, 957
  debriding of canal in, 957
  drying canal in, 957
  endodontic files in, 956–957
  gutta-percha in, 958
  sealing access opening in, 958–959
  sealing canal in, 957–958
Rotavirus infection, neonatal, 1331
Rotenone toxicosis, 105
Rottweiler dogs, neuroaxonal dystrophy
    and leukoencephalopathy in, IX:805

Salicylates. See also *Aspirin.*
  toxicity of, IX:524
Saline, hypertonic, dextran and, in
    shock, 328–329
Salmon poisoning disease, in dogs, 423
Salmonellosis, antimicrobial agents for,
    1363t
  due to turtles, 697–698
  in birds, VIII:637
Samoyed, hypomyelination in, 836
  juvenile renal disease in, 1168
Sample, statistical, 11–12
Saprolegniasis, in fish, 718–719
Scabies, ivermectin in, 561–562
  of pinnae, 623–624
Scaly face, in budgerigars, VIII:626
Schnauzer comedo syndrome, retinoids
    in, 558
Schnauzers, miniature, hyperlipidemia
    in, 1048
Scintigraphy, renal, IX:1108
Scleritis, nonsteroidal anti-inflammatory
    agents in, 643t
Scorpion sting, 183–184
Scotty cramp, VIII:702
Scyphidia, 712, 714
Sebaceous adenitis, retinoids in, 558
Seborrhea, ear margin, 623
  idiopathic, fatty acid supplements in,
    564
Seborrheic syndromes, retinoids in, 556–
    557

Sedative-hypnotics, in chemical restraint, 64–66
Seizures, in hypophosphatemia, 46
Semen, fresh, cold storage of, 1247–1248, 1248t
   frozen, IX:1243, 1247–1258
      acrosome morphology after thawing in, 1255
      AKC-approved collection and storage facilities for, 1257t
      collection and ejaculate fractionation for, 1250
      equilibration in cold of, 1251
      extenders for, 1249–1250, 1249t–1250t
      fertility testing of, 1253
      freezing format for, 1251–1252
      freezing rate for, 1252
      glycerol as cryoprotectant in, 1252–1253
      in vitro evaluation of, 1254
      insemination timing with, 1256–1257
      post-thaw motility measurements of, 1254, 1254–1255
      post-thaw thermoresistance of, 1255
      pregnancy success with, 1253–1254
         pellets and, 1253
         straws in, 1253
      registration of litters from, 1257–1258
      sperm numbers, concentration, dilution in extender, 1250–1251
      sperm numbers per insemination of, 1255
      thawing rate and temperature for, 1252
      vaginal vs uterine insemination in, 1255–1256, 1256
      variables affecting success rates with, 1248–1253, 1249t
Semen values, in dogs, 1345
Semilunar valve stenosis, echocardiography in, 208, 209
Senile hyperkeratosis, 619
Sensory neuropathy, 822–827
   acquired, 825–827, 826t
   clinical testing of, 823–824
   inherited, 824–825
      in boxers, 825
      in English pointers, 824
      in long-haired dachshunds, 824–825
      neuroanatomic basis of testing of, 822–823, 823
Sepsis, in total parenteral nutrition, 29
   insulin resistance in, 1018
Septic shock, 319, 328
   glucocorticoid therapy in, 61–62
   nonsteroidal anti-inflammatory drugs in, 52–53
Septicemia, acute neonatal hemorrhagic, herpesvirus, 1314
   neonatal, 1331
Septra, approximate doses of, 1379
Serum chemical constituents, in dogs and cats, 1340–1342
Serum samples, for endocrinology testing, 970–971, 971
Serum sickness, 540–541
Sex hormone–binding protein, 596
Sex steroids, physiology of, 595–596

Sexual development, 1261–1268
   chromosomal abnormalities in, 1262–1265
      hermaphrodite chimeras as, 1264–1265
      XO syndrome as, 1263–1264
      XX/XY chimera with testes as, 1265
      XXX syndrome as, 1264
      XXY syndrome as, 1263
      XY/XY chimera with testes as, 1265
   diagnosis of disorders of, 1262, 1263t
   gonadal abnormalities in, 1265–1266
      XX male syndrome as, 1266
      XX true hermaphroditism as, 1265–1266
   normal, 1261, 1262
   phenotypic abnormalities of, 1266–1268
      cryptorchidism as, 1268
      female pseudohermaphroditism as, 1266
      male pseudohermaphroditism as, 1266–1268
Sexual dysfunction, in male dogs, drugs causing, 1226
Sexual identification, in crocodiles, 801–802, 802
   in laboratory animals, 740t, 741, 741
   in lizards, 798, 798–801, 800–801
   in small mammals and reptiles, IX:764
   in snakes, 798–801, 800
   in tuatara, 802
   in turtles, 796–798, 797–798
Shaking puppy syndrome, 834–835, 835
Sheather's sugar centrifugal flotation, 1113, 1113t
Shell disease, in turtles and tortoises, IX:751
Shih tzu, juvenile renal disease in, 1168
Shock, 316–329
   acute stress response to, 317
   anaphylactic, 538–539, 539t
   cardiogenic, 318
   cardiorespiratory patterns in, 319t
   circulatory system in, 316, 317t
   classification of, 316, 317t
   compensatory mechanisms in, 317–318
   decompensatory mechanisms in, 319–320
   definition of, 316–317
   endotoxic, nonsteroidal anti-inflammatory drugs in, 52–53
   hemorrhagic, 318, 319t
      glucocorticoid therapy in, 61
   in disseminated intravascular coagulation, 453, 454
   monitoring in, 320–323
      clinical-pathophysiologic correlations in, 322–323
      laboratory data in, 322
      oxygen transport and tissue perfusion in, 320, 321t
      venous and arterial catheterization for, 321–322
   pathophysiology of, 317–320
   septic, 319, 328
      glucocorticoid therapy in, 61–62
      nonsteroidal anti-inflammatory drugs in, 52–53
   traumatic, 318–319

Shock (Continued)
   treatment of, 323–329
      antibiotics in, 328
      corticosteroids in, 327–328
      goals of, 323–324, 324t
      hypertonic saline and dextran solutions in, 328–329
      new concepts in, 328–329
      nutrition in, 328
      optimizing blood pressure and flow in, 325–326
      optimizing blood volume in, 324–325, 326t
      optimizing oxygen delivery in, 326–327
Siberian husky, laryngeal paralysis in, 346
Sick sinus syndrome, 288
Significance, statistical, 16t
Significance level, 16t
Silica gel toxicity, 112
Silver nitrate, antidote for, 120t
Sinus bradycardia, 286–287
Sinus tachycardia, 271, 272, 275
Sinuses, paranasal, neoplasms of, 399–402. See also Paranasal sinuses.
Skin. See also Dermatitis; Dermatology.
   histiocytosis of, 626
   in radiation therapy complications, 505–506
   mast cell tumors of, in cats, 627–628
   melanin pigmentation of, disorders of, 628–632. See also Hypermelanosis; Hypomelanosis.
   mycobacteriosis of, IX:529
   necrotizing disease of, VIII:473
   neoplasia of, retinoids in, 558–559
Skin bleeding time, 440
Skin cancer, photodynamic therapy in, 582
Skull fracture, 847–848
Smoke inhalation injury, 382–384
   complicating factors in, 384
   diagnosis of, 383–384
   pathophysiology of, 382–383
   stages of, 383t
   treatment of, 384
Smoke poisoning, 383
Snake bite, 177–181
   antidote for, 123t
   elapid (coral snakes), 180–181
   pit viper, 178–180
      clinical signs and diagnosis of, 179–180
      pathophysiology of, 178–179, 179
      treatment of, 180
   types of snakes in, 177–178
   venom yields and, 177t
Snakes, 697
   regurgitation in, IX:749
   sexual identification in, 798–801, 800
Sneezing, 337–342
   severe, 195
Soap toxicosis, 164
Sodium, in pet foods, 307t
Sodium bicarbonate, approximate doses of, 1379
   as antacid, 912
   in cardiopulmonary resuscitation, 333–334
   in chronic advanced renal failure, 1197

Sodium bicarbonate *(Continued)*
  in Fanconi's syndrome, 1165
Sodium chloride, approximate doses of, 1379
  in hypercalcemia of malignancy, 991
Sodium fluoroacetate, VIII:112
Sodium iodide, antifungal, 1104
Sodium iodine, approximate doses of, 1379
Sodium nitroprusside, approximate doses of, 1379
  in dilated cardiomyopathy, 248, 249t
Sodium restriction, homemade recipes for diet in, 304t
  in hypertension in renal failure, 1203
  in mitral and tricuspid regurgitation, 235
Sodium salicylate, pharmacology of, 50
Sodium sulfate, approximate doses of, 1379
Soft tissue, markers for, antigens as, 411t, 412
  tumors of, chemotherapy in, 489–493
Solar dermatitis, of pinnae, 623
Solar-induced lesions, of nose, 620
Somatostatin, 1021
  approximate doses of, 1379
Somatostatin analogue, in beta-cell tumors, 1021–1022, 1023t
  in gastrinoma, 1023–1024
Spectinomycin, approximate doses of, 1379
Sperm, frozen. See *Semen, frozen.*
  production of, endocrinology of, 1224
Spider bite, 182–183
  Latrodectus (black and red widow), 182–183
  Loxosceles (brown recluse and fiddle back), 183
Spinal cord, trauma of, glucocorticoid therapy for, 60
Spinal lesions, micturition and, VIII:722
Spironolactone, effects on male dog fertility of, 1226
  nutritional concerns with, 303
Splenomegaly, in ferret, 775
Spondylopathy, caudal cervical, 858
Sporotrichosis, clinical features of, 633
  diagnosis of, 633–634
  etiology of, 633
  public health considerations in, 633
  treatment of, 634
Sporozoans, of fish, *713*, 715–716
Springer spaniels, hypomyelination in, 834–835, *835*
Sputum analysis, in chronic bronchitis, 362, 364
Squamous cell carcinoma, of nose and footpads, 620
Stains, for blood smears, 413t, 415
  histologic, 410–411, 411t
Standard deviation, definition of, 10t
Stanozolol, approximate doses of, 1379
  in appetite stimulation, 24
  in pregnancy, 1296t
Staphage Lysate, in dermatology, 575–576
Staphylococcal antigens, in dermatology, 575–576
Staphylococcus, ecology of, 609–610
  heteroresistant, antimicrobial susceptibility testing of, 74

Staphylococcus *(Continued)*
  penicillin G resistance of, 74
Staphylococcus aureus, antimicrobial agents for, 1364t
Staphylococcus intermedius, 609–610
  bacteremia due to, 1081
Starvation, hepatic lipidosis in, 869–870
  nonstressed, 30–31
  pathophysiology of, 30–31
  stressed, 31
Statistical error, type I, 16t
  type II, 16t
Statistics, 8–9
  analytical, 11–13
    association between variables in, 12, 12t–13t
    data types in, 12, 12t
    differences between groups in, 12–13, 13t
    linear association in, 12, 13t
    population in, 11
    sample in, 11–12
    terminology in, 14t
  descriptive, 9
  flow diagram for, *15*
  in clinical studies, 8
  inferential, 9, 13–18
    confidence interval in, 14
    hypothesis test in, 15–18
      level of significance in, 16–17
      measure of reliability in, 17–18
      outcome in, 17
      terminology in, 16t
      test statistic in, 17
    point estimate in, 14
  summary, 9, 10t
  terminology in, 10t
Steroids, effects on male dog fertility of, 1224–1225
Stertor, 342, 342t
Sting, bee, wasp, hornet, ant, 184–185
  scorpion, 183–184
Stomatitis, IX:846
  in feline leukemia virus infection, 1071–1072
  in uremia, 1134
Stomatocytosis, 433, *434*
Strabismus, 691
Streptococcus, antimicrobial agents for, 1364t
Streptococcus A infection, in dogs and cats, 1094–1095
Streptococcus G infection, in kittens, 1091–1093
  clinical syndrome of, 1091–1092
  diagnosis in, 1092–1093
  necropsy findings in, 1092
  pathogenesis and immunity in, 1091
  public health significance of, 1093
  treatment and control of, 1093
Streptokinase, in aortic thromboembolism, in cats, 298
Streptomycin, in brucellosis, 1319
  in pregnancy, 1293t
Streptozotocin, in beta-cell tumors, 1022
Stress, effect of, on blood samples for endocrinology, 969–970
  in fish disease, 706
Stridor, 342t, 343
Stroke volume, 321t
Strontium, antidote for, 123t
Strychnine, antidote for, 123t

Strychnine toxicosis, VIII:98, 106
Stupor, myxedema in, 998–1000
Styrid Caricide, approximate doses of, 1379
Subaortic stenosis, breed and sex predilections for, 225t
  Doppler echocardiographic features of, 230t
  murmur in, 225, 227
Succinylcholine, in pregnancy, 1296t
Sucralfate, approximate doses of, 1379
  in gastrointestinal ulcer, 915–916
  in pregnancy, 1295t
  in reflux esophagitis, 909
Sudanophilic granules, in blood and bone marrow cells, 465, 466t
Sulfadiazine, approximate doses of, 1379, 1380
Sulfadimethoxine, approximate doses of, 1379
Sulfalazine, in dermatology, 572–573
Sulfamerazine, approximate doses of, 1379
Sulfamethazine, approximate doses of, 1379
Sulfamethizole, approximate doses of, 1379
Sulfasalazine, approximate doses of, 1379
  in plasmacytic-lymphocytic colitis, 943
  in pregnancy, 1295t
Sulfathalidine, approximate doses of, 1379
Sulfisoxazole, approximate doses of, 1379
Sulfonamide, in anaerobic infection, 1085
  in dermatology, IX:606
  in pregnancy, 1293t
Sulfones, in dermatology, IX:606
Sulindac, renal-sparing aspects of, 1160
Supraventricular tachycardia, re-entrant, 273, *273*
  drug therapy in, 277
Suramin, in feline leukemia virus infection, 1071
Surgery, prophylactic antimicrobial agents for, IX:24
Sutton's halo, 630
Symblepharon, conjunctival, 675
Synovial fluid analysis, 546–547
  in dogs and cats, 1344
Synovitis, plasmacytic-lymphocytic, diagnosis of, 549
  history and physical examination in, 544–545
  treatment of, 549–551
Système International conversion factors, 1339

Tachyarrhythmia, atrial, 271–278. See also *Atrial tachyarrhythmia.*
Tachycardia, atrial, 271–272, *273*
  re-entrant supraventricular, 273, *273*
  sinus, 271, 272, 275
  supraventricular, re-entrant, drug therapy in, 277
  ventricular, 278–280, *279*
  drug therapy in, 283–285
Talc, in pleurodesis, 407–408
Tamponade, cardiac, echocardiography in, *217*, 218
  in mitral regurgitation, 237

Tannic acid, approximate dose of, 1379
Tan-Sal, approximate doses of, 1379
Taurine, 254–256
    approximate dose of, 1379
    cat and, 255, 255t
    chemical structure of, 254, *254*
    deficiency, dietary recommendations
        in, 261–262
        in myocardial failure, 255–256
        treatment of, 260–261
    heart and, 255
    in parenteral nutrition, 26–27
    metabolic pathway of, 255, *255*
    physiologic functions of, 254–255
Telazol, in chemical restraint, 67–68
    of cats, 69
    of dogs, 69
Telogen defluxion, in intact female dogs,
    597
Temaril-P, approximate doses of, 1379
Temperature, body, in poisoning, 124
Teratogenesis, VIII:128
Terbutaline, adverse effects of, 313t
    approximate doses of, 1379
    in urinary incontinence, 1219t
Terrapin. See *Turtle.*
Test statistic, 16t
Testes, cryptorchid, alopecia in, 597–598
    neoplasia of, alopecia in, 598
    palpably normal, alopecia in, 599
    XX/XY chimera with, 1265
Testicular feminization, 1267–1268
Testosterone, approximate doses of, 1379
    in normal sexual development, 1261
    in pregnancy, 1296t
    in sperm production, 1224
    serum, ketoconazole in suppression of,
        83
        measurement of, 967
        samples of, 1284, *1284*
Testosterone cypionate, in urinary incon-
    tinence, 1219t
Testosterone propionate, in urinary in-
    continence, 1219t
Testosterone-responsive dermatosis,
    605–606
Tetanus, VIII:705
Tetanus antitoxin, approximate doses of,
    1379
Tetrachlorvinphos toxicosis, 102
Tetracycline, approximate doses of, 1379
    hepatic toxicity due to, 881
    in brucellosis, 1319
    in pleurodesis, 406–407
    in pregnancy, 1293t
    in pruritus, 568
    in urinary tract infection, 1206t
Tetrahymena pyriformis, 712, 714
Tetralogy of Fallot, breed and sex predi-
    lections for, 225t
    Doppler echocardiographic features of,
        230t
    murmur in, 227
    surgical correction of, 231
2,3,2–Tetramine, in copper toxicity, 893
Thallium, antidote for, 123t
Thenium, in pregnancy, 1294t
Thenium closylate, approximate doses of,
    1379
Theophylline, approximate doses of,
    1379
    in chronic bronchitis, 367

Theophylline *(Continued)*
    in pregnancy, 1295t
    in tracheal collapse, 355–356
    toxicities of, 313t, 314
Therapy by referral, IX:34
Thiabendazole, approximate doses of,
    1379
    in aspergillosis of nasal cavity, 1107
    in pregnancy, 1294t
Thiacetarsamide, 132–134
    algorithm for management of, 132, *133*
    approximate dose of, 1379
    chemistry and excretion of, 131
    evaluation before treatment with, 131–
        132
    hepatic toxicity due to, 880
    in heartworm disease, in cats, 270
        in dogs, 265–266
    in pregnancy, 1294t
    indications for, 131
    treatment with, 134
Thiamine, approximate doses of, 1379
    deficiency, in cats, 813
Thiamylal, approximate doses of, 1379
    in chemical restraint, 64–65
    in pregnancy, 1295t
Thiazide diuretics, adverse effects of,
    313t
    in calcium oxalate urolithiasis, 1187
    in diabetes insipidus, 977
    in pregnancy, 1295t
    nutritional concerns with, 303
Thiobarbiturates, in chemical restraint of
    cats, 69
6–Thioguanine, approximate doses of,
    1379
    in cancer therapy, 1368
Thiopental, in chemical restraint, 64–65
    in pregnancy, 1295t
ThioTEPA, approximate doses of, 1379
Thoracic duct ligation, in cat, 397–398
    in dog, 396–397, *397–398*
Thoracic duct lymph, 394t
Thoracic lymphangiectasia, 393, *394*
Thoracic radiography. See *Radiography,*
    thoracic.
Thoracotomy, in cardiopulmonary resus-
    citation, 332, 333
Thorax. See *Chest.*
Thrombin clotting time, 440–441
Thrombocythemia, 462
Thrombocytopenia, 458–461
    antiplatelet antibody in, 441
    chemotherapy modifications in, 472t
    classification by pathogenesis of, 458t
    deficient or ineffective thrombopoiesis
        in, 458–459, 459t
    due to destruction or abnormal distri-
        bution of platelets in, 459–461, 460t
    due to drugs, 459t
    immunologic, 459–461, 460t
        diagnosis of, 460, 460t
        idiopathic, 459, 460t
        rickettsial organisms in, 459–460
        therapy in, 460–461
    in chemotherapy-induced myelo-
        suppression, 495
    in feline leukemia virus infection, 1073
    isolated, causes of, 459t
    nonimmunologic, 461
Thrombocytopenic purpura, thrombotic,
    461

Thromboembolism, aortic, in cats, 295–
    302. See also *Aortic thromboembo-*
    lism, in cats.
    in glomerulonephropathy, 1176
    pulmonary, VIII:257
        in heartworm disease, 266–267
        pulmonary edema and, 387
Thrombopathia, in dogs, 463
    thrombasthenic, in dogs, 463
Thromboplastin time, partial, 440
Thrombopoiesis, ineffective, 459
Thrombosis, diagnosis and treatment of,
    IX:505
Thrombus, intracardiac, echocardiogra-
    phy in, 212, *214*
Thymosin, as biologic response modifier,
    510–511
Thyroarytenoid muscle, anatomy of, 344,
    345
Thyroid (desiccated), approximate doses
    of, 1380
Thyroid cartilage, anatomy of, 343, *344*
Thyroid function tests, 965–966
Thyroid hormone replacement therapy,
    IX:1018, 994t
Thyroid hormones, in dermatology, 602–
    603
Thyroid tumors, IX:1033
Thyroidectomy, 1005–1007
    anesthesia in, 1005–1006
    postoperative complications in, 1006–
        1007
    preoperative preparation in, 1005
    surgical considerations in, 1006
Thyroid-stimulating hormone, approxi-
    mate doses of, 1380
    stimulation test, 965–966
Thyrotoxicosis, 603
    in thyroid hormone replacement ther-
        apy, 995
Thyroxine, in pregnancy, 1296t
    plasma or serum, basal or resting, 965
L-Thyroxine, approximate doses of, 1380
Ticarcillin, in pregnancy, 1293t
Ticarcillin/calvulanic acid, 80–81, 80t, *81*
Tick bite, 185
Tiletamine, in chemical restraint, 67
Timolol, approximate doses of, 1380
    in glaucoma, 650
Tissue perfusion, in shock, 320, 321t
Tissue plasminogen activator, in aortic
    thromboembolism, in cats, 299
T-lymphotropic virus infection, in cats,
    530–534. See also *Feline T-lympho-*
    tropic virus infection.
Toad poisoning, VIII:160
Tobramycin, in pregnancy, 1293t
Tocainide, adverse effects of, 313t
    in dilated cardiomyopathy, 246, 249t
    in ventricular tachyarrhythmias, 284t
Toluene, approximate doses of, 1380
    toxicity, 110
Tooth extraction, 948–950. See also *Exo-*
    dontia.
Tortoise. See also *Turtle.*
    shell disease in, IX:751
Toxic conjunctivitis, 676
Toxic epidermal necrolysis, nose and
    footpad in, 619–620
Toxic gases, IX:203
Toxic milk syndrome, 1332
Toxic retinopathy, metabolic, 644–645

Toxicology. See also *Poisoning.*
  forensic, 114–115
  information resources for, IX:129
Toxicosis. See *Poisoning.*
Toxocara canis, in neonate, 1332
Toxocara cati, in neonate, 1332
Toxoplasma gondii, 1112
Toxoplasmosis, antimicrobial agents for,
    1364t
  due to carnivores, 702
  in cats, 1112–1115
    clinical signs of, 1112–1113
    diagnosis of, 1113–1114, 1113t
    etiology of, 1112
    prevention of, 1115, 1115t
    radiographic and laboratory values
      in, 1113
    therapy in, 1114–1115, 1114t–1115t
    transmission of, 1112
  in feline leukemia virus infection, 1071
Trachea, bronchoscopic anatomy of, 222
  cartilage of, demineralization of, 354
  culture of, in birds, 781
  in airway obstruction, 197
  neoplasms of, 403
Tracheal collapse, IX:303, 353–360
  diagnosis of, 354–355
  differential diagnosis of, 354
  etiology of, 353–354
  grading system for, 355, *355*
  medical management of, 355–356
  surgical management of, 356–360
    anesthetic considerations in, 356
    approach in, 356–357
    polypropylene spiral prosthesis tech-
      nique in, 357–359, *357–359*
    postoperative considerations in,
      359–360
    preoperative considerations in, 356
    total ring prosthesis technique in,
      359, *360*
Trachealis muscle weakness, 354
Tracheobronchial tree, cytology of,
    IX:243
  focal or generalized changes in, 222
  mucosa of, 222
  secretions of, 222
Tracheostomy, IX:262
  in respiratory emergencies, 200
Tracheotomy, IX:262
Tranquilizers, in chemical restraint, 63–
    64
Transfusion, blood, VIII:408
  in anemia, 428
  reactions to, in cats, IX:515
  granulocyte, in chemotherapy-induced
    myelosuppression, 497
Transplantation, bone marrow, 512–513,
    515–521
  organ, IX:114
Trauma, bleeding disorders and, 437
  blindness due to, 647
  brain, glucocorticoid therapy for, 60
  conjunctival, 674–675
  craniocerebral, 847–853
  epistaxis in, 195
  head, nervous system injury and,
    IX:830
  hematuria due to, 1119–1120
  nasal cavity, 196–197
  ocular emergencies in, 636–639. See
    also *Ocular emergencies.*

Trauma *(Continued)*
  pinnae, 624
  respiratory emergencies due to, 198–
    199
  self-inflicted, in periocular region,
    680
  spinal cord, glucocorticoid therapy for,
    60
  urinary tract, IX:1155
Traumatic shock, 318–319
Trematodes, in fish disease, *713*, 717
Tremblers, Bernese mountain dog, 836–
    837
Tremor syndrome, generalized, IX:800
Tresaderm, approximate doses of, 1380
Triamcinolone, approximate dose of,
    1380
Triamterene, nutritional concerns with,
    303
Trichlorfon, approximate doses of, 1380
  in pregnancy, 1294t
Trichodinids, 712, 714
Trichomoniasis, in birds, VIII:619
Trichophyton, antimicrobial agents for,
    1363t
Trichuris vulpis, in colitis, 940
Tricuspid dysplasia, breed and sex predi-
    lections for, 225t
  Doppler echocardiographic features of,
    230t
  murmur in, 225
Tricuspid regurgitation, ascites in, 237
  clinical signs of, 233–234
  diagnosis of, 234–235
  differential diagnosis of, 235
  in dogs, 232–237
  incidence and pathology of, 232
  medical management of, 235–237
    initial therapy in, 235
    inotropic drugs in, 235–236
    vasodilators in, 236–237, 236t
  myxomatous degeneration in, 232
  pathophysiology of, 233
Tricuspid valve, anatomy and function
    of, 232
Tricyclic antidepressants, in pruritus,
    567
Trientine, in copper toxicity, 893
Triethylenethiophosphoramide, in cancer
    therapy, 1367
Triiodothyronine, plasma or serum, basal
    or resting, 965
L-Triiodothyronine, approximate doses
    of, 1380
Trimethobenzamide, approximate doses
    of, 1380
Trimethoprim, in pregnancy, 1293t
Trimethoprim-sulfa, in urinary tract in-
    fection, 1206t
Trimethoprim-sulfadiazine, approximate
    dose of, 1380
  hepatic toxicity due to, 881
  in pregnancy, 1293t
Tripelennamine, approximate doses of,
    1380
Triple-X syndrome, 1264
Trisulfapyrimidine, approximate doses of,
    1380
Trypanosomiasis, due to carnivores, 702–
    703
  in dogs, 422–423
Trypsin, in reflux esophagitis, 907

Trypsin-like immunoreactivity, serum, in
    pancreatic insufficiency, 928–929,
    929
Tryptophan, in anorexia, 21
Tuatara, sexual identification in, 802
Tularemia, due to rabbits, 699–700
Tumor. See *Neoplasia.*
Tumor cell resistance, to antineoplastic
    agents, 473t
Tumor markers, immunologic, 411, 411t
Tumor necrosis factor, as biologic re-
    sponse modifier, 511
Tunica vasculosa lentis, persistent hyper-
    plastic, 667–668
Turner's syndrome, 1263–1264
Turpentine toxicity, 111–112
Turtle, hypervitaminosis A in, *793–794*,
    795
  hypovitaminosis A in, 791–795
  nutrition for, 791, 792t–793t
  salmonellosis due to, 697–698
  sexual dimorphism in, 797–798
  sexual identification in, 796–797, *797*–
    798
  shell disease in, IX:751
Tylosin, approximate doses of, 1380
  in plasmacytic-lymphocytic colitis, 943
  in pregnancy, 1293t
Tympanometry, 807, *808*
Tyrosinase deficiency, in chow chow,
    melanin disorder in, 629
Tyrosine crystalluria, 1132

Ulcer, corneal, 637–638, 656–658
  gastrointestinal, 911–918. See also
    Gastrointestinal ulcer.
Ulcerative colitis, histiocytic, 940
Ultrasonography, in pregnancy, 1240–
    1242, *1241*, 1241t
  in pyometra, 1307
  instrumentation in, 1240
  of birds, 788
  of fetus, 1241t
  of ovary, 1240, *1240*
  of prostate, 1227–1239
  of uterus, 1240–1242, *1241–1242*,
    1241t
  principles and applications of, IX:6,
    1238–1240
  real-time, in reproductive disorders,
    IX:1258
Ultrastructural studies, sample prepara-
    tion for, 412–413, 412t
Upper respiratory tract disease, in cats,
    341–342
  medical management of, 337–343. See
    also individual types.
  viral, nasal cavity in, 197
Urachus, 1153
  anomalies of, 1153, *1154*
Ureaplasma infertility, IX:1240
Uremia, 1133–1138
  acute, VIII:981
    parenteral nutrition in, VIII:994
  clinical manifestations of, 1134–1137,
    1135t
    cardiovascular and pulmonary, 1136
    gastrointestinal, 1134
    hemolymphatic, 1136
    integumentary, 1136–1137

Uremia (*Continued*)
  clinical manifestations of, laboratory
    findings in, 1137–1138
    musculoskeletal, 1136
    nervous system and ocular, 1137
    urinary, 1134–1136
  definition of, 1134
  fluid therapy in, VIII:989
  platelet disorders in, 463
Ureter, calculi of, hematuria due to,
    1121
  ectopic, 1214
Urethra, calculi of, hematuria due to,
    1121
  in cats, 1209–1210, *1210*
    obstruction of, 1210
    stricture of, after urethrostomy,
      1213
  papillitis of, hematuria due to, 1120–
    1121
  sphincter of, hypertonicity of, 1215,
    1221–1222
    hypotonicity of, 1215–1216, 1221
    urinary incontinence and, 1152
Urethral pressure profile, 1145–1147,
    1145–1148
Urethritis, granulomatous, 1161–1163
  diagnosis of, 1162
  treatment of, 1162–1163
  hematuria due to, 1120
  neoplasia in, 1161–1163
    diagnosis of, 1162
    treatment of, 1162–1163
Urethrostomy, in cats, 1209–1213
  bacterial urinary tract infections in,
    1211–1212, 1212t
  complications of, 1210–1213
  urethral stricture in, 1213
  urolithiasis in, 1212–1213
  vesicourachal diverticula and, 1156
Uric acid crystalluria, 1133
Urinalysis, in calcium oxalate urolithiasis,
    1186
  in ferret, 767t
  in hematuria, 1117–1118
  in laboratory animals, 746
  in uremia, 1137
  radiographic contrast media and,
    IX:1115
Urinary bladder, atonic, 1152
  hypercontractility of, 1215, 1217,
    1221
  hypocontractility of, 1215, 1216–1217
  infection of, hematuria due to, 1120
  neoplasia of, hematuria due to, 1121
Urinary catheterization, IX:1127
Urinary incontinence, 1214–1222
  causes of, 1214–1215
  classification by bladder and sphincter
    states in, 1215–1216
  in cats, IX:1159
  pharmacologic agents in, 1216–1222,
    1218t–1220t
    activities of, 1217t
    for bladder hypercontractility, 1217–
      1221
    for bladder hypocontractility, 1216–
      1217
    to decrease urethral tone, 1221
    to increase urethral tone, 1221
  urodynamics in, 1151–1152
  vulvar discharge due to, 1311

Urinary tract, abnormalities of, asympto-
    matic, hematuria due to, 1120
  parasites of, IX:1153
  trauma of, IX:1155
Urinary tract infection, 1204–1209
  ancillary therapy in, 1208
  antimicrobial therapy in, 1205–1208
    drugs and dosages in, 1206, 1206t
    frequent reinfection and, 1208
    in mixed infection, 1206
    length of, 1207–1208
    pathogen and, 1205, 1206t
    susceptibility testing in, 1206–1207
  bacteremia from, IX:1150
  bacterial, vesicourachal diverticula in,
    1156
  diagnosis and localization of, IX:1118,
    1204–1205
  host defense mechanisms in, 1205
  in cats, after urethrostomy, 1211–
    1212, 1212t
  management of, IX:1174
  neonatal, 1331
  prevention of, 1209
  uncomplicated vs complicated, 1205
Urination, normal, 1214
  pharmacologic manipulation of,
    IX:1207
  spinal lesions and, VIII:722
Urination disorders, cystometrogram in,
    1147–1149, *1149*
  urethral pressure profile in, 1145–
    1147, *1145–1148*
  urodynamics in, 1145–1150
  uroflowmetry in, 1149–1150
Urine, alkalinization of, in cystine uroli-
    thiasis, 1191
  collection of, 1117
    for laboratory animals, 746
    in acute toxicant–induced renal fail-
      ure, 127
  output, in shock, 326
  pH of, in poisoning, 123
    in urinary tract infection, 1208
  values, in dogs and cats, 1343–1344
  volume, in maintenance fluid therapy,
    40
Urine concentration tests, 1124–1125
Urodynamics, in micturition disorders,
    1145–1150
  in prostate disease, 1151–1152
Uroflowmetry, 1149–1150
Urogenital system, of llama, 735–736
Urolithiasis. See also *Crystalluria*.
  calcium oxalate, 1182–1188
    biologic behavior of, 1186
    breed distribution in, 1183t
    citrates in, 1187–1188
    clinical and laboratory findings in,
      1185
    diet in, 1186–1187
    epidemiology of, 1184
    etiopathogenesis of, 1184–1185
      hypercalcemic hypercalciuria in,
        1185
      normocalcemic hypercalciuria in,
        1184–1185
    medical treatment and prevention
      of, 1186–1188
    mineral composition in, 1182
    physical chemistry of, 1182–1184,
      1183

Urolithiasis (*Continued*)
  calcium oxalate, radiographic findings
    in, 1185–1186
    thiazide diuretics in, 1187
    urine chemistry in, 1186
  cystine, 1189–1192
    biologic behavior of, 1190
    dietary modification in, 1190–1191
    etiopathogenesis of, 1189
    mechanism and clinical manifesta-
      tions of, 1189–1190, *1190*
    medical management of, 1190–1192
    prevalence and mineral composition
      in, 1189
    prevention of, 1192
    thiol-containing drugs in, 1191–1192
    urine alkalinization in, 1191
  determination of mineral composition
    in, 1191t
  in cats, after urethrostomy, 1212–1213
    struvite, IX:1188
  in ferret, 775
  renal, hematuria due to, 1119, 1121
  struvite, in cats, IX:1188
    in dogs, IX:1177
  urate, 1178–1181
    chemical composition of, 1178–1179
    diagnosis of, 1179
    medical management of, 1179–1181
      in Dalmatian dogs, 1179–1180,
        1180t
      in portosystemic vascular anom-
        aly, 1180–1181
    prevention of, 1181
Urologic syndrome, in cats, IX:1196
Uropathy, obstructive, IX:1164
Urosepsis, IX:1150
Urticaria, 540
Uterus, hormonal regulation of, 1299–
    1302
  alpha-adrenergic and beta-adrener-
    gic agents in, 1301
  calcium in, 1300
  inhalation anesthesia and, 1301–
    1302
  oxytocin in, 1300–1301
  prostaglandins in, 1300, *1301*
  ultrasonography of, 1240–1242, *1241–
    1242*, 1241t
Uvea, anterior, disorders of, IX:649
Uveal tract, functional anatomy of, 652
Uveitis, 652–655
  acute, 638–639
  clinical signs of, 652–653
  etiology of, 653–654
  immunologic mechanisms of, 654
  nonsteroidal anti-inflammatory agents
    in, 643t
  systemic disease associations in, 654t
  treatment of, 654–655

Vaccination, for cats, 1356
  for dogs, 1354–1355
  for ferret, 767–768, 768t
  for humane society veterinary practice,
    87
  for nondomestic carnivores, 729t
  for wild animals, 1361–1362
Vaccine, anti-idiotype, 512
  canine DA2P, approximate doses of,
    1371

Vaccine (Continued)
  canine parvovirus, 1077, 1371
  feline leukemia, 1052–1064, 1075,
      1374. See also Feline leukemia virus
      infection.
  feline panleukopenia, 1374
  measles, 1375
  rabies, 1357, 1378
Vagina, electrical resistance of, in breed-
      ing management, 1281
  vaginoscopic appearance of, 1312
Vaginal cytology, epithelial cell types in,
      1276, 1276
  in breeding management, 1276–1278,
      1276–1279, 1286, 1287t
  stains for, 1276
Vaginal prolapse, 1302–1305
  clinical features of, 1302–1304, 1304t
  diagnosis of, 1304
  treatment of, 1305
  types of, 1302, 1303–1304
Vaginitis, hematuria due to, 1120
Vaginoscopy, in breeding management,
      1280, 1280–1281
  in vulvar discharge, 1311–1312
Vaginourethrography, 1142–1145
  complications of, 1144–1145
  indications for, 1142
  interpretation of, 1144, 1144
  preparation in, 1142–1143
  procedure in, 1143, 1143–1144
  technique in, 1142–1144
Valproic acid, approximate doses of, 1380
  in pregnancy, 1296t
Variable, statistical, 14t
Variance, analysis of (ANOVA), 14t
  definition of, 10t
Vascular resistance, pulmonary, 321t
  systemic, 321t
Vascularization, collateral, in aortic
      thromboembolism, 295, 296
Vasculature, glucocorticoid therapy ef-
      fects on, 57
Vasculitis, necrotizing, of central nervous
      system, 60
  nose and footpad in, 620
Vasodilator therapy, IX:329
  adverse effects of, 313t
  in congestive heart failure, 236–237,
      237t
  in hypertension in renal failure, 1203–
      1204
Vasopressin, physiology of, 973
Vasopressin tannate, approximate doses
      of, 1380
  in oil, in diabetes insipidus, 976
Venereal tumors, transmissible, VIII:413
Venipuncture, in laboratory animals, 742
  in llama, 734–735
  in whales, 724, 724
Venous catheterization, in shock, 321–
      322
Venous pressure, central, measurement
      of, 190
Venous pulse, in congenital heart dis-
      ease, 227
Ventilation. See also Breathing; Respira-
      tory.
  continuous positive pressure, in aspi-
      ration pneumonia, 381
  in cardiopulmonary resuscitation, 330–
      331

Ventilation (Continued)
  mechanical, in poisoning, 124
  short-term, IX:269
Ventricular afterload, in dilated cardio-
      myopathy, 244–245, 245t
Ventricular arrhythmia, 278–286
  causes of, 280, 281t
  identification of, 278–280, 279
  in congenital heart disease, 230
  patient evaluation and therapeutic
      guidelines in, 280–285, 281t–284t
  antiarrhythmic drugs in, 281–283,
      283t–284t
  in frequent ventricular premature
      contractions or tachycardia, 283–
      285
  in refractory arrhythmia, 285
  treatment of, 282
Ventricular contraction, premature, 278,
      279
  drug therapy in, 283–285
  in bronchoscopy, 221
Ventricular escape rhythm, 280
Ventricular fibrillation, 280
Ventricular flutter, 280
Ventricular preload, in dilated cardiomy-
      opathy, 244–245, 245t
Ventricular rhythm, accelerated, 280
Ventricular septal defect, breed and sex
      predilections for, 225t
  Doppler echocardiographic features of,
      230t
  murmur in, 225, 227
  surgical correction of, 230
Ventricular tachycardia, 278–280, 279
  drug therapy in, 283–285
Verapamil, adverse effects of, 313t
  approximate doses of, 1380
  in atrial tachyarrhythmia, 276
Vermiplex, approximate dose of, 1380
Vesicourachal diverticula, 1153–1157
  biologic behavior of, 1155–1156, 1155–
      1156
  diagnosis of, 1155
  macroscopic, 1153–1154, 1155t
  microscopic, 1153, 1154
  treatment of, 1156–1157
Vestibular disease, peripheral, in small
      mammals, IX:794
Vi-Sorbin, approximate dose of, 1380
Vinblastine, 473
  approximate dose of, 1380
  for cancer therapy, 1368
  preparation and administration of,
      477t
Vincristine, 473
  approximate dose of, 1380
  doxorubicin, cyclophosphamide and,
      protocol for soft tissue tumors, 490t,
      491
  effects of, on male dog fertility, 1225
  for cancer therapy, 1368
  in lymphoma, 485–486, 485t
  in pregnancy, 1294t
  preparation and administration of, 477t
Viokase, approximate doses of, 1380
Viral disease, of psittacine birds, IX:705
Viral infection, diagnosis of, VIII:1143
Viruses. See also individual types.
  disinfectants and, 92
Visceral larva migrans, due to carnivores,
      701

Vision loss, acute, 639, 644–647
  diagnosis of, 690–691
Visual pathway, 688, 688t
  lesions of, ocular signs of, 688t
Vitamin A, approximate doses of, 1380
  deficiency of, in turtles, 791–795
  excess of, in turtles, 793–794, 795
  in dermatology, 553–559. See also Re-
      tinoids.
Vitamin A–responsive dermatosis, in
      cocker spaniels, 554–556
Vitamin B complex, approximate doses
      of, 1380
  in appetite stimulation, 24
Vitamin B_{12}, approximate doses of, 1380
  deficiency of, in intestinal bacterial
      overgrowth, 935
  syndromes causing, 935
  malabsorption of, selective, 435
Vitamin D, approximate doses of, 1380
  in chronic advanced renal failure, 1197
  in hyperparathyroidism, 986–987
  toxicosis due to, 148–152. See also
      Cholecalciferol, toxicosis due to.
Vitamin E, approximate doses of, 1380
  in dermatology, 574–575
  in pruritus, 568
Vitamin K, absence or antagonists, pro-
      teins induced by, IX:513
  in coagulation, 143
  in parenteral nutrition, 27
  in rodenticide toxicity, 144t, 145–146
Vitamin K_1, approximate doses of, 1380
Vitamin supplementation, in pancreatic
      insufficiency, 931
  in parenteral nutrition, 27
  therapeutic use of, IX:40
Vitiligo, idiopathic, 619
  melanin disorder in, 629–630
Vitreous, diseases of, IX:660
  persistent hyperplastic primary, 667–
      668
Vogt-Koyanagi-Harada syndrome, in
      dogs, hypomelanosis in, 630
  of nose and footpads, 618–619
  periocular lesions in, 680
Vomiting, food aversion in cats and, 22
  food aversion in dogs and, 22
  in chemotherapy, 481
  in lymphocytic-plasmacytic enteritis,
      923
  in uremia, 1134
  induction of, 117
  maintenance fluid therapy in, 42
Von Willebrand factor, 446–447
Von Willebrand factor antigen, 441
Von Willebrand's disease, 446–450, 462–
      463
  buccal mucosal bleeding time in, 447–
      448, 448
  classification of, 448, 448–449, 448t
  dog breeds with, 446t
  laboratory and clinical assessment of,
      447–448, 448
  treatment of, 449–450, 450
VP16–213, preparation and administra-
      tion of, 477t
Vulvar discharge, IX:1229, 1310–1312
  cytologic examination in, 1310–1311
  history in, 1310
  physical examination in, 1310
  vaginoscopy in, 1311–1312

Waardenburg-Klein syndrome, melanin disorder in, 629
Wandering atrial pacemaker, 271
Warfarin, in aortic thromboembolism, in cats, 301
  in pregnancy, 1295t
Warfarin rodenticide toxicosis, 106
Wasp sting, 184–185
Water, aquarium, 704–706
  contaminated, IX:221
  total body, 37. See also under *Fluid*.
Water deprivation testing, in diabetes insipidus, 974–975
Water intake monitoring, in polydipsia, 1025
Weight, body, in maintenance fluid therapy, 40
  loss of, in uremia, 1134
Weight to body surface area conversion table, 1365
Weimaraners, hypomyelination in, 836
  immunodeficiency in, 524
Welsh Corgi, juvenile renal disease in, 1168
  recurring macroscopic hematuria of, 1120
West Highland white terriers, copper metabolism in, 889–890
Whale strandings, 721–727
  mass, 722
  medication dosages and, 725t
  orientation to, 721–722
  professional's response to, 723–726
    captivity as, 725
    euthanasia as, 725–726
    historical, 723–724
    immediate release as, 724–725

Whale strandings (*Continued*)
  mass, management of survivors in, 726
    pathobiologic considerations in, 726
    venipuncture in, 724, *724*
  public response to, 722–723
  single, 722
  success and release of survivors in, 726–727
  weight approximation according to length, 724t
Wheaten terrier, soft-coated, juvenile renal disease in, 1168–1169
Wheat-sensitive enteropathy, in Irish setters, IX:893
Wheeze, 189, 190
Whiskers, cat, sensitivity of, 22
White cells. See under *Leukocyte*.
White coat color, microphthalmia and ocular dysgenesis with, 666–667
Whole blood clotting time, 440
Wild animals, immunization of, 1361–1362
Wobbler syndrome, in Doberman pinscher, 858–862
  clinical management of, 859–860
  diagnosis of, 858–859
  history in, 858
  neurologic examination in, 858
  postoperative care in, 862
  prognosis in, 862
  radiology in, 859, *859*
  surgical management of, 860–862
    ventral decompression, bone graft, Lubra plate in, *859*, 860–861
    Steinmann's pins in, *861*, 861–862
  in dogs, IX:806
Wry bite, 952–953, *953*

XO syndrome, 1263–1264
XX male syndrome, 1266
XX sex reversal, 1265
XX true hermaphroditism, 1265–1266
XX/XY chimera, with testes, 1265
XXX syndrome, 1264
XXY syndrome, 1263
Xylazine, approximate doses of, 1379
  butorphanol and, in chemical restraint of dogs, 68–69
  in chemical restraint, 65–66
  uterine effects of, 1301
Xylazine stimulation test, 967
D-Xylose absorption test, in intestinal bacterial overgrowth, 936

Yersinia pestis, 1088, 1089–1090

Zidovudine, in feline leukemia virus infection, 1071
Zinc, in copper toxicity, 892
  in pruritus, 568
Zinc oxide toxicity, 108–109
Zinc-responsive dermatosis, 619
  periocular manifestations of, 679
Zolazepam, in chemical restraint, 63–64
Zollinger-Ellison syndrome, 1022–1024
Zoonoses, disinfectants and, 93
  of wild animals, 697–703, 697t–698t.
    See also specific species.
  pet-associated, potential and newly recognized, IX:1087